Leukemia

Leukemia

Seventh Edition

Edward S. Henderson, M.D.

Professor Emeritus of Medicine
State University of New York at Buffalo
Buffalo, New York

T. Andrew Lister, M.D.

Professor of Clinical Oncology
ICRF Department of Medical Oncology
St. Bartholomew's Hospital
London, England

Mel F. Greaves, Ph.D.

Professor of Cell Biology
Director, Leukemia Research Fund Centre
Institute of Cancer Research
London, England

SAUNDERS
An Imprint of Elsevier Science
Philadelphia   London   New York   St. Louis   Sydney   Toronto

SAUNDERS
An Imprint of Elsevier Science

The Curtis Center
Independence Square West
Philadelphia, Pennsylvania 19106

NOTICE

Pharmacology is an ever-changing field. Standard safety precautions must be followed, but as new research and clinical experience broaden our knowledge, changes in treatment and drug therapy may become necessary or appropriate. Readers are advised to check the most current product information provided by the manufacturer of each drug to be administered to verify the recommended dose, the method and duration of administration, and contraindications. It is the responsibility of the treating physician, relying on experience and knowledge of the patient, to determine dosages and the best treatment for each individual patient. Neither the Publisher nor the editor assumes any liability for any injury and/or damage to persons or property arising from this publication.

The Publisher

Library of Congress Cataloging-in-Publication Data

Leukemia / [edited by] Edward S. Henderson, T. Andrew Lister, Mel F. Greaves.—7th ed.
   p. ; cm.
  Includes bibliographical references and index.
  ISBN 0–7216–9060–2
   1. Leukemia. I. Henderson, Edward S. II. Lister, T. A. (Thomas Andrew) III.
Greaves, M. F. (Melvyn F.)
  [DNLM: 1. Leukemia. WH 250 L6519 2002]
RC643 .D32 2002
616.99′419—dc21   2002017018

Acquisitions Editor: Dolores Meloni
Project Manager: Natalie Ware

MD/MVY

Printed in the United States of America.

Last digit is the print number: 9 8 7 6 5 4 3 2 1

CONTRIBUTORS

H.J. Adriaansen, M.D., Ph.D.
Clinical Chemistry, Department of Clinical Chemistry, Gelre Hospitals, Apeldoorn, Netherlands
Immunobiology of Leukemia

Tiziano Barbui, M.D.
Chief, Division of Hematology, Ospedali Riuniti, Bergamo, Italy
Management of Bleeding and Thrombosis in Acute Leukemia and Chronic Myeloproliferative Disorders

Michael J. Barnett, B.M.
Professor of Transplantation Oncology, St. Bartholomew's Hospital and the Royal London School of Medicine and Dentistry, University of London, London, England
Chronic Myeloid Leukemia

Renato Bassan, M.D.
Consultant, Division of Hematology, Ospedali Riuniti, Bergamo, Italy
Management of Infections in Patients with Leukemia

Andrea Biondi, M.D., Ph.D.
Associate Professor of Pediatrics; Head, M. Tettamanti Research Centre, Pediatric Clinic University of Milano-Bicocca, Ospedale San Gerardo, Monza, Italy
Acute Promyelocytic Leukemia

Karl G. Blume, M.D.
Professor of Medicine, Stanford University School of Medicine, Stanford, California
Hematopoietic Cell Transplantation in the Leukemias

John D. Boice, Jr., Sc.D.
Professor of Medicine, Vanderbilt University Medical Center, Nashville, Tennessee; Scientific Director, International Epidemiology Institute, Rockville, Maryland
Radiation-Induced Leukemia

Michael A. Caligiuri, M.D.
Professor of Medicine; Chair, Cancer Research, John L. Marakas Nationwide Insurance Enterprise Foundation; Associate Director for Clinical Cancer Research, The Comprehensive Cancer Center, Ohio State University, Columbus, Ohio; Director, Division of Hematology/Oncology, Department of Internal Medicine, Ohio State University, Columbus, Ohio
Antisense and Gene Transfer as Therapeutic Strategies in Acute and Chronic Leukemia

Dario Campana, M.D., Ph.D.
Professor of Pediatrics, University of Tennessee College of Medicine; Member, Department of Hematology—Oncology and Pathology, St. Jude Children's Research Hospital, Memphis, Tennessee
Lymphopoiesis

Andrew Davies, M.D.
Clinical Research Fellow, Department of Medical Oncology, St. Bartholomew's Hospital, London, England
General Management of the Patient with Leukemia

Susan S. Devesa, Ph.D.
Chief, Descriptive Studies Section, National Cancer Institute, Division of Cancer Epidemiology and Genetics, Epidemiology and Biostatistics Program, Biostatistics Branch, Bethesda, Maryland
Epidemiology of Leukemia: Overview and Patterns of Occurrence

Connie J. Eaves, Ph.D.
Professor of Medical Genetics, University of British Columbia; Deputy Director, Terry Fox Laboratory, British Columbia Cancer Agency, Vancouver, British Columbia, Canada
Myelopoiesis; Chronic Myeloid Leukemia

Anna Falanga, M.D.
Associate Professor of Hematology, Ospedali Riuniti, Bergamo, Italy
Management of Bleeding and Thrombosis in Acute Leukemia and Chronic Myeloproliferative Disorders

Guido Finazzi, M.D.
Associate Professor of Hematology, Ospedali Riuniti, Bergamo, Italy
Management of Bleeding and Thrombosis in Acute Leukemia and Chronic Myeloproliferative Disorders

Arthur E. Frankel, M.D.
Professor of Cancer Biology and Medicine, Wake Forest University School of Medicine, Winston-Salem, North Carolina
Treatment of Leukemia with Monoclonal Antibodies, Immunotoxins, and Immunoconjugates

Paul S. Gaynon
Professor, Department of Pediatrics, Keck School of
    Medicine of the University of Southern California;
    Director, Clinical Oncology Research Program,
    Children's Hospital, Los Angeles, California
Childhood Acute Lymphoblastic Leukemia

Nicola Gökbuget, M.D.
Research Assistant, University of Frankfurt, Medical
    Clinic III, Frankfurt, Germany
Acute Lymphoblastic Leukemia in Adults

Jason Gotlib, M.D.
Senior Clinical Research Fellow in Hematology, Stanford
    University Medical Center, Stanford University,
    Stanford, California
Myelodysplastic Syndromes

Mel F. Greaves, Ph.D.
Professor of Cell Biology and Director, Leukemia
    Research Fund Centre, Institute of Cancer Research,
    London, England
Biology of Leukemia: An Overview

Peter L. Greenberg, M.D.
Professor of Medicine, Stanford University Medical
    Center, Stanford University, Stanford, California; Head,
    Hematology Section, Palo Alto Veterans Affairs Health
    Care System, Palo Alto, California
Myelodysplastic Syndromes

Edward S. Henderson, M.D.
Professor Emeritus of Medicine, State University of New
    York at Buffalo, Buffalo, New York
*History of Leukemia; Diagnosis, Classification, and
    Assessment of Response to Treatment*

Dieter Hoelzer, M.D., Ph.D.
Professor of Internal Medicine, University of Frankfurt,
    Medical Clinic III; Head, Medical Clinic III, University
    Hospital, Frankfurt, Germany
Acute Lymphoblastic Leukemia in Adults

Mark Hoffman, M.D.
Section Head, Hematology, Division of Hematology/
    Oncology, Long Island Jewish Medical Center, New
    Hyde Park, New York
Hairy Cell Leukemia

Simon P. Joel, Ph.D.
Barry Reed Oncology Laboratory, St. Bartholomew's
    Hospital, London, England
Pharmacology of Antileukemic Drugs

Michael J. Keating, M.B.B.S.
Professor of Medicine, University of Texas M.D.
    Anderson Cancer Center, Houston, Texas
Chronic Lymphocytic Leukemia

Beverly J. Lange, M.D.
Professor of Pediatrics, University of Pennsylvania
    School of Medicine; Medical Director, Division of
    Oncology, Children's Hospital of Philadelphia,
    Philadelphia, Pennsylvania
Acute Myeloid Leukemia in Children and Adolescents

Tucker W. LeBien, Ph.D.
Professor of Laboratory Medicine and Pathology,
    University of Minnesota Medical School; Deputy
    Director, Minnesota Cancer Center, Minneapolis,
    Minnesota
Lymphopoiesis

Martha S. Linet, M.D., M.P.H.
Chief, Population Studies Section, National Cancer
    Institute, Division of Cancer Epidemiology and
    Genetics, Epidemiology and Biostatistics Program,
    Radiation Epidemiology Branch, Bethesda, Maryland
*Epidemiology of Leukemia: Overview and Patterns of
    Occurrence*

T. Andrew Lister, M.D.
Professor of Clinical Oncology, ICRF Department of
    Medical Oncology, St. Bartholomew's Hospital,
    London, England
Acute Myelogenous Leukemia

Guido Marcucci, M.D.
Assistant Professor of Medicine, Division of Hematology/
    Oncology, Department of Internal Medicine, Ohio
    State University, Columbus, Ohio
*Antisense and Gene Transfer as Therapeutic Strategies
    in Acute and Chronic Leukemia*

Masao Matsuoka, M.D., Ph.D.
Professor, Institute for Virus Research, Kyoto University,
    Kyoto, Japan
Adult T-Cell Leukemia

James McArthur, M.D.
Professor Emeritus of Hematology and Medicine,
    University of Washington Medical School, Seattle,
    Washington
*Diagnosis, Classification, and Assessment of Response
    to Treatment*

Michael F. Murphy, M.D.
Senior Clinical Lecturer in Blood Transfusion, Oxford
    University; Consultant Hematologist, National Blood
    Service and Department of Hematology, Oxford
    Radcliffe Hospitals, Oxford, England
Management of Anemia in Patients with Leukemia

Robert S. Negrin, M.D.
Associate Professor of Medicine, Stanford University
    School of Medicine, Stanford, California
Hematopoietic Cell Transplantation in the Leukemias

James C. Neil, Ph.D.
Professor of Virology and Molecular Oncology, Head,
    Department of Veterinary Pathology, University of
    Glasgow, Scotland, United Kingdom
Viruses and Leukemia

Jens Pedersen-Bjergaard, M.D., Ph.D.
Head, Section Hematology/Oncology, Cytogenetics
    Laboratory, Juliane Marie Center, Rigshopitalet,
    Copenhagen, Denmark
Chemicals and Leukemia

Kanti Rai, M.D.
Chief, Division of Hematology/Oncology, Long Island
   Jewish Medical Center, New Hyde Park, New York
Hairy Cell Leukemia

Alessandro Rambaldi, M.D.
Head, Bone Marrow Transplant Unit, Division of
   Hematology, Ospedali Riuniti, Bergamo, Italy
Acute Promyelocytic Leukemia

Ama Rohatiner, M.D.
Professor of Hematology and Oncology, St.
   Bartholomew's and the Royal London School of
   Medicine and Dentistry University of London;
   Consultant Physician, Department of Medical
   Oncology, St. Bartholomew's Hospital, London,
   England
*General Management of the Patient with Leukemia;
Pharmacology of Antileukemic Drugs; Acute
Myelogenous Leukemia*

Thomas F. Schulz, M.D.
Professor of Virology, Hannover Medical School,
   Hannover, Germany
Viruses and Leukemia

Stuart E. Siegel, M.D.
Professor and Vice-Chair of Pediatrics, Keck School of
   Medicine of the University of Southern California;
   Director, Children's Center for Cancer and Blood
   Disorders, and Head, Division of Hematology-
   Oncology, Children's Hospital, Los Angeles, California
Childhood Acute Lymphoblastic Leukemia

Eric L. Sievers, M.D.
Assistant Professor of Pediatrics, University of
   Washington; Assistant Member, Fred Hutchinson
   Cancer Research Center, Seattle, Washington
*Treatment of Leukemia with Monoclonal Antibodies,
Immunotoxins, and Immunoconjugates*

T. Szczepański, M.D.
Department of Immunology, Erasmus MC, University
   Medical Center Rotterdam, Rotterdam, Netherlands
*Immunobiology of Leukemia; Detection of Minimal
Residual Disease*

Kiyoshi Takatsuki, M.D., Ph.D.
Professor Emeritus, Kumamoto University School of
   Medicine; Director, Kitano Hospital, Kumamoto, Japan
Adult T-Cell Leukemia

J.J.M. van Dongen, M.D., Ph.D.
Professor, Department of Immunology, Erasmus MC,
   University Medical Center Rotterdam; Medical
   Immunologist, Consultant in Immunology, Erasmus
   MC, University Medical Center Rotterdam, Rotterdam,
   Netherlands
*Immunobiology of Leukemia; Detection of Minimal
Residual Disease*

Bryan D. Young, Ph.D.
Professor of Molecular Oncology, St. Bartholomew's
   Hospital Medical School; ICRF Medical Oncology Unit,
   St. Bartholomew's Hospital, London, England
Molecular Cytogenetics of Leukemia

PREFACE

The first edition of this textbook appeared in 1958 as a monograph written entirely by William Dameshek and Frederick Gunz. It was authoritative and almost totally anecdotal. Very little science, preclinical or clinical, was included. Rather, there was extensive review of the "state of the art" concerning the diagnosis, pathogenesis, and treatment of the group of diseases under the rubric *leukemia*. As presented, it reflected both the extent of knowledge of the disease and the mode of medical education of that period. The two authors, a famed Boston professor and his not-yet famous associate (a visiting scholar from New Zealand), provided their readers with the sum of their knowledge and experience with the disease(s). The book was enthusiastically received, and it stimulated many young physicians to enter the then sparsely populated fields of hematology and oncology and young scientists to seek to unravel the mysteries of this poorly understood disorder.

The progress made since that time is the subject of the current volume. No two individuals could possibly provide the perspective and summarize the knowledge to the extent that Dameshek and Gunz succeeded in doing in 1958. The current seventh edition has three editors and 47 authors. Other differences are yet more striking. Virtually every chapter in this seventh edition contains data not available in 1958. Even much of the history chapter could not have been written then; it was in the process of being made. The clonal nature of leukemia was only speculative at that time, before the recognition of the Philadelphia chromosome. The existence of both T and B lymphocytes was not yet domesticated. Diagnosis depended solely on clinical features and stained blood smears. Treatment was based on a handful of drugs, and "cures" were so infrequent that a worldwide survey could identify fewer than 100 5-year survivors. As a consequence, most medical personnel, and to an even greater extent the public at large, considered the diagnosis of leukemia a death sentence, and whether to subject a patient to antileukemia drug thereapy was widely debated and heatedly contested. Even patients who achieved remission often found themselves ostracized by friends and schoolmates and were denied employment or admission to college. Surgical procedures were postponed or rejected on the basis of the poor prognosis perceived for the disease.

Currently for the majority of patients the situation is markedly different. Curative treatments exist, supportive measures ensure a degree of succor to almost all, and society recognizes and encourages the reintegration of leukemia patients into society. Over the last four decades, diagnostic, therapeutic, and prognostic maneuvers have been derived from rigorously controlled, prospective clinical studies of large numbers of patients. Recently there has been a second paradigm shift, from empirically based management to diagnosis and treatment plans derived directly from molecular genetic knowledge. Although these specifically targeted therapies are so far restricted to only a few forms of leukemia, their success encourages optimism for future progress in this group of diseases so recently regarded with despair.

This edition is dedicated to all those whose energies and dedication, or suffering and courage, have united to make this progress possible; and to those in the twenty-first century who continue to strive toward the goal of eradication or prevention of leukemia for all patients.

Edward S. Henderson, M.D.
T. Andrew Lister, M.D.
Mel F. Greaves, Ph.D.

PREFACE TO THE FIRST EDITION

LEUKEMIA, like cancer and poliomyelitis, has been classed as one of the "dread diseases." Without doubt, it represents the most important single problem in hematology. In the United States alone it kills at least 10,000 annually, many of them bright, active children or intelligent men and women in their prime of life. Most statistics indicate that the disease is on the increase, particularly in the last three decades of life. Whether or not this is actually true or due simply to more case studies and better recognition, there can be no question regarding the seriousness of the problem and the necessity to cope with it by all available means.

There have been many thousands of articles written about leukemia but the paucity of books on the subject is amazing. Forkner's text of 1938 was encyclopedic in its scope and for many years remained almost the only central source. The enormous resurgence of interest in the disease, brought about in large measure by the possibility of achieving at least temporarily beneficial results with various chemicals, has led to a quest for more precise knowledge of the disease: its character, the nature of the leukemic cell, the pathophysiology of such features as the anemia, hyperuricemia, the hemorrhagic state, etc. Etiologic factors, previously unknown, have come to the surface, and today there is great talk of the viruses and much statistical evidence for the leukemogenic effects of ionizing radiation. The empirical nature of most of our therapy, even that with the newer antimetabolic and cytotoxic agents, and its eventually unsatisfactory characteristics, have naturally led to an increasing inquiry into the more fundamental aspects of cellular growth and proliferation.

What is leukemia? Is it a reactive disturbance, or is it neoplastic? Does it represent a cellular reaction to an infectious or other agent, or does a harmful mutation take place, leading to an abnormal type of unusually rapid leukocyte proliferation? The leukemic cell seems to have some rather characteristic features as we examine it, but when one tries to analyze it feature by feature, chemical by chemical, the apparent differences between normal and leukemic cells become less and less pronounced. Perhaps this is why, in treating leukemia, we are always limited by what the chemical or other agent does to the *normal* cells; the action upon both leukemic and normal cells is so much alike.

This work on leukemia is limited almost entirely to a consideration of *human* leukemia. Not that mouse leukemia and fowl leukemia are not important; they are of utmost importance, particularly from the investigational aspect. We present in this monograph a rather personal account, not only of our own interests in this field but of what we think the practitioner (internist, pediatrician, pathologist and clinical pathologist) may be interested in. The work is by no means encyclopedic nor is it a textbook, although sometimes, as in the clinical descriptions, it must partake of some of the features of the latter. There is probably more emphasis on certain aspects than on others, again an indication of our special fields of interest: etiologic agents, the myeloproliferative syndromes, therapy. Nevertheless, we believe that there is presented in these pages a fairly comprehensive picture of the present state of our knowledge (some might say "ignorance") of leukemia. We realize full well that this is but an interim report and that perhaps in a short time, whether it be a year or a decade, a revolution in understanding and control of the disease may well take place. Actually, the fact that one has a difficult time in defining leukemia may in itself be somewhat hopeful. Since there is no complete certainty that the condition is malignant, nor even what "malignancy" is, it is altogether possible that leukemia may eventually turn out to be a deficiency state or an immunologic reaction or a response to an infectious agent. Again, what we learn from leukemia, with its readily available blood and tissue cells, should certainly be of considerable value in the understanding of neoplastic disease in general.

This work could never have been completed without the help of many individuals. From our patients we have learned a great deal, particularly in courage and forbearance. From out colleagues, who have come to work with us from many lands and many parts of this country, we have gleaned much valuable information, and the give-and-take of our daily discussions has been of utmost value. We may single out a few who have worked with us on specific problems in this field: Drs. Mario Baldini, Boston; Luis Bergna, Buenos Aires; Marvin Bloom, Buffalo; Edmund W. Campbell, Boston; Jyoti Chatterjea, Calcutta; William H. Crosby, Washington, D.C.; Solomon Estren, New York; Henry Goldenberg, Toronto; Norma Granville, Hartford; Zacharias Komninos, New York; William McFarland, U.S. Navy, Bethesda, Maryland; Carlos Mesa Arrau, Santiago, Chile; Enrique Perez Santiago, Santurce, Puerto Rico; Anthony Pisciotta, Milwaukee; Jack Rheingold, Washington, D.C.; Martin Rosenthal, New York; Fernando Rubio, Jr., Boston; Richard H. Saunders, Rochester; Laurence I. Schwartz, New York; Jay Silverberg, Pittsburgh; Karl Singer, deceased; Mario Stefanini, Boston; Asuman Unugur, Istanbul; Louis Weisfuse, Long Island, New York; Leda Zannos, Athens, Greece.

In addition, we wish to acknowledge with thanks the help of the following individuals, all of New Zealand: Drs. G. C. T. Burns, A. F. Burry, A. J. Campbell, A. M. Goldstein, R. F. Hough, J. B. Jameson, G. L. Rolleston, D. T. Stewart, and Messrs. S. E. Brooks and K. A. Donaldson.

Our secretarial staff headed by Miss Joyce Rock and including Mrs. Arlene Morris, Mrs. Mildred Seagraves and Miss Zelda Cushner, has somehow triumphed over a mountainous collection of drafts, copies, bibliographies, illustrations, made all the more complex by the half-world separating the two authors. Among our many technicians over the years, we must particularly note Mrs. Irma B. Mednicoff and Mrs. Louise D'esy Choinski.

Special thanks are due to Dr. H. Edward MacMahon, Professor of Pathology, Tufts University School of Medicine, and his staff for their cooperation in providing most of the photomicrographs of sections in the text (except those otherwise cited); Dr. Alice Ettinger, Radiologist, New England Center Hospital, for her continued interest in our work, and for supplying most of the x-ray illustrations used in the text; Dr. W. J. Mitus of our laboratory, for his aid in the histopathologic and histochemical sections; Professor Y. Kawakita of Kumamoto City, Japan, for his meticulous illustrations done while he was with us in Boston; Dr. Joseph Beard of Durham, North Carolina, who reviewed the section on viruses and with whom we had several profitable discussions on this important subject; Dr. Charles Congdon of Oak Ridge National Laboratories, Oak Ridge, Tennessee, who examined the section on reactions to x-rays and with whom we have collaborated in a bone marrow transplantation project; Dr. Wayne Rundles of Durham, North Carolina, who reviewed the sections on multiple myeloma and urethane and supplied several excellent electrophoretic patterns of serum and urine; Dr. Marcel Bessis, of Paris, who generously allowed the use of some of his extraordinary electron micrographs; and to Dr. Leon Dmochowski of Baylor University, Houston, Texas, who supplied electron micrographs showing viruses in leukemic cells from different animal species and humans. Mr. Tuckerman Day compiled the index.

We acknowledge with appreciation the help of our wives, Mrs. Ruddy Dameshek and Mrs. Joan P. Gunz, whose patience was undoubtedly strained at times while their husbands toiled over an ever-demanding manuscript. To our long-time secretary, Mrs. Edith M. Florentine, we extend thanks for her constant cooperation, particularly in unearthing pertinent clinical data.

Finally, we cannot fail to acknowledge the generous support throughout the years of the American Cancer Society, Inc., the American Cancer Society (Massachusetts Division), the National Cancer Institute of the United States Public Health Service, the Medical Research Branch (Division of Biology and Medicine) of the United States Atomic Energy Commission, the Damon Runyon Memorial Fund for Cancer Research, Inc., and of generous private donors. Among these may be listed Mr. E. Calvin Fowler, of Chattanooga, Tennessee (deceased May 29, 1958), Mr. E. Stanley Wright of Worcester, Massachusetts, the Greenbaum Family of Boston (in honor of Mrs. Sarah Greenbaum, deceased), and the Rho Pi Phi Ladies Auxiliary, of Boston. We are indebted to the Schering Corporation and to its Vice-President and Medical Director, Dr. Edward Henderson, for their generous contributions of large amounts of prednisone (Meticorten) and their financial aid in defraying the cost of the colored plates.

William Dameshek
Frederick Gunz

CONTENTS

Color Section

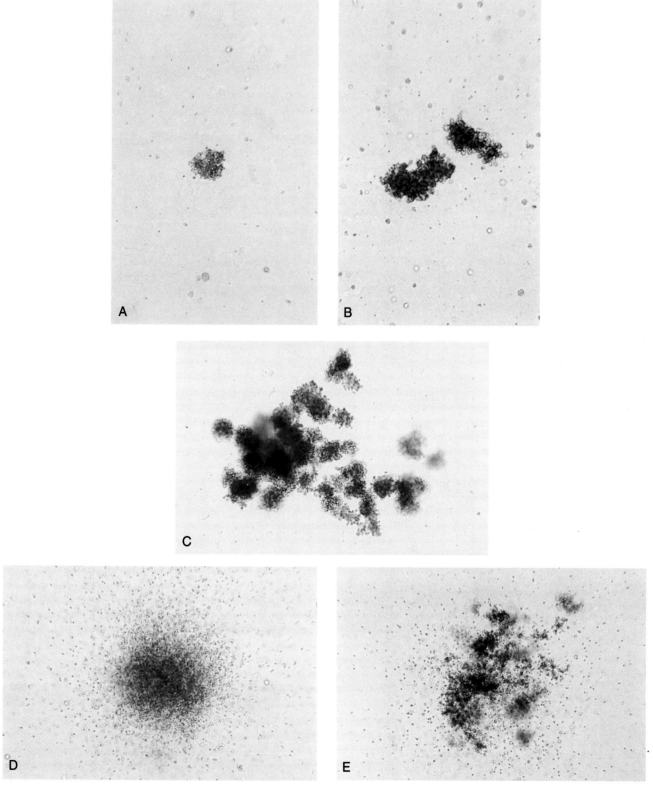

FIGURE 3–3. Photomicrographs of various types of hematopoietic colonies containing single or multiple lineages of differentiating blood cells. The colonies were photographed in the living state in the cultures in which they were generated. *A,* Typical CFU-E–derived colony. *B,* Typical BFU-E–derived colony. *C,* Typical primitive BFU-E–derived colony. *D,* Typical CFU-GM–derived colony. *E,* Typical CFU-GEMM–derived colony. All colonies shown at the same magnification.

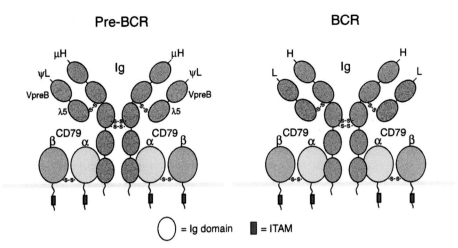

FIGURE 4–3. Molecular composition of the pre-B-cell receptor (pre-BCR) and B-cell receptor complexes. In the pre-BCR complexes, μH chains are associated with ψL chains. In BCR complexes, H chains are associated with L chains (either κ or λ). Signal transduction is mediated by CD79 molecules, which contain immunoreceptor tyrosine-based activation motifs in their cytoplasmic domains.

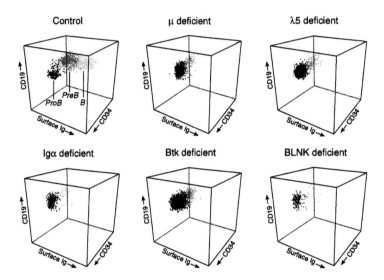

FIGURE 4–4. Block in B-cell differentiation in patients with agammaglobulinemia. Flow cytometric analysis of the immunophenotype of CD19+ B cells in a bone marrow of a healthy individual shows three distinct cell subpopulations: CD34+ surface Ig− (pro B), CD34− surface Ig− (pre-B), and CD34− surface Ig+ (immature and mature B). The immunophenotype of patients with agammaglobulinemia caused by different genetic abnormalities is shown. Note that the main block in B-cell differentiation in all patients is at the transition between pro-B and pre-B cells.[88, 101, 102, 154, 159]

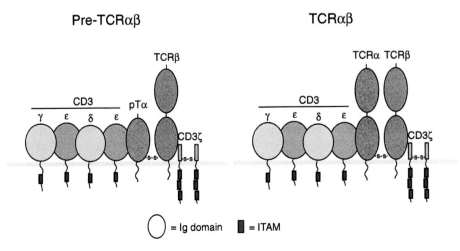

FIGURE 4–7. Molecular composition of the pre-T-cell receptor αβ (pre-TCRαβ) and T-cell receptor αβ (TCRαβ) complexes. TCRβ chains are associated with pTα chains in the pre-TCRαβ complexes and with TCRα chains in the TCRαβ complexes. Signal transduction is mediated by CD3 molecules, which contain immunoreceptor tyrosine-based activation motifs in their cytoplasmic domains.

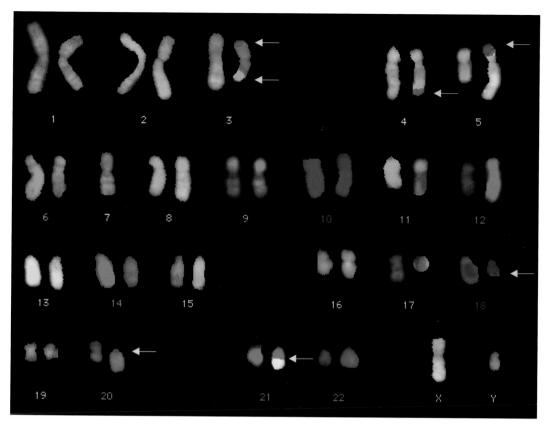

FIGURE 5–1. M-FISH analysis of a case of AML. The karyotype was analyzed as follows: 46,XY,del(5)(q22-q35),inv(8)(q13q24)/ 45,idem,-7/45,idem, -7,-12,+mar1/45,idem, der(3)(21qter->21q2::3p2->2q2::20?::5p1->5pter)der (4)(4pter->4q31::3p2->3pter) der(5)(5qter->5p1::20?::18q21->qter)-7der(18)(18pter->18q21::20?) der(20)(p10 or q10->q11 or p11::3q2->3pter)der(21)(21pter->21q2::4q31->4qter)/46,XY. (Courtesy of Deborah Lillington.)

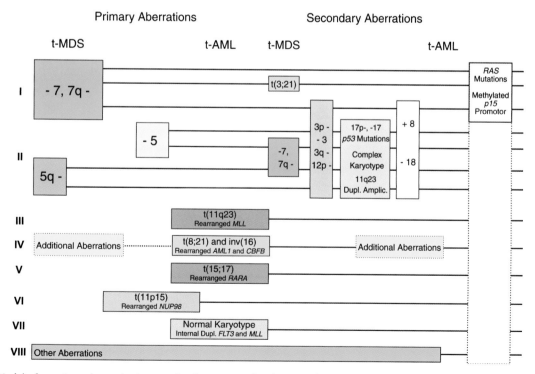

FIGURE 9–4. Model of genetic pathways in the genesis of treatment-related AML and MDS.

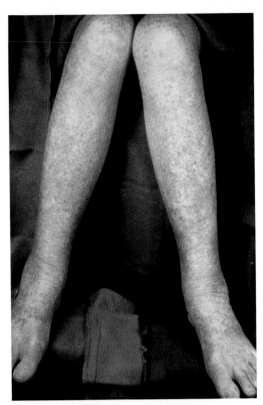

FIGURE 11–1. Petechial hemorrhages in a patient with severe thrombocytopenia.

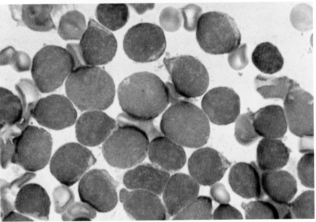

FIGURE 11–2. Acute lymphoblastic leukemia, FAB-L1 morphology. Note scant cytoplasm.

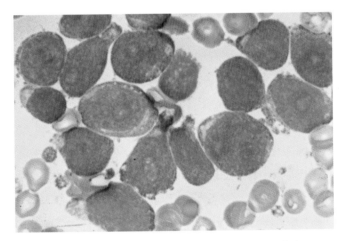

FIGURE 11–3. Acute lymphoblastic leukemia, FAB-L2 morphology. Cells have variable size and a lower nuclear-to-cytoplasmic ratio than L1 blasts.

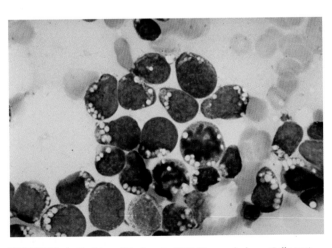

FIGURE 11–4. Burkitt cell leukemia, FAB-L3 morphology. Cells typically have deeply basophilic cytoplasm with numerous vacuoles. Most of these are cytoplasmic. Note the presence of a cell in metaphase, not an uncommon finding in this highly proliferative leukemia.

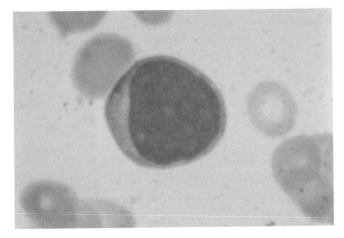

FIGURE 11–5. Type I myeloblast. Note nucleolus, noncondensed chromatin, and absence of cytoplasmic granules.

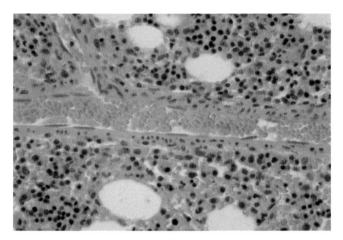

FIGURE 11–6. Bone marrow biopsy; type II myeloblast; similar to type I myeloblast but with slightly more cytoplasm containing a few azurophilic granules.

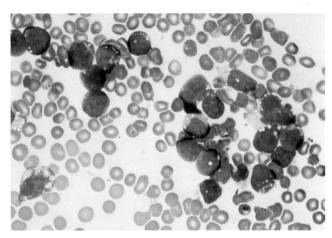

FIGURE 11–7. Undifferentiated acute myeloblastic leukemia (FAB-M0). Note the similarity to Burkitt cell leukemia (FAB-L3), ALL-L2, and acute megakaryocytic leukemia (FAB-M7). Diagnosis depends on the results of immunologic, cytogenetic, and molecular studies.

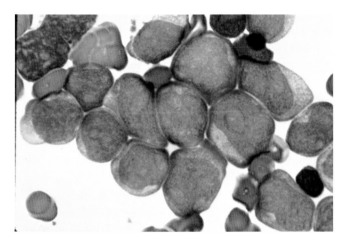

FIGURE 11–8. Acute myeloid leukemia, FAB-M1. Note many type I and few type II myeloblasts and little maturation in this bone marrow smear.

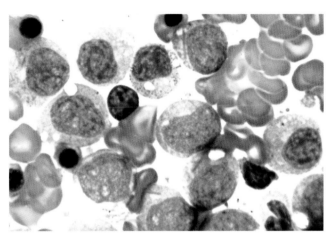

FIGURE 11–9. Acute myeloid leukemia with t(8;21)(q22;q21). This bone marrow exhibits FAB-M2 morphology with type II myeloblasts and some granulocytic maturation. Note the long, fine, and somewhat tubular-appearing Auer rods in four of the blasts characteristic of t(8;21) leukemia.

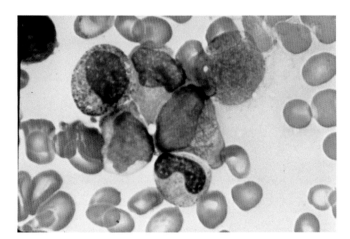

FIGURE 11–11. Hypergranular acute promyelocytic leukemia (FAB-M3). Note the indented nucleus, perinuclear clear zone ("haupt"); abundant cytoplasm containing abnormally large, "succulent" azurophilic granules; and multiple Auer rods, some appearing to be in bundles (faggots).

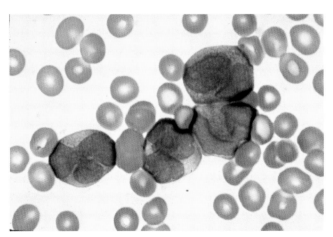

FIGURE 11–13. Microgranular acute promyelocytic leukemia, FAB AML-M3var. The large granules noted in Figure 11–11 are absent. The diagnosis can be suspected on the basis of the nuclear appearance with indentation and some chromatin condensation; however, it must be confirmed by cytogenetics or molecular detection of a translocation involving the *RARA* gene.

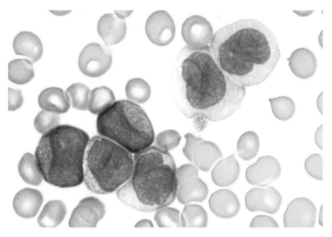

FIGURE 11–14. Acute myelocytic leukemia (FAB AML-M4) bone marrow. This category is typified by nearly equal numbers of myeloblasts and monoblasts plus promonocytes.

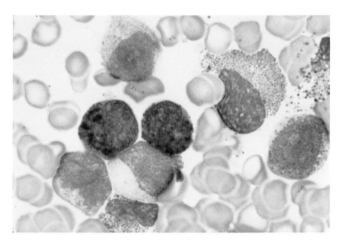

FIGURE 11–15. AML-M4 with abnormal eosinophils. This is classified as AML-M4Eo by the FAB Group. It is associated with cytogenetic aberrations involving chromosome 16, typically inv(16)(p13;q11).

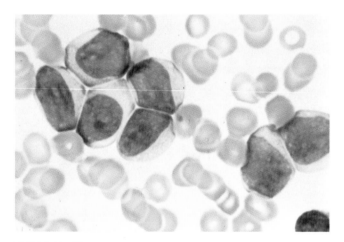

FIGURE 11–16. Acute monoblastic leukemia, FAB AML-M5a. Note the absence of mature monocytes and of granulocytic cells.

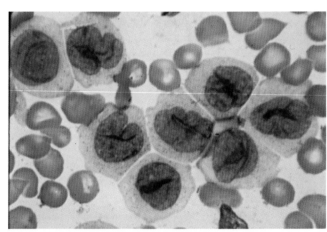

FIGURE 11–17. Acute monocytic leukemia, FAB AML-M5b. Smear consists primarily of partially differentiated monocytic cells, most promonocytes, with few blasts or granulocytic cells.

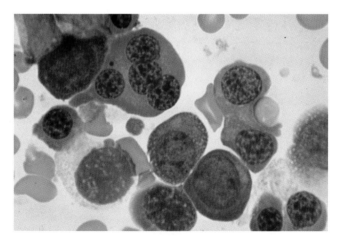

FIGURE 11–18. Acute erythroid leukemia, FAB AML-M6. Note the markedly dyspoietic erythroid precursor cells and the presence of excessive numbers of both erythroblasts and myeloblasts.

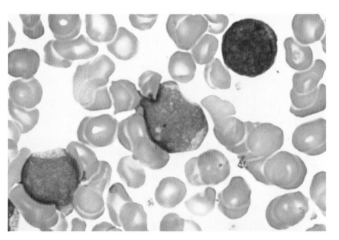

FIGURE 11–19. Acute megakaryocytic leukemia, FAB AML-M7. Peripheral blood smear containing a heterogeneous but poorly differentiated population of blast cells. Definite diagnosis depends on antigen phenotyping with use of antiplatelet membrane antigen reagents and/or platelet peroxidase staining and ultrastructural analysis (immunoelectron microscopy).

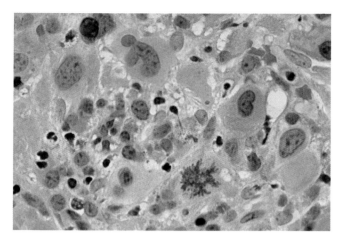

FIGURE 11–20. Acute megakaryocytic leukemia, bone marrow biopsy specimen revealing markedly increased numbers of megakaryocytes and fibrosis.

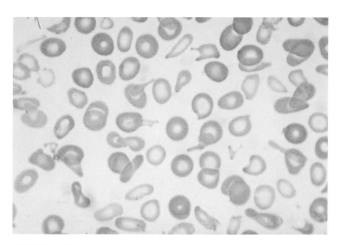

FIGURE 11–21. Peripheral blood smear from a patient with the refractory anemia form of myelodysplastic syndrome. Anisocytosis and poikilocytosis are striking, and neutrophils tend to be hypogranular.

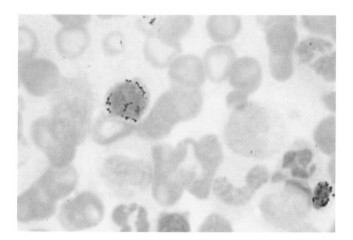

FIGURE 11–22. Refractory anemia with ring sideroblasts (iron stain of bone marrow aspirate).

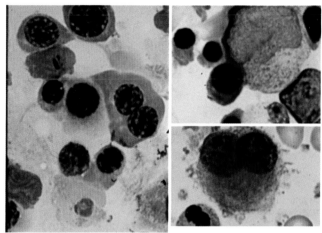

FIGURE 11–23. Composite of marrow cells from a patient with refractory cytopenia with multilineage dysplasia. Clockwise from top right: myelocyte, micromegakaryocyte, and multiple dysplastic erythroid precursors.

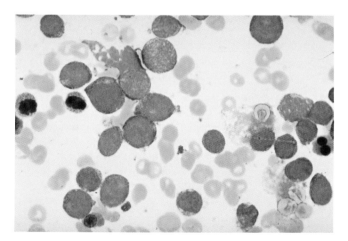

FIGURE 11–24. Refractory anemia with excess blasts. Both increased myeloblasts and dysplastic erythroid precursors are prominent.

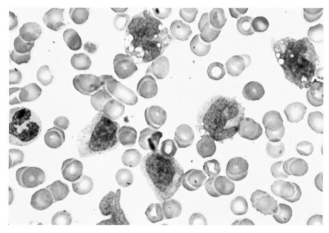

FIGURE 11–25. Chronic myelomonocytic leukemia. Note many monocytes and dysplastic mature neutrophils with hypogranulation. This is classed as a myelodysplastic syndrome by the FAB Group and as a myeloproliferative/myelodysplastic disorder by the WHO Committee.

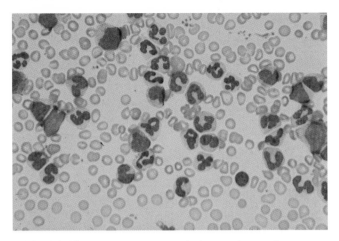

FIGURE 11–26. Chronic myelogenous leukemia, chronic phase. Myelocytes and banded and segmented neutrophils are present. Two Pelger-Huët cells (with bilobed nuclei) are also seen.

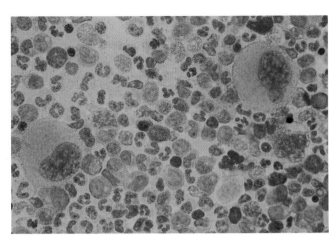

FIGURE 11–27. Chronic myelogenous leukemia, chronic phase, bone marrow biopsy specimen. Marked hypercellularity is seen with increased numbers of dysplastic megakaryocytes, and all stages of granulocytic differentiation are apparent.

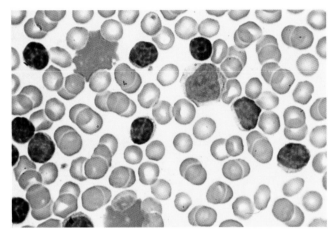

FIGURE 11–28. Chronic lymphocytic leukemia, B-cell type. Bone marrow aspirate shows small lymphocytes with condensed nuclear chromatin. Also present are several typical smudge cells. The T-cell type may resemble this or may have more T-cell characteristics.

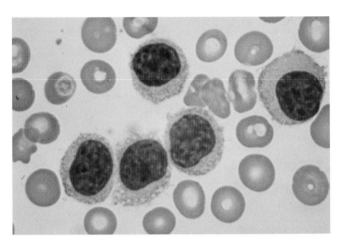

FIGURE 11–29. Hairy cell leukemia. Peripheral blood smear stained with Wright-Giemsa contains hairy cells.

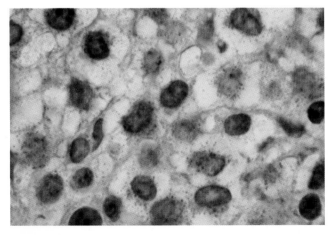

FIGURE 11–30. Hairy cell leukemia. Bone marrow biopsy specimen exhibits tartrate-resistant acid phosphatase staining of hairy cells. Note the wide separation of the hairy cells.

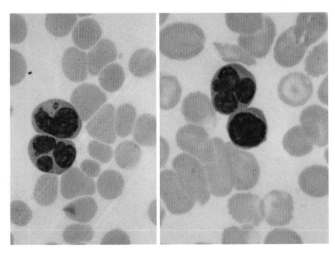

FIGURE 11–31. Adult T-cell leukemia/lymphoma. Peripheral blood contains characteristic malignant T cells with multilobed nuclei (cloverleaf or flower cells).

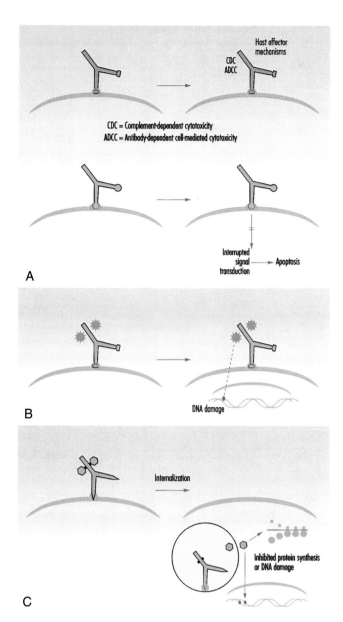

A

B

C

FIGURE 18–1. Antibody-targeted tumor killing, three mechanisms of action. *A*, Unconjugated monoclonal antibody: Binding of antibody initiates killing of target cells by complement-dependent cellular cytotoxicity or antibody-dependent cellular cytotoxicity in the top panel. Antibody binding (e.g., anti-CD20 antibody) interrupts cellular signal transduction, resulting in apoptosis in the lower panel. *B*, Monoclonal antibody linked with radioisotopes: Depending on the antigen targeted, radiolabeled antibody remains on the surface of the cell (CD45) or is internalized (CD33). Radiation induces DNA damage and cell death. In the instance of CD33, the radioisotope is delivered to the cell's interior. In the case of CD45, radiolabeled antibody remains on the cell surface. *C*, Both approaches damage DNA and lead to cell death. Monoclonal antibody linked with antitumor agents: Antibody-bound chemotherapy or toxin is internalized. Interaction with DNA or ribosomal protein synthesis results in cytotoxicity.

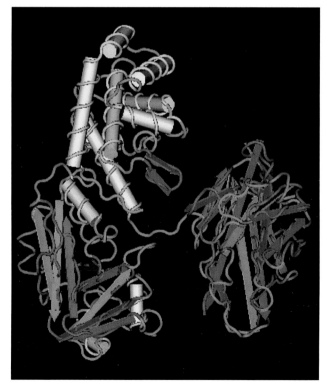

FIGURE 18–2. Ribbon drawing of α-carbon backbone of diphtheria toxin (DT) with domains in different colors. (From Choe S, Bennett MJ, Fujii G, et al: The crystal structure of diphtheria toxin. Nature 1992;357:216.)

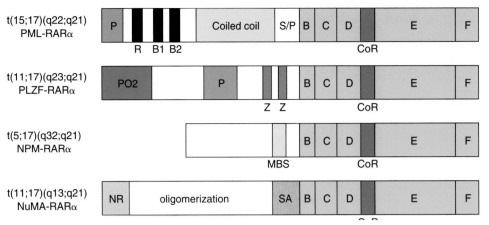

FIGURE 23–1. Chimeric fusion products arising from alternative APL associated translocations. Each of the chromosomal rearrangements disrupts *RARα* within the second intron, leading to the retention of the hormone receptor DNA-, RXR-, ligand-, and coactivator- and co-repressor-binding domain. *PML-RARα*:P: proline-rich domain; R, B1, and B2: cysteine-histidine–rich RING finger and B box domain; S/P: site of phosphorylation, nuclear localization signal. *PLZF-RARα*:POZ: repressor domain; P: proline-rich domain; Z: zinc fingers. *NPM-RARα*: MBS: potential metal binding site. *NuMA-RARα*:NR: nuclear assembly; SA: spindle association.

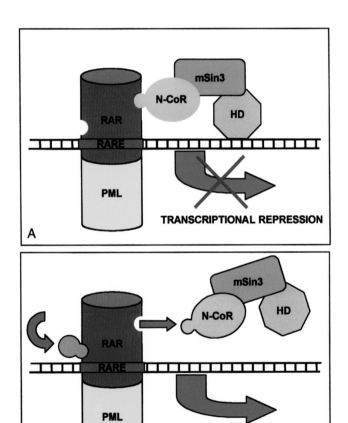

FIGURE 23–2. A schematic representation of the interaction of PML-RARα fusion protein with the N-CoR-mSin3-histone deacetylase (HD) complex. DNA-bound PML-RARα interacts with N-CoR (or SMRT) and recruits the m-Sin3-HD complex, decreasing histone acetylation and producing repressive chromatin organization and transcriptional repression *(A)*. ATRA induces dissociation of the N-CoR-mSin3-HD complex, recruitment of coactivators with acetyltransferase activity (not shown), increased levels of histone acetylation, chromatin remodeling, and transcriptional activation *(B)*.

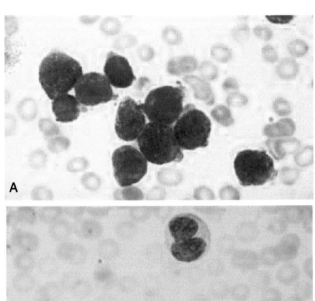

FIGURE 23–3. Representative morphology of M3-hypergranular *(A)* and M3v *(B)*. Bone marrow *(A)* and peripheral blood *(B)* smears were both stained with May-Grumwald-Giemsa ×1000-fold magnification. (Courtesy of Dr. A. Cantù-Rajnoldi, Milan, Italy.)

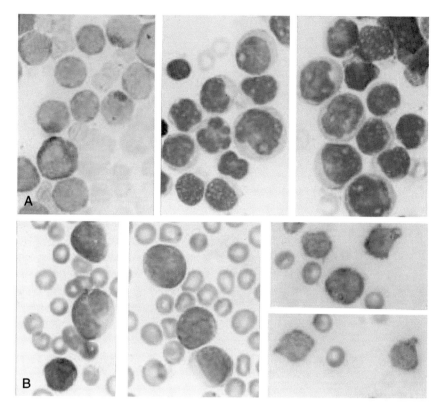

FIGURE 23–4. Representative morphology of atypical morphology in APL cases with *PML-RARα* fusion gene identified by FISH and molecular RT-PCR. Bone marrow smears were stained with May-Grumwald-Giemsa, ×1000-fold magnification. (Courtesy of Dr. D. Head, Vanderbilt University Medical School, Nashville, TN.)

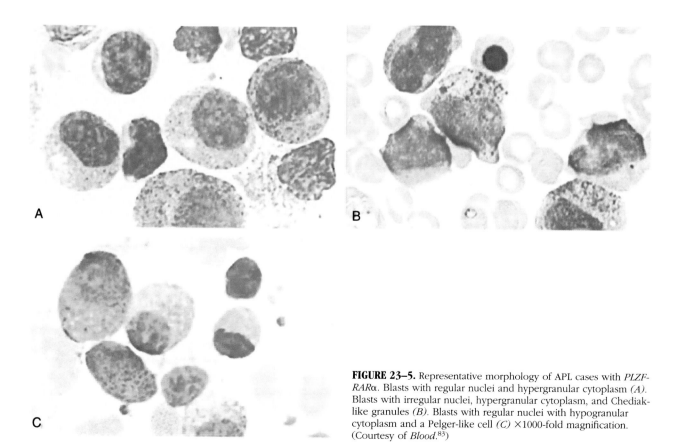

FIGURE 23–5. Representative morphology of APL cases with *PLZF-RARα*. Blasts with regular nuclei and hypergranular cytoplasm *(A)*. Blasts with irregular nuclei, hypergranular cytoplasm, and Chediak-like granules *(B)*. Blasts with regular nuclei with hypogranular cytoplasm and a Pelger-like cell *(C)* ×1000-fold magnification. (Courtesy of *Blood*.[83])

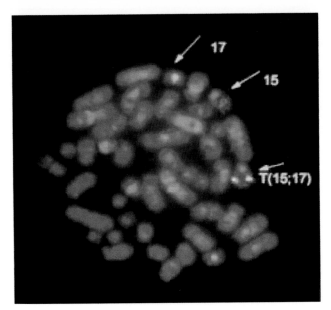

FIGURE 23–6. FISH analysis of an APL case. The result shown has been obtained by using the Vysis probe set, which is designed to detect only the *PML-RARα* fusion gene. It comprises a mixture of directly labeled probes: a *PML* probe, which begins in intron 7 and extends toward the centromere for 180 kb, and a *RARα* probe, which begins in intron 4 and extends toward the telomere for 400 kb. (Courtesy of Prof. A. Hagemeijer, Leuven, Belgium.)

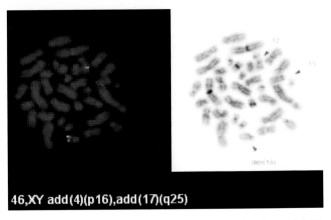

46,XY add(4)(p16),add(17)(q25)

FIGURE 23–7. FISH analysis of an APL case lacking the classic t(15;17) translocation, according to the full karyotype obtained by standard chromosomal banding techniques, but resulting positive for the presence of a *PML-RARα* fusion gene by FISH.

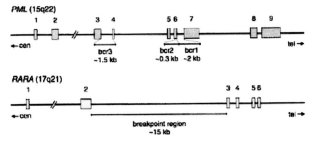

Genes' structures :

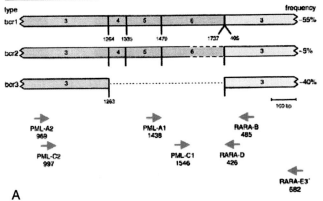

Fusion transcripts:

A

FIGURE 23–8. Schematic diagram of the exon/intron structure of the *PML* and *RARα* genes. The bcr1 and bcr2 breakpoint regions are juxtaposed in intron 6 and exon 6, respectively *(A)*. Schematic diagram of the three types of *PML-RARα* transcripts, related to the different *PML* breakpoint regions. The size of the bcr2 transcript is dependent on the position of the breakpoint in PML exon 6. Primers for RT-PCR analysis of the t(15;17) translocation with the *PML-RARα* fusion gene *(B)*. (Courtesy of *Leukemia*.[113])

Primer code	5' Position[a] (size)	Sequence (5'–3')
PML-A1	1438 (21)	CAGTGTACGCCTTCTCCATCA
PML-A2	969 (18)	CTGCTGGAGGCTGTGGAC
RARA-B	485 (20)	GCTTGTAGATGCGGGGTAGA
PML-C1	1546 (21)	TCAAGATGGAGTCTGAGGAGG
PML-C2	997 (19)	AGCGCGACTACGAGGAGAT
RARA-D	426 (20)	CTGCTGCTCTGGGTCTCAAT
RARA-E3'	682 (20)	GCCCACTTCAAAGCACTTCT

B

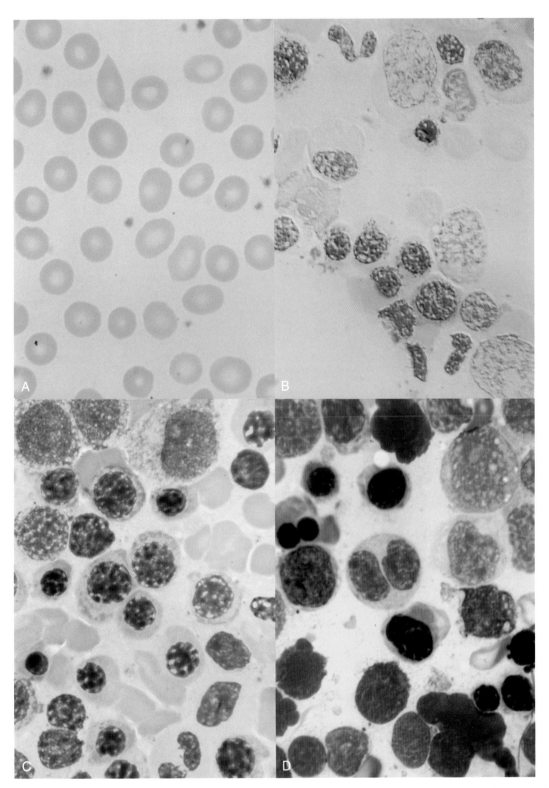

FIGURE 24–2. MDS: abnormal morphology mainly of the erythroid series. *A,* Peripheral blood smear shows macrocytic and macro-ovalocytic red blood cells in RAEB. *B,* Bone marrow aspirate shows ringed sideroblasts in RARS. *C,* Megaloblastoid dyserythropoiesis in RAEB. Atypical promyelocytes with nucleocytoplasmic asynchrony are seen here and in *D. D,* Bone marrow aspirate shows dyserythropoietic changes including nuclear budding (*bottom*) and a binucleate erythroid cell (*top*) in RARS. (All photographs ×64.)

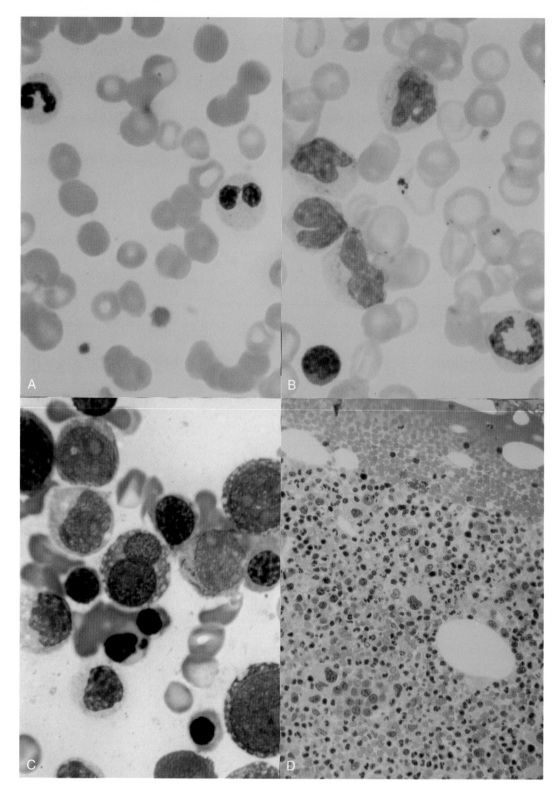

FIGURE 24–3. MDS: abnormal morphology mainly of the myeloid series. *A,* Peripheral blood smear shows dysplastic hypogranular neutrophil with a pseudo–Pelger-Huët anomaly in refractory anemia. *B,* Peripheral blood smear shows abnormal monocytes in CMML. Pappenheimer's bodies are seen in the red blood cells. *C,* Bone marrow aspirate shows a blast and atypical promyelocyte in RARS. *D,* Bone marrow biopsy shows ALIP. (All photographs ×64.)

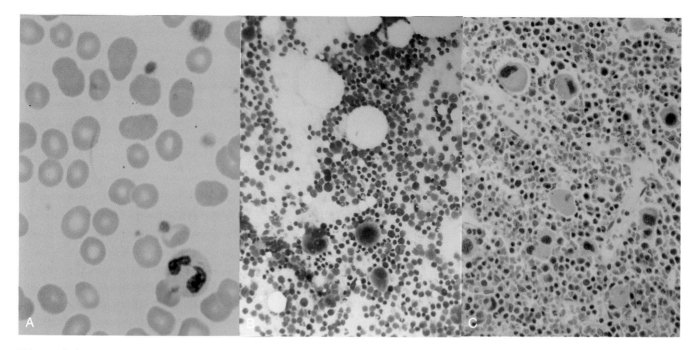

FIGURE 24–4. MDS: abnormal morphology mainly of the megakaryocyte series. *A,* Peripheral blood smear reveals large hypogranular platelets in RA in addition to a dysplastic neutrophil with a pseudo–Pelger-Huët anomaly. *B,* Bone marrow aspirate in RAEB. *C,* Bone marrow biopsy in RA shows hypolobated and micromegakaryocytes. (All photographs ×64.)

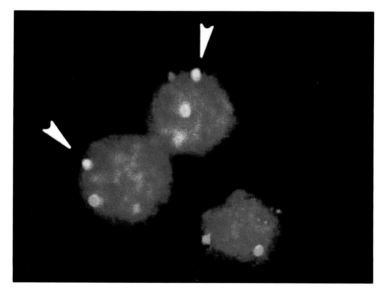

FIGURE 26–2. Fluorescence in situ hybridization (FISH) with a TEL/AML1 dual-color probe in the bone marrow cells of a child with ALL. The *TEL* gene labels with a green color, and the *AML1* gene labels with a red color. The arrows point to the *TEL/AML1* fusion gene (yellow color signals) in two interphase leukemic cells indicating the presence of t(12;21)(p13;q22). A single green signal *(TEL)* and red signal *(AML1)* from the uninvolved chromosomes may also be seen. A normal cell with two green signals (TEL genes) and two red cells (AML1 genes) is also present. (Courtesy Dr. Samual Wu, Childrens Hospital, Los Angeles, CA.)

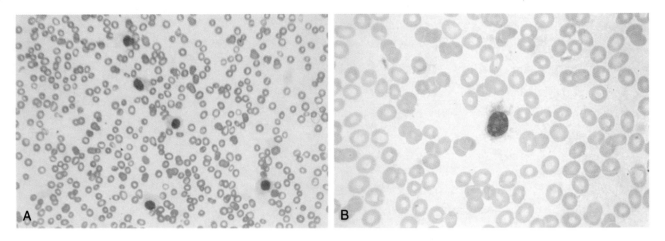

FIGURE 29–1. *A,* Light microscopy of typical hairy cells (Wright-Giemsa stain, × 200). *B,* Typical hairy cell with cytoplasmic projections (Wright-Giemsa stain, × 250).

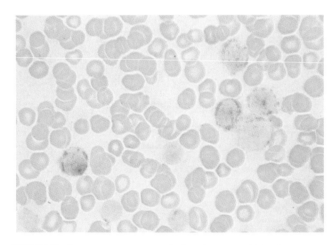

FIGURE 29–2. Tartrate-resistant acid phosphatase positivity in a case of HCL (× 250).

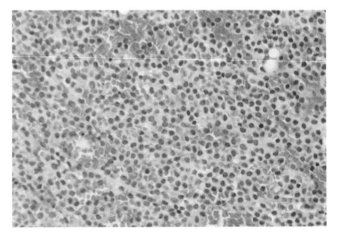

FIGURE 29–4. HCL in the bone marrow. Note the lymphoid cells with clear spaces surrounding each individual cell.

1

Edward S. Henderson

History of Leukemia

Unlike the history of many diseases, accounts and traces of leukemia are of a relatively recent origin. Before the middle of the nineteenth century, leukemia, unlike solid tumors, especially those of bone, was not perceived as an entity, but went undiagnosed, included in the numbers of patients whose diagnoses were recorded as infection, anemia, dropsy, and other conditions with protean causes and clinical manifestations. Not surprisingly, the earliest reports were made by pathologists, who recognized, first by gross observation and later through microscopy, that the blood was composed predominantly of white rather than red cells. The earliest report of the illness is generally considered to have been made by Velpeau in 1827, which was ignored until cited by Virchow some 20 years later.[1, 2]

The patient, a 63-year-old florist with a history of bibulousness and sexual intemperance, became ill in 1825 with fever, weakness, abdominal swelling, and urinary stones; he quickly expired. At autopsy he was found not to be luetic but to have marked hepatosplenomegaly and blood that was thick "like gruel . . . resembling in consistency and color the yeast of red wine . . . (resembling) laudable pus mixed with blackish coloring matter (rather) than blood." Similar cases were reported by Barth[3] and Craigie.[4] Fortunately, these later physicians referred their cases to microscopically trained pathologists for review, the former to Alexander Donné of Paris, the founder of French clinical microscopy, the latter to John H. Bennett, who had studied with Donné.

It is of historical interest that, although nearly two centuries had elapsed since Antonie van Leeuwenhoek described microscopic bacteria as "very little animalcules" in 1660, and despite the enthusiastic adoption of microscopy by protozoologists and entomologists, physicians had strenuously resisted including microscopy into the practice of medicine (doubtless it was costly, time-consuming, and not covered by the funding agencies of the time). Donné changed this attitude through a series of impressive studies, which included the discovery of *Trichomonas vaginalis*, the adaptation in collaboration with DaGuerre of photomicroscopy to medical education and research, and his discovery and description of blood platelets.[5] His lecture series at the Medical Faculty of Paris and his text *Cours de Microscopie*[6] popularized microscopic techniques and drew visitors such as Dr.

Bennett of Edinburgh to the continent to learn the techniques firsthand.

Of Barth's patient Donné wrote "the blood you sent me, my dear colleague, shows a remarkable and most conspicuous change. . . . More than half of the cells were mucous globules. This fact perhaps needs some explanation. You know that normal blood contains three types of cells: 1) red cells, 2) white cells or mucous cells, 3) the small globules (i.e., the platelets). It is the second variety which dominates so much that one wonders . . . whether this blood does not contain pus" (Dreyfus C., 1857 [quoted in Thorburn[5, 6]]). Bennett, in reviewing his own case and that of Craigie in 1845, had a similar impression: "I think there can be little doubt that (in both cases) pus in the blood was the cause of death, and that it produced the febrile symptoms." He added, "It is important to remember that there was no phlebitis, abscess, or purulent collection to which the appearances within the vessels could be ascribed."[7] (Donné later revised his initial view to state "the blood of (a later) patient showed such a number of white cells that I thought his blood was mixed with pus, but in the end, I was able to observe a clear-cut difference between these cells and the (normal, purulent) white cells."[8] However, it was the insights of Rudolf Virchow, the founder of the school of cellular pathology in Berlin, that led to the recognition of leukemia as a specific and distinct entity, a condition sui generis. Virchow's first publication on what he initially called "weisses Blut" appeared almost simultaneously with the co-publications of Craigie and Bennett.[9]

He described a patient who presented with a clinical picture similar to those described by Velpeau, Donné, Craigie, Bennett, and Fuller[10]; i.e., with fever, exhaustion, abdominal swelling, edema, and bleeding, leading to the patient's death. Autopsy revealed splenomegaly, uric acid stones, and whitish blood "looking like viscous pus." Microscopically, the proportion of colored (i.e., red) cells and colorless cells was dramatically altered so that "the proportion of the red and the colorless (in mass white) blood corpuscles is reversed without any noticeable admixture of foreign chemical or morphologic elements." The following year, using improved but still primitive techniques then available, he was able to state, "I have demonstrated that the morphologic characteristics of the changed blood do not justify the assumption of a suppura-

1

tive transformation. . . . I hereby claim for the colorless corpuscles a place in pathology."[2] In 1847 he used the term "leukemia" (leukämie) for the first time. He believed that the disease was "a primary autonomous disease of the spleen and lymphatic gland, and the direct cause for the increase in the number of colorless particles in the blood"[2]; he subsequently wrote that two types, a splenic and a lymphatic form, could be distinguished from each other on the basis of the morphologic similarities of the leukemia cells to the cells normally resident in, respectively, the spleen or lymph glands.

During this same fertile period, the distinction between acute and chronic forms of leukemia was appreciated.[11]

It was left to Neumann in 1868 to relate leukemia to changes in the bone marrow, in a case of the splenic form of leukemia.[12] He tentatively renamed this form of leukemia "myelogenous," a "provisional" term which quite successfully has withstood the test of time. Shortly thereafter, Mosler introduced bone marrow puncture as a means of antemortem diagnosis of leukemia.[13]

The neoplastic nature of leukemia and the origin of the disease in organs of blood formation having been established, the next advance in understanding its pathophysiology was provided by the introduction and application of aniline dyes to pathology. Although the first application of such stains to histopathology was reported by an American, Joseph Janvier Woodward, the use of stains in hematology was carried out, predictably, in Germany, in particular through the studies of Paul Ehrlich and his disciples.[14] During the century since Ehrlich's initial studies, identification of most of the major subcategories of leukemia was based on light microscopy: morphologic and cytohistochemical observations alone. Only relatively recently have molecular genetics and immunology taken the lead in identifying important new leukemia subtypes and in detecting residual foci of disease.

TREATMENT

Not long after leukemia was established as an entity, a treatment was discovered, and a modality was founded. In 1865, Lissauer administered arsenous oxide (Fowler's solution) as a tonic to a patient with chronic myelocytic leukemia, and surprisingly a complete remission was achieved.[15] Arsenicals quickly became the treatment of choice for leukemia, although remissions were unpredictably attained but predictably transient. The concept of chemotherapy for leukemia was thus, not surprisingly and quite appropriately, developed through the combination of serendipity and empiricism. The search for safer and more predictable methods of arsenic delivery led to the synthesis of organic arsenical compounds and to the discovery of important therapies for infectious diseases. If the field of infectious disease thereby benefited from the efforts of leukemia and cancer therapists, this debt was richly repaid in subsequent generations.

Roentgen rays were discovered in 1895. Their first application to the treatment of leukemia was reported in 1902 by Pusey[16] and in 1903 by Senn.[17] Roentgen rays quickly replaced arsenicals as the treatment of choice for leukemia; for nearly half a century, they remained the mainstay of therapy, particularly for the chronic forms of leukemia.

Like arsenicals, radiation therapy was only marginally effective in acute cases. Therapy remained ineffective until the mid-20th century. Indeed, acute leukemia was so universally held to be incurable that rare successes were ignored or scorned. In 1932, Dr. W. Gloor reported the successful treatment of an American businessman who in 1927 presented with acute myeloid leukemia while traveling in Europe. He arranged to be treated in Zurich at the celebrated clinic of Professor O. Naegeli, at which Dr. Gloor served. The patient received combination therapy that included radiation, arsenic, mesothorium, and two transfusions of whole blood donated by his sister. The results from the transfusions were dramatic. Immediately following the first, leukemic cells disappeared from the patient's blood, and his white cell count rose. He remained leukemia-free until his death from an unrelated cause at the age of 102, some 52 productive years since his successful combined-modality therapy.

In 1930, Gloor reported the case with a 3-year follow-up.[18] Far from receiving praise, he was charged with misrepresenting a benign condition as leukemia. Not long afterwards, he left Naegeli's clinic and academic medicine for unexplained reasons. It is possible that his attribution of at least part of the success of the therapy to the transfusions played some role in his dismissal. The importance of blood transfusions in the management of leukemia had been championed by the rival Viennese school but was held to be useless by Professor Naegeli.

Despite the exceptional case, leukemia remained virtually incurable and indifferently treatable until the 1940s. However, during this therapeutically fallow period, the foundations of cancer chemotherapy were being laid. Three major sources provided the bases for the subsequent rebirth of drug therapy for leukemia: the discovery of the hematologic effects of alkylating agents, the discovery and isolation of naturally occurring antibiotics, and the development of the theory and practice of antimetabolite therapy.

Clinically useful alkylating agents were the direct by-products of the two world wars. Cytotoxic gases were introduced with devastating effect into the trench battles toward the end of World War I. Pulmonary inflammation was the cause of acute morbidity and mortality rates, and pulmonary fibrosis and insufficiency crippled many of those who survived the initial injury. However, pathologic studies of mustard gas victims by Krumbhaar and Krumbhaar revealed that, in addition to pulmonary changes, these toxins regularly caused cytopenias and marrow hypoplasia in fatal cases.[19] When World War II began, it was feared these gases might be used again. In fact, no such gases were used, but terrible casualties resulted from the explosion of a mustard gas–laden munitions ship in Bari.[20] As a result, scientific investigations of their mechanisms of action were commissioned in the United States and Britain.[21] These confirmed that nitrogen mustards could destroy hematopoietic tissue in the marrow and lymphatics (Winternitz, cited by Zubrod).[21] Succeeding studies that showed that these agents could cause regression of transplanted murine lymphoma were promptly followed by clinical trials of mechlorethamine and tris(beta chloroethyl) amine hydrochloride in patients with lymphoma and leukemia.[22-25]

In 1946, Goodman and colleagues[23] reported that 6 of 12 patients with chronic leukemia responded with a degree of abnormal white blood cell reduction and lymph node regression comparable to that obtainable with radiation therapy. Results were less impressive with acute leukemia, although 3 of 7 patients showed some clinical and hematologic response. None of the responses in any disease were long-lasting. All the patients died and, in some cases, it was believed that "B-chloroethylene therapy may have accelerated the fatal termination." Nevertheless, the results of these preliminary trials, although of limited patient benefit, stimulated the development and evaluation of new alkylating agents with differing pharmacologic features, including drugs that could be given by mouth. Notable among these were busulfan,[26, 27] chlorambucil,[28] and cyclophosphamide,[29] which remain important drugs in the treatment of leukemia and in preparation of patients for bone marrow transplantation.

The development of programs for the discovery and/or synthesis and testing of drugs for the control of parasitic infections was the other major contributor to the development of effective antileukemia therapies. Paul Ehrlich had noted that synthetic dyes could localize and influence the growth of parasites. Methylene blue was shown to have marginal effectiveness against malaria. Later, trypan red proved therapeutic in mice infected with *Trypanosoma equiperdum*, the agent causing horse sleeping sickness.[30] Still later, Ehrlich's group was to bring the chemotherapy of infectious disease to world prominence through the demonstration of the effectiveness of the organic arsenical salvarsan (Preparation 606) in the treatment of *Treponema pallidum*, the causative organism in syphilis.[31]

Despite the successes in the treatment of protozoal infections, there remained great skepticism toward the prospect of developing a drug-based cure of bacterial infections (let alone neoplastic diseases). Nevertheless, programs were launched to develop therapies for tuberculosis and common bacterial pathogens. One notable program was conducted by the Bayer Division of I.G. Farben, which sought to develop and test dyes that might have utility in treating streptococcal infections, a leading cause of acute sepsis and of delayed cardiac and renal insufficiency. This program was led by the German chemist and pathologist Gerhard Domagk, whose team developed sulfamidochrysoidine (Prontosil), a red sulfanilamide.[32] Domagk was in the fortuitous position of being able to abet his own daughter's successful fight for life by administering Prontosil when she lay stricken with streptococcal septicemia.[33, 34] This and similar successes encouraged the discovery (and rediscovery) of other antibacterial agents, e.g., penicillin,[35-37] and led to mechanistic studies of the action of the sulfonamides. In 1940, Woods[38] and Fildes[39] postulated independently that sulfonamide acted through interference with normal metabolic reactions necessary for bacterial growth. This metabolite-antimetabolite concept provided the rationale for synthesis of biologically active compounds designed to competitively inhibit known metabolic pathways.

Infectious disease therapy has benefited from drugs such as additional sulfonamides, pyrimethamine, trimethoprim, acyclovir, and zidovudine. For cancer chemotherapy, the most immediate consequence of the new concept was the introduction of antagonists to folic acid. The vitamin activity of folic acid had been identified by Wills and Bilmoria[40] and subsequently by Mitchell and coworkers, who isolated it from leafy vegetables.[41] It was observed to be necessary for normal hematopoiesis and was also soon shown to accelerate the growth of leukemic tissue in mice and in people.[42] These observations quickly led to the synthesis and animal testing of antifolic acids.[43, 44] Of several candidates, pteropterin and aminopterin were selected for human trials by Farber and his colleagues.[45] The results were astonishing.

For the first time, the rapid progression of acute leukemia in children was regularly arrested, and in many cases hematopoiesis once again became normal. Unfortunately, these remissions could not be sustained, and all the young patients ultimately succumbed to recurrent disease. Nonetheless, these transitory successes, together with the responses to alkylating agents, were enough to encourage the tremendous scientific and clinical efforts in chemotherapy that continue to this day.

Almost concurrently, antimetabolites to purine and pyrimidine synthesis and DNA assembly were initiated, spearheaded most notably by George Hitchings and Gertrude Elion,[46-48] which led eventually to the introduction of 6-mercaptourine, 6-thioguanine, and allopurinol into clinical practice.[49, 50] Cytarabine was introduced in the 1960s.[51-53] The adenosine nucleoside analogs fludarabine and 2-chloroadenosine with broad antileukemic application are recent products from the cornucopia of antimetabolites.[54-56]

Natural products, such as enzymes, hormones, and toxins from animal, vegetable, and microbial sources, are a third major source of drugs of importance to leukemia therapists. These were first represented by adrenal hormones (and ACTH), shown in 1942 to cause lymphocyte death,[57, 58] an activity that was exploited promptly in the clinical treatment of both acute and chronic leukemias.[59, 60] In subsequent decades L-aparaginase,[61-63] vinca alkyloids,[64, 65] and antibiotics—most notably the anthracyclines[66, 67]—were noted in vitro and in animal drug screening systems to have a high level of anti–leukemia-cell activity and were successfully incorporated into clinical use.[68-72]

Since the mid-1970s, a different sort of natural product, the cytokines, entered the picture,[73] initially produced from lymphocytes and laboriously purified and, more recently, manufactured through recombinant gene techniques that proliferated during that era. These cell growth and development regulating factors were used either for their properties of tumor cell inhibition or their ability to stimulate normal hematopoiesis and thereby reduce the toxicity of then-conventional cytotoxic therapies.[74, 75] The most notable members of this class of compounds have been interferon-α, currently widely used in the treatment of chronic leukemias[76]; the various marrow stimulatory factors (granulocyte-stimulating factor, interleukin-3 [IL-3], and others); the immunostimulatory leukokines, notably interleukin-2 (IL-2); and in particular the differentiating vitamins, the most notable to date being all-*trans*-retinoic acid with its dramatic and mechanistically defined activity directed toward malignant promyelocytes.[77-81]

The new chemotherapeutic agents both established the importance of this modality of treatment and encouraged a new philosophy of caring for patients with leukemia. While skepticism persisted in some circles, in others enthusiasm of unknown proportions was kindled. Collaborating groups of clinical investigators were formed, and major public programs such as the National Cancer Institute's intramural and extramural programs of research support for leukemia therapy were established.

Cure was not only envisioned; in a small but growing fraction of patients, it was achieved. The pessimism that had pervaded all aspects of the care of leukemia patients began to be supplanted, in the face of demonstrable clinical gains, by guarded optimism. This was the direct result of the application to leukemia of lessons learned from the treatment of infectious disease.[82, 83] In addition to the exploitation of antimetabolites (and, later, antibiotics), the preclinical development and screening of candidate drugs in cell culture and animal disease models, the application of cell kinetics models, the appreciation of the parameters of cell killing, and the utility of combination chemotherapy were tested in infections and translated to leukemia (and then cancer) therapy.

From 1950 to 1960, many new drugs were introduced as well as programs with which to evaluate them. Methods of dealing with complications of leukemia, e.g., meningeal leukemia[84, 85] and thrombocytopenic bleeding,[86, 87] were developed.

The following decade witnessed the dramatic impact of the use of combination drug and modality therapy,[72, 88-90] high-dose therapy with "rescue,"[91-93] and treatment of the central nervous system in presymptomatic patients (adjuvant central nervous system drug and/or radiation therapy).[94, 95] Through these approaches, the 1960s witnessed the cure of acute lymphocytic leukemia in children evolve from an anecdotal wonder to a quantifiable reality.

During the same period, hematopoietic stem cell engraftment progressed from an uncertain and often dangerous curiosity to an important clinical modality. Bone marrow therapy had been attempted in the 19th century by Brown-Séquard and d'Arsonaval, who administered glycerol extracts of marrow by mouth to patients with leukemia[96] with an understandable lack of success. It was not until half a century later that a potentially efficacious route of stem cell administration was employed: intramuscular injection by Schretzenmayr in 1937,[97] intramedullary instillation by Rasjeck, and intravenous infusion by Osgood, Riddle, and Mathews.[98, 99] During the next 20 years, it was shown that living spleen and marrow cells could protect lethally irradiated mice and that this protection was due to the hematopoietic cells rather than to humoral factors.[100-104]

Subsequently, radiation chimeras were produced in dogs, goats, monkeys, and humans. The first marrow grafts for leukemia were transient and consistently fatal, with deaths due to marrow aplasia, recurrent disease, or so-called secondary disease as graft-versus-host disease

(GVHD) was then known.[105, 106] As GVHD became better understood, attempts were made to define human histocompatibility and to use related donors in the hopes of a fortuitous match. Grafts between identical twins proved that marrow engraftment could be successfully performed after myeloablative therapy to the leukemic recipient and that completely histocompatible marrow did not produce clinically significant GVHD. However, leukemia recurred in all these early cases.[107]

One transplant performed by Mathe and coworkers did, however, lead to a complete remission for 2½ years. The patient died of viral encephalitis in the setting of persistent chronic GVHD, but the absence of leukemia recurrence gave encouragement to transplanters that cure was possible with allogeneic marrow transplantation.[108] The elucidation of the genetics of human histocompatibilty[109] and the application of histocompatibility testing for organ transplantation led the way to frequent application of marrow grafting for leukemia and other marrow diseases in the United States, England, and continental Europe.[110-112]

In the early 1970s Thomas and his associates were able to accumulate and report a series of children with acute leukemia treated in relapse, of whom 20% were cured of their disease.[113] Thereafter, this experience was repeated in several centers worldwide and extended to patients in remission,[114] adults, and to patients with chronic myelogenous leukemia.[115] Improved control of transplant-related infections and of GVHD dramatically improved the frequency and quality of survival and broadened the applicability of the procedure to older individuals and cases with less favorable degrees of histocompatibility.

Underpinning these therapeutic advances (including technology with which to develop new treatments, identification of new targets for therapy, identification of prognostically significant subsets of leukemia, and provision of more sensitive means of monitoring treatment and identifying minimal foci of residual disease) were the remarkable advances in stem cell enumeration and culture,[116-119] immunology, genetics, and molecular biology.

Immunologic characterization as an important determinant of the outcome of therapy was emphasized in the late 1960s by Sen and Borella, using the rather primitive techniques available at that time.[120] The development of monoclonal antibodies[121] and automated cell analysis,[122] together with the extensive characterizations of cell surface antigens,[123-125] greatly augmented the diagnostic specification of leukemia.

Cytogenetics similarly provided not only the initial proof of the clonal origin of leukemic tissues[126] but also a means of subtype identification and minimal disease detection. Chromosomal banding studies led to the identification of the chromosomal translocations central to chronic myelogenous leukemia,[127] promyelocytic leukemia,[128] and Burkitt's lymphoma,[129-131] which in turn spurred the search for cancer gene involvement at or near the chromosome breakpoints. These studies led to the identification of new oncogenes,[132-138] repressor genes, and new targets for treatment interventions.[78-80, 139]

The development of molecular biology,[140] aided by advances in nucleoside sequencing[141-143] and the discovery of restriction endonucleases[144-146] and their application to

DNA and RNA analysis[147] and recombinant DNA production,[148] led to the appreciation of the physiologic role of DNA and RNA splicing[149-151] and identification of oncogenes; tumor suppression genes[152]; cell cycle regulatory,[153] apoptosis-stimulating, and apoptosis-inhibiting genes[154-157]; and the myriad nuclear-adhering proteins that influence their transcription and thus the regulation of proliferation, development, and death. The development of polymerase chain reaction technology[158, 159] helped bring these molecular events rapidly into clinical practice.

As we progress through the new millennium, the understanding of the nature of leukemia is expanding dramatically. Because of this, it is becoming possible to classify many types of leukemia based on their underlying genetic lesion rather than simply on their morphology or other phenotypic feature.[160] In some cases, it is also possible to direct therapy toward the specific biochemical lesion that drives and sustains the disease state and thus correct it by specific and minimally toxic means.[139]

With large-scale attempts to characterize all the various forms of hematopoietic malignancy, it is not unlikely that these successes will be extended to all forms of leukemia, myelodysplasia, and myeloproliferative and lymphoproliferative disease. If not in the next decade, certainly by the bicentennial of its discovery, leukemia will have become a curable and preventable disease.

REFERENCES

1. Velpeau A: Rev Med 1827, 2, 218.
2. Virchow R: Weisses Blut und Milztumoren: I. Med Z 1846, 15, 157; II. Med Z 1847, 16, 9.
3. Barth R: Alterations du sang remarquable par le predominance des globules blanc ou maqueux hypertrophie considerable de la rate. Bull Soc Med Hop (Paris), 1856, 3, 89.
4. Craigie D: Case of disease of the spleen in which death took place in consequence of the presence of purulent matter in the blood. Edinb Med Surg J 1845, 64 400.
5. Thorburn AL: Albert Francois Donne. 1801–1878. Discoverer of *Trichomonas vaginales* and leukemia. Br J Vener Dis 1974, 50, 377.
6. Seufert W, Seufert WD: The recognition of leukemia as a systemic disease. J History Med 1982, 37, 34.
7. Bennett JH. Case of hypertrophy of the spleen and liver, in which death took place from suppuration of the blood. Edinb Med Surg J 1845, 64 13.
8. Donné A. Cours de Microscopie. Paris, J.B. Bailliere, 1844.
9. Virchow RLK: Weisses Blut. N Notiz Geb Natur u Heilk 1845, 36, 151.
10. Fuller HW: Particulars of a case in which enormous enlargement of all the blood vessels of the body were found coincident with a peculiar altered condition of the blood. Lancet 1846, 2, 43.
11. Friedreich N: Ein neue Fall von Leukämie. Virchows Arch Path Anat 1857, 12, 37.
12. Neumann E: Ein Fall von Leukämie mit Erkränkung des Knochenmarkes. Arch Heilk (Lpz) 1870, 11, 1.
13. Mosler F: Klinische Symptome und Therapie des medullaren Leukämia. Berliner Klin Wschr 1876, 13, 702.
14. Ehrlich P, Lazarus P, Pinkus F: Leukemia, Pseudoleukemia, Haemoglobinemia. Vienna, A Hölder, 1901.
15. Lissauer H: Zwei Fälle von Leukämie. Berliner Klin Wschr 1865, 2, 403.
16. Pusey WA: Report of cases treated with Roentgen rays. JAMA 1902, 38, 911.
17. Senn N: The therapeutical value of the Roentgen ray in the treatment of pseudoleukemia. N York Med J 1903, 77, 665.
18. Gloor W: Ein Fall von geheiltes Myeloblastenleukemie. Münchner Med Wschr 1930, 77, 1096.
19. Krumbhaar EB, Krumbhaar HD. The blood and bone marrow in yellow cross (mustard) gas poisoning. Changes produced in bone marrow in fatal cases. J Med Res 1919, 40, 497.
20. Alexander AF: Medical report of the Bari Harbor mustard casualties. Milit Surg 1947, 101, 1.
21. Zubrod CG: Historic milestones in curative chemotherapy. Semin Oncol 1979, 6, 490.
22. Gilman A, Phillips FS: The biological action and therapeutic applications of the B-chloroethyl amines and sulfides. Science 1946, 103, 409.
23. Goodman LS, Wintrobe MW, Dameshek, W, et al: Nitrogen mustard therapy: Use of methyl-bis (beta-chloroethyl) amine hydrochloride and tris(beta-chloroethyl)amine hydrochloride for Hodgkin's disease, lymphosarcoma, leukemia, and certain allied and miscellaneous disorders. JAMA 1946, 105, 475.
24. Jacobson LO, Spurr CL, Barron ESG, et al: Nitrogen mustard therapy. JAMA 1946, 132, 263.
25. Rhoads CP: Nitrogen mustards in the treatment of neoplastic diseases. JAMA 1946, 131, 656.
26. Galton DAG: Myleran in chronic myeloid leukemia: Results of treatment. Lancet 1953, 264, 208.
27. Haddow A, Timmis GM: Myleran in chronic myeloid leukaemia: Chemical constitution and biological action. Lancet 1953, 1, 207.
28. Galton DAG, Israels LG, Nabarro JDN, et al: Clinical trials of p(D1–2-chloroethylamino)-phenylbutyric acid (CB1348) in malignant lymphoma. Brit Med J 1955, 2, 1172.
29. Brock N: Zur pharmakologischen Charakterisierung zyclischen NLost Phosphamidester als KrebsChemotherapeutica. Arzneim Forsch, 1958, 8, 1.
30. Ehrlich P, Shiga K. Farbentherapeutische Versache bei Trypanosomenerkränkung. Berliner Klin Wschr 1904, 41, 329.
31. Ehrlich P: Die Behandlung der Syphillis mit dem Ehrlichschen Präparat 606. Med Wschr (Lpz, Berl) 1910, 36, 1893.
32. Domagk G. Eine neue Klasse von Desinfektionsmitteln. Dtsch Med Wschr 1935, 61, 829.
33. Domagk G. Ein Beitrag zur Chemotherapie der bakteriellen Infektion. Dtsch Med Wsch 1935, 61, 250.
34. Richie-Calder, Lord: World health: An ethical-economic perspective. Bull N Y Acad Sci 1975, 51, 608.
35. Fleming A: On the antibacterial action of cultures of a penicillium, with special reference to their use in the isolation of *B. influenza*. Br J Exp Pathol 1929, 10, 226.
36. Chain E, Florey HW, Gardner AD, et al: Penicillin as a chemotherapeutic agent. Lancet 1940, ii, 226.
37. Waxman S, Woodruff HB: Bacteriostatic and bacteriocidal substances produced by soil *Actinomyces* 39. Proc Soc Exp Biol Med 1940, 45, 609.
38. Woods DD: The relationship of p-aminobenzoic acid to the mechanism of action of sulfanilamide. Br J Exp Pathol 1940, 21, 74.
39. Fildes P: A rational approach to research in chemotherapy. Lancet 1940, i, 955.
40. Wills L, Bilmoria HS: Studies in pernicious anemia of pregnancy: Production of macrocytic anemia in monkeys by deficient feeding. Indian J Med Res 1932, 20, 391.
41. Mitchell HK, Snell EE, Williams RJ: The concentration of "folic acid." J Am Chem Soc 1941, 63, 2284.
42. Heinle RW, Welch AD: Experiments with pteroylglutamic acid deficiency in human leukemia. J Clin Invest 1948, 27, 539.
43. Seeger DR, Smith JM Jr, Hultquist ME: Antagonist for pteroylglutamic acid. J Am Chem Soc 1947, 69, 2567.
44. Seeger DR, Consulich DB, Smith JM Jr, et al: Analogs of pteroylglutamic acid. III. 4-amino derivatives. J Am Chem Soc 1949, 71, 1753.
45. Farber S, Diamond LK, Mercer RD, et al: Temporary remissions in leukemia in children produced by folic acid antagonist 4-aminopteroyl-glutamic acid (aminopterin). N Engl J Med 1948, 238, 787.
46. Elion GB, Hitchings GH, Vander Wolff H: Antagonists of nucleic acid derivatives. VI. Purines. J Biol Chem 1951, 192, 505.
47. Elion GB, Burgi E, Hitchings GH. Studies on condensed pyrimidine systems. IX. The synthesis of some 6-substituted purines. J Am Chem Soc 1952, 74, 411.
48. Hitchings GH, Elion GB, Falco EH, et al: Studies on the analogs of purines and pyrimidines. Ann N Y Acad Sci 1950, 52, 1318.
49. Burchenal JH, Murphy ML, Ellison RR, et al: Clinical evaluation of a new antimetabolite, 6-mercaptopurine, in treatment of leukemia and allied diseases. Blood 1953, 8, 965.

50. Rundles RW, Wyngaarden JB, Hitchings GH, et al: Effects of the xanthine oxidase inhibitor, allopurinol, on thiopurine metabolism, hypruricemia, and gout. Trans Assoc Am Phys 1963, 176, 126.

51. Ellison RR, Holland JF, Weil M, et al: Arabinosyl cytosine, a useful agent in the treatment of acute leukemia in adults. Blood 1968, 32, 507.

52. Henderson ES, Burke PJ: Clinical experience with cytosine arabinoside. Proc Am Assoc Cancer Res 1965, 6, 26.

53. Howard JP, Albo V, Newton WA: Cytosine arabinoside: Results of a cooperative study in acute childhood leukemia. Cancer 1069, 21, 341.

54. Carson DA, Wasson DB, Taetle R, et al: Specific toxicity of 2-chlorodeoxy adenosine toward resting and proliferating human lymphocytes. Blood 1983, 62, 737.

55. O'Brien S, Kantarjian H, Beran M, et al: Results of FAMP and prednisone therapy in 264 patients with chronic lymphocytic leukemia with a multivariant analysis-derived prognostic model for response to treatment. Blood 1993, 82, 1695.

56. Piro LD, Carrera CJ, Carson DA, et al:. Lasting remissions in hairy cell leukemia induced by a single infusion of 2'-chlorodeoxy adenosine. N Engl J Med 1990, 323, 1117.

57. Dougherty TF, White A: Effect of pituitary adrenocorticotrophic hormones on lymphoid tissue. Proc Soc Exp Biol Med 1943, 53, 132.

58. Heilman FR, Kendall EC: The influence of 11-dihydro-17-hydroxy-corticosterone (compound E) on the growth of a malignant tumor in the mouse. Endocrine 1942, 34, 416.

59. Farber S: The effect of ACTH in acute leukemias in childhood. In Mote JR (ed): First Clinical ACTH Conference. New York, Blakiston, 1950, p 325.

60. Pearson OH, Eliel LP, Rawson RW, et al: ACTH and cortisone-induced regression of lymphoid tumors in man. Cancer 1949, 2, 943.

61. Broome JD: Evidence that the L-asparaginase of guinea pig serum is responsible for its antilymphoma effects. Nature 1961, 191, 1114.

62. Kidd JG: Regression of transplanted lymphoma induced in vivo by means of normal guinea pig serum. J Exp Med 1953, 98, 565.

63. Mashburn LT, Wriston JC Jr: Tumor inhibitory effect of L-asparaginase from Escherichia coli. Arch Biochem 1964, 105, 450.

64. Svoboda GH: Alkaloids of Vinca rosea. IX. Extraction and characterization of leurosidine and leurocristine. Lloydia 1961, 24, 173.

65. Johnson IS, Armstrong JG, Gorman M, et al: The vinca alkyloids: A new class of oncolytic agents. Cancer Res 1963, 23, 1390.

66. Arcamone F, DiMarco A, Gaetani M: Isolamento ad attivita antitumorale di un antibiotico da Streptomycies sp. Giorn Microbiol 1961, 9, 83.

67. Dubost M, Ganter P, Maral R, et al: Un nouvelle antibiotique a propriétés antitumorales. CR Acad Sci (Paris) 1963, 257, 1813.

68. Karon MR, Freireich, EJ, Frei E III: A preliminary report on vincristine sulfate: A new active agent for the treatment of acute leukemia. Pediatric 1962, 30, 791.

69. Tan C, Tasaka H, Dimarco A. Clinical studies of daunomycin. Proc Am Assoc Cancer Res 1965, 6, 64.

70. Hill JM, Roberts J, Loeb E, et al: L-asparaginase therapy for leukemia and other malignant neoplasms. JAMA 1967, 202, 882.

71. Oettgen HF, Old LJ, Boyse EA, et al: Inhibition of leukemia in man by L-asparaginase. Cancer Res 1967, 27, 2619.

72. Bernard J: Acute leukemia treatment. Cancer Res 1967, 27, 2565.

73. Morgan DA, Ruscetti FW, Gallo R: Selective in vitro growth of T-lymphocytes from normal human bone marrows. Science 1976, 193, 1007.

74. Metcalf D: The role of hematopoietic growth factors in the development and suppression of myeloid leukemia. Leukemia 1992, 6, 1875.

75. Moore MA: Clinical applications of + and − hematopoietc stem cell regulators. Blood 1991, 78, 1.

76. Quesada JR, Reuben J, Manning JT, et al: Alpha interferon for induction of remission in hairy-cell leukemia. N Engl J Med 1984, 310, 15.

77. Breitman T, Collins S, Keene B: Terminal differentiation of human promyelocytic leukemia cells in primary culture in response to retinoic acid. Blood 1981, 57, 1000.

78. Huang ME, Ye YC, Chen SR, et al: Use of all-trans retinoic acid in the treatment of acute promyelocytic leukemia. Blood 1988, 72, 567.

79. Castaigne S, Chomienne C, Daniel MT, et al: All-trans retinoic acid as a diffentiation therapy for acute promyelocytic leukemia. I. Clinical results. Blood 1990, 76, 1704.

80. Warrell RP Jr, Frankel SR, Miller WH, et al: Differentiation therapy of acute promyelocytic leukemia with tretinoin (all-transretinoic acid). N Engl J Med 1991, 324, 1385.

81. Tallman MS, Andersen JW, Schiffer CA, et al: All-trans retinoic acid in acute promyelocytic leukemia. N Engl J Med 1997, 337, 1021.

82. Goldin A, Venditti JM, Humphreys SM, et al: Modification of treatment schedules in the management of advanced mouse leukemia with amethopterin. J Natl Cancer Inst 1956, 17, 203.

83. Skipper HE, Schabel F Jr, Wilcox WS: Experimental evaluation of potential anticancer agents. XIII. On the criteria and kinetics associated with "curability" of experimental leukemia. Cancer Chemother Rep 1964, 35, 3.

84. Sansone G: Pathomorphosis of acute infantile leukemia treated with modern therapeutic agents: "Meningoleukemia" and Froehlich obesity. Ann Paediat 1957, 183, 33.

85. Whiteside JA, Phillips F, Dargeon HW, et al: Intrathecal amethopterin in neurological manifestations of acute leukemia. AMA Arch Int Med 1958, 101, 279.

86. Djerassi I, Farber S: Control and prevention of hemorrhage: Platelet transfusion. Cancer Res 1965, 25, 1499.

87. Freireich EJ, Karon M, Frei E III: Quadruple combination chemotherapy (VAMP) for acute lymphoblastic leukemia of childhood. Proc Am Assoc Cancer Res 1964, 5, 20.

88. Henderson ES, Freireich EJ, Henry PH, et al: Combination chemotherapy in acute lymphocytic leukemia of childhood. Proceedings of the Fifth International Congress of Chemotherapy, Vienna, Austria, 1967, 129.

89. Holland JF, Glidewell OJ: Chemotherapy of acute lymphocytic leukemia of childhood. Cancer 1972, 30, 1480.

90. Pinkel D: Five year follow-up of "total therapy" of childhood lymphocytic leukemia. JAMA 1971, 216, 648.

91. Goldin A, Venditti JM, Kline I, et al: Eradication of leukemia cells (L1210) by methotrexate and methotrexate plus citrovorum factor. Nature 1966, 212, 1548.

92. Djerassi I, Farber S, Abir E, et al: Continuous infusion of methotrexate in children with acute leukemia. Cancer 1967, 29, 233.

93. Rudnick SA, Cadman EC, Cappizzi RL, et al: High dose cytosine arabinoside (HDARAC) in refractory acute leukemia. Cancer 1979, 44, 1189.

94. George P, Pinkel D: Central nervous system radiation in children with acute lymphocytic leukemia in remission. Proc Am Assoc Cancer Res 1965, 6, 22.

95. Aur RJ, Simone J, Husto HO, et al: Central nervous system therapy and combination chemotherapy of childhood lymphocytic leukemia. Blood 1971, 37, 272.

96. Quine WE: The remedial application of bone marrow. JAMA 1896, 26, 1012.

97. Schretzenmayr A: Anämiebehandlung mit Knochenmarksinjectionen. Klin Wschr 1937, 16, 1010.

98. Osgood EE, Riddle MC, Mathews TJ: Aplastic anemia treated with daily transfusions and intravenous marrow. Ann Intern Med 1939, 13, 356.

99. Santos G: History of bone marrow transplantation. Clin Haematol 1983, 12, 611.

100. Barnes DWH, Loutit JF: Treatment of murine leukaemia with X-rays and homologous bone marrow. Br J Haematol 1957, 3, 241.

101. Jacobson LO, Marks EK, Gaston EO, et al: Effects of spleen protection on mortality following X-irradiation. J Lab Clin Med 1949, 34, 1538.

102. Lorenz E, Congden CC, Uphoff D. Modification of acute irradiation injury in mice and guinea pigs by bone marrow injections. J Natl Cancer Inst 1952, 12, 197.

103. Michison NA. The colonization of irradiated tissue by transplanted spleen cells. Br J Exp Pathol 1956, 37, 239.

104. Nowell PC, Cole LJ, Habermeyer JG, et al: Growth and continued function of rat marrow cells in X-irradiated mice. Cancer Res 1956, 16, 258.

105. Mathe G, Amiel JL, Schwarzenberg L, et al: Haemopoietic chimerism in man following allogeneic (homologous) bone marrow transplantation. Br Med J 1963, ii, 1633.

106. Thomas ED, Lochte HL Jr, Lu WC, et al: Intravenous infusion of bone marrow in patients receiving radiation and chemotherapy. N Engl J Med 1957, 257, 491.

107. Thomas ED, Herman EC Jr, Greenough WB II, et al: Irradiation and marrow infusion in leukemia. Arch Intern Med 1961, 107, 829.

108. Mathe G, Amiel JL, Schwarzenberg L, et al. Successful allogeneic bone marrow transplantation in man: Chimerism, induced specific tolerance and possible antileukemic effects. Blood 1965, 25, 179.

109. Dausset J: Iso-leuco-anticorps. Acta Haematologica (Basel) 1958, 20, 156.

110. Santos GW, Burke PJ, Sensenbrenner LL, et al: Marrow transplantation and graft-versus-host disease in acute monocytic leukemia. Exper Hematology 1969, 18, 20.

111. Graw RG, Brown JA, Yankee RA, et al: Transplantation of HLA-identical allogeneic bone marrow to a patient with acute lymphocytic leukemia. Blood 1970, 36, 736.

112. DeKoning J, van Bekkum DW, Dicke KA: Transplantation of bone-marrow cells and fetal thymus in an infant with lymphopenic immunological deficiency. Lancet 1969, i, 1223.

113. Thomas ED, Buckner CD, Rudolph RH, et al: Allogeneic marrow grafting for hematological malignancy using HLA-matched donor-recipient pairs. Blood 1971 38, 267.

114. Thomas ED, Buckner CD, Clift RA: Marrow transplantation for acute nonlymphoblastic leukemia in first remission. N Engl J Med 1979, 301, 597.

115. Fefer A, Cheever MA, Thomas ED, et al: Disappearance of Ph¹-positive cells in four patients with chronic granulocytic leukemia after chemotherapy, irradiation and marrow transplantation from an identical twin. N Engl J Med 1979, 300, 333.

116. Bradley TR, Metcalf D: The growth of mouse bone marrow cells in vitro. Aust J Exp Biol Med 1966, 44, 287.

117. Dexter TM, Allen TD, Lajtha LG: Conditions controlling proliferation of haemopoietic stem cells in vitro. J Cell Physiol 1977, 91, 335.

118. Pluznik DH, Sachs L: The cloning of normal "mast" cells in tissue culture. J Cell Comp Physiol 1965, 66, 319.

119. Till JE, McCulloch E: Direct measurement of the radiation sensitivity of normal mouse bone marrow. Radiat Res 1961, 14, 213.

120. Sen L, Borella L: Clinical importance of lymphoblasts with T markers in childhood acute leukemias. N Engl J Med 1975, 92, 828.

121. Koehler G, Milstein C: Continuous cultures of fresh cells secreting antibody of pre-defined specificity. Nature 1975, 256, 495.

122. Hulett HR, Bonner WA, Sweet RE, et al: Fluorescence-activated cell sorting. Rev Sci Inst 1972, 43, 404.

123. Greaves MF, Brown G, Rapson NT, et al: Antisera to acute lymphoblastic leukemia cells. Clin Immunol Immunopathol 1975, 4, 67.

124. Janossy G, Bollum FJ, Bradstock KF, et al: Cellular phenotypes of normal and leukemic hemopoietic cells determined by analysis with selected antibody combinations. Blood 1980, 56, 430.

125. Ritz J, Pesando M, Notis-McConarty J, et al: A monoclonal antibody to human acute lymphoblastic leukemia antigen. Nature 1980, 283, 583.

126. Nowell P, Hungerford DA: A minute chromosome in human granulocytic leukemia. Science 1960, 132, 1497.

127. Rowley JD: A new consistent chromosome abnormality in chronic myelogenous leukemia identified by quinacrine fluorescence and Giemsa staining. Nature 1973, 243, 290.

128. Golomb HM, Rowley JP, Vardiman JW, et al: Partial deletion of long arm of chromosome 17: A specific abnormality of acute promyelocytic leukemia? Arch Intern Med 1976, 136, 825.

129. Manolov G, Manolova Y: Marker band in one chromosome 14 from Burkitt lymphoma. Nature 1972, 237, 33.

130. Mitelman F, Anderrson-Anoret M, Brandt L, et al: Reciprocal 8;14 translocation in EBV-negative B-cell lymphocytic leukemia with Burkitt-type cells. Int J Cancer 1979, 24, 27.

131. Zech L, Haglund U, Nilsson K, et al: Characteristic chromosomal abnormalities in biopsies and lymphoid cell lines from patients with Burkitt and non-Burkitt lymphoma. Int J Cancer 1976, 17, 47.

132. Adams JM, Harris AW, Pinkert CA, et al: The c-myc oncogene driven by immunoglobulin enhancers induces lymphoid malignancy in transgenic mice. Nature 1985, 318, 533.

133. Canaani E, Gale RP, Steiner-Saltz D, et al: Altered transcription of an oncogene in chronic myeloid leukaemia. Lancet 1984, i, 593.

134. Dalla-Favera R, Bregni M, Erikson J, et al: Human c-myc oncogene is located on the region of chromosome 8 that is translocated to Burkitt lymphoma cells. Proc Natl Acad Sci U S A 1982, 79, 7824.

135. DeKlein A, van Kessel AG, Grosveld G, et al: A cellular oncogene is translocated to the Philadelphia chromosome in chronic myelocytic leukemia. Nature 1982, 300, 765.

136. Groffen J, Stephenson JR, Heisterkamp N, et al: Philadelphia chromosomal breakpoints are clustered within a limited region, bcr, on chromosome 22. Cell 1984, 36, 93.

137. Thirman MJ, Gill HJ, Burnett RC, et al: Rearrangement of the MLL gene in acute lymphoblastic and acute myeloid leukemia with 11q23 chromosomal translocation. N Engl J Med 1993, 329, 909.

138. Romana SP, Poerel H, LeCorniat M, et al: The t(12;21) in childhood B-lineage acute lymphoblastic leukemia results in a tel-AML1 gene fusion. Blood 1995, 85, 3662.

139. Drucker BJ, Talpaz M, Resta D, et al: Efficacy and safety of a specific inhibitor of the BCR-ABL tyrosine kinase in chronic myeloid leukemia. N Engl J Med 2001, 344:1031.

140. Kornberg A: Biologic synthesis of deoxyribonucleic acid. Science 1960, 131, 1503.

141. Fiers WF, Contreras G, Haaegeman R, et al: Complete nucleotide sequence of SV40 DNA. Nature 1978, 273, 113.

142. Maxam AM, Gilbert W: A new method of sequencing DNA. Proc Natl Acad Sci U S A 1977, 74, 560.

143. Sanger F, Coulson AR: A rapid method for determining sequences in DNA by primed synthesis with DNA polymerase. J Mol Biol 1975, 94, 444.

144. Linn S, Arber W: Host specificity of DNA produced by Escherichia coli. X. In vitro restriction of phage fd replicative form. Proc Natl Acad Sci U S A 1968, 59, 1300.

145. Mertz J, Davis RW: Cleavage of DNA by RI restriction endonuclease generates cohesive ends. Proc Natl Acad Sci U S A 1972, 69, 3370.

146. Smith HO, Wilcox KW: A restriction enzyme from Hemophilus influenzae. I. Purification and general properties. J Mol Biol 1970, 51, 379.

147. Southern EM: Detection of specific sequences among DNA fragments separated by gel electropheresis. J Molec Biol 1975, 98, 503.

148. Jackson D, Symons R, Berg P: Biochemical method for inserting new genetic information into DNA of simian virus 40: Circular SV40 DNA molecules containing lambda phage genes and the galactose operon of Escherichia coli. Proc Natl Acad Sci U S A 1972, 69, 2904.

149. Berger SM, Moore C, Sharp P: Spliced segments at the 5' termini of adenovirus-2 messenger RNA. Proc Natl Acad Sci U S A 1977, 74, 3171.

150. Hozumi H, Tonegawa S: Evidence for somatic rearrangement of immunoglobin genes coding for variable and constant regions. Proc Natl Acad Sci U S A 1976, 73, 3628.

151. Korsmeyer SJ, Arnold A, Bakhshi A, et al: Immunoglobulin gene rearrangements and cell surface antigen expression in acute lymphocytic leukemias of T cell and B cell precursor origins. J Clin Invest 1983, 71, 301.

152. Tokino T: The role of p53-target genes in human cancer. Crit Rev Oncol Haematol 2000, 33, 1.

153. Murray AW: Creative blocks: Cell cycle checkpoints and feedback controls. Nature 1992, 359, 599.

154. Askew DS, Ashmun RA, Simmons BC, et al: Constitutive cmyc expression in an IL3-dependent myeloid cell line suppresses cell cycle arrest and accelerates apoptosis. Oncogene 1991, 6, 1915.

155. Hockenbery D, Nunez G, Milliman C, et al: bcl2 is an inner mitochondrial membrane protein that blocks programmed cell death. Nature 1990, 348, 334.

156. Wylie AH, Kerr JFR, Carrie AR: Cell death: The significance of apoptosis. Int Rev Cytol 1980, 68, 251.

157. Yanish-Roauch E, Rosnitzky D, Lotem J, et al: Wild-type p53 induces apoptosis of myeloid leukemic cells that is inhibited by interleukin-6. Nature 1991, 352, 345.

158. Mullis K, Faloona F, Scharf S, et al: Specific enzymatic amplification of DNA in vitro: The polymerase chain reaction. Cold Spring Harb Symp Quant Biol 1986, 51, 263.

159. Heid CA, Stevens J, Livak KJ: Real time quantitative PCR. Meth Genome Res 1996, 6, 986.

160. Harris NL, Jaffe ES, Diebold J, et al: Conference report: The World Health Organization classification of neoplastic disease of the haematopietic and lymphoid tissues. Report of the Clinical Advisory Committee meeting, Airlie House, Virginia, November 1997. Histopathol 2000, 36, 69.

2

Mel Greaves

Biology of Leukemia: An Overview

CLONALITY OF LEUKEMIA

The leukemias have a number of consistent, abnormal biologic characteristics (Table 2-1) and these are reviewed. These are shared with almost all other types of cancer. A fundamental feature is clonality. The logic of monoclonality of leukemia is functional and statistical. The molecular events required to produce clinical disease are likely to be extraordinarily rare in relation to the number of "target" cells available, therefore, in the approximately 1% of individuals who will develop a hematologic malignancy, only 1 cell is likely to experience the essential rare mutant event or, as usually happens in cancer, a sequential series of mutational events (Fig. 2-1) (see also Color Section).

An origin of leukemia from a single cell was originally deduced from chromosome markers[1] and later by Fialkow and colleagues[2] who exploited X chromosome-linked glucose-6-phosphate dehydrogenase protein polymorphisms in females. A number of other constitutive X-linked polymorphisms amenable to DNA analysis have become available, with the added advantage of high-frequency heterozygosity in most patient populations[3-6] (Table 2-2). The "physiologic" clonal polymorphism of immunoglobulin and T-cell receptor genes also provides, with some caveats, valuable markers of clonality in lymphoid neoplasms[7] (see Table 2-2). Other acquired DNA markers linked to the leukemia process itself, i.e., chromosomal alterations, rearrangements, or mutations, have also been exploited as clonal markers. A striking example of the latter is the demonstration of the single cell origin in utero of concordant leukemia in monozygotic twins via the sharing of unique or clonotypic genomic fusion gene sequences, *MLL-AF4* or *TEL-AML1*.[8, 9] These various methods (see Table 2-2) have been used to demonstrate monoclonality of all types of acute and chronic leukemias as well as lymphomas and myelomas, other lymphoproliferative disorders, and a number of preleukemic myelodysplastic and myeloproliferative conditions, including chronic myelocytic leukemia (CML), polycythemia vera, and essential thrombocythemia. In addition, they have been exploited to analyze cell lineage involvement from which the stem cell or developmental origins of leukemic cells can be inferred[10] (Table 2-3), as well as for monitoring of minimal residual disease[11] (see Chapter 12).

MUTANT GENES IN LEUKEMIA

Our knowledge of mutant genes in leukemia originates from an extraordinary convergence of evidence from chromosome analysis (see Chapter 5), molecular virology (see Chapter 10), molecular cloning, and gene transfection and culminating in in vivo leukemia generated by transgenesis in mice.[12, 13] None of this would have been possible without recombinant DNA methods derived principally from bacterial studies. However, much credit is due to the recognition that chromosome alterations were nonrandom and likely to provide landmarks for the underlying culprit genes[14] (see Chapter 5). Exploitation of viral models of leukemia and cancer in chickens, leading to the discovery, via viral oncogenes, of human cellular proto-oncogenes, was also pivotal.[15] The list of chromosome changes and gene mutations in leukemia is now very extensive, involving more than 100 identified genes and including changes that are leukemia subtype-specific, e.g., transcription factor gene fusions in acute myelogenous leukemia (AML) and acute lymphoblastic leukemia (ALL) (see Chapter 5), and other alterations, e.g. *N-RAS*, mutation, CDK4 cyclin inhibitor deletion, *p53* mutations (or deletion) that are broader-based in leukemia associations. The majority of mutations in leukemia are acquired or nonconstitutive DNA alterations occurring in hemopoietic or lymphoid stem cells (see later). In rare cases (1% to 5% of acute leukemias), inherited mutant genes (e.g., *p53*, *ATM*, DNA ligase) or constitutive trisomy 21 (Down's) may be involved.

Genes can be altered in leukemia, resulting in loss or acquisition of function by multiple mechanisms, including illegitimate recombination (by chromosome transloca-

TABLE 2–1. Consistent Features of Leukemic Cells

Monoclonal origin.
Acquired gene mutations (1-n).
Genetic instability, clonal diversification, and progressive subclone selection (i.e., darwinian selection).
Dysregulation or uncoupling of critical cellular functions: proliferation, differentiation, cell death.
Net growth advantage, clonal dominance, vascular and extravascular spread, and compromise of normal tissue functions (territorial hijack).

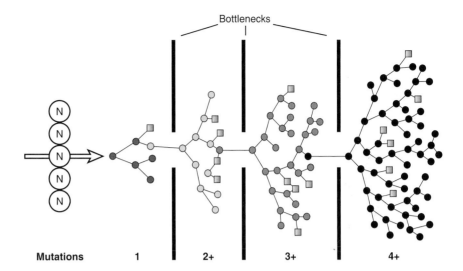

FIGURE 2–1. Clonal evolution of cancer.

tion, insertion, or inversion), loss (by deletion), or gain (by duplication or amplification) of genetic information or point mutation, i.e., single codon change. In other cases, genetic changes involve extra copies of particular chromosomes as exemplified by hyperdiploidy in child-hood ALL. This latter alteration is presumed to arise via chromosomal nondysjunction during mitosis, but its impact on gene expression (other than doubled dose) is uncertain.

Given the extraordinary number of blood cell divisions

TABLE 2–2. Molecular Markers of Clonality in Leukemia

Marker		Limitation	Advantages
X-Linked Gene Polymorphisms (in Females)*			
Glucose-6-phosphate dehydrogenase	(G6PD)	Relatively insensitive.	Stable marker for any leukemic subtype.
Hypoxanthine phosphoribosyl transferase	(HPRT)	False-positive result, skewed X chromosome expression; requirement for same patient non–blood tissue control.	Some (PGK, HUMARA) adaptable for PCR screening.
Phosphoglycerate kinase	(PGK)	Heterozygous ♀ only; most females homozygous for markers.	
DXS255 locus	(M27β)	Inconsistent methylation pattern for M27β.	
Androgen receptor	(HUMARA)		
Immunoglobulin and T-Cell Receptor Gene Rearrangements			
Protein products	IGH Igκ, λ	Lymphoid leukemias only.	Adaptable for PCR screening.
	TCR α, β, γ, δ, κ or λ idiotypes	Unstable markers: continuing rearrangements, mutations.	
		Clonal event (mutation) in lymphoid leukemia (ALL) may antedate IGH rearrangements.	
Acquired Chromosome Markers			
	e.g., Ph, t(9;22) (q34;q11)	May be secondary subclonal marker.	Usually stable marker.
	+8		Adaptable in some cases for FISH screening.
	5q⁻,9p⁻		
Acquired Molecular/DNA Changes			
	e.g., RAS, p53 mutations.	May be secondary subclonal marker.†	Stable markers.
	Fusion gene genomic sequences, e.g., MLL-partners, TEL-AMLI.		Adaptable for PCR screening.
	Viral integration pattern (e.g., HTLV-1).		Specificity.

*For review, see references 4 and 6. These methods exploit the fact that during embryogenesis, progenitor cells destined to form various tissues, including mesodermal derivatives such as blood, randomly inactivate one of the two parental X chromosomes (the Lyon hypothesis). All descendant cells therefore express genes from only one X chromosome, and normal populations of cells or tissue will be a mixture or mosaic of cells expressing either maternally or paternally derived X-linked genes. Differences or polymorphisms in parental and maternal copies of particular genes (alleles) can then be used as markers to determine which copy is active and hence whether a population of cells is polyclonal or derived from a single cell. The tests themselves exploit electrophoretic mobility of the protein product (G6PD), polymorphism in enzyme restriction sites (HPRT, PGK), or variation in the number of tandem repeats (VNTR, M27β). Tests using HPRT, PGK, and M27β as DNA clonal markers need to be adapted to distinguish active from inactive genes (both alleles will be detected in heterozygous females at the DNA level). This is achieved by the use of restriction enzymes that are methylation-sensitive.

†But probably primary initiating events in childhood leukemia.[8, 9, 38, 82]

PCR = polymerase chain reaction; FISH = fluorescence in situ hybridization.

TABLE 2–3. Applications of Clonal Markers in Leukemia

X-Linked Gene Polymorphisms
Multipotential stem-cell origin of CML[83] and MDS[83, 84] and variable myeloid lineage origins of AMI.[83, 85]
Lymphoid lineage restricted origins of ALL.[86]
Clonal remission in AMI.[85]
Clonality in chronic myeloproliferative disorders, idiopathic myelofibrosis, polycythemia vera, essential thrombocytopenia, myeloid metaplasia, and pancytopenia.[87-90]

Immunoglobulin and T-Cell Receptor Gene Rearrangements
Clonal (B or T) lineage restriction of all chronic lymphoid leukemias, non-Hodgkin's lymphomas, and myeloma.[7]
Minimal residual disease detection in ALL.[91, 92] See Chapter 12.
Clonal (lymphoid) origin of Richter's syndrome.[93]

Acquired Chromosome Markers/Gene Rearrangements and Mutations
Original definition of leukemia as a clone.[1]
Late relapse from original clone.[94]
Multimyeloid stem cell origins of AML.[95]
Multipotential or myeloid origins of Ph+ ALL.[96, 97]
Stem cell origins of idiopathic myelofibrosis (RAS mutations).[98]
Lymphoid lineage restricted origins of hyperdiploid ALL.[10]
Single cell origin in utero of concordant leukemia in monozygotic twins.[8, 9]
Backtracking of leukemic clone in childhood ALL to birth (presence of clonotypic marker in neonatal blood spots).[38, 82]

(i.e., cycles of DNA replication) that occur each day (about 10^{11}) (see Chapter 3) and the lack of complete fidelity of DNA replication and repair, it is likely that mutations in most, if not all, genes occur all the time (the chance of an "average"-size gene mutating in one cell cycle has been estimated at around 10^{-6}). Why we all do not have leukemia does require an explanation, and it is probably the following: most mutations either happen in irrelevant cells (i.e. dying cells, downstream of stem cells), or they are functionally neutral for the gene, or they kill the cell. Only very rarely will a mutation occur that has the required credentials: first, that it occurs in a hematopoietic cell with extensive self-renewal capacity and, second, that it is an "appropriate" gene that when altered in a particular sequence- or region-specific way, confers net growth and/or survival advantage on the clonal descendants of the cell in which it occurs. In many cases, there is a requirement for concurrent breakage of two independent genes on different chromosomes, followed by illegitimate recombination or fusion with severe structural constraints on which combinations will have a functional impact. In other cases, mutations or alterations in both parental alleles of the gene are necessary. Usually, an initiating mutation must be functionally complemented by other independent mutations in order to produce disease before the clone is exterminated by differentiation or other control mechanisms. Finally, such "cooperative" mutations may have to arise in a particular sequence or occur in particular pairings. A prediction that follows is that we probably all develop at some time a Ph chromosome or *RAS* mutations in cells that never achieve clonal dominance or produce overt disorder. Some evidence for this comes from the demonstration using the polymerase chain reaction (PCR) method and sequencing methods of *IGH-BCL-2* rearrangements in a high proportion of normal individuals that increase with age.[16]

FUNCTIONAL IMPACT OF ABERRANT GENES IN LEUKEMIA

The precise biochemical functions of the abnormal proteins encoded by many of the mutated genes in leukemia are the focus of intensive research. Many of them fit into generic functional categories or funnel into the same signaling pathways regulating the cell cycle, cell death, and DNA transcription. While all of this extraordinary molecular diversity is being unraveled, one way to rationalize its existence is via the Darwinian analogy.[17] What is likely to matter in the clonal evolution of leukemia, just as in the evolution of new species by germ cell mutation, is *net reproductive advantage* over time and under selective pressure or bottlenecks (see Fig. 2–1). Selective pressure comes from natural negative regulators of cell growth, competition among cells for limited nutrients, survival factors, space and, additionally, from cytotoxic therapy. Selection will be not only for genes that directly promote proliferation but also for those encoding other functions, albeit integrated with the cell cycle. Genes regulating programmed cell death (or apoptosis) play a key role, as may *p53* and other genes that regulate the detection and repair of DNA damage. Because many therapeutic agents (e.g., genotoxic drugs and ionizing radiation) rely on conserved mechanisms of apoptosis in target cells for their efficacy, it is now apparent why the "natural selection" of mutant genes abrogating this pathway in leukemia development (e.g., *p53*, *BCR-ABL*) can lead to therapeutic resistance.

Genes encoding transcriptional regulators or signaling kinases are frequently altered in acute leukemia often by illegitimate recombination or binary fusion, which overall, has a remarkably promiscuous pattern (Fig. 2–2) (see also Color Section) (see also Chapter 5). These key regulatory genes control developmental decisions of cells, and their disruption in leukemia probably accounts for the uncoupling of differentiation and proliferation. There is a striking link between transcriptional regulators that are essential for hemopoietic stem-cell differentiation, as revealed by knock-out experiments in mice, and frequent disruption of the genes encoding these same regulators in leukemia.[18] For example, the three genes encoding components of the CBF transcriptional complex are mandatory for hemopoiesis, and abnormalities of these genes constitute some of the most common molecular changes in leukemia (Fig. 2–3).

There is now some insight into the mechanisms by which these chimeric genes contribute to leukemogenesis. It appears that several fusion genes encoding hybrid transcription factors operate as *dominant negative* transcriptional deregulators.[19] They achieve this by recruitment of proteins that have a negative impact on transcription (e.g., NCOR), and of histone deacetylases that by alteration of DNA protein acetylation and chromatin assembly can silence gene transcription.[20, 21] For example, in the *TEL-AML1* and *AML1-ETO* fusion (in ALL and AML respectively), the partner gene for *AML1* (*TEL* or *ETO*) encodes a protein interaction domain that facilitates recruitment of transcriptional repressors that lead to inhibition of the activity of genes normally upregulated by

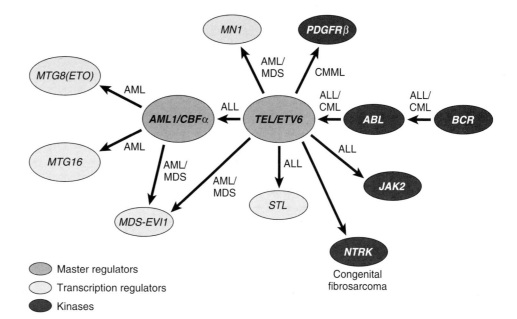

FIGURE 2–2. Promiscuous partner genes fuse in leukemia. Yellow: key transcriptional "master" genes *TEL* and *AML-1*. Orange: "partner" genes encoding kinase-signaling activity. Blue: "partner" genes encoding gene transcriptional regulatory activity.

AML1 itself. There is little information about target genes influenced by fusion genes in this way, but this problem is likely to be resolved soon by the use of microarrays to analyze gene expression patterns in leukemia in a comprehensive fashion.[22, 23]

Target Cells for Mutation in Leukemia

The cellular and molecular phenotypic diversity of leukemia suggests that the disease can be viewed as a clonal lesion originating at different developmental levels and lineage compartments of hematopoiesis. The phenotype of the leukemia at diagnosis will reflect the level of differentiation/maturation achieved by the dominant subclone, perhaps with deviations from normal counterparts imposed by the underlying leukemogenic mutations. Whereas this phenotype may be indicative of lineage origins and used as such for classification and treatment purposes, the issue of the precise cell type in which initiating and subsequent mutations arise is a more subtle question. This necessary complication arises because the majority of cells on a leukemic bone marrow smear are the descendants of a small-minority clonogenic cell population that may be less differentiated or antecedent in the developmental pathway.[24] Furthermore, the single clonogenic cell that produced the bulk leukemia may well be the descendant of an earlier clonogenic cell in which leukemia was initiated and which itself lies somewhere else (upstream) in the hematopoietic hierarchy (see Chapter 3). These points are well illustrated by CML and CML in blast crisis (see Chapter 25). This issue is not just one of biologic detail; the developmental levels at which mutations arise and clonogenic cells exist could have a significant impact on clinical response and attempts to eradicate the total leukemia clone.

Leukemias with multilineage phenotypes on individual cells pose a particular problem of interpretation. It is unclear whether this feature reflects aberrant differentiation and gene expression arising as a direct consequence of particular molecular abnormalities[25] or is a result of enforced self-renewal in the lymphomyeloid stem cells.[26] There is convincing molecular biologic evidence that normal multilineage progenitors or stem cells can coexpress genes that are, in descendent cells, lineage-restricted.[27, 28] Either way (and both interpretations may be partially correct), these leukemias probably originate primarily in multilineage stem cells. An origin in multilineage (e.g., lymphomyeloid) stem cells in hematopoiesis may be revealed by lineage switch (e.g., lymphoid to myeloid) following treatment but is formally demonstrated by clonal analysis (see earlier discussion) as first shown for the lymphomyeloid stem-cell origin of the Ph+ clone in CML. Single (clonal) colony analysis by PCR and single cell analysis by a combination of immunophenotype and interphase fluorescence in situ hybridization (FISH) offer powerful tools for evaluating lineage origins of mutant genes in leukemia.

Figure 2–4 illustrates a possible map of leukemic origins in this context. Some initiating mutations probably arise, albeit rarely, in the germ line or in embryonic

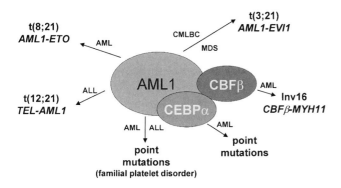

FIGURE 2–3. CBF transcriptional complex aberrations in leukemia. CBF, core binding factor.

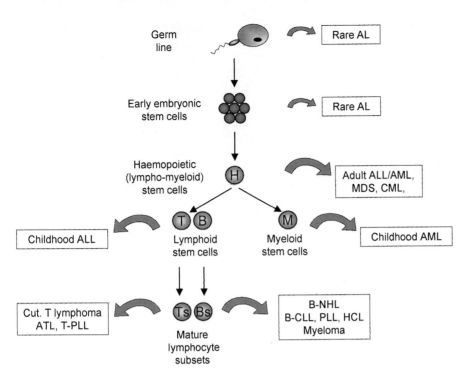

FIGURE 2–4. Developmental origins of hemopoietic malignancies. Hierarchical stem-cell origins of leukemia and related cancers. Arrows denote likely level of clonal selection for the majority of cases of leukemia of subtype listed. AL, acute leukemia; ALL, acute lymphoblastic leukemia; AML, acute myeloblastic leukemia; ATL, adult T-cell leukemia/lymphoma; cut, cutaneous; CLL, chronic lymphocytic leukemia; HCL, hairy cell leukemia; NHL, non-Hodgkin's lymphoma; PLL, prolymphocytic leukemia.

mesodermal/mesenchymal cells but, more commonly, multipotential or lymphoid- and myeloid-restricted stem cells will be the predominant targets. Hemopoietic stem cells arise during embryogenesis from mesodermal cells via a hemangioblast cell type that also gives rise to vascular endothelial cells and some stromal cells of the bone marrow microenvironment (see Chapter 3). It has been reported that the *BCR-ABL* fusion gene can be detected (by FISH) in endothelial cells generated from patients with CML.[29] One interpretation of this is that the common hemangioblast stem cell is the target for the Ph chromosomal translocation. Other interpretations are possible,[30] including the ability of otherwise committed hemopoietic stem cells to switch developmental options under particular conditions. This possibility is plausible given recent insights into the remarkably developmental plasticity of stem cells in different tissues, including those of blood, the central nervous system, and muscle.[31]

Note that mature lymphocyte subsets—the probable targets for chronic and prolymphocytic leukemias, hairy cell leukemia, and most lymphomas and myelomas—are unusual because mature cells in most other tissues seldom appear to provide cellular targets for cancer. The reason for this unfortunate vulnerability of lymphocytes is presumably their stem cell–like behavior, i.e., their longevity (in G_0) coupled with high proliferative potential exercised via clonal interaction with antigenic stimuli.

Although several developmental windows of leukemia risk in hematopoiesis clearly exist (see Fig. 2-2), in practice, risk may vary throughout life and in relation to lifestyle, and occupational or medical exposures (see Chapter 7). For example, lymphoid-restricted stem cells giving rise to common ALL (cALL) may be more at risk early in human life because of their extensive self-renewal during that period (see Chapter 4) and because of age-linked leukemogenic exposures such as infections (see

Chapter 7). Multipotential stem cells and germinal center B cells may, in common with epithelial cells, be more at risk throughout adult life, reflecting sustained selective pressure.

IMPLICATIONS FOR NATURAL HISTORY AND ETIOLOGY

Precisely how many sequential cooperating mutations (see Fig. 2-1) are required to produce overt, clinical leukemia is not entirely clear, but the relatively short latency, especially in infancy and childhood or following known genotoxic exposures, suggests only a few compared with most adult epithelial carcinomas that are thought to evolve over decades and that demonstrably can have an accumulated set of 5 to 15 mutations.[32] Experimentally, the minimum number of genetic events for such cancers appears to be three or four.[33] Leukemias arising in mobile stem cells with normal programming for circulatory spread of descendent progeny may require fewer genetic abnormalities in order to expand to the point of prompting diagnostic symptoms. Unlike epithelial cancers, they are less subject to the topographic constraints of tissue architecture.[34]

Without a complete genetic profile of leukemic clones, the number of mutations that usually accrue remains unknowable, but it is certainly plausible that two are sufficient and perhaps, exceptionally, one. In special cases, there are some data on the timing and sequence of these molecular events in leukemia. The most frequent chromosomal translocation in childhood ALL is the *TEL(ETV6) AML1(CBFα2)* fusion.[35, 36] Studies on monozygotic twins with concordant ALL[9, 37] and retrospective scrutiny by PCR of neonatal blood spots[38] have provided convincing evidence that this abnormality frequently arises before birth, in utero, to be followed by a variable but often protracted (1 to 14 years) postnatal latency. These data suggest therefore that chromosomal translocations can be very early or initiating events. Because twin concordance rates are around 5% to 10%, it is very likely that one or more additional postnatal genetic changes are required to complement the initial genetic abnormality. In the case of childhood ALL with *TEL-AML1* fusion, the most frequent additional chromosomal alteration is 12p$^-$ including deletion of the normal (nonrearranged) *TEL* allele.[39, 40] FISH and molecular studies[39, 41] indicate that this change is subclonal and therefore secondary to *TEL-AML1* fusion. On the basis of these data, a two-step pre/postnatal "minimal" model for the natural history of childhood common ALL has been proposed[34] (Fig. 2-5). On the assumption that *TEL-AML1* fusions and *TEL* deletions cooperatively block differentiation, it may be that additional genetic changes that promote proliferation (e.g., kinase activation) are also required for overt leukemia.[42]

This model is minimal in the sense that only very few mutations may be required for the clinical manifestation of ALL. Because the development of leukemia is a dynamic, ongoing, evolutionary process, it is inevitable that given time or lack of effective therapeutic intervention further genetic changes will occur and provide selective advantage for subclones. This phase can be regarded as *progression* of disease. The extent to which it occurs is likely to vary from patient to patient, with the same biologic type of disease depending on a number of factors, including the speed at which early diagnostic symptoms are noticed and acted on. A consequence of this is that, within the context of the natural history of the disease, there will be a variable diagnostic window. Delay in diagnosis might then be expected to incur a risk of more bulky disease, further genetic abnormalities, and increased therapeutic resistance.

This pattern of natural history has relevance to the possible role of exposures in the cause of leukemia, particularly if two independent genetic abnormalities that occur apart in time are necessary. The *TEL-AML1* fusion gene, along with several others in frame fusion genes in leukemias and sarcomas,[43, 44] has DNA sequence features indicating that it probably arises from nonhomologous

recombination and error-prone DNA repair following double-stranded DNA breaks.[45] This begs the question of how such breaks might occur. There are few, if any, unambiguous epidemiologic clues, i.e. to pregnancy/fetal exposures, that might explain this, though risk of such events may be influenced by folate intake and inherited polymorphisms in genes regulating folate metabolism.[46] In the absence of unambiguous associations with exposures it is possible that fusion genes arise relatively frequently as an accident of developmentally normal proliferation and oxidative stress. Certainly, these illegitimate gene fusions arise at a considerably higher frequency than that of the corresponding leukemias. For *TEL-AML1*, the accumulative risk (up to 15 years) of clinically diagnosed ALL with this particular fusion gene for any child is around 1 in 12,500. However, an in-frame *TEL-AML1* fusion gene is present in around 1% of normal newborn cord bloods, i.e., 100 times the leukemia rate.[47]

Environmental exposures could be important in the context of *promoting* critical postnatal secondary events in childhood leukemia. Many different categories of exposure have been considered as causative agents for ALL (see Chapter 7). The balance of evidence indicates that some of these—ionizing radiation and nonionizing electromagnetic fields, for example—are unlikely to be major causal factors. Infection remains a serious and plausible candidate, however. Although no specific microorganism has been implicated, there is circumstantial evidence that suggests that an abnormal immune response to some common infections may be involved[47] (see Chapter 7). This could arise in the context of population mixing as proposed by Kinlen[48] or as a result of delayed infection.[49, 50] In the latter case, any such role of infection would be seen as promoting the second, postnatal event (e.g., *TEL* deletion).[34] These important issues are being addressed by ongoing case/control epidemiologic studies.

Whatever the precise etiologic scenario for childhood ALL, it is unlikely to be the same for all leukemias. At least some biologically defined subtypes are likely to involve different causal pathways, and even within a single biologic or clinical entity, more than one etiologic mechanism is possible.

In infant ALL/AML with *MLL* gene fusions, for example, the very high rate of concordance in identical twins (50% to 100%?) and the remarkably short latency (in months) suggests that any required environmental exposures are likely to be confined to the prenatal period during pregnancy.[8] Exposure of pregnant mothers to chemicals inhibiting topo-isomerase II has been proposed as a possible mechanism based on the known association of topo II blocking cancer treatment drugs (epidophyllotoxins and anthracyclins; see Chapter 9) with secondary leukemia and *MLL* gene fusion.[51, 52] There is some preliminary epidemiologic support for this possibility.[53] The idea has also been endorsed by the observation that dietary bioflavonoid substances cause *MLL* breaks in vitro[54] and that individuals inheriting low-function alleles of NQ01—an enzyme involved in metabolism of some flavonoids (as well as benzene metabolites)—are at increased risk of infant leukaemia with *MLL* fusion.[55] A recent international case/control study has also identified a possible association between infant leukemias that have *MLL* gene fusions with maternal exposures during pregnancy to mosquitoi-

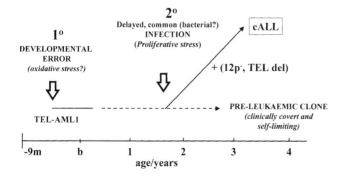

FIGURE 2–5. A "minimal" two-step model for the natural history and cause of childhood ALL.[34] (From Greaves M. Molecular genetics, natural history and the demise of childhood leukemia. Eur J Can. 1999;35: 173–185.)

TABLE 2–4. Inherited Genetic Variation and Leukemia Risk

Inherited Variation	Function	Impact on Risk of Leukemia	Occurrence in Population	Impact on Population Leukemia Load
Mutant genes	Highly penetrant (esp. in homozygous form)	Very high (= predisposition)	Rare	Low
Normal variants/alleles (SNP's)	Weak, poorly penetrant	Modest (= susceptibility)	Very common	High

dal insecticides, especially Baygon and the drug dipyrone.[56]

INHERITED GENETIC VARIATION AND LEUKEMIA

Although the great majority of genetic alterations observed in leukemia are acquired changes in blood cells, leukemia predisposition or susceptibility can be influenced by inheritance of mutant genes or normal gene variants respectively (Table 2–4).

Family studies in leukemia, in contrast to, i.e., prostate or breast/ovarian pedigrees, have not suggested the common involvement of highly penetrant mutant genes predisposing to leukemia. Although there are anecdotal reports of families with excess numbers of one or more types of leukemia,[57] chronic lymphocytic leukemia is the only type of hematological malignancy for which there is persuasive evidence for common familial clustering.[58] The gene involved has not been identified to date. When leukemia risk is highly elevated in families, it is almost invariably in the context of a syndrome that includes bone marrow failure or genetic instability (Table 2.5). These syndromes usually carry a considerably higher risk of several types of cancer, and this can be rationalized now that several of the genes involved have been identified: they all regulate the integrity of DNA or its repair after damage.[59, 60] Several of these genes operate as part of an integrated network of signals governing the recognition of damage to DNA and its repair (*p53*, ATM, FACC, DNA ligase).

The *AML1* gene encoding the transcriptional core binding factor (CBF) A2 subunit is frequently involved in acquired chromosomal translocations in ALL and AML. Normal function of the *AML1* gene is essential for hemopoiesis as revealed by knock-out experiments in mice.[61]

TABLE 2–5. Inherited Syndromes Predisposing to Leukemia and Other Cancers

Syndrome/Condition	Genes
Fanconi anemia	7 genes (*FAC* A-G)
Schwachmann–Diamond syndrome	?
Familial platelet disorder	*AML1*
Blackfan–Diamond syndrome	?
Ataxia telangiectasia	*ATM*
Bloom's syndrome	*BLM*
Li–Fraumeni syndrome	*p53*
Neurofibromatosis	*NF1*
Von-Hippel–Lindau syndrome	*VHS*

Mutations in *AML1* can also contribute to inherited predisposition to AML. Constitutive deletions or point mutations in *AML1* have been described in several pedigrees with familial platelet disorders (FPD) and AML.[62] This situation is unusual as loss of one allele of *AML1*, or haplo-insufficiency, appears to have been sufficient to strongly predispose towards FPD. However, other, acquired genetic abnormalities in the other *AML1* allele or other genes may be necessary for the development of AML in these families.

Leukemia risk is elevated some 30 times for individuals with constitutive trisomy 21 or Down syndrome.[63] Both AML and ALL appear to be increased but there is a striking (200×) elevated incidence of the FAB M7 megakaryocytic leukemia variant. To date, the relevant genes on chromosome 21 have not been elucidated. Abnormal expression of the *AML1* gene is one candidate, given its importance in hemopoietic stem cell development and in acquired chromosomal translocations in AML and ALL.

With the advent of the Human Genome Project coming to the first draft phase of its completion, we have a clearer picture of the extent of our inherent genetic diversity over and above what can be considered our mutation load. Somewhat surprisingly, the extent of normal variation in sequence is not great; in fact, it is considerably less than that for our chimpanzee and great ape cousins. This may reflect the relatively short time since the emergence of modern *H. sapiens* (~500,000 years) and perhaps a bottleneck that produced a small number of founders. Nevertheless, with nucleotide variations occurring on average at 10^{-3}, we have a total of approximately 1.4 million variant nucleotides or SNP's (single nucleotide polymorphisms), at least a minority of which influence function of an encoded protein.

The frequency of a gene/SNP or allele in any population can be determined (by PCR-based screening methods) and patients with leukemias (or other cancers) compared with controls. Such studies may be conducted where epidemiologic evidence already implicates a particular gene/environmental causal pathway; e.g., infection and immune response genes, chemical carcinogens, and genes encoding enzymes for carcinogen metabolism. Alternatively, gene screening and allelic or multigene (haplotype) association may, by way of 'reverse epidemiology', suggest potentially relevant exposures; e.g., MTHFR gene variants and folate uptake.[46, 64] Table 2.6 lists some of the genes whose variants may alter susceptibility to leukemia and reference to published studies. The latter are mostly preliminary or hypothesis generating, but encourage this line of investigation. By the time of the next edition of this book, we can anticipate a much more comprehensive analysis of the contribution of genetic

TABLE 2–6. Inherited Normal (Allelic) Gene Sequence Variation and Risk of Leukemia*

Gene	Function	Leukemia	Risk†	Reference
HLA DPB1 (0201)	Immune recognition	Childhood ALL	Increased	99
NAD(P)H:quinone oxidoreductase (NQ01)	Detoxification of benzoquinones and flavonoids	Infant leukemias with *MLL* gene fusions	Increased	55
		Adult AML and ALL	Increased	100
		Therapy related secondary leukemias	Increased	101
MTHFR (methylenetetrahydrofolate reductase)	Folate metabolism	Pediatric ALL of different molecular subtypes	Decreased	46
		Adult ALL	Decreased	64
		Myeloma	Decreased	102
Other phase I/II enzymes for carcinogen metabolism				
Phase I/CYP's	Carcinogen activation	Childhood ALL	Increased	103
Phase II/GST's	Carcinogen detoxification			
CYP3A		Therapy related secondary leukemias	Increased	104

*Preliminary data.
†i.e., change in relative risk (cases versus controls) for particular allele or SNP (single nucleotide polymorphism) tested.

variation to leukemia risk and, in particular, molecular epidemiological studies in which vulnerable genotype plus corresponding exposures are elucidated for particular subtypes of leukemia.

CLINICAL IMPLICATIONS

These biologic insights have radically changed our perceptions of the disease and have introduced into routine practice immunologic, cytogenetic, and molecular diagnostic tools combining specificity with sensitivity. The prognostic significance of particular biologic markers may depend on the therapy used, and some previous correlations disappear with improvements in treatment. Nevertheless, some striking associations have been demonstrated.[65] Foremost among these perhaps is the prognostic significance of the Ph chromosome or *BCR-ABL* fusion gene in ALL. This DNA rearrangement in either its p190 or p210 variant form increases in frequency with age and is an independent marker of very poor prognosis (see Chapters 26 and 27). The Ph chromosome may be missed by karyotypic screening at diagnosis; additional methods should be used such as reverse (RT) PCR or FISH (see Chapter 5). Although some studies suggest that Ph⁺ ALL in children may be successfully treated by intensive chemotherapy in some patients with modest white blood cell counts, for most patients a bone marrow transplant currently offers the most realistic chance of a cure.[66] This striking age association explains in large measure the marked difference in survival rates in pediatric versus adult ALL patients (see Chapters 26 and 27), mirrored by the reciprocal incidence rates of good-prognosis chromosome markers: hyperdiploidy and *TEL-AML1* fusion.[34] The long-recognized clinical difference in infant, childhood, and adult ALL can be seen to reflect the existence of leukemias that are distinct in terms of their cellular origins, molecular disorder, and drug responsiveness.

These associations raise another important question: why should leukemias with a similar immunophenotype or cell type (cALL) but with different molecular markers appear to behave so differently clinically with respect to overall clinical responsiveness, remission, duration, or cure rates, even in patients of the same age and with a similar total leukemic cell burden? It has been suggested that the responsiveness of most pediatric cALL patients to treatment may reflect an origin from clonogenic B-cell precursors that are intrinsically programmed for apoptosis in their normal development.[67] In most cases (including those with hyperdiploidy), this sensitivity is retained following leukemic transformation and, somewhat serendipitously, is exploited by genotoxic therapy. The latter will be successful *provided* the clone has not progressed genetically prior to diagnosis so as to include mutations that abrogate or lessen drug responsiveness (see Fig. 2–1). Hyperdiploidy in ALL may itself increase sensitivity to methotrexate and other antimetabolites,[68, 69] and B-cell precursor leukemic blasts with *TEL-AML* fusion appear to be very sensitive to L-asparaginase.[70] Ph⁺ cALL is, in contrast, much more intractable, possibly because of what might be called a "double burden." First, the disease may originate in many cases not in a B lymphoid progenitor cell but rather in a more primitive lymphomyeloid stem cell that is not so intrinsically susceptible to drug-induced apoptosis; second, the activated ABL kinase may itself influence drug sensitivity by blocking apoptosis and/or by regulating enzymes that can confer drug resistance.[71]

Much along the same lines, the finding that *p53* mutations are prevalent in relapsed ALL, blast crisis of CML, and other poor-prognosis hematologic malignancies is almost certainly linked to the normal function of *p53* as a cell cycle checkpoint for DNA damage and repair.

Hematopoietic cells lacking *p53* function are resistant to apoptosis induced by ionizing radiation and DNA strand-breaking drugs.

Moreover, *p53* null clonogenic cells surviving genotoxic therapy may be genetically unstable with a propensity to acquire additional mutations; i.e., treatment of such cells may be not only ineffective but may actually encourage molecular progression.[72] At least some of the many genes involved in clonal dysregulation, in particular those whose function is DNA damage detection and repair or regulation of programmed cell death, may therefore have a profound impact on the sensitivity of the clone to the many modalities of current treatment that operate via DNA damage and apoptosis. This in itself suggests a new way to look at drug responsiveness in leukemia and other cancers and may prompt new therapeutic strategies in which manipulation of apoptosis is a central theme.[73]

Given that the presence of molecular markers at diagnosis or relapse may have prognostic relevance, their systematic detection becomes a matter of some practical importance. The technology for routine diagnostic screening is still evolving with the demands of sensitivity, selectivity, speed, and cost having to be considered. Real-time quantitative PCR (TaqMan) machines provide a significant technical advance (e.g., for minimal residual disease detection) (see Chapter 12). There is a prospect that microarrays will provide a new level of incisive molecular prognostication as indicated by some studies in leukemia and lymphoma.[22, 23] Similarly, new FISH-based methods such as M-FISH and SKY offer a more detailed scrutiny of chromosome changes and reveal levels of complexity hitherto unsuspected.[74] Standard banded karyotypes provide an important first line or blind screen for gross chromosomal abnormalities, although they pose technical and logistic problems and may underestimate the frequency of many molecular abnormalities, including some that were originally uncovered via karyotype analysis (for example, *TAL* deletions in T-ALL, 9p deletions in ALL, 11q23 translocations in infant acute leukemia, trisomy 12 in CLL, *BCR-ABL* fusion in CML, and *TEL-AML1* fusion (t(12;21) in ALL). If and when such genetic markers or other genes altered by point mutations have known or suspected clinical relevance, they will have to be detected by molecular screening; e.g., FISH or PCR/RT-PCR.

In addition to their potential value at diagnosis, molecular markers by their clonal uniqueness and amenability to sensitive screening methods can be applied to the monitoring of treated patients for elimination, persistence, or reemergence of the leukemic clone. *IGH* and *TCRδ* genes and many of the unique rearrangements in leukemia are amenable to PCR screening at the mRNA or DNA level, permitting very–low-frequency cells to be detected with reliable specificity (see Chapters 6 and 12). Studies in ALL, acute promyelocytic leukemia, and transplanted CML and Ph⁺ ALL suggest that the results of serial screening of molecular markers by PCR (especially under quantitative conditions) do correlate with sustained remission or relapse and may therefore provide an important guide to patient management.

New insights into the biology and molecular pathogenesis of leukemia have also led to the possibility of novel therapeutic strategies. Prominent among these are immunologic manipulation of DNA vaccines (see Chapter 18), attempts to efficiently induce terminal differentiation in vivo (see Chapters 18 and 23) and, in particular, the various ways in which mutated genes or their products (mRNA, proteins) might be selectively targeted to provide potentially highly specific and nontoxic therapy.

There have been two very encouraging developments in this respect since the last edition of this book. The first is the development and application of a specific tyrosine kinase inhibitor (STI571) that inhibits *BCR-ABL* kinase activity and proliferation of Ph⁺ cells.[75] Early results of clinical trials in CML indicate a striking and perhaps surprising lack of toxicity and a substantial clinical benefit for a sizable fraction of patients.[76] Further clinical data on CML, CML in blast crisis, and Ph⁺ ALL are awaited with great interest. Also in transgenic models of *BCR-ABL* positive leukemia, specific inhibitors of farnesyl transferase have shown considerable promise.[77, 78] Finally, insight into the mechanisms of transcriptional repression by fusion genes (see earlier) have suggested that inhibitors of histone deacetylases might compromise fusion protein function and either by themselves or in combination with other drugs confer some clinical benefit.[79, 80] In vitro studies to model this approach[20] and preliminary clinical studies[81] have been encouraging.

REFERENCES

1. Nowell PC: The clonal evolution of tumor cell populations. Science 1976;194:23.
2. Fialkow PJ: Clonal origin of human tumors. Biochim Biophys Acta 1976;458:283.
3. Busque L, Gilliland DG: Clonal evolution in acute myeloid leukemia. Blood 1993;82:337.
4. Gale RE, Linch DC. Clonality studies in acute myeloid leukemia. Leukemia 1998;12:117.
5. Vogelstein B, Fearon ER, Hamilton SR, et al: Use of restriction fragment length polymorphisms to determine the clonal origin of human tumors. Science 1985;227:642.
6. Busque L, Gilliland DG: X-inactivation analysis in the 1990s: Promise and potential problems. Leukemia 1998;12:128.
7. Griesser H, Tkachuk D, Reis MD, et al: Gene rearrangements and translocations in lymphoproliferative diseases. Blood 1989; 73:1402.
8. Ford AM, Ridge SA, Cabrera ME, et al: *In utero* rearrangements in the trithorax-related oncogene in infant leukaemias. Nature 1993; 363:358.
9. Wiemels JL, Ford AM, Van Wering ER, et al: Protracted and variable latency of acute lymphoblastic leukemia after *TEL-AML1* gene fusion in utero. Blood 1999;94:1057.
10. Kasprzyk A, Harrison CJ, Secker-Walker LM: Investigation of clonal involvement of myeloid cells in Philadelphia-positive hyperdiploid acute lymphoblastic leukemia. Leukemia 1999;13:2000.
11. van Dongen JJM, MacIntyre EA, Gabert JA, et al: Standardized RT-PCR analysis of fusion gene transcripts from chromosome aberrations in acute leukemia for detection of minimal residual disease. Leukemia 1999;13:1901.
12. Adams JM, Cory S: Transgenic models of tumor development. Science 1991;254:1161.
13. Rowley JD: The critical role of chromosome translocations in human leukemias. Annu Rev Genet 1998;32:495.
14. Rowley JD: Identification of the constant chromosome regions involved in human hematologic malignant disease. Science 1982; 216:749.
15. Bishop JM: The molecular genetics of cancer. Science 1987;235: 305.
16. Liu Y, Hernandez AM, Shibata D, et al: *BCL2* translocation fre-

quency rises with age in humans. Proc Natl Acad Sci U S A 1994; 91:8910.

17. Greaves M: Cancer. The Evolutionary Legacy. Oxford: Oxford University Press; 2000.

18. Lutterbach B, Hiebert SW: Role of the transcription factor AML-1 in acute leukemia and hematopoietic differentiation. Gene 2000; 245:223.

19. Hiebert SW, Sun W, Davis JN, et al: The t(12;21) translocation converts AML-1B from an activator to a repressor of transcription. Mol Cell Biol 1996;16:1349.

20. Guidez F, Petrie K, Ford AM, et al: Recruitment of the nuclear receptor corepressor N-CoR by the TEL moiety of the childhood leukemia-associated TEL-AML1 oncoprotein. Blood 2000;96:2557.

21. Wang J, Hoshino T, Redner RL, et al: ETO, fusion partner in t(8;21) acute myeloid leukemia, represses transcription by interaction with the human N-CoR/mSin3/HDAC1 complex. Proc Natl Acad Sci U S A 1998;95:10860.

22. Golub TR, Slonim DK, Tamayo P, et al: Molecular classification of cancer: Class discovery and class prediction by gene expression monitoring. Science 1999;286:531.

23. Alizadeh AA, Eisen MB, Davis RE, et al: Distinct types of diffuse large B-cell lymphoma identified by gene expression profiling. Nature 2000;403:503.

24. Bonnet D, Dick JE: Human acute myeloid leukemia is organized as a hierarchy that originates from a primitive hematopoietic cell. Nat Med 1997;3:730.

25. Smith LJ, Curtis JE, Messner HA, et al: Lineage infidelity in acute leukemia. Blood 1983;61:1138.

26. Greaves MF, Chan LC, Furley AJW, et al: Lineage promiscuity in hemopoietic differentiation and leukemia. Blood 1986;67:1.

27. Hu M, Krause D, Greaves M, et al: Multilineage gene expression precedes commitment in the hemopoietic system. Genes Dev 1997;11:774.

28. Enver T, Greaves M: Loops, lineage, and leukemia. Cell 1998;94:9.

29. Gunsilius E, Duba H-C, Petzer AL, et al: Evidence from a leukaemia model for maintenance of vascular endothelium by bone-marrow-derived endothelial cells. Lancet 2000;355:1688.

30. Green AR: Haemangioblast origin of chronic myeloid leukaemia? Lancet 2000;355:1659.

31. Orkin SH: Stem cell alchemy. Nat Med 2000;6:1212.

32. Vogelstein B, Kinzler KW, eds: The Genetic Basis of Human Cancer. New York: McGraw-Hill Health Professions Division; 1998.

33. Hahn WC, Counter CM, Lundberg AS, et al: Creation of human tumour cells with defined genetic elements. Nature 1999;400:464.

34. Greaves M: Molecular genetics, natural history and the demise of childhood leukemia. Eur J Can 1999;35:173.

35. Romana SP, Poirel H, Leconiat M, et al: High frequency of t(12;21) in childhood B-lineage acute lymphoblastic leukemia. Blood 1995; 86:4263.

36. Shurtleff SA, Buijs A, Behm FG, et al: TEL/AML1 fusion resulting from a cryptic t(12;21) is the most common genetic lesion in pediatric ALL and defines a subgroup of patients with an excellent prognosis. Leukemia 1995;9:1985.

37. Ford AM, Bennett CA, Price CM, et al: Fetal origins of the TEL-AML1 fusion gene in identical twins with leukemia. Proc Natl Acad Sci U S A 1998;95:4584.

38. Wiemels JL, Cazzaniga G, Daniotti M, et al: Prenatal origin of acute lymphoblastic leukaemia in children. Lancet 1999;354:1499.

39. Raynaud S, Cavé H, Baens M, et al: The 12;21 translocation involving TEL and deletion of the other TEL allele: Two frequently associated alterations found in childhood acute lymphoblastic leukemia. Blood 1996;87:2891.

40. Raynaud SD, Dastugue N, Zoccola D, et al: Cytogenetic abnormalities associated with the t(12;21): A collaborative study of 169 children with t(12;21)-positive acute lymphoblastic leukemia. Leukemia 1999;13:1325.

41. Maia AT, Ford AM, Jalali GR, et al: Molecular tracking of leukemogenesis in a triplet pregnancy. Blood 2001;98:478.

42. Gilliland DG: Core binding factor mutations in leukemia. Blood 2000;96:70.

43. Gillert E, Leis T, Repp R, et al: A DNA damage repair mechanism is involved in the origin of chromosomal translocations t(4;11) in primary leukemic cells. Oncogene 1999;18:4663.

44. Zucman-Rossi J, Legoix P, Victor J-M, et al: Chromosome transloca-

tion based on illegitimate recombination in human tumors. Proc Natl Acad Sci U S A 1998;95:11786.

45. Wiemels JL, Greaves M: Structure and possible mechanisms of TEL-AML1 gene fusions in childhood acute lymphoblastic leukemia. Cancer Res 1999;59:4075.

46. Wiemels JL, Smith RN, Taylor GM, et al: Childhood Cancer Study Investigators. Methylenetetrahydrofolate reductase (MTHFR) polymorphisms and risk of molecularly defined subtypes of childhood acute leukemia. Proc Natl Acad Sci U S A 2001;98:4004.

47. Mori H, Xiao Z, Ford AM, et al: TEL-AML1 and AML1-ETO fusion sequences in normal newborn cord bloods. Blood 2000;96:88a.

48. Greaves MF, Alexander FE. An infectious etiology for common acute lymphoblastic leukemia in childhood? Leukemia 1993;7:349.

49. Kinlen LJ: Epidemiological evidence for an infective basis in childhood leukaemia. Br J Cancer 1995;71:1.

50. Greaves MF: Speculations on the cause of childhood acute lymphoblastic leukemia. Leukemia 1988;2:120.

51. Greaves MF: Aetiology of acute leukaemia. Lancet 1997;349:344.

52. Ross JA, Potter JD, Robison LL: Infant leukemia, topoisomerase II inhibitors, and the MLL gene. J Natl Cancer Inst 1994;86:1678.

53. Ross JA: Dietary flavonoids and the MLL gene: A pathway to infant leukemia? Proc Natl Acad Sci U S A 2000;97:4411.

54. Strick R, Strissel PL, Borgers S, et al: Dietary bioflavonoids induce cleavage in the MLL gene and may contribute to infant leukemia. Proc Natl Acad Sci U S A 2000;97:4790.

55. Wiemels JL, Pagnamenta A, Taylor GM, et al: A lack of a functional NAD(P)H:quinone oxidoreductase allele is selectively associated with pediatric leukemias that have MLL fusions. Cancer Res 1999; 59:4095.

56. Alexander FE, Patheal SL, Biondi A, et al: Transplacental chemical exposure and risk of infant leukaemia with MLL gene fusion. Cancer Res. In press.

57. Taylor GM, Birch JM: The hereditary basis of human leukemia. In: Henderson ES, Lister TA, Greaves MF, eds: Leukemia, 6th ed. Philadelphia: WB Saunders; 1996:210.

58. Gunz FW: Genetics of human leukaemia. Ser Haematol 1974; 7:164.

59. Malkin D, Li FP, Strong LC, et al: Germ line p53 mutations in a familial syndrome of breast cancer, sarcomas, and other neoplasms. Science 1990;250:1233.

60. Lavin MF, Shiloh Y: The genetic defect in ataxia telangiectasia. Ann Rev Immunol 1997;15:177.

61. Okuda T, van Deursen J, Hiebert SW, et al: AML1, the target of multiple chromosomal translocations in human leukemia, is essential for normal fetal liver hematopoiesis. Cell 1996;84:321.

62. Song W-J, Sullivan MG, Legare RD, et al: Haploinsufficiency of CBFA2 causes familial thrombocytopenia with propensity to develop acute myelogenous leukemia. Nat Genet 1999;23:166.

63. Malkin D, Brown EJ, Zipursky A: The role of p53 in megakaryocyte differentiation and the megakaryocytic leukemias of Down syndrome. Cancer Genet Cytogenet 2000;116:1.

64. Skibola CF, Smith MT, Kane E, et al: Polymorphisms in the methylenetetrahydrofolate reductase gene are associated with susceptibility to acute leukemia in adults. Proc Natl Acad Sci U S A 1999; 96:12810.

65. Kersey JH: Fifty years of studies of the biology and therapy of childhood leukemia. Blood 1997;90:4243.

66. Arico M, Valsecchi MG, Camitta B, et al: Outcome of treatment in children with Philadelphia chromosome–positive acute lymphoblastic leukemia. N Engl J Med 2000;342:998.

67. Greaves MF: Stem cell origins of leukaemia and curability. Br J Cancer 1993;67:413.

68. Whitehead VM, Vuchich MJ, Lauer SJ, et al: Accumulation of high levels of methotrexate polyglutamates in lymphoblasts from children with hyperdiploid (>50 chromosomes) B-lineage acute lymphoblastic leukemia: A Pediatric Oncology Group study. Blood 1992;80:1316.

69. Kaspers GJL, Smets LA, Pieters R, et al: Favorable prognosis of hyperdiploid common acute lymphoblastic leukemia may be explained by sensitivity to antimetabolites and other drugs: Results of an in vitro study. Blood 1995;85:751.

70. Ramakers-van Woerden NL, Pieters R, Loonen AH, et al: TEL/AML1 gene fusion is related to in vitro drug sensitivity for L-asparaginase in childhood acute lymphoblastic leukemia. Blood 2000;96:1094.

71. Nishii K, Kabarowski JHS, Gibbons DL, et al: BCR-ABL kinase

activation confers increased resistance to genotoxic damage via cell cycle block. Oncogene 1996;13:2225.

72. Griffiths SD, Clarke AR, Healy LE, et al: Absence of p53 permits propagation of mutant cells following genotoxic damage. Oncogene 1997;14:523.

73. Fisher DE: Apoptosis in cancer therapy: Crossing the threshold. Cell 1994;78:539.

74. Veldman T, Vignon C, Schröck E, et al: Hidden chromosome abnormalities in haematological malignancies detected by multicolour spectral karyotyping. Nat Genet 1997;15:406.

75. Druker B, Tamura S, Buchdunger E, et al: Effects of a selective inhibitor of the Abl tyrosine kinase on the growth of BCR-ABL-positive cells. Nat Med 1996;2:561.

76. Goldman JM: Tyrosine-kinase inhibition in treatment of chronic myeloid leukaemia. Lancet 2000;355:1031.

77. Reichert A, Heisterkamp N, Daley GQ, et al: Treatment of Bcr/Ab1-positive acute lymphoblastic leukemia in P190 transgenic mice with the farnesyl transferase inhibitor SCH66336. Blood 2001;97:1399.

78. Peters DG, Hoover RR, Gerlach MJ, et al: Activity of the farnesyl protein transferase inhibitor SCH66336 against BCR/ABL-induced murine leukemia and primary cells from patients with chronic myeloid leukemia. Blood 2001;97:1404.

79. Redner RL, Wang J, Liu J: Chromatin remodeling and leukemia: New therapeutic paradigms. Blood 1999;94:417.

80. Lin RJ, Egan DA, Evans RM: Molecular genetics of acute promyelocytic leukemia. Trends Genet 1999;15:179.

81. Warrell RP, He L-Z, Richon V, et al: Accelerated discovery. J Natl Cancer Inst 1998;90:1621.

82. Gale KB, Ford AM, Repp R, et al: Backtracking leukemia to birth: identification of clonotypic gene fusion sequences in neonatal blood spots. Proc Natl Acad Sci U S A 1997;94:13950.

83. Fialkow PJ: Clonal evolution of human myeloid leukemias. In Bishop JM, Rowley JD, Greaves MF, eds: Genes and Cancer. New York: Alan R Liss; 1984:215–226.

84. Tsukamoto N, Morita K, Maehara T, et al: Clonality in myelodysplastic syndromes: Demonstration of pluripotent stem cell origin using X-linked restriction fragment length polymorphisms. Br J Haematol 1993;83:589.

85. Fialkow PJ, Singer JW, Raskind WH, et al: Clonal development, stem-cell differentiation, and clinical remissions in acute non-lymphocytic leukemia. N Engl J Med 1987;317:468.

86. Dow LW, Martin P, Moohr J: Evidence for clonal development of childhood acute lymphoblastic leukemia. Blood 1985;66:902.

87. Ash RC, Detrick RA, Zanjani ED: In vitro studies of human pluripotential hematopoietic progenitors in polycythemia vera. J Clin Invest 1982;69:1112.

88. Raskind WH, Jacobson R, Murphy S, et al: Evidence for the involvement of B lymphoid cells in polycythemia vera and essential thrombocythemia. J Clin Invest 1985;75:1388.

89. Tsukamoto N, Morita K, Maehara T, et al: Clonality in chronic myeloproliferative disorders defined by X-chromosome linked probes: Demonstration of heterogeneity in lineage involvement. Br J Haematol 1994;86:253.

90. Van der Harst D, de Jong D, Limpens J, et al: Clonal B-cell populations in patients with idiopathic thrombocytopenic purpura. Blood 1990;76:2321.

91. Brisco MJ, Condon J, Hughes E, et al: Outcome prediction in childhood acute lymphoblastic leukaemia by molecular quantification of residual disease at the end of induction. Lancet 1994;343:196.

92. Yamada M, Wasserman R, Lange B, et al: Minimal residual disease in childhood B-lineage lymphoblastic leukemia. N Engl J Med 1990;323:448.

93. Nowell P, Finan J, Glover D, et al: Cytogenetic evidence for the clonal nature of Richter's syndrome. Blood 1981;58:183.

94. Zuelzer WW, Inoue S, Thompson RI, et al: Long-term cytogenetic studies in acute leukemia of children: The nature of relapse. Am J Hematol 1976;1:143.

95. Keinanen M, Griffin JD, Bloomfield CD, et al: Clonal chromosomal abnormalities showing multiple-cell-lineage involvement in acute myeloid leukemia. N Engl J Med 1988;318:1153.

96. Dow LW, Tachibana N, Raimondi SC, et al: Comparative biochemical and cytogenetic studies of childhood acute lymphoblastic leukemia with the Philadelphia chromosome and other 22q11 variants. Blood 1989;73:1291.

97. Kalousek DK, Dube ID, Eaves CJ, et al: Cytogenetic studies of haemopoietic colonies from patients with an initial diagnosis of acute lymphoblastic leukaemia. Br J Haematol 1988;70:5.

98. Buschle M, Janssen JW, Drexler H, et al: Evidence for pluripotent stem cell origin of idiopathic myelofibrosis: Clonal analysis of a case characterized by an N-ras gene mutation. Leukemia 1988;2:658.

99. Taylor GM, Robinson MD, Binchy A, et al: Preliminary evidence of an association between HLA-DPB1*0201 and childhood common acute lymphoblastic leukaemia supports an infectious aetiology. Leukemia 1995;9:440.

100. Smith MT, Wang Y, Kane E, et al: Low NAD(P)H:quinone oxidoreductase 1 activity is associated with increased risk of acute leukemia in adults. Blood 2001;97:1422.

101. Larson RA, Wang Y, Banerjee M, et al: Presence of the inactivating polymorphism in the NAD(P)H:quinone oxidoreductase (NQ01) gene in patients with primary and therapy-related myeloid leukemia. Blood 1999;94:803.

102. González Ordóñez AJ, Fernández Carreira JM, Fernández Alvarez CR, et al: Normal frequencies of the C677T genotypes on the methylenetetrahydrofolate reductase (MTHFR) gene among lymphoproliferative disorders but not in multiple myeloma. Leuk Lymphoma 2000;39:607.

103. Sinnett D, Krajinovic M, Labuda D: Genetic susceptibility to childhood acute lymphoblastic leukemia. Leuk Lymphoma 2000;38:447.

104. Felix CA, Walker AH, Lange BJ, et al: Association of CYP3A4 genotype with treatment-related leukemia. Proc Natl Acad Sci U S A 1998;95:13176.

3

Connie J. Eaves

Myelopoiesis

CELLULAR COMPARTMENTALIZATION OF THE HEMATOPOIETIC DIFFERENTIATION PROCESS

General Principles

Blood contains at least 10 different mature cell types, each with a unique set of specialized properties and, in most cases, important life-supporting functions. Most of the cells in the blood also have a relatively short life span. As a result, many billions of these cells are lost from the system each day. Nevertheless, their numbers are normally maintained at relatively constant levels throughout adulthood. This is achieved by the continuous production in the marrow and lymphoid tissue of new, mature blood cells from more primitive precursor cells through a complex, but balanced process in which the regulation of cell differentiation, proliferation, and death determines the rate of mature cell output. This process also provides for a remarkable degree of cell amplification and specialization, ultimately from a relatively small pool of self-maintaining pluripotent hematopoietic stem cells. Morphologically recognizable blood cells appear early in development, and any subsequent arrest or even severe perturbation of their production is rapidly life threatening. The process of hematopoiesis is thus essential as well as complex and, as such, has captured the interest and fascination of biologists and clinicians alike for many years.

A cardinal feature of normal hematopoiesis is the large number of cell generations over which coordinated changes in cellular properties can be observed. Of these, the latter three to five cell cycles have been the most extensively characterized because it is only during these terminal amplifying divisions that the differentiation programs of most lineages become readily apparent (morphologically) and the number of cells of a particular type is large enough to permit a variety of molecular and biochemical studies. Molecular changes occurring at this final stage of hematopoietic cell maturation have profound morphologic consequences and take place rapidly. As a result, sequential cell cycles can be readily distinguished with light microscopy, as originally shown by kinetic DNA labeling measurements.[1-3] In contrast, most types of more primitive hematopoietic cells look very similar to one another, at least when examined by conventional light microscopy, and in fact these cells resemble lymphoid blasts. Nevertheless, many subpopulations of primitive hematopoietic cells can now be reproducibly discriminated on the basis of their different functional properties, as well as by their differential expression of specific molecular features (e.g., expression of various cell surface markers) that are not accompanied by any obvious morphologic change. An association of specific changes in these latter properties with the display of a decreasing proliferative and differentiative potential has been repeatedly demonstrated and has led to a now widely accepted concept of hematopoiesis as the regulated passage of cells into and down individual pathways of a multilineage developmental hierarchy (Fig. 3-1).

We are now also beginning to understand these events in molecular terms. As with other developmental processes, a growing body of evidence indicates that hematopoietic cell differentiation involves the regulated and sequential activation and silencing of genes encoding various transcription factors. These include a number of members of the homeobox (*HOX*) gene family that regulate morphogenic changes and cell fate decisions in many tissues. Not surprisingly, many *HOX* genes are also common targets for leukemogenic changes.[4] Other transcription factors appear to have more unique roles in regulating the differentiation of hematopoietic cell development. Members of a family of transcription factors that specifically recognize the GATA sequence in the promoter region of genes expressed in differentiating hematopoietic cells[5] represent but one example of the latter. Gene knockout and forced gene overexpression experiments in mice have already identified a requirement for the expression of some of these genes to be upregulated or downregulated for hematopoiesis both to be initiated (e.g., AML1[6, 7] and SCL/tal-1[8, 9]) and to proceed along specific pathways (e.g., PU.1,[10-12] Pax5/BSAP,[13] ikaros,[14, 15] GATA-1,[16, 17] and GATA-3[18]). Such studies have further suggested lineage commitment to be a process involving separate molecular suppression of other lineage options in addition to the positive activation of a particular blood cell maturation program.[19-23] In addition, many data now indicate that some of the earliest steps in the hematopoietic cell differentiation process involve changes in either the expression and/or signaling capacity of cell surface receptors for different growth factors and cell adhesion molecules that participate in the regulation of hematopoiesis.[24]

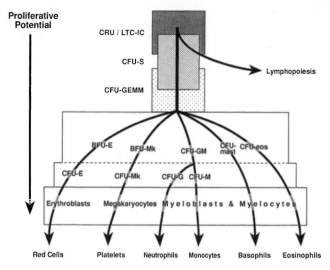

Proliferative Potential

CRU / LTC-IC

CFU-S

CFU-GEMM

Lymphopoiesis

BFU-E BFU-Mk CFU-GM CFU-mast CFU-eos

CFU-E CFU-Mk CFU-G CFU-M

Erythroblasts Megakaryocytes Myeloblasts & Myelocytes

Red Cells Platelets Neutrophils Monocytes Basophils Eosinophils

FIGURE 3–1. Hierarchical model of normal hematopoietic cell differentiation highlighting the continuous nature of the process (*arrows*) as well as attempts to define discrete stages or compartments (*boxes*) for distinguishing cells that differ significantly in their proliferative and differentiative potentialities.

As hematopoietic differentiation processes begin to be described in increasing molecular detail, they will need to account for and explain the variable (and even alternative) versions of particular programs that are known to be elicited under different biologic circumstances. Perhaps the most dramatic example of this situation is seen when the types of blood cells produced in fetal and adult life are compared. However, differences may also result from the types of external factors to which primitive hematopoietic cells are exposed, independent of their ontogenic status. This effect of external factors imposes other dimensions on the simple model shown in Figure 3-1 needs to be remembered in any discussion of how hematopoiesis is normally regulated. They are also relevant to any attempt to anticipate the consequences of specific perturbations of the processes regulating normal hematopoiesis as, for example, occurs in acute leukemia.

Historically, researchers have tended to investigate and consider the mechanisms controlling the output of lymphoid and myeloid cells separately. This separation is based in part on accumulating evidence that the lineages thus far associated with each of these two subdivisions of the hematopoietic system most frequently diverge from one another as a group early in the hematopoietic cell differentiation process in vivo.[25-28] However, evidence of variability in early hematopoietic commitment events obtained from analysis of multiple clonal populations[29-31] casts doubt on the universality of this concept. With a growing inventory of genomic information and more rapid input from functional analysis of differentially expressed genes, our understanding of these events is likely to change dramatically in the coming years. Nevertheless, at this point, separating discussion of the unique features of lymphopoiesis and myelopoiesis, as has been done in this book, provides a simple and practical solution to the problem of trying to review all the broad topics of hematopoiesis within a single chapter. It may also faci-

tate a review of the different types of leukemias that may arise in lymphoid as opposed to myeloid or totipotent precursors. Therefore, the focus of the present chapter has been restricted to the biology of pluripotent hematopoietic stem cells and the various myelopoietic progenitors that they generate, with the allocation of another full chapter to the specifics of lymphopoiesis and its regulation.

Detection and Quantitation of Primitive Hematopoietic Cells

Identification of Lymphomyeloid Stem Cells

Cells with the capacity to generate all types of mature blood cells, including those of both the lymphoid and myeloid systems, represent a small subpopulation of adult bone marrow cells that persist throughout normal life. Such cells were first demonstrated in mice in studies in which a variety of genetic marker strategies were used to distinguish large clonal populations of blood cells containing both lymphoid and myeloid elements regenerated in myeloablated or genetically anemic hosts.[32-36] The first evidence for an analogous type of primitive human hematopoietic cell with lymphomyeloid differentiation came from the demonstration of large neoplastic clones containing multiple types of mature blood cells in patients with various kinds of myeloproliferative[37] and myelodysplastic diseases.[38, 39] Subsequently, the occasional observation of donor-derived clonal blood cell populations (including both lymphocytes and granulocytes) in recipients of allogeneic marrow grafts provided more direct evidence of the existence of transplantable lymphomyeloid stem cells in normal adult human marrow.[40] More recently, the emergence of clonal hematopoiesis in otherwise normal older people has been documented.[41, 42]

These latter findings, as well as studies of serially transplanted stem cells in mice,[43-46] demonstrate the enormous proliferative potential that can be unleashed from some very primitive, but apparently normal hematopoietic cells; this is sufficient to enable the progeny of a single human hematopoietic stem cell to reconstitute the entire hematopoietic system of a person (10^{11} to 10^{12} cells) and sustain the production and turnover of mature blood cells at normal levels for several months ($>10^{11}$ cells/day $\times$ 100 days $= >10^{13}$ cells). However, the extent to which individual cells with this potential contribute to the daily output of mature blood cells under normal homeostatic conditions is still not clear. Several studies suggest the simultaneous and continuous activity in normal adults of multiple stem-cell–derived clones sufficient to give a picture of polyclonal hematopoiesis.[37, 40, 47] However, the actual number of such clones involved is not known and could be relatively small.[40, 46, 48, 49] This point is important, albeit unresolved, because clonal dominance in the human hematopoietic system is usually interpreted (perhaps mistakenly) as evidence of a neoplastic change (i.e., indicative of an abnormal outgrowth of cells from a primitive precursor that has been genetically altered).

Quantitation of In Vivo Repopulating Stem Cells

The existence of hematopoietic stem cells in the marrow of both normal adult mice and humans with a lifelong ability to generate all blood cell types is thus a well-established concept. The development of methodologies for quantitating these cells in a fashion that distinguishes them from other cells with more limited reconstituting activity and more restricted differentiation potentialities has been more of a challenge. This issue was first brought into focus in the 1960s and 1970s when functional assays for primitive murine cells with in vitro clonogenic potential were introduced, and it rapidly became clear that different types of apparently lineage-restricted progenitors and their more primitive pluripotent precursors could not be distinguished by using traditional morphologic approaches. Subsequently, in the 1980s, the discovery was made that even many of the primitive hematopoietic progenitors in mice that are functionally defined as CFU-S (colony-forming unit–spleen) because they are able to generate sufficient progeny to form a macroscopically visible colony in the spleen[50] (i.e., ~10^5 to 10^7 cells) actually produce only one lineage of daughter cells. Moreover, many CFU-S cells have lost demonstrable self-renewal activity.[51] These more "mature" CFU-S cells can now also be distinguished from cells with a long-term in vivo lymphomyeloid repopulating potential in terms of a number of other phenotypic characteristics that allow their isolation as separate populations.[52-55]

More recent emphasis has therefore focused on the development and validation of more specific assays for measuring transplantable stem cells with lifelong hematopoietic activity. Two approaches are now widely used. Both rely on transplantation of the test cells into recipients whose endogenous hematopoiesis has been suppressed to allow maximal stimulation of hematologic recovery. In the mouse, where syngeneic or congenic donor-recipient combinations are possible, prolonged (>4 months) post-transplant end points of test cell engraftment are required to ensure specificity of the read-out for stem cells with repopulating activity because the progeny of some types of transplantable cells with more restricted potentialities can be detected for periods of up to 4 months.[49, 56-58] Cotransplantation of equal numbers of genetically distinguishable but histocompatible test cells with a large "standard" competitor population and subsequent assessment of their separate contributions to one or more lineages more than 4 months later provides a sensitive measure of the *relative* stem-cell activity of the test cell population.[59] This determination can also be used to infer stem-cell *numbers* if the frequency of stem cells in the competitor population is known and if it is also assumed that the average output of mature cells by the test stem cells is the same as for those present in the competitor population.

An alternative approach is to measure the frequency of transplantable long-term repopulating cells directly by using limiting dilution analysis techniques. This latter procedure requires that recipients be given sufficient additional cells (or are sublethally conditioned) to ensure their survival independent of whether they receive any stem cells from the test innoculum. It also requires that

the number of other stem cells present in the recipients be kept to a minimum to maximize the sensitivity of the assay.[60-62] This assay is illustrated schematically in Figure 3-2. In recognition of the principles that it embodies, the cell that it detects has been assigned the operational term competitive repopulating unit (CRU).

However, not every cell with CRU potential would be expected to home to a hematopoietic tissue and be activated after injection in vivo.[63] For example, it has become apparent that proliferating CRUs acquire a marked, albeit reversible, inability to engraft intravenously transplanted recipients as they first enter G_1 from G_0 and then subsequently traverse the $S/G_2/M$ phases of the cell cycle.[64-69] Interestingly, the engraftment ability of hematopoietic cells with more restricted developmental capacities appears less sensitive to cell cycle transit.[70, 71] Thus, as in vitro assays able to *specifically* quantify cells with long-term in vivo lymphomyeloid output potential are refined and validated, they may offer the advantage of not being affected by cell cycle status for the detection of repopulating stem cells.[65, 72] Even in the absence of perturbations that reduce the ability of stem cells to engraft, it seems unlikely that CRUs would have a seeding efficiency of 100%. Thus, CRU measurements can be assumed to be underestimates of cells with stem-cell potential, and the extent of the underestimation may vary depending on the status and history of the cells being considered.

Murine CRUs are present in the bone marrow of normal adult mice at a frequency of approximately one per 10^4 nucleated cells,[60] and they can be enriched more than 1000-fold to achieve frequencies of at least 1 CRU in 10 cells,[57, 73, 74] even without considering the fact that these values would underestimate the actual number of stem cells in the highly purified populations isolated. Several lines of evidence point to the specificity of the

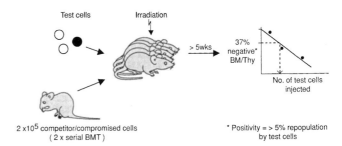

Quantitation Of "CRU" (Competitive Repopulating Units) By Limit Dilution Analysis

Test cells   Irradiation

> 5wks   37% negative* BM/Thy

No. of test cells injected

2 x10^5 competitor/compromised cells (2 x serial BMT)

* Positivity = > 5% repopulation by test cells

FIGURE 3–2. Original assay for murine CRUs. This procedure involves injecting limiting numbers of genetically distinguishable CRUs into myeloablated congenic recipient mice, together with sufficient numbers of another source of short-term progenitors that will ensure the survival of the recipients regardless whether they receive any CRUs in the test cell suspension (but not enough CRUs to reduce the detection of those in the test cell suspension). Alternatively, congenic sublethally irradiated and genetically compromised hosts can be used. To ensure detection of a cell with durable (lifelong) lymphomyeloid reconstituting activity, the presence of test cell–derived lymphoid and myeloid cells must be documented for at least 4 months post-transplant. This assay has been adapted for the detection of transplantable human cells with lymphomyeloid repopulating activity using sublethally irradiated NOD/SCID mice as hosts. For additional details, see reference 61.

murine CRU assay for cells with long-term lymphomyeloid system–reconstituting potential.[60, 75-77] The CRU assay has thus become the gold standard for the measurement of transplantable hematopoietic stem cells.

Recognition of the ability of intravenously injected, primitive *human* hematopoietic cells to enter the extravascular compartments of the marrow of highly immunocompromised mice[78-81] at high efficiency[82] has allowed the principles of the murine CRU assay to be applied to the detection and quantitation of human lymphomyeloid repopulating cells.[83, 84] For several years, the most popular genotype of mouse for such assays has been the non-obese diabetic (NOD)/severe combined immunodeficiency (NOD/SCID) mouse. In this case, their pretreatment with a sublethal dose of radiation is sufficient to maximize engraftment of transplanted human CRUs. However, because the latter represent a xenograft, coinjection of mature human T cells must be minimized to avoid graft-versus-host complications, which can be lethal. In addition, if the total number of human cells to be injected is small (e.g., as may be the case if purified subpopulations are being investigated), cotransplantation of other human cells is required to minimize nonspecific losses.[83, 85, 86]

Table 3-1 shows the frequency of CRUs in various human tissues detected by using end points that require the marrow of NOD/SCID mice transplanted at least 6 weeks previously to contain either more than 1% total human cells (DNA) or more than 0.25% human myeloid plus more than 0.25% human lymphoid cells. The term *SCID repopulating cell* (SRC) has also been used to identify these cells. However, the term *CRU* has the advantage that it implies the same defining properties and conditions that have been found to be useful for quantitating murine hematopoietic stem cells.[61] Most human CRUs

detected by their ability to engraft NOD/SCID mice appear to be AC 133+ [87, 88] and CD34+ CD38− .[83, 89] However, some may express detectable levels of CD38,[83] and some may not express CD34.[90] In adult mice, CD34− repopulating cells represent a significant fraction of the total CRU population,[91, 92] but the expression of CD34 on these cells is reversible and may be upregulated when they are activated.[93] In fact, heterogeneity in phenotypes of murine cells with long-term in vivo repopulating activity is an emerging theme[94-96] and hence one that is likely to find human parallels as xenograft models become more sensitive and able to support an increased output of all types of differentiated human myeloid and lymphoid cells.

Sheep injected in utero with human hematopoietic cells can also be efficiently engrafted and long-term multilineage chimerism established.[97, 98] This approach involves transplanting the fetus at a gestational stage when its immune system has not yet begun to develop. By using this model, a spectrum of phenotypes with variable engraftment durability have been identified in normal human marrow. These phenotypes include AC133+ cells[99] and CD34− CD38− [100] as well as CD34+ CD38− and CD34+ CD38+ populations.[101]

Both immunodeficient mice and fetal sheep engrafted with human hematopoietic cells support the generation of daughter cells with repopulating potential demonstrable in serial transplantation experiments.[101-104] As predicted from previous similar experiments in mice, greater numbers of daughter CRUs are obtained from fetal cells, and this self-renewal activity decreases progressively and dramatically during ontogeny.[103]

In Vitro Assays for Clonogenic Progenitors

The first successful attempts to develop in vitro assays for hematopoietic progenitors were undertaken in the early 1960s. These assays followed rapidly from the observation that murine granulopoietic cells could proliferate in suspension culture in the presence of fibroblast feeder cells[105] and exploited the potential of semisolid media to allow the number of responsive precursors present in the original suspension to be defined by their ability to generate discrete and visible colonies of daughter cells.[106-108] From a series of studies designed to investigate the relationship of CFU-S to murine cells that could generate colonies of granulocytes and macrophages in vitro, it was established that though closely related, these populations are largely distinct. The latter, called colony-forming cells (CFCs), proved to be mainly lineage-restricted granulocyte-macrophage progenitors[109, 110] (hence the terms colony-forming unit–granulocyte [CFU-G], CFU-M, and CFU-GM, which have subsequently been adopted).

These early observations provided the initial basis for formulating the type of hierarchic scheme of hematopoiesis shown in Figure 3-1. At the same time, they gave a strong impetus to the search for in vitro conditions that would allow the detection of putatively analogous populations of other types of lineage-restricted clonogenic progenitors. Such conditions are now well defined, and additional in vitro assays for cells that appear able to produce colonies of maturing erythroblasts only (from colony-

TABLE 3–1. Repopulating Stem-Cell (CRU) Numbers in Normal Human Tissues

Tissue	CRU Progeny Measured	Frequency*
Fetal liver—12–20 wk	CD19/20+ cells + CD15/66b+ cells	9
Cord blood	CD19/20+ cells + CD34+ CFCs	6
	CD45/71+ cells	29
	CD19/20+ cells + CD15/66b+ cells	6
	CD19/20+ cells + CD34+ CFCs	4
	CD45/71+ cells	27
	Human DNA	5†
Adult bone marrow	CD19/20+ cells + CD15/66b+ cells	0.8
	CD19/20+ cells + CD34+ CFCs	2
	CD45/71+ cells	2
	Human DNA	2†
G-CSF mobilized blood	Human DNA	1†

* Expressed per 10^5 CD34+lin− low-density (<1.077 g/mL) cells.

† Assuming that 2% of low-density cord blood and bone marrow cells are CD34+ (data from 84). The remaining data are from 103.

CFCs, colony-forming cells; CRU, competitive repopulating unit; G-CSF, granulocyte colony-stimulating factor.

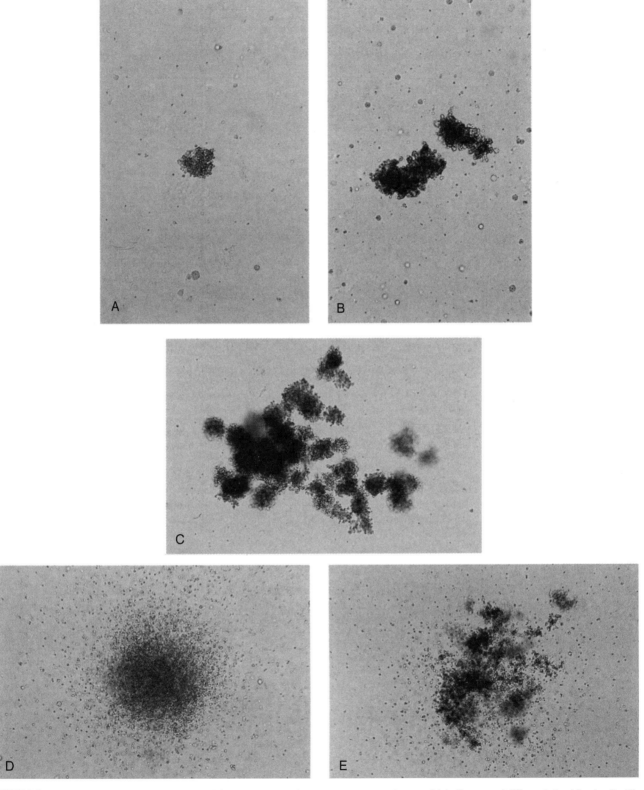

FIGURE 3–3. Photomicrographs of various types of hematopoietic colonies containing single or multiple lineages of differentiating blood cells. The colonies were photographed in the living state in the cultures in which they were generated. *A,* Typical CFU-E–derived colony. *B,* Typical BFU-E–derived colony. *C,* Typical primitive BFU-E–derived colony. *D,* Typical CFU-GM–derived colony. *E,* Typical CFU-GEMM–derived colony. All colonies shown at the same magnification. (See Color Section.)

forming or burst-forming units–erythroid [CFU-E and BFU-E]) or colonies of megakaryocytes (from colony-forming or burst-forming units–megakaryocyte [CFU-Mk and BFU-Mk]) have been described and standardized.[111-114]

Although the in vitro conditions required for the formation of granulopoietic, erythroid, and megakaryocytic colonies are not identical, they are also not mutually exclusive. It has thus been possible to also identify conditions that support the formation of colonies containing all of these myeloid lineages (i.e., from colony-forming unit–granulocyte, erythroid, megakaryocyte, and macrophage [CFU-GEMM]).[115] Typical examples of different types of human hematopoietic colonies are shown in Figure 3-3. In retrospect, it is interesting to note that the general in vitro growth requirements of the progenitors of these different types of hematopoietic colonies are very similar and can now be met with completely defined (serum-free) media.[116-119] The major differences required for stimulating the growth and differentiation of particular progenitor types thus appear to relate to their specific (though not necessarily unique) growth factor requirements.

It has now been formally shown that all the different types of hematopoietic colonies described can originate from single cells. In addition, assessment of colony formation from highly purified starting cell populations has demonstrated the very high plating efficiencies (up to 100%) that can be achieved when culture conditions are optimized. The further demonstration of a linear relationship between colony yield and the concentration of cells plated has helped validate the utility of these assays for quantitating progenitor numbers in patient samples or after various manipulations before plating.

The ultimate size, as well as the mature cell content, of the various types of hematopoietic colonies produced under "optimal" conditions in vitro are, generally speaking, indicative of the proliferative and the differentiative potential of each clonogenic progenitor originally present.[120, 121] The use of identical culture conditions to support the production of colonies that achieve very different sizes before undergoing terminal maturation along a particular pathway (e.g., as exemplified in Fig. 3-3 for the erythroid pathway) thus allows discrimination of a hierarchy of lineage-restricted progenitors with decreasing proliferative potential. (The later types of progenitors generate smaller colonies containing fewer mature cells, and these colonies appear sooner.) This phenomenon is particularly obvious for erythroid progenitors whose clonal progeny can be seen to undergo a sudden and dramatic change as hemoglobin synthesis is initiated in a semisynchronous fashion.[112] However, an analogous pattern is also evident from time course studies of other colony types.[122-124]

Results of multiparameter cell-sorting experiments have further shown that such functional discrimination of progenitor populations can be matched to changes in their surface phenotype (Fig. 3-4). These changes, in turn, have allowed the different types of progenitors to be physically separated and studied as discrete subpopulations.[117, 125, 126] In addition, many of the colony-stimulating factors (CSFs) that in early studies were contained in poorly characterized, albeit often potent conditioned me-

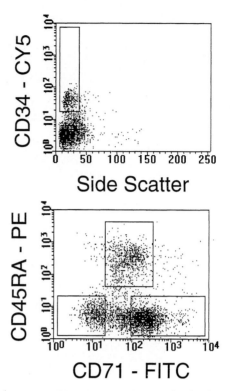

FIGURE 3–4. Representative FACS plot showing the distribution of cells within the CD34+ subpopulation *(top panel)* of normal light density human bone marrow cells according to the expression on each CD34+ cell of CD71 (the receptor for transferrin) and CD45RA (the high molecular weight form of CD45 *(bottom panel)*. The compartment of CD34+CD71−CD45RA− cells shown in the lower left region of the panel on the bottom contains most of the LTC-ICs and two-thirds of the CFU-GEMMs. The compartment of CD34+CD71±CD45+ cells shown in the upper middle region of this panel contains virtually no LTC-ICs or CFU-GEMMs or BFU-Es (or CFU-Es) but approximately half of the CFU-GMs. The compartment of CD34+CD71+D45 A− cells shown in the lower right region of this panel contains approximately two-thirds of the BFU-Es and virtually all CFU-Es but no LTC-ICs, very few CFU-GEMMs, and approximately half of the CFU-GMs.[126] Similar results are obtained with CD34+ cord blood cells.[117]

dia (e.g., media containing the secreted products of various cell types with or without their activation) are now available as purified recombinant proteins (see listing summarized in Table 3-2). Careful analysis of the actions of these factors on particular types of progenitors has revealed some specificity, as expected, but also unanticipated synergies and extensive redundancies. Moreover, even in the presence of different single factors or combinations of factors, the time course of development and the spectrum of colony types observed in semisolid cultures of hematopoietic cells have remained largely unchanged since their original description in assays that historically relied on less well defined mixtures.

Although there appears to be an upper limit to the number of divisions that lineage-restricted progenitors can execute before terminally differentiating, some evidence also suggests that this number can be varied by exposure to certain extrinsic modulators.[127-129] In addition, even under apparently identical conditions of exogenous stimulation, decisions that occur at the single-cell level may be characterized by a stochastic compo-

TABLE 3–2. The Hematopoietic Growth Factors — Genetically Cloned Cytokines with Major Effects on Hematopoietic Cells

Name(s)	Receptor(R)	Some Major Human Myeloid Target Cells and Responses
M-CSF (CSF-1)	CSF1R or FMS	Stimulation of CFU-Ms, survival and activation of monocytes/macrophages
G-CSF (CSF-β, pluripoietin)	G-CSFR	Stimulation of CFU-Gs, pluripotent cells; differentiation of some human leukemic cells
GM-CSF (CSF-α)	GM-CSFR-α + βc	Stimulation of CFU-GMs, BFU-Es, CFU-Mks, pluripotent cells; activation of neutrophils
Erythropoietin	EpoR	Stimulation of CFU-Es, BFU-Es; erythroblast survival
Interleukin-1 (hemopoietin-1)	IL-1R	Activation of macrophages, action on primitive human myeloid cells controversial
Interleukin-2 (T-cell growth factor)	IL-2Rα + β + γ	Action on myeloid cells controversial
Interleukin-3 (multi-CSF)	IL-3Rα + βc	Stimulation of CFU-GMs, BFU-Es, CFU-Mks, pluripotent cells
Interleukin-4 (B-cell–stimulating factor-1, B-cell growth factor)	IL-4R + IL-2Rγ	Stimulation of CFU-GMs, BFU-Es, pluripotent cells
Interleukin-5 (B-cell growth factor-2, eosinophil differentiation factor, T-cell–replacing factor)	IL-5Rα + βc	Stimulation of CFU-eos's
Interleukin-6 (interferon-β$_2$)	IL-6Rα + gp130(β)	Stimulation of CFU-GMs, CFU-Ms, CFU-Mks, pluripotent cells
Interleukin-7	IL-7R + IL-2Rγ	Stimulates cytokine production by monocytes
Interleukin-8 (neutrophil-activating peptide-1, one of CXC chemokines)	IL8-RA + B	Neutrophil chemoattractant, inhibition of neutrophil adhesion
Interleukin-9 (human homologue of murine T-cell growth factor p40)	IL-9R	Mast cell proliferation and activation, stimulation of CFU-Es, BFU-Es
Interleukin-10 (B cell–derived T-cell growth factor, cytokine synthesis inhibitory factor)		Inhibition of cytokine production by monocytes
Interleukin-11	IL-11Rα + gp130(β)	Stimulation of CFU-Mks; activation of fetal (but not adult) BFU-E, CFU-GM, CFU-GEMM cycling (but not colony formation)
Interleukin-12 (NK cell stimulatory factor, cytotoxic lymphocyte maturation factor)	IL-12R + ?	Activation of pluripotent cells
Steel factor (stem-cell factor, mast-cell growth factor, KIT ligand)	KIT	Stimulation of BFU-Es, CFU-GMs, CFU-Mks, pluripotent cells, human leukemic cells
FLK-2/FLT-3 ligand	FLK-2/FLT-3 (STK-1)	Stimulation of CFU-GMs, pluripotent cells
Thrombopoietin (c-mpl-ligand)	MPL	Stimulation of CFU-Mks, megakaryocytes, pluripotent cells
Leukemia inhibitory factor	LIF-R	Stimulation of pluripotent cells
Transforming growth factor-β	TGF-βR	Inhibition of primitive myeloid cells, stimulation of mature myeloid cells
Macrophage inflammatory protein-1 (one of the CC chemokines)	C-C CKR-1	Inhibition of primitive myeloid cells, stimulation of mature myeloid cells

BFU-E, burst-forming unit—erythroid; CFU-E/GM/GEMM/MK, colony-forming unit—erythroid/granulocyte-macrophage/granulocyte, erythroid, megakaryocyte, and macrophage/megakaryocyte; FLK, fetal liver kinase; FLT, FMS-like tyrosine kinase; G/M/GM-CSF, granulocyte/macrophage/granulocyte-macrophage colony-stimulating factor; MPL, proto-oncogene encoding a cell surface receptor corresponding to the myeloproliferative leukemia virus (MPLV)-transforming gene; NK, natural killer; STK, stem-cell tyrosine kinase.

nent.[130, 131] Either of these mechanisms could result in a larger or smaller than average output of mature cells being obtained from progenitor cells at a given stage and, hence, an apparent lengthening or shortening of the pathway that they would execute[120] (Fig. 3-5). Presumably, such variations reflect the existence within developmentally equivalent progenitor cells of intracellular mediators that can regulate the pace of further differentiation of these cells. One might then readily envisage that either unusual microenvironmental conditions or somatic mutations able to affect the probability of a particular response could have consequences relevant to both the genesis and treatment of leukemia.

Nevertheless, overall, the progenitor cell interrelationships portrayed in the model illustrated in Figure 3-1 have withstood the test of time and have proved useful in a period in which molecular correlates of specific hematopoietic differentiation steps are just beginning to be identified. However, as for the various in vivo assays for hematopoietic cells, it is important to remember that the end points used to detect different categories of

progenitors in vitro are usually insufficient to avoid overlap in the detection of closely related progenitor types. This issue may not be significant when assessing large effects on entire populations, but it could be critical to the investigation of minor or rare responses.

The ability of adherent marrow cells to stimulate cells capable of producing hematopoietic progeny for very long periods in vitro (see later) and the characterization of an ever-increasing number of growth factors able to synergistically stimulate very primitive hematopoietic progenitors have led to the development of "special" colony assays for detecting these cells. The progenitors thus detected are referred to as high–proliferative potential colony-forming cells (HPP-CFCs),[123, 132] colony-forming units type A (CFU-A),[133, 134] stroma-dependent or stroma-adherent blast colony-forming cells (Bl-CFCs),[135, 136] and blast colony-forming cells produced in response to defined factors[137, 138] to reflect the different clonal assay procedures used. The specificity required for exclusive identification of the small subset of colonies produced by each of these very primitive hematopoietic cell types is

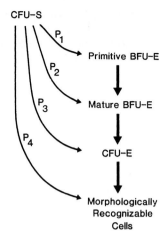

FIGURE 3–5. A model of hematopoietic progenitor cell differentiation that embodies the concept of a variable proliferative potential (pathway length) after pluripotent cells (CFU-S) commit to a single lineage. The example illustrated here is for the erythroid cell pathway. According to such a model, the number of divisions that intervene between commitment and terminal maturation events (e.g., hemoglobin production) is not fixed but is governed by probabilities (P_{1-4}), which are set by the properties of the stem-cell population or the environment in which the cells undergo commitment, or both. (From Eaves CJ, Eaves AC: Erythropoiesis. In Golde DW, Takaku F [eds]: Hematopoietic Stem Cells. New York, Marcel Dekker, 1985, p 19, by courtesy of Marcel Dekker, Inc.)

achieved in part by the use of either appropriate combinations of early-acting growth factors (HPP-CFCs, CFU-A, and blast colony-forming cells) or feeder layers of adherent marrow cells (B1-CFCs). These assays also use end points that include either a very large size criterion (e.g., a diameter of >0.5 to 1 mm or a content of >10^3 cells, which implies a proliferative potential of the original progenitor of >10 cell divisions; HPP-CFCs and CFU-A) or demonstration of the sustained production of conventionally defined clonogenic progenitors during the first 5 to 10 cell divisions in the development of the colony (B1-CFCs and blast colony-forming cells defined as described earlier). More recently, conditions for generating colonies containing murine B, T, and natural killer (NK) cells, as well as myeloid cells, have also been described,[139, 140] although extension of these conditions to human cells has not yet been reported.

In Vitro Assays for Precursors of Clonogenic Cells

In theory, it might be anticipated that any type of hematopoietic progenitor should be able to form a colony (in vitro) if the factors required for stimulating its proliferation and differentiation could be identified and an adequate supply of nutrients and oxygen were maintained during the interval required for these events to proceed. Why then, more than 30 years after the introduction of in vitro colony assay technology, has this approach still not been successfully adapted for the routine assessment of pluripotent cells with long-term in vivo repopulating potential? The explanation appears to be that the most primitive hematopoietic cells typically obtained from normal tissues in vivo are unable to proliferate in semisolid culture media even though they may do so in liquid

cultures.[141, 142] Interestingly, more recent studies indicate that this property can be rapidly and selectively modulated after exposure to high concentrations of certain growth factors in vitro.[143]

On the other hand, already by the late 1970s it had become clear that bone marrow adherent cells could support the output of murine CFCs and CFU-S in vitro for many weeks under so-called Dexter long-term culture (LTC) conditions,[144] and this system was subsequently shown to also be applicable to human cells[145-147] (Fig. 3–6). Furthermore, it was possible to show that the CFCs detectable in these LTCs were in a constant state of turnover as long as hematopoiesis was detectable (i.e., routinely for at least 8 weeks).[148, 149] Later studies showed that in spite of an overall net decline in their numbers, a proportion of murine CRUs will undergo extensive self-renewal within 4 weeks after being placed in LTC.[150] The LTC system thus appears to provide conditions that support both the proliferation and commitment of the most primitive types of hematopoietic stem cells, as well as the limited proliferation and differentiation of their granulopoietic progeny. Such a conclusion makes the correct prediction that after a sufficiently long interval, the total in vitro clonogenic cell content of these cultures might serve as a quantitative readout of a more primitive cell type present in the original input suspension—a cell therefore called an LTC-initiating cell (LTC-IC).[151, 152]

Just as the time taken by different types of clonogenic progenitors to produce colonies of mature progeny in vitro varies according to the differentiated state of the progenitor, so too does the timing and the duration of CFC production for different subpopulations of primitive hematopoietic precursors maintained in LTC.[151-154] Characterization and isolation of the input cells responsible for producing the more differentiated cells present after various periods have led to the adoption of a 4- or 5-week or longer interval to facilitate the measurement of rare input cells (LTC-ICs) in normal human (or mouse)

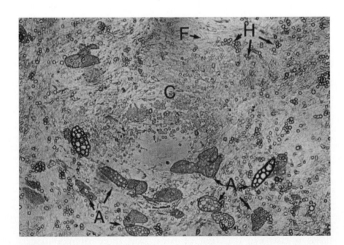

FIGURE 3–6. Photomicrograph of a typical field showing the adherent layer of a hematopoietically active 8-week-old LTC established from human bone marrow. Arrows indicate adipocytes (A), fibroblasts (F), and a cobblestone-like area of hematopoietic cells (C) in the adherent layer as well as other hematopoietic cells (H) floating in the nonadherent fraction.

marrow that differ from those identifiable directly as CFCs.[151, 155, 156]

Derivation of the absolute frequencies of LTC-ICs in specific test samples and examination of their individual properties are most rigorously done by using limiting dilution analysis procedures.[157-159] However, the generally high degree of consistency seen in the average clonogenic cell output per LTC-IC measured under standardized conditions (e.g., by using supportive cell lines as feeder layers[160] and the existence of a linear dose-response relationship between total CFC output and LTC-IC input over a wide range of LTC-IC input concentrations[157, 158] allow for LTC-IC numbers to be calculated from less labor-intensive bulk cultures for most routine applications. In this case, the number of input LTC-ICs is obtained simply by dividing the total number of CFCs detected by a predetermined (or simultaneously determined) value for the average output of CFCs per LTC-IC.

LTC-ICs determined represent a much rarer cell type than any type of lineage-restricted CFCs thus far defined, but like the different types of CFCs, they have also been found in all normal hematopoietic tissue examined to date. These include fetal[161-163] as well as neonatal[164, 165] and adult sources, the latter including blood from normal[159] and mobilized donors,[164, 166] in addition to marrow.[157, 167] Table 3-3 summarizes some of the properties of human LTC-ICs measured as originally described by using either human marrow LTC adherent layers or a murine fibroblast cell line as a feeder and a 5-week period of culture before assessing the number of CFCs present.

Several groups have found that the addition of various growth factors to human LTC can increase the number of CFCs produced for several months.[168-171] A similar effect can be obtained by using murine fibroblasts that have been genetically engineered to produce these growth factors constitutively.[160, 164] When such human growth factor–producing mouse fibroblasts are used as feeders in assays for human LTC-ICs, both the 6-week CFC output (per LTC-IC) and the number of input cells detectable as LTC-ICs are increased without a reduction in the specificity of the assay for very primitive cells.[164] However, it is important to note that the output of total CFCs in LTC (per LTC-IC), as well as the proportions of different types of CFCs produced, can vary according to

TABLE 3–4. Comparison of CFC Output from LTC-ICs Detected with Different Assay Conditions and Durations

Source of LTC-ICs	CFCs per LTC-IC		GM/E/GEMM	
	wk 5/6, No GF	wk 6, +GF	wk 5/6, No GF	wk 6, +GF
Fetal liver	36 ± 14*	72 ± 18	ND	81:17:2
Cord blood	17 ± 0.2	28 ± 2	ND	98:2:0.1
Bone marrow	7 ± 3	18 ± 6	90:9:1†	99:1:0.03
Mobilized blood	9 ± 2	25 ± 5	ND	ND

* Data from[163].
† Data from[159]. Remaining data from[164].
CFCs, colony-forming cells; GF, constitutively produced Steel factor, interleukin-3, and granulocyte colony-stimulating factor by the stromal feeder layer; GM/E/GEMM, granulocyte-macrophage/erythroid/granulocyte, erythroid, megakaryocyte, and macrophage; LTC-IC, long-term culture–initiating cell; ND, not done.

the ontogenic origin of the LTC-IC being assessed. Both total CFC output and the proportion of these cells that are erythropoietic are highest for fetal liver LTC-ICs, intermediate for cord blood LTC-ICs, and equivalently low for the LTC-ICs present in adult marrow or mobilized peripheral blood (Table 3-4).

It is still not clear what the factors are that stimulate the production of CFCs from LTC-ICs in the LTC system. A role of extracellular matrix has been demonstrated,[172] and undefined soluble factors,[173] as well as a delta-like notch ligand, have been implicated.[174] Several known factors, including interleukin-3 (IL-3), Steel factor (also known as kit ligand and stem-cell factor), and FLT-3 ligand, have each been shown to have the potential to mitogenically activate LTC-ICs.[175]

However, thus far, none of these growth factors are known to be essential to the mechanism by which "supportive" fibroblasts stimulate LTC-IC proliferation and differentiation.[176] On the other hand, systematic analysis of the effects of these and other growth factors on human populations that are highly enriched in LTC-IC content has shown that such defined growth factors alone can stimulate CD34+ CD38− cells to proliferate in vitro and generate daughter LTC-ICs (and CRUs).[83, 141, 177] However, whether the LTC-ICs and CRUs produced are actually derived from cells initially detectable as LTC-ICs (or CRUs) or are a closely related but distinct or partially overlapping subset has not yet been formally established.

It has also been possible to modify the LTC-IC assay to allow the detection in vitro of a subset of adult and fetal human LTC-ICs that have multiple lymphoid (B, T and NK cell) and myeloid differentiation potential.[161, 178-181] Initially, these cells were adapted from murine LTC-IC "switch" cultures in which the lymphopoietic activity of hydrocortisone-resistant cells produced during the first 4 weeks in culture was elicited by changing the culture conditions to those permissive to B lymphopoiesis.[182] With the subsequent identification of cytokines that enhance the proliferation of human lymphoid progenitors and the use of progenitor-enriched cell populations to initiate the cultures, obtaining a larger output of lymphoid cells has become easier and more efficient.

Many aspects of the assays for the various lineage-restricted CFCs, as well as for CFU-GEMMs and LTC-ICs,

TABLE 3–3. Frequencies and Properties of LTC-ICs$_{5\ Weeks}$ in Normal Adult Human Blood and Bone Marrow

Property	Blood	Bone Marrow
Total no. (assuming BM = 10^{12} cells)	15,000	20×10^6
Frequency	3000/L	1/50,000 cells
Low FLS (size)	94%	74%
CD34++	100%	100%
HLA-DR−	100%	54%
Rh−	88%	93%
4HC resistant	73%	60%

BM, bone marrow; FLS, forward light scatter; 4HC, 4 hydroperoxycyclophosphamide; LTC-ICs, long-term culture–initiating cells; Rh−, low retention of rhodamine 123.
Data summarized from 152, 157, 159.

TABLE 3–5. Progenitor Content of Normal Adult Human Blood and Marrow

Progenitor	Blood Number × 10³/L	Marrow Number per 10⁵ Cells
CFU-E	9 (1–100)	240 (4–120)
BFU-E	340 (93–1300)	97 (27–350)
CFU-GM	98 (28–340)	95 (48–190)
CFU-GEMM	19 (4–95)	4 (0.8–16)
LTC-IC$_{5 \text{ weeks}}$	0.4 (0.1–9)	0.4 (0.02–6.5)

Values shown are means ± 2 SD (95% confidence interval) of data from colony-forming cell (CFC) assays for 30 blood and 50 marrow samples from normal individuals. Data for long-term culture–initiating cells (LTC-ICs) are from a smaller subset of these samples.[454] CFC assays were performed in methylcellulose assays containing 50 ng/mL Steel factor; 20 ng/mL each of interleukin-3 (IL-3), IL-6, granulocyte-macrophage colony-stimulating factor (GM-CSF), and G-CSF; and 3 U/mL erythropoietin. LTC-IC data were measured by using the original 5-week protocol and then dividing by 7 to estimate the number of 6-week LTC-ICs expected to be present based on previous comparisons.[454]

BFU-E, burst-forming unit—erythroid; CFU-E/GM/GEMM, colony-forming unit—erythroid/granulocyte-macrophage/granulocyte, erythroid, megakaryocyte, and macrophage.

have now been analyzed and procedures for the detection of these progenitors standardized sufficiently to allow their application to the assessment of progenitor changes in patients with disease. Baseline values for the normal blood and marrow content of each of these cell types determined by using culture conditions that optimize their detection are shown in Table 3-5. These values form a useful reference for comparing data obtained from patients whose hematopoiesis is abnormal or from experiments with normal cells that have been variously manipulated. However, as discussed earlier, it is important to remember that assumptions inherent in relating the proliferative potential exhibited by a normal progenitor to its differentiated state (number of divisions separating it from its mature progeny) may not necessarily apply. Accordingly, appropriate caution needs to be exercised when interpreting such data.

Phenotypic Changes during Early Stages of Hematopoiesis

Although developmentally based (functional) assays have proved to be both quantitative and powerful in their ability to detect and discriminate different rare subpopulations of hematopoietic progenitor cells, such assays have two major drawbacks related to their retrospective nature. The first is that they take a long time (1 or more weeks) to be completed. In fact, the predictive value of having the progenitor data sought is, for many clinical applications, no longer useful by the time that it is available, precisely because the kinetics of mature blood cell production in vitro and in vivo is similar. A second drawback of functional assays for primitive hematopoietic cells relates to the fact that developmental assays require the cells being detected to proliferate and differentiate. As a result, the original cells are, of course, no longer present for further analysis or manipulation at the end of the procedure used to determine their initial presence.

More direct methods that allow discrete subpopulations of primitive hematopoietic cells to be identified and isolated without disturbing their viability or functional potentialities are therefore highly desirable. Bulk immunomagnetic and rosetting procedures, as well as multiparameter fluorescence-activated cell sorting (FACS), now allow highly purified populations of functionally similar cells to be obtained on a routine basis by using commercially available standardized antibodies and other fluorescent compounds taken up differentially by different types of hematopoietic cells. One cell surface antigen commonly used to discriminate primitive and mature hematopoietic cells is the sialomucin known as CD34.[183] CD34 is a ligand for L-selectin, a cell adhesion molecule involved in leukocyte–endothelial cell interactions.[184] In general, the extent of CD34 expression on human hematopoietic cells progressively decreases as the cells differentiate.[183] As a result, detectable differences can be seen between the average level of expression of CD34 on LTC-ICs and CFCs, and these differences are sufficient to allow their separation.[152] Not surprisingly, many other examples of heterogeneity among CD34$^+$ hematopoietic cells have also been defined, consistent with the extensively hierarchic nature of hematopoietic cell differentiation (see Fig. 3-1) and the initiation of commitment to specific hematopoietic lineages within the CD34$^+$ cell compartment. Thus, CD34$^+$ subpopulations that have begun to express markers associated with each of the major myeloid and lymphoid lineages have been described. This finding has been useful for obtaining selected subpopulations of CD34$^+$ hematopoietic cells believed to have started differentiating along particular blood cell pathways.[113, 117, 125, 185-188] Conversely, the CD34$^+$ precursors of these later types of CD34$^+$ cells are characterized by a lack of expression of these lineage-associated markers.[125, 161] The latter cells have also been uniquely characterized by their expression of Thy-1[161, 189] and AC133[88, 99] and lack of expression of CD38.[83, 178, 190, 191]

Recently, another property of very primitive hematopoietic cells has been identified and found to be useful for their selective purification. This characteristic is their verapamil-sensitive ability to efflux certain fluorescent dyes. Initial studies were undertaken with rhodamine 123 (Rh-123). These studies showed that murine repopulating cells and LTC-ICs could be largely separated from CFU-S and CFCs by their differential staining with Rh-123, the former being Rh-123 dull whereas many CFU-S and most CFCs are Rh-123 bright.[53, 151, 192, 193] Subsequent studies confirmed these differences for human cells[194] and showed that at least in mice, this property is largely regulated by expression of the ABC (ATP-binding cassette) transporter mdr-1a/1b.[195] Primitive hematopoietic cells also show a greater capacity to efflux Hoechst 33342. This property was originally attributed to their predominantly quiescent status.[196] However, it was later shown that this latter characteristic can be used to identify a rare subset of cells independent of their cell cycle status.[197] The cells thus identified are referred to as SP (side population) cells based on the unique FACS profile that they exhibit. SP cells containing primitive hematopoietic cells have subsequently been found in multiple species, including humans.[91, 198, 199] Interestingly, this phenotype appears to be controlled by an ABC transporter different from mdr1a/1b.[200]

Two observations suggest that the SP/Rh-123 dull phenotype (i.e., high transporter expression) may be functionally important to the preservation of stem-cell activity. The first is the finding that primitive cells from other tissues also have this phenotype.[201, 202] Importantly, these cells include those capable of generating hematopoietic as well as nonhematopoietic progeny.[201, 203] The second is that overexpression of P-glycoprotein (human MDR1) in murine stem cells can enhance their self-renewal and lead to a myeloproliferative syndrome in vivo.[204, 205]

An example of both the power and limitations of the direct immunophenotyping approach to primitive hematopoietic cell subclassification is illustrated in Figure 3–4. This figure shows how the combined use of several antibodies can allow different subpopulations of CD34$^+$ cells to be discriminated. One of these subpopulations contains most of the LTC-ICs.[164] Another defines a subset of granulocyte-macrophage precursors that can be largely separated from primitive erythroid progenitors, although such precursors are not confined to this subset. It can also be seen that developmentally indistinguishable erythroid progenitors can appear phenotypically heterogeneous with respect to one of the parameters used in this analysis (i.e., expression of CD71, the receptor for transferrin). Given the redundancy in the types of hematopoietic growth factors that may substitute for one another in supporting various stages of hematopoietic cell differentiation, it is possible that considerable additional heterogeneity will be encountered in the order or rate of many phenotypic changes that appear to characterize hematopoiesis in a normal adult. Such a possibility does not negate the theoretic potential of eventually using direct phenotype analysis to monitor primitive hematopoietic subpopulations, but it does highlight the need for continuing comparisons between phenotype and functional readouts. Indeed, numerous examples of a disassociation in the regulation of surface marker expression of primitive hematopoietic cell developmental status have been described for both murine[73, 75, 93, 96] and human cells.[206–208] In some cases, these changes appear to be related to cell activation,[93, 207] which, however, may be variably related to cell cycle progression, as indicated by other gene expression studies.[209]

Ontogeny of Hematopoiesis

Recognizable hematopoietic cells have been detected in the extraembryonic human yolk sac mesoderm as early as the 19th day of gestation, a time when the circulatory system is not yet complete.[210–213] Based on studies of both avian[214, 215] and murine cells,[216–221] it seems likely that the first hematopoietic cells to appear arise locally from more primitive precursors of both endothelial cells and hematopoietic cells. For many years, mammalian hematopoiesis was thought to originate in the yolk sac blood islands. However, it is now clear that the intraembryonic mesoderm in the para-aortic splanchnopleural region is also an important and independent coincident site of hematopoietic cell development in the embryo before the ap-

pearance of hematopoietic cells in the liver, both in mice[222–224] and in humans.[225]

The first mature human blood cells to appear both in the embryo and in the yolk sac include some myeloid and erythroid cells.[212] The erythroid cells are primarily of the primitive type, and they produce embryonic hemoglobin and remain nucleated.[226] The first phase of extraembryonic hematopoiesis is rapidly succeeded during the fifth to sixth week of gestation by a second phase characterized in part by a switch to the definitive erythroid differentiation program in which the red cells produce fetal rather than embryonic hemoglobin and extrude their nuclei.[227] The production of mature cells belonging to other myeloid lineages also becomes apparent at this time, and the major site of hematopoiesis shifts from the yolk sac to the fetal liver. Hematopoietic activity appears in the bone marrow by the 10th to 11th week, coincident with the onset of production of hemoglobin A, the adult form of hemoglobin.[130, 228] After 34 to 36 weeks of gestation, fetal hemoglobin production decreases along with a rapid rise in the number of erythroblasts synthesizing adult hemoglobin.[229] A small proportion of red blood cells containing fetal hemoglobin (F cells) continues to be produced in adults,[230] although this proportion is not fixed and may be increased in vivo under conditions of increased hematopoietic demand or in certain disease states.[231–234] Increased fetal hemoglobin production is also seen in vitro in conditions that stimulate erythropoiesis, particularly from more primitive cells.[235] These findings suggest some role of exogenous hematopoietic growth factor regulation in the control of this latter developmental program. Other cellular changes also accompany these developmentally related switches, at least some of which appear to be similarly initiated at the precursor cell level.[236]

Colony assay procedures developed for quantitating adult progenitors detect analogous cell types in the fetus.[162, 163, 213, 237, 238] This finding implies a similar hierarchic organization of lineage-restricted and pluripotent fetal progenitors that differentiate at approximately similar rates with each successive cell cycle. On the other hand, differences in the self-renewal potential (probability) of very primitive hematopoietic cell subpopulations in the fetus and adult have been suggested,[239, 240] and evidence of intermediate potentialities of cord blood progenitors support this concept.[103, 239, 241] Fetal cells also have reduced cell cycle times[177, 242–244] and hence generate larger colonies more quickly than their adult counterparts do. Interestingly, preliminary comparisons of the expression patterns of certain genes in CD34$^+$ CD38$^-$ cells from fetal versus adult sources also indicate that primitive fetal cells show signs of "activation" relative to their adult counterparts.[209]

REGULATION OF NORMAL MYELOPOIESIS

General Principles

The regulated production of mature cells to meet changing physiologic needs is a general feature of tissues characterized by continual cell turnover. For tissues in which acquisition of the specialized functions of the mature cell takes several cell cycles to complete, mechanisms must be in place to achieve an appropriate balance at the single-cell level between differentiation, proliferation, and maintenance of cell viability. Current evidence from studies of hematopoietic cells suggests that these responses may not necessarily be coordinately regulated[245-249] or that they require activation by the same growth factors,[31] inhibitors,[250, 251] or signal-transducing intermediates.[252, 253] An extreme example is provided by the demonstration that hematopoietic cell differentiation can proceed to completion from a stage before lineage commitment even in the complete absence of cell division.[254] Conversely, lineage switching or alterations in differentiation or viability can occur without specifically interfering with proliferation.[245, 246, 253, 255-258] Accordingly, it has been operationally useful to consider "self-renewal" at the single progenitor cell level as proliferation without further differentiation. How this property may relate to the mechanisms that maintain the most primitive cells in an undifferentiated state with all lineage options open is, however, not yet clear. Certainly, division without a change in differentiation status does appear to be an option that is compatible with continued viability in primitive normal hematopoietic cells, although this situation may not be the case for their progeny once they have reached the terminal stages of maturation. However, exactly if, when, or how such changes occur awaits delineation. Obviously, death of early-stage progenitors can have a potentially profound effect on subsequent cell output because of the large cell output potential of early hematopoietic cells even after their commitment to a specific lineage. Conversely, loss of cells by death at late stages of hematopoietic cell differentiation may have less potential impact but may nevertheless be a more physiologically significant mechanism for fine-tuning the final output of mature cells. Control of the rate of entry of cells into and out of a quiescent (G_0) state will have a potentially equivalent differential impact depending on the proliferative capacity of the progenitor cell. The permutations and combinations afforded by the differential operation of these three responses of hematopoietic cells at different stages thus provide an overall mechanism that embodies both the regenerative power and the flexibility for fine-tuning mature cell output that are hallmarks of the regulatory capacity of the hematopoietic system.

Table 3–2 lists a large array of cytokines that are believed to play important roles as intercellular molecular mediators of this regulation. These cytokines are often grouped roughly according to the responses that they elicit as those that either stimulate or inhibit proliferation (and differentiation) and those that either support cell viability or induce apoptosis (cell death). It is now recognized that the kind of response obtained may vary with the particular cell type being considered or the other factors to which the cell is being exposed. For example, the same factor may have either a stimulatory or an inhibitory effect on different progenitor targets, or the same target cell response may be stimulated by different cytokines.[251, 259, 260] Other cytokine classifications emphasize the degree and type of selectivity of a given factor for specific lineages or cells at early as opposed to later

stages of hematopoietic cell differentiation.[31, 261] Recently, new insights have emerged in this regard from the recognition of certain homologies in the chain composition, structure, and submolecular motifs characteristic of the receptors for groups of cytokines that are active on hematopoietic cells. In particular, these receptor similarities have helped explain some of the redundant or overlapping factor activities that have been described.[262-264] For a more detailed description of the signaling pathways used by these activated receptors, the reader is referred to other excellent reviews of this rapidly and continuously expanding field.[24, 265-267]

Control Mechanisms

Local versus Hormonal Mechanisms

Regulation of hematopoiesis is believed to involve a variety of extrinsic modulators. Some of these modulators are produced and act in a primarily local fashion within the bone marrow. Others (such as erythropoietin) are produced outside as well as within the bone marrow and operate as systemic hormones. An extreme example of the restricted type is provided by Steel factor, which is produced by fibroblasts in the bone marrow primarily in an obligate membrane-bound form,[268, 269] although a substantial level of soluble Steel factor (approximately 3 mg/L) is also normally found in blood.[270] Other factors, such as GM-CSF, are secreted exclusively as soluble molecules by a variety of cells within the hematopoietic system but are rarely found at detectable levels in serum. At least some of these factors, of which GM-CSF is a good example, can bind in a stable and reversible fashion to specific components of the extracellular matrix, in this case, to heparan sulfate.[271, 272] Other factors with potent effects on hematopoietic cells, such as M-CSF[273] and FLK-2/FLT-3 ligand,[274] appear to be made both as fixed components of the membrane of producer cells and as soluble factors.

A number of these cytokines are known to be produced by fibroblasts and endothelial cells, as well as macrophages and lymphocytes, all of which help form the unique, but locally heterogeneous microenvironment of the bone marrow. Moreover, in many instances, production of a cytokine is, in itself, a regulated activity of the producer cell, which provides an additional mechanism of local feedback control. In this way, the contributions of many cytokines to the regulation of hematopoiesis normally may involve only the transient and localized attainment of biologically effective concentrations in scattered regions throughout the bone marrow. Nevertheless, examples in which some of these factors can rise to significant concentrations in blood also exist, for example, after bone marrow transplantation.[275, 276] In addition, enhancement of hematopoiesis in response to the systemic administration of pharmacologic doses of hematopoietic growth factors is well documented.[277] Therefore, it is clear that most of these cytokines can act as hormones, although during normal adult life, homeostatic control of hematopoiesis appears for the most part to be achieved by the production of growth factors (and inhibitors) at levels that have negligible systemic consequences. Interestingly, this concept is one for which considerable experimental support was obtained long before the nature and diversity of the hematopoietic regulators now defined had begun to be dissected.[278, 279]

Over the last several years, the marrow-derived adherent layer of the LTC system has emerged as a useful in vitro model of the bone marrow microenvironment and, as such, has afforded a unique system for analyzing the nature and complexity of the multiple and interacting mechanisms that may actually regulate the turnover and survival of early as well as later stages of hematopoietic progenitors in vivo. The LTC adherent layer contains stromal fibroblasts, endothelial cells, and adipocytes, as well as many macrophages,[280-282] the same cell types that are thought to constitute the essential supportive and regulatory elements of the bone marrow.[283] In the adherent layer of the LTC system, these cells produce a variety of growth factors and inhibitors, some under constitutive control and others in response to a variety of manipulations of the culture medium.[284, 285] In the presence of these adherent cells, primitive hematopoietic progenitors and their differentiation into granulocytes and macrophages may be sustained for several months; in their absence, hematopoiesis eventually declines.[160]

Manipulations of the LTC medium that cause the levels of cytokines known to stimulate primitive hematopoietic cells to be increased (or that inhibit the growth of such cells) lead to predicted changes in the cycling activity of such cells when they are also contained within the adherent layer.[148, 284, 285] The ability of the LTC system to maintain very primitive hematopoietic cells as a viable but quiescent population has thus made it possible to experimentally determine whether a given cytokine can promote or block the cell cycle progression of primitive normal hematopoietic cells into S phase and, in some instances, whether it is an endogenous player in the system.[285-287]

Such studies have provided support for a minimal model of primitive hematopoietic cell regulation in vivo, specifically, one characterized by the production of various growth factors (such as Steel factor, G-CSF, GM-CSF, and IL-6) and inhibitors (such as transforming growth factor-β [TGF-β] and certain chemokines) at concentrations that on their own would rarely be effective but that in combination could elicit a significant alteration in progenitor response (either to exit from or remain in G_0). Such a model is of particular relevance to understanding how leukemic cells may acquire a sufficient proliferative advantage to explain their abnormal growth and yet remain apparently growth factor dependent. In an environment in which the effective level of progenitor stimulation is normally minimal, even slight increases in sensitivity to a growth factor or a slightly heightened response to its effects (or the converse for an inhibitor) might be enough for a cell with such a phenotype to outgrow its normal counterparts.

Although very little is yet understood about the intrinsic pathways that determine whether a hematopoietic stem cell will differentiate (further) or maintain its current status, a number of pieces of the puzzle are being identified. One important gene family that appears to be involved are the *HOX* genes. Stem-cell differentiation is accompanied by the downregulated expression of certain *HOX* genes,[126] and their expression can lead to a profound and selective expansion of the hematopoietic stem-cell compartment.[288, 289] Interestingly, related *HOX* genes and *HOX* cofactor genes are commonly involved in human leukemia,[4, 290, 291] and their overexpression can cause leukemic transformation in murine hematopoietic cell targets.[4] Other factors that appear to block stem-cell differentiation include the retinoic acid receptor agonist[292] (all-*trans*-retinoic acid) and certain notch ligands, including Jagged-1, Jagged-2, Delta-1, and Delta-like-1,[174, 293, 294] perhaps through accelerating the rate of passage through G_1.[295]

Cytokine Action

Most of our present understanding of the intracellular responses of hematopoietic progenitor cells to specific cytokines has been extrapolated from studies of immortalized factor–dependent (or factor-responsive) hematopoietic cell lines. Such studies have allowed a considerable body of information to be amassed that delineates a pattern of intracellular events that follow the binding of various growth factors (or inhibitors) to their specific cell surface receptors. A common early event is the dimerization of ligand-receptor complexes and the subsequent phosphorylation of tyrosine residues in the intracellular (cytoplasmic) portion of the signal-transducing chain of the receptor complex.[24, 264] For some receptors, this latter step is achieved by activation of the intrinsic tyrosine kinase activity of the receptor itself (e.g., as in the case of c-FMS and c-KIT—the receptors for M-CSF and Steel factor, respectively). For others, an associated cytoplasmic kinase (often a JAK kinase) is responsible.[24, 264, 266] The tyrosines phosphorylated by these activated kinases then serve as specific attachment sites for a variety of signal-transducing intermediates or linker molecules, or both. Eventually, the cascade of reactions thus triggered culminates in the initiation of DNA synthesis, the activation of a differentiative response, or the blocking of an apoptotic response. Apoptosis is a mechanism of cell death resulting from the rapid intracellular cleavage of nuclear DNA at internucleosomal sites by intrinsically activated DNases. This cleavage results in a characteristic laddered fragmentation pattern on gel electrophoresis of the isolated DNA.[296, 297]

Although it is recognized that the use of cell lines for delineating signal transduction pathways has inherent limitations, many of the intermediates involved have been found to be highly conserved over large evolutionary distances and to play a role in effecting a wide variety of cellular responses.[298] As yet, very little progress has been made in sorting out the particular molecular mechanisms that mediate the differential control of hematopoietic progenitor cell proliferation, differentiation, and retention of viability. However, the fact that these processes may involve the activation of separate signaling mechanisms by discrete regions of the same receptor[252, 263] provides an interesting starting point for further investigations.

As the molecular players in each of the pathways that mediate and regulate these different cellular responses are characterized and the corresponding genes cloned, their potential to serve as oncogenes is also emerging as a consistent theme. Examples of naturally arising oncogenes relevant to every level of the signaling networks that together regulate cell output have now been identified. For a more detailed analysis of these oncogenes, the reader is referred to Chapter 5.

Stem-Cell Homing and Mobilization

In vivo, hematopoiesis normally occurs in specific tissues, although the results of animal parabiosis[299] and partial-body irradiation experiments,[300, 301] as well as clinical experience with human bone marrow and mobilized peripheral blood transplants, provide clear evidence of the ability of primitive hematopoietic cells to enter and exit the circulation. The fact that murine CRU purities of greater than 1 in 10 can be achieved[57, 73, 74] indicates that for small numbers of CRUs in the circulation of lethally irradiated mice, at least 10% can home to a site where they will contribute to the regeneration of hematopoiesis in a substantial and sustained fashion. Direct measurements of murine LTC-IC and CFC homing efficiencies within 24 hours of intravenous injection have yielded values of approximately 20%.[302] These high seeding efficiencies support the concept that hematopoietic stem cells, like lymphocytes and granulocytes, express particular cell surface molecules that facilitate their exit from the circulation into the bone marrow. Conversely, these molecules may also play a role in facilitating the exit into the circulation of primitive hematopoietic cells resident in the extravascular space of the bone marrow.

Interestingly, analogous studies with human cells transplanted into sublethally irradiated NOD/SCID mice have shown that human LTC-ICs and CRUs home into the marrow of these xenogeneic hosts almost as efficiently (~5% to 10%).[82, 303] Although the molecular mechanisms regulating these processes are not well understood, several of the surface glycoproteins known to play a role in the adhesive interactions of lymphocytes and granulocytes with other cells have been demonstrated to also be present on primitive hematopoietic cells. These glycoproteins include ICAM-1(intercellular adhesion molecule-1)[304] CD44,[305, 306] VLA-4 (very late activation antigen-4),[307] VLA-5,[308] and CXCR4 (CXC chemokine receptor 4).[309] Evidence now also exists that some of these adhesion molecules can play a role in regulating hematopoietic stem-cell trafficking.[310-314]

A variety of toxic treatments that perturb hematopoiesis also stimulate the release of primitive hematopoietic cells into the peripheral blood, where they reach levels that are many times higher than normal.[315-320] A number of the growth factors that can act directly on primitive hematopoietic cells in vitro to stimulate their proliferation also cause (or enhance) the mobilization of these cells into the circulation after their injection in vivo.[84, 86, 166, 317, 321-323] Although the exact mechanism of this in vivo response is not known, it has been widely assumed that critical changes in the expression of key surface molecules on primitive hematopoietic cells are involved.[324-326] This concept is supported by the demonstration that injection of antibodies to the α_4 β_1 (VLA-4), but not the

β_2 integrins, are effective in mobilizing primitive hematopoietic cells into the circulation.[310, 311, 314]

In spite of the paucity of information about mechanisms that underlie either the homing or the release of primitive hematopoietic cells into and out of the marrow, it seems likely that both are commonly affected in certain types of leukemia. A feature of many leukemias is the presence of a large number of neoplastic progenitor cells in the circulation[327, 328] and the establishment of extramedullary sites of disease. Such mobilization occurs even in chronic leukemias such as chronic myelocytic leukemia (CML), in which in the chronic phase the neoplastic progenitors show few other alterations in their behavior. Interestingly, the latter have been shown to produce autocrine IL-3 and G-CSF,[329] which might be speculated to contribute to their mobilization. The ability to collect primitive normal hematopoietic cells that have been mobilized into the blood after chemotherapy for leukemia has made possible the use of these cells to ensure hematologic recovery after further treatments with myeloablative regimens.[330-332]

Turnover and Aging of Primitive Hematopoietic Cells

The results of studies of murine hematopoiesis indicate that the full hierarchy of progenitors shown in Figure 3–1 is maintained throughout adult life. Similar findings with human cells indicate that such maintenance of progenitor cells is also true for people. Analysis of telomere length in hematopoietic cells from healthy normal individuals suggests that the hematopoietic stem-cell population is nevertheless in a constant, albeit slow, state of turnover,[333, 334] unless perturbed.[335-337] In addition, the turnover of primitive hematopoietic cells during fetal life is much higher than in adult life.[64, 334] Hematopoiesis in older individuals has been reported to become oligoclonal,[41, 42] and this trend can be accelerated by exposure to anticancer chemotherapeutic regimens.[42, 338] However, whether this oligoclonality simply represents the random ascendancy of a single normal clone over time or the selective expansion of a minimally altered, preneoplastic population in either case is not yet clear.

Stem-Cell Plasticity

Several observations in the last few years have challenged the classic teachings of the sequential and irreversible changes in gene programming that constitute the developmental processes of tissue genesis during the formation of the embryo. These observations include the ability of cloned neural precursors to give rise to mature blood cells after their transplantation into myeloablated mice[339] and, more recently, to give rise to many other tissues after injection into blastocysts.[340] Conversely, cells isolated from marrow have been demonstrated to have neurogenic potential[341, 342] in addition to their ability to generate endothelial cells,[343] muscle cells,[201, 344] chrondroblasts, osteoblasts and adipocytes,[345, 346] and hepatocytes.[347] Evidence that the liver[348] and skeletal muscle[201, 203] are also both reservoirs of cells with pluripotent hematopoietic stem-cell potential has also recently been reported. Although formal evidence of adult cells with multiple tissue potentialities has been provided in only a few examples, these observations have clearly introduced the concept of persisting multipotent stem cells in multiple adult tissues and the possibility that these cells may be more "plastic" in their differentiation potential than previously thought.

Dysregulated Hematopoiesis

Dysregulation of hematopoiesis at the cellular level can be viewed in simplistic terms as the manifestation of alterations in the control of the three types of responses considered earlier: proliferation, differentiation, and viability. All three are well-known hallmarks of leukemia and account for the clonal expansion and production of nonfunctional blasts that characterize the most malignant forms of acute myeloid leukemia. With the development and refinement of quantitative methods to investigate most stages of normal hematopoietic cell development has come an increasing knowledge of the spectrum of factors to which these cells are responsive, as well as some understanding of the nature of those responses and the signaling intermediates that are involved in their activation. However, all these studies depend on the use of assays in which the initial progenitors are detected by virtue of their ability to complete normal differentiation programs. When these programs are themselves disrupted significantly, as occurs to varying degrees in different types of leukemia, the applicability of assays developed for normal cells becomes reduced or meaningless, and mechanisms of altered proliferation control are more difficult to analyze.

Therefore, it is not surprising that the best characterized examples of hematopoietic dysregulation that are intrinsically determined are those in which accompanying alterations in the differentiation process are minimal, a situation that characterizes the myeloproliferative disorders polycythemia vera, essential thrombocytosis, and CML. All three of these disorders represent clonal expansions of a neoplastic stem cell but are presumed to arise as a result of the activity of different gene mutations. The consequence of these mutations is to confer a general lineage-wide proliferative advantage to the early progenitors derived from the initially altered stem cell (see Chapter 2) and, at the same time, to selectively deregulate the output of a particular lineage of mature blood cells in a disease-specific (and hence presumably gene-specific) fashion.

Thus far, abnormalities in the dependence of committed progenitors that are normally responsive to erythropoietin,[349, 350] IL-3, GM-CSF,[351] and insulin-like growth factor[352] have been described as a common feature of the neoplastic cells from patients with polycythemia vera. Erythroid cells able to terminally differentiate in the absence of erythropoietin have also been documented to be common in patients with CML[353] and essential thrombocytosis.[354] How these abnormalities are explained at the level of alterations in the normal mechanisms of signaling by these growth factors is, however, still a mystery—even in the case of CML, in which both the

transforming genetic event and numerous details about the properties of the *BCR-ABL* oncogene product have already been identified.[355-359]

Another type of regulatory defect characteristic of primitive neoplastic progenitors from CML patients has been revealed from measurements of their cycling behavior in LTC. These measurements have demonstrated a failure of primitive CML clonogenic progenitors to respond to the inhibitory effect of both MIP-1α and MCP-1, chemokines that can block the growth factor–stimulated entry into S phase of primitive normal hematopoietic progenitors.[286, 287] This insensitivity to MIP-1 and MCP-1 is observed in spite of the normal responsiveness of the same types of primitive CML cells to TGF-β,[360] another selective inhibitor of primitive normal hematopoietic progenitor cycling.[251, 284] Recently, activation of an autocrine IL-3– and G-CSF–mediated mechanism of autonomous growth in CD34+ CML cells has also been demonstrated.[329]

In the more acute forms of myeloid leukemia, similar analyses of altered factor control of particular types of progenitors had to await the development and validation of suitable assays for primitive leukemic progenitor subpopulations.[328, 361] These assays allowed the demonstration of abnormal autocrine or paracrine mechanisms of growth stimulation of the leukemic blasts from many of these patients that may contribute to their uncontrolled amplification.[362, 363] Examples of abnormalities in the control of hematopoiesis resulting from alterations in the mechanism or mechanisms that regulate cell viability have also been documented.[364]

CLINICAL USES OF HEMATOPOIETIC CELLS

Marrow Rescue and Reconstitution

One of the major changes that has occurred in the treatment of malignancies in general and the hematologic malignancies in particular during the previous two decades has been the wider use of increasingly intensive chemotherapy regimens. Such regimens are sufficiently toxic to the hematopoietic system and the stem-cell population in particular to be life threatening. The rationale for such dose intensification is based on three assumptions. The first is that experimental data demonstrating a log linear relationship in tumor cell survival after exposure to increasing concentrations of drug are relevant to the response of malignant stem-cell populations in cancer patients. The second is that the toxic side effects of such treatments on the hematopoietic system can be overcome by transplanting back untreated normal stem cells obtained previously either from normal histocompatible (allogeneic) donors or from the patients themselves (autologous donors). The third is that a useful therapeutic advantage can be gained by increasing the dose of a drug or drugs without incurring unacceptable toxicity to other nonhematopoietic tissues or organ systems.

Initially, bone marrow was the primary source of cells used to rescue the hematopoietic system in patients being given myeloablative therapy. Approximately a liter of marrow containing a few times 10^{10} nucleated cells can routinely be aspirated from anesthetized adult donors, and such a harvest will typically contain sufficient precursors to rapidly reconstitute and sustain hematopoiesis after their intravenous infusion into individuals treated with what would otherwise be a lethal dose of chemotherapy (or radiotherapy, or both). More recently, it has been found that an effective allograft can be obtained by leukapheresis of normal individuals whose primitive cells have been mobilized to leave the marrow and enter the blood after growth factor (G-CSF) treatment.[332] Interestingly, the transplantation of peripheral blood harvests has, in most cases, been successful in providing not only durable hematopoiesis but also the initially unexpected and still biologically unexplained benefit of a usually more rapid recovery of neutrophils and platelets than is typically achievable with bone marrow transplants.

Another development in the hematopoietic stem-cell transplant field has been recognition of the clinical utility of cord blood as a source of primitive hematopoietic cells.[365-368] This recognition was prompted in part by early laboratory findings that not only is the concentration of primitive hematopoietic cells increased in cord blood (relative to that in normal adult blood), but the progenitors present may also have a greater proliferative capacity than their adult counterparts.[239, 241] In addition, careful attention to collection procedures has allowed larger volumes of cord blood to be harvested than was initially anticipated. Promising results have now been obtained in a large number of children who have received an allogeneic transplant, although hematologic recovery times have been slower than ideal and single-cord collections may be too small for effective widespread use in adults.[367, 368]

Much interest is also focused on the use of large doses of purified or enriched stem-cell populations to obtain engraftment in allogeneic hosts to overcome problems of rejection and yet minimize complications associated with graft-versus-host disease.[369, 370]

Therapeutic Applications of Ex Vivo–Manipulated Hematopoietic Cells

Purging

Leukemic progenitor cells have been found to be maintained poorly in culture in comparison to their normal counterparts.[371, 372] This poor maintenance in culture is likely to be explained, at least in part, by the fact that they need to be generated from a more primitive leukemic "stem-cell" population, which may be present at a paradoxically low concentration in the marrow, often even lower than the residual normal stem cells still present.[158, 373] However, a difference (defect) in the maintenance kinetics in vitro of certain types of leukemic stem cells (e.g., CML LTC-ICs) has also been documented,[158] and it has been possible to exploit this phenomenon to design clinical protocols to selectively remove leukemic stem cells from autologous stem cell harvests without deleteriously affecting their content of normal LTC-ICs.[374, 375]

Alternative approaches to the selective removal of leu-

kemic or other malignant cells from autografts have exploited differences in alcohol dehydrogenase levels[376] and differences observed in various antigens expressed on normal and malignant cells.[370, 377-379] Early transfusion studies with untreated white blood cell collections from CML donors,[380] inadvertent use of marrow from a donor with unrecognized acute leukemia,[381] and clinical retroviral marking studies with autotransplants[382, 383] all indicate that purging is important. However, at present, the greater problem of residual disease in the patient would outweigh the clinical significance of purging autografts in most instances.

Stem-Cell Expansion

Culture conditions have been described that readily support the generation of large numbers of committed progenitors from primitive precursors.[384-386] In general, these culture conditions followed from two technical advances. The first was the identification and cloning of specific growth factors subsequently shown to have potent growth stimulatory effects on primitive murine and human hematopoietic cells alike, particularly when present in combination. These growth factors include Steel factor, IL-6, IL-3, GM-CSF, and G-CSF.[75, 117, 268, 387-393] The second technical advance was the recognition that greater expansions could usually be achieved if the more mature cells were initially removed from the input innoculum and care was subsequently taken to ensure adequate dilution of the expanded cells and/or essential nutrients, growth factors, inhibitors, and O_2 kept above (or below) limiting concentrations.[394-397] However, the large expansions of CFCs achieved were frequently offset by absolute losses of CFCs during isolation of the primitive cell types used to initiate the cultures (e.g., LTC-ICs or CRUs) and equivalent expansions of the most primitive cell types were not obtained.

Subsequently, it became evident that the most primitive cell types require different factors for their mitogenesis and self-renewal.[31, 398-402] In addition, it was discovered that exposure to inappropriate combinations or concentrations of growth factors could efficiently stimulate the most primitive cells to divide, but without preservation of their stem-cell status. Such cell division resulted in a transient output of committed progenitors but failure to sustain stem-cell numbers. Examples of factors with such activity are IL-1, IL-3, and tumor necrosis factor.[143, 208, 403, 404] In addition, systematic analysis has revealed that the growth factor requirements for stimulating maximal expansions of analogous hematopoietic progenitor types from the precursors present in hematopoietic tissues at different stages of ontogeny are not identical.[405, 406] Nevertheless, conditions have now been defined that allow both murine and human long-term repopulating stem-cell numbers and their functional integrity to be reproducibly maintained or even slightly expanded ex vivo.[83, 399, 404, 407-410] The critical factors required to achieve this are FLT-3 ligand, Steel factor, IL-11 (or some other strategy for activating gp130), and thrombopoietin, some of which must be present in relatively high concentrations. However, it is also clear that the results obtained to date do not mimic the net expansions of long-term repopulating stem-cell numbers that can be shown to occur in mice both during ontogeny and after transplantation[103, 411, 412] This difference in stem-cell expansion suggests that additional factors or other modifications in the time and mode of their delivery remain to be discovered to improve results over those currently attainable.

Until recently, failure to demonstrate significant in vitro expansion of cells with long-term repopulating activity in rigorous quantitative assays casts doubt on whether these cells were even being stimulated to divide in the culture systems assessed. Careful dye tracking experiments that allow sequential generations of daughter cells to be reisolated and assayed in vivo for their engrafting potential have clearly eliminated this reservation.[177, 413, 414] On the other hand, more detailed studies of the properties of proliferating stem-cell populations have revealed a reversible engraftment defect that appears as these cells enter G_1 from G_0 and becomes even more pronounced as they transit $S/G_2/M$.[65, 67, 68] This deleterious effect of cell cycle transit on engraftment by the most primitive types of transplantable cells is much less pronounced in proliferating populations of later hematopoietic cells with short-lived engrafting activity.[70, 71, 415]

How and whether in vitro–expanded cells may be of use for various clinical applications are still under investigation and even under debate. The controversy arises from observations that highly purified populations of murine stem cells with long-term repopulating activity can give as rapid count recoveries in transplanted, myeloablated recipients as an equivalent volume of the unseparated marrow cells from which they were isolated.[416, 417] However, it is also clear that when sufficiently expanded numbers of murine cells with short-term repopulating activity are transplanted, white blood cell count recoveries can be accelerated.[418] Similar studies are under way with clinical transplants,[419] but definitive answers must await results from either allotransplanted cells (e.g., ex vivo–expanded cord blood cells[420, 421]) or retrovirally marked autologous cells.

Gene Transfer and Gene Therapy

Technologies developed almost two decades ago to enable the transfer of isolated genes into somatic cell targets are now being evaluated in a variety of clinical settings. The ease of transplanting hematopoietic stem cells, the durability of their engraftment, and the large experience worldwide with autografting procedures has focused particular interest on the clinical use of genetically modified hematopoietic stem cells. Early studies demonstrated the ability of retroviral vectors to efficiently transfer genes into primary hematopoietic cells, initially of murine[422] and subsequently of human[423-425] and nonhuman primate[426] origin. The creation of safe packaging cell lines to allow the reproducible production of the desired vector or vectors in the absence of helper virus (to prevent reinfection) was a significant step toward initiation of the first clinical gene transfer trials using retrovirally transduced hematopoietic cell transplants. Initial protocols sought to examine the durability of engraftment by ex vivo–manipulated cells and to determine whether autolo-

gous harvests used for hematologic rescue also contain malignant stem cells that later contribute to relapse.

The first such studies established the feasibility of this approach and were able to demonstrate the presence of both normal and malignant cells derived from the transduced cells transplanted many months previously.[382, 383, 427] However, subsequent attempts to reproduce these findings were plagued by much lower gene transfer efficiencies and an appreciation of the poor yield of stem cells at the end of the best transduction protocols,[428] as confirmed by follow-up studies in nonhuman primates[429, 430] and experiments in which human cells were transplanted into NOD/SCID mice.[431] This period of disappointment stimulated a systematic analysis of potential limiting parameters. Many of the earlier problems have now been overcome through an improved understanding of the unique properties of hematopoietic stem cells that are not necessarily shared by most of the CD34$^+$ cells or the more rapidly measured, but also less primitive, progenitors identified by CFC assays.

For standard retroviral vectors, optimization of gene transfer requires maximal exposure of the target cells to the vector in a receptive state just before entry of the cells into mitosis.[432, 433] Such optimization usually requires a minimum of 2 to 3 days' exposure to induce the stem cells into cycle and at the same time upregulate expression of the specific viral receptor.[434-437] Equally important is the use of strategies for increasing the probability of virus–target cell encounters once the cells are primed, for example, by colocalization of the cells and virus on fibronectin or its CH-296 fragment[438, 439] or simply on an inert but positively charged surface (such as a tissue culture dish[440]) in the presence of an anion (such as protamine sulfate, which is less toxic to very primitive hematopoietic cells than polybrene is[441]). Under such conditions, more than 10% of the transplantable stem cells from various human hematopoietic tissues are found to be reproducibly transduced when immunodeficient mice are used as hosts for their detection.[435, 442-446] The first indications that these improvements in gene transfer can be translated into larger-scale clinical protocols are also now beginning to emerge.[447-449]

Nevertheless, many challenges still lie ahead. The absolute yield of transduced human stem cells remains poor and would be greatly facilitated by better methods to expand stem-cell populations with full retention of the original engrafting properties of G_0 stem cells. Alternatively, it may be possible to circumvent these problems by using pseudotyped retroviral vectors whose entry into cells is not receptor limited[450, 451] or by using lentiviral vectors whose entry into the nucleus does not require passage of the target cell through mitosis.[452, 453] Other issues of sustained and controlled expression of the transduced gene will also need to be addressed. Finally, safe and effective strategies to achieve the selective expansion of transduced stem cells transplanted into patients who are not myeloablated will need to be developed to allow the application of stem-cell-based gene therapies to patients with gene disorders that are not themselves life threatening. Given the speed with which our understanding of hematopoietic stem cell regulation is increasing, we can expect that major progress in these exciting new areas should occur rapidly over the next decade.

Acknowledgment

The author thanks Amy Ahamed for excellent secretarial assistance in the preparation of this chapter and the National Cancer Institute of Canada (NCIC) and the NHLBI (NIH-PO1 55435) for grant support.

REFERENCES

1. Killmann SA, Cronkite EP, Fliedner TM, et al: Mitotic indices of human bone marrow cells. I. Number and cytologic distribution of mitoses. Blood 1962;19:743.
2. Killmann SA, Cronkite EP, Fliedner TM, et al: Mitotic indices of human bone marrow cells. III. Duration of some phases of erythrocytic and granulocytic proliferation computed from mitotic indices. Blood 1964;24:267.
3. Warner HR, Athens JW: An analysis of granulocyte kinetics in blood and bone marrow. Ann N Y Acad Sci 1964;113:523.
4. Buske C, Humphries RK: Homeobox genes in leukemogenesis. Int J Hematol 2000;71:301.
5. Orkin SH: GATA-binding transcription factors in hematopoietic cells. Blood 1992;80:575.
6. Okuda T, van Deursen J, Hiebert SW, et al: AML1, the target of multiple chromosomal translocations in human leukemia, is essential for normal fetal liver hematopoiesis. Cell 1996;84:321.
7. Wang Q, Stacy T, Binder M, et al: Disruption of the *Cbfa2* gene causes necrosis and hemorrhaging in the central nervous system and blocks definitive hematopoiesis. Proc Natl Acad Sci U S A 1996;93:3444.
8. Porcher C, Swat W, Rockwell K, et al: The T cell leukemia oncoprotein SCL/tal-1 is essential for development of all hematopoietic lineages. Cell 1996;86:47.
9. Robb L, Elwood NJ, Elefanty AG, et al: The *scl* gene is required for the generation of all hematopoietic lineages in the adult mouse. EMBO J 1996;15:4123.
10. Olson MC, Scott EW, Hack AA, et al: PU.1 is not essential for early myeloid gene expression but is required for terminal myeloid differentiation. Immunity 1995;3:703.
11. Scott EW, Simon MC, Anastasi J, et al: Requirement of transcription factor PU.1 in the development of multiple hematopoietic lineages. Science 1994;265:1573.
12. Voso MT, Burn TC, Wulf G, et al: Inhibition of hematopoiesis by competitive binding of transcription factor PU.1. Proc Natl Acad Sci U S A 1994;91:7932.
13. Urbanek P, Wang Z-Q, Fetka I, et al: Complete block of early B cell differentiation and altered patterning of the posterior midbrain in mice lacking Pax5/BSAP. Cell 1994;79:901.
14. Georgopolous K, Bigby M, Wang JH, et al: Early arrest in lymphocyte differentiation in Ikaros mutant mice. Cell 1994;78:143.
15. Georgopoulos K, Moore DD, Derfler B: Ikaros, an early lymphoid-specific transcription factor and a putative mediator for T cell commitment. Science 1992;258:808.
16. Fujiwara Y, Browne CP, Cunniff K, et al: Arrested development of embryonic red cell precursors in mouse embryos lacking transcription factor GATA-1. Proc Natl Acad Sci U S A 1996;93:12355.
17. Pevny L, Simon MC, Robertson E, et al: Erythroid differentiation in chimaeric mice blocked by a targeted mutation in the gene for transcription factor GATA-1. Nature 1991;349:257.
18. Hendriks RW, Nawijn MC, Engel JD, et al: Expression of the transcription factor GATA-3 is required for the development of the earliest T cell progenitors and correlates with stages of cellular proliferation in the thymus. Eur J Immunol 1999;29:1912.
19. Kulessa H, Frampton J, Graf T: GATA-1 reprograms avian myelomonocytic cell lines into eosinophils, thromboblasts, and erythroblasts. Genes Dev 1995;9:1250.
20. Nerlov C, Graf T: PU.1 induces myeloid lineage commitment in multipotent hematopoietic progenitors. Genes Dev 1998;12:2403.
21. Nutt SL, Heavey B, Rolink AG, et al: Commitment to the B-lymphoid lineage depends on the transcription factor Pax5. Nature 1999;401:556.
22. Rekhtman N, Radparvar F, Evans T, et al: Direct interaction of hematopoietic transcription factors PU.1 and GATA-1: Functional antagonism in erythroid cells. Genes Dev 1999;13:1398.
23. Takahashi T, Suwabe N, Dai P, et al: Inhibitory interaction of c-Myb and GATA-1 via transcriptional co-activator CBP. Oncogene 2000;19:134.
24. Ihle JN: Signal transduction in the regulation of hematopoiesis. In Pui CH, ed: Childhood Leukemias. Cambridge, UK, Cambridge University Press; 1999, p 89.
25. Akashi K, Traver D, Miyamoto T, et al: A clonogenic common myeloid progenitor that gives rise to all myeloid lineages. Nature 2000;404:193.
26. Matsuzaki Y, Gyotoku J, Ogawa M, et al: Characterization of c-kit positive intrathymic stem cells that are restricted to lymphoid differentiation. J Exp Med 1993;178:1283.
27. Kondo M, Weissman IL, Akashi K: Identification of clonogenic common lymphoid progenitors in mouse bone marrow. Cell 1997; 91:661.
28. Wu L, Antica M, Johnson GR, et al: Developmental potential of the earliest precursor cells from the adult mouse thymus. J Exp Med 1992;174:1617.
29. Ball TC, Hirayama F, Ogawa M: Lymphohematopoietic progenitors of normal mice. Blood 1995;85:3086.
30. Hirayama F, Lyman SD, Clark SC, et al: The *flt3* ligand supports proliferation of lymphohematopoietic progenitors and early B-lymphoid progenitors. Blood 1995;85:1762.
31. Ogawa M: Differentiation and proliferation of hematopoietic stem cells. Blood 1993;81:2844.
32. Dick JE, Magli MC, Huszar D, et al: Introduction of a selectable gene into primitive stem cells capable of long-term reconstitution of the hemopoietic system of W/Wv mice. Cell 1985;42:71.
33. Keller G, Paige C, Gilboa E, et al: Expression of a foreign gene in myeloid and lymphoid cells derived from multipotent haematopoietic precursors. Nature 1985;318:149.
34. Lemischka IR, Raulet DH, Mulligan RC: Developmental potential and dynamic behaviour of hematopoietic stem cells. Cell 1986; 45:917.
35. Mintz B, Anthony K, Litwin S: Monoclonal derivation of mouse myeloid and lymphoid lineages from totipotent hematopoietic stem cells experimentally engrafted in fetal hosts. Proc Natl Acad Sci U S A 1984;81:7835.
36. Wu AM, Till JE, Siminovitch L, et al: Cytological evidence for a relationship between normal hematopoietic colony-forming cells and cells of the lymphoid system. J Exp Med 1968;127:455.
37. Raskind WH, Fialkow PJ: The use of cell markers in the study of human hematopoietic neoplasia. Adv Cancer Res 1987;49:127.
38. Janssen JWG, Buschle M, Layton M, et al: Clonal analysis of myelodysplastic syndromes: Evidence of multipotent stem cell origin. Blood 1989;73:248.
39. Prchal JT, Throckmorton DW, Caroll AJ, et al: A common progenitor for human myeloid and lymphoid cells. Nature 1978;274:590.
40. Turhan AG, Humphries RK, Phillips GL, et al: Clonal hematopoiesis demonstrated by X-linked DNA polymorphisms after allogeneic bone marrow transplantation. N Engl J Med 1989;320:1655.
41. Champion KM, Gilbert JGR, Asimakopoulos FA, et al: Clonal haemopoiesis in normal elderly women: Implications for the myeloproliferative disorders and myelodysplastic syndromes. Br J Haematol 1997;97:920.
42. Gale RE, Fielding AK, Harrison CN, et al: Acquired skewing of X-chromosome inactivation patterns in myeloid cells of the elderly suggests stochastic clonal loss with age. Br J Haematol 1997; 98:512.
43. Harrison DE: Normal production of erythrocytes by mouse marrow continuous for 73 months. Proc Natl Acad Sci U S A 1973; 70:3184.
44. Harrison DE, Astle CM: Loss of stem cell repopulating ability upon transplantation. Effects of donor age, cell number, and transplantation procedure. J Exp Med 1982;156:1767.
45. Iscove NN, Nawa K: Hematopoietic stem cells expand during serial transplantation in vivo without apparent exhaustion. Curr Biol 1997;7:805.
46. Keller G, Snodgrass R: Life span of multipotential hematopoietic stem cells in vivo. J Exp Med 1990;171:1407.

47. Buescher ES, Alling DW, Gallin JI: Use of an X-linked human neutrophil marker to estimate timing of lyonization and size of the dividing stem cell pool. J Clin Invest 1985;76:1581.
48. Abkowitz JL, Linenberger ML, Newton MA, et al: Evidence for the maintenance of hematopoiesis in a large animal by the sequential activation of stem-cell clones. Proc Natl Acad Sci U S A 1990; 87:9062.
49. Jordan CT, Lemischka IR: Clonal and systemic analysis of long-term hematopoiesis in the mouse. Genes Dev 1990;4:220.
50. Till JE, McCulloch EA: A direct measurement of the radiation sensitivity of normal mouse bone marrow cells. Radiat Res 1961; 14:213.
51. Magli MC, Iscove NN, Odartchenko N: Transient nature of early haematopoietic spleen colonies. Nature 1982;295:527.
52. Johnson GR, Nicola NA: Characterization of two populations of CFU-S fractionated from mouse fetal liver by fluorescence-activated cell sorting. J Cell Physiol 1984;118:45.
53. Mulder AH, Visser JWM: Separation and functional analysis of bone marrow cells separated by rhodamine-123 fluorescence. Exp Hematol 1987;15:99.
54. Spangrude GJ, Smith L, Uchida N, et al: Mouse hematopoietic stem cells. Blood 1991;78:1395.
55. Visser JWM, de Vries P: Isolation of spleen-colony forming cells (CFU-s) using wheat germ agglutinin and rhodamine 123 labeling. Blood Cells 1988;14:369.
56. Miller CL, Rebel VI, Helgason CD, et al: Impaired steel factor responsiveness differentially affects the detection and longterm maintenance of fetal liver hematopoietic stem cells in vivo. Blood 1997;89:1214.
57. Morrison SJ, Weissman IL: The long-term repopulating subset of hematopoietic stem cells is deterministic and isolatable by phenotype. Immunity 1994;1:661.
58. Zhong R-K, Astle CM, Harrison DE: Distinct developmental patterns of short-term and long-term functioning lymphoid and myeloid precursors defined by competitive limiting dilution analysis in vivo. J Immunol 1996;157:138.
59. Harrison DE, Jordan CT, Zhong RK, et al: Primitive hemopoietic stem cells: Direct assay of most productive populations by competitive repopulation with simple binomial, correlation and covariance calculations. Exp Hematol 1993;21:206.
60. Szilvassy SJ, Humphries RK, Lansdorp PM, et al: Quantitative assay for totipotent reconstituting hematopoietic stem cells by a competitive repopulation strategy. Proc Natl Acad Sci U S A 1990; 87:8736.
61. Szilvassy SJ, Nicolini FE, Eaves CJ, et al: Quantitation of murine and human hematopoietic stem cells by limiting-dilution analysis in competitively repopulated hosts. In Methods in Molecular Medicine, vol 63: Klug CA, Jordan CT, eds: Hematopoietic Stem Cell Protocols. Totowa, NJ: Humana Press, 2001, p 167.
62. Trevisan M, Iscove N: Phenotypic analysis of murine long-term hemotopoietic reconstituting cells quantitated competitively in vivo and comparison with more advanced colony-forming progeny. J Exp Med 1995;181:93.
63. Siminovitch L, McCulloch EA, Till JE: The distribution of colony-forming cells among spleen colonies. J Cell Physiol 1963;62:327.
64. Fleming WH, Alpern EJ, Uchida N, et al: Functional heterogeneity is associated with the cell cycle status of murine hematopoietic stem cells. J Cell Biol 1993;122:897.
65. Glimm H, Oh I, Eaves C: Human hematopoietic stem cells stimulated to proliferate in vitro lose engraftment potential during their S/G$_2$/M transit and do not re-enter G$_0$. Blood 2000;96:4185.
66. Gothot A, Van der Loo JCM, Clapp W, et al: Cell cycle–related changes in repopulating capacity of human mobilized peripheral blood CD34$^+$ cells in non-obese diabetic/severe combined immune-deficient mice. Blood 1998;92:2641.
67. Habibian HK, Peters SO, Hsieh CC, et al: The fluctuating phenotype of the lymphohematopoietic stem cell with cell cycle transit. J Exp Med 1998;188:393.
68. Peters SO, Kittler ELW, Ramshaw HS, et al: Ex vivo expansion of murine marrow cells with interleukin-3 (IL-3), IL-6, IL-11, and stem cell factor leads to impaired engraftment in irradiated hosts. Blood 1996;87:30.
69. Rebel VI, Tanaka M, Lee J-S, et al: One-day ex vivo culture allows efficient gene transfer into human nonobese diabetic/severe combined immune-deficient repopulating cells using high-titer vesicu-
lar stomatitis virus G protein pseudotyped retrovirus. Blood 1999; 93:2217.
70. Monette FC, DeMello JB: The relationship between stem cell seeding efficiency and position in cell cycle. Cell Tissue Kinet 1979;12:161.
71. Szilvassy SJ, Meyerrose TE, Grimes B: Effects of cell cycle activation on the short-term engraftment properties of ex vivo expanded murine hematopoietic cells. Blood 2000;95:2829.
72. Ponchio L, Conneally E, Eaves C: Quantitation of the quiescent fraction of longterm culture–initiating cells (LTC-IC) in normal human blood and marrow and the kinetics of their growth factor-stimulated entry into S-phase in vitro. Blood 1995;86:3314.
73. Spangrude GJ, Brooks DM, Tumas DB: Long-term repopulation of irradiated mice with limiting numbers of purified hematopoietic stem cells: In vivo expansion of stem cell phenotype but not function. Blood 1995;85:1006.
74. Wolf NS, Kone A, Priestley GV, et al: In vivo and in vitro characterization of long-term repopulating primitive hematopoietic cells isolated by sequential Hoechst 33342–rhodamine 123 FACS selection. Exp Hematol 1993;21:614.
75. Rebel VI, Dragowska W, Eaves CJ, et al: Amplification of Sca-1$^+$ Lin$^-$ WGA$^+$ cells in serum-free cultures containing Steel factor, interleukin-6, and erythropoietin with maintenance of cells with long-term in vivo reconstituting potential. Blood 1994;83:128.
76. Smith LG, Weissman IL, Heimfeld S: Clonal analysis of hematopoietic stem-cell differentiation in vivo. Proc Natl Acad Sci U S A 1991;88:2788.
77. Szilvassy SJ, Fraser CC, Eaves CJ, et al: Retrovirus-mediated gene transfer to purified hemopoietic stem cells with long-term lympho-myelopoietic repopulating ability. Proc Natl Acad Sci U S A 1989; 86:8798.
78. Cashman JD, Lapidot T, Wang JCY, et al: Kinetic evidence of the regeneration of multilineage hematopoiesis from primitive cells in normal human bone marrow transplanted into immunodeficient mice. Blood 1997;89:4307.
79. Dick JE, Lapidot T, Pflumio F: Transplantation of normal and leukemic human bone marrow into immune-deficient mice: Development of animal models for human hematopoiesis. Immunol Rev 1991;124:25.
80. Nolta JA, Hanley MB, Kohn DB: Sustained human hematopoiesis in immunodeficient mice by cotransplantation of marrow stroma expressing human interleukin-3: Analysis of gene transduction of long-lived progenitors. Blood 1994;83:3041.
81. Pflumio F, Izac B, Katz A, et al: Phenotype and function of human hematopoietic cells engrafting immune-deficient CB17–severe combined immunodeficiency mice and nonobese diabetic–severe combined immunodeficiency mice after transplantation of human cord blood mononuclear cells. Blood 1996;88:3731.
82. Cashman JD, Eaves CJ: High marrow seeding efficiency of human lymphomyeloid repopulating cells in irradiated NOD/SCID mice. Blood 2000;96:3979.
83. Conneally E, Cashman J, Petzer A, et al: Expansion in vitro of transplantable human cord blood stem cells demonstrated using a quantitative assay of their lympho-myeloid repopulating activity in nonobese diabetic-*scid/scid* mice. Proc Natl Acad Sci U S A 1997; 94:9836.
84. Wang JCY, Doedens M, Dick JE: Primitive human hematopoietic cells are enriched in cord blood compared with adult bone marrow or mobilized peripheral blood as measured by the quantitative in vivo SCID-repopulating cell assay. Blood 1997;89:3919.
85. Bonnet D, Bhatia M, Wang JCY, et al: Cytokine treatment of accessory cells are required to initiate engraftment of purified primitive human hematopoietic cells transplanted at limiting doses into NOD/SCID mice. Bone Marrow Transplant 1999;23:203.
86. Van der Loo JCM, Hanenberg H, Cooper RJ, et al: Nonobese diabetic/severe combined immunodeficiency (NOD/SCID) mouse as a model system to study the engraftment and mobilization of human peripheral blood stem cells. Blood 1998;92:2556.
87. Gallacher L, Murdoch B, Wu DM, et al: Isolation and characterization of human CD34$^-$Lin$^-$ and CD34$^+$Lin$^-$ hematopoietic stem cells using cell surface markers AC133 and CD7. Blood 2000; 95:2813.
88. de Wynter EA, Buck D, Hart C, et al: CD34$^+$ AC133$^+$ cells isolated from cord blood are highly enriched in long-term culture–initiating cells, NOD/SCID-repopulating cells and dendritic cell progenitors. Stem Cells 1998;16:387.

89. Bhatia M, Wang JCY, Kapp U, et al: Purification of primitive human hematopoietic cells capable of repopulating immune-deficient mice. Proc Natl Acad Sci U S A 1997;94:5320.

90. Bhatia M, Bonnet D, Murdoch B, et al: A newly discovered class of human hematopoietic cells with SCID-repopulating activity. Nat Med 1998;4:1038.

91. Goodell MA, Rosenzweig M, Kim H, et al: Dye efflux studies suggest that hematopoietic stem cells expressing low or undetectable levels of CD34 antigen exist in multiple species. Nat Med 1997;3:1337.

92. Krause DS, Ito T, Fackler MJ, et al: Characterization of murine CD34, a marker for hematopoietic progenitor and stem cells. Blood 1994;84:691.

93. Sato T, Laver JH, Ogawa M: Reversible expression of CD34 by murine hematopoietic stem cells. Blood 1999;94:2548.

94. Jones RJ, Collector MI, Barber JP, et al: Characterization of mouse lymphohematopoietic stem cells lacking spleen colony-forming activity. Blood 1996;88:487.

95. Ortiz M, Wine JW, Lohrey N, et al: Functional characterization of a novel hematopoietic stem cell and its place in the c-kit maturation pathway in bone marrow cell development. Immunity 1999;10:173.

96. Randall TD, Weissman IL: Phenotypic and functional changes induced at the clonal level in hematopoietic stem cells after 5-fluorouracil treatment. Blood 1997;89:3596.

97. Zanjani ED, Pallavicini MG, Ascensao JL, et al: Engraftment and long-term expression of human fetal hemopoietic stem cells in sheep following transplantation in utero. J Clin Invest 1992;89:1178.

98. Zanjani ED, Srour EF, Hoffman R: Retention of long-term repopulating ability of xenogeneic transplanted purified adult human bone marrow hematopoietic stem cells in sheep. J Clin Lab Med 1995;126:24.

99. Yin AH, Miraglia S, Zanjani ED, et al: AC133, a novel marker for human hematopoietic stem and progenitor cells. Blood 1997;90:5002.

100. Zanjani ED, Almeida-Porada G, Livingston AG, et al: Human bone marrow CD34⁻ cells engraft in vivo and undergo multilineage expression that includes giving rise to CD34⁺ cells. Exp Hematol 1998;26:353.

101. Civin CI, Almeida-Porada G, Lee M-J, et al: Sustained, retransplantable, multilineage engraftment of highly purified adult human bone marrow stem cells in vivo. Blood 1996;88:4102.

102. Cashman J, Bockhold K, Hogge DE, et al: Sustained proliferation, multi-lineage differentiation and maintenance of primitive human haematopoietic cells in NOD/SCID mice transplanted with human cord blood. Br J Haematol 1997;98:1026.

103. Holyoake TL, Nicolini FE, Eaves CJ: Functional differences between transplantable human hematopoietic stem cells from fetal liver, cord blood, and adult marrow. Exp Hematol 1999;27:1418.

104. Srour EF, Zanjani ED, Cornetta K, et al: Persistence of human multilineage, self-renewing lymphohematopoietic stem cells in chimeric sheep. Blood 1993;82:3333.

105. Ginsburg H, Sachs L: Formation of pure suspensions of mast cells in tissue culture by differentiation of lymphoid cells from the mouse thymus. J Natl Cancer Inst 1963;31:1.

106. Bradley TR, Metcalf D: The growth of mouse bone marrow cells in vitro. Aust J Exp Biol Med Sci 1966;44:287.

107. Pluznik DH, Sachs L: The cloning of normal 'mast' cells in tissue culture. J Cell Comp Physiol 1965;66:319.

108. Senn JS, McCulloch EA, Till JE: Comparison of colony-forming ability of normal and leukaemic human marrow in cell culture. Lancet 1967;2:597.

109. Metcalf D: Hemopoietic Colonies. In Vitro Cloning of Normal and Leukemic Cells. Berlin: Springer-Verlag; 1977.

110. Till JE, McCulloch EA: Hemopoietic stem cell differentiation. Biochim Biophys Acta 1980;605:431.

111. Eaves CJ, Eaves AC: Fundamental control of hematopoiesis. In Fisher JW, ed: Biochemical Pharmacology of Blood and Bloodforming Organs. New Orleans, LA: Springer-Verlag; 1992, p 5.

112. Gregory CJ, Eaves AC: Human marrow cells capable of erythropoietic differentiation in vitro: Definition of three erythroid colony responses. Blood 1977;49:855.

113. Hogge D, Fanning S, Bockhold K, et al: Quantitation and characterization of human megakaryocyte colony-forming cells using a standardized serum-free agarose assay. Br J Haematol 1997;96:790.

114. Long MW, Heffner CH, Gragowski LL: In vitro differences in responsiveness of early (BFU-Mk) and late (CFU-Mk) murine megakaryocyte progenitor cells. In Levine RF, ed: Megakaryocyte Development and Function. New York: Alan R Liss; 1986, p 179.

115. Fauser AA, Messner HA: Identification of megakaryocytes, macrophages, and eosinophils in colonies of human bone marrow containing neutrophilic granulocytes and erythroblasts. Blood 1979;53:1023.

116. Guilbert LJ, Iscove NN: Partial replacement of serum by selenite, transferrin, albumin and lecithin in haemopoietic cell cultures. Nature 1976;263:594.

117. Mayani H, Dragowska W, Lansdorp PM: Characterization of functionally distinct subpopulations of CD34⁺ cord blood cells in serum-free long-term cultures supplemented with hematopoietic cytokines. Blood 1993;82:2664.

118. Migliaccio G, Migliaccio AR, Adamson JW: The biology of hematopoietic growth factors: Studies in vitro under serum-deprived conditions. Exp Hematol 1990;18:1049.

119. Sandstrom CE, Miller WM, Papoutsakis ET: Review: Serum-free media for cultures of primitive and mature hematopoietic cells. Biotechnol Bioeng 1994;43:706.

120. Eaves CJ, Eaves AC: Erythropoiesis. In Golde DW, Takaku F, eds: Hematopoietic Stem Cells. New York: Marcel Dekker; 1985, p 19.

121. Eaves CJ, Humphries RK, Eaves AC: In vitro characterization of erythroid precursor cells and the erythropoietic differentiation process. In Stamatoyannopoulos G, Nienhuis AW, eds: Cellular and Molecular Regulation of Hemoglobin Switching. New York: Grune & Stratton; 1979, p 251.

122. Bol S, Williams N: The maturation state of three types of granulocyte/macrophage progenitor cells from mouse bone marrow. J Cell Physiol 1980;102:233.

123. McNiece IK, Stewart FM, Deacon DM, et al: Detection of a human CFC with a high proliferative potential. Blood 1989;74:609.

124. Metcalf D, MacDonald HR: Heterogeneity of in vitro colony- and cluster-forming cells in the mouse marrow: Segregation by velocity sedimentation. J Cell Physiol 1975;85:643.

125. Lansdorp PM, Sutherland HJ, Eaves CJ: Selective expression of CD45 isoforms on functional subpopulations of CD34⁺ hemopoietic cells from human bone marrow. J Exp Med 1990;172:363.

126. Sauvageau G, Lansdorp PM, Eaves CJ, et al: Differential expression of homeobox genes in functionally distinct CD34⁺ subpopulations of human bone marrow cells. Proc Natl Acad Sci U S A 1994;91:12223.

127. Krystal G, Lam V, Dragowska W, et al: Transforming growth factor β1 is an inducer of erythroid differentiation. J Exp Med 1994;180:851.

128. Metcalf D: Clonal analysis of proliferation and differentiation of paired daughter cells: Action of granulocyte-macrophage colony-stimulating factor on granulocyte-macrophage precursors. Proc Natl Acad Sci U S A 1980;77:5327.

129. Panzenbock B, Bartunek P, Mapara MY, et al: Growth and differentiation of human stem cell factor/erythropoietin-dependent erythroid progenitor cells in vitro. Blood 1998;92:3658.

130. Leary AG, Ogawa M, Strauss LC, et al: Single cell origin of multilineage colonies in culture. J Clin Invest 1984;74:2193.

131. Suda T, Suda J, Ogawa M: Disparate differentiation in mouse hemopoietic colonies derived from paired progenitors. Proc Natl Acad Sci U S A 1984;81:2520.

132. McNiece IK, Williams NT, Johnson GR, et al: Generation of murine hematopoietic precursor cells from macrophage high-proliferative-potential colony-forming cells. Exp Hematol 1987;15:972.

133. Holyoake TL, Freshney MG, Konwalinka G, et al: Mixed colony formation in vitro by the heterogeneous compartment of multipotential progenitors in human bone marrow. Leukemia 1993;7:207.

134. Pragnell IB, Wright EG, Lorimore SA, et al: The effect of stem cell proliferation regulators demonstrated with an in vitro assay. Blood 1988;72:196.

135. Dowding CR, Gordon MY: Physical, phenotypic and cytochemical characterisation of stroma-adherent blast colony-forming cells. Leukemia 1992;6:347.

136. Gordon MY, Dowding CR, Riley GP, et al: Characterisation of stroma-dependent blast colony-forming cells in human marrow. J Cell Physiol 1987;130:150.

137. Leary AG, Ogawa M: Blast cell colony assay for umbilical cord blood and adult bone marrow progenitors. Blood 1987;69:953.

138. Nakahata T, Ogawa M: Identification in culture of a class of hemopoietic colony-forming units with extensive capability to self-renew and generate multipotential hemopoietic colonies. Proc Natl Acad Sci U S A 1982;79:3843.

139. Aiba Y, Ogawa M: Development of natural killer cells, B lymphocytes, macrophages, and mast cells from single hematopoietic progenitors in culture of murine fetal liver cells. Blood 1997;90:3923.

140. Hirayama F, Aiba Y, Ikebuchi K, et al: Differentiation in culture of murine primitive lymphohematopoietic progenitors toward T-cell lineage. Blood 1999;93:4187.

141. Petzer AL, Hogge DE, Lansdorp PM, et al: Self-renewal of primitive human hematopoietic cells (long-term-culture–initiating cells) in vitro and their expansion in defined medium. Proc Natl Acad Sci U S A 1996;93:1470.

142. Sitnicka E, Lin N, Priestley GV, et al: The effect of thrombopoietin on the proliferation and differentiation of murine hematopoietic stem cells. Blood 1996;87:4998.

143. Maguer-Satta V, Oostendorp R, Reid D, et al: Evidence that ceramide mediates the ability of TNF to modulate primitive human hematopoietic cell fates. Blood 2000;96:4118.

144. Dexter TM, Allen TD, Lajtha LG: Conditions controlling the proliferation of haemopoietic stem cells in vitro. J Cell Physiol 1977;91:335.

145. Coulombel L, Eaves AC, Eaves CJ: Enzymatic treatment of long-term human marrow cultures reveals the preferential location of primitive hemopoietic progenitors in the adherent layer. Blood 1983;62:291.

146. Gartner S, Kaplan HS: Long-term culture of human bone marrow cells. Proc Natl Acad Sci U S A 1980;77:4756.

147. Greenberg HM, Newburger PE, Parker LM, et al: Human granulocytes generated in continuous bone marrow culture are physiologically normal. Blood 1981;58:724.

148. Cashman J, Eaves AC, Eaves CJ: Regulated proliferation of primitive hematopoietic progenitor cells in long-term human marrow cultures. Blood 1985;66:1002.

149. Toksoz D, Dexter TM, Lord BI, et al: The regulation of hemopoiesis in long-term bone marrow cultures. II. Stimulation and inhibition of stem cell proliferation. Blood 1980;55:931.

150. Fraser CC, Szilvassy SJ, Eaves CJ, et al: Proliferation of totipotent hematopoietic stem cells in vitro with retention of long-term competitive in vivo reconstituting ability. Proc Natl Acad Sci U S A 1992;89:1968.

151. Ploemacher RE, Van Der Sluijs JP, Voerman JSA, et al: An in vitro limiting-dilution assay of long-term repopulating hematopoietic stem cells in the mouse. Blood 1989;74:2755.

152. Sutherland HJ, Eaves CJ, Eaves AC, et al: Characterization and partial purification of human marrow cells capable of initiating long-term hematopoiesis in vitro. Blood 1989;74:1563.

153. Hao QL, Thiemann FT, Petersen D, et al: Extended long-term culture reveals a highly quiescent and primitive human hematopoietic progenitor population. Blood 1996;88:3306.

154. Prosper F, Stroncek D, Verfaillie CM: Phenotypic and functional characterization of long-term culture–initiating cells present in peripheral blood progenitor collections of normal donors treated with granulocyte colony-stimulating factor. Blood 1996;88:2033.

155. Eaves CJ, Sutherland HJ, Udomsakdi C, et al: The human hematopoietic stem cell in vitro and in vivo. Blood Cells 1992;18:301.

156. Sutherland HJ, Eaves CJ: Long-term culture of human myeloid cells. In Freshney RI, Pragnell IB, Freshney MG, eds: Culture of Hematopoietic Cells. New York: John Wiley & Sons; 1994, p 139.

157. Sutherland HJ, Lansdorp PM, Henkelman DH, et al: Functional characterization of individual human hematopoietic stem cells cultured at limiting dilution on supportive marrow stromal layers. Proc Natl Acad Sci U S A 1990;87:3584.

158. Udomsakdi C, Eaves CJ, Swolin B, et al: Rapid decline of chronic myeloid leukemic cells in long-term culture due to a defect at the leukemic stem cell level. Proc Natl Acad Sci U S A 1992;89:6192.

159. Udomsakdi C, Lansdorp PM, Hogge DE, et al: Characterization of primitive hematopoietic cells in normal human peripheral blood. Blood 1992;80:2513.

160. Sutherland HJ, Eaves CJ, Lansdorp PM, et al: Differential regulation of primitive human hematopoietic cells in long-term cultures maintained on genetically engineered murine stromal cells. Blood 1991;78:666.

161. Baum CM, Weissman IL, Tsukamoto AS, et al: Isolation of a candidate human hematopoietic stem-cell population. Proc Natl Acad Sci U S A 1992;89:2804.

162. Nicolini FE, Holyoake TL, Cashman JD, et al: Unique differentiation programs of human fetal liver stem cells revealed both in vitro and in vivo in NOD/SCID mice. Blood 1999;94:2686.

163. Roy V, Miller JS, Verfaillie CM: Phenotypic and functional characterization of committed and primitive myeloid and lymphoid hematopoietic precursors in human fetal liver. Exp Hematol 1997;25:387.

164. Hogge DE, Lansdorp PM, Reid D, et al: Enhanced detection, maintenance and differentiation of primitive human hematopoietic cells in cultures containing murine fibroblasts engineered to produce human Steel factor, interleukin-3 and granulocyte colony-stimulating factor. Blood 1996;88:3765.

165. Hows JM, Bradley BA, Marsh JCW, et al: Growth of human umbilical-cord blood in longterm haemopoietic cultures. Lancet 1992;340:73.

166. Pettengell R, Luft T, Henschler R, et al: Direct comparison by limiting dilution analysis of long-term culture–initiating cells in human bone marrow, umbilical cord blood, and blood stem cells. Blood 1994;84:3653.

167. Miller CL, Eaves CJ: Long-term culture–initiating cell assays for human and murine cells. In Methods in Molecular Medicine, vol 63. Klug CA, Jordan CT, eds: Hematopoietic Stem Cell Protocols. Totowa, NJ, Humana Press, 2001, p 125.

168. Gabbianelli M, Pelosi E, Montesoro E, et al: Multi-level effects of flt3 ligand on human hematopoiesis: Expansion of putative stem cells and proliferation of granulomonocytic progenitors/monocytic precursors. Blood 1995;86:1661.

169. Hao Q-LH, Shah AJ, Thiemann FT, et al: A functional comparison of CD34 + CD38 − cells in cord blood and bone marrow. Blood 1995;86:3745.

170. Hogge DE, Cashman JD, Humphries RK, et al: Differential and synergistic effects of human granulocyte-macrophage colony-stimulating factor and human granulocyte colony-stimulating factor on hematopoiesis in human long-term marrow cultures. Blood 1991;77:493.

171. Otsuka T, Thacker JD, Eaves CJ, et al: Differential effects of microenvironmentally presented interleukin 3 versus soluble growth factor on primitive human hematopoietic cells. J Clin Invest 1991;88:417.

172. Verfaillie C, Hurley R, Bhatia R, et al: Role of bone marrow matrix in normal and abnormal hematopoiesis. Crit Rev Oncol Hematol 1994;16:201.

173. Gupta P, Oegema TRJ, Brazil JJ, et al: Structurally specific heparan sulfates support primitive human hematopoiesis by formation of a multimolecular stem cell niche. Blood 1998;92:4641.

174. Moore KA, Pytowski B, Witte L, et al: Hematopoietic activity of a stromal cell transmembrane protein containing epidermal growth factor–like repeat motifs. Proc Natl Acad Sci U S A 1997;94:4011.

175. Ponchio L, Eaves CJ: Very primitive hematopoietic cells (LTC-IC) in normal adult human blood and marrow show differences in the regulation of their cycling state [abstract]. Blood 1995;86:493.

176. Sutherland HJ, Hogge DE, Cook D, et al: Alternative mechanisms with and without Steel factor support primitive human hematopoiesis. Blood 1993;81:1465.

177. Glimm H, Eaves CJ: Direct evidence for multiple self-renewal divisions of human in vivo repopulating hematopoietic cells in short-term culture. Blood 1999;94:2161.

178. Berardi AC, Meffre E, Pflumio F, et al: Individual CD34 + CD38low CD19 − CD10 − progenitor cells from human cord blood generate B lymphocytes and granulocytes. Blood 1997;89:3554.

179. Miller JS, McCullar V, Punzel M, et al: Single adult human CD34 + /Lin − /CD38 − progenitors give rise to natural killer cells, B-lineage cells, dendritic cells, and myeloid cells. Blood 1999;93:96.

180. Punzel M, Wissink SD, Miller JS, et al: The myeloid-lymphoid initiating cell (ML-IC) assay assesses the fate of multipotent human progenitors in vitro. Blood 1999;93:3750.

181. Robin C, Pflumio F, Vainchenker W, et al: Identification of lymphomyeloid primitive progenitor cells in fresh human cord blood and in marrow of nonobese diabetic–severe combined immunodeficient (NOD-SCID) mice transplanted with human CD34 + cord blood cells. J Exp Med 1999;189:1601.

182. Lemieux ME, Rebel VI, Lansdorp PM, et al: Characterization and

purification of a primitive hematopoietic cell type in adult mouse marrow capable of lympho-myeloid differentiation in long-term marrow "switch" cultures. Blood 1995;86:1339.

183. Krause DS, Fackler MJ, Civin CI, et al: CD34: Structure, biology, and clinical utility. Blood 1996;87:1.

184. Baumhueter S, Singer MS, Henzel W, et al: Binding of L-selectin to the vascular sialomucin CD34. Science 1993;262:436.

185. Andrews RG, Singer JW, Bernstein ID: Precursors of colony-forming cells in humans can be distinguished from colony-forming cells by expression of the CD33 and CD34 antigens and light scatter properties. J Exp Med 1989;169:1721.

186. Loken MR, Shah VO, Dattilio KL, et al: Flow cytometric analysis of human bone marrow. II. Normal B lymphocyte development. Blood 1987;70:1316.

187. Lotzova E, Savary CA, Champlin RE: Genesis of human oncolytic natural killer cells from primitive CD34⁺ CD33⁻ bone marrow progenitors. J Immunol 1993;150:5263.

188. Schmitt C, Eaves CJ, Lansdorp PM: Expression of CD34 on human B cell precursors. Clin Exp Immunol 1991;85:168.

189. Craig W, Kay R, Cutler RL, et al: Expression of Thy-1 on human hematopoietic progenitor cells. J Exp Med 1993;177:1331.

190. Huang S, Terstappen LWMM: Lymphoid and myeloid differentiation of single human CD34⁺, HLA-DR⁺, CD38⁻ hematopoietic stem cells. Blood 1994;83:1515.

191. Terstappen LWMM, Huang S, Safford M, et al: Sequential generations of hematopoietic colonies derived from single nonlineage-committed CD34⁺ CD38⁻ progenitor cells. Blood 1991;77:1218.

192. Ploemacher RE, Brons RHC: Separation of CFU-S from primitive cells responsible for reconstitution of the bone marrow hemopoietic stem cell compartment following irradiation: Evidence for a pre-CFU-S cell. Exp Hematol 1989;17:263.

193. Spangrude GJ, Johnson GR: Resting and activated subsets of mouse multipotent hematopoietic stem cells. Proc Natl Acad Sci U S A 1990;87:7433.

194. Udomsakdi C, Eaves CJ, Sutherland HJ, et al: Separation of functionally distinct subpopulations of primitive human hematopoietic cells using rhodamine-123. Exp Hematol 1991;19:338.

195. Schinkel AH, Mayer U, Wagenaar E, et al: Normal viability and altered pharmacokinetics in mice lacking mdr1-type (drug-transporting) P-glycoproteins. Proc Natl Acad Sci U S A 1997;94:4028.

196. Baines P, Visser JWM: Analysis and separation of murine bone marrow stem cells by H33342 fluorescence-activated cell sorting. Exp Hematol 1983;11:701.

197. Goodell MA, Brose K, Paradis G, et al: Isolation and functional properties of murine hematopoietic stem cells that are replicating in vivo. J Exp Med 1996;183:1797.

198. Storms RW, Goodell MA, Fisher A, et al: Hoechst dye efflux reveals a novel CD7⁺ CD34⁻ lymphoid progenitor in human umbilical cord blood. Blood 2000;96:212.

199. Uchida N, Fujisaki T, Eaves A, et al: Transplantable hematopoietic stem cells in human fetal liver have a CD34⁺ side population (SP) phenotype. J Clin Invest 2001;108:1071.

200. Zhou S, Morris J, Bunting KD, et al: The ABC transporter B$_{crp1}$/ABCG2$_x$ is expressed in a wide variety of stem cells and is a molecular determinant of the side-population phenotype. Nat Med 2001;7:1028.

201. Gussoni E, Soneoka Y, Strickland CD, et al: Dystrophin expression in the *mdx* mouse restored by stem cell transplantation. Nature 1999;401:390.

202. Stingl J, Zandieh I, Eaves CJ, et al: Characterization of bipotent mammary epithelial progenitor cells in normal adult human breast tissue. Breast Cancer Res Treat 2001;67:93.

203. Jackson KA, Mi T, Goodell MA: Hematopoietic potential of stem cells isolated from murine skeletal muscle. Proc Natl Acad Sci U S A 1999;96:14482.

204. Bunting KD, Galipeau J, Topham D, et al: Transduction of murine bone marrow cells with an MDR1 vector enables ex vivo stem cell expansion, but these expanded grafts cause a myeloproliferative syndrome in transplanted mice. Blood 1998;92:2269.

205. Bunting KD, Zhou S, Lu T, et al: Enforced P-glycoprotein pump function in murine bone marrow cells results in expansion of side population stem cells in vitro and repopulating cells in vivo. Blood 2000;96:902.

206. Dorrell C, Gan OI, Pereira DS, et al: Expansion of human cord blood CD34⁺ CD38⁻ cells in ex vivo culture during retroviral transduction without a corresponding increase in SCID repopulating cell (SRC) frequency: Dissociation of SRC phenotype and function. Blood 2000;95:102.

207. Srour EF, Brandt JE, Leemhuis T, et al: Relationship between cytokine-dependent cell cycle progression and MHC class II antigen expression by human CD34 + HLA-DR − bone marrow cells. J Immunol 1992;148:815.

208. Zandstra PW, Conneally E, Petzer AL, et al: Cytokine manipulation of primitive human hematopoietic cell self-renewal. Proc Natl Acad Sci U S A 1997;94:4698.

209. Oh I-H, Lau A, Eaves CJ: During ontogeny primitive (CD34 + CD38 −) hematopoietic cells show altered expression of a subset of genes associated with early cytokine and differentiation responses of their adult counterparts. Blood 2000;96:4160.

210. Bloom W, Bartelmez GW: Hematopoiesis in young human embryos. Am J Anat 1927;67:21.

211. Gilmour JR: Normal haemopoiesis in intra-uterine and neonatal life. J Pathol 1941;52:25.

212. Kelemen E, Calvo W, Fliedner TM: Atlas of Human Hemopoietic Development. Berlin: Springer-Verlag; 1979.

213. Metcalf D, Moore MAS: Haematopoietic cells. In Neuberger A, Tatum EL, eds: Frontiers of Biology. Amsterdam: North-Holland Publishing; 1971, p 550.

214. Dieterlen-Lievre F: Hemopoietic cell progenitors in the avian embryo: Origin and migrations. Ann N Y Acad Sci 1987;511:77.

215. Eichmann A, Corbel C, Nataf V, et al: Ligand-dependent development of the endothelial and hemopoietic lineages from embryonic mesodermal cells expressing vascular endothelial growth factor receptor 2. Proc Natl Acad Sci U S A 1997;94:5141.

216. Choi K, Kennedy M, Kazarov A, et al: A common precursor for hematopoietic and endothelial cells. Development 1998;125:725.

217. Jaffredo T, Gautier R, Eichmann A, et al: Intraaortic hemopoietic cells are derived from endothelial cells during ontogeny. Development 1999;125:4575.

218. Medvinsky A, Dzierzak E: Definitive hematopoiesis is autonomously initiated by the AGM region. Cell 1996;86:897.

219. Nishikawa S-I, Nishikawa S, Kawamoto H, et al: In vitro generation of lymphohematopoietic cells from endothelial cells purified from murine embryos. Immunity 1998;8:761.

220. Shalaby F, Ho J, Stanford WL, et al: A requirement for Flk1 in primitive and definitive hematopoiesis and vasculogenesis. Cell 1997;89:981.

221. Shalaby F, Rossant J, Yamaguchi TP, et al: Failure of blood-island formation and vasculogenesis in Flk-1–deficient mice. Nature 1995;376:62.

222. Cumano A, Furlonger C, Paige CJ: Differentiation and characterization of B-cell precursors detected in the yolk sac and embryo body of embryos beginning at the 10- to 12-somite stage. Proc Natl Acad Sci U S A 1993;90:6429.

223. Godin IE, Garcia-Porrero JA, Coutinho A, et al: Para-aortic splanchnopleura from early mouse embryos contains B1a cell progenitors. Nature 1993;364:67.

224. Medvinsky AL, Samoylina NL, Muller AM, et al: An early pre-liver intra-embryonic source of CFU-S in the developing mouse. Nature 1993;364:64.

225. Tavian M, Coulombel L, Luton D, et al: Aorta-associated CD34 + hematopoietic cells in the early human embryo. Blood 1996;87:67.

226. Fantoni A, Farace MG, Gambari R: Embryonic hemoglobins in man and other mammals. Blood 1981;57:623.

227. Gale RE, Clegg JB, Huehns ER: Human embryonic haemoglobins gower 1 and gower 2. Nature 1979;280:162.

228. Kazazian HH Jr, Woodhead AP: Hemoglobin A synthesis in the developing fetus. N Engl J Med 1973;289:58.

229. Pataryas HA, Stamatoyannopoulos G: Hemoglobins in human fetuses: Evidence for adult hemoglobin production after the 11th gestational week. Blood 1972;39:688.

230. Boyer SH, Belding TK, Margolet L, et al: Fetal hemoglobin restriction to a few erythrocytes (F cells) in normal human adults. Science 1975;188:361.

231. Alter BP, Rappeport JM, Huisman THJ, et al: Fetal erythropoiesis following bone marrow transplantation. Blood 1976;48:843.

232. Boyer SH, Belding TK, Margolet L, et al: Variations in the frequency of fetal hemoglobin–bearing erythrocytes (F-cells) in well adults, pregnant women, and adult leukemics. Johns Hopkins Med J 1975;137:105.

233. Sheridan BL, Weatherall DJ, Clegg JB, et al: The patterns of fetal haemoglobin production in leukaemia. Br J Haematol 1976;32:487.

234. Wood WG, Stamatoyannopoulos G, Lim G, et al: F-cells in the adult: Normal values and levels in individuals with hereditary and acquired elevations of Hb F. Blood 1975;46:671.

235. Papayannopoulou TH, Brice M, Stamatoyannopoulos G: Hemoglobin F synthesis in vitro: Evidence for control at the level of primitive erythroid stem cells. Proc Natl Acad Sci U S A 1977;74:2923.

236. Papayannopoulou T, Chen P, Maniatis A, et al: Simultaneous assessment of i-antigenic expression and fetal hemoglobin in single red cells by immunofluorescence. Blood 1980;55:221.

237. Peschle C, Migliaccio AR, Migliaccio G, et al: Identification and characterization of three classes of erythroid progenitors in human fetal liver. Blood 1981;58:565.

238. Valtieri M, Gabbianelli M, Pelosi E, et al: Erythropoietin alone induces erythroid burst formation by human embryonic but not adult BFU-E in unicellular serum-free culture. Blood 1989;74:460.

239. Lansdorp PM, Dragowska W, Mayani H: Ontogeny-related changes in proliferative potential of human hematopoietic cells. J Exp Med 1993;178:787.

240. Micklem HS, Ford CE, Evans EP, et al: Competitive in vivo proliferation of foetal and adult haematopoietic cells in lethally irradiated mice. J Cell Physiol 1972;79:293.

241. Lu L, Xiao M, Shen R-N, et al: Enrichment, characterization and responsiveness of single primitive CD34^{+++} human umbilical cord blood hematopoietic progenitors with high proliferative and replating potential. Blood 1993;81:41.

242. Hassan MW, Lutton JD, Levere RD, et al: In vitro culture of erythroid colonies from human fetal liver and umbilical cord blood. Br J Haematol 1979;41:477.

243. Kubanek B, Rencricca N, Porcellini A, et al: The pattern of stem cell repopulation in heavily irradiated mice receiving transplants of fetal liver. Blood 1970;35:64.

244. Moore MAS, Williams N: Analysis of proliferation and differentiation of foetal granulocyte-macrophage progenitor cells in haemopoietic tissue. Cell Tissue Kinet 1973;6:461.

245. Borzillo GV, Ashmun RA, Sherr CJ: Macrophage lineage switching of murine early pre-B lymphoid cells expressing transduced fms genes. Mol Cell Biol 1990;10:2703.

246. Kato J-Y, Sherr CJ: Inhibition of granulocyte differentiation by G$_1$ cyclins D2 and D3 but not D1. Proc Natl Acad Sci U S A 1993;90:11513.

247. Metcalf D: Lineage commitment of hemopoietic progenitor cells in developing blast cell colonies: Influence of colony-stimulating factors. Proc Natl Acad Sci U S A 1991;88:11310.

248. Metcalf D: Lineage commitment in the progeny of murine hematopoietic preprogenitor cells: Influence of thrombopoietin and interleukin 5. Proc Natl Acad Sci U S A 1998;95:6408.

249. Metcalf D, Burgess AW: Clonal analysis of progenitor cell commitment to granulocyte or macrophage production. J Cell Physiol 1982;111:275.

250. Broxmeyer HE, Sherry B, Cooper S, et al: Comparative analysis of the human macrophage inflammatory protein family of cytokines (chemokines) on proliferation of human myeloid progenitor cells. J Immunol 1993;150:3448.

251. Keller JR, Jacobsen SEW, Dubois CM, et al: Transforming growth factor-β: A bidirectional regulator of hematopoietic cell growth. Int J Cell Cloning 1992;10:2.

252. Fukunaga R, Ishizaka-Ikeda E, Nagata S: Growth and differentiation signals mediated by different regions in the cytoplasmic domain of granulocyte colony-stimulating factor receptor. Cell 1993;74:1079.

253. Liboi E, Carroll M, D'Andrea AD, et al: Erythropoietin receptor signals both proliferation and erythroid-specific differentiation. Proc Natl Acad Sci U S A 1993;90:11351.

254. Fairbairn LJ, Cowling GJ, Reipert BM, et al: Suppression of apoptosis allows differentiation and development of a multipotent hemopoietic cell line in the absence of added growth factors. Cell 1993;74:823.

255. Chiba T, Nagata Y, Kishi A, et al: Induction of erythroid-specific gene expression in lymphoid cells. Proc Natl Acad Sci U S A 1993;90:11593.

256. Elefanty AG, Cory S: bcr-abl–Induced cell lines can switch from mast cell to erythroid or myeloid differentiation in vitro. Blood 1992;79:1271.

257. Klinken SP, Alexander WS, Adams JM: Hemopoietic lineage switch: v-raf oncogene converts Eμ-myc transgenic B cells into macrophages. Cell 1988;53:857.

258. Martin M, Strasser A, Baumgarth N, et al: A novel cellular model (SPGM 1) of switching between the pre-B cell and myelomonocytic lineages. J Immunol 1993;150:4395.

259. Broxmeyer HE, Sherry B, Lu L, et al: Enhancing and suppressing effects of recombinant murine macrophage inflammatory proteins on colony formation in vitro by bone marrow myeloid progenitor cells. Blood 1990;76:1110.

260. Hirayama F, Clark SC, Ogawa M: Negative regulation of early B lymphopoiesis by interleukin 3 and interleukin 1α. Proc Natl Acad Sci U S A 1994;91:469.

261. Metcalf D: Control of granulocytes and macrophages: Molecular, cellular, and clinical aspects. Science 1991;254:529.

262. Gearing DP, Ziegler SF: The hematopoietic growth factor receptor family. Curr Opin Hematol 1993;1:19.

263. Miyajima A, Mui ALF, Ogorochi T, et al: Receptors for granulocyte-macrophage colony-stimulating factor, interleukin-3, and interleukin-5. Blood 1993;82:1960.

264. Stahl N, Yancopoulos GD: The alphas, betas, and kinases of cytokine receptor complexes. Cell 1993;74:587.

265. Marshall CJ: Specificity of receptor tyrosine kinase signaling: Transient versus sustained extracellular signal–regulated kinase activation. Cell 1995;80:179.

266. Taniguchi T: Cytokine signaling through nonreceptor protein tyrosine kinases. Science 1995;268:251.

267. Weiss A, Schlessinger J: Switching signals on or off by receptor dimerization. Cell 1998;94:277.

268. Brandt J, Srour EF, van Besien K, et al: Cytokine-dependent long-term culture of highly enriched precursors of hematopoietic progenitor cells from human bone marrow. J Clin Invest 1990;86:932.

269. Flanagan JG, Chan DC, Leder P: Transmembrane form of the kit ligand growth factor is determined by alternative splicing and is missing in the Sl^d mutant. Cell 1991;64:1025.

270. Langley KE, Bennett LG, Wypych J, et al: Soluble stem cell factor in human serum. Blood 1993;81:656.

271. Gordon MY, Riley GP, Watt SM, et al: Compartmentalization of a haematopoietic growth factor (GM-CSF) by glycosaminoglycans in the bone marrow microenvironment. Nature 1987;326:403.

272. Roberts R, Gallagher J, Spooncer E, et al: Heparan sulphate bound growth factors: A mechanism for stromal cell mediated haemopoiesis. Nature 1988;332:376.

273. Rettenmier CW, Roussel MF, Ashmun RA, et al: Synthesis of membrane-bound colony-stimulating factor 1 (CSF-1) and downmodulation of CSF-1 receptors in NIH 3T3 cells transformed by cotransfection of the human CSF-1 and c-fms (CSF-1 receptor) genes. Mol Cell Biol 1987;7:2378.

274. Lyman SD, James L, Vanden Bos T, et al: Molecular cloning of a ligand for the flt3/flk-2 tyrosine kinase receptor: A proliferative factor for primitive hematopoietic cells. Cell 1993;75:1157.

275. Cairo MS, Suen Y, Sender L, et al: Circulating granulocyte colony-stimulating factor (G-CSF) levels after allogeneic and autologous bone marrow transplantation: Endogenous G-CSF production correlates with myeloid engraftment. Blood 1992;79:1869.

276. Yamasaki K, Solberg LA Jr, Jamal N, et al: Hemopoietic colony growth-promoting activities in the plasma of bone marrow transplant recipients. J Clin Invest 1988;82:255.

277. Singer JW, Nemunaitis J: Use of recombinant growth factors in bone marrow transplantation. In Forman SJ, Blume KG, Thomas ED, eds: Bone Marrow Transplantation. Boston: Blackwell; 1994, p 309.

278. Bernstein SE: Tissue transplantation as an analytic and therapeutic tool in hereditary anemias. Am J Surg 1970;119:448.

279. Gidali J, Lajtha LG: Regulation of haemopoietic stem cell turnover in partially irradiated mice. Cell Tissue Kinet 1972;5:147.

280. Andreoni C, Moreau I, Rigal D: Long-term culture of human bone marrow. I. Characterization of adherent cells in flow cytometry. Exp Hematol 1990;18:431.

281. Berneman ZN, Chen ZZ, Ramael M, et al: A quantitative and dynamic study of endothelial cells and megakaryocytes in human long-term bone marrow cultures. Leukemia 1989;3:61.

282. Simmons PJ, Przepiorka D, Thomas ED, et al: Host origin of marrow stromal cells following allogeneic bone marrow transplantation. Nature 1987;328:429.

283. Lichtman MA: The ultrastructure of the hemopoietic environment of the marrow: A review. Exp Hematol 1981;9:391.

284. Cashman JD, Eaves AC, Raines EW, et al: Mechanisms that regulate the cell cycle status of very primitive hematopoietic cells in long-term human marrow cultures. I. Stimulatory role of a variety of mesenchymal cell activators and inhibitory role of TGF-β. Blood 1990;75:96.

285. Eaves CJ, Cashman JD, Kay RJ, et al: Mechanisms that regulate the cell cycle status of very primitive hematopoietic cells in long-term human marrow cultures. II. Analysis of positive and negative regulators produced by stromal cells within the adherent layer. Blood 1991;78:110.

286. Cashman JD, Eaves CJ, Sarris AH, et al: MCP-1, not MIP-1α is the endogenous chemokine that cooperates with TGF-β to inhibit the cycling of primitive normal but not leukemic (CML) progenitors in long-term human marrow cultures. Blood 1998;92:2338.

287. Eaves CJ, Cashman JD, Wolpe SD, et al: Unresponsiveness of primitive chronic myeloid leukemia cells to macrophage inflammatory protein 1α, an inhibitor of primitive normal hematopoietic cells. Proc Natl Acad Sci U S A 1993;90:12015.

288. Sauvageau G, Thorsteinsdottir U, Eaves CJ, et al: Overexpression of HOXB4 in hematopoietic cells causes the selective expansion of more primitive populations in vitro and in vivo. Genes Dev 1995;9:1753.

289. Thorsteinsdottir U, Sauvageau G, Humphries RK: Enhanced in vivo regenerative potential of HOXB4-transduced hematopoietic stem cells with regulation of their pool size. Blood 1999;94:2605.

290. Golub TR, Slonim DK, Tamayo P, et al: Molecular classification of cancer: Class discovery and class prediction by gene expressing monitoring. Science 1999;286:531.

291. Kawagoe H, Humphries RK, Blair A, et al: Expression of HOX genes, HOX cofactors, and MLL in phenotypically and functionally defined subpopulations of leukemic and normal human hematopoietic cells. Leukemia 1999;13:687.

292. Purton LE, Bernstein ID, Collins SJ: All-trans retinoic acid enhances the long-term repopulating activity of cultured hematopoietic stem cells. Blood 2000;95:470.

293. Han W, Ye Q, Moore MA: A soluble form of human Delta-like-1 inhibits differentiation of hematopoietic progenitor cells. Blood 2000;95:1616.

294. Varnum-Finney B, Purton LE, Yu M, et al: The notch ligand, Jagged-1, influences the development of primitive hematopoietic precursor cells. Blood 1998;91:4084.

295. Carlesso N, Aster JC, Sklar J, et al: Notch1-induced delay of human hematopoietic progenitor cell differentiation is associated with altered cell cycle kinetics. Blood 1999;93:838.

296. Williams GT: Programmed cell death: Apoptosis and oncogenesis. Cell 1991;65:1097.

297. Williams GT, Smith CA: Molecular regulation of apoptosis: Genetic controls on cell death. Cell 1993;74:777.

298. Pawson T: Signal transduction—a conserved pathway from the membrane to the nucleus. Dev Genet 1993;14:333.

299. Brecher G, Cronkite EP: Post-radiation parabiosis and survival in rats. Proc Soc Exp Biol Med 1951;77:292.

300. Fujioka S, Hirashima K, Kumatori T, et al: Mechanism of hematopoietic recovery in the X-irradiated mouse with spleen or one leg shielded. Radiat Res 1967;31:826.

301. Hanks GE: In vivo migration of colony-forming units from shielded bone marrow in the irradiated mouse. Nature 1964;203:1393.

302. Van der Loo JCM, Ploemacher RE: Marrow- and spleen-seeding efficiencies of all murine hematopoietic stem cell subsets are decreased by preincubation with hematopoietic growth factors. Blood 1995;85:2598.

303. van Hennik PB, de Koning AE, Ploemacher RE: Seeding efficiency of primitive human hematopoietic cells in nonobese diabetic/severe combined immune deficiency mice: Implications for stem cell frequency assessment. Blood 1999;94:3055.

304. Arkin S, Naprstek B, Guarini L, et al: Expression of intercellular adhesion molecule-1 (CD54) on hematopoietic progenitors. Blood 1991;77:948.

305. Ghaffari S, Dougherty GJ, Lansdorp PM, et al: Differentiation-associated changes in CD44 isoform expression during normal hematopoiesis and their alteration in chronic myeloid leukemia. Blood 1995;86:2976.

306. Lewinsohn DM, Nagler A, Ginzton N, et al: Hematopoietic progeni-

tor cell expression of the H-CAM (CD44) homing-associated adhesion molecule. Blood 1990;75:589.

307. Simmons PJ, Masinovsky B, Longenecker BM, et al: Vascular cell adhesion molecule-1 expressed by bone marrow stromal cells mediates the binding of hematopoietic progenitor cells. Blood 1992;80:388.

308. van der Loo JC, Xiao X, McMillin D, et al: VLA-5 is expressed by mouse and human long-term repopulating hematopoietic cells and mediates adhesion to extracellular matrix protein fibronectin. J Clin Invest 1998;102:1051.

309. Peled A, Petit I, Kollet O, et al: Dependence of human stem cell engraftment and repopulation of NOD/SCID mice on CXCR4. Science 1999;283:845.

310. Craddock CF, Nakamoto B, Andrews RG, et al: Antibodies to VLA4 integrin mobilize long-term repopulating cells and augment cytokine-induced mobilization in primates and mice. Blood 1997;90:4779.

311. Papayannopoulou T, Nakamoto B: Peripheralization of hemopoietic progenitors in primates treated with anti-VLA₄ integrin. Proc Natl Acad Sci U S A 1993;90:9374.

312. Potocnik AJ, Brakebusch C, Fassler R: Fetal and adult hematopoietic stem cells require beta-l integrin function for colonizing fetal liver, spleen, and bone marrow. Immunity 2000;12:653.

313. Williams DA, Rios M, Stephens C, et al: Fibronectin and VLA-4 in haematopoietic stem cell–microenvironment interactions. Nature 1991;352:438.

314. Zanjani ED, Flake AW, Almeida-Porada G, et al: Homing of human cells in the fetal sheep model: Modulation by antibodies activating or inhibiting very late activation antigen-4–dependent function. Blood 1999;94:2515.

315. Barnes DWH, Loutit JF: Effects of irradiation and antigenic stimulation on circulating haemopoietic stem cells of the mouse. Nature 1967;213:1142.

316. Cline MJ, Golde DW: Mobilization of hematopoietic stem cells (CFU-C) into the peripheral blood of man by endotoxin. Exp Hematol 1977;5:186.

317. Pettengel R, Testa NG, Swindell R, et al: Transplantation potential of hematopoietic cells released into the circulation during routine chemotherapy for non-Hodgkin's lymphoma. Blood 1993;82:2239.

318. Richman CM, Weiner RS, Yankee RA: Increase in circulating stem cells following chemotherapy in man. Blood 1977;47:1031.

319. Sutherland HJ, Eaves CJ, Lansdorp PM, et al: Kinetics of committed and primitive blood progenitor mobilization after chemotherapy and growth factor treatment and their use in autotransplants. Blood 1994;83:3808.

320. To LB, Haylock DN, Thorp D, et al: The optimization of collection of peripheral blood stem cells for autotransplantation in acute myeloid leukaemia. Bone Marrow Transplant 1989;4:41.

321. Sheridan WP, Begley CG, Juttner CA, et al: Effect of peripheral-blood progenitor cells mobilised by filgrastim (G-CSF) on platelet recovery after high-dose chemotherapy. Lancet 1992;339:640.

322. Siena S, Bregni M, Bonsi L, et al: Increase in peripheral blood megakaryocyte progenitors following cancer therapy with high-dose cyclophosphamide and hematopoietic growth factors. Exp Hematol 1993;21:1583.

323. Socinski MA, Cannistra SA, Elias A, et al: Granulocyte-macrophage colony stimulating factor expands the circulating haemopoietic progenitor cell compartment in man. Lancet 1988;1:1194.

324. Griffin JD, Spertini O, Ernst TJ, et al: Granulocyte-macrophage colony stimulating factor and other cytokines regulate surface expression of the leukocyte adhesion molecule-1 on human neutrophils, monocytes, and their precursors. J Immunol 1990;145:576.

325. Ohsaka A, Saionji K, Sato N, et al: Granulocyte colony-stimulating factor down-regulates the surface expression of the human leucocyte adhesion molecule-1 on human neutrophils in vitro and in vivo. Br J Haematol 1993;84:574.

326. Socinski MA, Cannistra SA, Sullivan R, et al: Granulocyte-macrophage colony-stimulating factor induces the expression of the CD11b surface adhesion molecule on human granulocytes in vivo. Blood 1988;72:691.

327. Eaves CJ, Eaves AC: Cell culture studies in CML. In Hinton K, ed: Bailliere's Clinical Haematology. London: Bailliere Tindall/WB Saunders; 1987, p 931.

328. Minden MD, Buick RN, McCulloch EA: Separation of blast cell and

T-lymphocyte progenitors in the blood of patients with acute myeloblastic leukemia. Blood 1979;54:186.

329. Jiang X, Lopez A, Holyoake T, et al: Autocrine production and action of IL-3 and granulocyte colony-stimulating factor in chronic myeloid leukemia. Proc Natl Acad Sci U S A 1999;96:12804.

330. Carella AM, Simonsson B, Link H, et al: Mobilization of Philadelphia-negative peripheral blood progenitor cells with chemotherapy and rhuG-CSF in chronic myelogenous leukaemia patients with a poor response to interferon-alpha. Br J Haematol 1998; 101:111.

331. Klingemann H-G, Eaves CJ, Barnett MJ, et al: Transplantation of patients with high risk acute myeloid leukemia in first remission with autologous marrow cultured in interleukin-2 followed by interleukin-2 administration. Bone Marrow Transplant 1994;14: 389.

332. To LB, Haylock DN, Simmons PJ, et al: The biology and clinical uses of blood stem cells. Blood 1997;89:2233.

333. Bradford GB, Williams B, Rossi R, et al: Quiescence, cycling, and turnover in the primitive hematopoietic stem cell compartment. Exp Hematol 1997;25:445.

334. Rufer N, Brummendorf TH, Kolvraa S, et al: Telomere fluorescence measurements in granulocytes and T lymphocyte subsets point to a high turnover of hematopoietic stem cells and memory T cells in early childhood. J Exp Med 1999;190:157.

335. Brummendorf TH, Holyoake TL, Rufer N, et al: Prognostic implications of differences in telomere length between normal and malignant cells from patients with chronic myeloid leukemia measured by flow cytometry. Blood 2000;95:1883.

336. Notaro R, Cimmino A, Tabarini D, et al: In vivo telomere dynamics of human hematopoietic stem cells. Proc Natl Acad Sci U S A 1997;94:13782.

337. Wynn RF, Cross MA, Hatton C, et al: Accelerated telomere shortening in young recipients of allogeneic bone-marrow transplants. Lancet 1998;351:178.

338. Cachia PG, Culligan DJ, Clark RE, et al: Clonal haemopoiesis following cytotoxic therapy for lymphoma. Leukemia 1993;7:795.

339. Bjornson CRR, Rietze RL, Reynolds BA, et al: Turning brain into blood: A hematopoietic fate adopted by adult neural stem cells in vivo. Science 1999;283:534.

340. Clarke DL, Johansson CB, Wilbertz J, et al: Generalized potential of adult neural stem cells. Science 2000;288:1660.

341. Eglitis MA, Mezey E: Hematopoietic cells differentiate into both microglia and macroglia in the brains of adult mice. Proc Natl Acad Sci U S A 1997;94:4080.

342. Kopen GC, Prockop DJ, Phinney DG: Marrow stromal cells migrate throughout forebrain and cerebellum, and they differentiate into astrocytes after injection into neonatal mouse brains. Proc Natl Acad Sci U S A 2000;96:10711.

343. Shi Q, Rafii S, Wu MH-D, et al: Evidence for circulating bone marrow-derived endothelial cells. Blood 1998;92:362.

344. Ferrari G, Cusella-De Angelis G, Coletta M, et al: Muscle regeneration by bone marrow-derived myogenic progenitors. Science 1998;279:1528.

345. Horwitz EM, Prockop DJ, Fitzpatrick LA, et al: Transplantability and therapeutic effects of bone marrow-derived mesenchymal cells in children with osteogenesis imperfecta. Nat Med 1999; 5:309.

346. Pereira RF, Halford KW, O'Hara MD, et al: Cultured adherent cells from marrow can serve as long-lasting precursor cells for bone, cartilage, and lung in irradiated mice. Proc Natl Acad Sci U S A 1995;92:4857.

347. Petersen BE, Bowen WC, Patrene KD, et al: Bone marrow as a potential source of hepatic oval cells. Science 1999;284:1168.

348. Taniguchi H, Toyoshima T, Fukao K, et al: Presence of hematopoietic stem cells in the adult liver. Nat Med 1996;2:198.

349. Eaves AC, Krystal G, Cashman JD, et al: Polycythemia vera: In vitro analysis of regulatory defects. In Zanjani ED, Tavassoli M, Ascensao JL, eds: Regulation of Erythropoiesis. New York: PMA Publishing; 1988, p 523.

350. Prchal JF, Axelrad AA: Bone marrow responses in polycythemia vera. N Engl J Med 1974;290:1382.

351. Dai CH, Krantz SB, Dessypris EN, et al: Polycythemia vera. II. Hypersensitivity of bone marrow erythroid, granulocyte-macrophage, and megakaryocyte progenitor cells to interleukin-3 and granulocyte-macrophage colony-stimulating factor. Blood 1992; 80:891.

352. Correa PN, Eskinazi D, Axelrad AA: Circulating erythroid progenitors in polycythemia vera are hypersensitive to insulin-like growth factor-1 in vitro: Studies in an improved serum-free medium. Blood 1994;83:99.

353. Eaves AC, Henkelman DH, Eaves CJ: Abnormal erythropoiesis in the myeloproliferative disorders: An analysis of underlying cellular and humoral mechanisms. Exp Hematol 1980;8:235.

354. Turhan AG, Cashman JD, Eaves CJ, et al: Variable expression of features of normal and neoplastic stem cells in patients with thrombocytosis. Br J Haematol 1992;82:50.

355. Afar DEH, Goga A, McLaughlin J, et al: Differential complementation of Bcr-Abl point mutants with c-Myc. Science 1994;264:424.

356. Groffen J, Heisterkamp N: The BCR/ABL hybrid gene. In Hinton K, ed: Balliere's Clinical Haematology. London: Bailliere Tindall/ WB Saunders; 1987, p 983.

357. Pendergast AM, Quilliam LA, Cripe LD, et al: BCR-ABL-induced oncogenesis is mediated by direct interaction with the SH2 domain of the GRB-2 adaptor protein. Cell 1993;75:175.

358. Sattler M, Salgia R: Activation of hematopoietic growth factor signal transduction pathways by the human oncogene BCR/ABL. Cytokine Growth Factor Rev 1997;8:63.

359. Sawyers CL: Chronic myeloid leukemia. N Engl J Med 1999;340: 1330.

360. Cashman JD, Eaves AC, Eaves CJ: Granulocyte-macrophage colony-stimulating factor modulation of the inhibitory effect of transforming growth factor-β on normal and leukemic human hematopoietic progenitor cells. Leukemia 1992;6:886.

361. Nara N, McCulloch EA: The proliferation in suspension of the progenitors of the blast cells in acute myeloblastic leukemia. Blood 1985;65:1484.

362. Oster W, Mertelsmann R, Herrmann F: Role of colony-stimulating factors in the biology of acute myelogenous leukemia. Int J Cell Cloning 1989;7:13.

363. Young DC, Griffin JD: Autocrine secretion of GM-CSF in acute myeloblastic leukemia. Blood 1986;68:1178.

364. Wickremasinghe RG, Hoffbrand AV: Biochemical and genetic control of apoptosis: Relevance to normal hematopoiesis and hematological malignancies. Blood 1999;93:3587.

365. Broxmeyer HE, Douglas GW, Hangoc G, et al: Human umbilical cord blood as a potential source of transplantable hematopoietic stem/progenitor cells. Proc Natl Acad Sci U S A 1989;86:3828.

366. Gluckman E, Broxmeyer HE, Auerbach AD, et al: Hematopoietic reconstitution in a patient with Fanconi's anemia by means of umbilical-cord blood from an HLA-identical sibling. N Engl J Med 1989;321:1174.

367. Gluckman E, Rocha V, Boyer-Chammard A, et al: Outcome of cord-blood transplantation from related and unrelated donors. N Engl J Med 1997;337:373.

368. Rubinstein P, Carrier C, Scaradavou A, et al: Outcomes among 562 recipients of placental-blood transplants from unrelated donors. N Engl J Med 1998;339:1565.

369. Shizuru JA, Jerabek L, Edwards CT, et al: Transplantation of purified hematopoietic stem cells: Requirements for overcoming the barriers of allogeneic engraftment. Biol Blood Marrow Transplant 1996;2:3.

370. Berenson RJ, Bensinger WI, Hill RS, et al: Engraftment after infusion of CD34$^+$ marrow cells in patients with breast cancer or neuroblastoma. Blood 1991;77:1717.

371. Coulombel L, Eaves C, Kalousek D, et al: Long-term marrow culture of cells from patients with acute myelogenous leukemia. Selection in favor of normal phenotypes in some but not all cases. J Clin Invest 1985;75:961.

372. Coulombel L, Kalousek DK, Eaves CJ, et al: Long-term marrow culture reveals chromosomally normal hematopoietic progenitor cells in patients with Philadelphia chromosome-positive chronic myelogenous leukemia. N Engl J Med 1983;308:1493.

373. Eaves C, Udomsakdi C, Cashman J, et al: The biology of normal and neoplastic stem cells in CML. Leuk Lymphoma 1993;11:245.

374. Barnett MJ, Eaves CJ, Phillips GL, et al: Successful autografting in chronic myeloid leukaemia after maintenance of marrow in culture. Bone Marrow Transplant 1989;4:345.

375. Klingemann HG, Deal H, Reid D, et al: Design and validation of a clinically applicable culture procedure for the generation of interleukin-2 activated natural killer cells in human bone marrow autografts. Exp Hematol 1993;21:1263.

376. Yeager AM, Kaizer H, Santos GW, et al: Autologous bone marrow transplantation in patients with acute nonlymphocytic leukemia, using ex vivo marrow treatment with 4-hydroperoxycyclophosphamide. N Engl J Med 1986;315:141.

377. Gribben JG, Freedman AS, Neuberg D, et al: Immunologic purging of marrow assessed by PCR before autologous bone marrow transplantation for B-cell lymphoma. N Engl J Med 1991;325:1525.

378. Negrin RS, Atkinson K, Leemhuis T, et al: Transplantation of highly purified CD34$^+$ Thy-1$^+$ hematopoietic stem cells in patients with metastatic breast cancer. Biol Blood Marrow Transplant 2000; 6:262.

379. Shpall EJ, Jones RB, Bearman SI, et al: Transplantation of enriched CD34-positive autologous marrow into breast cancer patients following high-dose chemotherapy: Influence of CD34-positive peripheral blood progenitors and growth factors on engraftment. J Clin Oncol 1994;12:28.

380. Graw RG Jr, Buckner CD, Whang-Peng J, et al: Complication of bone-marrow transplantation: Graft-versus-host disease resulting from chronic-myelogenous-leukaemia leucocyte transfusions. Lancet 1970;2:338.

381. Niederwieser DW, Appelbaum FR, Gastl G, et al: Inadvertent transmission of a donor's acute myeloid leukemia in bone marrow transplantation for chronic myelocytic leukemia. N Engl J Med 1990;322:1794.

382. Brenner MK, Rill DR, Moen RC, et al: Gene-marking to trace origin of relapse after autologous bone-marrow transplantation. Lancet 1993;341:85.

383. Deisseroth AB, Zu Z, Claxton D, et al: Genetic marking shows that Ph$^+$ cells present in autologous transplants of chronic myelogenous leukemia (CML) contribute to relapse after autologous bone marrow in CML. Blood 1994;83:3068.

384. Scheding S, Kratz-Albers K, Meister B, et al: Ex vivo expansion of hematopoietic progenitor cells for clinical use. Semin Hematol 1998;35:232.

385. Williams DA: Ex vivo expansion of hematopoietic stem and progenitor cells—robbing Peter to pay Paul? Blood 1993;81:3169.

386. Zandstra PW, Eaves CJ, Piret JM: Environmental requirements of hematopoietic progenitor cells in ex vivo expansion systems. In Nordon R, Schindhelm K, eds: Ex Vivo Cell Therapy. Georgetown, TX: Landes Bioscience; 1999, p 245.

387. Bodine DM, Karlsson S, Nienhuis AW: Combination of interleukin 3 and 6 preserves stem cell function in culture and enhances retrovirus-mediated gene transfer into hematopoietic stem cells. Proc Natl Acad Sci U S A 1989;86:8897.

388. Brandt J, Briddell RA, Srour EF, et al: Role of c-kit ligand in the expansion of human hematopoietic progenitor cells. Blood 1992; 79:634.

389. Brugger W, Mocklin W, Heimfeld S, et al: Ex vivo expansion of enriched peripheral blood CD34$^+$ progenitor cells by stem cell factor, interleukin-1β (IL-β), IL-6, IL-3, interferon-γ, and erythropoietin. Blood 1993;81:2579.

390. Haylock DN, To LB, Dowse TL, et al: Ex vivo expansion and maturation of peripheral blood CD34$^+$ cells into the myeloid lineage. Blood 1992;80:1405.

391. Paul SR, Yang YC, Donahue RE, et al: Stromal cell–associated hematopoiesis: Immortalization and characterization of a primate bone marrow–derived stromal cell line. Blood 1991;77:1723.

392. Lansdorp PM, Dragowska W: Long-term erythropoiesis from constant numbers of CD34+ cells in serum-free cultures initiated with highly purified progenitor cells from human bone marrow. J Exp Med 1992;175:1501.

393. Migliaccio G, Migliaccio AR, Druzin ML, et al: Long-term generation of colony-forming cells in liquid culture of CD34$^+$ cord blood cells in the presence of recombinant human stem cell factor. Blood 1992;79:2620.

394. Caldwell J, Palsson BO, Locey B, et al: Culture perfusion schedules influence the metabolic activity and granulocyte-macrophage colony-stimulating factor production rates of human bone marrow stromal cells. J Cell Physiol 1991;147:344.

395. Koller MR, Emerson SG, Palsson BO: Large-scale expansion of human stem and progenitor cells from bone marrow mononuclear cells in continuous perfusion cultures. Blood 1993;82:378.

396. Schwartz RM, Palsson BO, Emerson SG: Rapid medium perfusion rate significantly increases the productivity and longevity of human bone marrow cultures. Proc Natl Acad Sci U S A 1991; 88:6760.

397. Zandstra PW, Petzer AL, Eaves CJ, et al: Cellular determinants affecting the rate of cytokine depletion in cultures of human hematopoietic cells. Biotechnol Bioeng 1997;54:58.

398. Dao MA, Hannum CH, Kohn DB, et al: Flt3 ligand preserves the ability of human CD34$^+$ progenitors to sustain long-term hematopoiesis in immune-deficient mice after ex-vivo retroviral-mediated transduction. Blood 1997;89:446.

399. Holyoake TL, Freshney MG, McNair L, et al: Ex vivo expansion with stem cell factor and interleukin-11 augments both short-term recovery posttransplant and the ability to serially transplant marrow. Blood 1996;87:4589.

400. Nordon RE, Ginsberg SS, Eaves CJ: High resolution cell division tracking demonstrates the Flt3-ligand-dependence of human marrow CD34$^+$ CD38$^-$ cell production in vitro. Br J Haematol 1997; 98:528.

401. Petzer AL, Zandstra PW, Piret JM, et al: Differential cytokine effects on primitive (CD34$^+$CD38$^-$) human hematopoietic cells: Novel responses to flt3-ligand and thrombopoietin. J Exp Med 1996; 183:2551.

402. Shah AJ, Smogorzewska EM, Hannum C, et al: Flt3 ligand induces proliferation of quiescent human bone marrow CD34$^+$ CD38$^-$ cells and maintains progenitor cells in vitro. Blood 1996;87:3563.

403. Yonemura Y, Ku H, Hirayama F, et al: Interleukin 3 or interleukin 1 abrogates the reconstituting ability of hematopoietic stem cells. Proc Natl Acad Sci U S A 1996;93:4040.

404. Yonemura Y, Ku H, Lyman SD, et al: In vitro expansion of hematopoietic progenitors and maintenance of stem cells: Comparison between Flt3/Flk-2 ligand and kit ligand. Blood 1997;89:1915.

405. Rebel VI, Lansdorp PM: Culture of purified stem cells from fetal liver results in loss of in vivo repopulating potential. J Hematother 1996;5:25.

406. Zandstra PW, Conneally E, Piret JM, et al: Ontogeny-associated changes in the cytokine responses of primitive human haematopoietic cells. Br J Haematol 1998;101:770.

407. Bhatia M, Bonnet D, Kapp U, et al: Quantitative analysis reveals expansion of human hematopoietic repopulating cells after short-term ex vivo culture. J Exp Med 1997;186:619.

408. Matsunaga T, Kato T, Miyazaki H, et al: Thrombopoietin promotes the survival of murine hematopoietic long-term reconstituting cells: Comparison with the effects of FLT3/FLK-2 ligand and interleukin-6. Blood 1998;92:452.

409. Miller CL, Eaves CJ: Expansion in vitro of adult murine hematopoietic stem cells with transplantable lympho-myeloid reconstituting ability. Proc Natl Acad Sci U S A 1997;94:13648.

410. Piacibello W, Sanavio F, Severino A, et al: Engraftment in nonobese diabetic severe combined immunodeficient mice of human CD34$^+$ cord blood cells after ex vivo expansion: Evidence for the amplification and self-renewal of repopulating stem cells. Blood 1999; 93:3736.

411. Eaves C, Miller C, Conneally E, et al: Introduction to stem cell biology in vitro: Threshold to the future. Ann N Y Acad Sci 1999; 872:1.

412. Pawliuk R, Eaves C, Humphries RK: Evidence of both ontogeny and transplant dose-regulated expansion of hematopoietic stem cells in vivo. Blood 1996;88:2852.

413. Oostendorp RAJ, Audet J, Eaves CJ: High-resolution tracking of cell division suggests similar cell cycle kinetics of hematopoietic stem cells stimulated in vitro and in vivo. Blood 2000;95:855.

414. Young JC, Lin K, Hansteen G, et al: CD34$^+$ cells from mobilized peripheral blood retain fetal bone marrow repopulating capacity within the Thy-1$^+$ subset following cell division ex vivo. Exp Hematol 1999;27:994.

415. Glimm H, Eisterer W, Lee K, et al: Distinct and previously undetected human hematopoietic cell populations with short term repopulating activity selectively engraft NOD/SCID–β$_2$ microglobulin–null mice. J Clin Invest 2001;107:199.

416. Uchida N, Aguila HL, Fleming WH, et al: Rapid and sustained hematopoietic recovery in lethally irradiated mice transplanted with purified Thy-1.1^{lo} Lin$^-$ Sca-1$^+$ hematopoietic stem cells. Blood 1994;83:3758.

417. Zijlmans JMJM, Visser JWM, Later Veer L, et al: The early phase of engraftment after murine blood cell transplantation is mediated by hematopoietic stem cells. Proc Natl Acad Sci U S A 1998; 95:725.

418. Szilvassy SJ, Weller KP, Chen B, et al: Partially differentiated ex

vivo expanded cells accelerate hematologic recovery in mye-loablated mice transplanted with highly enriched long-term repop-ulating stem cells. Blood 1996;88:3642.

419. Petz LD, Yam P, Wallace RB, et al: Mixed hematopoietic chimerism following bone marrow transplantation for hematologic malignan-cies. Blood 1987;70:1331.

420. Kogler G, Nurnberger W, Fischer J, et al: Simultaneous cord blood transplantation of ex vivo expanded together with non-expanded cells for high risk leukemia. Bone Marrow Transplant 1999;24:397.

421. McNiece I, Jones R, Cagnoni P, et al: Ex vivo expansion of hemato-poietic cells. In Ikeda Y, Hata J-I, Koyasu S, et al, eds: Cell Therapy. Hong Kong: Springer-Verlag; 2000, p 171.

422. Joyner A, Keller G, Phillips RA, et al: Retrovirus transfer of a bacterial gene into mouse haematopoietic progenitor cells. Nature 1983;305:556.

423. Gruber HE, Finley KD, Hershberg RM, et al: Retroviral vector-mediated gene transfer into human hematopoietic progenitor cells. Science 1985;230:1057.

424. Hogge DE, Humphries RK: Gene transfer to primary normal and malignant human hemopoietic progenitors using recombinant re-troviruses. Blood 1987;69:611.

425. Hughes PFD, Thacker JD, Hogge D, et al: Retroviral gene transfer to primitive normal and leukemic hematopoietic cells using clini-cally applicable procedures. J Clin Invest 1992;89:1817.

426. Kantoff PW, Gillio AP, McLachlin JR, et al: Expression of human adenosine deaminase in nonhuman primates after retrovirus-medi-ated gene transfer. J Exp Med 1987;166:219.

427. Brenner MK, Rill DR, Holladay MS, et al: Gene marking to deter-mine whether autologous marrow infusion restores long-term haemopoiesis in cancer patients. Lancet 1993;342:1134.

428. Dunbar CE, Cottler-Fox M, O'Shaughnessy JA, et al: Retrovirally marked CD34-enriched peripheral blood and bone marrow cells contribute to long-term engraftment after autologous transplanta-tion. Blood 1995;85:3048.

429. Kaptein LCM, van Beusechem VW, Riviere I, et al: Long-term in vivo expression of the MFG-ADA retroviral vector in rhesus mon-keys transplanted with transduced bone marrow cells. Hum Gene Ther 2000;8:1605.

430. Kiem H-P, Heyward S, Winkler A, et al: Gene transfer into marrow repopulating cells: Comparison between amphotropic and gibbon ape leukemia virus pseudotyped retroviral vectors in a competitive repopulation assay in baboons. Blood 1997;90:4638.

431. Larochelle A, Vormoor J, Hanenberg H, et al: Identification of primitive human hematopoietic cells capable of repopulating NOD/SCID mouse bone marrow: Implications for gene therapy. Nat Med 1996;2:1329.

432. Hanenberg H, Hashino K, Konishi H, et al: Optimization of fibro-nectin-assisted retroviral gene transfer into human CD34$^+$ hemato-poietic cells. Hum Gene Ther 1997;8:2193.

433. Miller DG, Adam MM, Miller AD: Gene transfer by retrovirus occurs only in cells that are actively replicating at time of infec-tion. Mol Cell Biol 1990;10:4239.

434. Crooks GM, Kohn DB: Growth factors increase amphotropic retro-virus binding to human CD34$^+$ bone marrow progenitor cells. Blood 1993;82:3290.

435. Hennemann B, Oh I-H, Chuo JY, et al: Efficient retrovirus-mediated gene transfer to transplantable human bone marrow cells in the absence of fibronectin. Blood 2000;96:2432.

436. Macdonald C, Walker S, Watts M, et al: Effect of changes in expression of the amphotropic retroviral receptor PiT-2 on trans-duction efficiency and viral titer: Implications for gene therapy. Hum Gene Ther 2000;11:587.

437. Orlic D, Girard LJ, Jordan CT, et al: The level of mRNA encoding the amphotropic retrovirus receptor in mouse and human hemato-poietic stem cells is low and correlates with the efficiency of retrovirus transduction. Proc Natl Acad Sci U S A 1996;93:11097.

438. Hanenberg H, Xiao XL, Dilloo D, et al: Colocalization of retrovirus and target cells on specific fibronectin fragments increases genetic transduction of mammalian cells. Nat Med 1996;2:876.

439. Moritz T, Patel VP, Williams DA: Bone marrow extracellular matrix molecules improve gene transfer into human hematopoietic cells via retroviral vectors. J Clin Invest 1994;93:1451.

440. Hennemann B, Chuo JY, Schley PD, et al: High-efficiency retroviral transduction of mammalian cells on positively charged surfaces. Hum Gene Ther 2000;11:43.

441. Flasshove M, Banerjee D, Mineishi S, et al: Ex vivo expansion and selection of human CD34$^+$ peripheral blood progenitor cells after introduction of a mutated dihydrofolate reductase cDNA via ret-roviral gene transfer. Blood 1995;85:566.

442. Hennemann B, Conneally E, Pawliuk R, et al: Optimization of retroviral-mediated gene transfer to human NOD/SCID mouse re-populating cord blood cells through a systematic analysis of proto-col variables. Exp Hematol 1999;27:817.

443. Marandin A, Dubart A, Pflumio F, et al: Retrovirus-mediated gene transfer into human CD34$^+$38^{low} primitive cells capable of recon-stituting long-term cultures in vitro and nonobese diabetic–severe combined immunodeficiency mice in vivo. Hum Gene Ther 1998; 9:1497.

444. Plavec I, Voytovich A, Moss K, et al: Sustained retroviral gene marking and expression in lymphoid and myeloid cells derived from transduced hematopoietic progenitor cells. Gene Ther 1996; 3:717.

445. Schilz AJ, Brouns G, Knöss H, et al: High efficiency gene transfer to human hematopoietic SCID-repopulating cells under serum-free conditions. Blood 1998;92:3163.

446. van Hennik PB, Verstegen MMA, Bierhuizen MFA, et al: Highly efficient transduction of the green fluorescent protein gene in human umbilical cord blood stem cells capable of cobblestone formation in long-term cultures and multilineage engraftment of immunodeficient mice. Blood 1998;92:4013.

447. Cavazzana-Calvo M, Hacein-Bey S, de Saint BG, et al: Gene therapy of human severe combined immunodeficiency (SCID)-X1 disease. Science 2000;288:669.

448. Abonour R, Williams DA, Einhorn L, et al: Efficient retrovirus-mediated transfer of the multidrug resistance 1 gene into autolo-gous human long-term repopulating hematopoietic stem cells. Nat Med 2000;6:652.

449. Kohn DB, Weinberg KI, Nolta JA, et al: Engraftment of gene-modified umbilical cord blood cells in neonates with adenosine deaminase deficiency. Nat Med 1995;1:1017.

450. Kelly PF, Vandergriff J, Nathwani A, et al: Highly efficient gene transfer into cord blood nonobese diabetic/severe combined im-munodeficiency repopulating cells by oncoretroviral vector parti-cles pseudotyped with the feline endogenous retrovirus (RD114) envelope protein. Blood 2000;96:1206.

451. Rebel VI, Tanaka M, Lee J-S, et al: One-day ex vivo culture allows effective gene transfer into human nonobese diabetic/severe com-bined immune-deficient repopulating cells using high titer vesicu-lar stomatitis virus G protein pseudotyped retrovirus. Blood 1999; 93:2217.

452. Case SS, Price MA, Jordan CT, et al: Stable transduction of quies-cent CD34$^+$CD38$^-$ human hematopoietic cells by HIV-1–based lentiviral vectors. Proc Natl Acad Sci U S A 1999;96:2988.

453. Miyoshi H, Smith KA, Mosier DE, et al: Transduction of human CD34$^+$ cells that mediate long-term engraftment of NOD/SCID mice by HIV vectors. Science 1999;283:682.

454. Eaves C, Cashman J, Eaves A: Defective regulation of leukemic hematopoiesis in chronic myeloid leukemia. Leuk Res 1998;22: 1085.

4

Dario Campana   Tucker W. LeBien

Lymphopoiesis*

INTRODUCTION

The mammalian immune system comprises three main populations of lymphocytes: B cells, T cells, and natural killer (NK) cells. Circulating B and T cells are morphologically identical and appear as small lymphocytes with no cytoplasmic granules, whereas most mature NK cells are larger, display cytoplasmic azurophilic granules, and are referred to as "large granular lymphocytes." The structure of lymphoid progenitors in the central lymphoid organs (i.e., fetal liver, bone marrow, and thymus) is heterogeneous and largely depends on the proliferative status of the cells. The structure ranges from that of a small lymphocyte to that of large cells with basophilic cytoplasm, fine chromatin, and multiple nucleoli. Immature and mature B, T, and NK cells express an array of surface and intracellular markers that allow their recognition, the assessment of their degree of maturation, and the identification of functionally distinct subsets. B cells recognize antigens through surface immunoglobulins (Ig) and T cells through surface T-cell receptors (TCR). NK cells express inhibitory receptors that recognize major histocompatibility complex (MHC) class I molecules and prevent the killing of healthy autologous cells. The hallmark of B-cell commitment is the rearrangement of Ig genes; that of T-cell commitment is the rearrangement of TCR genes. Neither set of genes is rearranged in NK cells.

Lymphoid leukemia results from the neoplastic clonal proliferation of lymphoid cells at different stages of maturation. Acute lymphoid leukemias are largely characterized by the immunophenotypic and antigen-receptor gene configuration of immature B or T cells; chronic leukemias and lymphoproliferative disorders appear to originate from mature lymphoid cells.[1] Although the morphologic and immunophenotypic features of leukemic cells generally resemble those of their normal counterparts, there are substantial differences. In addition to the genetic abnormalities associated with leukemogenesis (e.g., chromosomal translocations and gene fusions),[2] leukemic cells often express cell markers in combinations that are not found during normal lymphopoiesis; these

aberrant immunophenotypes can be exploited to monitor response to treatment and track residual leukemic cells in patients.[3] Moreover, the growth requirements and response to stimuli of leukemic cells are often markedly different than those of their normal counterparts.[4-6]

ONTOGENY OF LYMPHOID LINEAGES

Lymphoid Differentiation of Hematopoietic Stem Cells

The ontogeny of B, T, and NK cells is initiated by a putative common progenitor that ultimately differentiates into mature effector populations. The potential for multilineage differentiation is inherent to the definition of a stem cell, and experimental evidence of a hematopoietic stem cell with the capacity to differentiate into distinct lineages has been available for at least four decades.[7, 8] Studies employing transfected selectable genes have been instructive in defining ontogenic relationships between stem cells capable of engraftment and cells committed to the lymphoid lineages.[9-11] Studies of leukemia and myeloproliferative disorders have corroborated the notion of common hematopoietic stem cells. Thus, clonal analysis in chronic myelogenous leukemia has shown that the neoplastic process involves most hematopoietic lineages, including B lymphocytes.[12, 13] A proportion of blast crises of this disease resembles the proliferation of immature lymphoid cells and retains the multilineage genetic lesion, i.e., t(9;22)(q34;q11).[14-16] In idiopathic myelofibrosis, identical *N-ras* mutations were found in granulocytes, monocytes, and erythroblasts as well as in B and T lymphocytes.[17]

The immunophenotypic characterization of different subsets of lymphohematopoietic progenitors and their enrichment to a high degree of purity have clarified some aspects of lymphoid differentiation. Murine Thy-1^{low} Sca-1$^+$ cells that lack lineage-specific markers (Lin$^-$) represent less than 0.05% of adult mouse bone marrow cells but can repopulate the entire lymphohematopoietic system, including B and T lineages; injection of as few as 100 cells of this phenotype is sufficient to fully reconstitute the hematopoietic system of irradiated animals.[18, 19] An equally rare subset of human fetal bone marrow cells

* This work was supported by grants R01-CA58297, R01-CA31685, and P30-CA21765 from the National Cancer Institute, by the Apogee Enterprises Professorship in Cancer Research, and by the American Lebanese Syrian Associated Charities (ALSAC).

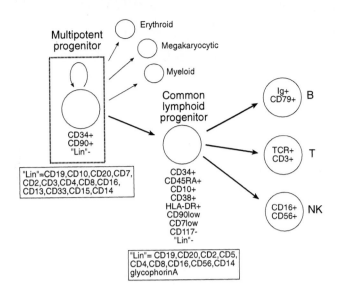

FIGURE 4–1. Proposed immunophenotypic features of human stem cells and common lymphoid progenitors.[20, 24] Lin = "lineage-associated markers." The definition of "Lin⁻" varies between different laboratories.

expressing CD34, CD90 (human Thy1) but lacking several lineage-associated markers can establish myelomonocytic and B-lymphoid cultures on mouse marrow stromal lines and can differentiate into T lymphocytes when placed in human fetal thymi transplanted into mice with severe combined immunodeficiency (SCID) (Fig. 4–1).[20] The subset of these cells that retains little of the fluorescent mitochondrial dye rhodamine 123 reportedly contains virtually all the cells that establish long-term cultures.[20] These results indicate either that cells of different lineages arise from a common CD34⁺CD90⁺Lin⁻ progenitor or that already committed progenitors of different lineages express homogeneous immunophenotypic features.

The existence of cells that have multilineage differentiation potential and can be isolated from human bone marrow has been demonstrated by limiting dilution and single cell sorting experiments. Plating human CD34⁺Lin⁻ cells on stroma under limiting dilution conditions led to the appearance of CD33⁺ myeloid and CD19⁺ B-lineage cells after 4 to 6 weeks of culture,[20] whereas single CD34⁺CD38⁻HLA-DR⁺ cells, when plated in a cytokine cocktail consisting of IL-3, IL-6, stem cell factor (SCF), granulocytic-monocytic colony-stimulating factor (GM-CSF), erythropoietin, basic fibroblast growth factor, and insulin-like growth factor-1, differentiated into myeloid and erythroid cells and CD10⁺CD19⁺ B-lineage cells.[21]

The progeny of murine stem cells includes cells whose differentiation potential is restricted to a few cell lineages[8]: common lymphocyte progenitors, which are restricted at a clonal level to give rise to B lymphocytes, T lymphocytes, and NK cells[22]; and myeloerythroid progenitors.[22] According to Kondo et al,[22] murine common lymphoid progenitors express the interleukin-7 (IL-7) receptor and display low levels of c-kit and Sca-1 on the cell surface. These progenitor cells lack Thy1.1 and several lineage-specific markers (CD3, CD4, CD8, CD45R,

CD11b, Gr-1, and TER-119). Putative common lymphoid progenitors have also been identified in humans; these cells reportedly express CD34, CD10, CD38, HLA-DR, and CD45RA and lack CD90, CD7, CD117, and various lineage-associated markers (see Fig. 4–1).[24] Such cells give rise only to B, T, NK, and lymphoid-dendritic cells.

Other investigators have described cells with the potential to differentiate to lymphoid and myeloid lineages, suggesting flexibility in the process of lineage commitment. Cumano et al and Hirayama et al[25, 26] identified bipotential precursors with the capacity to differentiate into myeloid or B-lineage cells in the murine fetal liver, and Bjorck and Kincade[27] described murine pro-B cells with the ability to differentiate into dendritic cells.

Transcription Factors and DNA Recombination Events Crucial for Lymphoid Differentiation

Studies of humans and mice with congenital immunodeficiencies and of mice with targeted disruption of genes have identified several molecules that are essential for normal lymphoid development. These include transcription factors (Table 4–1), molecules that participate in the recombination events leading to the rearrangements of Ig and TCR genes, and molecules mediating exogenous signals. Other sections in this chapter discuss the exogenous factors and signaling pathways influencing the development of lymphoid lineages.

Transcription Factors

Ikaros is a zinc finger DNA-binding protein that is involved at multiple stages of lymphohematopoiesis. There is experimental evidence indicating that Ikaros targets chromatin remodeling and deacetylation complexes and is involved in the restructuring of chromatin.[28] Georgopoulos and colleagues[29] evaluated the status of lymphocyte development in mice harboring a targeted disruption of the *Ikaros* gene. Mice homozygous for a germline mutation in the *Ikaros* gene, which produces a mutant protein acting as dominant-negative, lack B, T, and NK cells and

TABLE 4–1. Transcription Factors Crucial for Lymphoid Development

Transcription Factor	Family	Lymphoid Lineage Affected		
		B	T	NK
Ikaros	Zinc finger	√	√	√
PU.1	Ets	√	√	√
Ets-1	Ets	√	√	√
NF-κB/Rel	Rel	√	√	
E2A	bHLH	√	√	
TCF-1	HMG box		√	√
EBF	bHLH	√		
BSAP	Paired box	√		
SOX-4	HMG box	√		
OCT-2	POU	√		
OBF-1 (OCA-B,BOB1)	Coactivator	√		
GATA-3	Zinc finger		√	
IRF-1	IRF		√	

most of their defined progenitors, whereas the myeloid and erythroid lineages are essentially normal.[29] Therefore, the integrity of Ikaros is essential for stem-cell progression through the earliest stages of lymphoid development. In mice heterozygous for the mutation, thymocytes proliferate excessively; this proliferation precedes the development of T-cell leukemia and lymphoma.[30] The phenotype of mice carrying a null mutation is milder and CD4⁻CD8⁻ thymocytes can differentiate to CD4⁺CD8⁺ without expression of a TCR complex.[31] In these animals, Ikaros also regulates subsequent TCR-mediated events involving the transition of CD4⁺CD8⁺ cells to either CD4⁺CD8⁻ or CD4⁻CD8⁺ cells. T-cell malignancies invariably arise in the thymus of Ikaros-deficient mice.[31] Differences between the phenotypes resulting from the dominant-negative and the null mutation of *Ikaros* suggest that the Ikaros interacts with other factors. These factors include the Ikaros homologues Aiolos and Helios, which heterodimerize with Ikaros and may also participate in the regulation of lymphoid development.[32, 33] Ikaros-binding factors are also critical for the activity of hemopoietic stem cells, as mice homozygous for an *Ikaros*-null mutation display a reduction (>30-fold) in long-term hematopoietic repopulating activity, and mice homozygous for an *Ikaros* dominant-negative mutation have no measurable long-term repopulating activity.[34]

Other transcription factors that affect lymphoid development at various stages of maturation include PU.1 and Ets-1, members of the Ets protein family, as well as members of the Rel family of transcription factors (including the NF-κB subunits [p50 and p65] and RelB). Defective expression of the PU.1 transcription factor blocks B- and T-cell and myeloid development.[35, 36] Spleens of mice deficient in the transcription factor Ets-1 contained significantly reduced numbers of NK cells, and splenocytes of these mice displayed no detectable cytolytic activity against NK cell targets in vitro. Moreover, unlike wild-type animals, Ets-1–deficient mice developed tumors after they received subcutaneous injection of NK-susceptible RMA-S cells.[37] Ets-1 also affects proliferative responses of mature T lymphocytes and their propensity to apoptosis[38, 39] as well as the rate of differentiation of mature B cells to plasma cells.[39] Studies of mice with targeted mutation of *Rel* genes have demonstrated the crucial role of these factors at various stages of B-cell and thymic development.[40]

B-cell commitment depends on two basic helix-loop-helix proteins, E2A and early B-cell factor (EBF), and the paired box transcription factor Pax5 (also known as the B-cell–specific activator protein [BSAP]). Mice deficient in E2A and EBF lack B-lineage cells.[41-43] Loss of E2A activity also results in a partial block at the earliest stage of T-lineage development, which precedes the development of a T-cell lymphoma.[44] In the absence of Pax5, immature B cells are generated, but their differentiation and expansion progress only to the pro-B cell stage, with an apparent block at the junction between DJ and VDJ rearrangement of the Ig μ heavy (H)-chain gene.[45] Pro-B cells lacking Pax5 express genes associated with other lineages, including those encoding myeloperoxidase and the receptor for monocyte CSF (myeloid), GATA-1 (erythroid), perforin (NK), and pTα (T), and can differentiate into macrophages, osteoclasts, dendritic cells, granulocytes, and NK cells.[45] Moreover, Pax5-deficient pro-B cells transferred into mice lacking the recombination activating gene 2 *(RAG-2)* provide long-term reconstitution of the thymus and give rise to mature T cells expressing TCRαβ.[46] Restoration of Pax5 activity in *Pax5⁻/⁻* pro-B cells represses the expression of genes associated with other lineages, suggesting that one of the functions of this molecule is the suppression of the development of other hematopoietic lineages.[45] Other transcription factors directly involved in B-cell development include Oct-2 and OBF-1. Oct-2 is not required for the generation of B cells but is crucial for their maturation to Ig-secreting cells.[47] The transcriptional factor called Oct binding factor (OBF)-1 (or OCA-B or Bob1) is also not required for B-cell development but is essential for the response of B cells to antigens and the formation of germinal centers.[48, 49]

TCF-1 and SOX-4 are members of the "high mobility group box" transcription factors, which are involved in control of development in yeast, *Caenorhabditis elegans,* *Drosophila* species, and vertebrates. Disruption of the *Tcf-1* gene results in impairment of early T-cell differentiation before the rearrangement of the *TCRα* gene.[50] TCF-1 also determines the size of a subset of murine NK cells (defined by the expression of Ly49a).[51] SOX-4 deficiency causes a block in B-cell development at the pro-B cell stage.[52]

Other transcription factors that predominantly affect T-cell development include GATA-3, a member of the GATA family of transcription factors, and the interferon response factor 1 (IRF-1), a transcription factor involved in the induction of genes after interferon stimulation. GATA-3 deficiency causes failure to generate thymocytes or mature peripheral T cells, with a block in T cell differentiation at or before the earliest stage of thymocyte development.[53] A targeted mutation of IRF-1 allows generation of thymocytes but causes a reduction in the number of CD8⁺ thymocytes.[54, 55]

Effectors of Antigen-Receptor Gene Rearrangements

The differentiation of B cells is characterized by the genomic rearrangement of variable (V), diversity (D), and joining (J) regions of Ig genes, which eventually encode a μ H-chain protein. Similar rearrangements involving distinct V and J genes give rise to light (L)-chains (κ or λ). The human H-chain locus is located on chromosome 14, whereas the κ and λ L-chain loci are located on chromosomes 2 and 22, respectively.[56-58] The Ig rearrangement process uses a large number of distinct V-region genes that, in combination with a more limited number of D- and J-region genes, contribute substantially to the diversity of Ig receptor specificities.[56-58] Like the Ig molecule, the TCR molecules are encoded by distinct gene segments (V, D, J, and C) that undergo rearrangement during T-cell ontogeny. The human *TCRα* and *TCRδ* genes are located on chromosome 14, and the *TCRβ* and *TCRγ* genes are located on chromosome 7.[59] The *TCRδ* gene complex lies within the TCRα locus, between the Vα and Jα segments.[59]

RAG-1 and *RAG-2* encode proteins that are crucial to

the rearrangement of Ig and TCR genes.[60] RAG-1 and RAG-2 are expressed in lymphoid progenitors in which Ig and TCR gene rearrangements occur.[60] However, germinal center cells and mature B and T cells can reactivate *RAG* gene expression.[61-64] Secondary V(D)J rearrangements in mature cells are part of a revision mechanism that can further diversify the antigen receptors or induce tolerance. RAG-1–[65] and RAG-2–deficient mice[66] exhibit marked reductions in the number of mature B and T cells.

Another enzyme, terminal deoxynucleotidyl transferase (TdT), also expressed in B- and T-cell progenitors, catalyzes the addition of nontemplate-encoded nucleotides (N additions) between the recombining ends of Ig and TCR genes: these additions increase the potential diversity of these genes.[67] TdT-deficient mice have no substantial changes in the number of circulating lymphocytes but, as expected, the antigen-receptor gene segments in these animals lack N regions.[68]

The DNA-dependent protein kinase (DNA-PK), a serine-threonine kinase that is implicated in the repair of DNA double-strand breaks, DNA replication, transcription, and V(D)J recombination, also appears to be involved in lymphoid development.[69] The catalytic subunit of DNA-PK is involved in the joining of coding segments of antigen-receptor genes; impairment of DNA-PK activity is reportedly involved in generating defective B- and T-cell development in SCID mice.[70, 71] In mice with an altered DNA-binding subunit (Ku80) of DNA-PK, B- and T-lymphocyte development is arrested at early progenitor stages, with a profound deficiency in antigen-receptor gene rearrangements.[69] Mice deficient in the another subunit, (Ku70), lack mature B cells but develop small populations of thymic cells and have a significant incidence of thymic lymphomas.[72]

B-CELL DEVELOPMENT

The name "B cells" is derived from *b*ursa of Fabricius, the organ in birds where B cells were first identified and characterized. Antibody responses are initiated by surface Ig+ B cells, which receive a complex set of accessory signals from T cells, macrophages, and follicular dendritic cells and respond to these signals by undergoing clonal expansion and differentiating into Ig-secreting plasma cells. Before they mediate this critical function in host defense, B cells undergo an antigen-independent developmental phase in fetal tissue and adult bone marrow. Generally, the term "B-cell precursor" is used to indicate cells of all stages of B-cell development that occur before the expression of surface Ig, composed of μ chains and κ or λ chains. Precursor (pre)-B cells are distinguished by the presence of cytoplasmic μ H chains and the absence of L chains, whereas progenitor (pro)-B cells represent an earlier stage of development and lack cytoplasmic μ H chains and L chains (Fig. 4–2). B-cell precursors are the normal counterpart of B-lineage acute lymphoblastic leukemia (ALL) cells.[1]

Organs Involved in B-Cell Lymphopoiesis

The human fetal liver is a site of early hematopoiesis[73] and lymphopoiesis.[74] Pre-B cells are first detected in fetal

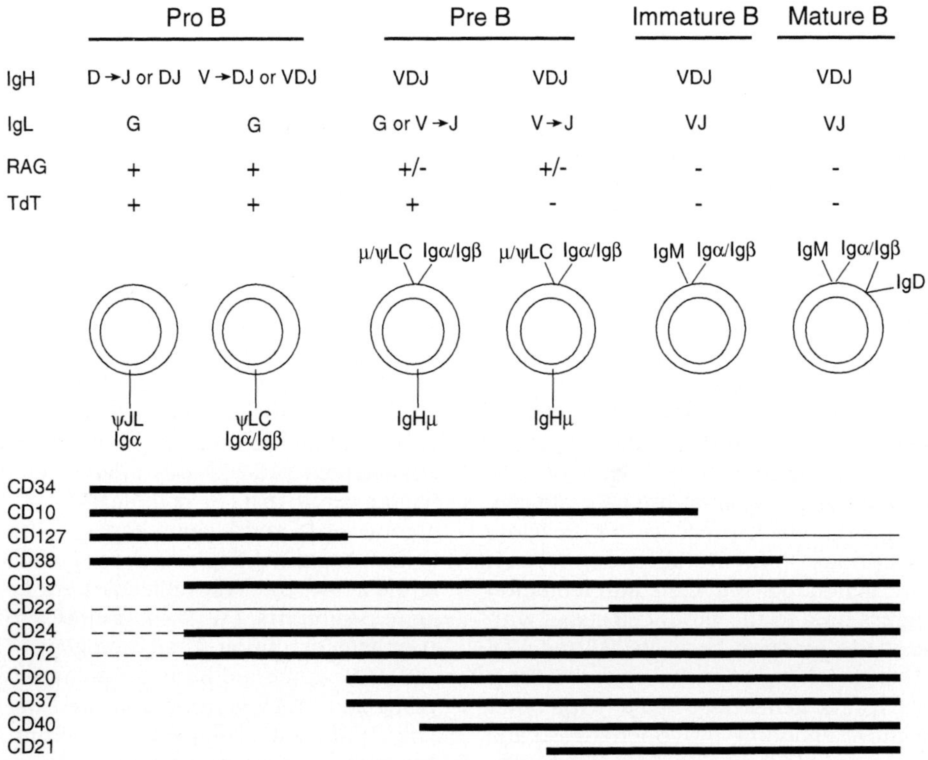

FIGURE 4–2. Schematic representation of human B-cell development.

liver and omentum at approximately 8 weeks of gestation.[74, 75] B-cell development continues in the liver and begins to shift to the bone marrow during 8 to 14 weeks of gestation. From the second trimester through neonatal and adult life, the bone marrow is the primary, if not exclusive, site of early B-cell development in humans. Although B cells are produced throughout life,[76] the percentage of B-cell progenitors in the total nucleated lymphohematopoietic cell pool is much higher in fetal bone marrow than in pediatric or adult bone marrow.[77, 78] Surface Ig$^+$ B cells, the differentiated progeny of pre-B cells, are readily detected in fetal spleen and lymph nodes at 14 weeks of gestation and subsequently throughout adult life in peripheral blood and secondary lymphoid tissues.[74]

Hepatic hematopoiesis is preceded by waves of hematopoiesis in two other sites: the yolk sac and the paraaortic splanchnopleure, which includes the aorta-gonad-mesonephros (AGM) region.[79] The AGM region, which has been identified at 5 weeks of human gestation,[79] contains multipotent hematopoietic stem cells and lymphoid and myeloid progenitors.[80, 81]

Ig Gene Rearrangements and Expression

Ig gene rearrangement during mammalian B-cell development generally follows an ordered progression, initiating at the H-chain locus and continuing at κ and then λ L-chain loci.[56-58] H-chain rearrangement begins at both alleles of the DH locus, which together include approximately 30 DH gene segments.[82-84] Rearrangement of one of the DH gene segments with one of the six JH elements creates a joined DJ element, which can be transcribed. Next, one of approximately 50 functional VH gene segments, located 5′ of the DH locus, undergoes rearrangement with the newly formed DJ element. In-frame rearrangement of a V segment to the DJ unit creates a sequence that encodes a complete Ig H-chain V domain.

Although the ordered pathway of H-chain to L-chain rearrangement is probably the most common mechanism of Ig gene recombination, alternative pathways of Ig gene rearrangement may be used during mouse[85] and human[86, 87] B-cell development. Nevertheless, mutations of

the μ H-chain gene that impair the expression of μ H chains are associated with a complete failure of B-cell development in both humans and mice.[88, 89]

Once a functional H-chain gene rearrangement has occurred in the pro-B cell, the cell has the capacity to differentiate to a pre-B cell. When H-chain gene rearrangement on both alleles fails to generate functional VDJ elements in a pro-B cell, the cell probably undergoes apoptosis and subsequent phagocytosis by macrophages in the bone marrow. The pre-B cell initiates L-chain rearrangement beginning at the κ locus.[56] A functional κ gene rearrangement results in the differentiation of the pre-B cell into an immature B cell, which expresses surface Ig consisting of μ and κ chains. Alternatively, if the κ gene rearrangements on one or both alleles are nonfunctional, the pre-B cell can rearrange gene segments within the λ locus, giving rise to an immature B cell expressing surface Ig comprising μ and λ.[56] Immature IgM$^+$ B cells do not proliferate or differentiate in response to antigen; exposure to self-antigen at this stage may lead to elimination of the cell clone or to tolerization.[57, 58] Editing of the Ig genes also occurs in response to receptor ligation by autoantigens. As a result of receptor editing, anti self-reactive cells are converted to non–self-reactive cells; self-reactive clones are thereby salvaged before negative selection.[90] Expression of surface IgD indicates that the cell is a mature B cell, which migrates to peripheral lymphoid organs. Mature B cells are short-lived unless they are exposed to antigen; exposure to antigen causes the mature B-cell to proliferate and differentiate into Ig-secreting plasma cells and memory B cells.

Ig-Associated Molecules

Several functionally important molecules associate physically with Ig chains (Fig. 4-3) (also see Color Section). Studies of pre-B cell lines showed that the μ H chain can be expressed on the cell surface in the absence of L-chain expression and that these μ H chains are associated with two surrogate (ψ) L chains named λ5 and Vpre-B.[56, 91] The genes encoding ψ L chains exhibit significant homology with conventional λL chains but do not un-

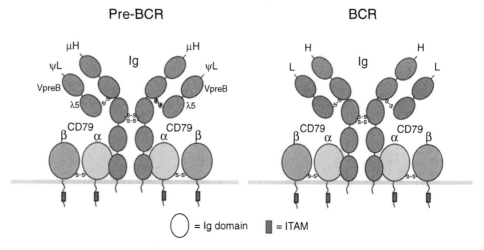

FIGURE 4–3. Molecular composition of the pre-B-cell receptor (pre-BCR) and B-cell receptor complexes. In the pre-BCR complexes, μH chains are associated with ψL chains. In BCR complexes, H chains are associated with L chains (either κ or λ). Signal transduction is mediated by CD79 molecules, which contain immunoreceptor tyrosine-based activation motifs in their cytoplasmic domains. (See Color Section.)

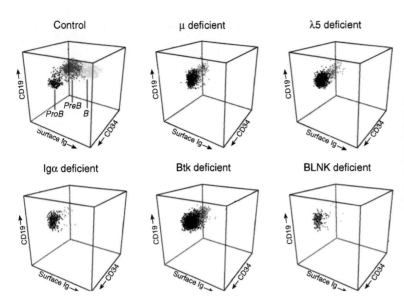

FIGURE 4–4. Block in B-cell differentiation in patients with agammaglobulinemia. Flow cytometric analysis of the immunophenotype of CD19+ B cells in a bone marrow of a healthy individual shows three distinct cell subpopulations: CD34+ surface Ig− (pro B), CD34− surface Ig− (pre-B), and CD34− surface Ig+ (immature and mature B). The immunophenotype of patients with agammaglobulinemia caused by different genetic abnormalities is shown. Note that the main block in B-cell differentiation in all patients is at the transition between pro-B and pre-B cells.[88, 101, 102, 154, 159] (See Color Section.)

dergo gene rearrangement.[56] In addition, two genes designated *mb-1* and *B29* encode molecules (called Igα or CD79α, and Igβ or CD79β) that are expressed specifically in B cells, are noncovalently associated with surface Ig, and have cytoplasmic domains containing immunoreceptor tyrosine-based activation motifs (ITAM), which are crucial for signal transduction.[92-94]

In humans and mice, the components of the surrogate λ chains and the Igα/Igβ heterodimer are expressed in the cytoplasm of B-cell precursors before the completion of V(D)J rearrangement.[95, 96] Surrogate light chains together with μ H chains and Igα and Igβ form the pre-B cell receptor (pre-BCR) complex.[97] In mice, the Igα/Igβ heterodimer is also expressed on the surface of pro-B cells in the absence of μ H chain.[98] Cross-linking of this receptor in mice that are unable to rearrange μ H-chain genes induces tyrosine and serine-threonine phosphorylation of cytoplasmic proteins and the differentiation of pro-B cells into pre-B cells.[98]

Mutations of murine λ5 result in a leaky phenotype with detectable humoral responses,[99] whereas mice that do not make the Igβ component have normal DJ rearrangement but impaired VDJ rearrangement.[100] In evaluating patients with agammaglobulinemia and markedly reduced numbers of B cells, Minegishi et al[101] identified patients with mutations of the λ5 gene. The same group also found defects in Igα in another patient.[102] The results of immunofluorescence analysis indicated that patients with λ5, Igα, or μ H-chain defects[88] had a complete block in B-cell development at the pro-B to pre-B transition, indicating that integrity of the pre-BCR is essential for progression beyond the pro-B stage in human B-cell ontogeny (Fig. 4–4) (also see Color Section).

Immunophenotypic Differentiation of B Cells

It is generally thought that the appearance of CD19 on the cell surface corresponds to commitment to the B lineage. However, the IgH locus was found to be active before surface expression of CD19, as indicated by the presence of germline Cμ and DH transcripts in bone marrow CD34+CD19− cells,[84] and partial DJ rearrangements were detected in bone marrow CD34+CD10+CD19− cells.[103] Therefore, transcription of unrearranged components of the IgH locus and DJ rearrangements can occur before the surface expression of CD19. Putative B-cell progenitors expressing CD34, CD10, and TdT but not CD19 have also been found in human bone marrow.[104, 105] Another pan-B marker, CD22, is expressed predominantly in the cytoplasm of pro-B and pre-B cells.[106, 107] Its expression is markedly increased on the surface of B cells expressing surface Ig.[106-108]

Pro-B cells can be distinguished from pre-B cells on the basis of their expression of CD34 and TdT. Unlike pro-B cells, pre-B cells generally express cytoplasmic μ H chain but do not express CD34 and TdT. However, the distinction between pro-B cells and pre-B cells is not absolute with respect to expression of TdT. A minor subpopulation of TdT+ cells (<10%) express cytoplasmic μ.[109] Most pro-B and pre-B cells as well as a fraction of surface Ig+ B lymphocytes in the bone marrow express CD10.[110, 111]

Mice[112] and humans[113] have a subpopulation of B cells that display CD5, a molecule expressed on the surface of most T cells. CD5+ B cells (commonly referred to as B-1 cells in the mouse) constitute a small percentage (<10%) of peripheral blood B cells but are highly enriched in fetal spleen and the adult peritoneal cavity.[112-114] CD5+ B cells have several characteristics that generally distinguish them from CD5− B cells, including origin during fetal ontogeny, relatively low rates of V-gene somatic mutation, and enrichment for cells producing so-called "natural autoantibodies."[115-118] Nevertheless, whether CD5+ B cells are truly a separate lineage of B cells is controversial.[119] CD5+ B cells are regarded as the normal counterparts of B-chronic lymphocytic leukemia cells.[120]

The precise function of many of the surface molecules expressed on immature B cells is unknown. CD19 and CD22 are transmembrane molecules that regulate the intensity of B-cell receptor signaling: signaling through CD19 in mature B cells lowers the threshold for signal transduction through the B-cell receptor complex (surface Ig plus Igα and Igβ), whereas signaling through CD22 raises it.[121] Deletion of CD19 in mice has no apparent effect on the generation of B cells in the bone marrow, although it reduces the number of B cells in peripheral lymphoid tissues.[122] In contrast, mice overexpressing CD19 had significant defects in early B-cell development in the bone marrow as well as augmented mitogenic responses and increased serum Ig levels.[122] Ablation of CD22 does not appear to affect B-cell development but causes a reduction in surface Ig levels and renders B cells hyper-responsive to B-cell receptor signaling.[123-125] Mice that do not express CD20, a tetraspan molecule involved in the regulation of Ca^{2+} flux, have no remarkable defect in B-cell development.[126]

Some surface molecules highly expressed in immature B cells have ectoenzymatic activity. For example, CD10 is a zinc metalloproteinase that can cleave a wide array of proteins,[127] and CD38 catalyzes the conversion of nicotinamide adenine dinucleotide (NAD) and NAD phosphate to the Ca^{2+}-mobilizing compounds cyclic adenosine diphosphate ribose and nicotinic acid ADP, respectively.[128, 129] However, the relation between the cellular function of these molecules and their enzymatic activity is unclear. In vivo treatment of mice with an inhibitor of the enzymatic activity of CD10 promoted B-cell reconstitution and maturation of splenic B cells.[130] Ligation of CD38 did not affect its enzymatic activity but induced apoptosis and inhibited the growth of human immature B-lymphoid cells.[131] CD38 ligation also caused rapid and transient tyrosine phosphorylation of intracellular tyrosine kinases and adaptor molecules,[132-135] and inhibitors of phosphatidyl inositol 3-kinase, activated by CD38 ligation, rescued cells from CD38-mediated suppressive effects.[133] Therefore, the cellular effects caused by CD38 ligation appear to be related to its signal transduction properties rather than to its ectoenzymatic potential.

Adhesion of Immature B Cells to the Microenvironment

B-cell ontogeny in the fetal liver and bone marrow is stringently regulated by a microenvironment consisting of other lymphohematopoietic cells, a complex structural network of nonlymphohematopoietic stromal cells, and the extracellular matrix. Adhesion of immature B cells to stromal cells is essential for their survival in vitro.[5, 136]

The association between immature B cells and stromal elements appears to require the engagement of the integrins VLA-4 and VLA-5.[4, 5, 137] One of the ligands of VLA-4 is vascular cell adhesion molecule-1 (VCAM-1), a member of the Ig superfamily.[138] Human bone marrow stromal cells that support the growth of normal B-cell progenitors express VCAM-1 constitutively.[139] A second ligand of VLA-4 is the CS-1 domain of fibronectin, one of the main components of the extracellular matrix.[140] The ligand of VLA-5 is the arginine–glycine–aspartic acid containing the central cell-binding domain of fibronectin.[140] VLA-4 is present on the microvilli and blebs that protrude from the surface of lymphoblasts and interact with fibroblasts and extracellular matrix (Fig. 4–5).[139] VLA-5 is distributed

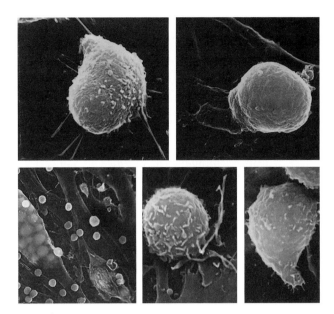

FIGURE 4–5. Scanning electron micrograph shows the interaction of normal and leukemic immature B cells with stromal layers. Top row illustrates B-lineage ALL cells; bottom row illustrates normal bone marrow CD19⁺ cells. B-lymphoid precursors adhere to stroma via filopods and pseudopods. (Modified from Manabe A, Murti KG, Coustan-Smith E, et al: Adhesion-dependent survival of normal and leukemic human B lymphoblasts on bone marrow stromal cells. Blood 1994;83,758–766.)

in a similar pattern, but it is also frequently expressed on the smoother part of the membrane.[139]

In vitro studies have demonstrated that B progenitors adhere to bone marrow stromal cells via a VLA-4/VCAM-1 interaction.[141, 142] Antibodies to VLA-4 markedly decrease murine B lymphopoiesis[137] and human B-lymphoid cell-survival in vitro,[5] but fibronectin by itself does not support the survival and growth of immature B cells (D. Campana, unpublished observations). Of note, integrin engagement not only promotes adhesion but also induces signal transduction in immature B cells.[143] Contact between B cells and stroma also induces tyrosine phosphorylation in stromal cells, followed by IL-6 secretion.[144] This effect, however, does not depend on VLA-4/VCAM-1 interactions.[145]

B-cell progenitors express other adhesion molecules potentially important for their interaction with the microenvironment, including CD31 (PECAM-1),[146] CD43 (leukosialin),[147] and the complex proteoglycan CD44.[4,148] CD31 and CD44 may bind multiple ligands, including heparan sulfate proteoglycans and hyaluronate, both of which exist in the extracellular matrix of the bone marrow.[149] CD44 is abundantly expressed in the regions of contact between lymphoid cells and fibroblasts.[139] Antibodies to CD44 inhibit B-cell development in mice,[148] but altered B-cell development has not been noted in mice lacking all CD44 isoforms.[150]

L-selectin (CD62L), which mediates binding of lymphocytes to endothelial cells, is expressed at relatively low levels during B-cell development and increases as B cells mature in the bone marrow.[151] The increased level of CD62L on the surface of immature B cells departing the bone marrow is consistent with a requirement for homing to secondary lymphoid tissues.

Signaling Molecules Critical for B-Cell Development

As outlined above, signaling through the pre-BCR is essential for B-cell development. Defective expression of its components causes a profound block in B-cell differentiation and agammaglobulinemia. Drastically reduced expression of molecules that participate in the transduction of pre-BCR signaling also impairs B-cell development. Indeed, the most common cause of agammaglobulinemia in humans is the defective production of Btk, a cytoplasmic tyrosine kinase expressed throughout B-cell and myeloid differentiation.[152, 153] Btk mutations result in a block of B-cell differentiation at the entry into the pre-B stage (see Fig. 4-4).[154, 155] Conley et al[156] analyzed 101 families in which affected males were diagnosed as having X-linked agammaglobulinemia (XLA) and identified mutations in the *Btk* gene in 38 of 40 families with more than one affected family member and in 56 of 61 families with sporadic disease. Mutations in *Btk* were identified in 43 of 46 patients with bona fide sporadic XLA. Two of the three remaining patients had defects in other genes required for normal B-cell development, and the third patient probably did not have XLA, as indicated by results of extensive *Btk* gene analysis. These studies indicate that 90% to 95% of males with presumed XLA have mutations in the *Btk* gene.

Another signaling molecule whose absence causes a block in B-cell development in humans and mice is BLNK, an adapter protein that links Btk and Syk kinases to the phosphoinositide and mitogen-activated kinase pathways.[157, 158] Similar to Btk deficiency, the lack of functional BLNK causes a block in B-cell differentiation at the entry of the pre-B stage (see Fig. 4-4).[159, 160]

Deficiency of the Src-family kinases Blk, Fyn, and Lyn does not affect B-cell development, whereas that of Syk does.[97] Studies of irradiated mice reconstituted with Syk-deficient fetal liver showed a block in B-cell development at the pro-B to pre-B cell transition.[161] Similarly, defective phosphatidyl inositol 3-kinase function leads to a block in B-cell development in mice.[162] Because Syk and phosphatidyl inositol 3-kinase are essential for survival, it is unlikely that the lack of expression of these molecules will emerge as a cause of selective agammaglobulinemia in humans.

Although IL-7 is essential for B-cell development in the mouse,[163] IL-7–mediated signaling does not appear to be crucial for human B-cell development.[164] For example, patients with X-linked SCID, caused by mutations in the γ chain common to IL-2, IL-4, IL-7, IL-9, and IL-15 receptors, have normal or increased numbers of peripheral blood B cells[165]; normal numbers of B cells are also found in patients with mutations of the IL-7 receptor α chain.[166]

T-CELL DEVELOPMENT

At least three stages in the ontogeny of T (thymus) cells can be defined: (1) T-cell progenitor development in fetal liver and in the fetal and postnatal bone marrow, (2) homing of progenitors to the thymus, and (3) intrathymic T-cell maturation. Positive selection (the process by which T cells recognizing foreign antigens in the context of self-MHC are selected) occurs when developing thymocytes interact with thymic epithelial cells; negative selection (the process by which T cells recognizing self-antigens are deleted) occurs when thymocytes interact with dendritic or interdigitating cells.[167-169] T-cell progenitors that successfully survive this odyssey develop into CD4+ helper and CD8+ cytotoxic/suppressor T cells. The TCR on the surface of mature T cells consists of αβ or γδ heterodimers associated with a complex of cell surface proteins designated CD3ε, CD3γ, and CD3δ, as well as two highly homologous polypeptides named CD3ζ and CD3η.[170] In general, the immunophenotypic and TCR gene rearrangement features of leukemic lymphoblasts in T-cell ALL resemble those of thymic T cells.[1]

Organs Involved in T-Cell Development

T-cell development is initiated when pluripotent stem cells or their immediate progeny migrate from the fetal liver or the bone marrow to the thymus. As early as 7 or 8 weeks of gestation, the human fetal liver contains lymphohematopoietic cells expressing CD7.[171, 172] At least some of these CD7+ cells can be classified as pro-T cells because they express the T-cell–restricted CD3ε protein in their cytoplasm.[171, 172] The CD7+, cytoplasmic CD3ε+ pro-T cells are present in fetal liver and fetal thorax just before cell colonization of the epithelial thymic rudiment.[171]

Reportedly, progenitor cells can be induced to differentiate into functional T cells expressing CD3 and TCR in the absence of an intact thymus. Thus, CD7− fetal liver hematopoietic cells, which express the genes encoding the γ, δ, ε, and ζ chains of CD3, can differentiate into T cells expressing CD3-TCR on their surface in vitro,[173] and fetal liver cells can proliferate and differentiate into T cells expressing functional TCRαβ or TCRγδ receptors, or CD3−CD16+ NK cells, depending on the culture conditions employed.[174] Others, however, have shown that, in the fetal liver, CD34+ cells can differentiate into NK cells but not into mature T cells.[175]

The subcapsular, cortical, and medullary regions and the corticomedullary junction of the thymus contain heterogenous populations of epithelial cells, macrophages, dendritic or interdigitating cells, and fibroblasts.[176] The human thymic microenvironment begins to develop at approximately 4 weeks of gestation, and T-cell development can be subsequently classified into at least three phases.[171, 176, 177] The first phase (4 to 8 weeks of gestation) is characterized by proliferation of endodermal- and ectodermal-derived thymic epithelial cells. The second phase (9 to 15 weeks of gestation) is characterized by the appearance of subcapsular, cortical, and medullary regions. Colonization by fetal liver–derived pro-T cells begins at about week 9. The third phase (beginning at 16 weeks of gestation) is characterized by a high rate of intrathymic T-cell maturation. In humans, the maximum size of the thymus is reached in the 1st year of life.

Thymic involution, with progressive decrease of the volume of the thymic epithelium (cortex and medulla), is continuous from the 1st year to the end of life.[178] However, the age-related involution may be more quantitative than qualitative; it has been shown that a substantial output of newly generated T lymphocyte and active TCR gene rearrangements can also occur in adults in their 50s and older.[179, 180]

Integrity of the thymic microenvironment is essential for T-cell development. Thus, mutations in RelB, a transcription factor that is important in the development of the thymic epithelium, indirectly impair murine T-cell development.[181] Likewise, patients with DiGeorge's syndrome have a severe impairment in T lymphopoiesis, possibly because of the defective development of the thymic microenvironment.[182] In turn, thymocyte maturation and development of at least some thymic microenvironmental cells (e.g., epithelium) appear to be interdependent because natural or experimentally induced depletion of developing thymocytes is associated with a reduction in the number of surrounding thymic epithelial cells.[183] Studies in mice with sequential blocks in T-cell differentiation have shown that the three-dimensional organization of thymic epithelial cells depends on the progression of thymocytes through the CD4⁻CD8⁻ stage and that the establishment of a thymic cortex is a prerequisite for the development of the thymic medulla.[184]

T-Cell Receptor Gene Rearrangements and Expression

Circulating T cells express clonally distributed heterodimeric protein products of either the *TCRαβ* or *TCRγδ*

genes. TCRαβ proteins are expressed on 90% to 95% of peripheral blood T cells,[185] whereas TCRγδ proteins are expressed on 5% to 10% of peripheral blood T cells.[186] TCRαβ-deficient mice exhibit normal development of TCRγδ cells.[187] Conversely, mice deficient in TCRγδ show no abnormalities in the development of TCRαβ cells.[188] These findings suggest that TCRαβ cells and TCRγδ cells originate in nonoverlapping progenitors.

During normal T-cell differentiation in the thymus, the synthesis and assembly of the CD3-TCR complex occur gradually (Fig. 4–6). The most immature thymic cells do not have detectable TCR chains but accumulate CD3ε, CD3δ and, possibly, CD3γ and CD3ζ in the cytoplasm.[170, 172, 189, 190] These CD3 molecules constitute a core onto which TCR proteins are added after the corresponding genes undergo productive rearrangements.[170] Productive TCRβ rearrangement is a rate-limiting step in the progression beyond the CD4⁻CD8⁻ stage. In TCRβ-deficient mice, CD4⁺CD8⁺ thymocytes are unable to undergo expansion, whereas disruption of the TCRα locus causes a block in the differentiation of CD4⁺CD8⁺ thymocytes into CD4⁺CD8⁻ or CD4⁻CD8⁺ cells.[187] TCRβ chains associate during early development with a substitute for TCRα, i.e., the pre-TCRα (pTα) chain, to form a functional pre-TCR complex (Fig. 4–7) (also see Color Section). It has been postulated that the formation of the complex triggers the transition of CD4⁻CD8⁻ to CD4⁺CD8⁺ thymocytes.[191] The pTα-TCRβ heterodimers have been shown to associate with CD3γ, CD3ε, CD3ζ, and CD3δ.[192] Pre-TCR and TCR signaling is transduced by the associated CD3 molecules, which contain ITAM in their cytoplasmic domains (see Fig. 4–7). In mice with a targeted mutation of the *CD3ε* gene that prevents the assembly of the pre-TCR, thymocyte development does

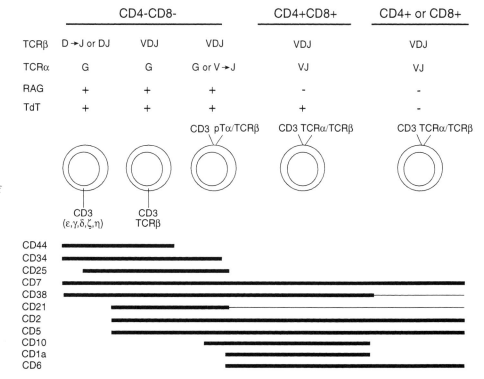

FIGURE 4–6. Schematic representation of human T-cell development.

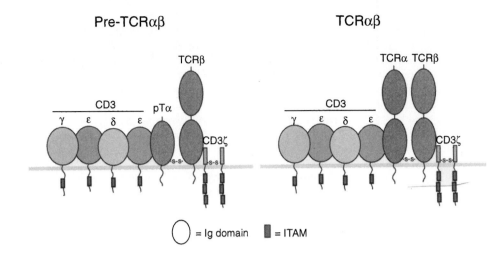

FIGURE 4–7. Molecular composition of the pre-T-cell receptor αβ (pre-TCRαβ) and T-cell receptor αβ (TCRαβ) complexes. TCRβ chains are associated with pTα chains in the pre-TCRαβ complexes and with TCRα chains in the TCRαβ complexes. Signal transduction is mediated by CD3 molecules, which contain immunoreceptor tyrosine-based activation motifs in their cytoplasmic domains. (See Color Section.)

not progress beyond the CD4$^-$CD8$^-$ stage.[193] In mice lacking all CD3 subunits, thymopoiesis is also arrested at early stages resembling that of *RAG$^{-/-}$* mice, but DJ and V(D)J recombination at the TCRβ locus was functional.[194] Human T-cell immunodeficiencies caused by lack of CD3ε and CD3γ expression have been described.[195, 196]

Human thymocytes express TCR proteins heterogeneously (see Fig. 4–5). Three subpopulations of cells can be distinguished on the basis of CD3 expression on the cell surface: CD3$^-$, CD3$^{+/-}$, and CD3$^+$.[197] Most CD3$^-$ thymocytes, however, express cytoplasmic CD3 molecules.[190, 198] The amount of TCRβ chains increases considerably as the cell matures. Large TdT$^+$ thymic blast cells appear to be mostly TCRβ-negative. TCRγδ-bearing cells are usually less than 1% of the fetal and infant thymocytes.[172, 186]

Immunophenotypic Differentiation of T Cells

A model of thymocyte maturation proposes that CD34$^+$ CD7$^+$ fetal liver or bone marrow pro-T cells migrate to the subcapsular area of the thymus and rapidly express CD2 and CD5.[199] These pro-T cells, which express cytoplasmic CD3 but lack CD4 and CD8,[190, 198] differentiate into cortical pre-T cells expressing CD4, CD8, CD1a, and low levels of CD3-TCRαβ on their surface (see Fig. 4–6). The stage represented by CD4$^-$CD8$^-$ cells and that represented by CD4$^+$CD8$^+$ populations may be separated by a CD4$^+$CD8$^-$ intermediate.[200, 201] The CD4$^+$CD8$^+$ pre-T cells constitute the majority of cortical thymocytes. TCRαβ pre-T cells differentiate into two main thymic medullary T-cell populations: CD4$^+$CD8$^-$ helper T cells and CD4$^-$CD8$^+$ cytotoxic/suppressor T cells. These populations are then exported to the peripheral blood and secondary lymphoid tissues where they participate in the functional T-cell immune response. CD4-deficient mice experience normal CD8$^+$ cell development,[202] whereas CD8-deficient mice develop normal numbers of CD4$^+$ cells.[203]

Adhesion of Immature T Cells to the Thymic Microenvironment

The adhesive interface between the developing thymocytes and the thymic microenvironment is highly complex.[183, 204-206] Contact of thymocytes with the thymic stromal cells is required for the generation of CD4$^+$CD8$^+$ thymocytes. Thymocytes express VLA-4,[199] and one microenvironmental component implicated in thymocyte differentiation is fibronectin. The presence of fibronectin in the perivascular space surrounding the thymus suggests a possible role for VLA-4 in the adhesion of prethymic T cells to the basement membrane of thymic epithelium.[207] In vitro, co-culture of murine CD4$^-$ CD8$^-$ thymocytes with thymic cell lines promotes expression of CD4 and CD8; this expression is blocked by antifibronectin antibodies.[208, 209] Thymocyte adhesion to epithelial cells is also mediated by VLA-3 and VLA-6[210] and by other receptor-counter-receptor pairs: CD2–CD58[211] and CD11a–CD54.[212] Other thymic stromal components, such as laminin-2 and laminin-5, influence thymocyte migration and differentiation.[213]

The role of other adhesion molecules that are highly expressed on the surface of thymocytes is unclear. L-selectin (CD62L), which mediates cell binding to endothelial cells, is expressed at high levels on putative bone marrow prothymocytes and recent thymic arrivals, and the levels are decreased on the surface of CD4$^+$CD8$^+$ cortical thymocytes.[199] Just before thymic export, mature T cells begin to express more L-selectin on their surface. L-selectin–deficient mice exhibit impaired migration of lymphocytes in peripheral lymphoid organs and primary T-cell responses.[214] The expression of CD44 is high in immature thymocytes lacking surface TCR and then downregulated in thymocytes expressing low or high levels of surface TCR.[215] Conceivably, the interaction between CD44 and its ligands hyaluronic acid and fibronectin is involved in the adhesion of thymocytes to the thymic microenvironment. In CD44-deficient mice, lymphocyte development is apparently unaltered, although the entry of precursor cells into the adult thymus is impaired,[150] consistent with the notion that high CD44 expression denotes precursor cells that have recently migrated to the thymus.

Signaling Molecules Critical for T-Cell Development

Cytokine stimulation is crucial for T-cell development (Fig. 4-8). In humans, the molecular basis of the most

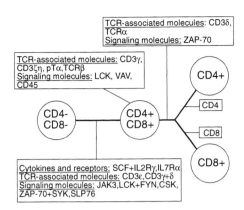

FIGURE 4–8. Signaling events crucial for T-cell development. The major blocks in differentiation caused by altered expression of the listed molecules are indicated.

frequent form of SCID (X-linked SCID) illustrates the roles played by some cytokines in early T lymphopoiesis. X-linked SCID is characterized by the absence of mature T and NK lymphocytes, and patients' thymi are almost completely devoid of T cells.[216] The SCID locus maps to Xq12–13.1 and encodes the common cytokine receptor γ chain, which, as mentioned earlier, is part of the receptors for IL-2, IL-4, IL-7, IL-9, and IL-15. Defective IL-7 signaling is likely to contribute to the T-cell defect of the X-linked SCID phenotype. In mice lacking the IL-7 receptor, TCRαβ-expressing T cells are generated at a greatly reduced rate, and TCRγδ-expressing cells are completely absent.[166, 217] Other cytokine signaling may also be important for T-cell development. For example, 4 to 5 weeks after birth, mice lacking IL-2 develop a progressive thymic disorder in which thymocyte maturation is disrupted, cellularity is reduced, immature CD4⁻CD8⁻ and CD4⁺CD8⁺ thymocytes are absent, and the thymic stroma is abnormal.[218]

Several molecules implicated in signal transduction are crucial for T-cell development. Mutations in Jak-3, a member of the Janus family of tyrosine kinases that is coupled to the cytokine receptor common γ chain and is required for its signaling, cause a phenotype indistinguishable from that of patients with X-linked SCID.[219] The Src tyrosine kinase Lck associates with the cytoplasmic domains of both CD4 and CD8 and interacts with the β chain of the IL-2 receptor. Thymic atrophy, with a marked reduction in CD4⁺CD8⁺ thymocytes and the absence of CD4⁺CD8⁻ and CD4⁻CD8⁺ thymocytes, is seen in Lck-deficient mice.[220] Humans and mice deficient in ZAP-70, a tyrosine kinase implicated in the transduction of early TCR signaling, have a defective transition of CD4⁺CD8⁺ to CD4⁺CD8⁻ and CD4⁻CD8⁺ thymocytes.[221, 222] The adaptor protein SLP-76 is a substrate of ZAP-70 and Syk. SLP-76–deficient mice have a profound block in thymic development; CD4⁺CD8⁺ thymocytes and peripheral T cells are absent.[223, 224] SOCS1 is a protein with a Src homology-2 (SH2) domain and is primarily expressed in thymocytes. Deletion of the *SOCS1* gene results in the loss of thymic cellularity and a decrease in the number of CD4⁺CD8⁺ thymocytes.[225] Finally, in the absence of the membrane tyrosine phosphatase CD45, there is a large increase in the thresholds of TCR stimulation required for positive and negative selection.[226]

The interaction between Notch receptors (1 through 4) and their ligands (Jagged-1, Jagged-2, and Delta) regulates cell-fate decisions during development.[227] Notch signaling influences multiple stages of T-cell development. Notch signaling appears to be essential for the initial commitment to progenitor cells of the T-cell lineage[228, 229] and may regulate subsequent steps of T-cell development in conjunction with signals from the pre-T and T-cell receptors.[230] A constitutively active Notch favors the development of CD8⁺ over CD4⁺ thymocytes[231] and the development of TCRαβ over TCRγδ T cells.[232]

NK CELL ONTOGENY

NK cells differ substantially from B and T lymphocytes because they do not express highly diverse antigen-recognition systems such as Ig or TCR on the cell surface. Nevertheless, NK cells have the capability to discriminate susceptible from nonsusceptible targets via surface receptors that recognize class I MHC-deficient target cells.[37, 233] Inhibitory signals mediated by these polymorphic inhibitory receptors, including killer inhibitory receptors (KIR), and the receptors CD94/NKG2 in humans and mice and Ly-49 in mice,[37, 233] prevent the lysis of healthy autologous cells. NK lymphoproliferative disorders are uncommon; they include NK large granular lymphocyte leukemia and NK chronic lymphocytosis.[234]

Unlike T cells, NK cells lack CD3 molecules on the cell surface and typically express CD56 and CD16.[235, 236] Cells with this immunophenotype can be found in the human fetal liver and spleen as early as 6 weeks of gestation.[235] These cells express CD3ε and CD3δ chains in the cytoplasm, perform characteristic NK cell functions (e.g., cytotoxicity against NK-sensitive tumor cells), respond to IL-2, and secrete interferon (IFN)-γ, GM-CSF, and tumor necrosis factor (TNF)-α after stimulation.[237] The cytoplasmic expression of CD3ε and CD3δ chains is characteristic of fetal NK cells and is not detectable in circulating NK cells in adults, although CD3ζ expression is typical, and CD3ε expression can be induced by activation.[235] Expression of CD94/NKG2 in NK-like cells of the fetal liver has also been described.[175]

The recombination mechanisms leading to antigen-receptor gene rearrangements are not required for the ontogeny of NK cells, which develop in SCID mice and in RAG-deficient mice, in which B- and T-cell production is impaired.[238] NK cells also develop normally in nude mice, which are athymic, and normal NK-cell function and numbers have been found in patients with DiGeorge's syndrome and thymic aplasia.[239] Thus, thymic integrity does not appear to be essential for NK-cell development. Very few NK cells are present in the thymus, and it is not clear whether these are resident or recirculating cells. Current models propose a thymic-independent development in which NK cells eventually develop from CD34⁺ progenitor cells of the fetal liver and bone marrow (in late fetal and postnatal life). Because murine cells expressing FγRIII give rise to T cells after thymic transfer or to NK cells after intravenous transfer, it was hypothesized that restricted NK–T cell progenitors are present in the fetal thymus.[240] Recent results suggest that the NK–T-cell precursors among this subset could be identified by their expression of CD117; mature NK cells do not express CD117, whereas precursor cells do.[241] Other studies have shown that human fetal thymocytes (16 to 22 weeks of gestation) cultured in methylcellulose in the presence of IL-7, IL-15, and SCF form colonies consisting of medium-to-large granular lymphocytes that express CD56 but not CD3 and exhibit cytolytic activity against K562 cells.[242] Colony-forming units-NK were enriched in CD34+Lin− subpopulations of fetal thymocytes. Spits et al[243] showed that in the thymus, the stem-cell progeny retain the ability to differentiate into T, NK, or dendritic cells. The induction of T-cell commitment is correlated with the appearance of CD1a, the loss of the ability of the progenitors to develop into NK or dendritic cells, and the initiation of *TCR* gene rearrangements.[243]

Bone marrow CD34+ cells expressing CD56 are rare, and the level of CD56 expression is low.[244] It has been postulated that CD7 expression is an early event in the commitment of hematopoietic progenitors to the NK lineage. Indeed, the number of NK cells that were derived from CD34+CD7+ cells was significantly higher than that of NK derived from other bone marrow cells, particularly cells with the highest levels of CD7 expression.[245]

IL-15 is required for NK cell development in vivo.[246, 247] IL-15 binds the IL-15 receptor on NK cells; this receptor is composed of an IL-15 receptor chain and the common IL-2 receptor β and γ chains. NK cell development is impaired in mice with homozygous mutations in either of the genes encoding the IL-2 receptor β or γ chains,[248, 249] and patients with X-linked SCID and common γ chain mutations have low numbers of NK cells.[165] However, NK cells develop normally in IL-2–deficient mice, a finding suggesting that the lack of response to IL-15 is the cause of the NK developmental defect in these animals.[248]

EXOGENOUS FACTORS INFLUENCING LYMPHOID CELL GROWTH

It is widely accepted that the interaction of progenitor cells with their microenvironment is crucial for lymphohematopoiesis. However, it is unclear whether the growth and differentiation of lymphohematopoietic cells are guided by external stimuli or whether they rely on an inherent cell program. If hematopoiesis is entirely directed by a genetic program, the microenvironment would simply play a permissive role by supporting cell survival. If, however, decisions about hematopoietic cell expansion and differentiation are directed by extracellular signals, the role of the microenvironment could be much more complex. The latter view is supported by observations in many developmental systems in which the differentiation of multipotent precursors is determined by microenvironmental cues.[250] This view has led some investigators to postulate the existence of specialized "niches" within the lymphohematopoietic microenvironment, with each niche producing distinct stimuli that drive the expansion and differentiation of stem cells and lineage-committed precursors.[251-253]

B-Cell Development and the Bone Marrow Microenvironment

The in vitro survival and growth of B-cell progenitors depend on functional bone-marrow stromal cells.[149, 254, 255] "Bone marrow stroma" is a general term that refers to cells anchored in the bone marrow cavity, including mesenchymal, endothelial, and reticular cells, fibroblasts, adipocytes, and macrophages.[149] These stromal cells grow readily in vitro, forming adherent layers essential for the long-term support of human and murine myelopoiesis and B lymphopoiesis.[251, 252, 256, 257]

Various combinations of stromal cell–secreted products and interactions of cell surface receptor with stroma surface molecules (e.g., VLA-4-VCAM-1) or extracellular matrix molecules (e.g., VLA-4 and VLA-5/fibronectin) probably promote self-renewal and differentiation of immature B cells. However, the precise combination of stroma-derived factors necessary for B-cell growth has not yet been identified. The survival of B-cell progenitors in vitro requires direct contact between these cells and stromal layers,[5] a finding suggesting that soluble factors are not sufficient by themselves to support the survival of immature B-lymphoid cells. Thus, cytokines may promote cell survival only when they are bound to plasma membranes or when they are highly concentrated in the extracellular matrix. Cytokines that stimulate the proliferation of murine and human early B-lineage cells in vitro include IL-3, IL-6, IL-7, insulin-like growth factor-1, SCF, and H + 3/HK − 2 ligand.[254, 255, 258, 259] However, none of these factors can replace stromal layers in maintaining human immature B cells in vitro.[260-262] Moreover, the addition of neutralizing antibodies to IL-7, SCF, TNFα, platelet-derived growth factor, and insulin-like growth factor-1 does not affect the growth of human immature B cells cultured on stromal layers.[263]

Stromal cell-derived factor-1 (SDF-1) is a chemotactic factor for many cells, including B-cell progenitors.[264] SDF-1, which binds the CXCR4 receptor,[265] probably regulates the migration and homing of progenitor cells. Gene inactivation studies have shown that both SDF-1[266] and CXCR4[265] are essential for B lymphopoiesis. In a study of human bone marrow B cells, expression of CXCR4 was found to be highest on the surface of pre-B cells, but expression decreased as cells developed into immature B cells.[267] As these cells entered the mature B-cell stage, expression of CXCR4 increased again. Somewhat unexpectedly, SDF-1 triggered migration responses only in early B cells that expressed low levels of CXCR4.[267]

A culture system for normal human B-cell progenitors includes mouse fibroblastic Ltk− cells transfected with the gene encoding the human Fc receptor CD32 onto which anti-CD40 antibody is added, or directly transfected with CD40 ligand.[268] Cross-linking CD40 using the Ltk− cell–CD40 system can, when coupled with the addition of exogenous IL-4, support the growth of B cells for 2 to 3 months.[268] Human B-cell progenitors will proliferate in the Ltk− cell–CD40 system when IL-3 is substituted for IL-4.[269, 270] Furthermore, it is the CD19+, CD34− pre-B-cell population that is uniquely responsive to IL-3 and anti-CD40.[269] Other results show that CD4+ T cells can exert a stimulatory effect on the proliferation of B-cell progenitors in vitro; this effect is apparently the result of the interaction between the CD40 ligand of the activated T cell and CD40 of the B cell.[271]

A culture system employing the murine S17 bone marrow stromal cell line can support the growth of human CD19[+] B-lineage cells from a starting population of cord blood CD34[+] mononuclear cells.[272] CD19[+] B-lineage cells emerge after an initial wave of myeloid cell growth,[272] reminiscent of the emergence of B-lineage cells in the original Whitlock-Witte culture system.[257] The CD19[+] cells coexpress CD10, but express little or no CD34 or TdT, and have germline Ig H-chain genes. If cord blood CD34[+] cells are first cultured on S17 cells and then on fibroblasts expressing human CD40 ligand in the presence of IL-10 and IL-4, mature B cells can develop[273]; these cells are capable of secreting Ig and undergo isotype switching.

These results point to a crucial role of CD40 signaling in early B-cell development. However, there is no apparent impairment in the early stages of B-cell differentiation in patients with defective expression of CD40 ligand or CD40 signaling. In these patients, the absence of CD40 signaling appears specifically to affect the ability of B lymphocytes to undergo Ig class switching.[274-278]

T-Cell Development and the Thymic Microenvironment

Growth and differentiation of T-cell precursors are regulated by the complex cell types that make up the thymic microenvironment and their secreted cytokines.[183, 204-206] Included among the secreted products of thymic epithelial cells are IL-1, IL-3, IL-6, IL-7, SCF, leukemia inhibitory factor, transforming growth factor-β and the colony-stimulating factors GM-CSF, G-CSF and M-CSF.[279-284] Production of some cytokines by the thymic epithelium can, in turn, be regulated by IL-1, IL-4, IFN-γ, epidermal growth factor, and transforming growth factor-β.[281-283]

T-cell differentiation is more effectively achieved in vitro in the presence of cellular elements of the thymic microenvironment. Human CD34[+] Lin[−] cells differentiate into T cells when injected into human fetal thymi that have been implanted into SCID mice[285] or when seeded onto thymic stromal monolayers.[286] In the presence of a thymic microenvironment, CD34[+] progenitors can differentiate into mature CD4[+]CD8[−] or CD4[−]CD8[+] T cells.[287, 288] The SCID-hu mouse has also been used as an in vivo microenvironment for the analysis of human thymocyte maturation[289] but, in this model, human thymic lobules must be implanted under the kidney capsule so that the lobules can serve as a microenvironment for developing thymocytes. IL-2,[173] IL-4,[173, 290] IL-7,[200] and SCF[291] reportedly regulate the growth and differentiation of thymocytes in vitro.

Exogenous Factors Influencing NK Cell Development

Human NK cells can be generated from bone marrow–derived CD34[+] cells cultured in the presence of IL-2 and a stroma feeder layer or in the presence of IL-2 and other hematopoietic growth factors such as SCF or IL-15.[292-295] Miller et al[292] reported that bone marrow CD34[+]HLA-DR[−] cells give rise to NK cells when the progenitors are plated on stromal layers and cultured with IL-2 and human serum. The same group also succeeded in deriving NK cells from human CD34[+], Lin[−], HLA-DR[−] progenitors in a culture system in which these cells are initially separated from the stroma by a microporous membrane and are grown with IL-3 and macrophage inflammatory protein-1α.[296] Cells are subsequently plated so they are in direct contact with the stroma, in the presence of hydrocortisone, IL-2, IL-7, and SCF. Later, hydrocortisone, IL-7, and SCF are replaced by human serum. The resulting cells are CD56[+]CD3[−] cells that exhibit cytotoxic activity against NK-sensitive K562 cells. Thymic stromal cells also support the generation of NK cells from CD34[+] bone marrow cells.[297]

Exogenous Factors Influencing the Survival and Growth of Leukemic Lymphoid Cells

Leukemic progenitor cells of patients have been difficult to maintain and study in vitro because of the lack of information about the survival requirements of lympho-hematopoietic cells. Efforts to culture primary leukemic cells in vitro have relied on factors such as fetal bovine serum, human plasma, "leukocyte-conditioned medium," and a variety of cytokines to support cell growth; with few exceptions, the number of viable cells decreases rapidly.[260, 298, 299]

The inability to maintain leukemic cells in vitro is an important constraint in developing robust in vitro drug cytotoxicity assays. This difficulty reduces the number of successful tests (those in which at least a few viable cells can be recovered from control cultures).[300] This difficulty also calls into question the reliability of results of drug cytotoxicity measurements that are performed on dying cells, a situation markedly different than that in vivo, where the number of leukemic cells increases relentlessly.

Despite these limitations, colony-forming assays, ^{3}H-thymidine incorporation assays, and cell cycle analysis have been used to evaluate the in vitro responsiveness of freshly isolated leukemic cells from patients with B-lineage ALL.[261, 299, 301-308] Studies using IL-3[301, 302] and IL-7[261, 302, 309] have demonstrated that a subset (generally <50%) of patients has growth-responsive B-lineage ALL cells. However, two studies involving a broad range of interleukins and CSFs concluded that no single cytokine or combination of cytokines delivered a substantive growth stimulus to the leukemic cells from a significant number of patients with B-lineage ALL.[303, 304]

Several laboratories have investigated the in vitro responsiveness of leukemic cells of patients with T-lineage ALL to various growth factors by using assays similar to those used in studies of B-lineage ALL.[309-313] IL-2, IL-7, or both exert growth-promoting effects in some cases, but some leukemic T cells do not respond to either IL-2 or IL-7. One significant variable that complicates the analysis of leukemic cells in T-lineage ALL is the fact that normal

T cells respond vigorously to IL-2 and IL-7. Because normal T cells frequently contaminate bone marrow and peripheral blood specimens of patients with ALL, formal proof that the leukemic T-cell clone is responding to a given growth stimulus must always be obtained by karyotypic or molecular (e.g., clonal rearrangement of TCR genes) analyses.

In our study of 125 cases of B-lineage ALL, the median cell recovery after 7 days of liquid culture was 1% of the cells originally seeded,[314] and studies of T-ALL and acute myeloid leukemia cells yielded similar results (D. Campana, unpublished observations). Cell loss was preceded by molecular and cellular changes characteristic of apoptosis. Because crucial survival signals for immature lymphohematopoietic cells are generated in the bone marrow microenvironment, we reasoned that bone marrow–derived stromal cells might provide a superior culture system for leukemic cells by preventing apoptosis and promoting long-term survival. Indeed, when leukemic cells were cultured on stroma, the median number of cells recovered after culture improved dramatically[298]; in a series of 131 cases, it was 91%.[314] Leukemic cell growth in vitro correlates well with treatment outcome[315] and is distinctly impaired in cases of B-lineage ALL with a modal chromosome number 51 to 65.[314]

Direct contact with stroma is essential for survival of ALL cells: separation results in the induction of apoptosis.[5] When single leukemic cells were placed in the stroma-coated wells of microtiter plates, the percentage of wells with leukemic cell growth after 2 to 5 months of culture ranged from 6% to 20% (median, 15%; five experiments).[316] The immunophenotypes and genetic features of cells recovered from these cultures were identical to those of ALL cells before culture, and cells maintained their stroma dependency and self-renewal capacity.[316] The development of ALL cell lines that depend on stroma for survival should prove useful in the elucidation of signaling events underlying the survival-promoting effect of the stroma.[317]

The supporting effects of stroma for the in vitro culture of malignant lymphoid cells extend to B-chronic lymphocytic leukemia (B-CLL). Bone marrow stromal cells suppress apoptosis of B-CLL cells in vitro.[318] In contrast to ALL cells, B-CLL cells can also be maintained, at least for a few days, in cultures containing IL-4, IFN-α, or IFN-γ.[319, 320]

CONCLUSION

The expansion of immunologic and molecular techniques over the last 2 decades has accelerated at great pace, resulting in an enormous increment in the understanding of the principles and mechanisms regulating lymphoid development. This progress has not only helped to elucidate the processes involved in normal and pathologic immune responses but has also significantly affected the study of lymphoid malignancies.

Immunophenotypic studies of normal lymphoid development have allowed the selection of specific cell markers for the classification of acute leukemias and lymphoproliferative disorders.[321] Comparative studies of normal and leukemic cell marker expression have identified marker combinations useful for monitoring submicroscopic disease.[3] The study of Ig and TCR gene rearrangements is also rapidly becoming a routine approach for the classification and monitoring of leukemia.[322] Finally, disruption of transcription factors crucial for normal development has been implicated in leukemogenesis.[2] Collectively, the gained knowledge should translate into improved clinical management practices and, hence, cure rates.

The realization that lymphohematopoietic cell growth depends on the interaction with the hematopoietic microenvironment has allowed the development of techniques to maintain leukemic lymphoid cells in vitro for prolonged periods, the study of their molecular interactions with the microenvironment, and the identification of factors that affect their survival and growth. One concept that has emerged from these studies is that the growth of leukemic lymphoblasts may be suppressed by triggering inhibitory signaling pathways via engagement of surface receptors. For example, IL-4 induces growth arrest and apoptosis of B-leukemic lymphoblasts in vitro[323-325] and suppresses the growth of human leukemic cells engrafted in immunodeficient mice.[326] IL-4 also induces apoptosis of normal B-lymphoid progenitors.[325] In contrast to the induction of normal B-cell proliferation by IL-7, this cytokine inhibits the growth of some leukemic B-cell lines.[6, 327] Ligation of CD38 induces apoptosis in leukemic lymphoblasts and markedly inhibits cell recovery after culture.[131] The understanding of the receptors and signaling pathways that suppress leukemia cell growth has obvious implications for the development of novel treatments for leukemia.

REFERENCES

1. Greaves MF: Differentiation-linked leukemogenesis in lymphocytes. Science 1986, 234, 697-704.
2. Look AT: Oncogenic transcription factors in the human acute leukemias. Science 1997, 278, 1059-1064.
3. Campana D, Coustan-Smith E: Detection of minimal residual disease in acute leukemia by flow cytometry. Cytometry 1999, 38, 139-152.
4. Ryan DH: Adherence of normal and neoplastic human B cell precursors to the bone marrow microenvironment. Blood Cells 1993, 19, 225-241.
5. Manabe A, Murti KG, Coustan-Smith E, et al: Adhesion-dependent survival of normal and leukemic human B lymphoblasts on bone marrow stromal cells. Blood 1994, 83, 758-766.
6. Pandrau-Garcia D, de Saint-Vis B, Saeland S, et al: Growth inhibitory and agonistic signals of interleukin-7 (IL-7) can be mediated through the CDw127 IL-7 receptor. Blood 1994, 83, 3613-3619.
7. Till JE, McCulloch EA: A direct measurement of the radiation sensitivity of normal bone marrow cells. Radiat Res 1961, 14, 213.
8. Weissman IL: Stem cells: Units of development, units of regeneration, and units in evolution. Cell 2000, 100, 157-168.
9. Dick JE, Magli MC, Huszar D, et al: Introduction of a selectable gene into primitive stem cells capable of long-term reconstitution of the hemopoietic system of W/Wv mice. Cell 1985, 42, 71-79.
10. Lemischka IR, Raulet DH, Mulligan RC: Developmental potential and dynamic behavior of hematopoietic stem cells. Cell 1986, 45, 917-927.
11. Brenner MK, Rill DR, Holladay MS, et al: Gene marking to determine whether autologous marrow infusion restores long-term haemopoiesis in cancer patients. Lancet 1993, 342, 1134-1137.
12. Fialkow PJ, Denman AM, Jacobson RJ, et al: Chronic myelocytic

leukemia: Origin of some lymphocytes from leukemic stem cells. J Clin Invest 1978, 62, 815–823.

13. Martin PJ, Najfeld V, Hansen JA, et al: Involvement of the B-lymphoid system in chronic myelogenous leukaemia. Nature 1980, 287, 49–50.

14. LeBien TW, Hozier J, Minowada J, et al: Origin of chronic myelocytic leukemia in a precursor of pre-B lymphocytes. N Engl J Med 1979, 301, 144–147.

15. Minowada J, Koshiba H, Janossy G, et al: A Philadelphia chromosome–positive human leukaemia cell line (NALM-1) with pre-B characteristics. Leuk Res 1979, 3, 261–266.

16. Vogler LB, Crist WM, Vinson PC, et al: Philadelphia-chromosome-positive pre-B-cell leukemia presenting as blast crisis of chronic myelogenous leukemia. Blood 1979, 54, 1164–1170.

17. Buschle M, Janssen JW, Drexler H, et al: Evidence for pluripotent stem cell origin of idiopathic myelofibrosis: Clonal analysis of a case characterized by a N-ras gene mutation. Leukemia 1988, 2, 658–660.

18. Uchida N, Weissman IL: Searching for hematopoietic stem cells: Evidence that Thy-1.1 Lin⁻ Sca-1⁺ cells are the only stem cells in C57BL/Ka-Thy-1.1 bone marrow. J Exp Med 1992, 175, 175–184.

19. Uchida N, Jerabek L, Weissman IL: Searching for hematopoietic stem cells. II: The heterogeneity of Thy-1.1 Lin⁻ Sca-1⁺ mouse hematopoietic stem cells separated by counterflow centrifugal elutriation. Exp Hematol 1996, 24, 649–659.

20. Baum CM, Weissman IL, Tsukamoto AS, et al: Isolation of a candidate human hematopoietic stem-cell population. Proc Natl Acad Sci U S A 1992, 89, 2804–2808.

21. Huang S, Terstappen LWMM: Lymphoid and myeloid differentiation of single human CD34⁺, HLA-Dr⁺, CD38⁻ hematopoietic stem cells. Blood 1994, 83, 1515–1526.

22. Kondo M, Weissman IL, Akashi K: Identification of clonogenic common lymphoid progenitors in mouse bone marrow. Cell 1997, 91, 661–672.

23. Akashi K, Traver D, Miyamoto T, et al: A clonogenic common myeloid progenitor that gives rise to all myeloid lineages. Nature 2000, 404, 193–197.

24. Galy A, Travis M, Cen D, et al: Human T, B, natural killer, and dendritic cells arise from a common bone marrow progenitor cell subset. Immunity 1995, 3, 459–473.

25. Cumano A, Paige CJ, Iscove NN, et al: Bipotential precursors of B cells and macrophages in murine fetal liver. Nature 1992, 356, 612–615.

26. Hirayama F, Shih JP, Awgulewitsch A, et al: Clonal proliferation of murine lymphohemopoietic progenitors in culture. Proc Natl Acad Sci U S A 1992, 89, 5907–5911.

27. Bjorck P, Kincade PW: CD19⁺ pro-B cells can give rise to dendritic cells in vitro. J Immunol 1998, 161, 5795–5799.

28. Kim J, Sif S, Jones B, et al: Ikaros DNA-binding proteins direct formation of chromatin remodeling complexes in lymphocytes. Immunity 1999, 10, 345–355.

29. Georgopoulos K, Bigby M, Wang JH, et al: The Ikaros gene is required for the development of all lymphoid lineages. Cell 1994, 79, 143–156.

30. Winandy S, Wu P, Georgopoulos K: A dominant mutation in the Ikaros gene leads to rapid development of leukemia and lymphoma. Cell 1995, 83, 289–299.

31. Winandy S, Wu L, Wang JH, et al: Pre-T cell receptor (TCR) and TCR-controlled checkpoints in T cell differentiation are set by Ikaros. J Exp Med 1999, 190, 1039–1048.

32. Morgan B, Sun L, Avitahl N, et al: Aiolos, a lymphoid restricted transcription factor that interacts with Ikaros to regulate lymphocyte differentiation. EMBO J 1997, 16, 2004–2013.

33. Kelley CM, Ikeda T, Koipally J, et al: Helios, a novel dimerization partner of Ikaros expressed in the earliest hematopoietic progenitors. Curr Biol 1998, 8, 508–515.

34. Nichogiannopoulou A, Trevisan M, Neben S, et al: Defects in hematopoietic stem cell activity in Ikaros mutant mice. J Exp Med 1999, 190, 1201–1214.

35. McKercher SR, Torbett BE, Anderson KL, et al: Targeted disruption of the PU.1 gene results in multiple hematopoietic abnormalities. EMBO J 1996, 15, 5647–5658.

36. Scott EW, Fisher RC, Olson MC, et al: PU.1 functions in a cell-autonomous manner to control the differentiation of multipotential lymphoid-myeloid progenitors. Immunity 1997, 6, 437–447.

37. Barton K, Muthusamy N, Fischer C, et al: The Ets-1 transcription factor is required for the development of natural killer cells in mice. Immunity 1998, 9, 555–563.

38. Muthusamy N, Barton K, Leiden JM: Defective activation and survival of T cells lacking the Ets-1 transcription factor. Nature 1995, 377, 639–642.

39. Bories JC, Willerford DM, Grevin D, et al: Increased T-cell apoptosis and terminal B-cell differentiation induced by inactivation of the Ets-1 proto-oncogene. Nature 1995, 377, 635–638.

40. Reya T, Grosschedl R: Transcriptional regulation of B-cell differentiation. Curr Opin Immunol 1998, 10, 158–165.

41. Bain G, Robanus Mandaag EC, te Riele HP, et al: Both E12 and E47 allow commitment to the B-cell lineage. Immunity 1997, 6, 145–154.

42. Lin H, Grosschedl R: Failure of B-cell differentiation in mice lacking the transcription factor EBF. Nature 1995, 637, 263–267.

43. O'Riordan M, Grosschedl R: Coordinate regulation of B-cell differentiation by the transcription factors EBF and E2A. Immunity 1999, 11, 21–31.

44. Bain G, Engel I, Robanus Mandaag EC, et al: E2A deficiency leads to abnormalities in alphabeta T-cell development and to rapid development of T-cell lymphomas. Mol Cell Biol 1997, 17, 4782–4791.

45. Nutt SL, Heavey B, Rolink AG, et al: Commitment to the B-lymphoid lineage depends on the transcription factor Pax5. Nature 1999, 401, 556–562.

46. Rolink AG, Nutt SL, Melchers F, et al: Long-term in vivo reconstitution of T-cell development by Pax5-deficient B-cell progenitors. Nature 1999, 401, 603–606.

47. Corcoran LM, Karvelas M, Nossal GJ, et al: Oct-2, although not required for early B-cell development, is critical for later B-cell maturation and for postnatal survival. Genes Dev 1993, 7, 570–582.

48. Schubart DB, Rolink A, Kosco-Vilbois MH, et al: B-cell–specific coactivator OBF-1/OCA-B/Bob1 required for immune response and germinal centre formation. Nature 1996, 383, 538–542.

49. Kim U, Qin XF, Gong S, et al: The B-cell–specific transcription coactivator OCA-B/OBF-1/Bob-1 is essential for normal production of immunoglobulin isotypes. Nature 1996, 383, 542–547.

50. Verbeek S, Izon D, Hofhuis F, et al: An HMG-box–containing T-cell factor required for thymocyte differentiation. Nature 1995, 374, 70–74.

51. Held W, Kunz B, Lowin-Kropf B, et al: Clonal acquisition of the Ly49A NK-cell receptor is dependent on the transacting factor TCF-1. Immunity 1999, 11, 433–442.

52. Schilham MW, Oosterwegel MA, Moerer P, et al: Defects in cardiac outflow tract formation and pro-B-lymphocyte expansion in mice lacking Sox-4. Nature 1996, 380, 711–714.

53. Ting CN, Olson MC, Barton KP, et al: Transcription factor GATA-3 is required for development of the T-cell lineage. Nature 1996, 384, 474–478.

54. Matsuyama T, Kimura T, Kitagawa M, et al: Targeted disruption of IRF-1 or IRF-2 results in abnormal type I IFN gene induction and aberrant lymphocyte development. Cell 1993, 75, 83–97.

55. Penninger JM, Mak TW: Thymocyte selection in Vav and IRF-1 gene-deficient mice. Immunol Rev 1998, 165, 149–166.

56. Melchers F, Haasner D, Grawunder U, et al: Roles of Ig H and L chains and of surrogate H and L chains in the development of cells of the B-lymphocyte lineage. Annu Rev Immunol 1994, 12, 209–225.

57. Burrows PD, Cooper MD: B-cell development and differentiation. Curr Opin Immunol 1997, 9, 239–244.

58. LeBien TW: B-cell lymphopoiesis in mouse and man. Curr Opin Immunol 1998, 10, 188–195.

59. Moss PA, Rosenberg WM, Bell JI: The human T-cell receptor in health and disease. Annu Rev Immunol 1992, 10, 71–96.

60. Agrawal A, Eastman QM, Schatz DG: Transposition mediated by RAG1 and RAG2 and its implications for the evolution of the immune system. Nature 1998, 394, 744–751.

61. Han S, Dillon SR, Zheng B, et al: V(D)J recombinase activity in a subset of germinal center B lymphocytes. Science 1997, 278, 301–305.

62. Papavasiliou F, Casellas R, Suh H, et al: V(D)J recombination in mature B cells: A mechanism for altering antibody responses. Science 1997, 278, 298–301.

63. Qin XF, Schwers S, Yu W, et al: Secondary V(D)J recombination in B-1 cells. Nature 1999, 397, 355–359.

64. Lantelme E, Palermo B, Granziero L, et al: Cutting edge: Recombinase-activating gene expression and V(D)J recombination in CD4+ CD3-low mature T lymphocytes. J Immunol 2000, 164, 3455–3459.

65. Mombaerts P, Iacomini J, Johnson RS, et al: RAG-1-deficient mice have no mature B and T lymphocytes. Cell 1992, 68, 869–877.

66. Shinkai Y, Rathbun G, Lam KP, et al: RAG-2-deficient mice lack mature lymphocytes owing to inability to initiate V(D)J re-arrangement. Cell 1992, 68, 855–867.

67. Desiderio SV, Yancopoulos GD, Paskind M, et al: Insertion of N regions into heavy-chain genes is correlated with expression of terminal deoxytransferase in B cells. Nature 1984, 311, 752–755.

68. Komori T, Okada A, Stewart V, et al: Lack of N regions in antigen receptor variable region genes of TdT-deficient lymphocytes. Science 1993, 261, 1171–1175.

69. Nussenzweig A, Chen C, da CS, V, et al: Requirement for Ku80 in growth and immunoglobulin V(D)J recombination. Nature 1996, 382, 551–555.

70. Roth DB, Menetski JP, Nakajima PB, et al: V(D)J recombination: Broken DNA molecules with covalently sealed (hairpin) coding ends in scid mouse thymocytes. Cell 1992, 70, 983–991.

71. Bogue MA, Jhappan C, Roth DB: Analysis of variable (diversity) joining recombination in DNA-dependent protein kinase (DNA-PK)–deficient mice reveals DNA-PK-independent pathways for both signal and coding joint formation. Proc Natl Acad Sci U S A 1998, 95, 15559–15564.

72. Gu Y, Seidl KJ, Rathbun GA, et al: Growth retardation and leaky SCID phenotype of Ku70-deficient mice. Immunity 1997, 7, 653–665.

73. Bloom W, Bartelmez GW: Hematopoiesis in young human embryos. Am J Anat 1940, 67, 21.

74. Gathings WE, Lawton AR, Cooper MD: Immunofluorescent studies of the development of pre-B cells, B lymphocytes and immunoglobulin isotype diversity in humans. Eur J Immunol 1977, 7, 804–810.

75. Solvason N, Kearney JF: The human fetal omentum: A site of B-cell generation. J Exp Med 1992, 175, 397–404.

76. Nunez C, Nishimoto N, Gartland GL, et al: B cells are generated throughout life in humans. J Immunol 1996, 156, 866–872.

77. Brashem CJ, Kersey JH, Bollum FJ, et al: Ontogenic studies of lymphoid progenitor cells in human bone marrow. Exp Hematol 1982, 10, 886–892.

78. Hokland P, Rosenthal P, Griffin JD, et al: Purification and characterization of fetal hematopoietic cells that express the common acute lymphoblastic leukemia antigen (CALLA). J Exp Med 1983, 157, 114–129.

79. Tavian M, Hallais MF, Peault B: Emergence of intraembryonic hematopoietic precursors in the pre-liver human embryo. Development 1999, 126, 793–803.

80. Medvinsky A, Dzierzak E: Definitive hematopoiesis is autonomously initiated by the AGM region. Cell 1996, 86, 897–906.

81. Ohmura K, Kawamoto H, Fujimoto S, et al: Emergence of T-, B-, and myeloid lineage–committed as well as multipotent hematopoietic progenitors in the aorta-gonad-mesonephros region of day 10 fetuses of the mouse. J Immunol 1999, 163, 4788–4795.

82. Schatz DG, Oettinger MA, Schlissel MS: V(D)J recombination: Molecular biology and regulation. Annu Rev Immunol 1992, 10, 359–383.

83. Cook GP, Tomlinson IM, Walter G, et al: A map of the human immunoglobulin VH locus completed by analysis of the telomeric region of chromosome 14q. Nat Genet 1994, 7, 162–168.

84. Bertrand FE, Billips LG, Burrows PD, et al: Ig D(H) gene segment transcription and rearrangement before surface expression of the pan-B-cell marker CD19 in normal human bone marrow. Blood 1997, 90, 736–744.

85. Ehlich A, Schaal S, Gu H, et al: Immunoglobulin heavy- and light-chain genes rearrange independently at early stages of B-cell development. Cell 1993, 72, 695–704.

86. Kubagawa H, Cooper MD, Carroll AJ, et al: Light-chain gene expression before heavy-chain gene rearrangement in pre-B cells transformed by Epstein-Barr virus. Proc Natl Acad Sci U S A 1989, 86, 2356–2360.

87. Pauza ME, Rehmann JA, LeBien TW: Unusual patterns of immuno-globulin gene rearrangement and expression during human B-cell ontogeny: Human B cells can simultaneously express cell surface kappa and lambda light chains. J Exp Med 1993, 178, 139–149.

88. Yel L, Minegishi Y, Coustan-Smith E, et al: Mutations in the mu heavy-chain gene in patients with agammaglobulinemia. N Engl J Med 1996, 335, 1486–1493.

89. Kitamura D, Rajewsky K: Targeted disruption of mu chain membrane exon causes loss of heavy-chain allelic exclusion. Nature 1992, 356, 154–156.

90. Nussenzweig MC: Immune receptor editing: Revise and select. Cell 1998, 95, 875–878.

91. Hollis GF, Evans RJ, Stafford-Hollis JM, et al: Immunoglobulin lambda light-chain–related genes 14.1 and 16.1 are expressed in pre-B cells and may encode the human immunoglobulin omega light-chain protein. Proc Natl Acad Sci U S A 1989, 86, 5552–5556.

92. Mason DY, Cordell JL, Tse AG, et al: The IgM-associated protein mb-1 as a marker of normal and neoplastic B cells. J Immunol 1991, 147, 2474–2482.

93. Nakamura T, Kubagawa H, Cooper MD: Heterogeneity of immunoglobulin-associated molecules on human B cells identified by monoclonal antibodies. Proc Natl Acad Sci U S A 1992, 89, 8522–8526.

94. Reth M, Wienands J: Initiation and processing of signals from the B cell antigen receptor. Annu Rev Immunol 1997, 15, 453–479.

95. Karasuyama H, Rolink A, Shinkai Y, et al: The expression of V pre-B/lambda 5 surrogate light chain in early bone marrow precursor B cells of normal and B-cell–deficient mutant mice. Cell 1994, 77, 133–143.

96. Lassoued K, Illges H, Benlagha K, et al: Fate of surrogate light chains in B-lineage cells. J Exp Med 1996, 183, 421–429.

97. Benschop RJ, Cambier JC: B-cell development: Signal transduction by antigen receptors and their surrogates. Curr Opin Immunol 1999, 11, 143–151.

98. Nagata K, Nakamura T, Kitamura F, et al: The Ig alpha/Ig beta heterodimer on mu-negative pro-B cells is competent for transducing signals to induce early B-cell differentiation. Immunity 1997, 7, 559–570.

99. Kitamura D, Kudo A, Schaal S, et al: A critical role of lambda 5 protein in B-cell development. Cell 1992, 69, 823–831.

100. Gong S, Nussenzweig MC: Regulation of an early developmental checkpoint in the B-cell pathway by Ig beta. Science 1996, 272, 411–414.

101. Minegishi Y, Coustan-Smith E, Wang YH, et al: Mutations in the human *lambda 5/14.1* gene result in B-cell deficiency and agammaglobulinemia. J Exp Med 1998, 187, 71–77.

102. Minegishi Y, Coustan-Smith E, Rapalus L, et al: Mutations in Ig alpha (CD79a) result in a complete block in B-cell development. J Clin Invest 1999, 104, 1115–1121.

103. Davi F, Faili A, Gritti C, et al: Early onset of immunoglobulin heavy-chain gene rearrangements in normal human bone marrow CD34+ cells. Blood 1997, 90, 4014–4021.

104. Ryan DH, Nuccie BL, Ritterman I, et al: Expression of interleukin-7 receptor by lineage-negative human bone marrow progenitors with enhanced lymphoid proliferative potential and B-lineage differentiation capacity. Blood 1997, 89, 929–940.

105. Dworzak MN, Fritsch G, Froschl G, et al: Four-color flow cytometric investigation of terminal deoxynucleotidyl transferase–positive lymphoid precursors in pediatric bone marrow: CD79a expression precedes CD19 in early B-cell ontogeny. Blood 1998, 92, 3203–3209.

106. Campana D, Janossy G, Bofill M, et al: Human B-cell development. I: Phenotypic differences of B lymphocytes in the bone marrow and peripheral lymphoid tissue. J Immunol 1985, 134, 1524–1530.

107. Dorken B, Moldenhauer G, Pezzutto A, et al: HD39 (B3), a B-lineage–restricted antigen whose cell surface expression is limited to resting and activated human B lymphocytes. J Immunol 1986, 136, 4470–4479.

108. Cyster JG, Goodnow CC: Tuning antigen receptor signaling by CD22: Integrating cues from antigens and the microenvironment. Immunity 1997, 6, 509–517.

109. Janossy G, Bollum FJ, Bradstock KF, et al: Terminal transferase-positive human bone marrow cells exhibit the antigenic phenotype of common acute lymphoblastic leukemia. J Immunol 1979, 123, 1525–1529.

110. Janossy G, Bollum FJ, Bradstock KF, et al: Cellular phenotypes of

normal and leukemic hemopoietic cells determined by analysis with selected antibody combinations. Blood 1980, 56, 430–441.

111. Villablanca JG, Anderson JM, Moseley M, et al: Differentiation of normal human pre-B cells in vitro. J Exp Med 1990, 172:, 325–334.

112. Kantor AB, Herzenberg LA: Origin of murine B-cell lineages. Annu Rev Immunol 1993, 11, 501–538.

113. Youinou P, Jamin C, Lydyard PM: CD5 expression in human B-cell populations. Immunol Today 1999, 20, 312–316.

114. Bofill M, Janossy G, Janossa M, et al: Human B-cell development. II: Subpopulations in the human fetus. J Immunol 1985, 134, 1531–1538.

115. Kipps TJ, Robbins BA, Carson DA: Uniform high-frequency expression of autoantibody-associated cross-reactive idiotypes in the primary B-cell follicles of human fetal spleen. J Exp Med 1990, 171, 189–196.

116. Kipps TJ, Duffy SF: Relationship of the CD5 B cell to human tonsillar lymphocytes that express autoantibody-associated cross-reactive idiotypes. J Clin Invest 1991, 87, 2087–2096.

117. Kasaian MT, Ikematsu H, Casali P: Identification and analysis of a novel human surface CD5-B lymphocyte subset producing natural antibodies. J Immunol 1992, 148, 2690–2702.

118. Schettino EW, Chai SK, Kasaian MT, et al: *VHDJH* gene sequences and antigen reactivity of monoclonal antibodies produced by human B-1 cells: Evidence for somatic selection. J Immunol 1997, 158, 2477–2489.

119. Arnold LW, McCray SK, Tatu C, et al: Identification of a precursor to phosphatidyl choline-specific B-1 cells suggesting that B-1 cells differentiate from splenic conventional B cells in vivo: Cyclosporin A blocks differentiation to B-1. J Immunol 2000, 164, 2924–2930.

120. Caligaris-Cappio F: B-chronic lymphocytic leukemia: A malignancy of anti-self B cells. Blood 1996, 87, 2615–2620.

121. Buhl AM, Cambier JC: Co-receptor and accessory regulation of B-cell antigen receptor signal transduction. Immunol Rev 1997, 160, 127–138.

122. Engel P, Zhou LJ, Ord DC, et al: Abnormal B-lymphocyte development, activation, and differentiation in mice that lack or overexpress the CD19 signal transduction molecule. Immunity 1995, 3, 39–50.

123. Otipoby KL, Andersson KB, Draves KE, et al: CD22 regulates thymus-independent responses and the lifespan of B cells. Nature 1996, 384, 634–637.

124. O'Keefe TL, Williams GT, Davies SL, et al: Hyperresponsive B cells in CD22-deficient mice. Science 1996, 274, 798–801.

125. Sato S, Miller AS, Inaoki M, et al: CD22 is both a positive and negative regulator of B-lymphocyte antigen receptor signal transduction: Altered signaling in CD22-deficient mice. Immunity 1996, 5, 551–562.

126. O'Keefe TL, Williams GT, Davies SL, et al: Mice carrying a CD20 gene disruption. Immunogenetics 1998, 48, 125–132.

127. Shipp MA, Look AT: Hematopoietic differentiation antigens that are membrane-associated enzymes: Cutting is the key! Blood 1993, 82, 1052–1070.

128. Howard M, Grimaldi JC, Bazan JF, et al: Formation and hydrolysis of cyclic ADP-ribose catalyzed by lymphocyte antigen CD38. Science 1993, 262, 1056–1059.

129. Aarhus R, Graeff RM, Dickey DM, et al: ADP-ribosyl cyclase and CD38 catalyze the synthesis of a calcium-mobilizing metabolite from NADP. J Biol Chem 1995, 270, 30327–30333.

130. Salles G, Rodewald HR, Chin BS, et al: Inhibition of CD10/neutral endopeptidase 24.11 promotes B-cell reconstitution and maturation in vivo. Proc Natl Acad Sci U S A 1993, 90, 7618–7622.

131. Kumagai M, Coustan-Smith E, Murray DJ, et al: Ligation of CD38 suppresses human B lymphopoiesis. J Exp Med 1995, 181, 1101–1110.

132. Silvennoinen O, Nishigaki H, Kitanaka A, et al: CD38 signal transduction in human B-cell precursors: Rapid induction of tyrosine phosphorylation, activation of syk tyrosine kinase, and phosphorylation of phospholipase C-gamma and phosphatidylinositol 3-kinase. J Immunol 1996, 156, 100–107.

133. Kitanaka A, Ito C, Nishigaki H, et al: CD38-mediated growth suppression of B-cell progenitors requires activation of phosphatidylinositol 3-kinase and involves its association with the protein product of the *c-cbl* proto-oncogene. Blood 1996, 88, 590–598.

134. Kitanaka A, Ito C, Coustan-Smith E, et al: CD38 ligation in human B-cell progenitors triggers tyrosine phosphorylation of CD19 and

135. Kitanaka A, Mano H, Conley ME, et al: Expression and activation of the nonreceptor tyrosine kinase Tec in human B cells. Blood 1998, 91, 940–948.

136. Takeda S, Gillis S, Palacios R: In vitro effects of recombinant interleukin-7 on growth and differentiation of bone marrow pro-B– and pro-T-lymphocyte clones and fetal thymocyte clones. Proc Natl Acad Sci U S A 1989, 86, 1634–1638.

137. Miyake K, Weissman IL, Greenberger JS, et al: Evidence for a role of the integrin VLA-4 in lymphohemopoiesis. J Exp Med 1991, 173, 599–607.

138. Elices MJ, Osborn L, Takada Y, et al: VCAM-1 on activated endothelium interacts with the leukocyte integrin VLA-4 at a site distinct from the VLA-4/fibronectin binding site. Cell 1990, 60, 577–584.

139. Murti KG, Brown PS, Kumagai M, et al: Molecular interactions between human B-cell progenitors and the bone marrow microenvironment. Exp Cell Res 1996, 226, 47–58.

140. Ruoslahti E: Fibronectin and its integrin receptors in cancer. Adv Cancer Res 1999, 76, 1–20.

141. Ryan DH, Nuccie BL, Abboud CN, et al: Vascular cell adhesion molecule-1 and the integrin VLA-4 mediate adhesion of human B-cell precursors to cultured bone marrow adherent cells. J Clin Invest 1991, 88, 995–1004.

142. Dittel BN, McCarthy JB, Wayner EA, et al: Regulation of human B-cell precursor adhesion to bone marrow stromal cells by cytokines that exert opposing effects on the expression of vascular cell adhesion molecule-1 (VCAM-1). Blood 1993, 81, 2272–2282.

143. Manie SN, Astier A, Wang D, et al: Stimulation of tyrosine phosphorylation after ligation of beta-7 and beta-1 integrins on human B cells. Blood 1996, 87, 1855–1861.

144. Jarvis LJ, LeBien TW: Stimulation of human bone marrow stromal cell tyrosine kinases and IL-6 production by contact with B lymphocytes. J Immunol 1995, 155, 2359–2368.

145. Jarvis LJ, Maguire JE, LeBien TW: Contact between human bone marrow stromal cells and B lymphocytes enhances very late antigen-4/vascular cell adhesion molecule-1–independent tyrosine phosphorylation of focal adhesion kinase, paxillin, and ERK2 in stromal cells. Blood 1997, 90, 1626–1635.

146. Watt SM, Williamson J, Genevier H, et al: The heparin binding PECAM-1 adhesion molecule is expressed by CD34+ hematopoietic precursor cells with early myeloid and B-lymphoid cell phenotypes. Blood 1993, 82, 2649–2663.

147. Hardy RR, Carmack CE, Shinton SA, et al: Resolution and characterization of pro-B and pre–pro-B-cell stages in normal mouse bone marrow. J Exp Med 1991, 173, 1213–1225.

148. Miyake K, Medina KL, Hayashi S, et al: Monoclonal antibodies to Pgp-1/CD44 block lymphohemopoiesis in long-term bone marrow cultures. J Exp Med 1990, 171, 477–488.

149. Dorshkind K: Regulation of hemopoiesis by bone marrow stromal cells and their products. Annu Rev Immunol 1990, 8, 111–137.

150. Protin U, Schweighoffer T, Jochum W, et al: CD44-deficient mice develop normally with changes in subpopulations and recirculation of lymphocyte subsets. J Immunol 1999, 163, 4917–4923.

151. Kincade PW: Cell interaction molecules and cytokines which participate in B lymphopoiesis. Baillieres Clin Haematol 1992, 5, 575–598.

152. Tsukada S, Saffran DC, Rawlings DJ, et al: Deficient expression of a B-cell cytoplasmic tyrosine kinase in human X-linked agammaglobulinemia. Cell 1993, 72, 279–290.

153. Vetrie D, Vorechovsky I, Sideras P, et al: The gene involved in X-linked agammaglobulinaemia is a member of the src family of protein-tyrosine kinases. Nature 1993, 361, 226–233.

154. Campana D, Farrant J, Inamdar N, et al: Phenotypic features and proliferative activity of B-cell progenitors in X-linked agammaglobulinemia. J Immunol 1990, 145, 1675–1680.

155. Conley ME, Parolini O, Rohrer J, et al: X-linked agammaglobulinemia: New approaches to old questions based on the identification of the defective gene. Immunol Rev 1994, 138, 5–21.

156. Conley ME, Mathias D, Treadaway J, et al: Mutations in btk in patients with presumed X-linked agammaglobulinemia. Am J Hum Genet 1998, 62, 1034–1043.

157. Fu C, Turck CW, Kurosaki T, et al: BLNK: A central linker protein in B-cell activation. Immunity 1998, 9, 93–103.

158. Hashimoto S, Iwamatsu A, Ishiai M, et al: Identification of the

SH2 domain-binding protein of Bruton's tyrosine kinase as BLNK: Functional significance of Btk-SH2 domain in B-cell antigen receptor-coupled calcium signaling. Blood 1999, 94, 2357-2364.

159. Minegishi Y, Rohrer J, Coustan-Smith E, et al: An essential role for BLNK in human B-cell development. Science 1999, 286, 1954-1957.

160. Pappu R, Cheng AM, Li B, et al: Requirement for B-cell linker protein (BLNK) in B-cell development. Science 1999, 286, 1949-1954.

161. Turner M, Mee PJ, Costello PS, et al: Perinatal lethality and blocked B-cell development in mice lacking the tyrosine kinase Syk. Nature 1995, 378, 298-302.

162. Fruman DA, Snapper SB, Yballe CM, et al: Impaired B-cell development and proliferation in absence of phosphoinositide 3-kinase p85-alpha. Science 1999, 283, 393-397.

163. von Freeden-Jeffry U, Vieira P, Lucian LA, et al: Lymphopenia in interleukin (IL)-7 gene-deleted mice identifies IL-7 as a nonredundant cytokine. J Exp Med 1995, 181, 1519-1526.

164. LeBien TW: Fates of human B-cell precursors. Blood 2000, 96:9-23.

165. Noguchi M, Yi H, Rosenblatt HM, et al: Interleukin-2 receptor gamma-chain mutation results in X-linked severe combined immunodeficiency in humans. Cell 1993, 73, 147-157.

166. Puel A, Ziegler SF, Buckley RH, et al: Defective IL7R expression in T(−)B(+)NK(+) severe combined immunodeficiency. Nat Genet 1998, 20, 394-397.

167. Goldrath AW, Bevan MJ: Selecting and maintaining a diverse T-cell repertoire. Nature 1999, 402, 255-262.

168. Laufer TM, Glimcher LH, Lo D: Using thymus anatomy to dissect T-cell repertoire selection. Semin Immunol 1999, 11, 65-70.

169. Marrack P, Kappler J: Positive selection of thymocytes bearing alpha beta T-cell receptors. Curr Opin Immunol 1997, 9, 250-255.

170. Malissen B, Ardouin L, Lin SY, et al: Function of the CD3 subunits of the pre-TCR and TCR complexes during T-cell development. Adv Immunol 1999, 72, 103-148.

171. Haynes BF, Martin ME, Kay HH, et al: Early events in human T-cell ontogeny: Phenotypic characterization and immunohistologic localization of T-cell precursors in early human fetal tissues. J Exp Med 1988, 168, 1061-1080.

172. Campana D, Janossy G, Coustan-Smith E, et al: The expression of T-cell receptor-associated proteins during T-cell ontogeny in man. J Immunol 1989, 142, 57-66.

173. Sanchez MJ, Gutierrez-Ramos JC, Fernandez E, et al: Putative prethymic T-cell precursors within the early human embryonic liver: A molecular and functional analysis. J Exp Med 1993, 177, 19-33.

174. Poggi A, Sargiacomo M, Biassoni R, et al: Extrathymic differentiation of T lymphocytes and natural killer cells from human embryonic liver precursors. Proc Natl Acad Sci U S A 1993, 90, 4465-4469.

175. Jaleco AC, Blom B, Res P, et al: Fetal liver contains committed NK progenitors, but is not a site for development of CD34+ cells into T cells. J Immunol 1997, 159, 694-702.

176. Haynes BF, Denning SM, Le PT, et al: Human intrathymic T-cell differentiation. Semin Immunol 1990, 2, 67-77.

177. Haynes BF, Heinly CS: Early human T-cell development: Analysis of the human thymus at the time of initial entry of hematopoietic stem cells into the fetal thymic microenvironment. J Exp Med 1995, 181, 1445-1458.

178. Steinmann GG, Klaus B, Müller-Hermelink HK: The involution of the aging human thymic epithelium is independent of puberty: A morphometric study. Scand J Immunol 1985, 22, 563-575.

179. Douek DC, McFarland RD, Keiser PH, et al: Changes in thymic function with age and during the treatment of HIV infection. Nature 1998, 396, 690-695.

180. Jamieson BD, Douek DC, Killian S, et al: Generation of functional thymocytes in the human adult. Immunity 1999, 10, 569-575.

181. Burkly L, Hession C, Ogata L, et al: Expression of relB is required for the development of thymic medulla and dendritic cells. Nature 1995, 373, 531-536.

182. Fischer A, Malissen B: Natural and engineered disorders of lymphocyte development. Science 1998, 280, 237-243.

183. Boyd RL, Tucek CL, Godfrey DI, et al: The thymic microenvironment. Immunol Today 1993, 14, 445-459.

184. van Ewijk W, Hollander G, Terhorst C, et al: Stepwise development of thymic microenvironments in vivo is regulated by thymocyte subsets. Development 2000, 127, 1583-1591.

185. Brenner MB, McLean J, Scheft H, et al: Characterization and expression of the human alpha beta T-cell receptor by using a framework monoclonal antibody. J Immunol 1987, 138, 1502-1509.

186. Groh V, Porcelli S, Fabbi M, et al: Human lymphocytes bearing T-cell receptor gamma/delta are phenotypically diverse and evenly distributed throughout the lymphoid system. J Exp Med 1989, 169, 1277-1294.

187. Mombaerts P, Clarke AR, Rudnicki MA, et al: Mutations in T-cell antigen receptor genes alpha and beta block thymocyte development at different stages. Nature 1992, 360, 225-231.

188. Itohara S, Mombaerts P, Lafaille J, et al: T-cell receptor delta-gene mutant mice: Independent generation of alpha beta T cells and programmed rearrangements of gamma delta TCR genes. Cell 1993, 72, 337-348.

189. Allison JP, Lanier LL: Structure, function, and serology of the T-cell antigen receptor complex. Annu Rev Immunol 1987, 5, 503-540.

190. Furley AJ, Mizutani S, Weilbaecher K, et al: Developmentally regulated rearrangement and expression of genes encoding the T-cell receptor-T3 complex. Cell 1986, 46, 75-87.

191. Hayday AC, Barber DF, Douglas N, et al: Signals involved in gamma/delta T-cell versus alpha/beta T-cell lineage commitment. Semin Immunol 1999, 11, 239-249.

192. Berger MA, Dave V, Rhodes MR, et al: Subunit composition of pre-T cell receptor complexes expressed by primary thymocytes: CD3 delta is physically associated but not functionally required. J Exp Med 1997, 186, 1461-1467.

193. Malissen M, Gillet A, Ardouin L, et al: Altered T-cell development in mice with a targeted mutation of the *CD3-epsilon* gene. EMBO J 1995, 14, 4641-4653.

194. Wang B, Wang N, Whitehurst CE, et al: T lymphocyte development in the absence of CD3 epsilon or CD3 gamma delta epsilon zeta. J Immunol 1999, 162, 88-94.

195. Soudais C, de Villartay JP, Le Deist F, et al: Independent mutations of the human CD3-epsilon gene resulting in a T-cell receptor/CD3 complex immunodeficiency. Nat Genet 1993, 3, 77-81.

196. Arnaiz-Villena A, Timon M, Corell A, et al: Brief report: Primary immunodeficiency caused by mutations in the gene encoding the CD3-gamma subunit of the T-lymphocyte receptor. N Engl J Med 1992, 327, 529-533.

197. Lanier LL, Weiss A: Presence of Ti (WT31)-negative T lymphocytes in normal blood and thymus. Nature 1986, 324, 268-270.

198. Campana D, Thompson JS, Amlot P, et al: The cytoplasmic expression of CD3 antigens in normal and malignant cells of the T-lymphoid lineage. J Immunol 1987, 138, 648-655.

199. Terstappen LW, Huang S, Picker LJ: Flow cytometric assessment of human T-cell differentiation in thymus and bone marrow. Blood 1992, 79, 666-677.

200. Hori T, Cupp J, Wrighton N, et al: Identification of a novel human thymocyte subset with a phenotype of CD3- CD4+ CD8 alpha+ beta-1: Possible progeny of the CD3- CD4- CD8- subset. J Immunol 1991, 146, 4078-4084.

201. Galy A, Verma S, Barcena A, et al: Precursors of CD3+CD4+CD8+ cells in the human thymus are defined by expression of CD34: Delineation of early events in human thymic development. J Exp Med 1993, 178, 391-401.

202. Rahemtulla A, Fung-Leung WP, Schilham MW, et al: Normal development and function of CD8+ cells but markedly decreased helper-cell activity in mice lacking CD4. Nature 1991, 353, 180-184.

203. Fung-Leung WP, Schilham MW, Rahemtulla A, et al: CD8 is needed for development of cytotoxic T cells but not helper T cells. Cell 1991, 65, 443-449.

204. Haynes BF: Human thymic epithelium and T-cell development: Current issues and future directions. Thymus 1990, 16, 143-157.

205. Kendall MD: Functional anatomy of the thymic microenvironment. J Anat 1991, 177, 1-29.

206. Muller-Hermelink HK, Wilisch A, Schultz A, et al: Characterization of the human thymic microenvironment: Lymphoepithelial interaction in normal thymus and thymoma. Arch Histol Cytol 1997, 60, 9-28.

207. Dunon D, Imhof BA: Mechanisms of thymus homing. Blood 1993, 81, 1-8.

208. Utsumi K, Sawada M, Narumiya S, et al: Adhesion of immature thymocytes to thymic stromal cells through fibronectin molecules and its significance for the induction of thymocyte differentiation. Proc Natl Acad Sci U S A 1991, 88, 5685-5689.

209. Meco D, Scarpa S, Napolitano M, et al: Modulation of fibronectin and thymic stromal cell-dependent thymocyte maturation by retinoic acid. J Immunol 1994, 153, 73-83.

210. Barda-Saad M, Rozenszajn LA, Ashush H, et al: Adhesion molecules involved in the interactions between early T cells and mesenchymal bone marrow stromal cells. Exp Hematol 1999, 27, 834-844.

211. Vollger LW, Tuck DT, Springer TA, et al: Thymocyte binding to human thymic epithelial cells is inhibited by monoclonal antibodies to CD-2 and LFA-3 antigens. J Immunol 1987, 138, 358-363.

212. Singer KH, Denning SM, Whichard LP, et al: Thymocyte LFA-1 and thymic epithelial cell ICAM-1 molecules mediate binding of activated human thymocytes to thymic epithelial cells. J Immunol 1990, 144, 2931-2939.

213. Vivinus-Nebot M, Ticchioni M, Mary F, et al: Laminin-5 in the human thymus: Control of T-cell proliferation via alpha-6 beta-4 integrins. J Cell Biol 1999, 144, 563-574.

214. Xu J, Grewal IS, Geba GP, et al: Impaired primary T-cell responses in L-selectin–deficient mice. J Exp Med 1996, 183, 589-598.

215. de la Hera A, Acevedo A, Marston W, et al: Function of CD44(Pgp-1) homing receptor in human T-cell precursors. Int Immunol 1989, 1, 598-604.

216. Leonard WJ: The molecular basis of X-linked severe combined immunodeficiency: Defective cytokine receptor signaling. Annu Rev Med 1996, 47, 229-239.

217. Kang J, Coles M, Raulet DH: Defective development of gamma/delta T cells in interleukin-7 receptor-deficient mice is due to impaired expression of T-cell receptor gamma genes. J Exp Med 1999, 190, 973-982.

218. Reya T, Bassiri H, Biancaniello R, et al: Thymic stromal-cell abnormalities and dysregulated T-cell development in IL-2–deficient mice. Dev Immunol 1998, 5, 287-302.

219. Macchi P, Villa A, Giliani S, et al: Mutations of *Jak-3* gene in patients with autosomal severe combined immune deficiency (SCID). Nature 1995, 377, 65-68.

220. Molina TJ, Kishihara K, Siderovski DP, et al: Profound block in thymocyte development in mice lacking p56lck. Nature 1992, 357, 161-164.

221. Arpaia E, Shahar M, Dadi H, et al: Defective T-cell receptor signaling and CD8$^+$ thymic selection in humans lacking zap-70 kinase. Cell 1994, 76, 947-958.

222. Negishi I, Motoyama N, Nakayama K, et al: Essential role for ZAP-70 in both positive and negative selection of thymocytes. Nature 1995, 376, 435-438.

223. Pivniouk V, Tsitsikov E, Swinton P, et al: Impaired viability and profound block in thymocyte development in mice lacking the adaptor protein SLP-76. Cell 1998, 94, 229-238.

224. Clements JL, Yang B, Ross-Barta SE, et al: Requirement for the leukocyte-specific adapter protein SLP-76 for normal T-cell development. Science 1998, 281, 416-419.

225. Marine JC, Topham DJ, McKay C, et al: SOCS1 deficiency causes a lymphocyte-dependent perinatal lethality. Cell 1999, 98, 609-616.

226. Mee PJ, Turner M, Basson MA, et al: Greatly reduced efficiency of both positive and negative selection of thymocytes in CD45 tyrosine phosphatase–deficient mice. Eur J Immunol 1999, 29, 2923-2933.

227. Artavanis-Tsakonas S, Rand MD, Lake RJ: Notch signaling: Cell fate control and signal integration in development. Science 1999, 284, 770-776.

228. Osborne B, Miele L: Notch and the immune system. Immunity 1999, 11, 653-663.

229. Pui JC, Allman D, Xu L, et al: Notch-1 expression in early lymphopoiesis influences B- versus T-lineage determination. Immunity 1999, 11, 299-308.

230. Yasutomo K, Doyle C, Miele L, et al: The duration of antigen receptor signalling determines CD4$^+$ versus CD8$^+$ T-cell lineage fate. Nature 2000, 404, 506-510.

231. Robey E, Chang D, Itano A, et al: An activated form of Notch influences the choice between CD4 and CD8 T-cell lineages. Cell 1996, 87, 483-492.

232. Washburn T, Schweighoffer E, Gridley T, et al: Notch activity influences the alphabeta versus gammadelta T-cell lineage decision. Cell 1997, 88, 833-843.

233. Long EO: Regulation of immune responses through inhibitory receptors. Annu Rev Immunol 1999, 17, 875-904.

234. Lamy T, Loughran TPJ: Current concepts: Large granular lymphocyte leukemia. Blood Rev 1999, 13, 230-240.

235. Spits H, Lanier LL, Phillips JH: Development of human T and natural killer cells. Blood 1995, 85, 2654-2670.

236. Raulet DH: Development and tolerance of natural killer cells. Curr Opin Immunol 1999, 11, 129-134.

237. Phillips JH, Hori T, Nagler A, et al: Ontogeny of human natural killer (NK) cells: Fetal NK cells mediate cytolytic function and express cytoplasmic CD3 epsilon, delta proteins. J Exp Med 1992, 175, 1055-1066.

238. Hackett JJ, Bosma GC, Bosma MJ, et al: Transplantable progenitors of natural killer cells are distinct from those of T and B lymphocytes. Proc Natl Acad Sci U S A 1986, 83, 3427-3431.

239. Sirianni MC, Businco L, Seminara R, et al: Severe combined immunodeficiencies, primary T-cell defects, and DiGeorge syndrome in humans: Characterization by monoclonal antibodies and natural killer cell activity. Clin Immunol Immunopathol 1983, 28, 361-370.

240. Rodewald HR, Moingeon P, Lucich JL, et al: A population of early fetal thymocytes expressing Fc gamma RII/III contains precursors of T lymphocytes and natural killer cells. Cell 1992, 69, 139-150.

241. Carlyle JR, Michie AM, Furlonger C, et al: Identification of a novel developmental stage marking lineage commitment of progenitor thymocytes. J Exp Med 1997, 186, 173-182.

242. Sato T, Laver JH, Aiba Y, et al: NK cell colony formation from human fetal thymocytes. Exp Hematol 1999, 27, 726-733.

243. Spits H, Blom B, Jaleco AC, et al: Early stages in the development of human T, natural killer and thymic dendritic cells. Immunol Rev 1998, 165, 75-86.

244. Coustan-Smith E, Behm FG, Hurwitz CA, et al: N-CAM (CD56) expression by CD34$^+$ malignant myeloblasts has implications for minimal residual disease detection in acute myeloid leukemia. Leukemia 1993, 7, 853-858.

245. Miller JS, Alley KA, McGlave P: Differentiation of natural killer (NK) cells from human primitive marrow progenitors in a stroma-based long-term culture system: Identification of a CD34$^+$7$^+$ NK progenitor. Blood 1994, 83, 2594-2601.

246. Ogasawara K, Hida S, Azimi N, et al: Requirement for IRF-1 in the microenvironment supporting development of natural killer cells. Nature 1998, 391, 700-703.

247. Liu I, Perussia I, Young JD: The emerging role of IL-15 in NK-cell development. Immunol Today 2000, 21, 113-116.

248. Suzuki H, Duncan GS, Takimoto H, et al: Abnormal development of intestinal intraepithelial lymphocytes and peripheral natural killer cells in mice lacking the IL-2 receptor beta chain. J Exp Med 1997, 185, 499-505.

249. DiSanto JP, Muller W, Guy-Grand D, et al: Lymphoid development in mice with a targeted deletion of the interleukin-2 receptor gamma chain. Proc Natl Acad Sci U S A 1995, 92, 377-381.

250. Conlon I, Raff M: Size control in animal development. Cell 1999, 96, 235-244.

251. Dexter TM, Spooncer E: Growth and differentiation in the hemopoietic system. Annu Rev Cell Biol 1987, 3, 423-441.

252. Muller-Sieburg CE, Deryugina E: The stromal cells' guide to the stem-cell universe. Stem Cells 1995, 13, 477-486.

253. Weissman IL: Developmental switches in the immune system. Cell 1994, 76, 207-210.

254. Kincade PW: B lymphopoiesis: Global factors, local control. Proc Natl Acad Sci U S A 1994, 91, 2888-2889.

255. Rolink A, Ghia P, Grawunder U, et al: In-vitro analyses of mechanisms of B-cell development. Semin Immunol 1995, 7, 155-167.

256. Lemischka IR: Microenvironmental regulation of hematopoietic stem cells. Stem Cells 1997, 15, 63-68.

257. Whitlock CA, Witte ON: Long-term culture of murine bone marrow precursors of B lymphocytes. Meth Enzymol 1987, 150, 275-286.

258. Ryan DH, Tang J: Regulation of human B cell lymphopoiesis by adhesion molecules and cytokines. Leuk Lymphoma 1995, 17, 375-389.

259. Hirayama F, Ogawa M: Cytokine regulation of early lymphohematopoietic development. Stem Cells 1996, 14, 369-375.

260. Eder M, Ottmann OG, Hansen-Hagge TE, et al: In vitro culture of common acute lymphoblastic leukemia blasts: Effects of interleukin-3, interleukin-7, and accessory cells. Blood 1992, 79, 3274-3284.

261. Eder M, Hemmati P, Kalina U, et al: Effects of Flt3 ligand and interleukin-7 on in vitro growth of acute lymphoblastic leukemia cells. Exp Hematol 1996, 24, 371-377.

262. McKenna HJ, Smith FO, Brasel K, et al: Effects of flt3 ligand on acute myeloid and lymphocytic leukemic blast cells from children. Exp Hematol 1996, 24, 378-385.

263. Pribyl JA, LeBien TW: Interleukin-7 independent development of human B cells. Proc Natl Acad Sci U S A 1996, 93, 10348-10353.

264. D'Apuzzo M, Rolink A, Loetscher M, et al: The chemokine SDF-1, stromal cell–derived factor-1, attracts early-stage B-cell precursors via the chemokine receptor CXCR4. Eur J Immunol 1997, 27, 1788-1793.

265. Zou YR, Kottmann AH, Kuroda M, et al: Function of the chemokine receptor CXCR4 in haematopoiesis and in cerebellar development. Nature 1998, 393, 595-599.

266. Nagasawa T, Hirota S, Tachibana K, et al: Defects of B-cell lymphopoiesis and bone-marrow myelopoiesis in mice lacking the CXC chemokine PBSF/SDF-1. Nature 1996, 382, 635-638.

267. Honczarenko M, Douglas RS, Mathias C, et al: SDF-1 responsiveness does not correlate with CXCR4 expression levels of developing human bone marrow B cells. Blood 1999, 94, 2990-2998.

268. Bancherau J, de Paoli P, Valle A, et al: Long-term human B-cell lines dependent on interleukin-4 and antibody to CD40. Science 1991, 251, 70-72.

269. Larson AW, LeBien TW: Cross-linking CD40 on human B-cell precursors inhibits or enhances growth depending on the stage of development and the IL co-stimulus. J Immunol 1994, 153, 584-594.

270. Saeland S, Duvert V, Moreau I, et al: Human B-cell precursors proliferate and express CD23 after CD40 ligation. J Exp Med 1993, 178, 113-120.

271. Renard N, Duvert V, Blanchard D, et al: Activated CD4+ T cells induce CD40-dependent proliferation of human B-cell precursors. J Immunol 1994, 152, 1693-1701.

272. Rawlings DJ, Quan S, Hao QL, et al: Differentiation of human CD34+CD38- cord blood stem cells into B-cell progenitors in vitro. Exp Hematol 1997, 25, 66-72.

273. Fluckiger AC, Sanz E, Garcia-Lloret M, et al: In vitro reconstitution of human B-cell ontogeny: From CD34(+) multipotent progenitors to Ig-secreting cells. Blood 1998, 92, 4509-4520.

274. Aruffo A, Farrington M, Hollenbaugh D, et al: The CD40 ligand, gp39, is defective in activated T cells from patients with X-linked hyper-IgM syndrome. Cell 1993, 72, 291-300.

275. Korthauer U, Graf D, Mages HW, et al: Defective expression of T-cell CD40 ligand causes X-linked immunodeficiency with hyper-IgM. Nature 1993, 361, 539-541.

276. DiSanto JP, Bonnefoy JY, Gauchat JF, et al: CD40 ligand mutations in X-linked immunodeficiency with hyper-IgM. Nature 1993, 361, 541-543.

277. Allen RC, Armitage RJ, Conley ME, et al: CD40 ligand gene defects responsible for X-linked hyper-IgM syndrome. Science 1993, 259, 990-993.

278. Conley ME, Larche M, Bonagura VR, et al: Hyper IgM syndrome associated with defective CD40-mediated B-cell activation. J Clin Invest 1994, 94, 1404-1409.

279. Dalloul AH, Arock M, Fourcade C, et al: Human thymic epithelial cells produce interleukin-3. Blood 1991, 77, 69-74.

280. Galy AH, Spits H: IL-1, IL-4, and IFN-gamma differentially regulate cytokine production and cell surface molecule expression in cultured human thymic epithelial cells. J Immunol 1991, 147, 3823-3830.

281. Galy AH, Spits H, Hamilton JA: Regulation of M-CSF production by cultured human thymic epithelial cells. Lymphokine Cytokine Res 1993, 12, 265-270.

282. Le PT, Lazorick S, Whichard LP, et al: Human thymic epithelial cells produce IL-6, granulocyte-monocyte-CSF, and leukemia inhibitory factor. J Immunol 1990, 145, 3310-3315.

283. Le PT, Lazorick S, Whichard LP, et al: Regulation of cytokine production in the human thymus: Epidermal growth factor and transforming growth factor-alpha regulate mRNA levels of interleukin-1 alpha (IL-1 alpha), IL-1 beta, and IL-6 in human thymic epithelial cells at a post-transcriptional level. J Exp Med 1991, 174, 1147-1157.

284. Mizutani S, Watt SM, Robertson D, et al: Cloning of human thymic subcapsular cortex epithelial cells with T-lymphocyte binding sites and hemopoietic growth factor activity. Proc Natl Acad Sci U S A 1987, 84, 4999-5003.

285. Gardner JP, Rosenzweig M, Marks DF, et al: T-lymphopoietic capac-

286. Galy AH, Webb S, Cen D, et al: Generation of T cells from cytokine-mobilized peripheral blood and adult bone marrow CD34+ cells. Blood 1994, 84, 104-110.

287. Yeoman H, Gress RE, Bare CV, et al: Human bone marrow and umbilical cord blood cells generate CD4+ and CD8+ single-positive T cells in murine fetal thymus organ culture. Proc Natl Acad Sci U S A 1993, 90, 10778-10782.

288. Plum J, De Smedt M, Defresne MP, et al: Human CD34+ fetal liver stem cells differentiate to T cells in a mouse thymic microenvironment. Blood 1994, 84, 1587-1593.

289. Peault B, Weissman IL, Baum C, et al: Lymphoid reconstitution of the human fetal thymus in SCID mice with CD34+ precursor cells. J Exp Med 1991, 174, 1283-1286.

290. Barcena A, Sanchez MJ, de la Pompa JL, et al: Involvement of the interleukin-4 pathway in the generation of functional gamma delta T cells from human pro-T cells. Proc Natl Acad Sci U S A 1991, 88, 7689-7693.

291. Tjonnfjord GE, Veiby OP, Steen R, et al: T-lymphocyte differentiation in vitro from adult human prethymic CD34+ bone marrow cells. J Exp Med 1993, 177, 1531-1539.

292. Miller JS, Verfaillie CM, McGlave PB: The generation of human natural killer cells from CD34+/DR- primitive progenitors in long-term bone marrow culture. Blood 1992, 80, 2182-2187.

293. Mrozek E, Anderson P, Caligiuri MA: Role of interleukin-15 in the development of human CD56+ natural killer cells from CD34+ hematopoietic progenitor cells. Blood 1996, 87, 2632-2640.

294. Shibuya A, Nagayoshi K, Nakamura K, et al: Lymphokine requirement for the generation of natural killer cells from CD34+ hematopoietic progenitor cells. Blood 1995, 85, 3538-3546.

295. Takenaka K, Mizuno SI, Harada M, et al: Generation of human natural killer cells from peripheral blood CD34+ cells mobilized by granulocyte colony-stimulating factor. Br J Haematol 1996, 92, 788-794.

296. Miller JS, McCullar V, Verfaillie CM: Ex vivo culture of CD34+/Lin-/DR- cells in stroma-derived soluble factors, interleukin-3, and macrophage inflammatory protein-1 alpha maintains not only myeloid but also lymphoid progenitors in a novel switch culture assay. Blood 1998, 91, 4516-4522.

297. Tjonnfjord GE, Steen R, Veiby OP, et al: Thymic stromal cells support differentiation of natural killer cells from CD34+ bone marrow cells in vitro. Eur J Haematol 1995, 54, 46-50.

298. Manabe A, Coustan-Smith E, Behm FG, et al: Bone marrow–derived stromal cells prevent apoptotic cell death in B-lineage acute lymphoblastic leukemia. Blood 1992, 79, 2370-2377.

299. Uckun FM, Gajl-Peczalska KJ, Kersey JH, et al: Use of a novel colony assay to evaluate the cytotoxicity of an immunotoxin containing pokeweed antiviral protein against blast progenitor cells freshly obtained from patients with common B-lineage acute lymphoblastic leukemia. J Exp Med 1986, 163, 347-368.

300. Kaspers GJ, Veerman AJ, Pieters R, et al: In vitro cellular drug resistance and prognosis in newly diagnosed childhood acute lymphoblastic leukemia. Blood 1997, 90, 2723-2729.

301. Findley HWJ, Zhou MX, Davis R, et al: Effects of low-molecular-weight B-cell growth factor on proliferation of leukemic cells from children with B-cell precursor acute lymphoblastic leukemia. Blood 1990, 75, 951-957.

302. Makrynikola V, Kabral A, Bradstock KF: Effects of recombinant human cytokines on precursor B acute lymphoblastic leukemia cells. Exp Hematol 1991, 19, 674-679.

303. Mirro JJ, Hurwitz CA, Behm FG, et al: Effects of recombinant human hematopoietic growth factors on leukemic blasts from children with acute myeloblastic or lymphoblastic leukemia. Leukemia 1993, 7, 1026-1033.

304. Touw I, Groot-Loonen J, Broeders L, et al: Recombinant hematopoietic growth factors fail to induce a proliferative response in precursor B acute lymphoblastic leukemia. Leukemia 1989, 3, 356-362.

305. Wormann B, Anderson JM, Ling ZD, et al: Structure/function analyses of IL-2 binding proteins on human B-cell precursor acute lymphoblastic leukemias. Leukemia 1987, 1, 660-666.

306. Wormann B, Mehta SR, Maizel AL, et al: Low-molecular-weight B-cell growth factor induces proliferation of human B-cell precursor acute lymphoblastic leukemias. Blood 1987, 70, 132-138.

307. Estrov Z, Freedman MH: Growth requirements for human acute lymphoblastic leukemia cells: Refinement of a clonogenic assay. Cancer Res 1988, 48, 5901-5907.

308. Roberts WM, Estrov Z, Ouspenskaia MV, et al: Measurement of residual leukemia during remission in childhood acute lymphoblastic leukemia. N Engl J Med 1997, 336, 317-323.

309. Touw I, Pouwels K, van Agthoven T, et al: Interleukin-7 is a growth factor of precursor B and T acute lymphoblastic leukemia. Blood 1990, 75, 2097-2101.

310. Makrynikola V, Kabral A, Bradstock K: Effects of interleukin-7 on the growth of clonogenic cells in T-cell acute lymphoblastic leukaemia. Leuk Res 1991, 15, 879-882.

311. Masuda M, Takanashi M, Motoji T, et al: Effects of interleukins 1-7 on the proliferation of T-lineage acute lymphoblastic leukemia cells. Leuk Res 1991, 15, 1091-1096.

312. Dibirdik I, Langlie MC, Ledbetter JA, et al: Engagement of interleukin-7 receptor stimulates tyrosine phosphorylation, phosphoinositide turnover, and clonal proliferation of human T-lineage acute lymphoblastic leukemia cells. Blood 1991, 78, 564-570.

313. Tomeczkowski J, Frick D, Schwinzer B, et al: Expression and regulation of c-kit receptor and response to stem cell factor in childhood malignant T-lymphoblastic cells. Leukemia 1998, 12, 1221-1229.

314. Ito C, Kumagai M, Manabe A, et al: Hyperdiploid acute lymphoblastic leukemia with 51 to 65 chromosomes: A distinct biological entity with a marked propensity to undergo apoptosis. Blood 1999, 93, 315-320.

315. Kumagai M, Manabe A, Pui CH, et al: Stroma-supported culture in childhood B-lineage acute lymphoblastic leukemia cells predicts treatment outcome. J Clin Invest 1996, 97, 755-760.

316. Nishigaki H, Ito C, Manabe A, et al: Prevalence and growth characteristics of malignant stem cells in B-lineage acute lymphoblastic leukemia. Blood 1997, 89, 3735-3744.

317. Shah N, Oseth L, LeBien TW: Development of a model for evaluating the interaction between human pre-B acute lymphoblastic leukemic cells and the bone marrow stromal cell microenvironment. Blood 1998, 92, 3817-3828.

318. Panayiotidis P, Jones D, Ganeshaguru K, et al: Human bone marrow stromal cells prevent apoptosis and support the survival of chronic lymphocytic leukaemia cells in vitro. Br J Haematol 1996, 92, 97-103.

319. Dancescu M, Rubio-Trujillo M, Biron G, et al: Interleukin-4 protects chronic lymphocytic leukemic B cells from death by apoptosis and upregulates Bcl-2 expression. J Exp Med 1992, 176, 1319-1326.

320. Buschle M, Campana D, Carding SR, et al: Interferon gamma inhibits apoptotic cell death in B-cell chronic lymphocytic leukemia. J Exp Med 1993, 177, 213-218.

321. Behm FG, Campana D: Immunophenotyping. In Pui CH (ed): Childhood Leukemias. New York, Cambridge University Press, 1999, pp 111-144.

322. van Dongen JJ, Langerak AW: Immunoglobulin and T-cell receptor gene rearrangements. In Pui CH (ed): Childhood Leukemias. New York, Cambridge University Press, 1999, pp 145-167.

323. Okabe M, Kuni-eda Y, Sugiwura T, et al: Inhibitory effect of interleukin-4 on the in vitro growth of Ph1-positive acute lymphoblastic leukemia cells. Blood 1991, 78, 1574-1580.

324. Pandrau D, Saeland S, Duvert V, et al: Interleukin-4 inhibits in vitro proliferation of leukemic and normal human B cell precursors. J Clin Invest 1992, 90, 1697-1706.

325. Srivannaboon K, Shanafelt AB, Todisco E, et al: An interleukin-4 variant (BAY 36-1677) selectively induces apoptosis in acute lymphoblastic leukemia. Blood 2001, 97, 752-758.

326. Mitchell PL, Clutterbuck RD, Powles RL, et al: Interleukin-4 enhances the survival of severe combined immunodeficient mice engrafted with human B-cell precursor leukemia. Blood 1996, 87, 4797-4803.

5

Bryan D. Young

Molecular Cytogenetics of Leukemia

The discovery of the Philadelphia chromosome in 1960 signaled the beginning of a new era in cancer genetics.[1] The realization that this small marker chromosome was the result of a t(9;22) chromosomal translocation[2] began a period of intensive study of the leukemic karyotype, revealing many more recurrent chromosomal abnormalities. Subsequently, many studies have confirmed that these abnormalities both assist in disease classification and represent significant prognostic factors. Today, no large-scale study of leukemia would be complete without karyotypic information. The leukemic cell can carry a variety of visible abnormalities including numerical changes, such as aneuploidy and trisomies, and structural changes, such as deletions, duplications, inversions, and reciprocal translocations. The identification of the *BCR* and *c-ABL* genes as the targets for the t(9;22) translocation represented another important landmark in establishing the genetic basis of leukemia.[3] Much subsequent work has established the underlying molecular basis of a range of recurrent chromosomal events in leukemia. In addition to providing clues as to the cause of leukemia, such advances have important implications for disease management: knowledge of the genes involved offers new possibilities for minimal residual disease detection.

Molecular biologic approaches also promise to radically change the analysis of the karyotype itself. Traditionally, karyotype analysis is performed on a Giemsa-banded karyotype and requires a fully trained cytogeneticist. In recent years, fluorescent in situ hybridization (FISH) has been so developed that each chromosome can be individually identified using techniques such as M-FISH[4] or spectral karyotyping.[5] The application of this technology, while not supplanting traditional methods, can yield extra information on the more complex karyotypes.[6] An example of M-FISH analysis of a leukemic cell is shown in Figure 5-1, in which a series of events are described that would not have been analyzable by conventional means.

Advances in the study of the human genome have offered a wealth of new tools and reagents that can be applied to the molecular analysis of the chromosomal abnormalities seen in leukemias. The most productive area for study has been chromosomal translocations, with more than 70 such events having been cloned molecularly. The molecular analysis of the other forms of abnormalities, such as deletions and trisomies, are more chal-

lenging technically because larger, less well defined, regions are usually involved. Knowledge of their genetic basis can allow these events to be grouped together according to previously unsuspected functional or structural similarities. An important further consequence is the new opportunity for rational therapeutic intervention.[7] An example of such an approach is the development and clinical use of a tyrosine kinase inhibitor specific for the BCR-ABL product of the t(9;22) translocation in chronic myeloid leukemia.[8] This chapter reviews the wealth of molecular information, particularly in regard to the genetic consequences of chromosomal translocations.

CHROMOSOMAL TRANSLOCATIONS

The presence of chromosomal translocations is a consistent feature of many types of leukemias, lymphomas, and certain solid tumors.[9] At the genetic level, these events can either deregulate an intact gene by disruption or removal and replacement of the adjacent controlling elements, or create a new fusion gene that expresses the N-terminus of one protein fused to the C-terminus of another protein. The former class of translocation is particularly found in rearrangements involving the immunoglobulin and T-cell receptor genes. The latter class usually involves breakage in intronic sequences within each gene and fusion in such a manner that the exons on either side of the junction are in-frame. Although many fusion translocations show a high degree of specificity between the two partner genes, for example between *BCR* and *ABL* in *CML,* there is an increasingly recognized number of fusion translocations that involve a particular chromosome region rearranging with multiple, different partner regions. A particularly important example of such a grouping involves the chromosome 11q23 region, which can be found rearranged with many different chromosomal regions in a wide variety of different leukemia subtypes.

Chromosome translocation is clearly an important oncogenic step in hematopoietic malignancy. Recently, however, a range of similar events has been discovered in solid tumors, principally in sarcomas.[10] In general, a different set of genes has been found to be rearranged in sarcomas when compared with hematopoietic malig-

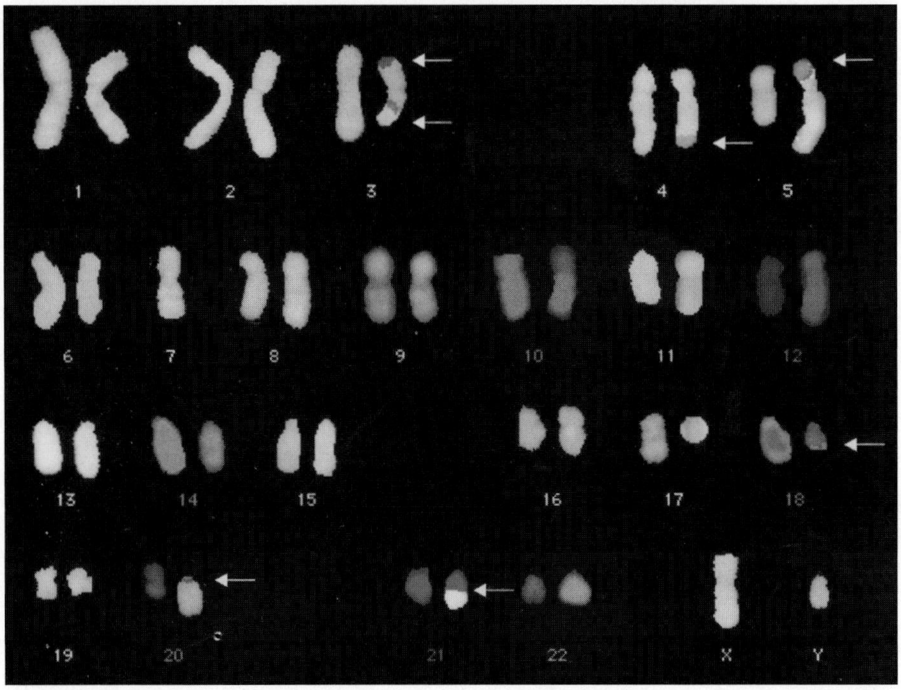

FIGURE 5–1. M-FISH analysis of a case of AML. The karyotype was analyzed as follows: 46,XY,del(5)(q22-q35),inv(8)(q13q24)/45,idem,-7/45,idem,-7,-12,+mar1/45,idem,der(3)(21qter->21q2::3p2->2q2::20?::5p1->5pter)der(4)(4pter->4q31::3p2->3pter) der(5)(5-qter->5p1::20?::18q21->qter)-7der(18)(18pter->18q21::20?) der(20)(p10 or q10->q11 or p11::3q2->3pter)der(21)(21pter->21q2::4q31->4qter)/46,XY. (Courtesy of Deborah Lillington.) (See Color Section.)

TABLE 5–1. The Immunoglobulin and T-Cell Receptor Gene-Associated Translocations

Translocation	Genes	Major Structures	Disease	Reference
t(8;14)(q24;q32)	*c-MYC* *IGH*	bHLH	ALL	18
t(2;8)(p12;q24)	*IGK* *C-MYC*	bHLH	ALL	118
t(8;22)(q24;q11)	*c-MYC* *IGL*	bHLH	ALL	119
t(14;19)(q32;13)	*IGH* *BCL-3*	IkB homology	B-CLL	120
t(5;14)(q31;q32)	*IL-3* *IGH*	Cytokine	pre–B-CLL	20
t(7;14)(q21;q32)	*THE (CDK6)* *IGH*	Cyclin-dependent kinase	B-CLL	22
t(9;14)(p21;q11)	*p16/p19 ARF* *TCRδ*	TS activity	B-ALL	21
t(7;19)(q35;p13)	*TCRβ* *LYL1*	bHLH	T-ALL	121
t(1;14)(p32;q11)	*TAL1/SCL* *TCRα*	bHLH	T-ALL	122
t(7;9)(q35;q34)	*TCRBβ* *TAL2*	bHLH	T-ALL	122
t(11;14)(p15;q11)	*LMO1/rbtn1/Tgt1* *TCR*	Lim domian	T-ALL	23
t(11;14)(p13;q11)	*LMO2/rbnt2/Tgt2* *TCR*	Lim domain	T-ALL	23
t(7;11)(q35;p13)	*TCRβ* *LMO2/rbnt2/Tgt2*	Lim domain	T-ALL	23
t(7;10)(q35;q24)	*TCRBβ* *HOX11*	Homeodomain	T-ALL	123
t(14;21)(q11;q22)	*TCRα* *BHLHB1*	bHLH	T-ALL	124
t(10;14)(q24;q11)	*HOX11* *TCRδ*	Homeodomain	T-ALL	123, 125, 126

nancy. The exceptions include the *FUS* gene, which was found fused with the *CHOP* gene in liposarcoma[11] and has subsequently been shown to be fused to a gene known as *ERG* in some cases of acute myeloid leukemia.[12] The *MN1* gene, which was found to be disrupted by a translocation in a meningioma,[13] is also a fusion partner for the *TEL/ETV6* gene in leukemias.[14] Finally, the *TEL/ETV6-TRKC* fusion has been found in leukemias[15] and in a congenital fibrosarcoma.[16] It remains an open question whether chromosomal translocations, such a prevalent feature of hematopoietic malignancy, will be found in the more common major epithelial tumors.

In order to facilitate discussion, the leukemia-specific translocations have been grouped functionally, where there are related structures or known protein-protein interactions in the affected proteins or where there is a single major target for these events (Tables 5-1 to 5-7). For the purposes of this description, the chromosome translocations found in lymphomas and myelomas have not been included (for a review, see Chesi, Kuehl, and Bergsagel[17]).

The *IGH* and *TCR* Groups of Translocations

A common feature of this group is that the breakpoints lie external to coding exons and the placing of the gene in a new chromosomal environment results in its inappropriate expression. One of the earliest genes to be identified through such a translocation was the *C-MYC* gene in t(8;14)(q24;q32), characteristic of Burkitt's lymphoma.[18] This translocation is also found in acute lymphoblastic leukemia of the L3 subtype and also results in the disruption of the *C-MYC* gene. Although the coding exons are usually intact in such translocations, it has been established that they are frequently mutated.[19] The process of

TABLE 5–2. *MLL*-Associated Translocations

Translocation	Genes	Major Structures	Disease	Reference
t(4;11)(q21;q23)	AF4	TA domain	ALL	38, 127
	MLL	AT hook, DNA MTase		
t(6;11)(q21;q23)	AF6q21	Forkhead domain	AML	128
	MLL	AT hook, DNA MTase		
t(9;11)(p22;q23)	AF9	TA domain, α helix	AML, ALL	127, 129
	MLL	AT hook, DNA MTase		
t(11;22)(q23;q11)	MLL	AT hook, DNA MTase	AML	130
	hCDCrel	CRE-like element		
t(11;17)(q23;q21)	MLL	AT hook, DNA MTase	AML	131
	AF17	AT hook, LZ		
t(10;11)(p12;q23)	AF10	AT hook, LZ	AML	132
	MLL	AT hook, DNA MTase		
t(11;19)(q23;p13)	MLL	AT hook, DNA MTase	AML	133
	ELL	RNA polII Elongation Factor		
t(1;11)(q21;q23)	AF1q	?	AML	134
	MLL	AT hook, DNA MTase		
t(11;19)(q23;p13)	MLL	AT hook, DNA MTase	AML, ALL	127, 135
	ENL	TA domain, α helix		
t(1;11)(p32;q23)	AF1p/eps15	α-helix	AML	136
	MLL	AT hook, DNA MTase		
t(11;17)(q23;q25)	MLL	AT hook, DNA MTase	tAML	137
	MSF	Septin like		
t(10;11)(p11.2;q23)	ABI1	SH3 domain, homeodomain	AML	138
	MLL	AT hook, DNA MTase		
t(11;16)(q23;p13.3)	MLL	AT hook, DNA MTase	tCMML	139
	CBP	Bromo domain, HAT		
t(3;11)(p21;q23)	AF3p21	Proline rich, SH3 domain	tAML	140
	MLL	AT hook, DNA MTase		
t(11;19)(q23;p13)	MLL	AT hook, DNA MTase	AML	141
	EEN	α-helix, SH3 domain		
t(X11)(q13;q23)	AFX	Forkhead domain	AML	142
	MLL	AT hook, DNA MTase		
ins(5;11)(q31;q13p23)	AF5q31	TA domain, AF4 related	ALL	143
	MLL	AT hook, DNA MTase		
t(6;11)(q27;q23)	AF6	α-helix, GLGF repeat	AML	144
	MLL	AT hook, DNA MTase		
t(11;17)(q23;p13)	MLL	AT hook, DNA MTase	tAML	145
	GAS7	OCT2 like motif		
t(11;22)(q23;q13)	MLL	AT hook, DNA MTase	AML	146
	p33	Bromo domain, HAT		
t(8;16)(p11;p13)	MOZ	PHD finger, HAT	AML	147
	CBP	Bromo domain, HAT		
inv(8)(p11;q13)	MOZ	PHD finger, HAT	AML	148
	TIF2	HAT		
t(10;11)(p12;q14)	AF10	AT hook, LZ	AML, T-ALL	54, 56
	CALM1	Clathrin assembly		

TABLE 5–3. *TEL/ETV6*- and *AML1*-Associated Translocations

Translocation	Genes	Major Structures	Disease	Reference
t(9;12)(q34;p13)	*ABL*	TK	CMML	149
	TEL/ETV6	PNT		
t(5;12)(q33;p13)	*PDGFRβ*	TK	CMML	95
	TEL/ETV6	PNT		
t(3;12)(q26;p13)	*MDS1/EVI1*	not known	MPD	150
	TEL/ETV6	PNT		
t(4;12)(q11–q12;p13)	*BTL*	BRX like	AML	151
	TEL/ETV6	PNT		
t(9;12)(p24;p13)	*JAK2*	TK	ALL, aCML	69, 152
	TEL/ETV6	PNT		
t(12;15)(p13;q25)	*TEL/ETV6*	PNT	AML, fibrosarcoma	15, 16, 153
	TREKC	TK		
t(12;22)(p13;q22)	*TEL/ETV6*	PNT	MPD, meningioma	13, 14
	MN1	glutamine repeat		
t(12;13)(p13;q12)	*TEL/ETV6*	PNT	AML	154
	CDX2	homeodomain		
t(6;12)(q23;p13)	*STL*	No open reading frame	ALL	155
	TEL/ETV6	PNT		
t(5;12)(q13;p13)	*ACS2*	acyl CoA synthetase 2	AML	156
	TEL/ETV6	PNT		
t(1;12)(q25;p13)	*ARG*	TK	AML	157, 158
	TEL/ETV6	PNT		
t(12;21)(p13;q22)	*TEL/ETV6*	PNT	ALL	159, 160
	AML1	runt		
t(8;21)(q22;q22)	*ETO/MTG8*	ZF	AML	73–75
	AML1	runt		
t(3;21)(q26;q22)	*EVI-1*	ZF	CML, MPD	150, 161
	AML1	runt		
t(3;21)(q26;q22)	*EAP*	ZF	MDS	162
	AML1	runt		
inv(16)(p13q22)	*MYH11*	myosin heavy chain	AML, M4Eo	82
t(16;16)(p13;q22)	*CBFβ*	CBFα binding		
t(16;21)(p11;q22)	*TLS/FUS*	GYSQ, RNA binding	AML, MLS	12, 163
	ERG	ETS DNA binding		

TABLE 5–4. The Tyrosine Kinase Group of Translocations

Translocation	Genes	Major Structures	Disease	Reference
t(9;22)(q34;q11)	*c-ABL*	TK	CML, ALL	3
	BCR	GRB2/SOS binding		
t(8;13)(p11;q12)	*FGFR1*	TK	MPD	87–89
	ZNF198/FIM/RAMP	Cysteine-rich MYM		
t(6;8)(q27;p11)	*GOP*	Leucine rich	MPD	90
	FGFR1	TK		
t(8;9)(p12;q33)	*FGFR1*	TK	MPD	91
	CEP110	LZ		
t(5;7)(q33;q11.2)	*PDGFRβ*	TK	CMML	164
	HIP1	Huntingtin interaction		
t(5;14)(q33;q32)	*PDGFRβ*	TK	AML	165
	CAV14	LZ		
t(5;10)(q33;q21)	*PDGFRβ*	TH	MPD	166
	H4/D10S170	LZ		

TABLE 5–5. The RARα Group of Translocations

Translocation	Genes	Major Structures	Disease	Reference
t(15;17)(q22;q21)	*PML*	Ring, B-box, α-helix	AML	96
	RARα	nuclear receptor		
t(11;17)(q23;q21)	*PLZF*	Zinc finger	AML	167
	RARα	nuclear receptor		
t(5;17)(q32;q21)	*NPM*	metal binding, NLS	AML	168
	RARα	nuclear receptor		
t(11;17)(q13;q21)	*NUMA*	Nucleosomal mitotic apparatus	AML	101
	Rarα	nuclear receptor		
der(17) only	*STAT5b*	DNA binding, SH2, SH3	AML	86
	RARα	nuclear receptor		
t(3;5)(q25;1;q34)	*MLF1*	no known homology	MDS, AML	100
	NPM	metal binding, NLS		

TABLE 5–6. The Nucleoporin Group of Translocations

Translocation	Genes	Major Structures	Disease	Reference
inv(11)(p15;q22)	NUP98	nucleoporin, GLGF	tAML	110
	DDX10	RNA helicase		
t(7;11)(p15;p15)	HOXA9	homeodomain	AML	110
	NUP98	nucleoporin, GLGF		
t(2;11)(q31;p15)	HOXD13	homeodomain	tAML	108
	NUP98	nucleoporin, GLGF		
t(11;20)(p15;q11)	NUP98	nucleoporin, GLGF	tMDS	111
	TOP1	topoisomerase I		
t(1;11)(q23;p15)	PMX1	homeodomain	AML	109
	NUP98	nucleoporin, GLGF		
t(4;11)(q21;p15)	RAP1GDS1	GEF	T-ALL	112
	NUP98	Nucleoporin, GLGF		
t(6;9)(p23;q34)	DEK	DNA binding	AML	106
	CAN/NUP214	nucleoporin		
Normal karyotype	SET	TAF-1 activity	AML	169
	CAN/NUP214	nucleoporin		

somatic hypermutation, which increases diversity in a normally rearranged immunoglobulin gene, is believed to be responsible for these mutations.

As indicated in Table 5–1, a series of genes has been identified by its involvement in translocations into immunoglobulin heavy-chain, κ and λ light-chain genes, and T-cell receptor genes (α, β, δ). A small but distinct subset of B-cell precursor ALL is characterized by eosinophilia and the presence of the t(5;14)(q31;q32) translocation. Molecular cloning has demonstrated the translocation results in the juxtaposition of the IL3 gene and the JH elements of the IGH locus in a head-to-head configuration.[20] The breakpoints are upstream of the IL3 promoter and result in overexpression of IL3 but not of GMCSF, the gene for which lies only 14 kb downstream from the breakpoints. In a single case of B-cell precursor ALL, the translocation t(9;14)(p21;q11) was found to have inactivated the p16/p19ARF gene by fusion to the T-cell receptor TCRδ locus.[21] This is a rare example of a translocation that results in inactivation of the target gene. This interpretation is supported by the fact that the CDKN2A/B tumor suppressor locus is known to undergo biallelic deletions in both B- and T-precursor ALL without translocation. The molecular cloning of the t(7;14)(q21;q32) in a case of B-CLL demonstrated the juxtaposition of the IGH locus with a human endogenous retroviral sequence of the transposable-like element (THE) family.[22] Subsequently, the molecular cloning of the t(2;7)(p12;q21) translocation in splenic lymphoma with villous lymphocytes (SLVL) showed that the target for this translocation is the cyclin dependent kinase (CDK)6 gene. The breakpoint on chromosome 2 involved an unrearranged

Vk gene. It is therefore possible that CDK6 was the actual target for the t(7;14)(q21;q32) reported in B-CLL. Disruption of CDK6 is likely to be of greater importance in SLVL because 7q22 breakpoints are recurrent in SLVL rather than in CLL.

Several genes have been discovered through their involvement in translocations to the T-cell receptor loci, usually in T-cell leukemias. The LMO1 gene, which encodes a small protein containing two copies of a particular type of zinc finger known as an LIM domain, was identified as the target for the t(11;14)(p15;q11) translocation.[23] Significantly, another member of the LMO family of genes, LMO2, was identified at the junction of the t(11;14)(p13;q11) translocation in T-cell leukemia. As reviewed,[24] the LMO family of proteins appears to be important during the very early stages of hematopoietic differentiation. A similar conclusion can be drawn for another target in T-cell translocations, the TAL1/SCL gene. Furthermore, it has been shown that there are not only direct interactions between the LIM proteins and the TAL1/SCL protein[25] but also with the GATA-1, E47, and Ldb/NLI proteins. These data suggest that the LMO and TAL1 proteins are part of a DNA binding complex that may regulate downstream genes and that their disruption through translocation may fundamentally change the differentiation program of the leukemic cell.

The MLL Group of Translocations

The first 11q23 abnormality to be described was the t(4;11) translocation.[26, 27] Since then, up to 30 transloca-

TABLE 5–7. The E2A Translocations

Translocation	Genes	Major Structures	Disease	Reference
t(17;19)(q23;p13)	HLF	LZ	B-ALL	170
	E2A	TA, bHLH		
t(1;19)(q23;p13)	PBX1	Homeodomain	B-ALL	171
	E2A	TA, bHLH		

tions involving 11q23 have been described, accounting for approximately 5% of all leukemias.[28] The 11q23 rearrangements have been documented in acute lymphoblastic leukemia, acute myeloblastic leukemia, biphenotypic leukemias, and myelodysplastic syndromes. Additionally, 11q23 abnormalities occur with a particularly high frequency in infant leukemias, with an overall prevalence of 60% to 80%.[29] Also of particular interest is the relatively frequent occurrence of 11q23 abnormalities in secondary or therapy-related leukemias,[30] particularly in patients with prior treatment with epipodophyllotoxins and other inhibitors of topoisomerase II. All the cytogenetic evidence, therefore, suggested that a critical genetic target, important for leukemogenesis, was disrupted by these events.

A European-wide study reviewed 550 cases of leukemia with 11q23 abnormalities.[31] Altogether, 30 distinguishable reciprocal translocations involving 11q23 were observed in 84% of samples. The remainder of cases involved additions, duplications, or inversions affecting 11q23. Although 11q23 abnormalities were found in approximately equal numbers of myeloid and lymphoid leukemias, certain translocations showed a marked association with a particular phenotype. For example, the two most frequent translocations, the t(4;11)(q21;q23) and the t(9;11)(p22;q23), were overwhelmingly associated with ALL and AML, respectively,[32, 33] confirming previous observations. Similarly, the t(11;19)(q23;p13.1), the t(6;11)(q27;q23), and the t(10;11)(p12;q23) translocations are mostly associated with AML with the M4/M5 FAB subtype.[34, 35] It was apparent that these associations were not absolute, however, as examples were found with phenotypes different from that of the majority, stressing the multilineage potential of these events. The t(11;19)(q23;p13.1) was exceptional in this study in that it showed a much more even distribution between AML and ALL.[36] Approximately 20% of the cases examined in this study were infant leukemias, and within this group the t(4;11)(q21;q23) predominated at 50%. The remainder of infant leukemias included significant numbers of the t(9;11)(p22;q23) and the t(11;19)(q23;p13.3). This study essentially confirmed and extended previous reports of the phenotypic associations of the various 11q23 translocations and strengthened the idea that disruption to 11q23 can lead to a variety of leukemic phenotypes.

Molecular cloning has demonstrated that the common target for all the above events is the *MLL* gene (also known as *ALL1, HRX, HTRX1*) located at 11q23.[37-39] The *MLL* gene, which consists of at least 36 exons spread over approximately 100 kb of DNA, encodes a large 4000–amino acid protein that contains several identifiable domains. These include (A) three adjacent "AT hooks" that contact DNA to bend it and stabilize its interactions with transcription factors,[40] (B) a cysteine-rich region that shares homology with DNA methyltransferases (MTase) and with the transcriptional repressor MeCP1,[41] (C) three PHD or LAP zinc fingers,[42, 43] and (D) a 130aa SET domain, which is conserved in evolution and present in proteins implicated in transcriptional activation or silencing and also in DNA repair and telomere function.[44, 45] Additionally, two small regions that confer a nuclear punctate distribution[46] and two sequences with transcriptional

transactivation and transrepression capacity have been identified.[47] Several lines of evidence indicate the importance of MLL protein for normal hematopoiesis. There are defects in yolk sac hematopoiesis in MLL-null embryos,[48] and there is a differentiation block in MLL-null embryonic stem cells.[49]

Molecular cloning of the 11q23 translocations has revealed that all of the breakpoints are clustered between exon 5 and exon 12 of the *MLL* gene, resulting in the retention of the sequences 5′ to the breakpoint and the replacement of the 3′ sequences with the equivalent sequences from the partner gene. It is evident that all the 11q23 breakpoints associated with acute leukemias in adults, children, and infants, whether in de novo or therapy-related disease, are clustered in this region. Significantly, all such translocations result in in-frame fusions at the mRNA level, and therefore the expression of a hybrid protein would be expected. It can also be predicted that the PHD zinc fingers and the SET domain would be disrupted or lost from the fusion proteins. At the time of writing, 20 translocations affecting 11q23 have been molecularly cloned and the partner genes identified (see Table 5–2, Bernard and Berger,[50] and Dimartino and Cleary[51]). It is evident that, although many of the fusion partners for *MLL* are unrelated to each other in terms of amino acid sequence, there are four pairs of related fusion partners. AF9, the fusion partner for the t(9;11)(p22;q23) translocation, is substantially related to ENL, the fusion partner for t(11;19)(q23;p13). Similarly, AF10, the fusion partner for t(10;11)(p12;q23), is related to AF17, the fusion partner for t(11;17)(q23;q21). AF17q25, the fusion partner for t(11;17)(q23;q25), is 46% identical to HCDCrel, the fusion partner for t(11;22)(q23;q11). Finally, the CREB binding protein (CBP) and p300 are both homologous transcriptional activators and are involved in *MLL* fusions in t(11;16)(q23;p13.3) and t(11;22)(q23;q13), respectively. Despite such similarities, the MLL fusion proteins seem to form a functionally diverse group. ENL, AF9, and AF4 activate transcription from synthetic reporter genes in vivo. AFX and AF6q21 are forkhead proteins known to have DNA binding and transcriptional control properties. ELL is an RNA polymerase II elongation factor. Partial tandem duplication is another form of disruption to the *MLL* gene that has been found particularly in association with trisomy 11 in adult AML.[52] Typically, exon 6 can be found linked to exon 2, resulting in the duplication of this region of *MLL*. It appears significant that this form of disruption is taking place in the same region affected by the translocations, i.e., in and around the PHD zinc fingers, and has been attributed to Alu-Alu recombination.[53]

The multiplicity of partner genes for *MLL* has raised questions about the role of these genes in the leukemic process. As out-of-frame fusions to *MLL* have never been reported, it appears unlikely that the loss of the C-terminal elements of *MLL* (PHD fingers and SET domain) alone represents a critical feature of these events. Also, the fact that several of the partner genes are related to each other suggests that they are not randomly selected and that their C-terminal elements may have a role in the transforming potential of the fusion protein. The possible leukemogenic role for the partners of *MLL* is emphasized by the fact that at least two of the *MLL* partner genes have been shown to be involved in translocations with genes other than *MLL*. These events are also listed in Table 5–2. Molecular cloning of the t(8;16)(p11;p13) translocation in *AML* demonstrated the fusion between *CBP* and *MOZ*, a gene encoding a protein with putative histone acetyl transferase activity that would be predicted to have been conserved in the MOZ-CBP fusion protein. Additionally, *MOZ* has been found fused to the gene-encoding TIF2 in the inv(8)(p11;q13) in AML. The t(10;11)(p12;q14) translocation in the U937 cell line has been shown to result in the fusion of the *AF10* gene with a gene called *CALM,* which encodes a new member of the AP-3 clathrin assembly protein family.[54] It has been subsequently shown that, in contrast to the *MLL-AF10* fusion, this translocation is associated with a wide range morphologic and immunologic phenotypes.[55-57] Studies of the fused transcripts have suggested that both the *CALM-AF10* and the *MLL-AF10* products are consistently expressed and could imply that features of the C-terminus of *AF10* are critical for leukemogenesis.

The transforming potential of the C-terminal component of the MLL fusion proteins has been investigated using two different experimental approaches. Homologous recombination has been used to create a germline in-frame fusion between the murine *MLL* gene and a C-terminal fragment of the human *AF9* gene.[58] Leukemias developed in both chimeric and heterozygous knock-in mice, the majority being acute myeloblastic in phenotype with a minority of lymphoid leukemias. These data support the concept that the MLL-AF9 protein preferentially results in myeloblastic leukemias, despite being expressed in many cell types and being in concordance with cellular phenotype of the human t(9;11) leukemias. Constructs in which the *AF9* component was replaced with *c-myc* did not result in leukemias. It was of particular interest that *MLL-AF9* expression resulted in a nonmalignant expansion of myeloid precursors soon after birth. The later onset of overt leukemia suggested that secondary mutations are necessary for malignancy associated with the *MLL-AF9* gene. Using a different approach, the *MLL-ENL* fusion cDNA was transduced by retroviral gene transfer into murine cell populations enriched in hematopoietic stem cells. The infected cells had a dramatically enhanced potential to generate myeloid colonies with primitive morphology in vitro. In contrast, wild-type ENL or a deletion mutant of *HRX-ENL* lacking the *ENL* component did not demonstrate in vitro transforming capabilities. Significantly, cells transduced with *MLL-ENL* induced myeloid leukemias in syngeneic and SCID recipients. Although both of the above studies demonstrated a requirement for the fusion partner protein in the generation of these experimental leukemias, the nature of the contribution remains uncertain. It was demonstrated that using a knock-in strategy, a fusion between *MLL* and the bacterial *lacZ* gene results in leukemias in chimeric mice, albeit with an increased latency when compared with *MLL-AF9* knock-in chimeric mice.[59] The lacZ protein is known to assume tetrameric conformation; it has been speculated that this could be a key feature of the partner proteins fused to *MLL*.

The *TEL/ETV6* and *AML1* Groups of Translocations

The t(12;21)(p13;q22) translocation results in the fusion of the *TEL/ETV6* gene at 12p13 with the *AML1* gene at 21q22. Although this translocation is difficult to observe by conventional means, apparent deletions of 12p were believed to involve translocations. It is now clear that this event is one of the most common translocations in childhood ALL, accounting for about 20% to 25% of cases.[60] This fusion has also been reported in adult ALL but at a much reduced frequency.[61, 62] It is now clear that, in addition to their involvement in t(12;21), both *TEL/ETV6* and *AML1* are involved independently (see Rubnitz, Pui, and Downing[63]) in a range of other translocations as summarized in Table 5–3.

The *TEL/ETV6* gene encodes a member of the Ets family of transcription factors. As such, it would be expected to function as a sequence-specific DNA-binding transcriptional regulator. *TEL/ETV6* contains a helix-loop-helix (HLH) N-terminal domain, also known as a PNT domain, which specifies a subgroup of Ets family members. The product of the *AML1* gene has been identified as one of three alternative DNA-binding α subunits of core binding factor (CBF), which has also been called PEBP2. CBF is a heterodimeric transcription factor that binds to the enhancer core motif TGT/cGGT. Transcriptional regulation by *AML1* through the enhancer core motif has been shown to be important for the tissue-specific expression of a number of hematopoietic-specific genes, including *IL3, GM-CSF, CSF-1R,* and myeloperoxidase.[64, 65] DNA-binding affinity is increased through heterodimerization with CBFβ, and both its DNA binding and interaction with CBFβ are mediated through a central domain with high homology to the *Drosophila* segmentation gene, *runt*. The structure of the TEL/ETV6-AML1 protein suggests that it would retain the ability to bind to the AML1 DNA target sequence and interact with CBFβ. Furthermore, the chimeric protein should retain the normal function of the HLH domain of TEL/ETV6. The ability of the TEL/ETV6-AML1 protein to directly repress AML1-mediated transcriptional activation is consistent with this hypothesis.[66] The observation that the HLH domain of TEL/ETV6 can mediate heterodimerization between TEL/ETV6-AML1 and TEL/ETV6 suggests that the chimeric protein may alter the normal function of TEL/ETV6. In this context, it is interesting that the nontranslocated TEL/ETV6 allele is frequently deleted in cases of ALL with t(12;21).[67] It appears that deletion of TEL/ETV6 may be a secondary event in leukemias that already have a TEL/ETV6-AML1 fusion. The importance of secondary events in the development of TEL/ETV6-AML1 leukemias has been further emphasized by the study of identical twins with leukemias. Identical TEL/ETV6-AML1 fusions have been shown for a pair of twins who developed leukemias at 3 years 6 months and 4 years 10 months, implying that the fusion was generated in utero.[68] Thus, the long latency implies that further secondary events are required for the full malignancy.

Among the other *TEL/ETV6* fusion partner genes, *PDGFRb, JAK2, ABL, TRKC,* and *ARG* encode tyrosine kinases, and the resultant fusion proteins are capable of dimerization, exhibit constitutive tyrosine kinase activity, and have transforming properties in cell lines and animal models.[69-72] It is believed that the HLH domain of *TEL/ETV6*, which is consistently present in the chimeric proteins, serves as a dimerization motif leading to constitutively activated tyrosine kinase.

The molecular cloning of t(8;21)(q22;q22) demonstrated that this event results in a fusion between *AML1* and a gene known as *ETO (CDR, MTG8)*.[73-75] The *ETO* gene encodes a putative transcription factor with two zinc fingers, a PEST region involved in intracellular degradation, and proline-rich transactivation domains. The *AML1-ETO* fusion gene is predicted to contain the promoter and *runt* homology domains of *AML1* fused to the *ETO* gene. It has been shown that the AML1-ETO fusion protein recognizes core binding sites in DNA. In particular, the AML1-ETO fusion protein and AML1 have been shown to synergistically upregulate the myeloid-specific macrophage colony-stimulating factor (M-CSF) receptor promoter.[76] Using knock-in strategies, it has also been shown that the *AML1-ETO* gene results in death during midgestation from central nervous system hemorrhage and impaired hematopoiesis in the fetal liver.[77] This indicates that the fusion protein blocks normal function of AML1 during hematopoiesis.

Evidence suggests that one of the ways in which the AML1-ETO protein can repress gene expression is through the aberrant recruitment of an N-CoR repressor complex (see Lutterbach and Hiebert[78]). It has been shown that the C-terminus of wild-type AML1 interacts with a p300-containing coactivator complex. This suggests that AML1 as part of the CBF complex activates transcription through local histone acetylation and nucleosomal remodeling. AML1-ETO is known to inhibit transcription of AML1-responsive genes. It is now apparent that wild-type ETO protein can repress transcription through its interaction with N-CoR and recruitment of an N-CoR/Sin3/ histone deacetylase (HDAC) 1 complex. As the region of ETO, which is known to interact with N-CoR, would be predicted to be retained in the AML1-ETO fusion protein, this could account for the gene repression demonstrated for the AML1-ETO protein.[79-81] It thus appears that AML1-ETO protein may actively repress transcription of AML1-responsive genes by maintaining the histones in the deacetylated conformation and thus making the DNA inaccessible to the transcriptional apparatus. In a manner analogous to the repressor effects of the PML-RARα protein, it may be surmised that the AML1-ETO protein results in a block in myeloid development and leukemic transformation of the maturing hematopoietic progenitor cells.

The inv(16)(p13;q22) is particularly associated with AML of the FAB M4Eo subtype. Molecular cloning has revealed that the inv(16) alters the β, or non-DNA binding subunit, of the CBF transcription factor complex by fusion of the *CBFB* gene at 16q22 to the smooth muscle myosin heavy-chain gene *MYH11* at 16p13.[82] The MYH11 protein includes an ATPase head, a hinge region, and a long tail of coiled-coil domains involved in filament assembly. There is heterogeneity in the breakpoints in both CBFB and MYH11. However, the relevant fusion messenger RNA appears to consist of 5′ CBFB-MYH11 3′. CBFB-MYH11 knock-in experiments have been shown to result in a blockage of definitive hematopoiesis during embryogenesis. This results in embryonic lethal hemorrhage in heterozygous knock-in mice and is similar to the phenotype obtained in the equivalent AML1-ETO knock-in mice. The CBFB-MYH11 fusion protein has also been shown to have gene repression activity by dominantly interfering with AML1-dependent transcriptional regulation.[78] It has been shown that the CBFB-MYH11 fusion protein cooperates with AML1 to repress gene transcription and can bind to AML-1B when it is associated with the mSin3A corepressor. It thus appears that both AML1-ETO and CBFB-MYH11 may result in aberrant repression of gene expression through inappropriate recruitment of histone deacetylase complexes.

The Tyrosine Kinase Group of Translocations

A significant group of chromosomal translocations involves disruption to genes encoding receptor and nonreceptor tyrosine kinases (see Table 5-4). A consistent feature of these events appears to be the fusion of N-terminal sequences to the C-terminal catalytic domains of a variety of tyrosine kinases, resulting in enhanced tyrosine kinase activity. Oligomerization mediated by the N-terminal moiety is believed to mimic normal tyrosine kinase signaling after binding of its normal cognate ligands. The partner component may also alter subcellular localization and result in phosphorylation of novel substrates. A notable and unexplained feature of this group of translocations is its strong association with myeloproliferative disorders. As this constitutes a heterogeneous group of diseases, molecular classification based on translocation events may offer a better understanding of their ontogeny.

The first example of such an event was provided by the molecular cloning of the t(9;22)(q34;q11) translocation, found in 90% of cases of chronic myeloid leukemia and in a proportion of cases of acute lymphoblastic leukemia. It was shown that this event results in a fusion between the *BCR* gene on chromosome 22q11 and the gene on chromosome 9q34, which encodes the ABL nonreceptor tyrosine kinase.[3] A variety of different breakpoints has been identified within the *BCR* gene, resulting in differently sized BCR-ABL products in CML and ALL but all with the common feature of activated tyrosine kinase activity.[83] Much subsequent work has demonstrated the transformation capacity of the BCR-ABL protein in cell lines and in animal models. Transformation by BCR-ABL appears to depend on multiple biochemical pathways. The activated tyrosine kinase activity phosphorylates a tyrosine residue within the BCR portion of the molecule, providing a docking site for the GRB2/SOS complex.[84] The resultant activation of p21-RAS and the RAF/MEK/ERK pathway contribute to cell proliferation. The transcription factor STAT5 is constitutively tyrosine phosphorylated in BCR-ABL transformed cells and appears to contribute to the growth and viability of these cells.[85] It is of interest that, in addition to being a target for BCR-ABL–mediated tyrosine phosphorylation, STAT5b has been found to be fused to RARα in rare APML cases.[86]

An emerging group of translocations is centered on the *FGFR1* gene, which is located at 8p12 and encodes one of the four tyrosine kinase receptors for the fibroblast growth factors. At the time this chapter was written, three such translocations had been molecularly cloned (see Table 5–4). The normal FGFR1 protein consists of three external immunoglobulin-like domains, a transmembrane domain, and an internal split tyrosine kinase domain. A consistent feature of these three translocations is the fusion of the C-terminal tyrosine kinase domain of FGFR1 to the different N-terminal portions of the partner protein. Such fusion proteins have been shown to have a constitutively activated tyrosine kinase activity.

The three known fusion partners for FGFR1 are unrelated and have different cellular locations, nuclear and nucleolar for FIM,[87-89] cytoplasmic for FOP,[90] and centrosomal for CEP110.[91] The deduced amino acid sequence of CEP110 has an extensive coiled-coil structure and four leucine zipper motifs, well characterized features of protein-protein interactions. The minimal region required for centrosomal location includes one of the leucine zippers and is predicted to be retained in the CEP110-FGFR1 fusion protein. Subcellular localization studies have shown that CEP110-FGFR1 is predominantly in the cytoplasm. Similar analysis has shown that the FIM-FGFR1 fusion protein also localizes to the cytoplasm. It is clear that the partner proteins FOP(6q27) and FIM(13q12) contribute potential oligomerization domains to the fusion proteins. Thus, a unifying feature of the FGFR1 fusions could be the continuous kinase stimulus, following dimerization mediated by components of the protein partner and inappropriate recruitment of signaling substrates in the cytoplasm.

It is of interest that another member of this family, FGFR3, is involved in chromosomal translocations in myeloma.[92, 93] The translocation t(4;14)(p16.3;q32.3) disrupts the *FGFR3* gene by fusion to the IGH locus and results in the expression of an activated mutated form of *FGFR3*. Also, a constitutively active form of *FGFR2* was identified in rat osteosarcoma cells.[94] This was caused by the C-terminal fusion to a gene called *FRAG1,* which resulted in a greatly increased transforming capability of *FGFR2*.

Another grouping involves translocations that affect the gene that encodes the platelet-derived growth factor receptor (PDGFRβ). The molecular cloning of t(5;12)(q33;p13) in a case of chronic myelomonocytic leukemia identified the *TEL/ETV6* gene fused to the *PDGFRβ* gene (see Table 5–3). This fusion placed the HLH domain of the *TEL/ETV6* N-terminal to the tyrosine kinase domain of *PDGFRβ*.[95] It has been established that the *PDGFRβ* gene is also disrupted in the t(5;7)(q33;q11.2), t(5;14)(q33;q32), and t(5;10)(q33;q21) translocations by fusion to the genes *HIP1, CEV14,* and *H4/D10S170,* respectively (see Table 5–4). Other examples of fusion partners for *TEL/ETV6* that would be expected to result in an

activated tyrosine kinase include ARG, JAK2, and TRKC (see Table 5–3).

The Retinoic Acid Receptor α Group of Translocations

Acute promyelocytic leukemia (APL) is one of the more common subtypes of myeloid leukemia, accounting for 10% to 15% of de novo cases in younger adults. This leukemia is characterized, in the majority of cases, by the t(15;17)(q22;q21) translocation. Molecular cloning demonstrated that this translocation disrupts a previously uncharacterized gene *PML* on chromosome 15 and the retinoic acid receptor α gene (RARα) on chromosome 17.[96] RARα is a member of the steroid hormone receptor superfamily and mediates the effect of retinoic acid at specific response elements. The t(15;17) translocation results in an in-frame fusion protein PML-RARα, which retains the retinoic acid ligand binding domain. It had been previously noticed that APL was unusually sensitive to differentiation by retinoids such as 9-*cis* RA and ATRA. The molecular cloning of the t(15;17) breakpoint, therefore, offered an insight into the unique sensitivity of APL to retinoids (see Grimwade[97]).

As indicated in Table 5–5, the RARα gene has been found to be rearranged in a total of five different chromosome translocations, each associated with acute promyelocytic leukemia. The different fusion partners for RARα are unrelated to each other in terms of amino acid sequence. The most frequent fusion partner for RARα, PML, is characterized by a tripartite motif consisting of a ring finger, two D boxes, and a coiled-coil domain. This structure is retained in the PML-RARα fusion protein. Normal PML protein is known to be present in discrete multiprotein nuclear structures known as PML nuclear bodies, MD10, KR bodies, or PML oncogenic domains. The function of these nuclear bodies is unknown, but it is of particular interest that these structures are disrupted in APL cases with the t(15;17) translocation. This raises the possibility that the disruption of these bodies could be a key feature of oncogenesis in APL.

PLZF, the fusion partner for RARα in the t(11;17)(q23;q21) translocation, is believed to function as a transcriptional repressor and is a member of the PLK (POZ and Kruppel) family of proteins. PLZF contains 9 zinc fingers and, in the cases characterized, the translocation leads to a disruption between the second and third zinc fingers. PLZF has been found to be expressed at highest levels in undifferentiated multipotential hematopoietic progenitor cells, with expression levels declining during lineage commitment and differentiation. This raises the possibility that PLZF may play a role in the maintenance of the phenotype of uncommitted hematopoietic progenitors. Although PML and PLZF are dissimilar, PLZF has also been localized to discrete nuclear bodies. Additionally, there is some evidence for at least partial co-localization of PML and PLZF within the nucleus,[98] raising the possibility that APL translocations could promote leukemogenesis through a common pathway involving the deregulation of components of PML nuclear bodies.

Nucleophosmin (NPM), the fusion partner for RARα in

the t(5;17)(q32;q21) translocation, is a highly conserved nuclear phosphoprotein that is believed to be involved with RNA processing, in particular transporting ribosomal ribonucleoproteins between the nucleolus and the cytoplasm during ribosome assembly. It is of interest that NPM is also disrupted by two other reciprocal translocations associated with hematologic malignancy. The t(2;5)(p23;q35) translocation associated with anaplastic large-cell lymphoma results in the fusion of the amino terminal region of NPM, including potential protein kinase C phosphorylation site and metal binding motif, to the tyrosine kinase catalytic domain encoded by ALK.[99] Also, the t(3;5)(q25.1;q35) translocation associated with myelodysplasia and AML results in the formation of a fusion involving a novel gene called *MLF1* with *NPM*.[100] The resulting fusion includes an additional 58 amino acids in comparison with NPM-ALK and NPM-RARα fusions. The molecular cloning of t(11;17)(q13;q21) identified a gene fusion between NUMA and RARα.[101] NUMA encodes a large, abundant coiled-coil protein that is believed to have a role in spindle function during mitosis and nuclear assembly during telophase. There is also evidence that NUMA plays a role in the interphase nucleus as a component of the nuclear matrix and may be involved in RNA processing. The t(11;17)(q13;q21) translocation was found to result in the fusion of the amino terminal 1883 amino acids of NUMA to the *RARα* gene. Recently, a novel gene fusion to the *RARα* gene has been reported that disrupts the *STAT5b* gene, which encodes a protein belonging to the Janus kinase (JAK/STAT) signaling pathway.[86] It was noted that the STAT5b component of the chimeric protein is de-localized from the cytoplasm to the nucleus where it displays a microspeckled pattern. It was therefore proposed that the APL in this case may result from disregulation of the JAK/STAT5 signal transducing pathways in the leukemic cells.

The sensitivity of the PML-RARα acute promyelocytic leukemias to ATRA is well established and forms the basis of current therapeutic protocols. This sensitivity contrasts with the resistance of APL leukemias that carry the PLZF-RARα fusion. There has been considerable interest in determining whether the different fusion proteins confer the apparent sensitivity or resistance to ATRA. Studies suggest that a key difference between the two fusion proteins is their ability to bind co-repressor molecules.[102] At physiologic levels of RA, PML-RARα fusion protein binds co-repressors that lead to the recruitment of sin3 and HDAC, a complex associated with deacetylation of histones and repression of gene expression. In the presence of pharmacologic levels of RA, binding of the ligand to the PML-RARα is associated with the displacement of the co-repressor complex from the retinoid receptor moiety. The result of this is the conformational change in the receptor induced by the ligand, permitting coactivator binding and activation of gene expression at retinoid response elements. A critical difference between PML-RARα and PLZF-RARα is that the PLZF moiety also has the capacity to bind the co-repressor complex. PLZF is unresponsive to pharmacologic levels of retinoic acid, and thus transcriptional activation is prevented. This model accounts for the sensitivity of the PML-RARα leukemias to retinoid treatment and the apparent resistance to

PLZF-RARα leukemias to similar treatment. Available data are limited, but it seems that APL cases with NPM-RARα and NUMA-RARα appear to be retinoid-responsive.[103]

The PML-RARα fusion protein has been strongly implicated in the pathogenesis of APL. It is now clear that the PML-RARα fusion protein is also critical in the differentiation induction in response to ATRA treatment. This is supported by the observation that APL NB4 cell lines that are resistant to ATRA treatment have mutations within the ligand-binding domain of PML-RARα and thus have an impaired hormone-binding capacity.[104] It has also been shown that resistance to retinoid treatment in relapsed APL patients is associated with mutations to the ligand-binding domain of PML-RARα.[105]

The Nucleoporin (NUP98, NUP214/CAN) Group of Translocations

The nucleoporins are components of the nuclear pore complex that promotes selective bidirectional transport of protein and RNA between the nucleus and cytoplasm. It is becoming clear that at least two members of this family can be targets for chromosomal translocation (see Table 5-6). The gene *CAN*, which was identified in the t(6;9)(p23;q34) translocation,[106] is now recognized as a component of the nuclear pore complex NUP214. CAN/NUP214 has also been infrequently found fused to a gene called *SET*. More recently, it has become clear that a gene called *NUP98*, which encodes another nucleoporin, is at the center of a series of translocations with six different partners (see Table 5-6). *NUP98* contains multiple phenylalanine-glycine (FG) repeats, a hallmark of the expanding nucleoporin family of proteins at the amino terminal side of all the known breakpoints. These peptide repeat motifs function as the docking sites for protein import at the nuclear pore. *NUP98* is expressed ubiquitously, and it has been suggested that the critical product in all the translocations is the amino terminal region of *NUP98* containing the FG repeats fused to a variety of different partner proteins. *NUP98* has been found to be fused to three different homeobox proteins, HOXA9, HOXD13, and PMX1, in such a manner that the FG repeats are fused to an uninterrupted homeodomain in each fusion protein.[107-109]

The remaining fusion partners for *NUP98* consist of a putative RNA helicase gene *DDX10*,[110] topoisomerase I (TOP1),[111] and guanine nucleotide exchange factor RAP1GDS1.[112] *DDX10* is ubiquitously expressed, contains a nuclear localization signal sequence, and has been predicted to be involved in ribosome assembly. The *NUP98-DDX10* fusions were found to include the FG repeats of *NUP98* fused to the putative RNA helicase domain of *DDX10*. The fusion with TOP1 can be predicted to contain most of the topoisomerase protein, including its core sequence, linker, and catalytic domain. Although the *RAP1GDS1* gene is expressed ubiquitously, only the NUP98-RAP1GDS1 product was found. The protein product RAP1GDS1 is usually referred to as smgGDS and has guanine nucleotide exchange factor activity (GEF). smgGDS is structurally unique among the GEFs because it consists largely of tandem repeats of the 43-amino-acid armadillo motif, a structure that has been suggested to mediate protein-protein interactions. This structure remains intact in the NUP98-RAP1GDS1 fusion protein. Most of the NUP98-based translocations have involved the myeloid lineage, some of the leukemias being secondary to previous therapy. The small number of NUP98-RAP1GDS1 fusions examined were found in T-cell ALL, consistent with previous studies showing the t(4;11)(q21; p15) translocation to be recurrent in T-ALL.

The potential importance of the FG repeats in the fusion proteins is further emphasized by the fact that similar repeats are present in CAN/NUP214 and would be predicted to be present also in the CAN/NUP214-DEK and CAN/NUP214-SET fusion proteins. Studies of the transforming ability of the NUP98-HOXA9 protein have demonstrated that the FG repeats can act as very potent transactivators of gene transcription.[113] Transactivation by FG repeat-rich segments of NUP98 correlated with their ability to interact functionally and physically with the transcriptional coactivators CREB binding protein and p300. It has therefore been suggested that the transactivation potential of the FG repeats in the fusion proteins may be a unifying feature of all NUP98- and NUP214-based translocations.

CONCLUSION

More than 70 chromosomal translocations in leukemia have been cloned molecularly and the affected genes identified (see Tables 5-1 to 5-7). A crucial question for future research is whether the identification of these proteins and the consequent effects offer any possibilities for novel therapeutic interventions. The regulation of gene expression through the process of histone acetylation and deacetylation appears to be a process that is disrupted by a number of fusion proteins (see Fenrick and Hiebert[114] and Redner, Wang, and Liu[115]). There is clear evidence that both the PML-RARα fusion proteins and the AML1-ETO fusion proteins are capable of aberrant recruitment of histone deacetylase complexes. It may be surmised reasonably that such fusion proteins are responsible for repression of genes critical in normal hematopoietic differentiation. It is possible that other fusion proteins created by chromosomal translocations may also have a direct or indirect role in the regulation of gene expression. For example, it is known that the SET domain of the MLL protein interacts with the INI1 protein, a component of the SWI/SNF chromatin remodeling complex.[116] All of the 11q23 chromosome translocations result in the loss of the SET domain from the fusion protein and its replacement by the C-terminus of the relevant partner proteins. Some of the proteins involved in fusion to MLL also have links to gene regulation through histone acetylation and deacetylation and to other chromatin remodeling systems. AF9 and ENL are homologous to a yeast protein known as ANC1, which has been shown to associate with the SWI/SNF chromatin remodeling complex.[117] Two other fusion partners for MLL—CBP and p300—are intimately involved in gene regulation as part of a coactivator complex and are known to have intrinsic histone acetyl transferase (HAT)

activity. It is possible, therefore, that MLL-CBP and MLL-p300 fusions result in abnormal chromatin remodeling through activation of HAT activity or recruitment of other acetyl transferase components of the coactivator complex. Another protein involved in translocations, which has HAT activity, is the MOZ protein. In the MOZ-CBP fusion, the zinc finger and catalytic domain of MOZ are fused to almost the entire CBP protein, the breakpoint in CBP being similar to that in the MLL-CBP fusion. The consequence is that the MOZ-CBP fusion protein is predicted to have two HAT domains.

The disruption of gene regulation through aberrant effects on chromatin may represent an underlying theme that could be amenable to therapeutic intervention. Future research will undoubtedly be directed at the elucidation of this process and the development of novel therapeutic agents capable of correcting the aberrant regulation of genes critical to the leukemogenic process.

REFERENCES

1. Nowell PC, Hungerford DA: A minute chromosome in human chronic granulocytic leukemia. Science 1960, 132, 1497.
2. Rowley JD: A new consistent chromosomal abnormality in chronic myelogenous leukemia identified by quinacrine fluorescence and Giemsa staining. Nature 1973, 243, 290.
3. Groffen J, Stephenson JR, Heisterkamp N, et al: Philadelphia chromosomal breakpoints are clustered within a limited region, bcr, on chromosome 22. Cell 1984, 36, 93.
4. Speicher MR, Gwyn Ballard S, Ward DC: Karyotyping human chromosomes by combinatorial multi-fluor FISH. Nat Genet 1996, 12, 368.
5. Schröck E, du Manoir S, Veldman T, et al: Multicolor spectral karyotyping of human chromosomes. Science 1996, 273, 494.
6. Veldman T, Vignon C, Schrock E, et al: Hidden chromosome abnormalities in haematological malignancies detected by multicolour spectral karyotyping. Nat Genet 1997, 15, 406.
7. Rabbitts TH: The clinical significance of fusion oncogenes in cancer. New Engl J Med 1998, 338, 192.
8. Druker BJ, Tamura S, Buchdunger E, et al: Effects of a selective inhibitor of the Abl tyrosine kinase on the growth of Bcr-Abl positive cells. Nat Med 1996, 2, 561.
9. Rabbitts TH: Chromosomal translocations in human cancer. Nature 1994, 372, 143.
10. de Alava E, Gerald WL: Molecular biology of the Ewing's sarcoma/primitive neuroectodermal tumor family. J Clin Oncol 2000, 18, 204.
11. Panagopoulos I, Hoglund M, Mertens F, et al: Fusion of the *EWS* and *CHOP* genes in myxoid liposarcoma. Oncogene 1996, 12, 489.
12. Kong XT, Ida K, Ichikawa H, et al: Consistent detection of TLS/FUS-ERG chimeric transcripts in acute myeloid leukemia with t(16;21)(p11;q22) and identification of a novel transcript. Blood 1997, 90, 1192.
13. Lekanne Deprez RH, Riegman PH, Groen NA, et al: Cloning and characterization of *MN1*, a gene from chromosome 22q11, which is disrupted by a balanced translocation in a meningioma. Oncogene 1995, 10, 1521.
14. Buijs A, Sherr S, van Baal S, et al: Translocation (12;22)(p13;q11) in myeloproliferative disorders results in fusion of the ETS-like *TEL* gene on 12p13 to the *MN1* gene on 22q11. Oncogene 1995, 10, 1511.
15. Eguchi M, Eguchi-Ishimae M, Tojo A, et al: Fusion of ETV6 to neurotrophin-3 receptor TRKC in acute myeloid leukemia with t(12;15)(p13;q25). Blood 1999, 93, 1355.
16. Knezevich SR, McFadden DE, Tao W, et al: A novel *ETV6-NTRK3* gene fusion in congenital fibrosarcoma. Nat Genet 1998, 18, 184.
17. Chesi M, Kuehl WM, Bergsagel PL: Recurrent immunoglobulin gene translocations identify distinct molecular subtypes of myeloma. Ann Oncol 2000, 11, 131.
18. Taub R, Kirsch I, Morton C, et al: Translocation of the *c-myc* gene

into the immunoglobulin heavy chain locus in human Burkitt lymphoma and murine plasmacytoma cells. Proc Natl Acad Sci U S A 1982, 79, 7837.

19. Rabbitts TH, Hamlyn PH, Baer R: Altered nucleotide sequences of a translocated *c-myc* gene in Burkitt lymphoma. Nature 1983, 306, 760.

20. Grimaldi JC, Meeker TC: The t(5;14) chromosomal translocation in a case of acute lymphocytic leukemia joins the interleukin-3 gene to the immunoglobulin heavy chain gene. Blood 1989, 73, 2081.

21. Duro D, Bernard O, Della Valle V, et al: Inactivation of the *P16INK4/MTS1* gene by a chromosome translocation t(9;14)(p21-22;q11) in an acute lymphoblastic leukemia of B-cell type. Cancer Res 1996, 56, 848.

22. Wahbi K, Hayette S, Callanan M, et al: Involvement of a human endogenous retroviral sequence (THE-7) in a t(7;14)(q21;q32) chromosomal translocation associated with a B cell chronic lymphocytic leukemia. Leukemia 1997, 11, 1214.

23. Sanchez-Garcia I, Rabbitts TH: LIM domain proteins in leukaemia and development. Semin Cancer Biol 1993, 4, 349.

24. Rabbitts TH, Bucher K, Chung G, et al: The effect of chromosomal translocations in acute leukemias: The LMO2 paradigm in transcription and development. Cancer Res 1999, 59, 1794.

25. Wadman I, Li J, Bash RO, et al: Specific in vivo association between the bHLH and LIM proteins implicated in human T cell leukemia. EMBO J 1994, 13, 4831.

26. Van den Berghe H, David G, Broeckaert-van Orshoven A, et al: A new chromosome anomaly in acute lymphoblastic leukaemia (ALL). Hum Genet 1979, 46, 173.

27. Oshimura M, Kakati S, Sandberg AA: Chromosomes and causation of human cancer and leukaemia: XXVII Possible mechanisms for the genesis of common chromosome abnormalities, including isochromosomes and the Ph1. Cancer Res 1977, 37, 3501.

28. Young BD: Cytogenetic and molecular analysis of chromosome-11q23 abnormalities in leukemia. Baillieres Clin Haematol 1992, 5, 881.

29. Rubnitz JE, Link MP, Shuster JJ, et al: Frequency and prognostic significance of HRX rearrangements in infant acute lymphoblastic leukemia: A Pediatric Oncology Group study. Blood 1994, 84, 570.

30. Felix CA: Secondary leukemias induced by topoisomerase-targeted drugs. Biochim Biophys Acta 1998, 1400, 233.

31. Secker-Walker LM: General Report on the European Union Concerted Action Workshop on 11q23, London, 1997. Leukemia 1998, 12, 776.

32. Johansson B, Moorman AV, Haas OA, et al: Hematologic malignancies with t(4;11)(q21;q23): A cytogenetic, morphologic, immunophenotypic and clinical study of 183 cases. European 11q23 Workshop participants. Leukemia 1998, 12, 779.

33. Swansbury GJ, Slater R, Bain BJ, et al: Hematological malignancies with t(9;11)(p21-22;q23): A laboratory and clinical study of 125 cases. European 11q23 Workshop participants. Leukemia 1998, 12, 792.

34. Lillington DM, Young BD, Berger R, et al: The t(10;11)(p12;q23) translocation in acute leukaemia: A cytogenetic and clinical study of 20 patients. European 11q23 Workshop participants. Leukemia 1998, 12, 801.

35. Martineau M, Berger R, Lillington DM, et al: The t(6;11)(q27;q23) translocation in acute leukaemia: A laboratory and clinical study of 30 cases. European 11q23 Workshop participants. Leukemia 1998, 12, 788.

36. Moorman AV, Hagemeijer A, Charrin C, et al: The translocations t(11;19)(q23;p13.1) and t(11;19)(q23;p13.3): A cytogenetic and clinical profile of 53 patients. European 11q23 Workshop participants. Leukemia 1998, 12, 805.

37. Tkachuk DC, Kohler S, Cleary ML: Involvement of a homolog of *Drosophila* trithorax by 11q23 chromosomal translocations in acute leukemias. Cell 1992, 71, 691.

38. Gu Y, Nakamura T, Alder H, et al: The t(4;11) chromosome translocation of human acute leukemias fuses the *ALL-1* gene, related to *Drosophila* trithorax, to the *AF-4* gene. Cell 1992, 71, 701.

39. Djabali M, Selleri L, Parry P, et al: A trithorax-like gene is interrupted by chromosome 11q23 translocations in acute leukaemias. Nat Genet 1992, 2, 113.

40. Thanos D, Maniatis T: Virus induction of human IFN-beta gene expression requires the assembly of an enhanceosome. Cell 1995, 83, 1091.

41. Cross SH, Meehan RR, Nan X, et al: A component of the transcriptional repressor MeCP1 shares a motif with DNA methyltransferase and HRX proteins. Nat Genet 1997, 16, 256.

42. Aasland R, Gibson TJ, Stewart AF: The PHD finger: Implications for chromatin-mediated transcriptional regulation. Trends Biochem Sci 1995, 20, 56.

43. Saha V, Chaplin T, Gregorini A, et al: The leukemia-associated-protein (LAP) domain, a cysteine-rich motif, is present in a wide range of proteins, including MLL, AF10, and MLLT6 proteins. Proc Natl Acad Sci U S A 1995, 92, 9737.

44. Corda Y, Schramke V, Longhese MP, et al: Interaction between Set1p and checkpoint protein Mec3p in DNA repair and telomere functions. Nat Genet 1999, 21, 204.

45. Jenuwein T, Laible G, Dorn R, et al: SET domain proteins modulate chromatin domains in eu- and heterochromatin. Cell Mol Life Sci 1998, 54, 80.

46. Yano T, Nakamura T, Blechman J, et al: Nuclear punctate distribution of ALL-1 is conferred by distinct elements at the N terminus of the protein. Proc Natl Acad Sci U S A 1997, 94, 7286.

47. Prasad R, Yano T, Sorio C, et al: Domains with transcriptional regulatory activity within the ALL1 and AF4 proteins involved in acute leukemia. Proc Natl Acad Sci U S A 1995, 92, 12160.

48. Hess JL, Yu BD, Li B, et al: Defects in yolk sac hematopoiesis in Mll-null embryos. Blood 1997, 90: 1799.

49. Fidanza V, Melotti P, Yano T, et al: Double knockout of the *ALL-1* gene blocks hematopoietic differentiation in vitro. Cancer Res 1996, 56, 1179.

50. Bernard OA, Berger R: Molecular basis of 11q23 rearrangements in hematopoietic malignant proliferations. Genes Chromosomes Cancer 1995, 13, 75.

51. Dimartino JF, Cleary ML: Mll rearrangements in haematological malignancies: Lessons from clinical and biological studies. Br J Haematol 1999, 106, 614.

52. Schichman SA, Caligiuri MA, Gu Y, et al: ALL-1 partial duplication in acute leukemia. Proc Natl Acad Sci U S A 1994, 91, 6236.

53. Schichman SA, Caligiuri MA, Strout MP, et al: ALL-1 tandem duplication in acute myeloid leukemia with a normal karyotype involves homologous recombination between Alu elements. Cancer Res 1994, 54, 4277.

54. Dreyling MH, Martinez-Climent JA, Zheng M, et al: The t(10;11)(p13;q14) in the U937 cell line results in the fusion of the *AF10* gene and CALM, encoding a new member of the AP-3 clathrin assembly protein family. Proc Natl Acad Sci U S A 1996, 93, 4804.

55. Kobayashi H, Hosoda F, Maseki N, et al: Hematologic malignancies with the t(10;11)(p13;q21) have the same molecular event and a variety of morphologic or immunologic phenotypes. Genes Chromosomes Cancer 1997, 20, 253.

56. Carlson KM, Vignon C, Bohlander S, et al: Identification and molecular characterisation of CALM/AF10 fusion products in T-cell acute lymphoblastic leukemia and acute myeloid leukemia. Leukemia 2000, 14, 100.

57. Bohlander SK, Muschinsky V, Schrader K, et al: Molecular analysis of the CALM/AF10 fusion: Identical rearrangements in acute myeloid leukemia, acute lymphoblastic leukemia and malignant lymphoma. Leukemia 2000, 14, 93.

58. Dobson CL, Warren AJ, Pannell R, et al: The *mll-AF9* gene fusion in mice controls myeloproliferation and specifies acute myeloid leukaemogenesis. EMBO J 1999, 18, 3564.

59. Dobson CL, Warren AJ, Pannell R, et al: Tumorigenesis in mice with a fusion of the leukaemia oncogene *mll* and the bacterial *lacZ* gene. EMBO J 2000, 19, 843.

60. Romana SP, Poirel H, Leconiat M, et al: High frequency of t(12;21) in childhood B-lineage acute lymphoblastic leukemia. Blood 1995, 86, 4263.

61. Raynaud S, Mauvieux L, Cayuela JM, et al: *TEL/AML1* fusion gene is a rare event in adult acute lymphoblastic leukemia. Leukemia 1996, 10, 1529.

62. Aguiar RC, Sohal J, van Rhee F, et al: TEL-AML1 fusion in acute lymphoblastic leukaemia of adults. MRC Adult Leukaemia Working Party. Br J Haematol 1996, 95, 673.

63. Rubnitz JE, Pui CH, Downing JR: The role of *TEL* fusion genes in pediatric leukemias. Leukemia 1999, 13, 6.

64. Shoemaker SG, Hromas R, Kaushansky K: Transcriptional regulation of interleukin-3 gene expression in T lymphocytes. Proc Natl Acad Sci U S A 1990, 87, 9650.

65. Takahashi A, Satake M, Yamaguchi-Iwai Y, et al: Positive and negative regulation of granulocyte-macrophage colony-stimulating factor promoter activity by AML1-related transcription factor, PEBP2. Blood 1995, 86, 607.

66. Hiebert SW, Sun W, Davis JN, et al: The t(12;21) translocation converts AML-1B from an activator to a repressor of transcription. Mol Cell Biol 1996, 16, 1349.

67. Romana SP, Le Coniat M, Poirel H, et al: Deletion of the short arm of chromosome 12 is a secondary event in acute lymphoblastic leukemia with t(12;21). Leukemia 1996, 10, 167.

68. Ford AM, Bennett CA, Price CM, et al: Fetal origins of the *TEL-AML1* fusion gene in identical twins with leukemia. Proc Natl Acad Sci U S A 1998, 95, 4584.

69. Lacronique V, Boureux A, Valle VD, et al: A TEL-JAK2 fusion protein with constitutive kinase activity in human leukemia. Science 1997, 278, 1309.

70. Golub TR, Goga A, Barker GF, et al: Oligomerization of the ABL tyrosine kinase by the Ets protein TEL in human leukemia. Mol Cell Biol 1996, 16, 4107.

71. Jousset C, Carron C, Boureux A, et al: A domain of TEL conserved in a subset of ETS proteins defines a specific oligomerization interface essential to the mitogenic properties of the TEL-PDGFR beta oncoprotein. EMBO J 1997, 16, 69.

72. Carroll M, Tomasson MH, Barker GF, et al: The TEL/platelet-derived growth factor receptor (PDGF beta R) fusion in chronic myelomonocytic leukemia is a transforming protein that self-associates and activates PDGF beta R kinase-dependent signaling pathways. Proc Natl Acad Sci U S A 1996, 93, 14845.

73. Miyoshi H, Shimizu K, Kozu T, et al: t(8;21) breakpoints on chromosome 21 in acute myeloid leukemia are clustered within a limited region of a single gene, AML1. Proc Natl Acad Sci U S A 1991, 88, 10431.

74. Erickson P, Gao J, Chang KS, et al: Identification of breakpoints in t(8;21) acute myelogenous leukemia and isolation of a fusion transcript, AML1/ETO, with similarity to *Drosophila* segmentation gene, *runt*. Blood 1992, 80, 1825.

75. Nisson PE, Watkins PC, Sacchi N: Transcriptionally active chimeric gene derived from the fusion of the *AML1* gene and a novel gene on chromosome 8 in t(8;21) leukemic cells. Cancer Genet Cytogenet 1992, 63, 81.

76. Rhoades KL, Hetherington CJ, Rowley JD, et al: Synergistic up-regulation of the myeloid-specific promoter for the macrophage colony-stimulating factor receptor by AML1 and the t(8;21) fusion protein may contribute to leukemogenesis. Proc Natl Acad Sci U S A 1996, 93, 11895.

77. Okuda T, Cai Z, Yang S, et al: Expression of a knocked-in *AML1-ETO* leukemia gene inhibits the establishment of normal definitive hematopoiesis and directly generates dysplastic hematopoietic progenitors. Blood 1998, 91, 3134.

78. Lutterbach B, Hiebert SW: Role of the transcription factor AML-1 in acute leukemia and hematopoietic differentiation. Gene 2000, 245, 223.

79. Gelmetti V, Zhang J, Fanelli M, et al: Aberrant recruitment of the nuclear receptor corepressor–histone deacetylase complex by the acute myeloid leukemia fusion partner ETO. Mol Cell Biol 1998, 18, 7185.

80. Wang J, Hoshino T, Redner RL, et al: ETO, fusion partner in t(8;21) acute myeloid leukemia, represses transcription by interaction with the human N-CoR/mSin3/HDAC1 complex. Proc Natl Acad Sci U S A 1998, 95, 10860.

81. Lutterbach B, Westendorf JJ, Linggi B, et al: ETO, a target of t(8;21) in acute leukemia, interacts with the N-CoR and mSin3 corepressors. Mol Cell Biol 1998, 18, 7176.

82. Liu P, Tarlé SA, Hajra A, et al: Fusion between transcription factor CBF beta/PEBP2 beta and a myosin heavy chain in acute myeloid leukemia. Science 1993, 261, 1041.

83. Walker LC, Ganesan TS, Dhut S, et al: Novel chimaeric protein expressed in Philadelphia positive acute lymphoblastic leukaemia. Nature 1987, 329, 851.

84. Tauchi T, Feng GS, Shen R, et al: SH2-containing phosphotyrosine phosphatase Syp is a target of p210bcr-abl tyrosine kinase. J Biol Chem 1994, 269, 15381.

85. Sillaber C, Gesbert F, Frank DA, et al: STAT5 activation contributes to growth and viability in Bcr/Abl-transformed cells. Blood 2000, 95, 2118.

86. Arnould C, Philippe C, Bourdon V, et al: The signal transducer and activator of transcription *STAT5b* gene is a new partner of retinoic acid receptor alpha in acute promyelocytic-like leukaemia. Hum Mol Genet 1999, 8, 1741.

87. Reiter A, Sohal J, Kulkarni S, et al: Consistent fusion of ZNF198 to the fibroblast growth factor receptor-1 in the t(8;13)(p11;q12) myeloproliferative syndrome. Blood 1998, 92, 1735.

88. Popovici C, Adélaüde J, Ollendorff V, et al: Fibroblast growth factor receptor 1 is fused to FIM in stem-cell myeloproliferative disorder with t(8;13). Proc Natl Acad Sci U S A 1998, 95, 5712.

89. Smedley D, Hamoudi R, Clark J, et al: The t(8;13)(p11;q11-12) rearrangement associated with an atypical myeloproliferative disorder fuses the fibroblast growth factor receptor 1 gene to a novel gene *RAMP*. Hum Mol Genet 1998, 7, 637.

90. Popovici C, Zhang B, Grégoire MJ, et al: The t(6;8)(q27;p11) translocation in a stem cell myeloproliferative disorder fuses a novel gene, *FOP*, to fibroblast growth factor receptor 1. Blood 1999, 93, 1381.

91. Guasch G, Mack GJ, Popovici C, et al: FGFR1 is fused to the centrosome-associated protein CEP110 in the 8p12 stem cell myeloproliferative disorder with t(8;9)(p12;q33). Blood 2000, 95, 1788.

92. Chesi M, Nardini E, Brents LA, et al: Frequent translocation t(4;14)(p16.3;q32.3) in multiple myeloma is associated with increased expression and activating mutations of fibroblast growth factor receptor 3. Nat Genet 1997, 16, 260.

93. Richelda R, Ronchetti D, Baldini L, et al: A novel chromosomal translocation t(4;14)(p16.3;q32) in multiple myeloma involves the fibroblast growth-factor receptor 3 gene. Blood 1997, 90, 4062.

94. Lorenzi MV, Horii Y, Yamanaka R, et al: *FRAG1*, a gene that potently activates fibroblast growth factor receptor by C-terminal fusion through chromosomal rearrangement. Proc Natl Acad Sci U S A 1996, 93, 8956.

95. Golub TR, Barker GF, Lovett M, et al: Fusion of PDGF receptor beta to a novel ets-like gene, *tel,* in chronic myelomonocytic leukemia with t(5;12) chromosomal translocation. Cell 1994, 77, 307.

96. de The H, Chomienne C, Lanotte M, et al: The t(15;17) translocation of acute promyelocytic leukaemia fuses the retinoic acid receptor alpha gene to a novel transcribed locus. Nature 1990, 347, 558.

97. Grimwade D: The pathogenesis of acute promyelocytic leukaemia: Evaluation of the role of molecular diagnosis and monitoring in the management of the disease. Br J Haematol 1999, 106, 591.

98. Koken MH, Reid A, Quignon F, et al: Leukemia-associated retinoic acid receptor alpha fusion partners, PML and PLZF, heterodimerize and colocalize to nuclear bodies. Proc Natl Acad Sci U S A 1997, 94, 10255.

99. Morris SW, Kirstein MN, Valentine MB, et al: Fusion of a kinase gene, *ALK*, to a nucleolar protein gene, *NPM*, in non-Hodgkin's lymphoma. Science 1995, 267, 316.

100. Yoneda-Kato N, Look AT, Kirstein MN, et al: The t(3;5)(q25.1;q34) of myelodysplastic syndrome and acute myeloid leukemia produces a novel fusion gene, *NPM-MLF1*. Oncogene 1996, 12, 265.

101. Wells RA, Catzavelos C, Kamel-Reid S: Fusion of retinoic acid receptor alpha to NuMA, the nuclear mitotic apparatus protein, by a variant translocation in acute promyelocytic leukaemia. Nat Genet 1997, 17, 109.

102. Grignani F, De Matteis S, Nervi C, et al: Fusion proteins of the retinoic acid receptor-alpha recruit histone deacetylase in promyelocytic leukaemia. Nature 1998, 391, 815.

103. Redner RL, Corey SJ, Rush EA: Differentiation of t(5;17) variant acute promyelocytic leukemic blasts by all-trans retinoic acid. Leukemia 1997, 11, 1014.

104. Rosenauer A, Raelson JV, Nervi C, et al: Alterations in expression, binding to ligand and DNA, and transcriptional activity of rearranged and wild-type retinoid receptors in retinoid-resistant acute promyelocytic leukemia cell lines. Blood 1996, 88, 2671.

105. Ding W, Li YP, Nobile LM, et al: Leukemic cellular retinoic acid resistance and missense mutations in the PML-RAR alpha fusion gene after relapse of acute promyelocytic leukemia from treatment with all-trans retinoic acid and intensive chemotherapy. Blood 1998, 92, 1172.

106. von Lindern M, Fornerod M, van Baal S, et al: The translocation

(6;9), associated with a specific subtype of acute myeloid leukemia, results in the fusion of two genes, *dek* and *can*, and the expression of a chimeric, leukemia-specific *dek-can* mRNA. Mol Cell Biol 1992, 12, 1687.

107. Borrow J, Shearman AM, Stanton VP Jr, et al: The t(7;11)(p15;p15) translocation in acute myeloid leukaemia fuses the genes for nucleoporin NUP98 and class I homeoprotein HOXA9. Nat Genet 1996, 12, 159.

108. Raza-Egilmez SZ, Jani-Sait SN, Grossi M, et al: *NUP98-HOXD13* gene fusion in therapy-related acute myelogenous leukemia. Cancer Res 1998, 58, 4269.

109. Nakamura T, Yamazaki Y, Hatano Y, et al: *NUP98* is fused to *PMX1* homeobox gene in human acute myelogenous leukemia with chromosome translocation t(1;11)(q23;p15). Blood 1999, 94, 741.

110. Arai Y, Hosoda F, Kobayashi H, et al: The inv(11)(p15q22) chromosome translocation of de novo and therapy-related myeloid malignancies results in fusion of the nucleoporin gene, *NUP98*, with the putative RNA helicase gene, *DDX10*. Blood 1997, 89, 3936.

111. Ahuja HG, Felix CA, Aplan PD: The t(11;20)(p15;q11) chromosomal translocation associated with therapy-related myelodysplastic syndrome results in an NUP98-TOP1 fusion. Blood 1999, 94, 3258.

112. Hussey DJ, Nicola M, Moore S, et al: The (4;11)(q21;p15) translocation fuses the NUP98 and RAP1GDS1 genes and is recurrent in T-cell acute lymphocytic leukemia. Blood 1999, 94, 2072.

113. Kasper LH, Brindle PK, Schnabel CA, et al: CREB binding protein interacts with nucleoporin-specific FG repeats that activate transcription and mediate NUP98-HOXA9 oncogenicity. Mol Cell Biol 1999, 19, 764.

114. Fenrick R, Hiebert SW: Role of histone deacetylases in acute leukemia. J Cell Biochem 1998, 30, 194.

115. Redner RL, Wang J, Liu JM: Chromatin remodeling and leukemia: New therapeutic paradigms. Blood 1999, 94, 417.

116. Rozenblatt-Rosen O, Rozovskaia T, Burakov D, et al: The C-terminal SET domains of ALL-1 and TRITHORAX interact with the INI1 and SNR1 proteins, components of the SWI/SNF complex. Proc Natl Acad Sci U S A 1998, 95, 4152.

117. Cairns BR, Henry NL, Kornberg RD: TFG/TAF30/ANC1, a component of the yeast SWI/SNF complex that is similar to the leukemogenic proteins ENL and AF-9. Mol Cell Biol 1996, 16, 3308.

118. Rappold GA, Hameister H, Cremer T, et al: c-myc and immunoglobulin kappa light chain constant genes are on the 8q+ chromosome of three Burkitt lymphoma lines with t(2;8) translocations. EMBO J 1984, 3, 2951.

119. Croce CM, Thierfelder W, Erikson J, et al: Transcriptional activation of an unrearranged and untranslocated c-myc oncogene by translocation of a C lambda locus in Burkitt. Proc Natl Acad Sci U S A 1983, 80, 6922.

120. Ohno H, Takimoto G, McKeithan TW: The candidate proto-oncogene bcl-3 is related to genes implicated in cell lineage determination and cell cycle control. Cell 1990, 60, 991.

121. Mellentin JD, Smith SD, Cleary ML: lyl-1, a novel gene altered by chromosomal translocation in T cell leukemia, codes for a protein with a helix-loop-helix DNA binding motif. Cell 1989, 58, 77.

122. Baer R: TAL1, TAL2 and LYL1: A family of basic helix-loop-helix proteins implicated in T cell acute leukaemia. Semin Cancer Biol 1993, 4, 341.

123. Kennedy MA, Gonzalez-Sarmiento R, Kees UR, et al: HOX11, a homeobox-containing T-cell oncogene on human chromosome 10q24. Proc Natl Acad Sci U S A 1991, 88, 8900.

124. Wang J, Jani-Sait SN, Escalon EA, et al: The t(14;21)(q11.2;q22) chromosomal translocation associated with T-cell acute lymphoblastic leukemia activates the BHLHB1 gene. Proc Natl Acad Sci U S A 2000, 97, 3497.

125. Dube ID, Kamel-Reid S, Yuan CC, et al: A novel human homeobox gene lies at the chromosome 10 breakpoint in lymphoid neoplasias with chromosomal translocation t(10;14). Blood 1991, 78, 2996.

126. Hatano M, Roberts CW, Minden M, et al: Deregulation of a homeobox gene, HOX11, by the t(10;14) in T cell leukemia. Science 1991, 253, 79.

127. Cimino G, Moir DT, Canaani O, et al: Cloning of ALL-1, the locus involved in leukaemias with the t(4;11)(q21;q23), t(9;11)(p22;q23), and t(11;19)(q23;p13) chromosome translocations. Cancer Res 1991, 51, 6712.

128. Hillion J, Le Coniat M, Jonveaux P, et al: AF6q21, a novel partner of the *MLL* gene in t(6;11)(q21;q23), defines a forkhead transcriptional factor subfamily. Blood 1997, 90, 3714.

129. Iida S, Seto M, Yamamoto K, et al: *MLLT3* gene on 9p22 involved in t(9;11) leukemia encodes a serine/proline–rich protein homologous to *MLLT1* on 19p13. Oncogene 1993, 8, 3085.

130. Megonigal MD, Rappaport EF, Jones DH, et al: t(11;22)(q23;q11.2) in acute myeloid leukemia of infant twins fuses MLL with *hCDCrel*, a cell division cycle gene in the genomic region of deletion in DiGeorge and velocardiofacial syndromes. Proc Natl Acad Sci U S A 1998, 95, 6413.

131. Prasad R, Leshkowitz D, Gu Y, et al: Leucine-zipper dimerization motif encoded by the *AF17* gene fused to ALL-1 (MLL) in acute leukemia. Proc Natl Acad Sci U S A 1994, 91, 8107.

132. Chaplin T, Ayton P, Bernard OA, et al: A novel class of zinc finger/leucine zipper genes identified from the molecular cloning of the t(10;11) translocation in acute leukemia. Blood 1995, 85, 1435.

133. Thirman MJ, Levitan DA, Kobayashi H, et al: Cloning of *ELL*, a gene that fuses to MLL in t(11;19)(q23;p13.1) in acute myeloid leukemia. Proc Natl Acad Sci U S A 1994, 91, 12110.

134. Tse W, Zhu W, Chen HS, et al: A novel gene, *AF1q*, fused to MLL in t(1;11) (q21;q23), is specifically expressed in leukemic and immature hematopoietic cells. Blood 1995, 85, 650.

135. Yamamoto K, Seto M, Komatsu H, et al: Two distinct portions of LTG19/ENL at 19p13 are involved in t(11;19) leukemia. Oncogene 1993, 8, 2617.

136. Bernard OA, Mauchauffe M, Mecucci C, et al: A novel gene, *AF-1p*, fused to HRX in t(1;11)(p32;q23), is not related to AF-4, AF-9, or ENL. Oncogene 1994, 9, 1039.

137. Osaka M, Rowley JD, Zeleznik-Le NJ: *MSF* (MLL septin-like fusion), a fusion partner gene of MLL, in a therapy-related acute myeloid leukemia with t(11;17)(q23;q25). Proc Natl Acad Sci U S A 1999, 96, 6428.

138. Taki T, Shibuya N, Taniwaki M, et al: ABI-1, a human homolog to mouse Abl-interactor 1, fuses the *MLL* gene in acute myeloid leukemia with t(10;11)(p11.2;q23). Blood 1998, 92, 1125.

139. Satake N, Ishida Y, Otoh Y, et al: Novel MLL-CBP fusion transcript in therapy-related chronic myelomonocytic leukemia with a t(11;16)(q23;p13) chromosome translocation. Genes Chromosomes Cancer 1997, 20, 60.

140. Sano K, Hayakawa A, Piao JH, et al: Novel SH3 protein encoded by the *AF3p21* gene is fused to the mixed lineage leukemia protein in a therapy-related leukemia with t(3;11)(p21;q23). Blood 2000, 95, 1066.

141. So CW, Caldas C, Liu MM, et al: EEN encodes for a member of a new family of proteins containing an Src homology 3 domain and is the third gene located on chromosome 19p13 that fuses to MLL in human leukemia. Proc Natl Acad Sci U S A 1997, 94, 2563.

142. Borkhardt A, Repp R, Haas OA, et al: Cloning and characterization of *AFX*, the gene that fuses to MLL in acute leukemias with t(X;11)(q13;q23). Oncogene 1997, 14, 195.

143. Taki T, Kano H, Taniwaki M, et al: *AF5q31*, a newly identified *AF4*-related gene, is fused to MLL in infant acute lymphoblastic leukemia with ins(5;11)(q31;q13q23). Proc Natl Acad Sci U S A 1999, 96, 14535.

144. Prasad R, Gu Y, Alder H, et al: Cloning of the ALL-1 fusion partner, the *AF-6* gene, involved in acute myeloid leukemias with the t(6;11) chromosome translocation. Cancer Res 1993, 53, 5624.

145. Megonigal MD, Cheung NK, Rappaport EF, et al: Detection of leukemia-associated MLL-GAS7 translocation early during chemotherapy with DNA topoisomerase II inhibitors. Proc Natl Acad Sci U S A 2000, 97, 2814.

146. Ida K, Kitabayashi I, Taki T, et al: Adenoviral E1A-associated protein p300 is involved in acute myeloid leukemia with t(11;22)(q23;q13). Blood 1997, 90, 4699.

147. Borrow J, Stanton VP Jr, Andresen JM, et al: The translocation t(8;16)(p11;p13) of acute myeloid leukaemia fuses a putative acetyltransferase to the CREB-binding protein. Nat Genet 1996, 14, 33.

148. Carapeti M, Aguiar RC, Goldman JM, et al: A novel fusion between MOZ and the nuclear receptor coactivator TIF2 in acute myeloid leukemia. Blood 1998, 91, 3127.

149. Papadopoulos P, Ridge SA, Boucher CA, et al: The novel activation of ABL by fusion to an ets-related gene, *TEL*. Cancer Res 1995, 55, 34.

150. Peeters P, Wlodarska I, Baens M, et al: Fusion of ETV6 to MDS1/

EVI1 as a result of t(3;12)(q26;p13) in myeloproliferative disorders. Cancer Res 1997, 57, 564.

151. Cools J, Bilhou-Nabera C, Wlodarska I, et al: Fusion of a novel gene, *BTL*, to ETV6 in acute myeloid leukemias with t(4;12)(q11–q12;p13). Blood 1999, 94, 1820.

152. Peeters P, Raynaud SD, Cools J, et al: Fusion of *TEL*, the ETS-variant gene 6 (ETV6), to the receptor-associated kinase JAK2 as a result of t(9;12) in a lymphoid and t(9;15;12) in a myeloid leukemia. Blood 1997, 90, 2535.

153. Rubin BP, Chen CJ, Morgan TW, et al: Congenital mesoblastic nephroma t(12;15) is associated with *ETV6-NTRK3* gene fusion: Cytogenetic and molecular relationship to congenital (infantile) fibrosarcoma. Am J Pathol 1998, 153, 1451.

154. Chase A, Reiter A, Burci L, et al: Fusion of ETV6 to the caudal-related homeobox gene *CDX2* in acute myeloid leukemia with t(12;13)(p13;q12). Blood 1999, 93, 1025.

155. Suto Y, Sato Y, Smith SD, et al: A t(6;12)(q23;p13) results in the fusion of ETV6 to a novel gene, *STL*, in a B-cell ALL cell line. Genes Chromosomes Cancer 1997, 18, 254.

156. Yagasaki F, Jinnai I, Yoshida S, et al: Fusion of TEL/ETV6 to a novel ACS2 in myelodysplastic syndrome and acute myelogenous leukemia with t(5;12)(q31;p13). Genes Chromosomes Cancer 1999, 26, 192.

157. Iijima Y, Ito T, Oikawa T, et al: A new ETV6/TEL partner gene, *ARG* (ABL-related gene or ABL2), identified in an AML-M3 cell line with a t(1;12)(q25;p13) translocation. Blood 2000, 95, 2126.

158. Cazzaniga G, Tosi S, Aloisi A, et al: The tyrosine kinase abl-related gene *ARG* is fused to ETV6 in an AML-M4Eo patient with t(1;12)(q25;p13): Molecular cloning of both reciprocal transcripts. Blood 1999, 94, 4370.

159. Romana SP, Mauchauffe M, Le Coniat M, et al: The t(12;21) of acute lymphoblastic leukemia results in a tel-AML1 gene fusion. Blood 1995, 85, 3662.

160. Golub TR, Barker GF, Bohlander SK, et al: Fusion of the *TEL* gene on 12p13 to the *AML1* gene on 21q22 in acute lymphoblastic leukemia. Proc Natl Acad Sci U S A 1995, 92, 4917.

161. Mitani K, Ogawa S, Tanaka T, et al: Generation of the *AML1-EVI-1* fusion gene in t(3;21)(q26;q22) causes blastic crisis in chronic myelocytic leukemia. EMBO J 1994, 13, 504.

162. Nucifora G, Begy CR, Erickson P, et al: The 3;21 translocation in myelodysplasia results in a fusion transcript between the *AML1* gene and the gene for EAP, a highly conserved protein associated with the Epstein-Barr virus small RNA EBER 1. Proc Natl Acad Sci U S A 1993, 90, 7784.

163. Shimizu K, Ichikawa H, Tojo A, et al: An ets-related gene, *ERG*, is rearranged in human myeloid leukemia with t(16;21) chromosomal translocation. Proc Natl Acad Sci U S A 1993, 90, 10280.

164. Ross TS, Bernard OA, Berger R, et al: Fusion of Huntingtin interacting protein 1 to platelet-derived growth factor beta receptor (PDGFbetaR) in chronic myelomonocytic leukemia with t(5;7)(q33;q11.2). Blood 1998, 91, 4419.

165. Abe A, Emi N, Tanimoto M, et al: Fusion of the platelet-derived growth factor receptor beta to a novel gene *CEV14* in acute myelogenous leukemia after clonal evolution. Blood 1997, 90, 4271.

166. Kulkarni S, Heath C, Parker S, et al: Fusion of H4/D10S1170 to the platelet-derived growth factor receptor β in BCR-ABL negative myeloproliferative disorders with t(5;10)(q33;q21). Cancer Res 2000 (in press).

167. Chen Z, Brand NJ, Chen A, et al: Fusion between a novel Kruppel-like zinc finger gene and the retinoic acid receptor-alpha locus due to a variant t(11;17) translocation associated with acute promyelocytic leukaemia. EMBO J 1993, 12, 1161.

168. Redner RL, Rush EA, Faas S, et al: The t(5;17) variant of acute promyelocytic leukemia expresses a nucleophosmin-retinoic acid receptor fusion. Blood 1996, 87, 882.

169. von Lindern M, Breems D, van Baal S, et al: Characterization of the translocation breakpoint sequences of two *DEK-CAN* fusion genes present in t(6;9) acute myeloid leukemia and a *SET-CAN* fusion gene found in a case of acute undifferentiated leukemia. Genes Chromosomes Cancer 1992, 5, 227.

170. Inaba T, Roberts WM, Shapiro LH, et al: Fusion of the leucine zipper gene *HLF* to the *E2A* gene in human acute B-lineage leukemia. Science 1992, 257, 531.

171. Nourse J, Mellentin JD, Galili N, et al: Chromosomal translocation t(1;19) results in synthesis of a homeobox fusion mRNA that codes for a potential chimeric transcription factor. Cell 1990, 60, 535.

6

J.J.M. van Dongen   T. Szczepański   H.J. Adriaansen

Immunobiology of Leukemia

INTRODUCTION

The various types of acute and chronic leukemias can be regarded as malignant counterparts of immature and more mature hematopoietic cells, respectively. This provides a good framework for applying basic immunobiologic knowledge of normal lymphopoiesis and myelopoiesis to the diagnosis and management of leukemia. This chapter first describes basic aspects of immunophenotyping of normal leukocytes and leukemias. This includes the cluster of differentiation (CD) nomenclature and immunophenotyping techniques as well as immunophenotyping for diagnosis and classification of leukemias. Then the chapter provides basic information about immunoglobulin (Ig) and T-cell receptor (TCR) gene rearrangement processes during normal lymphoid differentiation. Comparable Ig and TCR gene rearrangements also occur in leukemias. Based on this information, it is shown how these immunogenotypic characteristics of leukemias can be used to detect clonality with the Southern blot technique or the polymerase chain reaction (PCR).

IMMUNOPHENOTYPING OF LEUKEMIAS

Leukocytes and their malignant counterparts can be recognized on the basis of morphologic and cytochemical characteristics. Chapter 11 describes the classification of leukemias based on these characteristics. A more detailed characterization of leukocytes can be obtained by immunophenotyping.[1-5] For this purpose, antibodies are used to detect the expression of leukocyte antigens, either intracellularly or on the cell surface membrane. These leukocyte antigens concern proteins or glycoproteins. Because they are recognized by use of immunologic methods, they are also called immunologic markers. Following is a discussion of immunologic markers and their expression during hematopoiesis, techniques for immunophenotyping, and application of these markers for diagnosis and classification of the various types of leukemias.

Immunologic Markers and CD Nomenclature

For the detection of immunologic markers on hematopoietic cells, generally monoclonal antibodies (McAb) are used. During the last 20 years, many McAb have become available. An international nomenclature was designed in which a large part of the McAb against leukocyte antigens have been grouped into antibody clusters based on their reactivity with identical antigens (Table 6-1).[6-11] Each antibody cluster has its own code, part of the CD code. In principle, CD codes are assigned only if three or more McAb from different laboratories recognize the same antigen and if molecular mass and expression pattern of the antigen have been determined. If these criteria are not fulfilled completely, the nomenclature committee might decide for a preliminary clustering; in these cases the CD code is supplied with the letter w (workshop).[8, 9]

As a consequence of the CD nomenclature, the molecules and epitopes recognized by the clustered antibodies have been defined as CD molecules, CD antigens, and CD epitopes. In the literature, sometimes the confusing phrase "anti-CD-antibody" is used, which unintentionally refers to an antibody against a CD antibody, that is, an anti-idiotypic antibody; this use of the CD nomenclature should be avoided. It is recommended to place the name of the used McAb behind the CD code in parentheses.

Such a supplementation is important for optimal comparison of data from different laboratories, because McAb of the same cluster may differ slightly in their reaction pattern. For instance, the majority of CD3 antibodies recognize CD3-ε chains at the cell surface of viable cells,[12] but cytoplasmic CD3-ε chains (CyCD3-ε) in fixed cytocentrifuge preparations or frozen sections can be recognized by only a few CD3 antibodies, such as CD3 (Leu-4), CD3 (UCHT1), and CD3 (VIT-3).[12] Apparently not all epitopes on the CD3-ε chain are resistant to denaturation by acetone or ethanol fixation. Such information is important for leukemia diagnosis, because CyCD3 is an essential marker for immature T-cell leukemias (Fig. 6-1). Another example is the reactivity of the B1 and Leu-16 antibodies with extracellular epitopes of the CD20 molecule, whereas the L26 antibody recognizes an intracellular CD20 epitope.[13] This implies that application of the CD20 (L26) antibody needs permeabilization of cells, such as in frozen sections and cytocentrifuge preparations.[13]

During six Leukocyte Typing Conferences (Paris, 1982; Boston, 1984; Oxford, 1987; Vienna, 1989; Boston, 1993; Kobe, 1996), 166 CD codes were established.[6-11] A condensed summary of these clusters and the recognized antigens is given in Table 6-1.[10] Some clusters are subdi-

TABLE 6–1. CD Nomenclature, as Established During the Six Leukocyte Typing Conferences

CD Code	CD Antigen	CD Code	CD Antigen	CD Code	CD Antigen	CD Code	CD Antigen	CD Code	CD Antigen
CD1	T6 antigen	CD37	B-cell antigen	CD62P	P-selectin, PADGEM	CD95	APO-1/FAS	CD132	"common" γ chain
CD2	T11 antigen, LFA-2	CD38	T10 antigen	CD63	GP-53	CD96	TACTILE	CD133	not assigned
CD3	T3 antigen	CD39	gp80 antigen	CD64	FcγRI	CD97	CD55 ligand	CD134	OX-40 receptor
CD4	T4 antigen	CD40	gp50 antigen	CD65	fucoganglioside	CD98	4F2 antigen	CD135	Flt3/flk2
CD5	T1 antigen	CD41	platelet GPIIb	CD65s	sialylated CD65	CD99	MIC2 molecule	CDw136	MSPR
CD6	T12 antigen	CD42a	platelet GPIX	CD66a	BGP	CD100	activation antigen	CDw137	4-1BB
CD7	Tp41 antigen	CD42b	platelet GPIbα	CD66b	CGM6	CD101	T-cell antigen	CD138	syndecan-1
CD8	T8 antigen	CD42c	platelet GPIbβ	CD66c	NCA	CD102	ICAM-2	CD139	FCC marker
CD9	p24 antigen	CD42d	platelet GPV	CD66d	CGM1	CD103	HML-1, integrin αE chain	CD140a	PDGFR α chain
CD10	CALLA	CD43	leukosialin	CD66e	CEA	CD104	integrin β4 chain	CD140b	PDGFR β chain
CD11a	LFA-1, αL chain	CD44	Pgp-1, homing R	CD66f	PSG-1	CD105	endoglin	CD141	thrombomodulin
CD11b	MAC-1/CR3, αM chain	CD44R	CD44V9	CD67	canceled	CD106	VCAM-1	CD142	tissue factor
CD11c	p150,95/CR4, αX chain	CD45	LCA	CD68	Mφ-antigen	CD107a	LAMP-1	CD143	ACE
CDw12	myeloid antigen	CD45RO	restricted CD45	CD69	AIM	CD107b	LAMP-2	CD144	VE-cadherin
CD13	aminopeptidase N	CD45RA	restricted CD45	CD70	CD27-ligand	CDw108	adhesion molecule	CDw145	endothelial antigen
CD14	gp55 antigen	CD45RB	restricted CD45	CD71	transferrin-R	CD109	activation antigen	CD146	MUC-18/S-endo
CD15	X hapten, FAL	CD45RC	restricted CD45	CD72	CD5-ligand	CD110	not assigned	CD147	neurothelin/basigin
CD15s	sLe^x antigen	CD46	MCP	CD73	ecto-5-NT	CD111	not assigned	CD148	HPTP-eta/PEP-1
CD16	FcγRIII	CD47	gp47–52 antigen	CD74	invariant chain	CD112	not assigned	CDw149	MEM-133
CD16b	FcγRIIIB	CD48	gp41 antigen	CDw75	CD22 ligand	CD113	not assigned	CDw150	SLAM/IPO-3
CD17	lactosylceramide	CD49a	VLA-1, α1 chain	CD76	gp85/67 antigen	CD114	G-CSFR	CD151	PETA-3
CD18	integrin β2 chain	CD49b	VLA-2, α2 chain	CD77	Gb3 antigen	CD115	CSF-1R	CD152	CTLA-4
CD19	gp90 antigen	CD49c	VLA-3, α3 chain	CDw78	B-cell antigen	CD116	GM-CSFR αchain	CD153	CD30 ligand
CD20	p35 antigen	CD49d	VLA-4, α4 chain	CD79a	mb-1/Ig-α	CD117	SCFR/c-kit	CD154	CD40 ligand
CD21	CR2, EBV-R	CD49e	VLA-5, α5 chain	CD79b	B29/Ig-β	CDw118	IFNR/reserved	CD155	PVR
CD22	gp135 antigen	CD49f	VLA-6, α6 chain	CD80	B7/BB1	CD119	IFNγR αchain	CD156	ADAM8
CD23	FcεRII	CD50	ICAM-3	CD81	TAPA	CD120a	TNFRI	CD157	BST-1/MO-5
CD24	BA-1 antigen	CD51	VNR αchain	CD82	R2 molecule	CD120b	TNFRII	CD158a	p58.1/p50.1
CD25	IL2R αchain	CD52	Campath-1	CD83	HB15 molecule	CD121a	IL1RI	CD158b	p58.2/p50.2
CD26	DPP IV	CD53	gp32-40 antigen	CD84	2G7 molecule	CD121b	IL1RII	CD159	not assigned
CD27	p110 antigen	CD54	ICAM-1	CD85	VMP-55 molecule	CD122	IL2Rβ	CD160	not assigned
CD28	Tp44 antigen	CD55	DAF	CD86	FUN-1 molecule	CDw123	IL3R α-chain	CD161	NKRP1-A
CD29	integrin β1 chain	CD56	NCAM	CD87	urokinase-R	CD124	IL4R α-chain	CD162	PSGL-1
CD30	Ki-1 antigen	CD57	HNK1	CD88	C5aR	CDw125	IL5R α-chain	CD163	M130 antigen
CD31	platelet-GPIIa'	CD58	LFA-3	CD89	FcαR	CD126	IL6R α-chain	CD164	MGC-24
CD32	FcγRII	CD59	Ly-6 antigen	CD90	Thy-1 antigen	CD127	IL7R α-chain	CD165	AD2/gp37
CD33	gp67 antigen	CDw60	NeuAc-NeuAC-Gal	CD91	α2-macroglobulin-R	CDw128	IL8R	CD166	ALCAM
CD34	gp115 antigen	CD61	integrin β3 chain	CDw92	VIM-15 antigen	CDw129	IL9Rα-/reserved		
CD35	CR1	CD62E	E-selectin, ELAM-1	CD93	"single chain" gp	CD130	gp130		
CD36	platelet GPIV	CD62L	L-selectin, LECAM	CD94	Kp43 molecule	CDw131	"common" βchain		

ACE, angiotensin-converting enzyme; AIM, activation inducer molecule; ALCAM, activated leukocyte cell adhesion molecule; BGP, biliary glycoprotein; CALLA, common ALL antigen; CEA, carcinoembryonic antigen; CGM, CEA gene member; CR, complement receptor; CSF, colony stimulating factor; CTLA, cytotoxic T cell antigen; DAF, decay accelerating factor; DPP IV, dipeptidylpeptidase IV; EBV-R, Epstein-Barr virus receptor; FAL, fucosyl-N-acetyl-lactosamin; FcεR, Fc receptor for IgE; FcγR, Fc receptor for IgG; FCC, follicular center cell; Gb3, globotriaosylceramide; GM, granulocyte macrophage; GMP, granule membrane protein; GP, glycoprotein; HML, human mucosal lymphocyte; HNK, human natural killer cell; ICAM, intercellular adhesion molecule; IFN, interferon; IL, interleukin; LAMP, lysozyme associated membrane protein; LCA, leukocyte common antigen; LFA, leukocyte function antigen; LPS-R, lipopolysaccharide receptor; MCP, membrane cofactor protein; MGC, multi-glycosylated core; Mφ, macrophage; MSPR, macrophage stimulating protein receptor; NCA, non-cross reacting antigen; NCAM, neural cell adhesion molecule; NeuAc-NeuAc-Gal, disialosyl group; 5'-NT, 5'-nucleotidase; PDGFR, platelet derived growth factor receptor; PSG, pregnancy specific glycoprotein; PVR, polio virus receptor; R, receptor; RS, Reed Sternberg cell; SCFR, stem cell factor receptor; SLAM, surface lymphocyte activation marker; sLe x, sialyl-Lewis-X; TACTILE, T-cell activated increased late expression; TAPA, target for antiproliferative antibody; TNF, tumor necrosis factor; VCAM, vascular cell adhesion molecule; VLA, very late activation antigen; VNR, vitronectin receptor.

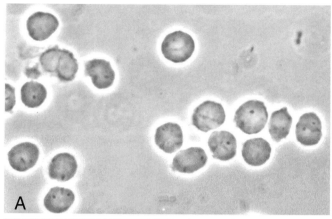
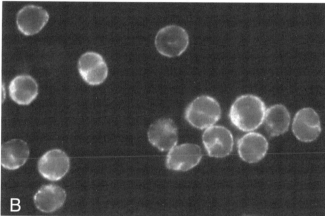

FIGURE 6–1. Immunofluorescence staining for cytoplasmic CD3 (CyCD3) on blood mononuclear cells from a patient with a T-cell acute lymphoblastic leukemia. *A,* Phase contrast morphology. *B,* CyCD3 (Leu-4)-positive cells (FITC labeled) with a typical intracellular staining pattern, also in nuclear clefts.

vided with letter codes. The antibodies of these clusters recognize antigens that are structurally or functionally homologous, or both, but not identical. The genes encoding these homologous protein molecules belong to the same gene complex (e.g. CD1, CD3, and CD11 clusters) or to the same gene family (e.g. CD49, CD62, and CD79 clusters).[14–17] In other clusters, division depends on the recognition of different splicing products from the same gene complex (e.g., CD45 cluster)[18] or reactivity with different protein chains from a protein complex (e.g., CD42 cluster).[10] However, not all antibodies against genetically, structurally, or functionally related antigens were grouped into the same clusters. For instance, antibodies against functionally and genetically related molecules for regulation of complement activation can be found in different clusters, that is, CD21, CD35, and CD55.[19] In addition, antibodies recognizing the α chain and β chain of the interleukin-2 (IL-2) receptor are clustered in the CD25 and CD122 clusters, respectively.[10]

Table 6–2 provides detailed information about clustered and nonclustered antibodies, which are useful for immunophenotyping of leukemias. This information concerns the function of the recognized antigen and its molecular mass and the reactivity of the antibodies with hematopoietic cells. For each cluster, a few typical exam-

ples of McAb are given. Several groups of leukocyte antigens are discussed in more detail.

Precursor Markers

Precursor cells of lymphopoiesis and myelopoiesis generally express the CD34 antigen, and a part of them also express the CD117 antigen, which is the receptor for the stem cell factor (c-kit).[20–23] The majority of normal bone marrow CD117[+] cells coexpress the HLA-DR and the myeloid associated CD33 antigen.[23] Terminal deoxynucleotidyl transferase (TdT) is a nuclear enzyme that is expressed in all immature lymphoid cells and a small fraction of precursor myeloid cells.[1, 4, 24, 25]

B-Cell Markers

During B-cell differentiation the CD19, CD22, and CD72 antigens are expressed on the cell surface membrane of both immature and mature differentiation stages.[2, 4, 9, 26–28] The CD79a and CD79b molecules (also known as mb-1 and B29, or Igα and Igβ respectively) are signal-transducing elements, associated with Ig molecules.[17] Expression of the CD79 molecules is only found in B-lineage cells: during precursor B-cell differentiation, both CD79 chains are expressed in the cytoplasm (CyCD79), whereas in the more mature differentiation stages, the CD79 chains are associated with surface membrane–bound immunoglobulin (SmIg) molecules (SmIg-CD79 complex).[29, 30] CyCD79a is one of the earliest B-lineage markers found in B-cell ontogeny, preceding surface expression of CD19.[31] Characterization of the various B-cell differentiation stages can be based on the expression of B-cell antigens (CD10, CD20, CD21, CD23, CD37, and FMC7) as well as on the various expression patterns of immunoglobulin (Ig) chains.[2, 4, 26, 32, 33] The characteristic feature of the pre–B-cell stage is the weak cytoplasmic expression of Igμ heavy chains in the absence of normal Ig light chains but in the presence of λ5/Vpre-B surrogate light chains (pre-B CyIgμ); these surrogate light chains are already found in the cytoplasm in earlier differentiation stages.[32, 34, 35] In part of the pre–B-cells, the incomplete pre-B Ig complex is also weakly expressed on the cell surface membrane (pre-B Igμ-CD79 or pre-B complex).[17, 36] Naïve immature B cells in bone marrow express on their surface SmIgμ and are CD27[−], whereas the majority of early immunocompetent B cells in peripheral blood are SmIgμδ[+].[37, 38] Positive B-cell selection in the germinal center is associated with Ig isotype switching, and most B cells then become SmIgγ[+], SmIgα[+], or SmIgε[+] and CD27[+].[37, 38] Plasma cells express high levels of cytoplasmic Ig (CyIg) and are often positive for the CD38 antigen and the CD138 (syndecan-1) molecule.[39, 40]

T-Cell Markers

Virtually all T-lineage cells express the CD2 antigen and the CD7 antigen.[12, 41, 42] Moreover, the T-cell–specific transcription factor TCF1 can be detected in the nuclei at all stages of T-cell differentiation except for resting mature T lymphocytes.[43] Comparable with the expression of the CD79 antigen during B-cell differentiation, the CD3 anti-

TABLE 6–2. Detailed Information Concerning Clustered and Nonclustered Antibodies for Immunophenotyping Leukemias

CD no.[1]	Antigen name(s)/function	mol mass (M_m) (kDa)	Reactivity with Hematopoietic Cells	Typical Examples of McAb (no complete listing)[2]
Precursor markers				
CD34	precursor antigen	gp105–120	lymphoid and myeloid progenitor cells	HPCA-1/My10, HPCA-2/8G12, BI-3C5
CD117	SCFR (stem cell factor receptor); c-kit; SLF (Steel's factor) receptor	gp145	hematopoietic progenitor cells, most colony-forming cells, and mast cells	17F11, YB5.B8
–	TdT/function in Ig and TCR gene rearrangement (insertion of nucleotides at junction sites)	p58	immature lymphoid cells, small fraction of myeloid precursor cells, virtually all ALL, and some AML	conventional antisera and HTdT-1 McAb
B-cell markers				
CD10	common ALL antigen (CALLA)/neutral endopeptidase (enkephalinase)	gp100	subset of precursor-B cells, subset of B lymphocytes (follicular center cells), subset of cortical thymocytes, granulocytes	J5, VIL-A1, BA-3
CD19	pan–B-cell antigen/function in B-cell activation; associates with CD21 antigen (CR2)	gp90	precursor-B cells and B lymphocytes	Leu-12, B4, HD37
CD20	B-cell antigen/function in B-cell activation	p35	subpopulation of precursor-B cells, all B lymphocytes, follicular dentritic reticulum cells	Leu-16, B1 L26 detects intracellular epitope (CD20-Cy Ab)
CD21	B-cell antigen/CR2 (C3d receptor); EBV receptor	gp140	subpopulations of B lymphocytes (e.g., follicular mantle cells), follicular dendritic reticulum cells subset of thymocytes	OKB7, B2
CD22	B-cell antigen/function in B-cell adhesion and B-cell activation	gp135	precursor-B cells and B lymphocytes	Leu-14/SHCL-1, RFB4, HD39
CD23	B-cell antigen/FcεRII (low affinity Fc receptor for IgE); two types of FcεRII exist, which differ in their cytoplasmic domain (FcεRIIa and FcεRIIb)	gp45	FcεRIIa is expressed by a subpopulation of B lymphocytes (e.g., follicular mantle cells) and B-CLL cells; FcεRIIb is expressed by subset of B lymphocytes, monocytes, eosinophils, dendritic cells	Leu-20/EBVCS-5, Tü1
CD24	B-cell/granulocytic antigen, heat stable antigen	gp35–45	subpopulation of (precursor) B cells mature granulocytes	OKB2, BA-1, ALB9, SN3
CD37	B-cell antigen (tetraspan molecule)	gp40–52	B lymphocytes; weak expression on T cells, monocytes and granulocytes	RFB7, Y29/55
CD72	B-cell antigen/ligand for CD5 antigen	gp43/39	precursor-B cells and B lymphocytes	J3-109
CD79a	mb-1; Igα (disulfide linked to CD79b and associated with SmIg)/signal transduction from SmIg to cytoplasm	gp32–33	precursor-B cells (cytoplasmic expression; CyCD79a) and SmIg+ B cells (membrane expression; SmCD79a)	HM57 detects intracellular epitopes of CD79a (CD79a-Cy Ab)
CD79b	B29; Igβ (disulfide linked to CD79a and associated with SmIg)/signal transduction from SmIg to cytoplasm	gp37–39	precursor-B cells (cytoplasmic expression; CyCD79b) and SmIg+ B cells (membrane expression; SmCD79b)	B29/123 detects intracellular epitope of CD79b (CD79b-Cy Ab)
CD138	Plasma cell antigen	gp20	plasma cells and multiple myeloma	B-B4
–	mature B-cell antigen	gp105	B lymphocytes	FMC7
–	pre-B CyIgμ (weak cytoplasmic expression of Igμ chain)	gp70	pre-B cells; only Ig-μ heavy chains are weakly expressed in the cytoplasma (no mature Ig light chains)	selected anti-Igμ antisera
–	λ5, distal part of the surrogate light chain	gp22	precursor-B cells	HSL11
–	VpreB, proximal part of the surrogate light chain	gp18	precursor-B cells	HSL96
–	SmIg (surface membrane immunoglobulin); IgM, IgD, IgG, IgA, IgE	M_m is dependent on Ig class	SmIg-positive cells; each B-cell clone expresses only one type of Ig light chain (κ or λ) but may express multiple IgH chains	conventional antisera and McAb
–	CyIg (cytoplasmic immunoglobulin)	M_m is dependent on Ig class	CyIg-positive cells (immunoblasts, immunocytes, and plasma cells)	conventional antisera and McAb

(continued)

TABLE 6–2. (Continued)

CD no.[1]	Antigen name(s)/function	mol mass (M_m) (kDa)	Reactivity with Hematopoietic Cells	Typical Examples of McAb (no complete listing)[2]
T-cell markers				
CD1	T6 antigen; common thymocyte antigen/MHC-like protein; can associate with β2-microglobulin	CD1a:gp49 CD1b:gp45 CD1c:gp43	cortical thymocytes, Langerhans' cells, subpopulation of dendritic cells, subpopulation of B lymphocytes	OKT6, NA 1/34 7C4/160/4G9 7C6/162/3B10
CD2	T11 antigen; SRBC receptor (= E rosette receptor); LFA-2/receptor for T-cell activation; ligand for CD58 (LFA-3)	gp50	all T cells, most NK cells; three different antigenic epitopes are known, of which one is the SRBC binding site	Leu-5b, OKT11, T11
CD3	T3 antigen (associated with TCR)/signal transduction from TCR to cytoplasm	gp16–25	immature T cells (cytoplasmic expression; CyCD3) and mature T cells (membrane expression)	Leu-4/SK7, OKT3, UCHT1, VIT-3
CD4	T4 antigen/involved in MHC-class-II-restricted antigen recognition; HIV receptor	gp59	subset of cortical thymocytes, helper/inducer T lymphocytes, subpopulation of monocytes and macrophages; some AML	Leu-3a, OKT4
CD5	T1 antigen/function in T-cell proliferation; ligand for CD72 antigen an B lymphocytes	gp67	thymocytes and mature T lymphocytes, subpopulation of B lymphocytes; B-CLL	Leu-1, T1
CD6	T12 antigen/related to CD5 antigen	gp120	thymocytes and mature T lymphocytes, subpopulation of B lymphocytes; B-CLL	OKT17, T12
CD7	Tp41 antigen/Fc receptor for IgM (FcμR)?	gp41	almost all T cells, NK cells, subpopulation of immature myeloid cells; some AML	Leu-9, 3A1, WT1
CD8	T8 antigen; the CD8 molecule consists of two disulfide linked chains: α-α homodimer or α-β heterodimer/involved in MHC class-I-restricted antigen recognition	CD8-α:gp32 CD8-β:gp32	subpopulation of cortical thymocytes, cytotoxic/suppressor T lymphocytes, subpopulation of NK cells	most CD8 antibodies detect CD8α chain: Leu-2a, OKT8
–	TCR-αβ (classical TCR;TCR2)	gp80 (44/40)	TCR-αβ is expressed by majority of mature CD3+ T cells	WT31, BMA031
–	TCR β chains	gp40	Intracellular TCR chains in most cortical thymocytes and many T-ALL	βF1
–	TCR-γδ (alternative TCR; TCR1)	gp75 (44/42 or 55/42)	TCR-γδ is expressed by minority of mature CD3+ T cells	anti-TCR-γ/δ-1, TCR1
–	Vβ domains	gp10	subpopulation of thymocytes and T cells	large panel of 20 to 25 Vβ McAb, recognizing 65%–75% of blood T lymphocytes
–	Vδ domains	gp10	subpopulation of thymocytes and T cells	Vδ1 (R9.12) Vδ2 (lmmu389, BB3) Vδ3 (p 11.5B)
–	Vγ domains	gp10	subpopulation of thymocytes and T cells	Vγ2/3/4 (23D12), Vγ3/5 (56.3), Vγ8 (R4.5) Vγ9 (Ti-A, Immu360)
–	TCF1, T-cell–specific transcription factor	p27	thymocytes, activated T cells	TCF1
NK-cell markers				
CD56	NCAM; PI-linked and transmembrane forms	gp120,140, 180	NK cells, some T lymphocytes (neuroectodermal cells)	Leu-19/My31, NKH-1
CD57	human natural killer cell antigen	gp110	subpopulation of NK cells, subpopulation of T lymphocytes, some B cells	Leu-7/HNK-1
CD94	kp43, HLA–class I inhibitory receptor for different HLA-A, -B or -C alleles.	gp43	NK cells, minor subset of T lymphocytes	Z199, Z270, NKH-3, HP-3B1
CD158a	p58.1, inhibitory NK-cell receptor specific for HLA-Cw4	gp58/50	NK cells, minor subset of T lymphocytes	EB6, HP-3E4
CD158b	p58.2, inhibitory NK-cell receptor specific for HLA-Cw3	gp58/50	NK cells, minor subset of T lymphocytes	GL183, CH-L
–	inhibitory NK-cell receptor specific for HLA-A allotypes	gp140	NK cells, minor subset of T lymphocytes	Q66, Q241
–	NKB-1, inhibitory NK-cell receptor specific for HLA-B	gp70	NK cells, minor subset of T lymphocytes	DX9, Z27
–	NKp46, natural cytotoxicity receptor	gp46	NK cells	BAB281

(continued)

TABLE 6–2. (Continued)

CD no.[1]	Antigen name(s)/function	mol mass (M_m) (kDa)	Reactivity with Hematopoietic Cells	Typical Examples of McAb (no complete listing)[2]
Pan-myeloid markers				
CD13	pan-myeloid antigen; amino-peptidase N; differential glycosylation generates different epitopes, detected by McAb	gp150	almost all myeloid cells, dendritic cells in the skin	My7, MCS2
CD33	pan-myeloid antigen	gp67	majority of myeloid and monocytic cells (weak expression on granulocytes)	My9, L4F3
CDw65	myelomonocytic antigen (fucoganglioside; ceramide-dodecasaccharide 40)	glycolipid	majority of myeloid and monocytes cells and a part of their precursors	VIM-2
–	MPO (myeloperoxidase); MPO consists of two subunits	gp60/12	majority of cells of the myeloid lineage (granulocytic and monocytic cells)	MPO-7, CLB-MPO-1
Myeloid-granulocytic markers				
CD15	Lewis-X (Le^x); X hapten; 3-FAL (3-fucosyl-N-acetyl-lactosamine)	variety of gp's	cells of the granulocytic lineage, weak expression by monocytes, Reed-Sternberg cells	Leu-M1, VIM-D5, 1G10
CD66b	CEA gene member 6 (CGM6) (PI-linked); previously clustered as CD67	gp95–100	granulocytes; increased expression upon activation	CLB-B13.9
CD66c	NCA	gp90	granulocytes and epithelial cells; some ALL	KOR-SA3544, 9A6
Monocytic-macrophage markers				
CD14	monocytic antigen; PI-linked protein/LPS receptor	gp55	monocytic cells, macrophages, follicular dendritic reticulum cells, B lymphocytes (weak); absent in patients with PNH	My4, Mo2, FMC17, UCHM1
CD68	macrophage antigen	gp110	macrophages (mainly cytoplasmic expression), activated platelets	Ki-M6, Ki-M7
–	macrophage antigen	gp25	macrophages	RFD9
Erythroid markers				
–	H antigen; backbone of ABO variable blood group proteins	variable	erythroid cells	CLB-eryH/1
–	GpA (glycophorin A)	gp41	erythroid cells	VIE-G4, CLB-ery/1
Megakaryocyte-platelet markers				
CD41	platelet GPIIb; integrin αIIb chain; platelet GPIIb consists of a large subunit and a small β subunit (disulfide linked) and is associated with platelet GPIIIa (CD61 antigen)/receptor for fibrinogen and von Willebrand factor	gp140(NR) gp125/22(R)	megakaryocytes, platelets; absent or reduced in patients with Glanzmann's thrombasthenia	CLB-thromb/7
CD42	consists of four subunits: CD42a: platelet GPIIb CD42b: platelet GPIbα subunit CD42c: platelet GPIbβ subunit CD42d: platelet GPV major receptor for von Willebrand factor and platelet adhesion	gp23 gp135(R) gp22(R) gp85	megakaryocytes, platelets; absent or reduced in patients with Bernard-Soulier syndrome	FMC25 AN51 GI27 CLB-SW16
CD61	integrin 3 chain (platelet GPIIIa; VNR-β chain); associated with platelet GPIIb (see CD41) or CD51 (VNR-α)	gp110	megakaryocytes, platelets	Y2/51, CLB-thromb/1 (C17)
Nonlineage restricted markers				
CD9	p24 antigen (tetraspan molecule)/induction of aggregation of platelets	p24	subpopulation of precursor-B cells, subpopulation of B lymphocytes (follicular center cells), monocytes, megakaryocytes, platelets, eosinophils, basophils	BA-2
CD11c	p150, 95 antigen (integrin αX chain); associated with CD18 antigen/adhesion molecule; CR4 (C3bi, C3dg receptor)	gp150	monocytes, macrophages, granulocytes, subpopulations of lymphocytes (e.g., HCL-like cells in the spleen and NK cells); no membrane expression in LAD-1 patients	Leu-M5/SHCL3

(continued)

TABLE 6–2. (Continued)

CD no.[1]	Antigen Name(s)/Function	mol mass (M$_m$) (kDa)	Reactivity with Hematopoietic Cells	Typical Examples of McAb (no complete listing)
CD16	FcγRIII (low-affinity Fc receptor for IgG); FcγRIIIA (transmembrane form) and FcγRIIIB (PI-linked form)	gp50–65	neutrophilic granulocytes, monocytes (weak), macrophages (weak), NK cells; FcγRIIIb is absent on granulocytes in patients with PNH	Leu-11b,CLB-FcR-gran/1: these antibodies recognize both FcγRIIIA and FcγRIIIB
CD24	B-cell–granulocytic antigen; PI-linked protein on granulocytes	gp42	subpopulation of (precursor) B cells, granulocytes; absent on granulocytes in patients with PNH	BA-1, VIB-C5
CD25	Tac antigen/α chain of the IL2 receptor (low affinity IL2R); high affinity IL-2R when associated with β chain (CD122 antigen) and/or γ chain	gp55	activated T cells, activated B lymphocytes, activated macrophages; HCL	2A3, ACT-1
CD27	TNF receptor superfamily, member 7/receptor for CD70 antigen	p120 (55/55)	mature T cells, activated T cells, memory B lymphocytes, and NK cells	L128, OKT18A, 1A4CD27
CD36	monocytic-thrombocytic antigen; thrombospondin receptor; platelet GPIV/role in cell signaling	gp90	monocytes, macrophages, early erythroid cells, megakaryocytes, platelets	OKM5, FA6.152, 5F1
CD38	T10 antigen	gp45	activated T and B cells, precursor cells (e.g., thymocytes), subpopulations of B cells (e.g. follicular center cells), plasma cells	Leu-17/HB7, OKT10
CD103	HML-1 (human mucosal lymphocyte 1 integrin); αE chain, which is associated with β7 chain	gp150,25	mucosa-associated T lymphocytes (especially intraepithelial CD8+ T cells) 2%–6% of blood lymphocytes; part of mucosal T-NHL (not other peripheral T-NHL) and HCL	B-ly7
–	granzyme B	p27	cytotoxic T lymphocytes, lymphokine activated killer (LAK), and NK cells	CLB-B11, GrB-7, MCA1645
–	TIA1 cytotoxic granule-associated RNA-binding protein	p15/40	cytotoxic T lymphocytes and activated NK cells	TIA1
–	perforin (PRF1, pore forming protein 1)	p70–75	cytoplasmic granules of natural killer and cytotoxic T cells	G9
–	HLA-DR, non-polymorphic antigen/MHC-class II molecule	gp29/34	hematopoietic precursor cells, B cells, activated T cells, monocytic cells, and macrophages	L243, OKDr

1. CD = cluster of differentiation, as described during the Leucocyte Typing Conferences (Paris, 1982; Boston, 1984; Oxford, 1986; Vienna, 1989; Boston, 1993; Kobe, 1996).

2. Complete list of all relevant clustered and non-clustered antibodies can be obtained via J.J.M. van Dongen, Dept. of Immunology, Erasmus University, PO box 1738, 3000 DR Rotterdam, the Netherlands.

ALL, acute lymphoblastic leukemia; AML, acute myeloid leukemia; CALLA, common ALL antigen; CEA, carcinoembryonic antigen; CGM, CEA gene member antigen; CyIg, cytoplasmic Ig; CLL, chronic lymphocytic leukemia; CR, complement receptor; EBV, Epstein Barr virus; FAL, fucosyl-N-acetyllactosamine; FcγR, Fc receptor for IgG; FcεR, Fc receptor for IgE; FcμR, Fc receptor for IgM; GP, glycoprotein; gp, glycoprotein; GpA, glycophorin; HCL, hairy cell leukemia; HIV, human immunodeficiency virus; HML, human mucosal lymphocyte; Ig, immunoglobulin; IL2, interleukin 2; LAD, leukocyte adhesion deficiency; Le^X, Lewis-X; LFA, leukocyte function antigen; LPS, lipopolysaccharide; McAb, monoclonal antibody/antibodies; MHC, major histocompatibility complex; MPO, myeloperoxidase; NCA, non-cross reacting antigen; NCAM, neural cell adhesion molecule; NK cell, natural killer cell; NR, non-reduced; PI, phosphatidyl-inositol glycan; PNH, paroxysmal nocturnal hemoglobinuria; R, reduced; SCFR, stem cell factor receptor; SLF, Steel factor; SmIg, surface membrane Ig; SRBC, sheep red blood cells; TCR, T-cell receptor; TNF, tumor necrosis factor; VNR, vitronectin receptor.

gen is expressed in the cytoplasm (CyCD3) of immature T cells, whereas mature T cells express this antigen on the cell surface membrane in association with the TCR (TCR-CD3 complex).[12, 17, 27] The other T-cell markers (CD1, CD4, CD5, CD6, and CD8) enable further characterization of the T cells.[12, 41, 42]

Natural Killer Cell Markers

Natural killer (NK) cells are positive for the pan–T-cell marker CD7 and often also for the CD2 antigen, but they are negative for the TCR-CD3 complex.[42, 44–46] Most NK cells are positive for the CD16 antigen (low-affinity Fc receptor for IgG) and the CD56 antigen, and a part of the NK cells express the CD57 antigen.[42, 44–46] Expression of the CD8 antigen can be found on a small fraction of the NK cells.[42] Several human NK cell receptors have been identified that trigger the process of natural cytotoxicity. These natural toxicity receptors (NCR) include NKp46, NKp44, and NKp30 proteins, which mediate cytolysis of allogeneic cells or tumor cells and induce cytokine production.[47] Moreover, NK cells differentially express various inhibitory receptors (killing inhibitory receptors [KIR]) specific for human leukocyte antigen

(HLA) class I molecules (e.g., CD94, CD158a, CD158b, and CD161) that prevent cytotocixity against autologous HLA class I positive cells.[48] NCR are exclusively expressed by NK cells, whereas other NK markers are not NK-cell specific. For example, T lymphocytes, especially CD8[+] T lymphocytes, can also be positive for CD16, CD56, and CD57 molecules as well as for KIRs.[42, 47, 48] Finally, the cytolytic granules of NK cells as well as cytotoxic, CD8[+] T cells contain several cytotoxic proteins, including perforins, granzymes, and T-cell "restricted" intracellular antigen (TIA1).[49-51]

Myeloid Markers

During myelopoiesis, most precursor cells and virtually all cells of the granulocytic and monocytic cell lineages express the panmyeloid markers CD13 and CD33.[52, 53] Only the most mature granulocytes are negative for the CD33 antigen.[53] In addition, most myeloid cells are positive for the CD65 antigen and myeloperoxidase.[54, 55] Monocytic cells express the CD14 antigen, and macrophages are generally positive for the CD68 antigen and RFD9.[56, 57] During granulopoiesis, the CD15 and CD66c antigens are expressed.[58, 59] More mature granulocytic cells are also positive for the CD16 and CD66b antigens.[8, 9]

Erythroid Markers and Megakaryocyte Platelet Markers

During erythropoiesis, glycophorin A and the H-antigen are expressed.[60] The CD41/CD61 antigens and the CD42 molecule are platelet glycoproteins, which can be used as megakaryocyte platelet markers.[61, 62]

Nonlineage Restricted Markers

Several useful immunologic markers are expressed in multiple differentiation lineages, such as the CD9 antigen, the CD11c antigen, the CD36 antigen, and HLA-DR. The expression patterns of these markers and a few other nonlineage restricted markers are summarized in Table 6-2.[2, 4, 8-10, 63]

Techniques for Immunophenotyping

Immunologic marker analysis can be performed on fresh or permeabilized cells in suspension and on fixed cells in cytocentrifuge preparations, smears, or tissue sections. The reactivity of antibodies is visualized by use of fluorochromes or enzymes as labels. In immunoenzyme techniques, the antibodies are labeled with an enzyme, such as peroxidase, alkaline phosphatase, or β-galactosidase.[64-66] Immunoenzyme stainings are generally applied on tissue sections or cytocentrifuge preparations. This technique allows a combined interpretation of histomorphologic or cytomorphologic information and immunophenotyping.

In immunofluorescence techniques antibodies are conjugated with a fluorochrome, such as fluorescein isothiocyanate (FITC), tetramethylrhodamine isothiocyanate, 7-amino 4-methylcoumarin acetate, phycoerythrin (PE),

peridinin chlorophyl (PerCP), and allophycocyanin (APC), or duochromes such as PE-Cy5 and PerCP-Cy5. A major advantage of fluorescence techniques is that double, triple, and quadruple stainings can be performed easily. This allows simultaneous evaluation of two, three, or four different immunologic markers; immunoenzyme techniques are not easily applicable for multiple marker analysis.[67]

The labeling technique of choice depends partly on the cell sample and the markers studied. Most clustered McAb against leukocyte antigens recognize surface membrane–bound molecules, but a few important differentiation markers are expressed intracellularly, e.g., CyCD3, CyCD79, TdT, and MPO. Immunophenotyping of leukemias is generally performed on cells in suspension; immunofluorescence techniques are used predominantly. Immunofluorescence stainings can be evaluated by microscopy or flow cytometry. The possibilities and limitations of both methods are compared next.

Fluorescence Microscopy

Most fluorescence microscopes use epi-illumination with a mercury lamp for the excitation of the fluorochromes. The filter combinations in the epi-illumination system consist of excitation filters, emission filters, and a dichroic mirror, which reflects the excitation light but allows the emission light to pass. For optimal evaluation of immunofluorescence stainings, the microscope should be equipped with phase contrast facilities. A major advantage of fluorescence microscopy is that it enables positive identification at the single-cell level, which is particularly important for detection of low frequencies of leukemic cells. Major drawbacks of fluorescence microscopy are that analysis of stained cells is laborious and that quantification of the fluorescence intensity is difficult, unless automated screening systems and automated data handling are used, but these systems are not yet routinely applied.[68] Traditionally, fluorescence microscopy was recommended for analysis of the typical staining patterns of intracellular antigens, such as CyCD3 (see Fig. 6–1) and TdT (Fig. 6–2).[12, 69] However, with the developments of flow cytometric detection of intracellular antigens, routine fluorescence microscopy is limited to detection of intracellular antigens for which McAb suitable for flow cytometry are not yet available (e.g., TCF1, c-MYC, TAL1). Fluorescence microscopy is also superior for the discrimination between intracellular staining patterns of wild-type proteins and leukemia-specific fusion proteins. This was demonstrated for the PG-M3 monoclonal antibody directed against amino terminal portion of human PML protein, producing characteristic microgranular pattern of PML-RARα fusion protein in AML-M3 with t(15;17) translocation, which was clearly different from the speckled fluorescence pattern of the PML protein in normal myeloid cells and t(15;17)-negative AML.[70]

Flow Cytometry

During the last two decades, major progress has been made in both flow cytometry and computer technology.[71] These developments have resulted in current fluorescence-activated flow cytometers for clinical practice. A

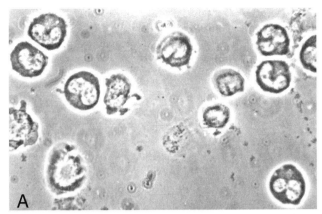

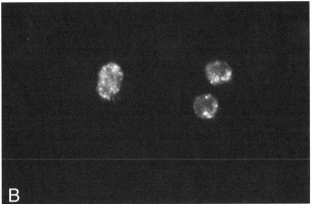

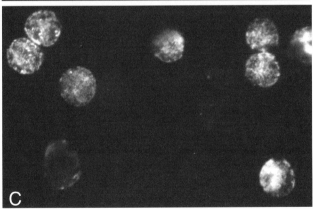

FIGURE 6–2. Immunophenotyping by use of fluorescence microscopy. Double immunofluorescence staining for TdT and the CD15 antigen on mononuclear bone marrow cells of a CML patient in early lymphoid blast crisis. Phase contrast morphology (*A*), TdT-positive cells (FITC labeled; *B*), and CD15- (VIM-D5) positive cells (TRITC labeled; *C*). The TdT-positive lymphoblasts do not express the granulocytic marker CD15.

typical instrument consists of an air-cooled 15-mW argonion laser light source that provides monochromatic light at 488 nm. The cells, which flow through the laser beam, refract the light and, if present, fluorochromes are excited and emit fluorescence. The refracted light is measured at two different angles, giving the scatter morphology. In forward direction of the laser beam, the forward scatter (FSC) or low-angle scatter is measured; at 90 degrees, the sideward scatter (SSC) is measured. The FSC signal depends primarily on the volume of the particles or cells, whereas the SSC signal provides a measure of internal

organization, cytoplasmic granularity, nuclear density, and external cell structure. The emitted fluorescence is collected by optics in the 90-degree angle. Depending on the wavelength of the emitted light, the light is separated by a series of dichroic mirrors into two or more beams. Most currently used single-laser flow cytometers allow the simultaneous detection of three fluorochromes: FITC, PE, and PerCP or the duochrome PE-Cy5.[71] Flow cytometers equipped with a second laser with 635-nm emission are being introduced increasingly into immunohematological laboratories, allowing the inclusion of a fourth fluorochrome, e.g., APC.[31, 72] The refracted light or fluorescence is measured by light detection devices, such as photodiodes and photomultiplier tubes, which convert light into an electric signal. The magnitude of the electric signal is proportional to the amount of light detected, which, in the case of fluorescence, is related to the number of fluorescent molecules. For each cell or particle, the signals produced by the different light detection devices are processed and sent as list mode data to the computer. Flow cytometry enables rapid acquisition of information about large numbers of cells (250–2500 cells/s).

The amount of information obtained during measurement is extensive, and sophisticated software programs are required for data processing and analysis.[71] Typically, 5000 to 10,000 cells are evaluated, and for each cell results on four to six different parameters are obtained.[67] The results of one parameter can be presented and analyzed by use of histogram analysis. However, it is more informative to plot two different parameters against each other in one graph, such as a dot plot diagram or contour plot diagram. Examples of dot plot analyses are given in Figure 6–3. A scatter diagram of FSC against SSC of lysed whole blood cells allows discrimination among lymphocytes, monocytes, and granulocytes. Analysis can be performed on all cells or on a specific subpopulation. In the latter case, the cells of interest are selected by gating on a specific subpopulation in a histogram or dot plot. Gating on scatter morphology in FSC/SSC dot plots is frequently used in immunophenotyping of normal and leukemic hematopoetic cells. The gated cells can be studied subsequently for various parameters (Fig. 6–3). For instance, the combination of SSC and weak-to-intermediate expression of the leukocyte common antigen (CD45) can identify a unique blast cell region in order to set gate on most immature leukemic cells.[73, 74] Modern flow cytometry enables multiparameter analysis of various cell populations.[67, 71] Because red blood cells can be lysed after leukocytes have been stained with an antibody, cell separation is no longer a prerequisite. The standardization of permeabilization/fixation solutions enables routine detection of intracellular antigens.[75] Another advantage of flow cytometry is that it enables quantification of fluorescence intensity. However, in contrast to fluorescence microscopy, analysis at the single cell level is not reliable.

Immunophenotypes of Leukemias

Four main categories of leukemias are recognized: (1) acute lymphoblastic leukemia (ALL), (2) acute myeloid leukemia (AML), (3) chronic lymphocytic leukemia (CLL), and (4) chronic myeloid leukemia (CML). Figure 6–4

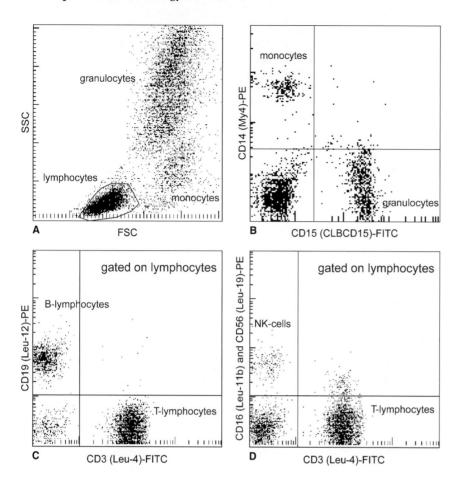

FIGURE 6–3. Immunophenotyping by use of flow cytometry. The figure shows dot plot analyses of three double stainings performed on lyzed whole blood cells obtained from a healthy volunteer. *A,* Scatter pattern (FSC versus SSC) of the blood leukocytes. Lymphocytes, monocytes, and granulocytes can be identified based on their scatter morphology. The gate for the lymphocyte population is indicated. *B,* CD15 (CLB-CD15)-FITC versus CD14 (My4)-PE staining of the total leukocyte population, allowing detection of CD15$^+$ granulocytes and CD14$^+$ monocytes. *C,* CD3 (Leu-4)-FITC versus CD19 (Leu-12)-PE staining gated on lymphocytes for detection of CD3$^+$ T lymphocytes and CD19$^+$ B lymphocytes. *D,* CD3 (Leu-4)-FITC versus CD16 (Leu-11c)-PE and CD56(Leu-19)-PE staining for detection of CD3$^+$ T lymphocytes and CD3$^-$/CD16$^+$-CD56$^+$ NK cells.

shows the age-related incidence of these four types of leukemias in the Netherlands.[76] Although the incidence of most malignancies increases with aging, the highest incidence of ALL occurs in early childhood. If all ages are taken into account, CLL and AML occur most frequently.

The cells in ALL and AML are generally regarded as malignant counterparts of immature lymphoid and myeloid cells, whereas the maturation arrest of CLL and CML generally occurs in more mature differentiation stages.[1-5] Most cells in non-Hodgkin's lymphomas (NHL)

are also arrested in the more mature differentiation stages.[1-5] Immunophenotyping enables the determination of the differentiation stage of normal and abnormal populations and subpopulations. Therefore, it allows identification and classification of most leukemias. Using immunophenotyping, it has been found that B-lineage leukemias dominate within the lymphoid leukemia groups (Table 6–3).[77-81]

Acute Lymphoblastic Leukemias

Using immunophenotyping, it is possible to discriminate at least seven different ALL subtypes.[2, 4, 79, 82] As has been

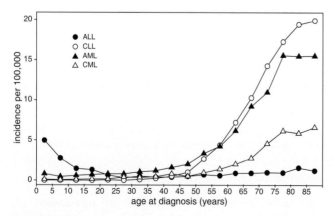

FIGURE 6–4. Age-related incidence of the four main types of leukemias in the Netherlands between 1991 and 1995. Data are from the Dutch Cancer Registry.

TABLE 6–3. B-lineage and T-lineage Origin of Lymphoid Leukemias

| | ALL | | Chronic Lymphoid Leukemias |
	Childhood	*Adult*	
B lineage	80%–85%	75%–80%	95% (B-CLL, T-PLL, HCL)
T lineage	15%–20%	20%–25%	5% (LGL, T-PLL, CTLL, ATLL)[1]

1. In Japan and Caribbean regions ATLL occurs in higher frequencies than in Europe and other Western countries.

CLL, chronic lymphocytic leukemia; PLL, prolymphocytic leukemia; HCL, hairy cell leukemia; LGL, large granular lymphocyte leukemia; CTLL, cutaneous T-cell leukemia lymphoma; ATLL, adult T-cell leukemia lymphoma.

TABLE 6–4. Immunophenotypic Characteristics of Precursor-B-ALL

Markers	pro–B-ALL	Common ALL	pre–B-ALL	Transitional pre–B-ALL[1]
TdT	++	++	++	++
CD10	−	++	++	++
CD19	++	++	++	++
CD20	−	+	+	+
CD22	++	++	++	++
CyCD79	++	++	++	++
Pre-B CyIgμ	−	−	++	++
SmVpre-B/λ5	−	−	−	++
SmIg-CD79	−	−	−	++
CD34	+	+	+	+
HLA-DR	++	++	++	++

1. 5% of pre–B-ALL patients have a "transitional pre–B-ALL," defined by both pre–B CyIgμ and surface membrane expression of the pre–B-cell complex (pre–B SmIgμ-CD79) without expression of mature κ or λ Ig light chains.[36]

−, <10% of the leukemias is positive; +, 25%–75% of the leukemias is positive; ++, >75% of the leukemias is positive.

drawn in Figure 6-5, these concern four types of B-lineage ALL and at least three types of T-ALL. The immunophenotypes of B-lineage ALL are summarized in Table 6-4. All four forms of precursor B-ALL (pro-B-ALL, common ALL, pre-B-ALL, and transitional pre–B-ALL) are TdT⁺. The previously recognized category of B-ALL is currently classified as Burkitt's leukemia and is TDT⁻. The B-lineage ALL types are positive for HLA-DR, CD19, CyCD79, and CD22. CD79 is completely B-cell–specific.[29, 30] Except for a small part of the pre-B-ALL, expression of the CD79 antigen in precursor B-ALL is restricted to the cytoplasm.[29, 30] CD10, pre-B CyIgμ, and SmIgμ are important markers for discrimination between the four subtypes of B-lineage ALL (see Table 6-4 and Fig. 6-5). An example of flow cytometric immunophenotyping of a common ALL is given in Figure 6-6. For the diagnosis of pre-B-ALL, expression of pre-B CyIgμ is a prerequisite: at least 10% to 20% of the ALL cells should express this marker.[35, 79, 83] The typical intracellular staining pattern of pre-B CyIgμ can be easily recognized by use of fluorescence microscopy, but weak CyIgμ expression can also be

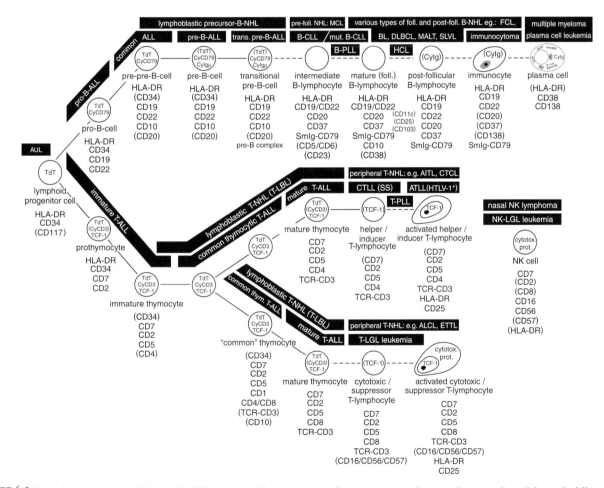

FIGURE 6–5. Hypothetical scheme of lymphoid differentiation. The expression of relevant immunologic markers is indicated for each differentiation stage; markers in parentheses are not always expressed. The bars represent the various types of leukemias and non-Hodgkin lymphomas (NHL) and indicate where these malignancies can be located according to their maturation arrest. AITL = angioimmunoblastic T-cell lymphoma, ALCL = anaplastic large cell lymphoma (of T-cell type), ALL = acute lymphoblastic leukemia, ATLL = adult T cell leukemia lymphoma, AUL = acute un-differentiated leukemia, CLL = chronic lymphocytic leukemia, CTCL = cutaneous T-cell lymphoma, CTLL = cutaneous T-cell leukemia lymphoma (mycosis fungoides/Sézary syndrome), DLBCL = diffuse large B-cell lymphoma, ETTL = enteropathy-type T-cell lymphoma, HCL = hairy cell leukemia, HTLV = human T cell leukemia virus, LGL = large granular lymphocyte, MALT = mucosa associated tissue lymphoma, NHL = non-Hodgkin's lymphoma, PLL = prolymphocytic leukemia (see reference 4).

TABLE 6–5. Immunophenotypic Characteristics of T-ALL

| Markers | Immature T-ALL | | Common Thymocytic T-ALL | | Mature T-ALL |
	Prothymocytic (pre–T-ALL)	Immature Thymocytic	SmCD3⁻	SmCD3⁺	
TdT	++	++	++	++	++
CD1	−	−	++	++	−
CD2	+	++	++	++	++
CyCD3	++	++	++	++	++
SmCD3	−	−	−	++	++
CD4⁻/CD8⁻	++	+	−	−	−
CD4⁺/CD8⁻	−	±	±	±	+
CD4⁻/CD8⁺	−	±	±	±	±
CD4⁺/CD8⁺	−	−	+	+	±
CD5	−	++	++	++	++
CD7	++	++	++	++	++
TCRαβ	−	−	−	60%–70%	
TCRγδ	−	−	−	30%–40%	
HLA-DR	+	−	−	−	−

−, <10% of the leukemias is positive; ±, 10%–25% of the leukemias is positive; +, 25%–75% of the leukemias is positive; ++, >75% of the leukemias is positive.

detected in CyIgμ/SmIgμ flow cytometric double labelings (Fig. 6-6). In about 5% of pre–B-ALL, faint expression of the Igμ-CD79 complex without normal Ig light chains is seen on the surface membrane (pre-B complex).[36] These ALLs have been defined as transitional pre–B-ALL.[36]

Virtually all T-ALL are positive for TdT, CD2, CD7, and CyCD3.[2, 4] Markers, which can be used for additional characterization, concern CD1, surface membrane CD3 (SmCD3), CD4, CD5, and CD8.[4, 12, 79, 82] In fact, using only CD1 and SmCD3, at least three types of T-ALL can be recognized: immature T-ALL (CD1⁻/SmCD3⁻), common thymocytic (cortical) T-ALL (CD1⁺/SmCD3⁻ ᵒʳ ⁺), and mature T-ALL (CD1⁻/SmCD3⁺) (Table 6-5; see Fig. 6-5).[4, 79] The immature T-ALLs concern either the rarely occurring prothymocytic T-ALL (pro–T-ALL) or the immature thymocytic T-ALL (pre–T-ALL).[4, 84] The common thymocytic T-ALL can be divided further in SmCD3⁻ and SmCD3⁺ types (see Table 6-5). The distinction between SmCD3⁻ T-ALL and SmCD3⁺ T-ALL is used widely; SmCD3 expression is found in approximately 35% of all T-ALL.[41] The CD3 antigen on the cell surface membrane is associated with TCR molecules. In approximately 30% to 40% of SmCD3⁺ T-ALL, this concerns TCRγδ.[41, 85] This frequency is essentially higher than in mature T-cell malignancies, which rarely express TCRγδ.[41, 42] SmCD3⁺ T-ALL could be further characterized with the monoclonal antibodies specific to particular β, γ, or δ gene segments.[86, 87] Our data indicate that approximately 65% of T-ALL is SmCD3⁻, approximately 20% is TCRαβ⁺, and approximately 15% is TCRγδ⁺.[41] Immunophenotypic classification of T-ALL gives significant prognostic information. The most immature T-ALL (CD1⁻/SmCD3⁻) is associated with unfavorable outcome, while CD1⁺ (and/or CD4⁺/CD8⁺) cortical T-ALL is a distinct subgroup with an excellent prognosis under intensive high-risk treatment.[82, 88-90] Within SmCD3⁺ T-ALL, event-free survival is significantly better in TCRγδ⁺ T-ALL when compared to TCRαβ⁺ T-ALL.[85]

The distribution of the immunophenotypic subgroups in ALL is age-related. Figure 6-7 summarizes the ALL subgroups in childhood.[91] In infants, pro–B-ALL predominates, whereas in young children (1 to 6 years old), high frequencies of CD10⁺ precursor-B-ALL (i.e., common ALL

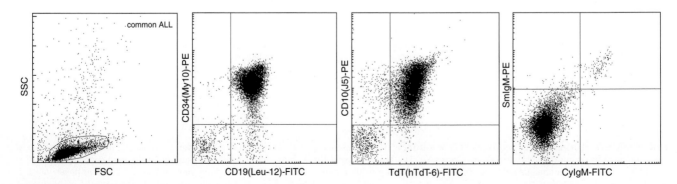

FIGURE 6-6. Flow cytometric immunophenotyping of mononuclear blood cells from a precursor-B-ALL patient at diagnosis. The CD19/CD34, CD10/TdT, and CyIg/SmIg double immunofluorescence stainings were analyzed within the indicated FSC/SSC gated cell population. The precursor-B-ALL cells expressed CD19, CD10, CD34 on the cell surface and TdT intracellularly, but they did not produce Ig protein. Such immunophenotype is typical for common ALL.

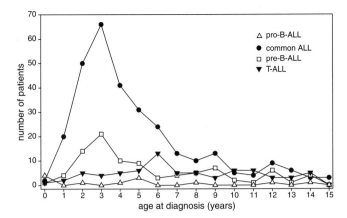

FIGURE 6–7. Age-related distribution of immunophenotypic subgroups in childhood ALL in the Netherlands (1986–1991), according to the Dutch Childhood Leukemia Study Group. (Adapted from Coebergh JWW et al.[91])

and pre–B-ALL) are found. Figure 6-7 illustrates that the relatively high incidence of ALL during early childhood (see Fig. 6-4) mainly concerns CD10[+] precursor-B-ALL. It has been proposed that altered patterns of infection due to an improved socioeconomic situation and hygiene may partly explain this high incidence in the developed countries (see Chapter 7).[92] In adults, there is also a predominance of B-lineage ALL, but T-ALL occurs more frequently than in childhood (see Table 6-3).[78, 79, 91, 93]

Burkitt's Leukemia/Lymphoma (B-ALL)

French-American-British (FAB) classification of ALL includes morphological type L3, which corresponds immunophenotypically to B-ALL.[94] Only rare cases of ALL-L3 have immunophenotype of T-ALL.[95] B-ALL is characterized by bright surface expression of IgM and negativity for TdT and CD34. Many cases are also CD10-positive. B-ALL comprises 2% to 3% of pediatric and adult ALL.[96] Based on its similar morphology, the presence of characteristic chromosomal aberrations involving *C-MYC* gene and clinical behavior, B-ALL is currently perceived as a leukemic form of Burkitt's lymphoma.[97, 98]

Chronic Lymphocytic Leukemias

Within the group of chronic lymphocytic leukemias, B-cell leukemias predominate (see Table 6-3).[77, 80, 81] T-cell chronic leukemias are uncommon in Europe and in the United States; these types of leukemias occur more frequently in Japan and in the Caribbean area, where they are related to the high prevalence of infections with human T-cell leukemia virus (HTLV)-type 1 (see Chapter 30).

Chronic B-Cell Leukemias

The majority of chronic B-cell leukemias express surface membrane Ig. Because a B-cell malignancy represents the clonal expansion of a single B cell, only one type of Ig light chain is expressed (κ or λ). The Igκ/Igλ ratio of the population of malignant B-cells is consequently deviant from the ratio characteristic for the population of reactive polyclonal B-cells (normal Igκ/Igλ ratio: 1.4; range: 0.8–2.4). Therefore, immunophenotyping is suitable for the detection of a B-cell malignancy (Fig. 6-8).[99–101] In addition, the differentiation stage of the leukemia can be determined by analysis of the various differentiation markers and the type of Ig-heavy chain expressed.[77, 80, 81] Table 6-6 summarizes the immunophenotypic characteristics of chronic B-cell leukemias.

In some types of B-cell NHL, involvement of blood and bone marrow is frequently seen. Especially if the number of leukemic NHL cells is high, discrimination between a chronic B-cell leukemia and a leukemic B-NHL may be difficult. In such cases, immunophenotyping may be helpful. Therefore, the immunophenotypes of the most common leukemic B-NHL are given in Table 6-6.[77, 80, 81]

B-cell chronic lymphocytic leukemia (B-CLL) is characterized by the weak (dim) expression of surface membrane Ig.[102, 103] In some B-CLL cases, SmIg expression cannot be detected by use of fluorescence microscopy or flow cytometry. The most prevalent type of Ig heavy chain is Igμ, followed by Igμδ or Igδ.[102, 103] An additional characteristic feature of B-CLL is the positivity for the CD5 and CD6 antigens (see Fig. 6-8).[102, 103] CD5 expression on B cells is not specific for B-CLL; CD5 is also found on some other B-cell malignancies (see Table 6-6).[77, 80, 81]

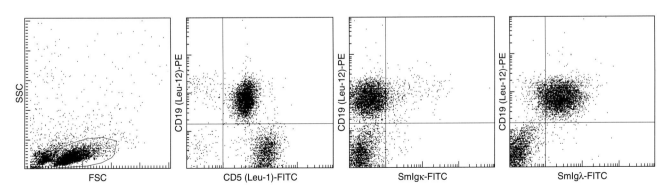

FIGURE 6–8. Flow cytometric analysis of peripheral blood mononuclear cells from a patient with B-CLL. The SmIgκ/SmIgλ expression pattern was analyzed on CD19[+] cells within the indicated FSC/SSC gated cell population. This figure shows that all CD19[+] B-CLL cells were CD5-positive and expressed SmIgλ on their surface.

TABLE 6–6. Immunophenotypic Characteristics of Chronic B-cell Leukemias and Leukemic B-NHL

Markers	Chronic B-cell Leukemias				Leukemic B-NHL		
	B-CLL	*B-PLL*	*HCL*	*HCLv*	*FCL*	*MCL*	*SLVL*
SmIg-expression	++w	++s	++	++	++s	++s	++
CyIg-expression	±	±	−	−	−	−	−
SmIgH-isotype	μ, μδ, δ (γ,α)	μ, μδ (γ,α)	μ, μδ, γ, α	γ	μ, μδ, γ	μ, μδ	μ, μδ, γ
CD19	++	++	++	++	++	++w	++
CD20	++w	++	++s	++	++	++s	++
CD22	+w	++s	++s	++	++	+	++s
CD23	++	−	−	±	±	−	±
CD24	++	++	−	−	++	++	++
CD5/CD6	++	±	−	−	±	++	±
CD10	−	±	±	−	+w	−	±
CD11c	+	−	++	+	−	−	+
CD25	+w	−	++	−	−	−	±
CD103	−	−	++	+	−	−	±
CD138	−	−	−	−	−	−	−
FMC7	±	++s	++	++	++	+	++

−, <10% of the leukemias is positive; ±, 10%–25% of the leukemias is positive; +, 25%–75% of the leukemias is positive; + +, >75% of the leukemias is positive; w, weak antigen expression; s, strong antigen expression.

B-CLL, B-cell chronic lymphocytic leukemia; B-PLL, B-cell prolymphocytic leukemia; HCL, hairy cell leukemia; HCLv, HCL variant; SLVL, splenic lymphoma with villous lymphocytes; MCL, mantle cell lymphoma; FCL, follicular cell lymphoma.

On the other hand, a few B-CLLs are CD5⁻ and generally occur in older patients, who present with lower lymphocyte counts but more advanced disease and therefore may have a shorter survival than patients with CD5⁺ B-CLL.[102-104] Most B-CLLs are positive for the CD23 antigen, which is not expressed by most other types of B-cell malignancies.[80, 102] Absence of the CD23 antigen or a weak expression of this antigen together with positivity for FMC7 is associated with a poor prognosis.[102] In these immunophenotypically atypical B-CLLs, there is often a high expression of SmIgM, which suggests an intermediate stage between B-CLL and B-cell prolymphocytic leukemia (B-PLL).[102] An immature subset of B-CLL has been identified, characterized by CD38 positivity on more than 30% of leukemic cells, which correlates with the prefollicular stage of transformed B cell (no somatic hypermutation of Ig genes).[105] Preliminary data suggest that patients with immature CD38⁺ B-CLL might respond poorly to continuous multiregimen chemotherapy and consequently have a shorter survival.[105] In some B-CLL patients during disease progression, the number of prolymphocytes increases. When this percentage is 10% to 55%, the diagnosis of prolymphocytic transformation of B-CLL is assumed.[106] However, such cases generally still have the typical B-CLL immunophenotype.

B-PLL is a rare type of chronic B-cell leukemia with more than 55% prolymphocytes, which show strong surface membrane Ig-expression, either Igμ or Igμδ.[77, 80, 81] In general B-PLL cells are negative for CD5, CD6, and CD23, whereas the CD22 antigen and FMC7 are strongly expressed (see Table 6-6).[81] The majority of hairy cell leukemias (HCL) is characterized by cytoplasmic projections that cause a typical light scatter morphology in flow cytometric analysis.[107] Due to high SSC signals, HCL cells might be missed if analyses are restricted to the cells with lymphocytic scatter morphology. The immunophenotype of HCL cells is unique.[77, 80, 81, 107, 108] They show a strong SmIg expression, sometimes Igμ or Igμδ, but frequently Igγ or Igα together with other Ig heavy chains; generally this concerns the Igγ3 subclass.[109] The expression of the CD20 antigen and the CD22 antigen is strong, and the cells are generally positive for the CD11c, CD25, and CD103 antigens.[63, 77, 80, 81, 107, 108] The last antigen, recognized by the B-Ly-7 antibody, is the most specific marker for HCL diagnosis because only a small fraction of splenic B lymphocytes and mucosa-associated T lymphocytes are CD103⁺.[10, 63] Interestingly, most HCL are negative for the B-cell marker CD24.[81]

HCL-variant has a higher nucleus/cytoplasm ratio, and the nucleus often contains a prominent nucleolus.[110] The main immunophenotypic difference between HCL and HCL-variant concerns the lack of CD25 expression (α-chain of IL-2 receptor) on HCL-variant cells.[108, 110] Interestingly, the β chain of the IL-2 receptor (CD122 antigen) is expressed by both HCL and HCL variant.[108]

Leukemic B-NHL

Some B-NHLs have a relatively high tendency to disseminate to blood and bone marrow, such as mantle cell lymphoma (MCL), follicular cell lymphoma (FCL), and splenic lymphoma with villous lymphocytes (SLVL). Leukemic presentation of SLVL is often misdiagnosed as B-CLL, B-PLL, or HCL.[77, 80, 81] However, most SLVL are negative for the CD5 antigen and the CD103 antigen (see Table 6-6).[77, 80, 81, 111] MCL is CD5⁺ and has a moderate-to-intense expression of surface Ig.[77, 80, 81, 112] In contrast to B-CLL, MCL strongly expresses the CD20 antigen, weakly expresses the CD19 antigen, and is usually CD23⁻.[112] FCL does not exhibit a characteristic immunophenotype, although frequently expression of the CD10 antigen is seen.[77, 81]

Chronic T-Lineage Leukemias

Chronic T-cell leukemias are also referred as post-thymic leukemias because they are negative for TdT and the CD1 antigen. They are relatively rare and consist of a group of disorders with marked heterogeneity in clinical, morphologic, and immunologic characteristics.[77, 80, 113-115] Immunophenotyping plays an essential role in the diagnosis of chronic T-cell leukemias. It enables differentiation between leukemias of T-cell origin (CD3[+]) and NK-cell origin (CD3[-], CD16[+], CD56[+]) and the subclassification of the former group.[42, 77, 80, 113-115] Aberrant CD4/CD8 ratios and the TCRαβ/TCRγδ ratios cannot be used to prove clonality. However, the currently available Vβ, Vγ, and Vδ antibodies allow detection of monotypic TCRβ or TCRγδ usage, which is suggestive of clonality.[86, 87, 116, 117] Formal proof can be obtained only by molecular studies (see later in this chapter). Furthermore, malignant cells of chronic T-cell leukemias may be deficient for one or more T-cell markers, or the expression of these markers may be low, but this is not a leukemia-specific characteristic, and it may also occur in reactive T-cell populations. The recently discovered NCR (particularly NKp46) can be used to further support the NK-cell origin,[47] whereas monotypic expression of KIR might serve as a surrogate clonality marker at the protein level.[48, 118] However the latter still needs to be proved.

Table 6-7 summarizes the immunophenotypic characteristics of the four main types of chronic T-cell leukemias, including the large granular lymphocyte (LGL) leukemia.[42, 46, 77, 80, 113-115, 119] T-cell prolymphocytic leukemia (T-PLL) has been defined as a clinically aggressive leukemia with marked lymphocytosis. In at least 70% of cases, these cells have a CD3[+]/CD4[+]/CD8[-] immunophenotype.[115] T-PLL can be differentiated immunologically from other CD4[+] chronic T-cell leukemias by its strong positivity for the CD7 antigen and by the lack of or weak reactivity with CD25 antibodies.[115] The immunophenotypes of adult T-cell leukemia lymphoma (ATLL) and cutaneous T-cell leukemia lymphoma (CTLL) have much in common: both T-cell malignancies generally express CD4.[80, 114] However, in contrast to a weak expression of the CD25 antigen by CTLL cells, ATLL shows a strong expression of this antigen. The diagnosis of ATLL requires confirmation by demonstration of infection with human T-cell leukemia lymphoma virus type 1 (HTLV-1) (see Chapter 30).

LGL leukemia forms a separate clinical disease entity, encompassing CD3[+] T-LGL and CD3[-] NK-LGL.[46, 113] In 85% to 90% of patients with LGL leukemia, this concerns a T-LGL leukemia; in 10% to 15% of cases, an NK-LGL leukemia can be found.[42, 46] Most T-LGL leukemias are CD4[-]/CD8[+]; sometimes coexpression of CD4 and CD8 can be observed. The majority of T-LGL is expressing the CD57 antigen, whereas positivity for CD16 and CD56 is observed in the minority of T-LGL patients (see Table 6-7). The majority of T-LGL patients are TCRαβ[+]; 10% to 15% of T-LGL patients express TCRγδ, almost exclusively utilizing the Vδ1 domain. NK-LGL is occasionally CD8[+], but most is negative for both CD4 and CD8 antigens. Virtually all NK-LGL has characteristic CD16[+]/CD56[+] immunophenotype, and approximately half is positive for CD57.[42, 46]

In the past, the recognition of LGL leukemia as a malignancy was hampered by the seemingly benign clinical course and the lack of techniques to demonstrate clonality. This has resulted in many names for the description of this disorder, such as T-γ lymphocytosis, chronic T-cell lymphocytosis, T-chronic lymphocytic leukemia, and lymphoproliferative disorder of granular lymphocytes.[46]

TABLE 6–7. Immunophenotypic Characteristics of Chronic T-cell Leukemias

				LGL Leukemias	
Markers	T-PLL	ATLL	CTLL	T-LGL (CD3[+])	NK-LGL (CD3[-])
TdT	−	−	−	−	−
CD1	−	−	−	−	−
CD2	++	++	++	++	++
CD3	++	++	++	++	−
TCRαβ	++	++	++	++	−
TCRγδ	−	−	−	±	−
CD4+/CD8−	+	++	++	−	−
CD4+/CD8+	±	−	−	±	−
CD4−/CD8+	±	−	−	++	±
CD4−/CD8−	−	−	−	−	++
CD5	++	++	++	++	−
CD7	++s	±	±	++	++
CD16	−	−	−	±/+	++
CD56	−	−	−	±	++
CD57	−	−	−	++	+
CD25	±w	++s	±	±	NR
HLA-DR	−	±	±	+	+

−, <10% of the leukemias is positive; ±, 10%–25% of the leukemias is positive; +, 25%–75% of the leukemias is positive; + +, >75% of the leukemias is positive; s, strong expression; NR, not reported; w, weak expression.
T-PLL, T-cell prolymphocytic leukemia; ATLL, adult T-cell leukemia lymphoma; CTLL, cutaneous T-cell leukemia lymphoma; LGL, large granular lymphocyte.

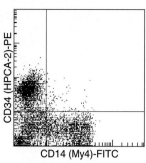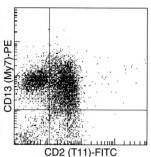

FIGURE 6–9. Flow cytometric analysis of CD14/CD34 and CD2/CD13 double immuno-fluorescence stainings on blood cells from a patient with AML-M4Eo. Both double stainings (middle and right panel) were analyzed within the indicated FSC/SSC gated cell population. The leukemic cells were CD13-positive, partly expressed the CD2 antigen, and contained CD14⁻/CD34⁺ and CD14⁺/C34⁻ subpopulations.

In most cases, the diagnosis of LGL leukemia can be made by using the following clinical and laboratory guidelines:

1) Lymphocytosis of more than 2 × 10⁹/L, or the immunophenotypic or molecular evidence for expansion of a discrete LGL population, persisting for 6 months or longer without an obvious cause.

2) Morphology of the peripheral blood lymphocytes (LGL cytomorphology) is not essential but can support the diagnosis.

3) Neutropenia or any other cytopenia in the absence of heavy bone marrow infiltration.

4) Predominance of a specific discrete T-cell subset by membrane marker analysis (e.g., CD8, CD16, CD56, CD57, and HLA-DR).[46, 114, 120]

Molecular techniques for detection of clonality in chronic T-cell leukemias are described later in this chapter.

Acute Myeloid Leukemia

AML is classified primarily by use of the morphologic FAB system.[94, 121] A few proposals for immunologic classification of AML have been made,[52, 122, 123] but they are not widely used. Both the morphologic FAB and the immunologic classifications are based on cell lineage and maturation characteristics. Nevertheless, no full concordance is found between the two types of classification.[124] This might be related to the fact that most AML exhibits heterogeneous immunophenotypes; i.e., most AML consists of several subpopulations (Fig. 6–9).[53, 125-127] This is in contrast to ALL, which generally shows homogeneous marker expression. Table 6–8 summarizes the immunophenotypic characteristics of AML. Virtually all are positive for the panmyeloid markers CD13 and CD33.[53, 124] In a minority of cases, the AML cells express only one of these antigens. MPO is the only panmyeloid marker fully specific for myeloid differentiation lineage. However, some AML-M0 and AML-M5 cases could be fully MPO⁻.[128, 129] Finally, approximately two-thirds of AML displays CD117 positivity, and this marker is exceptionally detected in ALL patients.[129, 130] In Table 6–8 the three myeloblastic leukemias as well as AML-M4 and AML-M5 are clustered; these AML types cannot be discriminated from each other based on their immunophenotype.[124, 131, 132] Markers that show a high correlation with the FAB classification are expression of the monocytic antigen CD14 in AML-M4 and AML-M5, glycophorin A expression in AML-M6, and expression of the platelet markers CD41/CD61 and CD42 in AML-M7.[60-62, 124, 131, 132] In AML-M4 and AML-M5 cases, monocytic differentiation can be confirmed by CD11c and/or CD36.[131] AML-M3 is characterized by a homogeneous immunophenotype with negativity for

TABLE 6–8. Immunophenotypic Characteristics of AML

Markers	AML-M0/M1/M2	AML-M3	AML-M4/M5a/M5b	AML-M6	AML-M7
CD13/CD33	++	++	++	+	++
CD65	±/+/++	+	++	±	±
MPO	−/+/++	++	++	+	−
CD11c	− or ±	−	++	−	−
CD14	−	−	+/+/++	−	−
CD15	±/±/++	±	−	−	−
CD36	−	−	+	++	+
H-antigen	−	−	−	++	+
GpA	−	−	−	+	−
CD41/CD61	−	−	−	−	++
CD42	−	−	−	−	+
CD34	++/++/+	±	±/+/±	+	+
CD117	++	+	+	+	+
HLA-DR	++/++/++	−	++	+	++
TdT	+	±	+	+	±

−, <10% of the leukemias is positive; ±, 10%–25% of the leukemias is positive; +, 25%–75% of the leukemias is positive; ++, >75% of the leukemias is positive; NR, not reported.

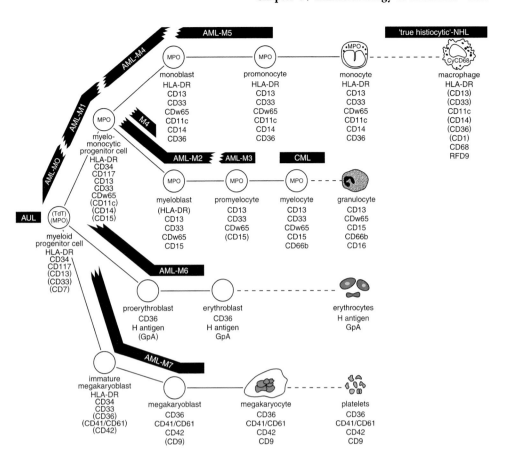

FIGURE 6–10. Hypothetical scheme of myeloid differentiation. The expression of relevant immunological markers is indicated for each differentiation stage; markers in parentheses are not always expressed. The bars represent the various types of leukemias and non-Hodgkin lymphomas (NHL) and indicate where these malignancies can be located according to their maturation arrest. It should be emphasized that most acute leukemias of the myeloid lineage have a heterogeneous phenotype, i.e., are composed of cells in multiple immature myeloid differentiation stages. To underline this phenotypic heterogeneity, several bars fade into each other. AML = acute myeloid leukemia, AUL = acute undifferentiated leukemia, CML = chronic myeloid leukemia (see reference 4).

HLA-DR and frequently also CD15, but positivity for CD13/CD33 as well as CD9.[133-135] Figure 6–10 summarizes the expression of relevant immunologic markers for each myeloid differentiation stage as well as the maturation arrest of the various types of AML.

The diagnosis of AML-M0 and AML-M7 cannot be made on morphologic criteria only.[136, 137] In these leukemias, the malignant cells lack the typical cytomorphologic characteristics of myeloid differentiation (including MPO activity), and it is often not possible to exclude ALL. To establish that such acute leukemias represent immature AML (AML-M0) or megakaryoblastic AML (AML-M7), immunophenotyping or ultrastructural microscopy should be performed.[136, 137] The application of these two techniques is included in the FAB criteria.[136, 137] For the AML-M0 diagnosis, leukemic cells should be positive for at least one myeloid antigen, such as CD13 or CD33, and the leukemic cells should be negative for lymphoid antigens (in this context CD2, CD4, and CD7 should not be regarded as lymphoid markers).[137] AML-M0 is also occasionally positive for MPO by use of ultrastructural microscopy.[138] AML-M7 diagnosis should be confirmed by ultrastructural demonstration of platelet peroxidase or by detection of platelet antigens, such as CD41, CD42, CD61, and factor VIII–related antigen.[136] Using these redefined FAB criteria together with the immunologic classification of ALL, only a very small group of acute leukemias is either classified as acute undifferentiated leukemia (AUL) or remains unclassifiable.

Immunophenotyping is a powerful tool for the characterization of the various subpopulations in phenotypically heterogeneous AML. Triple/quadruple immunologic marker analysis can be especially helpful discriminating the various immature and more mature subpopulations (see Fig. 6–9).[125, 127] Generally CD34, CD117, and TdT are markers for immature AML subpopulations.[24, 125, 126, 139, 140]

Myeloid/NK Cell Precursor Acute Leukemia

An unusual form of acute leukemia has been described with extramedullary involvement at initial presentation, characterized by immature cells with lymphoblastoid form and NK-like immunophenotype.[141] Such acute leukemias are negative for MPO and positive for CD7, CD33, CD34, CD56, and frequently also for HLA-DR. Some of these NK leukemias are positive for CyCD3ε. Although this immunophenotype can be classified as NK-like, such leukemias also display myeloid features like CD33 expression and sometimes positivity for MPO mRNA, which is sufficient for the diagnosis of AML-M0 according to FAB classification. It is not yet clear whether NK-like acute leukemias represent a separate disease entity. Only a few cases have been described so far. The prognosis of such leukemias is very poor: although the majority of patients reach clinical remission, most patients rapidly relapse and die of progressive disease.[141]

Cross-Lineage Marker Expression in Acute Leukemias

The expression of myeloid markers in ALL cells and the expression of lymphoid markers in AML have been de-

TABLE 6–9. Cross-lineage Market Expression in Acute Leukemias

Markers	Precursor B-ALL	T-ALL	AML
Myeloid markers			
CD13, CD14, CD15, CD33, CDw65	children 5–10% adults 10–20%	5%–10%	++
Lymphoid markers			
CD2	−	++	5%–15%
CD4	−	+	10%–30%
CD7	−	++	10%–20%
CD19	++	−	5%–15%
TdT	++	++	60%[1]

1. In AML, TdT is expressed in a part of the leukemic cell population, and the percentage of TdT+ AML depends on the cut-off value for defining positivity. In 60% of AML >1% of TdT+ leukemic cells are present. If the cut-off value is taken at 0.1%, 75% of AML is TdT+ (c.f. references 24 and 139).
−, <10% of the leukemias is positive; +, 25%–75% of the leukemias is positive; ++, >75% of the leukemias is positive.

fined as cross-lineage marker expression (Table 6-9).[24, 139, 140, 142-147] In ALL, this mainly concerns expression of CD13, CD14, CD15, CD33, and/or CD65 antigens in up to one-third of precursor-B-ALL and T-ALL patients.[142, 146, 148] In AML, this concerns expression of TdT, the B-cell marker CD19, and the T-cell markers CD2, CD4, and CD7.[24, 139, 143-145, 147] Such observations have been interpreted as lineage infidelity or lineage promiscuity. Terms such as hybrid acute leukemia, mixed lineage leukemia, biphenotypic acute leukemia, and biclonal acute leukemia have been used to describe acute leukemia with cross-lineage marker expression.[149] It has been suggested that these leukemias exhibit aberrant gene expression, but coexpression of lymphoid and myeloid genes may also occur in normal immature cells.[149] There are only a few lineage-specific antigens: CD79 and Ig molecules in B cells, CD3 and TCR molecules in T cells, and MPO in myeloid cells.[12, 29, 30, 54]

Chronic Myeloproliferative Disorders

For the diagnosis of chronic myeloproliferative disorders, immunophenotyping is not needed. The cells found in CML in chronic phase have a relatively mature immunophenotype, i.e. negative for CD34, CD117, TdT, and HLA-DR but positive for CD13, CD33, CD15, and MPO (see Fig. 6-10).[2] With standard chemotherapy, chronic-phase CML after an indolent course changes into an accelerated phase, which is characterized by an increase in the tumor burden and progressive resistance to treatment. When CML transforms into blast crisis, immunophenotyping is useful for discrimination between myeloid and lymphoid blast cells. Determination of the cell lineage of CML blasts is clinically important because lymphoid blast crisis is associated with a better response to chemotherapy and longer survival than blasts of other lineages.[150] Lymphoid blasts with immunophenotypic characteristics similar to common ALL or pre–B-ALL are found in 25% to 30% of cases.[2, 151, 152] In 60% to 70% of cases, the blast cells have an immature myeloid (AML-like) phenotype.[2, 151, 152] No specific immunophenotype is associated with myeloid blast crisis of CML. Compared with de novo AML, the blast cells often express erythroid or megakaryocytic markers, and in some cases the myeloid blast cells have complex immunophenotypes with coexpression of markers from several differentiation lineages.[2]

Applications of Immunophenotyping of Leukemias

Immunophenotyping is useful for diagnosing and classifying most leukemias (Table 6-10). In acute leukemias, the discrimination among ALL, AML, and acute undifferentiated leukemia is the most important step for initial selection of the effective treatment strategy; particularly, the diagnosis of AML-M0 and AML-M7 rely exclusively on immunophenotyping.[2, 4, 136, 137] Furthermore, immunophenotypic subclassification of ALL is clinically relevant, particularly the distinction between precursor-B-ALL and T-ALL. T-lineage immunophenotype of ALL is more fre-

TABLE 6–10. Applications of Immunophenotyping in Leukemia Diagnosis

Applications	Examples
Diagnosis and classification	discrimination between ALL, AML and AUL
	subclassification of ALL
	diagnosis of AML-M0 an AML-M7
	discrimination between B- and T-lineage leukemias and their subgroups
Defining prognostic features	poor prognosis in ALL: immature T-ALL, pro-B-ALL, and myeloid marker positivity in adult ALL
	poor prognosis in AML: CD7+ and CD34+
	poor prognosis in B-CLL: CD38+
Determination of clonality of SmIg+ B-cell leukemias (based on single Ig-light chain expression)	diagnosis of B-cell leukemias staging of B-cell lymphoma
Characterization of subpopulations	subpopulations in AML (occur frequently)
	early detection of blast crisis in CML
Correlation with cytogenetics	t(4;11) in CD15+, CD65+ and NG2+ pro-B-ALL
	hyperdiploidy in CD10+ precursor B-ALL
	t(1;19) in pre-B-ALL
	t(12;21) in CD66c−, CD9−/+, CD20−/+, My+ (CD13 and/or CD33) precursor B-ALL
	t(9;22) in CD25+, CD66c+ precursor B-ALL
	inv(14) in T-PLL
	t(8;21) in CD19+ AML-M2
	inv(16) in CD2+ AML-M4Eo
	t(15;17) in CD9+/HLA-DR AML-M3
Detection of minimal residual disease (see Chapter 12)	

quently associated with several high-risk features when compared with precursor-B-ALL. Inclusion of T-ALL patients into more intensive treatment protocols or even establishment of T-ALL phenotype-specific treatment regimens has been associated with significantly improved long-term survival.[153] Discrimination among the various types of chronic B- and T-cell leukemias is supported by immunophenotyping.[77, 80, 81] In fact, flow cytometric immunophenotyping of peripheral blood should be recommended for adults with persistent absolute lymphocytosis before carrying out more invasive procedures like bone marrow biopsy or lymph node biopsy.[154]

Detailed immunophenotyping can also be used for identification of leukemia subgroups with poor prognosis, such as pro-B-ALL, immature (CD1$^-$/CD3$^-$) T-ALL, and CD7$^+$ AML.[82, 88, 131, 132] Figure 6–11 illustrates event-free survival curves of various immunophenotypic subgroups of childhood ALL.[144] Myeloid marker expression

in adult ALL was traditionally associated with poor prognosis.[82, 142] In childhood ALL, this correlation was not clear because of conflicting data that were attributed to differences in treatment protocols (see Fig. 6–11).[82, 142, 144, 146] With the current intensive treatment protocols, myeloid antigen expression lacks prognostic significance both in adult and pediatric ALL.[93, 148, 155, 156] Although expression of CD7 and/or CD34 in AML is associated with poor prognosis,[131, 132, 157, 158] this has not been found for the precursor marker CD117 (*c-kit*).[140, 159] TdT expression was a marker of poor outcome in several studies on adult AML.[139, 158]

Clonality studies based on single Ig light chain expression are useful for diagnosis of chronic B-cell leukemias (see Fig. 6–8). However, determination of Igκ/Igλ distribution in blood and bone marrow B cells is suggested to be of limited value for staging in B-NHL patients when compared with morphologic assessment of bone marrow trephine biopsies.[160, 161] On the other hand, flow cytometric identification of lymphoma cells in bone marrow aspirate and particularly in peripheral blood may be sufficient to avoid bone marrow trephine biopsies.[154]

Detailed immunophenotyping also allows the detection of subpopulations within leukemia. The occurrence of multiple immature and more mature subpopulations is frequently seen in AML (up to 85% of patients) (see Fig. 6–9).[24, 125-127] Also, lymphoid or myeloid blast cells in early phases of CML blast crisis can be identified between the otherwise mature CML cells by use of double or triple labeling techniques (see Fig. 6–2).

Several studies indicate that particular chromosome aberrations are associated with specific immunophenotypes. The t(4;11) is seen in pro–B-ALL with cross-lineage expression of the myeloid markers CD15 and CD65 and ectopic expression of the NG2 antigen, i.e., human homologue of the rat chondroitin sulfate proteoglycan.[162-165] Hyperdiploidy especially occurs in CD10$^+$ precursor-B-ALL,[166] and t(1;19) seems to be restricted to CD10$^+$/CD19$^+$/CD34$^-$ precursor-B-ALL, especially pre-B-ALL.[167, 168] The t(12;21) occurring in more than 25% of pediatric precursor-B-ALL is characteristically CD66c$^-$, CD9 negative or partly positive, CD20 negative or partly positive, and frequently positive for myeloid antigens CD13, CD33, or both.[169-171] The most frequent aberration in adult ALL, i.e., t(9;22), is significantly linked with CD25 and CD66c positivity.[172, 173] Also in AML, distinctive immunophenotypic features are found to be associated with specific chromosome aberrations, such as CD19 expression in AML-M2 with t(8;21).[174, 175] Ectopic expression of NG2 antigen is also found in a proportion of AML with *MLL* gene rearrangements and is particularly restricted to AML-M4/M5 cases.[176-178] Additional examples are summarized in Table 6–10.[125, 133-135, 179] Because many chromosomal translocations are accompanied by fusion genes resulting in the production of chimeric proteins, monoclonal antibodies against such proteins would provide the most sensitive immunophenotypic proof for the particular chromosomal aberrations. Such antibodies have been reported with the specificity to E2A-PBX1 and CBFB-MYH11 chimeric proteins characteristic for t(1;19) and inv(16), respectively.[180, 181] Combined morphologic, immunophenotypic, molecular, cytogenetic, and clinical

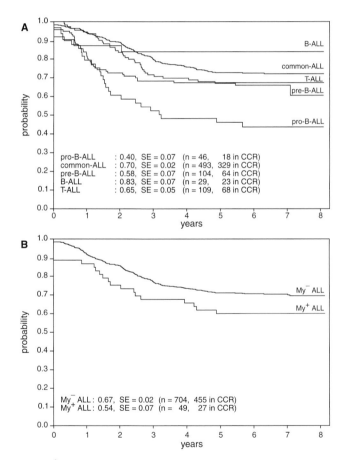

FIGURE 6–11. Event-free survival curves of immunophenotypic subgroups of childhood ALL. (Data from the ALL-BFM86 treatment protocol of the German ALL-BFM Study Group, with permission by Prof. dr. H. Riehm, Dr. Ch. Hüstebeck, and Dr. W.-D. Ludwig.[88]) *A*, Event-free survival of the five main immunophenotypic childhood ALL group (pro–B-ALL, common-ALL, pre–B-ALL, B-ALL, and T-ALL). *B*, Event-free survival of childhood ALL with myeloid antigen expression (My$^+$) and without myeloid antigen expression (My$^-$). Information for each immunophenotypic subgroup is given: probability of event-free survival with standard error of the mean (SE), number of patients (n) per subgroup and number of patients in continuous complete remission (CCR). The hatch in each curve indicates last patient of each subgroup.

data form the basis for delineation of biologically important subgroups within major leukemia and NHL categories. Such a combined approach resulted in new World Health Organization classification of neoplastic diseases of the hematopoietic and lymphoid tissues.[98]

Finally, immunologic marker analysis can be used in leukemia patients to study the effectiveness of treatment by monitoring bone marrow and blood samples for the occurrence of "minimal residual disease." This application is discussed in Chapter 12.

IMMUNOGENOTYPIC CHARACTERISTICS OF LEUKEMIAS

Lymphopoiesis results in the continuous production of mature B lymphocytes and T lymphocytes, which together form the antigen-specific immune system.[37, 182, 183] Both types of lymphocytes express unique receptors on their cell membrane that allow the specific recognition of antigens.[37, 183] The antigen-specific receptors are different on each lymphocyte, but each single lymphocyte or lymphocyte clone expresses thousands (approximately 10^5) of receptors with the same antigen specificity. Surface membrane-bound Ig molecules (SmIg) represent the antigen-specific receptors of B lymphocytes, whereas TCR molecules exhibit this function in T lymphocytes.[17, 37] Recognition of the matching antigen via the receptor molecule induces activation and proliferation of the involved lymphocytes. This results in maturation of B lymphocytes to B memory cells and plasma cells, which secrete antigen-specific Ig molecules, whereas the activated T-lymphocytes exhibit their specific regulatory and cytotoxic functions.[37, 182, 183]

This section describes the genetic basis of the extensive diversity of the antigen-specific receptors of lymphocytes; that is, the rearrangement processes in the genes that code for Ig and TCR molecules.[184] The various types of lymphoid leukemias can be regarded as clonal malignant counterparts of normal lymphoid cells.[1-5] Therefore, the information about Ig and TCR gene rearrangement processes can be used in the diagnosis of leukemias, especially for clonality studies.[185]

Rearrangement and Expression of Ig and TCR Genes

The immune system encounters millions of different antigens and antigenic epitopes. The ability to recognize specifically these antigens is based on the enormous diversity (at least 10^9) of antigen-specific receptors. If the entire repertoire of Ig and TCR molecules were to be encoded by separate genes, they would occupy a large part of the human genome. Instead, a limited number of gene segments is able to code for the receptor diversity owing to the fact that combinations of gene segments are made, which are different in each lymphocyte or lymphocyte clone.[182-184]

Immunoglobulin Molecules and Their Encoding Genes

Ig molecules consist of two Ig-heavy (IgH) chains and two Ig-light chains, held together by disulfide bonds. The

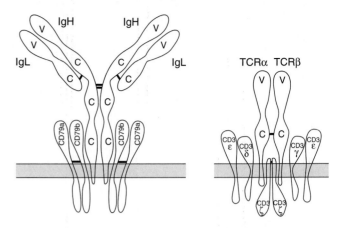

FIGURE 6–12. Schematic diagram of SmIg and TCR molecules on the surface membrane of a B lymphocyte and T lymphocyte, respectively. SmIg molecules are closely associated with disulfide-linked CD79 protein chains, whereas TCR molecules are associated with CD3 protein chains. V_H and C_H: variable and constant domain of IgH chains; V_L and C_L: variable and constant domains of Ig light chains; $V\alpha$ and $C\alpha$: variable and constant domains of TCRα chain; $V\beta$ and $C\beta$: variable and constant domains of TCRβ chain.

Ig class or subclass is determined by the isotype of the involved IgH chain and is independent of the Ig-light chain. Each B lymphocyte or B-lymphocyte clone expresses only one type of Ig-light chain (Igκ or Igλ), whereas multiple IgH chains can be expressed.[37] The majority of B lymphocytes in peripheral blood express IgM and IgD on the cell membrane, whereas a minority express IgG or IgA. In lymph nodes and other lymphoid tissues, higher frequencies of IgG- and/or IgA-bearing lymphocytes are present. SmIg molecules are closely associated with a disulfide-linked heterodimer, which consists of the CD79a protein chain (previously mb1 or Igα) and the CD79b chain (previously B29 or Igβ). In the SmIg-CD79 complex, the CD79 protein chains mediate the transmembrane signal transduction (Fig. 6–12).[17]

The Ig protein chains are composed of one variable domain, which is involved in antigen recognition, and one constant domain in case of Ig-light chains or three to four constant domains in case of IgH chains (Fig. 6–12). Each domain of an Ig chain is encoded by a separate exon (Fig. 6–13). The variable domain of an IgH chain is encoded by an exon, which consists of a combination of a V (variable), a D (diversity), and a J (joining) gene segment. A combination of a V and a J gene segment encodes the variable domain of an Ig-light chain.[37, 41] During B-cell differentiation, combinations of the available V, D, and J gene segments are made through a process of gene rearrangement.[184, 186] The constant domains of the Ig chains are encoded by C (constant) gene segments, depending on the isotype of the Ig chain (see Fig. 6–13).[187-194]

T-Cell Receptor Molecules and Their Encoding Genes

TCR molecules consist of two chains, which are generally disulfide-linked. Two types of TCR have been recognized: the "classical" TCR, which consists of a TCRα and a TCRβ chain (TCRαβ), and the "alternative" TCR, which

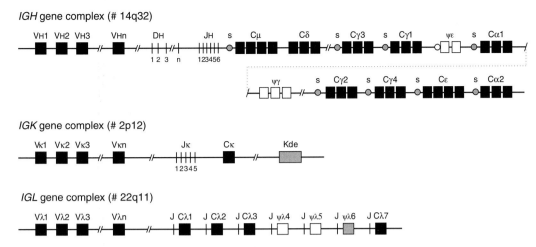

FIGURE 6–13. Schematic diagram of the human Ig gene complexes. The *IGH* gene complex consists of at least 40 functional VH gene segments, 27 DH gene segments, 6 functional JH gene segments, and several CH gene segments, which together encode the various IgH class and subclass constant domains. Most CH gene segments are preceded by a switch gene(s), which plays a role in IgH (sub)class switch. The *IGK* gene complex consists of approximately 35 functional Vκ gene segments, five Jκ gene segments, and a single Cκ gene segment. The Kde (kappa-deleting element) plays a role in the deletion of the Jκ-Cκ or Cκ-gene regions in B-cells, which rearrange their *IGL* genes. The *IGL* gene complex consists of approximately 30 Vλ gene segments and four functional Cλ genes, all of which are preceded by a Jλ gene segment. Pseudogenes (ψ) are indicated as open symbols.

is composed of a TCRγ and a TCRδ chain (TCRγδ).[41, 183] The majority of mature T-lymphocytes (85% to 98%) in peripheral blood and most lymphoid tissues express TCRαβ; a minority (2% to 15%) express TCRγδ.[41] Both types of TCR molecules are closely associated with the CD3 protein chains, which together form the TCR-CD3 complex (see Fig. 6–12). After antigen recognition by the TCR molecule, transmembrane signal transduction is mediated via the CD3 protein chains.[17]

Each TCR chain consists of two domains: a variable domain and a constant domain. Analogous to the Ig chains, the variable domain of a TCR chain is encoded by a combination of the available V and J gene segments, in case of TCRα and TCRγ chains, or by a combination of the available V, D, and J gene segments in case of TCRβ and TCRδ chains.[41, 183] The constant domains of the

TCR chains are encoded by C-gene segments: one C-gene segment for the constant domain of the TCRα chain and one for the TCRδ chain, and two C-gene segments are available for the constant domains of the TCRβ and TCRγ chains (Fig. 6–14).[195-203]

Gene Rearrangement: V-(D-)J joining

During early B- and T-cell differentiation, the germline V, (D), and J gene segments of the Ig and TCR gene complexes rearrange, and each lymphocyte thereby obtains a specific combination of V-(D)-J segments.[182-184] An example of an *IGH* gene rearrangement is illustrated in Figure 6–15: one of the J gene segments is joined to one of the D gene segments, and subsequently a V to D-J joining occurs, thereby deleting all intervening sequences. After

FIGURE 6–14. Schematic diagram of the four human TCR genes. The *TCRA* gene complex consists of >50 V gene segments, a remarkably long stretch of 61 functional J gene segments, and one C gene segment. The major part of the *TCRD* gene complex is located between the Vα and Jα gene segments and consists of eight V, three D, and four J gene segments and one C gene segment. The δRec and ψJα gene segments play a role in *TCRD* gene deletions, which precede *TCRA* gene rearrangements in developing T cells. The *TCRB* gene complex consists of 65 V gene segments and two C gene segments, both of which are preceded by one D and six or seven J gene segments. The *TCRG* gene complex consists of a restricted number of V gene segments (six functional V gene segments and nine pseudogene segments) and two C gene segments, each preceded by two Jγ1 or three Jγ2 gene segments. Pseudogenes (ψ) are indicated with open symbols.

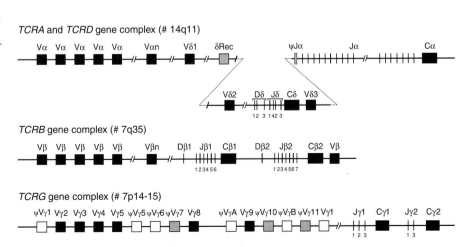

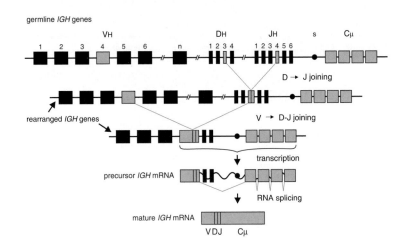

FIGURE 6–15. Schematic diagram of human *IGH* gene rearrangement. In this example DH3 is first joined to JH4, followed by VH4 to DH3-JH4 joining, thereby deleting all intervening sequences. The rearranged gene complex can be transcribed into precursor mRNA, which will be transformed into mature mRNA by splicing out all noncoding intervening sequences.

the process of rearrangement, the gene is transcribed into a precursor mRNA, which is transformed into mature mRNA by splicing and eliminating all noncoding intervening sequences. Comparable rearrangement and transcription processes occur in the other Ig and TCR gene complexes.

The gene rearrangement processes are mediated by a recombinase enzyme system, which probably contains several components, including the protein products of the so-called recombinase activating genes (*RAG-1* and *RAG-2*).[204, 205] The recombinase complex recognizes specific recombination signal sequences (RSS), which are well conserved during evolution and consist of a palindromic heptamer and nonamer sequence, separated by spacer regions of 12 or 23 base pairs.[206, 207] Complete RSS, starting with the heptamer, border the 3′ side of V gene segments, both sides of D gene segments, and the 5′ side of J gene segments.[206, 207] A gene rearrangement first involves a back-to-back fusion of the heptamer-nonamer RSS. This is followed by deletion of these RSS and all

intervening sequences in the form of a circular excision product and by joining of the two gene segments (Fig. 6–16).[206, 207] Although joining of two gene segments generally coincides with deletion of the intervening sequences, inversional rearrangements without deletion might also occur. These rearrangements occur especially in case of V gene segments with inverted orientation (e.g., Vδ3 gene segment and the upstream Vκ gene segments).[191, 202]

Secondary Gene Rearrangements

Ig and TCR gene rearrangements are complex processes in which the joining of the gene segments is imprecise.[183] Because of the triplet reading frame of DNA sequences, approximately two out of three joinings will be out of frame; that is, an mRNA is produced that cannot be transcribed into a complete protein.[183] The high frequency of out-of-frame rearrangements and the generation of stop codons at the joining sites may explain why

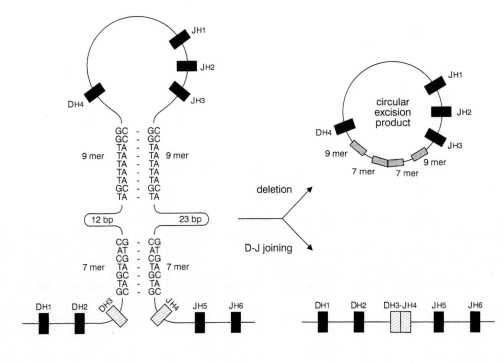

FIGURE 6–16. Schematic diagram of the role of heptamer-nonamer recombination signal sequences (RSS) during gene rearrangement. The downstream RSS of DH3 and upstream RSS of JH4 fuse back to back, followed by DH3-JH4 joining and deletion of the intervening sequences in the form of a circular excision product. The presented RSS are not the exact RSS of the DH3 and JH4 gene segments, but represent the consensus heptamer-nonamer RSS, which are well conserved in Ig and TCR genes.

TABLE 6–11. Occurrence of Secondary Rearrangements in Ig and TCR Genes

	Ig genes			TCR genes			
	IGH	*IGK*	*IGL*	*TCRA*	*TCRB*	*TCRG*	*TCRD*
D-J replacement	+	−	−	−	(+)	−	(+)
V-J replacement	−	+	(+)	+	−	+	−
V replacement	+	−	−	−	+	(+)	−

+, replacement reported to occur; (+), replacement can potentially occur, but not (yet) reported; −, replacement not likely to occur.

most B cells have rearranged both *IGH* alleles and why most T cells have biallelic rearrangements of their *TCRB* and *TCRG* genes.[184, 185]

In addition to the biallelic rearrangements, secondary gene rearrangements appear to occur that are assumed to rescue precursor B and T cells with nonproductive Ig or TCR genes. Three types of secondary rearrangements can occur, depending on the involved Ig or TCR gene complex and the type of preexisting rearrangement (Table 6–11). DH-JH replacements in B cells replace preexisting DH-JH complexes by joining an upstream DH gene segment to a downstream JH gene segment (Fig. 6–17).[208] D-J replacements can also potentially occur in *TCRB* and *TCRD* genes. In a comparable way, V-J replacements replace a preexisting V-J complex in *TCRA, TCRG,* and Ig-light chain genes.[209] Both types of replacements can occur repeatedly on the same Ig or TCR allele as long as germline V, (D), and J gene segments are available.

The third type of secondary rearrangement concerns V replacement in complete V(D)J complexes.[210, 211] The V gene segment of the V(D)J complex is replaced by a new upstream V gene segment (see Fig. 6–17). This process is mediated via an internal heptamer RSS in the 3′ part of the V gene segments in *IGH, TCRB,* and *TCRG* genes, but this heptamer RSS is not present in V gene segments of Ig-light chain, *TCRA,* and *TCRD* genes.[210-212]

So far, V replacements have especially been observed in *IGH* genes and have also been reported to occur in *TCRB* genes (see Table 6–11).

Secondary rearrangements have been found to replace not only preexisting nonproductive rearrangements but also productive rearrangements, such as productive Vα-Jα rearrangements.[213] This suggests that secondary rearrangements not only rescue precursor-B and T cells from nonproductive rearrangements but are also involved in selection processes, such as thymic selection of the T-cell repertoire.[209, 213]

Repertoire of Ig and TCR Molecules

The enormous diversity of antigen-specific receptors of lymphocytes is mediated by the described rearrangements of the gene segments that code for the variable domains of Ig and TCR molecules. The extent of the potential primary repertoire of antigen-specific receptors is based on the combinatorial diversity (i.e., the number of possible V-D-J combinations) and the junctional diversity (i.e., diversity due to imprecise joining of the V, D, and J gene segments).[182, 183]

The so-called combinatorial diversity can be calculated from the possible combinations of the available V, D, and J gene segments per gene complex and the pairing of two different protein chains per antigen-receptor molecule; i.e., IgH with Igκ or Igλ, TCRα with TCRβ, and TCRγ with TCRδ.[182, 183] For example, the *IGH* gene complex contains at least 40 functional VH gene segments, 25 functional DH gene segments, and 6 functional JH gene segments, resulting in at least 6000 possible VH-DH-JH combinations.[214-216] Together with the V-J combinations of the *IGK* and *IGL* genes, a potential combinatorial diversity of more than 2×10^6 can be obtained. A comparable diversity can be obtained for the TCRαβ molecules (Table 6–12). However the combinatorial diversity of TCRγδ molecules is less extensive due to the limited number of V,(D,) and J gene segments in the encoding gene complexes. Nevertheless, because of multiple Dδ gene usage, a combinatorial repertoire of potentially more than 5000 TCRγδ molecules can be produced.

The calculations in Table 6–12 are based on the assumption that the available functional V, D, and J gene segments are used randomly. This is not always the case. For instance, fetal B cells use a restricted set of VH gene segments, related to JH proximity.[217, 218] TCRαβ+ cells tend to use Jβ2 gene segments more frequently than Jβ1 gene segments.[219] Peripheral TCRγδ+ T lymphocytes exhibit preferential usage of Vγ9-Jγ1.2 and Vδ2-Jδ1 gene

D-JH replacement

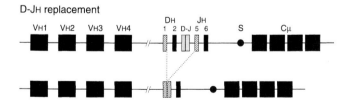

VH replacement

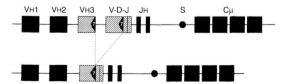

FIGURE 6–17. Examples of secondary gene rearrangements in *IGH* genes. *A,* DH-JH replacement: an upstream DH gene segment rearranges to a downstream JH gene segment, thereby replacing the preexisting DH-JH rearrangement. *B,* VH replacement: the VH gene segment in a complete V-D-JH rearrangement is replaced by an upstream VH gene segment via a rearrangement process, which is mediated via heptamer RSS (indicated as: 7) within the VH gene segments.

TABLE 6–12. Estimation of the Potential Primary Repertoire of Human Ig and TCR Molecules[a]

	Ig Molecules			TCRαβ Molecules		TCRγδ Molecules	
	IgH	**Igκ**	**Igλ**	**TCRα**	**TCRβ**	**TCRγ**	**TCRδ**
Number of functional gene segments:							
V gene segments	40–46	34–37	30–33	45	44–47	6	6
D gene segments	25[b]	—	—	—	2[b]	—	3[b]
J gene segments	6	5	4	50	13	5	4
Combinatorial diversity		$>2 \cdot 10^6$			$>2 \cdot 10^6$	>5000	
Junctional diversity	++	±	±	+	++	++	++++
Estimation of total repertoire		$>10^{12}$			$>10^{12}$	$>10^{12}$	

a. Based on the international IMGT (ImMunoGeneTics) Database.[258]

b. In *TCRD* gene rearrangements, multiple D segments might be used; this implies that the number of junctions can vary from one to four. In *IGH* and *TCRB* gene rearrangements, only one D gene segment is generally used.

segments.[220, 221] However, it might well be that the whole potential combinatorial repertoire is present but that particular receptor specificities dominate due to clonal selection and expansion.[222]

The junctional diversity of Ig and TCR genes is based on deletion of germline nucleotides by trimming the ends of the rearranging gene segments as well as by inserting nucleotides between the joined gene segments. Insertion of nucleotides (N region insertion) at the junction sites is mediated by TdT, which is able to add nucleotides to 3′ ends of DNA breakpoints without need for a template.[223, 224] The junctional regions of Ig and TCR genes encode for the so-called third complementarily determining region (CDR3), which contributes considerably to the antigen recognition site of the variable protein domains. Therefore, N-region insertion drastically increases the diversity of antigen receptors, especially when multiple junction sites occur in a junctional region, such as in *IGH, TCRB,* and especially *TCRD* genes (see Table 6–12). The random insertion and deletion of nucleotides at the junction sites of V,(D,) and J gene segments make the junctional regions into "fingerprint-like" sequences, which are most probably different in each lymphocyte (Fig. 6–18).

Absent or decreased TdT activity during Ig or TCR gene rearrangements leads to the absence of N-region insertion, as is found in fetal thymocytes and B-cell precursors in fetal liver.[225-227] Also, rearranged Ig-light chain genes in mature B cells lack N-region insertion,[182, 183, 228] suggesting that the Ig-light chain genes rearrange in the absence of TdT activity. This is in contrast to the junctional regions of postnatally rearranged TCR genes, all of which contain N regions. This discrepancy in N-region diversity between Ig and TCR genes is in line with the fact that SmIg⁺/TdT⁺ immature B cells are extremely rare, whereas TCR⁺/TdT⁺ T cells occur in a great amount in the thymus.[41, 229] Apparently TdT activity decreases early during B-cell differentiation (after *IGH* gene rearrangement), whereas TdT is expressed throughout thymic T-cell differentiation. The primary antibody repertoire can be further increased via antigen-induced somatic mutations in the VDJ exon region of rearranged Ig genes.[230-232] These point mutations occur in follicular center B lymphocytes and are not found in virgin B lymphocytes.[230-232] The mutations are assumed to promote affin-

ity maturation and clonal selection and to precede or coincide with IgH class switch. So far, somatic mutations have not been observed in rearranged TCR genes.

IgH Isotype Switch Rearrangement

Coexpression of IgM and IgD is mediated by alternative splicing processes of precursor mRNA, in which the same VDJ exon is joined to Cμ sequences or Cδ sequences, respectively.[233, 234] Coexpression of IgM and IgG and/or IgA also occurs and is assumed to be mediated via so-called trans-splicing processes of VDJ-Cμ and short "sterile" Cγ and/or Cα precursor mRNAs.[235, 236]

However, definitive switch to single isotype expression occurs via a rearrangement process, which replaces the Cμ gene segments by the appropriate CH gene segments. This rearrangement process is mediated via joining of so-called switch (s) sequences, which are located upstream of all CH genes except for Cδ (see Fig. 6–13; Fig. 6–19).[237] Joining of two switch sequences (s-s recombination) results in deletion of all intervening sequences (Fig. 6–19).[235, 237, 238] This second type of *IGH* gene rearrangement occurs during the course of antigen-induced B-cell activation and maturation and is regulated via T lymphocytes and interleukins.[235, 239]

Although IgH isotype switch is an important event during B-cell maturation, no evidence has been found for "TCR switch" in T lymphocytes.

Rearrangement and Expression of Ig and TCR Genes During Lymphoid Differentiation

Ig and TCR gene rearrangements start early during lymphoid differentiation and occur in a hierarchical order. One of the earliest events during normal B-cell differentiation is incomplete DH-JH rearrangement, which is already found in CD34⁺/CD19⁻/CD10⁺ precursor cells.[240, 241] Most of the more mature CD34⁺/CD19⁺/CD10⁺ B-lineage precursors contain at least one DH-JH rearranged allele and frequently also complete VH-(DH-)JH rearrangements.[241, 242] *IGH* gene rearrangements are followed by recombination in the *IGK* locus. If the latter rearrangements are nonfunctional, the *IGL* genes will rearrange.[182, 184] Generally, *IGL* gene rearrangements occur after or coincide with *IGK* gene deletions.[243, 244] All

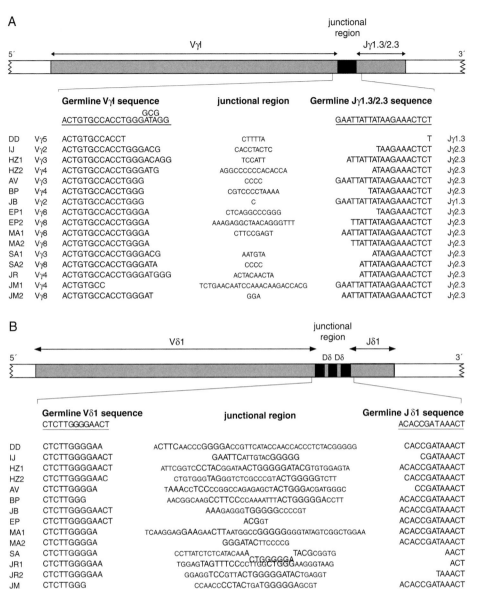

FIGURE 6–18. *A,* Schematic diagram of the VγⅠ gene segment joined to the Jγ1.3/2.3 gene segment via a junctional region. PCR-mediated amplification of the joined *TCRG* gene segments and subsequent sequencing of the junctional region in the obtained PCR products can be performed. The presented junctional region sequences are derived from T-ALL patients and illustrate the deletion of nucleotides from the germline sequences as well as the size and composition of the junctional regions. *B,* Schematic diagram of the Vδ1 gene segment joined to the Jδ1 gene segment via a junctional region. *TCRD* junctional regions may contain one, two, or three Dδ gene segments. The presented *TCRD* junctional region sequences are derived from the same T-ALL patients as in panel A and illustrate that deletion and insertion of nucleotides are more extensive than in the case of *TCRG* junctions, where they have much longer junctional regions. Dδ gene segments and inserted nucleotides are indicated by capital letters and small capital letters, respectively.

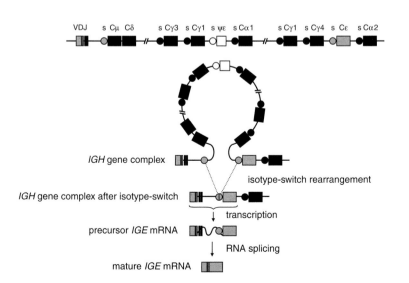

FIGURE 6–19. Schematic diagram of *IGH* isotype switch via gene rearrangement. *IGH* isotype switch rearrangements are mediated via the switch region sequences (s), which precede all functional Cʜ genes, except Cδ. The upstream part of Sμ is joined to the downstream part of another Sʜ, thereby deleting all intervening sequences (so-called looping-out with deletion).

IGK gene deletions are mediated via rearrangement of the so-called kappa-deleting element (Kde), which is located downstream of the Cκ gene segment (see Fig. 6–13).[245, 246] Kde rearranges to a heptamer RSS in the Jκ-Cκ intron, thereby deleting the Cκ gene segment, or to a Vκ gene segment, thereby deleting a large part of the *IGK* gene, including the Jκ and Cκ gene segments.[245, 247] Functional rearrangement of *IGH* and Ig-light chain genes results in SmIg+ B lymphocytes. After antigen-induced activation, somatic mutations and IgH isotype rearrangement can occur (Fig. 6–20).[184, 232]

During T-cell differentiation, *TCRD* genes rearrange followed by *TCRG* gene rearrangements, which might result in TCRγδ+ T lymphocytes if the rearrangements are functional. TCRαβ+ T lymphocytes most probably develop via a separate differentiation lineage with *TCRB* gene rearrangements prior to *TCRA* gene rearrangements.[184] *TCRA* rearrangements are preceded by deletion of the *TCRD* genes because the major part of the *TCRD* gene complex is located between the Vα and Jα gene segments[196, 201, 202, 248] and is flanked by the so-called δREC and ψJα gene segments (see Fig. 6–14).[249, 250] *TCRD* gene deletion is mediated via rearrangement of the δREC and

ψJα gene segments.[226, 249, 250] These rearrangement and deletion processes in the *TCRA/D* locus probably play a crucial role in the divergence of the TCRγδ and TCRαβ differentiation pathways.[41] It is not yet clear in which differentiation stage this divergence occurs, but it is remarkable that virtually all TCRαβ+ T lymphocytes have rearranged *TCRG* genes and that most TCRγδ+ T-lymphocytes have rearranged *TCRB* genes (see Fig. 6–20).[87, 184]

The SmIg-CD79 complex (see Fig. 6–12) is expressed on B cells as soon as functional *IGH* and Ig-light chain gene rearrangements are completed. However, in the pre–B-cell differentiation stage, the result of functional *IGH* gene rearrangement can be seen, i.e., the weak cytoplasmic expression of Igμ-heavy chain (pre-B-Cy-Igμ).[34, 35] In a part of the pre-B cells also, a weak membrane expression of the so-called pre-B cell complex (pre-B-SmIgμ-CD79) can be found.[17, 36] This pre–B-cell complex consists of CD79 and Igμ protein chains and a pseudo Ig-light chain, which is derived from nonrearranging Igλ-like gene segments.[251] The precise function of this transiently expressed pre–B-cell complex is still unclear, but it is assumed that it plays a role in the regulation of early B-cell development.[17] Maturation to the plasma cell

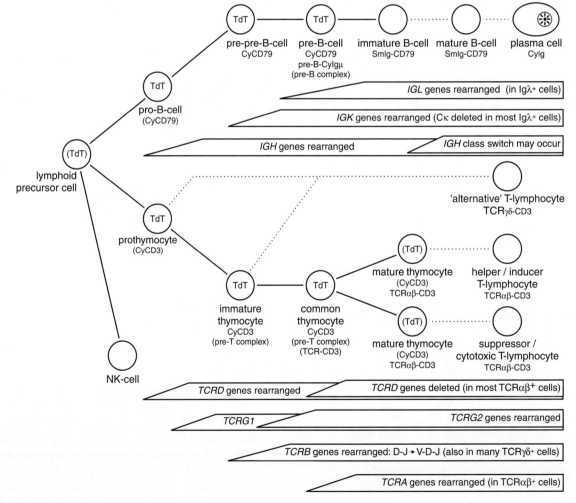

FIGURE 6–20. Hypothetical diagram of Ig and TCR gene rearrangements during lymphoid differentiation. The ordered rearrangement of Ig and TCR genes is indicated with bars. The expression of nuclear TdT, cytoplasmic CD3 (CyCD3), cytoplasmic CD79 (CyCD79), pre-B-Ig molecules (pre-B-CyIgμ and pre-B-SmIgμ-CD79), pre-T complex, and the mature SmIg-CD79 and TCR-CD3 antigen receptor complexes are indicated per differentiation stage.

stage is characterized by loss of the SmIg-CD79 complex and high levels of cytoplasmic Ig (CyIg) molecules (see Fig. 6–20).

Surface membrane expression of TCR-CD3 complexes depends on the functional rearrangement of *TCRD* and *TCRG* genes or *TCRB* and *TCRA* genes. Analogous to the pre–B-cell complex, the so-called pre–T-cell complex is weakly expressed on the surface membrane of immature thymocytes of the TCRαβ differentiation lineage.[252] In addition to CD3 and TCRβ protein chains, this pre–T-cell complex contains a second TCR chain.[252]

Already in the early stages of B- and T-cell differentiation, cytoplasmic expression of CD79 (CyCD79) and CD3 (CyCD3) is found.[12, 29, 30] This implies that these signal transduction protein chains are already available for assemblage and surface membrane expression together with Ig and TCR chains as soon as functional gene rearrangements have occurred.[17] Finally, all immature lymphoid cells express TdT in their nucleus.[25] TdT expression ceases in more mature differentiation stages with functionally rearranged Ig and TCR genes, which is in line with its role in N-region insertion.[223, 224] Although during T-cell differentiation, coexpression of TdT and TCR-CD3 complex is found, no coexpression of TdT and SmIg-CD79 is found during B-cell differentiation.[41, 229] This discrepancy may be related to the virtual absence of N regions in rearranged Ig-light chain genes of mature B cells.[182, 183, 228]

DETECTION OF CLONAL Ig AND TCR GENE REARRANGEMENTS

Rearrangements in Ig and TCR genes result in relocation and joining of gene segments with simultaneous deletion of the intervening gene segments. In principle, these rearrangements are assumed to be identical in all cells of a particular leukemia, because leukemias are clonal cell proliferations. The deletion-relocation-joining processes can be studied by Southern blotting and PCR-based techniques. Southern blotting allows detection of deletion and relocation of gene segments based on changes in distances between cleavage sites of restriction enzymes in the DNA. PCR analysis of Ig and TCR gene rearrangements is based on the (selective) amplification of junctional regions of rearranged Ig or TCR gene segments. Such amplification is possible only when the Ig or TCR gene segments are juxtaposed through rearrangement, as the distance between these gene segments in germline configuration is far too large for PCR amplification. It should be noted that clonality studies by Southern blotting take advantage of the combinatorial diversity, i.e., the relocation of gene segments, whereas clonality studies by PCR-based methods employ mainly the junctional diversity of Ig and TCR gene rearrangements.

Southern Blotting

In Southern blot studies the DNA samples are digested with restriction enzymes.[253] These are endonucleases that reproducibly cut DNA only at sites where they recognize a specific nucleotide sequence; e.g., the restriction enzyme *Eco*RI recognizes the sequence GAATTC, whereas *Bgl*II recognizes the sequence AGATCT. The obtained DNA fragments (restriction fragments) are size-separated by agar electrophoresis, transferred (blotted) onto a nitrocellulose or nylon membrane, and immobilized.[253] This membrane is incubated with a radiolabeled DNA probe that hybridizes to complementary sequences of Ig and TCR genes.[184] Unbound probe is washed away, and the location of the probe and thereby the size of the recognized restriction fragments can be detected by autoradiography or by phosphorimaging. If appropriate combinations of restriction enzymes and DNA probes are used, the detected restriction fragments of rearranged Ig or TCR genes will differ from those of germline genes.[184, 202, 254, 255] Figure 6–21 illustrates various aspects of Southern blot analysis of *IGH* genes: the germline restriction map of the JH-Cμ region with an appropriate JH probe (IGHJ6),

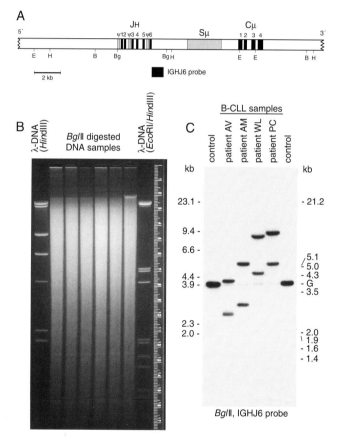

FIGURE 6–21. Southern blot analysis of *IGH* genes. *A,* Restriction map of JH-Cμ region. The position of the relevant *Eco*RI (E), *Hin*dIII (H), *Bam*HI (B), and *Bgl*II (Bg) restriction sites are indicated. Also the location of the hypervariable polymorphic (HVP) region upstream of the JH region as well as the switch region (Sμ) are indicated. The solid bar represents the JH probe (IGHJ6). *B,* Ethidium bromide-stained agarose gel with size-separated *Bgl*II restriction fragments of control DNA and four different B-CLL DNA samples. The two outer lanes contain size markers (*left: Hin*dIII-digested λDNA; *right: Eco*RI/*Hin*dIII-digested λ-DNA). The DNA fragments were blotted to a nylon filter. *C,* X-ray film after exposure to the nylon filter, which was hybridized to the ^{32}P-radiolabeled IGHJ6 probe. The size of the germline band (G) and the position of the size markers are indicated. The two control lanes contain the 3.9-kb germline band, whereas each of the four B-CLL lanes show two clonally rearranged bands, due to biallelic *IGH* gene rearrangements.

the separation of restriction fragments in an agarose gel, and the autoradiographic results of hybridization with the radiolabeled IGHJ6 probe.[184, 254]

Optimally designed Ig/TCR probes recognize sequences just downstream of the rearranging gene segments and should be used in combination with at least two different restriction enzyme digests, which result in germline restriction fragments that are not affected by polymorphisms and which are smaller than or the size of 10 kb. The latter is important for prevention of comigration of germline and/or rearranged bands.[184, 255-259]

Because Ig and TCR gene rearrangements in leukemias are identical, the (identical) restriction fragments give rise to a clearly visible rearranged band, which is different from the germline band.[184] Furthermore, two rearranged bands of comparable density will be visible if the clonal cell population has rearranged both Ig or TCR alleles (see Fig. 6-21). In contrast to clonal cell populations, reactive (polyclonal) lymphoid cell proliferations contain many different Ig and TCR gene rearrangements that are detectable as a characteristic background pattern or smear of multiple faint rearranged bands. Thus, Southern blot analysis of Ig and TCR genes allows discrimination between clonal rearrangements and polyclonal rearrangements.[184, 185] Leukemic cell populations can be detected with a sensitivity of approximately 5%, whereas the detection limit is 10% to 15% if a clonal cell population has to be identified within a background of polyclonal, reactive cells.

PCR Analysis

The PCR technique allows the selective amplification of a particular DNA region while it is still incorporated in the total genomic DNA.[260, 261] Knowledge of the precise nucleotide sequences, which flank the target DNA region, is a prerequisite for the PCR technique. Based on this information, two synthetic oligonucleotides are prepared that can hybridize to the flanking sequences of opposite strands (primer annealing), after the DNA has been denatured to single-stranded DNA.[260, 261] The two oligonucleotides serve as primers for the *Taq* polymerase-mediated DNA synthesis (primer extension), which proceeds across the target DNA region using this region as template (Fig. 6-22). The PCR process involves temperature-regulated cycles of DNA denaturation (94°C), primer annealing (55°-65°C), and primer extension (72°C). Because the PCR product of one primer can serve as a template for the other primer in subsequent cycles, each successive PCR cycle essentially doubles the number of PCR products (see Fig. 6-22). Continuation of the PCR procedure for 20-30 cycles theoretically results in $2^{20}-2^{30}$ times amplification of the target DNA region. In principle, the PCR technique can amplify target DNA sequences up to 10 kb, but preferably the PCR target should not be longer than 2 kb in routinely performed PCR analyses.[261, 262] The PCR primers for amplification of junctional regions are designed at opposite sides of the junctional region, generally within a distance of less than 500 bp (Fig. 6-23).

Because most PCR studies on Ig and TCR gene rearrangements in leukemias are performed at the DNA level, the primers are complementary to exon and/or intron sequences of V, D, and/or J gene segments, depending on the type and completeness of the rearrangement.[263-269] Also, mRNA of complete V-(D-)J-C transcripts can be used as target for the PCR technique after the mRNA has been transcribed into complementary (c)DNA by use of reverse transcriptase (RT-PCR). Such

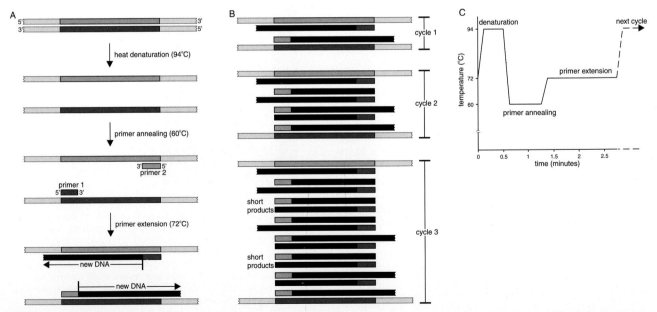

FIGURE 6–22. Schematic diagram of PCR. *A,* Temperature-regulated PCR cycle in which double-stranded DNA is heat denatured at 94°C, followed by primer annealing at 55°C, and primer extension by *Taq* polymerase at 72°C. In the first PCR cycle, synthesis of the new DNA proceeds across the target DNA, resulting in long PCR products. *B,* In subsequent cycles, the PCR products of the previous cycle(s) can serve as template, resulting in short PCR products. Each PCR cycle essentially doubles the number of PCR products. *C,* Temperature cycle for denaturation, primer annealing, and primer extension. Each cycle takes 5 to 10 minutes, depending on the size of the PCR product (i.e., the duration of primer extension).

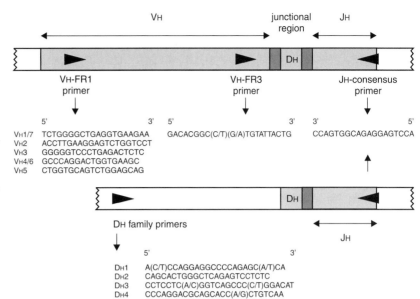

FIGURE 6-23. Schematic diagrams of VH-DH-JH and DH-JH junctional regions with primers for PCR analysis. The sequence, approximate position and orientation (5' 3') of the consensus VH-framework 3 (VH-FR3), VH-family specific framework 1 (VH-FR1), and DH-family specific primers as well as of JH-consensus primer are indicated.

studies generally use V exon primers in combination with a single C exon primer.[270-272] It is obvious that the choice of primers depends on the type of Ig or TCR gene and the type of rearranged gene segments. It may be possible to design general or consensus primers, which recognize virtually all V or J gene segments of a particular Ig or TCR gene complex; family-specific primers, which recognize families of V or J gene segments; or even member-specific primers, which recognize individual V or J gene segments (see Fig. 6-23).[263-269, 273, 274]

It should be noted that the Ig and TCR genes not only contain functional V, (D), and J gene segments but also nonfunctional (pseudo) gene segments. Such segments can be involved in gene rearrangements, provided they are flanked by a proper RSS. Table 6-13 summarizes the estimated number of gene segments and families of the three Ig genes and four TCR genes. For detection of all possible (functional and nonfunctional) Ig and TCR gene rearrangements, the primer sets should be able to recognize all V, (D), and J gene segments, implying that many different primer sets have to be designed.

Complete *IGH*, *TCRG*, and *TCRD* gene rearrangements can be analyzed relatively easily with the PCR technique,

because the *IGH* gene complex contains only seven VH families and six functional JH gene segments and because the *TCRG* and *TCRD* genes contain a limited number of V and J gene segments (see Table 6-12 and Fig. 6-14).[187, 189, 199, 202] This implies that only a restricted number of oligonucleotide primers is needed (see Fig. 6-23).[275, 276] In principle, PCR analysis of *IGK*, *IGL*, *TCRA*, and *TCRB* gene rearrangements is also possible, but it requires more primers, especially for the many different V and J gene segments in *TCRA* and *TCRB* gene complexes (see Fig. 6-14).[191, 194, 196, 197, 270-272, 277] RT-PCR analysis of *TCRA* and *TCRB* V-(D)-J-C transcripts still requires many different Vα or Vβ primers, although these can be used in combination with a single Cα or Cβ primer.[270-272]

One disadvantage of Ig or TCR gene analysis by PCR-based techniques, as compared with Southern blot analysis, is that the detectability of (clonal) rearrangements is limited by the choice of primers, raising the possibility of false-negative results. A more essential drawback is the risk of false-positive results owing to the fact that not only clonally rearranged Ig and TCR genes but also Ig and TCR rearrangements from normal, polyclonal cells are amplified. Because discrimination between clonal (leuke-

TABLE 6-13. Estimated Number of Human V, D, and J Gene Segments that can be Potentially involved in Ig or TCR Gene Rearrangements[a]

Gene segment	*IGH*	*IGK*	*IGL*	*TCRA*	*TCRB*	*TCRG*	*TCRD*
V (family)	~70 (7)	~60 (7)	~40 (11)	~60 (32)	~65 (30)	9 (4)	7[b]
D (family)	25 (7)	—	—	—	2	—	3
J (family)	6	5	5[c]	61[b]	13	5 (3)	4

a. The estimated numbers include nonfunctional (pseudo) gene segments with functional RSS, which allow rearrangement; orphan genes are excluded. The calculations are based on the international IMGT (ImMunoGeneTics) Database[358] and complete genomic sequences of *IGH*, *TCRB*, and *IGL*[215,359,360].

b. These numbers include the nonfunctional δREC gene segment (*TCRD* locus) and the ψJα gene segment (*TCRA* locus).

c. Two of the seven Jλ gene segments (Jλ4 and Jλ5) have never been observed in *IGL* gene rearrangements, probably because of their inefficient RSS (Tümkaya et al., unpublished results).

mia-derived) and polyclonal (reactive) PCR products is impossible by means of standard gel electrophoresis, an additional analysis of PCR-amplified rearranged gene products is mandatory for such distinction.

Analysis of PCR-Amplified Ig and TCR Gene Rearrangement Products

PCR-mediated detection of clonal Ig and TCR gene rearrangements is relatively easy if the percentage of leukemic cells is high (e.g., greater than 90%). In such cell samples, the background of Ig and TCR gene rearrangements in normal polyclonal cells generally does not hamper the PCR studies of leukemic cells. This is illustrated in Figure 6–24, which shows that PCR products of comparable clonal *TCRD* rearrangements in different T-cell leukemias are clearly different from each other, based on differences in the size of their junctional regions (compare with Fig. 6–18).[266] If many normal polyclonal B or T cells are present in the cell sample, many polyclonal PCR products will also be present. Discrimination between clonal (leukemia-derived) PCR products and polyclonal (normal) PCR products with standard gel electrophoresis is hampered by the fact that the clonal PCR products have to be identified as a dominant band within a background of multiple weaker bands of slightly different sizes, representing polyclonal PCR products.[267, 268] Because junctional regions are "fingerprint-like" sequences that differ between lymphocytes or lymphocyte clones, it is assumed that they represent specific markers for each individual leukemia.[263–266, 273, 274] Thus, strategies should be followed that employ the junctional regions of amplified rearranged Ig and TCR genes as PCR targets for discrimination between polyclonal and clonal cell populations.[263–266, 273, 274]

Methods that have been successfully applied to solve this background problem include direct sequencing of PCR products,[278, 279] single-strand conformation polymorphism analysis,[280, 281] denaturing gradient gel electropho-resis,[282, 283] heteroduplex analysis,[284, 285] temperature gradient gel electrophoresis,[286] high-resolution radioactive fingerprinting,[268, 287] and fluorescent gene scanning analysis.[288, 289] Of these, heteroduplex analysis is probably the simplest, fastest, and most cost-effective. Originally designed for the detection of mutations in genetic diseases,[290] heteroduplex analysis after modification can be applied for analysis of PCR-amplified Ig or TCR gene rearrangements. In the heteroduplex analysis, the double-strand PCR products are denatured at 94°C and subsequently renatured at 4°C for 1 hour to induce homoduplex formation (duplexes with identical, clonal junctions) or heteroduplex formation (duplexes with different junctional regions) (Fig. 6–25).[285] Homoduplexes and heteroduplexes can be separated from each other by polyacrylamide gel electrophoresis based on differences in conformation. Homoduplexes with perfectly matching junctional regions migrate more rapidly through the gel than do heteroduplex molecules with mismatches in the junctional regions. The latter form a background smear of more slowly migrating fragments because of less optimal duplex configuration at the site of the junctional region. As illustrated in Fig. 6–26, the heteroduplex analysis is capable of discrimination between PCR products derived from monoclonal and polyclonal cell populations, based on the presence of homoduplexes or (a smear of) heteroduplexes, respectively. Although heteroduplex PCR analysis is clearly a reliable technique for clonality assessment, being rapid, nonradioactive, and cost-effective, it cannot fully replace Southern blot analysis, which should be perceived as the "gold standard" for clonality assessment. Particularly in mature B-cell malignancies, the presence of somatic mutations can hamper primer annealing because of mismatches, leading to false-negative PCR results even when multiple primer sets are applied.[287]

Immunogenotype of Leukemias

As illustrated in Figure 6–20, Ig and TCR gene rearrangements start early during B- and T-cell differentiation, respectively, and probably occur in an hierarchical order. This implies that the majority of B-lineage and T-lineage leukemias have rearranged Ig and TCR genes, respectively.[185, 291–297] However, some leukemias exhibit unusual rearrangement patterns that are rare or absent in their normal counterparts. For example, TCR gene rearrangements can occur in non–T-cell leukemias, and Ig gene rearrangements can occur in non–B-cell leukemias.[149, 185, 298, 299] These so-called cross-lineage rearrangements are particularly prevalent in acute leukemias[298, 299] and probably result from the continuing activity of the recombinase enzyme system after malignant transformation.

Acute Leukemias

IG AND TCR GENE REARRANGEMENTS IN B-LINEAGE ALL

Based on their immunophenotypic characteristics, precursor B-ALL is generally regarded as a clonal malignant counterpart of normal precursor B cells. In line with this

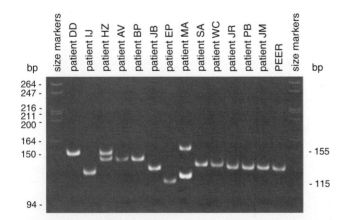

FIGURE 6–24. Vδ1-Jδ1 PCR products in cases of T-ALL with monoallelic or biallelic Vδ1-Jδ1 rearrangements. The PCR products were separated in a polyacrylamide gel, resulting in optimal size separation. The positions of the size markers are indicated in the left margin. The differences in size of the PCR products (115–155 bp) are due to differences in size of the junctional regions (see Figure 6–18B).

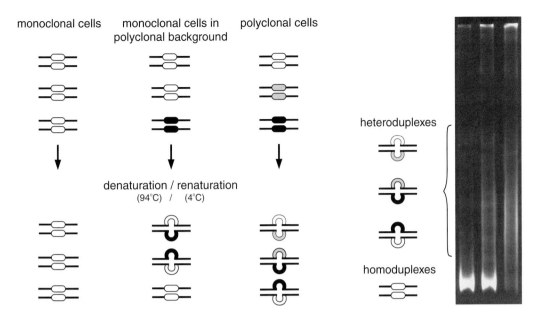

FIGURE 6–25. Schematic diagram of the heteroduplex PCR analysis, in which the junctional region heterogeneity of PCR products of rearranged Ig or TCR genes is employed to discriminate between PCR products derived from monoclonal and polyclonal lymphoid cell populations. In heteroduplex analysis, PCR products are heat-denatured and subsequently rapidly cooled to induce duplex (homo- or heteroduplex) formation. In cell samples consisting of clonal lymphoid cells, the PCR products of rearranged Ig or TCR genes give rise to homoduplexes after denaturation and renaturation, whereas in samples that contain polyclonal lymphoid cell populations, the single-strand PCR fragments will mainly form heteroduplexes upon renaturation (*left*). In case of an admixture of monoclonal cells in a polyclonal background, both hetero- and homoduplexes are formed. Because of differences in conformation, homo- and heteroduplexes can be separated from each other by electrophoresis in nondenaturing polyacrylamide gels. Homoduplexes with perfectly matching junctional regions migrate more rapidly through the gel than heteroduplex molecules with less perfectly matching junctional regions. The latter form a background smear of slower migrating fragments (*right*).

assumption, our studies indicate that more than 95% of precursor B-ALL has *IGH* gene rearrangements and that most of it contains *IGK* gene rearrangements (30%) or deletions (50%); even 20% of precursor B-ALL cases have *IGL* gene rearrangements (Table 6–14).[185, 255, 300, 301] Deletions in the *IGK* genes are predominantly mediated via

the Kde sequence, which implies that *IGK* gene deletions can be identified as Kde rearrangements, which occur on one allele or both alleles in 20% and 30% of precursor B-ALL cases, respectively.[255] Cross-lineage TCR gene rearrangements occur in high frequency in precursor-B-ALL cases: *TCRB*, *TCRG*, and *TCRD* gene rearrangements and/

FIGURE 6–26. *A,* Heteroduplex analysis of VγI-Jγ1.3/2.3 PCR products from several T-ALL and precursor–B-ALL patients in a nondenaturing 6% polyacrylamide gel. Following denaturation and renaturation of PCR products, the presence of homoduplexes in samples 96-130, 96-134A, 96-134B, and 96-136 proves the monoclonal character of these samples. The smear of heteroduplexes that is seen in 96-137 is indicative of a polyclonal cell population. The additional bands that are seen in samples 96-130, 96-134A, and 96-134B represent clonal heteroduplexes, resulting from renaturation of single-stranded fragments derived from biallelic rearrangements. The two homoduplexes from these biallelic rearrangements are easily seen in 96-134A and 96-134B (bone marrow and peripheral blood samples, respectively, from the same patient), but not in 96-130 owing to comigration. *B,* Heteroduplex PCR analysis of *IGH* in precursor–B-ALL patient. Malignant lymphoblasts at diagnosis contained a monoclonal VH1-JH gene rearrangement. Dilution of the diagnosis bone marrow DNA into polyclonal MNC DNA derived from healthy blood donors showed a sensitivity threshold of approximately 1%. The density of heteroduplex smears is related to the percentages of polyclonal CD19+ cells in the analyzed samples. he = heteroduplexes; ho = homoduplexes; Mw marker = 100-bp molecular weight marker.

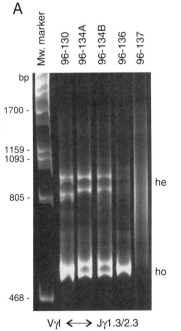

A

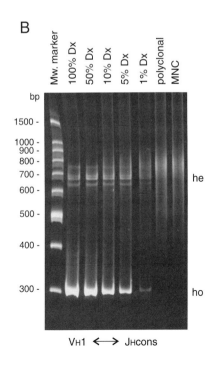

B

TABLE 6–14. Frequencies of Detectable Ig and TCR Gene Rearrangements and Deletions in Acute Leukemias

	IGH		*IGK*		*IGL*	*TCRB*	*TCRG*	*TCRD*	
	R	*D*	*R*	*D*	*R*	*R*	*R*	*R*	*D*
Precursor-B-ALL	96%	3%	30%[a]	50%[a]	20%	35%	60%	55%	35%
T-ALL									
CD3−	20%	0%		0%	0%	85%	90%	80%	10%
TCR-γδ+	50%	0%		0%	0%	95%	100%	100%	0%
TCR-αβ+	<5%	0%		0%	0%	100%	100%	35%	65%
AML	10%–15%	0%		0%	0%	5%	5%–10%	10%	0%

a. A total of ~60% of precursor-B-ALL have *IGK* gene rearrangements and/or deletions.[255]
R, at least one allele rearranged; D, both alleles deleted.

or deletions are found in 35%, 60%, and 90% of cases, respectively.[293, 299]

Several studies have shown that newly diagnosed precursor-B-ALL cases are frequently oligoclonal because they contain multiple *IGH* gene rearrangements (30% to 40% of cases) and even multiple *IGK* gene rearrangements (5% to 10% of cases).[300, 302] These multiple Ig gene rearrangements can result from continuing rearrangement processes (e.g., continuing Vн to Dн joining) and from secondary rearrangements (e.g., Dн-Jн replacements, Vн-Jн replacements, and Vκ-Jκ replacements), which result in one or more subclones.[302-306] Based on combined Southern blot and PCR data, the frequency of oligoclonality in the cross-lineage TCR gene rearrangements of precursor-B-ALL is approximately 20%.[299] This seems to be significantly lower as compared with *IGH*. However, when focusing on the group of patients with *TCRG* and *TCRD* gene rearrangements, the frequency of oligoclonality is comparable to that of the *IGH* gene.[299] Initially, subclone formation at diagnosis was thought to be less frequent for the *TCRD* gene complex, as indicated by Southern blot data.[202] However, 80% of all *TCRD* gene rearrangements in pre–B-ALL represents Vδ2-Dδ3 or Dδ2-Dδ3 rearrangements, so that subclone formation is difficult to detect by Southern blotting.[202, 307] Using heteroduplex PCR analysis and sequencing, substantial evidence has been obtained during the last years that Vδ2-Dδ3 and Dδ2-Dδ3 rearrangements in newly diagnosed precursor-B-ALL are often oligoclonal (Fig. 6–27).[299, 308] Furthermore, Vδ2-Dδ3 rearrangements are also prone to continuing rearrangements, particularly to Jα gene segments with concomitant deletion of the Cδ exons and subsequent Vα-Jα recombination.[309-311] In fact, 40% of *TCRD* gene deletions in precursor-B-ALL results from a Vδ2-Jα recombination, and the remaining 60% of Cδ deletions is caused most probably by Vα-Jα rearrangements.[299]

Analysis of a small group of adult precursor-B-ALL patients revealed several intriguing differences as compared with childhood patients.[312] First, a lower level of *IGH* oligoclonality (approximately 20%), despite a comparable incidence of *IGH* gene rearrangements, was observed. Second, all detected *IGK* gene deletions concerned rearrangements of the Kde to Vκ gene segments, which represent two-thirds of the Kde rearrangements in pediatric precursor-B-ALL and only half of the Kde rearrangements in mature B-cell leukemias.[255, 312] Finally, in adult precursor-B-ALL, a striking predominance of immature Dδ2-Dδ3 cross-lineage recombinations was observed (44%), whereas the more mature Vδ2-Dδ3 gene rearrangements occurred less frequently (38%). This is in contrast to the high frequency (>70%) of the more mature Vδ2-Dδ3 gene rearrangements in childhood precursor-B-ALL. Together with the characteristic *IGH* and *IGK* gene rearrangement patterns, this suggests that the Ig and TCR genotype of precursor-B-ALL is less mature in adults than in children.[312]

Comparative studies between cell samples taken at diagnosis and at relapse revealed that the ongoing rearrangements and secondary rearrangements can cause changes in the Ig and TCR gene configuration at the time of relapse.[305, 311, 313-315] Such changes are particularly prevalent in cases of precursor-B-ALL that already contain subclones at diagnosis.[313]

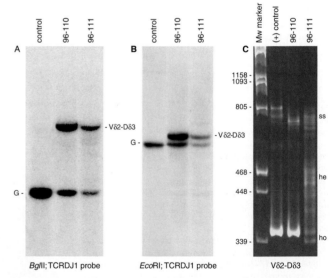

FIGURE 6–27. Clonality assessment via SB analysis and heteroduplex PCR analysis of *TCRD* genes in two precursor-B-ALL patients. *A,B,* DNA was digested with *Bgl*II and *Eco*RI. The filters were hybridized with the ³²P-labeled TCRDJ1 probe, and a monoallelic Vδ2-Dδ3 rearrangement was found in both patients. Additional weak rearranged bands were found in patient 96-111 (marked as *). *C,* Heteroduplex PCR analysis with a Vδ2 primer in combination with a Dδ3 primer showed a monoclonal rearrangement in patient 96-110 and an oligoclonal rearrangement pattern in patient 96-111 (as evidenced from the presence of several homo- and heteroduplexes). ss = single-strand fragments; he = heteroduplexes; ho = homoduplexes.

For 2 decades, B-ALL was assumed to be the most mature form of B-lineage ALL and to represent the leukemic stage of Burkitt's lymphoma. Recently, Burkitt's lymphomas were shown to have somatically mutated Ig genes, indicating that these tumors are derived from or related to (post)follicular center B cells.[316-318] The Ig gene rearrangement patterns in B-ALL are quite different from those in precursor-B-ALL, which is entirely in line with their SmIg expression. Comparable to Burkitt's lymphoma, the Ig genes of B-ALL contain somatic mutations. This observation fully justifies the replacement of the name "B-ALL" by "Burkitt's leukemia/lymphoma" as it is indicated by the WHO classification of neoplastic diseases of the hematopoietic and lymphoid tissues.[98]

TCR AND IG GENE REARRANGEMENTS IN T-ALL

The immunophenotype of T-ALL is fully comparable to those of cortical thymocytes. Subclassification of T-ALL into CD3$^-$, TCR$\gamma\delta^+$, and TCR$\alpha\beta^+$ subgroups also reveals major differences in TCR gene rearrangement patterns.[41, 185] Although the frequency of TCR gene rearrangements in the total group of T-ALL is very high, approximately 10% of CD3$^-$ T-ALL still has all TCR genes in germline configuration[41, 185]; this mainly concerns immature CD1$^-$/CD3$^-$ T-ALL of the prothymocytic/pre–T-ALL subgroup (see Table 6-5). The *TCRD* genes in CD3$^-$ T-ALL are rearranged in most cases (approximately 80%) and contain biallelic deletions in approximately 10% of cases.[41, 202] As expected, all TCR$\gamma\delta^+$ T-ALL have *TCRG* and *TCRD* gene rearrangements and the majority (approximately 95%) also contain *TCRB* gene rearrangements.[87, 202, 266] All TCR$\alpha\beta^+$ T-ALL contain *TCRB* and *TCRG* gene rearrangements and have at least one deleted *TCRD* allele (= *TCRA* rearrangement); the second *TCRD* allele is also deleted in two-thirds of cases.[185, 202] Analysis of the *TCRG* gene configuration in T-ALL showed that TCR$\gamma\delta^+$ T-ALL displays a less mature *TCRG* immunogenotype as compared with TCR$\alpha\beta^+$ and most CD3$^-$ cases. This is reflected by significantly more frequent usage of the more downstream Vγ genes and the upstream Jγ1 segments.[319] Cross-lineage Ig gene rearrangements occur at low frequency in T-ALL (approximately 20%) and involve only *IGH* genes (see Table 6–14).[185] Interestingly, cross-lineage *IGH* gene rearrangements occur more frequently in CD3$^-$ T-ALL (19%) and TCR$\gamma\delta^+$ T-ALL (50%) than in TCR$\alpha\beta^+$ T-ALL (less than 5%).[320] Heteroduplex PCR analysis showed a high frequency (approximately 80%) of incomplete D$_H$-J$_H$ rearrangements as well as preferential usage of D$_H$6-19 and the most downstream D$_H$7-27 gene segment together with the most upstream J$_H$1 and J$_H$2 gene segments. Complete V$_H$-J$_H$ recombinations comprised only 18% of cross-lineage *IGH* gene rearrangements in T-ALL patients. Furthermore, oligoclonality in the *IGH* locus was found in 27% of T-ALL patients with rearranged *IGH* genes.[320] These features suggest a predominance of immature *IGH* rearrangements in "immature" (non-TCR$\alpha\beta^+$) T-ALL.

Comparative studies at diagnosis and at relapse revealed that continuing and secondary TCR rearrangements could also occur in 40% to 50% of T-ALL patients.[313-315] Nevertheless, TCR oligoclonality is rarely seen at diagnosis in T-ALL cases,[185, 313] except for a few

CD3$^-$ cases that showed a faint band of δ_{REC}-ψJα rearrangements normally involved in *TCRD* gene deletions.[226] Detailed studies of these T-ALL cases revealed that the detected δ_{REC}-ψJα rearrangements were fully polyclonal but were derived from otherwise monoclonal T-ALL.[321] Interestingly, each case contained biallelic nonfunctional *TCRG* and/or *TCRD* gene rearrangements, which prevented TCR$\gamma\delta$ expression. Therefore, the δ_{REC}-ψJα rearrangements can be interpreted as continuous rearrangements in an attempt to produce functional *TCRA* gene rearrangement for TCR$\alpha\beta$ protein expression. Indeed, one of the analyzed CD3$^-$ T-ALL cases contained a leukemic TCR$\alpha\beta^+$ subpopulation that was detected by TCR$\alpha\beta$/TdT double immunofluorescence staining.[321]

It is clear that Ig and TCR gene rearrangement patterns in ALL display several unusual features as compared with normal lymphoid counterparts. Extensive molecular studies indicate that the unusual Ig and TCR gene rearrangements in ALL occur as an early postoncogenic event resulting from the continuing V(D)J recombinase activity on accessible gene loci. This hypothesis is supported by the absence of cross-lineage gene rearrangements in normal lymphocytes and mature lymphoid malignancies and by the presence of oligoclonality and secondary Ig and TCR gene rearrangements in ALL.[322]

Cross-lineage Ig and/or TCR gene rearrangements are also observed in 10% to 15% of AML cases.[298] This particularly concerns *IGH* and *TCRD* genes[298] and also *TCRB* and *TCRG* gene rearrangements,[298, 323, 324] and even a few cases with *IGK* gene rearrangements[298, 324] have been found.

Chronic Lymphoid Leukemias

Virtually all chronic B-lineage leukemias express SmIg molecules with either Igκ- or Igλ-light chains. They all contain *IGH* gene rearrangements, most of them on both alleles (see Fig. 6-21). All Igκ^+ B-lineage leukemias contain at least one rearranged *IGK* allele, whereas *IGL* gene rearrangements are rare (approximately 5% of cases).[185, 255, 294] *IGL* gene rearrangements are detectable by Southern blotting in virtually all (more than 95%) of Smλ^+ B-lineage leukemias; most of them have biallelic *IGK* deletions (see Table 6-15).[185, 255, 294]

The chronic T-lineage leukemias of ATLL, CTLL and T-PLL types probably all belong to the TCR$\alpha\beta$ lineage. This is in line with the finding that they all contain *TCRB* and *TCRG* gene rearrangements and that most of them have biallelic *TCRD* gene deletions.[185, 291, 297, 325-327]

The LGL leukemias can be divided into three subgroups: the major subgroup consists of TCR$\alpha\beta^+$ T-LGL, whereas the two minor subgroups consists of TCR$\gamma\delta^+$ T-LGL and NK-LGL.[46, 185] As expected, the TCR$\alpha\beta^+$ T-LGL contains *TCRB* and *TCRG* gene rearrangements and generally biallelic *TCRD* gene deletions.[46, 185] The TCR$\gamma\delta^+$ T-LGL contains *TCRG* and *TCRD* gene rearrangements, but most of them seem to have germline *TCRB* genes.[46, 185] The NK-LGL have all TCR genes in germline configuration, which is in line with the absence of TCR gene rearrangements in normal NK cells (Fig. 6-28; Table 6-15).[46, 185, 208, 210]

In contrast to acute leukemias, the chronic lymphoid

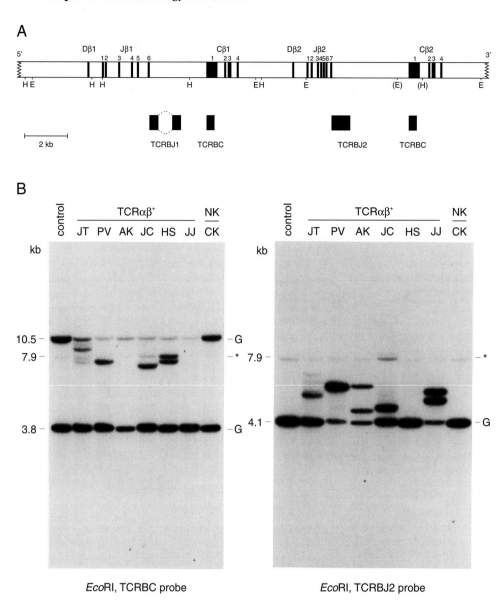

FIGURE 6–28. *A,* Restriction map of the human *TCRB* gene complex, i.e., the Dβ1-Jβ1-Cβ1 and Dβ2-Jβ2-Cβ2 regions. The position of the relevant *Eco*RI (E) and *Hin*dIII (H) restriction sites are indicated. The partly resistant *Eco*RI and *Hin*dIII restriction sites in the 2 region are given in brackets. The solid bars represent the *TCRB* genomic DNA probes: TCRBJ1, TCRBC, and TCRBJ2. The TCRBJ1 probe consists of two separate fragments, because the intervening sequences cause aspecific hybridization signals. The TCRBC probe recognizes the first exon of both Cβ regions. *B,* Southern blot analysis of *TCRB* genes in six patients with TCRαβ⁺ T-LGL leukemia and one patient with NK-LGL. The DNA samples were digested with *Eco*RI and the nylon filter was successively hybridized to the Cβ probe TCRBC (*left*) and the Jβ2 probe TCRBJ2 (*right*). The size of each germline band (G) is indicated in kilobases (kb); the 7.9 kb band (*) is due to incomplete digestion. As expected the TCRαβ⁺ T-LGL had rearrangements in their β1 and/or β2 loci, while the NK-LGL had germline *TCRB* genes. Interestingly, in the TCRαβ⁺ T-LGL of patient JT several faint rearranged bands are visible, indicating the presence of some small subclones.

TABLE 6–15. Frequencies of Detectable Ig and TCR Gene Rearrangments and Deletions in Chronic Lymphoid Leukemias

	IGH	*IGK*		*IGL*	*TCRB*	*TCRG*	*TCRD*	
	R	*R*	*D*	*R*	*R*	*R*	*R*	*D*
B-lineage								
Smκ⁺ B-CLL, B-PLL, and HCL	100%	100%	0%	<5%	<5%	<5%	0%	
Smλ⁺ B-CLL, B-PLL, and HCL	100%	25%	75%	>98%	<5%	<5%	0%	
T-lineage								
ATLL, CTLL, and T-PLLª	<5%	0%		0%	100%	100%	10%–25%	75%–90%
LGL leukemiaᵇ								
TCRαβ⁺ LGL	<5%	0%		0%	100%	100%	<25%	>75%
TCRγδ⁺ LGL	0%	0%		0%	~50%	100%	100%	0%
NK-LGL	0%	0%		0%	0%	0%	0%	0%

R at least one rearranged allele; D, both alleles deleted.
a. The majority of ATLL, CTLL, and T-PLL probably belong to the TCRαβ lineage.
b. Most LGL leukemias express TCRαβ (70%–80%), some express TCRγδ (10%–15%), and some belong to the NK-lineage (10%–15%) (see Table 6–7).

leukemias rarely contain cross-lineage Ig or TCR gene rearrangements.[185, 328, 329] It is obvious from Tables 6-14 and 6-15 that all ALL and all chronic lymphoid leukemias contain Ig and/or TCR gene rearrangements. Therefore, Southern blotting and/or PCR analysis can be used for clonality studies in the diagnosis and follow-up of lymphoid leukemias and suspect lymphoproliferations.[184, 185, 330-332]

Applications of Ig and TCR Gene Analysis for Diagnostic Clonality Studies

Our experience indicates that Southern blot analysis of *IGH, IGK,* and *TCRB* genes is relatively easy, results in unique rearrangement patterns in each clonal lymphoproliferation due to the extensive combinatorial repertoire of these genes, and is informative in the majority of cases.[184, 254, 255] The latter is in line with the high frequency of *IGH, IGK,* and *TCRB* gene rearrangements (see Tables 6-14 and 6-15). Southern blot analysis of *IGL, TCRG* and *TCRD* genes is less suitable for diagnostic clonality studies, because of the lower frequencies of *IGL* gene rearrangements[184] and because of the limited combinatorial repertoire and thereby the more limited number of differently rearranged bands in case of *TCRG* and *TCRD* genes (Table 6-12).[199, 202]

PCR-based diagnostic clonality studies focus largely on *IGH* and *TCRG* gene rearrangements[267-269, 279, 282, 284] because of the high frequency of these rearrangements in lymphoid leukemias and because of the relatively limited number of primer sets that are needed for the detection of rearrangements in these genes. This also implies that PCR analysis of *IGH* and *TCRG* genes can be readily performed on DNA level.

Cytomorphology and immunophenotyping are generally sufficient for making the appropriate diagnosis in suspect lymphoproliferations. However, diagnostic problems might arise, especially if the suspect cell population is small and if the proliferation concerns mature T cells. In such cases Ig and/or TCR gene clonality studies are very reliable for discrimination between polyclonal and monoclonal lymphoproliferations. Additional applications include detection of two or more subclones within a malignancy at diagnosis, detection of clonal evolution at relapse, analysis of the clonal origin of two lymphoid malignancies in a single patient, and analysis of the differentiation lineage of a malignancy (Table 6-16).[185]

Clonality studies can be very useful in diagnosing lymphoproliferative diseases, but it should be noticed that clonal cell populations do not always represent a clinically malignant disease. Furthermore, given the detection limits of the Southern blot and PCR analyses, small clonal cell populations might be missed if their relative size is less than 1% to 5% (see Table 6-16).[184, 185]

Discrimination Between Polyclonal and Monoclonal Lymphoproliferations

Immunophenotyping is generally sufficient to determine clonality in acute leukemias, except rare cases of smolder-

TABLE 6–16. Diagnostic Applications of Ig and TCR Gene Analysis

1. Discrimination between polyclonal and monoclonal lymphoproliferative diseases.
   Caution: monoclonality does not necessarily imply clinical malignancy (e.g., LGL leukemia and monoclonal or oligoclonal lymphoproliferations in immunodeficiency).
2. Detection of two or more subclones within one malignancy.
3. Analysis of lymphoid malignancies at diagnosis and subsequent relapses:
   Detection of identical Ig and TCR gene rearrangements
   Detection of differences: clonal evolution at first relapse and/or subsequent relapses.
4. Proof or exclusion of the common clonal origin of two malignant lymphoid cell populations.
   Caution: one should try to discriminate between two independent lymphoid malignancies and subclone formation within a malignancy.
5. Assignment or exclusion of the differentiation lineage of a malignancy.
   Caution: cross-lineage Ig and TCR gene rearrangements.
6. Detection of low numbers of malignant cells:
   Detection limit of the Southern blot technique is 1%–5%.
   Detection limit of PCR technique (in combination with heteroduplex analysis or gene scanning) is 0.1%–1%.[1]

1. The sensitivity of the PCR technique can be increased to 10^{-4} to 10^{-6}, if junctional region specific probes are used (see Chapter 12).

ing ALL, where a population of CD19[+]/CD10[+]/TdT[+] blasts comprises less than 25% of bone marrow cells.[333, 334] In such cases, molecular detection of clonal Ig or TCR gene rearrangements could be of final proof for a real preleukemic stage.[334, 335] In mature Ig[+] B-lineage leukemias, immunophenotypic markers for clonality are restricted to single Ig-light chain expression (i.e., Igκ/Igλ distribution). In other cases Ig and TCR gene analysis can be used for detection of clonality. This is especially important in Ig[-] B-cell proliferations and TdT[-] T-cell proliferations.[330-332] Figure 6-28 shows the analysis of *TCRB* genes for detection of clonality in blood samples of patients suspected of LGL leukemia.

Detection of Two or More Subclones in a Leukemia

IGH gene studies in precursor-B-ALL reveal that 30% to 40% of cases at diagnosis contain subclones, as deduced from the presence of multiple rearranged bands in Southern blot analysis (Fig. 6-29).[300] Such subclone formation might also be detectable at the *IGK* gene level, but cross-lineage TCR gene rearrangements generally confirm the clonal origin of the precursor-B-ALL.[300, 313] It has been demonstrated that the subclone formation is due to continuing rearrangements (e.g., VH to D-JH rearrangements) and secondary rearrangements, such as D-JH replacements and VH replacements.[302-304, 306]

Subclone formation has also been found by Southern blot analysis in follicular lymphomas and immunocytomas.[336-338] The Ig gene rearrangement patterns of the subclones in these lymphomas differ from those of the parental clone in some but not all restriction enzyme digests.[337, 338] This subclone formation is caused by somatic mutations, which effect some but not all restriction sites. This type of subclone formation has not been observed in ALL and chronic B-cell leukemias.[184, 300, 302, 339, 340]

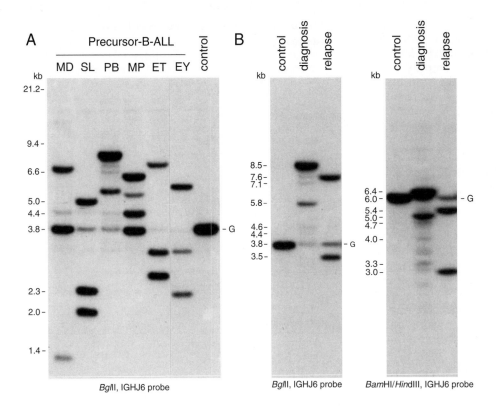

FIGURE 6–29. Southern blot analysis of *IGH* genes in precursor-B-ALL. *A,* Analysis at diagnosis with the restriction enzyme *Bgl*II and the IGHJ6 probe (see Figure 6–21). Multiple rearranged bands are present in each precursor-B-ALL lane. In patient SL, this is due to trisomy 14, but in all other cases subclone formation (biclonality or oligoclonality) is the cause. *B,* Comparative analysis of DNA samples of patient peripheral blood at diagnosis and relapse with *Bgl*II and *Bam*HI/*Hind*III digests and the IGHJ6 probe. Multiple rearranged bands of different density are present in both digests at diagnosis. However, at relapse only two rearranged bands are present, which probably have the same size as two faint rearranged bands at diagnosis.

Finally, biclonal and oligoclonal B-cell malignancies have been found in immunodeficient patients.[341-343] These are probably derived from Epstein-Barr virus–induced lymphoproliferations. Therefore, these patients probably suffer from multiple lymphomas; i.e., lymphomas that do not have a common clonal origin but that are caused by the same multistep oncogenic process.[344] It is unclear whether a comparable oncogenic mechanism causes biclonality in some B-CLL patients or whether some individuals are more prone to develop B-cell malignancies because of genetic factors.[345]

Analysis of Lymphoid Malignancies at Diagnosis and Subsequent Relapse

Analysis of Ig and/or TCR gene rearrangement patterns at diagnosis and subsequent relapse can prove whether the recurrence of a lymphoid malignancy represents a relapse or a secondary malignancy. Sometimes the histomorphologic and/or clinical characteristics of a B-cell malignancy are changed at relapse, whereas the *IGH* and Ig-light chain gene rearrangement patterns remain identical.[346] However, it should be noted that changes in Ig and/or TCR gene rearrangement patterns can occur at relapse in precursor-B-ALL and follicular-center-cell–derived lymphomas due to continuing/secondary rearrangements and somatic mutations, respectively (see Fig. 6–29).[302, 306, 313, 336-338]

Southern blot analysis has been considered the gold standard for the comparison of the Ig/TCR gene rearrangement patterns between diagnosis and recurrence of a lymphoid malignancy.[313] The finding of identically rearranged bands at diagnosis and at relapse reflects usage of identical gene segments, but not necessarily showing

identical junctional regions. For reliable proof of clonal identity, the identically sized rearranged bands should represent major gene rearrangements, and this should preferably be found for multiple Ig and TCR gene loci. This is particularly important for patients with oligoclonal Ig and TCR gene rearrangements, which are frequently found in ALL. When the only indication for clonal relationship is based on the identity of a single band, comparative analysis of junctional regions is mandatory. Such comparative junctional region analysis can be easily performed by mixing the PCR products of both disease stages and evaluating them by heteroduplex method. In case of relapsed leukemia, mixing will result in a single homoduplex band upon heteroduplex analysis, whereas in case of a secondary malignancy two distinct homoduplexes as well as two heteroduplexes will be found (Fig. 6-30). These heteroduplexes result from cross-renaturation of single-strand molecules of the two different malignant cell populations. Finally, when only nonidentical clonal PCR products at diagnosis and at relapse are detected with mixed heteroduplex PCR analyses, direct sequencing of clonal PCR products can be performed to exclude clonal evolution due to ongoing rearrangements; e.g., different VH to DH-JH rearrangements but with an identical preexisting DH-JH rearrangement.

Proof or Exclusion of the Common Clonal Origin of Two Malignant Lymphoid Cell Populations

In some patients with a B-cell malignancy, a second B-cell malignancy may develop, or sometimes two B-cell

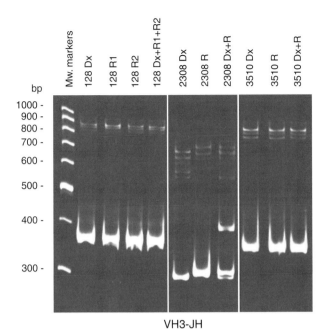

VH3-JH

FIGURE 6–30. Comparative heteroduplex analysis of VH3-JH PCR products in three precursor-B-ALL patients at diagnosis and at leukemia relapse. In two patients (0128 and 3510), identical clonal VH3-JH PCR products were found at both leukemia phases (identical size of homoduplexes and no heteroduplex formation after mixing and subsequent denaturation/renaturation). In patient 2308 monoclonal homoduplexes found at diagnosis and at relapse differed slightly in size. Mixing of the VH3-JH PCR products followed by heteroduplex PCR analysis demonstrated clear heteroduplex formation, proving that these VH3-JH gene rearrangements had different junctional regions.

malignancies occur simultaneously in the same patient.[185, 338, 346–349] Ig gene analysis can demonstrate whether such malignancies have a common clonal origin or represent two independent malignancies (Fig. 6–31).[185]

Determination of Differentiation Lineage

In some rare undifferentiated leukemias, immunophenotyping might not be sufficient to determine the differentiation lineage of the leukemic cells. It has been suggested that detection of Ig or TCR gene rearrangements can be used for lineage assignment. However, the cross-lineage Ig and TCR gene rearrangements in ALL and AML may hamper this application.[185, 293, 298, 299] However, the presence of germline Ig and TCR genes supports the non-lymphoid character or early (very immature) lymphoid character of a newly diagnosed malignancy.

Detection of Low Numbers of Malignant Cells

The detection limit of routinely performed Southern blot analysis is approximately 5%.[184] The PCR technique might be somewhat more sensitive if the "background" of normal polyclonal B and T cells is low.[267, 268, 279, 282] For many leukemias, such detection limits can also be reached with cytomorphology and immunophenotyping. Nevertheless, in some situations Ig and TCR gene analysis might be valuable; e.g., for discriminating between regenerating bone marrow with high frequencies of precursor B cells after withdrawal of cytotoxic treatment and an imminent relapse of precursor-B-ALL.[350–352]

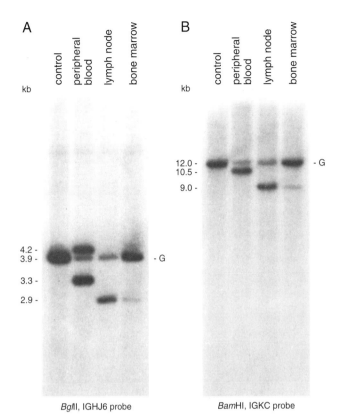

BglII, IGHJ6 probe   BamHI, IGKC probe

FIGURE 6–31. Southern blot analysis of *IGH* and *IGK* genes in a patient with three Igκ-positive B-cell malignancies. Peripheral blood mononuclear cells consisted of 80% SmIgκ⁺ B-CLL cells, the lymph node contained 60% SmIgκ⁺ B cell lymphoma cells, and bone marrow mononuclear cells consisted of 5% CyIgκ⁺ multiple myeloma cells. *A, Bgl*II-digested DNA samples were analyzed with the IGHJ6 probe. Two differently rearranged bands are visible in the peripheral blood lane, whereas a single identically rearranged band is present in the lymph node lane and bone marrow lane. *B, Bam*HI digested DNA samples were analyzed with the Cκ probe IGKC. In each lane one rearranged band is visible. The rearranged bands in the lymph node lane and bone marrow lane are identical. These results indicate that the B-cell lymphoma and multiple myeloma are related to each other, whereas the B-CLL is a second independent malignancy.

The sensitivity of the PCR technique can be increased to 10^{-4} to 10^{-6} (100 to 1 leukemic cells between 10^6 normal cells), if junctional–region specific oligonucleotide probes or primers are used for detection of the leukemia-derived PCR products.[263–266, 273, 274, 353–355] This approach proved to be valuable for evaluation of the effectiveness of the applied treatment, particularly in ALL patients.[356, 357] For this purpose the junctional regions of rearranged Ig and TCR genes of the leukemic cells at diagnosis have to be sequenced in order to design leukemia-specific junctional region probes (see Chapter 12).

CONCLUSION

Southern blotting and PCR analysis allow a detailed study of Ig and TCR gene rearrangements in leukemias based on the combinatorial diversity and junctional diversity of the gene rearrangements, respectively. Both techniques are suitable for diagnostic clonality studies, if appropriate probe/restriction enzyme combinations and appropriate primer sets are used. Routinely performed Southern blotting can generally be restricted to *IGH, IGK,* and *TCRB* gene analyses, whereas PCR analyses generally focus on junctional regions of rearranged *IGH* and *TCRG* genes. A reliable PCR-based method requires postamplification PCR product analysis to distinguish between polyclonality, oligoclonality, and monoclonality of the amplified Ig and TCR gene rearrangements.

REFERENCES

1. Janossy G, Bollum FJ, Bradstock KF, et al: Cellular phenotypes of normal and leukemic hemopoietic cells determined by analysis with selected antibody combinations. Blood 1980;56:430.
2. Foon KA, Todd RF: Immunologic classification of leukemia and lymphoma. Blood 1986;68:1.
3. Greaves MF: Differentiation-linked leukemogenesis in lymphocytes. Science 1986;234:697.
4. Van Dongen JJ, Adriaansen HJ, Hooijkaas H: Immunophenotyping of leukaemias and non-Hodgkin's lymphomas: Immunological markers and their CD codes. Neth J Med 1988;33:298.
5. Jennings CD, Foon KA: Flow cytometry: Recent advances in diagnosis and monitoring of leukemia. Cancer Invest 1997;15:384.
6. Bernard A, Boumsell L, Dausset J, et al, eds: Leucocyte Typing. Human Leucocyte Differentiation Antigens Detected by Monoclonal Antibodies. Berlin, Springer Verlag, 1984.
7. Reinherz EL, Haynes BF, Nadler LM, et al, eds: Leucocyte Typing II. Berlin, Springer Verlag, 1986.
8. McMichael AJ, Beverly PC, Gilks W, et al, eds: Leucocyte Typing III: White Cell Differentiation Antigens. Oxford, Oxford University Press, 1987.
9. Knapp W, Dörken B, Rieber EP, et al, eds: Leucocyte Typing IV. White Cell Differentiation Antigens. Oxford, Oxford University Press, 1989.
10. Schlossman SF, Boumsell L, Gilks W, et al, eds: Leucocyte Typing V: White Cell Differentiation Antigens. Oxford, Oxford University Press, 1994.
11. Kishimoto T, Kikutani H, Von dem Borne AEGK, et al, eds: Leucocyte Typing VI: White Cell Differentiation Antigens. New York & London, Garland Publishing, Inc. 1997.
12. Van Dongen JJM, Krissansen GW, Wolvers-Tettero IL, et al: Cytoplasmic expression of the CD3 antigen as a diagnostic marker for immature T-cell malignancies. Blood 1988;71:603.
13. Mason DY, Comans-Bitter WM, Cordell JL, et al: Antibody L26 recognizes an intracellular epitope on the B-cell–associated CD20 antigen. Am J Pathol 1990;136:1215.
14. Martin LH, Calabi F, Lefebvre FA, et al: Structure and expression of the human thymocyte antigens CD1a, CD1b, and CD1c. Proc Natl Acad Sci U S A 1987;84:9189.
15. Arnaout MA: Structure and function of the leukocyte adhesion molecules CD11/CD18. Blood 1990;75:1037.
16. Albelda SM: Role of integrins and other cell adhesion molecules in tumor progression and metastasis. Lab Invest 1993;68:4.
17. Borst J, Brouns GS, de Vries E, et al: Antigen receptors on T and B lymphocytes: Parallels in organization and function. Immunol Rev 1993;132:49.
18. Streuli M, Hall LR, Saga Y, et al: Differential usage of three exons generates at least five different mRNAs encoding human leukocyte common antigens. J Exp Med 1987;166:1548.
19. Rey-Campos J, Rubinstein P, Rodriguez de Cordoba S: A physical map of the human regulator of complement activation gene cluster linking the complement genes CR1, CR2, DAF, and C4BP. J Exp Med 1988;167:664.
20. Tindle RW, Nichols RA, Chan L, et al: A novel monoclonal antibody BI-3C5 recognises myeloblasts and non-B, non-T lymphoblasts in acute leukaemias and CGL blast crises, and reacts with immature cells in normal bone marrow. Leuk Res 1985;9:1.
21. Lerner NB, Nocka KH, Cole SR, et al: Monoclonal antibody YB5.B8 identifies the human c-kit protein product. Blood 1991;77:1876.
22. Bühring HJ, Ullrich A, Schaudt K, et al: The product of the proto-oncogene c-kit (P145c-kit) is a human bone marrow surface antigen of hemopoietic precursor cells which is expressed on a subset of acute non-lymphoblastic leukemic cells. Leukemia 1991; 5:854.
23. Macedo A, Orfao A, Martinez A, et al: Immunophenotype of c-kit cells in normal human bone marrow: Implications for the detection of minimal residual disease in AML. Br J Haematol 1995; 89:338.
24. Adriaansen HJ, van Dongen JJ, Kappers-Klunne MC, et al: Terminal deoxynucleotidyl transferase positive subpopulations occur in the majority of ANLL: Implications for the detection of minimal disease. Leukemia 1990;4:404.
25. Bollum FJ: Terminal deoxynucleotidyl transferase as a hematopoietic cell marker. Blood 1979;54:1203.
26. Campana D, Janossy G, Bofill M, et al: Human B cell development. I. Phenotypic differences of B lymphocytes in the bone marrow and peripheral lymphoid tissue. J Immunol 1985;134:1524.
27. Janossy G, Coustan-Smith E, Campana D: The reliability of cytoplasmic CD3 and CD22 antigen expression in the immunodiagnosis of acute leukemia: A study of 500 cases. Leukemia 1989; 3:170.
28. Boue DR, LeBien TW: Expression and structure of CD22 in acute leukemia. Blood 1988;71:1480.
29. Buccheri V, Mihaljevic B, Matutes E, et al: Mb-1: A new marker for B-lineage lymphoblastic leukemia. Blood 1993;82:853.
30. Verschuren MC, Comans-Bitter WM, Kapteijn CA, et al: Transcription and protein expression of mb-1 and B29 genes in human hematopoietic malignancies and cell lines. Leukemia 1993;7:1939.
31. Dworzak MN, Fritsch G, Froschi G, et al: Four-color flow cytometric investigation of terminal deoxynucleotidyl transferase-positive lymphoid precursors in pediatric bone marrow: CD79a expression precedes CD19 in early B-cell ontogeny. Blood 1998;92:3203.
32. Tsuganezawa K, Kiyokawa N, Matsuo Y, et al: Flow cytometric diagnosis of the cell lineage and developmental stage of acute lymphoblastic leukemia by novel monoclonal antibodies specific to human pre–B-cell receptor. Blood 1998;92:4317.
33. Zola H: The surface antigens of human B lymphocytes. Immunol Today 1987;8:308.
34. Gathings WE, Lawton AR, Cooper MD: Immunofluorescent studies of the development of pre-B cells, B lymphocytes and immunoglobulin isotype diversity in humans. Eur J Immunol 1977;7:804.
35. Vogler LB, Crist WM, Bockman DE, et al: Pre-B-cell leukemia: A new phenotype of childhood lymphoblastic leukemia. N Engl J Med 1978;298:872.
36. Koehler M, Behm FG, Shuster J, et al: Transitional pre-B-cell acute lymphoblastic leukemia of childhood is associated with favorable prognostic clinical features and an excellent outcome: A Pediatric Oncology Group study. Leukemia 1993;7:2064.
37. Rajewsky K: Clonal selection and learning in the antibody system. Nature 1996;381:751.
38. Küppers R, Klein U, Hansmann ML, et al: Cellular origin of human B-cell lymphomas. N Engl J Med 1999;341:1520.
39. Wijdenes J, Vooijs WC, Clement C, et al: A plasmocyte selective monoclonal antibody (B-B4) recognizes syndecan-1. Br J Haematol 1996;94:318.
40. Vooijs WC, Post J, Wijdenes J, et al: Efficacy and toxicity of plasmacell–reactive monoclonal antibodies B-B2 and B-B4 and their immunotoxins. Cancer Immunol Immunother 1996;42:319.
41. Van Dongen JJM, Comans-Bitter WM, Wolvers-Tettero ILM, et al: Development of human T lymphocytes and their thymus dependency. Thymus 1990;16:207.
42. Groeneveld K, Comans-Bitter WM, van den Beemd MWM, et al: Blood T-cell subsets in health and disease. J Int Fed Clin Chem 1994;6:84.
43. Castro J, van Wichen D, Comans-Bitter WM, et al: The human TCF-1 gene encodes a nuclear DNA-binding protein uniquely expressed in normal and neoplastic T-lineage lymphocytes. Blood 1995;86:3050.
44. Lanier LL, Le AM, Phillips JH, et al: Subpopulations of human natural killer cells defined by expression of the Leu-7 (HNK-1) and Leu-11 (NK-15) antigens. J Immunol 1983;131:1789.
45. Lanier LL, Le AM, Civin CI, et al: The relationship of CD16 (Leu-11) and Leu-19 (NKH-1) antigen expression on human peripheral blood NK cells and cytotoxic T lymphocytes. J Immunol 1986; 136:4480.
46. Loughran TP Jr: Clonal diseases of large granular lymphocytes. Blood 1993;82:1.

47. Moretta A, Biassoni R, Bottino C, et al: Natural cytotoxicity receptors that trigger human NK-cell–mediated cytolysis. Immunol Today 2000;21:228.

48. Moretta A, Biassoni R, Bottino C, et al: Major histocompatibility complex class I-specific receptors on human natural killer and T lymphocytes. Immunol Rev 1997;155:105.

49. Matutes E, Coelho E, Aguado MJ, et al: Expression of TIA-1 and TIA-2 in T-cell malignancies and T-cell lymphocytosis. J Clin Pathol 1996;49:154.

50. Anderson P, Nagler-Anderson C, O'Brien C, et al: A monoclonal antibody reactive with a 15-kDa cytoplasmic granule–associated protein defines a subpopulation of CD8 + T lymphocytes. J Immunol 1990;144:574.

51. Kummer JA, Kamp AM, Tadema TM, et al: Localization and identification of granzymes A and B–expressing cells in normal human lymphoid tissue and peripheral blood. Clin Exp Immunol 1995;100:164.

52. Griffin JD, Mayer RJ, Weinstein HJ, et al: Surface marker analysis of acute myeloblastic leukemia: Identification of differentiation-associated phenotypes. Blood 1983;62:557.

53. Sabbath KD, Ball ED, Larcom P, et al: Heterogeneity of clonogenic cells in acute myeloblastic leukemia. J Clin Invest 1985;75:746.

54. Van der Schoot CE, Daams GM, Pinkster J, et al: Monoclonal antibodies against myeloperoxidase are valuable immunological reagents for the diagnosis of acute myeloid leukaemia. Br J Haematol 1990;74:173.

55. Majdic O, Bettelheim P, Stockinger H, et al: M2, a novel myelomonocytic cell surface antigen and its distribution on leukemic cells. Int J Cancer 1984;33:617.

56. Radzun HJ, Kreipe H, Zavazava N, et al: Diversity of the human monocyte/macrophage system as detected by monoclonal antibodies. J Leukoc Biol 1988;43:41.

57. Munro CS, Campbell DA, Collings LA, Poulter LW: Monoclonal antibodies distinguish macrophages and epithelioid cells in sarcoidosis and leprosy. Clin Exp Immunol 1987;68:282.

58. Majdic O, Liszka K, Lutz D, et al: Myeloid differentiation antigen defined by a monoclonal antibody. Blood 1981;58:1127.

59. Boccuni P, Di Noto R, Lo Pardo C, et al: CD66c antigen expression is myeloid restricted in normal bone marrow but is a common feature of CD10 + early B-cell malignancies. Tissue Antigens 1998;52:1.

60. Villeval JL, Cramer P, Lemoine F, et al: Phenotype of early erythroblastic leukemias. Blood 1986;68:1167.

61. San Miguel JF, Gonzalez M, Canizo MC, et al: Leukemias with megakaryoblastic involvement: Clinical, hematologic, and immunologic characteristics. Blood 1988;72:402.

62. Breton-Gorius J, Villeval JL, Kieffer N, et al: Limits of phenotypic markers for the diagnosis of megakaryoblastic leukemia. Blood Cells 1989;15:259.

63. Visser L, Shaw A, Slupsky J, et al: Monoclonal antibodies reactive with hairy cell leukemia. Blood 1989;74:320.

64. Mason DY, Sammons R: Alkaline phosphatase and peroxidase for double immunoenzymatic labelling of cellular constituents. J Clin Pathol 1978;31:454.

65. Cordell JL, Falini B, Erber WN, et al: Immunoenzymatic labeling of monoclonal antibodies using immune complexes of alkaline phosphatase and monoclonal anti-alkaline phosphatase (APAAP complexes). J Histochem Cytochem 1984;32:219.

66. Leenen PJ, Melis ML, Van Ewijk W: Single-cell immuno-beta-galactosidase staining of heterogeneous populations: Practical application on limited cell numbers. Histochem J 1987;19:497.

67. Terstappen LW, Loken MR: Five-dimensional flow cytometry as a new approach for blood and bone marrow differentials. Cytometry 1988;9:548.

68. Steiner GE, Ecker RC, Kramer G, et al: Automated data acquisition by confocal laser scanning microscopy and image analysis of triple-stained immunofluorescent leukocytes in tissue. J Immunol Methods 2000;237:39.

69. Van Dongen JJM, Hooijkaas H, Comans-Bitter WM, et al: Triple immunological staining with colloidal gold, fluorescein and rhodamine as labels. J Immunol Methods 1985;80:1.

70. Falini B, Flenghi L, Fagioli M, et al: Immunocytochemical diagnosis of acute promyelocytic leukemia (M3) with the monoclonal antibody PG-M3 (anti-PML). Blood 1997;90:4046.

71. Carter NP, Meyer EW: Introduction to the principles of flow cytometry. In Ormerod MG ed: Flow Cytometry: A Practical Approach. New York, Oxford University Press, 1994.

72. Weir EG, Cowan K, LeBeau P, et al: A limited antibody panel can distinguish B-precursor acute lymphoblastic leukemia from normal B precursors with four-color flow cytometry: Implications for residual disease detection. Leukemia 1999;13:558.

73. Borowitz MJ, Guenther KL, Shults KE, et al: Immunophenotyping of acute leukemia by flow cytometric analysis: Use of CD45 and right-angle light scatter to gate on leukemic blasts in three-color analysis. Am J Clin Pathol 1993;100:534.

74. Lacombe F, Durrieu F, Briais A, et al: Flow cytometry CD45 gating for immunophenotyping of acute myeloid leukemia. Leukemia 1997;11:1878.

75. Groeneveld K, te Marvelde JG, van den Beemd MW, et al: Flow cytometric detection of intracellular antigens for immunophenotyping of normal and malignant leukocytes. Leukemia 1996;10:1383.

76. Visser O, Coebergh JWW, Schouten LJ, eds: Incidence of Cancer in the Netherlands: Second Report of the Netherlands Cancer Registry. Utrecht, The Netherlands Cancer Registry, 1994.

77. Bain B: Leukaemia diagnosis: A guide to the FAB classification. Philadelphia, JB Lippincott, 1990.

78. Van't Veer MB, van Putten WL, Verdonck LF, et al: Acute lymphoblastic leukaemia in adults: Immunological subtypes and clinical features at presentation. Ann Hematol 1993;66:277.

79. Ludwig WD, Raghavachar A, Thiel E: Immunophenotypic classification of acute lymphoblastic leukaemia. Baillieres Clin Haematol 1994;7:235.

80. General Haematology Task Force of BCSH: Immunophenotyping in the diagnosis of chronic lymphoproliferative disorders. J Clin Pathol 1994;47:871.

81. Litz CE, Brunning RD: Chronic lymphoproliferative disorders: Classification and diagnosis. Baillieres Clin Haematol 1993;6:767.

82. Pui CH, Behm FG, Crist WM: Clinical and biologic relevance of immunologic marker studies in childhood acute lymphoblastic leukemia. Blood 1993;82:343.

83. Van der Does-van den Berg A, Bartram CR, Basso G, et al: Minimal requirements for the diagnosis, classification, and evaluation of the treatment of childhood acute lymphoblastic leukemia (ALL) in the "BFM Family" Cooperative Group. Med Pediatr Oncol 1992;20:497.

84. Bene MC, Castoldi G, Knapp W, et al: Proposals for the immunological classification of acute leukemias: European Group for the Immunological Characterization of Leukemias (EGIL). Leukemia 1995;9:1783.

85. Schott G, Sperling C, Schrappe M, et al: Immunophenotypic and clinical features of T-cell receptor gammadelta + T-lineage acute lymphoblastic leukaemia. Br J Haematol 1998;101:753.

86. Van Dongen JJM, van den Beemd MWM, Schellekens M, et al: Analysis of malignant T cells with the Vβ antibody panel. Immunologist 1996;4:37.

87. Langerak AW, Wolvers-Tettero ILM, van den Beemd MWM, et al: Immunophenotypic and immunogenotypic characteristics of TCR gamma delta + T-cell acute lymphoblastic leukemia. Leukemia 1999;13:206.

88. Ludwig WD, Harbott J, Bartram CR, et al: Incidence and prognostic significance of immunophenotypic subgroups in childhood acute lymphoblastic leukemia: Experience of the BFM study 86. Recent Results Cancer Res 1993;131:269.

89. Niehues T, Kapaun P, Harms DO, et al: A classification based on T cell selection–related phenotypes identifies a subgroup of childhood T-ALL with favorable outcome in the COALL studies. Leukemia 1999;13:614.

90. Pullen J, Shuster JJ, Link M, et al: Significance of commonly used prognostic factors differs for children with T cell acute lymphocytic leukemia (ALL), as compared to those with B-precursor ALL: A Pediatric Oncology Group (POG) study. Leukemia 1999;13:1696.

91. Coebergh JWW, Van der Does A, Kamps WA, et al: Epidemiological studies of childhood leukaemia in the Netherlands since 1972: Experience of the Dutch Childhood Leukaemia Study Group (DCLSG). Medizinische Forschung 1993;6:235.

92. Greaves MF, Alexander FE: An infectious etiology for common acute lymphoblastic leukaemia in childhood? Leukemia 1993;7:349.

93. Czuczman MS, Dodge RK, Stewart CC, et al: Value of immunophenotype in intensively treated adult acute lymphoblastic leukemia: Cancer and Leukemia Group B study 8364. Blood 1999;93:3931.

94. Bennett JM, Catovsky D, Daniel MT, et al: Proposals for the classi-fication of the acute leukaemias: French-American-British (FAB) co-operative group. Br J Haematol 1976;33:451.

95. Gassmann W, Loffler H, Thiel E, et al: Morphological and cyto-chemical findings in 150 cases of T-lineage acute lymphoblastic leukaemia in adults: German Multicentre ALL Study Group (GMALL). Br J Haematol 1997;97:372.

96. Ludwig WD, Reiter A, Loffler H, et al: Immunophenotypic features of childhood and adult acute lymphoblastic leukemia (ALL): Expe-rience of the German Multicentre Trials ALL-BFM and GMALL. Leuk Lymphoma 1994;13:71.

97. Harris NL, Jaffe ES, Stein H, et al: A revised European-American classification of lymphoid neoplasms: A proposal from the Interna-tional Lymphoma Study Group. Blood 1994;84:1361.

98. Harris NL, Jaffe ES, Diebold J, et al: World Health Organization classification of neoplastic diseases of the hematopoietic and lymphoid tissues: Report of the clinical advisory committee meeting—Airlie House, Virginia, November 1997. J Clin Oncol 1999;17:3835.

99. Smith BR, Weinberg DS, Robert NJ, et al: Circulating monoclonal B lymphocytes in non-Hodgkin's lymphoma. N Engl J Med 1984; 311:1476.

100. Letwin BW, Wallace PK, Muirhead KA, et al: An improved clonal excess assay using flow cytometry and B-cell gating. Blood 1990; 75:1178.

101. Fukushima PI, Nguyen PK, O'Grady P, et al: Flow cytometric analysis of kappa and lambda light chain expression in evaluation of specimens for B-cell neoplasia. Cytometry 1996;26:243.

102. Geisler CH, Larsen JK, Hansen NE, et al: Prognostic importance of flow cytometric immunophenotyping of 540 consecutive patients with B-cell chronic lymphocytic leukemia. Blood 1991;78:1795.

103. Kurec AS, Threatte GA, Gottlieb AJ, et al: Immunophenotypic subclassification of chronic lymphocytic leukaemia (CLL). Br J Haematol 1992;81:45.

104. Shapiro JL, Miller ML, Pohlman B, et al: CD5 B-cell lymphoprolifer-ative disorders presenting in blood and bone marrow: A clinico-pathologic study of 40 patients. Am J Clin Pathol 1999;111:477.

105. Damle RN, Wasil T, Fais F, et al: Ig V gene mutation status and CD38 expression as novel prognostic indicators in chronic lymphocytic leukemia. Blood 1999;94:1840.

106. Rozman C, Montserrat E: Chronic lymphocytic leukemia. N Engl J Med 1995;333:1052.

107. Robbins BA, Ellison DJ, Spinosa JC, et al: Diagnostic application of two-color flow cytometry in 161 cases of hairy cell leukemia. Blood 1993;82:1277.

108. De Totero D, Tazzari PL, Lauria F, et al: Phenotypic analysis of hairy cell leukemia: "Variant" cases express the interleukin-2 re-ceptor beta chain, but not the alpha chain (CD25). Blood 1993; 82:528.

109. Kluin-Nelemans HC, Krouwels MM, Jansen JH, et al: Hairy cell leukemia preferentially expresses the IgG3 subclass. Blood 1990; 75:972.

110. Sainati L, Matutes E, Mulligan S, et al: A variant form of hairy cell leukemia resistant to alpha-interferon: Clinical and phenotypic characteristics of 17 patients. Blood 1990;76:157.

111. Matutes E, Morilla R, Owusu-Ankomah K, et al: The immunophe-notype of splenic lymphoma with villous lymphocytes and its relevance to the differential diagnosis with other B-cell disorders. Blood 1994;83:1558.

112. Molot RJ, Meeker TC, Wittwer CT, et al: Antigen expression and polymerase chain reaction amplification of mantle cell lympho-mas. Blood 1994;83:1626.

113. Bennett JM, Catovsky D, Daniel MT, et al: Proposals for the classi-fication of chronic (mature) B- and T-lymphoid leukaemias: French-American-British (FAB) Cooperative Group. J Clin Pathol 1989; 42:567.

114. Catovsky D, Matutes E: Leukemias of mature T cells. In Knowles DM, ed: Neoplastic Hematopathology. Baltimore, Williams & Wil-kins, 1992, p 1267.

115. Matutes E, Brito-Babapulle V, Swansbury J, et al: Clinical and laboratory features of 78 cases of T-prolymphocytic leukemia. Blood 1991;78:3269.

116. Brinkman K, van Dongen JJM, van Lom K, et al: Induction of clinical remission in T-large granular lymphocyte leukemia with cyclosporin A, monitored by use of immunophenotyping with Vbeta antibodies. Leukemia 1998;12:150.

117. Van den Beemd MWM, Boor PPC, Van Lochem EG, et al: Flow cytometric analysis of the Vβ repertoire in healthy controls. Cy-tometry 2000;40:336.

118. Haedicke W, Ho FCS, Chott A, et al: Expression of CD94/NKG2A and killer immunoglobulin-like receptors in NK cells and a subset of extranodal cytotoxic T-cell lymphomas. Blood 2000;95:3628.

119. Jaffe ES, Krenacs L, Raffeld M: Classification of T-cell and NK-cell neoplasms based on the REAL classification. Ann Oncol 1997;8:17.

120. Semenzato G, Zambello R, Starkebaum G, et al: The lymphoproli-ferative disease of granular lymphocytes: Updated criteria for diag-nosis. Blood 1997;89:256.

121. Bennett JM, Catovsky D, Daniel MT, et al: Proposed revised criteria for the classification of acute myeloid leukemia: A report of the French-American-British Cooperative Group. Ann Intern Med 1985;103:620.

122. San Miguel JF, Gonzalez M, Canizo MC, et al: Surface marker analysis in acute myeloid leukaemia and correlation with FAB classification. Br J Haematol 1986;64:547.

123. Drexler HG, Gignac SM, Minowada J: Routine immunophenotyp-ing of acute leukaemias. Blut 1988;57:327.

124. Drexler HG: Classification of acute myeloid leukemias: A compari-son of FAB and immunophenotyping. Leukemia 1987;1:697.

125. Adriaansen HJ, te Boekhorst PA, Hagemeijer AM, et al: Acute myeloid leukemia M4 with bone marrow eosinophilia (M4Eo) and inv(16)(p13q22) exhibits a specific immunophenotype with CD2 expression. Blood 1993;81:3043.

126. Terstappen LW, Safford M, Konemann S, et al: Flow cytometric characterization of acute myeloid leukemia. Part II. Phenotypic heterogeneity at diagnosis. Leukemia 1992;6:70.

127. Macedo A, Orfao A, Gonzalez M, et al: Immunological detection of blast cell subpopulations in acute myeloblastic leukemia at diagnosis: Implications for minimal residual disease studies. Leuke-mia 1995;9:993.

128. Nguyen PL, Olszak I, Harris NL, et al: Myeloperoxidase detection by three-color flow cytometry and by enzyme cytochemistry in the classification of acute leukemia. Am J Clin Pathol 1998;110: 163.

129. Khalidi HS, Medeiros LJ, Chang KL, et al: The immunophenotype of adult acute myeloid leukemia: High frequency of lymphoid antigen expression and comparison of immunophenotype French-American-British classification, and karyotypic abnormalities. Am J Clin Pathol 1998;109:211.

130. Bene MC, Bernier M, Casasnovas RO, et al: The reliability and specificity of c-kit for the diagnosis of acute myeloid leukemias and undifferentiated leukemias: The European Group for the Im-munological Classification of Leukemias (EGIL). Blood 1998;92: 596.

131. Solary E, Casasnovas RO, Campos L, et al: Surface markers in adult acute myeloblastic leukemia: Correlation of CD19+, CD34+ and CD14+/DR phenotypes with shorter survival. Groupe d'Etude Immunologique des Leucemies (GEIL). Leukemia 1992;6:393.

132. Del Poeta G, Stasi R, Venditti A, et al: Prognostic value of cell marker analysis in de novo acute myeloid leukemia. Leukemia 1994;8:388.

133. De Rossi G, Avvisati G, Coluzzi S, et al: Immunological definition of acute promyelocytic leukemia (FAB M3): A study of 39 cases. Eur J Haematol 1990;45:168.

134. Paietta E, Andersen J, Gallagher R, et al: The immunophenotype of acute promyelocytic leukemia (APL): An ECOG study. Leukemia 1994;8:1108.

135. Erber WN, Asbahr H, Rule SA, et al: Unique immunophenotype of acute promyelocytic leukaemia as defined by CD9 and CD68 antibodies. Br J Haematol 1994;88:101.

136. Bennett JM, Catovsky D, Daniel MT, et al: Criteria for the diagnosis of acute leukemia of megakaryocyte lineage (M7): A report of the French-American-British Cooperative Group. Ann Intern Med 1985;103:460.

137. Bennett JM, Catovsky D, Daniel MT, et al: Proposal for the recogni-tion of minimally differentiated acute myeloid leukaemia (AML-M0). Br J Haematol 1991;78:325.

138. Villamor N, Zarco MA, Rozman M, et al: Acute myeloblastic leuke-mia with minimal myeloid differentiation: Phenotypical and ultra-structural characteristics. Leukemia 1998;12:1071.

139. Drexler HG, Sperling C, Ludwig WD: Terminal deoxynucleotidyl transferase (TdT) expression in acute myeloid leukemia. Leukemia 1993;7:1142.

140. Reuss-Borst MA, Buhring HJ, Schmidt H, et al: AML: Immunophenotypic heterogeneity and prognostic significance of c-kit expression. Leukemia 1994;8:258.

141. Suzuki R, Yamamoto K, Seto M, et al: CD7+ and CD56+ myeloid/natural killer cell precursor acute leukemia: A distinct hematolymphoid disease entity. Blood 1997;90:2417.

142. Drexler HG, Thiel E, Ludwig WD: Review of the incidence and clinical relevance of myeloid antigen-positive acute lymphoblastic leukemia. Leukemia 1991;5:637.

143. Smith FO, Lampkin BC, Versteeg C, et al: Expression of lymphoid-associated cell surface antigens by childhood acute myeloid leukemia cells lacks prognostic significance. Blood 1992;79:2415.

144. Drexler HG, Thiel E, Ludwig WD: Acute myeloid leukemias expressing lymphoid-associated antigens: Diagnostic incidence and prognostic significance. Leukemia 1993;7:489.

145. Reading CL, Estey EH, Huh YO, et al: Expression of unusual immunophenotype combinations in acute myelogenous leukemia. Blood 1993;81:3083.

146. Wiersma SR, Ortega J, Sobel E, et al: Clinical importance of myeloid-antigen expression in acute lymphoblastic leukemia of childhood. N Engl J Med 1991;324:800.

147. Paietta E, Van Ness B, Bennett J, et al: Lymphoid lineage–associated features in acute myeloid leukaemia: Phenotypic and genotypic correlations. Br J Haematol 1992;82:324.

148. Pui CH, Rubnitz JE, Hancock ML, et al: Reappraisal of the clinical and biologic significance of myeloid-associated antigen expression in childhood acute lymphoblastic leukemia. J Clin Oncol 1998;16:3768.

149. Greaves MF, Chan LC, Furley AJ, et al: Lineage promiscuity in hemopoietic differentiation and leukemia. Blood 1986;67:1.

150. Kantarjian HM, Deisseroth A, Kurzrock R, et al: Chronic myelogenous leukemia: A concise update. Blood 1993;82:691.

151. Kantarjian HM, Keating MJ, Talpaz M, et al: Chronic myelogenous leukemia in blast crisis: Analysis of 242 patients. Am J Med 1987;83:445.

152. Khalidi HS, Brynes RK, Medeiros LJ, et al: The immunophenotype of blast transformation of chronic myelogenous leukemia: A high frequency of mixed lineage phenotype in "lymphoid" blasts and a comparison of morphologic, immunophenotypic, and molecular findings. Mod Pathol 1998;11:1211.

153. Amylon MD, Shuster J, Pullen J, et al: Intensive high-dose asparaginase consolidation improves survival for pediatric patients with T-cell acute lymphoblastic leukemia and advanced-stage lymphoblastic lymphoma: A Pediatric Oncology Group study. Leukemia 1999;13:335.

154. Davis BH, Foucar K, Szczarkowski W, et al: U.S.–Canadian consensus recommendations on the immunophenotypic analysis of hematologic neoplasia by flow cytometry: Medical indications. Cytometry 1997;30:249.

155. Uckun FM, Sather HN, Gaynon PS, et al: Clinical features and treatment outcome of children with myeloid antigen-positive acute lymphoblastic leukemia: A report from the Children's Cancer Group. Blood 1997;90:28.

156. Putti MC, Rondelli R, Cocito MG, et al: Expression of myeloid markers lacks prognostic impact in children treated for acute lymphoblastic leukemia: Italian experience in AIEOP-ALL 88-91 studies. Blood 1998;92:795.

157. Kita K, Miwa H, Nakase K, et al: Clinical importance of CD7 expression in acute myelocytic leukemia: The Japan Cooperative Group of Leukemia/Lymphoma. Blood 1993;81:2399.

158. Venditti A, Del Poeta G, Buccisano F, et al: Prognostic relevance of the expression of Tdt and CD7 in 335 cases of acute myeloid leukemia. Leukemia 1998;12:1056.

159. Smith FO, Broudy VC, Zsebo KM, et al: Cell surface expression of c-kit receptors by childhood acute myeloid leukemia blasts is not of prognostic value: A report from the Children's Cancer Group. Blood 1994;84:847.

160. Naughton MJ, Hess JL, Zutter MM, et al: Bone marrow staging in patients with non-Hodgkin's lymphoma: Is flow cytometry a useful test? Cancer 1998;82:1154.

161. Hanson CA, Kurtin PJ, Katzmann JA, et al: Immunophenotypic analysis of peripheral blood and bone marrow in the staging of B-cell malignant lymphoma. Blood 1999;94:3889.

162. Hagemeijer A, van Dongen JJM, Slater RM, et al: Characterization of the blast cells in acute leukemia with translocation (4;11):

163. Behm FG, Smith FO, Raimondi SC, et al: Human homologue of the rat chondroitin sulfate proteoglycan, NG2, detected by monoclonal antibody 7.1 identifies childhood acute lymphoblastic leukemias with t(4;11)(q21;q23) or t(11;19)(q23;p13) and MLL gene rearrangements. Blood 1996;87:1134.

164. Griesinger F, Elfers H, Ludwig WD, et al: Detection of HRX-FEL fusion transcripts in pre-B-ALL with and without cytogenetic demonstration of t(4;11). Leukemia 1994;8:542.

165. Ludwig WD, Rieder H, Bartram CR, et al: Immunophenotypic and genotypic features, clinical characteristics, and treatment outcome of adult pro-B acute lymphoblastic leukemia: Results of the German multicenter trials GMALL 03/87 and 04/89. Blood 1998;92:1898.

166. Pui CH, Raimondi SC, Dodge RK, et al: Prognostic importance of structural chromosomal abnormalities in children with hyperdiploid (greater than 50 chromosomes) acute lymphoblastic leukemia. Blood 1989;73:1963.

167. Borowitz MJ, Hunger SP, Carroll AJ, et al: Predictability of the t(1;19)(q23;p13) from surface antigen phenotype: Implications for screening cases of childhood acute lymphoblastic leukemia for molecular analysis: A Pediatric Oncology Group study. Blood 1993;82:1086.

168. Privitera E, Kamps MP, Hayashi Y, et al: Different molecular consequences of the 1;19 chromosomal translocation in childhood B-cell precursor acute lymphoblastic leukemia. Blood 1992;79:1781.

169. Borowitz MJ, Rubnitz J, Nash M, et al: Surface antigen phenotype can predict TEL-AML1 rearrangement in childhood B-precursor ALL: A Pediatric Oncology Group study. Leukemia 1998;12:1764.

170. Baruchel A, Cayuela JM, Ballerini P, et al: The majority of myeloid-antigen-positive (My +) childhood B-cell precursor acute lymphoblastic leukaemias express TEL-AML1 fusion transcripts. Br J Haematol 1997;99:101.

171. Hrusak O, Trka J, Zuna J, et al: Aberrant expression of KOR-SA3544 antigen in childhood acute lymphoblastic leukemia predicts TEL-AML1 negativity: The Pediatric Hematology Working Group in the Czech Republic. Leukemia 1998;12:1064.

172. Mori T, Sugita K, Suzuki T, et al: A novel monoclonal antibody, KOR-SA3544, which reacts to Philadelphia chromosome–positive acute lymphoblastic leukemia cells with high sensitivity. Leukemia 1995;9:1233.

173. Paietta E, Racevskis J, Neuberg D, et al: Expression of CD25 (interleukin-2 receptor alpha chain) in adult acute lymphoblastic leukemia predicts for the presence of BCR/ABL fusion transcripts: Results of a preliminary laboratory analysis of ECOG/MRC Intergroup Study E2993. Eastern Cooperative Oncology Group/Medical Research Council. Leukemia 1997;11:1887.

174. Hurwitz CA, Raimondi SC, Head D, et al: Distinctive immunophenotypic features of t(8;21)(q22;q22) acute myeloblastic leukemia in children. Blood 1992;80:3182.

175. Kita K, Nakase K, Miwa H, et al: Phenotypical characteristics of acute myelocytic leukemia associated with the t(8;21)(q22;q22) chromosomal abnormality: Frequent expression of immature B-cell antigen CD19 together with stem cell antigen CD34. Blood 1992;80:470.

176. Smith FO, Rauch C, Williams DE, et al: The human homologue of rat NG2, a chondroitin sulfate proteoglycan, is not expressed on the cell surface of normal hematopoietic cells but is expressed by acute myeloid leukemia blasts from poor-prognosis patients with abnormalities of chromosome band 11q23. Blood 1996;87:1123.

177. Hilden JM, Smith FO, Frestedt JL, et al: MLL gene rearrangement, cytogenetic 11q23 abnormalities, and expression of the NG2 molecule in infant acute myeloid leukemia. Blood 1997;89:3801.

178. Mauvieux L, Delabesse E, Bourquelot P, et al: NG2 expression in MLL rearranged acute myeloid leukaemia is restricted to monoblastic cases. Br J Haematol 1999;107:674.

179. Brito-Babapulle V, Pomfret M, Matutes E, et al: Cytogenetic studies on prolymphocytic leukemia. II. T-cell prolymphocytic leukemia. Blood 1987;70:926.

180. Sang BC, Shi L, Dias P, et al: Monoclonal antibodies specific to the acute lymphoblastic leukemia t(1;19)-associated E2A/PBX1 chimeric protein: Characterization and diagnostic utility. Blood 1997;89:2909.

181. Viswanatha DS, Chen I, Liu PP, et al: Characterization and use of

Report of eight additional cases and of one case with a variant translocation. Leukemia 1987;1:24.

an antibody detecting the CBFbeta-SMMHC fusion protein in inv(16)/t(16;16)-associated acute myeloid leukemias. Blood 1998; 91:1882.

182. Tonegawa S: Somatic generation of antibody diversity. Nature 1983;302:575.

183. Davis MM, Björkman PJ: T-cell antigen receptor genes and T-cell recognition. Nature 1988;334:395.

184. Van Dongen JJM, Wolvers-Tettero ILM: Analysis of immunoglobulin and T-cell receptor genes. Part I: Basic and technical aspects. Clin Chim Acta 1991;198:1.

185. Van Dongen JJM, Wolvers-Tettero ILM: Analysis of immunoglobulin and T-cell receptor genes. Part II: Possibilities and limitations in the diagnosis and management of lymphoproliferative diseases and related disorders. Clin Chim Acta 1991;198:93.

186. Chen J, Alt FW: Gene rearrangement and B-cell development. Curr Opin Immunol 1993;5:194.

187. Ravetch JV, Siebenlist U, Korsmeyer S, et al: Structure of the human immunoglobulin mu locus: Characterization of embryonic and rearranged J and D genes. Cell 1981;27:583.

188. Ichihara Y, Matsuoka H, Kurosawa Y: Organization of human immunoglobulin heavy chain diversity gene loci. EMBO J 1988; 7:4141.

189. Matsuda F, Shin EK, Nagaoka H, et al: Structure and physical map of 64 variable segments in the 3′0.8-megabase region of the human immunoglobulin heavy-chain locus. Nat Genet 1993;3:88.

190. Hieter PA, Max EE, Seidman JG, et al: Cloned human and mouse kappa immunoglobulin constant and J region genes conserve homology in functional segments. Cell 1980;22:197.

191. Schäble KF, Zachau HG: The variable genes of the human immunoglobulin kappa locus. Biol Chem Hoppe Seyler 1993;374:1001.

192. Vasicek TJ, Leder P: Structure and expression of the human immunoglobulin lambda genes. J Exp Med 1990;172:609.

193. Bauer TR Jr, Blomberg B: The human lambda L chain Ig locus: Recharacterization of JC lambda 6 and identification of a functional JC lambda 7. J Immunol 1991;146:2813.

194. Williams SC, Winter G: Cloning and sequencing of human immunoglobulin V lambda gene segments. Eur J Immunol 1993;23:1456.

195. Yoshikai Y, Clark SP, Taylor S, et al: Organization and sequences of the variable, joining and constant region genes of the human T-cell receptor alpha-chain. Nature 1985;316:837.

196. Griesser H, Champagne E, Tkachuk D, et al: The human T-cell receptor alpha-delta locus: A physical map of the variable, joining and constant region genes. Eur J Immunol 1988;18:641.

197. Toyonaga B, Yoshikai Y, Vadasz V, et al: Organization and sequences of the diversity, joining, and constant region genes of the human T-cell receptor beta chain. Proc Natl Acad Sci U S A 1985; 82:8624.

198. Quertermous T, Strauss WM, Van Dongen JJM, et al: Human T-cell gamma chain joining regions and T-cell development. J Immunol 1987;138:2687.

199. Lefranc MP, Rabbitts TH: The human T-cell receptor gamma (TRG) genes. Trends Biochem Sci 1989;14:214.

200. Zhang XM, Tonnelle C, Lefranc MP, et al: T-cell receptor gamma cDNA in human fetal liver and thymus: Variable regions of gamma chains are restricted to V gamma I or V9, due to the absence of splicing of the V10 and V11 leader intron. Eur J Immunol 1994; 24:571.

201. Takihara Y, Tkachuk D, Michalopoulos E, et al: Sequence and organization of the diversity, joining, and constant region genes of the human T-cell delta-chain locus. Proc Natl Acad Sci U S A 1988;85:6097.

202. Breit TM, Wolvers-Tettero ILM, Beishuizen A, et al: Southern blot patterns, frequencies and junctional diversity of T-cell receptor δ gene rearrangements in acute lymphoblastic leukemia. Blood 1993;82:3063.

203. Davodeau F, Peyrat MA, Hallet MM, et al: Characterization of a new functional TCR J-delta segment in humans: Evidence for a marked conservation of J-delta sequences between humans, mice, and sheep. J Immunol 1994;153:137.

204. Schatz DG, Oettinger MA, Baltimore D: The V(D)J recombination activating gene RAG-1. Cell 1989;59:1035.

205. Oettinger MA, Schatz DG, Gorka C, et al: RAG-1 and RAG-2, adjacent genes that synergistically activate V(D)J recombination. Science 1990;248:1517.

206. Lieber MR: The mechanism of V(D)J recombination: A balance of diversity, specificity, and stability. Cell 1992;70:873.

207. Lieber MR: The role of site-directed recombinases in physiologic and pathologic chromosomal rearrangements. In Kirsch IR, ed: The Causes and Consequences of Chromosomal Aberrations. CRC Press, 1993, p 240.

208. Reth MG, Jackson S, Alt FW: VHDJH formation and DJH replacement during pre-B differentiation: Non-random usage of gene segments. EMBO J 1986;5:2131.

209. Marolleau JP, Fondell JD, Malissen M, et al: The joining of germline V alpha to J alpha genes replaces the preexisting V alpha–J alpha complexes in a T-cell receptor alpha, beta–positive T-cell line. Cell 1988;55:291.

210. Reth M, Gehrmann P, Petrac E, et al: A novel VH to VHDJH joining mechanism in heavy-chain–negative (null) pre-B cells results in heavy-chain production. Nature 1986;322:840.

211. Kleinfield R, Hardy RR, Tarlinton D, et al: Recombination between an expressed immunoglobulin heavy-chain gene and a germline variable gene segment in a Ly 1 + B-cell lymphoma. Nature 1986; 322:843.

212. Covey LR, Ferrier P, Alt FW: VH to VHDJH rearrangement is mediated by the internal VH heptamer. Int Immunol 1990;2:579.

213. Fondell JD, Marolleau JP, Primi D, et al: On the mechanism of non-allelically excluded V alpha–J alpha T-cell receptor secondary rearrangement in a murine T-cell lymphoma. J Immunol 1990; 144:1094.

214. Cook GP, Tomlinson IM: The human immunoglobulin VH repertoire. Immunol Today 1995;16:237.

215. Matsuda F, Ishii K, Bourvagnet P, et al: The complete nucleotide sequence of the human immunoglobulin heavy chain variable region locus. J Exp Med 1998;188:2151.

216. Corbett SJ, Tomlinson IM, Sonnhammer ELL, et al: Sequence of the human immunoglobulin diversity (D) segment locus: A systematic analysis provides no evidence for the use of DIR segments, inverted D segments, "minor" D segments or D-D recombination. J Mol Biol 1997;270:587.

217. Alt FW, Blackwell TK, Yancopoulos GD: Development of the primary antibody repertoire. Science 1987;238:1079.

218. Schroeder HW Jr, Hillson JL, Perlmutter RM: Early restriction of the human antibody repertoire. Science 1987;238:791.

219. Leiden JM, Dialynas DP, Duby AD, et al: Rearrangement and expression of T-cell antigen receptor genes in human T-lymphocyte tumor lines and normal human T-cell clones: Evidence for allelic exclusion of Ti beta gene expression and preferential use of a J beta 2 gene segment. Mol Cell Biol 1986;6:3207.

220. Triebel F, Hercend T: Subpopulations of human peripheral T gamma delta lymphocytes. Immunol Today 1989;10:186.

221. Borst J, Wicherink A, Van Dongen JJM, et al: Non-random expression of T-cell receptor gamma and delta variable gene segments in functional T lymphocyte clones from human peripheral blood. Eur J Immunol 1989;19:1559.

222. Breit TM, Wolvers-Tettero IL, van Dongen JJ: Unique selection determinant in polyclonal V delta 2–J delta 1 junctional regions of human peripheral gamma delta T lymphocytes. J Immunol 1994; 152:2860.

223. Desiderio SV, Yancopoulos GD, Paskind M, et al: Insertion of N regions into heavy-chain genes is correlated with expression of terminal deoxytransferase in B cells. Nature 1984;311:752.

224. Landau NR, Schatz DG, Rosa M, et al: Increased frequency of N-region insertion in a murine pre-B-cell line infected with a terminal deoxynucleotidyl transferase retroviral expression vector. Mol Cell Biol 1987;7:3237.

225. Elliott JF, Rock EP, Patten PA, et al: The adult T-cell receptor delta chain is diverse and distinct from that of fetal thymocytes. Nature 1988;331:627.

226. Breit TM, Wolvers-Tettero IL, Bogers AJ, et al: Rearrangements of the human TCRD-deleting elements. Immunogenetics 1994;40:70.

227. Shiokawa S, Mortari F, Lima JO, et al: IgM heavy-chain complementarity-determining region 3 diversity is constrained by genetic and somatic mechanisms until two months after birth. J Immunol 1999;162:6060.

228. Victor KD, Capra JD: An apparently common mechanism of generating antibody diversity: Length variation of the VL-JL junction. Mol Immunol 1994;31:39.

229. Michiels JJ, Adriaansen HJ, Hagemeijer A, et al: TdT-positive B-cell acute lymphoblastic leukaemia (B-ALL) without Burkitt characteristics. Br J Haematol 1988;68:423.

230. Berek C, Milstein C: Mutation drift and repertoire shift in the maturation of the immune response. Immunol Rev 1987;96:23.

231. Rajewsky K, Forster I, Cumano A: Evolutionary and somatic selection of the antibody repertoire in the mouse. Science 1987;238:1088.

232. Klein U, Goossens T, Fischer M, et al: Somatic hypermutation in normal and transformed human B cells. Immunol Rev 1998;162:261.

233. Maki R, Roeder W, Traunecker A, et al: The role of DNA rearrangement and alternative RNA processing in the expression of immunoglobulin delta genes. Cell 1981;24:353.

234. Knapp MR, Liu CP, Newell N, et al: Simultaneous expression of immunoglobulin mu and delta heavy chains by a cloned B-cell lymphoma: A single copy of the VH gene is shared by two adjacent CH genes. Proc Natl Acad Sci U S A 1982;79:2996.

235. Esser C, Radbruch A: Immunoglobulin class switching: Molecular and cellular analysis. Annu Rev Immunol 1990;8:717.

236. Shimizu A, Nussenzweig MC, Han H, et al: Trans-splicing as a possible molecular mechanism for the multiple isotype expression of the immunoglobulin gene. J Exp Med 1991;173:1385.

237. Kataoka T, Miyata T, Honjo T: Repetitive sequences in class-switch recombination regions of immunoglobulin heavy-chain genes. Cell 1981;23:357.

238. Jäck HM, McDowell M, Steinberg CM, et al: Looping out and deletion mechanism for the immunoglobulin heavy-chain class switch. Proc Natl Acad Sci U S A 1988;85:1581.

239. Snapper CM, Mond JJ: Towards a comprehensive view of immunoglobulin class switching. Immunol Today 1993;14:15.

240. Bertrand FE III, Billips LG, Burrows PD, et al: Ig D(H) gene segment transcription and rearrangement before surface expression of the pan–B-cell marker CD19 in normal human bone marrow. Blood 1997;90:736.

241. Davi F, Faili A, Gritti C, et al: Early onset of immunoglobulin heavy-chain gene rearrangements in normal human bone marrow CD34+ cells. Blood 1997;90:4014.

242. Ghia P, ten Boekel E, Sanz E, et al: Ordering of human bone marrow B-lymphocyte precursors by single-cell polymerase chain reaction analyses of the rearrangement status of the immunoglobulin H and L chain gene loci. J Exp Med 1996;184:2217.

243. Hieter PA, Korsmeyer SJ, Waldmann TA, et al: Human immunoglobulin kappa light-chain genes are deleted or rearranged in lambda-producing B cells. Nature 1981;290:368.

244. Korsmeyer SJ, Hieter PA, Sharrow SO, et al: Normal human B cells display ordered light-chain gene rearrangements and deletions. J Exp Med 1982;156:975.

245. Siminovitch KA, Bakhshi A, Goldman P, et al: A uniform deleting element mediates the loss of kappa genes in human B cells. Nature 1985;316:260.

246. Klobeck HG, Zachau HG: The human CK gene segment and the kappa deleting element are closely linked. Nucleic Acids Res 1986;14:4591.

247. Graninger WB, Goldman PL, Morton CC, et al: The kappa-deleting element: Germline and rearranged, duplicated and dispersed forms. J Exp Med 1988;167:488.

248. Isobe M, Russo G, Haluska FG, et al: Cloning of the gene encoding the delta subunit of the human T-cell receptor reveals its physical organization within the alpha-subunit locus and its involvement in chromosome translocations in T-cell malignancy. Proc Natl Acad Sci U S A 1988;85:3933.

249. De Villartay JP, Hockett RD, Coran D, et al: Deletion of the human T-cell receptor delta gene by a site-specific recombination. Nature 1988;335:170.

250. Hockett RD, de Villartay JP, Pollock K, et al: Human T-cell antigen receptor (TCR) delta-chain locus and elements responsible for its deletion are within the TCR alpha-chain locus. Proc Natl Acad Sci U S A 1988;85:9694.

251. Melchers F, Karasuyama H, Haasner D, et al: The surrogate light chain in B-cell development. Immunol Today 1993;14:60.

252. Groettrup M, Ungewiss K, Azogui O, et al: A novel disulfide-linked heterodimer on pre-T cells consists of the T-cell receptor beta chain and a 33-kd glycoprotein. Cell 1993;75:283.

253. Sambrook J, Fritsch EF, Maniatis T: Molecular cloning, a laboratory manual. Cold Spring Harbor Laboratory, 1989.

254. Beishuizen A, Verhoeven MA, Mol EJ, et al: Detection of immunoglobulin heavy-chain gene rearrangements by Southern blot analysis: Recommendations for optimal results. Leukemia 1993;7:2045.

255. Beishuizen A, Verhoeven MA, Mol EJ, et al: Detection of immunoglobulin kappa light-chain gene rearrangement patterns by Southern blot analysis. Leukemia 1994;8:2228.

256. Tümkaya T, Comans-Bitter WM, Verhoeven MA, et al: Southern blot detection of immunoglobulin lambda light-chain gene rearrangements for clonality studies. Leukemia 1995;9:2127.

257. Tümkaya T, Beishuizen A, Wolvers-Tettero ILM, et al: Identification of immunoglobulin lambda isotype gene rearrangements by Southern blot analysis. Leukemia 1996;10:1834.

258. Moreau EJ, Langerak AW, van Gastel-Mol EJ, et al: Easy detection of all T-cell receptor gamma (TCRG) gene rearrangements by Southern blot analysis: Recommendations for optimal results. Leukemia 1999;13:1620.

259. Langerak AW, Wolvers-Tettero ILM, van Dongen JJM: Detection of T-cell receptor beta (TCRB) gene rearrangement patterns in T-cell malignancies by Southern blot analysis. Leukemia 1999;13:965.

260. Saiki RK, Scharf S, Faloona F, et al: Enzymatic amplification of beta-globin genomic sequences and restriction site analysis for diagnosis of sickle cell anemia. Science 1985;230:1350.

261. White TJ, Arnheim N, Erlich HA: The polymerase chain reaction. Trends Genet 1989;5:185.

262. Newton CR, Graham A: PCR. Oxford, BIOS Scientific Publishers, 1994.

263. Yamada M, Hudson S, Tournay O, et al: Detection of minimal disease in hematopoietic malignancies of the B-cell lineage by using third-complementarity-determining region (CDR-III)–specific probes. Proc Natl Acad Sci U S A 1989;86:5123.

264. d'Auriol L, MacIntyre E, Galibert F, et al: In vitro amplification of T-cell gamma gene rearrangements: A new tool for the assessment of minimal residual disease in acute lymphoblastic leukemias. Leukemia 1989;3:155.

265. MacIntyre EA, d'Auriol L, Duparc N, et al: Use of oligonucleotide probes directed against T-cell antigen receptor gamma delta variable-(diversity)-joining junctional sequences as a general method for detecting minimal residual disease in acute lymphoblastic leukemias. J Clin Invest 1990;86:2125.

266. Breit TM, Wolvers-Tettero ILM, Hählen K, et al: Extensive junctional diversity of γδ T-cell receptors expressed by T-cell acute lymphoblastic leukemias: Implications for the detection of minimal residual disease. Leukemia 1991;5:1076.

267. Deane M, Norton JD: Immunoglobulin heavy-chain variable region family usage is independent of tumor cell phenotype in human B-lineage leukemias. Eur J Immunol 1990;20:2209.

268. Deane M, Norton JD: Immunoglobulin gene 'fingerprinting': An approach to analysis of B-lymphoid clonality in lymphoproliferative disorders. Br J Haematol 1991;77:274.

269. Veelken H, Tycko B, Sklar J: Sensitive detection of clonal antigen receptor gene rearrangements for the diagnosis and monitoring of lymphoid neoplasms by a polymerase chain reaction–mediated ribonuclease protection assay. Blood 1991;78:1318.

270. Oksenberg JR, Stuart S, Begovich AB, et al: Limited heterogeneity of rearranged T-cell receptor V-alpha transcripts in brains of multiple sclerosis patients. Nature 1991;353:94.

271. Broeren CP, Verjans GM, Van Eden W, et al: Conserved nucleotide sequences at the 5′ end of T-cell receptor variable genes facilitate polymerase chain reaction amplification. Eur J Immunol 1991;21:569.

272. Doherty PJ, Roifman CM, Pan SH, et al: Expression of the human T-cell receptor V beta repertoire. Mol Immunol 1991;28:607.

273. Hansen-Hagge TE, Yokota S, Bartram CR: Detection of minimal residual disease in acute lymphoblastic leukemia by in vitro amplification of rearranged T-cell receptor delta chain sequences. Blood 1989;74:1762.

274. Jonsson OG, Kitchens RL, Scott FC, et al: Detection of minimal residual disease in acute lymphoblastic leukemia using immunoglobulin hypervariable region-specific oligonucleotide probes. Blood 1990;76:2072.

275. Aubin J, Davi F, Nguyen-Salomon F, et al: Description of a novel FR1 IgH PCR strategy and its comparison with three other strategies for the detection of clonality in B-cell malignancies. Leukemia 1995;9:471.

276. Pongers-Willemse MJ, Seriu T, Stolz F, et al: Primers and protocols for standardized MRD detection in ALL using immunoglobulin and T-cell receptor gene rearrangements and TAL1 deletions as PCR targets. Report of the BIOMED-1 Concerted Action: Investigation

of minimal residual disease in acute leukemia. Leukemia 1999; 13:110.

277. Wei S, Charmley P, Robinson MA, et al: The extent of the human germline T-cell receptor V–beta gene segment repertoire. Immunogenetics 1994;40:27.

278. Van Oostveen JW, Breit TM, de Wolf JT, et al: Polyclonal expansion of T-cell receptor-γδ + T lymphocytes associated with neutropenia and thrombocytopenia. Leukemia 1992;6:410.

279. Kneba M, Bolz I, Linke B, et al: Characterization of clone-specific rearranged T-cell receptor gamma-chain genes in lymphomas and leukemias by the polymerase chain reaction and DNA sequencing. Blood 1994;84:574.

280. Davis TH, Yockey CE, Balk SP: Detection of clonal immunoglobulin gene rearrangements by polymerase chain reaction amplification and single-strand conformational polymorphism analysis. Am J Pathol 1993;142:1841.

281. Koch OM, Volkenandt M, Goker E, et al: Molecular detection and characterization of clonal cell populations in acute lymphocytic leukemia by analysis of conformational polymorphisms of cRNA molecules of rearranged T-cell-receptor-gamma and immunoglobulin heavy-chain genes. Leukemia 1994;8:946.

282. Bourguin A, Tung R, Galili N, et al: Rapid, nonradioactive detection of clonal T-cell receptor gene rearrangements in lymphoid neoplasms. Proc Natl Acad Sci U S A 1990;87:8536.

283. Wood GS, Tung RM, Haeffner AC, et al: Detection of clonal T-cell receptor gamma gene rearrangements in early mycosis fungoides/Sezary syndrome by polymerase chain reaction and denaturing gradient gel electrophoresis (PCR/DGGE). J Invest Dermatol 1994; 103:34.

284. Bottaro M, Berti E, Biondi A, et al: Heteroduplex analysis of T-cell receptor gamma gene rearrangements for diagnosis and monitoring of cutaneous T-cell lymphomas. Blood 1994;83:3271.

285. Langerak AW, Szczepanski T, van der Burg M, et al: Heteroduplex PCR analysis of rearranged T-cell receptor genes for clonality assessment in suspect T-cell proliferations. Leukemia 1997;11:2192.

286. Linke B, Pyttlich J, Tiemann M, et al: Identification and structural analysis of rearranged immunoglobulin heavy-chain genes in lymphomas and leukemias. Leukemia 1995;9:840.

287. Derksen PW, Langerak AW, Kerkhof E, et al: Comparison of different polymerase chain reaction-based approaches for clonality assessment of immunoglobulin heavy-chain gene rearrangements in B-cell neoplasia. Mod Pathol 1999;12:794.

288. Linke B, Bolz I, Fayyazi A, et al: Automated high-resolution PCR fragment analysis for identification of clonally rearranged immunoglobulin heavy-chain genes. Leukemia 1997;11:1055.

289. Kneba M, Bolz I, Linke B, et al: Analysis of rearranged T-cell receptor beta-chain genes by polymerase chain reaction (PCR) DNA sequencing and automated high-resolution PCR fragment analysis. Blood 1995;86:3930.

290. Prosser J: Detecting single-base mutations. Trends Biotechnol 1993;11:238.

291. Williams ME, Innes DJ Jr, Borowitz MJ, et al: Immunoglobulin and T-cell receptor gene rearrangements in human lymphoma and leukemia. Blood 1987;69:79.

292. Korsmeyer SJ, Arnold A, Bakhshi A, et al: Immunoglobulin gene rearrangement and cell surface antigen expression in acute lymphocytic leukemias of T-cell and B-cell precursor origins. J Clin Invest 1983;71:301.

293. Felix CA, Wright JJ, Poplack DG, et al: T-cell receptor alpha, beta, and gamma genes in T-cell and pre–B-cell acute lymphoblastic leukemia. J Clin Invest 1987;80:545.

294. Foroni L, Catovsky D, Luzzatto L: Immunoglobulin gene rearrangements in hairy cell leukemia and other chronic B-cell lymphoproliferative disorders. Leukemia 1987;1:389.

295. Furley AJ, Mizutani S, Weilbaecher K, et al: Developmentally regulated rearrangement and expression of genes encoding the T-cell receptor-T3 complex. Cell 1986;46:75.

296. Van Dongen JJM, Quertermous T, Bartram CR, et al: T-cell receptor-CD3 complex during early T-cell differentiation: Analysis of immature T-cell acute lymphoblastic leukemias (T-ALL) at DNA, RNA, and cell membrane level. J Immunol 1987;138:1260.

297. Foroni L, Foldi J, Matutes E, et al: Alpha, beta and gamma T-cell receptor genes: Rearrangements correlate with haematological phenotype in T-cell leukaemias. Br J Haematol 1987;67:307.

298. Adriaansen HJ, Soeting PW, Wolvers-Tettero ILM, et al: Immuno-

globulin and T-cell receptor gene rearrangements in acute non-lymphocytic leukemias: Analysis of 54 cases and a review of the literature. Leukemia 1991;5:744.

299. Szczepanski T, Beishuizen A, Pongers-Willemse MJ, et al: Cross-lineage T-cell receptor gene rearrangements occur in more than ninety percent of childhood precursor–B-acute lymphoblastic leukemias: Alternative PCR targets for detection of minimal residual disease. Leukemia 1999;13:196.

300. Beishuizen A, Hählen K, Hagemeijer A, et al: Multiple rearranged immunoglobulin genes in childhood acute lymphoblastic leukemia of precursor B-cell origin. Leukemia 1991;5:657.

301. Beishuizen A, van Wering ER, Breit TM, et al: Molecular biology of acute lymphoblastic leukemia: Implications for detection of minimal residual disease. In Hiddeman W, Büchner T, Wörmann B, eds: Acute Leukemias V. Berlin, Springer Verlag, 1996, p 460.

302. Bird J, Galili N, Link M, et al: Continuing rearrangement but absence of somatic hypermutation in immunoglobulin genes of human B-cell precursor leukemia. J Exp Med 1988;168:229.

303. Kitchingman GR: Immunoglobulin heavy-chain gene VH-D junctional diversity at diagnosis in patients with acute lymphoblastic leukemia. Blood 1993;81:775.

304. Steenbergen EJ, Verhagen OJ, van Leeuwen EF, et al: Distinct ongoing Ig heavy chain rearrangement processes in childhood B-precursor acute lymphoblastic leukemia. Blood 1993;82:581.

305. Steward CG, Goulden NJ, Katz F, et al: A polymerase chain reaction study of the stability of Ig heavy-chain and T-cell receptor delta-gene rearrangements between presentation and relapse of childhood B-lineage acute lymphoblastic leukemia. Blood 1994;83:1355.

306. Wasserman R, Yamada M, Ito Y, et al: VH gene rearrangement events can modify the immunoglobulin heavy chain during progression of B-lineage acute lymphoblastic leukemia. Blood 1992; 79:223.

307. Biondi A, Francia di Celle P, Rossi V, et al: High prevalence of T-cell receptor V delta 2-(D)-D delta 3 or D delta 1/2-D delta 3 rearrangements in B-precursor acute lymphoblastic leukemias. Blood 1990;75:1834.

308. Ghali DW, Panzer S, Fischer S, et al: Heterogeneity of the T-cell receptor delta gene indicating subclone formation in acute precursor B-cell leukemias. Blood 1995;85:2795.

309. Hansen-Hagge TE, Yokota S, Reuter HJ, et al: Human common acute lymphoblastic leukemia–derived cell lines are competent to recombine their T-cell receptor delta/alpha regions along a hierarchically ordered pathway. Blood 1992;80:2353.

310. Yokota S, Hansen-Hagge TE, Bartram CR: T-cell receptor delta gene recombination in common acute lymphoblastic leukemia: Preferential usage of V delta 2 and frequent involvement of the J-alpha cluster. Blood 1991;77:141.

311. Steenbergen EJ, Verhagen OJ, van Leeuwen EF, et al: Frequent ongoing T-cell receptor rearrangements in childhood B-precursor acute lymphoblastic leukemia: Implications for monitoring minimal residual disease. Blood 1995;86:692.

312. Szczepanski T, Langerak AW, Wolvers-Tettero ILM, et al: Immunoglobulin and T-cell receptor gene rearrangement patterns in acute lymphoblastic leukemia are less mature in adults than in children: Implications for selection of PCR targets for detection of minimal residual disease. Leukemia 1998;12:1081.

313. Beishuizen A, Verhoeven MA, van Wering ER, et al: Analysis of Ig and T-cell receptor genes in 40 childhood acute lymphoblastic leukemias at diagnosis and subsequent relapse: Implications for the detection of minimal residual disease by polymerase chain reaction analysis. Blood 1994;83:2238.

314. Taylor JJ, Rowe D, Kylefjord H, et al: Characterisation of non-concordance in the T-cell receptor gamma chain genes at presentation and clinical relapse in acute lymphoblastic leukemia. Leukemia 1994;8:60.

315. Baruchel A, Cayuela JM, MacIntyre E, et al: Assessment of clonal evolution at Ig/TCR loci in acute lymphoblastic leukaemia by single-strand conformation polymorphism studies and highly resolutive PCR-derived methods: Implication for a general strategy of minimal residual disease detection. Br J Haematol 1995;90:85.

316. Klein U, Klein G, Ehlin-Henriksson B, et al: Burkitt's lymphoma is a malignancy of mature B cells expressing somatically mutated V-region genes. Mol Med 1995;1:495.

317. Tamaru J, Hummel M, Marafioti T, et al: Burkitt's lymphomas

express VH genes with a moderate number of antigen-selected somatic mutations. Am J Pathol 1995;147:1398.

318. Chapman CJ, Zhou JX, Gregory C, et al: VH and VL gene analysis in sporadic Burkitt's lymphoma shows somatic hypermutation, intraclonal heterogeneity, and a role for antigen selection. Blood 1996;88:3562.

319. Szczepanski T, Langerak AW, Willemse MJ, et al: T-cell receptor gamma (TCRG) gene rearrangements in T-cell acute lymphoblastic leukemia reflect "end-stage" recombinations: Implications for minimal residual disease monitoring. Leukemia 2000;14:1208.

320. Szczepanski T, Pongers-Willemse MJ, Langerak AW, et al: Ig heavy-chain gene rearrangements in T-cell acute lymphoblastic leukemia exhibit predominant DH6-19 and DH7-27 gene usage, can result in complete V-D-J rearrangements, and are rare in T-cell receptor αβ lineage. Blood 1999;93:4079.

321. Breit TM, Verschuren MCM, Wolvers-Tettero ILM, et al: Human T-cell leukemias with continuous V(D)J recombinase activity for TCR–delta gene deletion. J Immunol 1997;159:4341.

322. Szczepanski T, Pongers-Willemse MJ, Langerak AW, et al: Unusual immunoglobulin and T-cell receptor gene rearrangement patterns in acute lymphoblastic leukemias. Curr Top Microbiol Immunol 1999;246:205.

323. Schmidt CA, Oettle H, Neubauer A, et al: Rearrangements of T-cell receptor delta, gamma and beta genes in acute myeloid leukemia coexpressing T-lymphoid features. Leukemia 1992;6:1263.

324. Sanchez I, San Miguel JF, Corral J, et al: Gene rearrangement in acute non-lymphoblastic leukaemia: Correlation with morphological and immunophenotypic characteristics of blast cells. Br J Haematol 1995;89:104.

325. Waldmann TA, Davis MM, Bongiovanni KF, et al: Rearrangements of genes for the antigen receptor on T cells as markers of lineage and clonality in human lymphoid neoplasms. N Engl J Med 1985; 313:776.

326. Matsuoka M, Hagiya M, Hattori T, et al: Gene rearrangements of T-cell receptor beta and gamma chains in HTLV-I infected primary neoplastic T cells. Leukemia 1988;2:84.

327. Whittaker SJ, Smith NP, Jones RR, et al: Analysis of beta, gamma, and delta T-cell receptor genes in mycosis fungoides and Sezary syndrome. Cancer 1991;68:1572.

328. Kneba M, Bergholz M, Bolz I, et al: Heterogeneity of immunoglobulin gene rearrangements in B-cell lymphomas. Int J Cancer 1990; 45:609.

329. Szczepanski T, Langerak AW, van Dongen JJM, et al: Lymphoma with multi-gene rearrangement on the level of immunoglobulin heavy-chain, light-chain, and T-cell receptor beta chain. Am J Hematol 1998;59:99.

330. O'Connor N, Gatter KC, Wainscoat JS, et al: Practical value of genotypic analysis for diagnosing lymphoproliferative disorders. J Clin Pathol 1987;40:147.

331. Korsmeyer SJ: Antigen receptor genes as molecular markers of lymphoid neoplasms. J Clin Invest 1987;79:1291.

332. Van Dongen JJM: Analysis of immunoglobulin genes and T-cell receptor genes as a diagnostic tool for the detection of lymphoid malignancies. Neth J Med 1987;31:201.

333. Knulst AC, Adriaansen HJ, Hahlen K, et al: Early diagnosis of smoldering acute lymphoblastic leukemia using immunological marker analysis. Leukemia 1993;7:532.

334. Morley AA, Brisco MJ, Rice M, et al: Leukaemia presenting as marrow hypoplasia: Molecular detection of the leukaemic clone at the time of initial presentation. Br J of Haematol 1997;98:940.

335. Van Lochem EG, Wiegers YM, van den Beemd R, et al: Regeneration pattern of precursor–B-cells in bone marrow of acute lymphoblastic leukemia patients depends on the type of preceding chemotherapy. Leukemia 2000;14:688.

336. Raffeld M, Wright JJ, Lipford E, et al: Clonal evolution of t(14;18) follicular lymphomas demonstrated by immunoglobulin genes and the 18q21 major breakpoint region. Cancer Res 1987;47:2537.

337. Cleary ML, Galili N, Trela M, et al: Single-cell origin of bigenotypic and biphenotypic B cell proliferations in human follicular lymphomas. J Exp Med 1988;167:582.

338. De Jong D, Voetdijk BM, van Ommen GJ, et al: Alterations in immunoglobulin genes reveal the origin and evolution of monotypic and bitypic B-cell lymphomas. Am J Pathol 1989;134:1233.

339. Wagner SD, Martinelli V, Luzzatto L: Similar patterns of V kappa gene usage but different degrees of somatic mutation in hairy cell leukemia, prolymphocytic leukemia, Waldenström's macroglobulinemia, and myeloma. Blood 1994;83:3647.

340. Cannell PK, Amlot P, Attard M, et al: Variable kappa gene rearrangement in lymphoproliferative disorders: An analysis of V-kappa gene usage, VJ joining and somatic mutation. Leukemia 1994;8:1139.

341. Cleary ML, Sklar J: Lymphoproliferative disorders in cardiac transplant recipients are multiclonal lymphomas. Lancet 1984;2:489.

342. Shearer WT, Ritz J, Finegold MJ, et al: Epstein-Barr virus–associated B-cell proliferations of diverse clonal origins after bone marrow transplantation in a 12-year-old patient with severe combined immunodeficiency. N Engl J Med 1985;312:1151.

343. Pelicci PG, Knowles II DM, Arlin ZA, et al: Multiple monoclonal B-cell expansions and c-myc oncogene rearrangements in acquired immune deficiency syndrome–related lymphoproliferative disorders: Implications for lymphomagenesis. J Exp Med 1986;164: 2049.

344. Hanto DW, Frizzera G, Gajl-Peczalska KJ, et al: Epstein-Barr virus, immunodeficiency, and B cell lymphoproliferation. Transplantation 1985;39:461.

345. Fernhout F, Dinkelaar RB, Hagemeijer A, et al: Four aged siblings with B-cell chronic lymphocytic leukemia. Leukemia 1997;11: 2060.

346. Siegelman MH, Cleary ML, Warnke R, et al: Frequent biclonality and Ig gene alterations among B-cell lymphomas that show multiple histologic forms. J Exp Med 1985;161:850.

347. Van Dongen JJM, Hooijkaas H, Michiels JJ, et al: Richter's syndrome with different immunoglobulin light chains and different heavy-chain gene rearrangements. Blood 1984;64:571.

348. Downing JR, Grossi CE, Smedberg CT, et al: Diffuse large-cell lymphoma in a patient with hairy cell leukemia: Immunoglobulin gene analysis reveals separate clonal origins. Blood 1986;67:739.

349. Michiels JJ, van Dongen JJM, Hagemeijer A, et al: Richter's syndrome with identical immunoglobulin gene rearrangements in the chronic lymphocytic leukemia and the supervening non-Hodgkin lymphoma. Leukemia 1989;3:819.

350. Van Dongen JJM, Hooijkaas H, Adriaansen HJ, et al: Detection of minimal residual acute lymphoblastic leukemia by immunological marker analysis: Possibilities and limitations. In Hagenbeek A, Löwenberg B, eds: Minimal Residual Disease in Acute Leukemia. Dordrecht, M Nijhoff Publishers, 1986, p 113.

351. Smedmyr B, Bengtsson M, Jakobsson A, et al: Regeneration of CALLA (CD10+), TdT+ and double-positive cells in the bone marrow and blood after autologous bone marrow transplantation. Eur J Haematol 1991;46:146.

352. Van Wering ER, van der Linden-Schrever BE, Szczepanski T, et al: Regenerating normal B-cell precursors during and after treatment of acute lymphoblastic leukaemia: Implications for monitoring of minimal residual disease. Br J Haematol 2000;110:139.

353. Campana D, Yokota S, Coustan-Smith E, et al: The detection of residual acute lymphoblastic leukemia cells with immunologic methods and polymerase chain reaction: A comparative study. Leukemia 1990;4:609.

354. Van Dongen JJM, Breit TM, Adriaansen HJ, et al: Detection of minimal residual disease in acute leukemia by immunological marker analysis and polymerase chain reaction. Leukemia 1992; 6:47.

355. Pongers-Willemse MJ, Verhagen OJHM, Tibbe GJM, et al: Real-time quantitative PCR for the detection of minimal residual disease in acute lymphoblastic leukemia using junctional regions–specific TaqMan probes. Leukemia 1998;12:2006.

356. Van Dongen JJM, Seriu T, Panzer-Grumayer ER, et al: Prognostic value of minimal residual disease in acute lymphoblastic leukaemia in childhood. Lancet 1998;352:1731.

357. Cave H, van der Werff ten Bosch J, Suciu S, et al: Clinical significance of minimal residual disease in childhood acute lymphoblastic leukemia. N Engl J Med 1998;339:591.

358. Lefranc MP, Giudicelli V, Ginestoux C, et al: IMGT, the international ImMunoGeneTics database. Nucleic Acids Res 1999;27:209.

359. Slightom JL, Siemieniak DR, Sieu LC, et al: Nucleotide sequence analysis of 77.7 kb of the human V beta T-cell receptor gene locus: Direct primer-walking using cosmid template DNAs. Genomics 1994;20:149.

360. Kawasaki K, Minoshima S, Nakato E, et al: One-megabase sequence analysis of the human immunoglobulin lambda gene locus. Genome Res 1997;7:250.

7

Epidemiology of Leukemia: Overview and Patterns of Occurrence

Martha S. Linet   Susan S. Devesa

INTRODUCTION

Leukemia was first identified in 1845[16, 293] and given its current designation in 1847.[294] Since then, leukemia has been distinguished from other hematopoietic and lymphoproliferative neoplasms, although it was classified as a single entity until 1957.[308] Then, lymphoid and myeloid leukemias were designated as separate forms in the seventh revision of the International Classification of Diseases (ICD).[309] By 1967, the major cell-type categories (acute lymphoblastic leukemia [ALL], chronic lymphocytic leukemia [CLL], acute myeloid leukemia [AML], acute monocytic leukemia, and chronic myeloid leukemia [CML]) were distinguished in the eighth revision of the ICD.[310]

Morphologic codes, developed for the International Classification of Diseases for Oncology (ICD-O),[214] were derived clinically from the French-American-British (FAB) Cooperative Group classification scheme. The FAB and other working group expert hematologists have identified morphologic and cytochemical features characterizing ALL,[17, 49] AML,[18, 20, 56] and chronic B- and T-lymphoid leukemias,[55, 139] as well as distinct subtypes within each category. For example, the FAB-defined subtypes of AML include minimally differentiated (M0), myeloblastic (M1 and M2), promyelocytic (M3), myelomonocytic (M4), monocytic (M5), erythroid (M6), and megakaryoblastic leukemias (M7).[18, 20] The FAB Cooperative Group has also described 14 distinct types of CLL,[55] most derived from mature B lymphocytes. Subtypes include the rare forms of prolymphocytic leukemia, hairy cell leukemia, and adult T-cell leukemia/lymphoma (ATLL), the latter two designated as forms of non-Hodgkin's lymphoma in the proposed third revision of the ICD-O (ICD-O-3).

The proposed ICD-O-3 uses immunophenotypic features as well as morphology to classify leukemia and lymphoma subtypes. Mounting evidence supports the need for cytogenetic and molecular as well as morphologic and immunophenotypic characterization of subtypes comprising ALL,[111, 138, 236] CLL,[171, 180, 181, 223, 238] AML,[106, 198, 206] bilineage acute leukemias,[182] and CML.[280] But progress has lagged in systematically applying cytoge-

netic, molecular, and immunophenotypic assessment within clinical settings. Thus, newly diagnosed leukemia cases reported to population-based cancer registries can frequently be classified by morphologic features only. For these reasons, leukemia incidence data reported by population-based cancer registries are still restricted to major cell types.[207, 208] Leukemia mortality data are additionally complicated and difficult to interpret because at least 30% of death certificates do not report a specific leukemia cell type.[213]

Therefore, the classification used in this chapter includes four specific leukemia cell types (ALL, CLL, AML, and CML), a combined category of other and not-otherwise-specified (NOS) leukemias, and the combination of these five categories that the authors designate as total leukemia. Based on the FAB system approach, monocytic leukemia is subsumed under the broader myeloid category of AML, which is interchangeable with acute non-lymphocytic leukemia (ANLL). The relative rarity of the leukemias, particularly for specific subtypes, requires evaluation of large populations and/or data compiled over many years from smaller populations to generate sufficiently stable rate estimates. Despite these problems, many descriptive and analytic studies have been carried out using data from population-based general cancer registries,[207, 208, 224] specialized registries of hematopoietic disorders,[47] or pediatric tumor registries.[24]

Earlier epidemiologic studies focused primarily on mortality outcomes. For leukemia subtypes characterized by poor survival, mortality and incidence rates are similar. In contrast, there is a growing divergence between mortality and incidence for childhood ALL, a substantial fraction of CLL, and a growing proportion of other leukemia types, due to improved survival. In the last two decades, therefore, incidence-based leukemia data have been reported increasingly, although mortality data are still valuable for assessing the public health burden and trend patterns.

DESCRIPTIVE EPIDEMIOLOGY

Comparison of Rates

Clues to etiology may be obtained by comparing rates for total leukemia and specific subtypes among populations.

All material in this chapter is in the public domain, with the exception of any borrowed figures or tables.

Rates are calculated by dividing the number of cases (or deaths) by the product of the population at risk times years of observation, or by the sum of the annual population estimates. The resulting rate is usually expressed as cases (or deaths) per 100,000 person-years at risk. Because populations differ in age structure and leukemia rates vary considerably by age, one can compare rates for individuals in the same age group (age-specific rates) or weighted averages for all age groups among populations, using a common reference population to derive the weights (age-standardized rate). Age-standardized rate comparisons can also be made among population subgroups defined by gender, race, occupation, or other characteristics of interest.

Lack of accurate population census or leukemia occurrence data, particularly in developing countries, precludes meaningful population-based mortality and incidence rate estimates. In more developed regions, mortality data are generally available because of mandatory death certification. Regional or nationwide population-based cancer incidence data are increasingly available, but only the Connecticut, United States,[52, 112] and Danish Cancer Registry[33, 34] have been in operation for more than 50 years.

With these considerations, we have examined U.S. mortality data from the National Center for Health Statistics and the most recently published international incidence data.[208] We generally selected cancer registries that operated for at least 15 years, reported incidence for the six leukemia categories, included at least 100 total leukemia cases during 1988–1992, and covered a wide geographic area and a range of ethnic groups. The U.S. incidence data are from the National Cancer Institute's Surveillance, Epidemiology, and End Results (SEER) program, which includes information from five states and four cities (comprising approximately 10% of the U.S. population).[224] Rates were age-standardized, using the world standard.

Mortality Patterns and Trends: Total Leukemia

Internationally, the highest age-standardized mortality rates for total leukemia occur in the populations of Western Europe, Oceania, and North America, where rates generally ranged from 4.8 to 7.4/100,000 person-years for males and from 3.2 to 4.6/100,000 for females.[10] It is noteworthy that rates for both males and females in Israel and Costa Rica closely parallel those of the industrialized countries of Europe, Oceania, and North America. Lower rates (ranging from 3.7 to 4.5 for males and from 2.8 to 3.5 for females) characterize populations in Asia and Latin America.[10]

U.S. data from 1970–1994 reveal excess age-standardized leukemia mortality rates in the north and south-central regions for whites (Fig. 7-1), a pattern similar to that seen earlier (1950–1969) for both sexes.[68] Unfortunately, mortality data are too sparse in the north and south-central regions to evaluate patterns for African Americans.

U.S. age-standardized mortality trends since 1950 have shown a modest decline among whites and a slight increase among nonwhites (the latter comprising African Americans, Asian-Pacific Islanders, and Native Americans). Overall, the mortality trends demonstrate a convergence of rates within gender, although rates have been consistently higher among males than females. Age-specific mortality patterns reveal dramatic declines for white and nonwhite children and adolescents (ages 0–19 years) since the early 1960s, whereas a less rapid decline characterizes young adults (ages 20–44 years) (Fig. 7-2). There was little change in mortality during 1950–1996 among middle-aged persons. Rates rose among the elderly of both racial groups, although the rate of increase slowed substantially after 1960 among whites. The great decline among children and the increase in the elderly were similarly evident in other populations, although mortality rates leveled off in the 1960s and 1970s among whites in most developed countries.[143]

Survival: U.S. Population-Based Data

Total Leukemia. Overall, 5-year relative survival (adjusted for general population mortality) from all forms of leukemia combined has improved significantly (rising from 34.4% to 43.1%) in regions covered by the U.S. SEER Program registries (Table 7-1). In general, for total leukemia and subtypes occurring at all ages, white patients survive longer than African-American patients, but survival is similar for males and females.[217, 224]

Leukemia Subtypes. Based on SEER Program data, survival improved from 1974–1976 to 1989–1995 for patients with each form of leukemia (see Table 7-1). When survival data for 1989–1995 are evaluated according to age at diagnosis, ALL patients show the largest gradient, with 5-year relative survival ranging from 81.1% among children ages 0–14 years to 5.8% among those age 65 years and older. Progressive worsening in survival with increasing age has also been found in ALL patients in the United Kingdom.[53] Particularly notable has been the dramatic improvement in 5-year relative survival for childhood leukemia that began in the 1960s.[35, 54, 262] Between 1973–1974 and 1989–1995 SEER data demonstrate an increase in 5-year relative survival from 53.2% to 81.1% for children with ALL and from 13.7% to 42.6% for those with AML.[224] Survival for children with ALL depends heavily on age at diagnosis, with highest survival among those ages 1–4 years (85%) and 5–9 years (80%) and lowest survival among infants (37%).[264] For childhood ALL overall, 5-year survival rates were slightly better for females than males and notably better for whites than African Americans.[264] Survival is also poorer for other racial groups in the United States than for whites, particularly American Indians, due to worse prognostic features and problems with treatment compliance.[87]

The patterns for childhood AML patients demonstrate higher survival in those ages 5–9 years at diagnosis than for either younger or older children, better survival in females than males, but similar survival outcome in white and African-American children. For patients with either form of childhood leukemia, differences in survival by age, gender, and race mostly reflect underlying biologic factors, although socioeconomic factors and health care access may also contribute. The treatment-related improvements in survival of children diagnosed with ALL

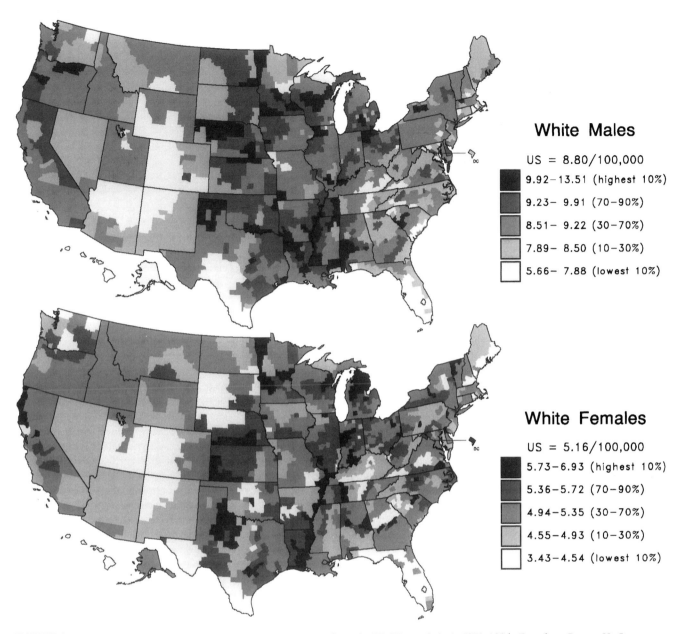

FIGURE 7–1. US leukemia mortality rates by state economic area (age-adjusted 1970 US population), 1970–1994. (Data from Devesa SS, Grauman DJ, Blot WJ, et al: Atlas of Cancer Mortality in the United States, 1950–94. Bethesda, Maryland: National Institutes of Health, National Cancer Institute, NIH Publication No. 99–4564, 1999.)

and AML have been responsible for the big declines in leukemia mortality among young people (see Fig. 7-2)[264]; some long-term survivors can be regarded as cured.[35]

CLL patients experienced a modest, although statistically significant, increase in 5-year relative survival between 1974–1976 and 1989–1995. Five-year relative survival was higher and similar among U.S. whites than among African Americans with CLL and higher in those younger than age 65 at diagnosis than older persons (see Table 7-1). Clinical trials, however, have shown little survival advantage for chemotherapy treatment of patients with indolent or early-stage CLL.[69, 139]

Among the four major leukemia cell types, prognosis is poorest for patients diagnosed with AML as adults; overall, 5-year relative survival is 14.5% in AML patients

of all ages combined during 1989–1995 (see Table 7-1). Unfortunately, results of clinical trials do not consistently support a survival advantage following treatment with autologous or allogeneic bone marrow transplantation compared with standard chemotherapy regimens.[48, 319] However, improved survival has been seen following response to early treatment with chemotherapy plus all-transretinoic acid among patients with acute promyelocytic leukemia (M3).[80]

CML is often indolent initially, with rising blood cell counts, sometimes resulting in early mortality from congestive heart failure or stroke (due to hyperviscosity associated with high blood cell counts). Between 1974–1976 and 1989–1995, 5-year relative survival rose significantly from 22.5% to 31.9%. African-American males have nota-

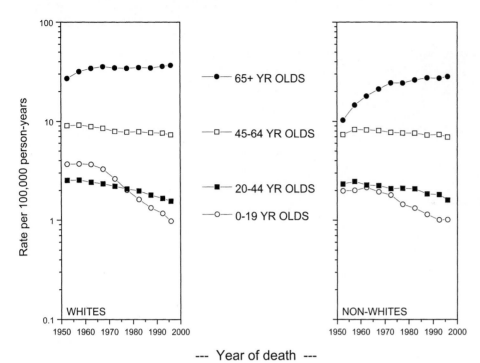

FIGURE 7–2. US trends in leukemia mortality (age-adjusted, world standard) by age group among whites and nonwhites 1950–1954 through 1995–1996.

bly lower survival (21.4%) than the 31% to 33% typical survival of white males and females; the small numbers of African-American women preclude meaningful comparisons (see Table 7-1). Early treatment with interferon alfa-2b (alone or in combination with other agents) may halt the progression,[113] but prognosis becomes grave subsequent to blast transformation.

Incidence Patterns and Trends

International Racial and Geographic Patterns

Total Leukemia. Within virtually all populations, total leukemia age-adjusted incidence rates are higher for males than for females (Fig. 7-3).[208] For leukemia patients of both sexes, there is a distinct racial and geographic gradient, with highest rates among white populations in North America, Australia, and New Zealand, followed by rates in populations in northern and western Europe, African Americans, and Hispanics in Los Angeles. Mid-level rates are observed for persons in southern Europe and Israeli Jews. Lowest rates occur (in descending order) in Japanese in Osaka, Chinese in Shanghai, and Indians in Bombay (see Fig. 7-3).

Leukemia Subtypes. For the worldwide registries shown in Fig. 7-3, other and NOS represents between 5% and 25% of total leukemia. Other and NOS comprise 10% or less of the total for both sexes in (ascending order or increasing proportion of other and NOS for males)

TABLE 7–1. 5-Year Relative Survival Rates for Leukemia in the U.S. Surveillance Epidemiology and End Results Program by Time Period, Race, Sex, Age, and Cell Type

	Leukemia Cell Type				
Period, Age, and Race/Sex Group	*CLL* (%)	*ALL* (%)	*Total* (%)	*CML* (%)	*AML* (%)
1974–1976, all ages, races, and sexes	68.2	38.4	34.4	22.5	5.7
1989–1995, all ages, races, and sexes	70.5*	58.8*	43.1*	31.9*	14.5*
White males	72.5*	57.7*	45.5*	31.2*	13.2*
White females	71.8	60.9*	43.0*	32.6	15.2*
A-A males	43.6	48.5	29.7	21.4	10.9
A-A females	53.7	54.6	37.5	47.6	15.6
Ages 0–14	N/C	81.1	74.0	N/C	42/6
Ages 0–64	78.8	63.4	51.2	40.9	25.1
Ages 65 +	65.9	5.8	33.9	21.7	2.8

*p<.05 for 1989-1995 versus 1974-1976.

A-A = African-American; N/C = not calculated.

From Ries LAG, Kosary CL, Hankey BF, et al (eds): Cancer Statistics Review, 1973-96 Bethesda, Maryland, National Cancer Institute, NIH Publication Number 99-2789, 1999.

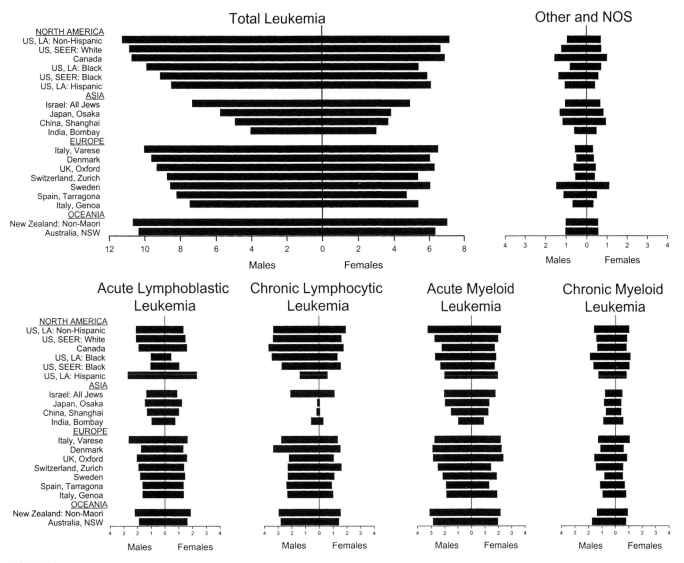

FIGURE 7–3. International variation in leukemia incidence (age-adjusted, world standard) by sex for total leukemia and by cell type. (Data from Parkin DM, Muir CS, Whelan SL, et al: Cancer Incidence in Five Continents, vol 7. Lyon, France, IARC Scientific Publication No. 143, 1997.)

Denmark, Switzerland, Italy (Varese), the United Kingdom, Los Angeles whites and African Americans (males only for the latter), Italy (Genoa), Australia, and New Zealand. Approximately 10% to 19% of total leukemia consists of other and NOS in (ascending order for men) SEER whites, Los Angeles Hispanics (less than 10% for women), Canada, Israel, Spain, SEER African Americans, India, and Sweden. Other and NOS comprise 20% or more of total leukemia (ascending for men) in Japan and China.

Similar to total leukemia, higher ALL age-standardized rates occur among populations in Northern and Western Europe, North America, and Oceania, and rates in Asian and black populations are lower. In contrast to international patterns for total leukemia, highest rates in Europe are reported from Varese, Italy, and the highest U.S. rates are described for Hispanics of both sexes in Los Angeles. Compared with other populations on the Asian landmass, Israeli Jews of both sexes have the highest total leukemia rates but lower ALL rates than those of other populations,

except for Indians in Bombay. Although common ALL accounts for virtually all of the early childhood incidence peak among most populations,[97] the distribution of ALL subtypes varies among populations.[97, 98]

Internationally, racial and geographic variation is greater for CLL than for any other form of leukemia, with the highest age-standardized rates in North American whites, followed by U.S. blacks and white populations in Oceania and northern and southern Europe. Lower rates occur among U.S. Hispanics, and significantly low rates occur among Asian populations (see Fig. 7–3).[102, 208] On the North American continent, there is a zone of high CLL incidence in the north-central United States (e.g., Iowa and Detroit) and also in the contiguous southern Canadian provinces (e.g., Saskatchewan, Quebec, Ontario, Alberta, and Manitoba).

ATLL, a mature T-cell neoplasm, is rare in most populations, except for endemic regions for human T-lymphotropic virus type I, which include southwestern parts of Japan, Jamaica and Trinidad, parts of West and Central

Africa, some regions in South America, and other restricted geographic areas.[81, 173] After a long latent period, ATLL is estimated to occur in 1 per 1000 carriers per year, for a total of an estimated 2500–3000 cases worldwide.[27] The age-standardized incidence rate of ATLL is estimated to range from 1.9 to 2.9 per 100,000 person-years, based on data from Jamaica and Trinidad,[57] and 2.6 to 4.0 based on data from Kyushu,[278] with highest risk among individuals who acquire the retrovirus during childhood. Those infected before age 20 years are estimated to have a cumulative lifetime risk of 4.0% for males and 4.2% for females.[197]

The international pattern for AML resembles that for total leukemia, with highest age-standardized incidence rates in Denmark, North American whites, Oceania, and African Americans (see Fig. 7–3). Midlevel rates are seen in Japanese, Israeli Jews, southern Europeans, and Hispanics in Los Angeles. Lowest rates occur in China and India. In most populations, AML incidence is higher for males than for females.

There is substantially less international variation for CML than is seen for any other cell type (see Fig. 7–3). For both males and females, rates are highest among the African-American population in Los Angeles, followed by whites in Australia and then by African Americans in the regions covered by the SEER registries. African Americans in Detroit and Los Angeles have the highest rates among females (see Fig. 7–3).[102] As with other leukemias, CML is more common among males than females.

U.S. Age-Standardized Rates and Time Trends

Total Leukemia. Age-standardized rates for total leukemia are higher for males of both races than for females and within each gender higher for whites than for African Americans (Fig. 7–4). Among whites, incidence changed little between 1973–1978 and 1985–1990, but declined somewhat thereafter. Incidence among African Americans rose between 1973–1978 and 1979–1984 and then declined slowly. Age-specific trends in the geographic regions covered by the U.S. SEER Program showed a slight increase in rates for children under age 15 years, mostly due to an abrupt jump up in rates between 1983 and 1984.[162] For leukemia patients younger than age 65 years at diagnosis, there was little overall change for whites during 1973–1996 and a small decline for African Americans (the latter greater for females than males). Declines were seen during 1973–1996 among leukemia patients diagnosed at age 65 years or older.[224] Internationally, leukemia incidence rates have been relatively stable since the 1960s for children, adolescents, young adults, and middle-aged persons, but rose among the elderly from the 1960s to the early 1970s.[75, 143]

Leukemia Subtypes. Other and NOS leukemias in the United States include acute NOS (ranging from 35% to 70% of all other and NOS leukemias), chronic NOS, lymphoid NOS, myeloid NOS, other NOS, and unspecified NOS (with either unspecified or myeloid NOS as the second largest contributor and generally ranging from 1%

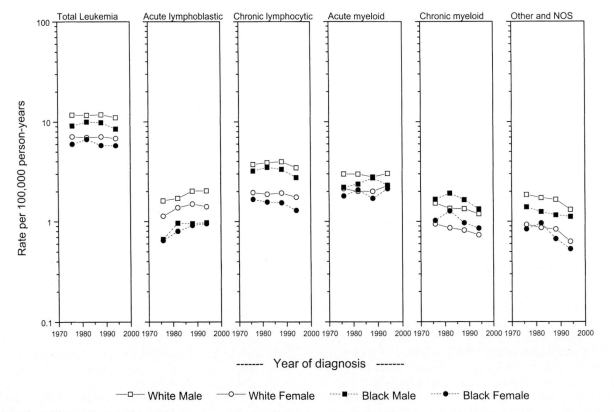

FIGURE 7–4. United States trends in leukemia incidence (age-adjusted, world standard) by race and sex for total leukemia and by cell type in the nine SEER areas. (Data from Ries LAG, Kosary CL, Hankey BF, et al: Cancer Statistics Review, 1973–96. Bethesda, Maryland: National Cancer Institute, NIH Publication No. 99-2789, 1999.)

to 40%). Other and NOS age-standardized rates, similar to that for total leukemia, are higher for males of both races than for females and higher for whites than African Americans within each gender. Rates for other and NOS in the United States declined for all four race-gender groups during the interval from 1973–1978 and 1991–1996. There was an acceleration of the rate of decline between 1985–1990 and 1991–1996 for whites and a steeper decline between 1979–1984 and 1991–1996 for African-American females (see Fig. 7-4).

For ALL, age-standardized incidence is higher for whites of both sexes than for African Americans. Incidence of ALL rose between 1973–1978 and 1985–1990 and then leveled off in all four race-sex groups (see Fig. 7-4).

Age-standardized CLL incidence rates are notably higher in males of both races than females; within each gender, rates are higher for whites than for African Americans (see Fig. 7-4), followed by Hispanics and American Indians, with very low and similar rates among Chinese Americans, Japanese Americans, and Filipinos.[84, 103] CLL age-standardized incidence in regions covered by SEER Program registries has declined in all four gender-race groups, commencing in 1973–1978 for females and in 1979–1984 for males (see Fig. 7-4).

For AML, age-standardized rates are modestly higher in males of both races than in females and within gender are higher in whites than in African Americans for males but similar for females of both races (see Fig. 7-4). Incidence was fairly stable during 1973–1978 through 1991–1996. A similar stable incidence trend pattern was seen for adults ages 15–64 years in the regions covered by a population-based specialist registry of hematologic diseases in the United Kingdom; however, significant decreases, estimated at 3% per year, occurred among the elderly.[47] This decline in AML among the elderly paralleled a highly significant increase of 6% per year for myelodysplastic syndromes among older persons. It is likely that the increasing recognition of myelodysplastic syndromes during the same period may have resulted in less misclassification of these disorders as AML.

Age-standardized incidence for CML is higher in males than in females of both races, with rates higher in African Americans than in whites within each gender, unique among the leukemias (see Fig. 7-4). Midlevel rates occur in Hispanics followed by progressively lower rates in Japanese Americans, Chinese Americans, Filipinos, and American Indians.[84, 103] Age-standardized incidence among whites declined steadily but slowly over time (see Fig. 7-4). Among African Americans, age-standardized incidence rose between 1973–1978 and 1979–1984 and then declined steadily thereafter at a more rapid rate than the decline observed in whites.

U.S. Age-Specific Rates and Racial/Ethnic Patterns

Total Leukemia. Approximately 1.5% of white males, 1.1% of white females, 0.8% of African-American males, and 0.7% of African-American females in the SEER populations will eventually develop some form of leukemia.[224] The racial and ethnic pattern for total leukemia in the United States parallels the findings observed in interna-

tional comparisons. For men, highest rates are found among white non-Hispanics (14.1 per 100,000 person-years, age-adjusted according to the 1970 U.S. population), followed by African Americans (10.7), and then white Hispanics (10.3). Progressively lower rates occur in Asian and Pacific Islanders (8.5) and American Indians (3.6).[224] For women, the pattern is similar, although rates are generally lower and differences less striking than those for males; high to midlevel rates were seen in female non-Hispanic whites (8.3) followed by African-American (6.9) and Hispanic whites (6.9), whereas low rates were seen in Asian/Pacific Islanders (5.8) and American Indians (3.1).

Leukemia Subtypes. Based on U.S. SEER Program data (1973–1996) for both genders and all races combined, lymphoid leukemias account for 47% of all leukemias (17.3% acute; 28.5% chronic; 1.2% lymphoid NOS); myeloid leukemias comprise 41.4% (25.3% acute; 13.2% chronic; 2.9% myeloid NOS); and other or unspecified types represent 11.7% (4.8% acute NOS, 0.3% chronic NOS, 6.6% other and NOS).[224] ALL is the predominant type before the age of 15 years (comprising 77.1% of total leukemia), and CLL is the most common type at age 65 years and older (40.2% of total leukemia).

For ALL, age-specific rates demonstrate a U-shaped pattern and are generally higher for whites of both sexes than for African Americans (Fig. 7-5). There is a notable peak in incidence between the ages of 2 and 3 years, which is also observed in most populations internationally,[159, 207] followed by declining rates during later childhood, adolescence, and young adulthood (see Fig. 7-5). Rates then rise, beginning in midlife, to reach a second peak (slightly lower than the peak in early childhood) among the elderly. Beginning in adolescence and continuing among all age groups, incidence among white males is consistently higher than among white females. A similar pattern is suggested in African Americans, although based on small numbers of cases (see Fig. 7-5).[102]

CLL incidence rates are consistently higher in males of both races than in females (sex ratios approach or exceed 2:1, the highest for any leukemia cell type), with little difference within gender until age 70, when rates for whites become somewhat higher than rates for African Americans (see Fig. 7-5). CLL almost never occurs before the age of 30 years and is predominantly a disease of the elderly (see Fig. 7-5). After age 30 years, CLL incidence rises exponentially and with a steeper slope than that for any leukemia cell type, achieving the highest incidence level among the elderly. Hairy cell leukemia is close to five times more common in males than in females, with higher rates in whites than in nonwhites.[22] Similar to CLL, hairy cell leukemia is unknown in childhood, but then rises in incidence beginning at age 30 years. Unlike CLL, hairy cell leukemia reaches a plateau at about age 60 years.

AML rates in infancy are higher among whites of both sexes than among African Americans, whereas in childhood there is some suggestion of higher rates in African Americans than in whites (see Fig. 7-5). Thereafter, rates are similar by sex and race in most age groups until late middle age, when incidence is higher in males of both races than among females, with rates within gender

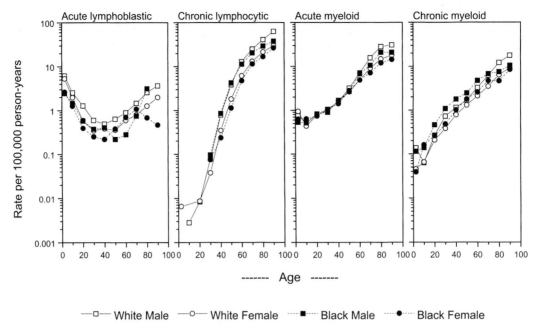

FIGURE 7–5. United States age-specific leukemia incidence rates according to leukemia cell type by race and sex in the nine SEER areas. (Data from Ries LAG, Kosary CL, Hankey BF, et al: Cancer Statistics Review, 1973–96. Bethesda, Maryland: National Cancer Institute, NIH Publication No. 99–2789, 1999.)

higher among whites than among African Americans (see Fig. 7-5). In one study from Los Angeles, Hispanics had a higher frequency of acute promyelocytic leukemia than non-Hispanics; this finding was observed among two series of patients with AML.[74] Among children, AML comprises about 15% to 25% of leukemia in most Western populations, with highest rates in infancy, followed by a decline in incidence until age 10 years when incidence begins to rise.[159, 264] After age 40 years, incidence rates increase at a more rapid rate until ages 70 to 80 years, after which the rates increase more slowly (see Fig. 7-5).

CML is the only leukemia subtype for which rates among African Americans are consistently higher than for those among whites in most age groups, except among the very young (see Fig. 7-5).[264] CML rarely occurs in children younger than 5 years of age, except for juvenile myelomonocytic leukemia in white males, who experience fourfold higher rates than females.[11, 202, 264] After age 5 years, rates are somewhat higher for males of both races than females. Between the ages of 5 and 65 years, incidence is higher in African-American males than in white males, whereas at age 75 years and older, the highest rates occur in white males. For females older than 5 years, rates are slightly higher in African Americans than in whites until age 80 years and older, when rates are slightly higher in whites than in African Americans. After early childhood, the rates rise log-linearly with increasing age (see Fig. 7-5).

Thus, ALL rates are notably higher among whites than among African Americans and have a distinct bimodal age distribution; CLL rates are notably higher among males than among females and rise more rapidly with age compared with other forms of leukemia; and CML is unique among the leukemias because of higher rates among African Americans than among whites.

ANALYTIC EPIDEMIOLOGY

Following the detailed consideration of the descriptive epidemiology of the leukemias, we now turn our attention to a brief overview of known and suspected risk factors. Although established and postulated risk factors are discussed individually, it must be recognized that etiology is clearly multifactorial. There are also likely to be different factors that induce or promote initial versus subsequent events in leukemogenesis. Given current limited understanding about the epidemiology of leukemia occurrence, there is little discussion of the role or timing of known or suspected risk factors acting at the specific steps.

Except for ionizing radiation, a few occupational and environmental chemical exposures, HTLV-I as the cause of ATLL, and a few genetic disorders, the risk factors for the leukemias are as yet poorly understood. Knowledge of leukemia risk factors is insufficient to explain the observed international variation in leukemia rates. Only during the last two decades have etiologic studies increasingly distinguished among the various forms of leukemia.

Radiation Exposure

Ionizing Radiation

Ionizing radiation is perhaps the best known and most studied risk factor for the leukemias, given the detailed prospective studies of populations exposed to environmental, occupational, military, and medically related sources of radiation. The relationship of this exposure to leukemia is described in more detail in Chapter 8.

Japanese Atomic Bomb Survivors. CLL has been the

only major leukemia cell type not linked with radiation exposure.[30, 229] Long-term follow-up studies of survivors of the bombing of Hiroshima and Nagasaki have provided much of the current understanding of the relation of estimated doses and dose-response function of ionizing radiation to mortality and incidence risks for ALL, AML, and CML.[216, 220, 254, 289] Leukemia was the first radiation-induced cancer reported among atomic bomb survivors. The dose-response pattern for total leukemia was consistent with a linear-quadratic relationship, with risks steadily increasing with dose up to approximately 3 to 4 Gy (1 gray or Gy = 100 rad), and then flattening somewhat at doses above this level. Based on mortality data, the summary excess relative risk estimate for leukemia among the atomic bomb survivors was 6.21 per Gy, and the absolute excess per 10^4 PY-Gy was 2.94.[254] Males had relative risks similar to those of females, but the former demonstrated absolute excess risks about twofold higher than the latter. For both forms of acute leukemia, persons younger than 20 years at exposure were characterized by absolute risks peaking within 10 years, and then falling rapidly. Population members ages 20 to 35 years at the time of the bomb had less pronounced peaks, followed by more gradual declines, whereas individuals older than 35 years demonstrated little variation in risk with time since exposure. CML was much less common among exposed survivors in Nagasaki than among those in Hiroshima (lower absolute risks), but there was no difference between the two cities in relative risks. For CML, those younger than 15 years at exposure experienced a sharp incidence peak and older persons a smaller peak at 5 years following exposure.[30, 289]

Workers Exposed to Ionizing Radiation. Workers in the medical fields of radiologic technology and diagnostic radiology comprise the largest category of persons exposed occupationally to ionizing radiation. Radiologists and x-ray technicians employed in the first half of the 20th century were reported to be at increased risk for leukemia. Physicians who were members of a professional radiologic society in Britain during 1897–1921 were characterized by a sixfold excess risk of mortality from leukemia, whereas there was no significant increase in leukemia among those joining the society after 1921.[268] U.S. radiologists who entered a professional specialty society during 1920–1929 had an 8.8-fold excess; those joining during 1930–1939 had a 3.4-fold excess (of primarily acute and myeloid leukemia); and those joining in 1940 or later had no significant excess mortality from leukemia.[178] Leukemia (except CLL) was significantly increased among 27,911 Chinese x-ray technicians who were monitored during 1950–1985.[295] However, leukemia was not significantly elevated among U.S. Army x-ray technicians monitored during 1946–1974[131] nor among U.S. civilian x-ray technologists who belonged to the American Registry of Radiation Technologists.[71]

Findings from many epidemiologic studies of cancer risk among nuclear energy workers have been reviewed extensively.[30, 158] A combined analysis of 95,673 U.S., U.K., and Canadian nuclear workers employed for 6 months or longer yielded a relative risk of 1.2 for leukemia mortality (excluding CLL), for a cumulative protracted dose of 100 mSv (1 sievert [Sv] = 100 rem) compared with 9 mSv

and an excess relative risk of 2.2 per Sv for leukemia.[45] Among 124,743 U.K. workers in industries with ionizing radiation exposure, a small, borderline significant excess relative risk was found for leukemia (excluding CLL), with 90% confidence limits (following adjustment for potential confounding factors) ranging from 0 to just under 4 times the risk estimated at low doses for Japanese atomic bomb survivors.[196] No significant excess risks for childhood leukemia were found among children of nuclear workers (39,557 male and 8,883 female workers) in nuclear plants in the United Kingdom although risks were significantly higher among children (based on three exposed childhood cases) whose fathers had a cumulative preconception dose of 100 mSv or more.[228] No excess risk of leukemia was found among children of parents residing in proximity to nuclear plants in Ontario, Canada, nor was there evidence of an elevated risk among offspring of those male residents who were radiation workers (based on linkage with the Canadian National Dose Registry).[185] Leukemia was not found in excess among cohorts of U.S.[270, 272] or U.K.[14] radium dial workers nor among uranium miners.[200] A borderline significant increase was reported among U.K. tin miners who had worked at least 10 to 20 years underground.[116] Whereas a 2.5-fold increase in leukemia (primarily AML and CML) was found among 3741 U.S. servicemen exposed to one aboveground nuclear detonation in 1957,[44] no increase was observed among 46,186 U.S. military participants in other nuclear atmospheric tests during 1951–1958.[226] However, leukemia mortality and incidence were elevated among 528 New Zealand military participants in British atomic weapons tests,[212] and excess mortality from leukemia and multiple myeloma (but not other radiation-related cancers) was found among 22,347 British military participants in nuclear tests.[64] It was noted, however, that the latter excess may have reflected a substantially lower rate of these two major categories of hematopoietic neoplasms among the unexposed comparison group when the comparison subjects were evaluated in relation to national mortality rates.[30]

Radiation Therapy: Malignant Conditions. Based on the findings of studies of atomic bomb survivors and other populations exposed at low to moderate doses of ionizing radiation, it is not surprising that acute leukemia and CML occur as second primary cancers in persons treated with radiation therapy for malignant[124] and benign conditions.[30, 158] Leukemia risks that are approximately two- to threefold increased have been linked consistently with radiation therapy treatments among adults treated for non-Hodgkin's lymphoma (treated with a range of doses to bone marrow),[99, 284, 285] breast cancer (estimated marrow doses ranged from less than 5 Gy to more than 9 Gy),[61] uterine cervix cancer (estimated marrow dose = 7 Gy),[29] and uterine corpus cancer (estimated marrow dose ranged from 1 to 15 Gy),[62] and in children treated for Ewing's sarcoma (estimated doses to affected bone ranged from 41 to 60 Gy)[152, 287] and Wilms' tumor (estimated doses to irradiated fields in the abdomen, and to a lesser extent the thorax, ranged from 6 to 40 Gy, although these patients are treated with radiotherapy less often now than previously).[36, 124, 157]

The elevated risks of secondary acute nonlymphocytic

leukemia associated with Hodgkin's disease and testicular cancer are most likely due to treatment with alkylating agents, whereas the consistently observed excess of secondary solid tumors in Hodgkin's disease (including breast, lung, thyroid, stomach, bone, connective tissue, and skin cancers) result from radiation therapy treatment.[135, 277, 286, 292] Results of a randomized clinical trial have shown a higher cumulative incidence of acute leukemia among patients with polycythemia vera treated with the radionuclide ^{32}P (6%) than among patients treated by phlebotomy alone (1%), but evidence is inconclusive about the potential leukemogenecity of high doses of ^{131}I for treating thyroid cancer.[124] Similar to results for the Japanese atomic bomb survivors, the excesses of leukemia subsequent to radiotherapy are generally apparent within the first 5 years following treatment, and most radiogenic leukemia arises within 10 to 15 years. Risk of radiation-induced leukemia appears to be greater when large volumes of bone marrow are treated with lower doses or dose fractions. It has been postulated that the low risk of secondary leukemia associated with high partial-body exposures to radiation is related to the ability of ionizing radiation to sterilize marrow stem cells.[124]

Radiation Therapy: Benign Conditions. Radiation therapy has also been used to treat benign conditions. Close to 14,000 patients treated with radiation therapy (mean total marrow dose = 4.38 Gy) for ankylosing spondylitis during 1935–1954 experienced an elevated mortality risk from leukemia (excluding CLL) that was greatest 1 to 5 years following treatment. In the most recent follow-up through 1991, the relative risk for leukemia in the period 1 to 25 years after exposure to a uniform dose of 1 Gy was estimated to be 7.0.[297] Leukemia excesses, ranging from 1.2- to 3.0-fold increases, have been reported in cohorts treated with radiotherapy for other benign conditions, including U.S. women with benign gynecologic disorders,[126] U.S.[127] and Scottish women[267] with menorrhagia not associated with malignancy, U.S. patients treated for peptic ulcer,[100] and Israeli[230] and U.S. children[255] treated for tinea capitis.

Thorotrast. Excess risks of leukemia and other hematologic disorders (as well as liver cancer and other tumors and cirrhosis of the liver) have been found in patients with neurologic disorders who received Thorotrast contrast material during cerebral angiography.[9, 73, 174, 291] The leukemias observed in patients who received Thorotrast are distinguished by long latency until onset and an increased proportion of erythroleukemias.

Diagnostic X-Ray Procedures. Prenatal exposure of the fetus to diagnostic x-rays has been linked in numerous case-control studies with a subsequent small excess of childhood leukemia (1.4- to 1.5-fold estimated increase),[289] but there has been long-standing debate about whether this association is causal.[31] The relationship of diagnostic x-ray exposure with adult leukemias and breast cancer has long been of interest, particularly for patients undergoing frequent evaluation, females evaluated repeatedly during puberty and early adolescence, those undergoing procedures involving substantial doses, and those evaluated before the 1980s, when radiation doses were higher. Whereas some investigators reported elevated risk of myeloid leukemia and CML,[104, 221] others found no

relationship or small increases confined to the few years immediately preceding diagnosis,[32, 78] suggesting that the diagnostic x-rays may have been obtained for early manifestations of leukemia.

Ionizing radiation induces DNA strand breaks, and most mutations caused by radiation are associated with chromosomal changes such as translocations and deletions.[164] A morphologic review of bone marrow in the mid-1980s affected by acute leukemia and CML among atomic bomb survivors and patients irradiated for cervical cancer revealed that these cases were similar to de novo leukemia cases, although the bone marrows of patients with ankylosing spondylitis more closely resembled occurring the morphologic and cytogenetic patterns seen among secondary leukemias after treatment with alkylating drugs.[21, 195] More research is needed to determine whether leukemia arising secondary to radiation exposures (from military, occupational, medically related, and environmental sources) is similar to or differs from de novo occurrence, using state-of-the-art morphologic, cytogenetic, and molecular assessment as part of a standardized protocol to evaluate all newly diagnosed secondary leukemia cases.

Nonionizing Radiation

In 1979 a report linked childhood leukemia and other forms of childhood cancer with residential exposure to nonionizing radiation in the form of extremely low frequency (ELF; 50 to 60 Hz) magnetic field exposures induced by nearby power lines.[298] Initial small studies appeared to support a 2- to 3-fold increase in risk associated with residential proximity to high-tension power lines.[82, 166, 247] However, more recent large studies with more extensive and direct measures of children's time-weighted average MF exposures have shown little evidence of elevated risks, except perhaps a very small percentage of children with high MF exposures.[160, 183, 188, 288] Experimental studies have shown no evidence of carcinogenesis associated with ELF MF exposures.[219]

Since 1982,[189] investigators using job title as a proxy measure of ELF MF exposures reported increased risks of AML, CLL, and brain tumors among adults employed in occupations believed to have high exposure (such as power linemen, utilities workers, electronics workers, and others).[219] Many of the studies used the dichotomous classification for "electrical jobs" versus "nonelectrical jobs" proposed by Milham.[190] Studies using a range of types of measurements, some in conjunction with job exposure matrices, have shown inconsistent findings.[83, 85, 134, 165, 175, 192, 240, 246, 283] Meta-analysis suggests nonsignificant small increases in odds ratios for medium (OR = 1.22) and high (OR = 1.15) exposure categories for total leukemia and overall estimated relative risks of 1.4 (95% CI = 1.2–1.7) for AML and 1.6 (95% CI = 1.1–2.2) for CLL.[140] A comprehensive review of data by a working group commissioned by the U.S. National Institute of Environmental Health Sciences concluded that, taken together, the studies suggest an association between exposure to magnetic fields and CLL.[219] This conclusion was based on small numbers of highly exposed cases from two Swedish studies[83, 85] and a French-Canadian investigation.[283]

Occupational Exposures

Various occupational and environmental chemical exposures have been implicated as causes of leukemia. The oldest and best-known chemical leukemogen is benzene.[67] Leukemia has been reported to be 1.9- to 10-fold increased in analytic studies of benzene-exposed painters, printers, and workers employed in petroleum refining and in chemical, rubber, Pliofilm, and shoe manufacturing.[205, 225, 304, 312] In a large study of Chinese benzene-exposed workers, the relative risk of the combined grouping of acute nonlymphocytic leukemia and myelodysplastic syndromes was 4.1 (3.0 for ANLL only) for "ever" versus "never" exposed. The grouping of acute nonlymphocytic leukemia and myelodysplastic syndromes was about threefold and significantly increased among workers with constant benzene exposure levels of less than 10 ppm, and risk rose to 7.1 for those exposed at constant levels of 25 ppm or higher.[109] Although benzene has been most strongly associated with AML and aplastic anemia, limited evidence suggests that CML, myelodysplastic syndromes, and non-Hodgkin's lymphoma may possibly be linked with exposure to this chemical.[109, 121, 129, 225, 245, 250, 312]

The dose-response pattern and the relevant exposure metric have been much debated.[59, 60, 211, 290] Peripheral blood lymphocyte counts appear to represent a sensitive marker of benzene exposure levels.[234, 296] Decreased lymphocyte counts, in conjunction with other forms of hematotoxicity (benzene poisoning), can serve as a biomarker to validate benzene exposure level estimates.[72] Total leukemia risk was not significantly increased overall or with higher cumulative benzene exposure among petroleum marketing and distribution workers in the United Kingdom or in Canada, although duration of exposure was more closely related to risk in both studies.[239, 249] Evidence from the U.K. study[239] suggested that the relevant benzene exposure metric (average dose, duration of exposure, etc.) may vary according to leukemia cell type. Data from the Chinese benzene workers study indicated that acute nonlymphocytic leukemia/myelodysplastic syndrome was significantly associated with more recent but not distant exposures, whereas non-Hodgkin's lymphoma was most strongly linked with exposures occurring at least 10 years before diagnosis.[109] If these findings are confirmed, then mechanistic studies should be undertaken to explain the results. A meta-analysis of cohort studies of petroleum workers in the United States and the United Kingdom (including refinery, production, pipeline, and distribution workers) revealed no excess of AML or other leukemia cell types.[222] Thus, the dose-response relationship for benzene requires further clarification, particularly for very low benzene exposure levels.

Other chemicals have been associated with leukemia in some investigations, but the results are not as consistent as the findings for benzene. Exposure to styrene and/or butadiene has been associated with increased risk of lymphomas, lymphatic leukemias, and total leukemia in some studies,[186, 204] but not in others,[305] perhaps due to confounding from other chemicals such as dithiocarbamates.[130] Recent investigations support the relationship between styrene-butadiene rubber production (but not exposure to the butadiene monomer alone) and leukemia risk and provide evidence of dose-response relationships with increasing levels of time-weighted average[176] or cumulative butadiene exposure.[168] Ethylene oxide has also been designated as a probable human carcinogen,[128, 271] based on leukemia and lymphoma excesses, although the findings are not consistent in all studies.[256, 281, 282, 306]

Data are more limited for other chemical exposures. Leukemia excesses have been observed among rubber workers,[233, 275] painters,[51, 179] embalmers,[108, 163] garage and transport workers,[120, 122] sawmill, wood, and furniture industry workers,[177, 193, 209] shoe workers,[42] hairdressers and cosmetologists,[167, 191] slaughterhouse and meat-packing industry workers,[187] seamen on tankers,[203] clinical laboratory, radiologic, and science technicians,[43] and other occupational and industrial populations.

The role of maternal and paternal occupational exposures in the causation of childhood leukemia has been evaluated for more than 25 years, but the findings have not been consistent. Recent studies have begun to link population-based cancer registry data and other computerized data sources; novel and more precise exposure assessment methods are also being used.[2, 151, 228] Risks of leukemia in offspring are being evaluated in relation to different exposure times, such as the preconception, prenatal, or postnatal periods.[133, 261]

Agricultural Exposures

Studies of farmers and farm workers have shown modest excesses of leukemia (risks ranging from 1.1- to 1.4-fold elevated) in some investigations and no increase in risk in others.[25, 137, 316] There is some variation in risks internationally, perhaps due to differences in agriculture-related exposures.[6, 13, 66, 150, 199, 302] Almost all leukemia types were increased among farmers in the studies demonstrating statistical associations. In addition to pesticides (particularly animal insecticides, but probably others as well), other suspected exposures include herbicides, fertilizers, diesel fuel and exhaust, infectious agents, and possibly others associated with livestock.[26] Although only a few of the earlier studies evaluated specific pesticide exposures in relation to leukemia risk,[38, 244] later studies have increasingly incorporated newer interview methods and biologic measurement components to evaluate specific pesticide and other agricultural exposures.[2, 273, 274]

Antineoplastic Treatments

Treatment with certain types of chemotherapeutic agents (primarily alkylating agents and, more recently, epipodophyllotoxins) prescribed for malignant and nonmalignant disorders (the latter including rheumatoid arthritis and other autoimmune diseases) is associated with increased risks of treatment-related myelodysplastic syndromes and/or secondary AML.[155] The myelodysplastic syndromes associated with alkylating agents are frequently characterized by a preleukemic phase, trilineage dysplasia, and frequent cytogenetic abnormalities involving partial deletions of chromosomes 5 and 7. The mean latency period between treatment and occurrence of the treatment-related hematologic disorder is 5 to 7 years. Treatment-related myelodysplastic syndromes and/or AML are more likely to occur following use of certain agents (e.g., melphalan poses higher risk than cyclophosphamide; stem cell priming with VP-16 has also been linked with high risks).[149] Therapy-related myelodysplastic syndromes and AML have been reported subsequent to treatment for Hodgkin's disease; non-Hodgkin's lymphoma; multiple myeloma; polycythemia vera; breast, ovarian, uterine cervix, uterine corpus, and testicular cancers; and other disorders. Risk is quantitatively related to cumulative alkylating drug dose.

Secondary leukemias related to therapy with topoisomerase II inhibitors (epipodophyllotoxins) have earlier onset than other forms of secondary leukemias and are not preceded by a preleukemic phase. These secondary leukemias frequently show balanced translocations involving 11q23 or, less often, t(8;21), t(3;21), inv(16), t(8;16), t(15;17), or t(9;22).[7, 79] In a study of 442 children treated with various regimens for germ cell tumors, no treatment-related AML occurred among patients treated with surgery or radiotherapy only, whereas 1% of those treated with chemotherapy and 4.2% of those treated with chemotherapy plus radiotherapy developed treatment-related AML.[251] In a review of multiple studies of patients treated with topoisomerase II inhibitors, the mean latency period between treatment and occurrence of treatment-related AML was approximately 2 years.[79]

Recent efforts have been directed to identifying factors that may influence risk of developing a secondary treatment-related AML, including polymorphisms of glutathione S-transferase[242, 307] and of NAD(P)H:quinone oxidoreductase (NQO1),[154] but limited data preclude firm conclusions. A detailed review of secondary leukemia associated with treatment of a wide variety of disorders is provided in Chapters 9 and 11.

Smoking, Alcohol, Diet, and Other Lifestyle Factors

Lifestyle risk factors have either been little studied or been found to play a limited role in the cause of the leukemias, with a few possible exceptions. A few large studies found small increases of adult ALL,[92, 136, 241] but cohort investigations have reported no excess leukemia associated with cigarette smoking.[1, 77] Summary assessments have concluded that cigarette smoking is weakly linked (relative risks estimated as 1.3–1.5) with elevated risks of adult myeloid leukemias.[40, 70] Maternal smoking during pregnancy appears to be unrelated to subsequent risk of childhood leukemia in the offspring,[37, 243, 252] but some evidence supports an association between paternal preconception smoking and subsequent childhood leukemia.[133, 269]

A few studies have evaluated the relationship of dietary factors[123, 153] or alcohol consumption[23, 39, 46, 114, 132, 248, 303] to the cause of the leukemias in adults, but overall there is little evidence supporting relationships. However, a small U.S. study reported a 10-fold excess risk of infant AML,

but not ALL, linked with increasing consumption during pregnancy of DNA topoisomerase II inhibitor–containing foods.[232] Recent findings from in vivo and in vitro experiments have shown topoisomerase II to be the target of dietary bioflavonoids and suggest a two-stage model for cellular processing of topoisomerase II inhibitors.[276] These results support the epidemiologic data and suggest that maternal ingestion of bioflavonoids may induce chromosomal translocations involving the MLL gene in utero, potentially leading to infant leukemia. Longer duration of breast-feeding was linked with reduced risks of childhood AML and ALL in a U.S. study,[259] whereas postnatal use of cod liver oil (containing vitamin D) was associated with reduced risk of ALL in Chinese children.[258] Two U.S. investigations have reported elevated risks of AML among infants and very young children in relation to maternal alcohol consumption during pregnancy.[253, 260] Experimental data suggest that calorie restriction may mitigate the leukemogenic effects of exposure to single, high-dose total body radiation.[313] These interesting leads deserve further exploration.

Infectious Agents

Retroviruses

Certain retroviruses have been associated with one or more forms of leukemia. Because many aspects, including the epidemiology, of these viruses are examined in greater detail in Chapter 10, they are only briefly mentioned here. HTLV-I is endemic in southwestern Japan, Jamaica, Trinidad, many regions in Africa, native ethnic groups in the Andes highlands, population subgroups in Brazil, and among Caribbean immigrants in Brooklyn, a borough of New York City.[12, 89, 156, 170, 173, 218, 311] Infection with HTLV-I is estimated to affect 10 to 20 million persons worldwide.[76] Most carriers remain asymptomatic, but some develop adult T-cell leukemia/lymphoma, whereas others experience HTLV-I-associated myelopathy/tropical spastic paraparesis.[173] In the endemic area of Nagasaki, Japan, a serosurvey of 18,485 persons for HTLV-I revealed an overall seroprevalence of 16.2%.[12] The age-standardized annual incidence rate of ATLL in persons age 30 years or older was 10.5 per 100,000 persons for men and 6.0 for women. Cumulative lifetime risk of developing ATLL was estimated as 6.6% for men and 2.1% for women. Between 1985 and 1995, 989 cases of ATLL, compared with 1745 cases of other non-Hodgkin's lymphoma, were registered at the Nagasaki Prefecture Cancer Registry. Molecular study has shown that isolates of HTLV-I from Brazilians of various ethnic origins (whites, blacks, mulattos, Japanese immigrants) resembled those of seropositive persons from other South American countries but differed from HTLV-I isolates from Africa and Japan.[311] The virus is spread vertically (from mother to child) during breastfeeding and horizontally (between adults) by sexual intercourse, intravenous drug use, and blood transfusions prior to routine screening of donor blood.[27]

Other Infectious Agents

Kinlen[141] described excesses of common ALL associated with population mixing, in which a higher incidence occurred among children born into relatively isolated populations subsequent to contact of adults from those communities with migrants from nonisolated communities. He hypothesized that childhood leukemia may be a rare response to an unidentified mild or subclinical infection (occurring in utero or postnatally). Transmission is facilitated by newly occurring proximity of infected persons to previously nonexposed persons residing in an isolated, nonendemic region following the population mixing. To date, Kinlen and colleagues have described a variety of examples of population mixing, all demonstrating elevated occurrence of childhood leukemia in the formerly isolated populations.[141, 142, 144-148] Although these studies are intriguing, no specific candidate organism has yet been identified.

Greaves and Alexander[95, 96] developed a hypothesis, based on several lines of evidence (including historical trend data, international rate comparisons, geographic variation, socioeconomic factors, and community characteristics), suggesting that the common form of ALL arises in affluent societies as a rare response to a common infection. A key element of the hypothesis is the role of the pattern and timing of infections in infancy and early childhood in relation to immune system development. Several aspects of lifestyle in developed countries (such as child rearing and social, breast-feeding, and hygiene practices) may affect the developing immune system. Specifically, the hypothesis proposes that the childhood common ALL peak is temporally related to a relative paucity of infections in infancy and early childhood, absence of or very limited breast-feeding, social isolation, and/or delayed exposure of the infant or young child to other children. Clinical leukemia arises as a result of an initial, spontaneous mutation in lymphoid tissue during fetal development that remains silent until delayed exposure to an infectious agent or other promoter causes an abnormal immune response, which is followed after a relatively brief interval by the onset of common ALL. Some epidemiologic data support the hypothesis,[215, 259, 265] but other studies provide only limited or little support.[101, 201]

Alexander and colleagues[3, 4] evaluated the hypothesis that population density may be linked with an increased risk of childhood leukemia using data for 13,551 incident cases of childhood leukemia in 17 European countries and population data for small census units. These investigators found modest but statistically significant evidence of clustering, with incidence showing a curvilinear association with population density. Incidence was highest in areas that were somewhat more densely populated (500 to 750 persons/km²). Statistically significant evidence of clustering was evident in areas of intermediate density (250 to 499 persons/km²). Among children 2 to 4 years old, risks were slightly increased for all population densities except the lowest density areas, but there was no evidence of any trends. As the authors[4] and others[231] conclude, such ecologic data cannot provide strong support for any specific hypothesis but may present some leads that should be explored in additional descriptive, ecologic, and analytic studies. Nevertheless, ecologic data are characterized by important limitations that must be acknowledged.

Genetics

Twin Studies

Several lines of epidemiologic evidence support an important role for genetic factors in the origins of the leukemias. A high degree of concordance has been observed for childhood leukemia among monozygotic twins,[125, 169, 194] although data from one twin study led to the conclusion that a strong constitutional genetic component for childhood leukemia and other cancers was lacking, except for retinoblastoma.[41] Molecular data also suggest that the leukemia concordance in twins is likely due to shared placental circulation rather than to an inherited genetic mutation.[86, 300]

Familial Aggregation

Epidemiologic studies have repeatedly confirmed familial occurrence of the leukemias, although only a small percentage of cases have affected close family members.[118] Familial leukemia is generally characterized by concordance of the leukemia cell types among the affected family members, particularly CLL. Among all types of familial cancer, familial CLL is one of the most common.[93] Recent studies of familial occurrence of CLL in parent and offspring have shown a substantially younger age at onset in the offspring compared with the affected parent (a genetic feature designated as "anticipation").[94, 119, 315] Only a small proportion of familial leukemia is characterized by discordance of the leukemia types.[105] More commonly, relatives of leukemia cases also appear to be at higher risk of developing other hematopoietic and lymphoproliferative neoplasms,[63, 161, 184] results postulated as consistent with a defect in the pluripotent hematopoietic stem cell.[257] The mode of inheritance of familial leukemia and/or other hematopoietic or lymphoproliferative neoplasms is unknown, although it has been hypothesized that an autosomal-dominant gene is responsible in pedigrees with multiple affected members. Postulated mechanisms for familial leukemia include inherited cytogenetic abnormalities, genetic mutations, or primary immunologic alterations; sharing of common haplotypes; and/or consanguinity, possibly in conjunction with leukemogenic environmental influences.

Germline Mutations and Genetic Syndromes

Childhood leukemia is part of the highly penetrant Li-Fraumeni cancer family syndrome, which also features sarcomas, breast cancer, brain tumors, and adrenal carcinoma as well as multiple primary cancers.[115] Some Li-Fraumeni families have inherited germline mutations in the TP53 gene. A report implicates mutations in the tumor suppressor hCHK2 gene, whose activation prevents cellular entry into mitosis.[15]

Approximately 5% of ALL and AML cases have been associated with inherited genetic syndromes, often involving genes functionally linked to DNA repair or other aspects of genomic stability.[279] Children with Down's syndrome (trisomy 21) are at increased risk of developing acute leukemia, particularly the M7 (megakaryoblastic) variant of AML,[107, 172, 318] perhaps due to a functional role of mutant p53 in the evolution from a transient form of leukemia to acute megakaryoblastic leukemia. It is also noteworthy that acquired trisomy 21 may occur in children and adults without Down's syndrome who develop certain forms of ALL or AML.[237] Another chromosomal syndrome that increases risk of leukemia is ataxia-telangiectasia, associated with ALL and non-Hodgkin's lymphoma.[110] Fanconi's anemia, linked with AML, is a congenital disorder in which morphologic myelodysplasia is frequent and associated with poor survival but is independent of the occurrence of cytogenetic clonal variation (including disappearance of clones, clonal evolution, and appearance of new clones).[5] Bloom's syndrome, associated with both ALL and AML, is a disorder in which the specific chromosome bands nonrandomly affected by spontaneous chromosomal aberrations are also significantly correlated with the fragile sites, breakpoints, and rearrangements characteristic of AML.[28, 90, 210] Other genetic bone marrow failure syndromes that appear to be linked with leukemia include Diamond-Blackfan and amegakaryocytic thrombocytopenia, and perhaps Klinefelter's syndrome and D trisomy.[88, 314, 320]

Cytogenetic Abnormalities and Oncogenes

The Philadelphia (Ph) chromosome was the first cytogenetic abnormality linked to a majority of cases with a disease entity, namely CML.[236] The Ph chromosome results from the transposition of part of the oncogene abl from chromosome 9 to an abbreviated gene within the breakpoint cluster region (bcr) at band q11 on chromosome 22, leading to the creation of a new gene with abnormal messenger RNA and a resultant abnormal protein product. Other oncogenes frequently implicated in the leukemias include h-ras and c-myc. A specific susceptibility to breakage at the centromere after exposure to alkylating agents is suggested as the explanation for the frequent loss of whole chromosomes (in particular, chromosomes 5 and 7) in therapy-related myelodysplastic syndromes and AML.[8] A few case-control studies of AML have reported associations of various other exposures (paints, cigarette smoking, alcohol use) with karyotypic abnormalities observed in myelodysplastic syndromes and AML such as 5/5q, 7/7q, +8, and t(8;21).[58, 65]

Studies of workers with high levels of benzene exposure (a known leukemogen) but no evidence of leukemia have shown similar types of cytogenetic abnormalities as have been observed in myelodysplastic syndromes (preleukemia) or AML. These include increased aneusomy and long-arm deletions of chromosomes 5 and 7 in lymphocytes[317] and translocations in chromosomes 8 and 21.[266]

Gale et al[91] demonstrated that unique or clonotypic MLL-AF4 genomic fusion sequences were present in neonatal blood spots of children diagnosed with ALL at ages 5 months to 2 years and thus must have arisen during fetal hematopoiesis in utero.[91] These data confirm the prenatal initiation of acute leukemia in very young children. In addition, Wiemels et al[299] identified TEL-AML1 gene fusion in neonatal blood spots of children newly diagnosed at ages 2 to 5 years with the common form of acute lymphoblastic leukemia characterized by this chromosomal translocation, thus demonstrating that the event initiating the chromosomal translocation must have occurred in utero. Yet, the delay in onset of common childhood ALL until years after the translocation also suggested that a postnatal promotional event was required.

Genetic Polymorphisms

For an unknown proportion of leukemia patients, certain polymorphisms of genes that encode metabolizing enzymes, detoxification of carcinogens, immune-related mechanisms, and other physiologic functions may modify (by increasing or reducing) leukemia risk associated with specific exposures. Individuals with specific polymorphisms in the methylenetetrahydrofolate reductase gene have been found to be at reduced risk of adult ALL.[263] Adult AML was weakly associated with both GST T1 null and GST M1 null polymorphisms, whereas adult ALL was linked with GST T1 null, even though no associations were found between smoking and disease risk in relation to GST T1 and GST M1 polymorphisms.[227] Benzene poisoning (hematotoxicity), a strong predictor for adult myelodysplastic syndromes and AML, was found to be associated with polymorphisms in genotypes of enzymes that activate (i.e., CYP2E1) and detoxify (i.e., NQO1) benzene and its metabolites among Chinese benzene-exposed workers.[235] Infants developing leukemia characterized by MLL gene rearrangements were more than twice as likely to have genotypes with low NQO1 function (a polymorphism in an enzyme that detoxifies quinones, which are a structural feature shared by many topoisomerase II–inhibiting drugs as well as other chemicals) than healthy children or childhood leukemia patients with TEL-AML1 gene fusions or with hyperdiploidy.[301] The subset of infants whose MLL gene rearrangement resulted in an MLL-AF4 gene fusion had an eightfold increased risk of low NQO1 function.[301] Chen and colleagues[50] reported a higher frequency of the double null genotype (lacking both glutathione S-transferase M1 (GSTM1) and GSTT1 genotypes) in African-American children with ALL, but this double-null genotype was not associated with prognosis. The relationship of this finding, if any, to the lower incidence of ALL in African-American rather than white children is unclear.

PROSPECTS FOR PREVENTION

In the absence of more substantial knowledge about major risk factors for leukemia, it does not appear that leukemia incidence can be substantially reduced in the near future. It is important to avoid unnecessary exposures to ionizing radiation, and the benefits of diagnostic and therapeutic medical radiation exposures must continue to be weighed against their risks. The ubiquitous exposure to benzene from environmental sources (cigarette smoking, automobile fuel and exhaust, and chemical contaminants) or industrial sources (occupational exposures in chemical manufacturing, petroleum refining, and other industrial plants) is now increasingly regulated throughout the industrialized world. However, the present state of knowledge is insufficient to recommend curtailing or modifying use of agricultural chemicals to prevent leukemia. Increasingly stringent measures are being used to prohibit smoking in public or work places, to prevent children from initiating smoking, and to limit smoking by a variety of public health and economic measures. The spread of HTLV-I can be disrupted by screening blood products, educating infected mothers not to breast feed, and discouraging needle sharing by parenteral drug users.

The principal risk factors for most forms of leukemia are as yet undiscovered. Thus, the prevention of leukemia awaits further advances in our knowledge of etiology. Variations in leukemia occurrence by subtype suggest that risk factors may not be identical for the different forms of leukemia. Future analytic studies should evaluate postulated host and environmental risk factors for homogeneous, biologically defined leukemia subtypes; improve the accuracy of exposure assessment; and incorporate detailed evaluation of a broad range of genetic factors that may affect the risk of developing leukemia.

Acknowledgments

We acknowledge the sustained high-quality operations of the individual registries participating in the SEER Program and the dedication of the NCI SEER staff. We are indebted to John Lahey (Information Management Systems, Rockville, MD) for expert programming assistance in figure development and to Dan Grauman (Biostatistics Branch, Division of Cancer Epidemiology and Genetics, National Cancer Institute) for producing the U.S. maps depicting geographic variation in leukemia mortality.

REFERENCES

1. Adami J, Nyren O, Bergstrom R, et al: Smoking and the risk of leukemia, lymphoma, and multiple myeloma. Cancer Causes Control 1998, 9, 49.
2. Alavanja MC, Sandler DP, McMaster SB, et al: The Agricultural Health Study. Environ Health Perspect 1996, 104, 362.
3. Alexander FE, Boyle P, Carli P-M, et al: Spatial clustering of childhood leukaemia: Summary results from the EUROCLUS project. Br J Cancer 1998, 77, 818.
4. Alexander FE, Boyle P, Carli P-M, et al: Population density and childhood leukaemia: Results of the EUROCLUS study. Eur J Cancer 1999, 35, 439.
5. Alter BP, Caruso JP, Drachtman RA, et al: Fanconi anemia: Myelodysplasia as a predictor of outcome. Cancer Genet Cytogenet 2000, 117, 125.
6. Amadori D, Nanni O, Falcini F, et al: Chronic lymphocytic leukaemias and non-Hodgkin's lymphomas by histological type in farming-animal breeding workers: A population case-control study based on job titles. Occup Environ Med 1995, 52, 374.
7. Andersen MK, Johansson B, Larsen SO, et al: Chromosomal abnormalities in secondary MDS and AML: Relationship to drugs and radiation with specific emphasis on the balanced rearrangements. Haematologica 1998, 83, 438.
8. Andersen MK, Pedersen-Bjergaard J: Increased frequency of dicentric chromosomes in therapy-related MDS and AML compared to de novo disease is significantly related to previous treatment with alkylating agents and suggests a specific susceptibility to chromosome breakage at the centromere. Leukemia 2000, 14, 105.
9. Andersson M, Carstensen B, Visfeldt J: Leukemia and other related hematological disorders among Danish patients exposed to Thorotrast. Radiat Res 1993, 134, 224.
10. Aoki K, Kurihara M, Hayakawa N, et al: Death rates for malignant neoplasms for selected sites by sex and five year age group in 33 Countries 1953-57 through 1983-87. Nagoya, Japan, University of Nagoya Press, 1992.
11. Arico M, Biondi A, Pui CH: Juvenile myelomonocytic leukemia. Blood 1997, 90, 479.
12. Arisawa K, Soda M, Endo S, et al: Evaluation of adult T-cell leukemia/lymphoma incidence and its impact on non-Hodgkin lymphoma incidence in southwestern Japan. Int J Cancer 2000, 85, 319.
13. Avnon L, Oryan I, Kordysh E, et al: Cancer incidence and risks in selected agricultural settlements in the Negev of Israel. Arch Environ Health 1998, 53, 336.
14. Baverstock DF, Papworth DG: The UK radium luminiser survey. In Gossner W, Gerber GB (eds): The Radiobiology of Radium. Munich, Urban, 1986, pp 22-28.
15. Bell DW, Varley JM, Szydlo TE, et al: Heterozygous germ line hCHK2 mutations in Li-Fraumeni syndrome. Science 1999, 286, 2528.
16. Bennett JH: Case of hypertrophy of the spleen and liver in which death took place from suppuration of the blood. Edinburgh Med Surg J 1845, 64, 413.
17. Bennett JM, Catovsky D, Daniel MT, et al: Proposals for the classification of the acute leukemias. Br J Hematol 1976, 33, 451.
18. Bennett JM, Catovsky D, Daniel MT, et al: Criteria for the diagnosis of acute leukemia of megakaryocyte lineage (M7): A report of the French-American-British Cooperative Group. Ann Intern Med 1985, 103, 460.
19. Bennett JM, Catovsky D, Daniel MT, et al: Proposal for the classification of chronic (mature) B and T lymphoid leukemias. J Clin Pathol 1989, 42, 567.
20. Bennett JM, Catovsky D, Daniel MT, et al: Proposal for the recognition of minimally differentiated acute myeloid leukemia (AMLMO). Br J Hematol 1991, 78, 325.
21. Bennett JM, Moloney WC, Greene MH, et al: Acute myeloid leukemia and other myelopathic disorders following treatment with alkylating agents. Hematol Pathol 1987, 1, 99.
22. Bernstein L, Newton P, Ross RK: Epidemiology of hairy cell leukemia in Los Angeles County. Cancer Res 1990, 50, 3605.
23. Blackwelder WC, Yano K, Rhoads GG, et al: Alcohol and mortality: The Honolulu Heart Study. Am J Med 1980, 68, 164.
24. Blair B, Birch JM: Patterns and temporal trends in the incidence of malignant disease in children I: Leukaemia and lymphoma. Eur J Cancer 1994, 30A, 1498.
25. Blair A, Zahm SH: Agricultural exposures and cancer. Environ Health Perspect 1995, 103, 205.
26. Blair A, Zahm SH, Pearce NE, et al: Clues to cancer etiology from studies of farmers. Scand J Work Environ Health 1992, 18, 209.
27. Blattner WA: Human retroviruses: Their role in cancer. Proc Assoc Am Physicians 1999, 111, 563.
28. Bloom GE, Warner S, Gerland PS, et al: Chromosome abnormalities in constitutional aplastic anemia. N Engl J Med 1966, 274, 8.
29. Boice JD, Blettner M, Kleinerman RA, et al: Radiation dose and leukemia risk in patients treated for cancer of the cervix. J Natl Cancer Inst 1987, 79, 1295.
30. Boice JD Jr, Land CE, Preston DL: Ionizing radiation. In Schottenfeld D, Fraumeni JF Jr (eds): Cancer Epidemiology and Prevention, 2nd edition. New York, Oxford University Press, 1996, pp 319-54.
31. Boice JD Jr, Miller RW: Childhood and adult cancer after intrauterine exposure to ionizing radiation. Teratology 1999, 59, 227.
32. Boice JD Jr, Morin MM, Glass AG, et al: Diagnostic x-rays and risk of leukemia, lymphoma, and multiple myeloma. J Am Med Assoc 1991, 265, 1290.
33. Boice JD Jr, Storm HH, Curtis RE, et al: Multiple primary cancers in Connecticut and Denmark. Bethesda, Maryland, USDHHS, PHS, NIH Publ. No. 85-2714, 1985.
34. Brasso K, Friis S, Kjaer SK, et al: Prostate cancer in Denmark: A 50-year population-based study. Urology 1998, 51, 590.
35. Brenner MK, Pinkel D: Cure of leukemia. Semin Hematol 1999, 36, 73.
36. Breslow NE, Takashima JR, Whitton JA, et al: Second malignant neoplasms following treatment for Wilms' tumor: A report from the National Wilms' Tumor Study Group. J Clin Oncol 1995, 13, 1851.

37. Brondum J, Shu XO, Steinbuch M, et al: Parental cigarette smoking and the risk of acute leukemia in children. Cancer 1999, 85, 1380.

38. Brown LM, Blair A, Gibson R, et al: Pesticide exposures and other agricultural risk factors for leukemia among men in Iowa and Minnesota. Cancer Res 1990, 50, 6585.

39. Brown LM, Gibson R, Burmeister LF, et al: Alcohol consumption and risk of leukemia, non-Hodgkin's lymphoma, and multiple myeloma. Leuk Res 1992, 16, 979.

40. Brownson RC, Novotny TE, Perry MC: Cigarette smoking and adult leukemia: A meta-analysis. Arch Intern Med 1993, 153, 469.

41. Buckley JD, Buckley CM, Breslow NE, et al: Concordance for childhood cancer in twins. Med Pediatr Oncol 1996, 26, 223.

42. Bulbulyan MA, Changuina OV, Zaridze DG, et al: Cancer mortality among Moscow shoe workers exposed to chloroprene (Russia). Cancer Causes Control 1998, 9, 381.

43. Burnett C, Robison C, Walker J: Cancer mortality in health and science technicians. Am J Ind Med 1999, 36, 155.

44. Caldwell GG, Kelley D, Heath CW Jr, et al: Mortality and cancer frequency among military nuclear test (Smoky) participants 1957 through 1959. JAMA 1983, 250, 620.

45. Cardis E, Gilbert ES, Carpenter L, et al: Effects of low doses and low dose rates of external ionizing radiation: Cancer mortality among nuclear industry workers in three countries. Radiat Res 1995, 142, 117.

46. Carstensen JM, Bygren LO, Hatschek T: Cancer incidence among Swedish brewery workers. Int J Cancer 1990, 45, 393.

47. Cartwright RA, McNally RJQ, Rowland DJ, et al: The Descriptive Epidemiology of Leukaemia and Related Conditions in Parts of the United Kingdom, 1984–1993. London, Leukaemia Research Fund, 1997.

48. Cassileth PA, Harrington DP, Appelbaum FR, et al: Chemotherapy compared with autologous or allogeneic bone marrow transplantation in the management of acute myeloid leukemia in first remission. N Engl J Med 1998, 339, 1649.

49. Catovsky D, Matutes E, Buccheri V, et al: A classification of acute leukemia for the 1990's. Ann Hematol 1991, 62, 16.

50. Chen CL, Liu Q, Pui CH, et al: Higher frequency of glutathione S-transferase deletions in black children with acute lymphoblastic leukemia. Blood 1997, 89, 1701.

51. Chen R, Seaton A: A meta-analysis of painting exposure and cancer mortality. Cancer Detect Prev 1998, 22, 533.

52. Chen YT, Zheng T, Chou MC, et al: The increase of Hodgkin's disease incidence among young adults: Experience in Connecticut, 1935–1992. Cancer 1997, 79, 2209.

53. Chessells JM, Hall E, Prentice HG, et al: The impact of age on outcome in lymphoblastic leukemia; MRC UKALL X and XA compared: A report from the MRC Paediatric and Adult Working Parties. Leukemia 1998, 12, 463.

54. Chessells JM, Richards SM, Bailey CC, et al: Gender and treatment outcome in childhood lymphoblastic leukaemia: Report from the MRC UKALL trials. Br J Haematol, 1995, 89, 364.

55. Cheson BD, Bennett JM, Grever M, et al: National Cancer Institute-sponsored Working Group guidelines for chronic lymphocytic leukemia: Revised guidelines for diagnosis and treatment. Blood 1996, 87, 4990.

56. Cheson BD, Cassileth PA, Head DR, et al: Report on the National Cancer Institute-sponsored workshop on definitions and response in acute myeloid leukemia. J Clin Oncology 1990, 8, 813.

57. Cleghorn FR, Manns A, Falk R, et al: Effect of human T-lymphotropic virus type I infections on non-Hodgkin's lymphoma incidence. J Natl Cancer Inst 1995, 87, 1009.

58. Crane MM, Strom SS, Halabi S, et al: Correlation between selected environmental exposures and karyotype in acute myelocytic leukemia. Cancer Epidemiol Biomarkers Prev 1996, 8, 639.

59. Crump KS: Risk of benzene-induced leukemia: A sensitivity analysis of the Pliofilm cohort with additional follow-up and new exposure estimates. J Toxicol Environ Health 1994, 42, 219.

60. Crump KS: Risk of benzene-induced leukemia predicted from the Pliofilm cohort. Environ Health Perspect 1996, 104, 1437.

61. Curtis RE, Boice JD, Stovall M, et al: Risk of leukemia after chemotherapy and radiation treatment for breast cancer. N Engl J Med 1992, 326, 1745.

62. Curtis RE, Boice JD, Stovall M, et al: Relation of leukemia risk to radiation dose after cancer of the uterine corpus. J Natl Cancer Inst 1994, 86, 1315.

63. Cuttner J: Increased incidence of hematologic malignancies in first-degree relatives of patients with chronic lymphocytic leukemia. Cancer Invest 1992, 10, 103.

64. Darby SC, Reeves G, Key T, et al: Mortality in a cohort of women given x-ray therapy for metropathia haemorrhagica. Int J Cancer 1994, 56, 793.

65. Davico L, Sacerdote C, Ciccone G, et al: Chromosome 8, occupational exposures, smoking, and acute nonlymphocytic leukemias: A population-based study. Cancer Epidemiol Biomarkers Prev 1998, 12, 1123.

66. Dean G: Deaths from primary brain cancers, lymphatic and haematopoietic cancers in agricultural workers in the Republic of Ireland. J Epidemiol Commun Health 1994, 48, 364.

67. Delore P, Borgomano C: Leukemia aigue un cour de l'intoxication benzenique, sur l'origine de certains leukemies aigues et leurs relations avec les anemies graves. J Med Lyon 1928, 9, 227.

68. Devesa SS, Grauman DJ, Blot WJ, et al: Atlas of cancer mortality in the United States. 1950–94. Bethesda, Maryland, NIH, NCI, NIH Publ. No. 99-4564, 1999.

69. Dighiero G, Maloum K, Desablens B, et al: Chlorambucil in indolent chronic lymphocytic leukemia: French Cooperative Group on Chronic Lymphocytic Leukemia. N Engl J Med 1998, 338, 1506.

70. Doll R: Cancers weakly related to smoking. Br Med Bull 1996, 52, 35.

71. Doody MM, Mandel JS, Lubin JH, et al: Mortality among United States radiologic technologists, 1926–90. Cancer Causes Control 1998, 9, 67.

72. Dosemeci M, Yin SN, Linet M, et al: Indirect validation of benzene exposure assessment by association with benzene poisoning. Environ Health Perspect 1996, 104, 1343.

73. dos Santos Silva I, Jones M, Malveiro F, et al: Mortality in the Portuguese Thorotrast study. Radiat Res 1999, 152, S88.

74. Douer D, Preston-Martin S, Chang E, et al: High frequency of acute promyelocytic leukemia among Latinos with acute myeloid leukemia. Blood 1996, 87, 308.

75. Draper GJ, Kroll ME, Stiller CA: Childhood cancer. Cancer Surv 1994, 19–20, 493.

76. Edlich RF, Arnette JA, Williams FM: Global epidemic of human T-cell lymphotropic virus type-I (HTLV-I). J Emerg Med 2000, 18, 109.

77. Engeland A, Andersen A, Haldorsen T, et al: Smoking habits and risk of cancers other than lung cancer: 28 years' follow-up of 26,000 Norwegian men and women. Cancer Causes Control 1996, 7, 497.

78. Evans JS, Wennberg JE, McNeil BJ: The influence of diagnostic radiography on the incidence of breast cancer and leukemia. N Engl J Med 1986, 315, 810.

79. Felix CA: Secondary leukemias induced by topoisomerase-targeted drugs. Biochim Biophys Acta 1998, 1400, 233.

80. Fenaux P, Chastang C, Chevret S, et al: A randomized comparison of all transretinoic acid (ATRA) followed by chemotherapy and ATRA plus chemotherapy and the role of maintenance therapy in newly diagnosed acute promyelocytic leukemia. The European APL Group. Blood 1999, 94, 1192.

81. Ferreira OC Jr, Planelles V, Rosenblatt JD: Human T-cell leukemia viruses: Epidemiology, biology, and pathogenesis. Blood Rev 1997, 11, 91.

82. Feychting M, Ahlbom A: Magnetic fields and cancer in children residing near Swedish high voltage power lines. Am J Epidemiol 1993, 138, 467.

83. Feychting M, Forssen U, Floderus B: Occupational and residential magnetic field exposure and leukemia and central nervous system tumors. Epidemiology 1997, 8, 384.

84. Finch SC, Linet MS: Chronic leukemias. In Fleming AF (ed): Epidemiology of Haematological Disease. Part I. London, Bailliere Tindall, 1992, pp 27–56.

85. Floderus B, Persson T, Stenlund C, et al: Occupational exposure to electromagnetic fields in relation to leukemia and brain tumors: A case-control study in Sweden. Cancer Causes Control 1993, 4, 465.

86. Ford AM, Ridge SA, Cabrera ME, et al: In utero rearrangements in the trithorax-related oncogene in infant leukemias. Nature 1993, 363, 358.

87. Foucar K, Duncan MH, Stidley CA, et al: Survival of children and adolescents with acute lymphoid leukemia: A study of American

Indians and Hispanic and non-Hispanic whites treated in New Mexico (1969 to 1986). Cancer 1991, 67, 2125.

88. Fraumeni JF, Miller RW: Epidemiology of human leukemia: Recent observations. J Natl Cancer Inst 1967, 38, 593.

89. Fujiyoshi T, Li HC, Lou H, et al: Characteristic distribution of HTLV type I and HTLV type II carriers among native ethnic groups in South America. AIDS Res Hum Retroviruses 1999, 15, 1235.

90. Fundia A, Gorla N, Larripa I: Non-random distribution of spontaneous chromosome aberrations in two Bloom syndrome patients. Hereditas 1995, 122, 239.

91. Gale KB, Ford AM, Repp R, et al: Backtracking leukemia to birth: Identification of clonotypic genefusion sequences in neonatal blood spots. Proc Natl Acad Sci U S A 1997, 94, 13950.

92. Garfinkel L, Boffetta P: Association between smoking and leukemia in two American Cancer Society prospective studies. Cancer 1990, 65, 2356.

93. Goldgar DE, Easton DF, Cannon-Albright LA, et al: Systematic population-based assessment of cancer risk in first-degree relatives of cancer probands. J Natl Cancer Inst 1994, 86, 1600.

94. Goldin LR, Sgambati M, Marti GE, et al: Anticipation in familial CLL. Am J Hum Genet 1999, 65, 265.

95. Greaves MF: Aetiology of acute leukaemia. Lancet 1997, 349, 344.

96. Greaves MF, Alexander F: An infectious etiology for common acute lymphoblastic leukemia in childhood? Leukemia 1993, 7, 349.

97. Greaves MF, Colman SM, Beard MEJ, et al: Geographical distribution of acute lymphoblastic leukemia subtypes: Second report of the collaborative group study. Leukemia 1993, 7, 27.

98. Greaves MF, Pegram SM, Chan LC: Collaborative group study of the epidemiology of acute lymphoblastic leukemia subtypes: Background and first report. Leuk Res 1985, 9, 715.

99. Greene MH: Interaction between radiotherapy and chemotherapy in human leukemogenesis. In Boice JD Jr, Fraumeni JF Jr (eds): Radiation Carcinogenesis: Epidemiology and Biological Significance. New York, Raven Press, 1984, pp 199–210.

100. Griem ML, Kleinerman RA, Boice JD Jr, et al: Cancer following radiotheraphy for peptic ulcer. J Natl Cancer Inst 1994, 86, 842.

101. Groves FD, Gridley G, Wacholder S, et al: Infant vaccinations and risk of childhood acute lymphoblastic leukemia in the USA. Br J Cancer 1999, 81, 175.

102. Groves FD, Linet MS, Devesa SS: Patterns of occurrence of the leukaemias. Eur J Cancer 1995, 31A, 941.

103. Groves FD, Linet MS, Devesa SS: Epidemiology of leukemia: Overview and patterns of occurrence. In Henderson ES, Lister TA, Greaves MF (eds): Leukemia, 6th ed. Philadelphia, WB Saunders, 1996, pp 145–159.

104. Gunz F, Atkinson H: Medical radiation and leukemia: A retrospective survey. Br Med J 1964, 5380, 389.

105. Gunz FW, Gunz JP, Veale AMO, et al: Familial leukemia: A study of 909 families. Scand J Haematol 1978, 15, 117.

106. Haferlach T, Bennett JM, Loffler H, et al: Acute myeloid leukemia with a translocation (8;21): Cytomorphology, dysplasia and prognostic factors in 41 cases. AJL Cooperative Group and ECOG. Leuk Lymphoma 1996, 23, 227.

107. Hasle H, Clemmensen IH, Mikkelsen M: Risks of leukemia and solid tumours in individuals with Down's syndrome. Lancet 2000, 355, 165.

108. Hayes RB, Blair A, Stewart PA, et al: Mortality of U.S. embalmers and funeral directors. Am J Ind Med 1990, 18, 641.

109. Hayes RB, Yin SN, Dosemeci M, et al: Benzene and the dose-related incidence of hematologic neoplasms in China. Chinese Academy of Preventive Medicine–National Cancer Institute Benzene Study Group. J Natl Cancer Inst 1997, 89, 1065.

110. Hecht F, Hecht BK: Cancer in ataxia telangectasia patients. Cancer Genet Cytogenet 1990, 46, 9.

111. Heerema NA: Cytogenetics of leukemia. Cancer Invest 1998, 16, 127.

112. Heston JF, Kelly JB, Meigs JW, et al: Forty-five years of cancer incidence in Connecticut, 1935-79. Bethesda, Maryland: USDHHS, PHS, NIH Publ. No. 86-2652, 1986.

113. Hill JM, Meehan KR. Chronic myelogenous leukemia: Curable with early diagnosis and treatment. Postgrad Med 1999, 106, 149.

114. Hinds MW, Kolonel LN, Lee T, et al: Associations between cancer incidence and alcohol and cigarette consumption among five ethnic groups in Hawaii. Br J Cancer 1980, 41, 929.

115. Hisada M, Garber JE, Fung CY, et al: Multiple primary cancers in families with Li-Fraumeni syndrome. J Natl Cancer Inst 1998, 90, 606.

116. Hodgson JR, Jones RD: Mortality of a cohort of tin miners 1941-86. Br J Ind Med 1990, 47, 665.

117. Horm JW, Devesa SS, Birhanstippanov L: Cancer incidence, mortality, and survival among racial and ethnic minority groups in the United States. In Schottenfeld D, Fraumeni JF (eds): Cancer Epidemiology and Prevention, 2nd ed. New York, Oxford University Press pp 192-235.

118. Horowitz M: The genetics of familial leukemia. Leukemia 1997, 11, 1347.

119. Horowitz M, Goode EL, Jarvik GP: Anticipation in familial leukemia. Am J Hum Genet 1996, 59, 990.

120. Hotz P, Lauwerys RR: Hematopoietic and lymphatic malignancies in vehicle mechanics. Crit Rev Toxicol 1997, 27, 443.

121. Huebner WW, Schnatter AR, Nicolich MJ, et al: Mortality experience of a young petrochemical industry cohort: 1979-1992 follow-up study of US-based employees. J Occup Environ Med 1997, 39, 970.

122. Hunting KL, Longbottom H, Kalavar SS, et al: Haematopoietic cancer mortality among vehicle mechanics. Occup Environ Med 1995, 52, 673.

123. Hursting SD, Margolin BH, Switzer BR: Diet and human leukemia: An analysis of international data. Prev Med 1993, 22, 409.

124. Inskip PD: Second cancers following radiotherapy. In Neugut AI, Meadows AT (eds): Multiple Primary Cancers, Philadelphia, Lippincott Williams & Wilkins, 1999, pp 91–135.

125. Inskip PD, Harvey EB, Boice JD Jr, et al: Incidence of cancer in twins. Cancer Causes Control 1991, 2, 315.

126. Inskip PD, Kleinerman RA, Stovall M, et al: Leukemia, lymphoma, and multiple myeloma after pelvic radiotherapy for benign disease. Radiat Res 1993, 135, 108.

127. Inskip PD, Monson RR, Wagoner JK, et al: Leukemia following radiotherapy for uterine bleeding. Radiat Res 1990, 122, 107.

128. International Agency for Research on Cancer: Monographs on the Evaluation of the Carcinogenic Risk of Chemicals to Man: Allyl Compounds, Aldehydes, Epoxides, and Peroxides, vol. 36. Lyon, France, IARC, 1985, pp 189-226.

129. Ireland B, Collins JJ, Buckley CF, et al: Cancer mortality among workers with benzene exposure. Epidemiology 1997, 8, 318.

130. Irons RD, Pyatt DW: Dithiocarbamates as potential confounders in butadiene epidemiology. Carcinogenesis 1998, 19, 539.

131. Jablon S, Miller RW: Army technologists: 29-year follow up for cause of death. Radiology 1978, 126, 677.

132. Jensen OM: Cancer morbidity and causes of death among Danish brewery workers. Int J Cancer 1979, 23, 454.

133. Ji BT, Shu XO, Linet MS, et al: Paternal cigarette smoking and the risk of childhood cancer among offspring of nonsmoking mothers. J Natl Cancer Inst 1997, 89, 238.

134. Johansen C, Olsen JH: Risk of cancer among Danish utility workers: A nationwide cohort study. Am J Epidemiol 1998, 147, 548.

135. Kaldor JM, Day NE, Clarke EA, et al: Leukemia following Hodgkin's disease. N Engl J Med 1990, 322, 7.

136. Kane EV, Roman E, Cartwright R, et al: Tobacco and the risk of acute leukaemia in adults. Br J Cancer 1999, 81, 1228.

137. Keller-Byrne JE, Khuder SA, Schaub EA: Meta-analysis of leukemia and farming. Environ Res 1995, 71, 1.

138. Khalidi HS, Chang KL, Medeiros LJ, et al: Acute lymphoblastic leukemia: Survey of immunophenotype, French-American-British classification, frequency of myeloid antigen expression, and karyotypic abnormalities in 210 pediatric and adult cases. Am J Clin Pathol 1999, 111, 467.

139. Khalil N, Cheson BD: Chronic lymphocytic leukemia. Oncologist 1999, 4, 352.

140. Kheifets LI, London SJ, Peters JM: Leukemia risk and occupational electric field exposure in Los Angeles County, California. Am J Epidemiol 1997, 146, 87.

141. Kinlen L: Evidence for an infective cause of childhood leukaemia: Comparison of a Scottish new town with nuclear reprocessing sites in Britain. Lancet 1988, ii, 1323.

142. Kinlen LJ: High-contact paternal occupations, infection and childhood leukaemia: Five studies of unusual population-mixing of adults. Br J Cancer 1997, 76, 1539.

143. Kinlen LJ: Leukemia. In Doll R, Fraumeni JF, Muir CS (eds): Trends in Cancer Incidence and Mortality. Cancer Surv 1994, 19/20, 475.

144. Kinlen LJ, Clarke K, Hudson C: Evidence from population mixing in British New Towns 1946–85 of an infective basis for childhood leukaemia. Lancet 1990, 336, 577.

145. Kinlen LJ, Dickson M, Stiller CA: Childhood leukaemia and non-Hodgkin's lymphoma near large rural construction sites, with a comparison with Sellafield nuclear site. Br Med J 1993, 310, 763.

146. Kinlen LJ, John SM: Wartime evacuation and mortality from childhood leukaemia in England and Wales in 1945–9. Br Med J 1994, 309, 1197.

147. Kinlen LJ, Petridou E: Childhood leukemia and rural population movements: Greece, Italy, and other countries. Cancer Causes Control 1995, 6, 445.

148. Kinlen LJ, Stiller C: Population mixing and excess of childhood leukemia. Br Med J 1993, 306, 930.

149. Krishnan A, Bhatia S, Slovak ML, et al: Predictors of therapy-related leukemia and myelodysplasia following autologous transplantation for lymphoma: An assessment of risk factors. Blood 2000, 95, 1588.

150. Kristensen P, Andersen A, Irgens LM, et al: Incidence and risk factors of cancer among men and women in Norwegian agriculture. Scand J Work Environ Health 1996, 22, 14.

151. Kristensen P, Andersen A, Irgens LM, et al: Cancer in offspring of parents engaged in agricultural activities in Norway: Incidence and risk factors in the farm environment. Int J Cancer 1996, 65, 39.

152. Kuttesch JF Jr, Wexler LH, Marcus RB, et al: Second malignancies after Ewing's sarcoma: Radiation dose dependency of secondary sarcomas. J Clin Oncol 1996, 14, 2818.

153. Kwiatkowski A: Dietary and other environmental risk factors in acute leukemias: A case-control study of 119 patients. Eur J Cancer Prev 1993, 2, 139.

154. Larson RA, Wang Y, Banerjee M, et al: Prevalence of the inactivating $^{609}C \rightarrow T$ polymorphism in the NAD(P)H:quinone oxidoreductase (NQO1) gene in patients with primary and therapy-related myeloid leukemia. Blood 1999, 94, 803.

155. Leone G, Mele L, Pulsoni A, et al: The incidence of secondary leukemias. Haematologica 1999, 84, 937.

156. Levine PH, Dosik H, Joseph EM, et al: A study of adult T-cell leukemia/lymphoma incidence in central Brooklyn. Int J Cancer 1999, 80, 662.

157. Li FP, Yan JC, Sallan S, et al: Second neoplasms after Wilms' tumor in childhood. J Natl Cancer Inst 1983, 71, 1205.

158. Linet MS, Cartwright RA: The leukemias. In Schottenfeld DM, Fraumeni JF (eds): Cancer Epidemiology and Prevention, 2nd ed. New York, Oxford University Press, 1996, pp 841–892.

159. Linet MS, Devesa SS: Descriptive epidemiology of childhood leukemia. Br J Cancer 1991, 63, 424.

160. Linet MS, Hatch EE, Kleinerman RA, et al: Residential exposure to magnetic fields and acute lymphoblastic leukemia in children. N Engl J Med 1997, 337, 1.

161. Linet MS, Pottern LM: Familial aggregation of hematopoietic malignancies and risk of non-Hodgkins' lymphoma. Cancer Res 1992, 52, 5468.

162. Linet MS, Ries LAG, Smith MA, et al: Cancer surveillance series: Recent trends in childhood cancer incidence and mortality in the United States. J Natl Cancer Inst 1999, 91, 1051.

163. Linos A, Blair A, Cantor KP, et al: Leukemia and non-Hodgkin's lymphoma among embalmers and funeral directors. J Natl Cancer Inst 1990, 82.

164. Little JB: Cellular, molecular, and carcinogenic effects of radiation. Hematol Oncol Clin North Am 1993, 7, 337.

165. London SJ, Bowman JD, Sobel E, et al: Exposure to magnetic fields among electrical workers in relation to leukemia risk in Los Angeles County. Am J Med 1994, 26, 47.

166. London SJ, Thomas DC, Bowman JD, et al: Exposure to residential electric and magnetic fields and risk of childhood leukemia. Am J Epidemiol 1991, 134, 923.

167. Lynge E: Danish Cancer Registry as a resource for occupational research. J Occup Med 1994, 36, 1169.

168. Macaluso M, Larson R, Delzell E, et al: Leukemia and cumulative exposure to butadiene, styrene and benzene among workers in the synthetic rubber industry. Toxicology 1996, 113, 190.

169. MacMahon B, Levy M: Prenatal origin of childhood leukemia: Evidence from twins. N Engl J Med 1964, 270, 1082.

170. Mahieux R, Ibrahim F, Mauclere P, et al: Molecular epidemiology of 58 new African human T-cell leukemia virus type 1 (HTLV-1) strains: Identification of a new and distinct HTLV-1 molecular subtype in Central Africa and in Pygmies. J Virol 1997, 71, 1317.

171. Maljaei SH, Brito-Babapulle V, Hiorns LR, et al: Abnormalities of chromosomes 8, 11, 14, and X in T-prolymphocytic leukemia studied by fluorescence in situ hybridization. Cancer Genet Cytogenet 1998, 103, 110.

172. Malkin D, Brown EJ, Zipursky A: The role of p53 in megakaryocyte differentiation and the megakaryocytic leukemias of Down syndrome. Cancer Genet Cytogenet 2000, 116, 1.

173. Manns A, Hisada M, La Grenade L: Human T-lymphotropic virus types I infection. Lancet 1999, 353, 1951.

174. Martling U, Mattson A, Travis LB, et al: Mortality after long-term exposure to radioactive Thorotrast: A forty-year follow-up survey in Sweden. Radiat Res 1999, 151, 293.

175. Matanoski GM, Elliott E, Breysse PN, et al: Leukemia in telephone linemen. Am J Epidemiol 1993, 137, 609.

176. Matanoski GM, Elliott E, Tao X, et al: Lymphohematopoietic cancers and butadiene and styrene exposure in synthetic rubber manufacture. Ann N Y Acad Sci 1997, 837, 157.

177. Matanoski GM, Kanchanaraksa S, Lees PS, et al: Industry-wide study of mortality of pulp and paper mill workers. Am J Ind Med 1998, 33, 354.

178. Matanoski GM, Sartwell P, Elliott E, et al: Cancer risks in radiologists and radiation workers. In Boice JD Jr, Fraumeni JF Jr (eds): Radiation Carcinogenesis: Epidemiology and Biological Significance. New York, Raven Press, 1984, pp 83–96.

179. Matanoski GM, Stockwell HG, Diamond EL, et al: A cohort mortality study of painters and allied tradesmen. Scand J Work Environ Health 1986, 12, 16.

180. Matutes E: Contribution of immunophenotype in the diagnosis and classification of haemopoietic malignancies. J Clin Pathol 1995, 48, 194.

181. Matutes E, Carrara P, Coignet L, et al: FISH analysis for BCL-1 rearrangements and trisomy 12 helps the diagnosis of atypical B cell leukaemias. Leukemia 1999, 13, 1721.

182. Matutes E, Morilla R, Farahat N, et al: Definition of acute biphenotypic leukemia. Haematologica 1997, 82, 64.

183. McBride ML, Gallagher RP, Theriault G, et al: Power-frequency electric and magnetic fields and risk of childhood leukemia in Canada. Am J Epidemiol 1999, 149, 831.

184. McKinney PA, Alexander FE, Roberts BE, et al: Yorkshire case control study of leukemias and lymphomas: Parallel multivariate analysis of seven disease categories. Leuk Lymph 1990, 2, 67.

185. McLaughlin JR, Clarke EA, Nishri ED, et al: Childhood leukemia in the vicinity of Canadian nuclear facilities. Cancer Causes Control 1993, 4, 51.

186. McMichael AJ, Spirtas R, Gamble JF, et al: Mortality among rubber workers: Relationship to specific jobs. J Occup Med 1976, 18, 178.

187. Metayer C, Johnson ES, Rice JC: Nested case-control study of tumors of the hematopoietic and lymphatic systems among workers in the meat industry. Am J Epidemiol 1998, 147, 727.

188. Michaelis J, Schuz J, Meinert R, et al: Childhood leukemia and electromagnetic fields: Results of a population-based case-control study in Germany. Cancer Causes Control 1997, 8, 167.

189. Milham S Jr: Mortality from leukemia in workers exposed to electrical and magnetic fields. N Engl J Med 1982, 307, 249.

190. Milham S Jr: Mortality in workers exposed to electromagnetic fields. Environ Health Perspect 1985, 62, 297.

191. Miligi L, Seniori Costantini A, Crosignani P, et al: Occupational, environmental, and life-style factors associated with the risk of hematolymphopoietic malignancies in women. Am J Ind Med 1999, 36, 60.

192. Miller AB, To T, Agnew DA, et al: Leukemia following occupational exposure to 60-Hz electric and magnetic fields among Ontario electric utility workers. Am J Epidemiol 1996, 144, 150.

193. Miller BA, Blair A, Reed EJ: Extended mortality follow-up among men and women in a U.S. furniture workers union. Am J Ind Med, 1994, 25, 537.

194. Miller RW: Deaths from childhood leukemia and solid tumors among twins and other sibs in the United States 1960-67. J Natl Cancer Inst 1971, 46, 203.

195. Moloney WC: Radiogenic leukemia revisited. Blood 1987, 70, 905.

196. Muirhead CR, Goodill AA, Haylock RG, et al: Occupational radiation exposure and mortality: Second analysis of the National Registry for Radiation Workers. J Radiat Prot 1999, 19, 3.

197. Murphy EL, Hanchard B, Figueroa JP, et al: Modeling the risk of adult T-cell leukemia/lymphoma in persons infected with human T-lymphotropic virus type I. Int J Cancer 1989, 43, 250.

198. Nagai K, Kohno T, Chen YX, et al: Diagnostic criteria for hypocellular acute leukemia: A clinical entity distinct from overt acute leukemia and myelodysplastic syndrome. Leuk Res 1996, 20, 563.

199. Nanni O, Amadori D, Lugaresi C, et al: Chronic lymphocytic leukaemias and non-Hodgkin's lymphomas by histological type in farming-animal breeding workers: A population case-control study based on a priori exposure matrices. Occup Environ Med 1996, 53, 652.

200. National Research Council: Health Effects of Exposure to Radon. BEIR VI. Washington, DC, National Academy of Sciences, 1999, pp 18-20.

201. Neglia JP, Linet MS, Shu XO, et al: Patterns of infection and day care utilization and risk of childhood acute lymphoblastic leukaemia. Br J Cancer 2000, 82, 234.

202. Neglia JP, Robison LL: Epidemiology of the childhood acute leukemias. Pediatr Clin North Am 1988, 35, 675.

203. Nilsson RI, Nordlinder R, Horte LG, et al: Leukaemia, lymphoma, and multiple myeloma in seamen on tankers. Occup Environ Med 1998, 55, 517.

204. Ott MG, Kolesar RC, Scharnweber HC, et al: A mortality survey of employees engaged in the development or manufacture of styrene-based products. J Occup Med 1980, 22, 445.

205. Ott MG, Townsend JC, Fishback WA, et al: Mortality among individuals occupationally exposed to benzene. Arch Environ Health 1978, 33, 3.

206. Paietta E, Racevskis J, Bennett JM, et al: Biologic heterogeneity in Philadelphia chromosome–positive acute leukemia with myeloid morphology: The Eastern Cooperative Oncology Group experience. Leukemia 1998, 12, 1881.

207. Parkin DM, Kramarova E, Draper GJ, et al: International Incidence of Childhood Cancer, vol. II. Lyon, France, IARC Scientific Publication No. 144, 1999.

208. Parkin DM, Muir CS, Whelan SL, et al: Cancer Incidence in Five Continents, vol. VII. Lyon, France, IARC Scientific Publication No. 143, 1997.

209. Partanen T, Kauppinen T, Luukkonen R, et al: Malignant lymphomas and leukemias, and exposures in the wood industry: An industry-based case-referent study. Int Arch Occup Environ Health 1993, 64, 593.

210. Passarge E: Bloom's syndrome: The German experience. Ann Genet 1991, 34, 179.

211. Paustenbach DJ, Price PS, Ollison W, et al: Reevaluation of benzene exposure for the Pliofilm (rubber worker) cohort (1936-1976). J Toxicol Environ Health 1992, 36, 177.

212. Pearce N, Prior I, Methven D, et al: Follow up of New Zealand participants in British atmospheric nuclear weapons tests in the Pacific. Br Med J 1990, 300, 1161.

213. Percy C, Stanek E 3d, Gloeckler L: Accuracy of cancer death certificates and its effect on cancer mortality statistics. Am J Publ Health 1981, 71, 242.

214. Percy C, Van Holten V, Muir C (eds): International Classification of Diseases for Oncology, 2nd ed. Geneva, World Health Organization, 1992.

215. Petridou E, Kassimos D, Kalmanti M, et al: Age of exposure to infections and risk of childhood leukaemia. Br Med J 1993, 307, 774.

216. Pierce DA, Shimizu Y, Preston DL, et al: Studies of the mortality of atomic bomb survivors—Report 12, Part I: Cancer: 1950-1990. Radiat Res 1996, 146, 1.

217. Pollock BH, DeBaun MR, Camitta BM, et al: Racial differences in the survival of childhood B-precursor acute lymphoblastic leukemia: A pediatric oncology group study. J Clin Oncol 2000, 18, 813.

218. Pombo De Oliveira MS, Loureiro P, et al: Geographic diversity of adult t-cell leukemia/lymphoma in Brazil: The Brazilian ATLL Study Group. Int J Cancer 1999, 83, 291.

219. Portier CJ, Wolfe MS: Assessment of health effects from exposure to power-line frequency electric and magnetic fields: Working group report. NIH Publ No. 98-3981. Research Triangle Park, North Carolina, NIEHS, NIH, DHHS, PHS.

220. Preston D, Kusumi S, Tomonaga M, et al: Cancer incidence in atomic bomb survivors—Part III: Leukemia, lymphoma, and multiple myeloma, 1950-1987. Radiat Res 1994, 137, S68.

221. Preston-Martin S, Thomas DC, Yu MC, et al: Diagnostic radiography as a risk factor for chronic myeloid and monocytic leukaemia (CML). Br J Cancer 1989, 59, 649.

222. Raabe GK, Wong O: Leukemia mortality by cell type in petroleum workers with potential exposure to benzene. Environ Health Perspect 1996, 194, 1381.

223. Reed JC: Molecular biology of chronic lymphocytic leukemia: Implications for therapy. Semin Hematol 1998, 35, 3:13.

224. Ries LAG, Kosary CL, Hankey BF, et al (eds): Cancer Statistics Review, 1973-96, Bethesda, Maryland, National Cancer Institute, NIH Publication Number 99-2789, 1999.

225. Rinsky RA, Smith AB, Hornung R, et al: Benzene and leukemia: An epidemiologic risk assessment. N Engl J Med 1987, 316, 1044.

226. Robinette CD, Jablon S, Preston TL: Mortality of Nuclear Weapons Test Participants. Medical Follow-Up Agency, National Research Council. Washington, DC, National Academy Press, 1985.

227. Rollinson S, Roddam P, Kane E, et al: Polymorphic variation within the glutathione S-transferase genes and risk of adult leukaemia. Carcinogenesis 2000, 21, 43.

228. Roman E, Doyle P, Maconochie N, et al: Cancer in children of nuclear industry employees: Report on children aged under 25 years from nuclear industry family study. Br Med J 1999, 318, 1443.

229. Ron E: Ionizing radiation and cancer risk: Evidence from epidemiology. Radiat Res 1998, 150, S30.

230. Ron E, Modan B, Boice JD Jr: Mortality after radiotherapy for ringworm of the scalp. Am J Epidemiol 1988, 127, 713.

231. Ross JA, Coppes MJ, Robison LL: Population density and risk of childhood acute lymphoblastic leukaemia. Lancet 1999, 532.

232. Ross JA, Potter JD, Reaman GH, et al: Maternal exposure to potential inhibitors of DNA topoisomerase II and infant leukemia (United States): A report from the Children's Cancer Group. Cancer Causes Control 1996, 7, 581.

233. Roth VS: Rubber industry epidemiology. Occup Med 1999, 14, 849.

234. Rothman N, Li GL, Dosemeci M, et al: Hematotoxicity among Chinese workers heavily exposed to benzene. Am J Ind Med 1996, 29, 236.

235. Rothman N, Smith MT, Hayes RB, et al: Benzene poisoning, a risk factor for hematological malignancy, is associated with the NQO1 ^{609}C → T mutation and rapid fractional excretion of chlorzoxazone. Cancer Res 1997, 57, 2839.

236. Rowley JD: The role of chromosome translocations in leukemogenesis. Semin Hematol 1999, 36, 59.

237. Rowley JD: Molecular genetics in acute leukemia. Leukemia 2000, 14, 513.

238. Rozman C, Montserrat E: Chronic lymphocytic leukemia. N Engl J Med 1995, 333, 1052.

239. Rushton L, Romaniuk H: A case-control study to investigate the risk of leukaemia associated with exposure to benzene in petroleum marketing and distribution workers in the United Kingdom. Occup Environ Med 1997, 54, 152.

240. Sahl JD, Kelsh MA, Greenland S: Cohort and nested case-control studies of hematopoietic cancers and brain cancer among electric utility workers. Epidemiology 1993, 4, 104.

241. Sandler DP, Shore DL, Anderson JR, et al: Cigarette smoking and risk of acute leukemia: Associations with morphology and cytogenetic abnormalities in bone marrow. J Natl Cancer Inst 1993, 85, 1994.

242. Sasai Y, Horiike S, Misawa S, et al: Genotype of glutathione S-transferase and other genetic configurations in myelodysplasia. Leuk Res 1999, 23, 975.

243. Sasco AJ, Vainio H: From in utero and childhood exposure to parental smoking to childhood cancer: A possible link and the need for action. Hum Exp Toxicol 1999, 18, 192.

244. Sathiakumar N, Delzell E: A review of epidemiologic studies of triazine herbicides and cancer. Crit Rev Toxicol 1997, 27, 599.

245. Savitz DA, Andrews KW: Review of epidemiologic evidence on benzene and lymphatic and hematopoietic cancers. Am J Ind Med 1997, 31, 287.

246. Savitz DA, Loomis DP: Magnetic field exposure in relation to leukemia and brain cancer mortality among electric utility workers. Am J Epidemiol 1995, 141, 123.

247. Savitz DA, Wachtel H, Barnes FA, et al: Case-control study of childhood cancer and exposure to 60-Hz magnetic fields. Am J Epidemiol 1988, 128, 21.

248. Schmidt W, Popham RE: The role of drinking and smoking in mortality from cancer and other causes in male alcoholics. Cancer 1981, 47, 1031.

249. Schnatter AR, Armstrong TW, Nicolich MJ, et al: Lymphohaematopoietic malignancies and quantitative estimates of exposure to benzene in Canadian petroleum distribution workers. Occup Environ Med 1996, 53, 773.

250. Schnatter AR, Theriault G, Katz AM, et al: A retrospective mortality study within operating segments of a petroleum company. Am J Ind Med 1992, 22, 209.

251. Schneider DT, Hilgenfeld E, Schwabe D, et al: Acute myelogenous leukemia after treatment for malignant germ cell tumors in children. J Clin Oncol 1999, 17, 3226.

252. Schuz J, Kaatsch P, Kaletsch U, et al: Association of childhood cancer with factors related to pregnancy and birth. Int J Epidemiol 1999, 28, 631.

253. Severson RK, Buckley JD, Woods WG, et al: Cigarette smoking and alcohol consumption by parents of children with acute myeloid leukemia: An analysis within morphological subgroups—a report from the Children's Cancer Group. Cancer Epidemiol Biomark Prev 1993, 2, 433.

254. Shimizu Y, Kato H, Schull WJ, et al: Studies of the mortality of A bomb survivors: Mortality, 1950–1985: Cancer mortality based on the recently revised doses (DS86). Radiat Res 1990, 122, 120.

255. Shore RE, Albert RE, Pasternack BS: Followup study of patients treated by x-ray epilation for tinea capitis: Resurvey of posttreatment illness and mortality experience. Arch Environ Health 1976, 31, 21.

256. Shore RE, Gardner MJ, Pannett B: Ethylene oxide: An assessment of the epidemiological evidence on carcinogenicity. Br J Ind Med 1993, 50, 971.

257. Shpilberg O, Modan M, Modan B, et al: Familial aggregation of haematological neoplasms: A controlled study. Br J Haematol 1994, 87, 75.

258. Shu XO, Gao YT, Brinton LA, et al: A population-based case-control study of childhood leukemia in Shanghai. Cancer 1988, 62, 635.

259. Shu XO, Linet MS, Steinbuch M, et al: Breast-feeding and risk of childhood acute leukemia. J Natl Cancer Inst 1999, 91, 1765.

260. Shu XO, Ross JA, Pendergrass TW, et al: Parental alcohol consumption, cigarette smoking, and risk of infant leukemia: A Children's Cancer Group study. J Natl Cancer Inst 1996, 88, 24.

261. Shu XO, Stewart P, Wen WQ, et al: Parental occupational exposure to hydrocarbons and risk of acute lymphocytic leukemia in offspring. Cancer Epidemiol Biomarkers Prev 1999, 8, 783.

262. Simone JV, Aur RJ, Hustu HO, et al: Combined modality therapy of acute lymphocytic leukemia. Cancer, 1975, 35, 25.

263. Skibola CF, Smith MT, Kane E, et al: Polymorphisms in the methylenetetrahydrofolate reductase gene are associated with susceptibility to acute leukemia in adults. Proc Natl Acad Sci U S A 1999, 96, 12810.

264. Smith MA, Gloeckler Ries LA, Gurney JG, et al: In Ries LAG, Smith MA, Gurney JG (eds): Cancer Incidence and Survival Among Children and Adolescents: United States SEER Program 1975–1995. Bethesda, Maryland National Cancer Institute, Pub. No. 99-4639, 1999, pp 17–34.

265. Smith MA, Simon R, Strickler HD, et al: Evidence that childhood acute lymphoblastic leukemia is associated with an infectious agent linked to hygiene conditions. Cancer Causes Control 1998, 9, 285.

266. Smith MT, Zhang L, Wang Y, et al: Increased translocations and aneusomy in chromosomes 8 and 21 among workers exposed to benzene. Cancer Res 1998, 58, 2176.

267. Smith PG, Doll R: Late effects of x irradiation in patients treated for metropathia haemorrhagica. Br J Radiol 1976, 49, 224.

268. Smith PG, Doll R: Mortality from cancer and all causes among British radiologists. Br J Radiol 1981, 54, 187.

269. Sorahan T, Prior P, Lancashire RJ, et al: Childhood cancer and parental use of tobacco: Deaths from 1971 to 1976. Br J Cancer 1997, 76, 1525.

270. Spiers FW, Lucas HF, Rundo J, et al: Leukemia incidence in U.S. dial workers. Health Physics 1983, 44, 65.

271. Stayner L, Steenland K, Greife A, et al: Exposure-response analysis of cancer mortality in a cohort of workers exposed to ethylene oxide. Am J Epidemiol 1993, 138, 787.

272. Stebbings JH, Lucas HF, Stenney AF: Mortality from cancers of major sites in female radium dial workers. Am J Ind Med 1984, 5, 435.

273. Stewart PA, Fears T, Kross B, et al: Exposure of farmers to phosmet, a swine insecticide. Scand J Work Environ Health 1999, 25, 33.

274. Stewart PA, Stewart WF, Heineman EF, et al: A novel approach to data collection in a case-control study of cancer and occupational exposures. Int J Epidemiol, 1996, 25, 744.

275. Straif K, Weiland SK, Werner B, et al: Workplace risk factors for cancer in the German rubber industry: Mortality from nonrespiratory cancers. Occup Environ Med 1998, 55, 325.

276. Strick R, Strissel PL, Borgers S, et al: Dietary bioflavonoids induce cleavage in the MLL gene and may contribute to infant leukemia. Proc Natl Acad Sci U S A 2000, 97, 4790.

277. Swerdlow AM, Douglass AJ, Vaughn Hudson G, et al: Risk of second primary cancers after Hodgkin's disease by type of treatment: Analysis of 2846 patients in the British National Lymphoma Investigation. Br Med J 1992, 304, 1137.

278. Tajima K: The 4th nation-wide study of adult T-cell leukemia/lymphoma (ATL) in Japan: Estimates of risk of ATL and its geographical and clinical features. The T- and B-cell Malignancy Study Group. Int J Cancer 1990, 45, 237.

279. Taylor GM, Birch JM: The hereditary basis of human leukemia. In Henderson ES, Lister TA, Greaves JF (eds): Leukemia, 6th ed. Philadelphia, WB Saunders, 1996, pp 210–245.

280. Tertian G, Avalos MR, Leonard C, et al: Additional translocation (9;12)(p13;q24.1) in newly diagnosed chronic myeloid leukemia: Complete cytogenetic remission after interferon therapy. Hematol Cell Ther 1996, 38, 269.

281. Teta MJ, Benson LO, Vitale JN: Mortality study of ethylene oxide workers in chemical manufacturing: A 10-year update. Br J Ind Med 1993, 50, 704.

282. Teta MJ, Sielken RL Jr, Valdez-Flores C: Ethylene oxide cancer risk assessment based on epidemiological data: Application of revised regulatory guidelines. Risk Anal 1999, 19, 1135.

283. Theriault G, Goldberg M, Miller AB, et al: Cancer risks associated with occupational exposure to magnetic fields among electric utility workers in Ontario and Quebec, Canada, and France 1970–1989. Am J Epidemiol 1994, 139, 550.

284. Travis LB, Curtis RE, Stovall M, et al: Risk of leukemia following treatment for non-Hodgkin's lymphoma. J Natl Cancer Inst 1994, 86, 1450.

285. Travis LB, Weeks J, Curtis RE, et al: Leukemia following low-dose total-body irradiation and chemotherapy for non-Hodgkin's lymphoma. J Clin Oncol 1996, 14, 565.

286. Tucker MA, Coleman CN, Cox RS, et al: Risks of second cancers after treatment for Hodgkin's disease. N Engl J Med 1988, 318, 76.

287. Tucker MA, Meadows AT, Boice JD Jr, et al: Late Effects Study Group: Cancer risk following treatment of childhood cancer. In Boice JD Jr, Fraumeni JF Jr (eds): Radiation Carcinogenesis: Epidemiology and Biological Significance. New York, Raven Press, 1984, pp 211–224.

288. UK Childhood Cancer Study Investigators: Exposure to power-frequency magnetic fields and the risk of childhood cancer. Lancet 1999, 354, 1925.

289. UNSCEAR: Sources and effects of ionizing radiation. United Nations Publ. No. E.94.IX.11. New York, United Nations Scientific Committee on the Effects of Atomic Radiation, 1994.

290. Utterback DF, Rinsky RA: Benzene exposure assessment in rubber hydrochloride workers: A critical evaluation of previous estimates. Am J Ind Med 1995, 27, 661.

291. van Kaick G, Dalheimer A, Hornik S, et al: The German Thorotrast study: Recent results and assessment of risks. Radiat Res, 1999, 152, S64.

292. van Leeuwen FE, Chorus AMJ, van den Belt-Dusebout AW, et al: Leukemia risk following Hodgkin's disease: Relation to cumulative dose of alkylating agents, treatment with teniposide combinations, number of episodes of chemotherapy, and bone marrow damage. J Clin Oncol 1994, 12, 1063.

293. Virchow R: Weisses Blut. Frorieps Notizen 1845, 36, 151.

294. Virchow R: Weisses Blut and Milztumoren. Med Z 1847, 16, 9.

295. Wang J-X, Inskip PD, Boice JD Jr, et al: Cancer incidence among medical diagnostic x-ray workers in China, 1950 to 1985. Int J Cancer 1990, 45, 889.

296. Ward E, Hornung R, Morris J, et al: Risk of low red or white

blood cell count related to estimated benzene exposure in a rubberworker cohort (1940–1975). Am J Ind Med 1996, 29, 247.

297. Weiss HA, Darby SC, Fears T, et al: Leukemia mortality after x-ray treatment for ankylosing spondylitis. Radiat Res 1995, 142, 1.

298. Wertheimer N, Leeper E: Electrical wiring configurations and childhood cancer. Am J Epidemiol 1979, 109, 273.

299. Wiemels JL, Cazzaniga G, Daniotti M, et al: Prenatal origin of acute lymphoblastic leukemia in children. Lancet 1999a, 354, 1499.

300. Wiemels JL, Ford AM, Van Wering ER, et al: Protracted and variable latency of acute lymphoblastic leukemia after TEL-AML1 gene fusion in utero. Blood 1999b, 94, 1057.

301. Wiemels JL, Pagnamenta A, Taylor GM, et al: A lack of a functional NAD(P)H:quinone oxidoreductase allele is selectively associated with pediatric leukemias that have MLL fusions. United Kingdom Childhood Cancer Study Investigators. Cancer Res 1999, 59, 4095.

302. Wiklund K, Holm LH: Trends in cancer risks among Swedish agricultural workers. J Natl Cancer Inst 1986, 77, 657.

303. Williams RR, Horm JW: Association of cancer sites with tobacco and alcohol consumption and socioeconomic status of patients: Interview study from the Third National Cancer Survey. J Natl Cancer Inst 1977, 58, 525.

304. Wong O: An industry-wide mortality study of chemical workers occupationally exposed to benzene II: Dose response analyses. Br J Ind Med 1987, 44, 382.

305. Wong O: A cohort mortality study and a case-control study of workers potentially exposed to styrene in the reinforced plastics and composites industry. Br J Ind Med 1990, 47, 753.

306. Wong O, Trent LS: An epidemiological study of workers potentially exposed to ethylene oxide. Br J Ind Med, 1993, 50, 308.

307. Woo MH, Shuster JJ, Chen C, et al: Glutathione S-transferase genotypes in children who develop treatment-related acute myeloid malignancies. Leukemia 2000, 14, 232.

308. World Health Organization (WHO): Manual of the International Statistical Classification of Diseases, Injuries, and Causes of Death, vol 1, 6th revision. Geneva, Switzerland, WHO, 1957.

309. World Health Organization (WHO): Manual of the International Statistical Classification of Diseases, Injuries, and Causes of Death, vol 1, 7th revision. Geneva, Switzerland, WHO, 1967.

310. World Health Organization (WHO): Manual of the International Statistical Classification of Diseases, Injuries, and Causes of Death, vol 1. 8th revision. Geneva, Switzerland, WHO, 1977.

311. Yamashita M, Veronesi R, Menna-Barreto M, et al: Molecular epidemiology of human T-cell leukemia virus type I (HTLV-I) Brazil: The predominant HTLV-Is in South American differ from HTLV-Is of Japan and Africa, as well as those of Japanese immigrants and their relatives in Brazil. Virology 1999, 26, 59.

312. Yin SN, Li GL, Tain FD, et al: Leukaemia in benzene workers: A retrospective cohort study. Br J Ind Med 1987, 44, 124.

313. Yoshida K, Inoue T, Nojima K, et al: Calorie restriction reduces the incidence of myeloid leukemia induced by a single whole-body radiation in C3H/He mice. Proc Natl Acad Sci U S A 1997, 94, 2615.

314. Young NS, Alter BP: Aplastic anemia, acquired and inherited. Philadelphia, WB Saunders, 1994.

315. Yuille MR, Houlston RS, Catovsky D: Anticipation in familial chronic lymphocytic leukaemia. Leukemia 1998, 12, 1696.

316. Zahm SH, Ward MH, Blair A: Pesticides and cancer. Occup Med 1997, 12, 269.

317. Zhang L, Rothman N, Wang Y, et al: Increased aneusomy and long arm deletion of chromosomes 5 and 7 in the lymphocytes of Chinese workers exposed to benzene. Carcinogenesis 1998, 19, 1955.

318. Zipursky A, Peters M, Poon A: Megakaryoblastic leukemia and Down's syndrome: A review. Pediatr Hematol Oncol 1987, 4, 211.

319. Zittoun RA, Mandelli F, Willemze R, et al: Autologous or allogeneic bone marrow transplantation compared with intensive chemotherapy in acute myelogenous leukemia: European Organization for Research and Treatment of Cancer (EORTC) and the Gruppo Italiano Malattie Ematologiche Maligne dell' Adulto (GIMEMA) Leukemia Cooperative Groups. N Engl J Med 1995, 332, 217.

320. Zuelzer WW, Thompson RI, Mastrangelo R: Evidence for a genetic factor related to leukemogenesis and congenital anomalies: Chromosomal aberrations in pedigree of an infant girl with partial D trisomy and leukemia. J Pediatr 1968, 72, 367.

8

John D. Boice, Jr.

Radiation-Induced Leukemia

HISTORICAL BACKGROUND

A new era began in 1895 when Röntgen discovered "a new kind of ray" that could penetrate the human body and reveal broken bones. The first x-ray film was taken in 1896, the same year that uranium was found by Becquerel to be naturally radioactive. The first radiation-induced skin cancer was reported in 1902 and appeared on the hand of a roentgenologist. Reports of excess leukemia among radiologists appeared in the 1940s, and radiation-induced leukemia is believed to have caused the death of Madame Curie and her daughter Irene. Patients treated with radiation for nonmalignant diseases in the 1930s to the 1950s were subsequently found to be at high risk for leukemia. The studies of Japanese atomic bomb survivors began in 1950 and have provided substantial knowledge on radiation effects.

Radiation is perceived by the public as a major carcinogen despite convincing evidence that it contributes only a small amount to the overall cancer burden. This perception probably comes from images of wartime uses of nuclear weapons and, more recently, reactor accidents such as Chernobyl. Although radiation is a nearly universal carcinogen (i.e., it causes many types of cancer), it is an ineffective carcinogen, in part because it is an especially good killer of cells. We live in a sea of low-level natural radiation from terrestrial and cosmic sources, and our bodies have developed repair mechanisms to correct damage after such exposures. Leukemia, although rare, is the most frequently reported malignant disease after radiation exposures.[142, 199, 201]

BASIC CONCEPTS

Energy emitted from a source is generally referred to as radiation. Examples include heat or light from the sun, radio signals from a transmitting antenna, microwaves from an oven, x-rays from an x-ray tube, and gamma rays from radioactive elements. Radiation of sufficient energy to remove electrons from atoms is called *ionizing* radia-

tion; it includes electromagnetic rays, such as x-rays and gamma rays, and energetic particles, such as protons, fission nuclei, and alpha and beta particles. Neutrons, unlike these other particles, have no charge and cannot ionize directly. Instead, they impart energy to protons through elastic collisions, and the protons then cause subsequent ionizations. Another way in which energy can be released in tissue is by *excitation,* whereby electrons are merely raised to a higher energy level within an atom but are not removed. The total amount of energy absorbed in matter as a result of radiation interactions is called the dose, which is measured in gray (Gy): 1 Gy = 1 joule per kilogram. In years past, the standard unit for dose was the rad (1 rad = 100 ergs per gram), but the conversion is simple: 1 Gy = 100 rad = 100 cGy. An acute whole-body dose of about 4 Gy (400 rad) is lethal about half of the time in humans; yet, this dose ionizes only about 1 of every 40 million molecules. Thus, permanent damage can be produced after a relatively small amount of energy is absorbed.

Radiation is absorbed randomly by atoms and molecules in cells and can alter molecular structure. These alterations can be amplified by biologic processes to result in observable effects. The biologic effects, however, depend not only on the total absorbed dose but also on the linear energy transfer (LET), or ionization density, of the type of radiation. LET is a measure of the energy loss per unit distance traveled and depends on the velocity, charge, and mass of a particle or on x-ray or gamma-ray energy. High-LET radiations, such as alpha particles (helium nuclei), release energy in short tracks of dense ionizations. They are not too penetrating and can often be stopped by the outer layers of skin. Low-LET or sparsely ionizing radiations, such as x-rays and beta particles, produce ionization events that are not close together. Ranges are generally greater than for high-LET radiation, leading to deposition of energy in a larger tissue volume. Depending on the biologic endpoint, the effect per gray may differ widely as a function of LET, but it is usually lower for low-LET radiation.

In experimental studies, the induction of many cancers after low-LET radiation appears to follow a nonlinear relationship with dose, with risk per unit dose being lower at low doses than at higher doses.[144, 200] Chronic exposures also result in fewer leukemias than do brief exposures of the same total dose.[204] The induction of cancer by exposure to high-LET radiation has generally appeared to follow a more linear dose response. Moreover, protraction and fractionation of dose from high-LET radiation tend not to decrease cancer risk but rather to increase it somewhat, especially at dose levels at which the competing effect of cell killing is likely.[200] Studies suggest that this enhancement of risk at lower dose rates may also occur at levels at which cell killing is minimal.

The relative biologic effectiveness of radiation characterizes its ability to produce a specific level of effect (e.g., increased frequency of chromosome aberration, cell death, or cancer) compared with a standard, usually x-rays or gamma rays. It is experimentally determined as the ratio of absorbed doses of different radiations to produce an identical effect. A relative biologic effectiveness of 20 for alpha particles at 10 cGy, for example, implies that the biologic effect from 10 cGy of alpha particles is the same as that from 200 cGy of gamma rays. The unit of biologic dose equivalence used in radiologic protection is the sievert (Sv), which has replaced the rem (1 Sv = 100 rem). The sievert represents the absorbed dose in grays, multiplied by a quality factor (or radiation weighting factor specific to the type of radiation) and other possible modifying factors. The sievert has also been applied to assess the effects of exposures to more than one type of radiation. For example, the dose equivalence of an exposure to 10 cGy of gamma rays plus 10 cGy of alpha particles, with gamma rays as the standard and a relative biologic effectiveness of 20 for alpha particles, is 2.1 Sv (210 rem).

SOURCES OF EXPOSURE

Background radiation from natural sources contributes the most to population exposure, about 2.9 mSv (290 mrem) per year[142, 199] (Table 8–1). These sources include cosmic rays (0.27 mSv/y), which vary by altitude; terrestrial radiations (0.28 mSv/y), which vary according to the

TABLE 8–1. Annual Population Exposures to Ionizing Radiation

Sources	Annual Effective Dose (mSv)*
Natural sources	
Cosmic, terrestrial, internal	0.94
Radon	2.00 (mainly to lung)
Medical	
X-ray diagnosis	0.39
Nuclear medicine	0.14
Consumer products	0.10
Other	
Occupational	<0.01
Nuclear fuel cycle	<0.01
Fallout	<0.01
Miscellaneous environmental sources	<0.01
Total (excluding radon)	1.6

*1 mSv = 0.1 rem, annual effective dose equivalent. From National Academy of Science: Health Effects of Exposure to Low Levels of Ionizing Radiation (BEIR V). Washington, DC: National Academy Press: 1990. Reprinted with permission from Health Effects of Exposure to Low Levels of Ionizing Radiation. Copyright 1990 by the National Academy of Sciences. Courtesy of the National Academy Press, Washington, DC.

distribution in soil and bedrock of radioactive elements such as uranium; internally deposited radionuclides such as potassium ^{40}K (0.39 mSv/y); and radon (2.0 mSv/y and confined mainly to lung). The greatest artificial source of radiation is medical procedures (0.53 mSv/y), and exposures increase directly with the patient's age. Nuclear medicine procedures are estimated to contribute 0.14 mSv/y average effective dose to the population. Occupation, nuclear power, fallout from testing of nuclear weapons, and consumer products make only a minor contribution (0.11 mSv/y). The average per capita dose from all sources of radiation, excluding radon, is thus about 1.6 mSv (160 mrem) per year. However, some individuals in the population can experience much higher exposures, for example, cancer patients treated with radiation.

On the basis of studies of Japanese atomic bomb survivors, the lifetime risk for development of leukemia after acute whole-body exposures of 1 Gy is estimated to be 85 per 10,000 persons (or 0.85%). Continuous lifetime exposure of 100,000 persons to 1 mSv/y has been estimated to induce about 65 leukemias.[142] If this is true, 3% to 5% of all leukemias might be attributable to all sources of radiation exposure (1.6 mSv/y). Although radiation has clearly been found to cause leukemia in humans, substantial uncertainties remain about the level of risk from low doses delivered at low dose rates. At doses below approximately 0.2 Gy, the risks appear too low to be detected, and extrapolations from high-dose studies are performed to estimate possible risks. The shape of the leukemia dose response among Japanese atomic bomb survivors is more consistent with a linear quadratic formulation than a linear one.

MECHANISMS

Ionizing radiation is relatively ineffective at inducing point mutations in DNA but is effective at inducing DNA strand breaks.[143] Most single-stranded breaks are rapidly repaired, but double-stranded breaks can result in chromosome rearrangements, including translocations, inversions, additions, and deletions. Such aberrations, if they are not lethal or if they are misrepaired, can lead to cancer through changes in expression of normal genes, the formation of new chimeric genes, and the loss or inactivation of genes inhibitory of tumorigenesis.[180]

Cytogenetic and molecular studies have demonstrated that many forms of leukemia and lymphoma are associated with specific chromosome rearrangements, at least some of which appear to result in the activation of proto-oncogenes and are believed to be central to the pathogenesis of these diseases[33, 167, 171, 180] (see Chapters 2 and 5 for details). This is in contrast to most epithelial cancers, for which the loss or inactivation of so-called tumor suppressor genes appears to be more generally important.[128] For leukemia, the paradigmatic case is the Philadelphia (Ph) chromosome, which is seen in leukemic cells of more than 90% of persons with chronic myelogenous leukemia (CML).[168] It results from a reciprocal translocation involving chromosomes 9 and 22.[148, 168] Part of the Abelson proto-oncogene, *ABL,* on chromosome 9 is cleaved and then fused with the *BCR* gene on the long arm of chromosome 22, resulting in the chimeric gene *BCRABL*. The protein product of the fused gene is a tyrosine kinase.[89] Molecular evidence of chimeric *BCRABL* genes was also seen in cytogenetically normal (Ph chromosome negative) patients with CML,[206] which lends credence to the view that this genetic change is causally involved in the pathogenesis of the disease rather than incidental to it. The Ph chromosome is also the most common cytogenetic abnormality seen in adults with acute lymphoblastic leukemia (ALL), although a variety of other rearrangements, including t(8;14) and t(4;11), have been noted in a high percentage of cases of ALL.[21] Different translocations have been associated with other forms of leukemia, including t(8;21) in acute myeloblastic leukemia, t(15;17) in acute promyelocytic leukemia, and t(10;11) and t(9;11) in acute monoblastic leukemia.[171]

The spectrum of chromosome abnormalities observed in leukemias is reported to differ between those arising after cytotoxic therapy and those arising de novo, that is, among persons lacking known exposure to a strong mutagenic agent. Partial or total losses of chromosomes 5 and 7 were seen in myeloid cells from a high percentage of persons who developed acute nonlymphocytic leukemia or myelodysplastic syndrome after combined radiotherapy and chemotherapy for a primary malignant neoplasm.[170] Growth factor and growth factor receptor genes are located on chromosome 5, but it is not known whether they play an etiologic role in leukemogenesis.[169] Moloney[135] reported that the mix of acute leukemia subtypes seen among irradiated cervical cancer patients and atomic bomb survivors was similar to the mix seen among patients with de novo disease; however, a different array of leukemic cell types was noted among persons previously irradiated for ankylosing spondylitis.

The relatively high frequency of nonrandom deletions (i.e., chromosomes 5q− and 7q−) associated with radiotherapy- or chemotherapy-induced acute myelogenous leukemia (AML)[171] is consistent with similar observations for radiation-induced AML among atomic bomb survivors.[88] In contrast, the frequency of the Ph chromosome associated with radiation-induced CML appears not to be related to the level of radiation exposure.[88] This argues against the notion that radiation initiates CML by inducing the Ph lesion.

Whether the nonrandom chromosome translocations, deletions, and other rearrangements seen for the different types of leukemia reflect the existence of fragile sites within the chromosomes[220] or selective clonal growth after randomly distributed damage is uncertain. Silver and Cox[176] reported evidence of a genetically determined predisposition to radiation-induced AML in a particular strain of mice. Susceptibility to AML appeared to be related to a polymorphism involving DNA sequences on chromosome 2 that are susceptible to breakage by ionizing radiation. Breckon and colleagues[22, 23] conjectured that fragile sites on the long arm of chromosome 5 might play a role in human radiation leukemogenesis analogous to the radiation-sensitive sites on the murine chromosome 2.

Lymphoid malignant neoplasms show a characteristic set of rearrangements.[33, 175, 171] B-cell and T-cell tumors often exhibit translocations that place cellular oncogenes

in the vicinity of immunoglobulin or T-cell receptor genes, resulting in proto-oncogene activation through transcriptional deregulation.[175] The best known example is the t(8;14) translocation in Burkitt's lymphoma, which results in the juxtaposition of the *MYC* proto-oncogene with immunoglobulin genes and consequent aberrant expression of *MYC*.[104] A high percentage of non-Burkitt's B-cell tumors, including chronic lymphocytic leukemia (CLL), diffuse lymphomas, and multiple myeloma, also show translocations involving the 14q band containing the locus for immunoglobulin heavy chains.[33] Interestingly, however, with the exception of ALL, cancers of lymphoid cells have not been convincingly linked to radiation exposure. In particular, CLL has not been found to be associated with irradiation in any major epidemiologic study.[12, 22, 27, 81, 159] Studies of the atomic bomb survivors also failed to detect an association between radiation dose and incidence of adult T-cell leukemia, a disease in which the human T-lymphotropic virus 1 is thought to play a causal role[159] (see Chapters 10 and 30). Whether radiation causes lymphoma and myeloma remains an unresolved question.[11]

In summary, ionizing radiation is a clastogen that deposits energy at random in tissues, and chromosome rearrangements appear to be causally involved in the pathogenesis of cancers of myeloid and lymphoid cells. Yet, susceptibility to radiation-induced cancer appears to vary widely among different subsets of marrow-derived cells. This underscores the importance of lineage-specific developmental processes and, perhaps, the heterogeneity of progenitor cell populations for blood cell malignant neoplasms[66] (see Chapter 2). Those cancers most closely associated with exposure to ionizing radiation, namely, CML, AML, and perhaps some types of ALL as well as several preleukemic syndromes, apparently originate in primitive, multipotential stem cells.[66] CLL, lymphoma, and multiple myeloma, on the other hand, are thought to arise from mature, differentiated lymphoid cells.[66] One would nonetheless expect radiation-induced genetic damage in a pluripotent stem cell to be propagated to descendants that differentiate along the lymphoid line. Why this would not be related to increased cancer risk is unclear. Perhaps the balance between cell transformation and inactivation as a function of radiation dose differs between lymphoid cells and those of other lineages. Alternatively, other genetic changes or developmental events, possibly immunologic in nature, might be rate limiting to cancer development in cells committed to this lineage.

In light of recent public concern about the possibility that *nonionizing* electromagnetic fields might also cause leukemia and other types of cancer, it should be noted that no evidence of chromosome breakage or other mutations has been found in experimental studies involving low-frequency electromagnetic fields.[150] If nonionizing radiation does indeed cause leukemia, and the evidence for this is far from persuasive, it seemingly must do so through a mechanism fundamentally different from that of ionizing radiations.

HUMAN STUDIES OF RADIOGENIC LEUKEMIA

Leukemia is the cancer most commonly identified after irradiation, probably because of its short minimal appear-

TABLE 8–2. Epidemiologic Studies of Populations Exposed to Ionizing Radiation and Subsequent Risk for Leukemia by Type of Exposure and Strength of Association[141, 142, 199, 201]

Type of Exposure	Study	Strength of Association*
Atomic bomb	Japanese survivors[159]	+ + +
Radiotherapy		
Malignant disease	Cervical cancer[12]	+ +
	Endometrial cancer[34]	+ +
	Breast cancer[35]	+ +
	Hodgkin's disease[196]	+
	Non-Hodgkin's lymphoma[193-195]	+
	Childhood cancer[73, 197]	±
	Retinoblastoma[218]	−
Nonmalignant disease	Ankylosing spondylitis[215]	+ + +
	Menstrual disorders[81]	+ + +
	Scalp ringworm[166]	+
	Peptic ulcer[69]	+
	Skin hemangioma	−
Diagnostic x-ray studies	Tuberculosis fluoroscopy[43]	−
	General radiography[15]	±
	Prenatal x-ray study[199]	±
Radionuclides	^{131}I[54, 70, 165]	±
	Thorotrast[3]	+ +
	Radium[147, 183, 216]	±
	^{32}P[6]	+
	Radon[103, 112]	−
	^{239}Pu[97, 152]	−
Occupation	Radiologists[212]	+ +
	X-ray technologists[48]	−
	Nuclear energy workers[26, 65, 90]	±
	Chernobyl[83, 161]	−
	Radon-exposed miners[42, 192]	−
Environmental contamination	Chernobyl[154, 155]	−
	Techa River[99]	+

*+ + +, highly significant finding; + +, meaningful association; +, suggested but unconfirmed; ±, equivocal; −, no evidence for an increased risk.

ance time, its relatively low natural incidence, and the high radiation sensitivity of active marrow. Radiogenic leukemia has an early onset; the minimal latency is about 2 years. The subsequent pattern of excess risk over time is wavelike. Excess leukemias have occurred among populations exposed as a result of military circumstances, occupational endeavors, medical care, and environmental situations[199, 201] (Table 8–2).

Nuclear Weapons Use and Testing

Japanese Atomic Bomb Survivors

For more than 50 years, the Radiation Effects Research Foundation (and its predecessor, the Atomic Bomb Casualty Commission) in Japan has studied the survivors of the atomic bomb detonations that occurred during World War II.[151, 157] This single study has provided more information on radiation risks than any other. The Leukemia Registry was established in 1948, and the first report of radiogenic leukemias appeared in 1952.[58] The most recent analyses in the Life Span Study sample include 253 cases of leukemia.[159] Compared with other tumors, leuke-

mia has one of the highest relative risk (RR) coefficients. At 1 Gy (100 rad) whole-body exposure, a sixfold risk is estimated, whereas it is 1.29 for all other cancers combined. More than half of leukemias occurring among the atomic bomb survivors are attributed to radiation.[157] It has been suggested that the temporal pattern of risk varies with age at exposure; those exposed at younger ages have a higher peak and a more rapid decline than do those exposed in later life[151] (Fig. 8–1).

More than 60% of the leukemia cases have been reclassified by use of the French-American-British nomenclature, and radiation risk is seen to vary by cell type. Few diagnoses of CLL have been made, and there is no evidence in this or any other study that radiation causes CLL. The risk for CML was high, and a wavelike time response was evident, especially in Hiroshima. CML has been thought to be the most characteristic leukemia of the atomic bomb survivors. The high risk in Hiroshima was once attributed to neutrons, but it is now thought to be related more to the higher naturally occurring rate in Hiroshima than in Nagasaki. AML, with more than 100 cases, is the most common leukemia, with excesses occurring at all ages. The radiation risk for ALL was somewhat higher than that for AML and decreased more rapidly; the excess of ALL also occurred predominantly among younger survivors. No association with radiation was found for the 30 cases of adult T-cell leukemia.

The risk for leukemia among atomic bomb survivors was also seen to increase with radiation dose[157] (Fig. 8–2). A suggested downturn after 4 Gy may be due to

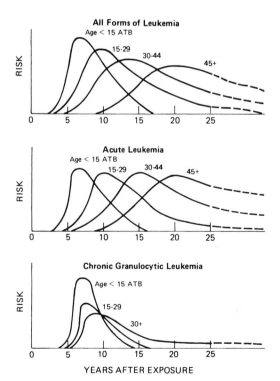

FIGURE 8–1. Schematic diagram of the temporal pattern of leukemia risk among atomic bomb survivors according to age at exposure and cell type. (From Okada S, Hamilton HB, Egami N, et al, eds: A review of thirty years of Hiroshima and Nagasaki atomic bomb survivors. J Radiat Res [Tokyo] 1975;16[suppl]:1.)

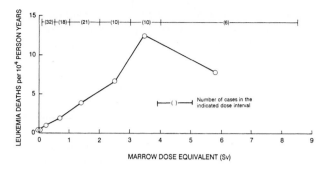

FIGURE 8–2. Leukemia dose-response relationship seen among Japanese atomic bomb survivors. (From Pierce DA, Shimizu Y, Preston DL, et al: Studies of the mortality of atomic bomb survivors. Report 12, Part I. Cancer: 1950–1990. Radiat Res 1996;146:1.)

cell killing of stem cells (or errors in dosimetry). The best-fitting dose-response model is linear quadratic, which implies that risk per unit exposure at low dose is less than that at higher doses. However, dose-response and risk estimates varied by subtype, age, time, and sex (Table 8–3), so that comparisons with other studies or generalizations to other populations must be done cautiously. Characterizing any single study population in terms of summary relative or absolute risk coefficients tends to obscure these important differences.

Leukemia has not been linked to in utero or preconception exposure in the atomic bomb study.[84, 146] Among the 1630 individuals exposed in utero, no childhood leukemias occurred; two cases of adult leukemia were diagnosed in individuals aged 18 and 29 years. Both patients received less than 0.05 Gy (5 rad) in utero, and there was no evidence of a dose-response relationship.[219] Later analyses are even more striking in that the dose response for leukemia was negative, albeit based on few cases,[45, 129] but they provide little direct evidence for a leukemia effect after in utero exposure.

With regard to possible germline effects, 44 cases of leukemia have been diagnosed among 76,000 offspring

of the atomic bomb survivors (F$_1$ cohort) as of 1985.[146] Only three cases of leukemia occurred among children born in 1946. These numbers were not in excess of expectation, and there was no evidence of a radiation effect in any of these groups. Thus, there was little evidence that parental exposure to radiation causes an increased susceptibility to leukemia in offspring among atomic bomb survivors. This is in contrast to a study in the United Kingdom, which reported an association of childhood leukemia with paternal exposure before conception at a nuclear fuel reprocessing plant in Sellafield, England. Subsequent studies around Scottish and Canadian nuclear plants, however, have failed to provide corroborative evidence of a preconception effect,[94, 125] and it has been concluded that paternal irradiation was not to blame.[46] Survivors of childhood cancer treated with radiotherapy and mutagenic chemicals have also not been reported to have offspring with an increased risk for childhood leukemia.[173]

Despite the singular importance of the Japanese atomic bomb survivor studies with respect to our understanding of radiation leukemogenesis and for radiation risk estimation, they provide no information on the effects of fractionated or low-dose exposures, such as experienced in occupational or medical settings, or about the effects of high-dose partial-body exposures, such as experienced in radiotherapy.

Fallout in Utah from Weapons Tests

Aboveground nuclear weapons testing in the 1950s and 1960s resulted in radioactive fallout exposures to populated areas in the United States. A case-control study of more than 1000 individuals who died of leukemia in southwestern Utah, near the Nevada Test Site, identified a weak positive association between estimated bone marrow dose and total leukemia, although the trend was not significant.[185] Significant risks were observed, however, for acute leukemia among those younger than 20 years when they were exposed to fallout, similar to estimates

TABLE 8–3. Relative Risk Estimates for Radiation-Induced Leukemia Among Atomic Bomb Survivors by Sex, Age at Exposure, and Time Since Exposure

| Characteristic | Exposed Cases | | | Relative Risk at 1 Gy | Excess Absolute Risk* |
	Observed	Expected	Mean Dose (Gy)		
Sex					
Male	71	35.3	0.26	4.91	3.35
Female	70	32.1	0.25	5.75	2.29
Age at exposure (yr)					
<20	46	17.9	0.26	7.11	2.28
≥20	95	49.5	0.25	4.70	3.06
Time since exposure (yr)					
5–10	29	5.1	0.25	19.7	5.87
11–20	45	40.3	0.25	1.46	0.50
21–30	34	18.5	0.25	4.32	2.21
31–42	33	28.1	0.25	1.70	0.75
All	141	67.4	0.25	5.37	2.73

*Excess leukemia cases per 10,000 persons per year per gray (10^4 person-years/Gy).
From Preston D, Kusumi S, Tomonaga M, et al: The incidence of leukemia, lymphoma, and myeloma among A-bomb survivors, 1950–87. Radiat Res 1994;137 (suppl):S68.

obtained from other studies of exposed populations. The increasing trends seen for CLL, a tumor not known to be elevated after irradiation, and the difficulty in estimating doses retrospectively are reasons for caution in interpretation.

Fallout in Nordic Countries

Secular trends in childhood leukemia within Nordic countries were evaluated for possible changes that might be related to fallout from atmospheric nuclear weapons testing in the 1950s and 1960s.[40] Estimates of fetal bone marrow exposure, primarily from cesium Cs 137, were about 0.14 mSv, and no increase in leukemia incidence could be tied to such levels. A 7-year cumulative exposure was estimated to be 1.5 mSv. There was no evidence for a preconception effect based on estimated paternal testicular dose. These data suffer the same uncertainties of all ecologic surveys in that doses to individuals are unknown and it is not possible to assign individual effects from group data.[68, 137] Further, there have been a great many other environmental and social changes since World War II other than low-level radioactive fallout that might influence the incidence, diagnosis, and reporting of leukemia over time.

Fallout in Marshall Islands

Residents of four atolls east of Bikini Island were exposed to nuclear fallout from a United States weapons test in 1954. Significant excesses of thyroid neoplasia have occurred. One case of AML was diagnosed in a 19-year-old man who was 1 year old when he was exposed.[30]

Participants at Nuclear Weapons Tests Conducted by the United States

No excess in total cancer mortality (112 versus 117.5) was found among 3017 of 3217 participants in military maneuvers during the 1957 nuclear test in Nevada called SMOKY.[25] Leukemia, however, was significantly elevated; 10 cases were observed, including the index case that prompted the investigation and one case that developed after radiation therapy and possibly chemotherapy for lymphoma, versus 4.0 expected on the basis of rates from the general population. Lower cancer frequencies were generally noted among the military units with the highest exposures based on film badge doses (mean, 0.46 cGy). A survey of 46,186 military participants in two weapons test series conducted at the Nevada Test Site and three in the Pacific Ocean also found no excess of nonleukemia deaths (990 versus 1187).[162] Excluding SMOKY, 46 leukemia deaths occurred versus 52.4 expected, suggesting that the leukemia excess among SMOKY participants was due either to chance or to circumstances peculiar to that shot (or its participants).

A mortality study was conducted of approximately 70,000 soldiers, sailors, and airmen who participated in at least one of five nuclear weapons test series at the Nevada Test Site or the Pacific Proving Ground.[191] Compared with the general population, the risks for dying of any leukemia (185 observed versus 250 expected) or

of leukemia excluding CLL (156 observed versus 208 expected) were significantly low. The leukemia risks in a nonexposed referent cohort of nearly 65,000 military personnel were even lower. A direct comparison suggested a slight elevation in leukemia risk among the exposed (RR about 1.15), which was not significant. This elevation, however, appeared to be related to a methodologic problem with the study. Causes of death among those known to have died were significantly less likely to be obtained for the referent group than for the exposed group (i.e., there were 1295 with unknown cause of death among the nonexposed versus 842 among the exposed). If these unknown causes of death are distributed proportionally over the known categories, the slight leukemia elevation disappears.

Participants at Nuclear Weapons Tests Conducted by the United Kingdom

Cancer mortality and incidence among 21,358 participants in the United Kingdom's atmospheric nuclear weapons tests in Australia and the Pacific Ocean between 1952 and 1967 and in 22,333 matched control subjects were evaluated.[39] Mortality from all causes and from all cancers was similar between the two study groups. Death due to leukemia occurred significantly more often among participants than among control subjects. Mortality from leukemia among participants, however, was equal to that predicted from national rates (RR = 1.0 based on 29 deaths) but was extremely low among control subjects (RR = 0.56 based on 17 deaths). Thus, the increased risk for leukemia was related more to a significant deficit among the control subjects than to an excess among the exposed.

Medical Irradiation

Studies of populations of patients irradiated for malignant[20] and nonmalignant diseases have provided valuable information on the influence of dose rate and partial-body exposure on leukemia risk. Scatter radiation to organs outside the treatment fields permits the evaluation of relatively low dose effects. Dosimetric and analytic methods have been developed to evaluate the complex nature of high-dose, nonuniform irradiation of bone marrow in a way that accounts for this heterogeneity. The ineffective ability of radiotherapy to induce leukemia is apparent from the relatively low rate of secondary leukemia seen after treatment of malignant disease.

Malignant Disease

CERVICAL CANCER

To evaluate the effects of high-dose radiation delivered to small volumes of tissue and low-dose scatter radiation received by other parts of the body, an international study was conducted of more than 100,000 women with cervical cancer who were treated in any of 15 countries. For the first time, a small but significant excess of leukemia was found after radiation therapy for cervical cancer.

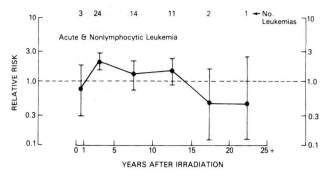

FIGURE 8–3. Characteristic wavelike pattern of leukemia risk over time since exposure seen among women treated with radiation for cervical cancer. (From Boice JD Jr, Day NE, Andersen A, et al: Second cancers following radiation treatment for cervical cancer. An international collaboration among cancer registries. J Natl Cancer Inst 1985;74:955.)

The wavelike pattern of risk over time was consistent with the study of atomic bomb survivors (Fig. 8–3), but the crude estimate of radiation risk was an order of magnitude lower.[13]

In a subsequent case-control study, CLL was not linked to radiation; but a twofold risk was seen for acute and chronic myelogenous leukemias.[12] Again, a relative risk of about 30 would have been predicted on the basis of the average dose received and risk estimates derived from the atomic bomb study. On the basis of actual radiotherapy records and simulated treatments involving measurements in anthropomorphic phantoms, estimates of dose to active bone marrow were made. Doses to 14 different bone marrow compartments were estimated and the risk for leukemia was modeled, taking into account the nonuniform dose distribution from this partial-body exposure. The leukemia risk increased up to doses of approximately 4 Gy (400 rad) and then decreased at higher levels, suggesting that cell killing might predominate over transformation at very high doses[12] (Fig. 8–4). A similar dose response was observed for radiation-induced chromosome aberrations in circulating lymphocytes among irradiated cervical cancer patients.[95] High-dose

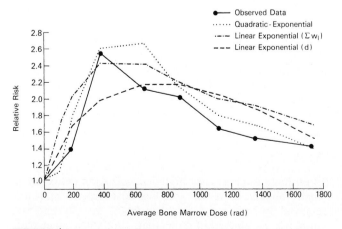

FIGURE 8–4. Leukemia dose-response relationship seen among women treated with radiation for cervical cancer. (From Boice JD Jr, Blettner M, Kleinerman RA, et al: Radiation dose and leukemia risk in patients treated for cancer of the cervix. J Natl Cancer Inst 1987;79:1295.)

cell killing seems a likely explanation as to why radiotherapy for cancer is so infrequently linked to secondary leukemia and, when it is, why it is usually at a very low level. In the most heavily irradiated marrow, potentially leukemic cells are inactivated or killed, and in marrow remote from the direct radiation field, relatively few cells are transformed.[78]

ENDOMETRIAL CANCER

In an attempt to replicate the cervical cancer study, more than 200 cases of leukemia occurring in a study population of 110,000 women with endometrial cancer were evaluated with similar methods.[34] Results were remarkably consistent with the cervical cancer findings. A nearly twofold risk was observed for the acute and myelogenous leukemias, and no risk was observed for CLL. Increased risks for leukemia were found among the elderly exposed after the age of 65 years. Overall, however, the pattern of risk by dose was erratic and consistent with a flat dose-response relationship. Interestingly, the risk after continuous exposures from brachytherapy at comparatively low doses and low dose rates (RR = 1.8; mean dose, 1.7 Gy) was similar to that after fractionated exposures at much higher doses and higher dose rates from external beam treatments (RR = 2.3; mean dose, 9.9 Gy). Again, the relationship of leukemia risk to radiation dose was complex and probably due to the competing processes of cell killing, transformation, and repair. At very high doses given at high rates, destruction of cells is likely to dominate, and the risk per unit dose is low. In the low dose range, at which dose was protracted and given at relatively low rates, the leukemia risk appears to be somewhat lower than that projected on the basis of the instantaneous whole-body exposures received by the atomic bomb survivors (Fig. 8–5).

BREAST CANCER

In a study of nearly 80,000 women with breast cancer, a twofold risk for leukemia was linked to adjuvant radiotherapy, which included substantial exposure to the chest wall, and there was evidence of a radiation dose response.[35] Chemotherapy was associated with a 10-fold risk, which supports the notion that alkylating agents are much more potent leukemogens than radiation. It appeared that the two treatment modalities interacted with each other in a more than additive manner, and the data were consistent with a multiplication of risks (i.e., RR = 17 if both radiotherapy and systemic chemotherapy were given).

LYMPHOMAS

The most serious consequence of curative therapies for lymphoma is the heightened risk for development of a new cancer.[10] However, only small increases in leukemia risk have been reported after radiotherapy alone for Hodgkin's disease.[87, 189, 196, 209] Radiotherapy for non-Hodgkin's lymphoma, however, has been correlated with excess leukemia.[194, 195] Total or hemibody irradiation for non-Hodgkin's lymphoma, a unique treatment that exposes

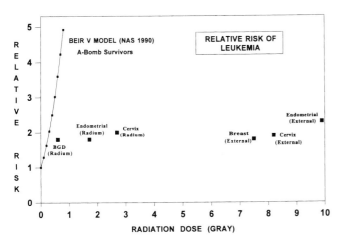

FIGURE 8–5. Risk for leukemia in several studies of medically irradiated populations compared with Japanese atomic bomb survivors according to average dose to bone marrow. (Data from National Academy of Science: Health Effects of Exposure to Low Levels of Ionizing Radiation [BEIR V]. Washington, DC: National Academy Press, 1990; Boice JD Jr, Blettner M, Kleinerman RA, et al: Radiation dose and leukemia risk in patients treated for cancer of the cervix. J Natl Cancer Inst 1987;79:1295; Inskip PD, Kleinerman RA, Stovall M, et al: Leukemia, lymphoma, and multiple myeloma after pelvic radiotherapy for benign disease. Radiat Res 1993;135:108; Curtis RE, Boice JD Jr, Stovall M, et al: Risk of leukemia after chemotherapy and radiation treatment for breast cancer. N Engl J Med 1992;326:1745; and Curtis RE, Boice JD Jr, Stovall M, et al: Relation of leukemia risk to radiation dose after cancer of the uterine corpus. J Natl Cancer Inst 1994;86:1315.)

large volumes of bone marrow to relatively low therapeutic doses, was also seen to heighten the subsequent risk for leukemia.[67] However, many of the patients studied also received chemotherapy, such as with cyclophosphamide, a known leukemogen, so that an independent leukemogenic effect for radiation was not clearly demonstrated.

CHILDHOOD CANCER

Radiotherapy was not found to increase the risk for leukemia in one study of children treated for cancer,[197] possibly because of the predominance of cell killing over oncogenic transformation at such high levels. A later study reported a leukemia risk after radiotherapy,[73] possibly due to associated or interactive effects with chemotherapeutic agents. Children treated for retinoblastoma are at high risk for radiogenic bone cancer because of an underlying genetic susceptibility, but no excess leukemia has been reported.[51, 55]

Nonmalignant Disease

BENIGN GYNECOLOGIC DISORDERS

In a cohort study of 12,955 women treated for benign gynecologic disease, a significant excess of leukemia death was observed after pelvic radiotherapy administered to stop uterine bleeding.[81] Such treatment was fairly common during the 1930s and 1940s. Most women were in their mid to late 40s at the time of treatment. Interestingly, the average bone marrow dose was a factor of 10 lower than that for uterine cancer treatment (about 0.7

Gy versus 7 Gy), but the relative risks were about the same, twofold. Again, this suggests the importance of cell killing or inactivation in defining dose-response relationships. Time-response patterns differed for CML and acute leukemia. Similar to the study of atomic bomb survivors (see Fig. 8–1), the excess mortality rate due to CML was concentrated within the first 15 years after irradiation, whereas the relative excess of acute leukemia was more evenly distributed over time. Another mortality study of 2067 women irradiated for menstrual conditions in Scotland also revealed a twofold risk for leukemia (n = 12) associated primarily with external beam therapy (mean dose, 1.3 Gy).[41] Risk remained elevated after 30 years of follow-up in both studies.

ANKYLOSING SPONDYLITIS

The mortality experience of 14,558 persons treated between 1935 and 1954 in 87 British radiotherapy clinics for ankylosing spondylitis, a rheumatoid condition of the spine, has been carefully evaluated.[38] Radiation doses were estimated for each leukemia fatality and for a 7% sample of the population and averaged about 3.8 Gy for the active bone marrow. Leukemia risk (47 observed versus 36.1 expected) peaked 3 to 5 years after radiotherapy and gradually declined but not to baseline levels; CLL was not increased (2 observed versus 2.4 expected). The dose-response relationship for leukemia was irregular and essentially flat, possibly reflecting reduced leukemogenesis in the most heavily irradiated portions of the marrow due to cell killing or to the fractionated nature of the exposures.[134, 177] Compared with general population rates, the relative risk for leukemia can be estimated as 1.53 at 1 Gy and the absolute excess risk as $0.38/10^4$ person-years/Gy. A follow-up of the spondylitis population has been published with slightly higher estimates of risk but still little evidence for a dose-response relationship.[215]

TINEA CAPITIS

In the 1940s and 1950s, radiation was often used to treat nonmalignant conditions, such as ringworm of the scalp. In this circumstance, estimated doses from ringworm treatments were on the order of 1 to 2 Gy to the cranium and 0.3 Gy averaged over marrow in the entire body. A small excess of leukemia mortality was found among 10,000 children exposed in Israel, indicating that partial-body, relatively low dose radiotherapy to the head can increase leukemia risk, at least after childhood exposures.[166]

PEPTIC ULCER

In a survey of 1831 patients with peptic ulcer treated with radiation (stomach dose, 16 Gy) and 1778 nonexposed ulcer patients, a small but significant increase in leukemia was based on 11 cases.[69]

OTHER THERAPY

Increases in leukemia (115 observed versus 95.5 expected) have been reported in patients treated for benign lesions of the locomotor system.[36] Doses averaged about 0.39 Gy to the bone marrow, and follow-up was complete with use of Swedish registry systems. Another large study of patients in Sweden observed children for late effects after radiotherapy for skin hemangioma right after birth. Doses were about 0.2 Gy, and no significant risk for leukemia was reported.[114] Still another cohort study in Sweden did not find an association between radiotherapy for benign conditions of the breast and leukemia, although once again, the estimated dose to bone marrow was low.[122]

Diagnostic Radiology

Studies of diagnostic radiology and leukemia risk include tuberculosis patients undergoing repeated chest fluoroscopy, patients receiving x-ray studies for diagnostic purposes, and children born after being exposed prenatally to x-rays. The doses associated with diagnostic procedures are generally small, and the possible risk is accordingly low and difficult to detect. It is estimated that only a small percentage of leukemias, if any, might be due to diagnostic radiography.[57]

Tuberculosis

In the 1940s, patients with tuberculosis frequently underwent chest fluoroscopy during treatment of lung collapse to monitor the extent of collapse and to estimate the amount of air needed to maintain the collapse. Such therapy could last 3 to 5 years. The average number of air injections and associated x-ray fluoroscopic examinations often approached 100. The radiation dose to the chest marrow has been estimated to be 0.7 Gy (70 rad), 0.09 Gy (9 rad) averaged over the body. No excess leukemia was observed among 6000 exposed patients with tuberculosis.[43] A relative risk of about 1.4 was predicted on the basis of the data from studies of atomic bomb survivors, suggesting that separating or splitting doses over time may lower the risk of radiation-induced leukemia, possibly by allowing cell repair mechanisms to operate. In contrast, radiogenic breast cancers continue to occur at a high rate in these women, which suggests that organs differ in their response to fractionated doses of radiation.[16]

General Radiography

Results from studies of diagnostic radiation and adult leukemia are inconsistent. An early report from England of a positive association was later retracted when the author attributed the concentration of x-ray studies within 5 years before leukemia diagnosis to symptoms related to preclinical disease, including an increased susceptibility to infection.[186] Excesses of CML in some studies appeared to be restricted to those who received an extremely large number of x-ray studies.[63] A study at the Mayo Clinic, which included accurate estimates of bone marrow doses, found no link between leukemia and diagnostic x-ray studies, but the numbers were small.[109] A report from California found an association between diag-nostic radiography, particularly x-ray studies of the lower back, and CML on the basis of personal interviews of 136 patients and 136 neighborhood control subjects.[160] The largest study of diagnostic x-ray exposures and leukemia risk in adults relied on medical records of prepaid health plans in two states.[15] Information on more than 25,000 x-ray studies was abstracted on 385 cases of leukemia and 1400 control cases. Overall, there was a hint that leukemia risk might increase with increasing numbers of x-ray studies, but the trend was not significant. When exposures near the time of leukemia diagnosis were excluded, the trend essentially disappeared. These data were interpreted as suggesting that persons with leukemia might undergo x-ray procedures frequently just before diagnosis for conditions related to the development or natural history of their disease and, again, that fractionated doses may carry a lower risk than single exposures for the same total dose. Multiple fluoroscopic chest x-ray studies did not increase the risk for leukemia among children undergoing heart catheterization.[181]

Prenatal Exposure

Most but not all studies of medical exposure to diagnostic x-ray studies during pregnancy are consistent with a 40% increased risk for childhood leukemia.[7, 117, 136, 187] As well as providing direct evidence of risk at relatively low doses between 1 and 10 cGy, such studies are important because of the possibility that the developing fetus may be more susceptible to the leukemogenic effects of radiation than the child is. These studies have been extensively reviewed.[142, 199, 202] It had been postulated that selection factors, related to the medical reasons that women receive prenatal x-ray studies, might be responsible for the increased leukemia risk and not the x-ray exposures themselves. The absence of any childhood leukemia (and only one childhood cancer) in atomic bomb survivors exposed in utero (mean uterine dose, 18 cGy)[84] supported the selection hypothesis, as did Miller's observation[130] that it was peculiar that diagnostic x-ray studies would increase all childhood malignant diseases by about the same percentage (50%) when there is such a remarkable degree of variability between tissues in their response to radiation at other ages and because childhood cancers are known to have dissimilar origins. Biologic plausibility was questioned because children younger than 10 years exposed to the atomic bombs were at high risk for childhood leukemia (n = 14), but no cases of other childhood cancers occurred. Animal experiments do not suggest an enhanced sensitivity to leukemia induction after irradiation during fetal stages.[200]

Evidence against the selection hypothesis comes from the demonstration of a dose-response relationship for childhood leukemia based on number of x-ray films taken and from the observation that the excess risk was as great among twins, for whom x-ray pelvimetry was far more frequent (55%) than for singletons (15%), simply because of a greater likelihood that pelvimetry will be used to determine fetal positioning before delivery.[133] This observation was confirmed in a case-control study of twins born in Connecticut.[72] Nonetheless, it is argued that the number of x-ray studies is not necessarily equivalent to fetal dose and that twin studies are difficult to interpret. For example, despite substantial population exposure to prenatal x-ray studies, cohort studies consistently find twins to be at significantly low risk for childhood leukemia compared with single births.[80, 199] In fact, it is notable that only case-control studies find increased leukemia risks after prenatal exposure and that not a single cohort investigation has reported convincing evidence of a positive effect.[31, 80, 84, 166] Although there is no reason to believe that the fetus should be immune to the leukemogenic effects of ionizing radiation, there is also little reason to believe that the risk should be substantially greater for exposures just before birth than for exposures in early childhood. Thus, although it is established that prenatal x-irradiation is associated with an increased risk for childhood cancer, the magnitude of the hazard and even the causal nature of the association remain uncertain.[116, 199]

Whether low-dose exposures can result in a detectable increase in cancer risk remains an issue that is highly debated, most recently by Doll and Wakeford[47] and Boice and Miller.[18] Reviewing the same data, they came up with different conclusions with regard to the strength of the evidence. Doll and Wakeford put more weight on the positive Oxford case-control study and consistency with other case-control studies, whereas Boice and Miller found the absence of risk in atomic bomb survivors (and all other cohorts) plus the peculiar similarity in the relative risks of all childhood cancers to be suggestive of an underlying bias in the case-control studies that tempers interpretation.

Radionuclide Exposures

Human studies of radioactive iodine I 131, phosphorus P 32, Thorotrast (a radioactive contrast agent containing thorium Th 232), and radium Ra 224 have been conducted and leukemia risk evaluated.

Radioactive Iodine

Several Swedish studies have addressed cancer risks among patients administered ^{131}I, including 35,000 patients given diagnostic doses, 10,000 patients treated for hyperthyroidism, and 800 patients treated for thyroid cancer.[70, 71, 77] The half-life of ^{131}I is about 8 days, and thus the dose is delivered at a low rate during a period of about 30 days. A wide range of bone marrow doses was observed, but no trend in the relative risk for leukemia was seen. Again, it seems possible that a radiation dose delivered gradually over time is less leukemogenic than a brief exposure delivering the same total dose. Similarly, no excess leukemia was seen in a large cooperative study conducted in the United States of patients treated with ^{131}I for hyperthyroidism.[165, 172] Other studies of patients treated with ^{131}I for hyperthyroidism have also failed to reveal an increase in leukemia risk.[44, 60] Small excesses of leukemia have been reported among cancer patients treated with very high doses, however. In a study of 258 persons given high-dose ^{131}I for inoperable thyroid cancer, 4 cases of leukemia were observed versus 0.08 ex-

pected on the basis of general population rates.[54] A slight excess of leukemia (4 versus 1.6) was reported among 834 patients treated with ^{131}I for thyroid cancer in Sweden.[71] The doses to the bone marrow and other organs in these series were large and likely to be between 0.5 and 1.0 Gy.

Polycythemia Vera

Among 1222 patients treated for polycythemia vera, a blood disease characterized by overproduction of red cells, leukemia developed in 11% of 228 patients treated with ^{32}P, 9% of 79 patients treated with x-rays, and 16% of 72 patients treated with both x-rays and ^{32}P, but in only 1% of 133 nonirradiated patients.[131] A randomized clinical trial found that leukemia developed in 9 of 156 patients (6%) treated with ^{32}P, in contrast to 1 of 134 patients (1%) treated by phlebotomy.[6] Patients treated with chlorambucil were at highest risk (16 of 141, 11%). It is possible that the bone marrow of patients with polycythemia vera may be unusually sensitive to radiation, and it is unclear what effect the natural history of polycythemia vera might have on leukemia development.[214]

Thorotrast

Patients given Thorotrast, a radiographic contrast medium containing thorium dioxide, are at increased risk for leukemia.[3, 49, 119, 138, 143, 207, 208] The cell types include erythrocytic leukemia, which is rare, and AML and CML. These data indicate that alpha particles can increase the risk for leukemia, at least those associated with a colloid of thorium oxide that is taken up in the red marrow. These data further suggest that the distribution of dose in bone marrow is important because leukemia excesses are not reported in radium dial painters, in which the dose of alpha particles is primarily to the bone surfaces and not the bone marrow.[183] In these instances of radium exposure, osteosarcoma develops, but not leukemia. Interestingly, the risk coefficient for alpha particle–induced leukemia seems close to that for exposure to the atomic bomb, indicating that the relative biologic effectiveness might be similar.[9]

Radium Ra 224

German patients with bone tuberculosis or ankylosing spondylitis were treated with [224]Ra during 1945 to 1955. Studies of patients treated with high-dose [224]Ra have failed to reveal an increased risk for leukemia, although high rates of osteosarcomas were observed.[147] Studies of 1577 patients with ankylosing spondylitis treated between 1948 and 1975 with much lower doses of [224]Ra than in the earlier study find an increased leukemia risk (13 observed cases versus 4.2 expected).[216] However, the absence of a dose-response analysis and the absence of an increased risk among the patients given much higher doses add caution to interpretation of the association as causal. Animal models provide mixed results; smaller mammals, such as the mouse, show a leukemia effect from radium injection, but large mammals, such as the beagle, do not. The mouse may be an inappropriate model because of its small size, that is, alpha particles from decaying ^{224}Ra in the bone could traverse the entire bone marrow; for larger mammals, the alpha particle would be unlikely to penetrate to the center of the marrow and damage stem cells.

Occupational Exposures

Leukemia that follows occupational exposures has been studied in radiologists and nuclear industry workers. Challenges of evaluating and quantifying the risks for radiogenic leukemia in worker studies include the uncertainties in the dosimetric data and the relatively low statistical power associated with low cumulative exposures.

Medical Radiation Workers

The first cancer attributed to ionizing radiation occurred on the hand of a radiologist in 1902,[142] and leukemia was first associated with chronic exposure in studies of radiologists.[118] Leukemia, aplastic anemia, and skin cancer were excessive among radiologists who practiced during the early part of this century before radiation protection guidelines were in use, but these risks appear to have disappeared among more recently employed radiologists.[105, 121, 178, 212] A report on 27,000 medical radiation workers in China found a significant excess of leukemia.[212] The average bone marrow dose was not known but may have been 1 Gy or more. Even today, it is not uncommon for x-ray workers in China to receive time off when their blood cell counts become severely depressed. These medical worker studies indicate that prolonged exposure of sufficient cumulative dose can result in leukemia, but the lack of dosimetry precludes quantification of risk. A study of 140,000 radiologic technologists should provide additional information on leukemia risks in the occupational setting.[14] The occupational doses were lower than those experienced by the pioneering radiologists, and there is little evidence to date to suggest an increase in leukemia mortality.[48]

Nuclear Industry Workers

The mortality experience of nearly 31,500 male and 12,600 female workers employed between 1944 and 1978 at the Hanford nuclear installation in Richland, Washington, has been reported by several investigators. The most recent analyses revealed a strong healthy worker effect; a significant deficit of cancer mortality, including leukemia; and no evidence of increasing risk with increasing film badge exposure for any cancer.[65]

Results from studies of workers at nuclear installations are generally inconsistent. The initial report of United Kingdom Sellafield workers revealed no leukemia excess, although a dose response was suggested when analysis included only exposures occurring 15 years or more before diagnosis.[179] Leukemia was elevated among persons employed at the Oak Ridge National Laboratory, but risk was inversely related to dose.[65] A previous analysis of data on workers at the Oak Ridge National Laboratory[217]

received considerable criticism.[64] An excess of leukemia, including CLL, was highlighted even though leukemia risk decreased with increasing level of exposure. Leukemia has not been found to be elevated among plutonium workers,[65, 152, 210] except in Russia, where high gamma-ray exposures (>1 Gy) were experienced in the early years of their weapons program.[97, 98]

A mortality study from a large registry of 95,000 radiation workers in the United Kingdom reported significantly increased risks for leukemia, excluding CLL.[90, 139] Risk estimates were consistent with atomic bomb survivor data but apparently not with the studies of United States workers, which were negative.[64] This report should be interpreted with some caution because the leukemia risk was evident only at one facility, Sellafield, where high cumulative exposures above 1 Gy have occurred and where exposure to leukemogenic chemicals during fuel reprocessing activities might have occurred. Further studies of nuclear facility workers are being conducted to validate risk estimates from high-dose studies, but the limited data available to date are sufficient only to rule out the possibility of unusually high risks from low-dose fractionated exposures.

Large-scale pooled analysis of workers from Canada, the United Kingdom, and the United States also finds small but significant risks for leukemia, due mainly to a few subjects who received greater than 0.4 Gy.[26, 79] Studies from Japan and Canada found no association between radiation and leukemia, but the numbers were relatively small, as were the doses.[4, 56]

Environmental Exposures

Studies of leukemia risk associated with environmental radiation have been largely noninformative because of the generally low doses involved and the associated low statistical power to detect an effect. This is not to say that low doses of radiation are without effect, just that epidemiologic methods are too crude to detect convincingly low-level excess risks on the order of 20% to 30%.[102] Analytic studies have been conducted of persons exposed to high levels of natural background radiation, persons living near nuclear installations, populations exposed as a result of nuclear reactor accidents, and persons exposed to radon.

Natural Background Radiation

Correlation studies attempting to link leukemia incidence or mortality with natural background radiation have generally been interpreted as negative[2, 32, 86, 120, 190, 211] but are fraught with uncertainties regarding dose levels, migration patterns, selection factors for place of residence, and geographic variations in the accuracy of cancer diagnoses.[158, 182] In England, childhood cancer was correlated with maternal irradiation from background sources,[96] but interpretation of a causal link is clouded by the serious limitations of ecologic correlation analyses.[142] The most extensive investigation of the possible health effects of naturally occurring radiation was conducted in China on a stable population of 73,000 persons who received three times the amount of background radiation (330 milliroentgens [mR]/y versus 110 mR/y) as 77,000 inhabitants of a comparison region. Differences in chromosome aberrations in circulating lymphocytes indicated that the background radiation levels were meaningfully different.[213] Leukemia, however, was not increased among residents of the high background area.[27, 190]

Surveys Around Nuclear Facilities

Reports of small clusters of childhood leukemia around nuclear installations in the United Kingdom in the 1980s prompted several large-scale systematic surveys. Lymphoid leukemia among persons younger than 25 years was found to be generally increased in populations living near nuclear fuel reprocessing or weapons production facilities in the United Kingdom but not in populations living near plants that generated electricity.[28, 59] Mortality from Hodgkin's disease at ages 0 to 24 years was also increased, whereas mortality from lymphoid leukemia at ages 25 to 64 years was significantly reduced. There was no overall increase in cancer mortality in the vicinity of nuclear installations.

Interestingly, a study from Britain evaluated residents of areas where construction of nuclear power stations had only been considered or just recently completed. Excesses of childhood leukemia and Hodgkin's disease, as well as deficits of adult leukemia, were reported that were similar to those previously identified in areas with operating nuclear facilities.[29] The authors concluded that the unexpected increases in some childhood cancers around nuclear installations are unlikely to be due to environmental radiation pollution but rather are due to other risk factors yet to be identified. An infectious agent associated with large immigrations of people into these areas, for example, has been proposed as one possible explanation.[93, 94]

In the largest ecologic survey to date, cancer mortality in 113 counties in the United States that contained or were adjacent to 62 nuclear facilities was compared with mortality in control counties with similar population and socioeconomic characteristics; 2,700,000 cancer deaths were included.[85] Overall, and for specific groups of nuclear installations, there was no evidence that mortality for any cancer, including childhood leukemia, was higher in counties with nuclear reactors than in the control counties. For childhood leukemia, the relative risk in the study counties versus their controls was 1.03 after plant start-up, whereas it was 1.08 before start-up. For all leukemia, the relative risks were 0.98 after start-up and 1.02 before. Systematic studies in France, Germany, and Canada also failed to identify excesses of childhood leukemia among populations residing near nuclear facilities.[75, 124, 127]

Clusters Around Nuclear Facilities

In 1983, a team of investigative television reporters from Yorkshire set out to evaluate the risk for cancer among workers at the Sellafield (Windscale) nuclear fuel reprocessing complex in West Cumbria, United Kingdom. Learning that neither cancer nor leukemia was excessive in these workers,[179] the reporters focused on an apparent cluster of seven young people who developed leukemia between 1950 and 1983 in Seascale, a village about 3 km south of Sellafield. A government report confirmed that childhood leukemia was elevated (4 observed versus 0.25 expected) in the region near Sellafield.[8] An assessment of total radiation exposure of the local population revealed that natural background contributed the greatest amount (66%), and Sellafield discharges only 16%. Thus, environmental pollution from radioactive releases seemed an unlikely culprit.[37] Additional studies found that the excess of leukemia occurred entirely among individuals born in Seascale (5 versus 0.53) and not among children born elsewhere (0 versus 0.54), suggesting that factors present in early life or before birth might be important.[61] A subsequent case-control study, discussed later, raised the possibility that parental occupational exposure among Sellafield workers might explain the cluster.[62] It was determined that a significant excess of leukemia also occurred among young people born in places other than Seascale, minimizing the possible role that preconception irradiation might have played overall.[91]

Other studies around nuclear facilities have failed to provide clear insights into the reasons for apparent clusterings of childhood cancer.[52, 115] In some investigations, findings depended entirely on the selection of particular geographic and calendar time groupings. Even the Seascale cluster might be considered suspect, because it was the *occurrence of the cases* that determined both the geographic boundary and the age definition of the cluster. Recall that the television reporters first went to Sellafield, not Seascale, and were seeking excesses of cancer among adult workers, not leukemia among young people in the general population.

Preconception Irradiation

The most provocative (and controversial) finding from the Seascale studies was the association between leukemia and preconception irradiation of the fathers working at Sellafield.[62] If this is true, the apparent cluster might be explained in terms of occupational rather than environmental radiation exposure. The study, however, is at odds with the prospective investigation of children of the atomic bomb survivors, for whom no excesses of cancer, chromosome aberrations, or genetic mutations in blood proteins were observed.[145, 146, 199] Other case-control studies in England, Scotland, and Canada have failed to confirm the association between paternal preconception irradiation and childhood leukemia.[94, 125, 164, 205] Further, a study of 10,363 children who were born to fathers who worked at Sellafield evaluated the geographic distribution in Cumbria of the paternal dose received before conception.[153] Paternal doses were consistently higher among fathers of children born outside Seascale. Because childhood leukemia was not increased in these areas of West Cumbria despite the higher preconception exposures, the authors concluded that paternal exposure to radiation before conception is, in itself, unlikely to be a sufficient causal factor for childhood leukemia. It is generally accepted that the cluster of childhood leukemia around Sellafield was not related to paternal irradiation before conception.[46]

An alternative hypothesis being pursued to explain the apparent clusters is that childhood leukemia may occur as a rare response to an unidentified infection whose transmission is facilitated when large numbers of people from different geographic areas come together, such as might occur when large industrial complexes are built in rural areas[92-94] (see also Chapters 2 and 7).

Nuclear Reactor Accidents and Environmental Contamination

The nuclear reactor accident at Three Mile Island released little radioactivity into the environment, much less than the annual population exposure to natural background. Any presumed increase in cancer at these levels would be negligible and undetectable,[203] and not surprisingly, no peculiar mortality patterns have been noted.[85] In contrast, the accident at Chernobyl resulted in a massive release of radioactivity.[199, 201] Studies of surrounding populations to date have not linked the release to increases in childhood leukemia,[154, 155] and it remains to be determined whether populations residing outside the immediate vicinity of the reactor complex have received sufficient exposure to result in a detectable increase in leukemia.[5, 76, 107] A study from Greece did suggest an ecologic correlation between Chernobyl fallout and selected subtype of childhood leukemia,[156] which was not confirmed in a similar analysis in Germany.[126] On the other hand, 600,000 workers were sent to Chernobyl after the accident to clean up the environment and entomb the reactor. Allowable occupational exposures for the workers were stated to be 0.35 Gy, suggesting that doses might have been high enough for future health studies to be informative. However, comprehensive studies of more than 4000 Chernobyl cleanup workers from Estonia failed to reveal an increase in leukemia incidence.[161] Larger studies of cleanup workers from Russia initially reported a leukemia excess,[82] but there were methodologic flaws that precluded meaningful interpretation,[19] and a more valid case-control investigation failed to find evidence of a leukemia dose-response relationship.[83] Comprehensive evaluation of chromosomes in blood lymphocytes by use of fluorescent in situ hybridization technologies also failed to find an increase in aberration yield among exposed cleanup workers (as opposed to accident workers or reactor personnel), suggesting that the doses received may have been too low to result in a detectable increase.[111]

An explosion in 1957 in a storage tank at the Chelyabinsk nuclear facility (the Kyshtym accident) in the former Soviet Union released large amounts of radioactive waste into the Techa River. High-level radioactive effluents had also been dumped into the river before the accident between 1949 and 1956.[99-101] Population doses among 28,000 residents were as high as 4 Gy, and leukemia was reported to be significantly increased on the basis of 37 cases.

Radon

Estimates of environmental radon exposures in England have been correlated with monocytic and other types of leukemia (but not with lung cancer).[53, 74, 113] The link was not confirmed, however, in a separate analysis using smaller geographic units.[140] The possibility that high levels of radon might be related to human leukemia seems unlikely because underground miners heavily exposed to radon have been found to be at high risk for lung cancer but not for leukemia.[42, 192] Case-control studies of indoor radon have not found associations for childhood leukemias[112] or adult leukemia.[103]

There was substantial criticism to the early ecologic studies and their interpretation.[24, 138, 219] The dosimetric model was questioned,[132] and it was noted that the estimated dose to red bone marrow from radon was only 1% of that to the lung.[24, 141, 149] The equivalent dose resulting from exposure to radon at 200 Bq m^{-3} for a year might be around 100 mSv for the lung and as high as 25 mSv for the skin, in contrast to the dose to red bone marrow of approximately 0.1 to 1.2 mSv.[141, 149] Concerns about confounding and biologic plausibility were raised, and it was further suggested that the observations might result from confounding by socioeconomic factors. Methodologic difficulties and intrinsic fallacies associated with ecologic analyses preclude firm conclusions on the importance of the descriptive correlations.[68, 137]

Nonionizing Electromagnetic Fields

Extremely low frequency electromagnetic fields (60 Hz) from household appliances or electrical power transmission lines do not possess enough energy to strip electrons from atoms. Although they are generating great public concern, exposures to nonionizing radiations have not been convincingly linked to leukemia in humans or animals, and the evidence to date is sufficient only to formulate hypotheses for testing in future studies.[150] Risk for childhood leukemia was evaluated in three Nordic studies.[1] An apparent excess of leukemia was based on a total of 13 cases that occurred during a period of more than 20 years. Associations were reported for estimated field strengths based on proximity to transmission lines and power consumption but not for measured magnetic fields. Differences in the methods used to estimate relevant electromagnetic field exposure, in the categorization of electromagnetic field exposure (cut points), and in the selected time relationships between exposure and leukemia diagnosis make interpretation of a causal association based on such small numbers tenuous at best. Thus, no causal relationship has been established between electromagnetic fields and childhood leukemia.[50] This conclusion is consistent with the results of comprehensive case-control studies in the United Kingdom, Canada, and the United States, which were all essentially negative.[108, 123, 198]

GENERALIZATIONS

Human studies of radiation-induced leukemia (see Table 8-2) have revealed the complex nature of the relationship between exposure and leukemia occurrence. Recognizing the differences in such studies, several generalizations can be made, nonetheless.

1. Radiation-induced leukemia is reported more frequently than any other cancer, owing largely to a short minimal latency period and a high relative risk coefficient.

2. The time response appears to be wavelike, peaking 3 to 10 years after exposure. Radiogenic leukemias occur much earlier than radiogenic solid tumors.

3. Age at exposure is an important determinant of risk. The young are apparently the most sensitive on a relative scale.

4. Different cell types vary in their response to radiation, and one common type of leukemia, CLL, has never been linked to radiation, nor has adult T-cell leukemia.

5. The exposure-response relationship appears to be nonlinear, with risk per unit dose being lower at low doses than at high doses.

6. At very high doses to limited volumes of tissues, cell killing may predominate over cell transformation. Secondary leukemia does not appear to be a common event after radiotherapy for cancer, but small excesses on the order of twofold have been observed. The excesses are much lower than predicted from studies of atomic bomb survivors.

7. The mechanism for radiation-induced leukemia is likely to involve chromosome rearrangements.

8. Fractionation or splitting of exposures over time may also lower risk appreciably, but more study is needed to clarify the magnitude of the risk reduction in humans.

9. The fetus appears vulnerable to the carcinogenic action of ionizing radiation, but whether the level of risk differs from that in young children is not entirely clear.

10. Alpha particles (helium nuclei) in some circumstances can cause leukemia, but the unusual distribution of dose from Thorotrast in the bone marrow may be a special case. Radium and radon have not been convincingly linked to leukemia.

11. Very low radiation doses received from environmental exposures are difficult to tie to increased leukemia risks because the anticipated excesses are so small in relation to natural occurrence.

12. The evidence that preconception irradiation increases leukemia risk in offspring is not convincing. The initial studies suggesting a link have not been confirmed.

FUTURE RESEARCH

The quantitative description of risk continues to present unique opportunities for research that may lead to a better understanding of the pathogenesis of cancer in humans, with implications for public health and the setting of radiation protection standards. Studies of populations exposed occupationally to ionizing radiations may provide valuable insights into the effects of low doses received at low dose rates. New biologic markers of exposure, such as the glycophorin A mutational assay for red blood cells and fluorescent in situ hybridization for chromosome aberration detection, may offer new possibilities for quantifying previous exposures.[188] It remains to be learned whether molecular mechanisms in radiation leukemogenesis are the same as for de novo leukemias. The interaction of radiation with other leukemogenic

exposures, such as chemotherapeutic agents, might reveal interesting mechanistic understandings. It remains puzzling why CLL, a common type of adult leukemia, has never been linked to ionizing radiation. It is unclear whether there are sensitive subgroups within the population who are at especially high risk for radiation-induced leukemia. New information about the human genome may permit a greater understanding of the genetic events leading to radiogenic leukemia.

REFERENCES

1. Ahlbom A, Feychting M, Koskenvuo M, et al: Electromagnetic fields and childhood cancer. Lancet 1993;342:1295.
2. Akiba S, Sun Q, Tao Z, et al: Infant leukemia mortality among the residents in high-background-radiation areas in Guangdong, China. In Wei L, Sugahara T, Tao Z, eds: High Levels of Natural Radiation, 1996: Radiation Dose and Health Effects. Amsterdam: Elsevier; 1997, p 255.
3. Andersson M, Carstensen B, Visfeldt J: Leukemia and other related hematological disorders among Danish patients exposed to Thorotrast. Radiat Res 1993;134:224.
4. Ashmore JP, Krewski D, Zielinski JM, et al: First analysis of mortality and occupational radiation exposure based on the National Dose Registry of Canada. Am J Epidemiol 1998;148:564.
5. Auvinen A, Hakama M, Arvela H, et al: Fallout from Chernobyl and incidence of childhood leukaemia in Finland, 1976–92. BMJ 1994;309:1514.
6. Berk PD, Goldberg JD, Silverstein MN, et al: Increased incidence of acute leukemia in polycythemia vera associated with chlorambucil therapy. N Engl J Med 1981;304:441.
7. Bithell JF, Stewart AM: Prenatal irradiation and childhood malignancy: A review of British data from the Oxford Survey. Br J Cancer 1975;31:271.
8. Black D: Investigation of the Possible Increased Incidence of Cancer in West Cumbria. Report of the Independent Advisory Group. London: Her Majesty's Stationery Office; 1984.
9. Boice JD Jr: Leukemia risk in Thorotrast patients. Radiat Res 1993; 136:301.
10. Boice JD Jr: Second cancer after Hodgkin's disease—the price of success. J Natl Cancer Inst 1993;85:4.
11. Boice JD Jr: Radiation and non-Hodgkin's lymphoma. Cancer Res 1992;52(suppl):5489s.
12. Boice JD Jr, Blettner M, Kleinerman RA, et al: Radiation dose and leukemia risk in patients treated for cancer of the cervix. J Natl Cancer Inst 1987;79:1295.
13. Boice JD Jr, Day NE, Andersen A, et al: Second cancers following radiation treatment for cervical cancer. An international collaboration among cancer registries. J Natl Cancer Inst 1985;74:955.
14. Boice JD Jr, Mandel JS, Doody MM, et al: A health survey of radiologic technologists. Cancer 1992;69:586.
15. Boice JD Jr, Morin MM, Glass AG, et al: Diagnostic x-ray procedures and risk of leukemia, lymphoma and multiple myeloma. JAMA 1991;265:1290.
16. Boice JD Jr, Preston D, Davis FG, et al: Frequent chest x-ray fluoroscopy and breast cancer incidence among tuberculosis patients in Massachusetts. Radiat Res 1991;125:214.
17. Boice JD Jr, Holm LE: Radiation risk estimates for leukemia and thyroid cancer among Russian emergency workers at Chernobyl. Radiat Environ Biophys 1997;36:213.
18. Boice JD Jr, Miller RW: Childhood and adult cancer after intrauterine exposure to ionizing radiation [review]. Teratology 1999;59: 227.
19. Boice JD Jr: Leukemia, Chernobyl and epidemiology. J Radiol Prot 1997;17:127.
20. Boivin JF, Hutchison GB, Evans FB, et al: Leukemia after radiotherapy for first primary cancers of various anatomic sites. Am J Epidemiol 1986;123:993.
21. Botti AC, Verma RS: The molecular biology of acute lymphoblastic leukemia [review]. Anticancer Res 1990;10:519.
22. Breckon G, Papworth D, Cox R: Murine radiation myeloid leukae-

mogenesis: A possible role for radiation sensitive sites on chromosome 2. Genes Chromosomes Cancer 1991;3:367.

23. Breckon G, Silver A, Cox R: Radiation-induced chromosome 2 breakage and the initiation of murine radiation acute myeloid leukaemogenesis. J Radiat Res 1991;32(suppl 2):46.

24. Butland BK, Muirhead CR, Draper GJ: Radon and leukaemia [letter]. Lancet 1990;335:1338.

25. Caldwell GG, Kelley D, Zack M, et al: Mortality and cancer frequency among military nuclear test (SMOKY) participants, 1957 through 1979. JAMA 1983;250:620.

26. Cardis E, Gilbert ES, Carpenter L, et al: Effects of low doses and low dose rates of external ionizing radiation: Cancer mortality among nuclear industry workers in three countries. Radiat Res 1995;142:117.

27. Chen D, Wei L: Chromosome aberration, cancer mortality and hormetic phenomena among inhabitants in areas of high background radiation in China. J Radiat Res 1991;32(suppl 2):46.

28. Cook-Mozaffari PJ, Ashwood FL, Vincent T, et al: Cancer incidence and mortality in the vicinity of nuclear installations, England and Wales, 1959–1980. OPCS Studies on Medical and Population Subjects 51. London: Her Majesty's Stationery Office; 1987.

29. Cook-Mozaffari P, Darby S, Doll R: Cancer near potential sites of nuclear installations. Lancet 1989;2:1145.

30. Conard RA: Acute myelogenous leukemia following fallout radiation exposure. JAMA 1975;232:1356.

31. Court-Brown WM, Doll R, Hill AB: Incidence of leukemia after exposure to diagnostic radiation in utero. Br Med J 1960;2:1539.

32. Court-Brown WM, Spiers FW, Doll R, et al: Geographical variation in leukaemia mortality in relation to background radiation and other factors. Br Med J 1960;1:1753.

33. Croce CM: Role of chromosome translocations in human neoplasia. Cell 1987;49:155.

34. Curtis RE, Boice JD Jr, Stovall M, et al: Relation of leukemia risk to radiation dose after cancer of the uterine corpus. J Natl Cancer Inst 1994;86:1315.

35. Curtis RE, Boice JD Jr, Stovall M, et al: Risk of leukemia after chemotherapy and radiation treatment for breast cancer. N Engl J Med 1992;326:1745.

36. Damber L, Larsson LG, Johansson L, et al: A cohort study with regard to the risk of haematological malignancies in patients treated with x-rays for benign lesions in the locomotor system. I. Epidemiological analyses. Acta Oncol 1995;34:713.

37. Darby SC, Doll R: Fallout, radiation doses near Dounreay, and childhood leukaemia. BMJ 1987;294:603.

38. Darby SC, Doll R, Gill SK, et al: Long term mortality after a single treatment course with x-rays in patients treated for ankylosing spondylitis. Br J Cancer 1987;55:179.

39. Darby SC, Kendall GM, Fell TP, et al: Further followup of mortality and incidence of cancer in men from the United Kingdom who participated in the United Kingdom's atmospheric nuclear weapon tests and experimental programmes. BMJ 1993;307:1530.

40. Darby SC, Olsen JH, Doll R, et al: Trends in childhood leukaemia in the Nordic countries in relation to fallout from atmospheric nuclear weapons testing. BMJ 1992;304:1005.

41. Darby SC, Reeves G, Key T, et al: Mortality in a cohort of women given x-ray therapy for metropathia haemorrhagica. Int J Cancer 1994;56:793.

42. Darby SC, Whitley E, Howe GR, et al: Radon and cancers other than lung cancer in underground miners: A collaborative analysis of 11 studies. J Natl Cancer Inst 1995;87:378.

43. Davis FG, Boice JD Jr, Hrubec Z, et al: Cancer mortality in a radiation-exposed cohort of Massachusetts tuberculosis patients. Cancer Res 1989;49:6130.

44. de Vathaire F, Schlumberger M, Delisle MJ, et al: Leukaemias and cancers following iodine-131 administration for thyroid cancer. Br J Cancer 1997;75:734.

45. Delongchamp RR, Mabuchi K, Yoshimoto Y, et al: Cancer mortality among atomic bomb survivors exposed in utero or as young children, October 1950–May 1992. Radiat Res 1997;147:385.

46. Doll R, Evans HJ, Darby SC: Paternal exposure not to blame [review]. Nature 1994;367:678.

47. Doll R, Wakeford R: Risk of childhood cancer from fetal irradiation [review]. Br J Radiol 1997;70:130.

48. Doody MM, Mandel JS, Lubin JH, et al: Mortality among United States radiologic technologists, 1926–90. Cancer Causes Control 1998;9:67.

49. dos Santos Silva I, Jones M, Malveiro F, et al: Mortality in the Portuguese thorotrast study. Radiat Res 1999;152(suppl):S88.

50. Draper G: Electromagnetic fields and childhood cancer. BMJ 1993;307:884.

51. Draper GJ, Sanders BM, Kingston JE: Second primary neoplasms in patients with retinoblastoma. Br J Cancer 1986;53:661.

52. Draper GJ, Stiller CA, Cartwright RA, et al: Cancer in Cumbria and in the vicinity of the Sellafield nuclear installation, 1963–1990. BMJ 1993;306:89.

53. Eatough JP, Henshaw DL: Radon and monocytic leukaemia in England. J Epidemiol Community Health 1993;47:506.

54. Edmonds CJ, Smith T: The long-term hazards of the treatment of thyroid cancer with radioiodine. Br J Radiol 1986;59:45.

55. Eng C, Li FP, Abramson DH, et al: Mortality from second tumors among long-term survivors of retinoblastoma. J Natl Cancer Inst 1993;85:1121.

56. Epidemiological Study Group of Nuclear Workers (Japan): First analysis of mortality of nuclear industry workers in Japan, 1986–1992. J Health Phys 1997;32:173.

57. Evans JS, Wennberg JE, McNeil BJ: The influence of diagnostic radiography on the incidence of breast cancer and leukemia. N Engl J Med 1986;315:810.

58. Folley J, Borges W, Yamawaki T: Incidence of leukemia in survivors of the atomic bomb in Hiroshima and Nagasaki, Japan. Am J Med 1952;13:311.

59. Forman D, Cook-Mozaffari P, Darby S, et al: Cancer near nuclear installations. Nature 1987;329:499.

60. Franklyn JA, Maisonneuve P, Sheppard M, et al: Cancer incidence and mortality after radioiodine treatment for hyperthyroidism: A population-based cohort study. Lancet 1999;353:2111.

61. Gardner MJ, Hall AJ, Downes S, et al: Followup study of children born to mothers resident in Seascale, West Cumbria (birth cohort). BMJ 1987;295:822.

62. Gardner MJ, Snee MP, Hall AJ, et al: Results of case-control study of leukaemia and lymphoma among young people near Sellafield nuclear plant in West Cumbria. BMJ 1990;300:423.

63. Gibson R, Graham S, Lilienfeld A, et al: Irradiation in the epidemiology of leukemia among adults. J Natl Cancer Inst 1972;48:301.

64. Gilbert ES, Cragle DL, Wiggs LD: Updated analyses of combined mortality data on workers at the Hanford Site, Oak Ridge National Laboratory, and Rocky Flats Weapons Plant. Radiat Res 1993;136:408.

65. Gilbert ES, Omohundro E, Buchanan JA, et al: Mortality of workers at the Hanford site: 1945–1986. Health Phys 1993;64:577.

66. Greaves MF: Stem cell origins of leukaemia and curability. Br J Cancer 1993;67:413.

67. Greene MH, Young RC, Merrill JM, et al: Evidence of a treatment dose response in acute nonlymphocytic leukemias which occur after therapy of non-Hodgkin's lymphoma. Cancer Res 1983;43:1891.

68. Greenland S, Robins J: Invited commentary: Ecologic studies—biases, misconceptions, and counterexamples. Am J Epidemiol 1994;139:747.

69. Griem ML, Kleinerman RA, Boice JD Jr, et al: Cancer following radiotherapy for peptic ulcer. J Natl Cancer Inst 1994;86:842.

70. Hall P, Boice JD Jr, Berg G, et al: Leukaemia incidence after iodine-131 exposure. Lancet 1992;340:1.

71. Hall P, Holm LE, Lundell G, et al: Cancer risks in thyroid cancer patients. Br J Cancer 1991;64:159.

72. Harvey EB, Boice JD Jr, Honeyman M, et al: Prenatal x-ray exposure and childhood cancer in twins. N Engl J Med 1985;312:541.

73. Hawkins MM, Kinnier-Wilson LM, Stovall MA, et al: Epipodophyllotoxins, alkylating agents, and radiation and risk of secondary leukaemia after childhood cancer. BMJ 1992;304:951.

74. Henshaw DL, Eatough JP, Richardson RB: Radon as a causative factor in induction of myeloid leukaemia and other cancers. Lancet 1990;335:1008.

75. Hill C, Laplanche A: Overall mortality and cancer mortality around French nuclear sites. Nature 1990;347:755.

76. Hjalmars U, Kulldorff M, Gustafsson G: Risk of acute childhood leukaemia in Sweden after the Chernobyl reactor accident. Swedish Child Leukaemia Group. BMJ 1994;309:154.

77. Holm LE, Hall P, Wiklund KE, et al: Cancer risk after iodine-131 therapy for hyperthyroidism. J Natl Cancer Inst 1991;83:1072.

78. Hutchison GB: Leukemia in patients with cancer of the cervix

uteri treated with radiation. A report covering the first five years of an international study. J Natl Cancer Inst 1968;40:951.

79. IARC Study Group on Cancer Risk Among Nuclear Industry Workers: Direct estimates of cancer mortality due to low doses of ionizing radiation: An international study. Lancet 1994;344:1039.

80. Inskip PD, Harvey EB, Boice JD Jr, et al: Incidence of childhood cancer in twins. Cancer Causes Control 1991;2:315.

81. Inskip PD, Kleinerman RA, Stovall M, et al: Leukemia, lymphoma, and multiple myeloma after pelvic radiotherapy for benign disease. Radiat Res 1993;135:108.

82. Ivanov VK, Tsyb AF, Gorsky AI, et al: Leukaemia and thyroid cancer in emergency workers of the Chernobyl accident: Estimation of radiation risks (1986–1995). Radiat Environ Biophys 1997; 36:9.

83. Ivanov VK, Tsyb AF, Konogorov AP, et al: Case-control analysis of leukaemia among Chernobyl accident emergency workers residing in the Russian Federation, 1986–1993. J Radiol Prot 1997;17:137.

84. Jablon S, Kato H: Childhood cancer in relation to prenatal exposure to atomic-bomb radiation. Lancet 1970;2:1000.

85. Jablon S, Hrubec Z, Boice JD Jr: Cancer in populations living near nuclear facilities. A survey of mortality nationwide and incidence in two states. JAMA 1991;265:1403.

86. Jacobson AP, Plato PA, Frigerio NA: The role of natural radiations in human leukemogenesis. Am J Public Health 1976;66:31.

87. Kaldor JM, Day NE, Clarke EA, et al: Leukemia following Hodgkin's disease. N Engl J Med 1990;322:7.

88. Kamada N, Tanaka K, Oguma N, et al: Cytogenetic and molecular changes in leukemia among atomic bomb survivors. J Radiat Res (Tokyo) 1991;2:257.

89. Kanopka JB, Watanabe SM, Witte ON: An alteration of the human cabl protein in K562 leukemia cells unmasks associated tyrosine kinase activity. Cell 1984;37:1035.

90. Kendall GM, Muirhead CR, MacGibbon BH, et al: Mortality and occupational exposure to radiation: First analysis of the National Registry for Radiation Workers. BMJ 1992;304:220.

91. Kinlen LJ: Can paternal preconceptional radiation account for the increase of leukaemia and non-Hodgkin's lymphoma in Seascale? BMJ 1993;306:1718.

92. Kinlen LJ, Clarke K, Balkwill A: Paternal preconceptional radiation exposure in the nuclear industry and leukaemia and non-Hodgkin's lymphoma in young people in Scotland. BMJ 1993;306:1153.

93. Kinlen LJ, Hudson CM, Stiller CA: Contacts between adults as evidence for an infective origin of childhood leukaemia: An explanation for the excess near nuclear establishments in West Berkshire. Br J Cancer 1991;64:549.

94. Kinlen LJ, O'Brien F, Clarke K, et al: Rural population mixing and childhood leukaemia: Effects of the North Sea oil industry in Scotland, including the area near Dounreay nuclear site. BMJ 1993; 306:743.

95. Kleinerman RA, Littlefield LG, Tarone RE, et al: Chromosome aberrations in peripheral lymphocytes and radiation dose to active bone marrow in patients treated for cancer of the cervix. Radiat Res 1989;119:176.

96. Knox EG, Stewart AM, Gilman EA, et al: Background radiation and childhood cancers. J Radiol Prot 1988;8:9.

97. Koshurnikova NA, Shilnikova NS, Okatenko PV, et al: The risk of cancer among nuclear workers at the "Mayak" production association: Preliminary results of an epidemiological study. In Boice JD Jr, ed: Implications of New Data on Radiation Cancer Risk. Proceedings No. 18. Bethesda, Md: National Council on Radiation Protection and Measurements; 1997, p 113.

98. Koshurnikova NA, Shilnikova NS, Okatenko PV, et al: Characteristics of the cohort of workers at the Mayak nuclear complex. Radiat Res 1999;152:352.

99. Kossenko MM, Degteva MO, Vyushkova OV, et al: Issues in the comparison of risk estimates for the population in the Techa River region and atomic bomb survivors. Radiat Res 1997;148:54.

100. Kossenko MM, Degteva MO: Cancer mortality and radiation risk evaluation for the Techa River population. Sci Total Environ 1994; 142:73.

101. Kossenko MM, Degteva MO, Petrushova NA: Estimate of the risk of leukemia to residents exposed to radiation as a result of a nuclear accident in the southern Urals. PSR Quarterly 1992;2:187.

102. Land CE: Estimating cancer risks from low doses of ionizing radiation. Science 1980;209:1197.

103. Law GR, Kane EV, Roman E, et al: Residential radon exposure and adult acute leukaemia. Lancet 2000;355:1888.

104. Leder P, Battey J, Lenoir G, et al: Translocations among antibody genes in human cancer. Science 1983;222:765.

105. Lewis EB: Leukemia, multiple myeloma, and aplastic anemia in American radiologists. Science 1963;142:1492.

106. Lindberg S, Karlsson P, Arvidsson B, et al: Cancer incidence after radiotherapy for skin haemangioma during infancy. Acta Oncol 1995;34:735.

107. Linet MS, Boice JD Jr: Radiation from Chernobyl and risk of childhood leukemia. Eur J Cancer 1993;29A:1.

108. Linet MS, Hatch EE, Kleinerman RA, et al: Residential exposure to magnetic fields and acute lymphoblastic leukemia in children. N Engl J Med 1997;337:1.

109. Linos A, Gray JE, Orvis AL, et al: Low-dose radiation and leukemia. N Engl J Med 1980;302:1101.

110. Little MP, Weiss HA, Boice JD Jr, et al: Risks of leukemia in Japanese atomic bomb survivors, in women treated for cervical cancer, and in patients treated for ankylosing spondylitis. Radiat Res 1999;152:280.

111. Littlefield LG, McFee AF, Salomaa SI, et al: Do recorded doses overestimate true doses received by Chernobyl cleanup workers? Results of cytogenetic analyses of Estonian workers by fluorescence in situ hybridization. Radiat Res 1998;150:237.

112. Lubin JH, Linet MS, Boice JD Jr, et al: Case-control study of childhood acute lymphoblastic leukemia and residential radon exposure. J Natl Cancer Inst 1998;90:294.

113. Lucie NP: Radon exposure and leukaemia. Lancet 1989;2:99.

114. Lundell M, Holm LE: Mortality from leukemia after irradiation in infancy for skin hemangioma. Radiat Res 1996;145:595.

115. MacMahon B: Leukemia clusters around nuclear facilities in Britain. Cancer Causes Control 1992;3:283.

116. MacMahon B: Some recent issues in low-exposure radiation epidemiology. Environ Health Perspect 1989;81:131.

117. MacMahon B: Prenatal x-ray exposure and childhood cancer. J Natl Cancer Inst 1962;28:1173.

118. March HC: Leukemia in radiologists. Radiology 1944;43:275.

119. Martling U, Mattsson A, Travis LB, et al: Mortality after long-term exposure to radioactive Thorotrast: A forty-year follow-up survey in Sweden. Radiat Res 1999;151:293.

120. Mason TJ, Miller RW: Cosmic radiation at high altitudes and U.S. cancer mortality, 1950–1969. Radiat Res 1974;60:302.

121. Matanoski GM, Seltser R, Sartwell PE, et al: The current mortality rates of radiologists and other physician specialists. Specific causes of death. Am J Epidemiol 1975;101:199.

122. Mattsson A, Hall P, Ruden BI, et al: Incidence of primary malignancies other than breast cancer among women treated with radiation therapy for benign breast disease. Radiat Res 1997;148:152.

123. McBride ML, Gallagher RP, Theriault G, et al: Power-frequency electric and magnetic fields and risk of childhood leukemia in Canada. Am J Epidemiol 1999;149:831.

124. McLaughlin JR, Clarke EA, Nishri D, et al: Childhood leukaemia in the vicinity of Canadian nuclear facilities. Cancer Causes Control 1993;4:51.

125. McLaughlin JR, King WD, Anderson TW, et al: Paternal radiation exposure and leukaemia in offspring: The Ontario case-control study. BMJ 1993;307:959.

126. Michaelis J, Kaletsch U, Burkart W, et al: Infant leukaemia after the Chernobyl accident. Nature 1997;387:246.

127. Michaelis J, Keller B, Haaf G, et al: Incidence of childhood malignancies in the vicinity of West German nuclear power plants. Cancer Causes Control 1992;3:255.

128. Mikkelsen T, Cavenee WK: Suppressors of the malignant phenotype. Cell Growth Differ 1990;1:201.

129. Miller RW, Boice JD Jr: Cancer after intrauterine exposure to the atomic bomb. Radiat Res 1997;147:396.

130. Miller RW: Delayed radiation effects in atomic-bomb survivors. Science 1969;166:569.

131. Modan B, Lilienfeld AM: Polycythemia vera and leukemia—the role of radiation treatment. A study of 1222 patients. Medicine (Baltimore) 1965;44:305.

132. Mole RH: Radon and leukaemia [letter]. Lancet 1990;335:1336.

133. Mole RH: Antenatal irradiation and childhood cancer: Causation or coincidence? Br J Cancer 1974;30:199.

134. Mole RH, Major IR: Myeloid leukaemia frequency after protracted

exposure to ionizing radiation: Experimental confirmation of the flat dose-response found in ankylosing spondylitis after a single treatment course with x-rays. Leuk Res 1983;7:295.

135. Moloney WC: Radiogenic leukemia revisited. Blood 1987;70:905.

136. Monson RR, MacMahon B: Prenatal x-ray exposure and cancer in children. In Boice JD Jr, Fraumeni JF Jr, eds: Radiation Carcinogenesis: Epidemiology and Biological Significance. New York: Raven Press; 1984, p 97.

137. Morgenstern H: Ecologic studies in epidemiology: Concepts, principles, and methods [review]. Annu Rev Public Health 1995;16:61.

138. Mori T, Kido C, Fukutomi K, et al: Summary of entire Japanese Thorotrast follow-up study: Updated 1998. Radiat Res 1999;152:S84.

139. Muirhead CR, Goodill AA, Haylock RG, et al: Occupational radiation exposure and mortality: Second analysis of the National Registry for Radiation Workers. J Radiol Prot 1999;19:3.

140. Muirhead CR, Butland BK, Green BM, et al: Childhood leukaemia and natural radiation. Lancet 1991;337:503.

141. National Academy of Science: Effects of Exposure to Radon (BEIR VI). Washington, DC: National Academy Press; 1999.

142. National Academy of Science: Health Effects of Exposure to Low Levels of Ionizing Radiation (BEIR V). Washington, DC: National Academy Press; 1990.

143. National Academy of Science: Health Risks of Radon and Other Internally Deposited Alpha-Emitters (BEIR IV). Washington, DC: National Academy Press; 1988.

144. National Council on Radiation Protection and Measurements: Influence of Dose and Its Distribution in Time on Dose-Response Relationships for Low-LET Radiations (Report No. 64). Washington, DC: NCRP; 1980.

145. Neel JV: Update on the genetic effects of ionizing radiation. JAMA 1991;266:698.

146. Neel JV, Schull WJ, eds: The Children of Atomic Bomb Survivors. A Genetic Study. Washington, DC: National Academy Press; 1991.

147. Nekolla EA, Kellerer AM, Kuse-Isingschulte M, et al: Malignancies in patients treated with high doses of radium-224. Radiat Res 1999;152:S3.

148. Nowell PC, Hungerford DA: A minute chromosome in chronic granulocytic leukemia. Science 1960;132:1497.

149. NRPB: Health Risks from Radon. Oxon: National Radiological Protection Board; 2000.

150. NRPB: Electromagnetic Fields and the Risk of Cancer. Report of an Advisory Group on Non-ionising Radiation (Documents of the NRPB, vol 3). Didcot: National Radiological Protection Board; 1992.

151. Okada S, Hamilton HB, Egami N, et al, eds: A review of thirty years of Hiroshima and Nagasaki atomic bomb survivors. J Radiat Res (Tokyo) 1975;16(suppl):1.

152. Omar RZ, Barber JA, Smith PG: Cancer mortality and morbidity among plutonium workers at the Sellafield plant of British Nuclear Fuels. Br J Cancer 1999;79:1288.

153. Parker L, Craft AW, Smith J, et al: Geographical distribution of preconception radiation doses at the Sellafield nuclear installation, West Cumbria. BMJ 1993;307:966.

154. Parkin DM, Cardis E, Masuyer E, et al: Childhood leukaemia following the Chernobyl accident: The European Childhood Leukaemia-Lymphoma Incidence Study (ECLIS). Eur J Cancer 1993;29A:87.

155. Parkin DM, Clayton D, Black RJ, et al: Childhood leukaemia in Europe after Chernobyl: 5 year follow-up. Br J Cancer 1996;73:1006.

156. Petridou E, Trichopoulos D, Dessypris N, et al: Infant leukaemia after in utero exposure to radiation from Chernobyl. Nature 1996;382:352.

157. Pierce DA, Shimizu Y, Preston DL, et al: Studies of the mortality of atomic bomb survivors. Report 12, Part I. Cancer: 1950–1990. Radiat Res 1996;146:1.

158. Pochin EE: Problems involved in detecting increased malignancy rates in areas of high natural radiation background. Health Phys 1976;31:148.

159. Preston D, Kusumi S, Tomonaga M, et al: The incidence of leukemia, lymphoma, and myeloma among A-bomb survivors, 1950–87. Radiat Res 1994;137(suppl):S68.

160. Preston-Martin S, Thomas DC, Yu MC, et al: Diagnostic radiography as a risk factor for chronic myeloid and monocytic leukemia (CML). Br J Cancer 1989;59:639.

161. Rahu M, Tekkel M, Veidebaum T, et al: The Estonian study of Chernobyl cleanup workers. II. Incidence of cancer and mortality. Radiat Res 1997;147:653.

162. Robinette CD, Jablon S, Preston TL: Mortality of Nuclear Weapons Test Participants. Washington, DC: National Academy Press; 1985.

163. Rodvall Y, Hrubec Z, Pershagen G, et al: Childhood cancer among Swedish twins. Cancer Causes Control 1992;3:527.

164. Roman E, Watson A, Beral V, et al: Case-control study of leukaemia and non-Hodgkin's lymphoma among children aged 0–4 years living in west Berkshire and north Hampshire health districts. BMJ 1993;306:615.

165. Ron E, Doody MM, Becker DV, et al: Cancer mortality following treatment for adult hyperthyroidism. Cooperative Thyrotoxicosis Therapy Follow-up Study Group. JAMA 1998;280:347.

166. Ron E, Modan B, Boice JD Jr: Mortality after radiotherapy for ringworm of the scalp. Am J Epidemiol 1988;127:713.

167. Rowley JD: Biological implications of consistent chromosome rearrangements in leukemia and lymphoma. Cancer Res 1984;44:3159.

168. Rowley JD: A new consistent chromosomal abnormality in chronic myelogenous leukemia identified by quinacrine fluorescence and Giemsa staining. Nature 1973;243:290.

169. Rowley JD, LeBeau MM: Cytogenetic and molecular analysis of therapy-related leukemia. Ann N Y Acad Sci 1989;567:130.

170. Rowley JD, Golomb HM, Vardiman JW: Nonrandom chromosome abnormalities in acute leukemia and dysmyelopoietic syndromes in patients with previously treated malignant disease. Blood 1981;58:759.

171. Rowley JD, Mitelman F: Principles of molecular cell biology of cancer: Chromosome abnormalities in human cancer and leukemia. In DeVita VT Jr, Hellman S, Rosenberg SA, eds: Cancer Principles and Practice of Oncology. Philadelphia: JB Lippincott; 1993, p 67.

172. Saenger EL, Thoma GE, Tompkins EA: Incidence of leukemia following treatment of hyperthyroidism. Preliminary report of the Cooperative Thyrotoxicosis Therapy Followup Study. JAMA 1968;205:855.

173. Sankila R, Olsen JH, Anderson H, et al: Risk of cancer among offspring of childhood-cancer survivors. Association of the Nordic Cancer Registries and the Nordic Society of Paediatric Haematology and Oncology. N Engl J Med 1998;338:1339.

174. Shimizu Y, Kato H, Schull WJ: Studies of the mortality of A-bomb survivors. 9. Mortality, 1950–1985. Part 2. Cancer mortality based on the recently revised doses (DS86). Radiat Res 1990;121:120.

175. Showe LC, Croce CM: The role of chromosomal translocations in B- and T-cell neoplasia. Annu Rev Immunol 1987;5:253.

176. Silver A, Cox R: Telomerelike DNA polymorphisms associated with genetic predisposition to acute myeloid leukemia in irradiated CBA mice. Proc Natl Acad Sci U S A 1993;90:1407.

177. Smith PG, Doll R: Mortality among patients with ankylosing spondylitis after a single treatment course with x-rays. BMJ 1982;284:449.

178. Smith PG, Doll R: Mortality from cancer and all causes among British radiologists. Br J Radiol 1981;54:187.

179. Smith PG, Douglas AJ: Mortality of workers at the Sellafield plant of British Nuclear Fuels. BMJ 1986;293:845.

180. Solomon E, Borrow J, Goddard AD: Chromosome aberrations and cancer. Science 1991;254:1153.

181. Spengler RF, Cook DH, Clarke EA, et al: Cancer mortality following cardiac catheterization: A preliminary followup study on 4,891 irradiated children. Pediatrics 1983;71:235.

182. Spiers FW: Background radiation and estimated risks from low-dose irradiation. Health Phys 1979;37:784.

183. Spiers FW, Lucas HF, Rundo J, et al: Leukaemia incidence in the U.S. dial workers. Health Phys 1983;44(suppl 1):65.

184. Spiess H, Mays CW, Chmelevsky D: Malignancies in patients injected with radium 224. In Taylor DM, Mays CW, Gerber GB, eds: Risks from Radium and Thorotrast. BIR Report 21. London: British Institute of Radiology; 1989, p 7.

185. Stevens W, Thomas DC, Lyon JL, et al: Leukemia in Utah and radioactive fallout from the Nevada test site. A case-control study. JAMA 1990;264:585.

186. Stewart A: The carcinogenic effects of low level radiation. A reappraisal of epidemiologists methods and observations. Health Phys 1973;24:223.

187. Stewart A, Webb J, Hewitt D: A survey of childhood malignancies. Br Med J 1958;1:1495.

188. Straume T, Lucas JN, Tucker JD, et al: Biodosimetry for a radiation worker using multiple assays. Health Phys 1992;62:122.

189. Swerdlow AJ, Douglas AJ, Hudson GV, et al: Risk of second primary cancers after Hodgkin's disease by type of treatment: Analysis of 2846 patients in the British National Lymphoma Investigation. BMJ 1992;304:1137.

190. Tao A-F, Kato H, Zha Y-R, et al: Study on cancer mortality among the residents in high background radiation area of Yangijang, China. In Wei L, Sugahara T, Tao Z, eds: High Levels of Natural Radiation, 1996: Radiation Dose and Health Effects. Amsterdam: Elsevier; 1997, p 249.

191. Thauls S, Page WF, Crawford H, et al: The Five Series Study. Mortality of Military Participants in U.S. Nuclear Weapons Tests. Washington, DC: National Academy Press; 2000.

192. Tomasek L, Darby SC, Swerdlow AJ, et al: Radon exposure and cancer other than lung cancer among uranium miners in West Bohemia. Lancet 1993;341:919.

193. Travis LB, Weeks J, Curtis RE, et al: Leukemia following low-dose total body irradiation and chemotherapy for non-Hodgkin's lymphoma. J Clin Oncol 1996;14:565.

194. Travis LB, Curtis RE, Boice JD Jr, et al: Second cancers following non-Hodgkin's lymphoma. Cancer 1991;67:2002.

195. Travis LB, Curtis RE, Glimelius B, et al: Second cancers among long-term survivors of non-Hodgkin's lymphoma. J Natl Cancer Inst 1993;85:1932.

196. Tucker MA, Coleman CN, Cox RS, et al: Risk of second cancers after treatment for Hodgkin's disease. N Engl J Med 1988;318:76.

197. Tucker MA, Meadows AT, Boice JD Jr, et al: Leukemia after therapy with alkylating agents for childhood cancer. J Natl Cancer Inst 1987;78:459.

198. UK Childhood Cancer Study Investigators: Exposure to power-frequency magnetic fields and the risk of childhood cancer. Lancet 1999;354:1925.

199. United Nations Scientific Committee on the Effects of Atomic Radiation: Sources and Effects of Ionizing Radiation (Publication E.94.IX.11). New York: United Nations; 1994.

200. United Nations Scientific Committee on the Effects of Atomic Radiation: Sources and Effects of Ionizing Radiation (Publication E.94.IX.2). New York: United Nations; 1993.

201. United Nations Scientific Committee on the Effects of Atomic Radiation: Sources and Effects of Ionizing Radiation (Publication E.00.IX.3). New York: United Nations; 2000.

202. United Nations Scientific Committee on the Effects of Atomic Radiation: Ionizing Radiation Levels and Effects, vol 2: Effects (Publication E.72.IX.18). New York: United Nations; 1972.

203. Upton AC: Health impact of the Three Mile Island accident. Ann N Y Acad Sci 1981;365:63.

204. Upton AC, Randolph ML, Conklin JW, et al: Late effects of fast neutrons and gamma-rays in mice as influenced by the dose rate of irradiation: Induction of neoplasia. Radiat Res 1970;41:467.

205. Urquhart JD, Black RJ, Muirhead MJ, et al: Case-control study of leukaemia and non-Hodgkin's lymphoma in children in Caithness near the Dounreay nuclear installation. BMJ 1991;302:687.

206. van der Plas DC, Hermans AB, Soekarman D, et al: Cytogenetic and molecular analysis in Philadelphia negative CML. Blood 1989; 73:1038.

207. van Kaick G, Wesch H, Lührs H, et al: The German Thorotrast Study—report on 20 years' followup. In Taylor DM, Mays CW, Gerber GB, Thomas RG, eds: Risks from Radium and Thorotrast. BIR Report 21. London: British Institute of Radiology; 1989, p 98.

208. van Kaick G, Dalheimer A, Hornik S, et al: The German Thorotrast study: Recent results and assessment of risks. Radiat Res 1999; 152:S64.

209. van Leeuwen FE, Somers R, Taal BG, et al: Increased risk of lung cancer, non-Hodgkin's lymphoma, and leukemia following Hodgkin's disease. J Clin Oncol 1989;7:1046.

210. Voelz GL: Health considerations for workers exposed to plutonium. Occup Med 1991;6:681.

211. Walter SD, Meigs JW, Heston JF: The relationship of cancer incidence to terrestrial radiation and population density in Connecticut, 1935–1974. Am J Epidemiol 1986;123:1.

212. Wang JX, Inskip PD, Boice JD Jr, et al: Cancer incidence among medical diagnostic x-ray workers in China, 1950 to 1985. Int J Cancer 1990;45:889.

213. Wang Z, Boice JD Jr, Wei L, et al: Thyroid nodularity and chromosome aberrations among women in areas of high background radiation in China. J Natl Cancer Inst 1990;82:478.

214. Wasserman LR: A cooperative study of polycythemia vera. Ann N Y Acad Sci 1985;459:328.

215. Weiss HA, Darby SC, Fearn T, et al: Leukemia mortality after x-ray treatment for ankylosing spondylitis. Radiat Res 1995;142:1.

216. Wick RR, Nekolla EA, Gossner W, et al: Late effects in ankylosing spondylitis patients treated with ^{224}Ra. Radiat Res 1999;152:S8.

217. Wing S, Shy CM, Wood JL, et al: Mortality among workers at Oak Ridge National Laboratory. Evidence of radiation effects in followup through 1984. JAMA 1991;265:1397.

218. Wong FL, Boice JD Jr, Abramson DH, et al: Cancer incidence after retinoblastoma: Radiation dose and sarcoma risk. JAMA 1997; 278:1262.

219. Wolff SP: Leukaemia risks and radon. Nature 1991;353:288.

220. Yoshimoto Y, Kato H, Schull WJ: Risk of cancer among children exposed in utero to A-bomb radiations, 1950–84. Lancet 1988; 2:665.

221. Yunis JJ, Soreng AL, Bowe AE: Fragile sites are targets of diverse mutagens and carcinogens. Oncogene 1987;1:59–69.

9

Jens Pedersen-Bjergaard

Chemicals and Leukemia

Based on the assumption that human cancer is often a result of exposure to well-defined chemical substances, much experimental research was previously devoted to chemical carcinogenesis. Subsequently, such an etiology was firmly established for only a limited number of chemicals and malignancies,[1] and it became possible in these cases to relate chemical structure and reactivity to chromosome abnormalities and to other genetic changes in the multistep process of malignant transformation.

OCCUPATIONAL CHEMICAL EXPOSURE

Different types of occupation and lifestyle with exposure to a number of more or less well-defined chemical substances have during the years been suggested to play a role in the epidemiology of leukemia as previously reviewed[2-4] (Table 9-1). The leukemias observed were in most cases acute myeloid leukemia (AML), often manifested as myelodysplasia (MDS), and the risk was shown to be only slightly increased in comparison to the risk of MDS and AML in the general population. In many instances, the results were not confirmed by subsequent studies.

Exposure to benzene was demonstrated almost a century ago to be a definitive occupational hazard because it could result in bone marrow toxicity and aplasia.[5-7] In some cases, the subsequent development of leukemia was observed.[8-14] In a 1988 review, 11 studies were identified that demonstrated a close association between benzene exposure and the development of leukemia.[15] Several years later, 18 community-based studies and 16 industry-based studies were identified,[16] all emphasizing the importance of the problem. The significance of benzene metabolism, the effects of benzene and its degradation products phenol and hydroquinone on normal hematopoiesis, and the role of benzene as a leukemogenic chemical have been reviewed in detail.[17, 18]

Not only shoemakers, as originally reported, but also other professions using benzene as a solvent may be at risk. Occupational exposure to the widely used petroleum products may likewise imply a risk because these substances regularly contain small amounts of benzene.[19] However, major studies have thus far not shown an increased risk of leukemia in gasoline service station workers.[20] In only a small proportion of heavily exposed refinery workers has an increased risk been demonstrated.[21] Epidemiologic risk assessment has suggested an exponentially increasing risk of leukemia by increasing cumulative doses of benzene.[22] Recently, not only an increased risk of MDS and AML but also other hematologic neoplasms such as non-Hodgkin's lymphomas has been suggested after exposure to benzene.[23]

A different individual susceptibility to benzene toxicity has been discussed, with an increased risk in individuals with high CYP2E1 enzyme activity, low reduced glutathione (GSH) transferase activity in the liver, and low or disturbed NQO1 reductase activity[24-26]; in addition, high myeloperoxidase activity in the bone marrow may increase the risk. Benzene must be considered a well-established leukemogenic chemical, and every effort should be taken to avoid any exposure in various occupations.

Epidemiologists have searched extensively for an increased risk of leukemia related to occupation and exposure to a wide variety of other chemical substances (see Table 9-1), generally with rather limited success. A slightly increased incidence of leukemia was observed in farmers[27, 28] related to exposure to herbicides[29] or pesticides.[30] These findings have not been confirmed by larger studies. The potential biases of this type of study have been summarized,[31] and the results are conflicting.[32]

In the rubber industry, exposure to solvents such as carbon tetrachloride and carbon disulfide[33] and to butadiene[34] has been in focus. In health care workers, ethylene oxide[35, 36] has been suggested as leukemogenic. A subsequent study, however, showed only a trend by duration of exposure, but no significant overall risk of leukemia in persons exposed to ethylene oxide.[37]

CHEMICAL EXPOSURE RELATED TO LIFESTYLE

Several lifestyle factors have been considered in relation to leukemogenesis. Smoking has consistently been shown to be a risk factor for the development of myeloid leukemia.[38-44] The relative risk of leukemia in smokers as compared with the general population, or the odds ratio, was in most studies only on the order of 2, with a marked dose-response effect. This finding indicates that approximately half the cases of leukemia observed in heavy smokers are tobacco induced, whereas the other half are incidental cases of de novo leukemia.

TABLE 9–1. Chemicals, Occupations, and Lifestyles That Have Been Related to an Increased Risk of Leukemia

	Chemicals	Exposed Risk Groups
Occupational exposure	Benzene	Shoemakers and gasoline handling
	Phenoxy herbicides	Farmers
	Organophosphates	Farmers
	Styrene-butadiene	Rubber workers
	Ethylene oxide	Medical supplies
Lifestyle	Smoking	
	Hair dye	
	Alcohol	Pregnant women
	Marijuana	Pregnant women
	Bioflavonoids in food	Pregnant women
Drugs	Chloramphenicol	Patients
	Phenylbutazone	Patients
	Cytostatic drugs	Patients

Other lifestyle exposure such as the use of permanent hair dye has been suggested to result in an increased risk of hematologic malignancies, including leukemia.[45] However, larger subsequent studies have not supported this observation.[46, 47] Other risk factors related to lifestyle such as increased intake of alcohol and the use of marijuana have been suggested to increase the risk of leukemia, but thus far in unconfirmed studies.

The increased incidence of leukemia in infants younger than 1 year has been related to exposure of mothers during pregnancy to different chemicals and to their lifestyle.[48] Maternal socioeconomic status, previous fetal loss, mothers' smoking, their abuse of marijuana and alcohol, and exposure to pesticides have all been evaluated for a role in the development of infant leukemia. Until recently, conflicting results have been obtained as previously reviewed.[48] In a recent study from Children's Cancer Group, increased maternal intake of agriculture products such as beans, fresh vegetables and fruit, all rich in bioflavonoids, was significantly associated with infant leukemia.[49] Subsequently, it was demonstrated that these bioflavonoids are topoisomerase II inhibitors and, in vitro and in vivo, induce the same cleavage of the *MLL* gene within the breakpoint cluster region (BCR) as the cytostatic agents etoposide and doxorubicin (see later).[50] A chemical structure shared by 20 bioflavonoids was identified as essential for the effect. This research was inspired by studies demonstrating that up to 80% of infant leukemias involve translocations to chromosome band 11q23 with chimeric rearrangement of the *MLL* gene. Furthermore, the clustering of breakpoints within the BCR region of the gene was the same for infant leukemia as for therapy-related AML (t-AML) after treatment with topoisomerase II inhibitors and was different from the clustering of breakpoints in de novo AML.[51-53] Lifelong exposure to phenol and hydroquinone derivatives from the diet and gastrointestinal flora activity has been considered a causal factor for leukemia.[54]

NONCYTOSTATIC DRUGS

For almost 50 years, case reports and smaller series of patients have indicated a general association between therapy with different noncytostatic drugs, bone marrow hypoplasia or aplasia, and the subsequent development of leukemia, most often AML. The two drugs most often implicated have been chloramphenicol[55] and phenylbutazone.[56] In a major 1976 review, Bloomfield and Brunning summarized 36 cases of chloramphenicol-related leukemia published in the literature.[57] The fact that patients with hereditary disorders characterized by insufficient hematopoiesis such as Fanconi's anemia and Kostmann's syndrome and patients with idiopathic aplastic anemia have an increased risk of AML[58, 59] supports the hypothesis that severely suppressed bone marrow function, though of a different etiology, may predispose to the development of AML.

CYTOGENETICS AND CHEMICAL EXPOSURE

The cytogenetic characteristics of AML have been studied and related to environmental and occupational exposure, and cytogenetic abnormalities of human blood cells exposed in vitro or in vivo to various chemicals have been studied in an effort to support a causal relationship between exposure to chemicals and the subsequent development of leukemia. A higher frequency of chromosome aberrations, particularly deletions or loss of the long arms or loss of whole chromosomes 5 and 7, was originally observed in four studies.[60-64] These studies included between 16 and 52 cases of AML with chemical exposure, and the patients were compared with nonexposed controls. In one recent study of 214 cases of MDS, only a nonsignificant excess of abnormalities of chromosomes 5 and 7 was observed in exposed patients,[65] and in another recent study of 213 patients with AML, patients with all types of chromosome abnormality were more likely to smoke and to use alcohol than were patients with a normal karyotype. However, other associations were not observed.[66]

In workers occupationally exposed to benzene, peripheral blood lymphocytes in one study showed a significantly increased number of breaks at chromosome band 7q22,[67] whereas another study showed an excess of trisomy 8 and 21, as well as translocations between these two chromosomes.[68] One in vitro experiment has demonstrated that normal human lymphocytes exposed to benzene metabolites have an excess of monosomy 5 and 7 and deletions of the long arms of these chromosomes,[69] whereas another study showed that hydroquinone, the main degradation product of benzene, induces an excess of monosomy 7 and trisomy 8 in human CD34$^+$ blood progenitors.[70] In conclusion, cytogenetic studies in vivo and in experimental systems emphasize that chemicals, particularly benzene, induce chromosome damage. However, until now, significant relationships between specific chemical exposure related to occupation or lifestyle and the development of t-AML with specific chromosome aberrations have not been definitively established. The many different chromosome aberrations observed in only a very small percentage of exposed and nonexposed patients, and sometimes in only a few cells, are a major problem in this type of study. Another problem relates to the fact that the frequency of abnormalities of chromosomes 5 and 7 in AML increases markedly with patient age, as does the likelihood of being exposed to chemicals.

CYTOSTATIC DRUGS

During the last 30 years, most research on chemical leukemogenesis has been devoted to studies of the increased risk of secondary or therapy-related myelodysplasia (t-MDS) and t-AML after chemotherapy for benign and malignant diseases as previously reviewed.[71-74] In numerous studies, this risk and risk factors have been evaluated, and in the clinic, leukemia has turned out to be the most serious long-term complication of cancer chemotherapy. In addition, from a scientific point of view, t-AML, often manifested as t-MDS, is of particular interest, inasmuch as this disease is induced by chemicals with a well-known mechanism of action. In series of intensively treated patients, almost all observed cases of t-MDS and t-AML must be considered to be directly chemotherapy induced because the relative risk of MDS and AML in comparison to the general population often exceeds 100. Furthermore, t-MDS progressing to t-AML represents an example of the multistep process of malignant transformation. Finally, most patients with t-MDS and t-AML have characteristic clonal chromosome aberrations that are related to the etiology of the disease and disclose some of its genetic abnormalities. Research on t-MDS and t-AML has mainly concentrated on three items: risk factors and risk estimates, cytogenetic abnormalities, and the molecular biology of the disease.

ROLE OF THE PRIMARY MALIGNANCY

t-AML, often manifested as t-MDS, was initially considered a specific phenomenon related to primary tumors such as multiple myeloma and Hodgkin's disease. Subsequently, it was realized that leukemic complications could occur in all patients treated with alkylating agents or topoisomerase II inhibitors. The most important diseases with a highly increased risk of t-MDS or t-AML demonstrated in well-defined cohort studies are shown in Table 9–2. AML may develop as part of the natural history of polycythemia vera,[75] essential thrombocythemia,[76] and germ cell tumors of mediastinal localization.[77, 78] For this reason, it is difficult, particularly in patients with polycythemia vera and essential thrombocythemia, to distinguish cases of AML related to intensive therapy with alkylating agents and other cytostatic drugs from sporadic cases of AML merely related to the primary disease. In all the other diseases shown in Table 9–2, the risk of t-MDS or t-AML has been exclusively related to chemotherapy.

LEUKEMOGENIC EFFECT OF ALKYLATING AGENTS

The first alkylating agents demonstrated to be leukemogenic were mechlorethamine administered together with radiotherapy in patients with Hodgkin's disease[79] and

TABLE 9–2. Primary Diseases with a Verified Increased Risk of t-MDS and t-AML after Chemotherapy

Hematologic neoplasms	Hodgkin's disease
	Non-Hodkin's lymphomas
	Multiple myeloma
	Polycythemia vera
	Essential thrombocythemia
	Acute lymphoblastic leukemia
Solid tumors	Breast cancer
	Ovarian cancer
	Lung cancer
	Testicular cancer
	Childhood solid tumors
	Gastrointestinal cancer
Nonmalignant diseases	Rheumatoid arthritis
	Psoriasis
	Wegener's granulomatosis

t-AML, therapy-related acute myeloid leukemia; t-MDS, therapy-related myelodysplasia.

melphalan used in combination with prednisone in patients with multiple myeloma.[80] Numerous subsequent studies have confirmed these observations as reviewed.[81-84] The studies have demonstrated that almost all alkylating agents in clinical use today are leukemogenic (Table 9–3). Only a few studies have addressed the question of the extent to which equitoxic doses of the different alkylating agents result in an identical risk for leukemia. The substitution in the MOPP combination (mechlorethamine, vincristin, procarbazine, and prednisone) of mechlorethamine for carmustine or lomustine[85] and the administration of lomustine at relapse[86] in patients with Hodgkin's disease have both been demonstrated to result in a particularly high risk of t-MDS and t-AML. In multiple myeloma and ovarian cancer, melphalan has been demonstrated to be more leukemogenic than cyclophosphamide,[87, 88] and busulfan was apparently more leukemogenic than cyclophosphamide in lung cancer.[89] The clinical choice of alkylating agent has not changed markedly to agents with a suggested lower risk of t-MDS and t-AML because other factors play a role in the clinical decision; for instance, therapy with cyclophosphamide has been shown to result in a substantially increased risk of transitional cell bladder cancer in addition to t-MDS and t-AML.[90-92]

LEUKEMOGENIC EFFECT OF TOPOISOMERASE II INHIBITORS

More recently, various topoisomerase II inhibitors have been demonstrated to be leukemogenic, in most cases administered in combination chemotherapy regimens including cisplatin or a classic alkylating agent. A leukemogenic effect of etoposide was first demonstrated when administered in combination with cisplatin and vindesine for non–small-cell lung cancer[93] and subsequently for etoposide or teniposide used in combination chemotherapy for acute lymphoblastic leukemia (ALL).[94] These results have been confirmed in patients with other malignancies such as germ cell tumors treated with etoposide and

TABLE 9–3. Cytostatic Drugs Associated with an Increased Risk of t-MDS and t-AML

Alkylating agents	Mechlorethamine
	Cyclophosphamide
	Ifosfamide
	Busulfan
	Dihydroxybusulfan
	Melphalan
	Chlorambucil
	Carmustine
	Lomustine
	Semustine
	Dacarbazine
	Dibromodulcitol
	Cisplatin
	Carboplatin
Topoisomerase II inhibitors	Etoposide
	Teniposide
	Doxorubicin
	Daunorubicin
	4-epidoxorubicin
	Mitoxantrone
	Razoxane
	Bimolane
Others	Procarbazine
	L-Asparaginase (together with etoposide)
	Dibromomannitol
	Hydroxyurea
	Pipobroman
	Fludarabine ?
	Paclitaxel ?
	Docetaxel ?
	Irinotecan ?
	Topotecan ?

t-AML, therapy-related acute myeloid leukemia; t-MDS, therapy-related myelodysplasia.

cisplatin,[95] various other tumors in adults,[96] and solid tumors in children.[97]

Likewise the anthracyclines, almost always administered in combination with other cytostatic drugs, have been demonstrated to be leukemogenic. In patients treated for non-Hodgkin's lymphomas,[98] ovarian cancer,[99] and childhood cancer,[100] doxorubicin has been shown to be leukemogenic. In patients treated for breast cancer with 4-epidoxorubicin plus cisplatin or cyclophosphamide,[101, 102] an increased risk of t-MDS and t-AML was partly ascribed to the anthracycline part of the combination. In addition, mitoxantrone administered to patients with breast cancer in various combination chemotherapy regimens has been demonstrated to result in an increased risk of t-MDS and t-AML.[103-105] An apparently lower risk of t-MDS and t-AML after therapy with the anthracyclines and mitoxantrone than after the epipodophyllotoxins may relate to the lower maximal cumulative dose of anthracyclines and mitoxantrone because of the risk of cardiotoxicity.

Finally, the dioxopiperazine derivatives razoxane and bimolane have been demonstrated to be leukemogenic as reviewed.[106] These drugs have been used as single-agent therapy for psoriasis, but as a result of British studies[107-110] and Chinese studies[111, 112] demonstrating their leukemogenic potential, these drugs have now been abandoned in the treatment of benign diseases. Dioxopiperazine deriva-

tives belong to the group of topoisomerase II inhibitors,[113, 114] although they have a different mechanism of action.[115] The fact that the leukemias observed after therapy with these drugs mainly have recurrent balanced translocations, primarily t(15;17), as also observed in the leukemias after therapy with epipodophyllotoxins, anthracyclines, and mitoxantrone (see later), supports the ability of dioxopiperazine derivatives to be leukemogenic.

RISK OF t-MDS AND t-AML AFTER HODGKIN'S DISEASE

Over the years, many single-institution and cooperative studies have examined the risk of t-MDS and t-AML after therapy for Hodgkin's disease with MOPP or MOPP-like regimens, and the cumulative risk has varied widely (Table 9-4). In many studies, the risk was related to the intensity of therapy or the cumulative dose of alkylating agents administered.[85, 121, 126, 127, 136, 138, 140, 146] Generally, the highest risks have been observed in single-institution studies, including cases of t-MDS diagnosed cytogenetically, and in studies including patients receiving multiple treatments for relapse of Hodgkin's disease. The risk has been higher in studies of adult patients than in studies of children, and most studies evaluating age as a risk factor have shown the risk to increase markedly by age.[85, 119-121, 127, 129, 135, 137, 147] In a single-institution study of patients treated very intensively, in some cases with chlorambucil as long-term maintenance chemotherapy, the cumulative dose of alkylating agents was evaluated for each patient. The risk of t-MDS and t-AML was shown to increase almost in direct proportion to the cumulative dose of alkylating agents and with the square of age.[126]

In many studies of Hodgkin's disease, high-voltage radiotherapy administered alone or in combination with chemotherapy was not a significant risk factor for t-MDS and t-AML.[85, 98, 118, 121, 124, 127, 132] The reason for this surprising observation is probably that most hematopoietic precursor cells within the irradiated fields cannot undergo leukemic transformation because they are killed by the therapy. In addition, statistical problems may play a role because the risk of t-MDS and t-AML after high-voltage radiotherapy is at least for 10-fold lower than the risk after intensive chemotherapy[127] and the standard error for most risk estimates is large in as much as only a few patients are alive and being monitored some years after the start of therapy.

The effect of splenectomy on the risk of t-MDS and t-AML has been studied repeatedly. Some studies have reported higher risks after splenectomy,[128, 129, 133, 148] whereas others have not observed such an effect.[135, 136, 144] Although the problem has been evaluated in multivariate analysis, the higher risk of splenectomized patients observed in some studies may relate to confounding factors. The major and recent British National Cooperative Study of 4576 patients treated for Hodgkin's disease showed no significant effect of splenectomy on the risk for t-MDS and t-AML,[149] and no substantial biologic evidence supports a higher risk of AML in asplenic individuals.

A low risk of t-MDS and t-AML has been observed after

TABLE 9–4. Cumulative Risk of t-MDS and t-AML in Patients Treated with MOPP-like Regimens for Hodgkin's Disease

Authors/Year	Institution	Cases of t-MDS/t-AML/ Treated	Cumulative Risk (%): Years from Start of Therapy	Significant Risk Factors/Remarks
Studies Mainly Including Adult Patients				
Coleman et al,[116] 1977	Stanford	RT: —/0/320 CT ± RT: —/6/360	— 1.5%–2.9%: 5 yr 2.0%–3.9%: 7 yr	CT + RT highest risk, MOPP
Valagussa et al,[117] 1980	Milan	ALL: —/9/528	1.4%: 5 yr 3.5%: 10 yr	MOPP
Baccarani et al,[118] 1980	Cooperative, Italy	RT: —/0/117 CT ± RT: —/7/496	— 3.0%: 8 yr	RT not a risk factor All AMLs manifested as MDS
Coltman et al,[119] 1982	SWOG	RT: —/0/95 CT ± RT: —/21/600	— 3.2%–6.2%: 5 yr 6.2%–7.7%: 7 yr	Age >40 yr: 20.7% at 7 yr, MOPP
Coleman et al,[120] 1982	Stanford	RT: —/1/441 CT ± RT: —/19/716	0.5%: 10 yr 3.5%–15.6%: 10 yr	CT versus RT, MOPP Age >40 yr
Glicksman et al,[85] 1982	CALGB	CT: —/6/369 CT ± RT: —/4/429	5.6%: 10 yr	BCNU and CCNU substit. in MOPP Maintenance with Clb: 26.2% at 10 yr Addition of RT not a risk factor Age >40 yr
Pedersen-Bjergaard et al,[121] 1982	Copenhagen	RT: 0/0/79 CT ± RT: 7/10/312	— 3.9%: 5 yr 4.9%: 9 yr	BCNU and CCNU substit. in MOPP Maintenance with Clb Addition of RT not a risk factor Intensity of CT Age >40 yr
Tester et al,[122] 1984	NCI, USA	RT: —/0/146 CT ± RT: —/9/327	— 2%–9%: 10 yr	CT versus RT, MOPP No effect of age
Valagussa et al,[123] 1986	Milan	RT: —/0/307 MOPP ± RT: —/19/1022 ABVD: —/0/180	— 1.4%–15.5%: 12 yr	Age ABVD not leukemogenic
Koletsky et al,[124] 1986	Yale	RT: —/0/253 CT ± RT: —/5/207	1.5%: 5 yr 5.9%: 10 yr	CT versus RT, MOPP-like regimens No effect of additional low-dose RT
Blayney et al,[125] 1987	NCI, USA	MOPP: 6/6/192	3%: 5 yr 10%: 10 yr	Peak incidence 5–7 yr from start of MOPP, no risk after 11 yr
Pedersen-Bjergaard et al,[126] 1987	Copenhagen	CT ± RT: 9/11/320	3.9%: 5 yr 13.0%: 10 yr	Risk increased proportional to cumulative dose of alkylating agents and with the square of age Risk leveled out beyond 7 yr after cessation of CT
Tucker et al,[127] 1988	Stanford	RT: —/2/535 CT ± RT: —/26/796	0.6%: 15 yr 4.9%–12.3%: 15 yr	CT versus RT Age >40 yr Alkylating agents, intensity RT in addition to CT: no effect
van der Velden et al,[128] 1988	Cooperative, international	All: —/18/1681	2.3%: 10 yr	Extensive RT, splenectomy MOPP
van Leeuwen et al,[129] 1989	Amsterdam	RT: 0/1/273 CT ± RT: 6/15/469	1.0%: 5 yr 6.3%: 15 yr	RT: no effect Age >40 yr Splenectomy
Lavey et al,[98] 1990	Durham	RT: —/1/75 CT ± RT: —/3/238	1.4%: 10 yr 2.0%: 10 yr	
Selby et al,[130] 1990	Royal Marsden	CT ± RT: —/2/284	2.7%: 10 yr	Me replaced by Clb and VCR replaced by Vlb: same risk
Devereux et al,[86] 1990	British National	RT: —/0/863 CT: —/4/852 CT ± RT: —/13/961	One treatment: 0.2%: 15 yr Two treatments: 2.3%: 15 yr Three or more: 8.1%: 15 yr Lomustine: 22.8%: 15 yr	
Cimino et al,[131] 1991	Cooperative, Italy	RT: —/0/115 CT ± RT: —/23/832	— 2.8%: 10 yr 10.2%: 19 yr	MOPP, RT not a risk factor

table continued on following page

TABLE 9–4. Cumulative Risk of t-MDS and t-AML in Patients Treated with MOPP-like Regimens for Hodgkin's Disease *Continued*

Authors/Year	Institution	Cases of t-MDS/t-AML/ Treated	Cumulative Risk (%): Years from Start of Therapy	Significant Risk Factors/Remarks
Swerdlow et al,[132] 1992	British National	RT: 0/1/935 CT ± RT: 1/14/1896	1.4%: 15 yr	Alkylating agents No additional effect of RT Me replaced by Clb in MOPP
Henry-Amar,[133] 1992	Cooperative, international	All: —/158/12411	1.8%: 10 yr 2.4%: 20 yr	Alkylating agents, age, splenectomy, and advanced stage
Abrahamsen et al,[134] 1993	Norway	RT: —/0/356 CT ± RT: —/9/773	— 1.5%: 12 yr	Alkylating agents in MOPP-like regimens No increase with age
Rodriguez et al,[135] 1993	M.D. Anderson	RT: 0/0/284 CT ± RT: 2/12/729	— 3%: 20 yr	Age and stage, alkylating agents Splenectomy and additional RT not risk factors
Biti et al,[136] 1994	Florence and Arezzo	RT: —/1/745 CT ± RT: —/10/376	0.2%: 15 yr 4.3%–11.1%: 15 yr	Intensity of CT RT and splenectomy not significant risk factors
van Leeuwen et al,[137] 1994	Cooperative, Netherland	RT: 0/1/552 CT ± RT: 12/30/1387	4.0%: 20 yr	CT, age >40 yr, splenectomy, advanced stage RT in addition to CT: no risk factor
Swerdlow et al,[138] 1997	Royal Marsden	All: —/12/1039	1.9%: 10 yr 2.3%: 20 yr	CT and its intensity Higher risk at younger age Clb = Me as substit. in MOPP
Swerdlow et al,[139] 2000	Cooperative, England	RT: —/1/1499 CT ± RT: —/43/4020	1.7%: 20 yr	Chemotherapy Younger age
Studies Mainly or Exclusively Including Children				
Tucker et al,[100] 1987	Late Effects Study Group	All: —/12/1036	4.2%: 20 yr	Increasing with age and score for alkylating agents RT not a risk factor
Meadows et al,[140] 1989	Late Effects Study Group	RT: —/0/281 CT ± RT: —/16/698	1%: 5 yr 4%: 15 yr	Increasing risk with stage and score for alkylating agents
Jenkin et al,[141] 1996	Toronto	All: —/6/343	2%: 10 yr 4%: 20 yr	All leukemias observed in patients treated with CT for relapse
Sankila et al,[142] 1996	Cooperative, Scandinavian	All: —/7/1641	0.8%: 30 yr	
Schellong et al,[143] 1997	Cooperative, German/Austrian	CT ± RT: 1/4/667	0.7%: 10 yr 1.1%: 15 yr	Low risk attributed to CT without alkylating agents or low-dose Ctx
Wolden et al,[144] 1998	Stanford	RT: —/0/178 CT ± RT: —/8/308	— 1.5%: 20 yr	CT with alkylating agents Age and splenectomy not risk factors
van Leeuwen et al,[145] 2000	Amsterdam, Rotterdam	All: —/15/1253	3.3%: 20 yr	Patients up to 40 yr old included

ABVD, Adriamycin (doxorubicin), bleomycin, vinblastine, and dacarbazine; BCNU, carmustine; CALGB, Cancer and Leukemia Group B; CCNU, lomustine; Clb, chlorambucil; CT, chemotherapy; Ctx, Cytoxan (cyclopharmide); Me, mechlorethamine; MOPP, mechlorethamine, vincristine, procarbazine, procarbazine, and prednisone; NCI, National Cancer Institute; RT, radiotherapy; SWOG, Southwestern Oncology Group; t-AML, therapy-related acute myeloid leukemia; t-MDS, therapy-related myelodysplasia; VCR, vincristine; Vlb, vinblastine.

treatment of Hodgkin's disease with ABVD (doxorubicin, bleomycin, vinblastine, and dacarbazine), an alternative regimen to MOPP in which the two most potent leukemogenic agents, mechlorethamine and procarbazine, have been replaced by doxorubicin and dacarbazine.[123, 150, 151] However, the ABVD combination is associated with other severe complications, so it has not totally replaced MOPP in the treatment of Hodgkin's disease. The introduction of doxorubicin, a topoisomerase II inhibitor, in the new regimen is possibly also the reason for a change in the cytogenetic characteristics of t-AML after ABVD.[152-154] A reduced risk of t-MDS and t-AML has been observed in children with Hodgkin's disease if mechlorethamine is excluded from MOPP or is replaced by low-dose cyclophosphamide.[143]

For many years, the risk of new cases of t-MDS and t-AML after, for instance, treatment of Hodgkin's disease was suggested to continue over prolonged periods. In 1987, however, two independent studies demonstrated that such is not the case. A study from the U.S. National Cancer Institute (NCI) showed a peak incidence of leukemia 5 to 7 years from the start of six cycles of MOPP,[125] with no further risk after 11 years. Our study from Copenhagen showed the risk of leukemia to level out beyond 7 years after cessation of chemotherapy.[126]

Besides the many studies of the actuarial risk of t-MDS and t-AML in well-defined, but often smaller cohorts of patients treated for Hodgkin's disease, larger epidemiologic studies have examined risk factors by evaluating the relative risk (RR) of t-MDS and t-AML. In these studies, the number of observed cases of t-AML has been compared with the expected number of de novo AML cases in the same group of patients, or the number of cases of t-AML observed after two different types of therapy has been compared.[148, 151, 155-158] In three studies, the RR was 66.2, 136, and 27.4 in comparison to the general population.[155, 157, 158] In two other studies, the RR was 9.0 and 14 for chemotherapy versus radiotherapy.[148, 151] Therapy with alkylating agents and the intensity of therapy were significant risk factors, but radiotherapy did not increase the risk after chemotherapy.[148, 155]

In summary, therapy with six cycles of MOPP or alternative regimens seems to result in a risk of t-MDS and t-AML of 1.5% to 4% after 6 to 8 years. More intensive therapy for relapse of Hodgkin's disease after initial chemotherapy and older patient age both result in cumulative risks on the order of 6% to 15% after 8 to 10 years, with a continuously increasing risk because of the extended period of treatment. High-voltage radiotherapy administered together with chemotherapy seems not to increase the risk of t-MDS and t-AML significantly.

RISK OF t-MDS AND t-AML AFTER NON-HODGKIN'S LYMPHOMAS

At least nine studies have analyzed the cumulative risk of t-MDS and t-AML in patients treated for non-Hodgkin's lymphomas (Table 9-5). Therapy has varied markedly over time, but because only a few patients with the indolent lymphomas are cured by chemotherapy and these lymphomas often remain sensitive to chemotherapy for years, many patients have received long-time chemotherapy. High cumulative doses of alkylating agents and the older age of patients with non-Hodgkin's lymphomas than with Hodgkin's disease are probably the reasons for a high cumulative risk of t-MDS and t-AML.[160-163, 165] In the early studies, peroral chlorambucil or cyclophosphamide was often combined with vincristine (Oncovin) and prednisone in the COP combination. Subsequently, doxorubicin (hydroxydaunorubicin) was also included in the so-called CHOP regimen. Finally, many and very complex regimens came into use that included etoposide, bleomycin, methotrexate, and/or cytosine arabinoside in the combinations. These regimens did not result in major improvements in the prognosis of the primary disease or marked changes in the cumulative risk of t-MDS or t-AML. As in patients treated for Hodgkin's disease, the lowest risks in patients treated for non-Hodgkin's lymphomas were observed in two studies not reporting cases of t-MDS separately.[98, 164] The risk has also been analyzed by a case-control study[167] showing that prednimustine, mechlorethamine plus procarbazine, and high cumulative doses of chlorambucil were all significant risk factors. Therapy with cyclophosphamide and radiotherapy alone were both associated with a small nonsignificant risk of

TABLE 9–5. Risk of t-MDS and t-AML in Patients Treated for Non-Hodgkin's Lymphomas

Authors/Year	Institution	Type of Treatment	Cases of t-MDS/t-AML/ Treated	Cumulative Risk (%): Years from Start of Therapy; Relative Risk	Significant Risk Factors/ Remarks
Harousseau et al,[159] 1980	Paris	RT/Clb, MOPP, CHOP	3/2/210	4.5%: 5 yr 8.6%: 6 yr	—
Gomez et al,[160] 1982	Roswell Park	RT/BCNU + Me + Ctx + VCR + Pred	2/3/117	20%: 41 mo 38%: 55 mo	Intensive CT with 3 alkylating agents
Greene et al,[161] 1983	NCI, USA	RT alone: 3 cases RT + COP: 6 cases	7/2/517	RR: 105 7.9%: 10 yr	RT + CT, relapsing indolent lymphomas
Pedersen-Bjergaard et al,[162] 1985	Copenhagen	RT COP ± RT	0/0/56 8/1/546	RR: 76 6.3%: 7 yr	RT: no effect CT and retreated with CT Maintenance Ctx
Ingram et al,[163] 1987	Cooperative, England	Ctx + Dox + CCNU + Mtx + VCR + Pred + Ara C + RT	1/5/261	7.8%: 7 yr (2 solid tumors included)	Intensively treated children
Lavey et al,[98] 1990	Durham	COP/Bleo CHOP	—/9/686	4.5%: 10 yr	RT not a risk factor Age >40 yr Doxorubicin
Lishner et al,[164] 1991	Toronto	RT/COP/MOPP COPP/BACOP	—/8/3021	1.3%: 12 yr RR: 6.9	—
Sugita et al,[165] 1993	Tochigi-ken, Japan	CHOP + Etop + Mtx + Ara C	0/5/38	18.4%: 4 yr	Children treated intensively with Etop twice weekly. M5 with 11q rearr. in 4/5 Low-dose TBI + CT
Travis et al,[166] 1996	NCI, Dana Farber, MD Anderson	Low-dose TBI/alkylating agents	1/4/61	17%: 15 yr	

Ara C, cytosine arabinoside; BACOP, bleomycin, Adriamycin, cyclophosphamide, Oncovin (vincristine), and prednisone; BCNU, carmustine; Bleo, bleomycin; CCNU, lomustine; CHOP, cyclophosphamide, hydroxydaunorubicin (doxorubicin), Oncovin, and prednisone; Clb, chlorambucil; COP, cyclophosphamide, Oncovin, and prednisone; COPP, Cytoxan (cyclophosphamide), Oncovin, procarbazine, prednisone; Ctx, Cytoxan; Dox, doxorubicin; Etop, etoposide; Me, mechlorethamine; MOPP, mechlorethamine, Oncovin, procarbazine, and prednisone; Mtx, methotrexate; NCI, National Cancer Institute; Pred, prednisone; RT, radiotherapy, t-AML, therapy-related acute myeloid leukemia; TBI, total body irradiation; t-MDS, therapy-related myelodysplasia; VCR, vincristine.

leukemia. Low-dose total body irradiation, with or without alkylating agents, is not used any longer because it has turned out to be particularly leukemogenic.[166] Although t-MDS has also been reported after purine nucleoside therapy for chronic lymphocytic leukemia.[168] A recent and comprehensive study does not support these drugs to be leukemogenic.[169]

RISK OF t-MDS AND t-AML AFTER MULTIPLE MYELOMA AND WALDENSTRÖM'S MACROGLOBULINEMIA

Multiple myeloma and Waldenström's macroglobulinemia were associated early with a high risk of t-MDS and t-AML related to long-term therapy with alkylating agents, often administered as a single agent or combined with prednisone as reviewed.[81] The high risk was first firmly demonstrated by a major case-control study from the Mayo Clinic.[80] Subsequently, at least four independent studies have analyzed the cumulative risk of t-MDS and t-AML in patients treated for myeloma (Table 9-6). In the three largest studies, the risk varied between 9.2% and 20% from 4 to 10 years after the start of chemotherapy. As in patients treated for non-Hodgkin's lymphomas, these high risks most probably relate to high cumulative doses of alkylating agents combined with an advanced age of most patients with multiple myeloma. The risk of t-MDS and t-AML has been shown to increase with patient age up to 75 years,[170] and melphalan has been demonstrated to be more leukemogenic than cyclophosphamide.[87]

MDS has been diagnosed in a few patients at evaluation for multiple myeloma and before chemotherapy was administered.[172] In addition, a case of acute leukemia evolving from multiple myeloma and co-expressing myeloid and plasma cell antigens has been reported.[173] For these reasons, rare cases of MDS and AML observed early in the course of multiple myeloma may be unrelated to therapy.

RISK OF t-MDS AND t-AML AFTER POLYCYTHEMIA VERA AND ESSENTIAL THROMBOCYTHEMIA

Major problems are associated with estimates of the risk of t-MDS and t-AML after chemotherapy for polycythemia vera and essential thrombocythemia.[174] The reason is that AML is a part of the natural history of these diseases and is repeatedly observed in untreated patients or in patients with polycythemia treated by phlebotomy only. The frequency of leukemias in untreated patients has not been definitively established, probably because of variation in the selection of patients from study to study. Some patients with polycythemia vera and essential thrombocythemia require only observation, phlebotomy, or intermittent low-dose single-agent chemotherapy and may not be referred to a hematologic center. Other patients require permanent, sometimes intensive combination therapy to control the disease, and such patients subsequently may have received several drugs. It is in this particular subgroup of patients that a high risk of t-AML is observed, a risk that may partially be a result of the natural history of the disease and partially a result of intensive therapy. Polycythemia and thrombocythemia are not easy to study because they are less common diseases and cooperative studies are therefore required. As shown in Table 9-7, ^{32}P and chlorambucil have been shown to increase the risk of t-AML in polycythemia as compared with phlebotomy alone.[75] Likewise, hydroxyurea increased the risk of t-AML in patients with thrombocythemia versus those not receiving cytoreduction.[76] Different studies indicate that not only busulfan and chlorambucil are leukemogenic but also pipobroman and hydroxyurea, particularly in multidrug-treated patients. The fact that deletions of the short arm of chromosome 17 and mutations in p53 are common in t-MDS and t-AML after therapy with hydroxyurea and pipobroman[178, 179] supports a leukemogenic effect of these drugs, with a cumulative risk of approxi-

TABLE 9–6. Risk of t-MDS and t-AML in Patients Treated for Multiple Myeloma

Authors/Year	Institution	Type of Treatment	Cases of t-MDS/t-AML/ Treated	Cumulative Risk (%): Years from Start of Therapy; Relative Risk	Significant Risk Factors/ Remarks
Kyle et al,[80] 1970	Mayo Clinic	Melphalan	—/3/250	RR: 240	
Bergsagel et al,[170] 1979	Canada + USA, cooperative	Melphalan + Ctx + BCNU	10/14/364	17.4%: 50 mo Crude risk: 6%	Risk increasing with age up to 75 yr
Wahlin et al,[171] 1982	Umeå, Sweden	Melphalan	—/4/71	2.5%: 5 yr	All four patients initially in MDS phase
Kyle et al,[83] 1984	Mayo Clinic	Melphalan and/or BCNU and/or Ctx	8/19/928	9.2%: 10 yr 3%: 5 yr	
Cuzick et al,[87] 1987	MRC, England cooperative	Melphalan Ctx	9/3/648	10%: 8 yr 20%: 10 yr	Melphalan more leukemogenic than Ctx Risk related to cumulative dose of melphalan

BCNU, carmustine; Ctx, Cytoxan; MRC, Medical Research Council; t-AML, therapy-related acute myeloid leukemia; t-MDS, therapy-related myelodysplasia.

TABLE 9–7. Risk of t-AML after Chemotherapy for Polycythemia and Essential Thrombocythemia

Authors/Year	Institution	Primary Tumor	Type of Treatment	Cases of t-MDS/t-AML/ Treated	Cumulative Risk (%): Years from Start of Therapy	Significant Risk Factors/ Remarks
Berk et al,[75] 1981	P.V. Study Group	Polycythemia vera	Phlebotomy Clb ^{32}P	—/1/134 —/16/141 —/9/156	1%: 7 yr 17%: 7 yr 10%: 7 yr	Highest risk and dose-dependent risk for Clb
Brusamolino et al,[175] 1984	Pavia, Italy	Polycythemia vera	Pipo alone Pipo + Bu Pipo + ^{32}P	—/5/73 —/1/16 —/0/11	6%: 5 yr; 9%: 7 yr	
Najean et al,[176] 1997	Cooperative, France	Polycythemia vera	Pipo HU	4/9/292	10%: 13 yr	All patients <65 yr old Risk identical for Pipo and HU
Najean et al,[177] 1997	Cooperative, France	Polycythemia vera	^{32}P alone ^{32}P + HU (low dose)	20/15/461	12.4%: 10 yr 22.3%: 10 yr	All patients >65 yr old Addition of HU significantly increased the risk of MDS/AML
Sterkers et al,[178] 1998	Cooperative, France	Essential thrombocythemia	^{32}P alone Bu alone HU alone Pipo alone Combined	—/2/29 —/1/35 —/7/201 —/0/12 —/7/80		No difference between single drugs HU combined with other agents: high risk Chromosome 17p deletions characteristic
Finazzi et al,[76] 2000	Cooperative, Italy	Essential thrombocythemia	HU No cytoreduction	—/7/56 —/1/58		Intent-to-treat study, HU + Bu; highest risk: —/5/15

Bu, busulfan; Clb, chlorambucil; HU, hydroxyurea; Pipo, pipobroman; t-AML, therapy-related acute myeloid leukemia; t-MDS, therapy-related myelodysplasia.

mately 10% to 20% 7 to 13 years after the start of chemotherapy (see Table 9-7).

RISK OF t-AML AFTER ACUTE LYMPHOBLASTIC LEUKEMIA

The development of t-AML as a secondary malignancy in patients treated for ALL was first reported more than 20 years ago.[180] During the last 10 years, increased attention has been paid to this problem, particularly after the introduction of topoisomerase II inhibitors such as the epipodophyllotoxins and anthracyclines in combination with other drugs in the treatment of ALL. An increased risk of AML in children treated for ALL with combination chemotherapy that included the epipodophyllotoxins was primarily established by studies from St. Jude's Hospital.[94] The leukemias were often myelomonocytic or monocytic with abnormalities of the long arm of chromosome 11 and thereby different from previous cases observed after chemotherapy with alkylating agents. Two other independent studies and two follow-up studies from St. Jude's Hospital have all confirmed that etoposide and teniposide increase the risk of t-AML after therapy for ALL (Table 9-8). The administration of epipodophyllotoxins twice weekly and L-asparaginase immediately before etoposide has been shown to increase the risk of t-AML.[181, 183, 184, 186] Only a single study from the Dana

Farber Institute could not confirm these findings. The cumulative risk 4 to 6 years after the start of therapy was on the order of 3.5% to 5.5%, depending on the schedule for etoposide and preceding administration of L-asparaginase.[184, 186] The cytogenetic characteristics, specifically, a change in karyotype from abnormalities characteristic of ALL to quite different abnormalities characteristic of t-AML with balanced translocations to chromosome band 11q23 (see later), support the interpretation of the development of a new type of leukemia.

RISK OF t-MDS AND t-AML AFTER OVARIAN CANCER

Therapy for ovarian cancer has over the years included surgery, radiotherapy, and chemotherapy administered alone or in various combinations. Previously, much attention was paid to the development of t-MDS and t-AML after single-agent therapy with an alkylating agent for this type of tumor, and the risk and risk factors were analyzed in at least five major studies (Table 9-9). Unfortunately, two of them provided only estimates of RR.[187, 190]

In all studies, the risk of t-MDS and t-AML was exclusively related to therapy with alkylating agents, most often melphalan. In four of the studies, indications of a dose-response effect could be found, and in one study, melphalan was shown to be more leukemogenic than

TABLE 9–8. Risk of t-AML in Children Treated for Acute Lymphoblastic Leukemia

Authors/Year	Institution	Cases of MDS/AML/ Treated	Cumulative Risk (%): Years from Start of Therapy	Significant Risk Factors/Remarks
Pui et al,[156] 1991	St. Jude	—/21/735	3.8%: 6 yr	Prolonged administration of Etop or Teni twice weekly, 12.4%: 4 yr Only 4/21 initially had t-MDS
Neglia et al,[182] 1991	Children's Cancer Study Group	—/2/9720	—	—
Winick et al,[183] 1993	Dallas/Fort Worth	—/10/205	5.9%: 4 yr	Alkylating agents not used High cumulative dose of Etop: 9.9 g/m^2 Only 2/10 initially had t-MDS
Pul et al,[184] 1995	St. Jude	—/4/154	5.4%: 2 yr	L-Asparaginase administered immediately before Etop a risk factor
Dalton et al,[185] 1998	Dana Farber	—/3/1597	—	None of 3 cases of t-AML had received alkylating agents or Etop

Etop, etoposide; t-AML, therapy-related acute myeloid leukemia; Teni, teniposide; t-MDS, therapy-related myelodysplasia.

cyclophosphamide.[88] The cumulative risks 5 to 10 years after the start of long-term chemotherapy were rather high, in the range of 7.5% to 11%.

Subsequently, two major case-control studies have both confirmed the significance of various alkylating agents for the increase risk of t-MDS and t-AML observed in patients treated for ovarian cancer.[99, 191] More recently, the leukemogenic potential of current combination chemotherapy for ovarian cancer has been analyzed,[192-194] and platin derivatives have turned out to be equally leukemogenic as the classic alkylating agents.

RISK OF t-MDS AND t-AML AFTER BREAST CANCER

Breast cancer, because it is one of the most common chemotherapy-sensitive solid tumors, has been studied extensively for the risk of t-MDS and t-AML (Table 9–10). The cumulative risk has varied widely in these studies, probably reflecting major variations in the intensity of chemotherapy and the accuracy of follow-up with cytogenetic bone marrow investigation in all patients in whom refractory and unexplained cytopenia developed. Initially, single–alkylating agent chemotherapy predominated. Subsequently, the CMF regimen (cyclophosphamide, methotrexate, and 5-fluorouracil) and the CAF modification (with methotrexate replaced by Adriamycin [doxorubicin]) were used extensively. Most recently, combination chemotherapy that included platinum derivatives and topoisomerase II inhibitors, primarily 4-epidoxorubicin or mitoxantrone, have been administered.

Chemotherapy, often with rather low cumulative doses, has been administered in larger scale as adjuvant therapy to women potentially cured of breast cancer.

TABLE 9–9. Risk of t-MDS and t-AML in Patients Treated for Ovarian Cancer

Authors/Year	Institution	Type of Treatment	Cases of t-MDS/t-AML/ Treated	Cumulative Risk (%): Years from Start of Therapy; Relative Risk	Significant Risk Factors/ Remarks
Reimer et al,[187] 1977	Cooperative, USA	All types	—/13/5455	RR: 9.3 after 2 yr: RR: 66.7	Alkylating agents
Pedersen-Bjergaard et al,[188] 1980	Copenhagen	Dihydroxybusulfan ± RT	3/4/553	RR: 175 7.6%: 5 yr	Long-term peroral therapy Additional RT not a risk factor
Greene et al,[189] 1982	Cooperative, USA	RT only RT ± CT	—/0/308 0/2/993	0 8.3%–12.1%: 7 yr	Initial drug dose
Einhom et al,[190] 1982	Stockholm	Melphalan	—/6/51	RR: 950	High cumulative doses of melphalan
Greene et al,[88] 1986	Cooperative, USA	RT only CT ± RT	—/2/955 7/26/1718	RR: 93 8.5%: 10 yr	Melphalan: 11.2%, 10 yr Ctx: 5.4%, 10 yr No effect of RT Dose-response effect for alkylating agents

CT, chemotherapy; Ctx, Cytoxan; RT, radiotherapy; t-AML, therapy-related acute myeloid leukemia; t-MDS, therapy-related myelodysplasia.

TABLE 9–10. Risk of t-MDS and t-AML in Patients Treated for Breast Cancer

Authors/Year	Institution	Type of Treatment	Cases of t-MDS/t-AML/ Treated	Cumulative Risk (%): Years from Start of Therapy; Relative Risk	Significant Risk Factors/ Remarks
Fisher et al,[195] 1985	NSABP, cooperative	RT only Melphalan ± RT	—/5/646 7/27/5299	1.4%: 10 yr 1.7%: 10 yr	No cases observed >5 yr from cessation of therapy
Valagussa et al,[196] 1987	NCI, Milano	Ctx ± Mtx ± 5-FU	—/0/666	—	No risk observed
Falkson et al,[197] 1989	Pretoria + Wisconsin	Mitolactol	11/12/1460	Crude risk: 1.6%	Dose dependent
Andersson et al,[103] 1990	Copenhagen	Prednimustine + Mit + Mtx + 5-FU	3/2/71	RR: 339 25.4%: 37 mo	Heavily treated patients
Curtis et al,[198] 1990	SEER, cooperative	Surgery only CT ± RT	—/7/7974 —/24/13,734	RR: 11.5 0.7%: 10 yr	Melphalan higher risk than Ctx
Pedersen-Bjergaard et al,[101] 1992	Copenhagen	4-epi ± Cis	0/5/151	RR: 668 16.0%: 33 mo	Heavily treated patients 3/5 with 11q23 rearrangements
Valagussa et al,[199] 1994	NCI, Milano	Ctx + Mtx + 5-FU	—/3/2465	RR: 2.3 0.23%: 12 yr	Low-intensity therapy
Cremin et al,[104] 1996	Dublin	Mit + Mtx ± Mito	1/2/59	Crude risk: 5%	
Diamandidou et al,[200] 1996	M.D. Anderson	Ctx + Dox + 5-FU	—/2/664 —/12/810	0.5%: 10 yr 2.5%: 10 yr	RT a significant risk factor
Chaplain et al,[105] 2000	Cooperative, Côte d'Or	Ctx + Dox + 5-FU + RT RT only CT including Mit CT including anthracycline	—/2/1759 —/7/449 —/1/341	0.1%: 4 yr 2.2%: 4 yr 0.4%: 4 yr	Dose dependent for Mit

Cis, cisplatin; CT, chemotherapy; CTX, Cytoxan; Dox, doxorubicin; 4-epi, 4-epidoxorubicin; 5-FU, 5-fluorouracil; Mit, mitoxantrone; Mito, mitomycin; Mtx, methotrexate; NCI, National Cancer Institute; NSABP, National Surgical Adjuvant Breast and Bowel Project; RT, radiotherapy; SEER, Surveillance, Epidemiology, and End Results Program; t-AML, therapy-related acute myeloid leukemia; t-MDS, therapy-related myelodysplasia.

Most studies have concentrated on this type of therapy, which has resulted in a nondetectable risk of leukemia[196] or low cumulative risks (see Table 9–10). In one study, melphalan was more leukemogenic than cyclophosphamide and exhibited a dose-response effect.[198, 201] More intensive chemotherapy for metastatic breast cancer, often in smaller but closely monitored series of patients, has resulted in a higher risk than adjuvant therapy has,[197, 200, 203] sometimes a very high risk.[101, 103]

Of particular interest in two of the larger studies is a low but significant risk related to radiotherapy.[194, 199] A dose-dependent and high risk of t-MDS and t-AML has been observed for mitoxantrone versus the anthracyclines.[105] A characteristic spectrum of balanced chromosome aberrations has also been observed in patients with t-MDS or t-AML after chemotherapy for breast cancer with topoisomerase II inhibitors,[101, 200, 203, 204] as further discussed later.

RISK OF t-MDS AND t-AML AFTER TESTICULAR CANCER

The first studies reporting single cases of t-AML after chemotherapy for testicular cancer were published more than 15 years ago,[205, 206] but most studies of patients treated for testicular cancer have appeared during the last decade (Table 9–11). In this period, intensive combination chemotherapy for a shorter duration and with a high potential for cure has been administered. This progress has been possible by introducing platinum derivatives and etoposide in combination with other drugs. When compared with the rather high cumulative risk of t-MDS and t-AML in patients receiving long-term chemotherapy for other diseases, the rather low risk observed after chemotherapy for testicular cancer possibly reflects the shorter duration of treatment and a low age of the patients. Two series[208, 209, 211, 214] observed a cumulative risk below 1%. In the remaining five series, cumulative risks of between 1% and 4.7% from 4 to 10 years after the start of treatment were observed. The reports of some cases of therapy-related ALL in these series are of interest.[215, 216] The results of the cohort studies have been confirmed by a major case-control study.[217] The important question, to what extent the cumulative dose of etoposide is of significance for the risk, is still not solved. Some studies have demonstrated a significantly higher risk of t-MDS and t-AML after a cumulative dose above 2 g/m^2,[210] analogous to the experience with alkylating agents. Other studies, however, have not been able to confirm these findings. A recent review of therapy-related malignancies after the treatment of germ cell tumors concluded that cumulative doses of etoposide above 2 g/m^2 administered at weekly intervals resulted in a higher risk of t-AML than did doses below 2 g/m^2 administered at longer intervals, thus suggesting that the frequency of administration may be more important for the risk than the dose.[214, 218] How-

TABLE 9–11. Risk of t-MDS and t-AML in Patients Treated for Testicular Cancer

Authors/Year	Institution	Type of Treatment	Cases of t-MDS/t-AML/ Treated	Cumulative Risk (%): Years from Start of Therapy; Relative Risk	Significant Risk Factors/ Remarks
Redman et al,[207] 1984	Solan-Kettering	RT only CT	0/1/132 1/2/376	RR: 7.1 RR: 50.1 1.8%: 5 yr	Combination CT including Ctx, Clb, and actinomycin-D
Pedersen-Bjergaard et al,[95] 1991	Copenhagen	Etop + Cis + Bleo	1/4/212	RR: 336	All received Etop, >2 g/m²
		Cis + VLB + Bleo	0/0/127	4.7%: 5.7 yr	Balanced transloc to 11q23 or 21q22: 3/5
Nichols et al,[208] 1993	Indiana	Etop + Cis + VLB + Bleo or Etop + Cis + Ifos	0/2/538	Crude risk: 0.4%	All received Etop, <2 g/m²
Bokemeyer et al,[209] 1993	Hanover, Germany	RT: 332 CT ± RT: 462	0/0/332 0/1*/462	Not provided	CT included Cis with or without Etop
Boshoff et al,[210] 1995	London	Ct including Etop and platinum derivatives	—/6/679	RR: 150 Crude risk: 1%	Only 25 patients received Etop, >2 g/m²; leukemia developed in 2 (significant)
Bokemeyer et al,[211] 1995b	Hanover, Germany	CT including Etop, >2 g/m², and Cis	0/1/128	0.8%: 4.5 yr	—
Kollmannsberger et al,[212] 1998	Cooperative, Germany	CT including Cis and Etop, >2 g/m², + ASCT	1/5/302	RR: 160 2%: 52 mo	—
Schneider et al,[213] 1999	Cooperative, Germany-Austria	Surgery only RT only CT only, VLB CT + RT	0/392 0/124 3/442 3/174	0 0 1.0%: 10 yr 4.2%: 10 yr	—

* Acute lymphoblastic leukemia.
ASCT, autologous stem-cell transplantation; Bleo, bleomycin; Cis, cisplatin; Clb, chlorambucil; CT, chemotherapy; Ctx, Cytoxan; Etop, etoposide; Ifos, ifosfamide; RT, radiotherapy; t-AML, therapy-related acute myeloid leukemia; t-MDS, therapy-related myelodysplasia; VCR, vincristine; VLB, vinblastine.

TABLE 9–12. Risk of t-MDS and t-AML in Adult Patients Treated for Various Solid Tumors

Authors/Year	Institution	Primary Tumor	Type of Treatment	Cases of t-MDS/t-AML/ Treated	Cumulative Risk (%): Years from Start of Therapy; Relative Risk	Significant Risk Factors/ Remarks
Stott et al,[89] 1977	London	Lung cancer	Busulfan Ctx	—/4/243 —/0/234	Crude risk: 1.6% 0	
Boice et al,[219] 1983	Cooperative, USA	Gastrointestinal cancer	Me-CCNU	7/8/3633	RR: 12.4 4.0%: 6 yr	Age and additional RT were not risk factors
Chak et al,[220] 1984	Stanford	Small-cell lung cancer	RT + Ctx + CCNU + Etop + Dox + Pro + Mtx + VCR	1/2/158	RR: 316 25%: 3.1 yr	Very intensive combination CT
Pedersen-Bjergaard et al,[221] 1985	Copenhagen	Small-cell lung cancer	Ctx + CCNU + Etop + Dox	4/2/796	RR: 77 14.0%: 4 yr	Very intensive combination CT
Ratain et al,[93] 1987	Chicago	Non–small-cell lung cancer	Etop + Cis + VDS	0/4/119	15%: 2 yr 44%: 2.5 yr	High-dose Etop
Rustin et al,[222] 1996	London	Gestational trophoblastic tumors	CT including Etop	0/4/372	RR: 64.8	Three out of 4 AML's cumulative dose of Etop, > 2.0 g/m²

CCNU, lomustine; Cis, cisplatin; CT, chemotherapy; Ctx, Cytoxan; Dox, doxorubicin; Etop, etoposide; Ifos, ifosfamide; Me-CCNU, semustine; Mtx, methotrexate; Pro, procarbazine; RT, radiotherapy; t-AML, therapy-related acute myeloid leukemia; t-MDS, therapy-related myelodysplasia; VCR, vincristine.

ever, other factors were also considered to play a role. A complete lack of a dose-response effect in leukemogenesis for the epipodophyllotoxins would be unique in chemical carcinogenesis. The experience from both testicular cancer and ovarian cancer indicates that both cisplatin and etoposide contribute to the increased risk of t-MDS and t-AML observed after therapy with the two drugs in combination.

RISK OF t-MDS AND t-AML AFTER OTHER SOLID TUMORS IN ADULTS

Cohorts of patients treated for other solid tumors with chemotherapy have also been evaluated for the risk of t-MDS and t-AML (Table 9–12). Four studies have focused on lung cancer, one study on gastrointestinal cancer, and one study on gestational trophoblastic tumors. A randomized study of patients resected for bronchial carcinoma observed 4 cases of leukemia in 243 patients treated with busulfan as single-agent chemotherapy versus no leukemias in 234 patients treated with cyclophosphamide.[89] Subsequently, three other studies demonstrated an extremely high cumulative risk of t-MDS and t-AML after intensive, prolonged combination chemotherapy for lung cancer, including etoposide, alkylating agents, or cisplatin in various drug combinations.[93, 220, 221]

Semustine was evaluated in an analysis of 3633 patients treated in nine randomized clinical trials for gastrointestinal cancer. A 6-year cumulative risk of 4.0% for t-MDS and t-AML was observed.[219] A subsequent analysis of the same cohort of patients demonstrated the risk of leukemia to increase significantly with an increasing cumulative dose of semustine.[223]

Finally, in 372 women treated with chemotherapy including etoposide at Charing Cross Hospital, London, for gestational trophoblastic tumors, leukemia developed in 5 patients, 3 of whom had the balanced translocations t(9;11), t(8;21), and t(9;22).[222] The relative risk of leukemia in this study was 64.8; unfortunately, the cumulative risk was not provided.

The rather uniform cumulative risk curves for adult patients treated intensively for different malignancies with an identical follow-up at our institution are shown in Figure 9–1. The very high risk estimates and the very short latency period in patients treated intensively for metastatic breast cancer and small-cell lung cancer with topoisomerase II inhibitors are remarkable.

RISK OF t-MDS AND t-AML AFTER CHILDHOOD SOLID TUMORS

Much attention has been paid to cases of t-MDS and t-AML developing after therapy for childhood solid tumors[224] (Table 9–13). Rather low cumulative risks of t-MDS and t-AML have been observed in children treated for Hodgkin's disease and non-Hodgkin's lymphomas as compared with adults (see also Tables 9-4, 9-5, and 9-11). The high cumulative risk observed in some studies of childhood solid tumors possibly relates to very intensive administration of topoisomerase II inhibitors. The highest risk was observed in a report from Sloan-Kettering, which included patients up to 40 years of age. A regimen including two alkylating agents, cyclophosphamide and ifosfamide, and two topoisomerase II inhibitors, doxorubicin and etoposide, resulted in a cumulative risk of 8.0% at 40 months.[227] Age older than 12 years was a significant risk factor in one of the studies,[225] and in another study, a dose-response effect was observed for the epipodophyllotoxins.[226]

Two findings in studies of solid tumors in childhood are of particular interest. The first is the consistent observation that cumulative doses of etoposide below 2 g/m² may also result in the subsequent development of leuke-

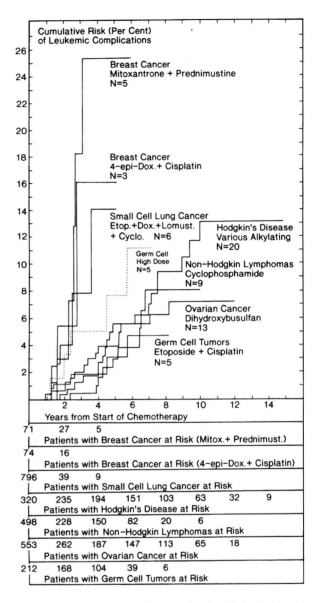

FIGURE 9–1. Cumulative risk of therapy-related myelodysplasia and acute myeloid leukemia in seven cohorts of patients treated for six different types of primary tumor (Kaplan-Meier estimates). Cyclo, cyclophosphamide; Dox, doxorubicin; 4-epi-Dox, 4-epidoxorubicin; Etop, etoposide; Lomust, lomustine; Mitox, mitoxantrone. (From Pedersen-Bjergaard J, Philip P, Larsen SO, et al: Leukemia 1993;7:1975.)

TABLE 9–13. Risk of t-MDS and t-AML in Patients Treated for Childhood Cancer

Authors/Year	Institution	Primary Tumor	Type of Treatment	Cases of t-MDS/t-AML/ Treated	Cumulative Risk (%): Years from Start of Therapy	Significant Risk Factors/ Remarks
Pui et al,[225] 1990	St. Jude	Hodgkin's	Not specified	1/5/447	1.3%: 10 yr	Treatment for relapse age >12 yr, and combined RT-CT all risk factors
		Non-Hodgkin's	—	1/2/420	1.3%: 10 yr	5/10 patients had balanced translocations, 2/10 patients had –7
		Neuroblastoma	—	0/3/440	1.2%: 10 yr	
Hawkins et al,[226] 1992	Cooperative, England	ALL	Not specified	—/4/4671	0.1%: 5 yr	Increasing risk with increasing exposure to alkylating agents, epipodophyllotoxins, and RT
		Hodgkin's	—	—/2/1046	0.2%: 5 yr	
		Non-Hodgkin's	—	—/6/699	1.4%: 5 yr	
		Astrocytoma	—	—/4/2258	0.2%: 5 yr	
		Neuroblastoma	—	—/1/712	0.2%: 5 yr	
Kushner et al,[227] 1998	Sloan-Kettering	Solid tumors	Ctx + Dox + VCR + Ifos + Etop + RT	2/3/86	8.0%: 40 mo	Patients up to 40 yr old included in the study
Smith et al,[97] 1999	CTEP,NCI, USA	Rhabdomyosarcoma	Combination CT			
		Medulloblastoma	Etop <1.5 g/m²	4/4/451	3.3%: 6 yr	No effect of cumulative dose of Etop
		Neuroblastoma	Etop 1.5–3.0 g/m²	4/2/1270	0.7%: 6 yr	
		Germ-cell tumors	Etop >3.0 g/m²	2/3/570	2.2%: 6 yr	
		ALL				
		Ewing's sarcoma				

CT, chemotherapy; CTEP, Cancer Therapy Evaluation Program; Ctx, Cytoxan; Dox, doxorubicin; Etop, etoposide; Ifos, ifosfamide; NCI, National Cancer Institute; RT, radiotherapy; t-AML, therapy-related acute myeloid leukemia; t-MDS, therapy-related myelodysplasia; VCR, vincristine.

mia.[213, 228] In fact, the Cancer Therapy Evaluation Program of the NCI observed the highest cumulative risk of t-MDS and t-AML in patients receiving a cumulative dose of etoposide below 1.5 g/m².[97] The study concluded, as demonstrated before,[181, 184, 186] that "factors other than epipodophyllotoxin cumulative dose seem to be of primary importance in determining the risk of secondary leukemia." The second finding of importance is the many cases of t-MDS and t-AML with recurrent balanced chromosome aberrations.[213, 225, 227, 228] This interesting phenomenon will be discussed in more detail later.

RISK OF t-MDS AND t-AML AFTER HIGH-DOSE CHEMOTHERAPY AND AUTOLOGOUS STEM-CELL TRANSPLANTATION

High-dose chemotherapy followed by autologous stem-cell transplantation as rescue has become widely used in the treatment of chemosensitive malignancies with a poor prognosis. A particularly high risk of t-MDS and t-AML has been observed after this type of therapy, as reviewed.[229–231] At least 18 studies have analyzed this problem (Table 9–14). Most patients had been treated intensively with alkylating agents or topoisomerase II inhibitors for malignant lymphoma before transplantation. This primary therapy has repeatedly been demonstrated to be the most important risk factor. In addition, the risk of t-MDS and t-AML has been demonstrated to increase with age.[233, 236, 237, 242, 243, 247] Furthermore, the transplantation procedure seems to play a role, though less markedly, in the risk of t-MDS and t-AML. First, the use of stem cells isolated from peripheral blood after chemotherapy

priming has been demonstrated to result in a higher cumulative risk of t-MDS and t-AML than has transplantation with stem cells isolated from the bone marrow without priming.[232, 233, 235, 248] Second, the use of whole-body irradiation in the preparative regimen for transplantation[236, 242] and the use of stem cell priming with etoposide[244] have both been demonstrated to result in a higher risk for leukemic complications. The predominant effect of chemotherapy administered before transplantation has recently been confirmed by a British cooperative study of patients treated for Hodgkin's disease.[149] In this study, patients treated with high-dose chemotherapy followed by autologous stem-cell transplantation were not at a significantly higher risk of t-MDS and t-AML than were patients with Hodgkin's disease treated conventionally without transplantation, if the intensity of previous chemotherapy was taken into consideration.

BONE MARROW PATHOLOGY OF t-MDS AND t-AML

The bone marrow pathology of t-MDS and t-AML has not been shown to differ markedly and can be classified in the same way as the pathology in de novo MDS and AML, as discussed elsewhere in this book. In t-AML, as in de novo AML, some characteristic associations can be noted between specific balanced chromosome aberrations and specific French-American-British (FAB) subtypes. Whereas in de novo MDS bone marrow pathology is in most cases diagnostic, hypoplasia and fibrosis are often prominent findings in t-MDS, for which reason dysplastic features may be difficult to identify. In addition, dysplastic changes

TABLE 9–14. Risk of MDS and AML after Autologous Stem-Cell Transplantation Results from the Literature

Authors/Year/ Institution	Primary Tumor	Cases of t-MDS/ t-MDS/ Number Treated	Cumulative Risk (%): Years from Start of Therapy; Relative Risk	Significant Risk Factors and Remarks	Cytogenetics Provided
Miller et al,[232] 1994, Minnesota	Hodgkin's Non-Hodgkin's	3/0/68 3/1/138	14.5%: 4 yr	PBSC/BMSC: 31% vs. 10.5%; P = 0.0035	Yes
Bhatia et al,[233] 1996 (follow-up)	Hodgkin's Non-Hodgkin's	9/1/258	13.5%: 6 yr	PBSC/BMSC; P = .004 Age >35 yr; P = .07	No
Traweek et al,[234] 1994, City of Hope	Hodgkin's Non-Hodgkin's	2/2/108 5/1/167	9%: 3 yr	5 patients with chromosome aberrations; no signs of MDS	Yes
Krishnan et al,[235] 1998 (follow-up)	Hodgkin's Non-Hodgkin's	24/612*	9.4%: 9 yr	PBSC/BMSC; P = .05 Topo II inhibitors — 11q23/21q22 transloc.	Yes
Darrington et al,[236] 1994, Nebraska	Hodgkin's Non-Hodgkin's	4/2/249 6/0/262	4%: 5 yr	Age ≥40 yr; P = .05 TBI; P = .06	Yes
Stone et al,[237] 1994, Dana Farber	Non-Hodgkin's	18/2/262	18%: 6 yr	Prolonged interval from diagnosis to ASCT; P = .003 Duration of previous CT; P = .019 Radiation of therapy; P = .032 Pelvic irradiation; P = .003 Age >38 yr and low platelet counts	Yes
Friedberg et al,[238] 1999 (follow-up)	Non-Hodgkin's	41/0/552	19.8%: 10 yr	Fewer no. of cells reinfused; P = .0003	Yes
Wheeler et al,[239] 1997, Dana Faber	Hodgkin's Non-Hodgkin's	6/300*	4.2%: 5 yr	Previous relapses; P = .009 Previous radiotherapy; P = .05	No
Taylor et al,[240] 1997, Newcastle	Hodgkin's Non-Hodgkin's	0/1/52 0/0/62	1.1%: 20 mo (+1 CML)	60% transplant. in 1st CR	Yes
Pedersen-Bjergaard et al,[241] 1997, Copenhagen	Hodgkin's Non-Hodgkin's	1/1/27 3/1/49	24.3%: 43 mo RR: 357	Multitreated Antecedent CT risk factor	Yes
Harrison et al,[149] 1999, British Cooperative	Hodgkin's	8/595*	1.9%: 10 yr 9.0%: 20 yr (3.1%: 5 yr after ASCT)	Quantity of previous therapy; P = .0001 MOPP; P = .0009 Lomustine; P = .001 Transplant versus non-transplant; P = .25	No
Milligan et al,[242] 1999, EBMT Cooperative	Hodgkin's Non-Hodgkin's	51/15/4998	4.6%: 5 yr 3.0%: 5 yr	Age at transplantation; P <.001 TBI at conditioning; P <.001 Number of transplants; P <.002 Years from diagnosis to transplantation; P <.001	No
Micallef et al,[243] 2000, London	Non-Hodgkin's	16/11/230	14.2%: 5 yr 36.5%: 10 yr	Previous fludarabine therapy; P = .009 Age at transplantation; P = .02 Interval from diagnosis to transplantation; P = .05	Yes
Krishnan et al,[244] 2000, City of Hope	Hodgkin's Non-Hodgkin's	16/6/612	8.6%: 6 yr	Stem-cell priming with Etop; P = .002 Etop related to 11q23 and 21q22 translocations	Yes
Govindarajan et al,[245] 1996, Little Rock, AK	Multiple myeloma (tandem transpl.)	0/0/71† 7/0/117‡	0% 12%: 4 yr	ASCT in 1st CR versus ASCT in multitreated; P = .02	Yes
Laughlin et al,[246] 1998, Duke University	Breast cancer	3/2/864§	1.6%: 4 yr		Yes
Kollmannsberger et al,[214] 1998, German/French Cooperative	Germ-cell tumors (advanced stage)	2/4/302	1.3%: 52 mo‖ RR: 160	Previous Etop, >2.4 g/m², + Cis + Ifos/Ctx	Yes

* Denotes no discrimination between t-MDS and t-AML.
† Previously received only one cycle of CT.
‡ Previously received more than one cycle of CT.
§ One case of acute lymphoblastic leukemia with t(1;11) included.
‖ Only four cases of overt AML are included, whereas 2 cases of MDS are excluded in the calculation.

ASCT, autologous stem-cell transplantation; BMSC, bone marrow stem cells; Cis, cisplatin; CML, chronic myeloid leukemia; CR, complete remission; CT, chemotherapy; Ctx, Cytoxan; EBMT, European Bone Marrow Transplant Registry; Etop, etoposide; Ifos, ifosfamide; MOPP, mechlorethamine, Oncovin (vincristine), procarbazine, and prednisone; PBSC, peripheral blood stem cells; t-AML, therapy-related acute myeloid leukemia; TBI, total body irradiation; t-MDS, therapy-related myelodysplasia; Topo, topoisomerase.

are sometimes observed during bone marrow recovery after intensive chemotherapy. As a result of these problems, much attention has been paid to cytogenetic abnormalities in the diagnosis of t-MDS, particularly because clonal chromosome aberrations are observed in approximately 90% of these patients.

CHROMOSOME ABNORMALITIES OF t-MDS AND t-AML AFTER ALKYLATING AGENTS

Although previously studied,[249] characteristic, clonal chromosome aberrations of t-MDS and t-AML were first demonstrated by Dr. Rowley and colleagues in 1977.[250] Eight of 10 patients with t-AML after radiotherapy and alkylating agents showed loss of a whole chromosome 5, and in 5 patients, a chromosome 7 was missing. The karyotypes were often complex, with many unidentified marker chromosomes and loss of chromosome material. These characteristics, as well as deletions of various parts or loss of the long arms of chromosomes 5 and 7, were subsequently confirmed as being highly characteristic of t-MDS and t-AML after therapy with alkylating agents.[251, 252] Eight subsequent studies demonstrated abnormalities of chromosomes 5 and 7 in approximately 70% of cases of t-MDS and t-AML and a normal karyotype in only 17%[253-260] (Table 9–15). The recurrent balanced chromosome aberrations frequently observed in de novo AML were seen rarely (4%) in these early studies, as previously reviewed.[261] Cases of t-AML with balanced translocations were considered by many investigators at that time to be incidental cases of de novo AML. Deletions or loss of 5q and 7q and monosomy 7 have subsequently been significantly related to manifestation of the disease as t-MDS, whereas monosomy 5 is observed equally often in t-MDS and overt t-AML.[262, 263]

Other unbalanced chromosome aberrations frequently observed in studies of t-MDS and t-AML include gain of a whole chromosome 8 and gain of the long arm of chromosome 1, deletions or loss of the short arm of chromosome 17, and loss of a whole chromosome 18, as demonstrated by our series of patients from Copenhagen[264] (Fig. 9–2). Deletions or loss of 12p and abnormalities of chromosome 3 have also been observed as recurrent abnormalities in t-MDS and t-AML. Because alkylating agents have been shown in vitro to induce chromosome damage in human lymphocytes that is the same type as observed in t-MDS and t-AML,[265] the chromosome aberrations in these diseases have been thought to be induced directly by the cytostatic drugs.

THE MOLECULAR BIOLOGY OF t-MDS AND t-AML AFTER ALKYLATING AGENTS

Despite much research, as discussed elsewhere in this book, the specific genetic abnormalities of MDS and AML directly cooperating with the cytogenetic defects of the long arms of chromosomes 5 and 7 in leukemogenesis still remain to be determined. More than one recurrently deleted chromosome region, the so-called critical regions, has been delineated on the long arm of chromosome 5[266-269] and on the long arm of chromosome 7.[270, 271] This finding indicates the possibility of mutations or other types of inactivation of more than one recessive gene on the long arm of the homologous, normal chromosome. Recently, the molecular biology of t-MDS and t-AML with deletions or loss of 5q was shown to differ markedly from that of t-MDS and t-AML with deletions or loss of 7q but normal chromosome 5. Whereas mutations of *p53* are rather rare in de novo AML,[272, 273] they are more common in t-AML.[274, 295] In t-MDS and t-AML, mutations of *p53* are closely associated with previous therapy with alkylating agents; with deletions or loss of 5q, they predict a very poor prognosis.[275] As in de novo AML,[276] the close association between *p53* mutations and abnormalities of chro-

TABLE 9–15. Cytogenetics in Larger Series of Patients with t-MDS and t-AML Published until 1989

Authors/Institution/Year	N Studied	−7 or del7q	−5 or del5q	Normal	Balanced Aberrations
French Collab,[253] 1984	55	27	19	6	1: t(15;17) 1: t(11;19)
Kantarjian et al,[255] 1986, M.D. Anderson	103	45		19	3: t(8;21) 1: t(15;17) 1: inv(16)
Le Beau et al,[254] 1986, Chicago	63	41	31	2	2: t(15;17)
Pedersen-Bjergaard et al,[256] 1987, Copenhagen	61	37	18	13	1: t(8;21) 1: t(9;22)
Zaccaria et al,[257] 1987, Europ. Cooperative	69	32	19	6	1: t(8;21) 1: t(15;17)
Whang-Peng et al,[258] 1988, NCI, USA	66	19	10	14	4: t(9;22) 2: inv(16) 1: t(15;17)
Arthur et al,[260] 1989, 6th Int. Workshop	55	26		16	2: t(15;17)
Iurlo et al,[259] 1989, Belgium + Italy	76	24	26	18	No cases
Total	548	180 (46%)	123 (32%)	94 (17%)	22* (4%)

* Five of 13 of these patients had received topoisomerase II inhibitors and another 5 patients only radiotherapy.
NCI, National Cancer Institute; t-AML, therapy-related acute myeloid leukemia; t-MDS, therapy-related myelodysplasia.

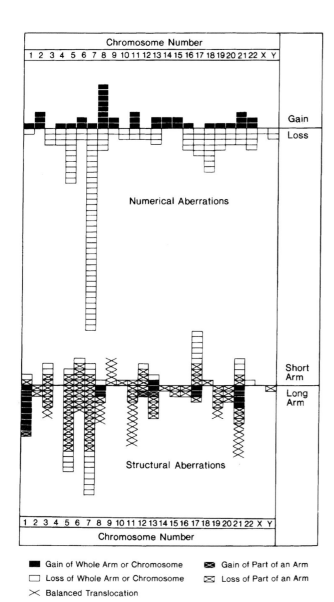

FIGURE 9–2. Chromosome aberrations in 115 consecutive cases of therapy-related myelodysplasia and acute myeloid leukemia. Only 17 patients presented a normal karyotype. (From Pedersen-Bjergaard J, Philip P, Larsen SO, et al: Leukemia 1993;7:1975.)

mosome 5 in t-MDS and t-AML suggests cooperation between deleted genes on 5q and mutations of *p53*, analogous to observations in some solid tumors.[277–279] Moreover, in patients with t-MDS and t-AML, an abnormal chromosome 5 and mutation of *p53* often present very complex karyotypes, with duplication or amplification of chromosome band 11q23, including the unrearranged *MLL* gene.[280] This observation is of interest because gene amplification, abnormal chromosome segregation, and chromosome instability have been experimentally associated with loss of function of *p53*. Patients with t-MDS and t-AML and deletions or loss of 7q but a normal chromosome 5, on the other hand, rarely have mutations of *p53*,[275] and they often show mutations of *RAS* genes[281, 282] and methylation of *p15* (Christiansen, personal communication).

CHROMOSOME ABNORMALITIES OF t-MDS AND t-AML AFTER TOPOISOMERASE II INHIBITORS

The first studies demonstrating that the epipodophyllotoxins are leukemogenic showed an excess of abnormalities of chromosome 11 in patients with t-AML after such therapy.[93, 94] This finding was subsequently confirmed in three single-institution studies of unselected cases of t-MDS and t-AML,[283–285] and in a multicenter study,[286] all demonstrating that only the balanced translocations to chromosome band 11q23 were associated with previous therapy with epipodophyllotoxins as well as with other topoisomerase II inhibitors such as the anthracyclines and mitoxantrone. Two of these studies also showed a significant association between previous therapy with the same drugs and t-AML with balanced translocations to chromosome band 21q22.[284, 285] The combined results of these two studies are shown in Table 9–16. Subsequent reviews suggested that other recurrent balanced chromosome aberrations, mainly observed in de novo AML, could also be characteristic of t-MDS and t-AML after therapy with topoisomerase II inhibitors.[287, 288] A 1998 review of the literature identified 422 cases of t-MDS and t-AML with balanced translocations and confirmed the hypothesis, inasmuch as patients with inv(16), t(15;17), and t(9;22) had also frequently been treated with topoisomerase II inhibitors.[280] An association with previous topoisomerase II inhibitor therapy has been discussed separately for t-MDS and t-AML with inv(16),[290, 291] t(15;17),[292–294] and t(9;22).[295]

An increasing number of cases of therapy-related ALL, primarily with t(4;11)(q21;q23), has been observed, all after previous treatment with topoisomerase II inhibitors.[106, 295, 296] This observation implies that such cases should also be included in calculations of the risk of therapy-related leukemia.

The changing pattern of chromosome abnormalities in adult patients with t-MDS and t-AML after the increased use of topoisomerase II inhibitors, from unbalanced aberrations of chromosomes 5 and 7 to the recurrent balanced aberrations, can be illustrated by two recently published studies from France.[203, 204] These two studies include a total of 20 cases of t-MDS or t-AML after breast cancer, mainly treated with mitoxantrone (Table 9–17). Only 1 of these 20 patients had defects of chromosomes 5 and 7, whereas 13 patients had various recurrent balanced chromosome aberrations.

Balanced translocations more specifically observed in t-MDS or t-AML after therapy with topoisomerase II inhibitors include t(3;21)(q26;q22), which is significantly associated with manifestation of the disease as t-MDS,[297, 298] t(16;21)(q24;q22),[299] t(8;16)(p11;p13),[290, 300] and various balanced translocations involving chromosome band 11p15 with involvement of the *NUP98* gene.[301, 302] The t(11;16)(q23;p13) translocation with chimeric rearrangement between the *MLL* and the *CBP* genes has thus far been observed predominantly in therapy-related disease.[303]

THE MOLECULAR BIOLOGY OF t-MDS AND t-AML AFTER TOPOISOMERASE II INHIBITORS

The molecular biology of de novo MDS and AML with the recurrent balanced chromosome aberrations, primar-

TABLE 9–16. Balanced Translocations to Chromosome Bands 11q23 and 21q22 in t-MDS and t-AML

	Topo II Inhib only	Topo II Inhib + AA	AA only	Other Treatment	Total
Balanced 11q23	4	6	1	0	11
Balanced 21q22	2	7	1	0	10
Unbalanced 11q23 or 21q22	0	4	10	2	16
Total patients	12	69	112	30	223

Balanced translocations to chromosome bands 11q23 and 21q22 were observed in 19 of 81 patients previously treated with topoisomerase II inhibitors (Topo II Inhib) with or without alkylating agents (AA) as compared with 2 of 142 patients treated with alkylating agents or other types of cytotoxic therapy, $P < .000001$, χ^2 test.
t-AML, therapy-related acute myeloid leukemia; t-MDS, therapy-related myelodysplasia.
Data from[284, 285].

ily the reciprocal translocations, has been studied extensively as discussed elsewhere in this book and reviewed previously.[304-306] These chromosome abnormalities often result in chimeric rearrangement between important regulatory genes and alternative partner genes (Fig. 9–3). The new fusion genes have in many cases been shown to experimentally induce leukemia in mice if transfected to bone marrow progenitors with an appropriate promotor. Whereas the origin of the balanced chromosome aberrations in de novo MDS and AML is completely unknown, the association with previous topoisomerase II inhibitor therapy in t-MDS and t-AML has inspired extensive research.[307-309]

The biologic effects of the enzyme topoisomerase II, as well as the effects of its inhibition by cytostatic drugs, in many ways support the fact that the characteristic balanced chromosome aberrations can be directly drug induced. Topoisomerase II induces transient 4–base pair-staggered double-stranded breaks of DNA for strand passage and unwinding. Many cytostatic drugs belonging to the topoisomerase II inhibitor group inhibit religation of these breaks, an effect that may subsequently result in apoptosis. Inhibition of DNA religation has been suggested to in some way facilitate illegitimate crossover recombination between two adjacent chromosomes.

Topoisomerase II preferentially localizes to the chromosomal scaffold.[310, 311] Experimentally, the enzyme interacts in particular with DNA crossovers.[312] The introduction of two DNA double-stranded breaks has been shown to provide a potent initiator of translocations,[313] and illegitimate recombinations have been linked to matrix associa-

TABLE 9–17. Cytogenetics in 20 Patients with t-MDS and t-AML after Chemotherapy, Mainly Mitoxantrone, for Breast Cancer

Finding	N
Normal karyotype	2
– 5, del5q, – 7, del7q	1
Balanced translocations to 11q23	4
Balanced translocations to 21q22	1
t(15;17)	5
inv(16)	3
Others or not evaluable	4
Total	20

t-AML, therapy-related acute myeloid leukemia; t-MDS, therapy-related myelodysplasia.
Data from[203, 204].

tion regions and to topoisomerase II.[314] Etoposide has been shown to induce illegitimate gene recombinations.[315]

The *MLL* gene at 11q23 is often chimerically rearranged in de novo AML, and it is the most frequently rearranged gene in t-AML. For this reason, its breakpoints have been studied in detail in both diseases. The breakpoints are clustered within a 8.3-kb BCR encompassing exons 5 to 11.[316, 317] In t-AML, the breakpoints have been shown to cluster at the telomeric part of the BCR region containing a high-affinity scaffold attachment region and several topoisomerase II consensus sites.[51-53, 318] In de novo AML, on the other hand, the breakpoints have been shown to cluster at the centromeric part of the BCR containing several Alu repeat sequences. Experimentally, topoisomerase II inhibitors have been shown to preferentially induce DNA breakage near the translocation breakpoints of the BCR.[319-321] In vivo, a topoisomerase II cleavage site colocalizes with a DNase I hypersensitive site near exon 9 in the BCR,[322] and it was suggested that the chromatin structure of the BCR could play a role in localization of the breakpoints within *MLL*.

Quite recently, the apoptotic process, induced not only by cytostatic agents but also by other chemicals, has been implicated in the development of rearrangements of the *MLL* gene. Several apoptosis-promoting chemicals have been shown to induce breakage at a site 3′ of the BCR.[323] Translocations involving *MLL* have been demonstrated at the molecular level in cells that evade apoptotic execution and survive, possibly related to the nonhomologous end-joining repair system.[324] The translocational rearrangements of the *MLL* gene thus seem to be complicated; many biologic mechanisms may be involved, and they may differ between t-AML and de novo AML.

The molecular biology of t-MDS and t-AML with the other recurrent balanced translocations has not been studied to the same extent. In t-AML and de novo AML with various balanced translocations to 21q22, the breakpoints within the *AML1* gene vary from translocation to translocation and possibly also differ between t-AML and de novo AML.[325] A fragile site for cleavage of the *AML1* gene by topoisomerase II inhibitors has been demonstrated.[326] In patients with t-AML and t(15;17)[294] and with inv(16),[291] the molecular biology has also been suggested to differ to some extent from that of de novo AML, although only a few cases have been studied thus far.

Chimeric gene fusions in acute myeloid leukaemia and related diseases with recurrent balanced chromsome aberrations

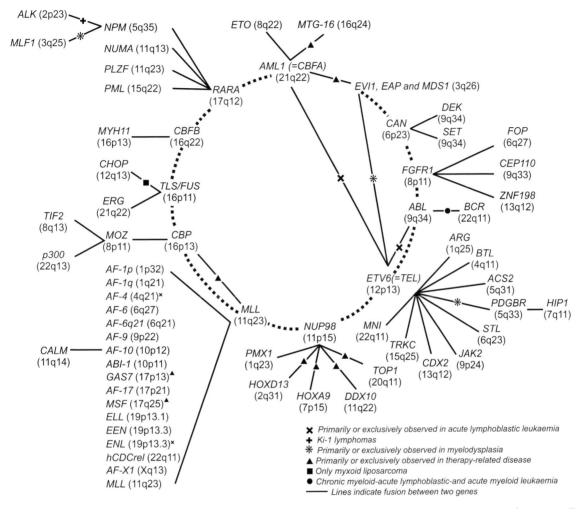

FIGURE 9–3. Chimeric gene fusions in acute myeloid leukemia and related diseases with recurrent balanced chromosome aberrations. (From Pedersen-Bjergaard J: Lancet 2001;357:491.)

OTHER CHROMOSOME CHANGES OBSERVED IN t-MDS AND t-AML

Cytogenetically unrelated clones are an interesting phenomenon in malignancy but are rarely observed in de novo MDS and AML. We recently observed cytogenetically unrelated clones in 12 of 180 consecutive cases of t-MDS and t-AML.[327] In some cases, one clone was shown to represent the leukemic cells, whereas the other clone originated from bone marrow involvement of the primary tumor, most frequently multiple myeloma. In other cases, two different defects of the long arm of chromosome 5 or the long arm of chromosome 7 were observed in two unrelated clones. Because these abnormalities in the two clones had different breakpoints on the same chromosome, they were considered to be of independent origin,

and the cytogenetic defects were supposed to arise secondary to a more important primary genetic change in the cell. Finally, some cases had secondary, uncharacteristic cytogenetic abnormalities in one or in both cytogenetically unrelated clones. Most likely, such cases are monoclonal, but their important general genetic abnormalities are not disclosed by their karyotype.

Dicentric chromosomes have for a long time been observed as being characteristic of t-MDS and t-AML.[256, 257] Recently, dicentric chromosomes were observed in 27 of 180 consecutive cases of t-MDS and t-AML versus only 7 of 231 consecutive cases of de novo MDS or AML ($P <$ .0001).[328] Dicentric chromosomes most often resulted in monosomy for 5q, 7q, or 17p and trisomy for 1q, and they were significantly associated with previous alkylating agent therapy. These results suggest that the centromeric or pericentromeric region of the chromosome may be particularly susceptible to damage and breakage by alkylation, which could explain the frequent loss of whole chromosomes in t-MDS and t-AML; if a centromeric breakage is not religated, the two chromosome fragments will undergo loss at a subsequent cell division.

Duplication or amplification of specific chromosome regions, particularly band 11q23, including an unrearranged *MLL* gene, is a newly observed phenomenon in leukemia.[280, 329, 330] Band 11q23 is often duplicated or amplified together with varying parts of the long arm of the chromosome in cases of t-MDS and t-AML. We recently observed duplication or amplification of the *MLL* gene in 12 of 70 unselected cases of t-MDS and t-AML.[280] The phenomenon was closely associated with previous therapy with alkylating agents and with mutations in *p53*. The levels of expression of the amplified *MLL* gene or other genes at 11q, the expression of similar, but rarer amplifications of the *ABL, AML1,* and *MYC* genes, and their more exact role in leukemic transformation remain to be determined.

DIAGNOSTIC AND PROGNOSTIC VALUE OF CHROMOSOME ABERRATIONS IN t-MDS AND t-AML

Cytogenetics, if characteristic, is of major importance in detecting early stages of t-MDS without diagnostic bone marrow cytology. Improved diagnostic accuracy is probably one of the main reasons for the generally higher risk of t-MDS and t-AML observed in most single-institute studies reporting cytogenetic details, as compared with larger cooperative studies not reporting such data. This point is exemplified by studies of the risk of t-MDS and t-AML after high-dose chemotherapy and autologous stem-cell transplantation (see Table 9–14 and Fig. 9–4).

The cytogenetic characteristics of t-MDS and t-AML are, as with the de novo subsets of the two diseases, important prognostic factors for the response to intensive antileukemic chemotherapy[263] and for survival.[254, 256, 331, 332] In particular, patients seen initially with t-MDS and deletions or loss of the long arms of chromosomes 5 and 7 or the whole chromosomes and a complex karyotype have an extremely poor prognosis. Few such patients obtain even a short remission after intensive chemotherapy, and new chemotherapy regimens and allogeneic bone marrow transplantation have not improved their outcome.[333-335] Patients with overt t-AML and balanced translocations or a normal karyotype often obtain complete remission after intensive chemotherapy, and in some cytogenetic subgroups such as inv(16) and t(15;17), almost half the patients become long-term survivors.[336] Patients with t-AML and balanced translocations to 11q23 often achieve complete remission after intensive chemotherapy, but they rarely become long-term survivors because of high relapse rate.[184, 337] Patients with t-MDS but

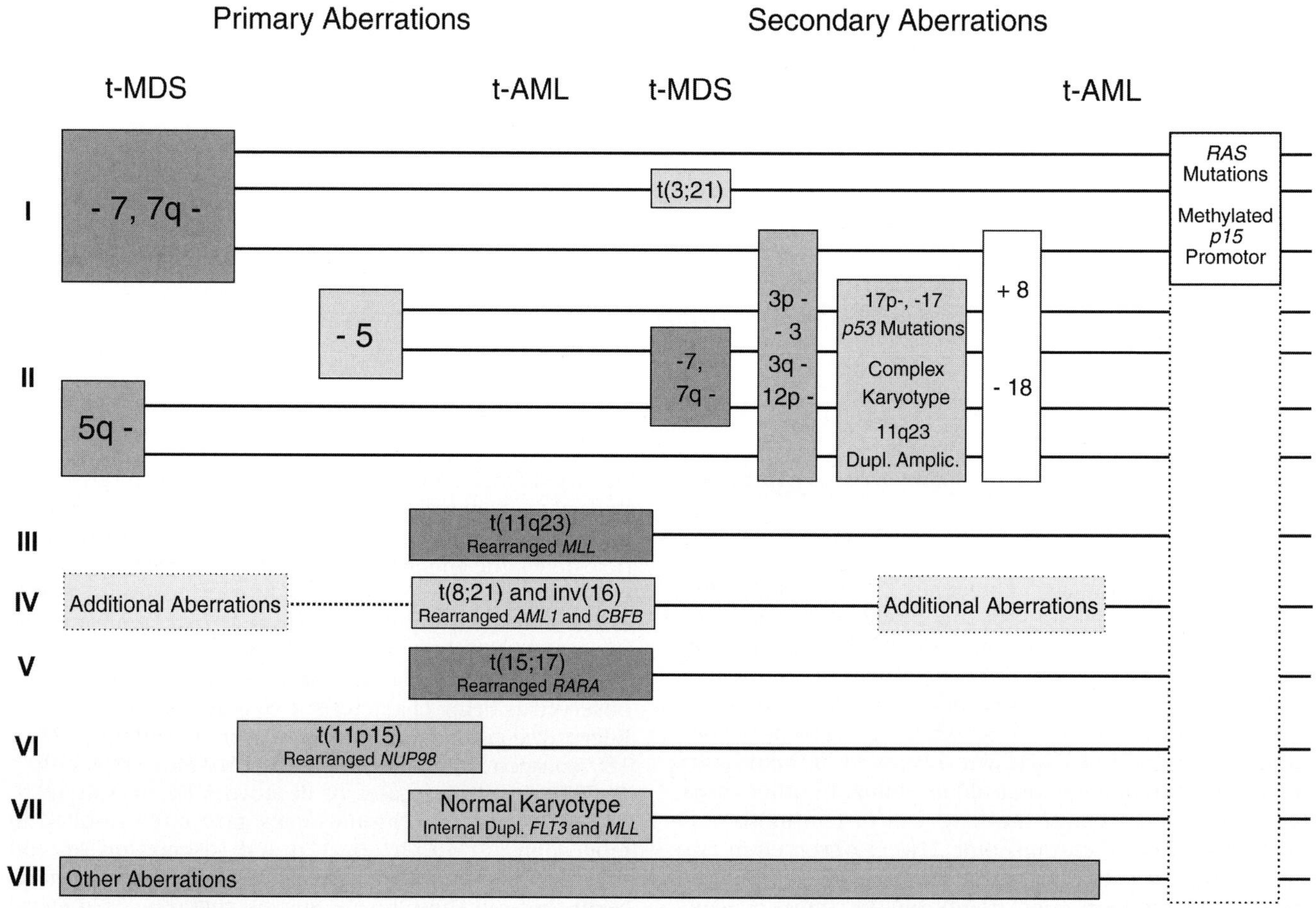

FIGURE 9–4. Model of genetic pathways in the genesis of treatment-related AML and MDS. (See Color Section.)

without severe cytopenia and with loss of a whole chromosome 7 as the only aberration seem to have a somewhat better outcome inasmuch as they may survive for years on supportive therapy only.[256]

PREDISPOSITION TO t-MDS AND t-AML

Like the situation for exposure to benzene, a different predisposition to t-MDS and t-AML from patient to patient after therapy with cytostatic drugs has been suggested, related to variations in the capacity to metabolize cytostatic drugs and to differences in DNA stability and DNA repair. The cytochrome P-450 enzymes degrade many anticancer drugs, and different CYP3A4 genotypes have been thought to result in variations in the risk of t-AML.[338] The risk of MDS in general[339] and the risk of t-AML[340] have been related to the null genotype of the glutathione transferase gene GSTT1, but this finding was not confirmed in a study of children with t-MDS and t-AML.[341] Quite recently, a polymorphism of another glutathione transferase gene, GSTP1, was shown to be overrepresented in 89 cases of t-AML.[342] Deletions of GSTT1 were not overrepresented in that study. Thiopurine methyltransferase, which catalyzes the S-methylation of 6-thioguanine, an antimetabolite used in therapy for ALL, tended to be lower[343] or was shown to be significantly lower[344] in patients with ALL in whom t-AML subsequently developed. An inactivating polymorphism in the NAD(P)H: quinone oxidoreductase NQO1 has also been observed in t-AML and in cases of de novo AML with deletions or loss of 5q and/or 7q as opposed to other patients with de novo AML.[345] This last observation is of interest because the same abnormality is selectively associated with pediatric leukemia with MLL fusions, mainly infants with t(4;11).[346] A mutator phenotype with microsatellite instability was observed in 15 of 16 patients with t-AML.[347] Although these studies indicate that patients may have different susceptibility to bone marrow damage that results in a different risk of t-MDS and t-AML from patient to patient, the results remain to be confirmed by larger prospective studies.

t-MDS AND t-AML AS MODELS FOR LEUKEMOGENESIS

For three main reasons, studies of patients with t-MDS and t-AML may be of importance in clarifying the molecular biology of MDS and AML in general. First, these diseases have almost the same cytogenetic and genetic abnormalities as de novo MDS and AML. Second, most cases of t-MDS and t-AML can be associated with a specific genotoxic exposure to cytostatic drugs with a known mechanism of action. Third, the distinction between cytogenetic and genetic abnormalities related to MDS and abnormalities related to AML can ideally be evaluated in t-MDS and t-AML. In de novo AML, information on a preceding phase of MDS is most often lacking, whereas most cases of t-MDS are diagnosed at an early stage of the disease because of close clinical follow-up with laboratory investigations after intensive radiotherapy or chemotherapy.

We have previously proposed different genetic pathways in t-MDS and t-AML based on characteristic chromosome aberrations.[263] The results of the many new studies now suggest a revised model.

Pathway I in the new model includes cases with deletion or loss of 7q or monosomy 7 but a normal chromosome 5. Most such patients have been treated with alkylating agents or radiotherapy. They present with t-MDS, and they sometimes have additional chromosome aberrations, in some cases t(3;21). These patients rarely show mutations of p53, and their prognosis is rather poor, except in patients without severe cytopenia and with loss of a chromosome 7 as the only abnormality. Such patients may survive for years on supportive therapy only.

Pathway II includes cases with deletions or loss of 5q or monosomy 5. These patients have characteristically been treated with alkylating agents, and patients with deletions or loss of 5q most often present with t-MDS. They often have very complex karyotypes with unidentified marker chromosomes, chromosome duplications, or amplifications. Mutations of p53 with loss of heterozygosity of the gene are very common in these patients, and their prognosis is extremely poor.

Pathway III includes cases with balanced translocations to chromosome band 11q23 and rearrangements of the MLL gene. These translocations are most commonly observed after therapy with topoisomerase II inhibitors, particularly in children with t-AML after epipodophyllotoxin therapy. The disease in this pathway is characteristically present as overt t-AML of FAB subtypes M4 or M5, and these patients respond favorably to intensive chemotherapy. However, long-term survival is poor because of a high relapse rate of leukemia.

Pathway IV includes cases with inv(16) and cases with balanced translocations to chromosome band 21q22 and chimeric rearrangement between the core-binding factor genes CBFB and AML1 and various partner genes. Such cases are characteristically observed in adult patients treated with topoisomerase II inhibitors, for instance, anthracyclines. The disease is manifested as overt t-AML of the FAB subtypes M4eo and M2, respectively. These patients respond favorably to intensive antileukemic chemotherapy, and they often become long-term survivors.

Pathway V includes cases with t(15;17) and rearrangement of the RARA gene. Such abnormalities have characteristically been observed in adult patients with t-AML after therapy with the dioxopiperazine derivatives and mitoxantrone. They respond favorably to intensive chemotherapy that includes retinoic acid, and they may become long-term survivors.

Pathway VI includes rather rare cases of t-AML with translocations to chromosome band 11p15 and rearrangement of the NUP98 gene. Cases in this pathway are most often observed after chemotherapy with topoisomerase II inhibitors.

Pathway VII includes patients with a normal karyotype. These cases seem unrelated to any specific type of previous therapy, they characteristically present as overt t-AML, and they often have internal tandem duplications of the FLT3 and MLL genes.[349] They probably often represent incidental cases of de novo AML, and if the *FLT3* and the *MLL* genes are not duplicated, they may respond rather favorably to intensive antileukemic therapy.

Pathway VIII includes cases with various other uncharacteristic, nonrecurrent chromosome aberrations. Some of them may turn out to be recurrent and characteristic of the disease when larger series of patients with t-MDS and t-AML are studied.

REFERENCES

1. Farber E: Chemical carcinogenesis. N Engl J Med 1981;305:1379.
2. Sandler DP: Epidemiology of acute myelogenous leukemia. Semin Oncol 1987;14:359.
3. Cartwright RA, Staines A: Acute leukaemias. Baillieres Clin Haematol 1992;5:1.
4. Sandler DP, Ross JA: Epidemiology of acute leukemia in children and adults. Semin Oncol 1997;24:3.
5. Selling L: A preliminary report of some cases of purpura haemorrhagica due to benzol poisoning. Bull Johns Hopkins Hosp 1910;21:33.
6. Selling L: Benzol as a leukotoxin. Studies on degeneration and regeneration of blood and hematopoietic organs. Bull Johns Hopkins Hosp 1916;17:83.
7. Bowditch M, Elkins HB: Chronic exposure to benzene (benzol). I. The industrial aspects. Ind Hyg Toxicol 1939;21:321.
8. Lignac GOE: Benzene induced leukemia in humans and white mice. Klin Wochenshr 1932;12:109.
9. Mallory TB, Gall EA, Brickley WJ: Chronic exposure to benzene (benzol). III. The pathogenic results. J Ind Hyg Toxicol 1939;21:355.
10. Vigliani EC, Saita G: Benzene and leukemia. N Engl J Med 1964;271:872.
11. Infante PF, Rinsky RA, Wagoner JK, et al: Leukaemia in benzene workers. Lancet 1977;2:76.
12. Aksoy M, Erdem S: Follow-up study on the mortality and the development of leukaemia in 44 pancytopenic patients with chronic exposure to benzene. Blood 1978;52:285.
13. Aksoy M: Benzene as a leukemogenic and carcinogenic agent. Am J Ind Med 1985;8:9.
14. Yin SN, Li GL, Tain FD, et al: Leukaemia in benzene workers: A retrospective cohort study. Br J Ind Med 1987;44:124.
15. Austin H, Deizell E, Cole P: Benzene and leukemia. A review of the literature and a risk assessment. Am J Epidemiol 1988;127:419.
16. Savitz DA, Andrews KW: Review of epidemiologic evidence on benzene and lymphatic and hematopoietic cancers. Am J Ind Med 1997;31:287.
17. Cronkite EP: Chemical leukemogenesis: Benzene as a model. Semin Hematol 1987;24:2.
18. Ross D: Metabolic basis of benzene toxicity. Eur J Haematol 1996;57:111.
19. Brandt L, Nilsson PG, Mitelman F: Occupational exposure to petroleum products in men with acute non-lymphocytic leukaemia. BMJ 1978;4:553.
20. Lynge E, Andersen A, Nilson R, et al: Risk of cancer and exposure to gasoline vapors. Am J Epidemiol 1997;145:449.
21. Rushton L, Alderson MR: A case-control study to investigate the association between exposure to benzene and deaths from leukaemia in our refinery workers. Br J Cancer 1981;43:77.
22. Rinsky RA, Smith AB, Hornung R, et al: Benzene and leukemia: An epidemiologic risk assessment. N Engl J Med 1987;316:1044.
23. Hayes RB, Yin SN, Dosemeci M, et al: Benzene and the dose-related incidence of hematologic neoplasms in China. J Natl Cancer Inst 1997;89:1065.
24. Nathaniel R, Smith MT, Hayes RB, et al: Benzene poisoning, a risk factor for hematological malignancy, is associated with the *NQO1*[609] C—T mutation and rapid fractional excretion of chlorzoxazone. Cancer Res 1997;57:2839.
25. Rothman N, Smith MT, Hayes RB, et al: Benzene poisoning, a risk factor for hematological malignancy, is associated with the *NQO1*[609] C—T mutation and rapid fractional excretion of chlorzoxazone. Cancer Res 1997;57:2839.
26. Snyder R: Issues in risk assessment of chemicals of concern to Department of Defense and other agencies session recent developments in the understanding of benzene toxicity and leukemogenesis. Drug Chem Toxicol 2000;23:13.
27. Pearce NE, Sheppard RA, Howard JK, et al: Leukemia among New Zealand agricultural workers. Am J Epidemiol 1986;124:402.
28. Meinert R, Schüz J, Kaletsch U, et al: Leukemia and non-Hodgkin's lymphoma in childhood and exposure to pesticides: Results of a register-based case control study in Germany. Am J Epidemiol 2000;151:639.
29. Timonen TTT, Palva P: Acute leukaemia after exposure to a weed killer, 2-methyl-4-chlorphenoxyacetic acid. Acta Haematol 1980;63:170.
30. Brown LM, Blair A, Gibson R, et al: Pesticide exposures and other agricultural risk factors for leukemia among men in Iowa and Minnesota. Cancer Res 1990;50:6585.
31. Lynge E: A follow-up study of cancer incidence among workers in manufacture of phenoxy herbicides in Denmark. Br J Cancer 1985;52:259.
32. Blair A: Cancer risks associated with agriculture: Epidemiologic evidence. Basic Life Sci 1982;21:93.
33. Checkoway H, Wilcosky T, Wolf P, et al: An evaluation of the associations of leukemia and rubber industry solvent exposures. Am J Ind Med 1984;5:239.
34. Santos-Burgoa C, Matanoski GM, Zeger S, et al: Lymphohematopoietic cancer in styrene-butadiene polymerisation workers. Am J Epidemiol 1992;136:843.
35. Hogstedt C, Aringer L, Gustavsson A: Epidemiologic support of ethylene oxide as a cancer-causing agent. JAMA 1986;255:1575.
36. Steenland K, Stayner L, Greife A, et al: Mortality among workers exposed to ethylene oxide. N Engl J Med 1991;324:1402.
37. Shore RE, Gardner MJ, Pannett B: Ethylene oxide: An assessment of the epidemiological evidence on carcinogenicity. Br J Ind Med 1993;50:971.
38. Kinlen LJ, Rogot E: Leukaemia and smoking habits among United States veterans. BMJ 1988;297:657.
39. McLaughlin JK: Cigarette smoking and leukemia. J Natl Cancer Inst 1989;81:1262.
40. Garfinkel L, Boffetta P: Association between smoking and leukemia in two American Cancer Society prospective studies. Cancer 1990;65:2356.
41. Mills PK, Newell GR, Beeson WL, et al: History of cigarette smoking and risk of leukemia and myeloma: Results from the Adventist Health Study. J Natl Cancer Inst 1990;82:1832.
42. Brown LM, Gibson R, Blair A, et al: Smoking and risk of leukemia. Am J Epidemiol 1992;135:763.
43. Pasqualetti P, Festuccia V, Acitelli P, et al: Tobacco smoking and risk of haematological malignancies in adults: A case-control study. Br J Haematol 1997;97:659.
44. Adami J, Nyrén O, Bergström R, et al: Smoking and the risk of leukemia, lymphoma, and multiple myeloma (Sweden). Cancer Causes Control 1998;9:49.
45. Cantor KP, Blair A, Everett G, et al: Hair dye use and risk of leukemia and lymphoma. Am J Public Health 1988;78:570.
46. Thun MJ, Altekruse SF, Namboodiri MM, et al: Hair dye use and risk of fatal cancers in U.S. women. J Natl Cancer Inst 1994;86:210.
47. Grodstein F, Hennekens CH, Colditz GA, et al: A prospective study of permanent hair dye use and hematopoietic cancer. J Natl Cancer Inst 1994;86:1466.
48. Ross JA, Davies SM, Potter JD, et al: Epidemiology of childhood leukemia, with a focus on infants. Epidemiol Rev 1994;16:243.
49. Ross JA, Potter JD, Reaman GH, et al: Maternal exposure to potential inhibitors of DNA topoisomerase II and infant leukemia (United States): A report from the children's cancer group. Cancer Causes Control 1996;7:581.
50. Strick R, Strissel PL, Borgers S, et al: Dietary bioflavonoids induce cleavage in the *MLL* gene and may contribute to infant leukaemia. Proc Natl Acad Sci U S A 2000;97:4790.
51. Domer PH, Head DR, Renganathan N, et al: Molecular analysis of 13 cases of *MLL*/11q23 secondary acute leukemia and identification of topoisomerase II consensus-binding sequences near the chromosomal breakpoint of a secondary leukemia with the t(4;11). Leukemia 1995;9:1305.
52. Broeker PLS, Super HG, Thirman MJ, et al: Distribution of 11q23

breakpoints within the *MLL* breakpoint cluster region in de novo acute leukemia and in treatment-related acute myeloid leukemia: Correlation with scaffold attachment regions and topoisomerase II consensus binding sites. Blood 1996;87:1912.

53. Cimino G, Rapanotti MC, Biondi A, et al: Infant acute leukemias show the same biased distribution of *ALL1* gene breaks as topoisomerase II related secondary acute leukemias, Cancer Res 1997; 57:2879.

54. McDonald TA, Holland NT, Skibola C, et al: Hypothesis: Phenol and hydroxyquinone derived mainly from diet and gastrointestinal flora activity are causal factors in leukemia. Leukemia 2001;15:10.

55. Lebon J, Messerschmidt J: Myélose aplastique d'origine médicamenteuse myéloblastose aigue terminale reflexions pathogéniques. Le Sang 1955;26:799.

56. Jensen MK, Roll K: Phenylbutazone and leukaemia. Acta Med Scand 1965;178:505.

57. Bloomfield CD, Brunning RD: Acute leukemia as a terminal event in nonleukemic hematopoietic disorders. Semin Oncol 1976;3:297.

58. de Planque MM, Kluin-Nelemans HC, van Krieken HJ, et al: Evolution of acquired severe aplastic anaemia to myelodysplasia and subsequent leukaemia in adults. Br J Haematol 1988;70:55.

59. Ohara A, Kojima S, Hamajima N, et al: Myelodysplastic syndrome and acute myelogenous leukemia as a late clonal complication in children with acquired aplastic anemia. Blood 1997;90:1009.

60. Mitelman F, Brandt L, Nilsson PG: Relation among occupational exposure to potential mutagenic/carcinogenic agents, clinical findings, and bone marrow chromosomes in acute nonlymphocytic leukemia. Blood 1978;52:1229.

61. Mitelman F, Nilsson PG, Brandt L, et al: Chromosome pattern, occupation, and clinical features in patients with acute nonlymphocytic leukemia. Cancer Genet Cytogenet 1981;4:197.

62. Golomb HM, Alimena G, Rowley JD, et al: Correlation of occupation and karyotype in adults with acute nonlymphocytic leukemia. Blood 1982;60:404.

63. Narod SA, Dubé ID: Occupational history and involvement of chromosomes 5 and 7 in acute nonlymphocytic leukemia. Cancer Genet Cytogenet 1989;38:261.

64. Fagioli F, Cuneo A, Piva N, et al: Distinct cytogenetic and clinicopathologic features in acute myeloid leukemia after occupational exposure to pesticides and organic solvents. Cancer 1992;70:77.

65. West RR, Stafford DA, White AD, et al: Cytogenetic abnormalities in the myelodysplastic syndromes and occupational or environmental exposure. Blood 2000;95:2093.

66. Crane MM, Strom SS, Halabi S, et al: Correlation between selected environmental exposures and karyotype in acute myelocytic leukemia. Cancer Epidemiol Biomarkers Prev 1996;5:639.

67. Sasiadek M: Nonrandom distribution of breakpoints in the karyotypes of workers occupationally exposed to benzene. Environ Health Perspect 1992;97:255.

68. Smith MT, Zhang L, Wang Y, et al: Increased translocations and aneusomy in chromosomes 8 and 21 among workers exposed to benzene. Cancer Res 1998;58:2176.

69. Zhang L, Wang Y, Shang N, Smith MT: Benzene metabolites induce the loss and long arm deletion of chromosomes 5 and 7 in human lymphocytes. Leuk Res 1998;22:105.

70. Smith MT, Zhang L, Jeng M, et al: Hydroquinone, a benzene metabolite increases the level of aneusomy of chromosome 7 and 8 in human CD34-positive blood progenitor cells. Carcinogenesis 2000;21:1485.

71. Grünwald HW, Rosner F: Acute leukemia and immunsuppressive drug use. A review of patients undergoing immunosuppresive therapy for non-neoplastic diseases. Arch Intern Med 1979;139:461.

72. Casciato DA, Scott JL: Acute leukemia following prolonged cytotoxic agent therapy. Medicine (Baltimore) 1979;58:32.

73. Park DJ, Koeffler HP: Therapy-related myelodysplastic syndromes. Semin Hematol 1996;33:256.

74. Thirman MJ, Larson RA: Therapy-related myeloid leukemia. Hematol Oncol Clin North Am 1996;10:293.

75. Berk PD, Goldberg JD, Silverstein MN, et al: Increased incidence of acute leukemia in polycythemia vera associated with chlorambucil therapy. N Engl J Med 1981;304:441.

76. Finazzi G, Ruggeri M, Rodeghiero F, Barbui T: Second malignancies in patients with essential thrombocythaemia treated with busulphan and hydroxyurea: Long-term follow-up of a randomised clinical trial. Br J Hematol 2000;110:577.

77. Nichols CR, Roth BJ, Heerema N, et al: Hematologic neoplasia associated with primary mediastinal germ-cell tumors. N Engl J Med 1990;322:1425.

78. Orazi A, Neiman RS, Ulbright TM, et al: Hematopoietic precursor cells within the yolk sac tumor component are the source of secondary hematopoietic malignancies in patients with mediastinal germ cell tumors. Cancer 1993;71:3873.

79. Lacher MJ, Sussman LN: Leukemia and Hodgkin's disease. Ann Intern Med 1963;59:369.

80. Kyle RA, Pierre RV, Bayrd ED: Multiple myeloma and acute myelomonocytic leukemia. Report of four cases possibly related to melphalan. N Engl J Med 1970;283:1121.

81. Rosner F, Grünwald HW: Multiple myeloma and Waldenström's macroglobulinemia terminating in acute leukemia. NY State J Med 1980;80:558.

82. Grünwald HW, Rosner F: Acute myeloid leukemia following treatment of Hodgkin's disease. Cancer 1982;50:676.

83. Kyle RA: Second malignancies associated with chemotherapeutic agents. Semin Oncol 1982;9:131.

84. Kyle RA: Second malignancies associated with chemotherapy. In: Perry MC, Yarbro JW, eds: Toxicity of Chemotherapy, New York: Grune & Stratton; 1984, p 479.

85. Glicksman AS, Pajak TF, Gottlieb A, et al: Second malignant neoplasms in patients successfully treated for Hodgkin's disease: A Cancer and Leukemia Group B study. Cancer Treat Rep 1982; 66:1035.

86. Devereux S, Selassie TG, Vaughan HG, et al: Leukaemia complicating treatment for Hodgkin's disease: The experience of the British National Lymphoma Investigation. BMJ 1990;301:1077.

87. Cuzick J, Erskine S, Edelman D, Galton DA: A comparison of the incidence of the myelodysplastic syndrome and acute myeloid leukaemia following melphalan and cyclophosphamide treatment for myelomatosis. Br J Cancer 1987;55:523.

88. Greene MH, Harris EL, Gershenson DM, et al: Melphalan may be a more potent leukemogen than cyclophosphamide. Ann Intern Med 1986;105:360.

89. Stott H, Fox W, Girling DJ, et al: Acute leukaemia after busulphan. BMJ 1977;2:1513.

90. Pedersen-Bjergaard J, Ersbøll J, Hansen VL, et al: Carcinoma of the urinary bladder after treatment with cyclophosphamide for non-Hodgkin's lymphoma. N Engl J Med 1988;318:1028.

91. Travis LB, Curtis RE, Glimelius B, et al: Bladder and kidney cancer following cyclophosphamide therapy for non-Hodgkin's lymphoma. J Natl Cancer Inst 1995;87:524.

92. Talar-Williams C, Hijazi YM, Walther MM, et al: Cyclophosphamide-induced cystitis and bladder cancer in patients with Wegener granulomatosis. Ann Intern Med 1996;124:477.

93. Ratain MJ, Kaminer LS, Bitran JD, et al: Acute nonlymphocytic leukemia following etoposide and cisplatin combination chemotherapy for advanced non–small cell carcinoma of the lung. Blood 1987;70:1412.

94. Pui C-H, Behm FG, Raimondi SC, et al: Secondary acute myeloid leukemia in children treated for acute lymphoid leukemia. N Engl J Med 1989;321:136.

95. Pedersen-Bjergaard J, Daugaard G, Hansen SW, et al: Increased risk of myelodysplasia and leukaemia after etoposide, cisplatin, and bleomycin for germ-cell tumours. Lancet 1991;338:359.

96. Whitlock JA, Greer JP, Lukens JN: Epipodophyllotoxin-related leukemia. Identification of a new subset of secondary leukemia. Cancer 1991;68:600.

97. Smith MA, Rubinstein L, Anderson JR, et al: Secondary leukemia or myelodysplastic syndrome after treatment with epipodophyllotoxins. J Clin Oncol 1999;17:569.

98. Lavey RS, Eby NL, Prosnitz LR: Impact on second malignancy risk of the combined use of radiation and chemotherapy for lymphomas. Cancer 1990;66:80.

99. Kaldor JM, Day NE, Pettersson F, et al: Leukemia following chemotherapy for ovarian cancer. N Engl J Med 1990;322:1.

100. Tucker MA, Meadows AT, Boice JD, et al: Leukemia after therapy with alkylating agents for childhood cancer. J Natl Cancer Inst 1987;78:459-464.

101. Pedersen-Bjergaard J, Sigsgaard TC, Nielsen D, et al: Acute monocytic or myelomonocytic leukemia with balanced chromosome

translocations to band 11q23 after therapy with 4-epi-doxorubicin and cisplatin or cyclophosphamide for breast cancer. J Clin Oncol 1992;10:1444.

102. Shepherd L, Ottaway J, Myles J, et al: Therapy-related leukemia associated with high-dose 4-epi-doxorubicin and cyclophospha-mide used as adjuvant chemotherapy for breast cancer. J Clin Oncol 1994;12:2514.

103. Andersson M, Philip P, Pedersen-Bjergaard J: High risk of therapy-related leukemia and preleukemia after therapy with prednimus-tine, methotrexate, 5-fluorouracil, mitoxantrone, and tamoxifen for advanced breast cancer. Cancer 1990;65:2460.

104. Cremin P, Flattery M, McCann SR, Daly PA: Myelodysplasia and acute myeloid leukemia following adjuvant chemotherapy for breast cancer using mitoxantrone and methotrexate with or with-out mitomycin. Ann Oncol 1996;7:745.

105. Chaplain G, Milan C, Sgro C, et al: Increased risk of acute leukemia after adjuvant chemotherapy for breast cancer: A population-based study. J Clin Oncol 2000;18:2836.

106. Pedersen-Bjergaard J: The dioxopiperazine derivatives, their leuke-mogenic potential and other biological effects. Leuk Res 1992; 11:1057.

107. Lakhani S, Davidson RN, Hiwaizi F, Marsden RA: Razoxane and leukaemia. Lancet 1984;2:288.

108. Caffrey EA, Daker MG, Horton JJ: Acute myeloid leukaemia after treatment with razoxane. Br J Dermatol 1985;113:131.

109. Gilbert JM, Hellmann K, Evans M, et al: Randomized trial of oral adjuvant razoxane (ICRF159) in resectable colorectal cancer: Five-year follow-up. Br J Surg 1986;73:446.

110. Bhavnani M, Wolstenholme RJ: Razoxane and acute promyelocytic leukaemia. Lancet 1987;2:1085.

111. Li YS, Zhao YL, Jiang QP, Yang CL: Specific chromosome changes and non-occupational exposure to potentially carcinogenic agents in acute leukemia in China. Leuk Res 1989;13:367.

112. Xue Y, Lu D, Guo Y, Lin B: Specific chromosomal translocations and therapy-related leukemia induced by bimolane therapy for psoriasis. Leuk Res 1992;16:1113.

113. Tanabe K, Ikegami Y, Ishida R, Andoh T: Inhibition of topoisomer-ase II by antitumor agents bis-2,6-dioxopiperazine derivatives. Can-cer Res 1991;51:4903.

114. Ishida R, Miki T, Narita T, et al: Inhibition of intracellular topoisom-erase II by antitumor bis(2,6-dioxopiperazine) derivatives: Mode of cell growth inhibition distinct from that of cleavable complex-forming type inhibitors. Cancer Res 1991;51:4909.

115. Roca J, Ishida R, Berger JM, et al: Antitumor bisdioxopiperazines inhibit yeast DNA topoisomerase II by trapping the enzyme in the form of a closed protein clamp. Proc Natl Acad Sci U S A 1994; 91:1781.

116. Coleman CN, Williams CJ, Flint A, et al: Hematologic neoplasia in patients treated for Hodgkin disease. N Engl J Med 1977;297:1249.

117. Valagussa P, Santoro A, Kenda R, et al: Second malignancies in Hodgkin's disease: A complication of certain forms of treatment. BMJ 1980;280:216.

118. Baccarani M, Bosi A, Papa G: Second malignancy in patients treated for Hodgkin's disease. Cancer 1980;46:1735.

119. Coltman CA Jr, Dixon DO: Second malignancies complicating Hodgkin's disease: A Southwest Oncology Group 10-year follow-up. Cancer Treat Rep 1982;66:1023.

120. Coleman CN, Kalan HS, Cox R, et al: Leukemias, non-Hodgkin's lymphomas and solid tumours in patients treated for Hodgkin's disease. Cancer Surv 1982;1:733.

121. Pedersen-Bjergaard J, Larsen SO: Incidence of acute nonlympho-cytic leukemia, preleukemia, and acute myeloproliferative syn-drome up to 10 years after treatment of Hodgkin's disease. N Engl J Med 1982;307:965.

122. Tester WJ, Kinsella TJ, Waller B, et al: Second malignant neoplasms complicating Hodgkin's disease: The National Cancer Institute Experience. J Clin Oncol 1984;2:762.

123. Valagussa P, Santoro A, Fossati-Bellani F, et al: Second acute leuke-mia and other malignancies following treatment for Hodgkin's disease. J Clin Oncol 1986;4:830.

124. Koletsky AJ, Bertino JR, Farber LR, et al: Second neoplasms in patients with Hodgkin's disease following combined modality therapy—the Yale Experience. J Clin Oncol 1986;4:311.

125. Blayney DW, Longo DL, Young RC, et al: Decreasing risk of leuke-mia with prolonged follow-up after chemotherapy and radiother-apy for Hodgkin's disease. N Engl J Med 1987;316:710.

126. Pedersen-Bjergaard J, Specht L, Larsen SO, et al: Risk of therapy-related leukaemia and preleukaemia after Hodgkin's disease. Lan-cet 1987;2:83.

127. Tucker MA, Coleman CN, Cox RS, et al: Risk of second cancers after treatment for Hodgkin's disease. N Engl J Med 1988;318:76.

128. van-der-Velden JW, van Putten WLJ, Guinee VF, et al: Subsequent development of acute non-lymphocyte leukemia in patients treated for Hodgkin's disease. Int J Cancer 1988;42:252.

129. van-Leeuwen FE, Somers R, Taal BG, et al: Increased risk of lung cancer, non-Hodgkin's lymphoma, and leukemia following Hodg-kin's disease. J Clin Oncol 1989;7:1046.

130. Selby P, Patel P, Milan S, et al: ChlVPP combination chemotherapy for Hodgkin's disease: Long term results. Br J Cancer 1990;62:279.

131. Cimino G, Papa G, Tura S, et al: Second primary cancer following Hodgkin's disease: Updated results of an Italian multicentric study. J Clin Oncol 1991;9:432.

132. Swerdlow AJ, Douglas AJ, Hudson GV, et al: Risk of second primary cancers after Hodgkin's disease by type of treatment: Analysis of 2846 patients in the British National Lymphoma Investigation. BMJ 1992;304:1137.

133. Henry-Amar M: Second cancer after the treatment for Hodgkin's disease: A report from the International Database on Hodgkin's disease. Ann Oncol 1992;3(Suppl 4):117.

134. Abrahamsen JF, Andersen AA, Hannisdal E, et al: Second malignan-cies after treatment of Hodgkin's disease: The influence of treat-ment, follow-up time, and age. J Clin Oncol 1993;11:255.

135. Rodriguez MA, Fuller LM, Zimmerman SO, et al: Hodgkin's disease: Study of treatment intensities and incidences of second malignan-cies. Ann Oncol 1993;4:125.

136. Biti G, Cellai E, Magrini SM, et al: Second solid tumors and leuke-mia after treatment for Hodgkin's disease: An analysis of 1121 patients from a single institution. Int J Radiat Oncol Biol Phys 1994;29:25.

137. van-Leeuwen FE, Klokman WJ, Hagenbeek A, et al: Second cancer risk following Hodgkin's disease: A 20-year follow-up study. J Clin Oncol 1994;12:312.

138. Swerdlow AJ, Barber JA, Horwich A, et al: Second malignancy in patients with Hodgkin's disease treated at the Royal Marsden Hospital. Br J Cancer 1997;75:116.

139. Swerdlow AJ, Barber JA, Hudson GV, et al: Risk of second malig-nancy after Hodgkin's disease in a collaborative British cohort: The relation to age at treatment. J Clin Oncol 2000;18:498.

140. Meadows AT, Obringer AC, Marrero O, et al: Second malignant neoplasms following childhood Hodgkin's disease: Treatment and splenectomy as risk factors. Med Pediatr Oncol 1989;17:477.

141. Jenkin D, Greenberg M, Fitzgerald A: Second malignant tumours in childhood Hodgkin's disease. Med Pediatr Oncol 1996;26:373.

142. Sankila R, Garwicz S, Olsen JH, et al: Risk of subsequent malignant neoplasms among 1,641 Hodgkin's disease patients diagnosed in childhood and adolescence: A population-based cohort study in the five Nordic countries. J Clin Oncol 1996;14:1442.

143. Schellong G, Riepenhausen M, Creutzig U, et al: Low risk of secondary leukemias after chemotherapy without mechloreth-amine in childhood Hodgkin's disease. J Clin Oncol 1997;15:2247.

144. Wolden SL, Lamborn KR, Cleary SF, et al: Second cancers following pediatric Hodgkin's disease. J Clin Oncol 1998;16:536.

145. van-Leeuwen FE, Klokman WJ, van't Veer MB, et al: Long-term risk of second malignancy in survivors of Hodgkin's disease during adolescence or young adulthood. J Clin Oncol 2000;18:487.

146. Canellos GP, DeVita VT, Arseneau JC, et al: Second malignancies complicating Hodgkin's disease in remission. Lancet 1975;947.

147. van-Leeuwen FE, Chorus AMJ, van den Belt-Dusebout AW, et al: Leukemia risk following Hodgkin's disease: Relation to cumulative dose of alkylating agents, treatment with teniposide combinations, number of episodes of chemotherapy, and bone marrow damage. J Clin Oncol 1994;12:1063.

148. Kaldor JM, Day NE, Clarke EA, et al: Leukemia following Hodgkin's disease. N Engl J Med 1990;322:7.

149. Harrison CN, Gregory W, Hudson GV, et al: High-dose BEAM chemotherapy with autologous haemopoietic stem cell trans-plantation for Hodgkin's disease is unlikely to be associated with a major increased risk of secondary MDS/AML. Br J Cancer 1999; 81:476.

150. Valagussa P, Santoro A, Fossati-Bellani F, et al: Absence of treat-ment-induced second neoplasms after ABVD in Hodgkin's disease. Blood 1982;59:488.

151. Boivin JF, Hutchison GB, Zauber AG, et al: Incidence of second cancers in patients treated for Hodgkin's disease. J Natl Cancer Inst 1995;87:732.

152. Amadori S, Papa G, Anselmo AP, et al: Acute promyelocytic leukemia following ABVD (doxorubicin, bleomycin, vinblastine and dacarbazine) and radiotherapy for Hodgkin's disease. Cancer Treat Rep 1983;67:603.

153. Narayanan MN, Morgenstern GR, Chang JC, et al: Acute lymphoblastic leukaemia following Hodgkin's disease is associated with a good prognosis. Br J Haematol 1994;86:867.

154. Gillis S, Sofer O, Zelig O, et al: Acute promyelocytic leukemia with t(15;17) following treatment of Hodgkin's disease: A report of 4 cases. Ann Oncol 1995;6:777.

155. Boivin JF, Hutchison GB, Lyden M, et al: Second primary cancers following treatment of Hodgkin's disease. J Natl Cancer Inst 1984; 72:233.

156. Coleman MP, Bell CMJ, Fraser P: Second primary malignancy after Hodgkin's disease, ovarian cancer and cancer of the testis: A population-based cohort study. Br J Cancer 1987;56:349.

157. Mauch PM, Kalish LA, Marcus KC, et al: Second malignancies after treatment for laparotomy staged IA-IIIB Hodgkin's disease: Long-term analysis of risk factors and outcome. Blood 1996;87:3625.

158. Metayer C, Lynch CF, Clarke EA, et al: Second cancers among long-term survivors of Hodgkin's disease diagnosed in childhood and adolescence. J Clin Oncol 2000;18:2435.

159. Harousseau JL, Andrieu JM, Dumont J, et al: Leucémies aiguës myéloblastiques survenant au cours de l'évolution de lymphomes malins non Hodgkiniens. Nouv Presse Med 1980;9:3513.

160. Gomez GA, Aggarwal KK, Han T: Post-therapeutic acute malignant myeloproliferative syndrome and acute nonlymphocytic leukemia in non-Hodgkin's lymphoma. Correlation with intensity of treatment. Cancer 1982;50:2285.

161. Greene MH, Young RC, Merrill JM, De Vita VT: Evidence of a treatment dose response in acute nonlymphocytic leukemias which occur after therapy of non-Hodgkin's lymphoma. Cancer Res 1983;43:1891.

162. Pedersen-Bjergaard J, Ersbøll J, Sørensen HM, et al: Risk of acute nonlymphocytic leukemia and preleukemia in patients treated with cyclophosphamide for non-Hodgkin's lymphomas. Ann Intern Med 1985;103:195.

163. Ingram L, Mott MG, Mann JR, et al: Second malignancies in children treated for non-Hodgkin's lymphoma and T-cell leukaemia with the UKCCSG regimens. Br J Cancer 1987;55:463.

164. Lishner M, Slingerland J, Barr J, et al: Second malignant neoplasms in patients with non-Hodgkin's lymphoma. Hematol Oncol 1991; 9:169.

165. Sugita K, Furukawa T, Tsuchida M, et al: High frequency of etoposide (VP-16)-related secondary leukemia in children with non-Hodgkin's lymphoma. Am J Pediatr Hematol Oncol 1993;15:99.

166. Travis LB, Weeks J, Curtis RE, et al: Leukemia following low-dose total body irradiation and chemotherapy for non-Hodgkin's lymphoma. J Clin Oncol 1996;14:565.

167. Travis LB, Curtis RE, Stovall M, et al: Risk of leukemia following treatment for non-Hodgkin's lymphoma. J Natl Cancer Inst 1994; 86:1450.

168. Van den Neste E, Louviaux I, Michaux JL, et al: Myelodysplastic syndrome with monosomy 5 and/or 7 following therapy with 2-chloro-2'-deoxyadenosine. Br J Haematol 1999;105:268.

169. Cheson BD, Vena DA, Barrett J, et al: Second malignancies as a consequence of nucleoside analog therapy for chronic lymphoid leukaemia. J Clin Oncol 1999;17:2454.

170. Bergsagel DE, Bailey AJ, Langley GR, et al: The chemotherapy of plasma-cell myeloma and the incidence of acute leukemia. N Engl J Med 1979;301:743.

171. Wahlin A, Ross G, Rudolphi O, Holm J: Melphalan-related leukemia in multiple myeloma. Acta Med Scand 1982;211:203.

172. Mufti CJ, Hamblin TJ, Clein GP, Race C: Coexistent myelodysplasia and plasma cell neoplasia. Br J Haematol 1983;54:91.

173. Stewart AK, Freedman J, Garvey MB: Acute leukemia evolving from multiple myeloma and co-expressing myeloid and plasma cell antigens. Am J Hematol 1990;34:210.

174. Murphy S, Peterson P, Iland H, et al: Experience of the polycythemia vera study group with essential thrombocythemia: A final report on diagnostic criteria, survival, and leukemic transition by treatment. Semin Hematol 1997;34:29.

175. Brusamolino E, Salvaneschi L, Canevari A, Bernasconi C: Efficacy trial of pipobroman in polycythemia vera and incidence of acute leukemia. J Clin Oncol 1984;2:558.

176. Najean Y, Rain J-D: Treatment of polycythemia vera: The use of hydroxyurea and pipobroman in 292 patients under the age of 65 years. Blood 1997;90:3370.

177. Najean Y, Rain J-D: Treatment of polycythemia vera: Use of ^{32}P alone or in combination with maintenance therapy using hydroxyurea in 461 patients greater than 65 years of age. Blood 1997; 89:2319.

178. Sterkers Y, Preudhomme C, Lai J-L, et al: Acute myeloid leukemia and myelodysplastic syndromes following essential thrombocythemia treated with hydroxyurea: High proportion of cases with 17p deletion. Blood 1998;91:616.

179. Merlat A, Lai JL, Sterkers Y, et al: Therapy-related myelodysplastic syndrome and acute myeloid leukemia with 17p deletion. A report on 25 cases. Leukemia 1999;13:250.

180. Mosijczuk AD, Ruymann FB: Second malignancy in acute lymphocytic leukemia. Am J Dis Child 1981;135:313.

181. Pui C-H, Ribeiro RC, Hancock ML, et al: Acute myeloid leukemia in children treated with epipodophyllotoxins for acute lymphoblastic leukemia. N Engl J Med 1991;325:1682.

182. Neglia JP, Meadows AT, Robison LL, et al: Second neoplasms after acute lymphoblastic leukemia in childhood. N Engl J Med 1991; 325:1330.

183. Winick NJ, McKenna RW, Shuster JJ, et al: Secondary acute myeloid leukemia in children with acute lymphoblastic leukemia treated with etoposide. J Clin Oncol 1993;11:209.

184. Pui C-H, Relling MV, Rivera GK, et al: Epipodophyllotoxin-related acute myeloid leukemia: A study of 35 cases. Leukemia 1995; 9:1990.

185. Dalton VMK, Gelber RD, Li F, et al: Second malignancies in patients treated for childhood acute lymphoblastic leukemia. J Clin Oncol 1998;16:2848.

186. Pui C-H, Relling MV, Behm FG, et al: L-Asparaginase may potentiate the leukemogenic effect of the epipodophyllotoxins. Leukemia 1995;9:1680.

187. Reimer RR, Hoover R, Fraumeni JF, et al: Acute leukemia after alkylating-agent therapy of ovarian cancer. N Engl J Med 1977; 297:177.

188. Pedersen-Bjergaard J, Nissen NI, Sørensen HM, et al: Acute non-lymphocytic leukemia in patients with ovarian carcinoma following long-term treatment with treosulfan (=dihydroxybusulfan). Cancer 1980;45:19.

189. Greene MH, Boice JD, Greer BE, et al: Acute nonlymphocytic leukemia after therapy with alkylating agents for ovarian cancer. N Engl J Med 1982;307:1416.

190. Einhorn N, Eklund G, Franzén S, et al: Late side effects of chemotherapy in ovarian carcinoma. Cancer 1982;49:2234.

191. Haas JF, Kittelmann B, Mehnert WH, et al: Risk of leukaemia in ovarian tumour and breast cancer patients following treatment by cyclophosphamide. Br J Cancer 1987;55:213.

192. Greene MH: Is cisplatin a human carcinogen? J Natl Cancer Inst 1992;84:306.

193. Colon-Otero G, Malkasian GD, Edmonson JH: Secondary myelodysplasia and acute leukemia following carboplatin-containing combination chemotherapy for ovarian cancer. J Natl Cancer Inst 1993; 85:1858.

194. Travis LB, Holowaty EJ, Bergfeldt K, et al: Risk of leukemia after platinum-based chemotherapy for ovarian cancer. N Engl J Med 1999;340:351.

195. Fisher B, Rockette H, Fisher ER, et al: Leukemia in breast cancer patients following adjuvant chemotherapy or postoperative radiation: The NSABP experience. J Clin Oncol 1985;3:1640.

196. Valagussa P, Tancini G, Bonadonna G: Second malignancies after CMF for resectable breast cancer. J Clin Oncol 1987;5:1138.

197. Falkson G, Gelman RS, Dreicer R, et al: Myelodysplastic syndrome and acute nonlymphocytic leukemia secondary to mitolactol treatment in patients with breast cancer. J Clin Oncol 1989;7:1252.

198. Curtis RE, Boice JD Jr, Moloney WC, et al: Leukemia following chemotherapy for breast cancer. Cancer Res 1990;50:2741.

199. Valagussa P, Moliterni A, Terenziani M, et al: Second malignancies following CMF-based adjuvant chemotherapy in resectable breast cancer. Ann Oncol 1994;5:803.

200. Diamandidou E, Buzdar AU, Smith TL, et al: Treatment-related

leukemia in breast cancer patients treated with fluorouracil-doxo-rubicin-cyclophosphamide combination adjuvant chemotherapy: The University of Texas M.D. Anderson Cancer Center Experience. J Clin Oncol 1996;14:2722.

201. Curtis RE, Boice JD Jr, Stovall M, et al: Risk of leukemia after chemotherapy and radiation treatment for breast cancer. N Engl J Med 1992;326:1745.

202. Bennett JM, Troxel AB, Gelman R, et al: Myelodysplastic syndrome and acute myeloid leukemia secondary to mitolactol treatment in patients with breast cancer. J Clin Oncol 1994;12:874.

203. Linassier C, Barin C, Calais G, et al: Early secondary acute myelogenous leukemia in breast cancer patients after treatment with mitoxantrone, cyclophosphamide, fluorouracil and radiation therapy. Ann Oncol 2000;11:1289.

204. Carli PM, Sgro C, Parchin-Geneste N, et al: Increase therapy-related leukemia secondary to breast cancer. Leukemia 2000;14:1014.

205. Wang SE, Fligiel S, Naeim F: Acute megakaryocytic leukemia following chemotherapy for a malignant teratoma. Arch Pathol Lab Med 1984;108:202.

206. Hoekman K, Huinink WWTB, Egbers-Bogaards MA, et al: Acute leukemia following therapy for teratoma. Eur J Cancer Clin Oncol 1984;20:501.

207. Redman JR, Vugrin D, Arlin ZA, et al: Leukemia following treatment of germ cell tumors in men. J Clin Oncol 1984;2:1080.

208. Nichols CR, Breeden ES, Loehrer PJ, et al: Secondary leukemia associated with a conventional dose of etoposide: Review of serial germ cell tumor protocols. J Natl Cancer Inst 1993;85:36.

209. Bokemeyer C, Schmoll H-J: Secondary neoplasms following treatment of malignant germ cell tumors. J Clin Oncol 1993;11:1703.

210. Boshoff C, Begent RHJ, Oliver RT, et al: Secondary tumours following etoposide containing therapy for germ cell cancer. Ann Oncol 1995;6:35.

211. Bokemeyer C, Schmoll H-J, Kuczyk MA, et al: Risk of secondary leukemia following high cumulative doses of etoposide during chemotherapy for testicular cancer. J Natl Cancer Inst 1995;87:58.

212. Kollmannsberger C, Beyer J, Droz J-P, et al: Secondary leukemia following high cumulative doses of etoposide in patients treated for advanced germ cell tumors. J Clin Oncol 1998;16:3386.

213. Schneider DT, Hilgenfeld E, Schwabe D, et al: Acute myelogenous leukemia after treatment for malignant germ cell tumors in children. J Clin Oncol 1999;17:3226.

214. Bokemeyer C, Schmoll H-J: Treatment of testicular cancer and the development of secondary malignancies. J Clin Oncol 1995; 13:283.

215. Pedersen-Bjergaard J: Acute lymphoid leukemia with t(4;11)(q21; q23) following chemotherapy with cytostatic agents targeting at DNA-topoisomerase II. Leuk Res 1992;16:733.

216. Andersen MK, Christiansen DH, Jensen BA, et al: Therapy-related acute lymphoblastic leukemia with *MLL* rearrangements following DNA topoisomerase II inhibitors, an increasing problem: Report on two new cases and review of the literature since 1992. Br J Haematol 2001;114:539.

217. Travis LB, Curtis RE, Storm H, et al: Risk of second malignant neoplasms among long-term survivors of testicular cancer. J Natl Cancer Inst 1997;89:1429.

218. Kollmannsberger C, Hartmann JT, Kanz L, Bokemeyer C: Therapy-related malignancies following treatment of germ cell cancer. Int J Cancer 1999;83:860.

219. Boice JD, Greene MH, Killen JY Jr, et al: Leukemia and preleukemia after adjuvant treatment of gastrointestinal cancer with semustine (methyl-CCNU). N Engl J Med 1983;309:1079.

220. Chak LY, Sikic BI, Tucker MA, et al: Increased incidence of acute nonlymphocytic leukemia following therapy in patients with small cell carcinoma of the lung. J Clin Oncol 1984;2:385.

221. Pedersen-Bjergaard J, Østerlind K, Hansen M, et al: Acute non-lymphocytic leukemia, preleukemia, and solid tumors following intensive chemotherapy of small cell carcinoma of the lung. Blood 1985;66:1393.

222. Rustin GJS, Newlands ES, Lutz JM, et al: Combination but not single-agent methotrexate chemotherapy for gestational trophoblastic tumors increases the incidence of second tumors. J Clin Oncol 1996;14:2769.

223. Boice JD, Greene MH, Killen JY Jr, et al: Leukemia after adjuvant chemotherapy with semustine (methyl-CCNU)—evidence of a dose-response effect. N Engl J Med 1986;314:119.

224. Meadows AT, Baum E, Fossati-Bellani F, et al: Second malignant neoplasms in children: An update from the Late Effects Study Group. J Clin Oncol 1985;3:532.

225. Pui C-H, Hancock ML, Raimondi SC, et al: Myeloid neoplasia in children treated for solid tumours. Lancet 1990;336:417.

226. Hawkins MM, Wilson LMK, Stovall MA, et al: Epipodophyllotoxins, alkylating agents, and radiation and risk of secondary leukaemia after childhood cancer. BMJ 1992;304:951.

227. Kushner BH, Heller G, Cheung NK, et al: High risk of leukemia after short-term dose-intensive chemotherapy in young patients with solid tumors. J Clin Oncol 1998;16:3016.

228. Stine KC, Saylors RL, Sawyer JR, Becton DL. Secondary acute myelogenous leukemia following safe exposure to etoposide. J Clin Oncol 1997;15:1583.

229. Stone RM: Myelodysplastic syndrome after autologous transplantation for lymphoma: The price of progress? Blood 1994;83:3437.

230. Deeg J, Socié G: Malignancies after hematopoietic stem cell transplantation: Many questions, some answers. Blood 1998;91:1833.

231. Pedersen-Bjergaard J, Andersen MK, Christiansen DH: Therapy-related acute myeloid leukemia and myelodysplasia after high-dose chemotherapy and autologous stem cell transplantation. Blood 2000;95:3273.

232. Miller JS, Arthur DC, Litz CE, et al: Myelodysplastic syndrome after autologous bone marrow transplantation: An additional late complication of curative cancer therapy. Blood 1994;83:3780.

233. Bhatia S, Ramsay NK, Steinbuch M, et al: Malignant neoplasms following bone marrow transplantation. Blood 1996;87:3633.

234. Traweek ST, Slovak ML, Nademanee AP, et al: Clonal karyotypic hematopoietic cell abnormalities occurring after autologous bone marrow transplantation for Hodgkin's disease and non-Hodgkin's lymphoma. Blood 1994;84:957.

235. Krishnan A, Bhatia S, Bhatia R, et al: Risk factors for development of therapy-related leukemia (t-MDS/t-AML) following autologous transplantation (ABMT) for lymphoma [abstract]. Blood 1998;92: 493.

236. Darrington DL, Vose JM, Anderson JR, et al: Incidence and characterization of secondary myelodysplastic syndrome and acute myelogenous leukemia following high-dose chemoradiotherapy and autologous stem-cell transplantation for lymphoid malignancies. J Clin Oncol 1994;12:2527.

237. Stone RM, Neuberg D, Soiffer R, et al: Myelodysplastic syndrome as a late complication following autologous bone marrow transplantation for non-Hodgkin's lymphoma. J Clin Oncol 1994;12: 2535.

238. Friedberg JW, Neuberg D, Stone RM, et al: Outcome in patients with myelodysplastic syndrome after autologous bone marrow transplantation for non-Hodgkin's lymphoma. J Clin Oncol 1999; 17:3128.

239. Wheeler C, Khurshid A, Elias JIA, et al: Low incidence of post-transplant myelodysplasia/acute leukemia (MDS/AML) in NHL patients autotransplanted after cyclophosphamide, carmustine and etoposide (CBV). Blood 1997;90:385.

240. Taylor PRA, Jackson GH, Lennard AL, et al: Low incidence of myelodysplastic syndrome following transplantation using autologous non-cryopreserved bone marrow. Leukemia 1997;11:1650.

241. Pedersen-Bjergaard J, Pedersen M, Myhre J, et al: High risk of therapy-related leukemia after BEAM chemotherapy and autologous stem cell transplantation for previously treated lymphomas is mainly related to primary chemotherapy and not to the BEAM-transplantation procedure. Leukemia 1997;11:1654.

242. Milligan DW, Ruiz de Elvira MC, Kolb HJ, et al: Secondary leukaemia and myelodysplasia after autografting for lymphoma: Results from the EBMT. Br J Haematol 1999;106:1020.

243. Micallef INM, Lillington DM, Apostolidis J, et al: Therapy-related myelodysplasia and secondary acute myelogenous leukemia after high-dose therapy with autologous hematopoietic progenitor-cell support for lymphoid malignancies. J Clin Oncol 2000;18:947.

244. Krishnan A, Bhatia S, Slovak ML, et al: Predictors of therapy-related leukemia and myelodysplasia following autologous transplantation for lymphoma: An assessment of risk factors. Blood 2000;95:1588.

245. Govindarajan R, Jagannath S, Flick JT, et al: Preceding standard therapy is the likely cause of MDS after autotransplants for multiple myeloma. Br J Haematol 1996;95:349.

246. Laughlin MJ, McGaughey DS, Crews JR, et al: Secondary myelodys-

plasia and acute leukemia in breast cancer patients after autologous bone marrow transplant. J Clin Oncol 1998;16:1008.

247. Bhatia R, Slovak ML, Arber D, et al: Risk factors for development of therapy-related leukemia (t-MDS/t-AML) following autologous transplantation (ABMT) for lymphoma [abstract]. Blood 1993;92:493.

248. André M, Henry-Amar M, Blaise D, et al: Treatment-related deaths and second cancer risk after autologous stem-cell transplantation for Hodgkin's disease. Blood 1998;92:1933.

249. Ezdinli EZ, Sokal JE, Aungst CW, et al: Myeloid leukemia in Hodgkin's disease: Chromosomal abnormalities. Ann Intern Med 1969;71:1097.

250. Rowley JD, Golomb HM, Vardiman J: Nonrandom chromosomal abnormalities in acute nonlymphocytic leukemia in patients treated for Hodgkin disease and non-Hodgkin lymphomas. Blood 1977;50:759.

251. Pedersen-Bjergaard J, Philip P, Mortensen BT, et al: Acute non-lymphocytic leukemia, preleukemia, and acute myeloproliferative syndrome secondary to treatment of other malignant diseases. Clinical and cytogenetic characteristics and results of in vitro culture of bone marrow and HLA typing. Blood 1981;57:712.

252. Rowley JD, Golomb HM, Vardiman JW: Nonrandom chromosome abnormalities in acute leukemia and dysmyelopoietic syndromes in patients with previously treated malignant disease. Blood 1981;58:759.

253. Groupe Français de Cytogénétique Hématologique: Chromosome analysis of 63 cases of secondary nonlymphoid blood disorders: A cooperative study. Cancer Genet Cytogenet 1984;12:95.

254. Le Beau MM, Albain KS, Larson RA, et al: Clinical and cytogenetic correlations in 63 patients with therapy related myelodysplastic syndromes and acute nonlymphocytic leukemia: Further evidence for characteristic abnormalities of chromosomes No. 5 and 7. J Clin Oncol 1986;4:325.

255. Kantarjian HM, Keating MJ, Walters RS, et al: Therapy-related leukemia and myelodysplastic syndrome: Clinical, cytogenetic and prognostic features. J Clin Oncol 1986;4:1748.

256. Pedersen-Bjergaard J, Philip P: Cytogenetic characteristics of therapy-related acute non-lymphocytic leukaemia, preleukaemia and acute myeloproliferative syndrome: Correlation with clinical data for 61 consecutive cases. Br J Haematol 1987;66:199.

257. Zaccaria A, Alimena G, Baccarani M, et al: Cytogenetic analysis in 89 patients with secondary hematologic disorders—results of a cooperative study. Cancer Genet Cytogenet 1987;26:65.

258. Whang-Peng J, Young RC, Lee EC, et al: Cytogenetic studies in patients with secondary leukemia/dysmyelopoietic syndrome after different treatment modalities. Blood 1988;71:403.

259. Iurlo A, Mecucci C, Van Orshoven A, et al: Cytogenetic and clinical investigations in 76 cases with therapy-related leukemia and myelodysplastic syndrome. Cancer Genet Cytogenet 1989;43:227.

260. Arthur DC, Berger R, Golomb HM, et al: The clinical significance of karyotype in acute myelogenous leukemia. Cancer Genet Cytogenet 1989;40:203.

261. Bloomfield CD: Chromosome abnormalities in secondary myelodysplastic syndromes. Scand J Haematol 1986;36(Suppl 45):82.

262. Johansson B, Mertens F, Heim S, et al: Cytogenetics of secondary myelodysplasia (sMDS) and acute nonlymphocytic leukemia (sANLL). Eur J Haematol 1991;47:17.

263. Pedersen-Bjergaard J, Pedersen M, Roulston D, et al: Different genetic pathways in leukemogenesis for patients presenting with therapy-related myelodysplasia and therapy-related acute myeloid leukemia. Blood 1995;86:3542.

264. Pedersen-Bjergaard J, Philip P, Larsen SO, et al: Therapy-related myelodysplasia and acute myeloid leukemia. Cytogenetic characteristics of 115 consecutive cases and risk in seven cohorts of patients treated intensively for malignant diseases in the Copenhagen series. Leukemia 1993;7:1975.

265. Mamuris Z, Prieur M, Dutrillaux B, Aurias A: The chemotherapeutic drug melphalan induces breakage of chromosome regions rearranged in secondary leukemia. Cancer Genet Cytogenet 1989;37:65.

266. Le Beau MM, Espinosa RE III, Neuman WL, et al: Cytogenetic and molecular delineation of the smallest commonly deleted region of chromosome 5 in malignant diseases. Proc Natl Acad Sci U S A 1993;90:5484.

267. Fairman J, Chumakov I, Chinault AC, et al: Physical mapping of

the minimal region of loss in 5q-chromosome. Proc Natl Acad Sci U S A 1995;92:7406.

268. Jaju RJ, Boultwood J, Oliver F, et al: Molecular cytogenetic delineation of the critical deleted region in the 5q− syndrome. Genes Chromosomes Cancer 1998;22:251.

269. Horrigan SK, Arbieva ZH, Xie HY, et al: Delineation of a minimal interval and identification of 9 candidates for a tumor suppressor gene in malignant myeloid disorders on 5q31. Blood 2000;95:2372.

270. Le Beau MM, Espinosa RE III, Davis EM, et al: Cytogenetic and molecular delineation of a region of chromosome 7 commonly deleted in malignant myeloid diseases. Blood 1996;88:1930.

271. Tosi S, Scherer SW, Giudici G, et al: Delineation of multiple deleted regions in 7q in myeloid disorders. Genes Chromosomes Cancer 1999;25:384.

272. Fenaux P, Jonveaux P, Quiquandon I, et al: p53 gene mutations in acute myeloid leukemia with 17p monosomy. Blood 1991;78:1652.

273. Lai JL, Preudhomme C, Zandecki M, et al: Myelodysplastic syndromes and acute myeloid leukemia with 17p deletion. An entity characterized by specific dysgranulopoiesis and a high incidence of p53 mutations. Leukemia 1995;9:370.

274. Horiike S, Misawa S, Kaneko H, et al: Distinct genetic involvement of the TP53 gene in therapy-related leukemia and myelodysplasia with chromosomal losses of nos 5 and/or 7 and its possible relationship to replication error phenotype. Leukemia 1999;13:1235.

275. Christiansen DH, Andersen MK, Pedersen-Bjergaard J: Mutations with loss of heterozygosity of p53 are common in therapy-related MDS and AML after exposure to alkylating agents, and significantly associated with deletion or loss of 5q, a complex karyotype and a poor prognosis. J Clin Oncol 2001;19:1405.

276. Castro PD, Liang JC, Nagarajan L: Deletions of chromosome 5q13.3 and 17p loci cooperate in myeloid neoplasms. Blood 2000;95:2138.

277. Tavassoli M, Steingrimsdottir H, Pierce E, et al: Loss of heterozygosity in chromosome 5q in ovarian cancer is frequently accompanied by TP53 mutation and identifies a tumor suppressor gene locus at 5q13.1–21. Br J Cancer 1996;74:115.

278. Tamura G, Ogasawara S, Nishizuka S, et al: Two distinct regions of deletion on the long arm of chromosome 5 in differentiated adenocarcinomas of the stomach. Cancer Res 1996;56:612.

279. Achille A, Baron A, Zamboni G, et al: Chromosome 5 allelic losses are early events in tumors of the papilla of Vater and occur at sites similar to those of gastric cancer. Br J Cancer 1998;78:1653.

280. Andersen MK, Christiansen DH, Kirchhoff M, Pedersen-Bjergaard J: Duplication or amplification of chromosome band 11q23, including the unarranged MLL gene, is a recurrent abnormality in therapy-related MDS and AML, is closely related to mutation of the tp53 gene and to previous therapy with alkylating agents. Genes Chromosome Cancer 2001;31:33.

281. Stephenson J, Lizhen H, Mufti GJ: Possible co-existence of RAS activation and monosomy 7 in the leukemic transformation of myelodysplastic syndromes. Leuk Res 1995;19:741.

282. Side L, Teel K, Wang P, et al: Activating RAS mutations in therapy-related myeloid disorders associated with deletions of chromosomes 5 and 7 [abstract 2252]. Blood 1996;88(Suppl 1):566.

283. DeVore R, Whitlock J, Hainsworth JD, et al: Therapy-related acute nonlymphocytic leukemia with monocytic features and rearrangement of chromosome 11q. Ann Intern Med 1989;110:740.

284. Pedersen-Bjergaard J, Philip P: Balanced translocations involving chromosome bands 11q23 and 21q22 are highly characteristic of myelodysplasia and leukemia following therapy with cytostatic agents targeting at DNA-topoisomerase II. Blood 1991;78:1147.

285. Larson RA, Le Beau MM, Ratain MJ, et al: Balanced translocations involving chromosome bands 11q23 and 21q22 in therapy-related leukemia. Blood 1992;79:1892.

286. Secker-Walker LM, Moorman AV, Bain BJ, Mehta AB: Secondary acute leukemia and myelodysplastic syndrome with 11q23 abnormalities. Leukemia 1998;12:840.

287. Pedersen-Bjergaard, Philip P: Two different classes of therapy-related and de-novo acute myeloid leukemia? Cancer Genet Cytogenet 1991;55:119.

288. Pedersen-Bjergaard J, Rowley JD: The balanced and the unbalanced chromosome aberrations of acute myeloid leukemia may develop in different ways and may contribute differently to malignant transformation. Blood 1994;83:2780.

289. Pedersen-Bjergaard J, Andersen MK, Johansson B: Balanced chromosome aberrations in leukemias following chemotherapy with DNA-topoisomerase II inhibitors. J Clin Oncol 1998;16:1897.

290. Quesnel B, Kantarjian H, Pedersen-Bjergaard J, et al: Therapy-related acute myeloid leukemia with t(8;21), inv(16), and t(8;16): A report on 25 cases and review of the literature. J Clin Oncol 1993;11:2370.

291. Dissing M, Le Beau MM, Pedersen-Bjergaard J: Inversion of chromosome 16 and uncommon rearrangements of the CBFB and MYH11 genes in therapy-related acute myeloid leukemia: Rare events related to DNA-topoisomerase II inhibitors? J Clin Oncol 1998;16:1890.

292. Detourmignies L, Castaigne S, Stoppa AM, et al: Therapy-related acute promyelocytic leukemia: A report on 16 cases. J Clin Oncol 1992;10:1430.

293. Hoffmann L, Möller P, Pedersen-Bjergaard J, et al: Therapy-related acute promyelocytic leukemia with t(15;17)(q22;q12) following chemotherapy with drugs targeting DNA topoisomerase II. A report of two cases and a review of the literature. Ann Oncol 1995; 6:781.

294. Kudo K, Yoshida H, Kiyoi H, et al: Etoposide-related acute promyelocytic leukemia. Leukemia 1998;12:1171.

295. Pedersen-Bjergaard J, Brøndum-Nielsen K, Karle H, et al: Chemotherapy-related—and late occurring—Philadelphia chromosome in AML, ALL and CML. Similar events related to treatment with DNA topoisomerase II inhibitors? Leukemia 1997;11:1571.

296. Pui C-H: Acute leukemias with the t(4;11)(q21;q23). Leuk Lymphoma 1992;7:173.

297. Rubin CM, Larson RA, Anastasi J, et al: t(3;21)(q26;q22): A recurring chromosomal abnormality in therapy-related myelodysplastic syndrome and acute myeloid leukemia. Blood 1990;76:2594.

298. Pedersen-Bjergaard J, Johansson B, Philip P: Translocation (3; 21)(q26;q22) in therapy-related myelodysplasia following drugs targeting DNA-topoisomerase II combined with alkylating agents, and in myeloproliferative disorders undergoing spontaneous leukemic transformation. Cancer Genet Cytogenet 1994;76:50.

299. Gamou T, Kitamaru E, Hosoda F, et al: The partner gene of AML1 in t(16;21) myeloid malignancies is a novel member of the MTG8(ETO) family. Blood 1998;11:4028.

300. Demuynck H, Verhoef GEG, Zachée P, et al: Therapy-related acute myeloid leukemia with t(8;16)(p11;p13) following anthracycline-based therapy for nonmetastatic osteosarcoma. Cancer Genet Cytogenet 1995;82:103.

301. Ahuja HG, Felix CA, Aplan PD: The t(11;20)(p15;q11) chromosomal translocation associated with therapy-related myelodysplastic syndrome results in an NUP98-TOPI fusion. Blood 1999;94: 3258.

302. Nishiyama M, Arai Y, Tsunematsu Y, et al: 11p15 translocations involving the NUP98 gene in childhood therapy-related acute myeloid leukemia/myelodysplastic syndrome. Genes Chromosomes Cancer 1999;3:215.

303. Rowley JD, Reshmi S, Sobulo O, et al: All patients with the t(11; 16)(q23;p13.3) that involves MLL and CBP have treatment-related hematologic disorders. Blood 1997;90:535.

304. Rabbitts TH: Chromosomal translocations in human cancer. Nature 1994;372:143.

305. Look TA: Oncogenic transcription factors in human leukemia. Science 1997;278:1059.

306. Rowley JD: The role of chromosome translocations in leukemogenesis. Semin Hematol 1999;36(Suppl 7):59.

307. Karp JE, Smith MA: The molecular pathogenesis of treatment-induced (secondary) leukemias: Foundations for treatment and prevention. Semin Oncol 1997;24:103.

308. Felix CA: Secondary leukemias induced by topoisomerase-targeted drugs. Biochim Biophys Acta 1998;1400:233.

309. Pui C-H, Relling MV: Topoisomerase II inhibitor-related myeloid leukaemia. Br J Haematol 2000;109:13.

310. Earnshaw WC, Halligan B, Cooke CA, et al: Topoisomerase II is a structural component of mitotic chromosome scaffolds. J Cell Biol 1985;100:1706.

311. Adachi Y, Kás E, Laemmli UK: Preferential, cooperative binding of DNA topoisomerase II to scaffold-associated regions. EMBO J 1989;8:3997.

312. Zechiedrich EL, Osheroff N: Eukaryotic topoisomerase recognizes nucleic acid topology by preferentially interacting with DNA crossovers. EMBO J 1990;4555.

313. Richardson C, Jasin M: Frequent chromosomal translocations induced by DNA double-strand breaks. Nature 2000;405:697.

314. Sperry AO, Blasquez VC, Garrard WT: Dysfunction of chromosomal loop attachment sites: Illegitimate recombination linked to matrix association regions and topoisomerase II. Proc Natl Acad Sci U S A 1989;86:5497.

315. Chen CL, Fuscoe JC, Liu Q, et al: Etoposide causes illegitimate V(D)J recombination in human lymphoid leukemic cells. Blood 1996;88:2210.

316. Hunger SP, Tkachuk DC, Amylon MD, et al: HRX involvement in de novo and secondary leukemias with diverse chromosome 11q23 abnormalities. Blood 1993;81:3197.

317. Gill Super HJ, McCabe NR, Thierman M, et al: Rearrangements of the MLL gene in therapy-related acute myeloid leukemia in patients previously treated with agents targeting DNA-topoisomerase II. Blood 1993;82:3705.

318. Negrini M, Felix CA, Martin C, et al: Potential topoisomerase II DNA-binding sites at the breakpoints of a t(9;11) chromosome translocation in acute myeloid leukemia. Cancer Res 1993;53: 4489.

319. Felix CA, Lange BJ, Hosler MR, et al: Chromosome band 11q23 translocation breakpoints are DNA topoisomerase II cleavage sites. Cancer Res 1995;55:4287.

320. Aplan PD, Chervinsky DS, Stanulla M, et al: Site-specific DNA cleavage within the MLL breakpoint cluster region induced by topoisomerase II inhibitors. Blood 1996;87:2649.

321. Lovett BD, Lo Nigro L, Rappaport EF, et al: Near-precise interchromosomal recombination and functional topoisomerase II cleavage sites at MLL and AF-4 genomic breakpoints in treatment-related acute lymphoblastic leukemia with t(4;11) translocation. Proc Natl Acad Sci U S A 2001;98:9802.

322. Strissel PL, Strick R, Rowley JD, Zeleznik-Le NJ: An in vivo topoisomerase II cleavage site and a DNase I hypersensitive site colocalize near exon 9 in the MLL breakpoint cluster region. Blood 1998; 92:3793.

323. Stanulla M, Wang J, Chervinsky DS, et al: DNA cleavage within the MLL breakpoint cluster region is a specific event which occurs as part of higher-order chromatin fragmentation during the initial stages of apoptosis. Mol Cell Biol 1997;17:4070.

324. Betti CJ, Villalobos MJ, Diaz MO, Vaughan AT: Apoptotic triggers initiate translocations within the MLL gene involving the nonhomologous end joining repair system. Cancer Res 2001;61:4550.

325. Roulston D, Espinosa R III, Nucifora G, et al: CBFA2 (AML1) translocations with novel partner chromosomes in myeloid leukemias: Association with prior therapy. Blood 1998;92:2879.

326. Stanulla M, Wang J, Chervinsky DS, Aplan PD: Topoisomerase II inhibitors induce DNA double-strand breaks at a specific site within the AML1 locus. Leukemia 1997;11:490.

327. Pedersen-Bjergard J, Timshel S, Andersen MK, et al: Cytogenetically unrelated clones in therapy-related myelodysplasia and acute myeloid leukemia: Experience from the Copenhagen series updated to 180 consecutive cases. Genes Chromosomes Cancer 1998;23:337.

328. Andersen MK, Pedersen-Bjergaard J: Increased frequency of dicentric chromosomes in therapy-related MDS and AML compared to de novo disease is significantly related to previous treatment with alkylating agents and suggests a specific susceptibility to chromosome breakage at the centromere. Leukemia 2000;14:105.

329. Felix CA, Megonial MD, Chervinsky DS, et al: Association of germline p53 mutation with MLL segmental jumping translocation in treatment-related leukemia. Blood 1998;12:4451.

330. Michaux L, Wlodarska I, Stul M, et al: MLL amplification in myeloid leukemias: A study of 14 cases with multiple copies of 11q23. Genes Chromosomes Cancer 2000;29:40.

331. Larson RA, Wernli M, Le Beau MM, et al: Short remission durations in therapy-related leukemia despite cytogenetic complete responses to high-dose cytarabine. Blood 1988;72:1333.

332. Kantarjian HM, Estey EH, Keating MJ: Treatment of therapy-related leukemia and myelodysplastic syndrome. Hematol Oncol Clin North Am 1993;7:81.

333. Anderson EA, Gooley TA, Schoch G, et al: Stem cell transplantation for secondary acute myeloid leukemia: Evaluation of transplantation as initial therapy or following induction chemotherapy. Blood 1997;89:2578.

334. Ballen KK, Gilliland DG, Guinan EC, et al: Bone marrow trans-

plantation for therapy-related myelodysplasia: Comparison with primary myelodysplasia. Bone Marrow Transplant 1997;20:737.

335. Yakoub-Agha I, de la Salmonière P, Ribaud P, et al: Allogeneic bone marrow transplantation for therapy-related myelodysplastic syndrome and acute myeloid leukemia: A long-term study of 70 patients—report of the French Society of Bone Marrow Transplantation. J Clin Oncol 2000;18:963.

336. Andersen MK, Larson RA, Mauritzson N, et al: Therapy-related MDS or AML with inv(16) or t(15;17), characteristics and relation to type of primary therapy. Preliminary results from the international workshop on leukemia karyotype and prior treatment [abstract 1995]. Blood 2000;96:463.

337. Sandler ES, Friedman DJ, Mahmoud MM, et al: Treatment of children with epipodophyllotoxin-induced secondary acute myeloid leukemia. Cancer 1997;79:1049.

338. Felix CA, Walker AH, Lange BJ, et al: Association of CYP3A4 genotype with treatment-related leukemia. Proc Natl Acad Sci U S A 1998;95:13176.

339. Chen H, Sandler DP, Taylor JA, et al: Increased risk for myelodysplastic syndromes in individuals with glutathione transferase theta/(GSTT1) gene defect. Lancet 1996;347:295.

340. Sasai Y, Horiike S, Misawa S, et al: Genotype of glutathione S-transferase and other genetic configurations in myelodysplasia. Leuk Res 1999;23:975.

341. Woo MH, Shuster JJ, Chen C, et al: Glutathione S-transferase geno-types in children who develop treatment-related acute myeloid malignancies. Leukemia 2000;14:232.

342. Allan JM, Wild CP, Rollinson S, et al: Polymorphism in glutathione S-transferase P1 is associated with susceptibility to chemotherapy-induced leukemia. Proc Natl Acad Sci U S A (in press).

343. Relling MV, Yanishevski Y, Nemec J, et al: Etoposide and antimetabolite pharmacology in patients who develop secondary acute myeloid leukemia. Leukemia 1998;12:346.

344. Thomsen JB, Schrøder H, Kristinsson J, et al: Possible carcinogenic effect of 6-mercaptopurine on bone marrow stem cells. Cancer 1999;86:1080.

345. Larson RA, Wang Y, Banerjee M, et al: Prevalence of the inactivating [609]C—T polymorphism in the NAD(P)H: Quinone oxidoreductase (NQ01) gene in patients with primary and therapy-related myeloid leukemia. Blood 1999;94:803.

346. Wiemels JL, Pagnamenta A, Taylor GM, et al: A lack of a functional NAD(P)H: Quinone oxidoreductase allele is selectively associated with pediatric leukemia that have MLL fusions. Cancer Res 1999;4095.

347. Ben-Yehuda D, Krichevsky S, Caspi O, et al: Microsatellite instability and p53 mutations in therapy-related leukemia suggest mutator phenotype. Blood 1996;88:4296.

348. Pedersen-Bjergaard J, Andersen MK, Christiansen DH, et al: Genetic pathways in therapy-related myelodysplasia and acute myeloid leukemia. Blood 2002.

10

Thomas F. Schulz   James C. Neil

Viruses and Leukemia

The first evidence that viruses can cause leukemia came in the early days of the 20th century, when Ellerman and Bang showed that chicken leukosis could be transmitted by a filterable agent.[1] This observation was followed over the following decades with further examples of naturally occurring tumors in chickens (sarcomas, myelocytomatosis) that could be passed on in similar fashion. In fact, emerging epidemics of infection with avian leukosis virus continue to present problems for the poultry industry despite the development of control measures.[2] However, for many years, tumor viruses seemed to be an idiosyncrasy of avian species, and it was not until several decades later, with the discovery of viruses that caused leukemias and lymphomas in mice, cats, and cattle, that it was appreciated that viruses could also be relevant to mammalian cancer.[3-5] The ensuing search for viral agents of human cancer has ultimately borne fruit, though perhaps not in a manner that could have been anticipated by the early pioneers. The viruses now known to play a role in human leukemia and lymphoma are generally slow-acting and inefficient leukemogens, but it seems highly probable that additional viral agents are yet to be discovered in human leukemia and that new epidemics will arise in the future. Efforts to identify and characterize viruses as leukemogenic agents are therefore highly relevant to the understanding and control of human leukemia and related diseases. For further detail the reader is referred to a recent compendium on retroviruses[6] or to earlier volumes that have more extensive coverage of the historical roots of RNA tumor viruses[7] and DNA tumor viruses.[8]

The study of viruses has been useful to oncology research in three quite different ways. First, viruses have provided general insight into the mechanisms by which cells are transformed to malignancy and the cellular genes that are the key targets for this process. This field of knowledge is predominantly the product of studies on animal retroviruses, and most of the principles were laid down before the known human retroviruses were discovered. Nevertheless, these discoveries made an immense contribution to our knowledge of human cancer inasmuch as the genes that act as oncogenic targets for animal retroviruses have proved to be highly conserved in evolution and, in many cases, their human homologues have been shown to be affected by nonviral oncogenic mechanisms that include chromosomal rearrangement,

gene amplification, and mutations induced by chemicals or radiation. The first part of this chapter presents a brief outline of the viral families involved and their mechanisms of action. We also consider in more detail two animal retroviruses that inspired the search for human retroviruses and have illuminated our understanding of the natural history of infection by their respective viral families.

The second major contribution of virology to cancer research has been in the identification of viruses that play an etiologic role in human disease. These discoveries raise the prospect of reducing the cancer burden through the identification of infected individuals, interruption of the transmission process by avoidance of infected blood products or immunization, and therapeutic intervention with antiviral drugs. Although these measures are in some cases difficult to achieved in practice, there is no doubt that control of oncogenic virus transmission has already contributed significantly to human health in populations at risk from infection. The bulk of the chapter is devoted to a description of the known human leukemia viruses and their modes of action. Several virus families with distinctive properties and modes of action have been implicated in the etiology of human leukemias or lymphomas and are considered individually. These families are the human T-cell leukemia virus (HTLV) group and two herpesviruses, Epstein-Barr virus (EBV/human herpesvirus-4 [HHV-4]) and Kaposi's sarcoma herpesvirus (KSHV/HHV-8).

Finally, viruses are now being harnessed in experimental cancer therapies both as vectors for gene delivery in vivo and for their capacity to infect and lyse cancer cells in a selective manner. In the case of the retroviruses, it is their ability to precisely integrate into host DNA and engage the host cell machinery for their expression, properties essential to their oncogenic activity, that is also fundamental to their use as therapeutic agents. This aspect of the virus-cancer relationship is covered in some detail in Chapter 19 and is therefore not discussed in detail here.

VIRUSES AND CANCER: GENERAL PRINCIPLES

Highly pathogenic viruses that deplete the numbers of their host species rapidly are short lived in nature; a more successful long-term strategy for a virus is to cause minimal disease and to leave reproductive fitness unimpaired. The oncogenic viruses conform to this general rule; the notable exception of human immunodeficiency virus (HIV) can be attributed to the recent nature of the acquired immunodeficiency virus (AIDS) epidemic and the fact that the balance between host and virus is far from equilibrium. HIV is also atypical because its major role is as a cofactor for other viruses rather than as a directly oncogenic agent. In AIDS-associated malignancies, tumor cells generally lack HIV sequences, and evidence of an etiologic role for this virus rests on the demonstration of epidemiologic associations between infection and the occurrence of the malignancy.[9] Another general principle that must be kept in mind when considering the role of viruses in malignant disease is that cancer development is a multistep process involving an accumulation of mutational changes to key regulatory genes. Viruses can be major or minor players in this process and generally act as risk factors, not as sufficient causes of neoplasia. Oncogenic viruses induce persistent infection and can reach high prevalence in host populations, but their replication is often suppressed by the host immune response. As a result, cell transformation may involve abortive or latent infection in which viral antigens need not be expressed on the tumor cells. This last feature complicates the search for unknown viruses in human cancers, and it can be difficult to establish their etiologic role. Table 10–1 lists viral agents known to play a role in leukemia/lymphoma.

VIRUSES AS MODEL LEUKEMOGENIC AGENTS

The first viruses to reveal the secrets of their leukemogenic mechanisms were the "simple" retroviruses of the alpharetrovirus (avian leukosis virus [ALV]) and gammaretrovirus (murine leukemia virus [MLV], feline leukemia virus [FeLV], gibbon ape leukemia virus [GaLV], reticuloendotheliosis virus [REV]) subfamilies (see Table 10–1 and Fig. 10–1). These RNA viruses replicate via a double-stranded DNA intermediate, the provirus, that becomes integrated into host cell DNA. The integrated provirus expresses viral RNA and proteins under the influence of the host cell transcriptional and translational machinery, and virus particles bud out from the host cell and acquire a host-derived outer membrane in the process. Replication of the simple retroviruses is generally noncytopathic and does not compromise host cell viability. The integrated provirus is therefore passed to daughter cells essentially as a cellular gene. The finding that eukaryotic genomes are littered with retrovirus-like proviruses and related elements, some of which can be shown to have entered the germline before the spread of present-day species, shows that interaction between retroviruses and their host genomes has been a regular feature throughout evolution.[10] Alternatively, when retroviral integration occurs in a nongermline cell, the provirus will be inherited as a somatically acquired mutation. The oncogenic potential of the simple retroviruses can be attributed in part to the accumulation of somatic mutations by this proc-

TABLE 10–1. Viral Agents of Leukemia and Lymphoma

Virus Group	Examples	Host	Hematopoietic Tumors
Retroviridae			
Alpharetrovirus	Avian leukosis virus	Chicken	Bursal lymphoma, myeloid leukemia, erythroblastosis
	Avian myeloblastosis virus		Myeloblastosis
	Myelocytomatosis virus MC29		Myelocytomatosis
	Avian erythroblastosis virus		Erythroblastosis
Betaretrovirus	Mouse mammary tumor virus	Mouse	T-cell lymphoma*
Gammaretrovirus	Murine leukemia virus	Mouse	T-cell lymphoma
	Friend murine leukemia virus		Erythroleukemia
	Moloney murine leukemia virus		T-cell lymphoma
	BXH2 leukemia virus		Myeloid leukemia
	Feline leukemia virus	Cat	T-cell lymphoma, myeloid leukemia, erythroleukemia
	Reticuloendotheliosis virus	Chicken, turkey	Reticuloendotheliosis, lymphoid leukosis
Deltaretrovirus	Bovine leukemia virus	Cattle	B-cell leukemia
	Human T-cell leukemia virus	Humans	Adult T-cell leukemia
Lentivirus†	Human immunodeficiency virus	Humans	B-cell lymphoma
	Simian immunodeficiency virus	Macaque‡	B-cell lymphoma
	Feline immunodeficiency virus	Cat	B-cell lymphoma
Herpesviridae			
Alphaherpesvirus	Marek's disease virus	Turkey, chicken	Lymphoproliferative disease, lymphoma
Gammaherpesvirus	Epstein-Barr virus (HHV-4)	Humans	Burkitt's lymphoma, transplant lymphoma, Hodgkin's disease
	Kaposi's sarcoma herpesvirus (HHV-8)	Humans	Primary effusion lymphoma, multicentric Castleman's disease, plasmablastic lymphoma
	Herpesvirus saimiri	Marmoset‡	T-cell lymphoma
	Herpesvirus ateles	Marmoset‡	T-cell lymphoma
	Murine gammaherpesvirus 68	Mouse	Lymphoproliferative disease

* Caused by an atypical MMTV variant.
† Indirect cause; this virus is not generally found in tumor cells.
‡ Non-native host.

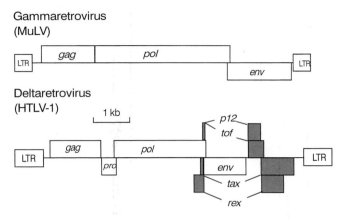

FIGURE 10–1. Genomic structure of oncogenic retrovirus types. The retroviral backbone structure includes (1) the long terminal repeats that carry *cis*-acting signals directing transcription and RNA processing of the viral genome and messenger RNA, as well as (2) three essential genes, *gag, pol,* and *env. Gag* encodes the internal virion proteins that are synthesized as a polyprotein precursor and cleaved to at least three nature virion proteins that are designated MA (matrix), CA (major capsid protein), and NC (nucleocapsid). The *pol* gene is expressed as a large precursor fused to *gag.* This is achieved in MuLV by occasional suppression of a stop codon and in HTLV by ribosomal frame-shifting. Minimally, *pol* encodes the reverse transcriptase (RT) and integrase (IN) enzymes. In some retroviruses, the aspartyl protease (PR) that processes the *gag* and *gag-pol* polyprotein precursors is located in *pol* (MuLV), while in others it is expressed with *gag* (e.g., in the alpharetrovirus ALV) or as a separate frame-shift product (HTLV). The *env* gene is expressed from a subgenomic mRNA as a precursor protein, which is cleaved to yield the major surface glycoprotein (SU) and a transmembrane anchor protein (TM). In addition, the complex retroviruses such as the deltaretroviruses (HTLV, BLV) encode a number of regulatory proteins, only some of which have clearly ascribed functions. The established regulatory functions include transcriptional transactivation (Tax) and regulation of transcript processing and export from the nucleus (Rex).

ess.[11, 12] Because the oncogenic retroviruses carry powerful transcriptional signals that drive expression of the integrated proviral form, they can disrupt the regulation of host cell genes close to the site of insertion (Fig. 10–2). The precise mechanism is variable and depends on the retrovirus, the target gene, and the individual tumor. In some instances, promoter elements in the provirus lead to read-through activation of a cellular gene (promoter insertion). In other cases, the proximity of enhancer elements in the provirus causes the unscheduled activity of endogenous promoter elements of the cellular gene (enhancer insertion). This mechanism may in some cases operate over 100 kilobases (Kb) or more of host cell DNA.[13–16]

More rarely, the retrovirus recombines with host cell DNA and picks up cellular gene-coding sequences at the expense of replicative genes (see Fig. 10–2). This process, known as transduction, is facilitated by the diploid nature of the retrovirus, which allows the propagation of a defective component in a mixed virus population that is sustained by the "helper" function of the replication-competent component. Although transduction is a complex process requiring several recombination events of low probability,[17] many examples have been found in nature, particularly in tumors induced by viruses such as ALV, MLV, and FeLV, which replicate very actively in a

persistently infected host.[18–20] The retroviruses that carry cell-derived oncogenes are among the most potent oncogenic agents known and can in some instances induce malignant disease within 1 or 2 weeks of establishing infection. Recognition of the molecular basis of this phenomenon in 1976 was a major milestone in cancer research.[21] The genes that act as targets for transduction or insertional activation are referred to as oncogenes to indicate that these genes can act in a dominant manner to confer the cancer cell phenotype. The term *proto-oncogene*[22] was coined to distinguish the wild-type version of these genes, many of which may play vital roles in the regulation of normal cellular growth and which encode a variety of growth factors, growth factor receptors, intracellular growth signaling molecules, cell cycle regulators, and transcription factors.[23]

The wider significance of retroviral oncogenes soon became evident from the study of their homologues in the human genome. Analysis of their chromosomal locations in the early 1980s led to the discovery that some of the nonrandom chromosomal rearrangements that were the hallmark of human leukemias (e.g., t[8;14] in Burkitt's lymphoma [BL][24] t[9;22] in chronic myeloid leukemia [CML][25]) involved the disruption and unscheduled expression of the very same proto-oncogenes. Moreover, the normal regulation of these genes can be disrupted by other processes such as gene amplification and point mutation. The list of somatic mutations of these genes in human cancers continues to grow. Table 10–2 lists genes that have been implicated as retroviral targets in leukemia and lymphoma and the human cancers in which they have been shown to be affected by other mechanisms. The information in this table has been distilled from a number of sources.[26–28]

It should be noted that retroviral insertion into a gene may result in loss of function rather than activation. The class of genes whose functions are lost in cancer cells are known as tumor suppressor genes. Eukaryotic cells are relatively resistant to tumor suppressor inactivation by retroviruses because of the very low probability of random integration at both alleles. Nevertheless, such integration can occur, and a number of examples of this phenomenon are well documented in retrovirus-induced cancers.[29, 30]

A distinct mechanism is involved in tumorigenesis by the deltaretroviruses HTLV and bovine leukemia virus (BLV). The oncogenicity of these complex retroviruses appears to rely on regulatory genes that are carried by these viruses, in addition to the basic retroviral complement of gag, pol, and env (see Fig. 10–1). The most important of these agents is the Tax protein, a regulator of viral gene expression that transactivates a wide range of cellular gene promoters and drives the proliferation of infected cells. However, the precise role of the Tax protein in tumor progression and maintenance of the transformed state is less clear-cut, as discussed later in this chapter.

The DNA tumor viruses have also made important contributions to leukemia research, although it is unusual to find viruses of this class that cause acute neoplastic disease in their natural host. For example, some simian herpesviruses cause malignant lymphoma when intro-

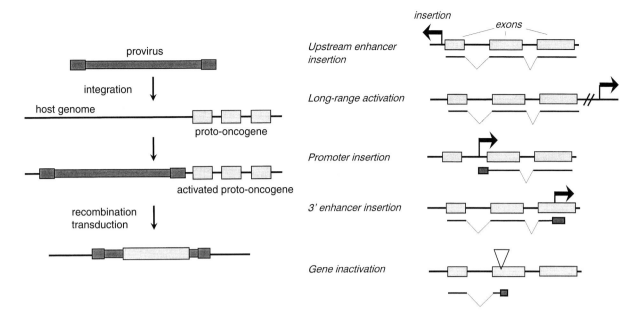

FIGURE 10–2. *Cis*-acting mechanisms of retroviral oncogenesis.
(a) Retroviruses integrate into host cell DNA as an obligatory step in their replication. This is a mutagenic process with consequences that vary according to the site of insertion, the host cell in which it occurs and the regulatory elements carried by the virus. While the integration of retroviruses and related elements is generally a random process, occasional insertion within or near a gene involved in control of cell growth (proto-oncogene) can lead to malignant disease. As a more extreme manifestation, a complex series of rearrangements occurs, resulting in the coding sequence of the cellular gene being captured as part of the viral genome (v-onc). This process is referred to as transduction. Although the resultant virus has lost replicative gene sequences, the diploid state of the retroviral particle helps to maintain it in a complex along with a replication-competent helper virus. Many examples of retroviral transduction of host cell genes have been found, especially in naturally occurring tumors of chickens, cats, and mice (see Table 10-2).
(b) A number of different mechanisms have been identified by which retroviral integration can influence the expression of a host gene in the cancer cell. The transcription unit need not be disrupted by integration if the virus carries powerful transcriptional enhancer elements that activate the cellular gene's own promoter. In some cases, this effect appears to be operative over very long distances (up to 300 kb). Alternatively, hybrid virus-cell transcripts are generated by the activation of the cryptic promoter in the 3′ LTR (promoter insertion). Finally, insertion may cause the disruption of gene function by interference with transcription or mutation of the normal gene product. The diagram depicts the exon structure of a putative target gene with arrows indicating the site and orientation of provirus insertion. The inverted triangle indicates that either orientation would suffice if gene inactivation is the selected outcome.

duced into non-native primate species but are effectively apathogenic in their natural hosts.[31, 32] An apparent exception to this rule is the agent of Marek's disease, a herpesvirus that caused widespread economic loss in poultry before the development of vaccines.[33] However, it could be argued that the extreme susceptibility of chicken flocks to these agents is an artifact of selective breeding for other useful traits.[34]

The most important insights into the molecular basis of cancer provided by the DNA tumor viruses have come from the polyomaviruses, a genus of small DNA viruses that cause a variety of tumors in laboratory rodents but cause few problems in their natural setting. They must be introduced into an inappropriate host species (simian virus 40 [SV40])[35] or the immunologically incompetent newborn (polyoma)[36] to manifest their oncogenic potential. Early studies on SV40-transformed cells revealed the p53 tumor suppressor protein to be a cellular protein that formed a complex with T antigen, the major viral transforming protein.[37, 38] SV40 induces quiescent cells to undergo DNA synthesis in the course of its lytic replication cycle,[39] and this synthesis is achieved in part by the binding and functional inactivation of p53 and Rb proteins by the viral T antigen. These interactions also prevent cells from undergoing apoptosis before productive

replication has occurred[40] and may therefore favor the survival of abortively infected cells expressing only the viral regulatory genes. Further studies have revealed frequent inactivation of the p53 and Rb tumor suppressor pathways in hematopoietic malignancies, and oncogenic viruses from different families appear to have evolved a series of distinct mechanisms of ablating these functions.[41]

LESSONS FROM THE ANIMAL RETROVIRUSES

Although no clear evidence can be found for epidemic infection of the human population by a virus belonging to the "simple" retrovirus classes, the presence of many vestigial proviruses as conserved elements in human DNA indicates the occurrence of many past epidemics.[10] Moreover, human leukemia clusters have been reported in the absence of any known viral involvement, which suggests that an as yet unknown infectious agent or agents may be involved.[42] It is therefore useful to summarize the biology and natural history of animal retroviruses that currently cause disease in their host populations and that provided the impetus to investigate the viral etiology of human leukemia and lymphoma.

TABLE 10–2. Retroviral Targets in Leukemia and Lymphoma

Locus	Tumor Lineage*	Product†	Retroviral Mechanism‡	Human Gene	Cancer	Mechanism§
Abl	B	NRTK	T	*ABL1*	CML, cALL	t(9;22), t(9;12)
Akt	T	SK	T	*AKT1*	Carcinoma	Amp
Bmi-1/flvi-2	B, T	TF	I	*BMI1*		
Cbl	B	A	T	*CBL*		
ErbA	E	NHR	T	*ERBA*		
ErbB	E	RTK	T, I	*ERBB*	Carcinoma	Amp
Evi-1/CB1/fim-3	M	TF	I	*EVI1*	AML	t(3:21)
Evi-2/NF1	M	TF	In	*NF1*	AML	Del
Ets-1/tpl-1	T, M	TF	T, I	*ETS1*		
Fli-1/sic-1	E	TF	I	*FLI1*	Ewing's sarcoma	t(11;22)
Fli-2	E	TF	In	*NFE2*		
Fms/fim-2	M, S	RTK	T, I	*FMS*	AML	PM
Gfi-1/pal1/evi-5	T, B	TF	I	*GFI1*		
Hoxa7	M	TF	I	*HOXA7*		
Kit	F	RTK	T	*KIT*	Mastocytoma	PM
Lck	T	NRTK	I	*LCK*	T-ALL	t(1;7)
Meis1	M	TF	I	*MEIS1*		
Mpl	M	R	T	*MPL*		
Myb	M, T	TF	T, I	*MYB*	AML, CML, ALL	Amp
Myc	T, M	TF	T, I	*MYC*	BL	t(8;14),t(8;2), or t(8;22)
N-myc	T	TF	I	*MYCN*	Neuroblastoma	Amp
Notch1	T	R	I	*NOTCH1*	T-ALL	t(7;9)
Notch2	T	R	T	*NOTCH2*		
Pim-1	T, B	SK	I	*PIM1*		
Pim-2	T, B	SK	I	*PIM2*	Many	PM, del
p53	E	TF	I	*P53*		
Raf/Mil	F, M	SK	T	*RAF*	NHL	inv(2)
Rel	M	TF	T	*REL*		
Sea	E	RTK	T	*SEA*		
Spi-1	E	TF	I	*PU.1*		
Til-1/Cbfal/Runx2	T	TF	I	*RUNX2*		
Tcr	T	R	T	*TCRB*		
Tpl-2	T	SK	I	*TPL2*		
Tiam-1	T	?	I	*TIAM1*	CLL, NHL	t(11;14)
Vin-1	T	C	I	*CCND1*		

* B, B-cell; E, erythroid; F, fibroblast; M, myeloid; T, T-cell.
† A, adapter; C, cyclin; NHR, nuclear hormone receptor; NRTK, non-receptor tyrosine kinase; R, receptor; RTK, receptor tyrosine kinase; SK, serine/threonine kinase; TF, transcription factor.
‡ I, insertional activation; In, insertional inactivation; T, transduction.
§ Amp, amplification; Del, deletion; Inv, inversion; PM, point mutation; T, translocation.
ALL, acute lymphoblastic leukemia; AML, acute myelogenous leukemia; BL, Burkitt's lymphoma; cALL, common acute lymphocytic leukemia; CLL, chronic lymphocytic leukemia; CML, chronic myelocytic leukemia; NHL, non-Holgkin's lymphoma; T-ALL, T-cell ALL.

Feline Leukemia Virus: Behavior of a Virus in a Natural, Outbred Population

Although much of the biochemistry of viral replication was elucidated in studies on other agents (ALV and MLV), FeLV has come to represent the paradigm for the behavior of a simple retrovirus in its natural setting. This virus has afflicted its host for a very long period inasmuch as FeLV-like replication-defective proviruses can be found in the genomes of the domestic cat and its near relatives that diverged an estimated 6 million years ago but are absent from the larger members of the feline species.[43]

FeLV is widespread in the domestic cat population worldwide. Free-ranging cats show serologic evidence of increasing rates of exposure with age.[44] However, susceptibility to infection is highest in young cats, which are most likely to become persistently infected after exposure.[45] Multiple-cat households harboring the virus show the greatest incidence of FeLV-associated disease, presumably because of the high-dose exposure of young cats.[46, 47]

Cats persistently infected with FeLV shed virus in saliva, urine, and milk, and infection often occurs by the oronasal route.[45] However, infection of the fetus across the placenta is highly efficient and is also important in FeLV pathogenesis.[48]

Pathogenesis of FeLV Infection

Initially, FeLV replication is concentrated in local lymphoid organs, but any of three different outcomes follow. Cats may mount an immune response and clear the infection, and this response is more likely to occur in older, immunocompetent animals. At the other extreme, the virus may spread to the bone marrow and then disseminate to multiple epithelial tissues, thereby leading to a lifelong, productive infection.[49] A third and intermediate outcome is also possible: the immune response may limit viral replication so that free virus is not detectable in blood but is readily observed in explanted bone marrow cultures where it is spontaneously activated.[50] This state of latent infection can lead to viral clearance and recovery in the absence of any further insult to the immune system.[51] However, administration of immunosuppressive agents during this phase will cause the infection to progress rapidly to persistent viremia.[52]

Although persistently infected cats can remain healthy for a period, the long-term prognosis is poor, and 85% succumb within 3.5 years. Most morbidity is due to degenerative disease, particularly immunosuppression secondary to virus-induced thymic atrophy.[53] However, neoplastic diseases are also common. Moreover, these diseases are diverse and include, in order of incidence, thymic and multicentric lymphosarcoma of T-cell origin, myeloproliferative disease and myeloid leukemia, alimentary lymphosarcomas of B-cell origin, and multicentric fibrosarcoma.[45]

Analysis of the molecular forms of FeLV in the terminal phases of disease shows that the virus evolves in the course of lifelong persistent infection. Because isolates taken from terminal disease generally reproduce the same limited disease spectrum but after a much reduced latent period, it is clear that this evolutionary process is driving pathogenicity, although the prototype infectious form (FeLV-A) invariably remains and presumably provides the helper virus function essential to sustain replication of the specific pathogenic forms. The variants are defective, not only for independent replication in vitro but also for transmission from cat to cat.[54] Thus, the evolution of variant viruses is important for the pathogenesis of FeLV infection in an individual animal but has little consequence for the epidemiology of viral infection because the variants die out with their hosts.

Subtle alterations to the *env* gene are responsible for variants that induce fatal immunosuppression and aplastic anemia.[55, 56] From cats with neoplastic diseases, three distinct types of change in the genome have been noted. One is sequence duplication within the long terminal repeat (LTR) enhancer elements that is associated with lymphoid tumors of rapid onset.[57] The effect of the sequence duplication may be to increase the efficiency of the virus as an insertional mutagen, and consistent with this model, several common insertion sites for FeLV have been found in feline lymphosarcomas, namely, c-myc, flvi-1, flvi-2, and fit-1.[18, 58-62] Another important source of variation in FeLV oncogenesis is recombination with host cell proto-oncogenes, where a large segment of viral coding sequence is replaced by the host-derived sequence. To date, nine different host cell genes have been found in natural isolates from thymic lymphosarcomas and multicentric fibrosarcomas (reviewed elsewhere[54]). Again, the variant viruses thus generated are capable of reproducing the disease from which they are isolated, but with a greatly reduced latent period.[63] A third type of change is driven by recombination with endogenous FeLV-related proviruses, which yields viruses with expanded host range and, in some cases, increased leukemogenic properties.[64-66]

Control of FeLV Infection

Before the development of prophylactic vaccines, the measures used to control FeLV infection were applied mainly to commercial breeding colonies and were limited to serologic testing for infection and removal of infected animals.[67] More recently, a number of prophylactic vaccines have shown efficacy under experimental conditions and have been licensed for field use, including FeLV-infected lymphoma cell extracts,[68] recombinant subunit vaccines based on the *env* gene product,[69] and recombinant poxviruses carrying FeLV structural genes.[70] The effect of these vaccines on the prevalence of FeLV infection in the field is not yet known.

Bovine Leukemia Virus: An Animal Model for Human T-Cell Leukemia Virus

The discovery of BLV in cattle with persistent lymphocytosis[71] long preceded identification of the HTLV family, but BLV now serves as an important animal model for the human virus because both agents can be grouped together unequivocally on the basis of sequence relatedness and many common features of replication, pathogenesis, and general biology. Together, these viruses comprise the deltaretrovirus subfamily.

Epidemiology and Transmission of BLV

The incidence of bovine leukemia varies markedly throughout the world, although it is one of the most common malignant tumors of cattle.[72] The highest incidence is seen where BLV infection is prevalent, in which case the disease is referred to as enzootic bovine leukosis. The host range of BLV is rather wide, and natural infection with BLV has been recorded in cattle, sheep, capybara, and water buffaloes. BLV can also be transmitted experimentally to goats, pigs, rabbits, rhesus macaques, and chimpanzees. Critical factors in transmission appear to be infected lymphocytes and the number of these cells transferred. The natural routes of transmission in cattle are less clear. In tropical zones, it appears that insect vectors are involved. In temperate zones, iatrogenic infection has also been a significant source in some cases, but infection can also be transferred to calves in utero.[73]

Pathogenesis of BLV Infection

The initial phase of infection with BLV is asymptomatic and detectable only by serology. Persistent lymphocytosis develops in some 30 to 35% of infected cattle within months of infection, whereas clonal tumors eventually develop in less than 5%.[73] In contrast, infected sheep progress more rapidly to the tumor phase, and virtually all succumb to neoplastic disease. In rabbits, BLV induces a wasting disease accompanied by severe neutropenia and lymphopenia.[74]

The major circulating target cells for BLV infection are surface immunoglobulin–bearing B cells that also express CD11c and CD5 markers, whereas BLV-induced tumors are composed of mature B cells.[75] In infected cattle, BLV is expressed in a small number of dividing lymphocytes. Even in persistent lymphocytosis, only a fraction of circulating lymphocytes harbor BLV, and at low copy number. Tumors in BLV-infected cattle and sheep contain integrated BLV proviruses, but these proviruses are not generally detectably expressed in the tumors. The tumors are of clonal origin and contain one or a few BLV proviruses, but no evidence has been presented for a preferred site of integration, which suggests that BLV oncogenesis does not operate by the insertional mutagenesis mechanism that is common to ALV and the gammaretroviruses.[76]

Like its human viral counterpart, BLV encodes regulatory gene products in addition to the basic retroviral complement of gag, pol, and env. The two major products from the 3' region of the genome (X) are p34tax and p18rex, which act in *trans* to regulate, respectively, the viral LTR promoter and the temporal switch from small, multiply spliced to full-length transcripts. Moreover, BLV tax protein can immortalize rat embryo fibroblasts in culture and can act in concert with the H-*ras* oncogene to promote tumorigenic conversion.[77] It is likely that these activities are due to the activation of cellular gene promoters by BLV tax protein, in a manner analogous to HTLV-I tax protein BLV tumor cells do not generally show detectable viral transcripts and sometimes contain only defective proviruses. However, the *tax* gene is invariably retained, thus suggesting that it plays an essential role at some stage of the leukemogenic process.

The role of BLV in tumor development remains unclear, but the low rate of progression to tumors and the lack of viral expression in the tumor cells suggest that it plays a rather inefficient initiating role, with nonviral mutations or cofactors completing and maintaining the malignant phenotype. In this respect, the relationship of BLV to its associated tumors is very similar to its human homologue HTLV.

Control of BLV Infection

In the United States and elsewhere, the high prevalence of BLV infection and relatively late onset of associated disease make control by slaughter of infected animals uneconomical. However, immunity to BLV can be conferred by purified antibodies from infected sheep serum or colostrum from sheep or cows, thereby offering the possibility of control by vaccination. Experimental vaccines based on the major viral glycoprotein gp51 have been promising, and the critical factor appears to be presentation of this glycoprotein in native configuration, where the glycoprotein induces a strong neutralizing antibody response.[78]

VIRUSES AND HUMAN LEUKEMIA

Human T-Lymphotropic Virus Types I and II

HTLV-I is the only human virus that has thus far been etiologically linked to a human leukemia. It causes adult T-cell leukemia (ATL). As discussed in more detail in Chapter 30, ATL was initially recognized as a distinct clinical entity on the basis of its aggressive nature and its geographic clustering in the southwestern parts of Japan.[79] B. Poiesz in R. Gallo's laboratory and I. Miyoshi in collaboration with Y. Hinuma independently discovered a novel human retrovirus in continuous T-cell lines established from patients with ATL.[80, 81]

Biology of HTLV-I

On the basis of electron micrographs, HTLV-I and its close relative HTLV-II were formerly classified as C-type retroviruses.[80, 81] However, HTLV-I virions show a rather inhomogeneous morphology (Fig. 10–3) and differ in this respect from other C-type retroviruses such as MLV and ALV. In addition, the genomic structure of HTLV-I is different from that of other C-type retroviruses (see later and Fig. 10–1), which has led to its classification in the delta-retrovirus group along with BLV (see Table 10–1). In contrast to other retroviruses, cell-free HTLV-I has only very low infectivity in vitro and requires close cell-cell contact for efficient spread.[82] Because epidemiologic evidence suggests that HTLV-I is mainly transmitted with infected cells (see later), HTLV-I virions seem to be poorly infectious in vivo as well. HTLV-I shares this characteristic trait with HTLV-II and BLV, and the reasons for it are unknown. HTLV-I infects cells by binding to a cell surface protein (receptor) that has thus far eluded identification.[83-85] In vitro studies have shown that a wide variety of human cells—as well as many cells from other species—express this receptor molecule.[83-85] In spite of this wide distribution of its cell surface receptor, infection by HTLV-I in vivo appears to involve mainly CD4+ T cells,[86] cells of the monocyte/macrophage series, including dendritic cells,[87] and cells from the synovial lining of arthritic joints.[88]

The genomic structure of HTLV-I is also different from that of the simple retroviruses (see Fig. 10–1). The genes encoding the structural proteins for the core (capsid) particle, the envelope protein, and the enzymes reverse

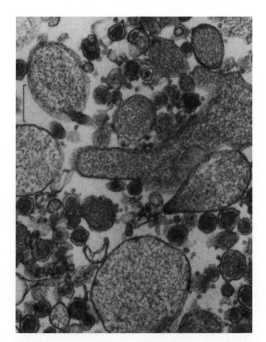

FIGURE 10–3. Electron micrograph of HTLV-I particle. Transmission electron micrograph of HTLV-I producing cells (IL-2-dependent ATL cells in vitro). Bar = 0.2 μm.

transcriptase, integrase, and protease are similar to those found in other retroviruses. In addition to these three structural genes, the HTLV-I genome contains an additional region encoding at least five other nonstructural proteins. One of these proteins, tax, is required for activating the viral promoter in the LTR[89-92] and is also responsible for the transactivation of a series of cellular genes in HTLV-I–infected cells.[93-101] The second of these proteins, rex, is involved in controlling the nuclear export and splicing of HTLV-I–encoded mRNA.[102-105] A detailed discussion of these nonstructural proteins is given in the sections on molecular biology and pathogenesis of ATL.

Epidemiology

HTLV-I is endemic in the southwestern area of Japan,[106, 107] the Caribbean,[108, 109] Africa,[110] South and Central America,[111-113] Melanesia,[114] and Papua New Guinea.[115] In addition, small foci of HTLV-I infection exist in other areas in the world, such as Iran[116] and Southern Italy,[117] and sporadic cases have been reported from many countries.[118, 119] In some of these countries, the epidemiologic link with endemic areas is clear (e.g., Afro-Caribbean immigrants in the United Kingdom); however, in others (e.g., isolated cases in countries of the former Soviet Union), the origin of the virus is still unclear. The sequences of HTLV-I isolates from different geographic regions are highly conserved and closely related to those of a similar simian virus, STLV-I, found in several Asian and African primate species. Likewise, the second human T-lymphotropic virus, HTLV-II, is related to STLV-II, a virus found in African pygmy chimpanzees. Together with STLV-L, a more distant lymphotropic retrovirus from a hamadryas baboon,[120] and a distinct member of the HTLV-II/STLV-II clade obtained from a Central African pygmy chimpanzee (bonobo, *Pan paniscus*), all primate lymphotropic retroviruses are grouped together as PTLV (reviewed elsewhere[120]). Members of the PTLV-I and PTLV-II lineage appear to have largely coevolved with their host species, although examples of possible cross-species transmission have been suggested.[121] It is thought that the common ancestor of the PTLVs may have originated in Africa, with subsequent divergence of the two main branches, as represented by HTLV-I and HTLV-II.[119, 121]

In spite of this high degree of conservation within the HTLV-I branch, three different HTLV-I clades can be distinguished. The first comprises strains from Central Africa, the second (termed the "cosmopolitan subtype") groups strains found in different parts of the world together, and the third represents the most divergent group of HTLV-I isolates and is found in the indigenous populations of Papua New Guinea, Australia, and Melanesia.[115, 120, 122-127] Analysis of HTLV-I sequences from different geographic regions has suggested that HTLV-I may have spread in association with certain populations. Thus, examples of closely related HTLV-I strains in Central or West Africa and the Caribbean support the notion that HTLV-I was brought to the Caribbean via the slave trade from Africa.[123]

HTLV-II has been found in pygmies from Zaire and Cameroon, some of the oldest inhabitants of Africa, and in Gabon and Mongolia and is endemic in several Amerindian populations in both North and South America.[128-134] It is therefore thought to have come to the Americas with the indigenous population during their migration from Asia across the Bering Strait. In addition, HTLV-II has spread to intravenous drug users, in whom it is responsible for most seroreactivity in HTLV-I/II serologic assays.[135, 136] Two closely related subtypes, HTLV-IIa and HTLV-IIb, can be distinguished by sequence analysis and restriction length polymorphism (RFLP).[131, 134, 137]

HTLV-I and HTLV-II are therefore very old viruses that have coexisted with and accompanied some human populations for many millenia. HTLV-I is mainly transmitted neonatally via breast milk and in adult life via sexual intercourse.[138-142] Its seroprevalence in women older than 30 years is higher than in men, thus indicating preferential male-to-female transmission.[140] HTLV-I–infected cells have been found in semen, which could account for the sexual transmission of HTLV-I.[141] Transmission in utero has been documented but seems to be relatively uncommon.[143] Parenteral transmission can occur by blood transfusions[138] and needle sharing, such as occurs among intravenous drug users, and this route is of particular importance for the spread of HTLV-II in intravenous drug users in several Western countries.[135, 136] HTLV-I has not been reported to be transmitted by noncellular blood products (e.g., fresh frozen plasma, factor VIII), thus highlighting the importance of virus-infected cells as vehicles for transmission.

Molecular Biology

In addition to the *gag, pol,* and *env* genes of other C-type retroviruses, HTLV-I and HTLV-II contain a region 3′ of the envelope gene, formerly called pX.[144] This region contains several reading frames and encodes six different nonstructural proteins—tax, rex, p21[rex], p12[I], p30[II], and p13[II]. These proteins are encoded by two exons joined together by multiple splicing of subgenomic mRNA.

The 40-kd tax protein is localized in the nucleus[145] and transactivates the viral promoter[89-91] by interacting with cellular transcription factors that bind to the U3 region of the HTLV-I LTR.[146] The U3 region contains three short 21–base pair (bp) repeats that have been identified as tax response elements (TREs).[146-149] The core of each of these elements is a sequence motif (cyclic adenosine monophosphate response element [CRE]) that is recognized by transcription factors belonging to the family of activating transcription factor/CRE-binding protein (ATF/CREB).[147, 150] Members of this family are characterized by a common structure (basic domain followed by a leucine zipper domain), and their DNA recognition sequence is present in a variety of viral and cellular promoters.[150] Tax achieves its transactivating effect by dimerizing several members of the ATF/CREB family, thus stabilizing the ATF/CREB-CRE interaction, and by recruiting the coactivator CREB-binding protein (CBP) into this complex.[151-153] Tax also binds to minor groove DNA sequences flanking the CRE, thereby forming a high-affinity binding site for the recruitment of ATF/CBP to the HTLV-I LTR.[154, 155]

Role of the Tax Protein in Cellular Transformation

Tax is thought to play a central role in HTLV-I–associated neoplasia. It has been shown to have transforming and tumorigenic properties in rodent fibroblast cultures.[156] Transduction of tax protein into peripheral blood T cells by a retroviral vector results in increased proliferation in the presence of interleukin-2 (IL-2) and anti-CD3 antibody.[157] Tax-transduced cells are still dependent on IL-2 but do not require periodic restimulation with antigen and feeder cells.[157] When a herpesvirus saimiri vector was used to transduce tax protein into cord blood T cells, tax was found to be necessary and sufficient for T-cell immortalization.[158] In transgenic models with different promoters and DNA constructs, tax protein has been reported to induce neurofibromas, mesenchymal tumors, and leukemia.[159-162]

At the molecular level, tax protein can activate or repress a number of cellular genes and interact with several pathways involved in the control of cellular proliferation (see Table 10–3; Figs. 10–4 and 10–5). By virtue of its ability to associate with members of the ATF/CREB family of transcription factors, tax can activate not only the HTLV-I LTR but also several cellular genes whose expression is controlled by members of the ATF/CREB family. An important example is E2F-1,[163] which itself controls the expression of cellular genes required for DNA and chromatin synthesis and cell cycle regulation. Tax also activates several signaling pathways and cellular genes under their control, such as the nuclear factor NFκB and the serum response factor.[164]

Stimulation of ATF/CREB-dependent genes, in particular E2F-1, is thought to play an important part in the permanent proliferation of tax-transduced human primary T cells.[165] In addition, tax protein may promote G_1/ S progression in transduced primary human T cells by stimulating the activity of the cyclin-dependent kinases CDK4 and CDK6 and thereby leading to hyperphosphorylation and thus inactivation of the central G_1/S regulator pRB.[166, 167] The exact basis for this tax-mediated stimulation of CDK4/CDK6 activity is not entirely clear. Tax has

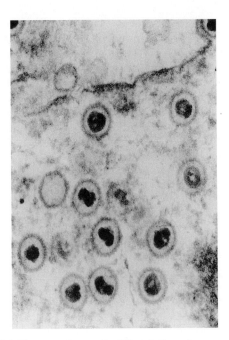

FIGURE 10–4. Electron micrograph of Epstein-Barr virus. Average diameter of viral particles is 120–150 nm (Courtesy of D. Crawford).

been shown to bind to at least two of the cellular CDK inhibitors, p16^INK4a and p15^INK4b, and to interfere with the ability of p16^INK4a to repress CDK4 activity.[168-170] In addition, tax protein represses expression of the p18^INK4c gene[170] (see Fig. 10–5). Moreover, tax can also stimulate CDK4 and CDK6 in a CDK inhibitor–independent pathway, possibly through increased phosphorylation of cyclin D3 in the presence of tax or transcriptional activation of the cyclin D2 gene.[167, 171] However, it is currently not entirely clear how tax protein stimulates cyclin D3 phosphorylation and whether it is indeed responsible for the increased phosphorylation and inactivation of pRB.[167]

Tax also represses the transcription of several cellular genes (see Table 10–3), among them the tumor suppressor p53.[172] On the other hand, the levels and half-life of p53 appear to be increased in HTLV-I-infected or tax-immortalized T cells,[173, 174] and tax protein abrogates the G_1 arrest and apoptosis induced by p53.[175] Many tumor viruses inhibit p53. However, unlike the p53-binding proteins of papillomavirus, adenovirus, and KSHV, tax does not seem to bind p53 directly, but may inactivate p53 by inducing its hyperphosphorylation.[176] It has also been suggested that tax protein could inhibit p53 function through competition for common transcriptional regulators such as CBP, which is involved in p53-mediated transcriptional activation.[177]

Tax also stimulates activation of the NFκB pathway. This activity seems to be required for its ability to transform rodent fibroblasts and confer IL-2 independence on a mouse T-cell line, as well as for its antiapoptotic properties seen in some, but not all experimental systems.[162, 178-180] Tax binds to and stimulates the activity of the IκB kinase complex and thus induces increased phosphorylation and inactivation of the NFκB inhibitor IκBα, which in turn leads to increased translocation of free NFκB to the nucleus[181, 182] (see Fig. 10–6).

TABLE 10–3. Cellular Genes Induced by Tax and Cellular Pathways Involved

Cellular Gene	Cellular Transcription Factor Involved
Cytokines and receptors	
GM-CSF, IL-1, IL-2, IL-6, IL2Rα (CD25), IL-8, IL-15, TNF-α, TNF-β	NF-κB
Transcription factors and proto-oncogenes	
c-*myc*, c-*rel*	NF-κB
c-*fos*, *erg*-1, *fra*-1	SRF
c-*sis*	EGR-1
Cell adhesion molecules	
gp34, ICAM-1, vimentin	NF-κB
OX-40	?
Inhibitors of apoptosis	
A-20	NF-κB
Genes repressed by Tax	
β-Polymerase, Bax, p53	
Lck	BHLH
Zap-70	?

Detailed references can be found in work by Sun et al., 1999.
GM-CSF, granulocyte-macrophage colony-stimulating factor; ICAM, intercellular adhesion molecule; IL, interleukin; NF, nuclear factor; TNF, tumor necrosis factor.

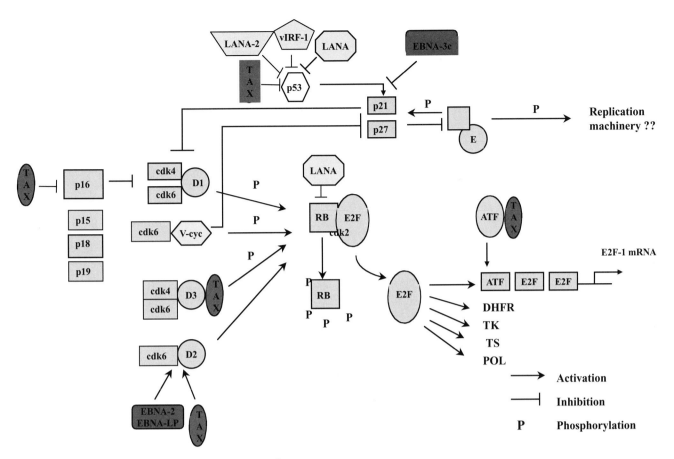

FIGURE 10–5. HTLV-I, EBV, KSHV and G1 checkpoint control.
Key players in the control of the G1/S checkpoint of the cell cycle are the retinoblastoma protein (RB), the cellular D-type cyclins D1, D2, D3, the cyclin-dependent kinases cdk4 and cdk6, the cdk-inhibitors p16, p15, p18, p19, and p53. During physiological G1/S transition RB is inactivated through phosphorylation by a complex of cdk4 or cdk6 and one of the cellular D-type cyclins. The cdk/cyclin complex is itself under negative control by the family of cdk inhibitors. P53 can arrest G1/S progression by activating p21, which has a negative regulatory effect on cdk4/6-D-type cyclin complex.

As outlined in the text, several viral proteins of the three human viruses involved in hematopoietic malignancies can interfere with these pathways and common themes have evolved for these three viruses. Thus HTLV-I Tax can inhibit p53 and the cdk inhibitors and can functionally interact with the cdk4–cyclin D3 complex as well as the cdk6-D2 complex. The net effect of these interactions would be to promote Rb phosphorylation and thus G1/S progression. EBV EBNA-2 and EBNA-LP induce cdk6-D2 activity and KSHV v-cyc interacts with cdk6 to phosphorylate Rb. LANA also inhibits p53 and pRB function. Two viral homologues of interferon regulatory factors (vIRF and LANA-2) also inhibit p53 function.

Although antiapoptotic properties have been described for tax protein in some experimental systems, it has also been reported to induce apoptosis in some T-cell lines, and such induction may, at least in part, involve the Fas/CD95 pathway and caspase function.[183, 184]

Among other reported properties of tax protein are its ability to bind to the human homologue of the *Drosophila* discs large tumor suppressor protein DLG.[185, 186] Tax blocks the inhibitory effect of DLG on proliferation.[185] The ability to bind DLG has also been reported for the human papillomavirus-18 E6 protein and an E4 region–derived adenoviral protein.[186] Tax also binds to TXBP151, a protein that blocks tumor necrosis factor α or CD95 (Fas/Apo-1)-induced apoptosis and is cleaved by caspases 3, 6, and 7.[187]

Other HTLV-I–Encoded Nonstructural Proteins

The 27-kd rex protein is localized in the nucleolus[188] and is involved in exporting unspliced (genomic RNA encoding gag/pol) or singly spliced (encoding env) viral RNA to the cytoplasm (reviewed by Cann and Chen[189]). p30[II] is a nuclear protein of as yet unidentified function that associates with mitochondria.[190, 191] p12[I] is associated with internal membranes, can cooperate with the transforming protein E5 of bovine papillomavirus in transforming cultured cells, and interacts with the β chain of the IL-2 receptor in T cells.[192-194] p12[I] is not needed for the ability of HTLV-I to transform T cells in vitro, but it is required for efficient viral replication in the rabbit model.[195]

Progression to Adult T-Cell Leukemia

In spite of these pleiotropic effects of tax and other proteins on different regulatory pathways and the tax-mediated deregulation of cellular gene expression, it is likely that additional events are required during the progression from HTLV-I–infected T cell to an ATL leukemic clone. ATL develops in only a small proportion of infected individuals, usually after a long latency period of several decades. It has been estimated that infection with HTLV-I in childhood carries a lifetime risk of development of ATL of around 4%.[196] However, very young children with ATL have been reported on a few occasions.[112]

Individuals infected with HTLV-I may harbor an oligoclonal population of HTLV-I–bearing T cells.[197] The size and clonality of this population are thought to be lower in asymptomatic individuals than in patients with tropical spastic paraparesis/HTLV-I–associated myelopathy (TSP/HAM) or, at the other end of the spectrum, in patients with "smouldering" or chronic ATL. Results of ex vivo cultures of HTLV-I–infected T cells suggest that these cells display an "activated" rather than a fully immortalized phenotype. Thus, HTLV-I–infected T-cell clones established from individuals with TSP/HAM resemble normal T-cell clones in being dependent on IL-2 and periodic restimulation by feeder cells, but they exhibit increased spontaneous proliferation in the absence of IL-2.[198] Infection of human T cells in vitro with HTLV-I can, however, lead to complete immortalization and IL-2 independence. HTLV-I–transformed T-cell lines express increased levels of Signal Transducers and Activators of Transcription (STAT) 1, STAT3, and STAT5, and this response has been attributed to tax.[199-201] Such activation has been suggested to render HTLV-I–infected cells more sensitive to the effects of IL-2, which induces the DNA-binding activity of STAT3 and STAT5, and to facilitate the early, still IL-2–dependent steps of HTLV-I–mediated T-cell transformation.[201] In contrast, transformation of T cells by HTLV-II does not appear to be linked to JAK/STAT activation.[201a]

HTLV-I–infected T cells are a target for virus-specific cytotoxic T lymphocytes (CTLs) in vivo. Recent immunogenetic studies suggest that particular major histocompatibility complex (MHC) class I alleles that allow the occurrence of a CTL epitope in tax are associated with better control of viral load in vivo and a lower risk of TSP/HAM.[202] Thus, an expanded population of HTLV-I–infected cells may represent an increased risk for the development of disease. Other HLA class I haplotypes are associated with an increased risk for TSP/HAM, as well as possibly ATL in as much as some HLA haplotypes have been linked to an increased risk for ATL.[203, 204]

The HTLV-I genome is integrated into the chromosomal DNA of infected cells, but no evidence has been found that integration occurs preferentially at particular sites in leukemic cells.[205] Recent observations suggest a slight preference for adenosine/thymidin (A/T)-rich regions of the human genome.[206] Insertional activation of cellular oncogenes does not therefore seem to play a role in most cases of ATL. In many cases, the integrated proviruses have undergone partial deletions; if such is the case, the X region, together with the 5′ LTR, is usually preserved.[207] Only very low levels of transcription of mRNA encoding tax, rex, p21, and p12^I can be detected by polymerase chain reaction (PCR) in a proportion of peripheral blood mononuclear cell (PBMC) from samples from patients with ATLL,[191] thus suggesting that in ATL cells, the virus genome is usually transcriptionally silent. It is therefore likely that other oncogenic events are responsible for the progression to a leukemic phenotype.

Components of the JAK/STAT pathway, in particular, JAK3, STAT1, STAT3, and STAT5, are constitutively active in ATL cells. This activity correlates with cell cycle progression.[208] Constitutive activation of the JAK/STAT pathway may thus represent a crucial step in the acquisition of IL-2 independence and progression to a leukemic phenotype.[199-201, 208] ATL cells have accumulated a series of chromosomal abnormalities, but so far no chromosomal abnormality has been found to be specific for ATL (see Chapter 30). Whether any of the cellular genes affected by these chromosomal abnormalities contribute to the characteristic features of ATL cells is therefore not currently known.

Association with Other Lymphomas

Starting with the patient from whom HTLV-I was first isolated, several reports have described an association of two other hematologic malignancies, Sézary's syndrome and mycosis fungoides, with HTLV-I.[81, 209, 210] Several studies have demonstrated the presence of deleted HTLV-I genomes in biopsy from patients with mycosis fungoides and other cutaneous T-cell lymphomas, but the reported proportions of HTLV-I–positive cases differ widely,[209, 210] and several groups have concluded that HTLV-I is not associated with most cases of Sézary's syndrome and mycosis fungoides outside HTLV-I–endemic regions (e.g., see Bazarbachi et al.[211]). Rarely, HTLV-I–associated T-cell lymphomas may occur in individuals lacking antibodies to HTLV-I.[212]

A few cases of B-cell chronic lymphocytic leukemia (B-CLL) in HTLV-I–positive individuals have been reported[213] without evidence for integration of HTLV-I in the leukemic cells. In two cases, the immunoglobulin synthesized by the leukemic cells was specific for two structural proteins of HTLV-I,[213] compatible with the notion that these cases resulted from the neoplastic transformation of an HTLV-I–specific B-cell clone whose proliferation was continuously stimulated by the presence of antigen. Continuous antigenic stimulation by a bacterial antigen may contribute to the development of B-cell gastric lymphomas.[214] However, no epidemiologic evidence has demonstrated an increased rate of CLL in HTLV-I–positive individuals from endemic countries.[215] These few CLL cases in HTLV-I–infected individuals are therefore either coincidental or occur rarely as a result of chronic antigenic stimulation by HTLV-I antigens.

Occasional cases of HTLV-I–associated Hodgkin's disease (HD) have been reported.[216]

Does HTLV-II Have a Role in Human Leukemia?

Although the first HTLV-II isolate was made from a patient with hairy-cell leukemia,[217] it has never been established that it was present in leukemic cells from this patient. A second isolate of HTLV-II[218] came from a patient with a B-cell hairy-cell leukemia and a coexisting malignant CD8$^+$ T-cell clone. The latter clone had the HTLV-II genome integrated.[218a] One case of mycosis fungoides in an HTLV-II–infected patient has been reported without evidence that the virus was present in the leukemic cell population.[210] A link between HTLV-II and occasional cases of large granular lymphocytic leukemia has been suggested.[128] Again, it is not clear from these studies whether HTLV-II was present in the leukemic cells or in other cell populations.

Association of HTLV-I/II with Other Diseases

In addition to ATL, HTLV-I is clearly associated with TSP and HAM.[219, 220] In addition, it has been linked to chronic inflammatory arthropathy, uveitis, polymyositis, and infective dermatitis.[88, 221-224] The involvement of HTLV-II in a rare chronic neurodegenerative condition has been suggested but remains unconfirmed.[225]

Epstein-Barr Virus

EBV (Fig. 10–6), one of the eight human herpesviruses known to date, is associated with several human malignancies, including endemic BL, nasopharyngeal carci-noma, large-cell B-lymphoblastic lymphoma in immuno-suppressed individuals, HD, and rare cases of T-cell lymphoma.

Epidemiology

EBV has a worldwide distribution, and seroprevalence in adults reaches 90%. Infection with EBV occurs during the first years of life in the developing world, but it is delayed into later childhood or adolescence in many individuals in Western society (reviewed elsewhere[226]). The most important route of transmission of EBV is via saliva.[226, 227] Although EBV has also been found in cervical secretions, no epidemiologic evidence of venereal transmission has been demonstrated.[228] Occasional reports of EBV transmission through blood transfusion have been reported.[229]

In adolescents, primary infection with EBV causes infectious mononucleosis (glandular fever), whereas it is asymptomatic or associated with only nonspecific symp-

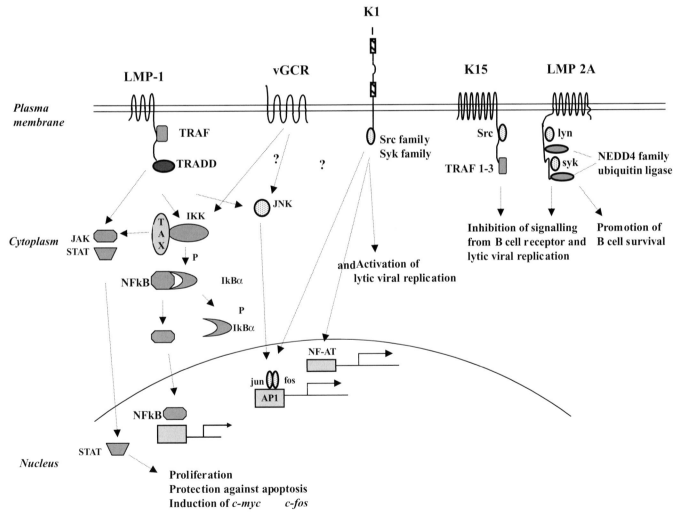

FIGURE 10–6. HTLV-I, EBV and KSHV interact with signalling pathways triggered by cellular membrane proteins. HTLV-I Tax, EBV LMP-1 and LMP2A, KSHV K1, K15 and vGCR interfere with intracellular signalling chains normally triggered by cellular membrane receptors. Thus LMP-1 and vGCR activate the NFkB and JNK pathways. LMP-1 and Tax can activate the JAK/STAT pathway. K1, K15 and LMP2A are phosphorylated on tyrosine residues and recruit members of the src and syk tyrosine kinase families. This can lead to the activation of cellular genes (KSHV K1, vGCR; EVB LMP-1), viral lytic replication (KSHV K1), the promotion of the survival of infected B cells (EBV LMP2A and LMP-1; perhaps KSHV K15/LAMP) and the expression of paracrine factors (vEGF induced by vGPCR; see text).

toms during the first years of life (reviewed by Rickinson and Kieff[226]).

Biology of EBV Infection

EBV is classified as a γ_1-herpesvirus, or lymphocryptovirus. Related viruses are found in many Old World primate species (reviewed elsewhere[230]). Two types of EBV, EBV-1 and EBV-2 (or EBV-A and EBV-B), circulate in many human populations, differ in their biologic properties, and can be distinguished on the basis of polymorphism in the EBV nuclear antigens (EBNA) 2, 3A, 3B, and 3C.[231-234] In most populations, type 1 strains predominate. Coinfection in one individual with both strains appears to be rare, but it does occur in HIV-1–infected homosexual men.[235] In dually infected individuals, recombination between types 1 and 2 can occur.[234, 236]

Like other herpesviruses, EBV has a double-stranded DNA genome of considerable size (172 kb) (for review, see Kieff[230]). Viral replication occurs in the oropharyngeal epithelium and the virus is shed into saliva, but viral shedding has also been reported for cervical secretions[227, 228, 237, 238] for review, see Rickinson and Kieff.[226] However, EBV persists mainly in B lymphocytes, where it adopts a latent (restricted) pattern of gene expression.

A total of six nuclear proteins (EBNA 1, 2, 3A, 3B, 3C, and 5), two latent membrane proteins (LMP 1 and 2), and two EBV-encoded, small, nonpolyadenylated RNAs (EBER 1 and 2) are expressed during latent viral persistence (reviewed elsewhere[226, 230]). Three patterns of latent gene expression can be distinguished. The most restricted pattern, latency pattern I, is adopted in BL cells and involves only the expression of EBNA-1 and the EBERs. Latency pattern II, found in nasopharyngeal carcinoma, HD, and EBV-associated T-cell lymphoma, consists of EBNA-1, EBERs, LMP-1, and LMP-2. In EBV-associated large-cell lymphoma in immunocompromised individuals, all six EBNAs, as well as the two LMPs and EBERs, are expressed (latency pattern III).

LMP-1 has oncogenic properties. LMP-1–transfected RAT-1 cells produce tumors in nude mice.[239] In transgenic mice, LMP-1 induces epidermal hyperplasia and aberrant keratin expression.[240] LMP-1 also inhibits the differentiation of epithelial cells and causes loss of contact inhibition.[239, 241] Biochemically, LMP-1 interacts with several pathways of intracellular signal transduction (see Fig. 10–5; reviewed elsewhere[226, 230]). It activates NFκB and the c-jun N-terminal kinase (JNK) and also triggers JAK/STAT activation.[242-244] LMP-1 expression also leads to expression of the antiapoptotic proteins Bcl-2 and A20 and the adherence molecules intercellular adhesion molecule-1 (ICAM-1), lymphocyte function-associated glycoprotein-1 (LFA-1), LFA-3, and in concert with EBNA-2, CD23.[245, 246]

EBNA-2 activates several viral (e.g., LMP-1) and cellular (e.g., CD23) promoters by binding to the transcriptional repressor CBF-1/RBP-Jk, as well as other modulators of transcription[247, 248]; for review, see Kieff.[230] Its ability to interact with CBF-1/RBP-Jk resembles that of the intracellular form of the developmental regulator Notch. However, it is likely that the role of EBNA-2 is more complex than that of notch.

EBNA-1 is a DNA-binding protein that recognizes a specific 30-bp sequence element occurring in three locations in the EBV genome. One of these locations represents the latent origin of replication, ori P, which is required for closed circular viral DNA molecules to replicate as episomes (reviewed by Kieff[230]). EBNA-1 is associated with human chromosomes during mitosis and may thus ensure the propagation of viral episomes during cell division. The EBNA-1 recognition element can act as an enhancer sequence, and in its presence EBNA-1 acts as a transcriptional activator.[249, 250] Lymphomas have been reported to develop in EBNA-1 transgenic mice.[251] When expressed in an EBV-negative cell line, EBNA-1 has been reported to inhibit differentiation and increase tumorigenicity.[252]

EBNA-3A and EBNA-3C are required for EBV-mediated B-cell transformation in vitro, whereas EBNA-3b is not needed.[253] EBNA-5 (also termed EBNA-LP), in concert with EBNA-2, activates the expression of cyclin D and progression through the G_1/S checkpoint of the cell cycle.[254]

EBV uses a complement receptor, CR2, as its receptor to enter its target cells.[255] This molecule is expressed on B cells, as well as on some epithelial cells of the nasopharynx and cervix. CR2 is expressed on circulating and noncommitted naive B cells of the germinal center and its expression is lost during the maturation to plasma cells. Noncommitted B cells normally have a short life span in vivo and are eliminated by programmed cell death (apoptosis). It is thought that expression of one or several of the "latent" EBV genes EBNA-2, EBNA-3ABC, EBNA-LP, and LMP-1/2 permits EBV to persist in human B cells by enabling them to escape apoptosis.[256] LMP-1–mediated activation of BCL-2, A20, or the NFκB pathway may play a role in this protection against apoptosis (see earlier).

When grown in vitro, EBV-infected normal human B cells are immortalized and show signs of a transformed phenotype (i.e., growth to high density in the presence of reduced serum concentrations, formation of cellular aggregates, tumor formation in severe combined immunodeficient mice). Some of the "latent" genes, in particular, EBNA-2 and LMP-1, contribute to this phenotype, which may, at least in part, be attributable to increased expression of the cell surface adherence molecules ICAM-1, LFA-1, LFA-3, and CD23 (reviewed elsewhere[226]).

Several lines of evidence indicate that in vivo, the proliferation of EBV-infected B cells is controlled by EBV-specific T cells. The EBV latent proteins EBNA-3A, EBNA-3B and EBNA-3C are frequently targets for such responses, but epitopes of EBNA-2, EBNA-LP, or the LMPs have also been shown to be recognized. By contrast, CTL responses against epitopes of EBNA-1 have not been observed (reviewed by Rickinson and Kieff[226]) because of an internal repeat sequence in EBNA-1 (Gly-Ala repeat) that inhibits its processing by the immunoproteasome to CTL-recognizable peptides.[257] As a consequence, latently infected human B cells, as well as tumor cells from EBV-positive large-cell lymphomas (see later) expressing the full set of "latent" EBV genes, are susceptible to lysis by EBV-specific CTLs. In contrast, EBV-associated BL cells, which express only EBNA-1, are not.[226] The importance of cellular immunity in controlling EBV in vivo is highlighted by the fact that it is possible to obtain EBV-transformed B cells from nearly all EBV-seropositive individuals by culturing their PBMCs after depleting T cells or by treating cultures with cyclosporine, a potent inhibitor of T-cell proliferation. Primary infection with EBV is controlled by EBV-specific T cells and can be life threatening in immunodeficient individuals.[226] Patients suffering from X-linked lymphoproliferation syndrome—an inherited immune deficiency—are unable to control EBV infections, and malignant EBV-associated lymphoma frequently develops during the course of primary EBV infections.[258] Finally, in immunocompromised transplant recipients, EBV is the main cause of large-cell immunoblastic lymphoma.

Lymphomas Associated with EBV

BURKITT'S LYMPHOMA

BL, first described by Denis Burkitt as a common childhood cancer in African children,[259] occurs in three settings: (1) endemic BL in areas of holoendemic malaria[260]; (2) sporadic BL, a rare tumor in Western countries; and (3) BL in AIDS patients. All three forms are histologically similar but may differ in their clinical features, in particular with regard to the anatomic sites involved. All three forms also share the hallmark translocation that involves the c-myc gene on chromosome 8q24 and either the immunoglobulin heavy-chain gene locus on chromosome 14 or one of the two light-chain loci on chromosomes 2 or 22.

EBV was first discovered in cultured BL cells.[261] It is virtually always found in the tumor cells of endemic BL but in only 15% to 25% of sporadic BL and 30% to 40% of cases of BL in AIDS patients.[226]

The high incidence of BL in regions of holoendemic malaria and in AIDS patients[262] points to the role of cofactors in the development of this disease. Unlike EBV-associated large B-cell lymphoma, BL is not more common in iatrogenically immunosuppressed patients, and the increased incidence in AIDS patients is therefore unlikely to be due to immune deficiency. In addition, as outlined earlier, the only EBV protein expressed in BL cells, EBNA-1, is not recognized by CTLs. In the absence of LMP-1 and EBNA-2, BL cells do not express cell surface adherence molecules such as LFA-1, ICAM-1, and LFA-3, which favor the interaction between CTLs and their targets.[263] BL cells would therefore not be expected to have a "survival advantage" in immunocompromised individuals. Infection with HIV-1—or another agent common in AIDS patients—may therefore act as a cofactor for the development of BL, similar to malaria or other cofactors in endemic BL in Africa. How these cofactors exert their effect is not clear. Children with acute malaria have higher numbers of EBV-producing peripheral blood B cells than do children without malaria infection.[264] HIV is known to cause polyclonal B-cell activation and hypergammaglobulinemia. It is therefore possible that the increased B-cell proliferation common to these two conditions might be a contributory factor. The phenotype of a BL cell (expression of CD10 and CD77; lack of activation markers such as CD23, CD30, CD39, and CD70 and adherence markers such as LFA-1, LFA-3, and ICAM-1) corresponds to that of a germinal center B cell.

Given that BL can occur in the absence of EBV infection and that BL cells lack many of the transactivating or transforming EBV proteins expressed in other EBV-associated malignancies (see later), the role of EBV in the pathogenesis of this tumor has been difficult to define. However, BL is strongly associated with EBV in all geographic regions with a BL incidence above the low rates seen in Western countries (reviewed elsewhere[226]), and EBV-positive BL cells harbor monoclonal EBV episomes, thus suggesting that EBV infection preceded emergence of the malignant clone.[265] These observations argue in favor of a causative role of EBV in the pathogenesis of this tumor.

EBV may increase the likelihood for the "hallmark" c-myc translocation by expanding the pool of proliferating B cells undergoing rearrangement of their immunoglobulin genes. However, it is also conceivable that EBV infects and expands B-cell clones that have suffered one of these translocations.[266] Because B-cell clones carrying c-myc translocations are no longer susceptible to apoptosis, expression of the latent EBV genes EBNA-2 and LMP would not be required in these cells.

EBV-ASSOCIATED IMMUNOBLASTIC LYMPHOMA IN IMMUNOSUPPRESSED INDIVIDUALS

EBV-positive large-cell immunoblastic lymphoma is a frequent complication in iatrogenically immunosuppressed individuals and in patients with AIDS.[262, 267] The spectrum of lymphoma associated with iatrogenic immunosuppression ranges from diffuse polymorphic B-cell hyperplasia to diffuse polymorphic B-cell lymphoma. Based on the pattern of immunoglobulin gene rearrangements, the B-cell proliferation may be oligoclonal as well as monoclonal.[268-270] Tumor cells express the most extensive pattern of latent genes (latency pattern III; see earlier), including all six EBNAs, LMP-1 and LMP-2, and the EBERs.[271-273] Their phenotype is therefore identical to that of B cells transformed in vitro with EBV. Because the main targets for EBV-specific CTLs are expressed in these tumors, it is thought that they originate from EBV-carrying B cells that proliferate in the presence of an impaired T-cell immunity.

EBV AND HODGKIN'S DISEASE

Evidence accumulated over the last years strongly suggests that EBV plays a role in the pathogenesis of some cases of HD. Many patients with HD have elevated antibody titers to EBV (reviewed by Jarrett and MacKenzie[274]). By Southern blot analysis and PCR, several laboratories have demonstrated the presence of EBV in biopsy samples from patients with HD. Up to 50% of patients in Western countries[275-278] and nearly all patients in some developing countries[279] carry EBV in Hodgkin/Reed-Sternberg (RS) cells, the neoplastic component of HD. By using Southern blot hybridization with probes to measure the number of terminal repeats in episomal (circular extrachromosomal) viral DNA, monoclonal EBV episomes have been documented in HD biopsy specimens, thus indicating that EBV infection precedes the emergence of a monoclonal tumor cell population.[275, 277, 280] In one study,[281] the same clonal episome was found in samples from different body sites, and in one report, the same terminal repeat pattern was found in the original tumor and after relapse.[282]

EBV adopts a latency II pattern in RS cells; that is, EBNA-1, EBERs, and LMP-1 and LMP-2 are expressed.[276, 283, 284] A few cases express BZLF-1,[284] which controls the switch between EBV latency and replication; therefore, a few cells may undergo productive viral replication. In view of the oncogenic properties of LMP-1 (see earlier), its expression in RS cells is taken as further evidence that EBV may contribute to the pathogenesis of HD.

Analysis of the immunoglobulin gene rearrangement pattern in single RS cells isolated by micromanipulation has revealed clonal V_H and/or V_L gene rearrangements.[285-287] In addition, evidence of somatic mutations was found in the variable regions of the rearranged immunoglobulin genes.[285] This observation suggests that RS cells are derived from germinal center B cells, specifically, B cells in which the normal process of immunoglobulin gene rearrangement and somatic hypermutation has taken place (for review, see Kuppers and Rajewsky[288]). In the case of HD of the mixed cellularity, nodular-sclerosing, and lymphocyte-depleted form, somatic mutations have been found that would "cripple" the antibody variable region such that the corresponding B cells would not normally be capable of recognizing antigen and thus be destined to undergo apoptosis. To explain their survival, these B cells would therefore have to be protected against apoptosis. It is conceivable that in the case of EBV-associated HD, LMP-1–mediated induction of BCL-2 and A20 or the NFκB pathway (see earlier) could allow these cells to escape apoptosis (see elsewhere[288] for review). NFκB has been found to be constitutively active in RS cells. In the case of EBV-negative HD, the nature of the antiapoptotic signal is not clear. However, recent observations suggest that IκBα, a key inhibitor of NFκB, might be mutated in at least some cases of EBV-negative HD, thus implying that constitutive activation of NFκB may also occur in the absence of EBV infection.[289-291]

In the case of lymphocyte-predominant HD, RS cells have also undergone clonal immunoglobulin gene rearrangements, but the pattern of somatic mutations suggests ongoing selection by antigen and intraclonal diversity.[285, 287, 292, 293] This phenotype resembles that of memory B cells, thus suggesting that lymphocyte-predominate RS cells, which often express κ or λ light chains, have been selected by antigen, can produce antibody, and therefore represent the developmental stage of B memory cells.

EBV AND OTHER LYMPHOMAS

Occasional reports have described T-cell lymphomas with latent EBV in the tumor cells, including nasal lymphomas of the natural killer (NK)/T-cell lineage, cutaneous lymphomas such as mycosis fungoides and Sézary's syndrome, T-cell lymphomas of a helper cell phenotype, angioimmunoblastic lymphadenopathy, and angiocentric T-cell lymphomas.[294-298] The clonal pattern of the episomal terminal repeats[294] would argue that infection with EBV occurred before monoclonal proliferation of the leukemic T-cell clone. In some cases, evidence of a latency II pattern of viral gene expression (LMP-1, LMP-2, EBNA-1, EBERs) can be found, similar to HD (see earlier).[297, 299] By analogy to HD and nasopharyngeal carcinoma, where EBV also adopts latency pattern II, this evidence would suggest a role for EBV in the pathogenesis of these lymphomas, but the mechanisms involved are not yet known.

Kaposi's Sarcoma–Associated Herpesvirus (Human Herpesvirus-8)

KSHV, or HHV-8, was first discovered in Kaposi's sarcoma (KS) lesions of AIDS patients[300] and plays an indispensable role in the pathogenesis of this tumor (reviewed elsewhere[301, 302]). It is also always found in primary effusion lymphoma (PEL), a rare B-cell lymphoma clinically characterized by primary malignant effusions in body cavities with tumor masses lining the endothelial surfaces.[303, 303a] This lymphoma is therefore also sometimes referred to as body cavity–based lymphoma. Furthermore, KSHV is associated with the plasma cell variant of multicentric Castleman's disease (MCD).[304] KSHV is classified as a γ₂-herpesvirus (rhadinovirus) and is thus distantly related to EBV, a γ₁-herpesvirus.[305]

Epidemiology of KSHV

Unlike most other herpesviruses and, in particular, EBV, KSHV is not ubiquitous, KSHV appears to be rare (seroprevalence, <5% to 10%) in northern Europe, the United States, and most parts of Asia. Its prevalence is somewhat higher in parts of Italy, in particular, in the south, and in Greece, Israel, and Egypt. In these regions, conservative but specific assays have estimated the seroprevalence to range from about 10% to 35%[306-310]; see elsewhere for review.[311] In contrast, KSHV appears to be highly prevalent in most parts of sub-Saharan Africa, with conservative assays indicating seroprevalence rates of about 30% to 60%.[306, 308, 312-314]

In endemic countries, much of the transmission and spread of KSHV appears to occur in childhood, in children 2 years or older, but evidence also indicates ongoing transmission among adults.[312, 313, 315] Transmission in childhood probably occurs within families.[312] Children from families with a KSHV-infected mother or sibling are at increased risk of becoming infected.[315] In contrast, KSHV transmission among homosexual men in Western countries is strongly associated with promiscuity and other sexually transmitted diseases, thus indicating transmission through sexual contact.[316-319] Although several epidemiologic studies have attempted to define the precise mode of transmission by analyzing the impact of different sexual behavior patterns on KSHV seroprevalence or incidence, no consensus has yet been achieved. Transmission via saliva and/or semen both appears possible.[316-319]

Cross-sectional and prospective serologic studies have provided firm evidence for KSHV being the cause of KS (reviewed elsewhere[301, 311]). It has, however, also become clear that KS is an extremely rare event in a KSHV-infected, HIV-negative, and otherwise healthy individual.[309, 310] This observation suggests that other cofactors may exist. Of these cofactors, infection with HIV-1 is the most important and is illustrated by the huge excess rate of KS in HIV-infected versus non–HIV-1–infected individuals.[262] Correlation may also be found between the incidence rates for "classic" KS and KSHV seroprevalence in different geographic regions.[309, 310]

Biology of KSHV Infection

A γ_2-herpesvirus, KSHV is distantly related to EBV but lacks all the EBV genes that are thought to play a role in pathogenesis (see earlier). Similar to EBV, KSHV can establish a latent infection in B cells and endothelial cells.[320-324] Lytic (productive) replication has been seen in macrophages, as well as in a small proportion of infected spindle cells, the neoplastic component of KS, and in B cells in MCD.[321, 325-328] KSHV therefore does not appear to be strictly latent in at least some tumors in vivo. It is thus conceivable that viral proteins expressed during either latent persistence or lytic replication could contribute to KSHV-associated pathology. Evidence has also been presented for the tissue-specific expression of individual viral genes.

Among the latent viral genes are those for the "latency-associated nuclear antigen" (LANA), a homologue of a cellular D-type cyclin (v-cyc), and an antiapoptotic protein (v-FLIP), as well as a group of small membrane proteins, "kaposin" A, B, C.[321-324] LANA is associated with nuclear heterochromatin and plays a role in maintenance of the viral genome as extrachromosomal, episomal circular DNA during latent persistence.[329, 330] It also inhibits transcriptional activity of the tumor suppressors p53[331] and Rb[331a] and may have yet other functions.[332] The viral cyclin homologue v-cyc can mediate the transition from the G_1 to the S phase of the cell cycle by mediating the phosphorylation, by cdk6, of the G_1 checkpoint control protein Rb and the cdk inhibitor p27[Kip].[333-335] The viral inhibitor of Fas-induced apoptosis, vFLIP, protects infected cells against CTLs.[336] "Kaposin A" has been shown to have transforming activity in rodent fibroblasts.[337] In addition to these latent genes, several nonstructural KSHV genes that are expressed after the onset of productive viral replication may play a role in pathogenesis. Among these genes are a homologue of interleukin-6 (vIL-6). Like cellular IL-6, vIL-6 can stimulate B-cell proliferation, but it appears to be less selective and may require only the β chain of the IL-6 receptor, which is shared by related interleukin receptors, to trigger signal transduction.[338] vIL-6 also has hematopoietic and angiogenic activity and induces plasma cell differentiation in vivo.[339] It is secreted from B cells in KSHV-associated PEL and MCD (see later) and may thus play a role in the pathogenesis of these neoplasms.

KSHV also encodes three chemokine homologues with angiogenic or chemotactic properties.[340] V-MIP-II is elaborated in lymphatic tissue and may be involved in the angiogenic changes sometimes seen in KSHV-infected lymphatic tissue.[341] A viral chemokine receptor, vGCR, can transform rodent fibroblasts to tumorigenicity and induce the secretion of vascular endothelial cell growth factor,[342] but its expression in tumor cells has thus far not been documented.[326] The membrane protein K1 has

similar transforming properties and is encoded in a similar region of the viral genome as LMP-1 in EBV,[343, 344] but unlike the latter, evidence of its expression in tumor cells in vivo has not been demonstrated. Another KSHV protein, K15/LAMP, has structural similarities to the two latent membrane proteins of EBV, LMP-1 and LMP-2A, and is expressed in PEL cell lines, but its expression in tumor cells in vivo is not yet known.[345-347]

Four homologues of interferon regulatory factors (vIRFs) have been identified. One of them, vIRF-1 (orf K9), can transform rodent fibroblasts to tumorigenicity and induces the c-myc oncogene by associating with p300, a component of the transcriptional activation complex.[348, 349] Immunohistochemical studies suggest that vIRF-1 is expressed in a small percentage of lytically infected B cells in MCD tissue.[327]

In vitro infection of endothelial cells with KSHV also leads to a mixture of persistently and lytically infected cells.[350, 351] Persistently infected cells have an extended life span and are able to grow in soft agar, but paracrine events in such cultures also seem to promote the growth of uninfected cells, in line with the indirect effects that some of the KSHV genes discussed in the preceding paragraph might have.[350, 351]

KSHV and Primary Effusion Lymphoma

PEL cells contain a large number (about 50 to 100 in cases in which it has been investigated) of KSHV genomes as circular episomal (extrachromosomal) DNA, characteristic of latent viral persistence.[303, 303a] These circular episomes appear to be of monoclonal origin, as shown by a constant (and for each tumor unique) number of terminal repeat subunits.[305, 352] As in EBV-associated lymphomas, this pattern indicates that viral infection preceded the emergence of a monoclonal B-cell clone. In many cases, PEL tumor cells are additionally infected with EBV, which is also present as monoclonal episomes.[303, 303a, 305] Some PEL tumors, however, contain only KSHV. Cell lines are easily established in vitro from PEL body cavity exudates and retain the same monoclonal terminal repeat pattern as the original tumor.[303a, 305] These observations and the similarity to EBV-associated lymphoma suggest a causative role of KSHV in the pathogenesis of this tumor.

In keeping with the presence of circular viral DNA in these tumor cells, KSHV adopts a restrictive gene expression pattern characteristic of latent infection. By immunohistochemistry, only LANA, one of the IRF homologues ("LANA-2"), and vIL-6 have thus far been found to be expressed.[306, 307, 322, 327, 340, 352a] On PEL-derived cell lines, mRNA for v-cyc, v-FLIP, and "kaposin" may be detected by Northern blot analysis.[323] However, the viral gene expression pattern in PEL cell lines is broader than for PEL cells in vivo, most likely as a result of culture-induced changes.[327]

KSHV and Multicentric Castleman's Disease

KSHV is found in many cases of the plasmacytic variant of MCD, mainly in HIV-1–infected individuals.[304, 352b] KSHV-infected B cells in these lesions are located in the perifollicular region. In addition to LANA these cells express vIL-

6, LANA–2, and, in a small proportion, also orf 50/Rta, the activator of the lytic replication cycle.[327, 352a, 353] It thus appears as though the KSHV gene expression pattern in MCD is not restricted to latent genes. The expression of vIL-6 suggests that this cytokine may play a role in the B-cell proliferation and plasma cell differentiation seen in this MCD variant.

Several case reports indicate that MCD may arise soon after primary KSHV infection. Thus, MCD-like features have been seen in an HIV-infected individual a few weeks after seroconverting to KSHV,[354] and MCD has also been seen in organ transplant recipients who contracted KSHV with the transplant.[355] Thus, MCD may represent the outcome of primary or reactivated KSHV in lymphatic tissue.

DO DIFFERENT TUMOR VIRUSES USE SIMILAR OR IDENTICAL PATHWAYS TO TRANSFORM THEIR TARGET CELLS?

As discussed in detail for each of the three human tumor viruses and summarized in Figures 10–5 and 10–6, common themes have begun to emerge. Thus, HTLV-I, EBV, and KSHV all target several control mechanisms of the G_1/S checkpoint and modify the function of p53 and/or some of the cdk inhibitors downstream of p53 (Fig. 10–5). Similarly, the NFκB pathway and the JAK/STAT, JNK, and src kinase signal transduction pathways are targeted by all three viruses (see Fig. 10–6). Other common "themes" include an interaction with CRB/p300 (HTLV-I tax, EBV EBNA-2, and KSHV vIRF-1[349]) and the targeting of apoptotic pathways by inducing cellular genes with antiapoptotic properties (BCL-2 by EBV LMP-1; NFκB by EBV LMP-1, HTLV-I tax, KSHV vGCR, and perhaps other KSHV genes) or the presence of viral genes with antiapoptotic properties (KSHV vFLIP, vBCL-2; EBV BHRF-1). Whereas the tax protein of HTLV-I appears to be involved in many different pathways, the two human herpesviruses have evolved several genes that assume individual functions.

The relative importance of targeting individual pathways for the ability of these viruses to cause cancer has not yet been fully resolved. It is likely that the primary reason for these viruses to target these pathways is related to their need to replicate the viral genome under "nonpermissive" conditions, for instance, when the infected cell is not programmed to replicate DNA. In addition, the need for the virus to survive in cell populations that are normally destined to die, as in the case of EBV and the germinal center B cell, or the need to counteract cellular surveillance mechanisms triggered by lytic viral infection or cellular interferons (as for KSHV vIRF-1) explains the need to evolve the ability to counteract apoptosis or interferon-induced pathways.

Some of the intracellular targets of these viruses are very suggestive with regard to a possible role in oncogenesis. Thus, the fact that all three target the G_1/S checkpoint, which is known to be affected in many cancers, suggests that this step may be important in virus-induced neoplasia. However, it is likely that the primary reason

for targeting of the G_1/S checkpoint by these viruses is related to the need to replicate the viral genome independently of cellular control mechanisms. Some "nononcogenic" viruses have the same requirement, and cellular cdks are, for example, recruited for replication of the genome of herpes simplex virus.[356] On the other hand, KSHV v-cyclin can induce G_1/S transition in resting fibroblast cultures, thus demonstrating that it can indeed control the cellular checkpoint, but it does not transform fibroblasts. Lymphoid malignancy develops in only a small minority of individuals infected with these three viruses and, in some cases, only after a long latency period. In the case of HTLV-I, the development of malignancy appears to involve the gradual expansion of infected T-cell populations, thereby increasing the chance of secondary oncogenic events. In spite of good evidence for a role of the cellular immune system in controlling HTLV-I viral load, no evidence currently suggests that HTLV-I–associated neoplasia is more common in immunosuppressed individuals. This observation and the lack of any good epidemiologic evidence for the involvement of another cofactor suggest that these secondary events may be of a stochastic nature.

In contrast, EBV-associated immunoblastic lymphoma is virtually only found in immunosuppressed individuals, thus highlighting the strong transforming potential of this virus. In addition, good evidence has been presented for the involvement of a dietary cofactor in nasopharyngeal carcinoma, another EBV-associated malignancy,[226] and for a role of other infections, for example, malaria or HIV, in the pathogenesis of BL (see earlier).

KSHV resembles EBV in that KS is strongly associated with immune suppression. Similarly, HIV infection is a strong cofactor in the pathogenesis of KSHV-associated lymphoid neoplasia, as well as KS, but HIV-negative cases of MCD and PEL have also been reported.

VIRUSES IN CHILDHOOD LEUKEMIA?

Several aspects of the epidemiology of childhood leukemia are compatible with the involvement of an infectious agent, most likely a virus, in the pathogenesis of childhood leukemia. Although the epidemiologic studies reported thus far do not normally address the phenotype of the leukemic cells, it is likely that these observations relate to common ALL. No convincing candidate agent has, however, been identified to date.

Thus, childhood leukemia is more common in families of higher socioeconomic status, in firstborn or single children, and in children who do not attend a daycare center. Such children are likely to be exposed to infectious agents at an older age than those who have older siblings or frequent contact with their peers.[357, 358] Clusters of childhood leukemia in the vicinity of nuclear installations and non-nuclear construction sites[42, 359, 360] could suggest that population mixing, accompanied by increased contact between infected and susceptible individuals, may increase the incidence of childhood leukemia. Furthermore, space-time clustering of childhood leukemia has been noted in Greece, again compatible with the involvement of an infectious agent.[361]

Both varicella and influenza infection during pregnancy have been associated with an increased risk of leukemia in children,[362, 363] but it is unclear whether these viruses explain the epidemiologic observations noted earlier.

Several observations suggest a relatively short interval between exposure to the putative infectious agent and development of this disease. Thus, childhood leukemia peaks in the 2- to 4-year-old age group, space-time clustering is strongest for children younger than 4 years,[361] and the excess in leukemia incidence after population mixing occurs within a year of the initiation of major construction works and is highest when building and operation phases overlap.[360] The currently available epidemiologic findings are compatible with the notion that the agent responsible is relatively common, with leukemia being a rare consequence of infection. However, other interpretations are also possible, and no good candidate agent has thus far been identified.

SUMMARY

Although only a few types of leukemia or lymphoma are thought to have a viral cause, the preceding sections illustrate the importance of viruses as the cause of leukemia or lymphoma. A number of different pathogenic mechanisms can be involved in the sequence of events that finally leads to a leukemic cell clone. In contrast to some animal leukemias, the role of viruses in human leukemia is a more subtle one, and malignant transformation remains a rare outcome of infection with the viruses involved. In fact, in view of the potent transformation potential of both EBV and HTLV-I in vitro, the fact that the development of lymphoma or leukemia is a rare event is a testimony to the efficiency of protective mechanisms, including the immune system.

Conversely, some diseases such as HD can occur in response to EBV, as well as perhaps other viruses. An example for an indirect role of a virus in the development of leukemia is provided by the emergence of a mature B-cell leukemia such as B-CLL in HTLV-I–positive individuals, presumably as a consequence of chronic antigenic stimulation (see earlier). Because B-cell proliferation in response to bacterial antigens can have a similar effect in the case of intestinal lymphomas, it could be envisaged that other viruses that are not usually considered leukemogenic may rarely be the cause of leukemias for similar reasons. Chronic antigenic stimulation has thus far been shown to be involved in leukemias of a mature B-cell phenotype. This model may therefore not apply to leukemias of an immature phenotype such as childhood (common) ALL.

REFERENCES

1. Ellerman V, Bang O: Experimentelle Leukamie bei Huhnern. Zentralb Bakteriol. 1908;046:595.
2. Witter RL: Avian tumor viruses: Persistent and evolving pathogens. Acta Vet Hung 1997;45:251.
3. Gross L: Spontaneous leukemia developing in C3H mice following inoculation, in infancy, with Ak-leukemic extracts, or Ak-embryos. Proc Soc Exp Biol Med 1951;76:27.
4. Jarrett WF, Martin WB, Crighton GW, et al: Leukemia in the cat. Transmission experiments with leukemia (lymphosarcoma). Nature 1964;202:566.
5. Van Der Maaten MJ, Boothe AD, Seger CL: Isolation of a virus from cattle with persistent lymphocytosis. J Natl Cancer Inst 1972;49:1649.
6. Coffin JM, Hughes SH, Varmus HE: Retroviruses. New York: Cold Spring Harbor Laboratory; 1997.
7. Weiss R, Teich N, Varmus H, et al: RNA Tumor Viruses. New York: Cold Spring Harbor Laboratory; 1982.
8. Tooze J: DNA Tumor Viruses. New York: Cold Spring Harbor Laboratory; 1980.
9. Levine AM: Acquired immune deficiency syndrome–related lymphoma. Blood 1992;80:8.
10. Boeke JD, Stoye JP: Retrotransposons, endogenous retroviruses and the evolution of retroelements. In Coffin JM, Hughes SH, Varmus HE, eds: Retroviruses. New York: Cold Spring Harbor Laboratory; 1997, p 343.
11. Neel B, Hayward WS, Robinson HL, et al: Avian leukosis virus-induced tumors have common proviral integration sites and synthesize discreet new RNAs: Oncogenesis by promoter insertion. Cell 1981;23:323.
12. Jonkers J, Berns A: Retroviral insertional mutagenesis as a strategy to identify cancer genes. Biochim Biophys Acta 1996;1287:29.
13. Lazo PA, Lee JS, Tsichlis PN: Long-distance activation of the *Myc* protooncogene by provirus insertion in Mlvi-1 or Mlvi-4 in rat T-cell lymphomas. Proc Natl Acad Sci U S A 1990;87:170.
14. Tsichlis PN, Lee JS, Bear SE, et al: Activation of multiple genes by provirus insertion in the Mlvi-4 locus in T-cell lymphoma induced by Moloney murine leukemia virus. J Virol 1990;64:2236.
15. Bartholomew C, Ihle JN: Retroviral insertions 90kb proximal to the evi-1 myeloid transforming gene activate transcription from the normal promoter. Mol Cell Biol 1991;11:1820.
16. Lammie GA, Smith R, Silver J, et al: Proviral insertions near cyclin D1 in mouse lymphomas: A parallel for BCL1 translocations in human B-cell neoplasms. Oncogene 1992;12:2381.
17. Swanstrom R, Parker RC, Varmus HE, et al: Transduction of a cellular oncogene: The genesis of Rous sarcoma virus. Proc Natl Acad Sci U S A 1983;80:2519.
18. Neil JC, Hughes D, McFarlane R, et al: Transduction and rearrangement of the *myc* gene by feline leukaemia virus in naturally occurring T-cell leukaemias. Nature 1984;308:814.
19. Langdon WY, Hartley JW, Holmes KL, et al: Identification of a transforming virus from a lymphoma of a mouse infected with a wild mouse retrovirus. Curr Top Microbiol Immunol 1984;113:241.
20. Nevins JR, Vogt PK: Cell transformation by viruses. In Fields BN, Knipe DM, Howley PM, eds: Fields Virology. Philadelphia: Lippincott-Raven; 1996, p 301.
21. Stehelin D, Varmus HE, Bishop JM, et al: DNA related to the transforming gene(s) of avian sarcoma viruses is present in normal avian DNA. Nature 1976;260:170.
22. Bishop JM: Cellular oncogenes and retroviruses. Annu Rev Biochem 1983;52:301.
23. Bishop JM: The rise of the genetic paradigm. Genes Dev 1995;9:1309.
24. Dalla-Favera R, Martinotti S, Gallo RC, et al: Translocation and rearrangements of the c-*myc* oncogene locus in human undifferentiated B-cell lymphomas. Science 1983;219:963.
25. Heisterkamp N, Stephenson JR, Groffen J, et al: Localization of the c-*abl* oncogene to a translocation break point in chronic myelocytic leukaemia. Nature 1983;306:239.
26. Hesketh R: The Oncogene and Tumour Suppressor Gene FactsBook. London: Academic Press; 1997.
27. Neil JC, Wyke JA: Viral oncogenicity. In Collier LH, Mahy BWJ, eds: Microbiology and Microbial Infections. London: Edward Arnold; 1996, p 211.
28. Rosenberg N, Jolicoeur P: Retroviral pathogenesis. In Coffin JM, Hughes SH, Varmus HE, eds: Retroviruses. New York: Cold Spring Harbor Laboratory; 1997, p 475.
29. Ben-David Y, Lavigueur A, Cheong GY, et al: Insertional inactivation of the p53 gene during leukemia: A new strategy for identifying tumor suppressor genes. New Biol 1990;2:1015.
30. Lu S-J, Rowan S, Bani MR, et al: Retroviral integration within the Fli-2 locus results in inactivation of the erythroid transcription

factor NF-E2 in Friend erythroleukemias: Evidence that NF-E2 is essential for globin expression. Proc Natl Acad Sci U S A 1994; 91:8398.

31. Melendez LV, Hunt RD, Daniel MD, et al: Acute lymphocytic leukemia in owl monkeys (*Aotus trivirgatus*) inoculated with herpesvirus saimiri. Science 1971;171:1161.

32. Melendez LV, Hunt RD, Kind NW, et al: Herpesvirus ateles, a new lymphoma virus of monkeys. Nature 1972;235:182.

33. Witter RL: Control strategies for Marek's disease: A perspective for the future. Poult Sci 1998;77:1197.

34. Lamont SJ: The chicken major histocompatibility complex in disease resistance and poultry breeding. J Dairy Sci 1989;72:1328.

35. Eddy BE, Borman GS, Grubbs GE, et al: Identification of the oncogenic substance in rhesus monkey kidney cell cultures as simian virus 40. Virology 1962;17:65.

36. Stewart SE, Eddy BE, Borgese N: Neoplasms in mice inoculated with a tumor agent carried in tissue culture. J Natl Cancer Inst 1958;20:1223.

37. Lane DP, Crawford LV: T antigen is bound to a host protein in SV40-transformed cells. Nature 1979;278:261.

38. Linzer DIH, Levine AJ: Characterization of a 54K dalton cellular SV40 tumour antigen in SV40-transformed cells and uninfected embryonal carcinoma cells. Cell 1979;17:43.

39. Acheson NH: Lytic cycle of SV40 and polyoma virus. In Tooze J, ed: DNA Tumor Viruses. New York: Cold Spring Harbor Laboratory; 1980, p 125.

40. McCarthy SA, Symonds HS, Van Dyke T: Regulation of apoptosis in transgenic mice by simian virus 40 T antigen-mediated inactivation of p53. Proc Natl Acad Sci U S A 1994;91:3979.

41. Neil JC, Baxter E, Cameron E: p 53 and tumour viruses: Catching the guardian off-guard. Trends Microbiol 1997;5:115.

42. Kinlen L: Evidence for an infective cause of childhood leukaemia: Comparison of a Scottish new town with nuclear reprocessing sites in Britain. Lancet 1988;2:1323.

43. Benveniste RE, Todaro GJ: Segregation of RD-114 AND FeLV-related sequences in crosses between domestic cat and leopard cat. Nature 1975;257:506.

44. Rogerson P, Jarrett W, Mackey L: Epidemiological studies on feline leukaemia virus infection. I. A serological survey in urban cats. Int J Cancer 1975;15:781.

45. Jarrett O: Pathogenesis of feline leukaemia virus-related diseases. In Goldman JM, Jarrett O, eds: Mechanisms of Viral Leukaemogenesis. Edinburgh: Churchill Livingstone; 1984, p 135.

46. Essex M, Cotter SM, Sliski AH, et al: Horizontal transmission of feline leukemia virus under natural conditions in a feline leukemia cluster household. Int J Cancer 1977;19:90.

47. Jarrett W, Jarrett O, Mackey L, et al: Horizontal transmission of leukemia virus and leukemia in the cat. J Natl Cancer Inst 1973; 51:833.

48. Hoover EA, Rojko JL, Quackenbush SL: Congenital feline leukemia virus infection. Leuk Rev Int 1983;1:7.

49. Rojko JL, Hoover EA, Mathes LE, et al: Pathogenesis of experimental feline leukemia virus infection. J Natl Cancer Inst 1979;63:759.

50. Rojko JL, Hoover EA, Quackenbush SL, et al: Reactivation of latent feline leukemia virus infection. Nature 1982;298:385.

51. Pacitti AM, Jarrett O: Duration of the latent state in feline leukaemia virus infections. Vet Rec 1985;117:472.

52. Kraut EH, Rojko JL, Olsen RG, et al: Effects of cobra venom factor treatment on latent feline leukemia virus infection. J Virol 1985; 54:873.

53. McClelland AJ, Hardy WD, Zuckerman EE: Prognosis of healthy feline leukemia virus infected cats. Hardy WD, Essex M, McClelland AJ, eds: Feline Leukemia Virus. New York: Elsevier/North-Holland; 1980, p 121.

54. Neil JC, Fulton R, Rigby M, et al: Feline leukaemia virus: Generation of pathogenic and oncogenic variants. Curr Top Microbiol Immunol 1991;171:67.

55. Overbaugh J, Donahue PR, Quackenbush SL, et al: Molecular cloning of a feline leukemia virus that induces fatal immunodeficiency disease in cats. Science 1988;239:906.

56. Rigby MA, Rojko JL, Stewart MA, et al: Partial dissociation of subgroup C phenotype and in vivo behaviour in feline leukaemia viruses with chimeric envelope genes. J Gen Virol 1992;73:2839.

57. Fulton R, Plumb M, Shield L, et al: Structural diversity and nuclear protein binding sites in the long terminal repeats of feline leukaemia virus. J Virol 1990;64:1675.

58. Forrest D, Onions D, Lees G, et al: Altered structure and expression of c-myc in feline T-cell tumours. Virology 1987;158:194.

59. Tsujimoto H, Fulton R, Nishigaki K, et al: A common proviral integration region, fit-1, in T-cell tumors induced by myc-containing feline leukemia viruses. Virology 1993;196:845.

60. Levy LS, Lobelle-Rich PA, Overbaugh J: Flvi-2, a target of retroviral insertional mutagenesis in feline thymic lymphosarcomas, encodes bmi-1. Oncogene 1993;8:1833.

61. Levesque KS, Bonham L, Levy LS: Flvi-1, a common integration domain of feline leukemia virus in naturally occurring lymphomas of a particular type. J Virol 1990;64:3455.

62. Tsatsanis C, Fulton R, Nishigaki K, et al: Genetic determinants of feline leukemia virus-induced lymphoid tumors: Patterns of proviral insertion and gene rearrangement. J Virol 1994;68:8294.

63. Onions D, Lees G, Forrest D, et al: Recombinant feline viruses containing the *myc* gene rapidly produce clonal tumours expressing T-cell antigen receptor gene transcripts. Int J Cancer 1987; 40:40.

64. Stewart MA, Warnock M, Wheeler A, et al: Nucleotide sequences of a feline leukemia virus subgroup A envelope gene and long terminal repeat and evidence for the recombinational origin of subgroup B viruses. J Virol 1986;58:825.

65. Sheets RL, Pandey R, Jen W-C, et al: Recombinant feline leukemia virus genes detected in naturally occurring feline lymphosarcomas. J Virol 1993;67:3118.

66. Tzavaras T, Stewart M, McDougall A, et al: Molecular cloning and characterisation of a defective recombinant feline leukaemia virus associated with myeloid leukaemia. J Gen Virol 1990;71:343.

67. Hardy WD Jr, McClelland AJ: Feline leukemia virus. Its related diseases and control. Vet Clin North Am 1977;7:93.

68. Lewis MG, Mathes LE, Olsen RG: Protection against feline leukemia by vaccination with a subunit vaccine. Infect Immunol 1981; 34:888.

69. Marciani D, Kensil CR, Beltz GA, et al: Genetically engineered subunit vaccine against feline leukemia virus. Vaccine 1991;9:89.

70. Tartaglia J, Jarrett O, Neil JC, et al: Protection of cats against feline leukemia virus by vaccination with a canarypox recombinant, ALVAC-FL. J Virol 1993;67:2370.

71. Miller J, Miller L, Olson C, et al: Virus-like particles in phytohemagglutinin-stimulated lymphocyte cultures with reference to bovine lymphosarcoma. J Natl Cancer Inst 1969;43:1297.

72. Ferrer JF: Bovine lymphosarcoma. Adv Vet Sci Comp Med 1980; 24:1.

73. Burny A, Bruck C, Cleuter Y, et al: Bovine leukemia virus, a versatile agent with various pathogenic effects in various animal species. Cancer Res 1985;45:4578.

74. Altanerova V, Ban J, Altaner C: Induction of immune deficiency syndrome in rabbits by bovine leukemia virus. AIDS 1989;3:755.

75. Depelchin A, Letesson J, Lostrie N, et al: Bovine leukemia virus (BLV) infected B cells express a marker similar to the CD5 T-cell marker. Immunol Lett 1989;20:69.

76. Gregoire D, Couez D, Deschamps J, et al: Different bovine leukemia virus-induced tumors harbor the provirus in different chromosomes. J Virol 1984;50:275.

77. Willems L, Heremans H, Chen G, et al: Cooperation between bovine leukemia virus transactivator protein and Ha-*ras* oncogene in cellular transformation. EMBO J 1990;9:1577.

78. Portetelle D, Callebaut I, Bex F, et al: Vaccination against animal retroviruses. In Pandey R, Hoglund S, Prasad G, eds: Progress in Vaccinology, vol 4, Veterinary Vaccines. Berlin: Springer-Verlag; 1993, p 87.

79. Uchiyama T, Yodoi J, Sagawa K, et al: Adult T-cell leukemia: Clinical and hematologic features of 16 cases. Blood 1977;50:481.

80. Miyoshi I, Yoshimoto S, Kubonishi I, et al: Transformation of normal human cord lymphocytes by co-cultivation with a lethally irradiated human T-cell line carrying type C virus particles. Gann 1981;72:997.

81. Poiesz BJ, Ruscetti FW, Gazdar AF, et al: Detection and isolation of type C retrovirus particles from fresh and cultured lymphocytes of a patient with cutaneous T-cell lymphoma. Proc Natl Acad Sci U S A 1980;77:7415.

82. Clapham P, Nagy K, Cheingsong PR, et al: Productive infection and cell-free transmission of human T-cell leukemia virus in a nonlymphoid cell line. Science 1983;222:1125.

83. Sommerfelt MA, Williams BP, Clapham PR, et al: Human T cell

leukaemia viruses use a receptor determined by human chromosome 17. Science 1988;242:1557.

84. Sutton RE, Littman DR: Broad host range of human T-cell leukemia virus type 1 demonstrated with an improved pseudotyping system. J Virol 1996;70:7322.

85. Trejo SR, Ratner L: The HTLV receptor is a widely expressed protein. Virology 2000;268:41.

86. Richardson JH, Edwards AJ, Cruickshank JK, et al: In vivo cellular tropism of human T-cell leukemia virus type 1. J Virol 1990; 64:5682.

87. Macatonia SE, Cruickshank JK, Rudge P, et al: Dendritic cells from patients with tropical spastic paraparesis are infected with HTLV-1 and stimulate autologous lymphocyte proliferation. AIDS Res Hum Retroviruses 1992;8:1699.

88. Kitajima I, Yamamoto K, Sato K, et al: Detection of human T cell lymphotropic virus type I proviral DNA and its gene expression in synovial cells in chronic inflammatory arthropathy. J Clin Invest 1991;88:1315.

89. Felber BK, Paskalis H, Kleinman-Ewing C, et al: The pX protein of HTLV-I is a transcriptional activator of its long terminal repeats. Science 1985;229:675.

90. Seiki M, Inoue J, Takeda T, et al: Direct evidence that p40x of human T-cell leukemia virus type I is a trans-acting transcriptional activator. EMBO J 1986;5:561.

91. Slamon DJ, Press MF, Souza LM, et al: Studies of the putative transforming protein of the type I human T-cell leukmia virus. Science 1985;228:1427.

92. Sodroski J, Rosen C, Goh WC, et al: A transcriptional activator protein encoded by the x-lor region of the human T-cell leukemia virus. Science 1985;228:1430.

93. Arai N, Nomura D, Villaret D, et al: Complete nucleotide sequence of the chromosomal gene for human IL-4 and its expression. J Immunol 1989;142:274.

94. Chan JY, Slamon DJ, Nimer SD, et al: Regulation of expression of human granulocyte/macrophage colony-stimulating factor. Proc Natl Acad Sci U S A 1986;83:8669.

95. Fujii M, Sassone-Corsi P, Verma IM: c-fos promoter trans-activation by the tax1 protein of human T-cell leukemia virus type I. Proc Natl Acad Sci U S A 1988;85:8526.

96. Green JE, Begley CG, Wagner DK, et al: Trans activation of granulocyte-macrophage colony-stimulating factor and the interleukin-2 receptor in transgenic mice carrying the human T-lymphotropic virus type 1 tax gene. Mol Cell Biol 1989;9:4731.

97. Greene WC, Leonard WJ, Wano Y, et al: Trans-activator gene of HTLV-II induces IL-2 receptor and IL-2 cellular gene expression. Science 1986;232:877.

98. Inoue J, Seiki M, Taniguchi T, et al: Induction of interleukin 2 receptor gene expression by p40x encoded by human T-cell leukemia virus type 1. EMBO J 1986;5:2883.

99. Kelly K, Davis P, Mitsuya H, et al: A high proportion of early response genes are constitutively activated in T cells by HTLV-I. Oncogene 1992;7:1463.

100. Miyatake S, Seiki M, Malefijt RD, et al: Activation of T cell–derived lymphokine genes in T cells and fibroblasts: Effects of human T cell leukemia virus type I p40x protein and bovine papilloma virus encoded E2 protein. Nucleic Acids Res 1988;16:6547.

101. Wano Y, Feinberg M, Hosking JB, et al: Stable expression of the tax gene of type I human T-cell leukemia virus in human T cells activates specific cellular genes involved in growth. Proc Natl Acad Sci U S A 1988;85:9733.

102. Bogerd HP, Huckaby GL, Ahmed YF, et al: The type I human T-cell leukemia virus (HTLV-I) Rex trans-activator binds directly to the HTLV-I Rex and the type 1 human immunodeficiency virus Rev RNA response elements. Proc Natl Acad Sci U S A 1991;88:5704.

103. Hidaka M, Inoue J, Yoshida M, et al: Post-transcriptional regulator (rex) of HTLV-I initiates expression of viral structural proteins but suppresses expression of regulatory proteins. EMBO J 1988;7:519.

104. Rimsky L, Hauber J, Dukovich M, et al: Functional replacement of the HIV-1 rev protein by the HTLV-1 rex protein. Nature 1988; 335:738.

105. Unge T, Solomin L, Mellini M, et al: The Rex regulatory protein of human T-cell lymphotropic virus type I binds specifically to its target site within the viral RNA. Proc Natl Acad Sci U S A 1991; 88:7145.

106. Hinuma Y, Nagata K, Hanaoka M, et al: Adult T-cell leukemia: Antigen in an ATL cell line and detection of antibodies to the antigen in human sera. Proc Natl Acad Sci U S A 1981;78:6476.

107. Hinuma Y, Komoda H, Chosa T, et al: Antibodies to adult T-cell leukemia-virus–associated antigen (ATLA) in sera from patients with ATL and controls in Japan: A nationwide sero-epidemiologic study. Int J Cancer 1982;29:631.

108. Blattner WA, Kalyanaraman VS, Robert GM, et al: The human type-C retrovirus, HTLV, in blacks from the Caribbean region, and relationship to adult T-cell leukemia/lymphoma. Int J Cancer 1982; 30:257.

109. Catovsky D, Greaves MF, Rose M, et al: Adult T-cell lymphoma-leukaemia in blacks from the West Indies. Lancet 1982;1:639.

110. Hunsmann G, Schneider J, Schmitt J, et al: Detection of serum antibodies to adult T-cell leukemia virus in non-human primates and in people from Africa. Int J Cancer 1983;32:329.

111. Merino F, Robert-Guroff M, Clark J, et al: Natural antibodies to human T-cell leukemia/lymphoma virus in healthy Venezuelan populations. Int J Cancer 1984;34:501.

112. de Oliveira MS, Matutes E, Famadas LC, et al: Adult T-cell leukaemia/lymphoma in Brazil and its relation to HTLV-I. Lancet 1990; 336:987.

113. Reeves WC, Saxinger C, Brenes MM, et al: Human T-cell lymphotropic virus type I (HTLV-I) seroepidemiology and risk factors in metropolitan Panama. Am J Epidemiol 1988;127:532.

114. Asher DM, Goudsmit J, Pomeroy KL, et al: Antibodies to HTLV-I in populations of the southwestern Pacific. J Med Virol 1988; 26:339.

115. Gessain A, Yanagihara R, Franchini G, et al: Highly divergent molecular variants of human T-lymphotropic virus type I from isolated populations in Papua New Guinea and the Solomon Islands. Proc Natl Acad Sci U S A 1991;88:7694.

116. Meytes D, Schochat B, Lee H, et al: Serological and molecular survey for HTLV-I infection in a high-risk Middle Eastern group. Lancet 1990;336:1533.

117. Manzari V, Gradilone A, Barillari G, et al: HTLV-I is endemic in southern Italy: Detection of the first infectious cluster in a white population. Int J Cancer 1985;36:557.

118. Wyld PJ, Tosswill JH, Mortimer PP, et al: Sporadic HTLV-I associated adult T-cell leukaemia (ATL) in the U.K. Br J Haematol 1990; 76:149.

119. Cunningham D, Gilchrist N, Jack A, et al: T-lymphoma associated with HTLV-I outside the Caribbean and Japan. Lancet 1985;ii:332.

120. Van Brussel M, Salemi M, Liu HF, et al: The discovery of two new divergent STLVs has implications for the evolution and epidemiology of HTLVs. Rev Med Virol 1999;9:155.

121. Franchini G, Reitz MSJ: Phylogenesis and genetic complexity of the nonhuman primate retroviridae. AIDS Res Hum Retroviruses 1994;10:1047.

122. Kelsey CR, Crandall KA, Voevodin AF: Different models, different trees: The geographic origin of PTLV-I. Mol Phylogenet Evol 1999; 13:336.

123. De BK, Lairmore MD, Griffis K, et al: Comparative analysis of nucleotide sequences of the partial envelope gene (5′ domain) among human T lymphotropic virus type I (HTLV-I) isolates. Virology 1991;182:413.

124. Gessain A, Gallo RC, Franchini G: Low degree of human T-cell leukemia/lymphoma virus type I genetic drift in vivo as a means of monitoring viral transmission and movement of ancient human populations. J Virol 1992;66:2288.

125. Komurian F, Pelloquin F, de The G: In vivo genomic variability of human T-cell leukemia virus type I depends more upon geography than upon pathologies. J Virol 1991;65:3770.

126. Komurian-Pradel F, Pelloquin F, Sonoda S, et al: Geographical subtypes demonstrated by RFLP following PCR in the LTR region of HTLV-I. AIDS Res Hum Retroviruses 1992;8:429.

127. Schulz TF, Calabro ML, Hoad JG, et al: HTLV-1 envelope sequences from Brazil, the Caribbean, and Romania: Clustering of sequences according to geographic origin and variability in an antibody epitope. Virology 1991;184:483.

128. Loughran TPJ, Coyle T, Sherman MP, et al: Detection of human T-cell leukemia/lymphoma virus, type II, in a patient with large granular lymphocyte leukemia. Blood 1992;80:1116.

129. Goubau P, Desmyter J, Ghesquiere J, et al: HTLV-II among pygmies [letter]. Nature 1992;359:201.

130. Goubau P, Liu HF, De Lange GG, et al: HTLV-II seroprevalence in

pygmies across Africa since 1970. AIDS Res Hum Retroviruses 1993;9:709.

131. Gessain A, Tuppin P, Kazanji M, et al: A distinct molecular variant of HTLV-IIB in Gabon, Central Africa. AIDS Res Hum Retroviruses 1994;10:753.

132. Heneine W, Kaplan JE, Gracia F, et al: HTLV-II endemicity among Guaymi Indians in Panama [letter]. N Engl J Med 1991;324:565.

133. Maloney EM, Biggar RJ, Neel JV, et al: Endemic human T cell lymphotropic virus type II infection among isolated Brazilian Amerindians. J Infect Dis 1992;166:100.

134. Hall WW, Takahashi H, Liu C, et al: Multiple isolates and characteristics of human T-cell leukemia virus type II. J Virol 1992;66:2456.

135. Lee H, Swanson P, Shorty VS, et al: High rate of HTLV-II infection in seropositive i.v. drug abusers in New Orleans. Science 1989; 244:471.

136. Tedder RS, Shanson DC, Jeffries DJ, et al: Low prevalence in the UK of HTLV-I and HTLV-II infection in subjects with AIDS, with extended lymphadenopathy, and at risk of AIDS. Lancet 1984; 2:125.

137. Dube DK, Sherman MP, Saksena NK, et al: Genetic heterogeneity in human T-cell leukemia/lymphoma virus type II. J Virol 1993; 67:1175.

138. Hino S, Kawamichi T, Funakoshi M, et al: Transfusion-mediated spread of the human T-cell leukemia virus in chronic hemodialysis patients in a heavily endemic area, Nagasaki. Gann 1984;75:1070.

139. Hirose S, Kotani S, Uemura Y, et al: Milk-borne transmission of human T-cell leukemia virus type I in rabbits. Virology 1988; 162:487.

140. Kajiyama W, Kashiwagi S, Hayashi J, et al: Intrafamilial clustering of anti-ATLA–positive persons. Am J Epidemiol 1986;124:800.

141. Nakano S, Ando Y, Ichijo M, et al: Search for possible routes of transmission of ATL virus. Jpn J Cancer Res 75:1044.

142. Tajima K, Tominaga S, Suchi T, et al: Epidemiological analysis of the distribution of antibody to adult T-cell leukemia-virus-associated antigen: Possible horizontal transmission of adult T-cell leukemia virus. Gann 1982;73:893.

143. Komuro A, Hayami M, Fujii H, et al: Vertical transmission of adult T-cell leukaemia virus [letter]. Lancet 1983;1:240.

144. Seiki M, Hattori S, Hirayama Y, et al: Human adult T-cell leukemia virus: Complete nucleotide sequence of the provirus genome integrated in leukemia cell DNA. Proc Natl Acad Sci U S A 1983; 80:3618.

145. Slamon DJ, Boyle WJ, Keith DE, et al: Subnuclear localization of the trans-activating protein of human T-cell leukemia virus type I. J Virol 1988;62:680.

146. Jeang KT, Boros I, Brady J, et al: Characterization of cellular factors that interact with the human T-cell leukemia virus type I p40x-responsive 21–base-pair sequence. J Virol 1988;62:4499.

147. Fujisawa J, Toita M, Yoshida M: A unique enhancer element for the trans activator (p40tax) of human T-cell leukemia virus type I that is distinct from cyclic AMP– and 12-O-tetradecanoylphorbol-13-acetate–responsive elements. J Virol 1989;63:3234.

148. Paskalis H, Felber BK, Pavlakis G: Cis-acting sequences responsible for the transcriptional activation of human T-cell leukemia virus type I constitute a conditional enhancer. Proc Natl Acad Sci U S A 1986;83:6558.

149. Shimotohno K, Takano M, Teruuchi T, et al: Requirement of multiple copies of a 21-nucleotide sequence in the U3 regions of human T-cell leukemia virus type I and type II long terminal repeats for trans-acting activation of transcription. Proc Natl Acad Sci U S A 1986;83:8112.

150. Hai TW, Liu F, Coukos WJ, et al: Transcription factor ATF cDNA clones: An extensive family of leucine zipper proteins able to selectively form DNA-binding heterodimers [published erratum appears in Genes Dev 1990 Apr;4(4):682]. Genes Dev 1989;3: 2083.

151. Wagner S, Green MR: HTLV-I Tax protein stimulation of DNA binding of bZIP proteins by enhancing dimerization. Science 1993; 262:395.

152. Yoshimura T, Fujisawa J, Yoshida M: Multiple cDNA clones encoding nuclear proteins that bind to the tax-dependent enhancer of HTLV-1: All contain a leucine zipper structure and basic amino acid domain. EMBO J 1990;9:2537.

153. Giebler HA, Loring JE, van Orden K, et al: Anchoring of CREB binding protein to the human T-cell leukemia virus type 1 promoter: A molecular mechanism of Tax transactivation. Mol Cell Biol 1997;17:5156.

154. Kwok RP, Laurance ME, Lundblad JR, et al: Control of cAMP-regulated enhancers by the viral transactivator Tax through CREB and the co-activator CBP. Nature 1996;380:642.

155. Lenzmeier BA, Giebler HA, Nyborg JK: Human T-cell leukemia virus type 1 Tax requires direct access to DNA for recruitment of CREB binding protein to the viral promoter. Mol Cell Biol 1998; 18:721.

156. Tanaka A, Takahashi C, Yamaoka S, et al: Oncogenic transformation by the tax gene of human T-cell leukemia virus type I in vitro. Proc Natl Acad Sci U S A 1990;87:1071.

157. Akagi T, Shimotohno K: Proliferative response of Tax1-transduced primary human T cells to anti-CD3 antibody stimulation by an interleukin-2–independent pathway. J Virol 1993;67:1211.

158. Grassmann R, Berchtold S, Radant I, et al: Role of human T-cell leukemia virus type 1 X region proteins in immortalization of primary human lymphocytes in culture. J Virol 1992;66:4570.

159. Hinrichs SH, Nerenberg M, Reynolds RK, et al: A transgenic mouse model for human neurofibromatosis. Science 1987;237:1340.

160. Nerenberg M, Hinrichs SH, Reynolds RK, et al: The tat gene of human T-lymphotropic virus type 1 induces mesenchymal tumors in transgenic mice. Science 1987;237:1324.

161. Grossman WJ, Kimata JT, Wong FH, et al: Development of leukemia in mice transgenic for the tax gene of human T-cell leukemia virus type I. Proc Natl Acad Sci U S A 1995;92:1057.

162. Coscoy L, Gonzalez-Dunia D, Tangy F, et al: Molecular mechanism of tumorigenesis in mice transgenic for the human T cell leukemia virus Tax gene. Virology 1998;248:332.

163. Lemasson I, Thebault S, Sardet C, et al: Activation of E2F-mediated transcription by human T-cell leukemia virus type I Tax protein in a p16(INK4A)-negative T-cell line. J Biol Chem 1998;273:23598.

164. Yoshida M, Suzuki T, Fujisawa J, et al: HTLV-1 oncoprotein tax and cellular transcription factors. Curr Top Microbiol Immunol 1995; 193:79.

165. Rosin O, Koch C, Schmitt I, et al: A human T-cell leukemia virus Tax variant incapable of activating NF-κB retains its immortalizing potential for primary T-lymphocytes. J Biol Chem 1998;273:6698.

166. Schmitt I, Rosin O, Rohwer P, et al: Stimulation of cyclin-dependent kinase activity and G1- to S-phase transition in human lymphocytes by the human T-cell leukemia/lymphotropic virus type 1 Tax protein. J Virol 1998;72:633.

167. Neuveut C, Low KG, Maldarelli F, et al: Human T-cell leukemia virus type 1 Tax and cell cycle progression: Role of cyclin D-cdk and p110Rb. Mol Cell Biol 1998;18:3620.

168. Low KG, Dorner LF, Fernando DB, et al: Human T-cell leukemia virus type 1 Tax releases cell cycle arrest induced by p16INK4a. J Virol 1997;71:1956.

169. Suzuki T, Kitao S, Matsushime H, et al: HTLV-1 Tax protein interacts with cyclin-dependent kinase inhibitor p16INK4A and counteracts its inhibitory activity towards CDK4. EMBO J 1996;15: 1607.

170. Suzuki T, Narita T, Uchida-Toita M, et al: Down-regulation of the INK4 family of cyclin-dependent kinase inhibitors by tax protein of HTLV-1 through two distinct mechanisms. Virology 1999;259: 384.

171. Santiago F, Clark E, Chong S, et al: Transcriptional up-regulation of the cyclin D2 gene and acquisition of new cyclin-dependent kinase partners in human T-cell leukemia virus type 1–infected cells. J Virol 1999;73:9917.

172. Uittenbogaard MN, Giebler HA, Reisman D, et al: Transcriptional repression of p53 by human T-cell leukemia virus type I Tax protein. J Biol Chem 1995;270:28503.

173. Reid RL, Lindholm PF, Mireskandari A, et al: Stabilization of wild-type p53 in human T-lymphocytes transformed by HTLV-I. Oncogene 1993;8:3029.

174. Akagi T, Ono H, Tsuchida N, et al: Aberrant expression and function of p53 in T-cells immortalized by HTLV-I Tax1. FEBS Lett 1997;406:263.

175. Mulloy JC, Kislyakova T, Ceresoto A, et al: Human T-cell lymphotropic/leukemia virus type 1 Tax abrogates p53-induced cell cycle arrest and apoptosis through its CREB/ATF functional domain. J Virol 1998;72:8852.

176. Pise-Masison CA, Radonovich M, Sakaguchi K, et al: Phosphorylation of p53: A novel pathway for p53 inactivation in human T-cell lymphotropic virus type 1–transformed cells. J Virol 1998;72:6348.

177. van Orden K, Giebler HA, Lemasson I, et al: Binding of p53 to the KIX domain of CREB binding protein. A potential link to human T-cell leukemia virus, type I–associated leukemogenesis. J Biol Chem 1999;274:26321.

178. Kitajima I, Shinohara T, Bilakovics J, et al: Abalation of transplanted HTLV-I Tax-transformed tumors in mice by antisense inhibition of NF-kappa-B. Science 1992;258:1792.

179. Iwanaga Y, Tsukahara T, Ohashi T, et al: Human T-cell leukemia virus type 1 tax protein abrogates interleukin-2 dependence in a mouse T-cell line. J Virol 1999;73:1271.

180. Kawakami A, Nakashima T, Sakai H, et al: Inhibition of caspase cascade by HTLV-I tax through induction of NF-κB nuclear translocation. Blood 1999;94:3847.

181. Yin MJ, Christerson LB, Yamamoto Y, et al: HTLV-I Tax protein binds to MEKK1 to stimulate IκB kinase activity and NF-κB activation. Cell 1998;93:875.

182. Sun SC, Ballard DW: Persistent activation of NF-1κB by the Tax transforming protein of HTLV-1: Hijacking cellular IκB kinases. Oncogene 1999;18:6948.

183. Chlichlia K, Busslinger M, Peter ME, et al: ICE-proteases mediate HTLV-I Tax-induced apoptotic T-cell death. Oncogene 1997;14:2265.

184. Ashkenazi A, Dixit VM: Death receptors: Signaling and modulation. Science 1998;281:1305.

185. Suzuki T, Ohsugi Y, Uchida-Toita M, et al: Tax oncoprotein of HTLV-1 binds to the human homologue of *Drosophila* discs large tumor suppressor protein, hDLG, and perturbs its function in cell growth control. Oncogene 1999;18:5967.

186. Lee SS, Weiss RS, Javier RT: Binding of human virus oncoproteins to hD1g/SAP97, a mammalian homolog of the *Drosophila* discs large tumor suppressor protein. Proc Natl Acad Sci U S A 1997;94:6670.

187. De Valck D, Jin DY, Heyninck K, et al: The zinc finger protein A20 interacts with a novel anti-apoptotic protein which is cleaved by specific caspases. Oncogene 1999;18:4182.

188. Kiyokawa T, Kawaguchi T, Seiki M, et al: Association of the pX gene product of human T-cell leukemia virus type-I with nucleus. Virology 1985;147:462.

189. Cann AJ, Chen ISY: Human T-cell leukemia virus types I and II. In Fields BN, Knipe DM, Howley PM, eds: Fields Virology. Philadelphia: Lippincott-Raven; 1996.

190. Ciminale V, Pavlakis GN, Derse D, et al: Complex splicing in the human T-cell leukemia virus (HTLV) family of retroviruses: Novel mRNAs and proteins produced by HTLV type I. J Virol 1992;66:1737.

191. Koralnik IJ, Gessain A, Klotman ME, et al: Protein isoforms encoded by the pX region of human T-cell leukemia/lymphotropic virus type I. Proc Natl Acad Sci U S A 1992;89:8813.

192. Koralnik IJ, Fullen J, Franchini G: The p12II, p13II, and p30II proteins encoded by human T-cell leukemia/lymphotropic virus type I open reading frames I and II are localized in three different cellular compartments. J Virol 1993;67:2360.

193. Franchini G, Mulloy JC, Koralnik IJ, et al: The human T-cell leukemia/lymphotropic virus type I p12I protein cooperates with the E5 oncoprotein of bovine papillomavirus in cell transformation and binds the 16-kilodalton subunit of the vacuolar H⁺ ATPase. J Virol 1993;67:7701.

194. Mulloy JC, Crownley RW, Fullen J, et al: The human T-cell leukemia/lymphotropic virus type 1 p12I proteins bind the interleukin-2 receptor beta and gamma chains and affects their expression on the cell surface. J Virol 1996;70:3599.

195. Collins ND, Newbound GC, Albrecht B, et al: Selective ablation of human T-cell lymphotropic virus type 1 p12I reduces viral infectivity in vivo. Blood 1998;91:4701.

196. Murphy EL, Hanchard B, Figueroa JP, et al: Modelling the risk of adult T-cell leukemia/lymphoma in persons infected with human T-lymphotropic virus type I. Int J Cancer 1989;43:250.

197. Wattel E, Vartanian JP, Pannetier C, et al: Clonal expansion of human T-cell leukemia virus type I–infected cells in asymptomatic and symptomatic carriers without malignancy. J Virol 1995;69:2863.

198. Hollsberg P, Wucherpfennig KW, Ausubel LJ, et al: Characterization of HTLV-I in vivo infected T cell clones. IL-2–independent growth of nontransformed T cells. J Immunol 1992;148:3256.

199. Migone TS, Lin JX, Cereseto A, et al: Constitutively activated Jak-STAT pathway in T cells transformed with HTLV-I. Science 1995;269:79.

200. Xu X, Kang SH, Heidenreich O, et al: Constitutive activation of different Jak tyrosine kinases in human T cell leukemia virus type 1 (HTLV-1) tax protein or virus-transformed cells. J Clin Invest 1995;96:1548.

201. Nakamura N, Fujii M, Tsukahara T, et al: Human T-cell leukemia virus type 1 Tax protein induces the expression of STAT1 and STAT5 genes in T-cells. Oncogene 1999;18:2667.

201a. Mulloy JC, Migone TS, Ross TM, et al: Human and simian T-cell leukemia viruses type 2 (HTLV-2 and STLV-2(pan-p)) transform T cells independently of Jak/STAT activation. J Virol 1998;72:4408.

202. Jeffery KJ, Usuku K, Hall SE, et al: HLA alleles determine human T-lymphotropic virus-I (HTLV-I) proviral load and the risk of HTLV-I–associated myelopathy. Proc Natl Acad Sci U S A 1999;96:3848.

203. Sonoda S, Fujiyoshi T, Yashiki S: Immunogenetics of HTLV-I/II and associated diseases. J Acquir Immune Defic Syndr Hum Retrovirol 1996;13(Suppl 1):119.

204. Manns A, Hanchard B, Morgan OS, et al: Human leukocyte antigen class II alleles associated with human T-cell lymphotropic virus type I infection and adult T-cell leukemia/lymphoma in a black population. J Natl Cancer Inst 1998;90:617.

205. Seiki M, Eddy R, Shows TB, et al: Nonspecific integration of the HTLV provirus genome into adult T-cell leukaemia cells. Nature 1984;309:640.

206. Leclercq I, Mortreux F, Cavrois M, et al: Host sequences flanking the human T-cell leukemia virus type 1 provirus in vivo. J Virol 2000;74:2305.

207. Malik KT, Even J, Karpas A: Molecular cloning and complete nucleotide sequence of an adult T cell leukaemia virus/human T cell leukaemia virus type I (ATLV/HTLV-I) isolate of Caribbean origin: Relationship to other members of the ATLV/HTLV-I subgroup. J Gen Virol 1988;69:1695.

208. Takemoto S, Mulloy JC, Cereseto A, et al: Proliferation of adult T cell leukemia/lymphoma cells is associated with the constitutive activation of JAK/STAT proteins. Proc Natl Acad Sci U S A 1997;94:13897.

209. Hall WW, Liu CR, Schneewind O, et al: Deleted HTLV-I provirus in blood and cutaneous lesions of patients with mycosis fungoides. Science 1991;253:317.

210. Zucker-Franklin D, Hooper WC, Evatt BL: Human lymphotropic retroviruses associated with mycosis fungoides: Evidence that human T-cell lymphotropic virus type II as well as HTLV-I may play a role in the disease. Blood 1992;80:1537.

211. Bazarbachi A, Soriano V, Pawson R, et al: Mycosis fungoides and Sézary syndrome are not associated with HTLV-I infection: An international study. Br J Haematol 1997;98:927.

212. el-Farrash MA, Salem HA, Kuroda MJ, et al: Isolation of human T-cell leukemia virus type I from a transformed T-cell line derived spontaneously from lymphocytes of a seronegative Egyptian patient with mycosis fungoides. Blood 1995;86:1842.

213. Mann DL, Desantis P, Mark G: HTLV-I–associated B-cell CLL: Indirect role for retroviruses in leukemogenesis. Science 1987;236:1103.

214. Wotherspoon AC, Doglioni C, Diss TC, et al: Regression of primary low-grade B-cell gastric lymphoma of mucosa-associated lymphoid tissue type after eradication of *Helicobacter pylori*. Lancet 1993;342:575.

215. Manns A, Cleghorn FR, Falk RT, et al: Role of HTLV-I in development of non-Hodgkin lymphoma in Jamaica and Trinidad and Tobago. The HTLV Lymphoma Study Group. Lancet 1993;342:1447.

216. Duggan DB, Ehrlich GD, Davey FP, et al: HTLV-I–induced lymphoma mimicking Hodgkin's disease. Diagnosis by polymerase chain reaction amplification of specific HTLV-I sequences in tumor DNA. Blood 1988;71:1027.

217. Kalyanaraman V, Sarngadharan M, Robert-Guroff M, et al: A new subtype of human T-cell leukemia virus (HTLV-2) associated with a T-cell variant of hairy cell leukemia. Science 1982;218:571.

218. Rosenblatt J, Goldie D, Wachsman W, et al: A second isolate of HTLV-2 associated with atypical hairy cell leukemia. N Engl J Med 1986;315:372.

218a. Rosenblatt JD, Giorgi JV, Golde DW, et al: Integrated human T-cell leukemia virus II genome in CD8⁺ T cells from a patient with "atypical" hairy cell leukemia: Evidence for distinct T and B cell lymphoproliferative disorders. Blood 1988;71:363.

219. Gessain A, Barin F, Vernant JC, et al: Antibodies to human T-lymphotropic virus type-I in patients with tropical spastic paraparesis. Lancet 1985;2:407.

220. Osame M, Usuku K, Izumo S, et al: HTLV-I associated myelopathy, a new clinical entity [letter]. Lancet 1986;1:1031.

221. LaGrenade L, Hanchard B, Fletcher V, et al: Infective dermatitis of Jamaican children: A marker for HTLV-I infection. Lancet 1990; 336:1345.

222. Mochizuki M, Watanabe T, Yamaguchi K, et al: HTLV-I uveitis: A distinct clinical entity caused by HTLV-I. Jpn J Cancer Res 1992; 83:236.

223. Morgan OS, Rodgers-Johnson P, Mora C, et al: HTLV-1 and polymyositis in Jamaica. Lancet 1989;2:1184.

224. Nishioka K, Maruyama I, Sato K, et al: Chronic inflammatory arthropathy associated with HTLV-I [letter]. Lancet 1989;1:441.

225. Hjelle B, Appenzeller O, Mills R, et al: Chronic neurodegenerative disease associated with HTLV-II infection. Lancet 1992;339:645.

226. Rickinson AB, Kieff E: Epstein-Barr virus. In Fields BN, Knipe DM, Howley PM, eds: Fields Virology. Philadelphia: Lippincott-Raven; 1996, p 2397.

227. Gerber P, Nonayama M, Lucas S, et al: Oral excretion of Epstein-Barr virus by healthy subjects and patients with infectious mononucleosis. Lancet 1972;2:988.

228. Sixbey JW, Lemon SM, Pagano JS: A second site for Epstein-Barr virus shedding: The uterine cervix. Lancet 1986;2:1122.

229. Gerber P, Walsh JH, Rosenblum EN, et al: Association of EB-virus infection with the post-perfusion syndrome. Lancet 1969;1:593.

230. Kieff E: Epstein-Barr virus and its replication. In Fields BN, Knipe DM, Howley PM, eds: Fields Virology. Philadelphia: Lippincott-Raven, 1996, p 2343.

231. Adldinger HK, Delius H, Freese UK, et al: A putative transforming gene of Jijoye virus differs from that of Epstein-Barr virus prototypes. Virology 1985;141:221.

232. Sample J, Young L, Martin B, et al: Epstein-Barr virus types 1 and 2 differ in their EBNA-3A, EBNA-3B, and EBNA-3C genes. J Virol 1990;64:4084.

233. Zimber U, Adldinger HK, Lenoir GM, et al: Geographical prevalence of two types of Epstein-Barr virus. Virology 1986;154:56.

234. Midgley RS, Blake NW, Yao QY, et al: Novel intertypic recombinants of Epstein-Barr virus in the Chinese population. J Virol 2000; 74:1544.

235. Yao QY, Tierney RJ, Croom-Carter D, et al: Frequency of multiple Epstein-Barr virus infections in T-cell–immunocompromised individuals. J Virol 1996;70:4884.

236. Yao QY, Tierney RJ, Croom-Carter D, et al: Isolation of intertypic recombinants of Epstein-Barr virus from T-cell–immunocompromised individuals. J Virol 1996;70:4895.

237. Miller G, Niederman JC, Andrews LL: Prolonged oropharyngeal excretion of Epstein-Barr virus after infectious mononucleosis. N Engl J Med 1973;288:229.

238. Yao QY, Rickinson AB, Epstein MA: A re-examination of the Epstein-Barr virus carrier state in healthy seropositive individuals. Int J Cancer 1985;35:35.

239. Wang D, Liebowitz D, Kieff E: An EBV membrane protein expressed in immortalized lymphocytes transforms established rodent cells. Cell 1985;43:831.

240. Wilson JB, Weinberg W, Johnson R, et al: Expression of the BNLF-1 oncogene of Epstein-Barr virus in the skin of transgenic mice induces hyperplasia and aberrant expression of keratin 6. Cell 1990;61:1315.

241. Dawson CW, Rickinson AB, Young LS: Epstein-Barr virus latent membrane protein inhibits human epithelial cell differentiation. Nature 1990;344:777.

242. Gires O, Kohlhuber F, Kilger E, et al: Latent membrane protein 1 of Epstein-Barr virus interacts with JAK3 and activates STAT proteins. EMBO J 1999;18:3064.

243. Huen DS, Henderson SA, Croom-Carter D, et al: The Epstein-Barr virus latent membrane protein-1 (LMP1) mediates activation of NF-kappa B and cell surface phenotype via two effector regions in its carboxy-terminal cytoplasmic domain. Oncogene 1995;10:549.

244. Eliopoulos AG, Young LS: Activation of the cJun N-terminal kinase (JNK) pathway by the Epstein-Barr virus–encoded latent membrane protein 1 (LMP1). Oncogene 1998;16:1731.

245. Wang F, Gregory CD, Rowe M, et al: Epstein-Barr virus nuclear antigen 2 specifically induces expression of the B-cell activation antigen CD23. Proc Natl Acad Sci U S A 1987;84:3452.

246. Henderson S, Rowe M, Gregory C, et al: Induction of bcl-2 expression by Epstein-Barr virus latent membrane protein 1 protects infected B cells from programmed cell death. Cell 1991;65:1107.

247. Zimber-Strobl U, Strobl LJ, Meitinger C, et al: Epstein-Barr virus nuclear antigen 2 exerts its transactivating function through interaction with recombination signal binding protein RBP-J kappa, the homologue of Drosophila Suppressor of Hairless. EMBO J 1994; 13:4973.

248. Laux G, Adam B, Strobl LJ, et al: The Spi-1/PU.1 and Spi-B ets family transcription factors and the recombination signal binding protein RBP-J kappa interact with an Epstein-Barr virus nuclear antigen 2 responsive cis-element. EMBO J 1994;13:5624.

249. Reisman D, Sugden B: Trans activation of an Epstein-Barr viral transcriptional enhancer by the Epstein-Barr viral nuclear antigen 1. Mol Cell Biol 1986;6:3838.

250. Sugden B, Warren N: A promoter of Epstein-Barr virus that can function during latent infection can be transactivated by EBNA-1, a viral protein required for viral DNA replication during latent infection. J Virol 1989;63:2644.

251. Wilson JB, Bell JL, Levine AJ: Expression of Epstein-Barr virus nuclear antigen-1 induces B cell neoplasia in transgenic mice. EMBO J 1986;15:3117.

252. Sheu LF, Chen A, Meng CL, et al: Enhanced malignant progression of nasopharyngeal carcinoma cells mediated by the expression of Epstein-Barr nuclear antigen 1 in vivo. J Pathol 1996;180:243.

253. Tomkinson B, Robertson E, Kieff E: Epstein-Barr virus nuclear proteins EBNA-3A and EBNA-3C are essential for B-lymphocyte growth transformation. J Virol 1993;67:2014.

254. Sinclair AJ, Palmero I, Peters G, et al: EBNA-2 and EBNA-LP cooperate to cause G_0 to G_1 transition during immortalization of resting human B lymphocytes by Epstein-Barr virus. EMBO J 1994;13: 3321.

255. Fingeroth JD, Weis JJ, Tedder TF, et al: Epstein-Barr virus receptor of human B lymphocytes is the C3d receptor CR2. Proc Natl Acad Sci U S A 1984;81:4510.

256. Gregory CD, Dive C, Henderson S, et al: Activation of Epstein-Barr virus latent genes protects human B cells from death by apoptosis. Nature 1991;349:612.

257. Levitskaya J, Sharipo A, Leonchiks A, et al: Inhibition of ubiquitin/proteasome-dependent protein degradation by the Gly-Ala repeat domain of the Epstein-Barr virus nuclear antigen 1. Proc Natl Acad Sci U S A 1997;94:12616.

258. Purtilo DT, Sakamoto K, Barnabei V, et al: Epstein-Barr virus–induced diseases in boys with the X-linked lymphoproliferative syndrome (XLP): Update on studies of the registry. Am J Med 1982;73:49.

259. Burkitt D: A sarcoma involving the jaws in African children. Br J Surg 1958;45:218.

260. Burkitt D: A children's cancer dependent upon climatic factors. Nature 1962;194:232.

261. Epstein MA, Achong BG, Barr YM: Virus particles in cultured lymphoblasts from Burkitt's lymphoma. Lancet 1964;1:702.

262. Beral V, Peterman T, Berkelman R, et al: AIDS-associated non-Hodgkin lymphoma. Lancet 1991;337:805.

263. Gregory CD, Murray RJ, Edwards CF, et al: Downregulation of cell adhesion molecules LFA-3 and ICAM-1 in Epstein-Barr virus-positive Burkitt's lymphoma underlies tumor cell escape from virus-specific T cell surveillance. J Exp Med 1988;167:1811.

264. Lam KM, Syed N, Whittle H, et al: Circulating Epstein-Barr virus-carrying B cells in acute malaria. Lancet 1991;337:876.

265. Neri A, Barriga F, Inghirami G, et al: Epstein-Barr virus infection precedes clonal expansion in Burkitt's and acquired immunodeficiency syndrome–associated lymphoma. Blood 1991;77:1092.

266. Lenoir GM, Bornkamm GW: Burkitt's lymphoma, a human cancer model for the study of the multistep development of cancer. Adv Viral Oncol 1987;7:173.

267. Obrams GI, Grufferman S: Epidemiology of HIV associated non-Hodgkin lymphoma. Cancer Surv 1991;10:91.

268. Cleary ML, Sklar J: Lymphoproliferative disorders in cardiac transplant recipients are multiclonal lymphomas. Lancet 1984;2:489.

269. Locker J, Nalesnik M: Molecular genetic analysis of lymphoid tumors arising after organ transplantation. Am J Pathol 1989; 135:977.

270. Swerdlow SH: Post-transplant lymphoproliferative disorders: A morphologic, phenotypic and genotypic spectrum of disease. Histopathology 1992;20:373.

271. Young L, Alfieri C, Hennessy K, et al: Expression of Epstein-Barr virus transformation-associated genes in tissues of patients with EBV lymphoproliferative disease. N Engl J Med 1989;321:1080.

272. Thomas JA, Hotchin NA, Allday MJ, et al: Immunohistology of Epstein-Barr virus–associated antigens in B cell disorders from immunocompromised individuals. Transplantation 1990;49:944.

273. Hamilton-Dutoit SJ, Rea O, Raphael M, et al: Epstein-Barr virus—latent gene expression and tumor cell phenotype in acquired immunodeficiency syndrome–related non-Hodgkin's lymphoma. Correlation of lymphoma phenotype with three distinct patterns of viral latency. Am J Pathol 1993;143:1072.

274. Jarrett RF, MacKenzie J: Epstein-Barr virus and other candidate viruses in the pathogenesis of Hodgkin's disease. Semin Hematol 1999;36:260.

275. Weiss LM, Movahed LA, Warnke RA, et al: Detection of Epstein-Barr viral genomes in Reed-Sternberg cells of Hodgkin's disease. N Engl J Med 1989;320:502.

276. Herbst H, Dallenbach F, Hummel M, et al: Epstein-Barr virus DNA and latent gene products in Ki-1 (CD30)-positive anaplastic large cell lymphomas. Blood 1991;78:2666.

277. Anagnostopoulos I, Herbst H, Niedobitek G, et al: Demonstration of monoclonal EBV genomes in Hodgkin's disease and Ki-1-positive anaplastic large cell lymphoma by combined Southern blot and in situ hybridization. Blood 1989;74:810.

278. Armstrong AA, Gallagher A, Krajewski AS, et al: The expression of the EBV latent membrane protein (LMP-1) is independent of CD23 and bcl-2 in Reed-Sternberg cells in Hodgkin's disease. Histopathology 1992;21:72.

279. Weinreb M, Day PJ, Niggli F, et al: The consistent association between Epstein-Barr virus and Hodgkin's disease in children in Kenya. Blood 1996;87:3828.

280. Stein H, Hummel M, Marafioti T, et al: Molecular biology of Hodgkin's disease. Cancer Surv 1997;30:107.

281. Boiocchi M, Dolcetti R, De Re V, et al: Demonstration of a unique Epstein-Barr virus–positive cellular clone in metachronous multiple localizations of Hodgkin's disease. Am J Pathol 1993;142:33.

282. Brousset P, Schlaifer D, Meggetto F, et al: Persistence of the same viral strain in early and late relapses of Epstein-Barr virus–associated Hodgkin's disease. Blood 1994;84:2447.

283. Jarrett RF, Gallagher A, Jones DB, et al: Detection of Epstein-Barr virus genomes in Hodgkin's disease: Relation to age. J Clin Pathol 1991;44:844.

284. Pallesen G, Hamilton-Dutoit SJ, Rowe M, et al: Expression of Epstein-Barr virus replicative proteins in AIDS-related non-Hodgkin's lymphoma cells. J Pathol 1991;165:289.

285. Kuppers R, Rajewsky K, Zhao M, et al: Hodgkin disease: Hodgkin and Reed-Sternberg cells picked from histological sections show clonal immunoglobulin gene rearrangements and appear to be derived from B cells at various stages of development. Proc Natl Acad Sci U S A 1994;91:10962.

286. Kanzler H, Hansmann ML, Kapp U, et al: Molecular single cell analysis demonstrates the derivation of a peripheral blood–derived cell line (L1236) from the Hodgkin/Reed-Sternberg cells of a Hodgkin's lymphoma patient. Blood 1996;87:3429.

287. Braeuninger A, Kuppers R, Strickler JG, et al: Hodgkin and Reed-Sternberg cells in lymphocyte predominant Hodgkin disease represent clonal populations of germinal center–derived tumor B cells [published erratum appears in Proc Natl Acad Sci U S A 1997 Dec 9;94(25):14211]. Proc Natl Acad Sci U S A 1997;94:9337.

288. Kuppers R, Rajewsky K: The origin of Hodgkin and Reed/Sternberg cells in Hodgkin's disease. Annu Rev Immunol 1998;16:471.

289. Jungnickel B, Staratschek-Jox A, Brauninger A, et al: Clonal deleterious mutations in the IκBα gene in the malignant cells in Hodgkin's lymphoma. J Exp Med 2000;191:395.

290. Emmerich F, Meiser M, Hummel M, et al: Overexpression of I kappa B alpha without inhibition of NF-kappaB activity and mutations in the I kappa B alpha gene in Reed-Sternberg cells. Blood 1999;94:3129.

291. Cabannes E, Khan G, Aillet F, et al: Mutations in the IκBα gene in Hodgkin's disease suggest a tumour suppressor role for IκBα. Oncogene 1999;18:3063.

292. Marafioti T, Hummel M, Anagnostopoulos I, et al: Origin of nodular lymphocyte-predominant Hodgkin's disease from a clonal expansion of highly mutated germinal-center B cells. N Engl J Med 1997;337:453.

293. Ohno T, Stribley JA, Wu G, et al: Clonality in nodular lymphocyte-predominant Hodgkin's disease. N Engl J Med 1997;337:459.

294. Su IJ, Hsieh HC, Lin KH, et al: Aggressive peripheral T-cell lymphomas containing Epstein-Barr viral DNA: A clinicopathologic and molecular analysis. Blood 1991;77:799.

295. Harabuchi Y, Yamanaka N, Kataura A, et al: Epstein-Barr virus in nasal T-cell lymphomas in patients with lethal midline granuloma. Lancet 1990;335:128.

296. Dreno B, Celerier P, Fleischmann M, et al: Presence of Epstein-Barr virus in cutaneous lesions of mycosis fungoides and Sézary syndrome. Acta Derm Venereol 1994;74:355.

297. Kagami Y, Nakamura S, Suzuki R, et al: Establishment of an IL-2-dependent cell line derived from 'nasal-type' NK/T-cell lymphoma of CD2+, sCD3−, CD3epsilon+, CD56+ phenotype and associated with the Epstein-Barr virus. Br J Haematol 1998;103:669.

298. Rivadeneira ED, Ferrari MG, Jarrett RF, et al: A novel Epstein-Barr virus–like virus, HV(MNE), in a *Macaca nemestrina* with mycosis fungoides. Blood 1999;94:2090.

299. Kanegane H, Miyawaki T, Yachie A, et al: Development of EBV-positive T-cell lymphoma following infection of peripheral blood T cells with EBV. Leuk Lymphoma 1999;34:603.

300. Chang Y, Cesarman E, Pessin MS, et al: Identification of herpesvirus-like DNA sequences in AIDS-associated Kaposi's sarcoma. Science 1994;266:1865.

301. Schulz TF: Kaposi's sarcoma–associated herpesvirus (human herpesvirus-8). J Gen Virol 1998;79:1573.

302. Boshoff C, Weiss RA: Kaposi's sarcoma–associated herpesvirus. Adv Cancer Res 1998;75:57.

303. Cesarman E, Chang Y, Moore PS, et al: Kaposi's sarcoma-associated herpesvirus-like DNA in AIDS-related body-cavity-based lymphomas. N Engl J Med 1995;332:1186.

303a. Cesarman E, Moore PS, Rao PH, et al: In vitro establishment and characterization of two acquired immunodeficiency syndrome-related lymphoma cell lines (BC-1 and BC-2) containing Kaposi's sarcoma–associated herpesvirus-like (KSHV) DNA sequences. Blood 1995;86:2708.

304. Soulier J, Grollet L, Oksenhendler E, et al: Kaposi's sarcoma-associated herpesvirus-like DNA sequences in multicentric Castleman's disease. Blood 1995;86:1276.

305. Russo JJ, Bohenzky RA, Chien MC, et al: Nucleotide sequence of the Kaposi sarcoma–associated herpesvirus (HHV8). Proc Natl Acad Sci U S A 1996;93:14862.

306. Gao SJ, Kingsley L, Hoover DR, et al: Seroconversion to antibodies against Kaposi's sarcoma–associated herpesvirus-related latent nuclear antigens before the development of Kaposi's sarcoma. N Engl J Med 1996;335:233.

307. Kedes DH, Operskalski E, Busch M, et al: The seroepidemiology of human herpesvirus 8 (Kaposi's sarcoma–associated herpesvirus): Distribution of infection in KS risk groups and evidence for sexual transmission [published erratum appears in Nat Med 1996 Sep;2(9):1041]. Nat Med 1996;2:918.

308. Simpson GR, Schulz TF, Whitby D, et al: Prevalence of Kaposi's sarcoma associated herpesvirus infection measured by antibodies to recombinant capsid protein and latent immunofluorescence antigen. Lancet 1996;348:1133.

309. Calabro ML, Sheldon J, Favero A, et al: Seroprevalence of Kaposi's sarcoma–associated herpesvirus/human herpesvirus 8 in several regions of Italy. J Hum Virol 1998;1:207.

310. Whitby D, Luppi M, Barozzi P, et al: Human herpesvirus 8 seroprevalence in blood donors and lymphoma patients from different regions of Italy. J Natl Cancer Inst 1998;90:395.

311. Schulz TF: Epidemiology of Kaposi's sarcoma–associated herpesvirus/human herpesvirus 8. Adv Cancer Res 1999;76:121.

312. Mayama S, Cuevas LE, Sheldon J, et al: Prevalence and transmission of Kaposi's sarcoma–associated herpesvirus (human herpesvirus 8) in Ugandan children and adolescents. Int J Cancer 1998;77:817.

313. Gessain A, Mauclere P, van Beveren M, et al: Human herpesvirus 8 primary infection occurs during childhood in Cameroon, Central Africa. Int J Cancer 1999;81:189.

314. Andreoni M, El-Sawaf G, Rezza G, et al: High seroprevalence of antibodies to human herpesvirus-8 in Egyptian children: Evidence of nonsexual transmission. J Natl Cancer Inst 1999;91:465.

315. Bourboulia D, Whitby D, Boshoff C, et al: Serologic evidence for mother-to-child transmission of Kaposi sarcoma–associated herpesvirus infection [letter]. JAMA 1998;280:31.

316. Melbye M, Cook PM, Hjalgrim H, et al: Risk factors for Kaposi's-sarcoma–associated herpesvirus (KSHV/HHV-8) seropositivity in a cohort of homosexual men, 1981-1996. Int J Cancer 1998;77:543.

317. Martin JN, Ganem DE, Osmond DH, et al: Sexual transmission and the natural history of human herpesvirus 8 infection. N Engl J Med 1998;338:948.

318. Dukers NH, Renwick N, Prins M, et al: Risk factors for human herpesvirus 8 seropositivity and seroconversion in a cohort of homosexual men. Am J Epidemiol 2000;151:213.

319. O'Brien TR, Kedes D, Ganem D, et al: Evidence for concurrent epidemics of human herpesvirus 8 and human immunodeficiency virus type 1 in US homosexual men: Rates, risk factors, and relationship to Kaposi's sarcoma. J Infect Dis 1999;180:1010.

320. Decker LL, Shankar P, Khan G, et al: The Kaposi sarcoma–associated herpesvirus (KSHV) is present as an intact latent genome in KS tissue but replicates in the peripheral blood mononuclear cells of KS patients. J Exp Med 1996;184:283.

321. Staskus KA, Zhong W, Gebhard K, et al: Kaposi's sarcoma–associated herpesvirus gene expression in endothelial (spindle) tumor cells. J Virol 1997;71:715.

322. Rainbow L, Platt GM, Simpson GR, et al: The 222 to 234-kilodalton latent nuclear protein (LNA) of Kaposi's sarcoma–associated herpesvirus (human herpesvirus 8) is encoded by orf73 and is a component of the latency-associated nuclear antigen. J Virol 1997;71:5915.

323. Sarid R, Flore O, Bohenzky RA, et al: Transcription mapping of the Kaposi's sarcoma–associated herpesvirus (human herpesvirus 8) genome in a body cavity–based lymphoma cell line (BC-1). J Virol 1998;72:1005.

324. Davis MA, Sturzl MA, Blasig C, et al: Expression of human herpesvirus 8–encoded cyclin D in Kaposi's sarcoma spindle cells. J Natl Cancer Inst 1997;89:1868.

325. Blasig C, Zietz C, Haar B, et al: Monocytes in Kaposi's sarcoma lesions are productively infected by human herpesvirus 8. J Virol 1997;71:7963.

326. Kirshner JR, Staskus K, Haase A, et al: Expression of the open reading frame 74 (G-protein–coupled receptor) gene of Kaposi's sarcoma (KS)–associated herpesvirus: Implications for KS pathogenesis. J Virol 1999;73:6006.

327. Parravicini C, Chandran B, Corbellino M, et al: Differential viral protein expression in Kaposi's sarcoma–associated herpesvirus-infected diseases: Kaposi's sarcoma, primary effusion lymphoma, and multicentric Castleman's disease. Am J Pathol 2000;156:743.

328. Cannon JS, Nicholas J, Orenstein JM, et al: Heterogeneity of viral IL-6 expression in HHV-8–associated diseases. J Infect Dis 1999;180:824.

329. Szekely L, Kiss C, Mattsson K, et al: Human herpesvirus-8–encoded LNA-1 accumulates in heterochromatin-associated nuclear bodies. J Gen Virol 1999;80:2889.

330. Ballestas ME, Chatis PA, Kaye KM: Efficient persistence of extrachromosomal KSHV DNA mediated by latency-associated nuclear antigen. Science 1999;284:641.

331. Friborg JJ, Kong W, Hottiger MO, et al: p53 inhibition by the LANA protein of KSHV protects against cell death. Nature 1999;402:889.

331a. Radkov SA, Kellam P, Boshoff C: The latent nuclear antigen of Kaposi's sarcoma. Associated herpesvirus targets the retinoblastoma-E2F pathway and with the oncogene h-ras transforms primary rat cells. Nat Med 2000;6:1121.

332. Platt GM, Simpson GR, Mittnacht S, et al: Latent nuclear antigen of Kaposi's sarcoma–associated herpesvirus interacts with RING3, a homolog of the *Drosophila* female sterile homeotic (fsh) gene. J Virol 1999;73:9789.

333. Ellis M, Chew YP, Fallis L, et al: Degradation of p27(Kip) cdk inhibitor triggered by Kaposi's sarcoma virus cyclin-cdk6 complex. EMBO J 1999;18:644.

334. Mann DJ, Child ES, Swanton C, et al: Modulation of p27(Kip1) levels by the cyclin encoded by Kaposi's sarcoma–associated herpesvirus. EMBO J 1999;18:654.

335. Swanton C, Mann DJ, Fleckenstein B, et al: Herpes viral cyclin/Cdk6 complexes evade inhibition by CDK inhibitor proteins. Nature 1997;390:184.

336. Djerbi M, Screpanti V, Catrina AI, et al: The inhibitor of death receptor signaling, FLICE-inhibitory protein defines a new class of tumor progression factors. J Exp Med 1999;190:1025.

337. Muralidhar S, Pumfery AM, Hassani M, et al: Identification of kaposin (open reading frame K12) as a human herpesvirus 8 (Kaposi's sarcoma–associated herpesvirus) transforming gene [published erratum appears in J Virol 1999 Mar;73(3):2568]. J Virol 1998;72:4980.

338. Molden J, Chang Y, You Y, et al: A Kaposi's sarcoma–associated herpesvirus-encoded cytokine homolog (vIL-6) activates signaling through the shared gp130 receptor subunit. J Biol Chem 1997;272:19625.

339. Aoki Y, Jaffe ES, Chang Y, et al: Angiogenesis and hematopoiesis induced by Kaposi's sarcoma-associated herpesvirus-encoded interleukin-6. Blood 1999;93:4034.

340. Moore PS, Boshoff C, Weiss RA, et al: Molecular mimicry of human cytokine and cytokine response pathway genes by KSHV. Science 1996;274:1739.

341. Boshoff C, Endo Y, Collins PD, et al: Angiogenic and HIV-inhibitory functions of KSHV-encoded chemokines. Science 1997;278:290.

342. Bais C, Santomasso B, Coso O, et al: G-protein–coupled receptor of Kaposi's sarcoma–associated herpesvirus is a viral oncogene and angiogenesis activator [published erratum appears in Nature 1998 Mar 12;392(6672):210]. Nature 1998;391:86.

343. Lee H, Guo J, Li M, et al: Identification of an immunoreceptor tyrosine-based activation motif of K1 transforming protein of Kaposi's sarcoma–associated herpesvirus. Mol Cell Biol 1998;18:5219.

344. Lee H, Veazey R, Williams K, et al: Deregulation of cell growth by the K1 gene of Kaposi's sarcoma–associated herpesvirus. Nat Med 1998;4:435.

345. Glenn M, Rainbow L, Aurad F, et al: Identification of a spliced gene from Kaposi's sarcoma–associated herpesvirus encoding a protein with similarities to latent membrane proteins 1 and 2A of Epstein-Barr virus. J Virol 1999;73:6953.

346. Poole LJ, Zong JC, Ciufo DM, et al: Comparison of genetic variability at multiple loci across the genomes of the major subtypes of Kaposi's sarcoma–associated herpesvirus reveals evidence for recombination and for two distinct types of open reading frame K15 alleles at the right-hand end. J Virol 1999;73:6646.

347. Choi JK, Lee BS, Shim SN, et al: Identification of the novel K15 gene at the rightmost end of the Kaposi's sarcoma–associated herpesvirus genome. J Virol 2000;74:436.

348. Gao SJ, Boshoff C, Jayachandra S, et al: KSHV ORF K9 (vIRF) is an oncogene which inhibits the interferon signaling pathway. Oncogene 1997;15:1979.

349. Jayachandra S, Low KG, Thlick AE, et al: Three unrelated viral transforming proteins (vIRF, EBNA2, and E1A) induce the MYC oncogene through the interferon-responsive PRF element by using different transcription coadaptors. Proc Natl Acad Sci U S A 1999;96:11566.

350. Flore O, Rafii S, Ely S, et al: Transformation of primary human endothelial cells by Kaposi's sarcoma–associated herpesvirus. Nature 1998;394:588.

351. Moses AV, Fish KN, Ruhl R, et al: Long-term infection and transformation of dermal microvascular endothelial cells by human herpesvirus 8. J Virol 1999;73:6892.

352. Judde JG, Lacoste CV, Bhere Z, et al: Monoclonality or oligoclonality of human herpesvirus 8 terminal repeat sequences in Kaposi's sarcoma and other diseases. J Natl Cancer Inst 2000;92:729.

352a. Rivas C, Thlick AE, Parravicini C, et al: Kaposi's sarcoma-associated herpesvirus LANA-2 is a B-cell specific latent viral protein that inhibits p53. J Virol 2002;75:429.

352b. Gessain A, Sudaka A, Briere J, et al: Kaposi sarcoma–associated herpes-like virus (human herpesvirus type 8) DNA sequences in multicentric Castleman's disease: Is there any relevant association in non–human immunodeficiency virus–infected patients? [letter]. Blood 1996;87:414.

353. Parravicini C, Corbellino M, Paulli M, et al: Expression of a virus-derived cytokine, KSHV vIL-6, in HIV-seronegative Castleman's disease. Am J Pathol 1997;151:1517.

354. Oksenhendler E, Cazals-Hatem D, Schulz TF, et al: Transient angiolymphoid hyperplasia and Kaposi's sarcoma after primary infection with human herpesvirus 8 in a patient with human immunodeficiency virus infection. N Engl J Med 1998;338:1585.

355. Parravicini C, Olsen SJ, Capra M, et al: Risk of Kaposi's sarcoma-associated herpes virus transmission from donor allografts among Italian posttransplant Kaposi's sarcoma patients. Blood 1997;90:2826.

356. Schang LM, Rosenberg A, Schaffer PA: Roscovitine, a specific inhibitor of cellular cyclin-dependent kinases, inhibits herpes simplex virus DNA synthesis in the presence of viral early proteins. J Virol 2000;74:2107.

357. MacMahon B: Is acute lymphoblastic leukemia in children virus-related? Am J Epidemiol 1992;136:916.

358. Petridou E, Kassimos D, Kalmanti M, et al: Age of exposure to infections and risk of childhood leukaemia. BMJ 1993;307:774.

359. Kinlen LJ, Clarke K, Hudson C: Evidence from population mixing in British New Towns 1946–85 of an infective basis for childhood leukaemia. Lancet 1990;336:577.

360. Kinlen LJ, Dickinson M, Stiller CA: Childhood leukaemia and non-Hodgkin's lymphoma near large rural construction sites, with a comparison with Sellafield nuclear site [published erratum appears in BMJ 1995 Apr 8;310(6984):911]. BMJ 1995;310:763.

361. Petridou E, Revinthi K, Alexander FE, et al: Space-time clustering of childhood leukaemia in Greece: Evidence supporting a viral aetiology. Br J Cancer 1996;73:1278.

362. Fine PE, Adelstein AM, Snowman J, et al: Long term effects of exposure to viral infections in utero. BMJ 1985;290:509.

363. Frederick J, Alberman EA: Reported influenza in pregnancy and subsequent cancer in the child. BMJ 1972;2:485.

11

Edward S. Henderson   James McArthur

Diagnosis, Classification, and Assessment of Response to Treatment

INTRODUCTION

Leukemia, myelodysplastic syndromes (MDS), and myeloproliferative diseases (MPD) are malignant, monoclonal proliferations of hematopoietic cells. The various entities result from genetic aberrations in cells of one or more hematopoietic lineages. Multipotent precursor cells are frequently involved, but more mature cells are involved primarily on occasion, and they are frequently the most plentiful malignant cells apparent at the time of diagnosis. The major categories of leukemia are described in terms of lineage and degree of maturation of the predominant malignant cells. Thus, there are lymphoid and myeloid leukemias, and each major subtype is in turn further divided into multiple subtypes on the basis of morphologic cell features and immunologic or genetic markers. Acute and chronic leukemias were originally distinguished by their clinical course, that is, by the rapidity with which the disease reached its deadly conclusion. With the introduction of adequate cell staining techniques,[1] the rapidity of progression was usually found to correlate with the degree of maturity of the predominant malignant cell, with blastic leukemia being the most rapidly fatal. The introduction of effective therapy has blurred the original meanings of acute and chronic, which are now determined by the morphologic, immunologic, and genetic characteristics of the leukemia cells at the time of diagnosis rather than by the rapidity of clinical progression.

During the first century after its discovery, the categorization, of leukemia depended on clinical observation and cytomorphologic evaluation; cytologic studies of first unstained and then polychromatic dye–stained blood and marrow cells led to the recognition of lymphoid and myeloid leukemias, polycythemia vera, and essential thrombocytosis. The myeloid leukemias were found to be those composed primarily of myeloblasts, promyelocytes, myelocytes and neutrophils, monoblasts and monocytes, or malignant erythroid precursors. Lymphoid leukemias could be separated into those with lymphoblasts and those with mature-appearing lymphocytes. With the advent of immunologic analysis, lymphoblastic leukemias could be further subdivided into early B-cell, pre–B-cell,

Burkitt cell, and precursor T-cell varieties. Similarly, immunophenotyping revealed some acute myeloid leukemias to actually be composed of megakaryoblasts, and many of what were previously considered to be undifferentiated blast cells (and often thought to be closely akin to lymphoblasts) in reality proved to be early myeloblasts.[2]

Acute leukemia and MDS may cause symptoms because of the accumulation of cells in the blood, spleen, and other tissues; but more often, the distress and the risks of these diseases stem from the failure of the leukemic bone marrow to produce adequate numbers of normally functioning blood cells. Thus, symptoms of anemia, bleeding, and infection are the common presenting complaints. Given such complaints, a peripheral blood cell count with white blood cell differential is called for. Leukemia cells may or may not be detected, but lower than normal red blood cell, platelet, and neutrophil counts will usually be noted in the peripheral blood.

Chronic leukemias and MPD, by contrast, usually present with evidence of blood cell overproduction manifested by splenomegaly, ruddiness of the skin in the case of polycythemia vera, thrombosis in polycythemia vera and essential thrombocytosis, and lymphadenopathy in chronic lymphocytic leukemia (CLL). Adequate numbers of normal blood cells are typically present when the patient is first seen. These illnesses are not infrequently detected on routine laboratory investigation at a time at which the patient has no complaints referable to the blood disease.

In all cases, the diagnosis of leukemia should be confirmed by examination of the bone marrow. A marrow aspiration and biopsy should be performed to determine the precise type of malignant cell, the extent of marrow involvement, and the cellularity of the marrow. Sufficient cells should be obtained to permit determination of the immune phenotype and for cytogenetic and molecular genetic studies. This work-up provides proof of the monoclonal nature of the proliferation, usually permits an estimate of the prognosis of the individual case, and assists in the selection of an optimal treatment program. No patient should be treated until a bone marrow specimen has been obtained and evaluated morphologically and appropriate additional studies have been initiated.

TABLE 11–1. Acute Leukemia with Specific Cytogenetic Abnormalities

Karyotype	Involved Genes	Types of Leukemia, FAB Designation
t(15;17)(q22;q21) t(5;17)(q32;q21) t(11;17)(q23;q21)	PML-RARA NPM-RARA PLZF-RARA	Acute promyelocytic (AML-M3)
t(8;21)(q22;q21)	AML1-ETO	Acute myeloid, with maturation (AML-M2)
inv(16)(p13;q22) t(16;16)(p13;q22)	CBFB-MYH11	Acute myelomonocytic with abnormal eosinophilia (AML-M4Eo)
t(v)(11q23)	Variable, MLL	Various; usually AML-M4 or AML-M5
t(8;14)(q24;q32) t(2;8)(p12;q24) t(8;22)(q24;q11)	MYC-IgH IGK-MYC MYC-IGL	Burkitt cell (ALL-L3)
t(9;22)(q34;q11)	BCR-ABL	Chronic myelogenous Acute lymphoblastic (ALL-L1/L2) Acute myeloid (any type)
t(12;21)(p12;q22)	TEL-AML1	Acute lymphoblastic (ALL-L1/L2)
t(2;20)(q23;p13)	E2A-PBX	Pre–B-lymphocytic (ALL-L1/L2)

The introduction of cytogenetics into hematology provided the first unique markers of a specific leukemia, the Philadelphia chromosome typical of chronic myelogenous leukemia (CML),[3, 4] and led to an appreciation of the role of abnormalities of the genome in the etiology of malignancy. Specific genetic abnormalities correlate with specific morphologic subtypes and determine response to treatment in certain instances[5-7] (Table 11-1).

This chapter briefly discusses the diagnosis of specific entities; detailed discussions are provided in the separate chapters devoted to the major subtypes of leukemia that follow in this text. This chapter focuses on the clinical circumstances that should lead to the consideration of the diagnosis of a malignant marrow disorder and outlines the approaches that must be taken to ensure the best possible outcome for the patient. The techniques and strategies of diagnostic methods are noted, and a general outline for the diagnosis and differentiation of leukemia subtypes is presented. At the conclusion, the classification proposed by the World Health Organization (WHO)[8] is discussed, and its relationship to the widely adopted classification developed by the French-American-British (FAB) Collaborative Group is reviewed.[2, 9-14]

DEFINITION OF LEUKEMIA

The operative definition of leukemia has traditionally been the presence of an identifiable clone of malignant leukocytes in the marrow and/or peripheral blood. When light microscopy was the sole means of detection, the diagnosis required either a superabundance of differentiated blood cells, as in CML and CLL, or the presence of increased numbers of primitive blood precursors in acute leukemia. The requisite proportion of primitive bone marrow cells was determined empirically to be more than

5% on the basis of the observation that the reduction, through therapy, of such cells to below that level resulted in a return of a relatively normal rate of blood cell production. This remains the most widely used definition of remission, and its obverse defines relapse, recurrence, and by analogy the first presentation of acute leukemia. In most patients, the extent of infiltration of the marrow at diagnosis substantially exceeds the 5% level. Accordingly, groups such as the FAB Collaboration and the National Cancer Institute have established 30% as the minimal level of blast cell (or, in acute promyelocytic leukemia [APL], malignant promyelocyte) infiltration required for the diagnosis of acute myeloid leukemia (AML).[9, 15] For acute lymphoblastic leukemia (ALL), the definition most frequently employed requires a 25% infiltration of the bone marrow to distinguish it from lymphoblastic lymphoma. For myeloid leukemia, there continues to be debate about the proper classification of cases in which the malignant nature of lesser numbers of immature cells can be ascertained by leukemia markers such as Auer bodies and, more recently, by cytogenetic or molecular abnormalities. This has led to the recognition of MDS, on the one hand, and the development of a new paradigm for definition of the hematopoietic malignant neoplasms, on the other, based on the increasing ability to identify, with near certainty, recurrent genetic abnormalities associated with and often causally related to leukemia, MDS, and MPD. Thus, when such a marker is detected in the setting of an alteration of blood cell production, the diagnosis of leukemia can be made independent of leukemia cell counts. In cases in which a marker cannot be demonstrated, diagnosis must depend on the detection of a clonal expansion of abnormal cells.

CLINICAL SETTING

Leukemia can occur at any age, from fetal life to old age. Overall, it appears with near equality between sexes and among races, although there are significant and as yet poorly understood differences in the frequencies among sexes and ethnic groups for certain subtypes of leukemia (see Chapter 7 for more details). Whereas ALL is the most frequently diagnosed malignant disease of childhood, the frequency of both acute and chronic leukemia and of MPD increases strikingly with increasing age. MDS are similarly more common in the elderly, but they are also seen with low frequency in pediatric patients.[16]

Whereas most cases of leukemia, MDS, and MPD appear without an identifiable preexistent cause, many conditions increase the risk for their development. Certain clinical disorders and genetic compositions carry an increased risk for leukemia and MDS (Table 11–2). Congenital disorders (Particularly Down's syndrome), genome instability states (such as Fanconi's anemia, ataxia-telangiectasia, Bloom's syndrome, and Diamond-Blackfan syndrome), immunodeficiency states exemplified by the Wiskott-Aldridge syndrome, inherited developmental defects, and multiple cancer syndromes (the Li-Fraumeni syndrome and others) carry a high risk for the development of leukemia and of MDS. Whereas the most common leukemia with most of these disorders is acute

TABLE 11–2. Conditions Predisposing to Leukemia

Older age
Congenital disorders
  Down's syndrome
  Monozygous twinning
Hereditary disorders
  Bloom's syndrome
  Fanconi's anemia
  Other constitutional bone marrow failure syndromes
  Neurofibromatosis, type 1
  Li-Fraumeni syndrome
  Ataxia-telangiectasia
  Wiskott-Aldrich syndrome
  Other immunodeficiency syndromes
Acquired illnesses
  Myeloproliferative diseases
  Systemic mastocytosis
  Urticaria pigmentosa
  Paroxysmal nocturnal hemoglobinuria
  Idiopathic sideroblastic anemia?
  Pernicious anemia?
Exposures
  Ionizing radiation
  Chemicals
  Cigarette smoke
  Viruses (HTLV-1, EBV?)
Occupation
  Farmers
  Miners?
  Petroleum workers?
  Rubber film workers

myeloid, Down's syndrome patients have a somewhat higher risk for lymphoblastic than for myeloid disease, and in ataxia-telangiectasia, the risk is restricted to lymphoid malignant neoplasms. Identical twins have a high risk for concordant ALL during childhood, but not thereafter. This has been shown to be the result of intrauterine transmission of leukemia cells arising in one twin into the other through their shared placental circulation.[17-19] In addition there are rare families in which a high incidence of hematologic malignant disease has been observed, including acute and chronic leukemia, especially CLL.[20] In part because of this, the incidence of leukemia is slightly greater for anyone who has a close family member afflicted with the disease. (See Chapter 2 for a comprehensive discussion of hereditary factors involved in the etiology of leukemia and allied diseases.)

A large variety of acquired hematologic disorders have a slight to moderate propensity for development of marrow malignant transformation. Paroxysmal nocturnal hemoglobinuria has been reported to transform into one or another form of AML in 9% of cases.[21] Megaloblastic anemia has also been reported to end in AML. In most of these cases, the anemia was not proved conclusively to be the result of folate or vitamin B_{12} deficiency and could well have been an early manifestation of MDS or leukemia. Similarly, acquired idiopathic sideroblastic anemia, which has a reported leukemia transformation rate of 10% to 26%, not infrequently exhibits cytogenetic abnormalities also seen with MDS. Such cases may in fact represent the "refractory anemia with ring sideroblasts" category of MDS.

Exposures to certain drugs and chemicals and to ioniz-

ing radiation have had the most significant impact of all known factors on the incidence of leukemia, MDS, and other cancers. The leukemogenic effect of radium and x-rays was suspected early on; Madame Curie died of CML, but it took the epidemic of leukemia among survivors of the Hiroshima and Nagasaki nuclear bombings to clarify the potency of ionizing radiation as a leukemogenic factor. The dose-response relationship of radiation risk is still a subject of research, but radiation exposure should always be assessed when a patient with suggestive signs and symptoms is evaluated (for a comprehensive discussion, see Chapter 8).

Similarly, benzene has clearly been shown to cause leukemia or MDS when the exposure has been prolonged, 10 to 30 years on average from the time of first exposure to the toxin (Table 11–3). The risk of other hydrocarbon solvents has not been established, although as a group, workers in industries in which solvent use is high have been shown to be at higher than normal risk. Pesticides have been implicated, and farm workers have been found to have a greater than average risk for development of lymphoproliferative neoplasms including ALL and CLL, although the susceptibility may be unrelated to drug exposure. There is also a modest increase in the incidence of leukemia (most often myelomonocytic) in patients with a history of significant cigarette smoking.[21-23]

The most common culprits in chemically induced leukemia are, ironically, the drugs used in the treatment of disseminated cancers, including leukemia. Of these, alkylating agents (e.g., cyclophosphamide, chlorambucil, melphalan) are the most notable offenders. Up to 20% of patients cured of lymphoma or Hodgkin's disease and ovarian cancer or in long remission control of multiple myeloma have development of AML or MDS within 8 years of treatment with drug regimens containing an alkylating agent.[24-27] Most of these leukemias have been myeloid, and most exhibit unfavorable cytogenic abnormalities. Their response to treatment is poor. The topoisomerase II inhibitors, notably epipodophyllins and anthracyclines, are the second class of leukemogenic cancer drugs.[27-29] The leukemia that ensues in up to 10% of cases can be either acute myeloid or acute lymphoblastic. The most common type has FAB-M2 morphology (i.e., myeloblastic leukemia with cellular maturation into promyelo-

TABLE 11–3. Chemical Exposure and Leukemia

Occupation related
  Benzene (chronic exposure)
  Toluene
  Other industrial solvents?
  Pesticides?
  Hair dyes?
Cancer chemotherapy related
  Alkylating agents
  Topoisomerase inhibitors
    Epipodophyllotoxins
    Anthracyclines
    Actinomycin D
    Anthracenediones
Recreational
  Cigarette smoke

cytes, myelocytes, and metamyelocytes) and has translocations involving 11q23 and the *MLL* gene, the (8; 21)(q23;q22) translocation leading to the fusion gene *AML1/ETO*, or t(15;17) forming *PML/RARA*. These cases usually manifest early (2 to 5 years) within the decade after exposure. Unlike the alkylating agent exposure cases, they tend to respond as well to leukemia therapy as do "de novo" cases of the same genotype and phenotype. MDS is rarely seen after topoisomerase treatment. (See Chapter 9 for a thorough discussion of chemically induced leukemia.)

Human T-lymphotropic virus type 1 (HTLV-1) is the only proven infectious cause of leukemia, in this case the adult T-cell leukemia. This is discussed in Chapter 10 and in Chapter 30. A history of residence in or travel to an endemic area, most often southwestern Japan, the Caribbean basin, or central Africa, and sexual relations with or transfusions of blood from a person with such a history should alert one to the possibility of adult T-cell leukemia in a person with marrow failure and lymphoproliferation. However, the average latency from exposure to overt disease is 40 to 50 years. A major differential diagnostic problem is with human immunodeficiency virus infection, particularly at an early stage. Immunologic or molecular assays for HTLV-1 will usually lead to the correct diagnosis.

Acute leukemia can evolve from any of the MPD and from MDS. Not all cases of MDS are preleukemic, and transformation of refractory anemia without excess myeloblasts is rare. Acute leukemia that relapses after an initial response to treatment may change phenotype, switching from lymphoblastic to myeloid and the reverse, or it may develop a mixed phenotype.

CLINICAL PRESENTATIONS

Bone Marrow Failure

The majority of patients with acute leukemia and MDS present with symptoms and signs reflecting inadequate hematopoiesis secondary to leukemia cell infiltration of the bone marrow. Anemia, although common, is not universal in acute leukemia, presumably because of the rapidity with which the disease progresses in some patients. By contrast, in MDS, anemia is almost invariably present at the clinical onset; it may be the only manifestation, and it is typically the chief complaint. Anemia is also present in most patients with chronic leukemia, either at diagnosis or during the course of the disease. In addition to anemia secondary to erythrocyte underproduction, antibody-mediated hemolytic anemia frequently complicates the course of CLL and may occur despite successful control of other manifestations of that disease.

Neutropenia and thrombocytopenia are usually present at diagnosis in both acute leukemia and MDS. The most telling finding in acute leukemia is the reduction of granulocytes with frequent or persistent infection. Next to anemia, infection is the most common feature of leukemia and MDS. Either repetitive infections or infections that do not respond to the administration of usually effective therapies should raise the possibility of malignant

proliferations that inhibit the production of normal phagocytes or immunocytes. The complete blood cell count will indicate whether there is significant neutropenia ($<1 \times 10^9$/L), marked lymphopenia, or (in the case of hairy cell leukemia) monocytopenia and whether there are circulating abnormal (leukemia) leukocytes. A serum immunoelectrophoresis will document a deficiency of or aberration in the immunoglobulins, which is common in CLL and may rarely occur in other forms of leukemia. Fever in patients with acute leukemia and MDS signifies the presence of an infection and requires both empirical treatment and a search for a source. Fever in chronic leukemia and other proliferative diseases is most often related to disease activity rather than to infection. In such cases, provided that blood neutrophil levels are adequate ($>1 \times 10^9$/L), treatment with antibiotics should not be instituted until the cause of the fever is determined.

Bleeding as the result of diminished platelets is also a common initial finding. This usually takes the form of petechial hemorrhages observable in the skin (Fig. 11–1), the mucous membranes, and the retina. Major internal hemorrhage is rare, although the unfortunate combination of leukemia with accidental injury or operative procedures can result in serious bleeding. Significant bleeding is uncommon at platelet counts above 20×10^9/L and is not a factor, even with surgery or trauma, when platelet levels are above 100×10^9/L. Two exceptions are (1) the bleeding that can occur with the high platelet levels sometimes seen in untreated CML polycythema vera or essential thrombocytosis and (2) hemorrhage sec-

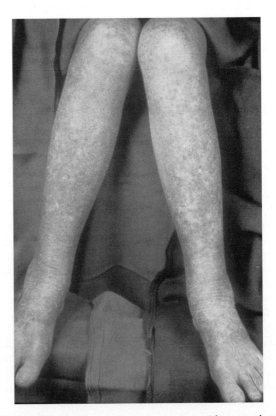

FIGURE 11–1. Petechial hemorrhages in a patient with severe thrombocytopenia. (See Color Section.)

ondary to leukostasis that may occur in the absence of thrombocytopenia.

Coagulopathy

Massive bleeding due to coagulopathy may be the presenting feature of some types of acute leukemia. Promyelocytic leukemia is the type most often causing this problem through the release of procoagulants and the reactive fibrinolysis, leading to major depletions of the labile coagulation proteins factor V, factor VIII, and fibrinogen. Other acute leukemias may occasionally present with similar coagulation abnormalities, particularly acute monocytic forms presenting with high white blood cell counts. Routine coagulation screens will reveal major coagulation deficits if the coagulopathy is far advanced. Fibrinogen levels are frequently above normal in leukemia and may remain within the normal range despite ongoing fibrinolysis or disseminated intravascular coagulation. Therefore, the diagnosis of abnormal plasma factor consumption requires the demonstration of fibrin degradation products and elevated D-dimers; lacking these assays, the accelerated lysis of clotted blood obtained from the patient is observed (see Chapter 15 for a fuller discussion of bleeding).

Organ Infiltration

The organ most consistently infiltrated is the bone marrow, but this is obviously not perceptible on physical examination. Lymphadenopathy and enlargement of the liver and spleen are the most common clinically assessable signs of leukemia, present in about 50% of patients with acute leukemia and 70% to 90% of patients with chronic leukemia. Any organ can be involved, but only those infiltrations that can be seen or palpated or that cause symptoms are recognized early. Of these, the central nervous system (CNS) leukemia is of the greatest concern because of the severity of its symptoms and the critical nature of its consequences. CNS leukemia is most common in precursor B-cell acute leukemia. Before the introduction of presymptomatic therapy to the CNS, meningeal leukemia occurred in 70% of patients with childhood leukemia and was a major cause of treatment failure in this group. CNS leukemia is also present in a high proportion of cases with Burkitt cell leukemia and with AML-M2 and AML-M4 Eo. Early treatment of the CNS in such cases has contributed in a major way to the remarkable progress made in the control of childhood leukemia during the last 40 years.

CNS leukemia usually consists of an infiltration of the meninges, which impairs egress of cerebrospinal fluid, creating a communicating hydrocephalus. The resultant increase in intracranial pressure can lead to medullary coning and death. Early symptoms include headache, blurred vision, and vomiting—often without associated nausea. The earliest physical signs may be cranial nerve palsies and diminished sensorium. Abducens palsy, leading to a lateral strabismus, is the most common cranial nerve abnormality. Eye examination may also reveal a hypopion, retinal infiltrates, and papilledema.

A less common but even more ominous form of CNS infiltration is leukostasis, in which small arterioles are packed with blasts that invade and disrupt the blood vessel walls. This can lead to massive hemorrhage, which is usually fatal and is always crippling. Leukostasis is associated with high and rapidly increasing numbers of blasts in the blood. Hemorrhagic strokes are rarely seen at blast cell counts below 200×10^9/L in acute leukemia; however, patients with the blast transformation of CML have suffered leukostasis-induced cerebrovascular accidents with blast cell counts of less than 100×10^9/L. Patients with chronic-phase CML or CLL almost never have problems with leukostasis, even with leukocyte counts above 1000×10^9/L. Leukostasis is not restricted to the CNS but can occur in any organ. The lung is especially sensitive to this condition. Pulmonary leukostasis occuring during response of APL to retinoid therapy may contribute to the highly dangerous retinoic acid syndrome seen in that disease (see Chapter 23).

Infiltration of all other organs occurs regularly but to varying degrees of clinical concern. Symptomatic enlargement of liver, spleen, and lymph nodes occurs most frequently with chronic leukemia, MDS, and MPD, particularly myelofibrosis. Gonad (both testes and ovary) and skin infiltration is more common in acute leukemia. Mucous membrane infiltration is seen most frequently with monoblastic acute leukemia. Leukemic tumors, so-called granulocytic or myeloid sarcomas, are limited to myeloid or monocytoid disease. They can affect any organ but are most common in subcutaneous tissues and may occur in the breast. They are most commonly seen at relapse or in the accelerated phases of CML, but they may occasionally be the first manifestation of the leukemia. Dermal infiltrates, so-called leukemids, are common and can be seen with all forms of leukemia. They are frequently purplish and may be associated with itching. Enlargement of the kidneys and infiltration of the gastrointestinal tract and of the heart occur regularly but rarely cause any dysfunction of the organ involved.

Bone and Joint Pain

Bone pain and joint pain are relatively common concomitants of ALL and may be the sole complaint initially in children with that disease. In the past, children have been misdiagnosed as having rheumatic fever because of pain and periarticular swelling of joints and have been treated with steroids, often with initial relief. Such a mistake may have drastic consequences because proper treatment that is highly curative must not be delayed. Bone pain is uncommon in AML and chronic leukemia. Standard radiographs often show growth arrest lines in children and may show periosteal elevation that can be correlated with local pain. Lytic lesions, often asymptomatic, can sometimes be seen in adults and children. Magnetic resonance imaging is useful in detecting dense masses of leukemia cells within bones.

Metabolic Abnormalities

Serum chemistry profiles obtained from patients with leukemia and MPD are frequently abnormal. Lactate dehydrogenase may be elevated in the blood, reflecting a large cell mass or rapid proliferation of leukemia cells. Elevated lactate dehydrogenase, occasionally with hyperbilirubinemia, is seen with red blood cell hemolysis, typically in patients with CLL. There is often modest elevation of transaminases, usually having little clinical significance, as well as a reduction of albumin, which is more ominous in terms of response to therapy. Creatinine and urea nitrogen may be elevated; this is usually a reflection of transient dehydration, which is rapidly reversed with fluid resuscitation, but azotemia can also be caused by intratubular precipitation of urate. A determination of uric acid level should always be included in the work-up of a leukemic patient, and appropriate measures are instituted if an increase in the uric acid pool is detected or is anticipated with therapy.

Other serious chemical disturbances include osteoclast-related hypercalcemia, which can occur with any leukemia but is a regular feature of adult T-cell leukemia; hypocalcemia; hyperkalemia, and hypokalemia; and hypomagnesemia. Lysozymemia and lysozymuria occur frequently with monocytic and monoblastic leukemias and may be helpful in supporting these diagnoses.

Fortuitous Discovery

The diagnosis of leukemia, MDS, or MPD is occasionally made through the discovery of infiltrates or minor hemorrhage on routine physical examination or from blood count abnormalities on routine blood testing of an asymptomatic individual. The presence of excess leukocytes can be manifested in a high "leukocrit" in a spun blood sample or by blood cell excesses or deficits on complete blood cell count examination. Such early detection does not change either the prognosis of the disease or the diagnostic and therapeutic maneuvers that must be undertaken. Rather, it provides an opportunity to complete the work-up and treatment planning with scrupulous care before instituting therapy.

DIAGNOSTIC PROCEDURES

Hematologic Tests

Peripheral Blood Examination. A standard complete blood cell count together with a careful differential count and morphologic evaluation of an adequate blood film usually provide the necessary information either to diagnose leukemia outright or to indicate the need to perform a bone marrow aspiration and biopsy. The blood film should be air dried (without fixative) and stained with a polychrome dye, such as May-Grünwald-Giemsa, and carefully scanned for morphologic abnormalities.

Bone Marrow Examination. Bone marrow can be obtained in adults from the sternum, anterior and posterior pelvis, ribs, or vertebrae; in children, bone marrow can be obtained from these areas plus the femur and proximal tibia. In practice, it is most convenient and safe to obtain the aspirate and biopsy sample from the posterior iliac crest, unless there is known disease of other type in the pelvis or unless the pelvis has been previously exposed to high doses of radiation. Because leukemia, MDS, and MPD are diffuse conditions, involving at diagnosis all areas of cellular marrow, evaluation of a single site is adequate for diagnosis. Aspiration and biopsy can be done consecutively at the same site. The aspiration is usually performed first, then the biopsy needle is introduced, at a slightly different angle, and a core of marrow is obtained for histopathologic analysis. Imprints should be made from the biopsy core, air dried, and stained in the same fashion as peripheral blood. Conversely, marrow particles obtained by aspiration may be concentrated by centrifugation, fixed, and examined as a tissue. Marrow aspirate should be spread on several slides and air dried. One or more slides should be stained with polychrome dyes. If morphologic examination is not adequate to specify the leukemia cell type, the remaining slides can be stained to look for myeloperoxidase, esterases, or other lineage-related features. One slide should be reserved for staining for intracellular iron. Whenever possible, sufficient cells should be obtained in sterile suspension for cytogenetic analysis, flow cytometric immunophenotyping and molecular analysis.

Cerebrospinal Fluid Examination. Cerebrospinal fluid should be checked at some time in the early management phase of all pediatric patients with ALL. This is particularly true for patients with the "common" CD10+ ALL of childhood, in which meningeal leukemia occurred in 70% of patients before effective CNS treatment, and for Burkitt cell leukemia, in which the highest rate of CNS disease occurs and for which treatment of the CNS should be a part of the remission induction plan (see Chapters 26 and 27 for details). For common ALL patients, the lumbar puncture should be deferred until the blood becomes free of lymphoblasts. With Burkitt cell leukemia, intrathecal medication is part of the induction therapy, and cerebrospinal fluid evaluation can be performed when the lumbar puncture is done for drug administration. In the absence of signs or symptoms of meningeal involvement, cerebrospinal fluid evaluation is less critical in AML, except in those cases with a monoblast/monocyte component or the t(8;21) form of AML-M2. Cerebrospinal fluid examination is not necessary in CLL, in MDS, or in MPD (including CML) until there is transformation to an acute leukemia. Standard lumbar puncture with use of a small-bore needle (e.g., 22-gauge) may be safely performed, even when there is evidence of increased intracranial pressure, provided that only a small amount of fluid is obtained and the patient is kept supine for 30 minutes to 1 hour after the tap. Bleeding or infection is rarely a clinical problem. The practice of introducing cytarabine or methotrexate after the sample is obtained is without clinical support, unless the decision to treat with intrathecal medication has already been made.

Analyses of Diagnostic Material

Morphology. Careful morphologic assessment of normal and abnormal cell components of peripheral blood and bone marrow remains essential to diagnosis and classification of hematologic malignant disease. In the majority of instances, the nature of the disease and its clinical aggressiveness and the urgency and often the specifics of initial treatment can be determined by evaluation of blood and marrow smears. In those cases in which uncertainty remains, the initial morphologic scan will suggest what types of further study need to be performed. Evaluation should be both qualitative and quantitative. Many of the important distinctions between leukemia subtypes, and the diagnosis of leukemia and MDS themselves, depend on accurate determinations of the proportion of blast cells, promyelocytes, and more mature granulocytic and lymphoid and erythroid progenitors.

Cytogenetics and Immunophenotyping. Cytogenetics is extensively discussed in Chapter 5, and immunologic phenotyping in Chapter 6. Both analyses are critical to the diagnosis of all but a few forms of leukemia. As noted earlier, the identification of specific recurrent chromosome abnormalities (or the fusion genes and transcripts that result therefrom) is the crux of diagnosis of an important handful of entities, notably t(15;17), t(8;14), t(8;21), inv(16), and translocations involving (11q23).

Molecular Studies. The development of polymerase chain reaction (PCR), reverse transcriptase–PCR, fluorescence in situ hybridization (FISH), and multicolor FISH (M-FISH) and extra-signal FISH techniques has led to the use of these approaches as part of the work-up of hematopoietic and lymphoid malignant neoplasms.[30-37] Multicolor flow cytometry is useful in discerning and confirming clonality and specific disease subtypes of both myeloid and lymphoid malignant neoplasms, and it is often available for prompt diagnosis when molecular techniques are not yet in place. Microarray technology is beginning to be applied to the study of normal hematopoiesis[38, 39] and of leukemia pathophysiologic mechanisms, and it can be expected to play an increasing role in diagnosis in the future.

DIAGNOSIS OF HEMATOLOGIC MALIGNANT DISEASE

Hematologic malignant disease is diagnosed by detecting a clonal population of abnormal cells within the blood and the blood cell–forming tissue. In leukemia, MDS, and MPD, this tissue is the bone marrow primarily, with secondary spillover into the blood and then to the spleen, lymphatics, and other organs. Diagnosis can be suspected if infiltrates of malignant blood cells, or particularly blood precursors, are found in tissues without obvious evidence of infection. However, the bone marrow must show an excess of these cells for the diagnosis to be confirmed.

Acute Leukemia

Acute Lymphoblastic Leukemia. For the diagnosis of ALL, more than 5% of bone marrow cells must be lymphoblasts, and 25% and 30% have been suggested as a requisite to distinguish ALL from lymphoblastic lym-

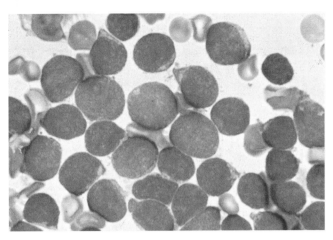

FIGURE 11–2. Acute lymphoblastic leukemia, FAB-L1 morphology. Note scant cytoplasm. (See Color Section.)

phoma. Most patients with ALL, however, present with a higher blast cell percentage in the marrow. Unlike in myeloid disease, there is no "preleukemic" or lymphodysplastic syndrome analogous to MDS for patients with 5% to 25% (or 30%) lymphoblasts. (See Figs. 11-2 through 11-4 for examples of typical ALL morphology; see also Color Section.)

Acute Myeloid Leukemia. For all categories of AML except acute promyelocytic, myeloblasts (types I and II, Figs. 11-5 and 11-27; see also Color Section) must account for more than 20% of the nonerythroid marrow cells. Patients with marrow myeloblast infiltrations of 5% to 20% are included in MDS according to WHO recommendations. This criterion is not accepted by all hematologists, many of whom broaden the scope of MDS to include patients with up to 30% myeloblasts in the bone marrow (see Chapter 24 for a fuller discussion). Suffice it to say that the criteria of MDS and AML remain in a period of evolution and refinement and will continue to change as newer information about pathophysiologic mechanisms and clinical response is accrued and compared.

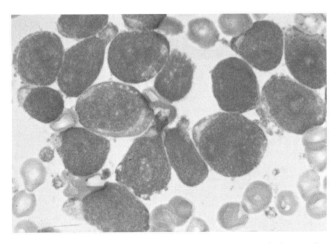

FIGURE 11–3. Acute lymphoblastic leukemia, FAB-L2 morphology. Cells have variable size and a lower nuclear-to-cytoplasmic ratio than L1 blasts. (See Color Section.)

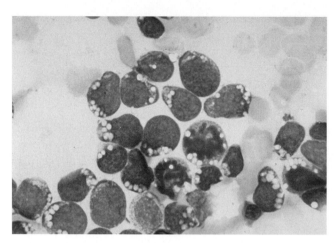

FIGURE 11–4. Burkitt cell leukemia, FAB-L3 morphology. Cells typically have deeply basophilic cytoplasm with numerous vacuoles. Most of these are cytoplasmic. Note the presence of a cell in metaphase, not an uncommon finding in this highly proliferative leukemia. (See Color Section.)

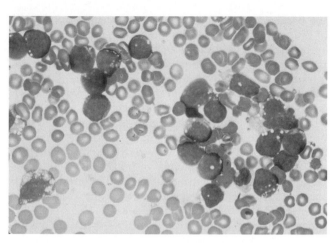

FIGURE 11–7. Undifferentiated acute myeloblastic leukemia (FAB-M0). Note the similarity to Burkitt cell leukemia (FAB-L3), ALL-L2, and acute megakaryocytic leukemia (FAB-M7). Diagnosis depends on the results of immunologic, cytogenetic, and molecular studies. (See Color Section.)

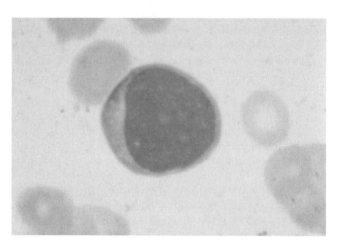

FIGURE 11–5. Type I myeloblast. Note nucleolus, noncondensed chromatin, and absence of cytoplasmic granules. (See Color Section.)

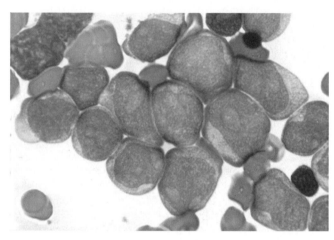

FIGURE 11–8. Acute myeloid leukemia, FAB-M1. Note many type I and few type II myeloblasts and little maturation in this bone marrow smear. (See Color Section.)

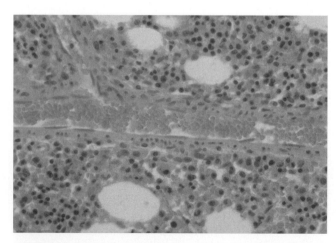

FIGURE 11–6. Bone marrow biopsy; type II myeloblast; similar to type I myeloblast but with slightly more cytoplasm containing a few azurophilic granules. (See Color Section.)

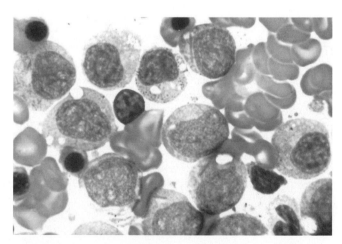

FIGURE 11–9. Acute myeloid leukemia with t(8;21)(q22;q21). This bone marrow exhibits FAB-M2 morphology with type II myeloblasts and some granulocytic maturation. Note the long, fine, and somewhat tubular-appearing Auer rods in four of the blasts characteristic of t(8;21) leukemia. (See Color Section.)

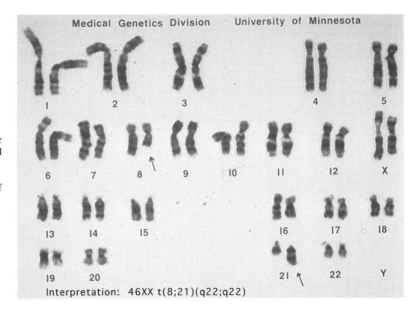

FIGURE 11-10. Karyotype of a leukemia cell from a patient with t(8;21)(q22;q22) acute myeloid leukemia. The arrows point to the abnormal chromosomes; the normal chromosomes 8 and 21 are on the left of the pair. This karyotype or the identification of the *AML/ETO* fusion gene or mRNA transcript is required for the diagnosis of this type of leukemia.

Acute Promyelocytic Leukemia. Patients with APL have increased promyelocytes and may or may not have an increased proportion of myeloblasts, but in no case are there more blasts than promyelocytes in the marrow. Most important, these cells exhibit karyotypic abnormalities involving the *RARA* gene of chromosome 17, the most common of which is the translocation (15;17)(q22; q11-12) (see Fig. 11-12; see also Color Section) resulting in the fusion gene *PML/RARA*. These genetic aberrations are detectable by use of molecular analyses widely available and usually by cytogenetics with banding. Under the WHO classification, patients with this genetic defect may be given the diagnosis of APL independent of the number of morphologically identifiable leukemia cells. APL cells have, in addition, a distinctive immunophenotype—CD9+ and CD68+ in conjunction with the usual myeloid markers CD13 and CD33—and are HLA-DR−. Immunophenotyping is particularly helpful in cases of microgranular

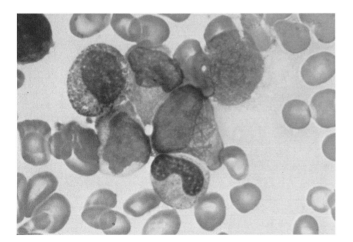

FIGURE 11-11. Hypergranular acute promyelocytic leukemia (FAB-M3). Note the indented nucleus, perinuclear clear zone ("haupt"); abundant cytoplasm containing abnormally large, "succulent" azurophilic granules; and multiple Auer rods, some appearing to be in bundles (faggots). (See Color Section.)

APL when molecular diagnosis is unavailable, the morphologic appearance is equivocal for diagnosis, and the urgency for treatment does not permit delay of intervention for cytogenetic studies to be completed. Results of a preliminary study suggest that APL resulting from the *PLZF/RARA* translocation gene may be morphologically distinguishable from classic APL with the *PML/RARA* gene. If confirmed, this will have great clinical significance because *PLZF/RARA* cells are resistant to the differentiating effects of all-*trans* retinoic acid[40] (see Chapter 23).

Acute Monoblastic and Myelomonocytic Leukemias. For acute monoblastic and myelomonocytic leukemias, the percentage of blasts (myeloblasts plus monoblasts) must equal or exceed 20% of marrow cells. When there is an abnormality of chromosome 16(p13q22), diagnosis can be made with fewer blasts; as with APL.

Acute Erythroleukemia. The diagnosis of acute erythroleukemia (FAB M6) requires that ≥50% of marrow nucleated cells are erythrocyte precursors and that ≥20% of the nonerythoid cells are myeloblasts.[12] In pure erythroid leukemia, the majority of cells are erythroblasts and other red blood cell precursors, and myeloblasts are absent.

Acute Megakaryocytic Leukemia. In this leukemia (AML-M7) ≥20% of the marrow cells are blasts, of which ≥20% are shown by immunotyping or ultrastructural studies to be of the megakaryocytic lineage.[11]

Biphenotypic Leukemia. Biphenotypic leukemia is a diagnosis made by immunophenotyping. The term encompasses clonal malignant neoplasms that express multiple features of two cell lineages, usually lymphoid and myeloid, but rarely including NK lineage characteristics. The morphologic cell features are usually uniform, but a cytologically distinct population of leukemia cells may occasionally coexist. The disease is diagnosed by identifying at least two disparate features in a population of lymphoid or myeloid cells (e.g., CD13 plus myeloperoxidase in a leukemia of lymphoblastic morphology and

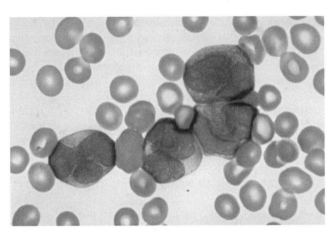

FIGURE 11–12. Classic karyotype of promyelocytic leukemia, t(15;17)(q22;q21). This translocation in present in both the hypergranular and the microgranular (variant) forms of the disease.

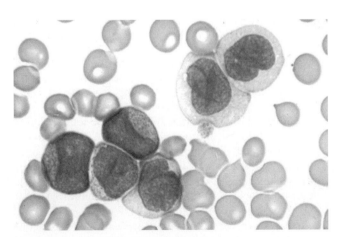

FIGURE 11–13. Microgranular acute promyelocytic leukemia, FAB AML-M3var. The large granules noted in Figure 11-11 are absent. The diagnosis can be suspected on the basis of the nuclear appearance with indentation and some chromatin condensation; however, it must be confirmed by cytogenetics or molecular detection of a translocation involving the *RARA* gene. (See Color Section.)

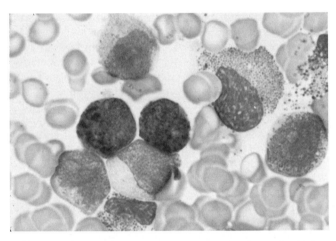

FIGURE 11–15. AML-M4 with abnormal eosinophils. This is classified as AML-M4Eo by the FAB Group. It is associated with cytogenetic aberrations involving chromosome 16, typically inv(16)(p13;q11). (See Color Section.)

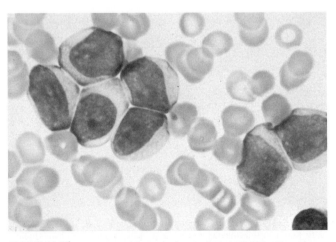

FIGURE 11–16. Acute monoblastic leukemia, FAB AML-M5a. Note the absence of mature monocytes and of granulocytic cells. (See Color Section.)

FIGURE 11–14. Acute myelocytic leukemia (FAB AML-M4) bone marrow. This category is typified by nearly equal numbers of myeloblasts and monoblasts plus promonocytes. (See Color Section.)

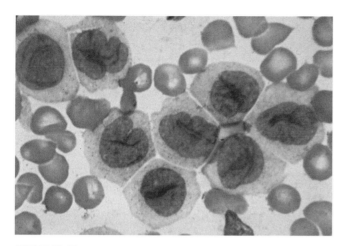

FIGURE 11–17. Acute monocytic leukemia, FAB AML-M5b. Smear consists primarily of partially differentiated monocytic cells, most promonocytes, with few blasts or granulocytic cells. (See Color Section.)

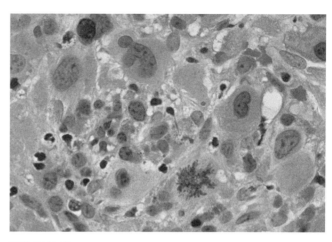

FIGURE 11–20. Acute megakaryocytic leukemia, bone marrow biopsy specimen revealing markedly increased numbers of megakaryocytes and fibrosis. (See Color Section.)

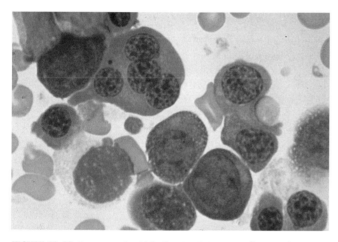

FIGURE 11–18. Acute erythroid leukemia, FAB AML-M6. Note the markedly dyspoietic erythroid precursor cells and the presence of excessive numbers of both erythroblasts and myeloblasts. (See Color Section.)

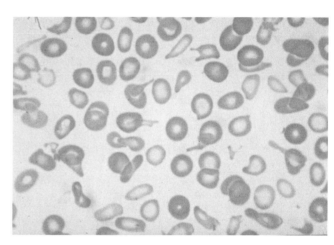

FIGURE 11–21. Peripheral blood smear from a patient with the refractory anemia form of myelodysplastic syndrome. Anisocytosis and poikilocytosis are striking, and neutrophils tend to be hypogranular. (See Color Section.)

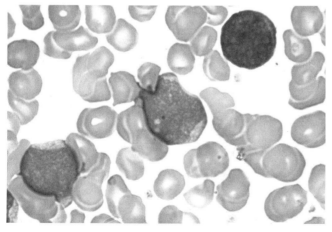

FIGURE 11–19. Acute megakaryocytic leukemia, FAB AML-M7. Peripheral blood smear containing a heterogeneous but poorly differentiated population of blast cells. Definite diagnosis depends on antigen phenotyping with use of antiplatelet membrane antigen reagents and/or platelet peroxidase staining and ultrastructural analysis (immunoelectron microscopy). (See Color Section.)

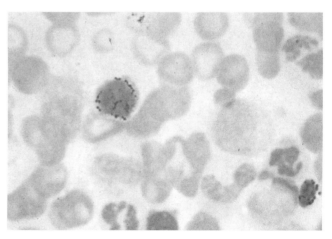

FIGURE 11–22. Refractory anemia with ring sideroblasts (iron stain of bone marrow aspirate). (See Color Section.)

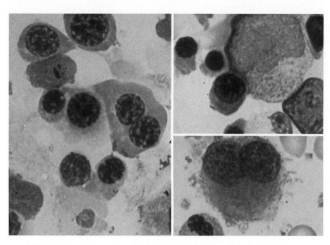

FIGURE 11–23. Composite of marrow cells from a patient with refractory cytopenia with multilineage dysplasia. Clockwise from top right: myelocyte, micromegakaryocyte, and multiple dysplastic erythroid precursors. (See Color Section.)

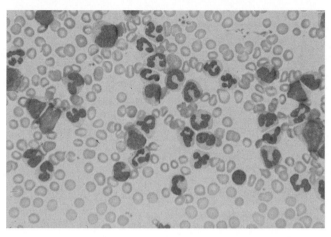

FIGURE 11–26. Chronic myelogenous leukemia, chronic phase. Myelocytes and banded and segmented neutrophils are present. Two Pelger-Huët cells (with bilobed nuclei) are also seen. (See Color Section.)

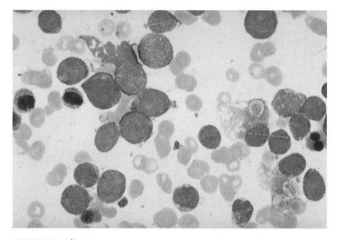

FIGURE 11–24. Refractory anemia with excess blasts. Both increased myeloblasts and dysplastic erythroid precursors are prominent. (See Color Section.)

lymphoid antigen profile (e.g., CD19⁺, CD20⁺). Biphenotypic leukemia should be distinguished from cases of AML or ALL with only one discordant antigen expressed. Several scoring systems have been proposed to clarify the diagnosis.[41, 42] They are based the grading of the lineage specificity of cell features, the presence of Auer rods being more specific for AML than the expression of CD13. One of these systems is presented in Table 11–4. Biphenotypic leukemias generally have a worse prognosis than do acute leukemias restricted to either of the lineages singly, especially when they occur in adults. They are frequently associated with unfavorable cytogenetics, especially translocations involving 11q23. Cases of this type can be distinguished by using gene expression multiple array technology.[42a]

Myelodysplastic Syndromes

Myelodysplastic syndromes are divided into five morphologic subtypes in the FAB schema (Table 11–5): refractory

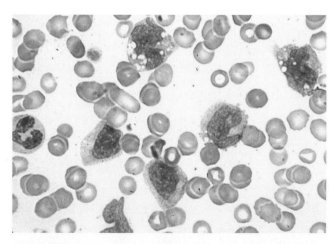

FIGURE 11–25. Chronic myelomonocytic leukemia. Note many monocytes and dysplastic mature neutrophils with hypogranulation. This is classed as a myelodysplastic syndrome by the FAB Group and as a myeloproliferative/myelodysplastic disorder by the WHO Committee. (See Color Section.)

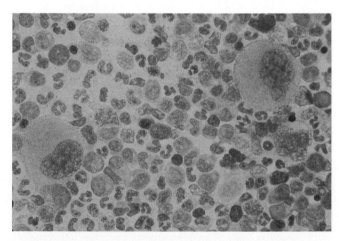

FIGURE 11–27. Chronic myelogenous leukemia, chronic phase, bone marrow biopsy specimen. Marked hypercellularity is seen with increased numbers of dysplastic megakaryocytes, and all stages of granulocytic differentiation are apparent. (See Color Section.)

TABLE 11–4. Criteria for the Diagnosis of Biphenotypic Leukemia (Royal Marsden Criteria)[42]

Score	B Lineage	T Lineage	Myeloid
2	cCD22 CD79a	cCD3	Myeloperoxidase
1	CD10 CD19	CD2 CD5	CD13 CD33
0.5	TdT	TdT CD7	CD11b/11c CD14 CD15

If more than 2 points are scored for two or more lineages, the case is classified as biphenotypic.

anemia with or without ring sideroblasts (RA, RARS), refractory anemia with excess blasts (RAEB), RAEB in transition to AML (RAEB-t), and chronic myelomonocytic leukemia (CMML)[13] RA and RARS have less than 5% myeloblasts and differ by the presence of more than 15% ring sideroblasts among the erythroblasts in the marrow of RARS. In the FAB schema, dysplasia is not restricted to the erythroid series; in the WHO classification for RA and RARS it is, and a new cateory, refractory cytopenia with multilineage dysplasia (RCMD), is added to include patients with RA and RARS with dysplasia of two or more lineages, as originally suggested by Rosati et al.[44] In RAEB the percentage of blasts may be 5% to 19%, multilineage dysplasia is seen, and frequent ring sideroblasts may be present. RAEB-t includes patients with more than 20% but less than 30% blasts. The WHO Committee recommends that this category be eliminated and that patients with this amount of marrow myeloblast infiltration be classified as AML. In CMML both marrow and blood contain increased numbers of promonocytes and monocytes. Blast cells are below 20% and usually less than 5%. As with RAEB, ring sideroblasts may be plentiful. This diagnostic category remains contentious, as there is major disagreement whether it is one or multiple entities, and whether it belongs in the realm of myeloproliferative or myelodysplastic disorders, or both. The FAB Committee suggested allotting the CMML to MPD or MDS based upon the white blood cell count (above or below 13,000/μl).[14] The WHO Committe recommends that one diagnosis should be used irrespective of the counts but places CMML in a category of combined MPD/MDS.[8] The ultimate classification of this group of disease will depend upon future clinical and laboratory observations. Chapter 24 should be consulted for additional insights and opinions regarding the controversy.

Chronic Leukemia

Chronic Lymphocytic Leukemia. Chronic lymphocytic Leukemia is diagnosed by the leukemic lymphocytosis ($>3 \times 10^9$/L) and the infiltration of malignant mature lymphocytes in the bone marrow (Table 11-6). The leukemia cells are typically small, with condensed chromatin, no observable nucleoli, and scanty cytoplasm (see Fig. 11-28; see also Color Section). They are fragile, and smudged or shattered cells (Gumprecht cells) are often seen on smears of blood and marrow. The CLL marrow is usually hypercellular and may be infiltrated with anything

TABLE 11–5. Myelodysplastic Syndromes

FAB Class	WHO Class	Characteristics
Refractory anemia (RA)	Refractory anemia (RA) (Fig. 11-21) 5q− syndrome	Erythroid dysplasia only. Less than 5% blasts. Resembles RA. Large megakaryocytes with uni- or bilobed nucleii.
	Refractory cytopenia with multilineage dysplasia (RCMD) (Fig. 11-23)*	Multilineage dysplasia. <5% myeloblasts.
Refractory anemia with ring sideroblasts (RARS)	Refractory anemia with ring sideroblasts (RARS) (Fig. 11-22)*	Same as RA, but with >15% of erythroblasts being ring sideroblasts.
	RCMD with ringed sideroblasts	Same as RARS, but with multilineage dysplasia.
Refractory anemia with excess blasts (RAEB)	Refractory anemia with excess blasts (RAEB) (Fig. 11-24)*	Multilineage dysplasia. Myeloblasts 5%–20%. RAEB-I: Blasts = 5%–9% of marrow cells. RAEB-II: Blasts = 10%–19% of marrow cells.
Refractory anemia with excess blasts in transition to acute leukemia (RAEB-t)	No such designation (patients have AML)	Multilineage dysplasia. Myeloblasts 20%–30%.
Chronic myelomonocytic leukemia (CMML)	CMML in separate category (see below)	Multilineage dysplasia. Monocytic cells >10% of nonerythroid cells; monoblasts <5%.

Myelodysplastic/Myeloproliferative Diseases (WHO Classification Only)

Name	Description
Chronic myelomonocytic leukemia	Monocytes >10%, nonerythroid blasts <5%. Included in FAB classification as a myelodysplastic syndrome (Fig. 11-25)*
Atypical chronic myelogenous leukemia	BCR/ABL negative. Included in FAB classification as a myeloproliferative disease.
Juvenile myelomonocytic leukemia	BCR/ABL negative. Usually in children <5 years of age. Moderate dysplasia. Increased fetal hemoglobin. Frequent skin rashes. Combined granulo- and monocytosis

*See also Color Section.

TABLE 11–6. Chronic Lymphoid Leukemias

Mature Lymphocyte Leukemia

B-Cell

B-cell chronic lymphocytic leukemia (small-cell lymphoma) (Fig. 11-28)*
B-cell prolymphocytic leukemia
Hairy cell leukemia (Figs. 11-29 and 11-30)*

T-Cell and NK-cell

T-Cell prolymphocytic leukemia
T-Cell granular lymphocyte leukemia
Aggressive NK-cell leukemia
Adult T-cell leukemia/lymphoma (HTLV⁺) (Fig. 11-31)*

*See also Color Section.

from scattered lymphocytes to nodules of lymphocytes to diffuse sheets of leukemia cells. Up to 10% of the peripheral and marrow B lymphocytes may be prolymphocytes. The diagnosis is usually unmistakable, but it should be confirmed by immune characterization, most conveniently performed by flow cytometry. CLL cells typically exhibit strong expression of CD19, CD20, and CD23 together with CD5 on their surface. CD22 and CD79b are typically negative. Surface immunoglobulin, usually IgM with or without IgD, is only weakly presented, in contrast to other "mature" B-cell malignant neoplasms. The clonality of the infiltrate can readily be demonstrated by flow cytometry, comparing κ and λ surface staining with use of separate fluorescent dyes.[45-47]

On the basis of genetic studies, B-CLL appears to be divisible into two forms distinguished by molecular definition of the maturation state of the transformed progenitor cell. One form is derived from a memory B cell, as evidenced by variable region hypermutation of the antigen receptor. The other has the characteristics of a "naive" B cell and lacks variable region hypermutation. These forms also have different cytogentics and a different clinical course with therapy. The naive cell type frequently contains trisomy 12 and responds poorly to therapy. The memory cell–derived leukemias often have a deletion of 13q14, often have a slow rate of progression, and have a favorable response to treatment. Thus, it is important to obtain cytogenetics and molecular studies in the optimal management (which includes education about therapy and prognosis) of the patient with CLL.[48]

T-Cell CLL. T-cell CLL has similar presenting signs, symptoms, and routine laboratory features, with some notable exceptions. Skin infiltrates are more common. Blood lymphocytes tend to be larger and more pleomorphic. Most critically, the leukemia cell immunophenotype is that of peripheral T cells, that is, CD4⁺ and CD7⁺.[49]

Large Granular Lymphocytosis. Large granular lymphocytosis is characterized by increased numbers of such cells in the marrow and blood. These cells can have one of two immunophenotypes: a peripheral T cell (CD3⁺, CD7⁺, and CD8⁺) or, alternatively, an NK cell (CD3⁺, CD16⁺, CD56⁺). Patients range in age from pediatric to elderly and are more frequently male. They typically have chronic anemia and neutropenia together with an enlarged spleen. Skin infiltrations are seen in about one quarter of cases. Rare cases have associated peripheral neuropathy. About half of the patients are asymptomatic when they are diagnosed. An association with rheumatoid arthritis has been noted consistently in a minority of patients.[50] Most T-cell large granular lymphocytosis and many NK cases run an indolent course.

Prolymphocytic Leukemia. Prolymphocytic Leukemia is diagnosed by increased blood and marrow prolymphocytes composing more than 10% of lymphoid cells. The more common B-cell type has a mature B-cell immunophenotype with CD19, CD20, and prominent surface immunoglobulin expression but CD5 negativity. Splenomegaly is usually present, and the clinical course is usually one of rapid progression in the absence of a response to therapy. The T-cell type is uncommon but has a clinical course similar to that of the B-cell type.

Hairy Cell Leukemia. In hairy cell leukemia, there is frequently no elevation of total blood leukocytes, but typical hairy cells (see Fig. 11-29; see also Color Section) are usually identifiable, provided that the search is careful enough.[51] Aspiration of marrow is often unsuccessful.

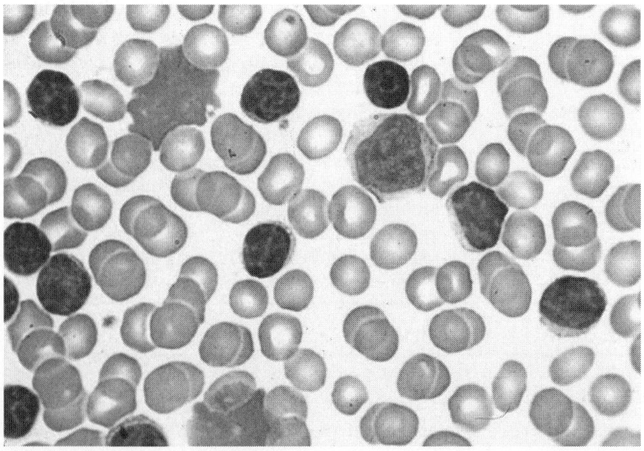

FIGURE 11–28. Chronic lymphocytic leukemia, B-cell type. Bone marrow aspirate shows small lymphocytes with condensed nuclear chromatin. Also present are several typical smudge cells. The T-cell type may resemble this or may have more T-cell characteristics. (See Color Section.)

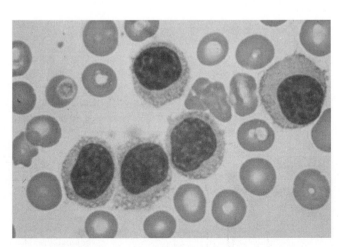

FIGURE 11–29. Hairy cell leukemia. Peripheral blood smear stained with Wright-Giemsa contains hairy cells. (See Color Section.)

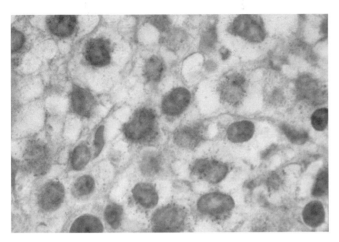

FIGURE 11–30. Hairy cell leukemia. Bone marrow biopsy specimen exhibits tartrate-resistant acid phosphatase staining of hairy cells. Note the wide separation of the hairy cells. (See Color Section.)

TABLE 11–7. WHO Classification: Myeloproliferative Diseases

WHO Classification	Classic/FAB Class
Chronic myelogenous leukemia, t(9;22) (q34;q11), BCR-ABL (Figs. 11–26 and 11–27)*	Chronic myelogenous leukemia
Chronic neutrophilic leukemia	—
—	Atypical chronic myelogenous Leukemia[a]
Polycythemia vera	Polycythemia vera
Essential thrombocytosis	Essential thrombocytosis
Chronic idiopathic myelofibrosis	Agnogenic myeloid metaplasia
Chronic eosinophilic leukemia	—
Myeloproliferative disease, unclassifiable	—
—	Juvenile myelogenous leukemia[a]

[a]These entities are included in the myelodysplastic/myeloproliferative disease category of the WHO classification.
*See also Color Section.

Marrow biopsy is required, and the histologic pattern is characteristic, the cells appearing to be separated from each other by a clear zone (see Fig. 11–30; see also Color Section). The immunophenotype of hairy cells is also characteristic and easily distinguished from CLL.[52] Typically, hairy cells strongly express surface immunoglobulin, CD19/20, CD25, and CD11c and are negative for CD5. Reaction to tartrate-resistant acid phosphatase is usually positive (see Fig. 11–30; see also Color Section). A variant form exists in which leukocytosis is prominent (see Chapter 29).

Chronic Myelogenous Leukemia. With chronic myelogenous leukemia in its chronic phase, there is an increase in all maturation steps of granulocytopoiesis except myeloblasts, which remain less than 5% of nucleated cells in the bone marrow (Table 11-7). As with other MPD, there is usually an initial increase in all blood cell lineages. Serum vitamin B_{12} and cyanocobalamin levels are usually elevated. Unlike in other MPD, the neutrophil alkaline phosphatase is low to absent in CML granulo-

cytes. The diagnosis is confirmed by the presence of the (9;22)(q34;q11) translocation and/or *BCR/ABL* transcripts in the leukemia cells. Without curative therapy, CML inevitably progresses to a more aggressive phase with fever, cytopenias, increased eosinophils and basophils, and often marrow fibrosis; finally, in more than 50% of cases, it evolves to become indistinguishable from an acute leukemia. The majority of cases of so-called blast crisis are of a myeloblastic phenotype, but cases of lymphoblastic and monoblastic disease also occur. In any case, the Philadelphia chromosome usually persists and is often accompanied by additional chromosome aberrations.

Atypical CML. Atypical CML is the terminology for cases presenting with a clinical picture similar to or identical with CML but in which neither the Philadelphia chromosome nor *BCR/ABL* transcription can be demonstrated. During the chronic phase, such patients frequently have lower blood leukocyte levels and more evidence of marrow failure than do those with Philadelphia chromosome–positive disease. There is often significant multiple lineage dysplasia, and there may be significant monocythemia. The clinical course to marrow failure and/or blastic transformation is shorter on the average in atypical CML than in standard CML. Differential diagnosis includes CML, chronic neutrophilic leukemia, CMML, and leukemoid reactions. CML is distinguished readily with molecular genetic studies. Differentiation from CMML is more difficult and largely arbitrary; atypical CML tends to have more myeloblasts and more frequent eosinophils and basophils. CML, atypical CML, and CMML each can evolve into a blastic leukemia.

Chronic Neutrophilic Leukemia. Chronic neutrophilic leukemia is a rare condition in which high numbers of mature neutrophils, often with toxic granulations, Döhle bodies, and ring-shaped nuclei, are seen in the absence of identifiable infection or lymphoproliferative disease. In contrast to CML, the peripheral blood does not contain excessive numbers of myeloid precursors, and the neutrophil alkaline phosphatase is usually normal to high. Myelodysplatic changes are usually minimal but may occur in some cases. As with CML, the serum vita-

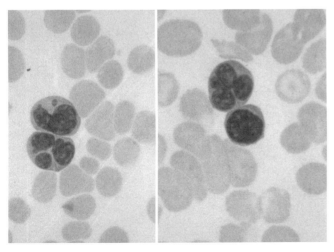

FIGURE 11–31. Adult T-cell leukemia/lymphoma. Peripheral blood contains characteristic malignant T cells with multilobed nuclei (cloverleaf or flower cells). (See Color Section.)

TABLE 11–8. Acute Leukemia Subtypes: French-American-British Cooperative Group Classification[9, 13]

Lymphoblastic

ALL-L1
Most common form in children
Small cells, high N/C; homogeneous nuclear chromatin; inconspicuous nucleolus inconspicuous nucleolus
Figure 11–2*

ALL-L2
"ALL with maturation"
Heterogeneous cell size and shape; usually large, low N/C; visible nucleoli
Figure 11–3*

ALL-L3
Burkitt cell leukemia
Large, uniform cells with diffuse chromatin, deeply basophilic cytoplasm, frequent vacuoles, prominent nucleoli
Figure 11–4*

Myeloid

AML-M0
Minimally differentiated AML
>30% blasts in marrow; <3% of blasts are positive by conventional techniques for MPO, SBB, or CAE
No cytoplasmic granules or Auer bodies
Diagnosed by ultrastructural studies, immunochemical demonstration of anti-MPO MoAb, or ultrastructural cytochemistry
Usually diagnosed $CD13^+$ and $CD33^+$ (but platelet antigens negative)
Figure 11–7*

AML-M1
AML without maturation
>30% blasts in marrow; <90% of nonerythroid cells are myeloblasts; ≥3% blasts MPO^+ or SBB^+
Maturing monocytes ≤10% and maturing granulocytes are each ≤10% of nonerythroid cells
Figure 11–8*

AML-M2
AML with (granulocytic) maturation
>30% blasts in marrow; blasts 30%-89% of nonerythroid cells
May have Auer rods (often thin, needle shaped)
Blasts are positive for CAE, MPO, SBB
Maturing granulocytic cells >10% and monocytic cells <10% of nonerythroid cells
Figures 11–9 and 11–10*

AML-M3
Hypergranular promyelocytic leukemia
Abnormal promyelocytes predominate
Blasts may be <30%
Frequent Auer rods, often multiple
Figures 11–11 and 11–12*
Nucleus folded, bilobed, or reniform, often obscured by dense large granules

AML-M3V
Microgranular variant of promyelocytic leukemia
Same characteristics as AML-M3, except for absence of large granules
May be confused with AML-M5b or M7
Diagnosed by cytogenetics, molecular genetics, immunophenotype ($CD14^-$, platelet antigen$^-$)
Figure 11–13*

AML-M4
Acute myelomonocytic leukemia
Blasts ≥30% of marrow cells and nonerythroid cells
Granulocytic (neutrophilic) component ≥20%
Monocytic component (blasts to mature) ≥20%, plus peripheral blood monocytes $≥5 \times 10^9$
NASDA or $ANAE^{2+}$
Figure 11–14*

AML-M4Eo
Acute myelomonocytic leukemia with eosinophilia
Same as M4, but with eosinophilic granulocytic maturation
Figure 11–15*

AML-M4Baso
Acute myelocytic leukemia with basophilia
Same as AML-M4, except with basophilic granulocytic maturation

AML-M5a
Acute monoblastic leukemia
Monoblasts are large with fine nuclear chromatin, basophilic extensive cytoplasm with fine pink granules and often with vacuoles
≥30% of marrow cells and nonerythroid marrow cells are monoblasts
Monocytic component ≥80% of nonerythroid marrow cells, and ≥80% of monocytic component is blasts
Auer rods are rare
NSE^+, lysozyme$^+$ usually, at least in maturing cells
Figure 11–16*

AML-M5b
Acute monocytic leukemia
Same as AML-M5a, except <80% of bone marrow monocytic cells are blasts
Figure 11–17*

AML-M6
AML with predominant erythroid differentiation (erythroleukemia)
Erythroblasts >50% of bone marrow cells
Blasts ≥30% of nonerythroid marrow cells
PAS^+, NSE^+
Figure 11–18*

AML-M7
Acute megakaryoblastic leukemia
Blasts ≥30% of marrow nucleated cells
Blasts are often pleomorphic, with basophilic cytoplasm; irregular, often multilobed nuclei with prominent, often multiple nucleoli
Blasts are platelet antigen$^+$ or shown to have PPO on ultrastructural studies
Figures 11–19 and 11–20*

*See also Color Section.

ANAE, α-naphthyl acetate esterase; CAE, chloroacetate esterase; MoAb, monoclonal antibody; MPO, myeloperoxidase; N/C, nuclear-to-cytoplasmic ratio; NASDA, naphthol AS-D acetate esterase; NSE, neuron-specific enolase; PAS, periodic acid–Schiff; PPO, platelet peroxidase; SBB, Sudan black B.

min B_{12} level is high. There may be associated hyperuricemia and hypercalcemia. The Philadelphia chromosome and *BCR/ABL* fusion is absent. When cytogenic abnormalities have been detected, the disease appears to be clonal. The most difficult distinction is between chronic neutrophilic leukemia and a leukemoid reaction. Demonstration of clonality provides a critical distinction. In the absence of markers, the clinical course provides the answer.[53]

CLASSIFICATION OF HEMATOLOGIC MALIGNANT DISEASE

The first described cases of leukemia most probably were chronic forms, with large volumes of malignant leukocytes and extensive organ infiltration. Virchow[54] distinguished a splenic (myeloid) form and a lymphatic form of the disease, and Friedreich,[55] in 1857, differentiated chronic from acute leukemia on the basis of clinical features and clinical course. After the introduction of metachromatic dyes by Ehrlich,[1] the varied morphologic features of the disease came to be appreciated. During the century that followed, all of the forms of leukemia recognized as distinct today as well as the myelodysplasias and myeloproliferative diseases were described. Despite this, until 1976, there was not general agreement about the number of entities that existed or the criteria for their recognition as distinct disorders. In that year, the FAB Cooperative Group of clinician-morphologists proposed a classification schema for acute leukemia[9]; with its revisions and additions,[2, 9-12] it has been widely used and accepted worldwide. The schema consisted originally of three subtypes of ALL plus six subtypes of AML; the more recent addition of undifferentiated AML (M0) and megakaryoblastic AML (M7) has brought the number of AMLs to eight (Table 11-8). In addition, an analogous classification for CML and MDS has been proposed and generally accepted.[10] Despite the extended use of these morphology-based classifications, their clinical utility was less than optimal. The distinction of B-cell from T-cell ALL was not possible on morphologic grounds, nor could morphology consistently distinguish leukemia with and without genetic abnormalities of relevance to prognosis and therapeutic choice.[6, 56, 57] With these limitations in mind, there have been a number of proposed classifications using, in addition to morphology and cytochemistry, immunologic characterization, cytogenetics, and molecular analysis.[43, 57, 58] These have culminated in proposals by the WHO for a comprehensive classification of hematologic malignant disorders.[8] The WHO classification is based largely on two sources, the International Lymphoma Study Group classification of lymphoid malignancy (REAL classification) and the revised FAB leukemia classifications. They recognize the merits of each but also the limitations. The most dependable and objective criteria are given preference in assigning subtypes. For example, the diagnosis of APL is primarily based on the karyotype and molecular genetics of its malignant cells, rather than on morphologic appearance, because they define not only the origin of the disease but also the response to therapy (Table 11-9).

TABLE 11–9. Acute Leukemia (WHO Recommendations[8])

Acute Lymphoid Leukemia

Precursor B-cell acute lymphoblastic leukemia
  Cytogenetic subgroups:
    Normal

t(9;22)(q34;q11)	*BCR-ABL*
t(variable;11q23)	*MLL* rearranged
t(1;19)(q23;p13)	*E2A-PBX*
t(12;21)(p12;q22)	*TEL-CBFA (AML1)*

Precursor T-cell acute lymphoblastic leukemia
Burkitt cell leukemia

Acute Myeloid Leukemia

Acute myeloid leukemia (AML) with recurrent cytogenetic translocations:
  AML with t(8;21)(q22;q22), AML *(CBFA-ETO)*
  Acute promyelocytic leukemia, AML with t(15;17)(q21;q11-12) and variants, *PML-RARA*
  AML with abnormal marrow eosinophils, AML with inv(16)(p13; q22) or t(16;16)(p13;q11), *CBFB-MYH11*
  AML with 11q23 abnormalities
  Cases with these abnormalities can be diagnosed independently of the proportion of blasts in the bone marrow.

Acute myeloid leukemia with multilineage dysplasia:
  With prior myelodysplastic syndrome
  Without prior myelodysplastic syndrome

Acute myeloid leukemia, therapy related:
  Alkylating agent related
  Epipodophyllotoxin related

Acute myeloid leukemia not otherwise categorized:

AML with minimal differentiation	FAB-M0 (Fig. 11-7)*
AML without maturation	FAB-M1 (Fig. 11-8)*
AML with granulocytic maturation	FAB-M2 (Fig. 11-9)*
Acute myelomonocytic leukemia	FAB-M4 (Fig. 11-14)*
Acute monoblastic leukemia	FAB-M5 (Figs. 11-16 & 11-17)*
Acute erythroid leukemia	FAB-M6 (Fig. 11-18)*
Acute megakaryocytic leukemia	FAB-M7 (Figs. 11-19 & 11-20)*
Acute basophilic leukemia	—
Acute panmyelosis with myelofibrosis	—

These categories require a minimum of 20% myeloblasts in the bone marrow.

Acute Biphenotypic Leukemia

This category requires a minimum of 20% blasts (other than erythroblasts) in the bone marrow.

*See also Color Section.

Similarly, t(9;22)(q34;q11) or *BCR/ABL* transcription determines CML and provides a target for therapy. The morphologic, cytochemical, immunologic, and clinical features of the disease should be consistent with the diagnosis, but in these cases, molecular genetics provides the most definitive diagnosis. By contrast, the clinical signs, clinical course, morphologic appearance, and typical immunophenotype are all more important than cytogenetics in the diagnosis of CLL or MDS. The WHO classification attempts to apply the most definitive criteria available for the diagnosis of each type of hematopoietic malignant disease, with the implicit understanding that as knowledge expands, both the classification itself and the criteria for each entity will necessarily change. Tables 11-5, 11-6, 11-7, and 11-9 list the WHO-designated entities relevant to a textbook on leukemia. When a congruent diagnosis in the FAB classification exists, it is noted. The tables also list the criteria for diagnosis and the more important clinical correlates to the diagnosis. Greater detail is provided in the chapters dedicated to each entity or group of diseases.

DIFFERENTIAL DIAGNOSIS

As noted earlier, the hematologic malignant diseases, collectively, can present a remakably varied array of clinical manifestations. Accordingly, they can be confused with a wide spectrum of other illnesses, including other malignant neoplasms. Some of the more common problems for differential diagnosis are listed in Table 11-10, together with the more important methods for their distinction from leukemia. The major underlying distinction depends on the identification of clonality and the search for markers of malignancy, infection, or other morbid conditions.

ANCILLARY STUDIES

In addition to correct diagnosis of the type and extent of the disease, several other assessments need to be made during the course of the disease. These are outlined in Table 11-11 and are also addressed in Chapter 13. These include identification of any leukemia-related or concordant physical or emotional problems that could complicate therapy or influence the type of treatment to be given, identification of potential donors in circumstances in which hematopoietic stem cell transplantation is a potential option (see Chapter 20), and monitoring of the toxic side effects of antileukemia therapy.

Although children have an advantage in terms of long-term disease control within almost all diagnostic groups, they are susceptible to alterations of physical and intellectual growth, which are less of a problem in adult populations. Accordingly, endocrinologic, neurologic, psychiatric, and educational testing and counseling should be considered for all children and young adults beginning as soon as possible after diagnosis.[59, 60]

TABLE 11-10. Differential Diagnosis of Leukemia

Leukemia Symptom/Signs Complex	Alternative Cause	Major Methods of Discrimination
Fever, malaise, granulocytosis, ± lymphadenopathy, ± hepatosplenomegaly	Infection (FUO), SBE, sepsis	Myeloid cell morphology, results of cultures, serology, bone marrow examination, cytogenetics
	Other tumors, especially Hodgkin's disease, lung cancer	Bone marrow biopsy, chest film, CT scans, node biopsy
Fever, malaise, lymphocytosis or monocytosis or both, ± lymphadenopathy, ± hepatosplenomegaly	Infectious mononucleosis syndrome, typhoidal phase of many infections, pertussis, tuberculosis, toxoplasmosis	Lymphocyte morphology, cultures and serologic tests for infectious agents (EBV,CMV), skin tests (PPD), bone marrow, chest film
	Chronic NK-cell lymphocytosis	Assess clonality (e.g., cytogenetics)
	Autoimmune lymphoproliferative syndrome	Check apoptosis, CD3$^+$/4$^-$/8$^-$ cells
	Non-Hodgkin's lymphoma, reticuloses	Biopsy of marrow, nodes, masses; morphology of lymphocytes; cytogenetics, immunophenotype
Arthralgias, bone pain	Flu syndrome, streptococcemia, rheumatic diseases, SLE, gout, myeloma, osteosarcoma, neuroblastoma, hemophilia, sicklemia	History; CBC with differential, ESR; serologies (RF, ANA, etc), cultures, SPEP, VMA and homovanillic acid, uric acid, coagulation profile, hemoglobin, electrophoresis; radiography
Pancytopenia	Aplastic anemia, megaloblastic anemia, PNH, Fanconi, AIDS, hepatitis	History (esp. drug, toxin, x-rays, diet, family history); B$_{12}$, folate, acid hemolysis; bone marrow with cytogenetics; HIV, hepatitis serology
Bleeding, hemorrhage	ITP, drug-induced thrombocytopenia, infection (esp. hepatitis, childhood exanthems, meningococcemia, HIV), scurvy, DIC, Henoch-Schönlein, Wiskott-Aldrich, Chédiak-Higashi	History (esp. drugs, toxins, x-rays, family, diet, infection [HIV, hepatitis] exposures), PE; CBC, blood cultures; LP if indicated, coagulogram; serologies for EBV, HIV, hepatitis
Palpable infiltrates	Lymphoma, infections, drug reactions, phenytoin (nodes)	History, PE; CBC with differential; serology for HIV, CMV; toxoplasmosis; needle aspiration or biopsy
Hepatosplenomegaly	Infection: mononucleosis, malaria, tuberculosis, kala-azar; lymphoma, cirrhosis, myelofibrosis, polycythemia, Gaucher's, hereditary or acquired hemolysis	History, PE; CBC (look at smear!); uric acid, liver function tests; chest film; abdominal CT; skin tests PPD; serology, serum B$_{12}$/transcobalamin, Coombs' test, LDH; liver biopsy, splenic FNA if necessary
Neurologic disorders	Trauma, migraine/other headache, encephalitis, toxoplasmosis, brain tumor, meningitis; drug reaction, overdose, toxicity (e.g., aminoglycoside)	History, PE including funduscopy, CBC with differential, serologies and cultures PRN, CT/MRI of head; LP with cytospin, culture
Testicular enlargement	Orchitis, epididymitis; seminoma/germ cell tumor; trauma; hydrocele, torsion	History, PE; CBC with differential; transillumination, α-fetoprotein, FSH; CT scan; biopsy

AIDS, acquired immunodeficiency syndrome; CBC, complete blood count; CMV, cytomegalovirus; CT, computed tomography; DIC, disseminated intravascular coagulation; EBV, Epstein-Barr virus; ESR, erythrocyte sedimentation rate; FNA, fine-needle aspiration; FSH, follicle-stimulating hormone; FUO, fever of unknown origin; HIV, human immunodeficiency virus; ITP, idiopathic thrombocytopenic purpura; LDH, lactate dehydrogenase; LP, lumbar puncture; MRI, magnetic resonance imaging; PE, physical examination; PNH, paroxysmal nocturnal hemoglobinuria; PPD, purified protein derivative tuberculin; SBE: subacute bacterial endocarditis; SLE, systemic lupus erythematosus; SPEP, serum protein electrophoresis; VMA, vanillylmandelic acid.

TABLE 11–11. Ancillary Studies in Hematopoietic Neoplasms

ALL	Serum uric acid, renal function, liver function, LDH
	Chest film, especially in childhood T-cell ALL, and in symptomatic patients
	LVEF, if anthracycline or mitoxantrone treatment is planned
	Lumbar puncture and cytospin cytology in children and high-risk adults
	HLA typing in high-risk patients up to 55 years of age
AML	Serum uric acid, tests of renal and hepatic function
	Coagulation screens, including fibrinogen and DIC work-up in APL and acute monoblastic leukemia
	LVEF if anthracycline or mitoxantrone treatment is planned
	Lumbar puncture and cytospin cytology in monocytoid morphologies (M4, M5) and M2
	Multidrug resistance gene or gene product in high-risk cases
	HLA typing in all except good-risk groups, i.e., t(15;17) and inv(16) or t(16;16) or patients >55 years of age
CML	Serum uric acid, LDH, tests of hepatic and renal function, vitamin B_{12}, transcobalamin, LDH
	HLA typing in patients <55 years of age
CLL	B_2-Microglobulin, LDH, serum iron/transferrin.
	Serum protein electrophoresis, quantitative immunoglobulins
	Serial stools for occult blood, colonoscopy or sigmoidoscopy
	HLA typing in patients <55 years of age
MDS	Serum iron, transferrin, ferritin, LDH, uric acid
	Serum protein electrophoresis
	HLA typing for patients with excess blasts <55 years of age

DIC, disseminated intravascular coagulation; LDH, lactate dehydrogenase; LVEF, left ventricular ejection fraction.

Renal and hepatic function should be monitored at regular intervals. Assessment of cardiac functions, particularly of the left ventrical, should be performed before each course of therapy that includes one of the cardiotoxic drug (e.g., anthracyclines and anthracenediones). Long-term effects on fertility should be discussed with patients who are desirous of children and are premenopausal, and their reproductive function should be assessed when appropriate.[60, 61]

At the time of diagnosis, it is also helpful to assess factors other than those inherent in the diagnosis itself that have prognostic significance. For example, the expression of the multidrug resistance gene (*MDR*, P-glycoprotein) should be determined when possible because it is associated with diminished drug sensitivity and survival and may be susceptible to pharmacologic modulation (see Chapter 17). Other tests may aid in diagnosis or in estimating prognosis. For example, the telomere length in CML progenitor cells has been reported to correlate with survival,[32] and the concentration of neovascular endothelial growth factor in leukemia marrows has been said to correlate with response to chemotherapy.

ASSESSING RESPONSE TO TREATMENT

Just as the goals of current treatment vary among the types of leukemia, so do the criteria for response. For acute leukemia of all subtypes and for CML and hairy cell leukemia, eradication of leukemia with resultant cure is

the appropriate goal. In such cases, cytoreduction is the key to long remission and cure. Therefore, serial assessment of residual disease is crucial, not only during treatment but for years after all therapy has been completed. The criteria for response in these cases are changing in response to increasing expectations of therapy and improvement in technology. Traditionally, a reduction of blasts cells (or, in the case of APL, malignant promyelocytes) to less than 5% together with return of marrow cellularity and function to normal levels and the disappearance of all extramedullary manifestations of leukemia infiltration constituted a complete remission.[15] In recent years, the criteria for complete remission have evolved from the disappearance of cytohistologically detectable leukemia cells from the blood and bone marrow to the absence of immunologically distinctive leukemia cells and cytogenetic abnormalities and to the disappearance of leukemia-specific genes or transcripts assessed by PCR or RT-PCR. These techniques are not universally applicable or available and on occasion can lead to clinically erroneous conclusions; correctly applied, they remarkably increase the ability to detect residual disease and have proved to be a useful adjunct to determining current and future management (see Chapter 12). Pui and Compana,[62] for example, have noted that patients with childhood ALL in whose remission marrows 10^5 leukemia cells can be detected are strikingly prone to relapse, whereas those with 10^4 cells and below almost always remain in long-lasting remission. Accordingly, for this group of patients, they suggest that these levels define a complete remission. Further experience should determine the value of this redefinition for ALL and other hematologic malignant neoplasms.

By contrast, for most patients with chronic leukemia or MDS, short of marrow transplantation, therapy does not aim for cure. Rather, stabilization of disease, diminution of symptoms, and improvement in quality of life are the major goals. In most instances, therapy to these ends does result in a reduction of the body's burden of malignant cells, but the extent of reduction is not an end in itself but one piece of the larger picture.

Defining response in patients with MDS has been attempted[63] (see Chapter 24). In general, evaluation of response and the success of treatment will remain highly subjective until improved therapies are developed. However, this in no way relieves the therapist of the responsibility of closely monitoring the extent of the disease and the occurrence of complications.

DEFINING RELAPSE

Relapse of leukemia is the reaccumulation of leukemia cells that, if left untreated, will lead to the clinical manifestations seen at diagnosis. Relapse may occur primarily in the bone marrow, in which case deficits in normal blood cell production lead to anemia, granulocytopenia, and thrombocytopenia. Alternatively, relapse may be localized primarily to extramedullary sites (e.g., the meninges, the skin, or the testes). These isolated relapses are almost always accompanied by disseminated disease, which will become apparent unless systemic treatment is instituted.

At relapse, the leukemia phenotype is usually but not always the same as it was at initial diagnosis. However, transitions of morphologic appearance from lymphoid to myeloid and immunologic alterations may occur. Cytogenetic and molecular studies will, however, reveal that the malignant cell population represents the initial clone, albeit sometimes with additional abnormalities. In cases in which genetic, immunologic, or other markers are absent, diagnosis of relapse can be made only by observing the progressive accumulation of leukemia cells over time.

Relapse of acute leukemia is traditionally defined as the presence of 5% or more blast cells in a marrow formerly in remission, or the appearance of leukemia cells in the circulation or extramedullary sites, on two or more occasions. In practice, the diagnosis is usually made on the basis of a single marrow examination revealing much more than a 5% infiltration of blasts. Alternatively, the presence of the markers seen earlier (e.g., Auer bodies, marker chromosomes, or antigen constellations) may identify relapse, often before it could be diagnosed on morphologic grounds.

For chronic leukemia or MDS, relapse is less well defined and practically consists of the increase in the cell burden of malignant cells as determined primarily by physical examination, blood counts, and marrow examination and secondarily by immunoglobulin levels, β_2-microglobulin, serum lactate dehydrogenase, and development of cytopenia unrelated to drug toxicity. Each entity has a different set of response and relapse criteria, detailed more extensively in the subsequent chapters.

LONG-TERM FOLLOW-UP

The extent and duration of active follow-up of hematopoietic malignant neoplasms will vary according to the factors that influence the chance of cure and those that predispose the patients to the long-term consequences of treatment. Cure—or at least long-term disease-free survival—depends chiefly on the specific diagnosis and on the age at which the diagnosis was established. For patients with acute leukemia, and for all other patients treated with curative intent (e.g., those receiving stem cell transplants), the risk for relapse is highest during the first years after diagnosis. By the end of the third year, the rate of relapse, and death, approaches but does not quite reach a plateau.[64, 65]

Assessment of continuing remission should therefore be performed frequently during the first 3 years, after which it can be spaced out, although never totally discontinued. Patients should be made knowledgeable about the signs and symptoms of recurrence and those of the major complications of their disease and its therapy. Above all, they should be advised to contact their therapy team whenever they experience fever, bleeding, neurologic difficulties, or an unexpected or unusual change in their condition. Patients who are potential candidates for transplantation (e.g., those with poor-risk ALL or AML in first remission) should be observed closely with frequent bone marrow examinations so that transplantation salvage therapy can be instituted at the first evidence of relapse.

Patients with incurable chronic leukemias and MDS often require less frequent monitoring for progression. These patients should be monitored for falling blood counts, the onset of fever, increases in splenomegaly, and lymphadenopathy. Hemolytic anemia can occur suddenly in CLL, often unrelated to the status of disease control. Treatment with fludarabine frequently precipitates autoimmune anemia or thrombocytopenia. Periodic checks of immunoglobulin production should be routine in CLL and other lymphoproliferative diseases.

PROSPECTUS

During the next decades, the detection and characterization of molecular aberrations intrinsic to leukemia and other blood cell malignant neoplasms will provide a quantitative basis for the diagnosis and subclassification of malignant diseases of the hematopoietic tissues. Not only will these subclassifications become the basis of cancer cell detection, but the molecular characterization will also provide guidelines for more effective (and less toxic) applications of "tailored" therapies. Multiarray plates will very likely be available in most laboratories for rapid screening of characteristic and clinically important gene expressions, on the basis of which therapeutic plans can be formulated. However, for the initial diagnosis of leukemia, MDS, and MPD, clinical acumen and knowledge of blood cell morphology will continue to play a primary role. Those who wish to be part of the management team will need to become, as is now the case, expert in bedside evaluation and laboratory microscopy as well as be well versed in the uses and limitations of molecular biologic approaches to diagnosis.

REFERENCES

1. Ehrlich P: Farbenanalytische Untersuchungen zur Histologie und Klinik des Bluts. Berlin: A Hirschwald; 1891.
2. Bennett JM, Catovsky D, Daniel MT, et al: Proposal for the recognition of minimally differentiated acute myeloid leukemia (AML M0). Br J Haematol 1991;78:325.
3. Nowell P, Hungerford DA: A minute chromosome in human chronic granulocytic leukemia [abstract]. Science 1960;132:1497.
4. Rowley J: A new consistent abnormality in chronic myelogenous leukemia identified by quinacrine fluorescence and Giemsa staining. Nature 1973;243:290.
5. Castaigne S, Chomienne C, Daniel MT, et al: All-*trans* retinoic acid is a differentiation therapy for acute promyelocytic leukemia. I. Clinical results. Blood 1990;76:1704.
6. Bloomfield CD, Lawrence D, Byrd JC, et al: Frequency of prolonged remission duration in acute myeloid leukemia varies by cytogenetic subtype. Cancer Res 1998;57:4173.
7. Drucker BJ, Talpaz M, Resta D, et al: Clinical efficacy and safety of an ABL specific tyrosine kinase inhibitor as targeted therapy for chronic myelogenous leukemia [abstract 1939]. Blood 1999; 94(suppl 1):368a.
8. WHO Classification of Tumors: Jaffe ES, Harris NL, Stein H, et al (eds): Pathology and genetics: Tumors of hematopoietic and lymphoid tissues. IARC Press, Lyon, 2001.
9. Bennett JM, Catovsky D, Daniel MT, et al: Proposals for the classifi-

cation of the acute leukaemias (FAB Cooperative Group). Br J Haematol 1976;33:451.

10. Bennett JM, Catovsky D, Daniel MT, et al: A variant form of acute hypergranular promyelocytic leukaemia (M3). Br J Haematol 1980; 44:169.

11. Bennett JM, Catovsky D, Daniel MT: Criteria for the diagnosis of acute leukemia of megakaryocytic lineage (M7): A report of the French-American-British Cooperative Group. Ann Intern Med 1985; 103:460.

12. Bennett JM, Catovsky D, Daniel MT, et al: Proposed revised criteria for the classification of acute myeloid leukemia. Ann Intern Med 1985;103:626.

13. Bennett JM, Catovsky D, Daniel MT, et al: Proposals for the classification of the myelodysplastic syndromes. Br J Haematol 1982; 51:189.

14. Bennett JM, Catovsky D, Daniel MT, et al: The chronic myeloid leukaemias: Guidelines for distinguishing chronic granulocytic, atypical chronic myeloid, and chronic myelomonocytic leukaemia. Proposals by the French-American-British Cooperative Leukaemia Group. Br J Haematol 1994;87:746.

15. Cheson BD, Cassileth PA, Head DR, et al: Report of the National Cancer Institute–sponsored workshop on definitions of diagnosis and response in acute myeloid leukemia. J Clin Oncol 1990;8:813.

16. Emanuel PD: Myelodysplasia and myeloproliferative disorders in childhood: An update [review]. Br J Haematol 1999;105:852.

17. Clarkson BD, Boyse EA: Possible explanation of the high concordance for acute lymphoblastic leukemia in monozygotic twins. Lancet 1971;1:699.

18. Chaganti RSK, Miller DR, Meyers PA, et al: Cytogenetic evidence of the intrauterine origin of acute leukemia in monozygotic twins. N Engl J Med 1979;300:1032.

19. Hartley SE, Sainsbury C: Acute leukaemia and the same chromosomal abnormality in monozygotic twins. Hum Genet 1981;58:408.

20. Gunz FW, Gunz JP, Veale AMO, et al: Familial leukaemia. A study of 909 families. Scand J Haematol 1975;15:117.

21. Devine DV, Gluck WL, Rosse W, et al: Acute myeloblastic leukemia in paroxysmal nocturnal hemoglobinuria. Evidence of evolution from the abnormal paroxysmal nocturnal hemoglobinuria clone. J Clin Invest 1987;79:1987.

22. Garfinkel L, Boffetta P: Association between smoking and leukemia in two American Cancer Society studies. Cancer 1990;68:2356.

23. Mills PK: History of cigarette smoking and the risk of leukemia and myeloma. Results from the Adventist Health Study. J Natl Cancer Inst 1990;89:1832.

24. Arseneau JC, Sponzo RW, Levin DL, et al: Non-lymphomatous malignant tumors complicating Hodgkin's disease. Possible association with intensive therapy. N Engl J Med 1972;287:1119.

25. Greene MH, Boice JD, Green BE, et al: Acute nonlymphocytic leukemia after therapy with alkylating agents for ovarian cancer. A study of five randomized trials. N Engl J Med 1982;307:1416.

26. Rosner F, Grünwald HW: Cytotoxic drugs and leukaemogenesis. Clin Haematol 1980;9:663.

27. Pedersen-Bjergaard J, Philip P: Therapy-related malignancies: A review. Eur J Haematol 1988;42(suppl 48):39.

28. Pui CH, Behm FG, Raimondi SC, et al: Acute myeloid leukemia in children treated for acute lymphoid leukemia. N Engl J Med 1989; 321:136.

29. Pui CH, Hancock ML, Raimondi SC, et al: Myeloid neoplasia in children treated for solid tumors. Lancet 1990;336:417.

30. Macintyre EA, Delbesse F: Molecular approaches in the diagnosis and evaluation of lymphoid malignancies. Semin Hematol 1999; 36:373.

31. Kozu T, Miyoshi H, Shimizu K, et al: Junctions of the AML1/MTG8 (ETO) fusion are constant in t(8;21) acute myeloid leukemia detected by reverse transcription polymerase chain reaction. Blood 1993;83:1270.

32. Downing JR, Head DR, Cùrcio-Brint AM, et al: An AML1/ETO fusion transcript is consistently detected by RNA-based polymerase chain reaction in acute myelogenous leukemia containing the (8;21)(q22; q22) translocation. Blood 1999;81:2860.

33. LeGouill S, Talmant P, Milspied N, et al: Fluorescence in situ hybridization on peripheral blood specimens is a reliable method to evaluate response in chronic myeloid leukemia. J Clin Oncol 2000; 18:1533.

34. Park KU, She CJ, Shin HY et al: Low incidence of TEL/AML fusion and TEL deletion in Korean childhood acute leukemia by extra-signal fluorescence in situ hybridization. Cancer Genet Cytogenet 1999;110:7.

35. Corlando C, Penzani P, Pazzagli M: Developments in quantitative polymerase chain reaction [review]. Clin Chem Lab Med 1998; 36:256.

36. Brummendorf TH, Holyoke TL, Rufer N, et al: Prognostic implication of differences in telomere length between normal and malignant cells from patients with chronic myeloid leukemia measured by flow cytometry. Blood 2000;95:1883.

37. Marschhauser F, Cayuela JM, Martini S, et al: Evaluation of minimal residual disease using reverse-transcription polymerase chain reaction in t(8;21) acute leukemia: A multicenter study of 51 patients. J Clin Oncol 2000;18:788.

38. Staudt LM, Brown PO: Genomic views of the immune system. Annu Rev Immunol 2000;18:829.

39. Shena M, Shalon D, Davis RN, et al: Quantitative monitoring of gene expression patterns with complementary DNA microassay. Science 1996;270:467.

40. Sainty D, Liso V, Cantù-Rajnoldi A, et al: A new morphologic classification system for acute promyelocytic leukemia distinguishes cases with underlying PLZF/RARA gene rearrangements. Blood 2000;96:1287.

41. Mirro J, Kitchingman GP: The morphology, cytochemistry, molecular characteristics and clinical significance of acute mixed-lineage leukemia. In Scott CS (ed): Leukemia Cytochemistry: Principles and Practice. Chichester: Ellis Horwood Limited; 1989; p 155.

42. Matutes E, Morilla R, Farahat N, et al: Definition of biphenotypic leukemia. Haematologica 1997;82:64.

42a. Armstrong SA, Staunton JE, Silverman LB, et al: MLL translocations specify a distinct gene expression profile that distinguishes a unique leukemia. Nat Genet 2002 Jan; 30(1):41–7.

43. European Group for Immunological Characterization of Leukemias [EGIL], Bene MC, Castoldi G, Knapp W, et al: Proposals for the immunological classification of acute leukemias. Leukemia 1995; 9:1783.

44. Rosati S, Mick R, Xu F, et al: Refractory cytopenias with multilineage dysplasia: Further characterization of an "unclassifiable" myelodysplastic syndrome. Leukemia 1996;10:20.

45. Foon KA, Todd RF III: Immunologic classification of leukemia and lymphoma. Blood 1986;68:1.

46. Baldini L, Cro L, Cortelezzi R, et al: Immunophenotypes in "classical" B-cell chronic lymphocytic leukemia. Correlation with normal cellular counterparts and clinical findings. Cancer 1990;66:1738.

47. Zwiebal JA, Cheson BD: Chronic lymphocytic leukemia. Staging and prognostic factors. Semin Oncol 1998;25:42.

48. Stevenson F, Sahota S, Zhu D, et al: Insight into the origin and clonal history of B-cell tumors as revealed by analysis of immunoglobulin variable region genes. Immunol Rev 1998;162:247.

49. Hoyer JD, Ross CW, Li CY, et al: True T-cell chronic lymphocytic leukemia: A morphologic and immunophenotypic study of 25 cases. Blood 1995;86:1163.

50. Rabbini GR, Phyliky RL, Tefferi A: A long-term study of patients with chronic natural killer cell lymphocytosis. Br J Haematol 1999; 106:960.

51. Pettitt AR, Zuzel M, Cawley JC: Hairy-cell leukaemia: Biology and management [review]. Br J Haematol 1999;106:2.

52. Robbins BA, Ellison DH, Spinosa HC, et al: Diagnostic applications of two color cytofluorometry in 161 cases of hairy cell leukemia. Blood 1993;82:1272.

53. Hasle H, Oleson G, Kundrup G, et al: Chronic neutrophil leukaemia in adolescence and young adulthood. Br J Haematol 1996;94:628.

54. Virchow R: Weisses Blut. Neve Notiz Geb Natur Heilk 1845;36:151.

55. Friedreich N: Eine neue Fall von Leukämie. Virchows Arch Pathol Anat 1857;12:37.

56. Hoelzer D, Thiel E, Löffler H, et al: The German multicenter trials for treatment of acute lymphoblastic leukemia in adults. Leukemia 1992;6(suppl 3):175.

57. Bain BJ: The classification of acute leukaemias: The necessity for incorporating cytogenetic and molecular genetic information. J Clin Pathol 1998;51:420.

58. First MIC Cooperative Study Group: Morphologic, immunologic, and cytogenetic (MIC) working classification of acute lymphoblastic leukemia. Cancer Genet Cytogenet 1986;23:189.

59. Ochs J, Mulhern R: Late effects of antileukemic treatment. Pediatr Clin North Am 1989;35:815.

60. Brown RT, Madan-Swain A, Pais R, et al: Chemotherapy for acute lymphocytic leukemia: Cognitive and academic sequelae. J Pediatr 1992;121:855.

61. Byrne J, Mulvihill J, Myers MH, et al: Effect of treatment on fertility of long term survivors of adolescent cancer. N Engl J Med 1987; 317:1315.

62. Pui CH, Compana D: New definition of remission in childhood acute lymphoblastic leukemia. Leukemia 2000;14:783.

63. Cheson B, Bennett J, Kantarjian H, et al: Report of an international workshop group to standardize response criteria for myelodysplastic syndromes. Blood 2000;96:3671.

64. Estey E, de Lima M, Strom S, et al: Long-term follow-up of patients with newly diagnosed acute myeloid leukemia treated at the University of Texas M. D. Anderson Cancer Center. Cancer 1997; 80(suppl):2176.

65. Applebaum FR, Kopecky KJ: Long-term survival after chemotherapy for acute myeloid leukemia. The experience of the Southwest Oncology Group. Cancer 1997;80(suppl):2199.

12

T. Szczepański   J.J.M. van Dongen

Detection of Minimal Residual Disease

Current cytotoxic treatment protocols induce complete remission in most acute leukemia patients, in some patients with chronic lymphocytic leukemia (CLL), and in most patients with non-Hodgkin's lymphoma (NHL). The introduction of allogeneic and autologous bone marrow transplantation (BMT) into treatment protocols has further increased the remission rates in acute leukemias and NHL. Nevertheless, many of these patients relapse. Apparently, the treatment protocols are not capable of killing all clonogenic malignant cells in these patients, although they reached complete remission according to cytomorphologic criteria. The detection limit of cytomorphologic techniques is not lower than 1% to 5% of malignant cells, which implies that these techniques can provide only superficial information about the effectiveness of the treatment. More sensitive techniques are required for the detection of low frequencies of malignant cells during and after treatment, specifically, the detection of minimal residual disease (MRD). MRD techniques should reach sensitivities of at least 10^{-3} (1 malignant cell within 1000 normal cells), but sensitivities of 10^{-4} to 10^{-6} are preferred. Moreover, reliable MRD techniques should be characterized by leukemia specificity (discrimination between malignant and normal cells without false-positive results), reproducibility, and feasibility (easy standardization and rapid collection of results for clinical application). Such characteristics allow "true" MRD detection and thereby evaluation of the effectiveness of the total treatment and assessment of the contribution of each treatment phase[1-3] (Fig. 12–1).

The application of MRD techniques is especially valuable in malignancies that can potentially be cured by the use of cytotoxic therapy and/or BMT, including acute leukemias, several types of NHL, and chronic myeloid leukemia (CML). In these disease categories, MRD information might be used for adaptation of treatment.

During the last 15 years, several methods of MRD detection have been developed and evaluated. Most of these techniques appeared to have limited sensitivity, specificity, and/or applicability:

- *Cytogenetics:* sensitivity of 10^{-2} and applicability limited to microscopically detectable chromosome aberrations. Cytogenetics is dependent on the possibility to obtain cells in metaphase.[4-6] Low mitosis frequency and preferential growth of normal cells might further decrease its sensitivity and reproducibility.

- *Cell culture systems:* variable sensitivity. Standardized application on a routine basis is difficult.[7-10]
- *Fluorescence in situ hybridization (FISH) techniques:* sensitivity of 10^{-2} and application restricted to malignancies with a well-defined chromosome aberration for which suitable FISH probes are available.[11-13] The sensitivity of interphase FISH for translocations, inversions, and deletions is limited to 1% to 5%. The limited sensitivity of the classic fusion signal FISH is caused by artifactual colocalization of two independent (unlinked) breakpoint probe signals in normal cells, which might cause false positivity.[12, 13] The sensitivity can be slightly increased by the application of metaphase FISH, which does not produce false-positive results but, like conventional cytogenetics, is dependent on the availability of cells in metaphase.[14] Another possibility to increase the sensitivity of MRD detection is the application of "split-signal" FISH, in which two differently labeled FISH probes are positioned at opposite sides of the breakpoint area, but sufficiently close to give a fusion signal in normal cells, whereas the signal is split in case of a breakpoint.[15, 16] The split-signal FISH technique will in principle not produce false-positive results and therefore has an essentially higher sensitivity (10^{-2} to 10^{-3}) than fusion-signal FISH does. Finally, FISH can be performed on fluorescence-activated cell-sorted (FACS) subpopulations of hematopoietic cells, such as myeloid precursors in acute myeloid leukemia (AML) or myelodysplastic syndromes (MDSs).[17]
- *Southern blotting:* sensitivity of 10^{-1} to 10^{-2} and application in virtually all lymphoid malignancies with rearranged immunoglobulin (Ig) or T-cell receptor (TCR) genes, as well as in malignancies with well-defined chromosome aberrations for which suitable DNA probes are available.[18-20]

Thus far, only two techniques are sufficiently sensitive and specific and have relatively broad applicability: immunophenotyping techniques and polymerase chain reaction (PCR) techniques (Table 12–1 and Fig. 12–1). Application of immunophenotyping techniques is based on the occurrence of aberrant, unusual, or ectopic phenotypes, whereas PCR techniques can be used for the detection of tumor-specific sequences, such as junctional regions of rearranged Ig and TCR genes or breakpoint fusion regions of chromosome aberrations.[1-3] These techniques

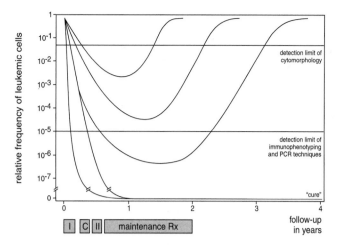

FIGURE 12–1. Diagram of the putative relative frequencies of leukemic cells in peripheral blood or bone marrow of acute leukemia patients during and after chemotherapy and during development of relapse. The detection limit of cytomorphologic techniques is indicated, as well as the detection limit of immunophenotyping and polymerase chain reaction techniques. Con-Rx, consolidation treatment; I-Rx, induction treatment; M-Rx, maintenance treatment.

can reach sensitivities of 10^{-3} to 10^{-6}, depending on the immunophenotype and genotype of the hematopoietic malignancy. In acute leukemias, both immunophenotyping and PCR techniques can be used for MRD detection. However, in chronic leukemias, immunophenotyping techniques are not generally sufficiently sensitive to reach 10^{-3} levels. Nevertheless, PCR analysis of Ig and TCR genes can be used for detection of MRD in CLL, and reverse transcription–PCR (RT-PCR) analysis of *BCR-ABL* transcripts can be used to detect MRD in CML.[21-23] In this chapter we will initially discuss the technical aspects of immunophenotyping and PCR analysis for MRD detection. Subsequently, we will summarize the clinical applications of these MRD techniques and discuss their clinical relevance in particular categories of hematopoietic malignancies.

TECHNIQUES FOR MINIMAL RESIDUAL DISEASE MONITORING

MRD Detection by Immunophenotyping

Aberrant Immunophenotypes as Targets for MRD Detection

Acute and chronic leukemias can be regarded as malignant counterparts of cells in immature and more mature stages of hematopoiesis, respectively.[24-28] Most ALL cells indeed have immunophenotypes comparable to those of normal immature lymphoid cells, and CLL cells resemble mature B or T lymphocytes. The same applies to immunophenotypes of myeloid leukemias. This similarity implies that the presence of normal hematopoietic cells limits the immunophenotypic detection of leukemic cells.[1-3, 29, 30] In principle, immunologic markers allow detection of only leukemic cells if the positive cells occur at higher frequencies than in normal cell samples. Despite this

inherent limitation to detect malignant cells, MRD detection is still possible because hematopoietic malignancies might display aberrant or unusual antigen expression (Fig. 12–2) or clonal patterns of Ig or TCR expression.[31-34]

Aberrant or unusual immunophenotypes are the result of cross-lineage antigen expression, maturational asynchronous expression of antigens, antigen overexpression, absence of antigen expression, and/or ectopic antigen expression.[1-3, 30, 35] The latter refers to the expression of particular antigens on cells outside their normal breeding sites or homing areas or to the expression of antigens that are normally expressed only on nonhematopoietic cells. Cross-lineage antigen expression represents the expression of typical myeloid antigens on lymphoid cells or vice versa and the presence of B-lineage antigens on T-lineage cells or vice versa.[1-3]

Clonal Ig molecules can be found in most chronic B-cell leukemias and B-NHL; they are detectable as single Ig light-chain expression, specifically, Igκ or Igλ.[31, 33] In chronic T-cell leukemias and in T-NHL, expression of clonal TCRαβ molecules is detectable with antibodies against the variable (V) domains of TCRβ chains; virtually no antibodies against variable domains of TCRα chains are available (Van Dongen et al., unpublished results).[34] Antibodies against the various V domains of TCRγ and TCRδ chains might contribute to clonality assessment of suspect TCRγδ⁺ T-cell proliferations.[36]

PRECURSOR–B-CELL ACUTE LYMPHOBLASTIC LEUKEMIA

Most precursor–B-cell acute lymphoblastic leukemia (B-ALL) cells express the CD10 antigen and terminal deoxynucleotidyl transferase (TdT). However, detection of low frequencies of precursor–B-ALL cells with CD10/TdT double-immunofluorescence (IF) staining is hampered by the background of normal TdT⁺ precursor B cells in bone marrow (BM) (generally <10% of mononuclear cells) and peripheral blood (PB) (generally <0.4%).[29, 37, 38] Moreover, detection of small numbers of CD10⁺TdT⁺ leukemic cells in regenerating BM after chemotherapy or BMT is even more difficult because levels of precursor B cells can be as high as 50% in these samples.[29, 39] Substantial expansion of normal precursor B cells in regenerating BM takes place not only after maintenance therapy but also during treatment.[40, 41] At the end of short intervals after intensive induction and consolidation blocks, regeneration of B-cell development occurs in BM with a large fraction of immature CD34⁺TdT⁺ B cells (Fig. 12–3). In contrast, in regenerating BM after cessation of maintenance treatment, the more mature TdT⁻CD19⁺CD10⁺ B cells are significantly increased, whereas the fraction of immature CD34⁺TdT⁺ B cells is essentially smaller[40, 41] (Fig. 12–3). The extent of B-lineage regeneration in BM also differs per treatment protocol and seems to be dependent on the intensity of the preceding treatment.[40] Interestingly, a substantial proportion (10% to 30%) of the blood B cells after maintenance treatment coexpress CD10. These percentages are markedly higher than normal values of CD10⁺ blood B cells thus indicating that CD10⁺ B cells are easily released from regenerating BM after cessation of therapy.[41] Only atypical features of blast cells such as CD10 overexpres-

TABLE 12–1. Detection of Minimal Residual Disease in Cell Samples from Leukemia Patients

Technique	Detection Limit	Applicability	Requirements, Limitations, and Pitfalls
Immunologic marker analysis			
Multiparameter flow cytometry (scatter pattern and double or triple labeling of membrane markers)	10^{-2} to 10^{-4}	70%–80% of childhood precursor–B-ALL 80%–90% of adult precursor–B-ALL 90% of T-ALL and lymphoblastic T-NHL 70%–80% of AML	Only applicable in cases with unusual or aberrant immunophenotype (including ectopic and tumor-specific antigen expression) Normal cell populations (especially in BM) will influence the detection limit
T-cell marker/TdT double IF staining (fluorescence microscopy)	10^{-4} to 10^{-5}	>95% of T-ALL	Experience with fluorescence microscopy and TdT staining patterns is advised
Single Ig light-chain expression: Igκ/Igλ ratio (double or triple IF staining in B-cell populations or specific B-cell subsets)	10^{-1} to 10^{-3}	All Ig light-chain–positive B-cell malignancies	Weak SmIg light-chain expression on leukemic cells (e.g., in B-CLL) may hamper their detectability Occurrence of normal SmIg light-chain–positive B cells will influence the detection limit
Vβ, Vγ, and Vδ expression: excess of TCR-V gene expression (double or triple IF staining in T-cell population or specific T-cell subsets)	10^{-1} to 10^{-3}	All TCR-positive T-cell malignancies	Occurrence of normal T cells will influence the detection limit Oligoclonal T-cell subsets might occur in the elderly
PCR techniques			
Junctional regions of rearranged Ig and TCR genes (DNA level)	10^{-3} to 10^{-6}	>90% of precursor–B-ALL >95% of T-ALL >95% of chronic lymphoid leukemias 60%–80% of B-NHL >95% of T-NHL 10%–15% of AML	Rearrangements have to be detected and identified precisely by use of well-designed PCR primers The occurrence of somatic hypermutation of Ig genes in B-NHL might prevent proper primer annealing and thereby inhibit detection and identification of Ig gene rearrangements at diagnosis and during follow-up Junctional regions have to be sequenced to design junctional region–specific probes for each individual patient Oligoclonality and clonal evolution at Ig or TCR gene level may cause false-negative results Occurrence of normal cells with rearrangements of the same gene segments as the malignant cells influences sensitivity
Chromosome aberrations with well-defined breakpoints at the DNA level	10^{-4} to 10^{-6}	20%–25% of T-ALL 25%–40% of B-NHL	Availability of well-designed PCR primers Fusion region oligonucleotide probes are useful for identification of PCR products from different patients
Chromosome aberrations resulting in leukemia-specific fusion genes and fuson mRNA (PCR analysis after reverse transcription into cDNA: RT-PCR analysis)	10^{-4} to 10^{-6}	30%–35% of childhood precursor–B-ALL 35%–40% of adult precursor–B-ALL 15%–20% of T-ALL 20%–25% of childhood NHL <5% of adult NHL 25%–40% of AML >95% of CML	Availability of well-designed RT-PCR primers Cross-contamination of RT-PCR products is the main pitfall (even cross-contamination between samples from different patients appears to occur) Detection limit is dependent on the abundance of fusion gene transcription and the efficiency of the reverse transcription step

AML, acute myeloid leukemia; B-ALL, B-cell acute lymphoblastic leckemia; BM, bone marrow; IF, immunofluorescence; Ig, immunoglobulin; SmIg, surface membrane Ig; TCR, T-cell receptor; TdT, terminal deoxynucleotidyl transferase; T-NHL, T-cell non-Hodgkin's lymphoma.

sion on precursor–B-ALL cells or molecular clonality analysis can support the discrimination between normal and malignant precursor B cells. On one hand, moderately increased frequencies of CD19+CD10+TdT+ BM cells should never be directly interpreted as relapse of ALL, particularly during the high-dose treatment phases. On the other hand, a substantial increase in B-cell precursors after chemotherapy, particularly with a homogeneous immunophenotype, may herald a relapse of the disease. Vervoordeldonk et al[42] analyzed CD10+CD19+ and CD20-CD22+ fractions of CD34+ cells in remission BM and found that increased percentages of these immature B-cell precursors within the first year of treatment indicated a likelihood of relapse. However, it would be diffi-

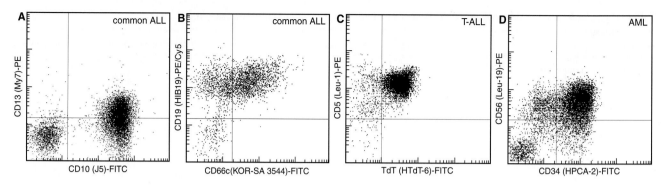

FIGURE 12–2. Examples of uncommon, aberrant, and ectopic antigen expression in acute leukemias. *A,* Weak CD13 expression on CD10⁺ precursor–B-cell acute lymphoblastic leukemia (B-ALL) cells. *B,* Cross-lineage expression of CD66c (KOR-SA3544) antigen on CD19⁺ precursor-B-ALL cells. *C,* Combined expression of the CD5 antigen and terminal deoxynucleotidyl transferase constitutes a typical characteristic of T-ALL and is normally found only in cortical thymocytes, not in extrathymic locations such as bone marrow or peripheral blood. *D,* Asynchronous expression of CD34 and CD56 in a patient with acute myeloid leukemia.

cult to have clinically relevant cutoff values for the frequencies of these subsets of CD34⁺ B-cell precursors.

Alternatively, in many ALL patients, the malignant cells can be distinguished from normal early B-lineage cells by their atypical immunologic characteristics. Aberrant antigen expression in precursor–B-ALL might be used for MRD detection in multiparameter flow cytometry (Table 12-2 and Fig. 12-2). Such aberrant expression includes cross-lineage expression of T-lineage antigens (e.g., CD5, CD7) or myeloid antigens (CD13, CD15, CD33, CD66c), maturational asynchronous expression of antigens (e.g., CD20 on CD45⁻ cells), lack of expression of CD45 (particularly the isoform CD45RA), and antigen overexpression (e.g., CD10 overexpression).[29, 30, 35, 43-48] The finding of NG2 expression on the surface membrane of precursor–B-ALL cells carrying the t(4;11) or t(11;19) translocation represents an example of true ectopic antigen expression.[49, 50] Application of such aberrant antigen expression in multiparameter flow cytometry is an attractive method that can distinguish malignant from normal B-cell precursors.[38, 48, 51-54] Flow cytometric investigation based on double/triple antigen staining has shown the presence of leukemia-associated phenotypes in 50% to 95% of patients with precursor-B-ALL.[48, 54-56] Recently, investigation of normal BM B-lineage precursors has en-

abled establishment of multiparameter templates for normal B-cell development, whereas malignant precursor B lymphoblasts frequently display aberrant immunophenotypic features and thereby fall into so-called empty spaces outside the normal B-lineage pathways[52, 53, 57] (Fig. 12-4). Preliminary data indicate that such an approach, preferably with quadruple antigen staining, reveals leukemia-associated phenotypes in virtually all patients.[53] Together, this frequency may further increase when specific antibodies become available to the fusion proteins or ectopic antigens that are observed in precursor-B-ALL with translocations such as t(1;19) or t(12;21).[58] Moreover, in cases of hyperdiploid precursor–B-ALL, which represents about one third of patients, simultaneous immunophenotyping and flow cytometric DNA content analysis could detect residual aneuploid cells with a sensitivity of at least 10⁻³.[59]

One important pitfall of immunophenotypic MRD detection in precursor–B-ALL is the occurrence of immunophenotypic shifts during the course of the disease. Differences in immunologic marker expression are found in up to two thirds of patients with precursor-B-ALL.[60] Although the differences usually concern single markers, they lead to an intralineage shift in 10% to 15% of cases.[60, 61] However, at least one leukemia-specific marker combi-

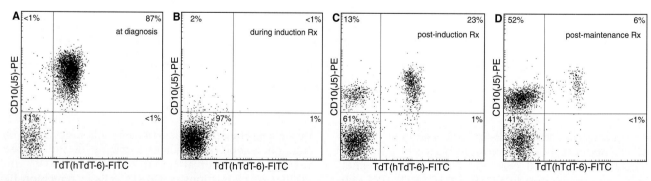

FIGURE 12–3. Representative examples of CD10/terminal deoxynucleotidyl transferase double staining on bone marrow mononuclear cells of a patient with precursor–B-cell acute lymphoblastic leukemia. *A,* Primary diagnosis. *B,* During remission induction treatment. *C,* During regeneration after a 2-week therapy stop following induction treatment. *D,* During regeneration after cessation of treatment. Cell populations were analyzed within a life gate on lymphocytes, as defined by the light scatter characteristics. (See ref. 40 for details.)

TABLE 12–2. Leukemia-Associated Immunophenotypes in Acute Leukemia

Leukemia-Associated Phenotype	Precursor –B-ALL	T-ALL	AML
Cross-lineage antigen expression (%)	~70	~50	~70
Asynchronous antigen expression (%)	~10	~25	~40
Overexpression or absence of antigen (%)	~60	0	~15
Ectopic phenotype (%)	~5	~90	~10
Total	80–90	90–100	70–80

AML, acute myeloid leukemia; ALL, acute lymphoblastic leukemia.

nation is retained by leukemic cells at relapse in over 80% of patients,[35] which implies that at least two marker combinations per patient should be used for immunophenotypic MRD monitoring.

T-CELL ACUTE LYMPHOBLASTIC LEUKEMIA AND LYMPHOBLASTIC T-CELL NON-HODGKIN'S LYMPHOMA

Nearly all T-ALL cells express TdT as well as the pan–T-cell antigens CD2, cytoplasmic CD3 (CyCD3), CD5, and CD7. Additional T-cell antigens such as CD1, CD3, CD4, and/or CD8 are also often expressed. In healthy individuals, the combination of T-cell marker and TdT expression is found in the cortical thymus, but this immunophenotype is absent or rare in extrathymic locations such as BM or PB (<0.3% and <0.02%, respectively). Moreover, if T-cell marker+TdT+ cells are found in BM or PB, they express only CD2 and/or CD7 and no other T-cell antigens such as CD3, CD4, or CD8. Dilution experiments have

demonstrated that the microscopic T-cell antigen/TdT double IF staining technique (Figs. 12–5 and 12–6) has a detection limit of 10^{-4} to 10^{-5} and that detection of such ectopic double-positive cells by this technique can be used for evaluating the effectiveness of the applied cytotoxic treatment.[1, 29] Furthermore, T-cell marker/TdT combinations are stable throughout the disease course and are retained at relapse in the vast majority of T-ALL cases.[60] After the introduction of flow cytometric detection of TdT, it is now also possible to perform routine flow cytometric T-cell marker/TdT staining, which allows MRD detection in 90% of cases of T-ALL[3, 62] (see Table 12–2 and Fig. 12–7).

Lymphoblastic T-NHL cells are fully comparable to T-ALL cells in that they express TdT in combination with one or more T-cell antigens. Therefore, T-cell antigen/TdT staining can also be used for MRD detection in lymphoblastic T-NHL.

Flow cytometric analysis based on cross-lineage myeloid antigen expression, asynchronous antigen expression (e.g., CD34+ CD3+), and antigen overexpression (e.g., CD7++) can also be used for MRD detection in T-ALL.[3, 62] Similar to precursor–B-ALL, multiparameter flow cytometry in T-ALL reveals "empty spaces" outside the templates for the normal T-cell compartment in BM and PB.[62] Together, the various leukemia-associated immunophenotypes can be used for MRD detection in all cases of T-ALL and lymphoblastic T-NHL.[3, 62] The presence of tumor-specific antigens resulting from chromosome aberrations may further increase the number of immunophenotypic MRD targets per T-ALL patient. One important candidate is the TAL1 protein that is ectopically expressed in T-ALL with the *SIL-TAL* fusion gene.[63-65]

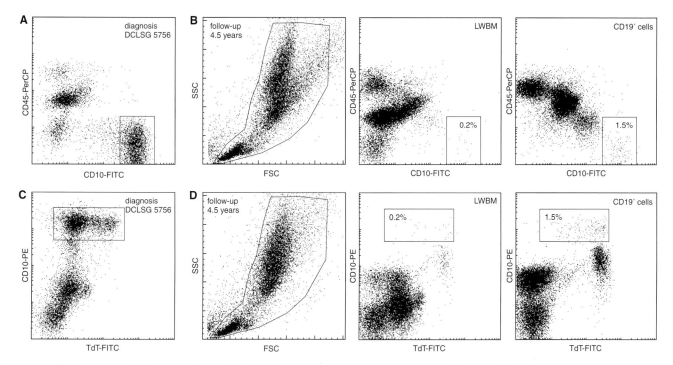

FIGURE 12–4. Flow cytometric detection of minimal residual disease in a precursor–B-ALL patient 5756 by use of the CD45/CD10/CD19 (*A* and *B*) and TdT/CD10/CD19 (*C* and *D*) triple labelings. The leukemia-specific immunophenotypic detection was based on CD10 overexpression and CD45 negativity. In the follow-up BM sample, taken 4.5 years from the diagnosis of ALL, the population of cells with leukemia-specific immunophenotype comprised 0.2% of BM cells: i.e., 1.5% of CD19+ cells. At that time the patient was in complete clinical remission of the leukemia. However, he underwent the overt hematological relapse of precursor–B-ALL nine months after this positive MRD test. (Courtesy of E.G. van Lochem et al.)

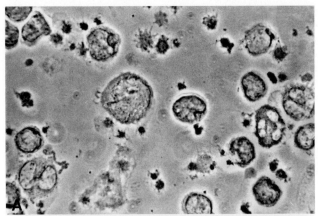
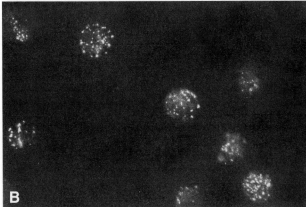
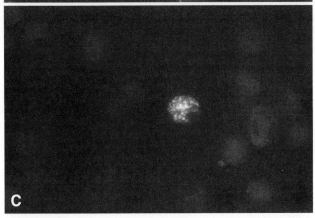

FIGURE 12–5. Double labeling for a T-cell antigen and terminal deoxynucleotidyl transferase (TdT) on bone marrow mononuclear cells of a patient with T-cell acute lymphoblastic leukemia (T-ALL) 20 weeks after diagnosis. *A,* Phase-contrast morphology. *B,* T-cell antigen–positive cells. *C,* TdT-positive cell. One cell expresses both the T-cell antigen and TdT and most probably is a T-ALL cell, whereas the other T-cell antigen–positive cells probably represent normal peripheral blood T lymphocytes.

CHRONIC LYMPHOCYTIC LEUKEMIA AND NON-HODGKIN'S LYMPHOMA

The relatively high frequency of mature lymphoid cells in BM and PB hampers immunophenotypic MRD detection in patients with CLL of B or T lineage. In an analogous manner, immunophenotypic MRD detection in B-NHL or T-NHL can also be hampered by the presence of mature lymphoid cells in lymph nodes and in potentially involved

BM or PB compartments. Because of the normal background of lymphoid cells, low levels of MRD ($<10^{-3}$) will be detectable only if tumor-related aberrant phenotypes can be used.

Chronic B-Cell Leukemias and B-Cell Non-Hodgkin's Lymphoma

Single Ig light-chain (Igκ or Igλ) expression can be used for detection of Ig$^+$ B-cell leukemias and Ig$^+$ B-NHL because normal and malignant B lymphocytes express only one type of Ig light chain.[31, 33] The distribution of Igκ$^+$ versus Igλ$^+$ cells (Igκ/Igλ ratio) can be accurately determined by analysis of Igκ and Igλ expression within the B-cell population by double or triple staining with CD19, CD20, CD22, or CD37 as pan–B-cell antigens. In normal B-cell populations, the Igκ/Igλ ratio is approximately 1.4 (range, 0.8 to 2.5). The size of the normal B-cell population in BM, PB, and lymph nodes obviously influences the detectability of malignant B cells by analysis of the Igκ/Igλ ratio. Because of this normal background, the detection limit of routinely performed Ig light-chain/B-cell marker double or triple staining in BM and PB is 10^{-1} to 10^{-2} (see Table 12–1 and Fig. 12–8).[31, 33]

The use of additional antigens in triple or quadruple staining allows detection of MRD at levels of around 10^{-3} (see Table 12–1). Such additional markers may involve antigens that are normally expressed only on a subpopulation of B cells. Examples include the CD103 antigen in hairy-cell leukemia and the CD5 antigen in B-CLL and mantle-cell lymphoma (MCL).[66-71] The sensitivity of detection might be further increased by using differences in expression levels between normal and malignant B cells, for instance, bright CD19 expression or increased CD5 expression in B-CLL patients.[72] Furthermore, protein products from particular chromosome aberrations may also be used as additional markers in triple or quadruple staining. For example, BCL2/B-cell antigen/Ig light chain triple IF staining may be used for MRD detection in patients with follicular center lymphomas because BCL2 overexpression is observed in this type of B-NHL with t(14;18) and in a subset of B-CLL.[73] Malignant cells overexpressing BCL2 can be also detected with a sensitivity of at least 1% by immunostaining of BM trephine biopsy samples combined with computed image analysis.[74] Similarly, the overexpression of cyclin D1 (BCL1) in MCL with t(11;14) or the overexpression of MYC in Burkitt's lymphomas with t(2;8), t(8;14), or t(8;22) may be used for MRD detection in these types of B-NHL.[75]

Chronic T-Cell Leukemias and T-Cell Non-Hodgkin's Lymphoma

The relatively high frequency of T lymphocytes and natural killer (NK) cells in normal BM and PB samples and T lymphocytes in lymph nodes hampers the immunophenotypic detectability of leukemic T cells and T-NHL cells. Even expression of the less common CD3$^+$CD4$^-$CD8$^-$, CD3$^+$CD4$^+$CD8$^+$, or TCRγδ$^+$ phenotypes, as well as antigen loss (absence of particular T-cell antigens), will generally result in a limited sensitivity of only 10^{-1} to 10^{-2}.

The vast majority of chronic T-cell leukemias and

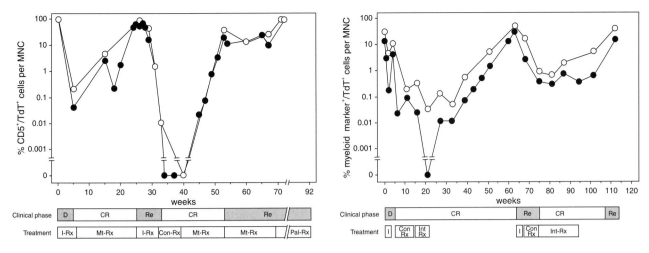

FIGURE 12–6. Detection of minimal residual disease during follow-up of patient CJ (8-year-old girl) with T-cell acute lymphoblastic leukemia (T-ALL) by the use of CD5/terminal deoxynucleotidyl transferase (TdT) double labeling (*left*) and TdT$^+$ patient PZ (3-year-old boy) with acute myeloid leukemia (AML) by the use of myeloid marker/TdT double labeling (*right*). ●-●, blood samples; ○-○, bone marrow samples; Con-Rx, consolidation treatment; CR, complete remission; D, diagnostic phase; Int-Rx, intensification treatment; I-Rx or I, induction treatment; MNC, mononuclear cells; Mt-Rx, maintenance treatment; Pal-Rx, palliative treatment; Re, relapse. The doubling time of the leukemic cells during imminent relapse was 6.5 days in the T-ALL patient and 17 days in the TdT$^+$ AML patient.

T-NHL belong to the TCRαβ differentiation lineage, whereas only a minor fraction (<5%) express TCRγδ. During the last decade, a large series of antibodies against the protein products of V gene segments of most *TCRBV* gene families have been produced. Together these Vβ antibodies recognize 65% to 70% of normal and malignant T cells with TCRβ chain expression.[34, 76] Also, antibodies against most Vγ and Vδ domains of TCRγδ molecules have become available. These Vγ and Vδ antibodies might be useful for detection and monitoring of malignant (clonal) TCRγδ$^+$ T cells,[36] although the presence of normal TCRγδ$^+$ T lymphocytes might interfere with this application. In this context, one should be aware that most normal TCRγδ$^+$ T lymphocytes have the Vγ9/Vδ2$^+$ phenotype, which is rare (or absent) in malignant T cells.[77, 78] Application of the Vβ, Vγ, and Vδ antibodies in well-chosen triple and quadruple staining can result in sensitivity levels of approximately 10^{-2} (Table 12–1). For example, CD3 can be used for life gating together with CD4 (or CD8), leukemia-specific Vβ antibody, and addi-

tional leukemia-specific antigen (e.g., CD7 in T-cell prolymphocytic leukemia, CD25 in adult T-cell leukemia, CD16 in T-cell large granular lymphocytic [LGL] leukemia, etc.). Sensitivities around 10^{-2} do not allow true MRD detection but may enable monitoring of T-cell leukemia patients during treatment (Fig. 12–9) or predicting the possible outgrowth of a dominant subclone in case of oligoclonal T-cell proliferation.

Detection of lower MRD levels ($\sim10^{-3}$) in chronic T-cell leukemia or T-NHL is possible only by analysis of tumor-associated antigens or translocation-specific fusion gene proteins. For example, antibodies against ALK epitopes of the *NPM-ALK* (anaplastic lymphoma kinase/nucleolar protein nucleophosmin) fusion gene protein might be used in large-cell anaplastic lymphomas with t(2;5).[79]

ACUTE MYELOID LEUKEMIA

Leukemia-associated immunophenotypes can be identified in 70% to 80% of AML patients.[3, 80, 81] Cross-lineage

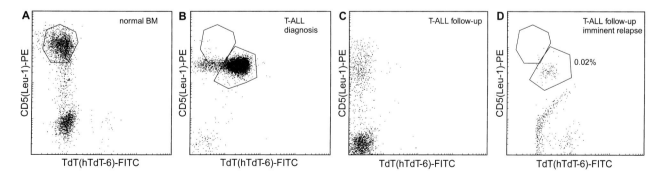

FIGURE 12–7. Flow cytometric detection of minimal residual disease in a patient with T-cell acute lymphoblastic leukemia (T-ALL) by the use of terminal deoxynucleotidyl transferase (TdT)/CD5/CD7 triple labeling. *A,* Normal bone marrow (BM). *B,* T-ALL at primary diagnosis. *C,* Follow-up BM sample. *D,* The same follow-up BM sample measured after live gating on TdT$^+$ cells. A TdT$^+$, weak CD5$^+$ T-cell subpopulation was clearly detectable and accounted for approximately 0.02% of BM cells (with courtesy to E.G. van Lochem et al).

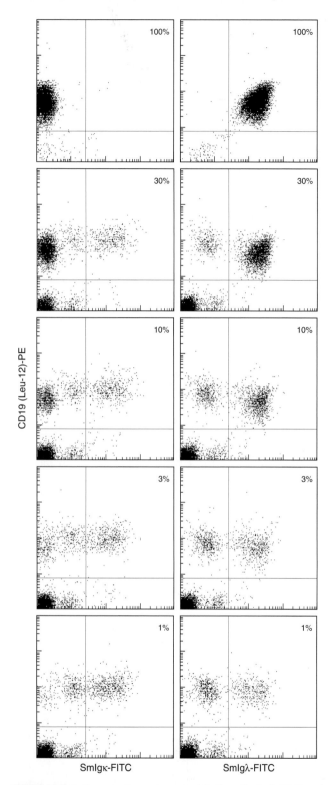

FIGURE 12–8. Surface membrane immunoglobulin κ (SmIgκ) CD19 and SmIgλ/CD19 double labeling on serial dilutions of SmIgλ⁺ B-cell non-Hodgkin's lymphoma (B-NHL) cells into peripheral blood mononuclear cells of a healthy individual. The percentages of B-NHL cells that are present in each dilution step are indicated. The detection limit of the SmIg/CD19 double labeling is clearly influenced by the frequency of normal polyclonal B lymphocytes.

antigen expression, especially TdT expression and expression of the T-cell antigens CD2, CD4, and CD7 and the B-cell antigen CD19,[82-87] is found in 40% to 70% of cases of AML. Also, maturational asynchronous antigen expression can be frequently found in AML, for example, coexpression of CD15 and CD34, CD56 and CD34, and CD15 and CD117, combinations that are not seen in normal bone marrow.[44, 45, 86, 88-91] Antigen overexpression can involve CD13, CD14, CD15, and CD33.[80, 81] Comparable to ALL with 11q23 translocations, ectopic NG2 expression is also found in a proportion of AML cases with 11q23 abnormalities and most probably represents an excellent leukemia marker.[50] In contrast to most cases of ALL, immunophenotypic subpopulations can be identified in the majority of AML patients.[90, 92, 93] This presence of subpopulations also applies to cross-lineage and asynchronous antigen expression. For instance, in 60% of cases of AML, coexpression of a pan-myeloid marker (CD13 and/or CD33) and TdT is found in 1% to 50% of mononuclear cells.[82]

Multiparameter flow cytometric detection of unusual or aberrant immunophenotypes can in principle be used for MRD detection in 70% to 80% of patients with AML[3, 80, 81] (see Table 12–2). The sensitivity of such multiparameter analysis is dependent on the normal flow cytometric background and is estimated to be 10^{-3} to 10^{-4}, depending on the type of triple labeling. In this context, it should also be noted that immunophenotypic MRD studies in AML are hampered by the fact that generally only one subpopulation of AML blast cells is monitored.[93, 94] However, in most cases of AML, multiple aberrant marker combinations can be used for MRD monitoring, and no major changes in aberrant immunophenotypes are found in AML at relapse.[95]

An alternative immunophenotypic approach relies on the ratio between CD34⁺ myeloid and CD34⁺ lymphoid precursors in BM, which reflects the balance in the precursor compartment of the hematopoietic system. Persistence of abnormally high ratios in AML patients at the end of chemotherapy was significantly correlated with an increased risk of relapse.[96]

CHRONIC MYELOID LEUKEMIA

Immunophenotyping will not contribute to MRD detection in CML patients. However, transformation of CML into a blast crisis might be detectable by the use of immunologic marker analysis, especially in patients with a lymphoid blast crisis. The large majority of lymphoid blast crises express a CD10⁺ TdT⁺ precursor–B-cell phenotype. Therefore, CD10/TdT double IF staining can be used for early detection of lymphoid blast crisis in CML patients.[37]

MRD Detection by the Use of PCR Techniques

Specific amplification of a particular DNA segment or mRNA by the use of PCR technology allows the detection of low frequencies of malignant cells if the target DNA or mRNA sequences are tumor specific. Two types of PCR targets can be used for MRD detection in leukemia

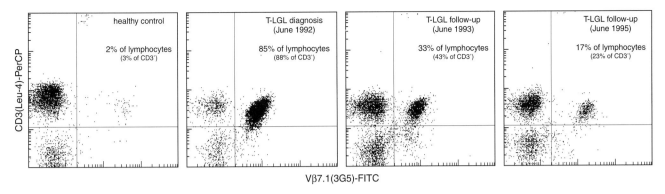

FIGURE 12–9. Monitoring of a T-cell large granular lymphocytic (T-LGL) leukemia patient by use of a Vβ antibody. In a healthy individual, only a minor subpopulation of CD3⁺ T cells express Vβ7.1, whereas in a T-LGL leukemia patient at diagnosis, virtually all CD3⁺ T lymphocytes expressed Vβ7.1. This single Vβ gene expression was in line with the clonally rearranged *TCRB* genes. Vβ7.1/CD3 double labeling during follow-up allowed rapid and precise monitoring of the Vβ7.1⁺ T-LGL cells, which decreased to 43% and 23% of CD3⁺ T lymphocytes during follow-up.

patients: junctional regions of rearranged Ig and TCR genes and breakpoint fusion regions of chromosome aberrations (see later).[1, 3, 97–100] Because of the high sensitivity of PCR techniques, all possible precautionary measures should be taken to prevent cross-contamination of PCR products between patient samples in PCR-mediated MRD studies.[101]

MRD Detection by PCR Analysis of Rearranged Ig and TCR Genes

JUNCTIONAL REGIONS AS PCR TARGETS FOR MRD DETECTION

As explained in Chapter 6, the junctional regions of rearranged Ig and TCR genes are unique *"fingerprint-like"* sequences that are assumed to be different in each lymphoid cell and thus also in each lymphoid malignancy.[1, 18] Therefore, junctional regions can serve as tumor-specific targets for MRD-PCR analysis with the use of primers at opposite sides.[102–107] For this purpose, the various Ig and/or TCR gene rearrangements have to be identified in each leukemia at initial diagnosis by using the various PCR primer sets. It should be determined whether the PCR products obtained are derived from the malignant cells and not from contaminating normal cells with similar Ig or TCR gene rearrangements. For this purpose, the PCR products are analyzed for their clonal origin, such as by heteroduplex analysis or by gene scanning. Subsequently, the precise nucleotide sequence of the junctional regions should be determined. This sequence information allows the design of junctional region–specific oligonucleotides. These oligonucleotides can be used to detect malignant cells among normal lymphoid cells during follow-up of patients in two different ways. One possibility is use of the oligonucleotides as patient-specific junctional region probes in hybridization experiments to detect PCR products derived from the malignant cells (Figs. 12-10 and 12-11). The other possibility is to use the junctional region–specific oligonucleotide as a primer in the second step of a nested PCR to specifically amplify the rearrangements of the malignant clone.

SENSITIVITY OF PCR ANALYSIS OF JUNCTIONAL REGIONS

Theoretically, the detection limit of the PCR technique is approximately 10^{-6} if a DNA segment is used as the PCR target. This figure is based on the assumption that 1 million cells, equivalent to about 6.25 μg of DNA, can be tested in one reaction tube, although generally only 0.5 to 1.0 μg of DNA is used per tube (i.e., 1.5 to 3.0 μg in the case of triplicate testing). This detection limit can indeed be reached, but it generally varies between 10^{-4} and 10^{-6} (Figs. 12-10 and 12-11).[1, 3, 97, 108] The sensitivity of MRD-PCR analysis of junctional regions is dependent on the type of rearrangement and on the "background" of normal lymphoid cells with comparable Ig or TCR gene rearrangements. Junctional regions of complete V-D-J rearrangements are extensive, whereas junctional regions of V-J rearrangements are three to four times smaller. Normal cells can contain the same rearranged gene segments as the leukemic cells. For instance, Vδ1-Jδ1 rearrangements frequently occur in T-ALL, but also in a small fraction (0.1% to 2%) of normal blood T cells; Vγ1-Jγ1.3 and Vγ1-Jγ2.3 rearrangements occur in many precursor–B- and T-cell malignancies, but they are also found in a large fraction (70% to 90%) of normal blood T cells. Therefore, it can be expected that MRD-PCR analysis of long Vδ1-Jδ1 junctional regions in PB samples is more sensitive (10^{-5} to 10^{-6}) than MRD-PCR analysis of short Vγ-Jγ junctional regions (10^{-3} to 10^{-4}),[1, 109] although in practice straightforward prediction of sensitivity does not appear to be possible.

MRD-PCR ANALYSIS OF JUNCTIONAL REGIONS IN ACUTE LYMPHOBLASTIC LEUKEMIA

Junctional regions of *IGH*, *IGK* (especially Kde), *TCRG*, and *TCRD* gene rearrangements are convenient MRD-PCR targets because they require only a limited number of PCR primer sets[110] (Fig. 12-12). Furthermore, the vast majority (>90%) of precursor–B-ALL patients contain *IGH*, *IGK*, *TCRG*, and/or *TCRD* gene rearrangements with identifiable junctional regions[111, 112] (Table 12-3).

Ig and TCR gene rearrangements in precursor–B-ALL and T-ALL might be prone to subclone formation as a result of continuing rearrangements or secondary re-

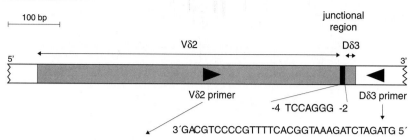

100 bp

junctional region

Vδ2

Dδ3

5′   3′

Vδ2 primer

Dδ3 primer

-4 TCCAGGG -2

3′GACGTCCCCGTTTTCACGGTAAAGATCTAGATG 5′

5′CGCGTCGACCAAACAGTGCCTGTGTCAATAGG 3′

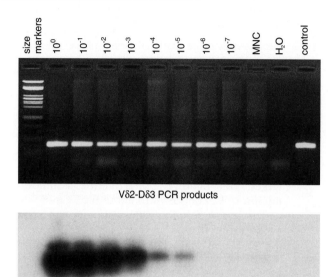

V δ2-Dδ3 PCR products

hybridization with junctional region probe (CTGTGA<u>TCCAGGG</u>TGGGGGA)

FIGURE 12–10. Precursor–B-ALL with a Vδ2-Dδ3 rearrangement as the polymerase chain reaction (PCR) target for detection of minimal residual disease. The specificity of the junctional region is based on the deletion of six nucleotides and the random insertion of seven nucleotides. This sequence information was used for the design of a patient-specific junctional region probe. DNA from the ALL cells was diluted into DNA from normal blood mononuclear cells (MNCs) and subjected to PCR analysis with Vδ2 and Dδ3 primers. PCR products were separated by size in an agarose gel, blotted onto a nylon membrane, and hybridized with the junctional region probe. In all dilution steps and in the MNCs, Vδ2-Dδ3 PCR products were found, but only the first five dilution steps appeared to contain leukemia-derived PCR products; that is, a sensitivity of 10^{-5} was reached.

arrangements caused by the active recombinase enzyme system in these immature lymphoid malignancies.[115-123] In particular, *IGH* gene rearrangements are known to change in the period between diagnosis and relapse. In fact, at diagnosis, multiple *IGH* gene rearrangements are already found in 30% to 40% of cases of precursor–B-ALL,

thus indicating the presence of biclonality or oligoclonality.[124] The problem of oligoclonality at diagnosis is the uncertainty of which clone is going to emerge at relapse and should thus be monitored by MRD-PCR analysis (see Table 12-1). Frequently, continuing or secondary *IGH* gene rearrangements represent VH to DH-JH re-

FIGURE 12–11. A VκII-Kde rearrangement of a precursor–B-cell acute lymphoblastic leukemia as a sensitive minimal residual disease–polymerase chain reaction (MRD-PCR) target. The patient-specific junctional region probe was designed according to the junctional region sequence with deletion of five nucleotides and insertion of only three nucleotides. Tenfold dilutions were made from DNA of the leukemic cells into DNA from mononuclear cells. PCR analysis with VκII and Kde primers was performed on the dilution samples. The PCR products were blotted in duplicate on a nylon membrane and hybridized with the junctional region probe. This specific MRD-PCR target reached a sensitivity of 10^{-6} without background signals despite the relatively short junctional region.

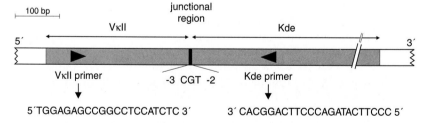

100 bp

junctional region

VκII

Kde

5′   3′

VκII primer

Kde primer

-3 CGT -2

5′TGGAGAGCCGGCCTCCATCTC 3′

3′ CACGGACTTCCCAGATACTTCCC 5′

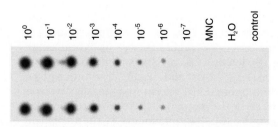

dot blot hybridization with junctional region probe (CAATTTCCC<u>CGT</u>AGCCCTAGT)

TABLE 12–3. Frequencies of Identifiable Ig and TCR Gene Rearrangements as MRD-PCR Targets in ALL

Gene	Rearrangement Type	Precursor –B-ALL (%)	T-ALL (%)
IGH	VH-JH	93	5
	DH-JH	20	23
	Total IGH	98	23
IGK	Vκ-Kde	45	0
	Intron RSS-Kde	25	0
	Total Kde	50	0
TCRG	Vγ-Jγ	55	95
TCRD	Vδ1-Jδ1 or Dδ-Jδ1	0	50
	Vδ2-Dδ3 or Dδ2-Dδ3	40	5
	Total TCRD	40	55
	At least 1 PCR target	~95	>95
	At least 2 PCR targets	~90	~90
	At least 3 PCR targets	~65	~50

ALL, acute lymphoblastic leukemia; Ig, immunoglobulin; MRD, minimal residual disease; PCR, polymerase chain reaction; TCR, T-cell receptor.

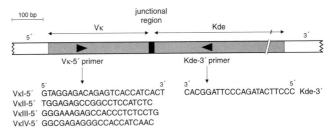

FIGURE 12–12. Schematic diagram of Vκ-Kde rearrangements and forward and reverse primers for polymerase chain reaction (PCR) analysis of diagnosis and follow-up samples. Kde gene rearrangements within the IGK gene locus are stable PCR targets for detection of minimal residual disease in precursor–B-cell acute lymphoblastic leukemia.[111]

arrangements or VH replacements, respectively.[118, 119] During these rearrangements, the DH-JH junctional region remains unaffected, which has led to the concept of designing the primers around the relatively stable DH-JH region to prevent false-negative PCR results.[118, 119]

Subclone formation at diagnosis was thought to be less frequent for the TCRD gene complex based on Southern blot information.[113] However, PCR amplification followed by heteroduplex analysis or sequencing has demonstrated that Vδ2-Dδ3 and Dδ2-Dδ3 rearrangements in precursor-B-ALL are oligoclonal at diagnosis in 30% to 40% of cases.[112, 120, 125] Vδ2-Dδ3 rearrangements are also prone to continuing rearrangements, especially to Jα gene segments with deletion of the Cδ exons.[120, 123]

Rearrangements of the TCRG genes in T-ALL tend to be more stable, and oligoclonality at diagnosis is rare.[114] In contrast, approximately 40% of cross-lineage TCRG gene rearrangements in precursor–B-ALL are oligoclonal.[112]

At present, the Kde rearrangements of IGK genes are considered to be the most stable MRD-PCR targets, probably because Kde rearrangements are end-stage rearrangements and do not allow continuing or secondary rearrangements.[126]

False-negative results caused by clonal evolution are a major drawback of using Ig/TCR gene rearrangements as PCR targets for MRD detection. Changes in IGH gene rearrangement patterns at relapse occur at high frequency in precursor-B-ALL, especially when subclone formation is already present at diagnosis.[115, 117] Changes in TCRG and TCRD gene rearrangements at relapse are found in both precursor-B-ALL and T-ALL, but they generally involve only one allele.[115, 121, 122] The risk of changes in rearrangement patterns increases with time (i.e., with remission duration).[115, 117] However, in relapse patients, further clonal evolution is not usually observed at second or third relapse.[123] Despite the high frequency of immunogenotypic changes in ALL at relapse, at least one rearranged IGH, TCRG, and/or TCRD allele remains stable in 75% to 90% of cases of precursor–B-ALL and in 90% of patients with T-ALL.[115, 117, 121, 122] More importantly, in most ALL patients at least two suitable PCR targets are available (Table 12-3). Therefore, it can be anticipated that MRD-PCR studies with at least two targets per patient will result in a major reduction of false negativity.

PCR ANALYSIS OF IG GENES IN MATURE B-CELL MALIGNANCIES

The Ig gene rearrangements in most mature B-cell malignancies provide several PCR targets for MRD studies (Table 12-4). Indeed, in most chronic B-cell leukemias, the Ig gene rearrangements can easily be detected and

TABLE 12–4. Frequencies of Identifiable Ig and TCR Gene Rearrangements and Deletions as Potential MRD-PCR Targets in Mature Lymphoid Malignancies

	IGH	IGK		IGL	TCRB	TCRG	TCRD	
	R*	R	D	R	R	R	R	D
B-lineage chronic lymphoid malignancies								
SmIgκ+ (%)	100	100	0	0	5	<5	<5	0
SmIgλ+ (%)	100	25	75	>98	<5	<5		0
T-lineage chronic lymphoid malignancies (%)	<5	0		0	>98	>98	10–25	75–90
NK-LGL leukemia† (%)	0	0		0	0	0	0	0

* R, at least one rearranged allele; D, both alleles deleted.

† Most LGL leukemias express TCRαβ (70% to 80%), some express TCRγδ (10% to 15%), and some belong to the NK lineage (10% to 15%).

LGL, large granular lymphocytic; MRD, minimal residual disease; NK, natural killer; PCR, polymerase chain reaction; SmIg, surface membrane immunoglobulin; TCR, T-cell receptor.

used as MRD-PCR targets because the majority of them do not contain somatic mutations.[127-129] However in many cases of B-NHL, especially follicular and postfollicular B-NHL, somatic mutations in the Ig genes may lead to false-negative results because of the inability of proper PCR primer annealing.[130, 131] This problem can only partly be overcome by the use of multiple V and J consensus primer sets in the hope that at least one primer set will not be hampered by the somatic mutations. Such an approach is successful in 70% to 90% of cases.[132]

The somatic mutation process tends to focus on the V-D-J exon of the rearranged *IGH, IGK,* and *IGL* genes from the leader sequences onward, whereas further downstream sequences are progressively less affected. Therefore, the leader sequences upstream of the V-D-J exon and the constant (C) gene segments at the downstream side are probably not affected by somatic mutations. Therefore, it would be worthwhile to use V leader primers and C primers for RT-PCR analysis of Ig gene transcripts. At the DNA level, this approach will not work easily because of the large intervening distance between the V leader primer and the C primer: 8 to 10 kilobases (kb) for rearranged *IGH* genes, 3.5 to 5 kb for rearranged *IGK* genes, and 2 to 2.5 kb for rearranged *IGL* genes. Sequencing of the V-D-J exons in the RT-PCR products obtained should allow the design of patient-specific V

and J primers and junctional region probes for MRD-PCR studies at the DNA level. Nevertheless, it should be noted that false-negative results could still be obtained in follicular B-NHL, which may have active somatic mutation machinery leading to subclones that are not recognized anymore by the patient-specific primers and/or probes.[133]

PCR ANALYSIS OF TCR GENES IN MATURE T-CELL MALIGNANCIES

TCRG gene rearrangements are found in virtually all mature T-lineage malignancies (Table 12–4), except for NK-LGL leukemias.[134] In fact, all Ig and TCR genes are in germline configuration in NK-LGL leukemias.[134, 135] Southern blot analysis has also shown that all malignancies belonging to the TCRαβ lineage have *TCRB* gene rearrangements and most of them have biallelic *TCRD* gene deletions. Thus, MRD studies in mature T-cell malignancies can generally use junctional regions of rearranged *TCRG* genes as PCR targets. Alternatively, *TCRB* genes can be used as MRD-PCR targets, but the number of Vβ and Jβ primer combinations is rather high for efficient detection of all Vβ-Jβ gene rearrangements. Therefore, it might be necessary to determine the precise *TCRB* gene rearrangement by RT-PCR analysis of *TCRB* gene transcripts with the use of multiple Vβ family primers in

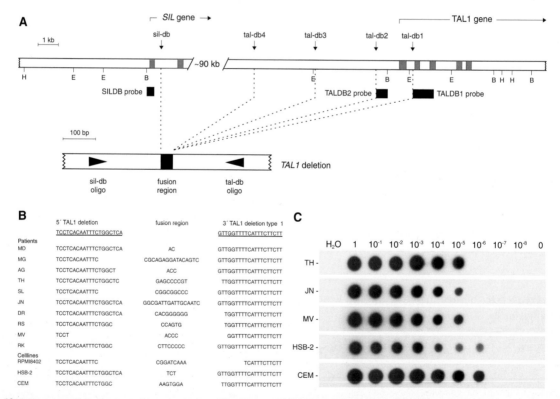

FIGURE 12–13. Polymerase chain reaction (PCR) analysis of *TAL1* deletions for detection of minimal residual disease. *A,* Schematic diagram of four types of *TAL1* deletions. The *arrows* indicate the four breakpoints in the upstream region of the *TAL1* gene (*TAL1*-db) and the single breakpoint in the *SIL* gene (*SIL*-db). The relevant probes (*solid bars*) and relevant restriction sites for Southern blot analysis are indicated: *Hin*dIII (H), *Eco*RI (E), and *Bam*HI (B). *B,* Fusion region sequences of 10 patients with T-cell acute lymphoblastic leukemia (T-ALL) and three T-cell lines with type 1 *TAL1* deletions are aligned with the germline sequences (*underlined*) at the *SIL* side (5′ *TAL1* deletion) and the *TAL1* side (3′ *TAL1* type 1 deletion). The fusion region sequences are different in each case because of the deletion and insertion of nucleotides. *C,* Dot-blot PCR analysis of serial dilutions of T-ALL DNA or T-cell line DNA into DNA from the peripheral blood mononuclear cells of a healthy individual. The blotted PCR products were hybridized with a general *TAL1* deletion probe (patient TH) or with a fusion region–specific probe in the case of patients JN and MV and the cell lines HSB-2 and CEM. In all cases, hybridization signals were detected down to 10^{-5} or 10^{-6} dilution mixtures.

combination with a single Cβ primer. As soon as the involved Vβ and Jβ gene segments as well as the junctional region are identified by sequencing, suitable primers and patient-specific junctional region probes can be used for MRD-PCR studies at the DNA level.

In contrast to mature B-cell malignancies, TCR genes are not affected by somatic mutations. For this reason, it should be relatively easy to monitor mature T-cell malignancies during and after treatment.

MRD Detection by PCR Analysis of Chromosome Aberrations

CHROMOSOME ABERRATIONS AS PCR TARGETS FOR MRD DETECTION

Breakpoint fusion regions of chromosome aberrations can be used as unique tumor-specific PCR targets for MRD detection if the chosen PCR primers are at opposite sides of the breakpoint fusion region. PCR-mediated amplification of breakpoint fusion sequences at the DNA level can be used only for chromosome aberrations in which the breakpoints of different patients cluster in a relatively small breakpoint area of preferably less than 2 kb inasmuch as PCR products should not exceed about 2 kb in routine MRD-PCR analysis. Such is the case in t(14;18) in FCL, where most breakpoints are clustered in a few relatively small regions of the *BCL2* gene that are juxtaposed to one of the JH gene segments of the *IGH* locus. Other examples include T-ALL–associated aberra-

tions such as t(11;14)(p13;q11), t(1;14)(p34;q11), t(10;14)(q24;q11), and *TAL1* deletions. Despite clustering of the breakpoints, the nucleotide sequences of the breakpoint fusion regions of the aforementioned chromosome aberrations differ per patient. Therefore, these breakpoint fusion regions represent unique patient-specific and sensitive PCR targets for MRD detection[64, 136] (Fig. 12-13).

In most translocations, however, breakpoints of different patients are more widespread and result in breakpoint regions larger than 2 kb, which implies that in each individual patient the exact breakpoint has to be determined for PCR primer design, a laborious and time-consuming process. However, several malignancies with chromosome aberrations have characteristic tumor-specific fusion genes that are transcribed into fusion gene mRNA molecules that are similar in individual patients despite distinct breakpoints at the DNA level. After reverse transcription into cDNA, these fusion gene mRNA molecules can therefore be used as appropriate targets for MRD-PCR analysis. Examples include *BCR-ABL* transcripts in the case of CML or precursor–B-ALL with t(9;22), *TEL-AML1* transcripts in the case of precursor–B-ALL with t(12;21), *E2A-PBX1* mRNA in most pre–B-ALL with t(1;19), *MLL-AF4* transcripts in pro–B-ALL with t(4;11), *PML-RARA* mRNA in acute promyelocytic leukemia (APL) with t(15;17), *AML1-ETO* mRNA in AML with t(8;21), and *NPM-ALK* mRNA in large-cell anaplastic lymphoma with t(2;5)[137-140] (Table 12–5).

Recently, simplified strategies were developed to deter-

TABLE 12–5. Chromosome Aberrations as Major PCR Targets for MRD Detection in Acute Leukemias*

Aberration	Target (mRNA or DNA)	Frequency of Applicability[†] (%)	
		Children	*Adults*
Precursor–B-ALL			
t(9;22)(q34;q11)	*BCR-ABL* (mRNA)	5–8	30–35
t(1;19)(q23;p13)	*E2A-PBX1* (mRNA)	5–8[‡]	3–4
t(4;11)(q21;q23)	*MLL-AF4* (mRNA)	3–5	3–4
11q23 aberrations	Aberrant *MLL* (mRNA)	5–6	<5
t(12;21)(p13;q22)	*TEL-AML1* (mRNA)	~30	1–3
Total		40–45	40–45
T-ALL			
TAL1 deletion	*SIL-TAL1* (DNA)	10–25	5–10
t(8;14)(q24;q11)	*c-MYC-TCRA/D* (DNA)	2–4	
t(11;14)(p15;q11)	*RHOM1-TCRD* (DNA)	1	
t(11;14)(p13;q11)	*RHOM2-TCRD* (DNA)	3–7	
t(1;14)(p34;q11)	*TAL1-TCRD* (DNA)	1–3	
t(10;14)(q24;q11)	*HOX11-TCRD* (DNA)	1–3	
Total		25–30	10–15
AML[§]			
t(8;21)(q22;q22)	*AML1-ETO* (mRNA)	10–14	6–8
t(15;17)(q23;q21)	*PML-RARA* (mRNA)	8–10	5–15[‖]
inv(16)(p13q22)	*CBFB-MYH11* (mRNA)	5–7	5–6
11q23 aberrations	Aberrant *MLL* (mRNA)	~1.0	~1.0
t(9;22)(q34;q11)	*BCR-ABL* (mRNA)	<1	<1
Total		25–30	20–25

* The detection limit of PCR analysis of chromosome aberrations is 10^{-3} to 10^{-5}.

† The indicated percentages represent frequencies within the precursor–B-ALL, T-ALL, and AML groups.

‡ In infant ALL, the frequency of t(4;11) can be as high as 70%.

§ The indicated percentages mainly concern adult AML patients younger than 60 years. In AML patients older than 60 years, the total frequency of detectable fusion genes is only 10% to 15%.

‖ In southern European regions, the frequency of t(15;17) with *PML-RARA* is essentially higher than in northern European regions.

ALL, acute lymphoblastic leukemia; AML, acute myelogenous leukemia; MRD, minimal residual disease; PCR, polymerase chain reaction.

mine precise DNA breakpoint sequences in ALL patients with t(4;11) and t(12;21) based on multiple long-range PCR and long-range inverse PCR, respectively, followed by cloning and sequencing.[141, 142] Further studies should confirm the sensitivity, specificity, and clinical value of MRD monitoring based on such DNA targets. An advantage of using chromosome aberrations as tumor-specific PCR targets for MRD detection is their stability during the disease course. However, MRD detection of chromosome aberrations by PCR is not always applicable because in most hematopoietic malignancies, no specific chromosome aberrations have been found yet. Depending on the type of tumor-specific PCR target, detection limits of 10^{-3} to 10^{-6} can be reached by using chromosome aberrations as MRD targets in nested PCR reactions (see Table 12-5). However, because of the high sensitivity of PCR techniques, cross-contamination of RT-PCR products between patient samples is a major pitfall in PCR-mediated MRD studies. Such cross-contamination is difficult to recognize because leukemia-specific fusion gene mRNA PCR products are not patient specific, in contrast to PCR products obtained from breakpoint fusion regions at the DNA level, such as in t(14;18) and *TAL1* deletions, which can be identified by the use of patient-specific oligonucleotide probes. Furthermore, very low levels of fusion transcripts, particularly *BCR-ABL* mRNA, have also been found in healthy individuals and may occasionally be the source of false-positive results in leukemia patients in long-term remission.[143, 144] Also, t(14;18)-positive B cells have been observed in healthy individuals and occur with increasing frequency during aging.[145, 146]

ACUTE LYMPHOBLASTIC LEUKEMIA

MRD detection is possible in several types of childhood and adult precursor–B-ALL because of the presence of particular leukemia-specific fusion gene transcripts that can be used as MRD-PCR targets. Examples are *BCR-ABL* fusion transcripts, which are especially observed in adult ALL cases with t(9;22) (Fig. 12-14); *E2A-PBX1* mRNA in most pre-B-ALL with t(1;19); *MLL-AF4* transcripts, which are found at high frequency in infant pro–B-ALL with t(4; 11); and *TEL-AML1* fusion mRNA in childhood precursor–B-ALL with t(12;21).[137, 139, 147] In this way, RT-PCR analysis of leukemia-specific fusion gene mRNA for detection of low levels of MRD ($<10^{-3}$) can be applied in 40% to 45% of cases of childhood precursor–B-ALL and 35% to 40% of adult precursor–B-ALL (Table 12-5).

In contrast, MRD-PCR analysis of chromosome aberrations is possible in only 15% to 25% of T-ALL cases and mainly concerns *TAL1* deletions and to some extent t(1; 14), t(10;14), and t(11;14) (see Table 12-5). Similar to chromosome aberrations in precursor–B-ALL, *TAL1* deletions can be detected at the mRNA level by means of *SIL-TAL1* fusion gene transcripts.[139, 148] However, the T-ALL–associated chromosome aberrations can also be analyzed at the DNA level. This latter approach has the advantage that the breakpoint fusion regions can be used for sensitive patient-specific MRD detection with the use of patient-specific oligonucleotide probes[64, 136] (see Fig. 12-13). Other potential sensitive targets for MRD monitoring in T-ALL are deletions in multiple tumor suppressor

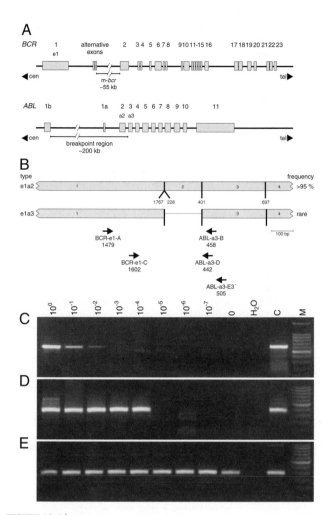

FIGURE 12–14. Reverse transcription–polymerase chain reaction (RT-PCR) analysis of *BCR-ABL* fusion gene transcripts for detection of minimal residual disease. *A,* Schematic diagram of the exon/intron structure of the *BCR* and *ABL* genes involved in t(9;22)(q34;q11) with a focus on the minor breakpoint cluster region (m-*bcr*). The centromeric (cen) and telomeric (tel) orientation, exon numbering, and relevant breakpoint regions are indicated. The old nomenclature for BCR exon 1 and ABL exons 2 and 3 is also indicated. *B,* Schematic diagrams of the *BCR-ABL* p190-type fusion gene transcripts. The *numbers* under the fusion gene transcript refer to the first (5′) nucleotide of the involved exon, except when the last (3′) nucleotide of the upstream gene is indicated. The *arrows* indicate the relative position of the primers, and the *numbers* refer to the 5′ nucleotide position of each primer. The outer primers A and B (BCR-e1-A and ABL-a3-B) are used for first-round amplification, and the internal primers C and D (BCR-e1-C and ABL-a3-D) are used for the nested RT-PCR reaction. Primer E is the so-called shifted primer used exclusively to confirm the positive results obtained with A↔B primers. The five primers were developed by the PCR laboratories participating in the BIOMED-1 Concerted Action "*Investigation of minimal residual disease in acute leukemia: International standardization and clinical evaluation.*"[139] *C,* Agarose gel electrophoresis of first-round amplification of serially diluted leukemic cells derived from a patient with precursor–B-cell acute lymphoblastic leukemia, patient, as well as undiluted cDNA from the MIK-ALL cell line as a control. In the first round, RT-PCR products can be detected down to 10^{-2} dilution mixtures. *D,* Agarose gel electrophoresis of a nested RT-PCR reaction of the same serially diluted samples and the undiluted MIK-ALL control sample. RT-PCR products can be detected down to 10^{-4} dilution mixtures in a nested RT-PCR reaction. *E,* Agarose gel electrophoresis of a control RT-PCR amplification with primers used for the constitutively expressed *ABL* gene. M, size marker.

1 *(MTS1/p16)* genes, which occur in 80% of T-ALL patients, most probably resulting from illegitimate V-D-J recombinase activity.[149, 150] Despite the clustering of the deletion breakpoints, the nucleotide sequences of each breakpoint differ per patient, similar to the junctional regions of Ig and TCR gene rearrangements.[150]

CHRONIC LYMPHOID MALIGNANCIES

In CLL, MRD detection by (RT-)PCR analysis of chromosome aberrations is virtually impossible because of a lack of frequently occurring, well-defined chromosome aberrations that can be used as PCR targets. In B-NHL, chromosomal aberrations frequently involve Ig genes. For example, in FCL with t(14;18), the *BCL2* gene is joined to J$_H$ gene segments,[151, 152] whereas in MCL with t(11;14), the *BCL1* gene is joined to *IGH* gene segments.[153, 154] Furthermore, in Burkitt's lymphoma with t(8;14), t(2;8), and t(8;22), one of the Ig loci (*IGH, IGK,* and *IGL,* respectively) is coupled to the *MYC* gene.[155] In all these B-NHL types the breakpoints generally occur far outside coding regions, thus implying that these translocations are not amenable to RT-PCR analysis for MRD detection but should be studied at the DNA level. Therefore, the detectability of these chromosome aberrations is dependent on clustering of the breakpoints of different patients in relatively small DNA regions. Southern blotting can scan essentially larger DNA regions (10 to 15 kb) than PCR analysis can (1 to 2 kb) and therefore detects higher frequencies of particular chromosome aberrations in B-NHL. Nevertheless in about 30% of B-NHL patients, chromosome aberrations can potentially be used for MRD-PCR studies at the DNA level. The t(14;18) translocation has already proved to be an important and sensitive PCR target for MRD studies in 90% of follicular center lymphomas because of the presence of a patient-specific breakpoint fusion region by coupling of the *BCL2* and *IGH* genes.[156, 157] Comparably, in approximately 30% of cases of MCL with t(11;14), the *BCL1-IGH* fusion gene is detectable by PCR.[158]

In peripheral T-NHL, only a few well-defined translocations are known thus far, including the *NPM-ALK* fusion gene, which is observed in large-cell anaplastic lymphoma with t(2;5) and can potentially be used for RT-PCR analysis.[140] Furthermore, lymphoblastic T-NHL in childhood might have the same chromosome aberrations as found in T-ALL, such as *TAL1* deletions.

ACUTE MYELOID LEUKEMIA

MRD detection by applying leukemia-specific fusion gene transcripts in RT-PCR assays is possible in several types of childhood and adult AML. In virtually all APL cases, fusion gene products can be identified, typically *PML-RARA* mRNA associated with t(15;17) in over 90% of APL patients and, in the remaining cases, mostly *PLZF-RARA* mRNA associated with t(11;17).[159] Other examples of leukemia-specific fusion genes include *AML1-ETO* mRNA in AML (usually M2) with t(8;21), *CBFB-MYH11* mRNA in AML-M4Eo with inv(16) or t(16;16), and numerous fusion transcripts resulting from translocations involving the gene *MLL* on chromosome 11q23 (mostly AML M4

and M5).[137-140] In this way, RT-PCR analysis of leukemia-specific fusion gene mRNA for detection of low levels of MRD ($<10^{-3}$) can be used in 25% to 30% of AML patients (see Table 12-5).

In conclusion, multiparameter immunophenotyping, PCR analysis of Ig and TCR gene rearrangements, and RT-PCR detection of fusion genes resulting from chromosomal translocations are sensitive techniques for MRD detection in patients with hematopoietic malignancies (see Table 12-1). In some disease categories such as ALL with t(9;22), all three methodologies can be effectively applied, and in the vast majority of leukemias and NHL, at least one of the techniques is applicable (Table 12-6). Selection of a particular MRD technique depends on target availability (preferably in virtually all patients), sensitivity (at least 10^{-3}), specificity (patient-specific targets should be preferred over leukemia-specific targets), and stability. Reliable MRD monitoring should take into account all specific biologic limitations and technical pitfalls to prevent, on the one hand, false-negative results from insufficient sensitivity or clonal evolution and, on the other hand, false-positive results caused by limited target specificity or intralaboratory contamination.

Quantification of MRD by Use of PCR Analysis

MRD quantification by PCR analysis is a complex process that is essential for reliable disease monitoring. First, the quality and amplifiability of isolated DNA should be ensured. In RT-PCR-based MRD monitoring, the number of fusion mRNA transcripts should be normalized to the number of transcripts of a housekeeping gene. Second, minor variations in RT efficiency, primer annealing, and primer extension may lead to major variations after 30 to 35 PCR cycles. The disadvantages of PCR end point quantification might (partly) be overcome by using serial dilutions of DNA or RNA isolated from the leukemic cell sample at diagnosis into the DNA (RNA) of normal mononuclear cells. The same dilution series of diagnosis DNA is generally used to determine the tumor load in a follow-up sample in a semiquantitative manner by comparison of the hybridization signals. This approach gives an indication of the tumor burden in the follow-up sample. A more precise but also more laborious quantification method is based on limiting dilution of MRD-positive remission samples.[160, 161] To make this assay reliable, it is necessary to perform replicate experiments to determine the level of MRD positivity. Another less tedious strategy for quantitative PCR uses an internal standard that is co-amplified with the target of interest. Quantification by competitive PCR is performed by comparing the PCR signal of the specific target DNA with that of known concentrations of an internal standard, the competitor.[162-164]

Recently, a novel technology has become available, "real-time" quantitative PCR (RQ-PCR).[165] In contrast to the previously described PCR end point quantification techniques, RQ-PCR permits accurate quantification during exponential PCR amplification. The first available RQ-PCR technique was based on TaqMan technology (Fig. 12-15). This assay exploits the $5' \rightarrow 3'$ nuclease activity

TABLE 12–6. Applicability of MRD Techniques in Hematopoietic Malignancies*

	Flow Cytometric Immunophenotyping		PCR Analysis	
	Aberrant Immunophenotypes $(10^{-3}–10^{-4})$	*Igκ/Igλ Distribution or TCR-V Analysis* $(10^{-1}–10^{-2})$†	*Junctional Regions of Ig/TCR Genes* $(10^{-3}–10^{-6})$	*Chromosome Aberrations* $(10^{-4}–10^{-6})$
Precursor–B-ALL (%)				
Children	40–50	—	~95	40–45
Adults	70–80	—	~95	40–45
T-ALL (%)				
Children	~95	30–35‡	>95	25–30
Adults				10–15
Chronic B-cell leukemias (%)	—	>95	>95	—
Chronic T-cell leukemias (%)	—	60–65§	~95	—
B-NHL (%)	—	>95	70–80‖	25–30
T-NHL (%)	20–25¶	50–60	~95	10–15
AML (%)	60–90	—	10–15	25–40
CML (%)	—	—	—	>95

* The percentages indicate the applicability of the MRD techniques per category of hematopoietic malignancy; J.J.M. van Dongen, unpublished results.

† The sensitivity of flow cytometric detection of the Igκ/Igλ distribution or TCR-V gene usage can be improved to around 10^{-3} in triple labelings with specific markers such as BCL2, cytoplasmic CD3, or ALK proteins.

‡ Based on the expression of TCRαβ molecules (20% of cases) and TCRγδ molecules (~10% of cases).

§ TCR-V antibodies recognize 65% to 70% of TCRαβ molecules and most TCRγδ molecules.

‖ Somatic mutations hamper primer annealing in patients with B-NHL or B-CLL.

¶ Based on T-ALL–like immunophenotype in lymphoblastic T-NHL and NPM-ALK expression in about ~50% of large-cell anaplastic lymphomas of T-cell lineage.

ALL, acute lymphoblastic leukemia; AML, acute myeloid leukemia; CML, chronic myeloid leukemia; Ig, immunoglobulin; MRD, minimal residual disease; NHL, non-Hodgkin's lymphoma; PCR, polymerase chain reaction; TCR, T-cell receptor.

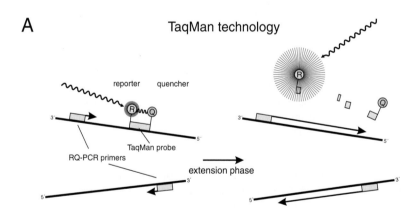

A   TaqMan technology

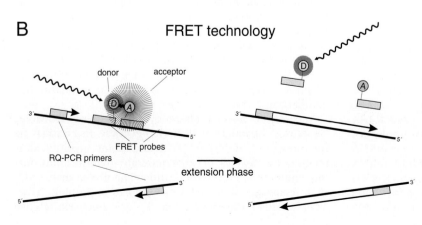

B   FRET technology

FIGURE 12–15. Real-time quantitative polymerase chain reaction (PCR) analysis by use of the TaqMan technique *(A)* and the fluorescence resonance energy transfer technique (FRET) *(B)*. In the TaqMan technique, the TaqMan probe contains a reporter dye (R) and a quencher dye (Q) that prevents emission of the reporter dye as long as the reporter dye and the quencher dye are closely linked. During the extension phase of each PCR cycle, the annealed TaqMan probe is digested by the exonuclease activity of the *Taq* polymerase, thereby separating the reporter dye from the quencher dye. This process results in a fluorescent signal, which further increases during each subsequent PCR cycle. In the FRET technique, the FRET probe consists of two separate oligonucleotides that should anneal closely to each other so that the donor dye of one oligonucleotide can excite the acceptor dye of the other oligonucleotide. In this case, the fluorescent signal of the acceptor dye is visible only during the annealing phase of the PCR cycle and the intensity of the fluorescence signal is directly related to the amount of PCR product.

of *Taq* polymerase to detect and quantify specific PCR products as the reaction proceeds.[166] On amplification, an internal target-specific TaqMan probe conjugated with a reporter and a quencher dye is degraded with subsequent emission of a fluorescent signal by the reporter dye that accumulates during the consecutive PCR cycles. Because of the real-time detection, the method has a very large dynamic detection range over five orders of magnitude, thereby eliminating the need for performing serial dilutions of follow-up samples (Fig. 12–16). Quantitative data can be accumulated in a short time because post-PCR processing is not necessary. Several groups have

shown that RQ-PCR based on the TaqMan technology can be used for the quantitative detection of MRD, with leukemia-specific chromosome aberrations used as PCR targets, as well as junctional regions of Ig and TCR gene rearrangements.[167-173] Another type of RQ-PCR exploits the so-called fluorescence resonance energy transfer (FRET) technology (see Fig. 12–15). This method requires two hybridization probes complementary to neighboring sequences, one labeled with a fluorescent dye at the 3′ end and the other carrying a fluorochrome at the 5′ end. One dye is a donor fluorochrome, whereas the other fluorochrome (acceptor) emits light if it is positioned close to the donor dye. Fluorescence is measured during each annealing step, when both probes hybridize to adjacent target sequences on the same strand.[174, 175] Another possibility for RQ-PCR is detection of SYBR green (DNA intercalating dye) fluorescence during PCR conducted with patient-specific primers.[176] Although this approach is the most cost-effective and potentially sensitive,[176] further studies should show whether SYBR green–based detection of all double-stranded DNA during PCR ensures satisfactory specificity.

CLINICAL VALUE OF DETECTION OF MINIMAL RESIDUAL DISEASE DURING AND AFTER TREATMENT

Acute Lymphoblastic Leukemia

MRD in ALL During Cytotoxic Treatment

Most MRD studies in ALL have focused on childhood ALL. The initial retrospective and small prospective studies with short follow-up indicated that the degree of MRD in ALL in childhood has potent clinical value, although the results of these clinical studies were not fully concordant.[30, 54, 56, 100, 106, 107, 164, 177-195] This incomplete concordance of results was attributed to differences in intensity of cytotoxic treatment protocols, as well as differences in the methodology and sensitivity of MRD monitoring. Recently published results of several large prospective studies have confirmed the clinical value of MRD monitoring, thereby justifying incorporation of the MRD information to refine risk assignment in current childhood ALL treatment protocols.[55, 196-198]

The most significant application of MRD monitoring in ALL is estimation of the initial response to single or multiagent therapy. Traditionally, a good clinical response with a blast count in PB of less than 1000/μL after a week of single-agent steroid therapy or the absence of circulating blasts after 7 days of multiagent induction chemotherapy was found to be an important prognostic factor. As a logical continuation of these clinical findings, low levels or absence of MRD after completion of induction therapy seems to predict a good outcome, as found by flow cytometric immunophenotyping and PCR studies.[55, 56, 181, 185, 192, 193, 196-199] Meta-analysis of published MRD studies has shown that approximately 50% of children with ALL are MRD positive at the end of induction treatment and approximately 45% of these MRD-positive patients will ultimately relapse.[200] The risk of relapse is

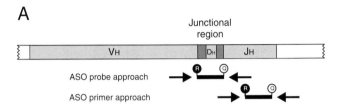

A

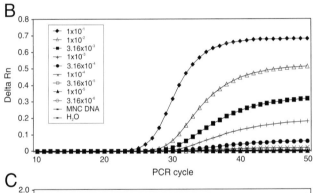

B

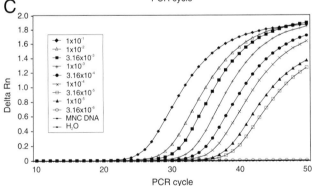

C

FIGURE 12–16. *A,* Schematic diagram of an *IGH* gene rearrangement and allele specific oligonucleotide (ASO) probe and ASO primer RQ-PCR approaches. For the ASO probe approach, TaqMan probes were designed complementary to the junctional region (VH-DH or the DH-JH), in combination with two germline VH and JH primers. For the ASO primer approach, TaqMan probes were designed at the 3′ end of the JH gene segments, in combination with one ASO primer complementary to the junctional region and one primer complementary to the germline sequence downstream of the JH gene segments. Primers are indicated by arrows and probes are indicated by bars.

Real-time amplification plots of the serial diagnosis DNA dilutions into MNC DNA in precursor-B-ALL patient 6480.[173] RQ-PCR analysis by use of the TaqMan technique was performed using an *IGH* gene rearrangement with both ASO probe approach, *B,* and ASO primer approach, *C.* The ASO primer approach resulted in higher PCR product yield (δRn), a larger reproducible range, and a higher maximal sensitivity than the ASO probe approach.

proportional to the levels of MRD detected.[185, 192, 196, 198] Furthermore, the presence of MRD at the end of induction treatment, as measured by immunophenotyping, is significantly correlated with the presence of particular chromosomal aberrations, such as t(9;22) or *MLL* rearrangements, that are associated with an unfavorable outcome.[55] On the other hand, preliminary results of RT-PCR studies in patients with the prognostically favorable *TEL-AML1* aberration suggest that MRD levels at the end of induction therapy are generally below the threshold associated with a bad outcome.[201, 202] The level of MRD-PCR positivity or the percentage of cells with an aberrant "leukemia-specific" immunophenotype after induction therapy is the most powerful prognostic factor. Multivariate analysis has shown that this prognostic value is independent of other clinically relevant risk factors, including age, blast count at diagnosis, immunophenotype at diagnosis, presence of chromosome aberrations, response to prednisone, and classic clinical risk group assignment, provided that accurate MRD quantification on adequate BM samples is performed.[55, 196-198] Results from the large prospective MRD study of the International BFM Study Group have indicated that analysis of MRD at a single time point is not sufficient for the recognition of patients with a poor prognosis, as well as patients with a good prognosis.[198] In contrast, combined information on the kinetics of the decrease in tumor load at the end of induction treatment and before consolidation treatment is highly informative in this regard. This combined MRD information distinguishes patients at low risk with MRD negativity at both time points (3-year relapse rate of 2%), patients at high risk with an intermediate (10^{-3}) or high ($\geq 10^{-2}$) degree of MRD at both time points (3-year relapse rate of 75%), and the remaining patients at intermediate risk (3-year relapse rate of 23%)[198] (Fig. 12-17). The MRD-based low-risk patients make up a group of

substantial size (approximately 45%), comparable to the frequency of survivors of childhood ALL before treatment intensification was introduced.[203, 204] Within the MRD-based low-risk group, half of the patients already have low ($\leq 10^{-4}$) or undetectable MRD levels after 2 weeks of treatment.[205] This group might particularly profit from treatment reduction. On the other hand, the group of patients at MRD-based high risk is larger than any previously identified high-risk group (approximately 15%) and has an unprecedented high 3-year relapse rate of 75%. This group might benefit from further intensification of treatment protocols, including BMT during first remission or novel treatment modalities, such as antibodies conjugated with immunotoxins or tyrosine kinase inhibitors.[198]

Continuous MRD monitoring in childhood ALL has shown that a steady decrease in MRD levels to negative PCR results during treatment is associated with a favorable prognosis,[179, 184, 186] whereas persistence of high MRD levels or a steady increase in MRD levels generally leads to clinical relapse* (Figs. 12-18 and 12-19). Therefore, persisting MRD levels during treatment can be regarded as the best indicator of treatment resistance. PCR-based MRD monitoring was shown to be able to select the group of "poor responders" with early relapse during maintenance treatment.[55, 164, 196-198] This predictive value of MRD monitoring is particularly clear after the first relapse.[187] Sequential sampling generally shows positive MRD-PCR results before clinical relapse (Fig. 12-20), unless false-negative results are obtained because of continuing or secondary Ig or TCR gene rearrangements (clonal evolution). Such false-negative results can generally be prevented by using two Ig/TCR targets per patient (see earlier).[198]

Low levels of MRD after therapy might be associated with the late development of relapse, but absence of MRD at the end of treatment is not sufficient to ensure that the patient is cured.[183, 193] Despite the high sensitivity of most MRD techniques, it should be noted that MRD negativity does not exclude the presence of leukemic cells in the patient because each MRD test screens only a minor fraction of all BM and PB leukocytes. Curiously, it has been reported that multiple PCR analyses (testing a higher cell number) give evidence of residual leukemia at very low levels in approximately 90% (15/17) of patients remaining in long-term clinical remission.[189] In 7 of these 15 patients, this PCR result was confirmed in a blast colony assay. Thus far, these data have not been confirmed by other investigators. In contrast, large prospective studies have shown 0% to 10% of patients being positive at the end of treatment; most of these MRD-positive patients later relapsed.[55, 193, 198]

A striking correlation was found between a high initial white blood cell count in precursor–B-ALL and persisting high levels of immunophenotypically detected MRD; this correlation was not found in T-ALL,[30] in line with the clinical evidence of an association between a high leukocyte count and unfavorable clinical outcome in precursor–B-ALL and lack of such a correlation in T-ALL.[206] The MRD data from a single study suggest slower kinetics

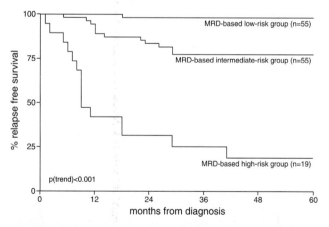

FIGURE 12–17. Relapse-free survival of the three minimal residual disease (MRD)-based risk groups treated with International BFM Study Group chemotherapy protocols, as defined by combined MRD information at the end of induction treatment (time point 1) and before consolidation treatment (time point 2).[198] Patients in the low-risk group have MRD negativity at both time points (43% of patients), patients in the high-risk group have MRD levels of 10^{-3} or greater at both time points (15% of patients), and the remaining patients form the MRD-based intermediate-risk group (43% of patients). The numbers of patients at risk are given in parentheses for each group at 24 and 48 months after time point 2.

---

*See references 1, 3, 29, 31, 42, 54, 55, 178, 180, 182, 193, 195, 198.

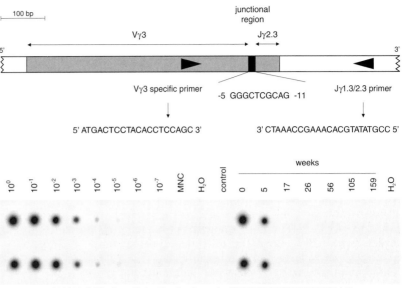

FIGURE 12–18. A patient with precursor–B-cell acute lymphoblastic leukemia was monitored for the presence of minimal residual disease (MRD) in bone marrow (BM) follow-up samples with a Vγ3-Jγ2.3 polymerase chain reaction (PCR) target. PCR analysis with Vγ3 and Jγ1.3/2.3 primers was performed on 10-fold dilutions of the DNA isolated at diagnosis into mononuclear cell DNA and on DNA extracted from BM samples during follow-up (time points in weeks). The junctional region sequence had a deletion of 16 germline nucleotides and a random insertion of 10 nucleotides. Hybridization with the patient-specific probe resulted in a sensitivity of 10^{-5}. The follow-up sample at week 5 (end of induction therapy) was found to be MRD positive, and the tumor load was estimated to be 10^{-2} based on comparison of the signal with the dilution series of the diagnosis DNA. Subsequent time points were MRD negative.

of leukemia clearance in patients with T-ALL than in precursor–B-ALL patients.[191] Virtually all (16 of 17) patients were found to be MRD positive at the end of induction treatment, whereas a later time point at the beginning of maintenance treatment carried the most significant prognostic information. All but one (seven of eight) patient MRD positive at this later time point subsequently relapsed, whereas all 8 MRD-negative patients remained in continuous complete remission.[191]

The preliminary results of MRD studies in adult ALL in which junctional regions were used as MRD-PCR targets showed a molecular response to chemotherapy similar to that in childhood ALL, but with a higher frequency of

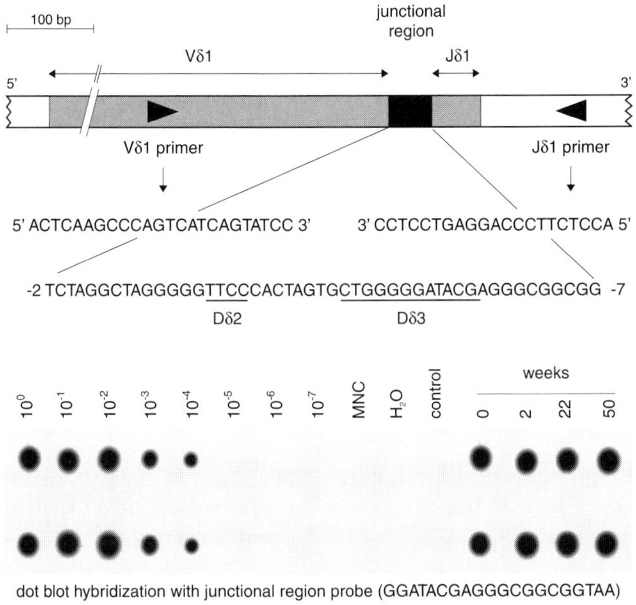

FIGURE 12–19. A complete *TCRD* rearrangement was used to monitor minimal residual disease (MRD) in a patient with T-cell acute lymphoblastic leukemia. The large junctional region of the Vδ1-Jδ1 rearrangement contained Dδ2 and Dδ3 sequences. The size of the junctional region was 48 nucleotides, including the Dδ2 and Dδ3 sequences. Polymerase chain reaction (PCR) amplification was performed with Vδ1 and Jδ1 primers on DNA from the diagnosis dilution series and from bone marrow follow-up samples (time points in weeks). Hybridization of the spotted PCR products with the junctional region probe resulted in a sensitivity of 10^{-4}. All follow-up time points tested gave a signal representative of a high tumor load of 10^{-2} or greater based on comparison with the signals from the diagnosis dilution series. This patient had a clinical relapse 50 weeks after diagnosis. According to molecular MRD detection, this patient never reached remission.

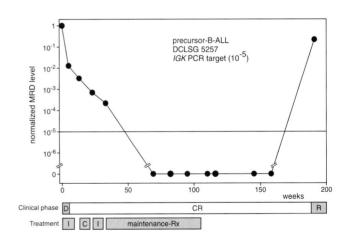

FIGURE 12–20. MRD detection during follow-up of precursor–B-ALL patient 5257 by use of the *IGK* (VκIII-Kde) gene rearrangement. Hybridization with the patient specific probe resulted in a sensivity of 10^{-5}. The follow-up sample at week 5 (I-BFM time point one; i.e., end of induction therapy) was found to be MRD positive and the tumor load was estimated to be 10^{-2}. The tumor load at week 12 (I-BFM time point two; i.e., before consolidation therapy) was estimated at 10^{-3}. Based on MRD information this patient was classified as MRD high-risk patient (3-year relapse rate of 75%). Although the patient became MRD–negative during the maintenance therapy, he relapsed one year after maintenance treatment cessation.

persistent MRD positivity in adults.[190, 207] Not only the frequencies of MRD positivity but also the MRD levels in adult patients were significantly higher than in comparably treated children; this finding points toward more frequent in vivo drug resistance in adult ALL.[190, 208]

MRD Detection in ALL Patients Undergoing BMT

High levels of MRD positivity (10^{-2} to 10^{-3}) before allogeneic BMT are invariably associated with relapse after transplantation, whereas the 2-year event-free survival rate in patients with a low level of MRD positivity (10^{-3} to 10^{-5}) approximated 36%.[209] In contrast, MRD-negative status before allogeneic transplantation significantly correlated with better outcome and a 2-year event-free survival rate of 73%.[209] Therefore, patients with a high MRD burden before BMT might be offered alternative treatment (e.g., further cytoreduction before BMT, intensified conditioning, and/or early post-BMT immunotherapy) to improve their generally dismal outcome.[209]

MRD-PCR positivity in ALL patients after BMT is suggestive of impending relapse.[210, 211] This finding is true both for high-risk patients who received transplants in first remission and for patients subjected to BMT in second remission after leukemia relapse. MRD was shown to occur in post-BMT samples in 88% of patients who subsequently relapsed, whereas only 22% of patients in long-term complete remission showed MRD at any time after BMT, mostly at low levels.[211] Patients with persistent MRD after BMT might be candidates for early treatment with immunotherapy, including donor lymphocyte infusions to increase the graft-versus leukemia effect.[211]

MRD Detection in Poor-Risk ALL with t(9;22) and t(4;11)

Philadelphia chromosome–positive (Ph$^+$) ALL with t(9; 22) is characterized by high drug resistance and a very poor prognosis.[212, 213] This leukemia subtype is also associated with an increased percentage of MRD-positive patients and increased MRD levels at the end of induction treatment.[55, 214] Chemotherapy can lower the degree of MRD as measured by *BCR-ABL* transcript levels by only 2 to 3 logs in most patients, which is not enough for prolonged hematologic remission.[215] Nevertheless, in some patients with favorable prognostic features (e.g., low initial leukocyte count or good prednisone response), the disease can be controlled with intensive chemotherapy.[213, 216, 217] Long-term disease-free survival after intensive chemotherapy and/or BMT was observed in ALL patients with t(9;22) after the eradication of *BCR-ABL*$^+$ cells below the level of RT-PCR detectability.[212, 218–220] Positivity for *BCR-ABL* transcripts by RT-PCR analysis seems to be a significant predictor of impending post-transplant relapse, independent of other clinical and biologic factors. This relationship appears to be particularly true for patients with detectable *BCR-ABL* transcripts of the p190 type.[221] However, because of the poor prognosis of ALL with t(9;22) and the very low frequency of complete cure in this patient group, the aforementioned results should be confirmed by large multicenter studies.

The requirement of RT-PCR negativity as a sine qua non for a patient's cure was found in preliminary studies on MRD in ALL with t(4;11) and t(1;19).[222–224] Prospective MRD monitoring in ALL patients with t(4;11) showed persistent RT-PCR positivity in more than 50% of patients preceding overt hematologic relapse at a median time of 6 months from diagnosis.[225] In 20% of patients, conversion to PCR positivity was observed during the treatment, followed by relapse of disease. However, a small subgroup of t(4;11)-positive patients rapidly achieved molecular remission after intensive chemotherapy and/or allogeneic BMT and persistent PCR negativity in long-term complete remission.[225, 226] Therefore, prospective MRD monitoring can be used for assessment of treatment response and individualization of therapy to further improve the outcome of high-risk, t(4;11)-positive leukemia, including infant ALL patients.[227]

Can Blood Sampling Replace BM Sampling for MRD Detection in ALL?

Replacement of BM sampling by PB sampling has been a topic of debate in MRD studies for the last 15 years. Initial immunophenotypic studies in T-ALL indicated that MRD in PB is generally less than 10-fold lower than in BM.[29] Nevertheless, particularly in precursor–B-ALL, a proportion of patients have detectable leukemic cells in follow-up BM but not PB.[35] The data from a single PCR study showed an 11.7-fold difference between BM and PB during induction treatment of precursor–B-ALL patients,[228] which implies that MRD techniques need to be at least 10-fold more sensitive (i.e., $\leq 10^{-5}$) when PB samples are monitored.[198] The difference between BM and PB might be lower in Ph$^+$ precursor–B-ALL, most probably because of a generally higher degree of MRD than in other ALL subtypes.[215, 229, 230] Undoubtedly, the differences in MRD levels between BM and PB are additionally influenced by the degree of dilution of BM aspirates with PB. This effect of dilution is suggested by the finding of a 4.1-fold greater mean MRD level in trephine BM biopsy samples than in BM aspirates.[231] More information is needed to decide whether and to what extent the more traumatic BM sampling can be replaced by PB sampling.

In conclusion, detection of MRD in ALL has proved to be of clinical importance and is currently being incorporated into stratification of ALL treatment protocols. Several different methodologic approaches for MRD monitoring are currently available; they yield comparable results and guarantee a clinically relevant sensitivity of at least 10^{-4}.[232, 233] Further studies should prove whether it would be possible, based on MRD data, to individualize treatment protocols and thereby improve treatment outcome for high-risk patients on the one hand and prevent unnecessary treatment-related toxicity in low-risk ALL patients on the other hand.

B-Cell Chronic Lymphocytic Leukemia

B-CLL typically occurs at an advanced age, is characterized by an indolent course, and frequently requires no specific treatment.[234] However, in a subgroup of young patients with high-risk B-CLL, intensive treatment (including BMT) should be considered. Immunophenotypic monitoring of residual disease in B-CLL is based on overexpression of the CD5 antigen on CD20$^+$ cells or an abnormal Igκ/Igλ ratio in a B-cell–enriched population or on CD37$^+$-gated B cells.[33, 235, 236] In this way (sensitivity, ~10^{-2}), residual leukemic cells were detected in most (56%) B-CLL patients in cytomorphologic remission after chemotherapy.[235] Moreover, virtually all these patients (93%) were MRD positive with clonal IGH gene rearrangements demonstrated by Southern blotting.[235]

In contrast, immunophenotypic MRD analysis after treatment of B-CLL with fludarabine plus prednisone showed that the vast majority of patients in complete clinical remission had no immunophenotypically aberrant cells.[237] Relapse-free survival in this group was significantly longer than in patients with detectable MRD by flow cytometry. The reappearance of cells with a B-CLL immunophenotype preceded overt clinical relapse by 3 to 14 months.[237] Similarly, in the study of Brugiatelli and colleagues,[238] immunophenotypic remission after chemotherapy was associated with significantly longer relapse-free survival of patients, but this remission was not related to prolonged overall survival. Persistence of immunophenotypic MRD was associated with more rapid progression of B-CLL.[72]

PCR analysis of IGH junctional regions was able to detect malignant cells with a sensitivity of 10^{-3} to 10^{-5} in advanced-stage B-CLL patients referred for BMT.[239] None of the patients reached molecular remission after conventional or salvage chemotherapy.[239, 240] In the study of Provan and associates[239] the vast majority of patients remained disease free without PCR-detectable MRD after allogeneic or B-cell–purged BMT. Persistence of MRD positivity after BMT was almost unequivocally associated with impending relapse. No evidence of clonal evolution was noted during progression of the disease, which is in line with the absence of secondary rearrangements and the rare occurrence of somatic mutations in B-CLL.[239] In contrast to the latter study, other investigators reported MRD positivity for several months or even several years in B-CLL patients in complete clinical remission after stem-cell (SC) transplantation.[240, 241]

In conclusion, MRD data in B-CLL are preliminary and mostly retrospective, and the clinical value of MRD in this leukemia type should be fully established. It is clear that MRD kinetics in B-CLL differs per treatment protocol. Nevertheless, patients with high-risk B-CLL in particular should definitely profit from more precise treatment monitoring.

Follicular Cell Lymphoma with t(14;18) and BCL2-IGH Fusion Genes

MRD Detection in FCL Patients Treated with Chemotherapy

MRD detection might be especially important in the subgroup of high- and intermediate-grade lymphomas, where circulating lymphoma cells are frequently found in BM and PB. The vast majority of clinical studies concentrated on FCL with t(14;18) and used the BCL2-IGH fusion gene as a DNA target for PCR-based MRD analysis.[242-253] Most of the patients suffering from this disease harbor lymphoma cells in BM or PB at diagnosis, with BM being more informative for MRD monitoring than PB.[243-245] More than half of the patients convert to MRD negativity during the first year of cytotoxic treatment, which is associated with longer relapse-free survival.[246] In patients with advanced t(14;18)-positive NHL (stage III/IV) treated with conventional induction therapy, no obvious correlation was found between the presence or absence of MRD positivity and relapse-free survival.[247] Recently, a combination of chemotherapy and chimeric (mouse-human) CD20 antibody treatment was shown to produce durable clinical remission in a subgroup of FCL patients with PCR negativity.[248]

MRD Detection in FCL Patients Treated with Autologous BMT

MRD studies for the presence of BCL2-IGH fusion genes in patients treated with purged autologous BMT showed that none of the patients in continuous molecular remission relapsed, as opposed to most patients with persistent PCR positivity.[249, 250] In another group of patients treated with autologous peripheral blood stem-cell (PBSC) transplantation, reappearance of PCR positivity at any time post-transplantation was associated with an increased relapse risk.[251] Diametrically different conclusions were drawn from another study: most patients after purged autologous BMT remained MRD positive, and no correlation was found between MRD-PCR status and relapse-free survival.[252]

Technical Pitfalls of MRD Detection in FCL

Circulating t(14;18)-positive cells were also detected in patients in long-term clinical remission after radiation therapy for localized FCL.[253] It should be noted that positive results in sensitive BCL2-IGH PCR studies should be interpreted with caution because the presence of t(14;18)-positive B cells has also been reported in healthy individuals.[145, 146] Also, an international multicenter study revealed high variability of BCL2-IGH PCR results between different laboratories with an unexpectedly high frequency of false-positive results.[254] Such false-positive results from normal t(14;18)$^+$ cells or intralaboratory contamination can be prevented by routine design of patient-specific oligonucleotides directed against the fusion region sequence of the BCL2-IGH junction.[255] Moreover, several discrepancies in MRD kinetics between BM and PB in FCL might be clarified when quantitative PCR data become available. For this purpose, RQ-PCR is particularly attractive, with preliminary results showing good concordance with clinical remission status.[168, 256] Further investigations and standardization on a multicenter level are required to establish quantitative criteria for molecular remission in FCL and potential applicability of MRD information for clinical decision making.

MRD Detection in Non-Hodgkin's Lymphomas by *IGH*-Based PCR Analysis

PCR-based MRD detection by use of fusion genes as DNA targets is possible in only 20% to 30% of NHL patients (see Table 12–6). In contrast, *IGH* gene rearrangements could be successfully identified in the vast majority (70% to 90%) of NHL cases.[132]

With *IGH* gene rearrangements and *BCL1-IGH* fusion genes used as DNA targets, MCL patients were found to be continuously MRD positive in BM and/or PB during chemotherapy.[257, 258] In most MCL patients, MRD levels in BM and PB vary between 10^{-2} and 10^{-3}, indicative of significant resistance to conventional chemotherapy schemes.[258]

PCR analysis of *IGH* gene junctional regions was used to assess the efficacy of the purging process in autologous BM harvests of B-NHL patients.[259] The purging appeared to be ineffective in patients with diffuse B-NHL but was successful in 50% of FCL cases. Persistence of MRD positivity in BM after autologous BMT was invariably associated with impending clinical relapse, whereas all patients with eradication of PCR-detectable lymphoma cells remained in continuous clinical remission.[259] Nevertheless, persistence of patient-specific *IGH* gene rearrangements in patients in long-term complete remission has also been reported.[260] MRD was investigated with patient-specific PCR techniques in a group of patients with advanced-stage FCL or MCL.[261] After high-dose sequential chemotherapy it was possible to harvest MRD-negative autologous BM grafts in most FCL patients. None of the patients who received an MRD-negative BM graft relapsed at a median follow-up of 24 months.[261] These combined MRD studies indicate that transplantation with MRD-negative autologous BM or PBSC grafts is a promising treatment modality in patients with FCL. In contrast, it is virtually impossible to harvest MRD-negative BM or PBSC grafts in MCL.[257, 258, 261] Reinfusion of MRD-positive grafts is uniformly associated with relapse of MCL.[257] For patients with advanced disease, allogeneic BMT currently remains the only effective treatment regimen, and preliminary data show conversion to MRD negativity after BMT, which is related to long-term hematologic remission.[257, 262]

Acute Myeloid Leukemia

Immunophenotypic MRD Detection in AML

The only technique of MRD monitoring available for the vast majority of AML patients is multiparameter immunophenotyping. Initial attempts were based on the cross-lineage expression of TdT in AML.[30, 94] Control studies revealed that normal counterparts of myeloid marker$^+$TdT$^+$ cells are rare in BM ($<10^{-3}$) and PB ($<10^{-4}$), if they occur at all.[263, 264] The microscopic myeloid marker/TdT double IF staining technique was used for monitoring TdT$^+$ leukemic cells in 14 AML patients during treatment. These investigations revealed that effectiveness of treatment can be monitored in TdT$^+$ AML patients if TdT positivity at diagnosis encompasses at least 1% of the leukemic cells[1, 94, 264] (see Fig. 12–6). Depending on the frequency of BM and PB sampling, myeloid marker/TdT

double IF staining allows detection of relapse 3 to 9 months earlier than with the use of cytomorphology.[94] However, in some cases, false-negative results might be obtained because of a phenotypic shift to TdT negativity at relapse.[94]

Multiparameter flow cytometry studies have indicated that persistence and/or an increase in cells with leukemia-associated immunophenotypes precedes hematologic relapse.[45] Immunophenotypic analysis at the time of first cytomorphologic remission has shown the presence of MRD in at least half of patients.[265] Two studies demonstrated the strong prognostic significance of MRD levels at the end of induction treatment and the risk of AML relapse, with the cutoff point ranging from 2×10^{-3} to 5×10^{-3} residual cells at the first cytomorphologic remission.[86, 266] In an extensive study by San Miguel et al,[266] the risk of relapse was significantly increased in patients bearing 5×10^{-3} or more residual cells at the end of induction treatment (67% incidence of relapse), whereas only 20% of patients with less than 5×10^{-3} residual cells relapsed. At the end of intensification treatment, the threshold value of 2×10^{-3} residual cells also identified two distinct groups with relapse rates of 69% and 36%. Increased levels of MRD at the end of induction and intensification treatment correlated with multidrug resistance as measured by the rhodamine 123 efflux assay.[266] Multivariate analysis showed that this type of MRD information is independent of other known prognostic factors such as cell counts at diagnosis, age, or multidrug resistance.[266]

The preliminary results of MRD monitoring in AML patients after BMT showed an unequivocal association between the finding of cells with an abnormal phenotype and subsequent relapse. Multiparameter flow cytometry was also shown to be an effective tool for discrimination between normal blasts transiently present in PB after BMT and leukemic blasts heralding medullary relapse.[267] Furthermore, in AML patients subjected to autologous BMT, detection of leukemia-specific phenotypes in harvested bone marrow was associated with treatment failure secondary to relapse.[199] Accordingly, MRD levels of 10^{-3} or greater in autologous PBSC harvests were found to be associated with AML relapse post-transplantation at a median time of 6 months.[268]

RT-PCR–Based MRD Detection in APL with t(15;17) and PML-RARA Fusion Transcripts

The most extensive MRD studies in AML involved RT-PCR monitoring of *PML-RARA* fusion mRNA in APL patients with t(15;17). The results of several retrospective and prospective RT-PCR studies in APL patients showed several distinct molecular characteristics of this AML subtype,[269–282] and these characteristics led to the first successful treatment intervention protocol based on MRD information.[283] First, MRD is typically present 1 month after diagnosis, probably because of remaining mature leukemic cells; this finding does not correlate with outcome.[269] Treatment with all-*trans*-retinoic acid (ATRA) alone never eliminates all leukemic cells.[271, 272, 274] Rapid loss of MRD positivity during the first 3 months of ATRA and cytotoxic treatment correlates well with a good outcome, whereas continuous positivity is associated with relapse.[275, 277] Patients with refractory APL are RT-PCR positive even at the end of treatment intensification.[277] On one hand, *PML-RARA* positivity after consolidation treatment is a strong predictor of subsequent hematologic relapse; on the other hand, PCR negativity after completion of treatment does not exclude relapse.[282] Patients in long-term remission after chemotherapy or BMT do not usually have detectable levels of *PML-RARA* fusion mRNA,[273, 278] although one study suggested that with increased sensitivity of RT-PCR assays, trace levels of *PML-RARA* could be found in a proportion of patients in long-term remission.[284] With modern treatment protocols combining ATRA with consolidation chemotherapy, PCR negativity is achieved at the end of treatment in virtually all patients, although 20% to 30% of patients will still suffer from APL relapse.[280] To obtain clinically relevant information, continuous prospective MRD monitoring is required during the first 6 to 12 months after consolidation treatment for early identification of patients at increased risk of relapse.[159] Reappearance of detectable MRD usually precedes hematologic relapse at a median time of 2 to 3 months.[272, 274, 276, 281] This information led to the definition of molecular relapse in APL, which is manifested by conversion from RT-PCR negativity to positivity in two successive BM samplings during follow-up.[281] Lo Coco and associates[283] demonstrated that patients treated at the time of molecular relapse have a much better 2-year event-free survival rate than do patients treated with the same salvage therapy at the time of hematologic relapse (92% versus 44%). For patients in the second remission of APL, one of the treatment options is allogeneic or autologous SC transplantation. Autologous BM or PBSC grafts with PCR positivity for *PML-RARA* fusion mRNA carry an increased risk of subsequent relapse of disease.[279, 285, 286] For APL patients in second remission with MRD-positive autologous grafts, alternative aggressive treatment approaches should be seriously considered, including unrelated donor allogeneic BMT. Conversely, preliminary data show that autologous BMT with MRD-negative grafts results in long-term clinical remission in most patients.[285]

RT-PCR–Based MRD Detection in AML with t(8;21) and AML1-ETO Fusion Transcripts

The clinical value of MRD-PCR studies in AML patients with t(8;21) is less certain. Several RT-PCR studies indicate that *AML1-ETO* fusion mRNA remains detectable in the blood and BM of patients in long-term remission after chemotherapy or allogeneic/autologous BMT,[287-291] whereas other reports showed disappearance of *AML1-ETO* mRNA in long-term survivors of leukemia in complete remission over 10 years.[292, 293] It is not clear whether the detectability of *AML1-ETO* mRNA in these long-term remission patients implies that the aberrant fusion protein is expressed and whether this situation is equivalent to the presence of in vivo clonogenic leukemic cells.[287-290] Nevertheless, in vitro analysis indicates that residual *AML1-ETO*–positive cells in patients in long-term remission have multipotent clonogenic potential.[291, 294] Preliminary results from several quantitative RT-PCR and/or RQ-PCR studies indicate that a gradual reduction to very low *AML1-ETO* mRNA levels or to PCR negativity throughout the disease course is associated with durable clinical remission.[295-297] In contrast, markedly increased MRD levels during treatment are associated with subsequent hematologic relapse.[169, 295-297] Moreover, the levels of *AML1-ETO* transcripts in PB, though at least 10-fold lower than in BM, yield fully concordant MRD information.[297]

In the vast majority of t(8;21)-positive AML patients, PBSC harvests are contaminated with leukemic cells expressing *AML1-ETO* fusion gene transcripts. This contamination is, however, not necessarily associated with relapse after conditioning chemotherapy and autologous SC support.[298]

RT-PCR–Based MRD Detection in AML with inv(16) and CBFB-MYH11 Fusion Transcripts

Several small studies have analyzed MRD kinetics in AML-M4Eo patients with inv(16) or t(16;16) by RT-PCR monitoring of *CBFB-MYH11* fusion transcripts.[299-304] MRD positivity was observed for several months after achieving hematologic remission.[299, 300] Although *CBFB-MYH11* mRNA was usually absent in patients in long-term remission,[299, 302, 303] a single study showed the presence of such fusion transcripts in long-term survivors.[301] Molecular positivity for *CBFB-MYH11* mRNA was typically found in pretransplant BM, which did not have any influence on survival after SC transplantation.[303] In contrast, rapid conversion to PCR negativity after transplantation was associated with an excellent outcome.[303] Quantitative RT-PCR studies showed a gradual decrease in MRD levels by at least four orders of magnitude within the first year of treatment in patients in complete hematologic remission, whereas persistently high MRD levels were associated with subsequent relapse.[302, 304]

MRD Detection in AML with Other Chromosomal Aberrations

A single MRD study in AML patients with t(9;11) that used *MLL-AF9* fusion transcripts as a molecular target showed rapid clearance of MRD in patients in long-term complete remission and persistence of MRD in patients who subsequently relapsed.[305] Also, a single MRD study involving interphase FISH analysis of FACS-sorted myeloid precursors was reported in AML patients with numeric chromosomal aberrations, including monosomy 7, trisomy 8, and so on. The finding of more than 3% FISH-positive sorted cells at the first complete remission sample (3 to 4 weeks from diagnosis) was significantly correlated with shorter remission duration.[17]

In conclusion, immunophenotypic and PCR-based MRD studies in AML have yielded significant information on disease kinetics during and after treatment. Moreover, quantitative flow cytometry and RT-PCR assays allow the identification of patients at high risk of hematologic relapse, patients who might profit from early treatment reintensification.[159, 306] Serial quantitative MRD monitoring might also be useful to select more aggressive treatment strategies (including BMT) in drug-resistant patients with otherwise chemosensitive AML (e.g., t[15;17], t[8;21], or inv[16] positive leukemias), for which SC transplantation is not always recommended in first complete remission.

Chronic Myeloid Leukemia

High-dose chemotherapy and interferon alfa (IFN-α) therapy have to be followed by allogeneic BMT to cure patients with CML in chronic phase.[307] Long-term survival rates after allogeneic BMT range from 55% to 70%, with relapse rates of 15% to 20%.[307] Unfortunately, such treatment is available for only a minority of patients. RT-PCR detection of *BCR-ABL* fusion mRNA is possible in virtually all (>95%) CML patients. As a consequence, numerous MRD studies have been performed in patients after allogeneic BMT in an attempt to identify those at risk for relapse.[162, 163, 308-313] The initial RT-PCR studies, performed with different sensitivities, used patient groups treated with different pre-BMT cytoreductive regimens and consequently produced not fully concordant but biologically significant results. Such discordant results created substantial skepticism regarding whether MRD information in CML patients could have any clinical value.[314] Some authors reported conversion to negative RT-PCR results, which indeed seemed to indicate cure of leukemia, whereas PCR positivity after allogeneic BMT was associated with an increased risk of relapse.[308, 315-317] However, several studies showed that positive RT-PCR results were frequently observed in CML patients in long-term clinical remission after BMT, without being predictive of imminent relapse.[308, 311] Persistent PCR positivity seemed to be significantly related to absent or less severe graft-versus-host disease.[318, 319] These seemingly discordant results could be explained when precise quantification of MRD levels in CML was introduced, which was proved to be of clinical value, particularly for identifying patients at risk for recurrence of leukemia.[162, 163, 310, 320-322]

Based on the currently available quantitative RT-PCR data in CML patients after allogeneic BMT, it has been concluded that the vast majority of patients are PCR positive in the first 6 to 9 months after BMT, thus indicating that the conditioning regimens before BMT cannot eradicate all leukemic cells.[323, 324] In vitro experiments have shown that at least a proportion of *BCR-ABL*–positive cells have clonogenic potential.[325] Sustained PCR negativity within 1 year after BMT is associated with cure, whereas patients with PCR positivity after 1 year or more post-BMT have a significantly greater risk of relapse than do patients with PCR negativity.[323] However, not all patients with persistent PCR positivity relapse.[319] The group of high-risk patients could be identified by serial quantitative PCR analysis, which generally shows increasing MRD levels several months before hematologic or cytogenetic relapse.[320, 322, 323, 326] A rapid increase in MRD levels before relapse is an indication of more aggressive disease, such as relapse into accelerated phase or blast crisis.[320, 322, 323, 327] Patients who remain in remission generally have decreasing or persistently low MRD levels, with some patients being *BCR-ABL* mRNA positive even 10 years after allogeneic BMT.[313]

Quantitative MRD studies in CML have enabled definition of molecular relapse after allogeneic BMT, which is equivalent to rising or persistently high MRD levels (*BCR-ABL/ABL* ratio of >0.02%) in two consecutive specimens more than 4 months after BMT.[328] Preliminary data indicate that the incidence of molecular relapse (followed by cytogenetic or hematologic relapse) is significantly lower after allogeneic PBSC transplantation than after allogeneic BMT.[329] Quantitative MRD analysis was also used for monitoring the response to immunotherapy, specifically, donor lymphocyte infusions for patients relapsing after allogeneic BMT.[170, 322, 330, 331] Preliminary data indicate that the outcome after immunotherapy is more favorable when donor lymphocyte infusions are administered at the phase of cytogenetic or molecular relapse.[330, 331] In some responders, such early treatment results in conversion to sustained PCR negativity.[330]

For patients who are not eligible for allogeneic BMT, IFN-α remains the current first-line therapy, with 25% to 30% of patients experiencing complete or partial cytogenetic remission.[307] Levels of MRD are significantly correlated with the degree of response to IFN-α treatment as measured by cytogenetics.[332-334] Interestingly, the vast majority of patients demonstrating a complete response to IFN-α have variable detectable levels of *BCR-ABL* transcripts,[332, 335, 336] with a mean *BCR-ABL/ABL* ratio of 0.045% at the time of maximal response.[337] At this time point, the *BCR-ABL/ABL* ratio was significantly higher in patients who subsequently relapsed than in patients remaining in complete remission.[337] In vitro analysis showed that some of these *BCR-ABL* mRNA–positive cells demonstrate clonogenic potential.[338, 339] Sequential MRD monitoring of patients during IFN-α therapy showed a gradual decline in MRD levels over time.[337, 340] A study by Kurzrock et al[340] suggested the possibility of conversion to PCR negativity in patients in long-term complete remission after IFN-α treatment, whereas others have detected very low MRD levels in all patients more than 5 years in remission.[337]

In conclusion, qualitative MRD studies in CML are insufficient for prediction of the disease course in individual patients.[324, 328, 341] In contrast, recent developments in quantitative PCR assays for the detection of *BCR-ABL* mRNA have proved their clinical value. Quantitative PCR enables identification of patients at high risk of relapse after allogeneic BMT at a point when the burden of disease is relatively low (molecular relapse) and restarting treatment is more effective.[342] Moreover, MRD monitoring in patients with sequential PCR negativity 6 to 9 months after BMT might be substantially reduced, with virtually all such patients remaining in long-term remission.[342] In patients with a complete response to IFN-α, MRD monitoring indicating low levels of *BCR-ABL* transcripts might be helpful to determine the precise time for treatment discontinuation.[337] Finally, several studies have indicated that MRD levels in CML patients are comparable in both BM and PB.[332, 334, 343]

SPECIFIC CLINICAL APPLICATIONS OF DETECTION OF MINIMAL RESIDUAL DISEASE

Detection of Central Nervous System Involvement in Acute Lymphoblastic Leukemia Patients

The incidence of central nervous system (CNS) involvement in ALL patients at diagnosis is relatively low according to classic cytomorphologic criteria, such as the presence of distinct blasts and/or an increased cerebrospinal fluid (CSF) leukocyte count (>5 cells/μL). However, before the introduction of CNS prophylaxis, up to 50% of ALL patients suffered from meningeal relapse, thus indicating the high frequency of asymptomatic CNS involvement in ALL patients.[344] Therefore, the introduction of therapy for prevention of meningeal leukemia is regarded to be a milestone in the progress of leukemia treatment.[204, 345]

Normal CSF does not contain TdT$^+$ or CD34$^+$ progenitor cells, which implies that their presence provides evidence of meningeal infiltration. Microscopic immunophenotyping of CSF samples at diagnosis showed the presence of TdT$^+$ cells in approximately 25% (11/43) of children with ALL, whereas only 1 of the 11 positive cases had overt CNS leukemia according to cytomorphologic criteria.[346] During follow-up, CNS leukemia developed in six children, all belonging to the group with TdT$^+$ CSF at diagnosis. This finding implies that TdT staining of CSF samples has high prognostic value and should be used to supplement classic cytomorphology.[346] Monitoring of MRD in the CSF samples of more than 100 patients with a TdT$^+$ malignancy during a 5-year follow-up period showed the development of overt CNS involvement in 70% of the patients with repeated detection of TdT$^+$ cells in CSF despite normal cytomorphology.[346] On the other hand, patients with an elevated CSF leukocyte count or "suspicious" morphology but TdT negativity (probably activated lymphocytes) had no evidence of subsequent CNS disease.[199, 346]

Incomplete *TCRD* rearrangements have been used as a PCR target for detection of CNS involvement in childhood precursor–B-ALL.[347] Identical rearrangements were found in both BM and CSF in 43% of the patients analyzed, which confirms the clinical assumption that asymptomatic CNS involvement occurs much more frequently than diagnosed on the basis of classic cytomorphologic criteria.[347]

Early Diagnosis of Leukemia/Lymphoma in Patients with Unexplained Cytopenia

Hypoplastic bone marrow in ALL patients at initial evaluation is a rare phenomenon that occurs in about 2% of childhood ALL cases and is rarely seen in adult ALL.[348, 349] In contrast to aplastic anemia, the presence of relatively high frequencies of CD10$^+$TdT$^+$ cells in BM and PB is a distinct feature in hypoplastic bone marrow with smoldering leukemia.[37] A few published case reports have demonstrated the presence of identical clonal cell populations during the hypoplastic phase, the subsequent recovery phase, and overt leukemia when patient-specific gene rearrangements were used as PCR targets.[350, 351] In contrast, monoclonal gene rearrangements could not be detected in patients with idiopathic hypoplastic anemia.[351]

In a proportion of patients, unexplained cytopenia might mask underlying malignancies. In a comprehensive multiparameter flow cytometry study of 121 patients with pancytopenia and/or refractory anemia, Wells et al[352] showed the presence of an abnormal cell population

in 17 cases. Further immunophenotyping confirmed the diagnosis of hairy-cell leukemia in eight patients, NHL in two patients, and AML/MDS in the remaining seven patients. Importantly, the diagnosis of a lymphoid malignancy in six patients that was previously diagnosed as MDS resulted in a major treatment modification and deferral of BMT.[352]

Detection of Bone Marrow Involvement During "Isolated" Extramedullary Relapse of Acute Lymphoblastic Leukemia

"Isolated" extramedullary relapse (e.g., in the CNS or testes) in ALL patients is usually associated with detectable MRD levels in BM.[29, 198, 353-356] This finding is in concordance with the clinical observation that full systemic reinduction therapy is required in these patients to prevent impending hematologic relapse. Nevertheless, some ALL patients with isolated CNS relapse were reported without detectable MRD levels in BM.[164, 177, 198, 353] MRD positivity of histologically normal end-of-treatment testicular biopsy specimens was shown to be followed by overt testicular relapse.[356] Nevertheless, in some patients, testicular relapse did occur despite MRD negativity in testicular biopsy samples. Moreover, PCR-based MRD assays allow reliable exclusion of occult leukemic blasts in the histologically normal contralateral testis at the time of unilateral testicular relapse.[356]

Detection of Bone Marrow Involvement During Initial Staging of Non-Hodgkin's Lymphoma

Immunophenotypic and molecular detection of BM involvement has not yet been implemented into clinical staging of NHL. Initial evaluation of the tumor burden is based on cytomorphologic findings, with a requirement for bilateral bone marrow aspiration and biopsy in high-grade lymphoma.[357] Several studies have demonstrated the presence of aberrant CD5$^+$ TdT$^+$ cells in the BM of children with lymphoblastic T-NHL.[29, 358] Similarly, BM involvement detected by PCR analysis of *BCL2-IGH* is a constant feature of not only advanced-stage FCL with t(14;18) but also localized stages I and II.[243, 244] Preliminary results of a PCR-based MRD study of *IGH* genes in B-NHL have demonstrated a higher incidence of BM involvement than suggested by cytomorphologic findings.[359] Further prospective studies should reveal whether detection of BM involvement with sensitivities of 10^{-3} to 10^{-5} would improve the clinical outcome in lymphoma patients if MRD-positive patients receive more intensive treatment, including BMT.

MRD Detection in Autologous Stem-Cell Grafts

MRD in Autologous SC Grafts in ALL

Autologous purged BMT and autologous PBSC transplantation after intensified chemotherapy are currently being evaluated as new treatment modalities in aggressive lymphoproliferative diseases.[360] These treatment strategies are used in high-risk patients—for instance, in second complete remission of ALL when an allogeneic donor is not available. PCR studies have shown that MRD positivity of autologous BM grafts before purging is the most predictive factor of treatment failure in ALL, regardless of a successful purging procedure (MRD-negative graft).[361-363] In fact, the duration of remission after autologous BMT significantly correlates with MRD levels before the purging procedure. Study of *BCR-ABL*–positive ALL patients has revealed that autologous BM grafts are more heavily contaminated with leukemic cells than are autologous PBSC grafts.[364] Although the purging procedure might be more effective for autologous BM grafts, the chance of obtaining an MRD-negative autologous BM graft after purging is significantly lower than achieving an MRD-negative PBSC graft.[364] Detection of MRD in autologous BM or PBSC grafts is associated with an increased risk of relapse in ALL patients after transplantation.[188] In addition, ex vivo gene marking of autologous BM grafts suggests that residual malignant clonogenic cells in the autologous grafts are responsible for relapse after transplantation.[365]

MRD in Autologous SC Grafts in NHL

Several studies have focused on autologous BMT in B-NHL with t(14;18), where BM infiltration is common at the time of diagnosis.[243] Also, PBSC harvests are frequently contaminated by lymphoma cells, with MRD levels comparable to MRD in BM.[366, 367] Even CD34+CD19+ progenitors with t(14;18) could be identified in BM and PB.[251, 368] In fact, mobilization regimens before PBSC harvest might result in increased PB contamination with tumor cells, which was clearly shown for MCL.[258] With the currently available techniques, it is possible to effectively purge autologous grafts of FCL cells, as assessed by the disappearance of clonal *BCL2-IGH* PCR products.[369-371] In contrast, the purging procedure in MCL is generally unsuccessful.[257, 258, 371] Patients who received MRD-negative autologous grafts showed significantly longer disease-free survival than did those whose marrow contained residual clonal lymphoma cells after purging.[371, 372]

MRD in Autologous SC Grafts in CML

Autologous PBSC grafts in Ph+ CML patients that are negative by conventional cytogenetics usually demonstrate variable levels of *BCR-ABL* transcripts, with the two first aphereses containing the lowest degree of MRD.[373] Further studies should demonstrate whether any relationship exists between the degree of leukemic cell contamination of PBSC grafts and outcome after autologous transplantation in CML patients.

CONCLUSION

Several immunophenotyping and PCR techniques are available for MRD detection in patients with hematopoietic malignancies, as summarized in Table 12-6. Espe-

cially in precursor-B-ALL and T-ALL, multiple sensitive MRD techniques can be used. Each MRD technique has advantages and disadvantages, which have to be weighed carefully to make an appropriate choice (see Table 12-1). On the one hand, false-positive and false-negative results should be prevented, but on the other hand, the MRD techniques should be sufficiently sensitive. These requirements can generally be met with PCR analysis of chromosome aberrations if adequate precautionary measures are taken to prevent cross-contamination of the PCR products. Speed and relatively low cost will also play a role in the choice of MRD technique and can be achieved with flow cytometric MRD analysis. PCR analysis of junctional regions of Ig/TCR gene rearrangements has the advantage of broad applicability in all categories of lymphoid malignancies, as well as the advantage of high sensitivity levels (Table 12-6). Finally, numerous studies have shown that reliable MRD techniques should allow precise quantification of residual leukemic cells. Such quantification is an inherent feature of immunophenotyping, whereas the advent of quantitative PCR techniques, particularly RQ-PCR, has enabled not only precise quantification of levels of clonal PCR products but also their relationship to the single-cell level.

Although most MRD techniques are relatively sensitive, one should realize that MRD negativity does not exclude the presence of malignant cells.[374] Each MRD test screens only 10^5 to 10^6 cells, a minor fraction of the total amount of hematopoietic cells. In addition, it might well be that the distribution of low numbers of malignant lymphoid cells throughout the body is not homogeneous and that the cell sample investigated is therefore not fully representative.[375, 376]

Finally, the clinical impact of MRD detection in the various categories of hematopoietic malignancies is not identical. In ALL, the main application of MRD data was shown to be evaluation of the early response to treatment, with precise measurement of the reduction in tumor load during remission induction therapy. This approach can substantially improve treatment risk group stratification, which might be translated in the near future into a higher cure rate with less treatment-related toxicity. In contrast, the value of MRD detection in APL and CML relies on continuous monitoring, with possibilities of gauging the treatment based on MRD results. This application of MRD is also most probably the case in other subtypes of AML and mature lymphoid malignancies, but further studies are required to fully define the need and clinical significance of MRD monitoring in AML, CLLs, and NHL.

REFERENCES

1. Van Dongen JJM, Breit TM, Adriaansen HJ, et al: Detection of minimal residual disease in acute leukemia by immunological marker analysis and polymerase chain reaction. Leukemia 1992; 6:47.
2. Campana D, Pui CH: Detection of minimal residual disease in acute leukemia: Methodologic advances and clinical significance. Blood 1995;85:1416.
3. Van Dongen JJM, Szczepanski T, de Bruijn MAC, et al: Detection of minimal residual disease in acute leukemia patients. Cytokines Mol Ther 1996;2:121.

4. Sonta SI, Sandberg AA: Chromosomes and causation of human cancer and leukemia: XXVIII. Value of detailed chromosome studies on large numbers of cells in CML. Am J Hematol 1977;3:121.

5. Hittelman WN, Tigaud JD, Estey E, et al: Premature chromosome condensation in the study of minimal residual disease. Bone Marrow Transplant 1990;6:9.

6. Freireich EJ, Cork A, Stass SA, et al: Cytogenetics for detection of minimal residual disease in acute myeloblastic leukemia. Leukemia 1992;6:500.

7. Estrov Z, Grunberger T, Dube ID, et al: Detection of residual acute lymphoblastic leukemia cells in cultures of bone marrow obtained during remission. N Engl J Med 1986;315:538.

8. Gerhartz HH, Schmetzer H: Detection of minimal residual disease in acute myeloid leukemia. Leukemia 1990;4:508.

9. Uckun FM, Kersey JH, Vallera DA, et al: Autologous bone marrow transplantation in high-risk remission T-lineage acute lymphoblastic leukemia using immunotoxins plus 4-hydroperoxycyclophosphamide for marrow purging. Blood 1990;76:1723.

10. Miller CB, Zehnbauer BA, Piantadosi S, et al: Correlation of occult clonogenic leukemia drug sensitivity with relapse after autologous bone marrow transplantation. Blood 1991;78:1125.

11. Anastasi J, Thangavelu M, Vardiman JW, et al: Interphase cytogenetic analysis detects minimal residual disease in a case of acute lymphoblastic leukemia and resolves the question of origin of relapse after allogeneic bone marrow transplantation. Blood 1991; 77:1087.

12. Heerema NA, Argyropoulos G, Weetman R, et al: Interphase in situ hybridization reveals minimal residual disease in early remission and return of the diagnostic clone in karyotypically normal relapse of acute lymphoblastic leukemia. Leukemia 1993;7:537.

13. Nylund SJ, Ruutu T, Saarinen U, et al: Detection of minimal residual disease using fluorescence DNA in situ hybridization: A follow-up study in leukemia and lymphoma patients. Leukemia 1994;8:587.

14. El-Rifai W, Ruutu T, Vettenranta K, et al: Follow-up of residual disease using metaphase-FISH in patients with acute lymphoblastic leukemia in remission. Leukemia 1997;11:633.

15. Van der Burg M, Beverloo HB, Langerak AW, et al: Rapid and sensitive detection of all types of MLL gene translocations with a single FISH probe set. Leukemia 1999;13:2107.

16. Mancini M, Cedrone M, Diverio D, et al: Use of dual-color interphase FISH for the detection of inv(16) in acute myeloid leukemia at diagnosis, relapse and during follow-up: A study of 23 patients. Leukemia 2000;14:364.

17. Engel H, Drach J, Keyhani A, et al: Quantitation of minimal residual disease in acute myelogenous leukemia and myelodysplastic syndromes in complete remission by molecular cytogenetics of progenitor cells. Leukemia 1999;13:568.

18. Van Dongen JJM, Wolvers-Tettero ILM: Analysis of immunoglobulin and T cell receptor genes. Part I: Basic and technical aspects. Clin Chim Acta 1991;198:1.

19. Wright JJ, Poplack DG, Bakhshi A, et al: Gene rearrangements as markers of clonal variation and minimal residual disease in acute lymphoblastic leukemia. J Clin Oncol 1987;5:735.

20. Katz F, Ball L, Gibbons B, et al: The use of DNA probes to monitor minimal residual disease in childhood acute lymphoblastic leukaemia. Br J Haematol 1989;73:173.

21. Billadeau D, Blackstadt M, Greipp P, et al: Analysis of B-lymphoid malignancies using allele-specific polymerase chain reaction: A technique for sequential quantitation of residual disease. Blood 1991;78:3021.

22. Morgan GJ, Hughes T, Janssen JW, et al: Polymerase chain reaction for detection of residual leukaemia. Lancet 1989;1:928.

23. Gabert J, Thuret I, Lafage M, et al: Detection of residual bcr/abl translocation by polymerase chain reaction in chronic myeloid leukaemia patients after bone-marrow transplantation. Lancet 1989;2:1125.

24. Janossy G, Bollum FJ, Bradstock KF, et al: Cellular phenotypes of normal and leukemic hemopoietic cells determined by analysis with selected antibody combinations. Blood 1980;56:430.

25. Foon KA, Todd RF: Immunologic classification of leukemia and lymphoma. Blood 1986;68:1.

26. Greaves MF: Differentiation-linked leukemogenesis in lymphocytes. Science 1986;234:697.

27. Van Dongen JJ, Adriaansen HJ, Hooijkaas H: Immunophenotyping of leukaemias and non-Hodgkin's lymphomas. Immunological markers and their CD codes. Neth J Med 1988;33:298.

28. Jennings CD, Foon KA: Flow cytometry: Recent advances in diagnosis and monitoring of leukemia. Cancer Invest 1997;15:384.

29. Van Dongen JJM, Hooijkaas H, Adriaansen HJ, et al: Detection of minimal residual acute lymphoblastic leukemia by immunological marker analysis: Possibilities and limitations. In Hagenbeek A, Löwenberg B, eds: Minimal Residual Disease in Acute Leukemia. Dordrecht, Germany: Martinus Nijhoff; 1986, p 113.

30. Campana D, Coustan-Smith E, Janossy G: The immunologic detection of minimal residual disease in acute leukemia. Blood 1990; 76:163.

31. Van Dongen JJM, Adriaansen HJ, Hooijkaas H: Immunological marker analysis of cells in the various hematopoietic differentiation stages and their malignant counterparts. In Ruiter DJ, Fleuren GJ, Warnaar SO, eds: Application of Monoclonal Antibodies in Tumor Pathology. Dordrecht, Germany: Martinus Nijhoff; 1987, p 87.

32. Letwin BW, Wallace PK, Muirhead KA, et al: An improved clonal excess assay using flow cytometry and B-cell gating. Blood 1990; 75:1178.

33. Peters RE, Janossy G, Ivory K, et al: Leukemia-associated changes identified by quantitative flow cytometry. III. B-cell gating in CD37/kappa/lambda clonality test. Leukemia 1994;8:1864.

34. Van Dongen JJM, van den Beemd MWM, Schellekens M, et al: Analysis of malignant T cells with the Vβ antibody panel. Immunologist 1996;4:37.

35. Campana D, Coustan-Smith E: Detection of minimal residual disease in acute leukemia by flow cytometry. Cytometry 1999;38:139.

36. Langerak AW, Wolvers-Tettero ILM, van den Beemd MWM, et al: Immunophenotypic and immunogenotypic characteristics of TCRγδ+ T cell acute lymphoblastic leukemia. Leukemia 1999; 13:206.

37. Knulst AC, Adriaansen HJ, Hahlen K, et al: Early diagnosis of smoldering acute lymphoblastic leukemia using immunological marker analysis. Leukemia 1993;7:532.

38. Farahat N, Lens D, Zomas A, et al: Quantitative flow cytometry can distinguish between normal and leukaemic B-cell precursors. Br J Haematol 1995;91:640.

39. Smedmyr B, Bengtsson M, Jakobsson A, et al: Regeneration of CALLA (CD10+), TdT+ and double-positive cells in the bone marrow and blood after autologous bone marrow transplantation. Eur J Haematol 1991;46:146.

40. Van Lochem EG, Wiegers YM, van den Beemd R, et al: Regeneration pattern of precursor–B-cells in bone marrow of acute lymphoblastic leukemia patients depends on the type of preceding chemotherapy. Leukemia 2000;14:688.

41. Van Wering ER, van der Linden-Schrever BE, Szczepanski T, et al: Regenerating normal B-cell precursors during and after treatment of acute lymphoblastic leukaemia: Implications for monitoring of minimal residual disease. Br J Haematol 2000;110:139.

42. Vervoordeldonk SF, Merle PA, Behrendt H, et al: Triple immunofluorescence staining for prediction of relapse in childhood precursor B acute lymphoblastic leukaemia. Br J Haematol 1996;92:922.

43. Smith RG, Kitchens RL: Phenotypic heterogeneity of TDT+ cells in the blood and bone marrow: Implications for surveillance of residual leukemia. Blood 1989;74:312.

44. Macedo A, Orfao A, Ciudad J, et al: Phenotypic analysis of CD34 subpopulations in normal human bone marrow and its application for the detection of minimal residual disease. Leukemia 1995; 9:1896.

45. Drach J, Drach D, Glassl H, et al: Flow cytometric determination of atypical antigen expression in acute leukemia for the study of minimal residual disease. Cytometry 1992;13:893.

46. Hurwitz CA, Gore SD, Stone KD, et al: Flow cytometric detection of rare normal human marrow cells with immunophenotypes characteristic of acute lymphoblastic leukemia cells. Leukemia 1992;6:233.

47. Mori T, Sugita K, Suzuki T, et al: A novel monoclonal antibody, KOR-SA3544 which reacts to Philadelphia chromosome–positive acute lymphoblastic leukemia cells with high sensitivity. Leukemia 1995;9:1233.

48. Dworzak MN, Fritsch G, Fleischer C, et al: Comparative phenotype mapping of normal vs. malignant pediatric B-lymphopoiesis unveils leukemia-associated aberrations. Exp Hematol 1998;26:305.

49. Behm FG, Smith FO, Raimondi SC, et al: Human homologue of the rat chondroitin sulfate proteoglycan, NG2, detected by mono-

clonal antibody 7.1, identifies childhood acute lymphoblastic leukemias with t(4;11)(q21;q23) or t(11;19)(q23;p13) and MLL gene rearrangements. Blood 1996;87:1134.

50. Smith FO, Rauch C, Williams DE, et al: The human homologue of rat NG2, a chondroitin sulfate proteoglycan, is not expressed on the cell surface of normal hematopoietic cells but is expressed by acute myeloid leukemia blasts from poor-prognosis patients with abnormalities of chromosome band 11q23. Blood 1996;87:1123.

51. Wells DA, Sale GE, Shulman HM, et al: Multidimensional flow cytometry of marrow can differentiate leukemic from normal lymphoblasts and myeloblasts after chemotherapy and bone marrow transplantation. Am J Clin Pathol 1998;110:84.

52. Lucio P, Parreira A, van den Beemd MW, et al: Flow cytometric analysis of normal B cell differentiation: A frame of reference for the detection of minimal residual disease in precursor–B-ALL. Leukemia 1999;13:419.

53. Weir EG, Cowan K, LeBeau P, et al: A limited antibody panel can distinguish B-precursor acute lymphoblastic leukemia from normal B precursors with four color flow cytometry: Implications for residual disease detection. Leukemia 1999;13:558.

54. Griesinger F, Piró-Noack M, Kaib N, et al: Leukaemia-associated immunophenotypes (LIAP) are observed on 90% of adult and childhood acute lymphoblastic leukaemia: Detection in remission marrow predicts outcome. Br J Haematol 1999;105:241.

55. Coustan-Smith E, Behm FG, Sanchez J, et al: Immunological detection of minimal residual disease in children with acute lymphoblastic leukaemia. Lancet 1998;351:550.

56. Ciudad J, San Miguel JF, Lopez-Berges MC, et al: Prognostic value of immunophenotypic detection of minimal residual disease in acute lymphoblastic leukemia. J Clin Oncol 1998;16:3774.

57. Ciudad J, San Miguel JF, Lopez-Berges MC, et al: Detection of abnormalities in B-cell differentiation pattern is a useful tool to predict relapse in precursor–B-ALL. Br J Haematol 1999;104:695.

58. Sang BC, Shi L, Dias P, et al: Monoclonal antibodies specific to the acute lymphoblastic leukemia t(1;19)-associated E2A/PBX1 chimeric protein: Characterization and diagnostic utility. Blood 1997; 89:2909.

59. Nowak R, Oelschlaegel U, Schuler U, et al: Sensitivity of combined DNA/immunophenotype flow cytometry for the detection of low levels of aneuploid lymphoblastic leukemia cells in bone marrow. Cytometry 1997;30:47.

60. Van Wering ER, Beishuizen A, Roeffen ET, et al: Immunophenotypic changes between diagnosis and relapse in childhood acute lymphoblastic leukemia. Leukemia 1995;9:1523.

61. Abshire TC, Buchanan GR, Jackson JF, et al: Morphologic, immunologic and cytogenetic studies in children with acute lymphoblastic leukemia at diagnosis and relapse: A Pediatric Oncology Group study. Leukemia 1992;6:357.

62. Porwit-MacDonald A, Bjorklund E, Lucio P, et al: BIOMED-1 concerted action report: Flow cytometric characterization of CD7+ cell subsets in normal bone marrow as a basis for the diagnosis and follow-up of T cell acute lymphoblastic leukemia (T-ALL). Leukemia 2000;14:816.

63. Brown L, Cheng JT, Chen Q, et al: Site-specific recombination of the tal-1 gene is a common occurrence in human T cell leukemia. EMBO J 1990;9:3343.

64. Breit TM, Mol EJ, Wolvers-Tettero ILM, et al: Site-specific deletions involving the tal-1 and sil genes are restricted to cells of the T cell receptor alpha/beta lineage: T cell receptor delta gene deletion mechanism affects multiple genes. J Exp Med 1993;177:965.

65. Delabesse E, Bernard M, Meyer V, et al: TAL1 expression does not occur in the majority of T-ALL blasts. Br J Haematol 1998;102:449.

66. Visser L, Shaw A, Slupsky J, et al: Monoclonal antibodies reactive with hairy cell leukemia. Blood 1989;74:320.

67. Geisler CH, Larsen JK, Hansen NE, et al: Prognostic importance of flow cytometric immunophenotyping of 540 consecutive patients with B-cell chronic lymphocytic leukemia. Blood 1991;78:1795.

68. Kurec AS, Threatte GA, Gottlieb AJ, et al: Immunophenotypic subclassification of chronic lymphocytic leukaemia (CLL). Br J Haematol 1992;81:45.

69. Robbins BA, Ellison DJ, Spinosa JC, et al: Diagnostic application of two-color flow cytometry in 161 cases of hairy cell leukemia. Blood 1993;82:1277.

70. Molot RJ, Meeker TC, Wittwer CT, et al: Antigen expression and polymerase chain reaction amplification of mantle cell lymphomas. Blood 1994;83:1626.

71. Lenormand B, Bizet M, Fruchart C, et al: Residual disease in B-cell chronic lymphocytic leukemia patients and prognostic value. Leukemia 1994;8:1019.

72. Cabezudo E, Matutes E, Ramrattan M, et al: Analysis of residual disease in chronic lymphocytic leukemia by flow cytometry. Leukemia 1997;11:1909.

73. Hermine O, Haioun C, Lepage E, et al: Prognostic significance of bcl-2 protein expression in aggressive non-Hodgkin's lymphoma. Blood 1996;87:265.

74. Gala JL, Guiot Y, Delannoy A, et al: Use of image analysis and immunostaining of bone marrow trephine biopsy specimens to quantify residual disease in patients with B-cell chronic lymphocytic leukemia. Mod Pathol 1999;12:391.

75. De Boer CJ, Schuuring E, Dreef E, et al: Cyclin D1 protein analysis in the diagnosis of mantle cell lymphoma. Blood 1995;86:2715.

76. Van den Beemd MWM, Boor PPC, Van Lochem EG, et al: Flow cytometric analysis of the Vβ repertoire in healthy controls. Cytometry 2000;40:336.

77. Triebel F, Hercend T: Subpopulations of human peripheral T gamma delta lymphocytes. Immunol Today 1989;10:186.

78. Borst J, Wicherink A, Van Dongen JJM, et al: Non-random expression of T cell receptor gamma and delta variable gene segments in functional T lymphocyte clones from human peripheral blood. Eur J Immunol 1989;19:1559.

79. Pulford K, Lamant L, Morris SW, et al: Detection of anaplastic lymphoma kinase (ALK) and nucleolar protein nucleophosmin (NPM)-ALK proteins in normal and neoplastic cells with the monoclonal antibody ALK1. Blood 1997;89:1394.

80. San Miguel JF, Gonzalez M, Orfao A: Detection of minimal residual disease in myeloid malignancies. In Degos L, Linch D, Löwenberg B, eds: Textbook of Malignant Haematology. London: Martin Dunitz; 1998, p 871.

81. Macedo A, Orfao A, Vidriales MB, et al: Characterization of aberrant phenotypes in acute myeloblastic leukemia. Ann Hematol 1995;70:189.

82. Adriaansen HJ, van Dongen JJ, Kappers-Klunne MC, et al: Terminal deoxynucleotidyl transferase positive subpopulations occur in the majority of ANLL: Implications for the detection of minimal disease. Leukemia 1990;4:404.

83. Drexler HG, Thiel E, Ludwig WD: Acute myeloid leukemias expressing lymphoid-associated antigens: Diagnostic incidence and prognostic significance. Leukemia 1993;7:489.

84. Drexler HG, Sperling C, Ludwig WD: Terminal deoxynucleotidyl transferase (TdT) expression in acute myeloid leukemia. Leukemia 1993;7:1142.

85. Paietta E, Van Ness B, Bennett J, et al: Lymphoid lineage–associated features in acute myeloid leukemia: Phenotypic and genotypic correlations. Br J Haematol 1992;82:324.

86. Reading CL, Estey EH, Huh YO, et al: Expression of unusual immunophenotype combinations in acute myelogenous leukemia. Blood 1993;81:3083.

87. Smith FO, Lampkin BC, Versteeg C, et al: Expression of lymphoid-associated cell surface antigens by childhood acute myeloid leukemia cells lacks prognostic significance. Blood 1992;79:2415.

88. Coustan-Smith E, Behm FG, Hurwitz CA, et al: N-CAM (CD56) expression by CD34+ malignant myeloblasts has implications for minimal residual disease detection in acute myeloid leukemia. Leukemia 1993;7:853.

89. Macedo A, Orfao A, Martinez A, et al: Immunophenotype of c-kit cells in normal human bone marrow: Implications for the detection of minimal residual disease in AML. Br J Haematol 1995; 89:338.

90. Macedo A, Orfao A, Gonzalez M, et al: Immunological detection of blast cell subpopulations in acute myeloblastic leukemia at diagnosis: Implications for minimal residual disease studies. Leukemia 1995;9:993.

91. Nakamura K, Ogata K, An E, et al: Flow cytometric assessment of CD15+CD17+ cells for the detection of minimal residual disease in adult acute myeloid leukaemia. Br J Haematol 2000;108:710.

92. Adriaansen HJ, te Boekhorst PA, Hagemeijer AM, et al: Acute myeloid leukemia M4 with bone marrow eosinophilia (M4Eo) and inv(16)(p13q22) exhibits a specific immunophenotype with CD2 expression. Blood 1993;81:3043.

93. Terstappen LW, Safford M, Konemann S, et al: Flow cytometric characterization of acute myeloid leukemia. Part II. Phenotypic heterogeneity at diagnosis. Leukemia 1992;6:70.

94. Adriaansen HJ, Jacobs BC, Kappers-Klunne MC, et al: Detection of residual disease in AML patients by use of double immunological marker analysis for terminal deoxynucleotidyl transferase and myeloid markers. Leukemia 1993;7:472.

95. Macedo A, San Miguel JF, Vidriales MB, et al: Phenotypic changes in acute myeloid leukaemia: Implications in the detection of minimal residual disease. J Clin Pathol 1996;49:15.

96. Martinez A, San Miguel JF, Vidriales MB, et al: An abnormal CD34 + myeloid/CD34 + lymphoid ratio at the end of chemotherapy predicts relapse in patients with acute myeloid leukemia. Cytometry 1999;38:70.

97. Campana D, Yokota S, Coustan-Smith E, et al: The detection of residual acute lymphoblastic leukemia cells with immunologic methods and polymerase chain reaction: A comparative study. Leukemia 1990;4:609.

98. Negrin RS, Blume KG: The use of the polymerase chain reaction for the detection of minimal residual malignant disease. Blood 1991;78:255.

99. Sklar J: Polymerase chain reaction: The molecular microscope of residual disease. J Clin Oncol 1991;9:1521.

100. Potter MN, Steward CG, Oakhill A: The significance of detection of minimal residual disease in childhood acute lymphoblastic leukaemia. Br J Haematol 1993;83:412.

101. Kwok S, Higuchi R: Avoiding false positives with PCR. Nature 1989;339:237.

102. Breit TM, Wolvers-Tettero ILM, Hählen K, et al: Extensive junctional diversity of γδ T-cell receptors expressed by T-cell acute lymphoblastic leukemias: Implications for the detection of minimal residual disease. Leukemia 1991;5:1076.

103. Yamada M, Hudson S, Tournay O, et al: Detection of minimal disease in hematopoietic malignancies of the B-cell lineage by using third-complementarity-determining region (CDR-III)-specific probes. Proc Natl Acad Sci U S A 1989;86:5123.

104. d'Auriol L, Macintyre E, Galibert F, et al: In vitro amplification of T cell gamma gene rearrangements: A new tool for the assessment of minimal residual disease in acute lymphoblastic leukemias. Leukemia 1989;3:155.

105. Hansen-Hagge TE, Yokota S, Bartram CR: Detection of minimal residual disease in acute lymphoblastic leukemia by in vitro amplification of rearranged T-cell receptor delta chain sequences. Blood 1989;74:1762.

106. Jonsson OG, Kitchens RL, Scott FC, et al: Detection of minimal residual disease in acute lymphoblastic leukemia using immunoglobulin hypervariable region specific oligonucleotide probes. Blood 1990;76:2072.

107. Macintyre EA, d'Auriol L, Duparc N, et al: Use of oligonucleotide probes directed against T cell antigen receptor gamma delta variable-(diversity)-joining junctional sequences as a general method for detecting minimal residual disease in acute lymphoblastic leukemias. J Clin Invest 1990;86:2125.

108. Bartram CR: Detection of minimal residual leukemia by the polymerase chain reaction: Potential implications for therapy. Clin Chim Acta 1993;217:75.

109. Van Dongen JJM, Szczepanski T, Langerak AW, et al: Detection of minimal residual disease in lymphoid malignancies. In Degos L, Linch D, Löwenberg B, eds: Textbook of Malignant Haematology. London: Martin Dunitz; 1998, p 685.

110. Pongers-Willemse MJ, Seriu T, Stolz F, et al: Primers and protocols for standardized MRD detection in ALL using immunoglobulin and T cell receptor gene rearrangements and TAL1 deletions as PCR targets. Report of the BIOMED-1 CONCERTED ACTION: Investigation of minimal residual disease in acute leukemia. Leukemia 1999; 13:110.

111. Beishuizen A, de Bruijn MAC, Pongers-Willemse MJ, et al: Heterogeneity in junctional regions of immunoglobulin kappa deleting element rearrangements in B cell leukemias: A new molecular target for detection of minimal residual disease. Leukemia 1997; 11:2200.

112. Szczepanski T, Beishuizen A, Pongers-Willemse MJ, et al: Cross-lineage T-cell receptor gene rearrangements occur in more than ninety percent of childhood precursor–B-acute lymphoblastic leukemias: Alternative PCR targets for detection of minimal residual disease. Leukemia 1999;13:196.

113. Breit TM, Wolvers-Tettero ILM, Beishuizen A, et al: Southern blot patterns, frequencies and junctional diversity of T-cell receptor δ

gene rearrangements in acute lymphoblastic leukemia. Blood 1993;82:3063.

114. Szczepanski T, Langerak AW, Willemse MJ, et al: T cell receptor gamma (TCRG) gene rearrangements in T cell acute lymphoblastic leukemia reflect "end-stage" recombinations: Implications for minimal residual disease monitoring. Leukemia 2000;14:1208.

115. Beishuizen A, Verhoeven MA, van Wering ER, et al: Analysis of Ig and T-cell receptor genes in 40 childhood acute lymphoblastic leukemias at diagnosis and subsequent relapse: Implications for the detection of minimal residual disease by polymerase chain reaction analysis. Blood 1994;83:2238.

116. Bird J, Galili N, Link M, et al: Continuing rearrangement but absence of somatic hypermutation in immunoglobulin genes of human B cell precursor leukemia. J Exp Med 1988;168:229.

117. Wasserman R, Yamada M, Ito Y, et al: V_H gene rearrangement events can modify the immunoglobulin heavy chain during progression of B-lineage acute lymphoblastic leukemia. Blood 1992; 79:223.

118. Kitchingman GR: Immunoglobulin heavy chain gene V_H-D junctional diversity at diagnosis in patients with acute lymphoblastic leukemia. Blood 1993;81:775.

119. Steenbergen EJ, Verhagen OJ, van Leeuwen EF, et al: Distinct ongoing Ig heavy chain rearrangement processes in childhood B-precursor acute lymphoblastic leukemia. Blood 1993;82:581.

120. Ghali DW, Panzer S, Fischer S, et al: Heterogeneity of the T-cell receptor delta gene indicating subclone formation in acute precursor B-cell leukemias. Blood 1995;85:2795.

121. Steward CG, Goulden NJ, Katz F, et al: A polymerase chain reaction study of the stability of Ig heavy-chain and T-cell receptor delta gene rearrangements between presentation and relapse of childhood B-lineage acute lymphoblastic leukemia. Blood 1994;83: 1355.

122. Taylor JJ, Rowe D, Kylefjord H, et al: Characterisation of non-concordance in the T-cell receptor gamma chain genes at presentation and clinical relapse in acute lymphoblastic leukemia. Leukemia 1994;8:60.

123. Steenbergen EJ, Verhagen OJ, van Leeuwen EF, et al: Frequent ongoing T-cell receptor rearrangements in childhood B-precursor acute lymphoblastic leukemia: Implications for monitoring minimal residual disease. Blood 1995;86:692.

124. Beishuizen A, Hählen K, Hagemeijer A, et al: Multiple rearranged immunoglobulin genes in childhood acute lymphoblastic leukemia of precursor B-cell origin. Leukemia 1991;5:657.

125. Szczepanski T, Langerak AW, Wolvers-Tettero ILM, et al: Immunoglobulin and T cell receptor gene rearrangement patterns in acute lymphoblastic leukemia are less mature in adults than in children: Implications for selection of PCR targets for detection of minimal residual disease. Leukemia 1998;12:1081.

126. Beishuizen A, Verhoeven MA, Mol EJ, et al: Detection of immunoglobulin kappa light-chain gene rearrangement patterns by Southern blot analysis. Leukemia 1994;8:2228.

127. Wagner SD, Martinelli V, Luzzatto L: Similar patterns of V kappa gene usage but different degrees of somatic mutation in hairy cell leukemia, prolymphocytic leukemia, Waldenström's macroglobulinemia, and myeloma. Blood 1994;83:3647.

128. Cannell PK, Amlot P, Attard M, et al: Variable kappa gene rearrangement in lymphoproliferative disorders: An analysis of V kappa gene usage. VJ joining and somatic mutation. Leukemia 1994;8:1139.

129. Hamblin TJ, Davis Z, Gardiner A, et al: Unmutated Ig V(H) genes are associated with a more aggressive form of chronic lymphocytic leukemia. Blood 1999;94:1848.

130. Rajewsky K, Forster I, Cumano A: Evolutionary and somatic selection of the antibody repertoire in the mouse. Science 1987;238: 1088.

131. Berek C, Milstein C: Mutation drift and repertoire shift in the maturation of the immune response. Immunol Rev 1987;96:23.

132. Derksen PW, Langerak AW, Kerkhof E, et al: Comparison of different polymerase chain reaction–based approaches for clonality assessment of immunoglobulin heavy-chain gene rearrangements in B-cell neoplasia. Mod Pathol 1999;12:794.

133. Cleary ML, Meeker TC, Levy S, et al: Clustering of extensive somatic mutations in the variable region of an immunoglobulin heavy chain gene from a human B cell lymphoma. Cell 1986;44:97.

134. Van Dongen JJM, Wolvers-Tettero ILM: Analysis of immunoglobulin

and T cell receptor genes. Part II: Possibilities and limitations in the diagnosis and management of lymphoproliferative diseases and related disorders. Clin Chim Acta 1991;198:93.

135. Biondi A, Allavena P, Rossi V, et al: T cell receptor delta gene organization and expression in normal and leukemic natural killer cells. J Immunol 1989;143:1009.

136. Breit TM, Beishuizen A, Ludwig WD, et al: tal-1 deletions in T-cell acute lymphoblastic leukemia as PCR target for detection of minimal residual disease. Leukemia 1993;7:2004.

137. Rabbitts TH: Chromosomal translocations in human cancer. Nature 1994;372:143.

138. Pallisgaard N, Hokland P, Riishoj DC, et al: Multiplex reverse transcription–polymerase chain reaction for simultaneous screening of 29 translocations and chromosomal aberrations in acute leukemia. Blood 1998;92:574.

139. Van Dongen JJM, Macintyre EA, Gabert JA, et al: Standardized RT-PCR analysis of fusion gene transcripts from chromosome aberrations in acute leukemia for detection of minimal residual disease. Report of the BIOMED-1 CONCERTED ACTION: Investigation of minimal residual disease in acute leukemia. Leukemia 1999;13:1901.

140. Morris SW, Kirstein MN, Valentine MB, et al: Fusion of a kinase gene, ALK, to a nucleolar protein gene, NPM, in non-Hodgkin's lymphoma. Science 1994;263:1281.

141. Wiemels JL, Cazzaniga G, Daniotti M, et al: Prenatal origin of acute lymphoblastic leukaemia in children. Lancet 1999;354:1499.

142. Reichel M, Gillert E, Breitenlohner I, et al: Rapid isolation of chromosomal breakpoints from patients with t(4;11) acute lymphoblastic leukemia: Implications for basic and clinical research. Cancer Res 1999;59:3357.

143. Biernaux C, Loos M, Sels A, et al: Detection of major bcr-abl gene expression at a very low level in blood cells of some healthy individuals. Blood 1995;86:3118.

144. Bose S, Deininger M, Gora-Tybor J, et al: The presence of typical and atypical BCR-ABL fusion genes in leukocytes of normal individuals: Biologic significance and implications for the assessment of minimal residual disease. Blood 1998;92:3362.

145. Limpens J, Stad R, Vos C, et al: Lymphoma-associated translocation t(14;18) in blood B cells of normal individuals. Blood 1995;85:2528.

146. Liu Y, Hernandez AM, Shibata D, et al: BCL2 translocation frequency rises with age in humans. Proc Natl Acad Sci U S A 1994;91:8910.

147. Look AT: Oncogenic transcription factors in the human acute leukemias. Science 1997;278:1059.

148. Delabesse E, Bernard M, Landman-Parker J, et al: Simultaneous SIL-TAL1 RT-PCR detection of all tal(d) deletions and identification of novel tal(d) variants. Br J Haematol 1997;99:901.

149. Cayuela JM, Madani A, Sanhes L, et al: Multiple tumor-suppressor gene 1 inactivation is the most frequent genetic alteration in T-cell acute lymphoblastic leukemia. Blood 1996;87:2180.

150. Cayuela JM, Gardie B, Sigaux F: Disruption of the multiple tumor suppressor gene MTS1/p16(INK4a)/CDKN2 by illegitimate V(D)J recombinase activity in T-cell acute lymphoblastic leukemias. Blood 1997;90:3720.

151. Cleary ML, Sklar J: Nucleotide sequence of a t(14;18) chromosomal breakpoint in follicular lymphoma and demonstration of a breakpoint-cluster region near a transcriptionally active locus on chromosome 18. Proc Natl Acad Sci U S A 1985;82:7439.

152. Tsujimoto Y, Croce CM: Analysis of the structure, transcripts, and protein products of bcl-2, the gene involved in human follicular lymphoma. Proc Natl Acad Sci U S A 1986;83:5214.

153. De Boer CJ, Loyson S, Kluin PM, et al: Multiple breakpoints within the BCL-1 locus in B-cell lymphoma: Rearrangements of the cyclin D1 gene. Cancer Res 1993;53:4148.

154. Williams ME, Meeker TC, Swerdlow SH: Rearrangement of the chromosome 11 bcl-1 locus in centrocytic lymphoma: Analysis with multiple breakpoint probes. Blood 1991;78:493.

155. Leder P, Battey J, Lenoir G, et al: Translocations among antibody genes in human cancer. Science 1983;222:765.

156. Lee MS, Chang KS, Cabanillas F, et al: Detection of minimal residual cells carrying the t(14;18) by DNA sequence amplification. Science 1987;237:175.

157. Crescenzi M, Seto M, Herzig GP, et al: Thermostable DNA polymerase chain amplification of t(14;18) chromosome breakpoints and detection of minimal residual disease. Proc Natl Acad Sci U S A 1988;85:4869.

158. De Boer CJ, van Krieken JH, Schuuring E, et al: Bcl-1/cyclin D1 in malignant lymphoma. Ann Oncol 1997;8:109.

159. Lo Coco F, Diverio D, Falini B, et al: Genetic diagnosis and molecular monitoring in the management of acute promyelocytic leukemia. Blood 1999;94:12.

160. Sykes PJ, Neoh SH, Brisco MJ, et al: Quantitation of targets for PCR by use of limiting dilution. Biotechniques 1992;13:444.

161. Ouspenskaia MV, Johnston DA, Roberts WM, et al: Accurate quantitation of residual B-precursor acute lymphoblastic leukemia by limiting dilution and a PCR-based detection system: A description of the method and the principles involved. Leukemia 1995;9:321.

162. Lion T, Izraeli S, Henn T, et al: Monitoring of residual disease in chronic myelogenous leukemia by quantitative polymerase chain reaction. Leukemia 1992;6:495.

163. Cross NC, Feng L, Chase A, et al: Competitive polymerase chain reaction to estimate the number of BCR-ABL transcripts in chronic myeloid leukemia patients after bone marrow transplantation. Blood 1993;82:1929.

164. Cave H, Guidal C, Rohrlich P, et al: Prospective monitoring and quantitation of residual blasts in childhood acute lymphoblastic leukemia by polymerase chain reaction study of delta and gamma T-cell receptor genes. Blood 1994;83:1892.

165. Heid CA, Stevens J, Livak KJ, et al: Real time quantitative PCR. Genome Res 1996;6:986.

166. Holland PM, Abramson RD, Watson R, et al: Detection of specific polymerase chain reaction product by utilizing the 5′ → 3′ exonuclease activity of *Thermus aquaticus* DNA polymerase. Proc Natl Acad Sci U S A 1991;88:7276.

167. Kreuzer KA, Lass U, Bohn A, et al: LightCycler technology for the quantitation of bcr/abl fusion transcripts. Cancer Res 1999;59:3171.

168. Luthra R, McBride JA, Cabanillas F, et al: Novel 5′ exonuclease-based real-time PCR assay for the detection of t(14;18)(q32;q21) in patients with follicular lymphoma. Am J Pathol 1998;153:63.

169. Marcucci G, Livak KJ, Bi W, et al: Detection of minimal residual disease in patients with AML1/ETO-associated acute myeloid leukemia using a novel quantitative reverse transcription polymerase chain reaction assay. Leukemia 1998;12:1482.

170. Mensink E, van de Locht A, Schattenberg A, et al: Quantitation of minimal residual disease in Philadelphia chromosome positive chronic myeloid leukaemia patients using real-time quantitative RT-PCR. Br J Haematol 1998;102:768.

171. Pallisgaard N, Clausen N, Schroder H, et al: Rapid and sensitive minimal residual disease detection in acute leukemia by quantitative real-time RT-PCR exemplified by t(12;21) TEL-AML1 fusion transcript. Genes Chromosomes Cancer 1999;26:355.

172. Pongers-Willemse MJ, Verhagen OJHM, Tibbe GJM, et al: Real-time quantitative PCR for the detection of minimal residual disease in acute lymphoblastic leukemia using junctional region specific TaqMan probes. Leukemia 1998;12:2006.

173. Verhagen OJHM, Willemse MJ, Breunis WB, et al: Application of germline *IGH* probes in real-time quantitative PCR for the detection of minimal residual disease in acute lymphoblastic leukemia. Leukemia 2000;14:1426.

174. Eckert C, Landt O, Taube T, et al: Potential of LightCycler technology for quantification of minimal residual disease in childhood acute lymphoblastic leukemia. Leukemia 2000;14:316.

175. Emig M, Saussele S, Wittor H, et al: Accurate and rapid analysis of residual disease in patients with CML using specific fluorescent hybridization probes for real time quantitative RT-PCR. Leukemia 1999;13:1825.

176. Nakao M, Janssen JW, Flohr T, et al: Rapid and reliable quantification of minimal residual disease in acute lymphoblastic leukemia using rearranged immunoglobulin and T-cell receptor loci by LightCycler technology. Cancer Res 2000;60:3281.

177. Yamada M, Wasserman R, Lange B, et al: Minimal residual disease in childhood B-lineage lymphoblastic leukemia. Persistence of leukemic cells during the first 18 months of treatment. N Engl J Med 1990;323:448.

178. Yokota S, Hansen-Hagge TE, Ludwig WD, et al: Use of polymerase chain reactions to monitor minimal residual disease in acute lymphoblastic leukemia patients. Blood 1991;77:331.

179. Nizet Y, Martiat P, Vaerman JL, et al: Follow-up of residual disease

(MRD) in B lineage acute leukaemias using a simplified PCR strategy: Evolution of MRD rather than its detection is correlated with clinical outcome. Br J Haematol 1991;79:205.

180. Neale GA, Menarguez J, Kitchingman GR, et al: Detection of minimal residual disease in T-cell acute lymphoblastic leukemia using polymerase chain reaction predicts impending relapse. Blood 1991;78:739.

181. Wasserman R, Galili N, Ito Y, et al: Residual disease at the end of induction therapy as a predictor of relapse during therapy in childhood B-lineage acute lymphoblastic leukemia. J Clin Oncol 1992;10:1879.

182. Biondi A, Yokota S, Hansen-Hagge TE, et al: Minimal residual disease in childhood acute lymphoblastic leukemia: Analysis of patients in continuous complete remission or with consecutive relapse. Leukemia 1992;6:282.

183. Ito Y, Wasserman R, Galili N, et al: Molecular residual disease status at the end of chemotherapy fails to predict subsequent relapse in children with B-lineage acute lymphoblastic leukemia. J Clin Oncol 1993;11:546.

184. Nizet Y, Van Daele S, Lewalle P, et al: Long-term follow-up of residual disease in acute lymphoblastic leukemia patients in complete remission using clonogeneic IgH probes and the polymerase chain reaction. Blood 1993;82:1618.

185. Brisco MJ, Condon J, Hughes E, et al: Outcome prediction in childhood acute lymphoblastic leukaemia by molecular quantification of residual disease at the end of induction. Lancet 1994; 343:196.

186. Kitchingman GR: Residual disease detection in multiple follow-up samples in children with acute lymphoblastic leukemia. Leukemia 1994;8:395.

187. Steenbergen EJ, Verhagen OJ, van Leeuwen EF, et al: Prolonged persistence of PCR-detectable minimal residual disease after diagnosis or first relapse predicts poor outcome in childhood B-precursor acute lymphoblastic leukemia. Leukemia 1995;9:1726.

188. Seriu T, Yokota S, Nakao M, et al: Prospective monitoring of minimal residual disease during the course of chemotherapy in patients with acute lymphoblastic leukemia, and detection of contaminating tumor cells in peripheral blood stem cells for autotransplantation. Leukemia 1995;9:615.

189. Roberts WM, Estrov Z, Ouspenskaia MV, et al: Measurement of residual leukemia during remission in childhood acute lymphoblastic leukemia. N Engl J Med 1997;336:317.

190. Foroni L, Coyle LA, Papaioannou M, et al: Molecular detection of minimal residual disease in adult and childhood acute lymphoblastic leukaemia reveals differences in treatment response. Leukemia 1997;11:1732.

191. Dibenedetto SP, Lo Nigro L, Mayer SP, et al: Detectable molecular residual disease at the beginning of maintenance therapy indicates poor outcome in children with T-cell acute lymphoblastic leukemia. Blood 1997;90:1226.

192. Gruhn B, Hongeng S, Yi H, et al: Minimal residual disease after intensive induction therapy in childhood acute lymphoblastic leukemia predicts outcome. Leukemia 1998;12:675.

193. Goulden NJ, Knechtli CJ, Garland RJ, et al: Minimal residual disease analysis for the prediction of relapse in children with standard-risk acute lymphoblastic leukaemia. Br J Haematol 1998;100:235.

194. Evans PA, Short MA, Owen RG, et al: Residual disease detection using fluorescent polymerase chain reaction at 20 weeks of therapy predicts clinical outcome in childhood acute lymphoblastic leukemia. J Clin Oncol 1998;16:3616.

195. Farahat N, Morilla A, Owusu-Ankomah K, et al: Detection of minimal residual disease in B-lineage acute lymphoblastic leukemia by quantitative flow cytometry. Br J Haematol 1998;101:158.

196. Cave H, van der Werff ten Bosch J, Suciu S, et al: Clinical significance of minimal residual disease in childhood acute lymphoblastic leukemia. N Engl J Med 1998;339:591.

197. Jacquy C, Delepaut B, Van Daele S, et al: A prospective study of minimal residual disease in childhood B-lineage acute lymphoblastic leukaemia: MRD level at the end of induction is a strong predictive factor of relapse. Br J Haematol 1997;98:140.

198. Van Dongen JJM, Seriu T, Panzer-Grumayer ER, et al: Prognostic value of minimal residual disease in acute lymphoblastic leukaemia in childhood. Lancet 1998;352:1731.

199. Campana D: Applications of cytometry to study acute leukemia: In vitro determination of drug sensitivity and detection of minimal residual disease. Cytometry 1994;18:68.

200. Foroni L, Harrison CJ, Hoffbrand AV, et al: Investigation of minimal residual disease in childhood and adult acute lymphoblastic leukaemia by molecular analysis. Br J Haematol 1999;105:7.

201. Cayuela JM, Baruchel A, Orange C, et al: TEL-AML1 fusion RNA as a new target to detect minimal residual disease in pediatric B-cell precursor acute lymphoblastic leukemia. Blood 1996;88:302.

202. Nakao M, Yokota S, Horiike S, et al: Detection and quantification of TEL/AML1 fusion transcripts by polymerase chain reaction in childhood acute lymphoblastic leukemia. Leukemia 1996;10:1463.

203. Stiller CA, Bunch KJ: Trends in survival for childhood cancer in Britain diagnosed 1971–85. Br J Cancer 1990;62:806.

204. Rivera GK, Pinkel D, Simone JV, et al: Treatment of acute lymphoblastic leukemia. 30 years' experience at St. Jude Children's Research Hospital. N Engl J Med 1993;329:1289.

205. Panzer-Grumayer ER, Schneider M, Panzer S, et al: Rapid molecular response during early induction chemotherapy predicts a good outcome in childhood acute lymphoblastic leukemia. Blood 2000; 95:790.

206. Rivera GK, Raimondi SC, Hancock ML, et al: Improved outcome in childhood acute lymphoblastic leukaemia with reinforced early treatment and rotational combination chemotherapy. Lancet 1991; 337:61.

207. Scholten C, Fodinger M, Mitterbauer M, et al: Kinetics of minimal residual disease during induction/consolidation therapy in standard-risk adult B-lineage acute lymphoblastic leukaemia. Ann Hematol 1995;71:155.

208. Brisco MJ, Hughes E, Neoh SH, et al: Relationship between minimal residual disease and outcome in adult acute lymphoblastic leukemia. Blood 1996;87:5251.

209. Knechtli CJ, Goulden NJ, Hancock JP, et al: Minimal residual disease status before allogeneic bone marrow transplantation is an important determinant of successful outcome for children and adolescents with acute lymphoblastic leukemia. Blood 1998;92: 4072.

210. Radich J, Ladne P, Gooley T: Polymerase chain reaction-based detection of minimal residual disease in acute lymphoblastic leukemia predicts relapse after allogeneic BMT. Biol Blood Marrow Transplant 1995;1:24.

211. Knechtli CJ, Goulden NJ, Hancock JP, et al: Minimal residual disease status as a predictor of relapse after allogeneic bone marrow transplantation for children with acute lymphoblastic leukaemia. Br J Haematol 1998;102:860.

212. Roberts WM, Rivera GK, Raimondi SC, et al: Intensive chemotherapy for Philadelphia-chromosome-positive acute lymphoblastic leukaemia. Lancet 1994;343:331.

213. Arico M, Valsecchi MG, Camitta B, et al: Outcome of treatment in children with Philadelphia chromosome-positive acute lymphoblastic leukemia. N Engl J Med 2000;342:998.

214. Brisco MJ, Sykes PJ, Dolman G, et al: Effect of the Philadelphia chromosome on minimal residual disease in acute lymphoblastic leukemia. Leukemia 1997;11:1497.

215. Mitterbauer G, Nemeth P, Wacha S, et al: Quantification of minimal residual disease in patients with BCR-ABL-positive acute lymphoblastic leukaemia using quantitative competitive polymerase chain reaction. Br J Haematol 1999;106:634.

216. Ribeiro RC, Broniscer A, Rivera GK, et al: Philadelphia chromosome-positive acute lymphoblastic leukemia in children: Durable responses to chemotherapy associated with low initial white blood cell counts. Leukemia 1997;11:1493.

217. Schrappe M, Arico M, Harbott J, et al: Philadelphia chromosome-positive (Ph+) childhood acute lymphoblastic leukemia: Good initial steroid response allows early prediction of a favorable treatment outcome. Blood 1998;92:2730.

218. Mitterbauer G, Fodinger M, Scherrer R, et al: PCR-monitoring of minimal residual leukaemia after conventional chemotherapy and bone marrow transplantation in BCR-ABL-positive acute lymphoblastic leukaemia. Br J Haematol 1995;89:937.

219. Miyamura K, Tanimoto M, Morishima Y, et al: Detection of Philadelphia chromosome-positive acute lymphoblastic leukemia by polymerase chain reaction: Possible eradication of minimal residual disease by marrow transplantation. Blood 1992;79:1366.

220. Keil F, Kalhs P, Haas OA, et al: Relapse of Philadelphia chromosome positive acute lymphoblastic leukaemia after marrow transplantation: Sustained molecular remission after early and dose-escalating infusion of donor leucocytes. Br J Haematol 1997;97:161.

221. Radich J, Gehly G, Lee A, et al: Detection of bcr-abl transcripts in Philadelphia chromosome–positive acute lymphoblastic leukemia after marrow transplantation. Blood 1997;89:2602.

222. Privitera E, Rivolta A, Ronchetti D, et al: Reverse transcriptase/polymerase chain reaction follow-up and minimal residual disease detection in t(1;19)-positive acute lymphoblastic leukaemia. Br J Haematol 1996;92:653.

223. Cimino G, Elia L, Rivolta A, et al: Clinical relevance of residual disease monitoring by polymerase chain reaction in patients with ALL-1/AF-4 positive-acute lymphoblastic leukaemia. Br J Haematol 1996;92:659.

224. Janssen JW, Ludwig WD, Borkhardt A, et al: Pre-pre-B acute lymphoblastic leukemia: High frequency of alternatively spliced ALL1-AF4 transcripts and absence of minimal residual disease during complete remission. Blood 1994;84:3835.

225. Cimino G, Elia L, Rapanotti MC, et al: A prospective study of residual-disease monitoring of the ALL1/AF4 transcript in patients with t(4;11) acute lymphoblastic leukemia. Blood 2000;95:96.

226. D'Sa S, Verfuerth S, Vyas P, et al: Early PCR-negativity after allogeneic BMT in adults with t(4;11) ALL in the absence of acute or chronic GVHD. Bone Marrow Transplant 1999;23:695.

227. Szczepanski T, Pongers-Willemse MJ, Hahlen K, et al: Intensified therapy for infants with acute lymphoblastic leukemia: Results from the Dana-Farber Cancer Institute Consortium. Cancer 1998;83:1055.

228. Brisco MJ, Sykes PJ, Hughes E, et al: Monitoring minimal residual disease in peripheral blood in B-lineage acute lymphoblastic leukaemia. Br J Haematol 1997;99:314.

229. Van Rhee F, Marks DI, Lin F, et al: Quantification of residual disease in Philadelphia-positive acute lymphoblastic leukemia: Comparison of blood and bone marrow. Leukemia 1995;9:329.

230. Martin H, Atta J, Bruecher J, et al: In patients with BCR-ABL-positive ALL in CR peripheral blood contains less residual disease than bone marrow: Implications for autologous BMT. Ann Hematol 1994;68:85.

231. Sykes PJ, Brisco MJ, Hughes E, et al: Minimal residual disease in childhood acute lymphoblastic leukaemia quantified by aspirate and trephine: Is the disease multifocal? Br J Haematol 1998;103:60.

232. Neale GAM, Coustan-Smith E, Pan Q, et al: Tandem application of flow cytometry and polymerase chain reaction for comprehensive detection of minimal residual disease in childhood acute lymphoblastic leukemia. Leukemia 1999;13:1221.

233. Dworzak MN, Stolz F, Froschl G, et al: Detection of residual disease in pediatric B-cell precursor acute lymphoblastic leukemia by comparative phenotype mapping: A study of five cases controlled by genetic methods. Exp Hematol 1999;27:673.

234. Rozman C, Montserrat E: Chronic lymphocytic leukemia. N Engl J Med 1995;333:1052.

235. Brugiatelli M, Callea V, Morabito F, et al: Immunologic and molecular evaluation of residual disease in B-cell chronic lymphocytic leukemia patients in clinical remission phase. Cancer 1989;63:1979.

236. Lavabre-Bertrand T, Janossy G, Exbrayat C, et al: Leukemia-associated changes identified by quantitative flow cytometry. II. CD5 over-expression and monitoring in B-CLL. Leukemia 1994;8:1557.

237. Robertson LE, Huh YO, Butler JJ, et al: Response assessment in chronic lymphocytic leukemia after fludarabine plus prednisone: Clinical, pathologic, immunophenotypic, and molecular analysis. Blood 1992;80:29.

238. Brugiatelli M, Claisse JF, Lenormand B, et al: Long-term clinical outcome of B-cell chronic lymphocytic leukaemia patients in clinical remission phase evaluated at phenotypic level. Br J Haematol 1997;97:113.

239. Provan D, Bartlett-Pandite L, Zwicky C, et al: Eradication of polymerase chain reaction–detectable chronic lymphocytic leukemia cells is associated with improved outcome after bone marrow transplantation. Blood 1996;88:2228.

240. Mattsson J, Uzunel M, Remberger M, et al: Minimal residual disease is common after allogeneic stem cell transplantation in patients with B cell chronic lymphocytic leukemia and may be controlled by graft-versus-host disease. Leukemia 2000;14:247.

241. Magnac C, Sutton L, Cazin B, et al: Detection of minimal residual disease in B chronic lymphocytic leukemia (CLL). Hematol Cell Ther 1999;41:13.

242. Corradini P, Ladetto M, Pileri A, et al: Clinical relevance of minimal residual disease monitoring in non-Hodgkin's lymphomas: A critical reappraisal of molecular strategies. Leukemia 1999;13:1691.

243. Gribben JG, Freedman A, Woo SD, et al: All advanced stage non-Hodgkin's lymphomas with a polymerase chain reaction amplifiable breakpoint of bcl-2 have residual cells containing the bcl-2 rearrangement at evaluation and after treatment. Blood 1991;78:3275.

244. Lambrechts AC, Hupkes PE, Dorssers LC, et al: Translocation (14;18)-positive cells are present in the circulation of the majority of patients with localized (stage I and II) follicular non-Hodgkin's lymphoma. Blood 1993;82:2510.

245. Gribben JG, Neuberg D, Barber M, et al: Detection of residual lymphoma cells by polymerase chain reaction in peripheral blood is significantly less predictive for relapse than detection in bone marrow. Blood 1994;83:3800.

246. Lopez-Guillermo A, Cabanillas F, McLaughlin P, et al: The clinical significance of molecular response in indolent follicular lymphomas. Blood 1998;91:2955.

247. Lambrechts AC, Hupkes PE, Dorssers LC, et al: Clinical significance of t(14;18)-positive cells in the circulation of patients with stage III or IV follicular non-Hodgkin's lymphoma during first remission. J Clin Oncol 1994;12:1541.

248. Czuczman MS, Grillo-Lopez AJ, White CA, et al: Treatment of patients with low-grade B-cell lymphoma with the combination of chimeric anti-CD20 monoclonal antibody and CHOP chemotherapy. J Clin Oncol 1999;17:268.

249. Gribben JG, Neuberg D, Freedman AS, et al: Detection by polymerase chain reaction of residual cells with the bcl-2 translocation is associated with increased risk of relapse after autologous bone marrow transplantation for B-cell lymphoma. Blood 1993;81:3449.

250. Von Neuhoff N, Dreger P, Suttorp M, et al: Comparison of different strategies of molecular genetic monitoring following autologous stem cell transplantation in patients with follicular lymphoma. Bone Marrow Transplant 1998;22:161.

251. Moos M, Schulz R, Martin S, et al: The remission status before and the PCR status after high-dose therapy with peripheral blood stem cell support are prognostic factors for relapse-free survival in patients with follicular non-Hodgkin's lymphoma. Leukemia 1998;12:1971.

252. Johnson PW, Price CG, Smith T, et al: Detection of cells bearing the t(14;18) translocation following myeloablative treatment and autologous bone marrow transplantation for follicular lymphoma. J Clin Oncol 1994;12:798.

253. Finke J, Slanina J, Lange W, et al: Persistence of circulating t(14;18)-positive cells in long-term remission after radiation therapy for localized-stage follicular lymphoma. J Clin Oncol 1993;11:1668.

254. Johnson PW, Swinbank K, MacLennan S, et al: Variability of polymerase chain reaction detection of the bcl-2–IgH translocation in an international multicentre study. Ann Oncol 1999;10:1349.

255. Galoin S, al Saati T, Schlaifer D, et al: Oligonucleotide clonospecific probes directed against the junctional sequence of t(14;18): A new tool for the assessment of minimal residual disease in follicular lymphomas. Br J Haematol 1996;94:676.

256. Mandigers CM, Meijerink JP, Raemaekers JM, et al: Graft-versus-lymphoma effect of donor leucocyte infusion shown by real-time quantitative PCR analysis of t(14;18). Lancet 1998;352:1522.

257. Andersen NS, Donovan JW, Borus JS, et al: Failure of immunologic purging in mantle cell lymphoma assessed by polymerase chain reaction detection of minimal residual disease. Blood 1997;90:4212.

258. Jacquy C, Lambert F, Soree A, et al: Peripheral blood stem cell contamination in mantle cell non-Hodgkin lymphoma: The case for purging? Bone Marrow Transplant 1999;23:681.

259. Zwicky CS, Maddocks AB, Andersen N, et al: Eradication of polymerase chain reaction detectable immunoglobulin gene rearrangement in non-Hodgkin's lymphoma is associated with decreased relapse after autologous bone marrow transplantation. Blood 1996;88:3314.

260. Scholten C, Hilgarth B, Hilgarth M, et al: Predictive value of clone-specific CDR3 PCR in high-grade non-Hodgkin's lymphoma: Long-term persistence of a clone-specific rearrangement in a patient with secondary high-grade NHL in remission after high-dose therapy. Br J Haematol 1997;97:246.

261. Corradini P, Astolfi M, Cherasco C, et al: Molecular monitoring of minimal residual disease in follicular and mantle cell non-Hodg-

kin's lymphomas treated with high-dose chemotherapy and peripheral blood progenitor cell autografting. Blood 1997;89:724.

262. Corradini P, Ladetto M, Astolfi M, et al: Clinical and molecular remission after allogeneic blood cell transplantation in a patient with mantle-cell lymphoma. Br J Haematol 1996;94:376.

263. Bradstock KF, Kerr A, Kabral A, et al: Coexpression of p165 myeloid surface antigen and terminal deoxynucleotidyl transferase: A comparison of acute myeloid leukaemia and normal bone marrow cells. Am J Hematol 1986;23:43.

264. Adriaansen HJ, Hooijkaas H, Kappers-Klunne MC, et al: Double marker analysis for terminal deoxynucleotidyl transferase and myeloid antigens in acute nonlymphocytic leukemia patients and healthy subjects. Haematol Blood Transfus 1990;33:41.

265. Sievers EL, Lange BJ, Buckley JD, et al: Prediction of relapse of pediatric acute myeloid leukemia by use of multidimensional flow cytometry. J Natl Cancer Inst 1996;88:1483.

266. San Miguel JF, Martinez A, Macedo A, et al: Immunophenotyping investigation of minimal residual disease is a useful approach for predicting relapse in acute myeloid leukemia patients. Blood 1997; 90:2465.

267. Shulman HM, Wells D, Gooley T, et al: The biologic significance of rare peripheral blasts after hematopoietic cell transplantation is predicted by multidimensional flow cytometry. Am J Clin Pathol 1999;112:513.

268. Reichle A, Rothe G, Krause S, et al: Transplant characteristics: Minimal residual disease and impaired megakaryocytic colony growth as sensitive parameters for predicting relapse in acute myeloid leukemia. Leukemia 1999;13:1227.

269. Lo Coco F, Avvisati G, Diverio D, et al: Molecular evaluation of response to all-trans-retinoic acid therapy in patients with acute promyelocytic leukemia. Blood 1991;77:1657.

270. Lo Coco F, Diverio D, Pandolfi PP, et al: Molecular evaluation of residual disease as a predictor of relapse in acute promyelocytic leukaemia. Lancet 1992;340:1437.

271. Miller WH Jr, Kakizuka A, Frankel SR, et al: Reverse transcription polymerase chain reaction for the rearranged retinoic acid receptor alpha clarifies diagnosis and detects minimal residual disease in acute promyelocytic leukemia. Proc Natl Acad Sci U S A 1992; 89:2694.

272. Miller WH Jr, Levine K, DeBlasio A, et al: Detection of minimal residual disease in acute promyelocytic leukemia by a reverse transcription polymerase chain reaction assay for the PML/RAR-alpha fusion mRNA. Blood 1993;82:1689.

273. Diverio D, Pandolfi PP, Biondi A, et al: Absence of reverse transcription–polymerase chain reaction detectable residual disease in patients with acute promyelocytic leukemia in long-term remission. Blood 1993;82:3556.

274. Huang W, Sun GL, Li XS, et al: Acute promyelocytic leukemia: Clinical relevance of two major PML-RAR alpha isoforms and detection of minimal residual disease by retrotranscriptase/polymerase chain reaction to predict relapse. Blood 1993;82:1264.

275. Laczika K, Mitterbauer G, Korninger L, et al: Rapid achievement of PML-RAR alpha polymerase chain reaction (PCR)-negativity by combined treatment with all-trans-retinoic acid and chemotherapy in acute promyelocytic leukemia: A pilot study. Leukemia 1994; 8:1.

276. Korninger L, Knobl P, Laczika K, et al: PML-RAR alpha PCR positivity in the bone marrow of patients with APL precedes haematological relapse by 2–3 months. Br J Haematol 1994;88:427.

277. Fukutani H, Naoe T, Ohno R, et al: Prognostic significance of the RT-PCR assay of PML-RARA transcripts in acute promyelocytic leukemia. Leukemia 1995;9:588.

278. Martinelli G, Remiddi C, Visani G, et al: Molecular analysis of PML-RAR alpha fusion mRNA detected by reverse transcription-polymerase chain reaction assay in long-term disease-free acute promyelocytic leukemia patients. Br J Haematol 1995;90:966.

279. Takatsuki H, Umemura T, Sadamura S, et al: Detection of minimal residual disease by reverse transcriptase polymerase chain reaction for the PML/RAR alpha fusion mRNA: A study in patients with acute promyelocytic leukemia following peripheral stem cell transplantation. Leukemia 1995;9:889.

280. Mandelli F, Diverio D, Avvisati G, et al: Molecular remission in PML/RAR alpha–positive acute promyelocytic leukemia by combined all-trans retinoic acid and idarubicin (AIDA) therapy. Gruppo Italiano-Malattie Ematologiche Maligne dell'Adulto and Associazione Italiana di Ematologia ed Oncologia Pediatrica Cooperative Groups. Blood 1997;90:1014.

281. Diverio D, Rossi V, Avvisati G, et al: Early detection of relapse by prospective reverse transcriptase–polymerase chain reaction analysis of the PML/RAR alpha fusion gene in patients with acute promyelocytic leukemia enrolled in the GIMEMA-AIEOP Multicenter "AIDA" Trial. GIMEMA-AIEOP Multicenter "AIDA" Trial. Blood 1998;92:784.

282. Burnett AK, Grimwade D, Solomon E, et al: Presenting white blood cell count and kinetics of molecular remission predict prognosis in acute promyelocytic leukemia treated with all-trans retinoic acid: Result of the Randomized MRC Trial. Blood 1999;93:4131.

283. Lo Coco F, Diverio D, Avvisati G, et al: Therapy of molecular relapse in acute promyelocytic leukemia. Blood 1999;94:2225.

284. Tobal K, Liu Yin JA: RT-PCR method with increased sensitivity shows persistence of PML-RARA fusion transcripts in patients in long-term remission of APL. Leukemia 1998;12:1349.

285. Meloni G, Diverio D, Vignetti M, et al: Autologous bone marrow transplantation for acute promyelocytic leukemia in second remission: Prognostic relevance of pretransplant minimal residual disease assessment by reverse-transcription polymerase chain reaction of the PML/RAR alpha fusion gene. Blood 1997;90:1321.

286. Roman J, Martin C, Torres A, et al: Absence of detectable PML-RAR alpha fusion transcripts in long-term remission patients after BMT for acute promyelocytic leukemia. Bone Marrow Transplant 1997;19:679.

287. Nucifora G, Larson RA, Rowley JD: Persistence of the 8;21 translocation in patients with acute myeloid leukemia type M2 in long-term remission. Blood 1993;82:712.

288. Kusec R, Laczika K, Knobl P, et al: AML1/ETO fusion mRNA can be detected in remission blood samples of all patients with t(8; 21) acute myeloid leukemia after chemotherapy or autologous bone marrow transplantation. Leukemia 1994;8:735.

289. Saunders MJ, Tobal K, Keeney S, et al: Expression of diverse AML1/MTG8 transcripts is a consistent feature in acute myeloid leukemia with t(8;21) irrespective of disease phase. Leukemia 1996;10:1139.

290. Jurlander J, Caligiuri MA, Ruutu T, et al: Persistence of the AML1/ETO fusion transcript in patients treated with allogeneic bone marrow transplantation for t(8;21) leukemia. Blood 1996;88:2183.

291. Miyamoto T, Nagafuji K, Akashi K, et al: Persistence of multipotent progenitors expressing AML1/ETO transcripts in long-term remission patients with t(8;21) acute myelogenous leukemia. Blood 1996;87:4789.

292. Satake N, Maseki N, Kozu T, et al: Disappearance of AML1-MTG8(ETO) fusion transcript in acute myeloid leukaemia patients with t(8;21) in long-term remission. Br J Haematol 1995;91:892.

293. Morschhauser F, Cayuela JM, Martini S, et al: Evaluation of minimal residual disease using reverse-transcription polymerase chain reaction in t(8;21) acute myeloid leukemia: A multicenter study of 51 patients. J Clin Oncol 2000;18:788.

294. Saunders MJ, Brereton ML, Adams JA, et al: Expression of AML1/MTG8 transcripts in clonogenic cells grown from bone marrow of patients in remission of acute myeloid leukaemia with t(8;21). Br J Haematol 1997;99:921.

295. Muto A, Mori S, Matsushita H, et al: Serial quantification of minimal residual disease of t(8;21) acute myelogenous leukaemia with RT-competitive PCR assay. Br J Haematol 1996;95:85.

296. Krauter J, Wattjes MP, Nagel S, et al: Real-time RT-PCR for the detection and quantification of AML1/MTG8 fusion transcripts in t(8;21)-positive AML patients. Br J Haematol 1999;107:80.

297. Tobal K, Newton J, Macheta M, et al: Molecular quantitation of minimal residual disease in acute myeloid leukemia with t(8;21) can identify patients in durable remission and predict clinical relapse. Blood 2000;95:815.

298. Miyamoto T, Nagafuji K, Harada M, et al: Quantitative analysis of AML1/ETO transcripts in peripheral blood stem cell harvests from patients with t(8;21) acute myelogenous leukaemia. Br J Haematol 1995;91:132.

299. Hebert J, Cayuela JM, Daniel MT, et al: Detection of minimal residual disease in acute myelomonocytic leukemia with abnormal marrow eosinophils by nested polymerase chain reaction with allele specific amplification. Blood 1994;84:2291.

300. Poirel H, Radford-Weiss I, Rack K, et al: Detection of the chromosome 16 CBF beta-MYH11 fusion transcript in myelomonocytic leukemias. Blood 1995;85:1313.

301. Tobal K, Johnson PR, Saunders MJ, et al: Detection of CBFB/MYH11 transcripts in patients with inversion and other abnormalities of chromosome 16 at presentation and remission. Br J Haematol 1995;91:104.
302. Evans PA, Short MA, Jack AS, et al: Detection and quantitation of the CBFbeta/MYH11 transcripts associated with the inv(16) in presentation and follow-up samples from patients with AML. Leukemia 1997;11:364.
303. Elmaagacli AH, Beelen DW, Kroll M, et al: Detection of CBFbeta/MYH11 fusion transcripts in patients with inv(16) acute myeloid leukemia after allogeneic bone marrow or peripheral blood progenitor cell transplantation. Bone Marrow Transplant 1998;21:159.
304. Laczika K, Novak M, Hilgarth B, et al: Competitive CBFbeta/MYH11 reverse-transcriptase polymerase chain reaction for quantitative assessment of minimal residual disease during postremission therapy in acute myeloid leukemia with inversion(16): A pilot study. J Clin Oncol 1998;16:1519.
305. Mitterbauer G, Zimmer C, Fonatsch C, et al: Monitoring of minimal residual leukemia in patients with MLL-AF9 positive acute myeloid leukemia by RT-PCR. Leukemia 1999;13:1519.
306. Liu Yin JA, Tobal K: Detection of minimal residual disease in acute myeloid leukaemia: Methodologies, clinical and biological significance. Br J Haematol 1999;106:578.
307. Sawyers CL: Chronic myeloid leukemia. N Engl J Med 1999;340:1330.
308. Roth MS, Antin JH, Bingham EL, et al: Detection of Philadelphia chromosome–positive cells by the polymerase chain reaction following bone marrow transplant for chronic myelogenous leukemia. Blood 1989;74:882.
309. Lee M, Khouri I, Champlin R, et al: Detection of minimal residual disease by polymerase chain reaction of bcr/abl transcripts in chronic myelogenous leukaemia following allogeneic bone marrow transplantation. Br J Haematol 1992;82:708.
310. Thompson JD, Brodsky I, Yunis JJ: Molecular quantification of residual disease in chronic myelogenous leukemia after bone marrow transplantation. Blood 1992;79:1629.
311. Miyamura K, Tahara T, Tanimoto M, et al: Long persistent bcr-abl positive transcript detected by polymerase chain reaction after marrow transplant for chronic myelogenous leukemia without clinical relapse: A study of 64 patients. Blood 1993;81:1089.
312. Miyamura K, Barrett AJ, Kodera Y, et al: Minimal residual disease after bone marrow transplantation for chronic myelogenous leukemia and implications for graft-versus-leukemia effect: A review of recent results. Bone Marrow Transplant 1994;14:201.
313. Van Rhee F, Lin F, Cross NC, et al: Detection of residual leukaemia more than 10 years after allogeneic bone marrow transplantation for chronic myelogenous leukaemia. Bone Marrow Transplant 1994;14:609.
314. Faderl S, Talpaz M, Kantarjian HM, et al: Should polymerase chain reaction analysis to detect minimal residual disease in patients with chronic myelogenous leukemia be used in clinical decision making? Blood 1999;93:2755.
315. Roth MS, Antin JH, Ash R, et al: Prognostic significance of Philadelphia chromosome–positive cells detected by the polymerase chain reaction after allogeneic bone marrow transplant for chronic myelogenous leukemia. Blood 1992;79:276.
316. Radich JP, Gehly G, Gooley T, et al: Polymerase chain reaction detection of the BCR-ABL fusion transcript after allogeneic marrow transplantation for chronic myeloid leukemia: Results and implications in 346 patients. Blood 1995;85:2632.
317. Drobyski WR, Endean DJ, Klein JP, et al: Detection of BCR/ABL RNA transcripts using the polymerase chain reaction is highly predictive for relapse in patients transplanted with unrelated marrow grafts for chronic myelogenous leukaemia. Br J Haematol 1997;98:458.
318. Pichert G, Roy DC, Gonin R, et al: Distinct patterns of minimal residual disease associated with graft-versus-host disease after allogeneic bone marrow transplantation for chronic myelogenous leukemia. J Clin Oncol 1995;13:1704.
319. Gaiger A, Lion T, Kalhs P, et al: Frequent detection of BCR-ABL specific mRNA in patients with chronic myeloid leukemia (CML) following allogeneic and syngeneic bone marrow transplantation (BMT). Leukemia 1993;7:1766.
320. Lion T, Henn T, Gaiger A, et al: Early detection of relapse after bone marrow transplantation in patients with chronic myelogenous leukaemia. Lancet 1993;341:275.
321. Lion T: Clinical implications of qualitative and quantitative polymerase chain reaction analysis in the monitoring of patients with chronic myelogenous leukemia. The European Investigators on Chronic Myeloid Leukemia Group. Bone Marrow Transplant 1994;14:505.
322. Lin F, van Rhee F, Goldman JM, et al: Kinetics of increasing BCR-ABL transcript numbers in chronic myeloid leukemia patients who relapse after bone marrow transplantation. Blood 1996;87:4473.
323. Cross NC, Hughes TP, Feng L, et al: Minimal residual disease after allogeneic bone marrow transplantation for chronic myeloid leukaemia in first chronic phase: Correlations with acute graft-versus-host disease and relapse. Br J Haematol 1993;84:67.
324. Hochhaus A, Weisser A, La Rosee P, et al: Detection and quantification of residual disease in chronic myelogenous leukemia. Leukemia 2000;14:998.
325. Pichert G, Alyea EP, Soiffer RJ, et al: Persistence of myeloid progenitor cells expressing BCR-ABL mRNA after allogeneic bone marrow transplantation for chronic myelogenous leukemia. Blood 1994;84:2109.
326. Preudhomme C, Revillion F, Merlat A, et al: Detection of BCR-ABL transcripts in chronic myeloid leukemia (CML) using a 'real time' quantitative RT-PCR assay. Leukemia 1999;13:957.
327. Gaiger A, Henn T, Horth E, et al: Increase of bcr-abl chimeric mRNA expression in tumor cells of patients with chronic myeloid leukemia precedes disease progression. Blood 1995;86:2371.
328. Cross NC: Minimal residual disease in chronic myeloid leukaemia. Hematol Cell Ther 1998;40:224.
329. Elmaagacli AH, Beelen DW, Opalka B, et al: The risk of residual molecular and cytogenetic disease in patients with Philadelphia-chromosome positive first chronic phase chronic myelogenous leukemia is reduced after transplantation of allogeneic peripheral blood stem cells compared with bone marrow. Blood 1999;94:384.
330. Van Rhee F, Lin F, Cullis JO, et al: Relapse of chronic myeloid leukemia after allogeneic bone marrow transplant: The case for giving donor leukocyte transfusions before the onset of hematologic relapse. Blood 1994;83:3377.
331. Raanani P, Dazzi F, Sohal J, et al: The rate and kinetics of molecular response to donor leucocyte transfusions in chronic myeloid leukaemia patients treated for relapse after allogeneic bone marrow transplantation. Br J Haematol 1997;99:945.
332. Hochhaus A, Lin F, Reiter A, et al: Quantification of residual disease in chronic myelogenous leukemia patients on interferon-alpha therapy by competitive polymerase chain reaction. Blood 1996;87:1549.
333. Tchirkov A, Giollant M, Tavernier F, et al: Interphase cytogenetics and competitive RT-PCR for residual disease monitoring in patients with chronic myeloid leukaemia during interferon-alpha therapy. Br J Haematol 1998;101:552.
334. Branford S, Hughes TP, Rudzki Z: Monitoring chronic myeloid leukaemia therapy by real-time quantitative PCR in blood is a reliable alternative to bone marrow cytogenetics. Br J Haematol 1999;107:587.
335. Malinge MC, Mahon FX, Delfau MH, et al: Quantitative determination of the hybrid Bcr-Abl RNA in patients with chronic myelogenous leukemia under interferon therapy. Br J Haematol 1992;82:701.
336. Hochhaus A, Lin F, Reiter A, et al: Variable numbers of BCR-ABL transcripts persist in CML patients who achieve complete cytogenetic remission with interferon-alpha. Br J Haematol 1995;91:126.
337. Hochhaus A, Reiter A, Saussele S, et al: Molecular heterogeneity in complete cytogenetic responders after interferon-alpha therapy for chronic myelogenous leukemia: Low levels of minimal residual disease are associated with continuing remission. German CML Study Group and the UK MRC CML Study Group. Blood 2000;95:62.
338. Talpaz M, Estrov Z, Kantarjian H, et al: Persistence of dormant leukemic progenitors during interferon-induced remission in chronic myelogenous leukemia. Analysis by polymerase chain reaction of individual colonies. J Clin Invest 1994;94:1383.
339. Reiter A, Marley SB, Hochhaus A, et al: BCR-ABL–positive progenitors in chronic myeloid leukaemia patients in complete cytogenetic remission after treatment with interferon-alpha. Br J Haematol 1998;102:1271.
340. Kurzrock R, Estrov Z, Kantarjian H, et al: Conversion of interferon-

induced, long-term cytogenetic remissions in chronic myelogenous leukemia to polymerase chain reaction negativity. J Clin Oncol 1998;16:1526.

341. Lion T: Monitoring of residual disease in chronic myelogenous leukemia by quantitative polymerase chain reaction and clinical decision making. Blood 1999;94:1486.

342. Goldman JM, Kaeda JS, Cross NC, et al: Clinical decision making in chronic myeloid leukemia based on polymerase chain reaction analysis of minimal residual disease. Blood 1999;94:1484.

343. Lin F, Goldman JM, Cross NC: A comparison of the sensitivity of blood and bone marrow for the detection of minimal residual disease in chronic myeloid leukaemia. Br J Haematol 1994;86:683.

344. Pinkel D, Woo S: Prevention and treatment of meningeal leukemia in children. Blood 1994;84:355.

345. Mahmoud HH, Rivera GK, Hancock ML, et al: Low leukocyte counts with blast cells in cerebrospinal fluid of children with newly diagnosed acute lymphoblastic leukemia. N Engl J Med 1993;329:314.

346. Hooijkaas H, Hahlen K, Adriaansen HJ, et al: Terminal deoxynucleotidyl transferase (TdT)-positive cells in cerebrospinal fluid and development of overt CNS leukemia: A 5-year follow-up study in 113 children with a TdT-positive leukemia or non-Hogdkin's lymphoma. Blood 1989;74:416.

347. Januszkiewicz DA, Nowak JS: Molecular evidence for central nervous system involvement in children with newly diagnosed acute lymphoblastic leukemia. Hematol Oncol 1995;13:201.

348. Escudier SM, Albitar M, Robertson LE, et al: Acute lymphoblastic leukemia following preleukemic syndromes in adults. Leukemia 1996;10:473.

349. Sills RH, Stockman JA: Preleukemic states in children with acute lymphoblastic leukemia. Cancer 1981;48:110.

350. Ishikawa K, Seriu T, Watanabe A, et al: Detection of neoplastic clone in the hypoplastic and recovery phases preceding acute lymphoblastic leukemia by in vitro amplification of rearranged T-cell receptor delta chain gene. J Pediatr Hematol Oncol 1995;17:270.

351. Morley AA, Brisco MJ, Rice M, et al: Leukaemia presenting as marrow hypoplasia: Molecular detection of the leukaemic clone at the time of initial presentation. Br J Haematol 1997;98:940.

352. Wells DA, Hall MC, Shulman HM, et al: Occult B cell malignancies can be detected by three-color flow cytometry in patients with cytopenias. Leukemia 1998;12:2015.

353. Goulden N, Langlands K, Steward C, et al: PCR assessment of bone marrow status in 'isolated' extramedullary relapse of childhood B-precursor acute lymphoblastic leukaemia. Br J Haematol 1994;87:282.

354. Neale GA, Pui CH, Mahmoud HH, et al: Molecular evidence for minimal residual bone marrow disease in children with 'isolated' extra-medullary relapse of T-cell acute lymphoblastic leukemia. Leukemia 1994;8:768.

355. O'Reilly J, Meyer B, Baker D, et al: Correlation of bone marrow minimal residual disease and apparent isolated extramedullary relapse in childhood acute lymphoblastic leukaemia. Leukemia 1995;9:624.

356. Lal A, Kwan E, al Mahr M, et al: Molecular detection of acute lymphoblastic leukaemia in boys with testicular relapse. Mol Pathol 1998;51:277.

357. Sandlund JT, Downing JR, Crist WM: Non-Hodgkin's lymphoma in childhood. N Engl J Med 1996;334:1238.

358. Bradstock KF, Kerr A: Immunological detection of covert leukaemic spread in mediastinal T-cell lymphoblastic lymphoma. Leuk Res 1985;9:905.

359. Kurokawa T, Kinoshita T, Ito T, et al: Detection of minimal residual disease B cell lymphoma by a PCR-mediated RNase protection assay. Leukemia 1996;10:1222.

360. Toren A, Rechavi G, Nagler A: Minimal residual disease post–bone marrow transplantation for hemato-oncological diseases. Stem Cells 1996;14:300.

361. Uckun FM, Kersey JH, Haake R, et al: Pretransplantation burden of leukemic progenitor cells as a predictor of relapse after bone marrow transplantation for acute lymphoblastic leukemia. N Engl J Med 1993;329:1296.

362. Vervoordeldonk SF, Merle PA, Behrendt H, et al: PCR-positivity in harvested bone marrow predicts relapse after transplantation with autologous purged bone marrow in children in second remission of precursor B-cell acute leukaemia. Br J Haematol 1997;96:395.

363. Mizuta S, Ito Y, Kohno A, et al: Accurate quantitation of residual tumor burden at bone marrow harvest predicts timing of subsequent relapse in patients with common ALL treated by autologous bone marrow transplantation. Bone Marrow Transplant 1999;24:777.

364. Atta J, Fauth F, Keyser M, et al: Purging in BCR-ABL–positive acute lymphoblastic leukemia using immunomagnetic beads: Comparison of residual leukemia and purging efficiency in bone marrow vs peripheral blood stem cells by semiquantitative polymerase chain reaction. Bone Marrow Transplant 2000;25:97.

365. Brenner MK, Rill DR, Holladay MS, et al: Gene marking to determine whether autologous marrow infusion restores long-term haemopoiesis in cancer patients. Lancet 1993;342:1134.

366. Hardingham JE, Kotasek D, Sage RE, et al: Molecular detection of residual lymphoma cells in peripheral blood stem cell harvests and following autologous transplantation. Bone Marrow Transplant 1993;11:15.

367. Leonard BM, Hetu F, Busque L, et al: Lymphoma cell burden in progenitor cell grafts measured by competitive polymerase chain reaction: Less than one log difference between bone marrow and peripheral blood sources. Blood 1998;91:331.

368. Macintyre EA, Belanger C, Debert C, et al: Detection of clonal CD34 + 19 + progenitors in bone marrow of BCL2-IgH–positive follicular lymphoma patients. Blood 1995;86:4691.

369. Gribben JG, Saporito L, Barber M, et al: Bone marrows of non-Hodgkin's lymphoma patients with a bcl-2 translocation can be purged of polymerase chain reaction–detectable lymphoma cells using monoclonal antibodies and immunomagnetic bead depletion. Blood 1992;80:1083.

370. Di Nicola M, Siena S, Corradini P, et al: Elimination of bcl-2-IgH–positive follicular lymphoma cells from blood transplants with high recovery of hematopoietic progenitors by the Miltenyi CD34+ cell sorting system. Bone Marrow Transplant 1996;18:1117.

371. Tarella C, Corradini P, Astolfi M, et al: Negative immunomagnetic ex vivo purging combined with high-dose chemotherapy with peripheral blood progenitor cell autograft in follicular lymphoma patients: Evidence for long-term clinical and molecular remissions. Leukemia 1999;13:1456.

372. Gribben JG, Freedman AS, Neuberg D, et al: Immunologic purging of marrow assessed by PCR before autologous bone marrow transplantation for B-cell lymphoma. N Engl J Med 1991;325:1525.

373. Corsetti MT, Lerma E, Dejana A, et al: Quantitative competitive reverse transcriptase–polymerase chain reaction for BCR-ABL on Philadelphia-negative leukaphereses allows the selection of low-contaminated peripheral blood progenitor cells for autografting in chronic myelogenous leukemia. Leukemia 1999;13:999.

374. Morley A: Quantifying leukemia. N Engl J Med 1998;339:627.

375. Beishuizen A, Verhoeven MA, Hahlen K, et al: Differences in immunoglobulin heavy chain gene rearrangement patterns between bone marrow and blood samples in childhood precursor B-acute lymphoblastic leukemia at diagnosis. Leukemia 1993;7:60.

376. Martens AC, Schultz FW, Hagenbeek A: Nonhomogeneous distribution of leukemia in the bone marrow during minimal residual disease. Blood 1987;70:1073.

13

Andrew Davies   Ama Rohatiner

General Management
of the Patient with Leukemia

The management of the person with leukemia begins with the establishment of the diagnosis. Although this is essentially morphologic, based on findings in the peripheral blood and bone marrow, diagnostic precision and prognostic factors have been augmented by immunologic, cytogenetic, and molecular genetic techniques. The physician and a team of allied health care professionals will support not only the patient but the patient's relatives and friends throughout the disease and during diagnosis, treatment, and follow-up. This relationship may come to an end only with the death of the patient. However, increasing numbers of individuals remain disease free many years after completion of therapy. They continue to require regular follow-up for the purposes of surveillance for recurrence and management of complications that may have resulted from either disease or therapy.

During the course of the disease, the patient will be confronted with a large amount of new information and may be required to make difficult choices at emotionally demanding times. The health care professional must have detailed knowledge of disease biology and potentially available therapeutic options to be able to inform the individual appropriately and accurately. Those options depend on the specific subtype of leukemia; whether it is newly diagnosed, recurrent, or refractory; and the patient's co-morbidity. A range of care from simple support through modest or more intensive chemotherapeutic regimens may be considered.

There continue to be rapid advances in both supportive care and therapies. This must be the most compelling argument for referring newly diagnosed patients to tertiary centers. Such centers not only provide the full range of support services and expertise required for management of the patient but also may provide access to clinical trials and novel agents unavailable to the primary physician. Although accrual of knowledge continues at a phenomenal rate, we should try to learn from every individual being treated, and whenever possible, patients should be entered into peer-reviewed clinical trials. The invitation to participate in a trial may be a difficult and unwelcome decision for the patient, and should the patient decline entry, this must be respected. Many centers may request the collection and storage of additional clinical material (e.g., blood or bone marrow) for research purposes; this serves an important role as we endeavor to understand more about the disease. The clinician at the interface with the patient should gain consent for collection of samples because only with a continued supply of such material may important projects continue.

Information is increasingly available to the patient through the media, particularly with widespread access to health information and interest groups through the Internet. This may influence a patient's preference and prejudices. The treating physician must take this into account when discussing therapeutic options and individualizing a patient's therapy.

This chapter deals with the issues surrounding symptoms as well as with specific organ and metabolic dysfunction in leukemia. Specific options for chemotherapy, transplantation, and treatment of infective complications are dealt with in other chapters of this text. Even if no specific antileukemic therapy is considered appropriate, much can be done to provide both physiologic and psychological support for the individual with leukemia.

SYMPTOMS AND SIGNS AT PRESENTATION

In acute and chronic leukemias, there is failure of normal hematopoiesis; this occurs at different rates dependent on disease biology. However, the failure of normal bone marrow function results in certain symptoms common to all leukemias, that is, anemia, infection, and bleeding. These may occur individually or in combination with one feature predominating. The clinical features of leukemia have been extensively reviewed and are discussed in Chapter 13.

Failure of erythropoiesis due to marrow infiltration largely accounts for the anemia seen in leukemia. However, acute and chronic bleeding, hypersplenism, and, particularly in chronic lymphocytic leukemia (CLL), hemolysis may play an important role. Bleeding due to thrombocytopenia may manifest as spontaneous bruising, purpura, epistaxis, menorrhagia, or hematuria. Again, thrombocytopenia is usually a result of marrow failure, although autoimmune phenomena and hypersplenism may be contributory. There may be coagulopathy associated with disseminated intravascular coagulation, most frequently in promyelocytic leukemia (AML M3), although it may occur in other subtypes of acute myelogenous leukemia (AML) and rarely in acute lymphoblastic leukemia (ALL). Disseminated intravascular coagulation may also result from severe sepsis.

Infection may present in many ways, although fever is the most common. In acute leukemias, myelodysplastic syndromes, and CLL, fever should be presumed to be infective in origin and prompt empirical treatment initiated. By contrast, chronic myelogenous leukemia (CML) and rarely CLL may present with fever and night sweats in the absence of infection.

Lymphadenopathy is common in patients with CLL[1-4] and may be detected in up to 50% of those with ALL at presentation.[5-8] In those with myeloid leukemias, lymphadenopathy is less common, although it is sometimes seen in AML M5 and the juvenile form of CML (juvenile chronic myelomonocytic leukemia) and in CML in accelerated phase or at blastic transformation.[9-11]

Splenomegaly may be massive in CML at presentation, causing considerable abdominal discomfort and features of hypersplenism. The majority of individuals with CML, CLL, and chronic myelomonocytic leukemia will have splenomegaly, with or without hepatomegaly. It is relatively uncommon in AML and ALL.

SUPPORTIVE CARE

Together with advances in and refinement of cytotoxic therapies have come improvements in supportive care techniques. These have been of significant benefit to the individual with leukemia.

Indwelling Venous Catheters

A welcome advance in the supportive care of the patient with leukemia has been the evolution of the indwelling central venous catheter, providing access for blood sampling and the administration of blood products, fluids, and antimicrobials. Although different catheters are available, two main types are in common use: the subcutaneously tunneled Hickman and Groshong catheters, which may have one to three lumens (most commonly two), and the fully implantable venous catheter systems (e.g., Port-a-cath) with a subcutaneous reservoir. Numerous complications have been associated with their insertion, including pneumothorax, hemothorax, and chylothorax. Phrenic nerve palsies have occurred along with the problem of catheter displacement. Central venous catheters should be inserted by a skilled operator with the benefit of radiologic screening. The type of device employed should depend on locally available expertise. Although differing superiorities have been reported,[12-17] familiarity with use of a single system in one institution should minimize complications. A complication rate of 0.28 per 100 days has been reported for indwelling catheters;

72% of these problems were attributed to catheter-related sepsis or exit site infections.[14]

The increased use of indwelling catheters has been paralleled by an increase in the incidence of gram-positive infections. The most commonly identified organism is *Staphylococcus epidermidis*, with *Staphylococcus aureus* and streptococci often being isolated.[12] Catheter-related sepsis may be successfully treated on an outpatient basis with antibiotic therapy, achieving salvage rates of 74%.[18, 19]

Thrombotic complications are also common; mural thrombi have been identified in 38% of catheterized veins at postmortem examination.[20] Clinical thrombosis of the axillary vein, subclavian vein, or superior vena cava may be managed by anticoagulation. Bern and colleagues[21] reported that the use of low-dose continuous warfarin at a dose of 1 mg/day may protect against thrombotic complications without inducing a hemorrhagic state. Caution is advised, however, in view of thrombocytopenia and coagulopathies associated with leukemia and its treatment.

Cutaneous infiltration at relapse has been described at the point of a previous Hickman line exit site.[22] Examination at follow-up is therefore recommended. In patients who have undergone allogeneic bone marrow transplantation, the skin changes associated with chronic graft-versus-host disease may predispose to infective complications from the retained Dacron cuff, which may often be left in situ on removal of the Hickman line. It is therefore recommended that the Dacron cuff be removed in all patients who have undergone transplantation.[23]

Blood Product Support

Regular clinical examination, including ophthalmoscopy, of the patient with thrombocytopenia is mandatory for detection of occult bleeding. Prophylactic platelet transfusions are typically administered to maintain the platelet count above 10×10^{12}/L. Higher levels should be achieved in those with sepsis, as platelets are consumed, and in those with evidence of bleeding. Alloantibodies may develop with multiple transfusions, necessitating the use of HLA-matched platelets.

The management of bleeding complications is discussed extensively in Chapter 17. It is important to correct coagulopathies with fresh frozen plasma, cryoprecipitate, and factor concentrate as appropriate. At St. Bartholomew's Hospital, red blood cells are transfused to maintain the hemoglobin level above 9.0 g/dL to improve oxygen delivery to tissues. Care should be taken, however, to avoid precipitating leukostasis in those with high white blood cell counts.

Antimicrobial Prophylaxis

Gram-negative bacterial infections occur commonly in the patient with marrow aplasia after chemotherapy. The use of prophylactic quinolone antibiotics with and without nonabsorbable antibiotics has been investigated. Although there appears to be no impact on mortality, the incidence of and morbidity from gram-negative sepsis may be reduced.[24, 25] Infective complications are discussed in Chapter 14.

Psychological Issues

Special attention to the individual's psychological need is required throughout the management of the patient with leukemia. Many units are now able to provide the services of a psychologist or psychiatrist with a particular interest in the care of these individuals and their families. It is important for health care professionals to be able to recognize the times when this is imperative. Critical events, such as at the time of diagnosis, during outcome assessment, and at the end of therapy, will require particular attention. There should also be a high index of suspicion for psychological problems so that preventive measures may be employed. This may be time-consuming because long, difficult conversations are required, and the contents of these often need repeating on several occasions. These conversations are best held in a quiet, comfortable room specifically reserved for this purpose. Other members of the professional team (usually the patient's nurse) and any relation or friend should be present so that they may have input into the discussion. The situation and its implications should be carefully explained. Patients need to be given support to adjust to their circumstances in ways that are most appropriate to themselves. The health care team should also be alert to specific cultural issues that may concern an individual, and independent translators should also be available for those not conversing in their own language.

The patient's confidentiality is of importance, and the person may not wish details of the illness to be discussed with family members or friends. This group, however, may themselves require support, and the patient should be encouraged to be as open as possible about the illness. The children of patients need special attention; understanding of the illness, long absences of the parent, disruption of their lifestyle, and possible death of a parent may result in behavioral difficulties. Support of a specialist should be offered.

Children and adolescents diagnosed with leukemia present a difficult problem. They may have to consider the possibility of premature death; there may be problems with relationships, altered body image as a result of therapy, and alterations in activity. There may also be the issue of infertility to consider and concerns about future sexual function. Anger and rebellion may be natural responses, and professionals should support and manage them appropriately.

Symptom Control

Although many symptoms may be attributable to the underlying disease, many are iatrogenic. It is imperative to provide prompt relief for the patient's comfort while the underlying cause is attended to.

Nausea and Vomiting

These are perhaps the most distressing side effects of modern chemotherapy and may be ameliorated to a large extent by careful selection of antiemetics. Most units now have a protocol for appropriate choice of these agents based on the perceived emetogenicity of the cytotoxic agent employed. Although these act as a good starting point, therapy should be tailored to the individual and modified in light of the patient's previous experiences of therapy.

The cause of nausea and vomiting should be actively searched out because many possible etiologic factors other than chemotherapy alone may be contributing. These include gastric stasis, intestinal obstruction, biochemical disturbances, adrenal dysfunction and, rarely, raised intracranial pressure. These should be corrected. Prokinetic antiemetics (e.g., metoclopramide) or those acting on the vomiting center (e.g., cyclizine) are usually sufficient, although their action may be augmented by corticosteroids. After chemotherapy, there is massive release of 5-hydroxytryptamine (5-HT) from enterochromaffin cells and platelets; the 5-HT$_3$ receptor antagonists have been revolutionary in the management of chemotherapy-induced nausea and vomiting, being particularly valuable during the first 72 hours after therapy.[26]

Anorexia

Anorexia with associated weight loss is common. It is usually multifactorial, caused not only by nausea but by biochemical disturbances (e.g., uremia and hypercalcemia), dyspepsia, altered taste, mucositis, and pain. In the hospital environment, food is often unappetizing and timings are regimented, with depression exacerbating the anorexia. It is a difficult symptom to manage, and patients should be encouraged to eat food of their choice and at times suited to them. The provision of a ward kitchen may help to achieve this in the hospital environment. Although corticosteroids often used in management have an appetite-stimulatory effect, their role is minor.

Pain

Pain is an uncommon feature of leukemia in adults, and causal factors should be clearly identified. Analgesics should be prescribed according to the World Health Organization analgesic ladder, although prescription of nonsteroidal anti-inflammatory agents may be precluded as a result of thrombocytopenia or renal impairment.

Morphine and its analogues are the mainstay of the analgesic armamentarium. They may be administered in different formulations, and the dose should initially be titrated with use of an immediately available oral preparation. Steady state should be achieved before conversion to a slow-release formulation, which provides convenience. About 30% of patients experience significant nausea requiring the co-administration of an antiemetic, and a laxative should be prescribed at the initiation of opiate therapy to avoid drug-induced constipation.

Diamorphine is widely used in Europe, although it is not available in the United States; a more soluble prodrug of morphine, it is preferred for the subcutaneous or parenteral route of administration. Fentanyl, long used in anesthetic practice, is now available by the transdermal route; it has the advantages of less constipation and ease of administration.

Corticosteroids are frequently used in the management of splenic capsular pain and the bone pain occasionally seen in refractory disease. Likewise, tricyclic antidepressants and anticonvulsants have a special role in neuropathic pain.

Constipation and Diarrhea

Constipation may be a result of opiate analgesia, immobility, drugs, biochemical disturbances, and dietary changes. The choice of laxative largely depends on the physician's preference.

A cause of diarrhea should be identified before antimotility agents are prescribed. Factors associated with diarrhea include broad-spectrum antibiotics, *Clostridium difficile*–associated colitis, mucositis, infection, and drugs.

Admission to Intensive Care Unit

The mortality of patients with hematologic malignant neoplasia admitted to the intensive care unit is high. In one series of 92 patients, only 23% survived to leave the hospital, with a median survival in that group of 23 months.[27] Other authors have reported short-term mortality rates of 69% to 80%.[28-30] These poor outcomes are achieved at considerable expense, and several factors have been identified to predict poor outcomes. These have been found to include the requirement of mechanical ventilation, hypotension requiring inotropic and/or vasopressor support, persistent neutropenia, relapsed or refractory disease, and multiorgan failure.[31] The development of respiratory failure is associated with a particularly poor outlook, with mortality rate in excess of 80%.[30] In recipients of bone marrow transplants, the outcomes are worse; only 6% of those requiring mechanical ventilation survive for 30 days after extubation,[32] with higher rates (17%) reported by Jackson and coworkers[33] in 1998. Those recipients who are mechanically ventilated and either receive vasopressors or develop hepatic or renal insufficiency do not survive.[32]

The decision to admit a patient with leukemia is influenced by these factors; however, few would dispute admission for the young individual undergoing remission induction therapy. In individuals with relapsed disease, the issue is much less clear. The increasing use of continuous positive airway pressure and noninvasive ventilation may enable patients to remain in a high-dependency area. Early input from the intensive care physician may avoid admission and also allow more electively planned admissions to the intensive care unit.

It is clear that for individuals admitted to the intensive care unit with these poor prognostic factors, the decision should be made to limit or withdraw supportive therapy on the basis of a daily assessment by all involved. This will avoid futile supportive attempts. For those undergoing bone marrow transplantation, guidelines have been proposed to avoid prolonged life support,[32] although in the context of such a planned procedure, these issues may be discussed during counseling before transplantation. The opportunity to have such frank discussions with the patient newly diagnosed with leukemia may not be so apparent.

METABOLIC DISORDERS ASSOCIATED WITH LEUKEMIA

Numerous metabolic complications are encountered in leukemias, particularly in the acute forms. Many of these are associated with the underlying pathologic process; however, they are commonly iatrogenic. The changes are summarized in this section.

Tumor Lysis Syndrome

Acute tumor lysis is a syndrome caused by a rapid destruction of tumor cells, resulting in a release of cellular breakdown products. Spontaneous occurrence has been reported in some leukemias[34] and in the context of persistent high fevers.[35] More usually, however, it follows the administration of cytotoxic therapies. There have been case reports after administration of methotrexate by the intrathecal route.[36] Those conditions particularly associated with this syndrome are the B-cell and T-cell acute lymphoblastic leukemias, particularly in those individuals with a very high white blood cell count and elevated lactate dehydrogenase. These are obvious markers of a high disease burden.

The classic features are those of hyperuricemia, hyperkalemia, hyperphosphatemia, and hypocalcemia.[37] Renal failure is a consequence of the high urate load, with hyperphosphatemia contributing to this by inducing hypocalcemia through precipitation of phosphate with calcium, producing insoluble salts. These metabolic changes are commonly seen in patients undergoing induction therapy for acute leukemias; but with a high index of suspicion, careful monitoring, and prophylactic therapy, renal failure may be avoided, although its development may occasionally be inevitable.

Strategies to minimize acute tumor lysis syndrome include adequate hydration and the establishment of a forced diuresis.[38] The maintenance of a high glomerular filtration rate and urine output is achieved by fluid loading, often augmented by diuretics. This should be performed with extreme care in those with cardiac dysfunction and the elderly. Monitoring of central venous pressures is recommended, as is assessing the pulmonary artery capillary wedge pressure through a Swan-Ganz catheter in some circumstances. The use of mannitol to induce a diuresis is favored over loop diuretics because they may decrease tubular urine pH. The addition of sodium bicarbonate either orally or to the intravenous fluid regimen results in alkalization of urine and thus reduces precipitation of urate (see later). Allopurinol reduces urate production and should be continued until leukemic blasts have been cleared from the peripheral blood. The administration of cytotoxic agents should be avoided until an adequate diuresis is achieved and urate levels are normalized. This may result in a delay in their administration for several days. Spreading the first days of therapy over a longer period may reduce the risk for tumor lysis.

Inevitably, oliguric renal failure, hyperkalemia, or fluid overload may develop, and hemodialysis should be instigated. Renal failure is commonly reversible when the tumor bulk has been attended to[39]; in some pediatric settings, prophylactic continuous veno-venous hemofiltration has been employed during and immediately after chemotherapy administration.[40]

Hyperuricemia and Urate Nephropathy

Nucleic acid catabolism results in the production of uric acid. This is a particular problem when there is high cell turnover. After cytotoxic therapy, uric acid levels rise dramatically. In situations in which the concentrations of uric acid are high, urate may be precipitated in the renal tubules (urate nephropathy), resulting in renal failure. This may be exacerbated by dehydration, commonly seen in the context of febrile episodes. Uric acid is relatively insoluble in the acid environment of urine, and the urine pH may be decreased further by cell products released at the time of tumor lysis. This will contribute to urate precipitation.

High urine flow rates (>100 mL/hr) should be achieved by a forced diuresis and the urine alkalized by the administration of sodium bicarbonate. The xanthine oxidase inhibitor allopurinol should be administered to reduce the production of uric acid, and therapy is delayed until uric acid levels are normal.

Urate oxidase (uricozyme), a naturally occurring proteolytic enzyme of nonhuman origin, is now available. It is capable of oxidizing human uric acid to allantoins. These are highly soluble at renal tubular pH (5 to 10 times more than urate). It has been used successfully to treat urate nephropathy associated with the tumor lysis syndrome.[41] Studies of its prophylactic use have shown a greater and more rapid reduction in serum urate levels with lower serum creatinine concentration than in those historical control subjects managed according to the conventional modalities described before.[42] However, being a biologic product, allergic reactions have been documented.

Potassium Metabolism

Careful attention should be paid to potassium homeostasis in the leukemic patient. In the acutely unwell individual, cardiac arrhythmias may be associated with significant morbidity and mortality. Serum potassium concentration should be regularly monitored and appropriate action taken to correct abnormalities.

Hypokalemia may be caused by a number of mechanisms. Diarrhea associated with the use of broad-spectrum antibiotics and gut losses from chemotherapy-induced mucositis may result in loss of large amounts of potassium. Excessive vomiting and ileus likewise deplete

potassium. The nephropathy associated with nephrotoxic antibiotics and antifungal agents may result in tubular wasting of potassium, which may be reduced by prophylactic prescription of a potassium-sparing agent (e.g., amiloride). Care should be taken in the use of potassium-losing diuretics to correct iatrogenic fluid overload; these may exacerbate losses, resulting in large depletions of intracellular potassium. Potassium frequently needs to be replaced intravenously at high concentrations for correction of depletion. This should be undertaken in a closely monitored environment through a central vein.

Hyperkalemia is less commonly encountered, although it may occur during tumor lysis syndrome (see earlier) or as a result of renal failure. The acidosis associated with sepsis may result in a transmembrane flux of potassium from the intracellular environment, increasing serum levels although total body amounts are normal. Iatrogenic hyperkalemia in the replacement of lost potassium should be avoided. A pseudohyperkalemia may be seen in individuals with a very high white blood cell count. Cell breakdown in vitro releases potassium, which is measured in the serum. Care should be taken to distinguish this from a true hyperkalemia so that inappropriate treatment is avoided.

Sodium Metabolism

A syndrome of inappropriate antidiuretic hormone secretion (SIADH) may occur in the context of therapy for leukemia. The agents most commonly implicated are cyclophosphamide and vincristine.[43-47] The diagnosis may be difficult to establish. The patient is euvolemic with hyponatremia and a low plasma osmolality. The urine is relatively concentrated compared with the plasma, and adrenal, hepatic, and thyroid function is normal. SIADH may also be secondary to pneumonia, central nervous system disease, and other drugs used during the patient's treatment. The underlying cause should be established and corrected, and fluid restriction is commenced.

Sodium may be lost as a result of renal tubular wasting (aminoglycosides) and from excessive diarrhea and vomiting. Careful assessment of volume status and fluid balance may indicate the cause.

Hypernatremia is less common but may result from dehydration, particularly during sepsis or excessive use of fluids containing sodium. Diabetes insipidus with hypernatremic dehydration may result from leukemic infiltration of the pituitary or hypothalamus. This may be corrected by the administration of desmopressin.

Calcium and Magnesium Metabolism

Unlike in other hematologic malignant diseases, hypercalcemia is a rare feature of leukemia.[48, 49] However, it does commonly occur in human T-lymphotropic virus type 1 (HTLV-1)–associated adult T-cell leukemia, in which calcium levels may be very high.[50, 51] It is usually symptomatic with lethargy, nausea, vomiting, abdominal pain, constipation, and dehydration secondary to marked polyuria. Other leukemias associated with hypercalcemia include

ALL and blastic transformation of CML.[52-57] Hypercalcemia has been documented in AML.[58] Hypercalcemia constitutes a medical emergency, and rehydration with a saline diuresis should be commenced urgently. A loop diuretic increases calcium loss in the urine and may be employed once volume deficits have been corrected. Fluids and diuretics are temporizing measures, and an agent to reduce bone resorption should be employed. The osteoclastic inhibitors of the diphosphonate family (e.g., pamidronate and etidronate) are now in common use. Corticosteroids are a useful adjunct, although they are now used less frequently.

The mechanism of hypercalcemia is not entirely clear. There may be enhanced 1α-hydroxylase activity, increasing the production of 1,25-dihydroxyvitamin D_3 that induces bone resorption.[59] The presence of parathyroid hormone–related peptides may also be contributory.[50] There have been case reports of hypercalcemia induced by all-trans retinoic acid use in the treatment of acute promyelocytic leukemia.[60, 61]

Hypocalcemia may have a wide variety of clinical manifestations, including tetany, seizures, and cardiovascular failure. However, symptoms may be markedly decreased in the leukemic patient because of coexistent acidosis (e.g., from sepsis), which may reduce neuromuscular irritability. When rapid falls in calcium concentration occur from tumor lysis syndrome, however, the symptoms may be marked.[62]

Hypomagnesemia contributes to hypocalcemia by inducing a functional hypoparathyroidism. The most common reasons for low magnesium concentration are renal losses due to antibiotics/antifungals and protracted diarrhea. The hypocalcemia resulting from magnesium deficit is resistant to calcium replacement, and the magnesium deficit must be corrected first. Other factors contributing to hypocalcemia are sepsis, the administration of large amounts of blood products that contain citrate, and some chemotherapeutic agents (including methotrexate). A case of profound hypocalcemia associated with osteoblastic bone formation has been described in an individual with AML,[63] a phenomenon more commonly recognized in lung and breast malignant neoplasms.

Protein and Carbohydrate Metabolism

Leukemia results in a catabolic state, which is exacerbated by chemotherapy. Maintaining an adequate protein intake may be difficult, and muscle bulk is lost. Attention should be paid to dietary intake, which may require supplementation. A specially trained oncology dietitian may undertake the supervision of the patient's dietary requirements. Parenteral nutrition is required rarely in cases in which there is severe mucositis or complications precluding gastrointestinal absorption. The complications of this modality are numerous, not least of which is infection.

Hyperglycemia may be associated with the use of glucocorticoids and L-asparaginase in induction regimens for ALL. Blood glucose levels should be monitored, particularly in the elderly, at regular intervals during therapy.

SITE-SPECIFIC PROBLEMS

Although it is a disease originating in the bone marrow, leukemia may involve or result in complications at any organ or site. Those most commonly involved and the complications that are particularly a problem are outlined here. Some sites of involvement may be specific to a disease or subtype.

Gastrointestinal Tract

The oral cavity is frequently the site of problems in the leukemic patient. Oral candidiasis is common at presentation and throughout therapy. It may be treated with oral antifungal agents including nystatin, amphotericin, miconazole, and fluconazole. Nystatin and amphotericin are not absorbed by the gastrointestinal tract, whereas absorption of fluconazole is good (miconazole occupies an intermediate position). Mucosal ulceration may occur in the context of neutropenia and as a side effect of cytotoxic therapy. This disruption of the normal mucosal barrier may allow entry of potentially pathogenic oral flora into the circulation. Bleeding gums and petechial hemorrhage may result from thrombocytopenia, and the oral cavity should be inspected regularly for evidence of this. Leukemic cells, particularly those with a monocytic component (AML M4 and M5), may infiltrate the gums.

Careful attention to oral hygiene is essential, and patients should be encouraged to maintain a program of good oral toilet; this may reduce the risk for bacterial infection, particularly with anaerobes. A dental assessment, if circumstances permit, is recommended before therapy; however, the ability to perform corrective dental work may be limited by cytopenias. Tranexamic acid mouthwash may help problems of bleeding within the oral cavity.

Esophageal involvement with Candida infection is common and may present with odynophagia, dysphagia, and bleeding. Diagnosis is made endoscopically and confirmed microbiologically from brushings and biopsy specimens.[64] Gastric and intestinal involvement is less common. Use of an oral antifungal agent is usually sufficient, although intravenous administration is more appropriate in those with swallowing difficulties.

Perhaps surprisingly, gastrointestinal symptoms are relatively common at presentation, although the etiology is often unclear. It is often multifactorial, although leukemic infiltration of the digestive tract may be seen in approximately 25% of new presentations and may go some way toward accounting for these symptoms.[65]

Typhlitis is a neutropenic enterocolitis seen in patients with leukemia. There is an association with cytosine arabinoside therapy, and it typically occurs during induction therapy. Typical clinical features are pyrexia, abdominal pain, and distention with or without bloody diarrhea. Blood cultures may be positive for intestinal flora, and radiologic investigations may show a range of features from nonspecific bowel gas patterns to frank colonic pneumatosis. These may be followed by serial abdominal radiography, ultrasonography, or computed tomography. The pathologic findings may be confined to the cecum;

however, more extensive involvement of the ileum and other areas of the colon may be seen. Primary treatment is with bowel rest (nothing by mouth and parenteral nutrition) and broad-spectrum antimicrobials; however, surgical intervention may be required if there is persistent gastrointestinal bleeding, perforation, or the presence of shock requiring inotropic support.[66-69] Surgery in the leukemic patient is obviously high risk, but this should not be a deterrent to intervention. In some situations, surgery may be required to exclude other causes of the symptoms.

Vincristine therapy may induce constipation and occasionally a syndrome of adynamic bowel. This again is managed conservatively, although metoclopramide may have a role in expediting recovery.[70] Pancreatitis may be induced by L-asparaginase in ALL induction therapy. The physician should be mindful of this and monitor the serum amylase concentration during its use. There may be disturbances of liver function as a result of cytotoxic and antimicrobial therapy, although they may result directly from leukemic infiltration or infection.

Skin Manifestations

The skin may be affected in many ways in the individual with leukemia. Cutaneous lesions should be carefully examined, with note taken of the temporal relationship of their development to the stage of therapy. The clinician should have a low threshold for biopsy of lesions (a punch biopsy is easily performed on the ward or in ambulatory surgery), and the dermatologist should be involved at an early stage when any doubt exists concerning diagnosis.

Cutaneous infiltration with leukemia is seen typically in the acute myelogenous leukemias with a monocytic component (FAB M4 and M5); however, they may be seen in myeloid blast crisis of CML and are common in HTLV-1–associated T-cell leukemia/lymphoma. They typically present as mauve papules or nodules and may be singular or multiple, may occur at any site, and are typically itchy. They appear to be more common at relapse than at initial presentation. Bruising and purpura are common manifestations of marrow failure and are frequently seen at presentation.

In the context of neutropenia, cutaneous manifestations of bacterial infection may be seen. Staphylococcal skin infections are common, and cutaneous pseudomonal lesions of pyoderma gangrenosum may be extensive and require skin grafting. Viral infection is less common, but herpes zoster infections, particularly in CLL and after myeloablative regimens, are associated with considerable morbidity. These may be reduced by the use of prophylactic acyclovir, which should be continued for 1 year after transplantation. There is also an increased frequency of herpes simplex in the immunocompromised individual. Fungal skin lesions may also be seen and are readily diagnosed by skin scrapings or biopsy.

Drug reactions with cutaneous manifestations are common. The specific offender may be difficult to identify because patients are typically receiving a large combination of medications. The most frequently implicated drugs are allopurinol, antibiotics, and cytarabine (causing an erythroderma palmaris et plantaris syndrome). Careful scrutiny of the drug chart may aid diagnosis.

Central Nervous System

Neurologic symptoms and signs should be carefully evaluated in the patient with leukemia. Leukemic involvement in the central nervous system may present as headache, dizziness, focal neurologic symptoms, back pain, or drowsiness. There may be leukemic blasts in the cerebrospinal fluid, which may be readily identifiable on a fresh cytospin preparation. Complications of a diagnostic lumbar puncture performed by an experienced physician, with the appropriate platelet cover, are low, and the information obtained is invaluable. Peripheral neuropathy may also be caused by infiltration of cranial or spinal nerve roots by leukemic cells, although this is notoriously difficult to demonstrate by any radiologic technique. A therapeutic trial of irradiation may be required to relieve the symptoms and confirm the diagnosis.

In contrast to the case in both lymphoma and myeloma, extradural compression of the spinal cord is an unusual clinical event. A solid localized mass of leukemic cells known as a chloroma, seen in AML and blastic transformation of CML, may result in extradural compression, however. Chloromas may be visualized by magnetic resonance imaging and can be treated by standard cytotoxic agents or radiotherapy.

Chemotherapeutic agents may themselves cause neurologic problems. The vinca alkaloid vincristine regularly causes peripheral neuropathy; autonomic neuropathies have also been described.[71-74] A usually reversible cerebellar syndrome may be seen with the use of cytarabine (particularly at higher doses).[75-77] Fludarabine has also been associated with neurologic toxicity,[78] although this complication is rare in the lower doses now commonly used in CLL.

Ocular involvement is most commonly seen with ALL. In this setting, meningeal leukemia is associated with infiltration of the choroid and optic nerve. Infiltration of the retina may occur in both childhood AML and ALL.[79] Chloromas may form in the orbit, and visual loss may result from thrombocytopenic hemorrhage.

Cardiovascular and Respiratory Systems

Although there may be leukemic involvement of the heart and lungs, it is typically asymptomatic.[80-83] Cardiac abnormalities are infrequently detected clinically on physical examination, although when precordial murmurs are elicited, they are usually a result of altered flow characteristics from anemia or fever and not a result of new structural abnormalities. One should be mindful, however, of infective endocarditis in the septic patient with a murmur and repeatedly positive blood cultures. Abnormal electrocardiograms have been recorded in about 35% of patients with acute leukemia. The most common finding is sinus tachycardia, although nonspecific ST segment changes, T wave changes, and premature atrial and ventricular contractions are also common.[83] Cardiac abnormalities are largely clinically silent and detected post mortem. There may be hemorrhage and direct infiltration by leukemic cells, affecting all four chambers. Disease of the pericardium may result in effusions from either thrombocytopenia or infection. These may manifest as cardiac tamponade and should be managed in the usual way by drainage once the platelet count has been corrected.

Pulmonary infiltrates on a chest radiograph are typically infective in origin, but they may represent leukemic infiltration or be a manifestation of leukostasis.[81] They may also represent pulmonary hemorrhage. High-resolution computed tomography and bronchoscopy may help diagnostic accuracy. Indeed, high resolution computed tomography may aid diagnosis in those with a normal chest radiograph.[84] Leukostasis must be treated promptly with leukapheresis while the underlying disease is managed with cytotoxic agents (see later). T-cell ALL is frequently associated with a mediastinal mass.[85, 86] This may cause superior vena caval obstruction, which again should be treated promptly.

Urogenital System

Renal failure is an uncommon presenting manifestation of leukemia; however, it is commonly encountered during therapy. This is typically a result of nephrotoxic agents, acute tubular necrosis secondary to hypotensive episodes, and hyperuricemia (dealt with earlier in this chapter). The physician should frequently monitor renal function and observe fluid balance so that prompt steps may be taken to reverse etiologic factors.

The kidneys may be directly infiltrated by leukemia, although this is rarely in itself a problem. It may be detected on plain radiography or by ultrasonography. Hematuria may be frank or microscopic and is common in the context of thrombocytopenia. It may be ameliorated by platelet transfusion. Hemorrhagic cystitis complicates cyclophosphamide therapy and may cause problems ranging from microscopic hematuria with minimal urinary symptoms to life-threatening hemorrhage requiring cystectomy. To reduce the risk of this, it is important to maintain a high urine output with intravenous fluids and to consider employing the uroepithelial protective agent mesna when cyclophosphamide-containing therapies are given.

Testicular involvement is classically associated with ALL in children and adults. It typically presents as painless unilateral testicular enlargement, although it may occur bilaterally.[87-90] It is typically a site of relapse and may precede marrow relapse.[85, 86] Infiltration is diagnosed by biopsy or aspiration of the testes. The ovaries may rarely be involved in female patients. Leukostasis-induced priapism may occur in patients with CML and less commonly with acute leukemias.[91-93]

Skeletal System

Bone pain is common at presentation in childhood ALL (30% of patients) but is infrequent in adult leukemias.[94-96]

The cause may be either infiltration or bone infarction. Treatment with cytotoxic agents results in improvement; however, steroids may be helpful in resistant disease.

The awareness of hyperuricemia and the use of allopurinol have now made gout rare. Avascular necrosis, particularly of the femoral heads, may be seen as a late sequela of the use of corticosteroids.

SPECIAL SITUATIONS

Leukostasis

Leukostasis is the clinical manifestation of hyperleukocytosis. It is seen most commonly in the patient with AML but also in those with CML in myeloid blast crisis and in those patients presenting with very high white blood cell counts. The two most susceptible sites are the lungs and the brain. This accounts for the high early mortality, in excess of 20%, observed in those presenting with white blood cell counts of greater than 100×10^9/L.[97]

Myeloblasts are relatively inelastic, causing plugging of vascular channels. As a result, leukocyte aggregation and thrombus formation occur. With the resulting capillary distention, leakage, and capillary rupture, myeloblasts move into the surrounding parenchyma. There they may release procoagulants and inflammatory factors, exacerbating local organ damage.[98] Those patients with a monocytic leukemia (FAB M4 and M5) appear particularly vulnerable.[81]

Respiratory distress is a common clinical manifestation. There may be significant hypoxemia with local or diffuse pulmonary infiltrates on the chest radiograph. Urgent organ support with mechanical ventilation may be required. Septal thickening from accumulation of parenchymal myeloblasts produces a classic diffusion block, with lung injury exacerbated by hemorrhage from vascular injury and thrombocytopenia. Ventilation/perfusion mismatching contributes to hypoxia.[98]

In the central nervous system, leukostasis is associated with a particular type of intracerebral hemorrhage found in the white matter.[99] Hemorrhage occurs at platelet counts not normally associated with spontaneous bleeding, suggesting the relative importance of endothelial damage. Neurologic symptoms include headache, dizziness, visual disturbance, and impairment in the level of consciousness. The bleeding can be massive, leading to severe neurologic deficits and frequently to death.

Other important manifestations of leukostasis are priapism and cardiac failure.

Patients with hyperleukocytosis are protected somewhat from marked increases in blood viscosity by a relative anemia. Transfusion of red blood cells may result in a rise in viscosity, precipitating leukostasis.

Urgent measures are required to lower the circulating blast count, and success in this seems to predict clinical improvement in the symptomatic individual.[81] Action should be taken before symptoms develop; it is often too late to prevent morbidity and death once symptoms occur. Hydroxyurea rapidly lowers the blast count before commencement of definitive induction therapy.[100] Leukapheresis is also beneficial,[97, 101] as is cranial radiotherapy in those with central nervous system disease.[102] An inverse relationship exists between the height of the presenting white blood cell count and survival in acute nonlymphocytic leukemia.[97] The long-term outlook for those individuals who may be successfully supported through leukostasis is poor; those with hyperleukocytosis have difficulty achieving remission[103, 104] and have a reduced duration of remission.[97, 103, 104]

Pregnancy

Information about leukemia in pregnancy is sparse. Virtually all antileukemic agents cross the placenta, and concern about their teratogenicity may result in a recommendation to terminate the pregnancy. In the context of pancytopenia, however, this may be hazardous. With close multidisciplinary management, successful outcomes for both patient and fetus have been achieved. In cases in which pregnancy has been continued, response to treatment and survival appear to be equivalent to those of women who are of comparable age and who are not pregnant.[105]

It has been demonstrated that leukemic cells may cross the placenta,[106] but no evidence exists of transfer of leukemia from mother to child. The administration of standard remission induction chemotherapy to patients with acute leukemia has been reported during the second and third trimesters.[107, 108] At this stage, remission may be achieved in the patient with no adverse effects on the fetus. For patients who elect to continue with a pregnancy when leukemia is diagnosed in the first trimester, the rate of fetal abnormalities is high because of drug-induced teratogenicity.[109, 110] However, there appears to be no increased risk for birth defects in children of parents who have completed chemotherapy or in those whose fathers were receiving chemotherapy at the time of conception.[105, 111, 112]

The timing of delivery may be a problem because thrombocytopenia and granulocytopenia may be disastrous for the mother during delivery. Case reports suggest that at the time of delivery, active leukemia presents more of a hazard to the mother than if she were in remission.[113] It may not be possible to achieve remission before delivery, however, because of resistant disease or the unpredictable timing of delivery, particularly with presentation in the third trimester.[114] In these circumstances, it may be beneficial to delay commencement of specific therapy until after delivery. Granulocyte colony-stimulating factor has been used in the third trimester in a patient with AML, resulting in a significant clinical and hematologic improvement that allowed sufficient time for maturation of the fetus in utero and safe delivery before induction therapy.[115]

When it is possible, CML in pregnancy should be managed with leukapheresis because it avoids the potential teratogenic effects of chemotherapy[116, 117]; however, there have been successes with busulfan[118] (although there may be an excess of fetal abnormalities) and interferon alfa.[119] Interferon alfa does not inhibit DNA synthesis and has also been used successfully in the management of hairy cell leukemia during pregnancy. However, because experience is still limited, a specific recommendation cannot be made. Hydroxyurea has been reported to control the maternal blood count, with successful outcomes when conception has occurred during its administration.[120] It has been suggested that a combination of leukapheresis and hydroxyurea, beginning after the first trimester, is an appropriate method of management.[121]

Fetal marrow suppression has been documented after maternal chemotherapy[122]; thus, at the time of delivery, the hematologic status of the fetus should be taken into account. Long-term follow-up of children born to mothers who have received cytotoxic chemotherapy for hematologic malignant disease in pregnancy has revealed no physical, psychologic, neurologic, or cytogenetic abnormalities,[123] although some series have reported congenital abnormalities.[124]

Completion of Therapy

Apparent successful completion of antileukemic therapy, although a welcome milestone, may result in the individual's having difficulty adjusting to activity that was previously considered normal. With a reduced frequency of hospital visits, the security of knowing that close observation is being made may be lost, and there may be ongoing concern about disease recurrence and long-term health. The patient may find it difficult to consider himself or herself a healthy person and no longer in the "sick role."

Other people's perception of the individual may be altered, and the individual may continue to be seen as ill. Employers may be unwilling to allow resumption of previous tasks, and there may be problems associated with a future employer's concerns about the diagnosis of leukemia.

Most people are able to adjust to these difficulties, although no one can forget that he or she has had leukemia. Return outpatient visits for regular follow-up will serve as a reminder of this and may be associated with significant anxiety.

Long-term Follow-up

It is now more than 30 years since the first papers described the use of combination cytotoxic therapies to induce remission in acute leukemias.[125] There is now a sizable proportion of individuals who are living in good health an excess of 10 years from diagnosis. These individuals are of interest not only because they represent the success of therapeutic modalities but also because they may demonstrate the long-term harmful effects these treatments may have caused, which may restrict a return to complete health. At St. Bartholomew's Hospital, 12% of those diagnosed with acute leukemia survived for more than 10 years from diagnosis.[126] Although survival at 3 years from diagnosis appears to represent a plateau, late recurrences develop and have been documented more than 20 years or longer from the end of treatment.

For long-term adult survivors, infertility may be an important issue. Standard combination therapy for AML may not necessarily cause azoospermia, although by contrast, ALL therapy usually does.[112] This is usually a result of end-organ gonadal failure and not of hypothalamic/pituitary dysfunction secondary to cranial radiotherapy. Gonadal dysfunction in female survivors of ALL is a result of direct radiotherapy to the ovaries from craniospinal radiotherapy, compared with cranial therapy alone.[127] In the St. Bartholomew's series, 39% of long-term survivors have either become pregnant or fathered children. There was no increase in the incidence of congenital abnormalities above that expected in the normal population.[126] For those women who do undergo a premature menopause, the benefits of hormone replacement therapy should be discussed.

The issue of a secondary malignant neoplasm should be considered in the context of long-term follow-up. In survivors of childhood cancer, the risk for development of malignant disease is 6 to 10 times higher than the risk for development of a first malignant neoplasm in the general population.[128] With a median time to occurrence of 6.7 years and a cumulative incidence of 2.7% at 18 years,[128] and the 10-year actuarial incidence of 3.5% in studies of bone marrow transplant recipients,[129] it is important to be mindful of these secondary malignant neoplasms in the design of new therapeutic modalities. The St. Bartholomew's series reported a cumulative incidence of 27% at 20 years, although this may reflect the older age of patients in this group.[126]

Treatment Failure

Many individuals with leukemia will die of the disease, either at the outset or after the achievement of remission. Recurrent and secondary therapy-related leukemias may bring shock and disappointment followed by death. People vary in their willingness to discuss the mode of death, but fear is common. Pain is not usually a feature of death from leukemia, and catastrophic bleeding fortunately occurs infrequently. This is often a concern of caregivers of those patients wishing to die at home.

Unlike in many other malignant diseases, the time during which the patient deteriorates is often very short, and expectations should be openly discussed. The individual's wish to choose an appropriate place to die should be acceded to whenever possible. With such support, many choose to die at home, although others may elect to stay in the hospital where they have built up relationships with staff and feel secure. In areas where they are available, hospices may provide a suitable alternative. The assistance of palliative care physicians and nursing staff may aid the transition from intensive therapeutic interventions to a focus on symptom control.

Whatever choice is made, the caregivers have a duty to provide, whenever possible, a dignified end to their patients' lives.

REFERENCES

1. Binet JL, Auguier A, Dighiero G, et al: A new prognostic classification of chronic lymphocytic leukemia derived from a multivariate survival analysis. Cancer 1981;48:198.

2. Catovsky D, Fooks J, Richards S: Prognostic factors in chronic lymphocytic leukaemia: The importance of age, sex and response to treatment in survival. Br J Haematol 1989;72:141.
3. Karmiris T, Rohatiner AZ, Love S, et al: The management of chronic lymphocytic leukemia at a single centre over a 24 year period: Prognostic factors for survival. Hematol Oncol 1994;12:29.
4. Rai KR, Sawitsky A, Eugene P, et al: Clinical staging of chronic lymphocytic leukemia. Blood 1975;46:219.
5. Bloomfield CD, Goodman AL, Alimena G, et al: Chromosomal abnormalities identify high-risk and low-risk patients with acute lymphoblastic leukemia. Blood 1986;67:415.
6. Borella L, Sen L: T-cell surface markers on lymphoblasts from acute lymphoblastic leukemia. J Immunol 1973;11:1257.
7. Brouet JC, Preud'homme JL, Penit C, et al: Acute lymphoblastic leukemia with pre B-cell characteristics. Blood 1979;54:269.
8. Vogler LB, Crist WM, Bockman DE, et al: Pre-B-cell leukemia. A new phenotype of childhood lymphoblastic leukemia. N Engl J Med 1978;298:872.
9. Mutz TD, Humphrey GB, Henderson ES: Chronic myelogenous leukemia of juvenile type. Eur J Pediatr 1976;121:227.
10. Smith KL, Johnson W: Classification of chronic myelocytic leukemia in children. Cancer 1974;43:670.
11. Tan KH, Tan TS: Chronic myeloid leukemia in children. Singapore Med J 1968;9:39.
12. Mueller BU, Skelton J, Callender DP, et al: A prospective randomized trial comparing the infectious and noninfectious complications of externalized catheter versus a subcutaneously implanted device in cancer patients. J Clin Oncol 1992;10:1943.
13. Kappers-Klunne MC, Degener JE, Stijnen T, et al: Complications from long-term indwelling central venous catheters in hematologic patients with special reference to infection. Cancer 1989;64:1747.
14. Mullan FJ, Hood JM, Barros D'Sa AA: Use of the Hickman catheter for central venous access in patients with haematological disorders. Br J Clin Pract 1992;42:167.
15. Shaw JH, Douglas R, Wilson T: Clinical perfromance of Hickman and Portacath atrial catheters. Aust N Z J Surg 1988;58:657.
16. Sharpe PC, Morris TC: Complications associated with central venous catheters in a haematology unit. Ulster Med J 1994;63:144.
17. Sariego J, Bootorabi B, Matsumoto T, et al: Major long term complications in 1,422 permanent venous access devices. Am J Surg 1993;165:249.
18. Kinsey SE: Experience with teicoplanin in non-inpatient therapy in children with central line infections. Eur J Haematol 1998;62(suppl):11.
19. Ketley NJ, Kelsey SM, Newland AC: Teicoplanin and oral ciprofloxacin as outpatient treatment of infective episodes in patients with indwelling central venous catheters and haematological malignancy. Clin Lab Haematol 1995;17:71.
20. Raad II, Luna M, Khalil SA, et al: The relationship between thrombotic and infective complications of central venous catheters. JAMA 1994;271:1014.
21. Bern MM, Lokich JJ, Wallach SR, et al: Very low doses of warfarin can prevent thrombosis in central venous catheters. A randomized prospective trial. Ann Intern Med 1990;112:423.
22. Martino R, Sureda A, Sitjas D, et al: Leukemic dermal infiltrate at the exit site of a central venous catheter. Haematologica 1993;78:132.
23. Ruppel LJ, Brown RA, Borsin RA, et al: Retained Hickman catheter cuff as an infection source following allogeneic bone marrow transplant. Bone Marrow Transplant 1994;14:169.
24. Karp JE, Merz WG, Hendricksen C, et al: Oral norfloxacin for prevention of gram-negative bacterial infections in patients with acute leukemia and granulocytopenia. A randomized, double-blind, placebo-controlled trail. Ann Intern Med 1987;106:1.
25. Arning M, Wolf HH, Aul C, et al: Infection prophylaxis in neutropenic patients with acute leukemia—a randomized, comparative study with ofloxacin, ciprofloxacin and co-trimoxazole/colistin. J Antimicrob Chemother 1990;26(suppl D):137.
26. Twycross R: Anorexia, cachexia, nausea and vomiting. Medicine (Baltimore) 2000;28:7.
27. Yau E, Rohatiner AZ, Lister TA: Long term prognosis and quality of life following intensive care for life-threatening complications of haematological malignancy. Br J Cancer 1991;64:938.
28. Lloyd-Thomas AR, Wright I, Lister TA, et al: Prognosis of patients receiving intensive care for life-threatening medical complications of haematological malignancy. BMJ 1988;296:1025.

29. Peters SG, Meadows JA, Gracey DRE: Outcome of respiratory failure in hematologic malignancy. Chest 1988;94:99.

30. Estopa R, Torres-Marti A, Kastanos N, et al: Acute respiratory failure in severe hematological disorders. Crit Care Med 1984;12:26.

31. Hinds CJ, Martin R, Quinton P: Intensive care for patients with medical complications of haematological malignancy: Is it worth it? Schweiz Med Wochenschr 1998;128:1467.

32. Rubenfeld GD, Crawford SE: Withdrawing life support from mechanically ventilated recipients of bone marrow transplants: A case for evidence-based guidelines. Ann Intern Med 1996;125:625.

33. Jackson SR, Tweeddale MG, Barnett MJ, et al: Admission of bone marrow transplant recipients to the intensive care unit: Outcome, survival and prognostic factors. Bone Marrow Transplant 1998;21:697.

34. Lofti M, Brandwein JM: Spontaneous acute tumor lysis syndrome in acute myeloid leukemia? A single case report with discussion of the literature. Leuk Lymphoma 1998;29:625.

35. Levin M, Cho S: Acute tumor lysis in high grade lymphoblastic lymphoma after a prolonged episode of fever. Med Pediatr Oncol 1996;26:417.

36. Benekli M, Güllü IH, Savas MC, et al: Acute tumor lysis syndrome following intrathecal methotrexate. Leuk Lymphoma 1996;22:361.

37. Silverman P, Distelhorst C: Metabolic emergencies in clinical oncology. Semin Oncol 1989;16:504.

38. Razis E, Arlin ZA, Ahmed T, et al: Incidence and treatment of tumor lysis syndrome in patients with acute leukemia. Acta Haematol 1994;91:171.

39. Arrambide K, Toto RD: Tumor lysis syndrome. Semin Nephrol 1993;13:273.

40. Saccente SL, Kohaut EC, Berkow RL: Prevention of tumor lysis syndrome using continuous veno-venous hemofiltration. Pediatr Nephrol 1995;9:569.

41. Leach M, Parsons RM, Reilly JT, et al: Efficacy of urate oxidase (uricozyme) in tumour lysis induced urate nephropathy. Clin Lab Haematol 1998;20:169.

42. Pui CH, Relling MV, Lascombe F, et al: Urate oxidase in prevention and treatment of hyperuricemia associated with lymphoid malignancies. Leukemia 1997;11:1813.

43. Cutting HO: Inappropriate secretion of antidiuretic hormone secondary to vincristine therapy. Am J Med 1971;51:269.

44. Meriweather WD: Vincristine toxicity with hyponatraemia and hypochloremia in an adult. Oncology 1971;25:234.

45. Nicholson RG, Feldman W: Hyponatremia in association with vincristine therapy. Can Med Assoc J 1972;106:356.

46. Slater LM, Weiner RA, Serpick AA: Vincristine neurotoxicity with hyponatremia. Cancer 1969;23:122.

47. Stuart MM, Cuaso C, Miller M, et al: Syndrome of recurrent increased secretion of antidiuretic hormone following multiple doses of vincristine. Blood 1975;45:315.

48. Canellos GP: Hypercalcemia in malignant lymphoma and leukemia. Ann N Y Acad Sci 1974;230:240.

49. Frolich D, Lohrmann P, Ziegler R, et al: Hypercalcemia and kidney failure as early symptoms of acute leukemias. Verh Dtsch Ges Inn Med 1972;78:117.

50. Haratake J, Ishii N, Horie A, et al: Adult T-cell leukemia complicated by hypercalcemia. Report of three autopsy cases with special reference to etiologic factor of hypercalcemia. Acta Pathol Jpn 1985;35:437.

51. Fujihira T, Eto S, Sato K, et al: Evidence of bone resorption-stimulating factor in adult T-cell leukemia. Jpn J Clin Oncol 1985;15:385.

52. Aach R, Kissane J: Hypercalcemia and an elevated alkaline phosphatase level. Am J Med 1973;54:751.

53. Gewirtz A, Stewart AF, Vignery A, et al: Hypercalcaemia complicating acute myelogenous leukaemia: A syndrome of multiple aetiologies. Br J Haematol 1983;54:133.

54. Kinsley RE: Hypercalcemia associated with leukemia. Arch Intern Med 1966;118:14.

55. Mwadsley C, Holman RL: Hypercalcaemia in acute leukaemia. Lancet 1957;1:78.

56. Stein RC: Hypercalcemia in leukemia. J Pediatr 1971;78:861.

57. O'Regan S, Carson S, Chesney RW, et al: Electrolyte and acid-base disturbances in the management of leukemia [editorial review]. Blood 1977;49:345.

58. Kronfield SJ, Reynold TB: Leukemia and hypercalcemia. N Engl J Med 1964;271:399.

59. Fetchick DA, Bertolin DR, Sarin PS, et al: Production of 1,25-dihydroxyvitamin D_3 by human T-cell lymphotrophic virus–transformed lymphocytes. J Clin Invest 1986;78:592.

60. Suzumiya J, Asahara, Katakami H, et al: Hypercalcaemia caused by all-*trans* retinoic acid treatment of acute promyelocytic leukaemia; case report. Eur J Haematol 1994;53:126.

61. Lemez P: Hypercalcaemia caused by all-*trans* retinoic acid (ATRA) treatment in a case of acute promyelocytic leukaemia was manageable after decreasing the ATRA dose to 27 mg/m^2/day. Eur J Haematol 1995;55:275.

62. Abramson EC, Gajardo H, Kukreja SC: Hypocalcemia in cancer. Bone Miner 1990;10:161.

63. Schenkein DP, O'Neill WC, Shapiro J, et al: Accelerated bone formation causing profound hypocalcemia in acute leukemia. Ann Intern Med 1986;105:375.

64. Trier JS, Bjorkman DJ: Esophageal, gastric and intestinal candidiasis. Am J Med 1984;77:39.

65. Boggs DA, Wintrobe MM, Cartwright GE: The acute leukemias. Analysis of 322 cases and review of the literature. Medicine (Baltimore) 1962;41:163.

66. Varki AP, Armitage JO, Feagler JR: Typhlitis in acute leukemia: Successful treatment by early surgical intervention. Cancer 1979;43:695.

67. Moir CR, Scudamore CH, Benny WB: Typhlitis: Selective surgical management. Am J Surg 1986;151:563.

68. Katz JA, Wagner ML, Gresik MV, et al: Typhlitis. An 18-year experience and post mortem review. Cancer 1990;65:1041.

69. Shamberger RC, Weinstein HJ, Delorey MJ, et al: The medical and surgical management of typhlitis in children with acute non-lymphocytic (myelogenous) leukemia. Cancer 1986;57:603.

70. Garewal HS, Dalton WS: Metoclopramide in vincristine-induced ileus. Cancer Treat Rep 1985;69:1309.

71. Bradley WB, Lassman LP, Pearce GW, et al: The neuromyopathy of vincristine in man. Clinical, electrophysiological and pathological studies. J Neurol Sci 1970;10:107.

72. Caccia MR, Comotti B, Ubali E, et al: Vincristine polyneuropathy in man. A clinical and electrophysiological study. J Neurol 1977;216:21.

73. Casey EB, Jelliffe AM, LeQuesne PM, et al: Vincristine neuropathy. Clinical and electrophysiological observations. Brain 1973;96:69.

74. Raphaelson MI, Stevens JC, Newman BP: Vincristine neuropathy with bowel and bladder atony mimicking spinal cord compression. Cancer Treat Rep 1983;67:604.

75. Barnett MJ, Richards MA, Ganesan TS, et al: Central nervous system toxicity of high dose cytosine arabinoside. Semin Oncol 1985;2(suppl 3):227.

76. Capizzi RL, Poole M, Cooper MR, et al. Treatment of poor risk acute leukemia with sequential high dose ARA-C and asparaginase. Blood 1984;63:694.

77. Herzig RH, Lazarus HM, Wolff SN, et al: High-dose cytosine arabinoside therapy with and without anthracycline antibiotics for remission reinduction of acute nonlymphoblastic leukemia. J Clin Oncol 1985;3:992.

78. Spriggs DR, Stopa E, Mayer RJ, et al: Fludarabine phosphate (NSC 312887) infusion for the treatment of acute leukemia: Phase I and neuropathological study. Cancer Res 1986;46:5953.

79. Robb RM, Ervin LD, Sallan SE: An autopsy study of eye involvement in acute leukemia of childhood. Med Pediatr Oncol 1979;6:171.

80. Jenkins PF, Ward MJ, Davies P, et al: Non-Hodgkin's lymphoma, chronic lymphocytic leukaemia and the lung. Br J Dis Chest 1981;175:22.

81. Lester JJ, Johnson JW, Cuttner J: Pulmonary leukostasis. The single worst prognostic factor in patients with acute myelocytic leukemia and hyperleukocytosis. Am J Med 1985;70:43.

82. Nathan DJ, Sanders M: Manifestations of acute leukemia in the parenchyma of the lung. N Engl J Med 1955;252:797.

83. Roberts WC, Bodey GP, Wertlake PT: The heart in acute leukemia. A study of 420 autopsy cases. Am J Cardiol 1966;21:388.

84. Heussel CP, Kauczor HU, Heussel GE, et al: Pneumonia in febrile neutropenic patients and in bone marrow and blood stem-cell transplant recipients: Use of high-resolution computer tomography. J Clin Oncol 1999;17:796.

85. Hoelzer D, Thiel E, Löffler H, et al: Prognostic factors in a multicenter study for treatment of acute lymphoblastic leukemia in adults. Blood 1988;71:123.

86. Linker CA, Levitt LJ, O'Donnell M, et al: Treatment of acute lymphoblastic leukemia with intensive cyclical chemotherapy. A follow-up report. Blood 1991;78:2814.

87. Eden OB, Hardisty RM, Innes EM, et al: Testicular disease in acute lymphoblastic leukaemia in childhood. BMJ 1978;1:334.

88. Husto HO, Aur RJA: Extramedullary leukaemia. Clin Haematol 1978;7:313.

89. Finkelstein JZ, Dyment PA, Hammond GD: Leukemic infiltrates of the testes during bone marrow remission. Pediatrics 1969; 43:1042.

90. Pavlovsky S, Salazar C, Eppinger-Heift M, et al: Incidence of testicular infiltration in acute lymphoblastic leukemias. Sangre (Barc) 1979;24:559.

91. Craver LF: Priapism in leukemia. Surg Clin North Am 1933;13:472.

92. Graw RG, Skeel RT, Carbonne PP: Priapism in a child with chronic granulocytic leukemia. J Pediatr 1969;74:788.

93. Vadakan VV, Ortega J: Priapism in acute lymphoblastic leukemia. Cancer 1972;50:373.

94. Kundel DW, Brecher G, Bodey GP, et al: Reticulin fibrosis and bone infarction in acute leukemia. Implications for prognosis. Blood 1964;23:526.

95. Masera G, Carnelli V, Ferrari M, et al: Prognostic significance of radiological bone involvement in childhood ALL. Arch Dis Child 1979;54:73.

96. Nies BA, Kundel DW, Thomas LB, et al: Leucopenia, bone pain, and bone necrosis in patients with acute leukemia. A clinicopathological complex. Ann Intern Med 1965;62:698.

97. Dutcher JP, Schiffer CA, Wiernick PH: Hyperleukocytosis in adult nonlymphoblastic leukemia: Impact on remission rate and duration of survival. J Clin Oncol 1987;5:1964.

98. Prakash UB, Divertie MB, Banks PM: Aggressive therapy in acute respiratory failure from pulmonary infiltrates. Chest 1979;75:559.

99. Freireich EJ, Louis B, Thomas LB, et al: A distinctive type of intracerebral hemorrhage associated with blastic crisis in patients with leukemia. Cancer 1960;13:146.

100. Grund FM, Armitage JO, Burns CP: Hydroxyurea in the prevention of the effects of leukostasis in acute leukemia. Arch Intern Med 1977;137:1246.

101. Cuttner J, Holland JF, Norton L, et al: Therapeutic leukapheresis for hyperleukocytosis in acute myelocytic leukemia. Med Pediatr Oncol 1983;11:76.

102. Wiernik PH, Serpick AA: Factors affecting remission and survival in adult acute non-lymphoblastic leukemia (ANLL). Medicine (Baltimore) 1970;49:505.

103. Rohatiner AZ, Gregory WM, Bassan R, et al: Short term therapy for acute myelogenous leukemia. J Clin Oncol 1988;6:218.

104. Hug V, Keating M, McCredie K, et al: Clinical course and response to treatment of patients with acute myelogenous leukemia presenting with a high leukocyte count. Cancer 1983;52:773.

105. Nicholson HO: Cytotoxic drugs in pregnancy: Review of reported cases. J Obstet Gynaecol Br Commonw 1968;75:307.

106. Rigby PG, Hanson TA, Smith RS: Passage of leukemic cells across the placenta. N Engl J Med 1964;271:124.

107. Estin M: Successful pregnancy in leukaemia. Lancet 1977;1:433.

108. Volkenandt M, Buchner T, Hiddemann W, et al: Acute leukaemia during pregnancy [letter]. Lancet 1988;1:1404.

109. Myers AM, McCaskill T, Belliveau J, et al: Severe teratogenic effects of second trimester antileukemic chemotherapy. Proc Am Soc Clin Oncol 1984;3:22.

110. Sieber SM, Adamson RH: Toxicity of anti-neoplastic agents in man: Chromosomal aberrations, anti-fertility effects, congenital abnormalities and carcinogenic potential. Adv Cancer Res 1975; 22:57.

111. Blatt J, Mulvihill JJ, Ziegler JL, et al: Pregnancy outcome following cancer chemotherapy. Am J Med 1980;69:828.

112. Waxman J, Terry Y, Rees LH, et al: Gonadal function in men treated for acute leukaemia. BMJ 1983;287:1093.

113. Murray JA, Gee H: Acute leukaemia during pregnancy [letter]. Lancet 1988;1:243.

114. Griffiths M: Acute leukaemia during pregnancy [letter]. Lancet 1988;1:586.

115. Cavenagh JD, Richardson DS, Cahill MR, et al: Treatment of acute myeloid leukaemia in pregnancy [letter]. Lancet 1995;346:441.

116. Caplan SN, Coco FV, Berkman EM: Management of chronic myelocytic leukemia in pregnancy by cell phoresis. Transfusion 1978; 18:120.

117. Fitzgerald D, Rowe JM, Heal J: Leukapheresis for control of chronic myelogenous leukemia during pregnancy. Am J Hematol 1986; 22:213.

118. Dugdale M, Fort AT: Busulfan treatment of leukemia during pregnancy. Case report and review of the literature. JAMA 1967;199: 131.

119. Baer MR, Ozer H, Foon KA: Interferon alpha therapy during pregnancy in chronic myelogenous leukaemia and hairy cell leukaemia. Br J Haematol 1992;82:783.

120. Jackson N, Shukri A, Ali K: Hydroxyurea treatment for chronic myeloid leukaemia during pregnancy. Br J Haematol 1993;85:203.

121. Fitzgerald JM, McCann SR: The combination of hydroxyurea and leukapheresis in the treatment of chronic myeloid leukaemia in pregnancy. Clin Lab Haematol 1993;15:63.

122. Murray NA, Acolet D, Deane M, et al: Fetal marrow suppression after maternal chemotherapy for leukaemia. Arch Dis Child Fetal Neonatal Ed 1994;71:F209.

123. Aviles A, Diaz-Maqueo JC, Talavera A, et al: Growth and development of children of mothers treated with chemotherapy during pregnancy: Current status of 43 children. Am J Hematol 1991; 36:243.

124. Reynoso EE, Shepherd FA, Messner HA, et al: Acute leukemia during pregnancy; the Toronto Leukemia Study Group experience with long-term follow-up of children exposed to chemotherapeutic agents. J Clin Oncol 1987;5:1098.

125. Scott RB: Leukaemia. Lancet 1957;1:1053.

126. Micallef INM, Rohatiner AZ, Carter M, et al: Long-term outcome of patients surviving more than ten years following treatment for acute leukaemia. Br J Haematol 2001;113:443.

127. Hamre MR, Robison LL, Nesbit ME, et al: Effects of radiation on ovarian function in long-term survivors of childhood acute lymphoblastic leukemia: A report from the Childrens Cancer Study Group. J Clin Oncol 1987;5:1759.

128. Kimball Dalton VM, Gelber RD, Li F, et al: Second malignancies in patients treated for childhood acute lymphoblastic leukemia. J Clin Oncol 1998;16:2848.

129. Kolb HJ, Socie G, Duell T, et al: Malignant neoplasms in long-term survivors of bone marrow transplantation. Ann Intern Med 1999; 131:738.

14

Renato Bassan

Management of Infections in Patients with Leukemia

ETIOLOGY AND PATHOGENESIS

The relationship between people and microorganisms is very old. Whereas the genus *Homo* appeared relatively recently in the evolutionary time scale (about 2.3 million years ago),[1] protobacteria and bacteria are possibly the earliest known forms of life and are detectable in fossil specimens as old as 3.5 billion years, as in the case of the stromatolites associated with growth of earliest cyanobacteria.[2] Many ancestral bacterial species required iron for growth and proliferation. This characteristic has been retained and helps explain why the blood iron concentration is sensibly reduced as a result of the activation of monocytes and macrophages in response to infection.

Bacteria exhibit the most spectacular diversification among all living species (representing more than two thirds of all those known) and show an exceptional adaptive capacity to extreme environmental circumstances (*Methanococcus, Pyrobaculum, Lyngbya, Eoentophysalis.*)[3] Moreover, in living cells, fundamental cellular structures such as mitochondria and chloroplasts (in plant cells) are thought to have originated from early phylogenetic integration (endosymbiosis) between eukaryotic cells and bacteria specialized in the production of energy. Other microorganisms grow in symbiosis and have become essential for survival of the host species, as occurs with the intestinal bacteria producing vitamin K. Globally, the commensals provide a protective effect against other pathogens through a competitive local growth mechanism.

Etiology

Infections are caused by bacteria, viruses, fungi, and protozoa. In patients with leukemia, all types of infections can occur, either being present at diagnosis or arising during antileukemic treatment and subsequent follow-up. The types of pathogens are listed in Table 14-1.[4-6]

Mode of Acquisition

Microorganisms are normally present in the environment and can be acquired by patients after hospitalization. Others are already present in the host as commensals and become more pathogenic by reason of changes in patient defenses.[6-11] Among bacteria and fungi, most of those found to cause serious infections are normally detectable in the skin and body orifices or belong to *Escherichia coli, Klebsiella pneumoniae,* anaerobic bacteria such as *Clostridium difficile,* and *Candida* species. For infections caused by *Pseudomonas aeruginosa* and *Aspergillus* species, on the other hand, transmission from an exogenous source is more usual, although a transient colonization phase can precede the overt spread of infection. The mode of acquisition of viral infections follows a different path.[6] In children, primary exogenous infection with herpes simplex virus type 1 (HSV-1), cytomegalovirus (CMV), and varicella-zoster virus (VZV) occurs through the air by being in proximity to infected people. In adults, reactivation of endogenous latent disease is much more common for HSV-1, HSV-2, and VZV infections and is possible for CMV. CMV infection is frequent in leukemia patients who undergo allogeneic hematopoietic stem-cell (HSC) transplantation. In this setting, the rate of infection is significantly higher in seronegative recipients who receive blood products from seropositive subjects or transplants from seropositive siblings. CMV is present in the white blood cells of asymptomatic seropositive subjects and can be transmitted via blood products to those who are seronegative. Transmission of infection by transfusion also occurs with hepatitis C virus (HCV), although screening methods are becoming increasingly effective in the prevention of this infection.

Multifactorial Pathogenesis and Risk Class

In healthy subjects, despite heavy environmental and endogenous contamination with several types of pathogens, the occurrence of life-threatening infections is uncom-

TABLE 14–1. Principal Microorganisms Causing Infections in Leukemic Patients

Pathogens	Frequency	
	Very Common/Common	*Occasional/Rare*
Bacteria		
Gram-negative	*Pseudomonas aeruginosa, Escherichia coli, Klebsiella* spp.	*Enterobacter* spp., *Proteus* spp., *Salmonella* spp., *Haemophilus influenzae, Alcaligenes* spp., *Legionella* spp., *Neisseria* spp., *Acinetobacter* spp., *Shigella* spp., *Citrobacter* spp., *Serratia marcescens, Aeromonas* spp., *Capnocytophaga* spp., *Stenotrophomonasmaltophilia*
Gram-positive	*Staphylococcus aureus* and *epidermidis; Streptococcus pneumoniae, viridans,* and *pyogenes; Enterococcus faecalis*	*Corynebacterium* spp., *Listeria* spp., *Leuconostoc* spp.
Anaerobes		*Bacteroides* spp., *Clostridium* spp., *Fusobacterium* spp.
Mycobacteria		*Mycobacterium tuberculosis,* atypical mycobacteria
Fungi	*Candida* spp., *Aspergillus* spp.	*Fusarium* spp., *Mucor* spp., *Torulopsis glabrata, Trichosporon* spp., *Curvularia, Alternaria, Exserohilum, Bipolaris* spp., *Scedosporium* spp.
Protozoa	*Pneumocystis carinii*	*Toxoplasma gondii, Strongyloides stercoralis, Cryptococcus neoformans, Histoplasma capsulatum, Coccidioides immitis*
Viruses	Varicella-zoster, herpes simplex, cytomegalovirus	Epstein-Barr virus enteroviruses, human herpesvirus-6, BK virus adenovirus, respiratory syncytial virus, live virus vaccines, hepatitis viruses B and C, influenza/parainfluenza viruses, HIV-1
Other		*Chlamydia* spp., *Mycoplasma* spp.

mon. Normally, several bacterial species (and some fungi, but not viruses and protozoa) inhabit the upper aerodigestive tract, the skin, the mucosal surface of the outer genitalia, and the large bowel. Apart from that, infections are prevented by the anatomic integrity of mucocutaneous barriers and fought by the humoral (immunoglobulin-producing B cells: opsonins, lysins, and the complement system) and cellular branches (phagocytes, T cells, natural killer [NK] cells) of the immune system. All these branches act in a highly coordinated fashion and express a vast array of cell-to-cell and cell-to–humoral factor interactions whose ultimate goal is rapid reconaissance of the foreign pathogen and isolation and destruction of it by means of integrated defense mechanisms.[6] Thus, when infection arises in leukemic patients, a multifactorial pathogenesis is likely, and profound alterations occur in these systems, as shown in Table 14–2. The general mechanisms by which leukemic patients may become infected

during progression and management of their disease are shown in Table 14-3. As a result of the type and stage of leukemia, the characteristics of the patients, and the type and intensity of treatment, the risk of development of serious infectious complications is highly variable, as summarized in Figure 14-1. First, many patients are always at relatively high risk, and the risk is aggravated further by aggressive therapeutic choices and by progression of disease. Second, several other pathogenetic cofactors can significantly add to this risk, as illustrated in Figure 14-2. The final, simplified model identifies two different risk classes calling for risk-oriented prophylactic and therapeutic measures (Fig. 14-3). Low- and high-risk patients with characteristics like those indicated in Figure 14-3 have been recognized by most authorities,[12-15] so this distinction should be applied whenever possible to define individual risk and improve the conduct and interpretation of clinical studies.

TABLE 14–2. Host Defense Mechanisms against Infections

Branch	Description	Function
Anatomic	Integrity of skin and mucosal surfaces, production of mucus, activity of cilia	Anatomic/functional barriers
	Spleen	Protection from blood-borne pathogens, opsonization
Humoral	Immunoglobulins (IgG, IgA, IgM; total, >0.5 g/dL) by B cells	Antigen recognition, opsonization, complement activation
	Lysozyme, complement interleukins, colony-stimulating factors, interferon (soluble factors)	Chemotaxis, pathogen lysis, generation, and propagation of an immune response
Cellular	T cells (CD4+ and CD8+ subset)	Adaptive immune system, cooperate with B cells and soluble factors
	Neutrophils, monocytes, natural killer cells, tissue phagocytes	Innate immune system, cooperate with soluble factors
Commensals	Colonizing oropharyngeal and fecal flora	Competitive growth

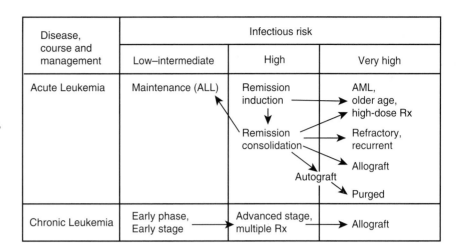

FIGURE 14–1. Infectious risk according to the type of leukemia, treatment phase and intensity, and selected host features. ALL, acute lymphocytic leukemia; AML, acute myelogenous leukemia.

TABLE 14–3. Mechanisms of Reduced Resistance to Infections in Leukemia

Mechanisms	Primary Effects	Secondary Effects
Leukemia	Reduction/inhibition of normal hematopoiesis	Granulocytopenia, monocytopenia, lymphocytopenia
	Altered immunoglobulin synthesis	Hypogammaglobulinemia
	T-cell defects	Defective adaptive immunity
	Neutrophil/monocyte dysfunction	Defective innate immunity
Chemo/radiotherapy	Myelosuppression	Blood cytopenia
	Mucosal damage	Disruption of the anatomic barrier
	Immune suppression	B-/T-cell deficiency
Hospitalization (air, food, water, personal contact)	Altered colonization of endogenous flora	Nosocomial infections
Cathethers, drainage tubes, etc.	Skin/mucosal damage	Disruption of the anatomic barrier

FIGURE 14–2. Details of concurrent pathogenetic risk factors for infections. CLL, chronic lymphocytic leukemia; GVHD, graft-versus-host disease.

Pathogenetic cofactors	Infectious risk		
	Low–intermediate	High	Very high
Neutropenia	$0.5–1\times10^9$/L, <8 days	$0.1–0.5\times10^9$/L, 8–14 days	0.1×10^9/L, >14 days
Mucositis	Absent, mild (grade I)	Severe (grade II)	Diffuse, ulcerative (grade III)
Immune impairment	Hypogamma-globulinemia (<0.5 g/L, CLL)	CD4 cytopenia, (<200–50/mL)	GVHD, T cell depletion, unrelated/mismatch (allograft)
Drugs (other than neutropenia and mucositis)	Antineoplastics (general), Antibiotics (fungal)	Purine nucleoside analogs (CLL), corticosteroids (*Aspergillus* spp.)	
Environment	Moist, wet	Active construction, season (*Aspergillus* spp.)	

Main pathogenetic cofactors	Infectious risk	
	Standard	High
Neutropenia	>0.5×10⁹/L; <0.5×10⁹/L, <8 days	<0.1×10⁹/L; <0.5×10⁹/L, >8 days
Mucositis	Nonsevere	Severe
Disease	Chronic leukemia, early phase, responsive	Acute leukemia, advanced phase, nonresponsive
Treatment	Conventional-dose, first-line, maintenance, outpatient	High-dose, autograft, allograft

FIGURE 14–3. Simplified risk model for infections according to principal risk factors.

Myelosuppression and Neutropenia

Neutropenia is the most important factor predisposing to infection in leukemic patients.[4, 6, 15-19] Neutropenia and severe neutropenia are defined by an absolute polymorphonuclear cell count of less than 1.5×10^9/L and 0.5×10^9/L, respectively. The mechanism leading to absolute neutropenia in untreated leukemia patients is variable and does not always relate to physical substitution of normal marrow cellularity by leukemic cells. Although it varies with subtype, time elapsed from the onset of symptoms to diagnosis, and administration of chemotherapy to suppress further bone marrow activity, neutropenia is constant in acute leukemia patients. Neutropenia is common in patients with the most advanced form of myelodysplastic disorder, refractory anemia with excess myeloblasts before acute transformation. In chronic leukemias, neutropenia is most often encountered in hairy-cell leukemia (HCL) at onset[20] and in advanced-stage chronic lymphocytic leukemia (CLL), in hypersplenomegalic variants, or in the rare cases producing antineutrophil antibodies. Autoimmune neutropenia is relatively rare in CLL,[21, 22] but it is one of the dominant clinical features of the chronic lymphoproliferative disorder sustained by large granular lymphocytes with immunophenotypic and functional characteristics of either cytotoxic T lymphocytes or NK cells of non T-cell lineage.[23-25] With few exceptions, the initial treatment of leukemia generally entails the administration of cytotoxic and hence myelotoxic chemotherapy and/or radiotherapy.[6, 26] It is expected that leukemia patients undergoing cytotoxic treatment will become and remain neutropenic, the length of the neutropenic period depending on the administrative schedule and time necessary for myelosuppressive activity to subside after bone marrow regeneration. Myelosuppression by antineoplastic drugs is dose dependent and aggravated by concomitant radiotherapy.[27] Vincristine, bleomycin, and L-asparaginase are virtually devoid of this most unwanted effect. Anthracycline derivatives, mitoxantrone, m-AMSA, alkylating agents, cytosine arabinoside, hydroxyurea, and nitrosoureas are potent depressants of marrow function. Thus, many of the drugs associated with the best therapeutic outcomes in patients with newly diagnosed disease, especially acute leukemias, are strongly myelotoxic. Epipodophyllotoxins and methotrexate used without folinic acid rescue confer an intermediate degree of myelotoxicity. Whatever the primary cause and pathogenesis, neutropenia favors infections by gram-negative bacteria such as the classic triad of *E. coli*, *K. pneumoniae*, and *P. aeruginosa*: Infection by gram-positive bacteria and anaerobes is also facilitated, in addition to infection with *Candida* and *Aspergillus* species. The risk of acquiring these infections is inversely correlated with the neutrophil count; it is high at counts less than 0.5×10^9/L and extremely high at counts less than 0.1×10^9/L. Another important corollary is that the longer the duration of neutropenia, the greater the frequency of infections. In early studies, the maximal risk of infection occurred after 10 to 14 days with a neutrophil count less than 0.5×10^9/L.[16, 17] That these thresholds are critical and affect survival was confirmed recently. In a large series of 2276 patients undergoing HSC transplantation,[28] the risk ratio of mortality before day 100 fluctuated between 2.01 and 5.78 in patients with a neutrophil count lower than 0.1×10^9/L after day 14.

In another series involving 444 cancer patients (17% with acute leukemia) with febrile neutropenia ($<0.5 \times 10^9$/L), the incidence of serious, life-threatening complications was significantly increased (36% versus 16%, $p < 0.00001$) when the absolute neutropenic period lasted ≥ 7 days.[28a]

Mucositis and Altered Anatomic Integrity

Chemotherapeutic agents and radiation therapy are toxic not only to blood cells and their precursors but also to many other tissues.[29, 30] The skin and mucosal surfaces are effective anti-infective barriers in healthy subjects. Drug-related upper and lower gastrointestinal mucositis is common, and the skin is often disrupted for diagnostic or therapeutic procedures (marrow aspiration, venipuncture, lumbar puncture, insertion of indwelling intravenous catheters), thereby permitting the entry and dissemination of pathogens. Mucositis is subjectively one of the worst aspects of leukemia therapy, yet its contribution to infectious complications will never be stressed enough. Both drugs and radiotherapy can cause mucositis of the upper and lower aerodigestive tracts, the effects of which are highly unpleasant to patients and they offer potential pathogens almost ideal access to the blood stream. The combination of mucosal ulcers, neutropenia, and altered local microbial flora can lead to the most devastating and life-threatening infections in patients with acute leukemia who are receiving intensive therapy. Mucosal damage with high-dose cytarabine occurs early,[31] 24 to 48 hours from the start of treatment, and is associated with a high incidence of *Streptococcus viridans* septicemia.[32] Mucositis associated with myeloablative treatment and HSC transplants is usually very severe and results in an increased risk of morbidity and mortality from infections.[33, 34] Although breakdown of mucosal barriers is

TABLE 14–4. MUCPEAK: A Mucositis Scoring System Predicting the Incidence and Severity of Mucositis-Associated Infections

A. MUCPEAK	Denotes peak oral mucositis score based on the University of Nebraska Oral Assessment Score, which assigns a numeric score (1–3) to the 8 separate clinical aspects listed below. Scoring is to be performed daily. The range of possible scores is 8–24. At least mild mucositis is associated with a score >12. Severe mucositis is defined by scores ≥18 and was associated with higher incidence of positive blood cultures ($P = .001$) and early mortality ($P = .001$)		
B. Scoring system C. Evaluation	1 = normal	2 = mild/moderate abnormality	3 = severe abnormality
1. Voice quality	Normal	Deep/raspy	Difficulty talking/painful
2. Swallowing	Normal	Painful	Unable to swallow
3. Lips	Smooth/pink/moist	Dry/cracked	Ulcerated/bleeding
4. Tongue	Pink/moist/papillated	Coated/without papillae/shiny	Blistered/cracked
5. Saliva	Watery	Thick/ropy	Absent
6. Mucosae	Pink/moist	Reddened/coated	Ulcerated
7. Gingiva	Pink/stipled/firm	Edematous	Bleeding
8. Teeth	Clean/no debris	Localized plaque/debris	Diffuse plaque/debris

Adapted from[33].

easily detectable at the oropharyngeal and other accessible sites, similar damage must be assumed to occur throughout the entire digestive channel and may affect the respiratory and genitourinary systems as well. Because of its pathogenetic importance (see Figs. 14–2 and 14–3), scoring systems have been developed to allow more objective measurement of mucositis and correlation with major clinical events.[33, 35, 36] In these studies, severe mucositis correlated significantly with a higher incidence of infections and infection-related mortality, gastrointestinal symptoms (diarrhea), dysmetabolic changes (weight loss, hypoalbuminemia), and longer duration of total parenteral nutrition. Functional methods such as the D-xylose absorption test are also available, but they are more cumbersome and expensive than direct clinical evaluation. Because of its prognostic value and ease of performance, even in critically ill subjects, the MUCPEAK score system[33] is presented as an example in Table 14–4. Apart from drug and radiation-induced injury to mucosal surfaces, widely used intravenous indwelling catheters, both the tunneled and nontunneled types, and other infusion or drainage equipment break normal anatomic barriers and can therefore facilitate local and then disseminated infections not only with gram-positive *Streptococcus* and *Staphylococcus* species but also with *Pseudomonas, Corynebacteria, Klebsiella,* and *Candida.*[6, 37–43] Neutropenia on the day of insertion is correlated with a risk of catheter-related infection, regardless of whether the catheter is inserted in the operating room or radiology suite.[44] Contamination during marrow aspiration for transplants occurs rarely.[45]

Impaired Immunity

In patients with leukemia, whether neutropenic or not, the functional capabilities of phagocytic cells may be intrinsically defective and result in decreased microbial killing even in the presence of adequate numbers of cells. In this case, the pattern of infections closely resembles that observed in neutropenic patients, with few differences. In patients with myeloid leukemias and particularly those with myelodysplastic syndromes, several defects in chemotaxis, oxidative and energy metabolism,

enzymatic activity, including myeloperoxidase activity, cytokine secretion, and membrane receptors have been reported.[46–49] Because laboratory testing of these defects is complex and has little impact on practical management of the disease, in most cases these dysfunctional lesions can be hypothesized, but seldom proved in patients with neutrophil/monocyte counts in the low-normal range who suffer from frequent infectious complications. These defects are very likely present if morphologic and histochemical changes in neutrophils, such as cytoplasmic hypogranularity, nuclear hyposegmentation, and reduced myeloperoxidase or alkaline phosphatase staining, are detected on examination of peripheral blood smears. Humoral and cellular immune mechanisms mediated by B and T lymphocytes, respectively, can be profoundly altered in patients with leukemia. B cells produce immunoglobulins, which in concert with complement proteins and phagocytes, act primarily in the opsonization, lysis, and neutralization of bacteria. T cells, other than cooperating with all components of the immune system, are predominantly involved in recognizing intracellular microrganisms and activating macrophages. NK cells of non–T-cell lineage have proven antiviral activity.[50] Thus, any quantitative or qualitative derangement of these systems from baseline may facilitate the occurrence of infections, though in a less clear fashion than neutropenia. Hypogammaglobulinemia, defined as a total gamma globulin concentration less than 0.5 g/dL, is especially frequent in late-stage CLL, but it can be observed in any other leukemia patient treated with immunosuppressive drugs. Notably, the T-cell and NK cell systems are intrinsically altered in many subtypes of leukemia, and the abnormalities sometimes involve the network of hematopoietic growth factors.[20, 47, 51–56] A complex defect of all aspects of the immune system, aggravated by the prolonged immunosuppressive therapy, characterizes HSC transplant procedures. A low immunoglobulin level predisposes to infections by both gram-positive and gram-negative bacteria and by *Giardia lamblia.* The clinical spectrum of infections is more complex in the case of abnormal cell-mediated immunity and ranges from bacterial infections caused by intracellular organisms *(Legionella, Nocardia asteroides, Mycobacterium)* to fungal infections *(Candida, Cryptococcus neoformans, Histoplasma capsula-*

tum), viral diseases (VZV, HSV, CMV, Epstein-Barr virus [EBV]), and protozoal diseases *(Pneumocystis carinii, Strongyloides stercoralis, Cryptosporidium, Toxoplasma gondii)*.

Drug-Related Effects Other than Neutropenia and Mucositis

In addition to myelosuppression and mucositis, most drugs useful in the treatment of leukemias can induce functional impairment of phagocytes, and some selectively depress cell-mediated immunity.[6, 57] Among others, methotrexate, cyclophosphamide, and corticosteroids are potent immunosuppressive agents, but additional problems are emerging with new drugs. For example, a severe cellular immunodeficiency with very low levels of circulating CD4$^+$ T lymphocytes develops in many patients with CLL and HCL who are treated with the new purine nucleoside analogues fludarabine, 2-chloro-2'deoxyadenosine, and 2'-deoxycoformycin.[58-66] The immune defect can persist for 1 year and longer, even in patients with responsive disease. The infections described in these patients are typically related to T-cell dysfunction and are observed at increased frequency when the absolute CD4$^+$ cell count is less than 50/μL *(Listeria monocytogenes, P. carinii*, CMV, HSV, VZV, mycobacteria). However, quite often, no causative agent can be identified during the course of the febrile episode. It has been calculated that one third to one half of patients who are treated with these drugs suffer from some infectious complication. The concomitant use of corticosteroids, extensive previous therapy, neutropenia, hypogammaglobulinemia, older age, worse performance status, elevated serum creatinine, and poor treatment response are factors that aggravate the risk and the related death rate.[20, 47, 51-57] With regard to other drugs, corticosteroids are routinely used in the treatment of lymphoid malignancies and may have a place in the general management of patients with gram-negative sepsis,[66] bacterial meningitis, *P. carinii* pneumonia, and autoimmune problems or when immunosuppression is specifically required to manipulate immune reactions after allogeneic HSC transplants. These effects are obtained through inhibition of activation and migration of phagocytes, suppression of cytotoxic functions, and a general anti-inflammatory action that reduces fever and other usual clinical signs and symptoms of infection.[67-69] Conversely, corticosteroids may exert a strong proinfective action in certain fungal infections. Pharmacologic concentrations of hydrocortisone accelerate the growth of *Aspergillus* species, shorten the doubling time to approximately 48 minutes, and induce hyphal extension of 1 to 2 cm/hr.[70] Cyclosporine is another immunosuppressive drug used in HSC transplant patients. This drug selectively inhibits cell-mediated immunity. Despite this potent immunosuppressive effect, there is no certainty that cyclosporine adds significantly to the infectious risk in these patients,[6, 71] but data regarding new potent immunosuppressants (FK-506, tacrolimus) are still lacking. Other drugs interfering with the normal function of immunocompetent cells are allopurinol, some antibiotics, and nonsteroidal anti-inflammatory drugs, but it is

unknown precisely how they contribute to infections in specific situations. Among biologic response modifiers, interleukin-2 (IL-2) is being tested as a means of immunotherapy for some forms of leukemia.[72] Altered phagocyte and lymphocyte function and increased susceptibility to infection with *Staphylococcus aureus* and *Staphylococcus epidermidis* have been described with IL-2.[73] The use of recombinant human interferon alfa (IFN-α) in patients with different types of leukemia has been associated with several hematologic and immune function changes, the most relevant of which is reversible neutropenia.[74] Although some degree of activation of NK cells was observed in cancer patients,[75, 76] interferon therapy has been found to aggravate myelosuppression when given after bone marrow transplants.[77] Serotherapy for B- or T-cell malignancies with monoclonal antibodies conjugated with cellular toxins or radionuclides is another promising therapy being developed.[78] Although immunotoxins and immunoradiotoxins are harmful to normal residual B/T lymphocytes, no apparent increase in infectious risk has been noted.[79, 80] Paradoxically, the use of drugs fundamental to the management of infected leukemic patients can sometimes also favor the opposite effect. Antibiotic-related infections may arise primarily, as second episode, or as a component of multiple infections. A rather common occurrence is the development of infections with microorganisms not covered by the drug in question when patients are given prophylactic antibiotics.[6] This mechanism is typical of streptococcal and other gram-positive infections in patients treated prophylactically with oral quinolones.[81] Another example is enterocolitis by *C. difficile,* an anaerobic organism normally present in the colon. Overgrowth of *C. difficile* is facilitated by long-term antibiotic therapy and concomitant suppression of other commensals.[6, 82-85] Prolonged administration of antibiotics and corticosteroids as well predisposes to infections by *Aspergillus* species.[6, 86, 87] In turn, antifungal therapy with amphotericin B (AmB) and fluorocytosine appears to slow neutrophil recovery after intensive chemotherapy and can thus contribute to the onset of other infections.[88]

Environmental Factors

The problem of mucositis is compounded by the fact that the oral cavity and distal part of the digestive tract normally harbor several microorganisms and the normal colonizing flora can be partially replaced by more virulent microorganisms from the environment.[7-9, 89] Of great concern is the fact that hospitalization of leukemic patients is followed by the acquisition or predominance in the oropharyngeal and fecal flora of *E. coli, Pseudomonas* species, *K. pneumoniae, Enterobacter* species, and anaerobes, even without the concomitant administration of antibiotics. As previously shown, some of the most pathogenic bacterial and fungal species are predominantly exogenous and acquired after a transient phase of colonization following admission to the hospital.[6, 10, 11] Air, water, most surfaces (bathrooms, lavatories, and floors), uncooked food, fresh vegetables and fruit, and staff or visitors may all be contaminating sources of *Aspergillus, Pseudomonas, Staphylococcus, Enterobacter,* and *Kleb-*

TABLE 14–5. Factors Associated with an Increased Risk of Infection in Patients Receiving HSC Transplants

Treatment Phase	Factors	Effects (at HSC Transplantation)
Pretransplant	Any unresolved infection	Aggravation
	HBV, HCV	Aggravation if hepatitis is still active
	CMV, VZV, HSV, HBV, HCV	Reactivation of latent virus
At transplant	Chemo/radiotherapy	High-grade mucositis
		Lung and gastrointestinal toxicity
		Immune suppression
	Purged autograft	Delayed neutrophil recovery
	Acute GVHD	Aggravation of tissue damage and immune suppression
Post-transplant	Slow immune system recovery	Humoral and cellular immune deficiency
	Immunosuppressive therapy	Delayed immune reconstitution
	Chronic GVHD	Delayed immune reconstitution, functional asplenia

CMV, cytomegalovirus; GVHD, graft-versus-host disease; HBV, hepatitis B virus; HCV, hepatitis C virus; HSC, hematopoietic stem cell; HSV, herpes simplex virus; VZV, varicella-zoster virus.

siella. Transmission of these pathogens to immunocompromised hosts is therefore very likely. For *Aspergillus* infections, an association with active construction in the ward and hospital area has been confirmed,[70] and sometimes seasonal variation is reported, with a higher incidence in the spring and autumn.

Hematopoietic Stem-Cell Transplants

HSC bone marrow or peripheral blood transplantation has become a standard procedure in leukemia therapy. Autologous HSC transplantation is often used as consolidation treatment in patients with acute leukemia in first remission, whereas allogeneic HSC transplantation is generally offered as a curative option to younger patients with advanced primary myelodysplasia or chronic myelogenous leukemia, to those with recurrent or high-risk acute leukemia, and sometimes to all these patients provided that a family donor can be found. The use of allogeneic HSC transplants from unrelated volunteer donors is increasing, particularly in high-risk situations where no other available therapeutic option appears to be curative. During and after HSC transplantation particularly allogeneic transplantation and the use of unrelated donors, the risk of infection is very high and the clinical spectrum is the widest.[90-95] The number of predisposing factors, their variable prevalence over the subsequent treatment phases, and the complexity of their interactions explain the characteristic pattern of infections associated with HSC transplants and deserve detailed analysis (Tables 14-5 and 14-6).

Problems before HSC Transplantation

FUNGAL INFECTIONS

Pretransplant, some patients might have suffered from infections related to the specific disease and its primary treatment. Normally, transplantation is discouraged in patients with active infection of any kind, unless it appears to be the only lifesaving treatment, in which case the risk could be taken after detailed discussion with the patient and relatives. Patients who have completely recovered from a previous fungal infection are eligible, provided

that elimination of the infection is confirmed by a thorough clinical search. High-resolution computed tomography (HRCT), examination and culturing of bronchoalveolar fluid, and respiratory function tests are useful aids in those who had lung infiltrates. Because reactivation of latent infection may have disastrous consequences, prophylactic surgical excision of isolated lung lesions caused by *Aspergillus* species has been advocated.[96] This approach, however, necessitates considerable surgical skill and may not be required if the lesions are quiescent

TABLE 14–6. Cofactors and Type of Prevailing Infections in Relation to Time of HSC Transplantation

	Transplant Phase		
	Before Engraftment (First Month)	Early after Engraftment (Second and Third Months)	Late Period
Cofactors			
Conditioning toxicity	+++	+	–
Skin/mucosal damage	+++	++	–
Slow hematologic recovery	+	+++	–
T-cell depletion	++	++	+/–
Intravascular devices	+	+	+
Reactivation of viruses	+	+++	+
Cytomegalovirus	–	+++	–
Humoral immunodeficiency	–	++	++
Cellular immunodeficiency	–	++	++
Acute GVHD	+	+++	–
Chronic GVHD	–	+	+++
Prevailing infections			
Bacteria (gram-positive and gram-negative)	+++	+	+/–*
Herpes simplex	+++	–	–
Epstein-Barr virus			
Cytomegalovirus	–	+++	+
Varicella-zoster virus	–	+	++
BK virus	–	+	–
Hepatitis C virus	–	–	+
Candida spp.	++	+/–	–
Aspergillus spp.	+†	++	+
Pneumocystis carinii	–/+	++	–

* *P. pneumoniae.*
† T-cell–depleted autograft.

and effective antifungal prophylaxis is given.[97-100] In patients with previous fungal disease who undergo allogeneic HSC transplantation, the average risk of reactivation is around 30%, but it is significantly higher in those who receive allografts from unrelated/mismatched donors, after T-cell depletion, in those in whom severe graft-versus-host disease (GVHD) develops, or in patients who are taking corticosteroids (>7 mg/kg/wk). These patients, if they receive allografts, have a very high risk of death from disseminated fungal infection.[101] Surgery appears to be justified in patients with unresolved infection or recurrent hemoptysis and infiltrates surrounding major vessels or other vital structures that put them at risk of sudden death from hemorrhage.[102] Likewise, disseminated candidiasis is not an absolute contraindication to HSC transplantation when adequate therapy is continued.[103]

HEPATITIS VIRUS INFECTIONS

Another source of great concern in the preparative phase for HSC transplantation is the detection of hepatitis B or C virus antigenemia or active hepatitis in the recipient or, alternatively, in the case of an allogeneic HSC transplant, in the donor. New hepatitis G and TT viruses have been identified and associated with the occurrence of liver dysfunction after conventional therapy for leukemia or after HSC transplantation. However, these recently discovered pathogens do not appear to induce very severe or long-lasting and potentially fatal degrees of liver injury as hepatitis B and C viruses (HBV, HCV) can do.[104-108] Most, if not all leukemia patients given myelosuppressive therapy are regularly transfused with packed red cells and platelet concentrates, so the risk of post-transfusion hepatitis and chronic sequelae in those who are initially seronegative is increased.[109-112] Transplant patients infected with HBV and, seemingly, HCV are at risk for veno-occlusive disease (occurring in the early post-transplant phase) and hepatitis reactivation, which can subsequently evolve to liver failure and death. Reactivation of hepatitis occurs in the mid to late post-transplant period, after initial reduction or withdrawal of immunosuppressive drugs and restoration of the immune response in the host, and in turn leads to recognition and destruction of infected hepatocytes.[113-115] Healthy people are normally at some risk of being infected with these viruses, but more so patients with leukemia. In some places, the risk of infection with HBV is endemic. In an European survey,[115] the prevalence of HBV infection (hepatitis B surface antigen [HBsAg] positive, with HBV DNA positivity indicating active infection) and HCV infection (presence of anti-HCV antibodies, with HCV RNA positivity indicating active infection) in candidates for HSC allografting was 3.5% and 5%, respectively. The overall mortality from liver failure post-transplant was 4.5%, with no difference between patients with normal or elevated transaminase values. The attitude toward transplantation varied widely among the 63 participating centers: in only 17 institutions was HSC transplantation carried out irrespective of liver function test results. In summary, carrier status may not represent an absolute contraindication to transplantation, but transplant-related morbidity and mortality are

expected to increase. For this reason, it is important to recognize which patients will be at greatest risk and/or the subgroups for which additional diagnostic and therapeutic steps are necessary before a final decision is made. Furthermore, seronegative patients can obviously receive an HSC graft from a seropositive patient; with HBsAg+ donors, 22% of HBsAg− patients converted to seropositivity (43% if previously anti-HBs−), 21% suffered from subacute hepatitis or veno-occlusive disease, but only 5.5% became chronic carriers.[116] The risk appears higher in anti-HBs− patients who receive transplants from HBeAg+/anti-HBe+ donors and in those who are HBeAg−, anti-HBe+, HBV DNA+; HBsAg− and anti-HBs+ patients have a very low risk of persisting hepatitis developing but can occasionally progress very rapidly to acute liver failure.[113, 114, 116] Altogether, the risk of severe liver failure and death could range from 20% to 50% in patients who receive allografts from seropositive donors and varies according to the serologic marker profile, the risk of death from HBV infection in previously HBsAg− recipients is about 12%,[114] and the risk of both severe liver disease and early death from HCV infection is lower. Whatever the situation, simultaneous evaluation of liver function test results, serologic markers, and HBV DNA or HCV RNA tests by polymerase chain reaction (PCR) in patients (and suitable donors) provides a means to assess the general risk for hepatitis reactivation, transmission, and severity during and after the HSC transplant phase. In patients with uncertain status, it is mandatory to perform a wedge liver biopsy to exactly quantitate the extent of the liver damage. Patients with documented cirrhosis or advanced portal fibrosis plus active viral replication appear to share the highest risk of post-transplant complications and fulminant liver failure. Current knowledge and indications for HSC-based therapy in patients with previous HBV/HCV infection or after the use of infected donors are summarized in Table 14-7. In the allogeneic setting, special additional problems may arise when both the patient and donor are HBV or HCV seropositive. In this case, diagnostic and prophylactic therapeutic measures can be taken in both the patient and donor, but the risk of post-transplant liver disease is the highest, and the decision to perform a HSC procedure must be highly individualized. Drugs useful in the management of infected HSC transplant candidates and/or donors are ganciclovir, famciclovir/penciclovir, and lamivudine for HBV and INF-α/alfacon-1 with or without ribavirin for HCV.[114] These drugs can be given before HSC transplantation to minimize the load of actively replicating viruses and/or thereafter as preemptive treatment when HBV DNA levels start rising. Because HCV infection is associated with a significant risk of late chronic liver disease, prolonged postgraft antiviral treatment may be indicated in all HCV-infected patients with signs of active infection (elevated transaminases, serologic markers, HCV RNA). Liver biopsy is often indicated to differentiate organ damage caused by viral hepatitis from graft-versus-host reactions.

Problems during and after HSC Transplantation

During HSC transplantation, the type and timing of infections are influenced by the intensity and toxicity of the

TABLE 14–7. HSC Transplants for Patients or from Donors with Hepatitis B and C Virus Infection

Group, Infection	Risk Group*	Clinical Risk†	HSC Transplant, Other Measures
A. Patients, HBV	Negative, anti-HBs+	None, protected	Not contraindicated
	Anti-HBc+, HBsAg−, anti-HBs−	Hepatitis reactivation	Not contraindicated; after transplant, add antiviral therapy if HBV DNA–positive
	HBsAg+	VOD, hepatitis reactivation	Contraindicated if cirrhosis/fibrosis (biopsy); before transplant, add antiviral therapy if HBV DNA–positive, monitor if HBV DNA–negative
	HBsAg+, HBeAg−, anti-HBe+, HBV DNA+; HBsAg−, anti-HBs+, anti-HBc+/−	Very high-risk subsets	Add antiviral therapy before transplant: decision to transplant made on an individual basis
B. Patients, HCV	Anti-HCV+, HCV RNA−	Low-intermediate	Contraindicated only if cirrhosis/marked fibrosis (biopsy); otherwise, not contraindicated
	Anti-HCV+, HCV RNA+	Intermediate-high	Not strictly contraindicated; long-term monitoring for antiviral therapy
C. Donors, HBV	Anti-HBs+	None	Not contraindicated
	Anti-HBc+, HBsAg−, anti-HBs−	Variable (HBV DNA status)	Treat with antiviral therapy if HBV DNA–positive
	HBsAg+	High	Consider alternative donor, antiviral treatment; monitor recipient for HBV DNA
D. Donors, HCV	HCV RNA+	Intermediate-high	Consider alternative donor or antiviral treatment

* Based on serum hepatitis markers.
† Significant risk for liver complications after very high-dose therapy with an HSC transplant.
‡ Associated with abnormal liver function tests and/or positive HBV DNA test.
HBc, hepatitis B core; HBe, hepatitis B "early"; HBsAg, hepatitis B surface antigen; HBV, hepatitis B virus; HCV, hepatitis C virus; HSC, hematopoietic stem cell; VOD, veno-occulusive disease.

conditioning regimen, time to engraftment, occurrence and severity of GVHD, administration of contaminated blood products (mainly by CMV), reactivation of endogenous infections (mainly VZV and CMV), immunosuppressive treatments, and long-term immune reconstitution (see Tables 14-5 and 14-6).[6, 90, 94, 117, 118] The problems related to previous invasive mycosis and hepatitis virus infection have been reviewed. As regards other infections, clinical syndromes and possible prophylaxis and treatment will be presented in the sections devoted to specific diseases. The difference between allogeneic and autologous HSC transplantation is essentially the relevance of GVHD, the need for post-transplant immunosuppressive therapy, and the usually longer hematologic recovery time in the latter. In the early transplant period, infections are principally caused by the absence of phagocytes and the mucocutaneous damage secondary to high-dose chemotherapy and radiotherapy. Bacterial infections caused by gram-positive and sometimes gram-negative organisms are common, with a high incidence of *S. viridans*-positive blood cultures and an increased risk of associated early fungal infections.[119-122] Indeed, a very early peak of invasive infections by *Aspergillus* species is currently recognized, even in patients without neutropenia.[123] Later, after hematologic engraftment and resolution of mucositis, the effects of abnormal humoral and cellular immunity prevail, together with the tissue damage produced by GVHD. Transmission of CMV infection with blood products, reactivation of VZV, and a high incidence of fungal infections are observed in this period. In autopsy studies, most infection-related deaths are in fact caused by CMV and fungi.[124] Patients receiving T-cell–depleted HSC transplants from matched unrelated donors frequently suffer from invasive fungal infections.[125] The prevalence is higher in those with bacteremia and viral infections, possibly because of worsened immune dysfunction, mucosal damage, and antibiotic use.[121, 125] Apart from the most common pathogens indicated in Table 14-6, other causative agents can occasionally cause significant problems. Reports have described the transmission or reactivation of infection by *Plasmodium* species[126-128]; *Legionella*[129]; *Listeria*[130]; *T. gondii*[131, 132]; *Trypanosoma cruzi*[133]; *Mycobacterium* species[134, 135]; adenovirus and polyomavirus, which can induce hemorrhagic cystitis[136]; and community-acquired respiratory viruses, including respiratory syncytial virus (RSV), influenza A virus, parainfluenza virus, rhinovirus, and picornavirus.[137-139] The latter group of infections is characterized by a mild upper respiratory tract illness, but these infections can be complicated by severe, life-threatening pneumonia in up to half of patients. With regard to pathogenetic cofactors, in HSC recipients, the duration of neutropenia varies and depends on the HSC source (marrow versus peripheral blood), but the severity of the mucositis is almost always in the highest range. In the allogeneic setting, patients who receive an adequate number of cells usually have rapid engraftment and recover from deep neutropenia in 2 to 3 weeks. Engraftment with autotransplants is slower and requires up to 4 weeks or longer, particularly when the harvested marrow was incubated ex vivo with cytotoxic drugs such as mafosfamide or myeloid-specific monoclonal antibodies.[140-145] During allotransplantation, mucosal and tissue damage is aggravated by acute and chronic GVHD, the management or prevention of which in turn entails the use of strong immunosuppressants. The ensuing result is that both humoral and cellular immune mechanisms remain defective for a long time, which favors infections even after resolution of the neutropenia and healing of mucosal ulcers. Several studies have shown that reconstitution of B-cell, T-cell, and NK cell function may take up to 1 year or more postgrafting.[146-149] Immune reconstitution is particularly slow in people in whom chronic GVHD develops because the functional asplenia contributes to the development of late bacterial infections.[150] Studies considering late infection, specifically, infection from day 50 to 90 onward[151-153] in allogeneic or autologous HSC transplant recipients have shown a high incidence of adverse events causing readmission to the hospital and non–relapse-related mortality. All known causative agents were involved, but the fatality rate was high in patients with pneumococcal infection, in those with pneumonia secondary to *P. carinii* or *Pseudomonas* species, and in patients who received grafts from unrelated donors.

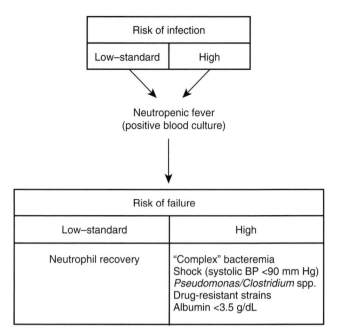

FIGURE 14–4. Risk of treatment failure at onset of bacteremic infection. The outcome is influenced by the indicated clinical and diagnostic characteristics. BP, blood pressure. (Adapted from[12].)

DETERMINANTS OF THE CLINICAL COURSE AND OUTCOME

Risk of Treatment Failure

Patients with leukemia have a variable risk of infection several times during the course of their illness (see Figs. 14-1 to 14-3). Before reviewing the crude data on incidence and mortality, three other pathogenetic aspects contributing to the clinical course and final outcome need to be considered: the risk of treatment failure, the emergence of new pathogens, and drug resistance. In the first place, all patients in whom an infection actually develops regardless of the initial risk class, have an obvious risk of treatment failure and eventually death from this complication. The attendant risk of an adverse outcome is also variable. For instance, in patients with acute leukemia who receive remission induction chemotherapy (representing a homogeneous and predefined risk class), the risk of subsequent treatment failure is higher in those in whom pneumonia develops early, within the first 2 weeks of treatment.[154] A first assessment model from Dana-Farber Cancer Institute[29] identified the following factors as those independently associated with an increased likelihood of mortality in high-risk neutropenic cancer patients: short latency (<10 days) from chemotherapy to onset of febrile complication; patient age ≥40 years; and (surprisingly) absence of mucosal damage or inflammation at oropharyngeal and perineal areas. Mortality increased from 9% in cases with none of these features to 39% and 64%, respectively, in those with a cumulative incidence of two or three factors ($p<0.001$).[155] In a broader context, according to a landmark study from M.D. Anderson Cancer Center in which 909 bacteremic episodes in 799 neutropenic cancer patients were analyzed,[12] the outcome can be significantly worse, in a multivariate model, in the presence of any of the following determinants: systolic blood pressure lower than 90 mm Hg (shock is a preeminent prognostic factor); isola-

tion of *Pseudomonas, Clostridium,* or drug-resistant microorganisms; a low serum albumin level; and the occurrence of "complex" bacteremia. This adverse risk applies to infections involving major organs and tissues (lungs, liver, spleen, kidney, colon, bones, joints, veins, heart, meninges), as well as to abscesses or cellulitis with a diameter larger than 5 cm and to soft-tissue infections of any size with necrosis (thus excluding cystitis, bacteriuria, nonsuppurative otitis and pharyngitis, and soft-tissue infection without necrosis). On the other hand, rapid neutrophil recovery was associated with the best outcome. Though thus far restricted to hematogenous bacterial infections, early identification of groups of patients at greatest risk for treatment failure (Fig. 14-4) can be crucial in the interpretation of clinical trials involving antimicrobials and in assessment of the cost-effectiveness of new expensive drugs such as hematopoietic growth factors, lipid formulations of AmB (with extrapolation of the same concept to fungal infections), and others.

Changing Etiologic Pattern

Bacteria

The prevalence of infections has changed over time, and drug resistance to commonly used drugs is being reported with increased frequency as a consequence of the increasing intensity of antileukemic programs, the emergence of new epidemiologic patterns, the use of prophylactic measures exerting a selective growth pressure on a variety of pathogens, and the use of antacids and H_2 blockers (predisposing to infection by gram-positive bacteria).[155] Prophylactic antibiotic and antiviral drugs have often resulted in a dramatic change in previously recognized patterns. Early infections by herpesviruses, *P. carinii,* and gram-negative bacteria have all been significantly reduced, if not almost totally eliminated by large-scale administration of acyclovir, trimethoprim-sulfamethoxazole (TMP-SMX), and oral quinolones, respectively, to at-risk patients.[6] In many studies, bacterial infections by gram-positive rods have become numerically predominant, and infections by fungi have also increased alarmingly. In a large series from the U.S. National Cancer Institute, 63% of the early infectious episodes were caused by gram-positive rods.[156] Similar data regarding an increasing rate of infections by *S. aureus,* coagulase-negative staphylococci, enterococci, and *Candida* species have been provided by analysis of nosocomial blood stream infections in the years 1980 to 1989.[157] In other series considering both induction and variably intensive consolidation treatments, transplants included, the rate of infection by gram-positive and gram-negative bacteria ranged from 36% to 47% and from 30% to 50%, respectively.[158-162] Infections by viridans streptococci in transplant patients were observed in 13% to 22% of cases.[163] Again, 20% to 44% of all patients had fever of unknown or undetermined significance that was managed as though infectious in nature.[164, 165] In the experience of the European Organization for Research and Treatment of Cancer (EORTC), the incidence of documented gram-positive bacterial isolates increased from 28% to 40% in four consecutive studies, whereas infections by gram-negative bacteria decreased from 68% to 57%.[166] In a subsequent update of eight EORTC studies conducted between 1973 and 1994,[167] the rate of gram-positive infections peaked at 69% (1993–1994), whereas gram-negative bacteria were responsible for only 31% of the isolates. Among these microorganisms, *Streptococcus* species have become an increasing problem in that they represent almost 40% of the total gram-positive isolates. Thus, infections by gram-positive bacteria are currently responsible for about 70% of all primary febrile episodes in neutropenic patients,[55] with *S. aureus* and other coagulase-negative staphylocci being the leading organisms.[167] New bacterial isolates are relatively frequent with both gram-positive (*Leuconostoc, Streptococcus mitis* and *milleri, Corynebacterium jeikeium* and *urealyticum, Rhodococcus, Stomatococcus, Lactobacillus, Bacillus cereus, Clostridium septicum* and *tertium*) and gram-negative (*Stenotrophomonas, Alteromonas, Legionella pneumophila* and *micdadei, Vibrio parahaemolyticus, Capnocytophaga, Alcaligenes, Chryseobacterium, Burkholderia, Fusobacterium, Leptotrichia, Methylobacterium, Moraxella*) rods.[155]

Fungi

Fungal infections have increased as well and tend to occur earlier during the course of the disease. A review of data again from M.D. Anderson Cancer Center demonstrated an increase over the years from 11% to 20%, paralleled by a rise from 8% to 40% of all fatal infections.[86, 168, 169] Fungal infections are expected to be fatal in up to 80% of cases.[86] Data from other sources have indicated an incidence of fungal infections of 3% to 27% (>10% in five of nine reports) and have confirmed the high lethality rate.[160-163, 165, 166, 170-172] In autopsy studies, fungal infections by *Aspergillus* species (30%) and by

Candida species (58%) were identified in 25% of patients with leukemia.[173] Similarly, *Candida* species accounted for two thirds of the fungal isolates from nosocomial infections in the years 1980 to 1990,[174-176] but infections by *Aspergillus* species are common in patients undergoing very high-dose treatment with HSC transplantation.[70, 123] *Aspergillus fumigatus* accounts for about 90% of cases of invasive aspergillosis; other cases are due to the *Aspergillus* species *flavus, niger, terreus, nidulans,* and several other very rare species. Emerging fungal infections are those caused by *Candida* species other than *Candida albicans: tropicalis, glabrata, parapsilosis, krusei, stellatoidea, lusitaniae, guilliermondii,* and *pseudotropicalis*[177]; zygomycosis, hyalohyphomycosis, and phaeohyphomycosis caused by molds resident in soil and plants (*Fusarium, Mucorales, Mucor, Rhizomucor, Absidia, Cunninghamella, Pseudallescheria, Scedosporium, Bipolaris, Exophiala, Xylohypha, Aureobasidium, Acremonium, Penicillium, Scytalidium, Paecilomyces, Sporothrix, Curvularia, Exserohilum,* and *Scopulariopsis*); and those caused by previously nonpathogenic non-*Candida* species (*Trichosporon, Blastoschizomyces, Malassezia, Hansenula,* and *Rhodotorula*).[178, 179] Some of these organisms are associated with peculiar clinical syndromes, and invasive and rapidly progressive candidemia appears to be increasingly associated with non–*C. albicans* species that display a reduced sensitivity to currently available antifungal agents.[175, 180, 181]

Viruses

Infections by HSV and VZV in patients not covered with prophylactic acyclovir were reported with variable frequency, from less than 5% during conventional induction/consolidation therapy,[163, 165] to 10% to 21% during autotransplants,[159, 172, 183] to greater than 50% during allotransplants. In patients who undergo HSC transplants, new viruses causing clinical problems other than CMV are community respiratory viruses, adenovirus, polyomavirus, HH-V6, HH-V7, HH-V8, and EBV.[137-140, 184-188] Rather than an infectious picture, EBV and HH-V8 appear to induce a post-transplant lymphoproliferative disease, and HH-V6 can be associated with severe encephalitis.[89]

Changing Patterns of Drug Susceptibility

The acquisition and overexpression of drug resistance through several possible mechanisms is a way that leukemic cells commonly adopt to escape the effects of curative-intent chemotherapy. Not surprisingly, many infectious agents can be driven into a similar drug-resistant status by selective circumstances represented by use and overuse of prophylactic and therapeutic antimicrobials. Drug resistance genes are transmissable among various bacteria by conjugation of plasmids and transposons. The major types and mechanisms of antimicrobial drug resistance are the following[90]: the emergence of extended-spectrum beta-lactamases in gram-negative bacilli (in response to the widespread use of beta-lactam antibiotics; requiring treatment with a combination of beta-lactamase inhibitor and beta-lactam antibiotic; this may in turn elicit the hyperproduction of beta-lactamases); the emergence of resistance to glycopeptide antibiotics vancomycin and sometimes teicoplanin in gram-positive cocci, among them the ascendant nosocomial pathogens enterococci (VRE, vancomycin-resistant enterococci) and recently *S. aureus*,[191] through decreased affinity of the cell wall structure (in *S. viridans, Enterococcus faecium, faecalis,* and *gallinarum;* requiring highly individualized therapy supported by in vitro susceptibility tests); the emergence of penicillin-resistant streptococci; the development of fluoroquinolone resistance in staphylococci and virtually all gram-negative pathogens including *E. coli* through alteration in DNA topoisomerase (a significant problem in view of the diffusion of these drugs in prophylactic regimens); and the emergence of other resistance mechanisms to macrolides, aminoglycosides, and TMP-SMX. Both resistant bacteria and new species are being isolated at increasing frequency.[156] Data of drug susceptibility patterns derived from clinical studies in large numbers of neutropenic febrile patients (Table 14–8) clearly indicate that many currently employed drugs are losing their initial therapeutic activity against the most common pathogens.[168] Ceftazidime for instance is presently often of little value because of the increasing prevalence of resistant streptococci and staphylococci, whereas the low activity of older fluoroquinolones against many gram-posi-

tive isolates can be improved with administration of the newer extended-spectrum agents trovafloxacin and levofloxacin. Some changes in current empiric prophylactic and therapeutic regimens are therefore advisable in light of these results. With regard to invasive fungal infections, the problem of antifungal resistance is aggravated by the shortage of available active antifungal drugs and by the severity of these infections in neutropenic patients. Resistance of *C. albicans* to ketoconazole is rather common (about 30%), and resistance to fluconazole or even AmB is sometimes being reported.[179] It has been calculated that between 1988 and 1993, more than 15 million patients have been exposed worldwide to fluconazole.[191] These data emphasize the degree of general selective pressure exerted by fluconazole on *Candida* species. In patients with candidemia, non-*C. albicans* species are being increasingly associated with resistance to either fluconazole (*C. parapsilosis, C. krusei*) or AmB (*T. glabrata*) administered both prophylactically and therapeutically.[180] The rate of resistance of *A. fumigatus* to itraconazole is low, but that of other species can be variable. Other azoles are not usually effective against aspergillosis.[192] Unfortunately, tests of in vitro resistance to AmB are poorly predictive of the clinical course and outcome.[70] It is possible that new lipid formulations of AmB and the

TABLE 14–8. In Vitro Drug Resistance Rates (Expressed as a Percentage of Resistant Cases) in Bacterial Isolates from Neutropenic Cancer Patients

Drugs	Gram Positive				
	Staphylococcus aureus	*Coagulase-Negative Staphylococci*	*Enterococci*	*Streptococcus viridans*	*Streptococcus pneumoniae*
Cefepime	26	71	98	8	7
Gentamicin	12	41	29	–	–
Imipenem	26	71	29	–	–
Ciprofloxacin	24	37	46	57	38
Trovafloxacin	10	22	42	1	0.2
Piperacillin/tazobactam	26	71	25	–	–
Amoxicillin/ampicillin	91	88	20	8	14
Erythromycin	60	74	94	32	12
Trimethoprim-sulfamethoxazole	9	43	38	2	18
Vancomycin	0	0	11	3	0.1

	Gram Negative				
	Pseudomonas aeruginosa	*Escherichia coli*	*Klebsiella*	*Enterobacter*	*Serratia*
Ceftazidime*	13	3	6	22	7
Cefepime	10	0	1	0.5	4
Ceftriaxone	46	2	5	13	9
Gentamicin	12	3	3	6	7
Imipenem	8	0.1	0.2	0.5	2
Aztreonam	19	3	6	19	7
Ciprofloxacin	13	2	3	4	7
Trovafloxacin	24	2	3	6	12
Ampicillin	98	43	89	91	88
Piperacillin	11	37	13	21	17
Piperacillin/tazobactam	9	2	4	11	11
Trimethoprim-sulfamethoxazole	95	24	10	12	10

* Not tested in the gram-positive category because of potency known to be less than that of other β-lactams.
Adapted from[167].

new azole voriconazole and caspofungin may be more effective against some of the resistant strains of *Aspergillus*. Furthermore, some therapeutic synergy can be obtained by combining AmB with either flucytosine or rifampicin.[98] With regard to viral infections, drug resistance to front-line antivirals can also develop.[193] Similar to fungal infections, the repertoire of active drugs for highly resistant cases is limited. For acyclovir-resistant herpetic infections and ganciclovir-resistant CMV disease, the drug of choice appears to be foscarnet.[194]

INCIDENCE AND MORTALITY

Acute Myelogenous Leukemia

It has long been known that early death from infection is the major determinant of failure of the initial therapy for acute leukemias, and such infection is responsible for up to 73% of all initial treatment failures.[4, 154, 195] In addition, infections have become very frequent during postremission treatment and lead to readmission, protracted hospitalization, and occasionally death of remission patients. Obviously, both the incidence of infection and mortality are significantly increased in patients with refractory and recurrent acute leukemia as a result of the cumulative effects of retreatment, uncontrolled disease, and toxicity from previous therapy. From comprehensive analysis of studies published before 1994,[6] the estimated cumulative incidence of documented infections and neutropenic fever in patients with acute myelogenous leukemia (AML) was 22% to 96% (greater than 50% in four of six studies examined) during induction, 25% to 60% (greater than 50% in three of five studies) during consolidation courses, 63% to 100% during autologous marrow transplantation, and 24% to 100% (greater than 50% in three of four studies) during allogeneic bone marrow transplantation, with an incidence of transplant-related interstitial pneumonia of 7% to 27%. The incidence of death from infections of any etiology was 1.5% to 21.9% (mean of 14.6%) during induction, 0% to 17% (mean of 5.6%) during conventional consolidation, 0% to 12% (mean of 5%) during autologous bone marrow transplantation, and 0% to 30.4% (mean of 17.2%) during allogeneic marrow transplantation, the latter case including interstitial pneumonia. Death rates from interstitial pneumonia alone were between 5.6% and 23.8% (mean of 14%), a figure reflecting the diagnostic, prophylactic, and therapeutic improvements recently obtained in this field. The proportion of deaths from infection was lower in children, with fatality rates generally under 5%, regardless of the treatment phase. In contrast, the worst results were observed in the elderly, with early death rates from infection of 0% to 42.3% (mean of 22%). Infectious death rates in the postremission period did not differ greatly from those reported in younger patients, but many elderly patients do not receive very intensive postremission consolidation. In patients treated with high-dose cytarabine-containing regimens, life-threatening infections are commonly seen in conjunction with high-grade mucositis and heavy, long-lasting myelosuppression. Because of the increasing importance of cytarabine in the management of

patients with AML, data from recent studies providing sufficient detail on infectious complications with this specific therapeutic modality, as well as other high-dose treatments with allografts or autografts (mainly phase III trials), are reported separately in Table 14–9.

Acute Lymphocytic Leukemia

In a previous analysis,[6] the incidence of infections in patients with acute lymphocytic leukemia (ALL) ranged from 30% to 100% during induction, but it was somewhat lower during standard consolidation and maintenance therapy (3.4% to 75%, less than 50% in three of five studies) and generally lower in children. Infectious death rates during induction therapy for adult patients were 0% to 20% (mean of 5.8%, greater than 10% in 3 of 12 studies), 0% to 7.1% (mean of 2.8%) during consolidation chemotherapy, 0% to 10% (mean of 4.8%) during autologous bone marrow transplantation, and 11% to 25.6% (mean of 17.8%) during allogeneic bone marrow transplantation. The fatality rate for patients in whom interstitial pneumonia developed after allotransplantation was 3.7% to 17.9% (mean of 10.3%). In children, infection and death from *P. carinii* pneumonia became very infrequent during intensive induction, consolidation, and autotransplantation after the introduction of prophylactic TMP-SMX. In the elderly, the reported mortality was 6.7% from two published series of patients receiving intensive induction therapy, whereas data are very scanty concerning postremission therapy. Patients who are infected at diagnosis still have a significantly worse outlook.[208] Data from the most recent and representative clinical studies in adult patients are shown in Table 14–10.

Chronic Leukemias and Preleukemic Myelodysplasia

Despite the fact that morphologic cytochemical, and functional abnormalities of neutrophils have been frequently reported in Philadelphia chromosome–positive chronic myelogenous leukemia,[47, 52] such patients do not appear to suffer from an increased incidence of infections, at least while in the chronic phase. The infection pattern is otherwise similar to that observed in acute leukemia when blastic transformation supervenes and is aggravated by the prolonged exposure to myelotoxic drugs and often by therapeutic refractoriness. Because chronic myelogenous leukemia is incurable by conventional treatments, all patients with a histocompatible sibling or an unrelated bone marrow donor are usually considered for allogeneic bone marrow transplantation. In studies of allogeneic bone marrow transplants from siblings, the overall incidence of infections ranged from 59.6% to 100%,[231-234] and in one of these studies, 1.54 infectious episodes per patient were reported.[231] Death rates from infection and from interstitial pneumonia were 6.2% to 17% and 16.6% to 25%, respectively. For patient receiving an allotransplant from unrelated donors, the probability of death by viral infection was increased.[233] In general, as reviewed previously, transplants from volun-

TABLE 14–9. Incidence and Death Rates from Infections in Recently Published (1991–1999), Selected (Total >100 Initial Patients) Phase II/III Adult Acute Myeloid Leukemia Studies Using Intermediate/High-Dose Cytarabine for Remission Induction and/or Postremission Consolidation Therapy

Study (1st Author, Year)	Remission Induction Phase				Postremission Phase			
	Type*	No.	Incidence	Deaths	Type*	No.	Incidence	Deaths
Harousseau, 1991[196]	Std	115	NR	NR	HD	57	32 (56%)	3 (5%)
Schiller, 1992[197]	Std	51	NR	2 (4%)	HD (all cases)		NR	NR
	ID	50	NR	4 (8%)				
Cassileth, 1992[198]	Std	449	NR	NR	HD	87	22 (5%)†	17 (19.5%)
					Std	83	0†	0
					BMT	54	41 (76%)	13 (24%)
Mayer, 1994[199]	Std	1088	NR	NR	HD	187	71%‡	9 (5%)
					ID	206	59%‡	12 (6%)
					Std	203	16%‡	2 (1%)
Estey, 1994[200]	HD	112	102 (91%)	25 (22%)	—	—	—	—
Zittoun, 1995[201]	Std	941	NR	NR	ID1§	75	NR	6 (8%)
					ID2§	501	NR	23 (4.5%)
					HD	126	NR	9 (7%)|
					ABMT	95	NR	12 (9%)|
					BMT	168	NR	29 (17%)|
Bishop, 1996[202]	HD	149	109 (73%)	NR	Std	106	92 (88%)	4 (4%)
	Std	152	96 (63%)	NR	Std	112	40 (35%)	0
Weick, 1996[203]	HD	228	37 (16%)	33 (14%)	HD	212	NR	2%-4%¶
	Std	490	47 (9.5%)	30 (6%)	Std	126	NR	NR
Sierra, 1996[204]	Std	159	NR	4 (2.5%)	HD**	118	NR	2 (2%)
					BMT	47	NR	3 (6%)
					ABMT	68	NR	0
Harousseau, 1997[205]	Std	504	NR	NR	HD	228	NR	6 (2.5%)
Bassan, 1998[206]	Std	153	NR	NR	ID	24	16 (67%)	2 (8%)
					ABMT	41	28 (68%)	3 (7%)
Büchner, 1999[207]	HD	365	146 (40%)	NR	Std	171	19 (11%)	NR
	Std	360	119 (33%)	NR	Std	147	17 (11%)	NR

* Std, standard intensity; ID, intermediate dose, cytarabine based (400 to 1000 mg/m² per dose); HD, high dose, cytarabine based (>1000 mg/m² per dose); BMT, allogeneic bone marrow transplant; ABMT, autologous BMT; NR, not reported.

† Only severe/life-threatening cases reported.

‡ Figures refer to the number of courses requiring readmission for neutropenic fever (four courses planned per patient).

§ All cases undergoing consolidation 1: ID1, cytarabine, 1000 mg/m² per dose; ID2, cytarabine, 500 mg/m² per dose.

| Figures refer to total death rates in patients who actually underwent consolidation 2 (therapy given).

¶ By patient age and cytarabine dose (2 versus 3 g/m²).

** Before BMT/ABMT.

teer unrelated donors in this and other hematologic neoplasms carry a probability of death from infection and interstitial pneumonia of about 25% and 15%, respectively.[235] In addition, patients with chronic lymphoid leukemias have an increased risk of infection. Reported infection rates for CLL and HCL were 0.51 and 1.13 infections per patient per year, respectively.[236] Besides the rare lymphoproliferative disorder of large granular lymphocytes associated with severe neutropenia, these two chronic lymphoid leukemias confer the highest risk for infection. In CLL, infection can be directly responsible for the patient's death in the most advanced stages, when granulopoiesis is severely impaired, hypogammaglobulinemia develops, and drug-related toxicity (use of purine nucleoside analogues) is more pronounced. In HCL, neutropenic bacterial infections are common at diagnosis, whereas other infections by intracellular microorganisms such as *Toxoplasma, Histoplasma,* and mycobacteria are typically secondary to defective cellular immunity and tend to occur later. In chronic leukemias, splenectomy aggravates the risk of infection by certain pathogens.

Preleukemic myelodysplasia is another distinct and clinically heterogeneous chronic pancytopenic syndrome typical of elderly patients and predisposes to infection by means of neutropenia and functional abnormalities of granulocytes and lymphocytes.[45, 48, 237] The infection rate in myelodysplastic syndromes is high, on average around one documented episode per patient per year, but it increases up to three to five episodes per patient per year in the diagnostic subtypes with bone marrow excess of blast cells, in patients with fewer than 1×10^9/L neutrophils, and in those given corticosteroids or antileukemic treatment.[237, 238] More frequently, these patients suffer from bacterial infections of the lungs, skin, and urinary tract and from sepsis, infections very much resembling those seen in acute leukemia. Other types of infections are rare, each accounting for less than 10% of all episodes. Overall, the importance of infections in patients with primary myelodysplastic states is stressed by the fact that infection was the proximate cause of death in 20% to 64% of cases, depending on whether transformation to acute leukemia was considered.[237, 238]

TABLE 14–10. Incidence and Death Rates from Infections in Recently Published (1990–2000), Selected (>50 Patients) Adult Acute Lymphocytic Leukemia Studies

Study (1st Author, Year)	Remission Induction Phase			Postremission Phase		
	No.	Incidence	Deaths	No.	Incidence	Deaths
Kantarjian, 1990[182]	105	44 (42%)	3 (3%)*	88	7%-35%†	6 (7%)
Rohatiner, 1990[209]	54	NR	11 (20%)‡	36	NR	3 (8%)‡
Linker, 1991[210]	109	69 (63%)	3 (3%)	96	NR	1 (1%)
Ellison, 1991[211]	277	NR	24 (9%)*	151	15%-82%†	4 (3%)
Bassan, 1991[212]	82	NR	5 (6%)*	66	NR	2 (3%)
Fière, 1993[213]	572	NR	22 (4%)	436	NR	NR
Hoelzer, 1993[214]	841	NR	48 (6%)	696	NR	NR
Durrant, 1993[215]	281	NR	NR	232	NR	6 (2.5%)
Wiernik, 1993[216]	55	36 (65%)	4 (7%)	42	13 (13%)	4 (9.5%)
Evensen, 1994[217]	79	NR	NR	65	NR	2 (3%)
Todeschini, 1994[218]	86	NR	NR	68	NR	4 (6%)
Wernli, 1994[219]	63	NR	3 (5%)	51	NR	1 (2%)
Larson, 1995[220]	197	107 (54%)	14 (7%)	167	82 (49%)	7 (4%)
Thomas, 1995[221]	57	29 (51%)	0	51	NR	1 (2%)
Bosco, 1995[222]	74	NR	2 (3%)	54	NR	NR
Attal, 1995[223]	135	NR	3 (2%)	126	NR	NR
Dekker, 1997[224]	130	NR	12 (9%)	86	53 (62%)	1 (1%)
Ludwig, 1998[225]	57	NR	5 (9%)	42	NR	NR
Daenen, 1998[226]	66	49 (74%)‡	3 (4.5%)	58	NR	NR (0?)
Todeschini, 1998[227]	60	19 (32%)	3 (5%)	56	NR	2 (3.5%)
Bassan, 1999[228]	96	44 (46%)	15 (16%)*	79	10 (13%)	2 (2.5%)
Bassan, 1999[229]	88	42 (48%)	6 (7%)	76	NR	NR
Kantarjian, 2000[230]	204	112 (55%)	12 (6%)	185	15%–23%†	11 (6%)
Cumulative data	3768	502/971 (52%)§	206/3408 (6%)∣	2919	289/981 (29%)¶	57/1459 (4%)**

* Total deaths from myelosuppression.
† By treatment type and/or phase.
‡ Total induction plus consolidation data (excluded from cumulative data analysis).
§ Nine evaluable studies (out of a total of 23).
∣ Twenty-one evaluable studies.
¶ Seven evaluable studies.
** Sixteen evaluable studies.
NR, not reported.

CLINICAL PICTURE

Bacterial Infections

Acute Leukemias

In patients with acute leukemia, early infection by gram-negative rods is less frequent than in the past. Sepsis resulting from gram-negative bacteria that produce endotoxins can be extremely serious when caused by *P. aeruginosa,* in which case extensive tissue necrosis and rapidly fatal pneumonia with hypotension, renal failure, and septic shock can supervene. Lately, gram-positive bacteria have emerged as the predominant etiology. Sepsis caused by these organisms is generally less dangerous in the short term, except for acute respiratory distress syndrome secondary to α-hemolytic streptococci, infections by *S. viridans,* septic shock from *S. aureus,* and necrotizing soft-tissue infection by *Streptococcus pyogenes.*[6, 19, 163, 239-241] Gram-positive sepsis prevails in patients bearing indwelling venous devices, in which case it can be complicated by pneumonia and endocarditis. Other catheter-related infections diagnosed with increasing frequency are listed in Table 14–11. Catheter-related infections can involve the exit site or the subcutaneous tunnel and spread easily to other organs through the blood stream.

Infections by anaerobes are less common, perhaps accounting for only 5% to 10% of cases, and they generally become manifested as peritonitis or another deep intra-abdominal infection, marginal necrotizing gingivitis, and soft-tissue infection, including perianal cellulitis.[82, 241, 242] Fulminant sepsis by *Clostridium perfringens* is known. A different case can be made for *C. difficile,* a toxin-producing anaerobe whose acquisition and colonic overgrowth in hospitalized neutropenic patients can lead to a diarrheal illness of variable severity from mild gastroenteritis to pseudomembranous colitis. Localized bacterial infections include sinusitis, otitis and otomastoiditis, upper respiratory tract infections, and obviously, pneumo-

TABLE 14–11. Pathogens Frequently Associated with Infections of Indwelling Venous Catheters

Type of Infection	Isolated Pathogens
Bacterial	*Streptococcus* spp., *Staphylococcus* spp., *Corynebacterium* JK, *Bacillus* spp., *Pseudomonas aeruginosa* and others, *Mycobacterium fortuitum* and *chelonei*
Fungal	*Candida* spp., *Malassezia furfur*

nia. Patients with acute leukemia and pneumonia or other infections at diagnosis have a reduced probability of survival.[154, 208] Focal lung infiltrates can be related to any known bacterial pathogen if the patient is neutropenic. In non-neutropenic cases, atypical species are more common.

Chronic Leukemias

Patients with neutropenic myelodysplasia or chronic leukemia show a rather similar pattern of infections, except that neither the effects of disrupted mucocutaneous integrity nor those of a central venous line are prominent unless chemotherapy is initiated and a permanent venous catheter is in place. Other infections are more specific to peculiar disease entities or therapy-related conditions. Patients with HCL have been found to be susceptible to a variety of infections and characteristically had an increased incidence of atypical mycobacterial infections (*Mycobacterium kansasii, fortuitum, chelonei, avium-intracellulare* complex) that was related to the absolute monocytopenia and cell-mediated immunity defects typical of this disease.[243, 244] Patients with chronic lymphoid leukemias who undergo treatment with purine nucleoside analogues suffer from infection by opportunistic microorganisms, as reviewed.[61-63] Patients undergoing therapeutic splenectomy or in whom a functional asplenic state (bone marrow transplants) develops are at risk for infection by *Streptococcus pneumoniae, Neisseria* species, and *Haemophilus influenzae*. These infections are unpredictable, occur even years after splenectomy, and are characterized by a very rapid or fulminant course with shock, signs of neurologic involvement, acute adrenal insufficiency, and necrotizing skin lesions. Infection by these encapsulated microorganisms, usually less clinically aggressive than in splenectomized patients, is also a feature of patients with B-cell CLL because of a decreased level of IgG. These patients also frequently suffer from gram-positive and gram-negative infections involving the lungs and the urinary tract.

Fungal Infections

Fungal infections cause substantial morbidity and mortality in patients with leukemia and tend to occur earlier during the course of the disease than previously recognized.[6, 86, 163, 168, 170] Because of their protean clinical features and ominous prognosis when not promptly recognized and properly treated, these infections are a major critical issue in the management of leukemia patients. The usual setting of fungal infections is that of hospitalized patients with long-lasting neutropenia; patients heavily pretreated with antineoplastic drugs, antibiotics, or corticosteroids; those with refractory disease; patients undergoing marrow transplantation; and patients with permanent intravenous or bladder devices.[6, 86, 168, 170, 172, 245-249] Two main types of pathogens predominate, *Candida* and *Aspergillus* species both of which cause a variety of clinical syndromes* (Table 14-12). Infections by

*See references 4, 6, 70, 102, 103, 168, 170, 173, 181, 250-252.

TABLE 14-12. Fungal Infections in Leukemia Patients

Pathogens	Clinical Syndromes
Common	
Candida spp.	Oral thrush, esophagitis, candidemia, urinary tract infection, hepatosplenic candidiasis, catheter-related infection
Aspergillus spp.	Acute invasive pulmonary disease, chronic invasive pulmonary disease, tracheobronchitis, sinusitis, disseminated cutaneous (catheter-related) infection, cerebal infection
Uncommon	
Cryptococcus neoformans	Central nervous system and pulmonary cryptococcosis
Mucor	Rhinocerebral and pulmonary mucormycosis
Fusarium spp.	Disseminated infection with skin lesions
Trichosporon	Disseminated infection

Mucor, Fusarium, and *Trichosporon* are occasionally reported but may be increasing in transplant and other heavily treated patient groups.[253, 254] Infection with *C. neoformans* is common only in patients with defective cell-mediated immunity.

Infections by Candida *Species*

Candida infections are the most common fungal infections. *C. albicans* is a normal component of the gastrointestinal and cutaneous flora. Local overgrowth and dissemination of this pathogen are favored by the conditions examined earlier. Colonization of the oral cavity and the urinary tract may precede invasive *Candida* infection, so surveillance cultures to detect early colonization at superficial sites can be helpful in guiding prophylactic and treatment decisions.[255] Notably, *Candida* species adhere very avidly to the plastic surfaces of indwelling venous and urinary catheters, where replication and shedding of the microorganism can lead to systemic dissemination. Oral and esophageal candidiasis are very common, but usually manageable. Esophagitis must be suspected in patients with retrosternal burning pain and difficult swallowing, particularly when oral thrush was previously diagnosed. The diagnosis can be established with certainty only by endoscopy plus mucosal biopsy. The distal part of the esophagus is the initial and sometimes the only involved site. The most severe form of *Candida* infection is candidemia, which is characterized by high-grade fever that does not respond to a protracted antibiotic course, embolic skin lesions, myalgia, respiratory distress, collapse, and multiple visceral manifestations with a prevalence of liver, spleen, eye, and lung nodulation. The diagnosis is established by a positive blood culture for *Candida* species, which should be performed as soon as candidemia is suspected. Unrecognized and untreated, candidemia evolves rapidly and is invariably fatal. Unfortunately, drug-resistant non-*albicans Candida* species are emerging as causative agents of many candidemic episodes. The lung is often affected by

Candida infections and is the most frequently involved organ in autopsy studies.[173] The next most common sites are the gastrointestinal tract, spleen, and kidney. Candidal endophthalmitis is relatively rare but may result in permanent blindness. A complete ophthalmic evaluation is mandatory in patients with extensive *Candida* infection and visual disturbances. A serious complication is hepatosplenic candidiasis, now called chronic disseminated candidiasis, and it often occurs late in patients who have already recovered from neutropenia but remain febrile.[2, 6,168, 170, 256] Suggestive symptoms, other than fever of unknown origin unresponsive to antibiotics, are persistent leukocytosis, elevated serum alkaline phosphatase, and abdominal pain. Characteristically, these patients can be treated with chemotherapy or even undergo HSC transplantation with continuous antifungal treatment.[103, 252]

Infections by Aspergillus Species

The second fungal organism most frequently encountered is *Aspergillus*.[6, 86, 168, 170, 257] This pathogen is not a component of the normal human flora but is acquired from the environment by hospitalized patients. Air is the usual route of transmission, and inhalation of conidia with colonization of the upper respiratory tract generally precedes overt invasive infection. Thus, the growth of *Aspergillus* species from nasal swabs may have a predictive value for the development of invasive infection in high-risk patients. Leukemia patients with a history of smoking seem to be at greatest risk. Other predisposing factors have been reviewed. Hematogenous dissemination does not usually occur but can be observed in highly immunocompromised patients. The main characteristic of *Aspergillus* infection is localized growth of destructive lesions. The histopathologic changes observed in the organs involved consist of invasion of blood vessels, infarction, and necrosis. Spread by contiguity with surrounding tissues and adjacent bones and cartilage is frequent but occurs in a rather unpredictable fashion. The lung is the preferred target of invasive aspergillosis. Invasive, acute pulmonary aspergillosis consists of unifocal or multifocal, infarctive parenchymal lesions that grow rapidly, cause pleuritic chest pain and hemoptysis, and can extend to the pleura and chest wall. Sometimes, in the early phase and particularly in patients who are receiving corticosteroids, fever and other clinical symptoms are absent[70] and hemoptysis may occur abruptly as the first sign of infection.[102] In symptomatic cases, fever, cough, and chest pain are common symptoms. Aspergillomas are fungal masses in lung cavities colonized by *Aspergillus* species that occur after a rise in the neutrophil count and the formation of a reactive inflammatory wall. Aspergillomas predispose to hemoptysis, depending on their anatomic proximity to larger vessels. A concurrent or antecedent infection of the upper airways is frequent. Typically, the maxillary sinuses and nasal spaces are very frequently affected, with nasal discharge, mucocutaneous ulcers, pain, and local hemorrhage often present. These lesions can extend to the hard palate inferiorly or to the orbit and other basal skull bones.

Other Fungal Infections

Mucormycosis was recently reviewed in marrow transplant recipients and patients with blood malignancies.[250, 258] The disease is clinically aggressive and resembles a more malignant infection of *Aspergillus* species; it invades the vascular walls and causes tissue necrosis, but it differs from invasive aspergillosis in that it may involve the bones, muscles, or kidney or be manifested as disseminated infection and have a rapidly fatal course if the patient is neutropenic and the AmB dose is low. *Fusarium* is another emerging pathogen.[253, 254] This agent causes skin infection (Fig. 14-5), arthritis, and ophthalmitis. Cryptococcosis is observed more commonly in lymphoma patients. The central nervous system is involved, but dissemination can occur.[6] Other infections by fungi are occasionally reported (*Histoplasma, Trichosporon, Alternaria, Penicillium, Curvularia, Hansenula, Saccharomyces*) in the form of a disseminated or localized aggressive disease (brain, sinusitis).[31]

Viral Infections

Herpes Simplex and Varicella-Zoster

Viruses cause definite clinical syndromes in leukemic patients (Table 14-13). The chronology of viral infections

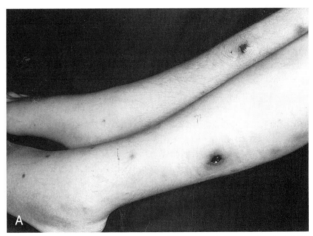

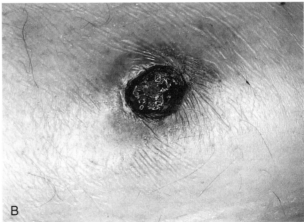

FIGURE 14–5. Disseminated skin infection by *Fusarium* spp. (biopsy proven) in a young patient with refractory acute lymphoblastic leukemia who relapsed after high-dose treatment with a hematopoietic stem-cell autograft. Partial clinical improvement was observed with liposome-associated amphotericin B.

TABLE 14–13. Viral Infections in Leukemia Patients

Patogens	Clinical Syndromes
Common	
HSV	Localized mucocutaneous infection (oropharyneal, esophagitis, anogenital)
	Disseminated visceral infection
VZV	Disseminated primary infection (children)
	Zoster or shingles (adults)
	Meningoencephalitis
CMV	Interstitial pneumonia, esophagitis, gastroenteritis
Uncommon	
HHV-6	Pneumonia, encephalitis
Adenovirus	URTI, pneumonia
Influenza/parainfluenza	URTI, pneumonia
BK virus	Hemorrhagic cystitis
RSV	URTI, pneumonia
HHV-8, EBV	Post-transplant lymphoproliferative disease

CMV, cytomegalovirus; EBV, Epstein-Barr virus; HHV, human herpesvirus; HSV, herpes simplex virus; RSV, respiratory syncytial virus; URTI, upper respiratory tract infection; VZV, varicella-zoster virus.

is peculiar and follows the induction of severe cellular immunodeficiency by protracted cytotoxic treatment or by marrow transplant regimens and related immunosuppressive therapies. The HSC transplant setting, moreover, is typically complicated by CMV infection. HSV infection is usually localized and very rarely disseminated.[6, 259] Early mucocutaneous lesions (oral cavity and perioral skin, esophagus, genital and perianal area) are very painful and vesicular in appearance, but they soon become indistinguishable from ulcerative infections of another nature or even chemotherapy- or radiotherapy-induced mucositis. Often, in acutely ill and intensively treated patients, mucosal ulcers are of multifactorial origin and favor secondary bleeding and bacterial superinfection. Unusual HSV infections have been reported. HSV lymphadenitis is a rare complication that should be differentiated from leukemic lymphadenopathy.[260] HSV infection of the jejunum has been described after bone marrow transplantation.[261] Primary infection with VZV, or chickenpox, can be a deadly disease in severely immunocompromised children with leukemia. Death usually follows the onset of pneumonia, which generally appears a few days after the typical skin lesions.[6, 262, 263] The liver and brain can be other sites of dissemination. Secondary infection by VZV, known as zoster or shingles, represents reactivation of latent disease and is thus more common in adults after intensive treatment. The early cutaneous lesions resemble those of chickenpox but tend to be confluent and have a characteristic dermatomal distribution that may vary greatly in extent. Pain of moderate to severe intensity is present and sometimes precedes appearance of the rash. Dissemination is much rarer than with primary infection, but extensive visceral (lungs, liver, central nervous system) VZV disease may develop in as many as one third of patients undergoing high-dose therapy supported by autologous or allogeneic HSC transplantation.[264, 265]

Cytomegalovirus Infection and Disease in HSC Transplants

CMV is another member of the human herpesvirus (HHV) family that can cause significant morbidity and mortality in leukemia patients; those most vulnerable are HSC transplant recipients, particularly when receiving an allogeneic transplant after conditioning by total body irradiation and when GVHD develops.[90-95, 163, 266, 267] Transfusion of seropositive blood products to seronegative patients is one pathogenetic mechanism, the other being reactivation of dormant infection in seropositive cases. The rate of seropositivity in healthy adults is high and ranges from 40% to 90%, as for HSV-1 and VZV. Infection of HSCs, monocytes/macrophages, and marrow stromal cells is possible,[268-271] and both marrow progenitor cells and circulating monocytes can be sites of CMV persistence.[272] Vascular endothelial cells can be an additional reservoir.[273] CMV immunity is mediated by subsets of specific CD4+ helper T cells and CD8+ cytotoxic T lymphocytes[274, 275] that in allogeneic HSC transplants are transferred from donor to patient. Thus, T-cell depletion during allogeneic HSC transplantation may aggravate the risk of CMV reactivation and disease, whereas donor lymphocyte infusions could exert a protective effect.[276] An increased incidence of CMV disease has also been noted after allogeneic HSC transplantation from unrelated donors.[277] The risk is not apparently increased in recipients of peripheral blood HSC transplants.[278] Although overt CMV infection develops relatively early after HSC transplantation (see Table 14–6), late infections (>100 days) are not uncommon and may be responsible for a number of deaths within the first year after grafting.[279-281] The possibility of late infection underlines the need for prolonged diagnostic surveillance. The clinical spectrum of CMV infection is considerably wide, yet interstitial pneumonia with respiratory insufficiency is the most dramatic occurrence with high mortality rates. Incidence rates have been reduced in recent years because of widespread use of prophylactic ganciclovir.[282] In autologous HSC transplants, the median incidence of CMV interstitial pneumonia is 0.8% (range, 0% to 8.6%).[283] Infection of the entire gastrointestinal tract is also frequent and results in a painful, mixed diarrheic and hemorrhagic syndrome of variable severity; in addition pancreatitis, hepatitis, cholecystitis, retinitis, and rarely encephalitis are seen with some frequency.[6] The symptoms are respiratory distress, gastroenteritis with irregular bowel movements, abdominal pain, cystitis, elevated transaminase levels, fluid retention, and neurologic dysfunction. Sometimes, localized gastrointestinal CMV disease is the predominant complication[284, 285] and must be differentiated from an episode of intestinal GVHD. Problems involving blood counts and bone marrow activity are frequent and may be exacerbated by the concomitant use of myelotoxic drugs, including some effective antiviral agents (ganciclovir). Delayed recovery of platelets and neutrophils can be noted,[286] whereas unexplained neutropenia/thrombopenia or reversal of blood counts can be an isolated sign of CMV disease.[287] Bone marrow hypoplasia after HSC transplantation could result from CMV-induced release of IL-2 with activation of NK cells able to damage the bone marrow microenvironment.[288] Death from CMV-induced myelosuppression is possible as a result of the extreme damage to early CD34+ stem cells[289] and would be more likely with infection by the gB3 and gB4 genotypes of CMV.[290]

Other Viruses

Community-acquired viruses causing upper respiratory tract infection may be responsible for outbreaks of pneumonia associated with respiratory failure in the setting of HSC transplantation.[137-139] In transplanted patients, adenovirus and polyomavirus BK can induce severe hemorrhagic cystitis.[136, 291] HHV-6 can cause a diffuse maculopapular rash and encephalopathy and has been associated with the development of severe GVHD in allograft recipients.[186, 188, 292] Enteroviruses can be isolated from some patients with gastrointestinal symptoms and are occasionally the underlying cause of death.[293]

Interstitial Pneumonia

Interstitial pneumonia is relatively common in HSC recipients. Although it may be caused by *P. carinii, Legionella,* or viruses (Table 14-14), it is typically associated with CMV infection.[294-301] Patients in whom symptoms and signs of respiratory insufficiency develop after a mean of 2 months post-transplant are often, but not exclusively those undergoing allogeneic transplantation. The coexistence of GVHD is common. Shortness of breath is typical, but physical examination of the lungs is often unrewarding. Fever is sometimes absent, especially when patients are receiving steroids, as frequently occurs. Sputum is very scarce or absent because the alveoli are usually spared by the inflammatory reaction. An isolated, decreased partial arterial O_2 pressure is an early sign indicating interstitial damage. CO_2 pressure increases later. Metabolic changes induced by respiratory hypoxemia can eventually lead to a mixed respiratory and metabolic acidosis. The chest radiograph shows interstitial markings involving different, but usually multiple lung areas, with shadows prevailing in the bases and the perihilar area (Fig. 14-6). The process can extend to involve the entire lung fields, up to a complete whiteout of lung images. The disease should be differentiated from fluid overload within a capillary leaky syndrome or veno-occlusive dis-

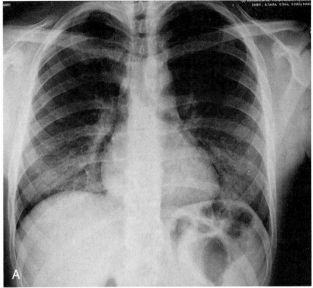

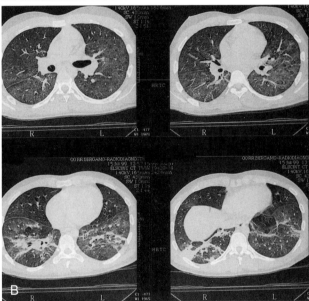

FIGURE 14-6. Interstitial pneumonia in a patient with acute leukemia who was receiving mercaptopurine plus methotrexate low-dose oral maintenance. The chest film (*top*) shows the characteristic bilateral interstitial shadowing prevailing in the lower lung fields; high-resolution computed tomography (*bottom*) highlights the degree and extent of inflammatory changes in affected tissues. *Pneumocystis carinii* could be isolated from bronchoalveolar lavage fluid (see Fig. 14-10).

ease, which can be determined by a short trial with diuretics. Other disseminated infections that may be characterized by respiratory failure and a chest radiographic picture resembling interstitial pneumonitis are candidemia and acute respiratory distress syndrome secondary to gram-positive bacteria. In these conditions, however, the picture of septicemia is predominant.

Parasites

Except for HSC transplants, infection with *P. carinii* is now relatively uncommon. The infection results from

TABLE 14-14. Causes of Interstitial Pneumonitis

Etiology	Pathogenic Agents
Infectious, viral	CMV, HSV, VZV, adenovirus, RSV, measles virus
Infectious, nonviral	*Pneumocystis carinii, Legionella pneumophilia, Chlamydia,* tuberculosis, fungi, *Toxoplasma gondii*
Noninfectious	Irradiation and drugs (total body irradiation, cyclophosphamide, busulfan, methotrexate)
Idiopathic	Not identified

CMV, cytomegalovirus; HSV, herpes simplex virus; RSV, respiratory syncytial virus; VZV, varicella-zoster virus.

reactivation of cysts acquired early in life and is observed in patients with an underlying defect in cellular immunity, mainly children with ALL who are receiving corticosteroids and intensive chemotherapy with immunosuppressive drugs and not receiving adequate prophylaxis.[302-304] An acute, bilateral pulmonary infection with alveolar infiltrates spreading from the hili to the peripheral lung tissue is a common clinical manifestation. Infections by *T. gondii, S. stercoralis,* and *Cryptosporidium* are definitely rare.

CLINICAL EVALUATION AND DIAGNOSIS

Fever and Other Symptoms

In evaluating leukemia patients at risk, special attention must be paid to the occurrence of fever and other clinical signs of infection and to the degree of neutropenia. The leading concept is that fever is common in neutropenic patients with leukemia and that most of the time it is caused by infection. A corollary with prognostic relevance is that infections are aggravated by neutropenia. From a clinical standpoint, neutropenia hinders the evaluation process by diminishing the usual symptoms and signs of infection, which may be minimal.[4, 6, 305] However, fever, erythematous changes, and pain are generally preserved in neutropenic states. An oral temperature of 38°C (100.4°F) or higher for 1 hour or a single measurement over 38.3°C (101°F) indicates a serious febrile state.[13] Localized tenderness and/or skin or mucosal erythema suggest infection, even in the absence of a temperature higher than 38°C. Thus, pleuritic chest pain, painful bowels or perianal discomfort, and tenderness above the facial sinuses may be the only detectable signs of infection in these sites. Similarly, clinicians should be alerted by minimal skin changes at the exit site of an indwelling venous catheter or by a dry cough, although it is often difficult to ascribe such a cough to pneumonia without other concomitant symptoms. Meningitis can be heralded by disturbed consciousness and a modest headache rather than by the classic signs of meningeal irritation with pleocytosis. Essentially, all the clinical signs directly attributable to the accumulation and metabolic activation of neutrophils may be diminished in the neutropenic states of severely immunocompromised patients. Therefore, swelling and drainage from the infected area, exudation, and fluctuance are reduced in comparison to non-neutropenic states. This distinction must be born in mind when examining the traditional risk sites, specifically, the whole oropharyngeal cavity, the axillae, the skin, the fingernails, and the perineal area. Conversely, it must also be considered that fever may be due to the leukemia itself or to the administration of cytotoxic drugs through a mechanism involving tumor lysis and release of cellular pyrogens. Some patients with acute leukemia are indeed febrile when initially seen but do not have infection. Although this possibility does not alter the practical management of patients, it may have prognostic relevance. The use of corticosteroids can complicate patient evaluation. In both truly infected and noninfected neutropenic patients, corticosteroids may further diminish all inflammatory signs, including fever. Performing a careful, day-to-day, infection-oriented clinical review is mandatory in patients receiving significant amounts of corticosteroids, such as those with ALL. A high index of suspicion of infection must always be maintained in ill patients with leukemia if the temperature is as high as 38°C.

Initial Evaluation

Infection by gram-positive or gram-negative bacteria in the form of either a febrile bacteremia, sepsis with or without pneumonia, or localized infection and infection by fungi and some viruses are expected to develop in patients in whom leukemia is recently diagnosed and treated. Clinical evaluation of these patients at early risk involves an expeditious, detailed analysis of their medical history, immune status, subjective complaints, and objective findings and performance of selected clinicolaboratory investigation[4, 6, 305] (Table 14-15). Sepsis is present when the patient has any two or more of the following symptoms: fever or hypothermia, leukocytosis or leukopenia (both rare as a secondary event in these patients), and tachycardia and tachypnea or supranormal minute ventilation.[306] Febrile patients in whom an infection of the major organs develops are defined as having complex bacteremia[12] (see Fig. 14-4). Shock secondary to sepsis is defined as a systolic pressure less than 90 mm Hg that is unresponsive to fluids or requires vasoactive drugs. Frequently associated symptoms are ileus, lactic acidosis, oliguria, acute lung injury, and high protein and calorie

TABLE 14-15. Initial Evaluation of Leukemia Patients with Fever and/or Other Signs of Infection

Medical history	Previous bacterial/fungal infections, viral hepatitis, herpes infection
Laboratory	Neutrophil count, monocytes, lymphocyte subsets, complement, immunoglobulin level
	Immunization to CMV, HSV, VZV; serology for hepatitis B and C virus infection (if indicated)
	Urinalysis and liver and kidney function tests
Physical examination	Blood pressure, heart respiratory rates. High-risk sites: oral cavity, catheter exit sites, skin, perineum, anus
X-ray examination	Chest film (two projections), facial sinuses if symptoms are present (pain, nasal discharge)
Culture studies	Two sets of blood cultures from peripheral veins and the catheter as well as one from each lumen to examine for bacteria and fungi. Culturing of draining and exuding fluids, stool, and urine if specific symptoms are present
Reassessment	Repeat analysis when indicated and reassessment of the patient's condition daily
Miscellaneous	Computed tomography, ultrasound scan (chest, abdomen, brain) if indicated (especially if early fungal infection is suspected)

requirements. Practice guidelines for diagnostic tests, including detailed methodology for measurement of temperature were recently presented for critically ill patients admitted to intensive care units.[307] Many of these recommendations could well apply to patients with leukemia. Noninfectious causes of fever must be considered and may be due to any drug through a hypersensitivity mechanism, but such fever is usually associated with antimicrobials (especially β-lactams), antiepilectic drugs (phenytoin), antiarrhythmics (quinidine, procainamide), antihypertensives (methyldopa), transfusions of red blood cells and platelets, and noninfectious inflammatory states (chemical thrombophlebitis, pulmonary infarction, pancreatitis, myocardial infarction, hyperthyroidism). The aim of the initial evaluation is to assess the extent and degree of the damage induced by infection and identify the pathogen responsible and its chemosensitivity pattern to select the most appropriate therapeutic strategy. No delay in obtaining these facts is justifiable. Culturing of blood, urine, and other body fluids suspected of contamination is mandatory, with special techniques as requested for the identification of unusual pathogen.[307] Periodic reevaluation of patients is mandatory, and it may be necessary to repeat some investigations more than once, always guided by evolution of the clinical picture and by the response to empiric therapy and exclusively on a patient-to-patient basis.

Radiologic Investigations

As far as the lungs are concerned, the plain chest film is often normal initially, but it must nevertheless be obtained to serve as a baseline for future comparisons. If parenchymal infiltrates are detected, they may be limited (less than a lobe) or diffuse and include nodular, reticular, congestive, and alveolar radiologic patterns.[308] Radiology and CT or magnetic resonance imaging are used to define the extent of the lesions in the lungs, abdomen, maxillary sinuses, other craniofacial structures, and brain. Recent studies have indicated that especially in neutropenic patients, pneumonia is detectable in the early phase only by means of HRCT, which has a sensitivity of 87%, specificity of 57%, and negative predictive value of 88%.[309] HRCT is particularly valuable in the early detection of pulmonary invasive aspergillosis in neutropenic states. The halo sign (masslike infiltrate with a surrounding halo of ground-glass attenuation) and the air crescent sign (air cavitation) are the characteristic diagnostic findings.[96] HRCT can significantly reduce the time to diagnosis (and hence to start of treatment) and is therefore indicated in patients who have a normal chest radiograph but are nevertheless at risk for pneumonia of both fungal and nonfungal etiology[98] (Fig. 14–7). The diagnosis of hepatosplenic candidiasis is supported by imaging studies (CT and nuclear magnetic resonance) that show peculiar,

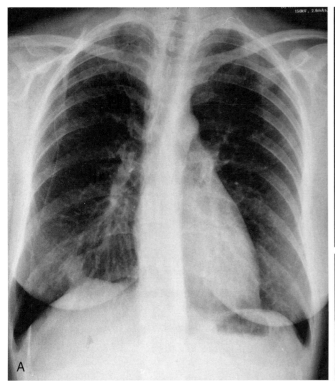
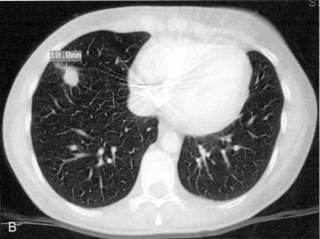
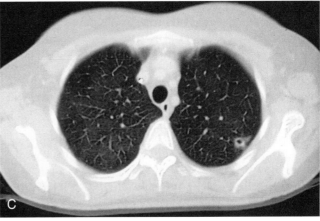

FIGURE 14–7. Persistent fever in a patient with acute myelogenous leukemia and a normal chest film (*left panel*) could be attributed to suspected fungal infection after demonstration of pulmonary infiltrates with cavitation on high-resolution computed tomography (*right panels, top and bottom*). Empiric treatment with systemic antifungals was successful.

"bulls-eye"–like lesions, and it is confirmed by a liver biopsy with histologic and culture studies. In patients with interstitial pneumonia or pneumonia caused by opportunistic organisms, an additional CT scan may be helpful to better define the extent and severity of the lesions (see Fig. 14-6).

Surveillance Cultures

Routine surveillance cultures of the nose, throat, urine, and stool were advocated in the past as a means of predicting the subsequent spread of infection by colonizing microorganisms, particularly *Pseudomonas* and *Aspergillus* species. Because of the cost and the lower than expected diagnostic power, surveillance cultures are no longer recommended,[6, 19, 310, 311] with the possible exception of patients exposed to abnormally prolonged neutropenia (longer than 2 weeks) and in institutions with a high incidence of virulent or antibiotic-resistant strains of gram-positive bacteria, *Pseudomonas,* and *Aspergillus* and *Candida* species.[13, 255, 310]

Laboratory Tests

At least two to three cultures of blood (from a peripheral vein and from each lumen of a central venous line, if in place) for bacteria and fungi must be obtained. Cultures from other sites are obtained if clinically indicated (nasal discharge, urine, cerebrospinal fluid, abdominal cavity, pleura, skin, etc.). Among laboratory tests, determination of C-reactive protein levels is preferable to determination of the erythrocyte sedimentation rate and other methods to monitor infection-related acute phase protein changes during evolution of the illness.[312, 313] Diarrheal stools are tested for *C. difficile* toxin, other bacteria (*Salmonella, Shigella, Campylobacter, Aeromonas, Yersinia*), viruses (rotavirus, CMV), and *Cryptosporidium. C. difficile* colitis is confirmed by isolation from the stool of *C. difficile* toxins A and B with a cytotoxin tissue culture assay or an enzyme-linked immunoassay; more than one sample is often necessary. Associated clinical features are semi-formed stools, use of antibiotics (cephalosporin) for at least 6 days before onset of the symptoms, and the presence of fecal leukocytes.[314]

Diagnosis of Fungal Infections

A. fumigatus and *flavus* can be grown from sputum or from bronchial lavage fluid obtained during bronchoscopy (Fig. 14-8). The diagnosis of hepatosplenic candidiasis is confirmed by a liver biopsy with histologic and culture studies (Fig. 14-9). *Mucor, Fusarium,* and all other fungal species should be cultured from biopsy material. Often, in acutely ill patients, biopsy or bronchoscopy may be impossible to perform,[315] and early introduction of an antifungal agent appears to be mandatory. A presumptive diagnosis of fungal infection based on clinical judgment, evaluation of cumulative risk factors, and HRCT or another imaging technique is therefore accept-

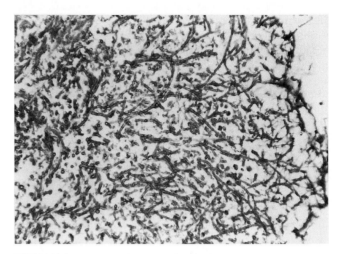

FIGURE 14-8. A mass of *Aspergillus*-like organisms obtained at bronchoscopy in a patient with leukemia (periodic acid–Schiff staining, 400×).

able. A powerful aid is offered by antigen detection tests.[168, 316] Antigen detection by a variety of methods is available for both *Candida*[317-319] and *Aspergillus* species.[98, 320, 321] With serial evaluation over time, these methods can also help predict the response to treatment and the final outcome of the infection. For invasive aspergillosis, detection of the galactomannan antigen appears to be highly sensitive and specific and can reveal early infection well before the onset of any other clinical sign.[322] False-positive results from transient antigenemia in neutropenic patients should prompt caution in interpreting these tests.[323] However, the combination of a positive antigen test (obtained twice weekly and confirmed on the next day of positivity) and a positive HRCT result is considered proof of early invasive aspergillosis in high-risk patients with hematologic malignancies.[324, 325]

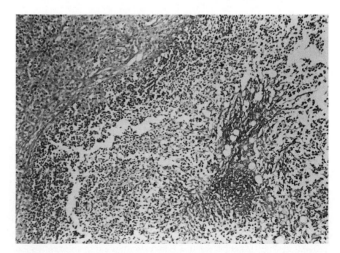

FIGURE 14-9. Transcutaneous liver biopsy demonstrating a fungal abscess. Within the context of normal liver (*upper left corner*), a mass of inflammatory cells and necrotic material is surrounding fungal hyphae (periodic acid–Schiff staining, 100×). This picture is highly suggestive of hepatosplenic candidiasis.

Diagnosis of Viral Infections

The diagnosis of HSV infection is established by culturing the fluid obtained from vesicular lesions, by isolating the virus from affected tissues, or by performing PCR.[326] Disseminated primary VZV infection is diagnosed by performing the Tzanck test on scraping of skin lesions, by immunostaining, and by serial determination of serum antibody titer. However, these tests are seldom required because of the relatively well defined clinical picture in most instances. Exceptions occur with clinical entities for which the precise etiology must be known to optimize treatment, such as interstitial pneumonia and CMV infection in allografted patients. Lung biopsy has long been the preferred modality to confirm interstitial pneumonitis, but it is no longer required if other tests (DNAemia by PCR, antigenemia, examination for immunostaining of bronchoalveolar fluid) are informative. Histologically, fluid accumulation with mononuclear cell infiltration is prominent in the interstitium. Giant cells with characteristic viral inclusion bodies are seen in CMV-associated cases; however, viruses other than CMV can induce similar inclusion bodies in lung cells. The diagnosis is made by specific immunofluorescence techniques or PCR for viral nucleic acid. The final diagnosis of CMV-associated interstitial pneumonitis, however, rests on additional investigations, as detailed later.[327] Assays for detecting viral DNA (HHV-6, HHV-7, EBV, polyomavirus BK) in biologic samples are available and may be successfully used to confirm infection by other viruses.[186, 188, 291, 292]

Early Diagnosis of CMV Infection in HSC Transplants

Because of the potentially fatal clinical course of CMV disease, the early diagnosis of CMV infection in recipients of allogeneic HSC transplants is a powerful clinical tool to implement antiviral strategies. Accurate and sensitive tests based on detection of virus antigen and PCR allow rapid diagnosis and post-therapeutic monotoring of CMV infection in various body fluids, including bronchoalveolar lavage fluid, and in cells.[328-333] The start of effective, preemptive treatment at the time of occult CMV infection, before the development of overt CMV disease, is made possible by currently available sensitive and rapid assays for detection of the CMV pp65 antigen in leukocytes (immunostaining) and CMV DNA (PCR and quantitative PCR). The results of both antigenemia assay (detecting more than two to four antigen-positive leukocytes) and PCR assay (detecting CMV DNAemia, number of genomes per milliliter) from blood samples correlate well with subsequent CMV disease and transplant-related mortality,[334-337] are more sensitive, and permit earlier recognition of impending CMV disease than standard culture assays[338-340] or surveillance bronchoscopy does in patients at risk.[341] Antigenemia and/or PCR assays are performed weekly or biweekly, starting from the day of transplantation or later according to the study protocol. Because of the lower incidence and morbidity of CMV infection and disease, respectively, the use of these methods in patients undergoing autologous HSC transplantation has been questioned.[287]

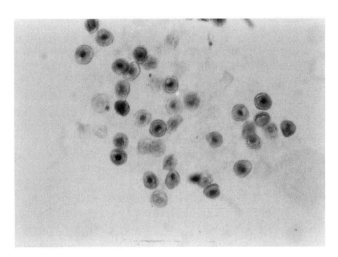

FIGURE 14–10. *Pneumocystis carinii* isolated from bronchoalveolar lavage fluid in the case presented in Figure 14–6 (silver staining, 1000×).

Diagnosis of Parasitic Infections

Diagnosis of *P. carinii* infection is made possible by the observation of characteristic cysts in tissue sections with the use of specific stains or in bronchoalveolar lavage fluid (Fig. 14–10). The histologic diagnosis can be supported by more specific immunofluorescence staining with monoclonal antibody.

Unresolving or Late Fever and Infection

Additional investigations are required when the first-line evaluation is inconclusive and no microorganisms are isolated, when the febrile state endures despite broad-spectrum empiric antibiotic or antifungal therapy, when a new episode occurs, and generally when the patient's clinical status deteriorates (Table 14–16). Patients in this

TABLE 14–16. Evaluation of Leukemia Patients with Unresolving or Late Fever and Infection

General	Repeat the general evaluation (Table 14–15)
Culture studies	Draining fluids, stool, cerebrospinal fluid, fine-needle aspirates as indicated. Search to include anaerobes, *Clostridium difficile* toxin, protozoa, fungi, viruses
Imaging	Computed tomography and nuclear magnetic resonance of the chest, abdomen, pelvis, bone (repeat as indicated)
Endoscopy	Bronchial tree, gastrointestinal tract (as indicated) with biopsy and complete culture study
[111]In-IgG scanning	Help localize deep-seated infections
Serology and molecular biology studies	Immunofluorescence, ELISA, polymerase chain reaction (for CMV, HCV, fungal antigens, etc.)

CMV, cytomogalovirus; ELISA, enzyme-linked immunosorbent assay; HCV, hepatitis C virus.

situation are those who are heavily pretreated and have recurrent or late febrile episodes and in whom the neutropenia has often resolved and thus bacterial infections appear to be less probable.[6, 342] Drug-related and other noninfectious-type fevers should be considered in well-looking non-neutropenic patients and the hypothesis tested by discontinuing the use of all antibiotics, antifungals, and other drugs not essential to survival.[307] In non-neutropenic recipients of an HSC transplant, fever caused by engraftment syndrome/T-lymphocyte recovery must be considered if accompanied by rash and fluid overload. At this stage, in all other cases it is justified to look for deep-seated bacterial infections and to search for fungal, viral, or other atypical infections.[4-6, 19, 166, 168, 305, 343-345] Vascular devices must be carefully examined. Concomitant and sequential infections are not uncommon.[13] However, in many cases no pathogen can be isolated and the interpretation remains empiric. CT or nuclear magnetic resonance of the brain, chest, abdomen, and pelvis are valuable aids for detecting occult foci of infection and determining their extent. Deep-seated infections in neutropenic patients can be localized by indium 111–labeled IgG scanning.[346] Fine-needle biopsy of the identified lesion should be performed whenever anatomically possible and provided that the platelet count and coagulation tests are not contraindications to the procedure. In patients with the air crescent sign or other lung opacities suggesting invasive pulmonary aspergillosis, HRCT and transtracheal aspiration or bronchoscopy with either biopsy of abnormal-looking mucosal surfaces or sampling of bronchoalveolar lavage fluid can be rewarding.[347-349] Patients eligible for these procedures are those who are unresponsive to standard empiric treatment and in whom great therapeutic benefit is expected to follow the documentation of a specific infectious etiology. The material should be sent for complete microbiologic analysis and histologic review. Second-line investigations are often time and money consuming, yet the benefit to the patient can be immeasurable when an exact diagnosis is made, the infection is controlled, and antileukemic therapy can proceed safely. Therefore, the decision regarding the most appropriate tests entails a continuing and critical review of the patient's condition and must be complemented by clinical competence.

PREVENTION

A Multistep Process

Limiting infections in leukemic patients at high risk is an essential component of their management. Optimal prevention of infections is difficult because of their multifactorial etiology and pathogenesis and heterogeneous institutional epidemiologic data. Basically, prevention is a multistep process. Reduction of the burden of foreign pathogens transmissible to the patient from inanimate environmental and other living sources is a first step and should be integrated with the activation of measures able to minimize the entry of microorganisms into the patient's body. These measures can be as simple as hand washing or as extreme and expensive as keeping the patient in a totally protective and sterile environment. Limiting the degree and duration of therapy-induced mucositis is another rational objective that deserves further investigation. Second, effort can be directed at reducing the burden of endogenous infectious microorganisms. Several prophylactic drug regimens have been developed over the years, and debate is still continuing regarding their efficacy and indications in different risk groups. With regard to prophylaxis, present state-of-the-art therapy is far from ideal: no prophylactic agent is fully effective, some are toxic or even very toxic, issues of cost-effectiveness are poorly defined, and promotion of drug resistance is likely. A recent extension of prophylaxis is preemptive therapy, or the institution of specific treatment at the earliest signs of infection, usually detectable through laboratory investigations before the occurrence of overt disease. Finally, attempts are made to restore or accelerate the recovery of host immune defenses, primarily an adequate neutrophil count, by a variety of methods ranging from the administration of vaccines or immunoglobulin to grafting with peripheral blood stem cells (PBSCs) and/or the administration of hematopoietic growth factors. The two latter methods have been under clinical investigation for over a decade and are now a cornerstone for the prevention and, to some extent, the management of many infections in severely cytopenic patients. A comprehensive overview of both established and novel developmental prophylactic maneuvers is presented in Figure 14–11. Although it is clearly not possible to combine all these aspects in a single patient and although for many of these patients it remains to be unequivocally demonstrated which method is better or even just worthwhile, both the complexity of this matter and the potential seriousness of infections arising in patients with leukemia should motivate evaluation of prophylactic guidelines for different risk classes. Details are presented of the most promising approaches on which final decisions are usually taken.

Reducing the Acquisition of Pathogens

Direct transmission of pathogens from the environment is possible from inanimate structures, particularly floors and moist surfaces, air ventilation systems, or food, and of course they may be transmitted by personal contact. Whatever the source, acquisition and dissemination of pathogens are greatly facilitated by skin and mucosal damage induced by chemotherapy or radiotherapy, venipuncture, and indwelling cathethers. Microorganisms of almost all types are transmitted on the hands. General prophylactic measures (Table 14–17) should always include thorough hand washing of both staff and visitors after and before every contact with a high-risk patient.[5-7, 350] This simple but effective measure must be followed by all the people caring for the patient and by all incoming relatives. The significance of this basic rule should be firmly reminded to inadvertent offenders. Daily antiseptic rinses of floors, baths, and lavatories are part of this program.

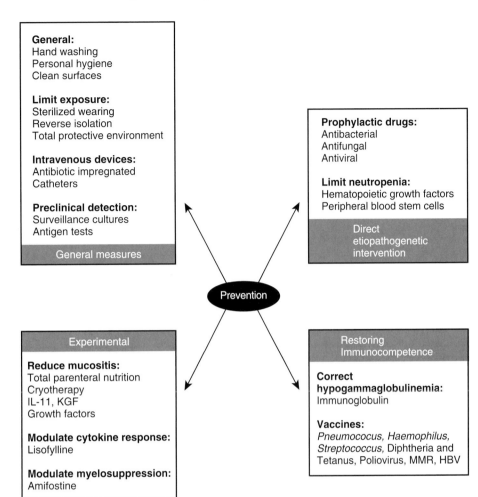

FIGURE 14–11. A summary of measures able to prevent infection in patients with leukemia.

Role of Early Diagnosis

The role of local colonization (upper aerodigestive tract, large bowel) by some pathogens was presented earlier. Cultures performed sequentially from risk sites in asymptomatic subjects and serial antigen studies or nucleic acid studies (by PCR) may facilitate the early identification of patients at high risk of invasive infections. In this case, treatment is applied prophylactically (or preemptively), on the basis of the initial evidence for infection but before the onset of overt disease. The indications for this helpful approach, as already discussed, are restricted to CMV infection, *Aspergillus* infection and other invasive mycoses in high-risk patients (high-dose therapies, HSC

transplants), and possibly infections caused by drug-resistant bacterial strains such as vancomycin-resistant enterococci (VRE)[351] and when local epidemiologic data suggest an increased incidence of a given microbial species.

Medicated Intravenous Devices

Indwelling cathethers must be handled with great care and flushed daily with heparin to maintain the lumen viable and clean. Even so, infections associated with the use of these devices are relatively frequent and clinically serious because of bacteremic dissemination. Therefore, studies were initiated to determine whether the introduc-

TABLE 14–17. Prevention of the Exogenous Acquisition of Pathogens

Main Topics	Possible Interventions	Indications
Patient	Personal hygiene, care of catheters, antiseptic washing	Always
	Sterile food and beverages	In total protective environment
Staff/visitor	Hand washing	Always: most important rule
	Wearing of gown, glove, mask	Selected circumstances
Environment	Washing/disinfection of floors, walls, toilets, items	Always
	Filtered air and sterile rooms (LAF/HEPA)	Selected circumstances (high-risk allografts)

HEPA, high-efficiency particulate air filter; LAF, laminar airflow.

tion of new antiseptic catheters, specifically, those impregnated with antimicrobials on either the luminal or both the luminal and external surfaces, would significantly lower this risk. Controlled studies have shown antiseptic catheters to be safe with no adverse side effects and to be clinically advantageous over traditional catheters. Lower risk was demonstrated with both chlorhexidine–silver sulfadiazine impregnation (reduced risk of colonization at removal, $P = .005$; fewer blood stream infections, $P = .03$)[352] and minocycline-rifampin impregnation (reduced colonization, $P < .001$; fewer blood stream infections, $P < .01$).[353] Minocyclin-rifampin-impregnated catheters proved superior when the two antiseptic methods were directly compared (reduced colonization, $P < .001$; fewer blood stream infections, $P < .002$).[354] The insertion location (radiology suite versus operating room) apparently has no effect on the rate of subsequent catheter-associated infections.[44]

Modulating Myelosuppression

Recent advances allow a reduction in myelosuppression after high-intensity chemotherapy or radiotherapy. Such a reduction translates into a net prophylactic effect because of a reduced rate or severity of infectious complications. The primary supportive role of granulocyte (G-CSF) and granulocyte-macrophage (GM-CSF) colony-stimulating factors and PBSC infusions is considered separately later in this section. Other substances have shown potential for clinical use. These agents, collectively called chemotherapy and radiotherapy protectants,[355] would essentially limit the damage to HSCs (and possibly other cells) and shorten the length of neutropenia. Interpretation of the results of trials with protectants is difficult, so firm rules on their use cannot be presently given.[356] The SCI/rhMIP1α protein might protect marrow blood stem cells[357] and provide improved neutrophil recovery after myelosuppressive therapies. Another agent attracting attention in patients with hematologic malignancies is amifostine. This drug, in untreated patients with cytopenic myelodysplasia, may significantly increase both neutrophil and platelet counts.[358] Data regarding the use of amifostine after chemotherapy are still scanty, except for its use in preventing myelosuppression from alkylating agents (in which case amifostine can provide protection).[355] Other studies are ongoing, and further developments in the whole issue of protectants are needed.

Modulating Cytokine Response

It is known that regimen-related toxicity from high-dose therapy can be mediated by the release of proinflammatory and/or marrow inhibitory cytokines (HPODE, tumor necrosis factor α, IL-1β, macrophage inhibitory factor 1α, transforming growth factor β). These factors cause myelosuppression and mucositis and, in patients with allogeneic HSC transplants, contribute to the development of GVHD and immune derangement. Infections are therefore facilitated. Abrogation of the abnormal cytokine response can be viewed as a broad prophylactic intervention against these phenomena. Cytokine response inhibitors used in clinical trials in patients with leukemia were lisofylline and pentoxifylline. In a first lisofylline randomized study,[359] regimen-related toxicity, survival, and the incidence of infections after allogeneic bone marrow transplantation were significantly improved in the group receiving lisofylline, 3-mg/kg (every 6 hours), versus the lisofylline, 2 mg/kg, and placebo arms, but neither neutrophil nor platelet recovery times were affected. In another randomized trial,[360] however, lisofylline administered at the same dose to patients with AML and high-risk myelodysplasia who were receiving front-line chemotherapy was unable to modify both myelosuppression and the rate of infectious complications. In a pentoxifylline-ciprofloxacin-prednisone phase II study,[361] once again no effect was detected, and the rate of infectious complications was increased, possibly because of the early use of steroids. Modulation of cytokine response therefore remains a matter for additional clinical studies in selected risk classes.

Reducing Mucositis

The problem of mucositis is closely related to the aforementioned factors, given that proinflammatory cytokines are implicated in its pathogenesis and also determine its severity. Presently, no effective, large-scale means is available for preventing radiotherapy/chemotherapy-induced mucosal breakage. In some studies, the formation of oral ulcers and the incidence of infection were lowered by chlorhexidine rinses or by oral cryotherapy with ice chips.[362, 363] Pentoxyfilline, as reported, and prostaglandins were not effective.[364, 365] Pentoxifylline can additionally promote replication of CMV, an effect that would clearly offset any other benefit in patients at risk for viral reactivation.[366] Several other studies using heterogeneous strategies for prevention and treatment of mucositis were recently reviewed, with pertinent conclusions and suggestions.[367] In spite of occasional claims of efficacy, no method has achieved general agreement. According to the study conclusions, it is possible that some methods may be preferable in a particular context (local cryotherapy for high-dose methotrexate and melphalan; propantheline for high-dose etoposide) and that hematopoietic growth factors could stimulate epithelial and mucosal cell proliferation as well. Further advancement may be at hand with the use of keratinocyte growth factor and IL-11[368, 369] and probably through the institution of new comparative clinical trials.

Protected Environments

The most obvious way to minimize exposure to pathogens is isolating the patient in a germ-free environment, usually with concomitant administration of antibacterial prophylaxis.[6, 370] Mechanical isolation can be achieved by two means. One is a strict or "reverse" isolation of the patient while deeply neutropenic, with all staff members and visitors wearing sterile gowns, gloves, and masks and only cooked food or food and beverages with a low bacterial content being allowed. This approach has not inarguably resulted in a decreased risk of infections, although the burden of exogenously transmitted pathogens is theoretically reduced. However, it might indirectly be of benefit because it heightens the attention of both staff and visitors to hand washing and other general hygienic rules.[6] Of greater interest are total protective environments. In these rooms, the air is made sterile by high-efficiency particulate air (HEPA) filtration, laminar positive airflow (LAF) is maintained, and all objects and items are sterilized. The patient is given only sterilized food and beverages. Oral prophylactic antibiotic decontamination is prescribed, and daily washing of the skin, mouth, and all body orifices with antiseptic solutions is carried out. A significant benefit of this approach was initially reported and confirmed in patients with newly diagnosed acute leukemia: the incidence of infection and the mortality rate were reduced by approximately 25% in comparison to patients treated in open wards.[6, 370-372] The system is expensive, however, and requires a larger staff and longer assistance times, but because of recent improvements in both prophylaxis and treatment of infections, it is no longer regarded as necessary for the routine management of patients with acute leukemia[6] or those undergoing high-dose therapy with an HSC autograft.[373] Nevertheless, HEPA/LAF isolation may still be of value in some selected, very high-risk conditions. Several studies reported a reduction in invasive fungal and other severe infections in allografted patients treated in total protective environments. An International Bone Marrow Transplantation Registry survey[374] published in 1998 and reporting on 5068 leukemia patients receiving HSC allografts between 1988 and 1992 underlined the superiority of HEPA/LAF isolation over conventional isolation in reducing the risk of death, mainly from infection, within the first 100 days ($P = .009$ and $P = .003$ for HLA-identical sibling and alternative donor transplants, respectively). HEPA/LAF isolation is recommended in the high-risk transplant setting, especially when invasive fungal infections are more likely to develop (T-cell–depleted and unrelated donor HSC allografts).

Antibacterial Prophylaxis

First Attempts and Trimethoprim-Sulfamethoxazole

Several prophylactic antibacterial regimens have been developed for severely neutropenic leukemia patients. The underlying concept is that suppression of the endogenous flora would result in a limitation of infections by these bacteria, particularly by gram-negative organisms resident in the alimentary tract. In addition, credit was given to the concept of selective decontamination, that is, a preferential inhibition of the more pathogenic aerobic flora with relative sparing of the protective anaerobic bacteria. Prophylactic regimens have usually been administered as oral preparations of either nonabsorbable or absorbable drugs (Table 14–18). Initially, multiagent prophylaxis with nonabsorbable antibiotics (and antifungals) was attempted as a means of achieving total intestinal decontamination despite the fact that patients were not nursed in a bacteria-sterile environment. Oral gentamicin, vancomycin, colistin, framycetin, nystatin, and polymyxin were given in various combinations.[5, 343, 370, 375] Efficacy was documented in some, but not all the reports; however, these regimens suffered from a low to very low compliance rate because of the unpleasant taste of the drugs and relative difficulty in administration. Low compliance and exposure to antibiotics caused resistance to develop in some cases. In the light of their unproven efficacy and problematic tolerability, these regimens have now been almost completely abandoned, but they must be remembered as the first rationale attempt to develop effective antibacterial prophylaxis for patients with leukemia at risk of infection. The prophylactic use of oral TMP-SMX can be regarded as the prototypic, selectively decontaminating regimen in that this drug eliminates most enteric gram-negative microorganisms (excluding *P. aeruginosa*) but appears to preserve the majority of anaerobes. Many controlled studies have documented a reduction in infection rates in patients receiving the drug as compared with untreated controls.[5, 6, 376-378] One additional advantage of prophylactic TMP-SMX is its value against *P. carinii* infection. Thus, TMP-SMX is indicated when the risk of infection by this latter organism is high, as in children with ALL treated with intensive, prolonged, and strongly immunosuppressive consolidation therapy.[302, 303, 379] Patients intolerant to it can be given atovaquone.[380] Conversely, TMP-SMX should not be used in institutions or clinical studies in which a rather high incidence of infection by *Pseudomonas* species is expected. Adverse effects from TMP-SMX are known but rarely encountered. Among others, myelosuppression appears to be of some concern in these patients because the length of the neutropenic period can be prolonged

TABLE 14–18. Prophylactic Regimens for Bacterial Infections (All Drugs Intended for Oral Administration) and *Pneumocystis carinii* Infection

Regimen/Drugs	Dosage	Notes/Indications
Oral nonabsorbable combinations (gentamicin, colistin, framycetin, nystatin, vancomycin, polymyxin B)	Variable, not reported	Historical interest, low compliance, induction of resistance
Trimethoprim-sulfamethoxazole	150–750 mg/m²/day*	Highly active with *P. carinii*, does not cover *Pseudomonas* spp., myelotoxic, induction of resistance
Fluorinated quinolones (ciprofloxacin, ofloxacin, pefloxacin, levofloxacin)	500 mg every 12 hr†	Best available option against gram-negative bacteria, well tolerated, possible induction of resistance

* Intermittent use: two to three times weekly or 3 consecutive days for *P. carinii*.
† Ciprofloxacin in adults; levofloxacin, 500 mg/day.

and thus predispose to superinfections and other infections by *C. difficile* and fungi.[381, 382] Altogether, the only currently accepted indication for the prophylactic use of TMP-SMX is that of *P. carinii* infection, whereas better and less toxic drugs are available for other eventualities. In at-risk patients (neutropenic patients with CLL who are receiving fludarabine plus prednisone or similarly immunosuppressive drugs; childhood ALL), TMP-SMX should be administered on an intermittent schedule at least twice weekly.

Fluoroquinolones

Oral fluorinated quinolones are the drugs investigated most in recent years.[81] These drugs are well tolerated, do not affect the bone marrow regenerative capability,[383] and share a very broad spectrum of antibacterial activity against gram-negative bacteria but still retain the capacity of decontaminating the gut in a selective manner[384-388] Recent studies have confirmed that oral quinolones, when given prophylactically, reduce the incidence of infection by gram-negative pathogens to a significant extent and shorten the duration of antibacterial treatment when fever occurs. Tolerability is almost absolute, if one excludes the problem of oral administration during mucositis, in which case erratic absorption is bypassed by intravenous administration. The activity of quinolones in preventing gram-negative sepsis was demonstrated to be superior when directly compared with that of nonabsorbable antibiotics and TMP-SMX–containing combinations.[383, 384, 389-392] Among the available drugs, ciprofloxacin was more effective than norfloxacin.[393] One interesting finding with ciprofloxacin was a reduction in myelotoxicity in sublethally irradiated mice.[394] Two recent meta-analyses[395, 396] examining 19 and 18 trials confirmed quinolones to be highly active in preventing gram-negative bacteremias and related infections, but not gram-positive infections and the overall risk of infection-related deaths. These data cast some doubt on the usefulness of quinolones in low-risk patients, but they remain effective against gram-negative bacteria in high-risk situations.[382, 397] The main problem with quinolones is indeed an increasing prevalence of infections by gram-positive rods, against which their activity is largely insufficient. To obviate this problem, attempts were undertaken to test prophylaxis with quinolones plus anti–gram-positive drugs, either vancomycin or a macrolide,[384, 392, 398, 399] rifampin,[400] penicillin,[397] and most recently, newer extended-spectrum agents (levofloxacin and others). Interestingly, the addition of metronidazole to quinolones in HSC transplant recipients significantly reduced the incidence of acute GVHD as a result of the suppression of endogenous anaerobic flora.[401] Because resistant strains of staphylococci can be induced by these approaches, for the time being, the quinolone-vancomycin combination must be considered investigational and not routinely used.[81] In a similar vein, quinolones can induce the emergence of gram-negative and coagulase-negative staphylococcal resistant strains, though at a lower rate than with other antibiotics given prophylactically. Induction of resistant strains can have a negative therapeutic impact at the onset of the febrile episode, when quinolones themselves cannot

be used.[81] For these reasons and the fact that overall mortality rates by infections were not generally affected by quinolones in the published studies, their use as prophylaxis has been questioned, if not openly discouraged.[13] The final decision regarding their use should be made after evaluation of the infectious risk in specific patient categories and previous institutional data. If this review indicates the need for an antibiotic prophylaxis but the attendant risk for *P. carinii* pneumonia is low, oral quinolones should be the preferred drugs (Fig. 14-12).

Antifungal Prophylaxis

Old Drugs

The increasing incidence of fungal infections in leukemia patients, their clinical gravity, and the availability of active new compounds to be administered orally have led to renewed interest in antifungal prophylaxis[6, 168, 192, 402] (Table 14-19). As for the early use of antibacterial agents, the first step in this direction addressed the administration of oral nystatin, AmB, miconazole, ketoconazole, or clotrimazole.[6, 168, 246, 403] The principal antifungal agent is AmB, a polyene that binds to a cell membrane component (ergosterol), eventually increasing its permeability and leading to cell death. Unfortunately, AmB has a narrow therapeutic index and is frequently associated, at therapeutic doses, with acute effects (chills, fever) and nephrotoxicity. Most of the early prophylaxis studies focused on the fact that inhibiting the growth of colonizing fungal species in the gut and upper aerodigestive tract would theoretically result in a decreased incidence of invasive infections. The spectrum of action of these drugs, with the exception of AmB, was generally restricted to *Candida* species, whereas *Aspergillus* species and other less frequent pathogens were excluded. Another limitation was that although colonization by potentially pathogenic species, mainly *C. albicans,* was reduced, it was accompanied by recolonization with more resistant and pathogenic types such as *C. tropicalis* and by *Aspergillus* species. Eventually, this approach was demonstrated to reduce the frequency of colonizing species but not to significantly decrease the incidence of invasive fungal infections; hence it was abandoned, at least in high-risk patients. Because *Aspergillus* organisms are known to transiently colonize the nasal spaces and are exquisitely sensitive to AmB, attempts were made to assess the prophylactic role of intranasal nebulized AmB preparations.[404-406] Results indicated that invasive infections developed less frequently, even when no attempt was made to reduce environmental contamination by fungal spores. Clearly, this approach deserves further study with large patient numbers because of its effect on invasive disease, as well as its good tolerability profile and the low cost of the treatment schedule.[407] AmB can additionally be considered for systemic prophylaxis via the intravenous route at a low to intermediate dosage of 0.1 mg/kg/day or 0.5 mg/kg three times per week.[168, 388, 407, 408] At this dosage, the drug is relatively well tolerated.

New Drugs

With the advent of the new oral triazoles (fluconazole, itraconazole),[192] the issue of effective antifungal preven-

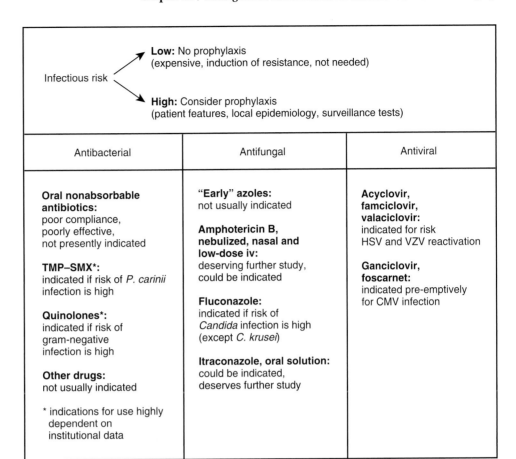

FIGURE 14–12. Drug prevention of bacterial, fungal, and viral infections.

tion gained momentum. These drugs bind to cytochrome P-450 enzymes and affect lanosterol demethylation, which in turn reduces the synthesis of membrane ergasterol. Fungal cell death eventually follows through a mechanism similar to that of AmB. A characteristic of these drugs, especially itraconazole, is their interaction with the metabolism of other drugs, as occurs frequently with cyclosporine in the HSC allograft setting. Periodic monitoring of cyclosporine levels and adjustments of drug doses are thus necessary in allografted patients taking itraconazole. Prophylactic fluconazole was demonstrated in some early studies to reduce the incidence of all fungal infections exept those by *C. krusei*.[249, 409] A number of subsequent randomized trials have confirmed that fluconazole, given orally or intravenously at a total dose of 200

to 400 mg/day is equivalent or superior to prophylaxis with either AmB[410-412] or other drugs[413] or to no prophylaxis or placebo[414-418] and that it significantly reduces the incidence of documented fungal infections from 16% to 35% to 3% to 17%,[411, 413-416] except those by *C. krusei*, with an associated survival benefit ascertained in only a few of the studies.[413, 416] When compared with AmB, fluconazole was better tolerated and induced fewer toxic side effects. In one study,[418] fluconazole was particularly effective in the management of intensively treated patients with AML. In contrast, in a different report[419] the drug was no better than oral AmB. Other new antifungal agents available for prophylactic use are itraconazole (a new azole with an extended spectrum of activity against *Aspergillus* species) and the lipid formulations of AmB.

TABLE 14–19. Antifungal Prophylaxis

Drugs	Dosage/Schedule	Notes
Nystatin, amphotericin B, miconazole, clotrimazole	Variable (orally)	Decreased colonization, recolonization by resistant species, lack of overall benefit
Amphotericin B	Intranasal or nebulized 0.5 mg/kg IV on alternate days or 0.1 mg/kg/day	Seemingly effective, not very toxic, further studies needed As above
Fluconazole	200–400 mg/day PO or IV	Active against non-*krusei Candida* spp., nontoxic, expensive
Itraconazole	5 mg/kg/day PO	Promising agent, expensive, oral solution better, frequent drug interactions, further studies needed

The use of itraconazole oral solution (400 mg/day or 5 mg/kg/day), which improved bioavailability even in transplanted patients,[420] conferred some advantage in two randomized trials,[421, 422] with a reduced incidence of invasive aspergillosis and fungal deaths in one.[422] Finally, liposomal AmB (AmBisome) was tested as prophylactic measure in a placebo-controlled trial.[423] The study results did not support a definite prophylactic role for this drug. It is not yet clear, in summary, how best to prevent invasive fungal infections in neutropenic patients with leukemia because with only few exceptions, none of the new drugs eventually reduced the incidence of fungal deaths and the need for therapeutic AmB. Moreover, the cost-benefit ratio thus far ascertained for the new azoles does not presently allow their widespread use in an unselected patient population. As for antibacterial prophylaxis, the cost is high or very high and the generalized use of these drugs favors the selection of drug-resistant molds or yeasts. Different antifungal approaches may be justified in different risk classes, as determined by local epidemiologic data (prevalence of invasive *Candida* or *Aspergillus* infections), data from surveillance laboratory tests in high-risk patients (serial antigen determinations, throat and stool cultures), and controlled study programs[31, 407] (Fig. 14–12).

Antiviral Prophylaxis

HSV and VZV

Antiviral prophylaxis is another complex matter ranging from the optional use of nontoxic drugs given orally to prevent HSV infection in low-risk patients to the extremely critical setting of HSC transplant recipients at risk for the lethal complications of CMV infection (Table 14–20). Intravenous or oral acyclovir is highly effective in preventing disease reactivation by HSV.[6, 163, 424–427] Success rates close to 100% have been reported. Notably, in one placebo-controlled trial conducted on 80 HSV-seropositive adult patients with AML,[428] prophylactic acyclovir significantly postponed the development of fever and initiation of systemic antibiotics and significantly reduced the incidence of nonfungal oral infections localized outside the soft palate. Other recently developed drugs with increased oral bioavailability are valacyclovir and famciclovir.[193] Because with prophylactic regimens drug dosages are lower than those used therapeutically, in general, patient compliance is excellent and the incidence of toxic side effects is negligible. Prophylaxis against HSV infection should be considered for patients at high risk of activation, such as those with an earlier episode or a significant antibody titer of greater than 1:16 and exposure to high-dose chemotherapy or radiotherapy regimens or other intensive acute leukemia treatment is foreseeable. Prevention of primary infection by VZV, or chickenpox, chiefly involves isolation of the infected patient and recent contacts because the disease is transmitted through the air even during the incubation period before the typical skin lesions become manifested. The prophylactic administration of immunoglobulin to low-titer patients at risk for chickenpox significantly reduces the morbidity and mortality of the disease in immunocompromised hosts and must be considered after exposure. Virus reactivation in the form of zoster is frequent after HSC transplantation or other intensive antileukemic treatments. Both intravenous and oral long-term acyclovir given for 6 months is highly effective in preventing reactivation during this period.[429, 430] However, infections developed after withdrawal of the drug, but they were usually manageable with reinstitution of intravenous therapy and were very rarely clinically severe. Longer prophylaxis, up to 1 year, could reduce late reactivation rates. Because fatal disseminated zoster is equally rare in subjects not given prophylactic acyclovir, as long as such patients are treated promptly at the onset of symptoms, there is no direct proof that prophylactic acyclovir improves survival in patients at risk. However, because reactivation of dis-

TABLE 14–20. Prophylaxis for Common Viral Infections and Preemptive Therapy for CMV

Infection	Drugs and Schedule	Indications and Notes
HSV	Acyclovir, 400 mg PO q8 h Valacyclovir, 500 mg PO q12 h Famciclovir, 250–500 mg PO q12 h	High-risk patients (high antibody titer)
VZV		
Chickenpox	Isolate patient and contacts, zoster immunoglobulin	High-risk patients (low antibody titer)
Zoster	Acyclovir, 400–800 mg PO q6 h (3–12 mo)*	High-risk patients (history, treatments)
CMV		
Seronegative	CMV-negative or filtered blood products	Always
Seropositive	Immunoglobulin	Questionable efficacy
	Intravenous acyclovir → oral acyclovir	Intermediate efficacy
	Ganciclovir, 5–6 mg/kg/day IV for 5–7 days/wk for 100–120 days	Effective, neutropenia possible
Preemptive	Ganciclovir, 5 mg/kg/day IV for 2 wk, then 5 mg/kg/day for 5 days/wk for 2 wk†	When positive antigenemia/PCR assay, monitor during preemptive therapy
	Foscarnet, 90 mg/kg/day IV for 2 wk then 90 mg/kg/day for 2 wk‡	If ganciclovir resistant or as alternative

* Variable schedules, consider famciclovir/valacyclovir as an alternative drug.
† Other schedules reported, including 10 mg/kg/day for initial therapy; if positive/increasing antigenemia PCR results after 3 to 4 weeks (equals resistance), shift to foscarnet.
‡ Preferable in T-cell-depleted allografts (cyclosporine not given equals low risk of nephrotoxicity) and in patients with slow hematologic recovery.
CMV, cytomegalovirus; HSV, herpes simplex virus; PCR, polymerase chain reaction; VZV, varicella-zoster virus.

ease is subjectively very unpleasant and can lead to readmission of patients shortly after discharge, oral prophylaxis appears to be justified, at least in patients with a proven history of recurrent infection.

CMV

In patients undergoing HSC transplantation, CMV infection is associated with a severe clinical picture, so an effective preventive strategy is thus necessary (Table 14-20). Two distinct clinical situations may arise, one regarding seronegative and, the other seropositive patients. First, evidence suggests that seronegative patients should always receive transfusions of blood products obtained from seronegative donors to eliminate the risk of blood-borne transmission.[431-434] Filtration of leukocytes from blood products might be equally effective because the viable virus resides mostly in the mononuclear cell fraction removed by filtration.[435] Receiving a transplant from a seropositive donor is another possible source of infection in these subjects, a situation in which cell filtration is obviously not possible. In this case, as well as in that of seronegative patients not given seronegative blood products, the prophylactic administration of immunoglobulin could be useful to prevent CMV-related syndromes and decrease severe GVHD and, in turn, interstitial pneumonitis.[433, 434, 436-438] Others consider the use of immunoglobulin controversial,[439] so presently, this method alone is not recommended to prevent CMV disease. In seropositive recipients, the disease is usually a consequence of endogenous reactivation. Among historical antiviral agents, high-dose intravenous acyclovir, 500 mg/m^2 three times a day for 5 days before to 30 days after transplantation, followed by 800 mg four times a day orally for 6 months, demonstrated appreciable activity in decreasing the incidence of overt CMV disease, in addition to having a very good toxicity profile.[440, 441] These findings led to implementation of a two-step strategy consisting of acyclovir given first and until evidence of prophylaxis failure.[442] Subsequently, prophylactic ganciclovir emerged as a highly effective drug. Ganciclovir significantly abated the incidence of both detectable CMV infection and related diseases from 24% to 70% to 0% to 25%, and it also contributed to improved overall survival in most published studies.[282, 433, 443-449] Ganciclovir is expected to be less effective during T-cell–depleted or unrelated donor HSC allografting and in conjunction with very heavy immunosuppressive treatment.[439, 449-452] Neutropenia resulting from myelotoxicity was the predominant toxic effect and put patients at an increased risk of bacterial infections, fungal infections, and an occasional aplastic death.[290, 340, 453] The use of prophylactic ganciclovir can be recommended for seropositive recipients of allogeneic bone marrow transplants and in general for patients at high risk for CMV disease.

PREEMPTIVE THERAPY, NEW DRUGS, NOVEL APPROACHES

Preemptive treatment at the first signs of infection (before overt clinical disease) is being evaluated as a new modality to prevent CMV disease (see Table 14-20). This strategy means that antiviral drugs are given only to pa-

tients showing early evidence of systemic viral spread. The latter information can be obtained through CMV pp65 antigen and/or nucleic acid detection tests (PCR for CMV DNA appears to be most sensitive) performed serially during the period of high risk as previously detailed. In this manner, patients in whom CMV disease is not going to develop are initially spared drug exposure, with avoidance of myelosuppression (with ganciclovir) and a reduction in treatment costs. On the other hand, those with antigen- or PCR-positive results can be identified approximately 1 to 4 weeks before overt disease and treated according.[338-340, 454] Moreover, foscarnet has been recently introduced to substitute for ganciclovir because it is non–cross-resistant and not myelotoxic. Foscarnet, which is mainly nephrotoxic, has been successfully used for both prophylaxis and preemptive therapy and as a first-line, alternative, or combination drug.[339, 450, 455, 456] To summarize, both drugs appear to be substantially and equally effective, with different toxic side effects that are usually manageable by appropriate dose reductions; preemptive treatment is safe and generally as effective or nearly as effective as prophylactic drugs. A word of caution is necessary about the augmented incidence of early CMV disease sometimes reported in preemptive therapy groups as a result of failure to detect early disease and in highly immunocompromised hosts.[340, 450, 457] On the other hand, early prophylaxis with ganciclovir (from engraftment day) will aggravate neutropenia and facilitate fungal infections and late CMV disease. Studies are in progress to precisely define the role of preemptive versus prophylactic ganciclovir and/or foscarnet and to improve the specificity and sensitivity of diagnostic tests for early preemptive therapy, along with the introduction of quantitative PCR for CMV DNA and detection of CMV mRNA. Other novel approaches include the possibility of developing a CMV vaccine[458] and/or elicit and then boost an immune response from CMV-specific T-cell clones isolated from HLA-compatible HSC donors.[274, 275] The latter would be useful in patients at risk for late CMV disease (T-cell–depleted and/or unrelated donor HSC allografts). An oral formulation of ganciclovir is also being studied.[193]

Prevention of Rare Pathogens

It may occasionally be indicated, in patients with a history of previous infection or at high risk for other reasons, to initiate prophylaxis against parasites or mycobacteria. The role of intermittent TMP-SMX for the prevention of *P. carinii* infection has been discussed. Pyrimethamine/sulfadoxine may be effective in preventing both pneumocystosis and toxoplasmosis.[459] In patients at risk of progression of tuberculosis, as identified by a positive purified protein derivative test, prophylactic isoniazid is appropriate. Among rare viral diseases, prophylaxis of RSV and influenza A virus can be achieved with RSV-enriched immunoglobulin plus aerosolized ribavirin and with amantadine/rimantadine, respectively.[31, 460]

Immunoglobulin

The passive immunization of subjects lacking an adequate humoral immune response to certain pathogens can limit the incidence and virulence of infections. In patients with leukemia, two groups seem likely to benefit from the prophylactic administration of immunoglobulin. First, for patients undergoing allogeneic HSC transplantation, the administration of human immune or hyperimmune gamma globulin products led in several studies to a significant reduction in overall mortality as a result of a decreased incidence of not only fatal CMV infections (see earlier) but also intersitial pneumonitis and infections from other causes.[461-464] Hyperimmune globulin preparations are also available for VZV and RSV infections; however, routine use is not indicated, partly because of effective therapy being promptly available for at least VZV infection and because of uncertain therapeutic benefit. Some evidence has indicated a favorable effect of immunoglobulin on GVHD. Indeed, a 1994 review of published randomized studies indicated the latter as the dominant clinical effect of immunoglobulin prophylaxis.[465] Dosages are usually high in relation to the increased protein catabolism post-transplant, in the range of 0.5 to 1 g/kg intravenously every 1 to 2 weeks starting from the initiation of cytotoxic therapy or postgrafting and until the resolution of neutropenia or for a limited period of some months. Extension of the prophylactic period until 1 year post-transplant was prompted by the recognition of a long-lasting deficiency of IgG2 and IgG4 subclasses, which predisposes to late infections by encapsulated microorganisms, and such extension of prophylaxis sometimes resulted in a decreased incidence of these infections.[464, 466] Patients undergoing autografting do not appear to benefit from immunoglobulin administration,[467] but indications for the use of immunoglobulin in selected cases cannot be categorically excluded beforehand. Another potential application of immunoglobulin in bone marrow transplant patients is administration by the oral route, which is under investigation as a means of limiting the rate and severity of gastrointestinal infections.[466, 468] In summary, some evidence suggests that immunoglobulin prophylaxis can be viewed as an integral part of the management program to prevent a variety of infections in allogeneic HSC recipients. For patients receiving other types of intensive treatment, the gamma globulin serum concentration should be monitored longitudinally and immunoglobulin administered when hypogammaglobulinemia is documented in the presence of other factors predisposing to infection (mucositis, neutropenia, use of immunosuppressants). The second point of interest concerns patients with CLL. Approximately half of these patients show variable degrees of hypogammaglobulinemia that correlate with the stage and course of the disease. Although not solely attributable to hypogammaglobulinemia, infections are more frequent when hypogammaglobulinemia is present, thus suggesting a pathogenetic role.[469] Patients with CLL and hypogammaglobulinemia, as defined by a concentration of 50% or less of the lower normal limit of IgG, or a history of infection were treated by periodic infusion of gamma globulin (400 mg/kg every 3 weeks for 1 year) and showed a significant advantage over the control group in terms of the incidence of bacterial infections and a longer interval to the first infection.[470] Hypogammaglobulinemia-associated infections in patients with CLL typically affect

the upper aerodigestive tract and the lungs and are mainly due to reduced concentrations of the IgG3 (also predisposing to herpetic infections) and IgG4 subclasses. Subsequently, the issue was reassessed with a decision-analysis model to determine the cost-effectiveness ratio and the overall clinical benefit to patients. This study did not suggest a survival benefit with prophylactic immunoglobulin in CLL and showed this approach to be extraordinarily expensive in comparison with other therapies.[471] When prophylactic gamma globulin administration is being considered, CLL patients should be evaluated individually in the light of their history of infections, activity of the disease, the therapeutic program (especially if it includes the new purine analogue), and the presence of cofactors that aggravate the risk of infections, such as neutropenia or splenectomy.

Vaccines

Active immunization with vaccines is an effective way of preventing infections in subjects at high risk. Many patients with leukemia, particularly the older age groups, have already been immunized against several viral disorders before the development of leukemia. The immunosuppressive effects of chemotherapy, radiotherapy, and corticosteroids include a decline in antibody production previously elicited by active immunization. Because complete seronegativity can develop after intensive treatment, particularly marrow transplants, reinduction of immunity may be necessary in patients at risk. Traditionally, the administration of live attenuated vaccines was discouraged in patients recently exposed to chemotherapy or radiotherapy because of the possible induction of disseminated disease in immunocompromised hosts.[6, 472] Moreover, intensively treated patients may require months to reconstitute an immune system able to produce significant amounts of antibodies to foreign antigens. After allogeneic-HSC transplantation, for instance, this process takes no less than 6 months and usually much more. In this case, B cells of donor origin are the source of newly formed antibodies, and the immune response can be enhanced by active immunization of both the donor and recipient.[473-475] Seronegative HSC transplant patients not showing severe GVHD and not needing immunosuppressive therapy may be considered for vaccination 6 to 12 months post-transplant.[476-479] More specific guidelines suggested recently by some authorities are summarized in Table 14–21.[480-483] The prevailing indication is that most allografted as well as the majority of autografted patients would benefit from restoration of the immune response through vaccination and that only live attenuated vaccines (measles-mumps-rubella, bacille Calmette-Guérin, oral poliovirus, VZV, adenovirus) should not be administered before the second year postgraft and on individual basis thereafter. Household contacts likely to acquire or transmit any of these infectious agents should be vaccinated along with patients. The case of late infection from encapsulated bacteria is a special one and is discussed in the next section on asplenic states. Outside HSC transplants, patients not receiving chemotherapy for a minimum of 3 months or receiving only

TABLE 14-21. Suggested Guidelines for Vaccine Reimmunization of Transplanted Leukemic Patients

Category and Context	Somani and Larson[481]	Singhal and Mehta[482]	Ljungman for EBMT[480, 483]
Type HSC transplant	Allogeneic	Allogeneic/autologous	Allogeneic/autologous
Vaccines, postgraft timing, notes			
Pneumococcal	7 and 24 mo	24 mo	6–12 mo
Haemophilus influenzae type b (Hib)	Hib conjugate at 7 mo, × 3 (every 6 mo)	4 and 10 mo	Allogeneic (all)/autologous (risk group), season dependent
Diphtheria toxoid	After 12 mo	12, 13, 14 mo	6–12 mo
Tetanus toxoid	>12 mo	12, 13, 14 mo	6–12 mo
Poliovirus*	>12 mo, × 3 (monthly, no GVHD)	12, 13, 14 mo	6–12 mo
Hepatitis B virus	Schedule as for eIPV	6, 7–8, 10–12 mo	Individual basis/epidemiology, 6–12 mo
Influenza virus†	Every autumn	6 mo, annually	Season dependent
MMR‡	>2 yr (no GVHD)	Individual basis, >2 yr	Individual basis, >2 yr

* Enhanced inactivated (eIPV); avoid oral polio vaccine.
† Currently inactivated.
‡ Mumps-measles-rubella live attenuated vaccine.
GVHD, graft-versus-host disease.

low-dose corticosteroids can be safely considered for immunization, even with live vaccines. Children appear to lose their immune status more commonly than adults do,[472] in whom the natural immunity elicited by infection is often preserved. Therefore, prophylactic reimmunization may be necessary after highly immunosuppressive regimens in children and adults who become entirely and persistently seronegative, even after autologous transplants, and such reimmunization has been variously advocated for poliovirus, measles, rubella, mumps, *Haemophilus, Pneumococcus,* tetanus, diphtheria, hepatitis B, and influenza.[6, 472, 484]

Asplenic States

Splenectomy is sometimes performed in patients with idiopathic myelofibrosis, HCL, and splenomegalic CLL variants. Moreover, functional asplenia occurs after HSC transplantation with total body irradiation–based regimens. Because asplenia, whether anatomic or functional, predisposes to late, unpredictable, but clinically very severe infections by *S. pneumoniae* and *H. influenzae,* prophylactic reimmunization with the 14- or 23-valent pneumococcal vaccine and the *H. influenzae* conjugate vaccine is indicated, together with prolonged (2 years to lifelong) administration of penicillin V (250 mg twice daily orally) or, in penicillin-intolerant subjects, erythromycin (250 mg twice daily orally), clarithromycin (250 mg daily orally), or TMP-SMX.[480, 482] Prophylactic antibiotics are required with vaccination because the available pneumococcal vaccines are poorly immunogenic, particularly in patients with GVHD and/or those receiving immunosuppressants.

Use of Hematopoietic Growth Factors: Characteristics and Types

In recent years, factors stimulating the growth of HSC, have been cloned and fully characterized. Globally known as colony-stimulating factors (CSFs) by virtue of their capability of supporting the proliferative and maturation potential of stem-cell colonies in vitro, these peptides correspond to the cytokines that normally regulate blood cell production in bone marrow in vivo and have been obtained for clinical use by means of recombinant DNA technology.[485, 486] Granulocyte (G-), macrophage (M-), and granulocyte-macrophage (GM-) CSFs are potent inducers of proliferation and differentiation of myeloid precursor cells to mature granulocytes and/or monocytes. Activation of the metabolic and phagocytic functions of terminal nondividing cells occurs in parallel. After G- or GM-CSF administration, therefore, the number of granulocytes or monocytes increases greatly and rapidly in the circulating blood, and their antimicrobial killing capacity is highly enhanced. Different types of G- and GM-CSFs are known and are available for clinical use (Table 14–22). Glycosylated (lenograstim) and nonglycosylated (filgrastim) G-CSFs appear to be fundamentally equivalent. In contrast, marked differences may be noted among the available types of GM-CSF: sargramostim (yeast derived, glycosylated), molgramostim (*E. coli* derived, nonglycosylated), and regramostim (hamster ovary cell derived, glycosylated). Nonglycosylated GM-CSF is distributed rather quickly in the body and induces fast leukotriene biosynthesis. This characteristic may be responsible for the high rate of clinical side effects (fluid retention, fever, myalgia), relatively high dropout rates, and perhaps the lack of clinical benefit sometimes reported in studies with molgramostim.[487, 488] For other CSFs, the information is still limited. Some data, reviewed previously, suggest a role for stem-cell factor (SCF/c-kit ligand), IL-3, and IFN-γ.[6]

Activities of G-CSF, GM-CSF, M-CSF, and Other Cytokines

With G-CSF, the mitogenic activity of neutrophil bone marrow precursors (all stages from immature $CD34^+CD33^-$ cells to myelocytes) is greatly increased, the transit time of mature cells from the bone marrow to peripheral blood is decreased from 6 to approximately 3 days, the metabolic and functional capability of mature

TABLE 14–22. Cytokines for Leukemia Patients at Risk of Infection

Drug (Dosage)	Activity, Effects
IL-3 (max, 1000 µg/m²/day)	Stimulates early pluripotent stem cells, to be used with other CSFs
G-CSF (5–32 µg/kg/day)	Stimulates neutrophil lineage committed stem cells, activates neutrophil phagocytic functions, accelerates neutrophil recovery, and mobilizes peripheral blood stem cells after chemotherapy; synergy with IL-3 and stem-cell factor
GM-CSF (5–32 µg/kg/day 250 mg/m²/day)	As for G-CSF; stimulates multilineage and macrophage progenitors and activates monocyte/macrophage functions, stimulates T cells, protects neutrophils from adrenal steroids; side effects possible (by type/source)
Stem-cell factor	Synergy with G-CSF (investigational)
Interferon-γ	Neutrophil activation, synergy with other CSFs (investigational)

G-CSF, granulocyte colony-stimulating factor; GM-CSF, granulocyte-macrophage CSF; IL-3, interleukin-3.

cells is stimulated, and their life span is increased as a result of antiapoptotic effects.[489] Relevant functional changes include an upward regulation of chemotaxis and phagocytosis with increased expression of complement (CD11b/CD18b, CD35), immunoglobulin (CD64, CD32, CD16), and integrin (LAM-1, CD14) receptors and simultaneous activation of the respiratory oxidative burst. Divergent results have been observed in recent studies. In one, G-CSF adversely affected neutrophil chemotaxis and bacterial cell killing.[490] A shift toward an anti-inflammatory cytokine response was observed in another.[491] Direct stimulation of *K. pneumoniae* growth by G-CSF has been reported.[492] GM-CSF, in addition to stimulating neutrophil production and activity in a fashion similar to G-CSF, exerts a powerful induction of proliferation and functional activation of cells of the monocyte-macrophage lineage and also stimulates immunocompetent T-cell subsets and dendritic cells.[493] Thus, GM-CSF plays a central role as a physiologic upregulator of many immune functions and may therefore be useful in the treatment (or prevention) of infections broadly related to an immunodeficient status and not caused by neutropenia alone. In particular, CSFs and primarily GM-CSF may have a justified role as antifungal agents.[494–496] Improved control of growth and subsequent destruction of several fungal (*Aspergillus, Candida, Crypococcus*) and bacterial (*Staphylococcus, Mycobacterium*) species by GM-CSF–stimulated neutrophils and monocytes-macrophages have been documented in preclinical and clinical studies.[488, 493, 497, 498] The role of M-CSF in regard to fungal infections may be comparable to that of GM-CSF.[499] With respect to other cytokines, experimental data in animal models have documented a significant myelostimulatory effect and reduction of mortality from streptococcal sepsis by SCF/c-kit

ligand plus G-CSF.[500] IFN-γ does enhance the oxidative metabolism of phagocytes in response to fungal infection and also stimulates some NK, T-, and B-cell subsets.[487, 497] Moreover, like GM-CSF but not G-CSF, IFN-γ prevents the detrimental effect of corticosteroids on neutrophil activity against *Aspergillus* species. IL-3 primarily stimulates the proliferation of early pluripotent stem cells, but it has no maturation effect. Accordingly, IL-3 can be used to rapidly expand the pool of early stem cells, after which the subsequent administration of G-/GM-CSF promotes further differentiation and quantitative expansion of activated granulocytes and monocytes. It is possible that the combined use of G- and GM-CSF could result in a comparably high output from the marrow of both early and mature myeloid and monocytic cells.[493]

CSFs in Neutropenic Patients

Early studies demonstrated the feasibility and safety of both intravenous and subcutaneus administration of CSFs and determined effective and relatively nontoxic dosages.[501] Theoretically, all the biologic features of G-, GM-, and M-CSF can be of benefit to leukemia patients receiving myelosuppressive treatment or in whom infectious complications develop (Table 14–22). However, there is no simple way, with very few exceptions, to predict which patient will eventually benefit from the administration of CSFs. The uncertainty stems from the multifactorial pathogenesis of infectious complications, neutropenia being the major but not the sole determinant. Table 14–23 reports general recommendations on the use of CSFs adopted by the American Society of Clinical Oncology.[502] It is evident that different risk groups are recognized and that for high-risk categories (defined by an expected incidence of febrile neutropenia of >40%), the

TABLE 14–23. Use of Hematopoietic CSFs: A Summary of Recommendations from the American Society of Clinical Oncology (1996)[502]

Intervention with CSFs	Guidelines and Notes
Primary prophylaxis	Reserve for patients with an expected incidence of febrile neutropenia of ≥40%, identify patients at high risk
Secondary prophylaxis	Consider if neutropenia causes treatment delay
Therapy	Inadequate data on afebrile patients, consider in high-risk patients (sepsis, hypotension, fungal infection, pneumonia)
Adjunct to hematopoietic transplants	Consider as an adjunct to allogeneic and autologous progenitor stem cell transplants
Use in AML and MDS	No significant harm, consider in high-risk patients (age ≥55 yr), consider intermittent application in myelodysplasia patients with neutropenia and recurrent infections
Dose and route	G-CSF, 5 µg/kg/day; GM-CSF, 250 µg/m²/day either SC or IV

AML, acute myelogenous leukemia, CSFs, colony-stimulaing factors; G-CSF, granulocyte CSF; GM-CSF, granulocyte-macrophage CSF; MDS, myelodysplastic syndrome.

use of CSFs has no contraindications. Three distinct clinical situations that extend the role of CSFs from prophylaxis to treatment need detailed evaluation: infections in a non-neutropenic patient, neutropenia without fever and infection, and use of a CSF at the onset of fever in conjunction with antibiotics. Regarding the first point, the effects of G-CSF in 756 nonleukemic (non-neutropenic) hospitalized patients with community-acquired pneumonia were analyzed in a recent phase III trial.[503] Although overall cure rates and failure rates were identical, G-CSF accelerated radiologic improvement and significantly reduced the rate of serious complications (acute respiratory distress syndrome, empyema, disseminated intravascular coagulation) and improved the outcome of the patients with multilobar pneumonia. By extrapolation, the use of a CSF (G-CSF) could be indicated in a patient with leukemia and a serious infectious complication (complex infection), even when non-neutropenic, to accelerate recovery from the acute phase and minimize the risk of chemotherapy delay. Regarding the second topic, in another randomized trial, G-CSF was given to cancer patients with severe chemotherapy-induced afebrile neutropenia.[504] Although the time to increase the neutrophil count was significantly shorter in the G-CSF group, no other clinical benefit was observed. However, the median duration of severe neutropenia was short in both groups (2 days with G-CSF versus 4 days with placebo), which excluded these patients from the high-risk category with an estimated neutropenic period of 10 days and greater. This study illustrates one possible pitfall in the use of CSFs for the prevention of infectious complications. The final investigation,[505] relative to the third point, compared the outcome of 107 cancer patients (only a proportion of whom had leukemia) who were given, at the onset of neutropenic fever, antibiotics alone or antibiotics plus GM-CSF. The response rate was higher with GM-CSF (96% versus 82%, $P = .03$), but survival was similar and side effects were common (with molgramostim).

First Studies with CSFs in Patients with Leukemia

Early studies conducted in patients with leukemia confirmed with few exceptions the safety and usefulness of CSFs during remission induction and autologous or allogeneic HSC transplantation in patients with ALL. Albeit with some differences relating to the protocol used and the type of patients, the advantages demonstrated were a faster leukocyte and sometimes platelet recovery, a reduced incidence of infections, shorter hospitalization, and a lower overall mortality.[506-512] The possibility of a stimulatory effect on the disease itself represented an obstacle for the use of CSFs in myeloid lineage leukemia. Attempts to address this important question were initiated, first by using CSFs in AML patients at very high risk of infection or death to conveniently cope with ethical issues. High-risk patients were those older than 60 years and those with recurrent or refractory disease. In such an instance, the administration of CSFs after chemotherapy was not associated with an increased likelihood of progressive disease and resulted in a greater than expected proportion of patients entering remission, with

reduced neutropenic periods and infection rates.[513, 514] By inference, studies in patients with myelodysplastic preleukemic syndromes showed that only a minority of cases progressed to more aggressive disease after CSFs whereas positive effects on granulopoiesis were documented by both GM-CSF and IL-3.[49, 515-517] Most recently, a complete and durable response was obtained with G-CSF alone in some patients with leukemia of myeloid origin relapsing after an allogeneic bone marrow transplant.[518] Other observations from previous in vitro studies suggested that leukemic cell growth is not inevitably stimulated by CSFs.[519]

CSFs in ALL and Other Lymphoid Leukemias

The main results from representative phase III clinical studies in adults and children with untreated ALL are summarized in Table 14-24. In general, the use of G-CSF ameliorated the duration of severe neutropenia and reduced the incidence of infections and fever and days in the hospital. In the largest study to date,[524] the early use of G-CSF together with intensive induction chemotherapy was safe and effective and allowed completion of early chemotherapy courses with less delay. Tighter adherence to planned treatment schedules was reported by others,[520, 521] unfortunately without improving the long-term outcome. No clear-cut clinical benefit was noted in the single study with GM-CSF (molgramostim, E. coli derived).[525] These results appear to confirm the clinical safety of G-CSF in adult[520, 522, 524] and childhood[521, 523] ALL, the benefits being confined to a lower incidence of febrile neutropenia and better treatment compliance. Several points remain to be addressed. It is possible that the benefits from CSFs may vary with the intensity of the chemotherapy regimen, as well as the timing of CSF administration. Indeed, the more positive effects (including reduced early mortality), were observed with G-CSF started soon after heavy therapy with cyclophosphamide, anthracyclines at substantial doses and high-dose cytarabine.[521, 524] With regard to high-dose cytarabine, the outcome improves in patients receiving additional G-CSF.[526] With regard to anthracyclines and the timing of G-CSF, the early administration of G-CSF (from treatment day 4) after an idarubicin-based regimen was similarly associated, in comparison to late administration of G-CSF, with a quicker neutrophil increase and a reduced incidence of infectious complications and use of antibiotics and antifungals[527] (Fig. 14-13). Just as in another study,[525] GM-CSF added after aggressive induction with doxorubicin did not exert any appreciable effect.[528] In summary, G-CSF given early could limit the hematologic toxicity of intensive induction regimens for ALL. CSF treatment is safe, with minimal toxic side effects, and stimulation of ALL cell growth has never been described. The issue of cost-effectiveness remains open,[523, 527] but compliance with treatment and rates of postremission treatment adherence are improved. On the other hand, the limited experience thus far accumulated with GM-CSF (molgramostim) is far less satisfactory. The alternative use of sargramostim, earlier administration, and direct comparison between G- and GM-CSF warrant further studies. Relatively few data are available for chronic lymphoid

TABLE 14–24. Randomized Clinical Trials with CSFs (G-CSF, GM-CSF) in Acute Lymphocytic Leukemia

Study (1st Author, Year)	No.	Study Arms and Medications	Main Results and Comments (CSF Group)
Ottmann, 1995[520]	37 39	G-CSF in induction phase II Control group	Shorter neutropenia of $<1 \times 10^9$/L ($P < .002$), trend to fewer infections, more rapid completion of chemotherapy ($P = .008$)
Welte, 1996[521]	17 17	G-CSF in induction (from day 7) Control group	Reduced febrile neutropenia ($P = .07$), fewer documented infections ($P = .04$), higher adherence to planned therapy ($P = .007$)
Geissler, 1997[522]	25 26	G-CSF in induction (from day 2) Control group	Shorter neutropenia of $<1 \times 10^9$/L ($P < .001$), reduced febrile neutropenia ($P < .05$) and documented infections ($P = .05$)
Pui, 1997[523]	73 75	G-CSF after induction Placebo	Fewer days in the hospital ($P = .011$) and documented infections ($P = .009$)
Larson, 1998[524]	102 96	G-CSF in induction (from day 4) Placebo	Shorter neutropenia of $<1 \times 10^9$/L ($P < .001$), and thrombocytopenia, fewer days in the hospital ($P = .02$), fewer induction deaths ($P = .04$)
Ifrah, 1999[525]	35 29	GM-CSF after induction (from day 7) Placebo	Reduced severe mucositis ($P = .03$) and fewer days with fever ($P = .07$)

G-CSF, granulocyte colony-stimulating factor; GM-CSF, granulocyte-macrophage colony-stimulating factor.

leukemias. In HCL, the use of filgrastim after cladribine did not lower the incidence of infectious complications, but the duration of severe neutropenia was reduced from 22 days in historical controls to 9 days in study patients.[529] In patients with CLL who are receiving fludarabine, G-CSF ameliorated the duration of neutropenia and reduced the incidence of pneumonia.[61] Larger studies are needed in patients at high-risk for neutropenic complications who are being treated with purine nucleoside analogues.

CSFs in AML and Related Disorders

Recombinant human CSFs can directly stimulate the proliferation of AML cells. When G-CSF or GM-CSF is given to patients with untreated AML, blood blasts, bone marrow blasts, and the percentage of blast cells in S phase are variably increased in virtually all cases.[530-533] Terminal differentiation of immature myelomonocytic cells is induced and may occasionally prevail on the proliferative stimulus and thereby lead to a transient remission status.[534] Indeed, in all the studies cited, the neutrophil count was modestly increased. Therefore, G- and GM-CSF have been used to recruit blast cells into S phase to enhance their sensitivity to chemotherapeutic agent,[535, 536] but many investigators have long been reluctant to give these agents to accelerate hematopoietic recovery. Results from the initial studies, which documented no harm from CSF administration to patients with AML, as well as some clinical advantage, are available in excellent review articles.[487, 537-541] Many randomized clinical trials were closed and published in the mid to late 1990s, so it is now possible to attempt to draw even better conclusions. The studies carried out in AML and closely related entities such as secondary AML, myelodysplasia-associated AML, and high-risk primary myelodysplasia are summarized in Table 14–25. The results are grouped according to the type and subtype of CSF used, along with the inclusion of pertinent patient characteristics and primary treatment end points. G-CSF and GM-CSF can shorten the period of neutropenia and/or monocytopenia after chemotherapy for AML and can exert an additive functional stimulus that is not detectable in these studies because of a different design. Whether this activity is sufficient to significantly lower the incidence and the length of severe myelosuppression and related complications from current anti-AML therapy is a central matter of

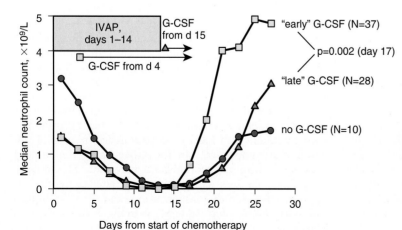

FIGURE 14–13. Effects on neutrophil recovery of early (from day 4) or late (from day 15) granulocyte colony-stimulating factor (G-CSF) administration during induction chemotherapy (IVAP: idarubicin, vincristine, L-asparaginase, prednisone) for adult acute lymphocytic leukemia. Patients treated early with G-CSF suffered from fewer documented infectious episodes and required less intravenous antimicrobials and antifungals ($p < .05$). (Adapted from[527].)

TABLE 14–25. Randomized Clinical Studies with CSFs in AML and Allied Disorders

Study (1st Author, Year)	Patient Age (yr) and Diagnosis*	No.	Study Arms†	Main Results in CSF Group(s)
With nonglycosylated G-CSF (filgrastim)				
Ohno, 1990[542]	13–69, AML, BC, MDS-/Re-/s-AML‡	48 / 50	−/+ (course I) / Control group	Shorter time to neutrophils >0.5 × 10⁹/L (median, 20 vs. 28 days; $P = .0002$), fewer infections ($P = .028$)
Heil, 1997[543]	≥16, AML	259 / 262	−/+ (courses I–III) / Placebo	Shorter time to neutrophils >0.5 × 10⁹/L (median, 20 vs. 25 days; $P = .0001$) reduced duration of fever ($P = .009$), and use of antibiotics ($P = .0001$) and antifungals ($P = .04$), shorter hospital stay ($P = .0001$)
Bernasconi, 1998[544]	< 70, HR-MDS, MDS-AML	53 / 52	−/+ (courses I–III) / Control group	Shorter neutropenia of <1 × 10⁹/L ($P < 0.05$), higher response rate ($P < .05$)
Godwin, 1998[545]	≥56, AML, s-/MDS-AML	106 / 105	−/+§ (course I) / Placebo	Shorter time to neutrophils >1 × 10⁹/L (median, 24 vs. 27 days; $P = .014$), trend to fewer days with fever and days receiving antibiotics
Ossenkoppele, 1999[546]	16–76, HR-MDS	33 / 31	+/+ (courses I–III) / Control group	Shorter time to neutrophils >1 × 10⁹/L (median, 23 vs. 35 days; $P = .015$), trend to higher response rate, shorter intercycle interval
Estey, 1999[547]	>71, HR-MDS	107 / 108	+/+ (courses I–V) / Control group	Trend to higher remission rate ($P = .087$), shorter time to neutrophils >1 × 10⁹/L (median, 24 vs. 29 days; $P < .001$)|
Harousseau, 2000[548]	47.5, AML	100 / 94	Consolidation (× 2) / Control group	Shorter time to neutrophils >0.5 × 10⁹/L (median, 12 vs. 19 days; $P < .001$), reduced hospitalization ($P = .001$) and duration of antibiotic and antifungal therapy
With glycosylated G-CSF (lenograstim)				
Dombret, 1995[549]	64–83, AML	88 / 85	−/+ (course I) / Placebo	Shorter neutropenia of <1 × 10⁹/L (median, 21 vs. 27 days; $P < .001$), higher remission rate ($P = .002$)
With nonglycosylated GM-CSF (mogramostim)				
Heil, 1995[550]	17–73, AML	41 / 39	+/+ (courses II–IV) / Placebo	No significant effect detected
Stone, 1995[551]	≥60, AML	193 / 195	−/+ (course I) / Placebo	Shorter neutropenia of <0.5 × 10⁹/L (median, 15 vs. 17 days; $P = .02$)
Zittoun, 1996[552]	17–59, AML	24 / 27 / 25 / 26	+/+ (course I) / −/+ / +/− / Control group −/−	Decreased remission rate in +/+ and −/+ groups ($P = .008$), trend to shorter neutropenia
Löwenberg, 1997[553]	15–60, AML	69 / 67 / 69 / 69	+/+ (courses I–III) / −/+ / +/− / Control group −/−	Shorter neutropenia of <1 × 10⁹/L (median, 26 vs. 30 days; $P < .001$) and monocytopenia ($P < .005$)
Löwenberg, 1997[554]	>60, AML	157 / 161	+/+ (courses I–II) / Control group −/−	Shorter neutropenia of <0.5 × 10⁹/L (median, 23 vs. 25 days; $P = .0002$)
Witz, 1998[555]	55–75, AML	110 / 122	+/+ (course I) / Placebo	Shorter time to neutrophils >0.5 × 10⁹/L (median, 24 vs. 29 days; $P < .001$), reduced use of antibiotics ($P = .018$), improved disease-free survival ($P = .003$)
With glycosylated GM-CSF (sargramostim)				
Rowe, 1995[556]	55–70, AML	60 / 57	−/+¶ (course I) / Placebo	Trend to higher remission rate ($P = .08$), reduced infections ($P = .015$) and treatment toxicity ($P = .049$), shorter time to neutrophils >0.5 × 10⁹/L (median, 13 vs. 17 days; $P = .001$)
With M-CSF (mirimostim)				
Ohno, 1997[557]	≥15, AML	97 / 101	−/+ (consolidation × 3) / Placebo	Reduced incidence and duration of febrile neutropenia ($P = .02$ and .002, respectively), shorter time to complete therapy ($P = .005$) faster neutrophil/platelet recovery ($P < .05$), reduced use of systemic antimicrobials ($P < .05$)

* AML, primary acute myelogenous leukemia; s-AML secondary AML; MDS-, myelodysplasia-associated AML; HR-MDS, high-risk MDS; Re-, recurrent/refractory AML; BC, blast crisis of chronic myelogenous leukemia.
† Start of CSF administration in relation to indicated chemotherapy course(s): +/+, during and after; +/−, only during; −/+, only after; −/−, never.
‡ Includes 27 patients with ALL (27.5%).
§ From day 10 if bone is hypocellular with less than 5% blasts.
| Data pooled from four-arm trial of chemotherapy with or without G-CSF and all-*trans*-retinoic acid.
¶ From day 11 if bone marrow on day 10 is aplastic without leukemia.

investigation. Remission rates, overall survival, and disease-free survival are obvious primary treatment end points, but they may not be adequate to assess the contribution of CSFs because any improvement in these parameters attributable to CSFs may be marginal or, instead, affect only selected risk groups. Assuming that about 10% of patients do not enter remission because of lethal infectious complications, both remission and survival rates would not improve significantly in most studies as a result of insufficient statistical power of the sample size. Moreover, although severe and prolonged neutropenia is common in AML, it is not the only factor pathogenic for infections. In some studies, CSFs were given as both a chemotherapy primer and a hematopoietic growth factor, and this use is taken into account in Table 14-25. Altogether, whatever the CSF type and the modality of administration, neither overall survival nor disease-free survival rates were substantially improved. However, though sporadically reported,[552] stimulation of AML cell growth has not been a clinical problem, whereas the improved neutrophil recovery times, most often a median of 3 to 7 days earlier than in control/placebo arms, led to a reduced incidence and duration of febrile neutropenia and better compliance with treatment, especially in the larger trials and in patients at a relatively younger age and with de novo AML.[543, 545, 547, 555] The results obtained with G-CSF tended to be better than with GM-CSF (most of the latter studies used molgramostim). In the single trial with sargramostim,[556] however, the results were improved in the study arm, where GM-CSF–treated patients did better and had a significantly reduced incidence of serious fungal infections.[488, 498] These data suggest that sargramostim may be preferable to E. coli–derived, nonglycosylated GM-CSF and are in agreement with previous preclinical and clinical observations on the role of GM-CSF against fungal pathogens. A randomized investigation of sargramostim is therefore being conducted by the International Oncology Study Group to further test this hypothesis. All things considered, the administration of CSFs to patients with AML, after chemotherapy, can lead to faster recovery from the neutropenic nadir without any detrimental effect on the likelihood of response to chemotherapy. The use of CSFs does not normally confer a definite survival advantage, is highly expensive, and does not (or not always) reduce the total cost of supportive care. Administration of a CSF during chemotherapy does not appear to be advantageous in terms of protection from myelosuppressive effects and may be more toxic as observed in some of the cited studies and others,[558] especially with molgramostim. This modality can therefore be abandoned unless cellular priming for chemotherapy is a concurrent objective in an investigational study. All the documented benefits concerned so-called secondary end points, such as the incidence and length of febrile neutropenia, the systemic use of antimicrobials, and possibly, the length of hospitalization. In some but not all studies,[542, 546, 559] tolerance to intensive postremission consolidation was improved, again without obtaining a parallel increase in disease-free survival. The groups likely to benefit most from CSFs remain poorly defined despite several hundred patients who have been treated to date. Likewise, because of the adoption of conventional-dose treatment in nearly all the studies reviewed, current limited knowledge[514] on the role of CSFs after high-dose cytarabine-based regimens must be expanded in view of the high efficacy as well as the high myelotoxic power of this form of treatment (see Table 14-9). In summary, if the largest G-CSF study[543] is representative of an unselected adult AML patient population and the single sargramostim study[556] truly depicts the value of glycosylated GM-CSF (pending confirmation from a larger collaborative trial), both agents could have a definite place in reducing the rate of neutropenic complications in AML.

CSFs and Myeloablative Therapy with HSC Support

CSFs were demonstrated to be effective in reducing the duration of absolute neutropenia after myeloablative procedures supported by either allogeneic or autologous HSC transplantation in a variety of lymphoid and myeloid malignancies. Their use was associated with improved patient outcome and reduced morbidity after transplantation,[493, 498, 506-508, 511, 560-564] improved regeneration of immunocompetent cell subsets,[560, 563] and sometimes longer survival.[560] Short-course administration of CSFs (G- or GM-CSF) after transplantation appears to be safe and can contribute to reduce the rate of infectious complications. CSFs can be recommended at least for patients with or at high-risk of long-lasting neutropenia (bone marrow source of HSCs, low progenitor cell content in the graft) and immunosuppression-related complications (allografts, T-cell depletion).[502]

Conclusions about CSFs

Evidence is now accumulating that some clinical benefit can be obtained with CSFs in high-risk categories. This benefit appears to outweigh the risk of potential stimulation of residual leukemic cells, which is rarely observed in AML and allied diseases and never in lymphoid malignancies. Physicians should have no reluctance to administer CSFs to critically ill and severely neutropenic patients and those likely to face life-threatening infections, provided that substantial prolongation of survival is foreseeable on resolution of the episode. The definition of high-risk patients can be rather broad in view of the strongly myelosuppressive effects exerted by modern treatment strategies and should encompass all patients who will undergo sufficiently intensive therapy to induce a prolonged (>7 days) severe neutropenia (<0.5 × 10^9/L), which in turn is associated with a high risk of febrile complications. This definition includes patients undergoing high-dose or myeloablative treatments and those with a severe or complicated infection of either bacterial or fungal etiology that is not responding satisfactorily to standard therapies, regardless of the neutrophil count. Of interest is that CSFs, especially GM-CSF, were found to accelerate the resolution of invasive fungal infections and that they could act synergically with prophylactic antibiotics.[565] Whether GM-CSF should be preferred over G-CSF, or vice versa, and in which situations remains investigational. A similar issue may concern the different types of G- and GM-CSF and the correct positioning of CSFs within specific chemotherapy programs. In view of the high cost of the treatment, CSFs should not be prescribed for patients receiving only palliative care for their disease and those who experience short neutropenic periods and have a low risk of infections.

Role of Peripheral Blood Stem-Cell Transplants

Supporting myeloablative treatment with CSF-primed PBSCs (defined as such by positive CD34 surface antigen expression and by the ability to form blood cell cultures in vitro and in vivo and to rescue lethally irradiated/treated individuals) is a rapidly expanding technique that is nearly becoming a technique of first choice for leukemia patients eligible for these procedures.[566-569] The key feature with PBSC transplantation is that neutrophil recovery is significantly faster than with marrow transplants and early morbidity and mortality from infections is therefore diminished. In early clinical studies after experiments in animal models,[570] autotransplants with PBSCs obtained from patients in remission demonstrated that permanent restoration of hematopoiesis was possible.[566, 571] Other reported advantages correlating with improved postgraft outcome and survival were a general cost savings, faster recovery of immune lymphocyte function, less blood product support, reduced mucositis, and reduced discomfort to patients not having their bone marrow harvested under general anesthesia.[569, 572-578]

Characteristics and Harvesting of PBSCs

Normally, low levels of PBSCs can be detected in the blood of healthy subjects and leukemia patients in remission. These cells can be identified immunologically in as much as they consistently express a varying amount of the very early CD34 surface antigen and several other antigens to a variable extent (Thy-1, HLA-DR, CD7, CD33, CD38) and can also be identified by in vitro culture.[579-581] About 1% to 3% of bone marrow cells are CD34$^+$, and among them, 10% express high levels of CD34 antigen together with a characteristic phenotypic profile, including negative expression of lineage-specific antigens (CD34^{bright}lin$^-$Thy-1$^+$CD38$^-$CD45RO$^+$ ^{123}Rh^{dull}). These cells are thought to be very early precursor cells and represent a very small fraction of circulating CD34$^+$ cells. The ability of circulating CD34$^+$ cells to give rapid rise to erythroid, myeloid, and megakaryocytic colonies[582] has been confirmed, and differences from true multipotent bone marrow stem cells have been identified.[583] In patients treated with chemotherapy, PBSCs are significantly increased at the time of marrow recovery and resolution of leukopenia when compared with baseline values. A further several-fold increase can be obtained by the administration of CSFs, usually G-CSF or GM-CSF. Thus, chemotherapy plus CSFs was shown to mobilize enough PBSCs to support prompt hematopoietic regeneration after a myeloablative program.[567, 568, 584-586] A variety of regimens involving chemotherapy plus CSF have been successfully developed as a means to promote large-scale collection of peripheral CD34$^+$ cells. From the data available, it appears that after chemotherapy in patients or in healthy volunteer donors, GM-CSF can mobilize an equal

or greater number of blood stem cells than G-CSF can, that glycosylated G-CSF (lenograstim) is better than nonglycosylated G-CSF (filgrastim), and that the association of G-CSF plus GM-CSF can be highly effective.[493, 569, 585, 587, 588] Furthermore, CD34$^+$ cell–containing preparations can undergo selective decontamination of putative leukemia/lymphoma cells by several techniques without compromising the quality of the graft and the subsequent recovery of hematopoiesis,[589, 590] or it can be manipulated ex vivo for quantitative expansion.[591] Because PBSCs can be precisely enumerated in a cytofluorometric assay by CD34 antigen expression, attempts have been made to define the minimal threshold of cells associated with a clinical benefit in patients (rapid engraftemt with trilineage hematopoiesis) and the optimal timing for their collection. The administration of at least 1×10^6 CD34$^+$ cells per kilogram is considered the minimal threshold, with an optimum between 3.5 and 5×10^6/kg.[592-594] In a study consisting of 48 patients infused with 1.17 to 2.40 $\times 10^6$ CD34$^+$ cells per kilogram, all patients achieved an absolute neutrophil count of greater than 0.5×10^9/L at a median of day 11, but platelet recovery was delayed in 30%.[595] Patients with AML or myelodysplastic syndromes may sometimes require higher PBSC counts.[596] These numbers of CD34$^+$ cells can be harvested with a single leukapheresis procedure in most cases with an absolute CD34$^+$ cell count of 20×10^6/L or more on the preceding day (approximately on days 10 to 12 of CSF administration).[597] The probability of microbial contamination of PBSC collections is very low and ranged from 0.23% to 2.2% in two reports.[598, 599] This rate was not greater than with bone marrow (3.8% reported) and was not associated with serious clinical infections.

Clinical Use of PBSCs

Despite the fact that (autologous) PBSCs, with or without additional G- or GM-CSF, have been successfully used to support consecutive, high-dose nonmyeloablative chemotherapy cycles in patients with both solid cancers and lymphoma,[600-605] most, if not all studies in patients with leukemia focused instead on autologous or allogeneic CD34$^+$ cell rescue after permanently myeloablative treatment. The use of PBSC transplants was clearly safe in these patients, with few associated significant toxic side effects and faster recovery from the pancytopenic phase. In an early report comparing the clinical outcome after autografting or allografting with marrow or peripheral blood in different hematologic tumors,[574] the median time to reach a neutrophil count greater than 0.5×10^9/L was 11 days after a PBSC autograft, 22 days after a bone marrow autograft, and 24.5 days after a bone marrow allograft. These differences were highly significant and were associated with an increasing incidence of infectious complications. Similar data were confirmed in larger surveys[606] and in patients at very high risk for severe infections.[607] One problem associated with PBSC transplants (and sometimes with CSF-supported bone marrow transplants) that should be differentiated from an infectious complication is the so-called engraftment syndrome. The clinical picture is reminiscent of the syndrome of T-lymphocyte recovery after GM-CSF,[558] and similar to an acute GVHD reaction, it is probably mediated by the release of cytokines by expanding T-cell subsets and monocytes. The symptoms can initiate abruptly at the first signs of hematologic engraftment, specifically when the leukocyte count starts rising, and consist of high fever, rash, pulmonary infiltrates, and diarrhea from capillary leak. It can be observed in about 5% of cases, particularly in those who are infused with very high CD34[+] cell numbers or receive additional CSFs.[608, 609] Clinical examination and culture assays clearly exclude infections. The illness can respond to corticosteroid treatment. Fatalities are rare and involve acute respiratory distress and alveolar hemorrhage. With regard to patients with leukemia, most published or continuing studies concern PBSC autografts in chronic myelogenous leukemia (mainly to promote a partially Philadelphia chromosome–negative hematopoiesis) and autografts/allografts in AML. It is especially in the latter condition, as well as in preliminary studies in ALL, that a strongly positive impact on the duration of severe neutropenia and the incidence of febrile neutropenia is expected and is therefore presented in detail.

PBSC TRANSPLANTATION IN PATIENTS WITH LEUKEMIA

Because an HSC autograft or allograft is often a planned step in the treatment of many patients with acute leukemia, reduction of treatment-associated morbidity is essential to improve disease-free survival, particularly in the allogeneic setting, where the cumulative burden of toxicity and attendant infections is still very high. In AML, autografting with PBSCs has not been associated with an increased risk of relapse,[610] and it accelerates hematopoietic recovery with a reduction in life-threatening infectious complications.[611] In the most representative studies, the period of absolute neutropenia of less than $0.5 \times 10^9/L$ ranged from 10 to 15 days as compared with 25 days and longer with bone marrow (see Table 14-26). The rapid granulocyte recovery and the low incidence of severe infectious complications have been confirmed by many others,[586, 616-619] and PBSC autografting has recently been tested in patients in very unfavorable risk catego-

ries.[620] Initially, PBSCs were sometimes used in conjunction with marrow-derived cells.[613] This approach is no longer required since the demonstration of sustained long-term hematopoiesis after PBSC reinfusion. Therefore, CD34[+] stem cells can be procured with one or more apheresis sessions in 80% to 90% of patients with AML in remission after several different chemotherapy plus CSF-priming protocols.[621, 622] Rapid and complete hematopoietic engraftment is expected to occur in nearly all cases and allow early hospital discharge and minimize transfusional needs and the incidence of severe, life-threatening infections. In rare instances, PBSC autografting fails and additional backup marrow is needed. It should be noted, however, that although lethal events and fungal infections were only occasionally reported, the incidence of acute bacterial infections, including difficult organisms such as *C. difficile* and *S. viridans,* was not reduced in comparison to marrow transplantation.[606, 623-625] This similarity in the frequency of acute infections emphasizes the pathogenetic role of other cofactors (toxicity of the conditioning regimen, mucositis, the use of corticosteroids and antibiotics). Therefore, the issue of antibacterial and antifungal prophylaxis remains important. The use of PBSC transplantation in patients with ALL might result in similarly improved neutrophil and recovery rates.[626] As in the autologous setting, early data from both phase III studies and retrospective evaluations of PBSC versus bone marrow allografting demonstrate improvements in engraftment time, complication rate, and duration of hospital stay (Table 14-27).

TREATMENT

Therapeutic Strategy

Untreated infections in neutropenic patients with leukemia are almost always fatal as a result of the lack of an adequate immune response against the invading microorganism. A mortality rate of 90% was reported for patients with gram-negative sepsis and an underlying malignant illness with neutropenia. Though clinically less severe at initial evaluation, untreated infections by gram-positive

TABLE 14–26. Neutrophil Recovery Data and Rate of Lethal Infectious Complications after PBSC versus BM (Historical Control) Autografting in AML

Study (1st Author, Year)	Patient Age and Diagnosis*	No. and Type of Transplant	Median Days to Granulocytes $>0.5 \times 10^9/L$	Deaths from Infection	Other Significant Findings†
Korbling, 1991[612]	41, CR1	20 PBSC	10 ($P = .0001$)	0	Quicker platelet recovery ($P = .05$), earlier discharge ($P = .0005$)
	23	23 BM	28	1	
Demirer, 1995[613]	49, CR1/Re/>CR	14 PBSC + BM	13 ($P < .0001$)	0	Quicker platelet recovery ($P < .0001$), fewer transfusions ($P < .0001$)
	34	158 BM	29	NR	
Vellenga, 1999[614]	44.5, CR1	28 PBSC	17 ($P < .0001$)	NR	Quicker platelet recovery ($P < .0001$)
	NR	41 BM	37	NR	
Visani, 1999[615]	44, CR1	23 PBSC	17 ($P = .01$)	NR	Quicker platelet recovery ($P = .001$), fewer transfusions ($P = .01$), earlier discharge ($P = .001$)
	47	21 BM	36	NR	

 * Median in years; disease phase in PBSC/BM autografted patients and historical controls: CR (first complete remission), Re (at relapse/refractory), >CR (second or later remission).
 † In favor of PBSC autografting.
 AML, acute myelogenous leukemia; BM, bone marrow; NR, not reported; PBSC, peripheral blood stem cell.

TABLE 14–27. Neutrophil Recovery Data and Rate of Lethal Infectious Complications after PBSC versus BM Allograftings in AML

Study (1st Author, Year)	Patient Age* and Diagnosis	No. and Type of Transplant	Median Days to Granulocytes >0.5 × 10⁹/L	Deaths from Infection	Other Significant Findings†
Bensinger, 1996[627]	38, advanced L/Ly	37 PBSC 37 BM	14 ($P = 0.006$) 16	2 9	Quicker platelet recovery ($P = .001$), fewer transfusions ($P = .0005$)
Russell, 1996[628]	40, L/Ly	26 PB 26 BMT	16 ($P = .0002$) 21.5	NR NR	Quicker platelet recovery ($P = .0003$), fewer transfusions ($P = .015$), earlier discharge ($P = .02$)
Blaise, 2000[629]	37, AML/ALL/CML	48 PB 53 BM	15 ($P < 10^{-5}$) 21	3 1	Quicker platelet recovery ($P < 10^{-4}$), earlier discharge ($P < .03$) reduced cost ($P = .004$)
Powles, 2000[630a]	36, AML/ALL/CLL CML/NHL/MM	20 PB 19 BM	17.5 ($P = .002$) 23	NR NR	Quicker platelet recovery ($P < .0001$), earlier discharge ($P = .01$), quicker lymphocyte recovery ($P = .05$)

* Median in years.
† In favor of PBSC allografting.
ALL, acute lymphocytic leukemia; AML, acute myelogenous leukemia; BM, bone marrow; CLL, chronic lymphocytic leukemia; CML, chronic myelogenous leukemia; L/Ly, different types of leukemias and lymphomas; MM, multiple myeloma; NHL, non-Hodgkin's lymphoma; NR, not reported; PBSC, peripheral blood stem cell.

rods and invasive fungal diseases are equally dangerous. Notably, because fever and other signs of infection can be absent or minimal and prophylactic antibiotics are often used, all diagnostic investigations, including culture studies, can be initially negative in such patients or require days to give a positive result. The rate of positive microbiologic isolates is variable and depends on several local factors, not least of which is the ability of the microbiologic laboratory. However, it is highly illogical to wait for such results in view of the incomplete success rates from culture studies, the time necessary to obtain an answer, and the rapid course of an untreated infection. Accordingly, the first rule is that fever must always be investigated and managed as infectious in nature, even when apparently attributable to a drug reaction, transfusions, or disease. A second rule is that because of the diminished inflammatory response, the application of both diagnostic and empiric therapeutic steps is mandatory even without fever if any of the alterations that can be associated with a potentially serious infection develops (described previously) (see Table 14-15). The last rule is that treatment must be immediate. The initial diagnostic evaluation should be performed expeditiously and empiric treatment started without delay.

Underlying Principles and Flexibility of Empirical Therapy

The scope of empiric antibiotic therapy is to provide effective antimicrobial coverage to neutropenic patients who are at increased risk of life-threatening infections by certain microorganisms. The most dangerous species are gram-negative rods capable of rapidly inducing bacteremic shock. Infection by gram-positive bacteria is much more frequent, but it is usually characterized by a less aggressive course. Infections by other microorganisms tend to occur later during the illness, but early atypical infections can occur, as in the case, for instance, of candidemia. Nevertheless, determination of a specific etiology for every single early or late infectious episode is

often difficult, and treatment may remain empiric long-term. In essence, early anti-infective therapy is lifesaving in intent and directed primarily against a group of highly toxic gram-negative rods with extension, in selected clinical situations, to other, gram-positive rods and *Candida* species. Later, the pattern of infections is more heterogeneous and necessitates a more critical and diagnosis-oriented therapeutic approach. In addition, the intensity of first-line treatment can be modulated according to the patient's risk class (for treatment failure), which for low-risk categories means cost saving and reduced drug-induced selection of resistant strains. For all these reasons, flexible treatment programs that take into account the likelihood of a given etiology over time in selected risk classes were developed and are currently recommended.

Intensified Care for Patients in Critical Condition

General diagnostic criteria for classifying low- and high-risk patients and for monitoring their clinical status at the onset of neutropenic fever were given before (see Figs. 14-1 to 14-4, Tables 14-4 to 14-6). General supportive measures are instituted to prevent or manage septic shock and may thus include, on a patient-to-patient basis, the use of assisted ventilation to maintain arterial blood oxygen saturation over 95%, fluid replacement without overloading (monitoring lung perfusion, central venous pressure, urinary output), adrenergic stimulation with dopamine or another inotropic agent, correction of acidosis, and nutritional support.[306] The role of systemic adrenocorticosteroids in neutropenic cancer patients is uncertain when supportive care is correctly initiated.[66] It is expected that the clinical benefits, if any, might be manifested only during the first few hours and that patients with gram-negative sepsis will respond better. An exception might concern those with evidence of infectious meningitis; in this case, dexamethasone can reduce local signs of inflammation and intracranial pressure, thereby improving the clinical course.[630] When general intensive measures fail and acute respiratory failure develops, the patient can be transferred to an intensive care unit. Some patients are rescued, but mortality at this stage remains high because of persistent neutropenia and multiorgan failure.[631, 632]

Toward a Simplified Treatment for Low-Risk Patients

All that was said about patient risk classes is applicable to the therapeutic strategy. A low-risk patient is one with an absolute neutropenia of less than 0.5×10^9/L lasting less than 8 to 10 days, with leukemia in remission. For the same reasons as those leading to short neutropenia, the risk of a neutrophil count less than 0.1×10^9/L, high-grade mucositis, and other severe regimen-related toxicity developing is similarly low (see Figs. 14–1 to 14–3). These patients, as well as non-neutropenic ones, have a low chance of development of life-threatening infections, "complex" bacteremias, and early fungal infections (see Figs. 14–3 and 14–4). According to the results of some clinical trials,[633–639] low-risk patients are eligible, at the onset of febrile complications and after thorough clinical and microbiologic evaluation, to receive gentle, outpatient management consisting of monotherapy and/or oral drugs in different combinations as appropriate[13–15] (Fig. 14–14) and without the additional use of CSFs. Clearly, if any prophylaxis was given previously, treatment is not simple because of the risk of drug-resistant bacteria being responsible for the febrile episode. For the remainder, therapy can be commenced on an inpatient basis and continue after discharge (step-down). Patients selected for home treatment must live within miles from hospital (<2 hours' travel) and not alone and must be able to understand properly, feed themselves, and report

on the phone about their status and the progression of therapy. If the clinical picture ameliorates, treatment continues until about day 7. By this time, with the normalization of neutrophil counts, the patient is assumed to be cured. If the patient deteriorates or does not respond after a trial lasting 48 to 72 hours, in-hospital evaluation is mandatory, at which point treatment is generally shifted to an intravenous broad-spectrum antibiotic. The studies cited confirmed the validity of this approach: readmission rates were 7% to 30%; death rates, 0% to 7%; and success rates, 59% to 89%, with no gross differences between the study and control arms (intravenous antibiotics, inpatient therapy). This strategy, when carefully applied, contributes to reduce cost and improves quality of life. High-risk patients or low-risk patients treated with quinolone prophylaxis are best suited for traditional therapy based on continuing hospitalization and broad-spectrum intravenous antibiotics.

Empiric Antibiotic Treatment

The Option of Monotherapy

The ideal antibiotic, when used empirically, should possess a broad spectrum of bactericidal activity in the blood and tissues regardless of the neutrophil count. Moreover, induction of resistant strains should be minimal, the toxicity acceptable, and the cost low. No antibiotic satisfies all these requirements, but some highly effective drugs and combinations have been selected over the years by numerous clinical studies. Sensible recommendations for the initial management of high-risk patients were presented by panels of experts[12–15, 31] (Fig. 14–15). The Infectious Diseases Society of America (IDSA) published updated therapeutic recommendations in 1997.[13] More

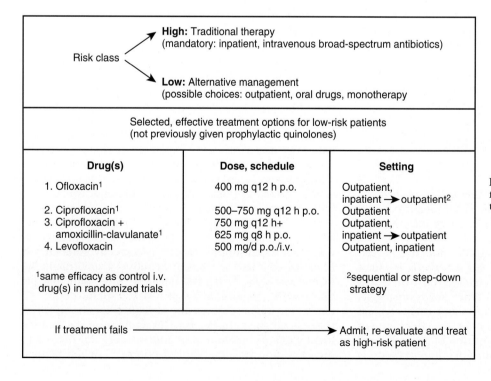

Drug(s)	Dose, schedule	Setting
1. Ofloxacin[1]	400 mg q12 h p.o.	Outpatient, inpatient → outpatient[2]
2. Ciprofloxacin[1]	500–750 mg q12 h p.o.	Outpatient
3. Ciprofloxacin + amoxicillin-clavulanate[1]	750 mg q12 h+ 625 mg q8 h p.o.	Outpatient, inpatient → outpatient
4. Levofloxacin	500 mg/d p.o./i.v.	Outpatient, inpatient

[1]same efficacy as control i.v. drug(s) in randomized trials

[2]sequential or step-down strategy

If treatment fails ⟶ Admit, re-evaluate and treat as high-risk patient

FIGURE 14–14. Possible oral and/or simplified antibiotic regimens for low-risk patients with febrile neutropenia.

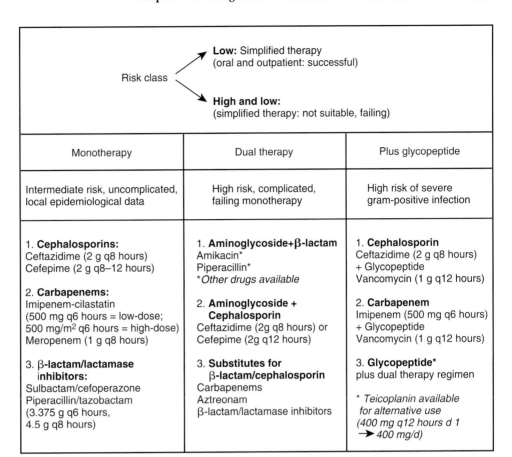

FIGURE 14–15. Intravenous drugs and combinations for first-line therapy for neutropenic fever in patients not eligible for simplified/oral treatment (see Fig. 14–4).

information can be obtained from the IDSA website at *http://www.idsociety.org*. Early empiric treatment is primarily directed at controlling gram-negative infections, although some of the drugs used exert a desirable, though moderate anti–gram-positive effect. β-Lactams, including penicillins and third-/fourth-generation cephalosporins, have significant activity against the most dangerous member of the gram-negative family, *P. aeruginosa*. An emerging concept is that some of the new antibiotics can be used initially as monotherapy with exactly the same degree of efficacy as dual- or multiple-therapy programs. These agents must be active against the vast majority of gram-negative rods and partially against *S. viridans*, but resistance of coagulase-negative staphylococci, enterococci, and other gram-positive agents is still a problem (up to 25% of isolates). The drugs selected for initial monotherapy are mainly fourth-generation cephalosporins (cefepime, cefpirome),[31, 640] carbapenems (imipenem, meropenem),[641-644] or β-lactamase inhibitor conjugates (sulbactam/cefoperazone, piperacillin/tazobactam).[645, 646] Monotherapy but not oral therapy[633, 634] is indicated for the early management of low- to intermediate-risk, uncomplicated patients with neutropenic fever who are unable to take oral medications because of mucositis, even when discharged home.[640, 647] In monotherapy studies, early success rates ranged from 48% to 88%, with final success rates close to 90%, and the incidence of treatment modifications (caused by nonresponse, superinfection) ranged from 16% to 48%. The final choice must be guided by local analysis of the type, frequency, and

antibiotic susceptibility pattern of bacterial isolates.[13] In general, in view of these issues, ceftazidime appears to be losing its potential for use as monotherapy,[167] whereas imipenem and other carbapenems, the most active single antibiotics to date, should be used with great care as primary therapy because of possible induction of resistance and loss of therapeutic activity in subsequent episodes. A clinical trial comparing the response rates of single-agent imipenem or ceftazidime versus either agent plus amikacin validated the assumption that ceftazidime alone may be inadequate.[648]

Dual Therapy

The synergistic effect provided by the addition of an aminoglycoside (gentamicin, tobramycin, amikacin) compound to a third- or fourth-generation cephalosporin or extended-spectrum penicillin forms the basis of several two-drug empiric broad-spectrum combinations.[5, 19, 166, 343, 644, 649-655] Dual treatment is still considered the standard regimen for high-risk patients by many clinical investigators and is recommended as an alternative schedule for low-risk patients for whom primary monotherapy fails. To simplify treatment, interestingly, one report documented an equivalence between single and multiple daily administrations of cephalosporin and an aminoglycoside.[654] Others found continuous infusion preferable.[656] With regard to cephalosporins (ceftazidime, ceftriaxone, cefoperazone), ceftriaxone should not be used against *P. aeruginosa* because it is barely active.[13] The fluorinated quinolones can be considered an alternative to cephalosporins in patients not previously given these drugs as prophylaxis. Equally effective is a double β-lactam combination, that is, a third-generation cephalosporin plus an extended-spectrum penicillin.[5] This approach should be discouraged in centers in which infections by species producing inducible β-lactamase (*Serratia, Enterobacter, Citrobacter*) occur; it does not protect against anaerobes and most gram-positive bacteria and therefore is less frequently adopted. The new β-lactam/β-lactamase inhibitor conjugate antibiotics provide a means of overcoming resistance in organisms producing inducible β-lactamase (sulfabactam/cefoperazone, ticarcillin/clavulanic acid, piperacillin/tazobactam) and are being considered as both monotherapy and components of dual therapy. β-Lactamase–resistant and/or highly active antipseudomonal drugs include carbapenems and similar agents (imipenem-cilastatin, aztreonam, meropenem). Imipenem-cilastatin is a member of the carbapenem family and probably the most powerful antibiotic known in that it provides full coverage of gram-negative bacteria, anaerobes, most *Streptococcus* species, and coagulase-positive methicillin-sensitive staphylococci.[641, 648] Imipenem is highly active in polymicrobial sepsis and in complicated severe infections, where it should be used at high dosage (500 mg/m^2 every 6 hours).[644, 657] Aztreonam is a monobactam with potent, but restricted antipseudomonal activity that can be used instead of β-lactams in patients allergic to this latter class, but always in conjunction with another anti–gram-negative agent. These new drugs are sometimes used empirically, but again, one has to balance the weight of their activity against the risk of loss of efficacy from induction of resistance. The success rate with any empiric combination (or monochemotherapy) should approach 70% or more against gram-negative bacteria. Inferior results dictate a careful search for the emergence and spread of drug-resistant strains and mandate subsequent modification of the empiric schedule. Suggested dual regimens are presented in Figure 14–15.[13, 31]

Addition of a Glycopeptide and Vancomycin-Resistant Enterococci

A central issue surrounds gram-positive bacteria, the incidence of which is highest at the first febrile episode. Although dual regimens share some activity against these rods, none provides extended coverage. For this reason, some authors have advocated the early adjunctive use of the glycopeptide drug vancomycin. It is not yet entirely clear whether this addition represents an advantage or not in light of the low mortality rate (around 5%) associated with gram-positive bacteria and the risk of inducing subsequent resistance (see VRE and related arguments in previous sections) and because these infections, with rare exceptions, do not cause rapid clinical deterioration and respond well to specific antibiotic therapy once the pathogen is identified by culture. Although some studies have demonstrated a beneficial trend with the inclusion of vancomycin into a front-line empiric regimen,[156, 658] current recommendations do not favor early empiric use of this drug because of its toxicity.[5, 6, 166, 659–661] Exceptions are selected epidemiologic and clinical situations, such as high infection rates with methicillin-resistant *S. aureus* or *S. viridans,* rapid induction of septic shock, catheter-related pyogenic infections, sepsis after the use of prophylactic quinolones, or ulcerative mucositis from high-dose cytarabine. When vancomycin-related toxicity is of concern, as in bone marrow transplant patients receiving concomitant cyclosporine, which may increase the risk for renal damage, the non-nephrotoxic antibiotic teicoplanin can provide similar activity.[662, 663] Useful vancomycin regimens consist of monotherapy or a dual regimen that includes the drugs illustrated in Figure 14–15. Treatment of VRE infections and other vancomycin-resistant gram-positive rods is highly individualized and entails both a degree of empiricism and the results of chemosensitivity tests.[31, 189] In sensitive cases, teicoplanin is the drug of choice; otherwise, one must consider the use of high-dose ampicillin (20 g/day), an ampicillin/β-lactamase inhibitor conjugate, chloramphenicol plus an aminoglycoside, or other combinations as dictated from in vitro susceptibility studies. Sources must be identified and sterilized, along with disinfection of environmental surfaces, strict isolation of patients and contacts, and the use of materials reserved for such patients.

Modifications of Empiric Antibiotic Therapy

Several problems can arise after empiric therapy is started. Daily patient re-evaluation is required for modifications of the chosen protocol (Fig. 14–16). Apart from the occurrence of rapid clinical deterioration mandating immediate therapeutic changes, the key point for deciding whether the patient is responding to a given therapy is after day 3.[13] If on the day of examination the patient is afebrile, no etiology has been documented, and the neutropenia is likely to subside soon (low-risk patient), treatment could be simplified by changing to oral antibiotics and/or monotherapy and monitoring the patient closely at home until completion of a full 7-day course.[12, 13, 31] In patients initially treated with a glycopeptide who show clinical improvement and do not have gram-positive isolates, use of the drug can be discontinued after 5 total days. This strategy reduces toxicity and the likelihood of priming vancomycin resistance. In other patients, the fever may continue and/or cultures may become positive. In these cases, treatment must continue unmodified for a minimum of 7 days and obviously adjusted according to the microbiologic results only. Persistence of fever for up to 7 days is not considered sufficient evidence of treatment failure if the patient is otherwise well,[13, 14] and the use of vancomycin is not necessary, outside the situations explained earlier, if blood cultures are persistently negative. From the fifth to the seventh day onward, treatment choices for nonresponsive patients are dictated by the course of the neutrophil count, clinical reassessment, and epidemiologic considerations. Because of an increased incidence of second infections and superinfections by gram-positive agents and fungi, treatment changes must include, with few but notable exceptions as reported later, the addition of a glycopeptide or an antifungal drug[5–7, 19, 163, 166, 305, 343, 653, 664] On the other hand, if vancomycin was already part of the initial empiric treatment, lack of clinical progress after 5 to 7 days again suggests

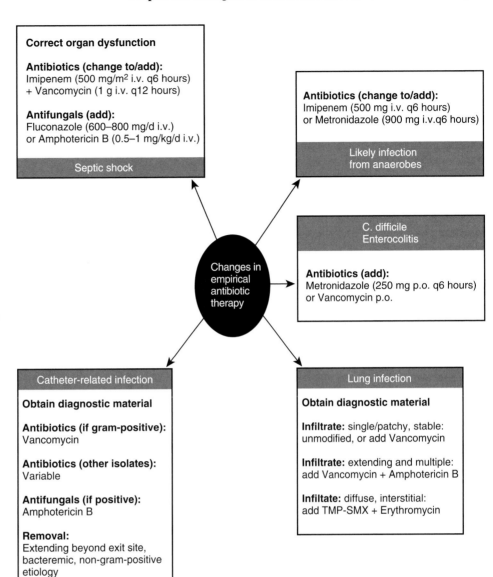

Correct organ dysfunction

Antibiotics (change to/add):
Imipenem (500 mg/m² i.v. q6 hours)
+ Vancomycin (1 g i.v. q12 hours)

Antifungals (add):
Fluconazole (600–800 mg/d i.v.)
or Amphotericin B (0.5–1 mg/kg/d i.v.)

Septic shock

Antibiotics (change to/add):
Imipenem (500 mg i.v. q6 hours)
or Metronidazole (900 mg i.v.q6 hours)

Likely infection
from anaerobes

C. difficile
Enterocolitis

Antibiotics (add):
Metronidazole (250 mg p.o. q6 hours)
or Vancomycin p.o.

Changes in empirical antibiotic therapy

Catheter-related infection

Obtain diagnostic material

Antibiotics (if gram-positive):
Vancomycin

Antibiotics (other isolates):
Variable

Antifungals (if positive):
Amphotericin B

Removal:
Extending beyond exit site,
bacteremic, non-gram-positive
etiology

Lung infection

Obtain diagnostic material

Infiltrate: single/patchy, stable:
unmodified, or add Vancomycin

Infiltrate: extending and multiple:
add Vancomycin + Amphotericin B

Infiltate: diffuse, interstitial:
add TMP-SMX + Erythromycin

FIGURE 14–16. Changes in empiric therapy according to selected clinical conditions.

that the drug should be discontinued because of the unlikelihood of a gram-positive etiology.[13] A last choice is withdrawal of all drugs, followed by continuing diagnostic re-evaluation. Any empiric modification chosen is susceptible to further refinement as soon as the results of laboratory and microbiologic studies are known.

Modifications in Selected Clinical Conditions

From a practical standpoint, when one must decide how to modify empiric treatment, the best indicators are the patient's general status, fever, and the presence of specific symptoms suggesting a given etiology (see Fig. 14-16). In patients who become hypotensive and whose clinical condition quickly worsens breakthrough bacteremia by aggressive or drug-resistant strains (*P. aeruginosa*, α-hemolytic and viridans streptococci, staphylococci) or even a disseminated candidemic infection should always be suspected and looked for. This situation calls for an immediate switch to an alternative antibiotic regimen and/or the addition of systemic fluconazole or AmB (when

fluconazole was used prophylactically). Imipenem, aztreonam, and β-lactam/lactamase inhibitor conjugates are the drugs of choice to substitute for ceftazidime, and vancomycin should always be empirically added if gram-positive rods could be the causative agents. Granulocyte transfusions can be lifesaving in the short term, although they are very rarely used. In the same line, some have advocated the use of G-CSF or GM-CSF to hasten neutrophil and macrophage cell recovery.[12] This proposal is rational and should be investigated in depth, although these agents could be better suited for prophylactic than therapeutic use (see the earlier sections on CSFs). To obtain the best therapeutic chance, however, it is essential to know in detail the past institutional experience and chemosensitivity patterns in similar cases. In patients in whom severe mucositis ulcers of the upper aerodigestive tract with necrotizing features (especially marginal gingivitis) and deeply localized cellulitis develop, one should suspect superinfection by anaerobes, with possible associated reactivation of HSV and fungal infection. After performing the appropriate diagnostic tests, careful review of symptoms, and local examination, treatment with antianaerobic agents, systemic antifungals, acyclovir, or combinations thereof should be instituted. Antianaerobic coverage should be strongly considered in patients with clinical symptoms suggestive of perianal or abdominal infection. Treatment of anaerobic infections is possible with imipenem, clindamycin, or intravenous metronidazole, 500 to 900 mg every 6 hours.[6, 31, 665] Documented *C. difficile* enterocolitis must be treated with vancomycin given orally. When oral drug intake is not possible, prolonged-course intravenous metronidazole can be an effective alternative. Surgery plus intensive postsurgical care can be considered in neutropenic patients with acute abdominal complications.[666] CT and ultrasound scans have been reported to be useful in revealing hemoperitoneum and localizing the site of complication. Other common infections are those related to intravenous catheters. Current recommendations are that exit site infections by gram-positive or gram-negative bacteria can be managed by protracted antibiotic therapy without removal of the catheter. Removal is indicated when infections are localized in the subcutaneous tunnel or are caused by *Bacillus, Candida, Aspergillus,* and *Mycobacterium* species. Catheter exchange by guidewire could be attempted before removal in patients with positive blood culture unresponsive to antibiotics.[667] Therapeutic decisions about lung lesions are more complex, at least in the absence of a positive isolate from diagnostic procedures. As a rule, documentation of infiltrative lesions after an initially negative radiographic evaluation and during the increase in granulocytes is still compatible with maintenance of the original empiric schedule because the lesions might represent only the delayed appearance of a previously undetectable infection. In this case, progressive clearing of lung opacities is expected as the neutrophil count increases. If such clearing occurs and the patient's clinical condition remains stable, the patient can be managed expectantly. Patients with increasing lung opacities and/or those expected to remain profoundly granulocytopenic and patients in whom a central venous line was inserted must always be given additional AmB and/or vancomycin. In the case of diffuse or interstitial pneumonitis in patients not at risk of CMV infection, it is customary to add TMP-SMX (for at least 2 weeks) and erythromycin (at least 3 weeks) or another macrolide to the broad-spectrum antibiotic regimen.

Unresolving Fever

In all other cases not thus far considered, if after day 3 from the start of empiric treatment the infection site is not detected, fever continues, the neutropenia is unresolved, and no microorganism has been grown from the cultured samples or detected by antigen studies, modification of the empiric regimen is also required. Some useful therapeutic algorithms that take into account the duration of the febrile episode (>5 to 7 days), the duration of severe neutropenia less than 0.5×10^9/L, and the increased likelihood of gram-positive infections and late fungal infections have been developed to deal with this common occurrence.[5, 6, 13, 31, 166] Basically, the addition or substitution of vancomycin is again the first step. A

change to antibiotics different from those used as frontline agents must be considered and based on the results of microbiologic analysis and the patient's course. The patient is then re-evaluated in depth between days 5 and 7, by which time AmB can be added if fever and other signs of infection have not subsided, regardless of the previous demonstration of a bacterial infection and whether a positive fungal isolate was obtained. In these circumstances, a high incidence of fungal infections is common, independent of a positive diagnostic isolate, and mortality is higher if antifungal therapy is not instituted.[6, 166, 168, 343, 653] When used empirically, AmB has been given at a dosage that varies between 0.5 and 1 mg/kg/day until resolution of the febrile episode or neutropenia or a specific nonfungal etiology has been convincingly demonstrated.[6, 166, 168] Oral ketoconazole was found to be inferior to AmB in one randomized study,[668] but fluconazole might be as effective.

Duration of Antibiotic Therapy

The duration of the afebrile period and neutropenia were the parameters used in predicting the probability of recurrent fever or infection developing and therefore determined the optimal time for stopping antibiotic therapy. Treatment can be safely stopped in responsive low-risk patients after 7 days. Preliminary data suggest discontinuation of all antibiotics even after 24 hours from the demonstration of defervescence in these cases.[31] Some believe this approach to be much too precipitous and hazardous and do not recommend it for routine use.[14] It appears that antibiotic therapy should never last less than 10 to 14 days in patients remaining severely neutropenic and should be continued for at least 5 to 7 days after defervescence.[6, 13, 31, 168, 344] Treatment should not be stopped, regardless of its duration, in very severely neutropenic (<0.1×10^9/L) patients with fever and those with unstable vital signs and extensive mucosal damage. One possibility for neutropenic and persistingly febrile patients with no documented infection is changing to a prophylactic regimen after 14 days of empiric treatment. In febrile patients with recovery of granulocytes to more than 0.5×10^9/L, discontinuation of empiric antibiotic therapy is permitted after 5 days to facilitate the diagnostic program. Great interpatient variation is to be expected in the latter categories, and the risk of recurrent infection and fever is high.

Empiric Antifungal Treatment

Indications for empiric antifungal treatment were previously given. AmB had long remained the only drug available in this setting until less toxic, better tolerated and more effective azoles became available. Current antifungal therapies are listed in Table 14–28. Intravenous or oral fluconazole, in particular, was tested in controlled trials of empiric antifungal therapy. The results were encouraging because response rates were essentially comparable in the fluconazole and AmB arms: 75% with fluconazole, 6 mg/kg/day, versus 66% with AmB[669] and 56% with fluconazole, 400 mg/day, versus 46% with AmB.[670]

TABLE 14–28. Treatment of Common Fungal Infections

Type of Infection	Drugs	Schedule
Candida spp.		
Oral thrush/mild esophagitis	Nystatin, clotrimazole, ketoconazole, fluconazole, amphotericin B	PO, 1–2 wk to healing
Extensive esophagitis	Fluconazole	PO 200–400 mg/day
Candidemia, endophthalmitis	Amphotericin B (previous fluconazole therapy)	IV 0.5 mg/kg/day to healing
Hepatosplenic, renal candidiasis	Fluconazole*	IV/PO 400–800 mg/day
	Amphotericin B (previous fluconazole therapy) +/− 5-fluorocytosine	IV ≥0.7–1 mg/kg/day minimum of 2 g IV 100–150 mg/kg/day
Aspergillus spp.		
Invasive aspergillosis	Amphotericin B	IV 1–1.25 mg/kg/day minimum of 2 g
	Itraconazole (second line)	PO 400–600 mg/day

For the role of surgery, amphotericin B lipid formulations, new drugs, and hematopoietic growth factors, see the text.
* Except for *Candida krusei*.

The favorable treatment outcome was accompanied by significantly less toxicity and improved compliance. Thus, fluconazole (or the more toxic AmB), given empirically to neutropenic and persistingly febrile cancer patients with no discernible fungal disease, appears to improve the clinical course in approximately half these patients and is therefore recommended. As shown earlier (see Fig. 14-16), the fluconazole dose is increased (600 to 800 mg/day) in patients with breakthrough septicemia who are at risk of candidemia.[31]

Candida *Infections*

Nonsevere oral thrush caused by *Candida* species in non-neutropenic patients can be effectively managed with the use of oral clotrimazole, nystatin, ketoconazole, fluconazole, and AmB preparations. If the patient is granulocytopenic and suffering from mucosal ulcers, which increase the risk for dissemination, the use of systemic drugs at low dosage (AmB, 0.3 to 0.5 mg/kg/day intravenously, fluconazole, 200 to 400 mg/day intravenously) is preferable.[6, 168] *Candida* esophagitis can be managed in the same way for a period of 1 to 2 weeks and until the neutrophil count has recovered and the ulcers have healed. Some patients with limited disease and an adequate neutrophil count can benefit from oral therapy with fluconazole.[6, 192] For the management of either suspected or proven severe candidal infection (candidemia, renal candidiasis, endophthalmitis, and hepatosplenic or other visceral infection), AmB and fluconazole are the drugs of choice. In patients with candidemia but without concomitant neutropenia, fluconazole, 400 mg/day, and AmB, 0.5 to 0.6 mg/kg/day were equally effective (70% to 80% success rate).[671] These results were later confirmed in similar patients, even if neutropenic, with superimposable success rates (66% and 64% in a retrospective study, 73% and 71% in a prospective study) reported for both fluconazole, 200 to 600 mg/day, and AmB, 0.3 to 1.2 mg/kg.[672, 673] The incidence of toxicity and the tolerance profile were again in favor of fluconazole, which should therefore be preferred as the first-line drug for invasive candidiasis, unless *C. krusei* infection is documented. In a recent international consensus conference,[674] fluconazole at a dose ranging from 400 to 800 mg/day, depending on

the patient's clinical status was recommended as initial treatment for patients with candidemia, along with removal of central venous lines, if not previously exposed to the drug as prophylaxis. In cases treated prophylactically, AmB should be used at a dose of 0.7 to 1.2 mg/kg/day or greater according to the patient's response until complete resolution of the neutropenia and to a total dose varying with type of infection[6, 343] (see Table 14-28). Because of the high mortality and morbidity rates, intravenous 5-fluorocytosine, 100 to 150 mg/kg/day, is sometimes combined with AmB in treating candidemia and hepatosplenic candidiasis in unstable deteriorating patients.[6, 88, 343, 674] Those with hepatosplenic candidiasis may require an abnormally high AmB cumulative dosage to achieve a cure, up to greater than 5 total g. Antileukemic chemotherapy can be administered simultaneously under strict control when delay is deemed unwise.[675]

Aspergillus *Infections*

Documented invasive *Aspergillus* infections in neutropenic patients are commonly treated with AmB at dosages slightly higher than for *Candida* infections, specifically, between 1 and 1.25 mg/kg/day, at least for the first 10 to 14 days.[6, 98, 343] A total dose of at least 2 g is usually required, and long-term secondary prophylaxis is often indicated with an active oral azole (itraconazole and not fluconazole).[70] Itraconazole would also appear useful as a primary therapeutic choice for systemic aspergillosis[192] because it achieves a cure in a consistent fraction of cases, even among nonresponders to AmB, but incomplete oral absorption limits wider use of it in patients with frequent gastroenteric complications.[676] If oral drug intake is preserved, itraconazole can be administered at a dose of 200 mg every 6 hours for 4 days and then 200 mg every 12 hours daily.[70] Because of drug interaction problems through cytochrome P-450 metabolism, cyclosporine levels should be strictly monitored in allografted patients and immunosuppressive therapy reduced accordingly. Rifampicin was shown to be synergistic to AmB in in vitro studies, but it is rarely considered.[98] Surgery is indicated for resection of lung lesions that puts the patient at risk of bleeding[96]; before HSC transplants to remove possible sites of disease reactivation, superinfection, and bleeding; and in the case of rhinosinusal aspergillosis with necrotizing features. These interventions are very often difficult and greatly depend on local surgical skills, but surgery must be considered a matter of urgency if the lung disease appears to involve the proximal, larger lung vessels. Alternative strategies based on early demonstration of *Aspergillus* antigen, HRCT scanning, and radionuclide imaging should reduce the interval from diagnosis to treatment and allow more patients to be cured with fewer complications.[96, 322, 325, 677]

Rare Infections, New Drugs and Formulations

AmB is also the appropriate therapy for cryptococcosis, mucormycosis, fusariosis, and all other less common types of fungal infections. In mucormycosis, as for aspergillosis, surgical débridement is indicated in patients with infiltration of risk sites.[250] The possible adjunctive role of hematopoietic growth factors in the treatment of fungal infections, including rare subtypes,[253] may be an important developmental aspect and is reviewed elsewhere in this chapter. As a general statement, both G-CSF and GM-CSF are strong candidates to support treatment of invasive fungal infections. New antifungal drugs include caspofungin, new triazoles (voriconazole) and new formulations (itraconazole oral suspension) that increase intestinal absorption and drug bioavailability.[192, 420, 678] The most notable advancement concerns lipid formulations of AmB: in liposomes (AmBisome), complexed with lipids (ABLC, Abelcet), and as a colloidal dispersion (ABCD).[679] Patients with fungal infections who are not responsive to or do not tolerate intravenous AmB can be effectively rescued by the new lipid formulations.[6, 168, 680, 681] Tolerance is generally good, even if severe, acute toxic side effects are reported.[682] Not all studies, however, have reported improved results.[683] Rescue rates for patients failing or intolerant to conventional AmB given for suspected or confirmed invasive mycoses were 61% with AmBisome[684] and 57%,[685] 66%,[686] and 69%[687] for ABLC. Experience with ABCD is more limited.[680] In most of these studies and others,[688] acute side effects were more frequent with ABLC. The principal results from a number of comparative trials investigating standard versus lipid-associated AmB and/or different AmBisome doses are presented in Table 14-29. The information being accrued is that AmBisome and ABCD or ABLC are therapeutically at least as effective as conventional AmB. The benefits could be substantial with AmBisome in selected risk categories (breakthrough fungal infection),[693] and treatment tolerance is certainly improved, with fewer infusion-related effects and less renal function damage. The latter conclusion may facilitate treatment of fungal infections in HSC recipients receiving other nephrotoxic drugs.[695] Keeping the AmBisome dose low (1 mg/kg/day) might not adversely affect treatment outcome and is less expensive.[692] In summary, AmB lipid formulations preferably AmBisome, 1 to 3 mg/kg/day) could be reserved for patients intolerant of or refractory to conventional AmB and those undergoing HSC transplantation. More studies are needed to precisely define the optimal dosage and the likelihood of a therapeutic response in the various clinical and diagnostic disease subtypes.

Established Viral Infections

Acyclovir and ganciclovir are the mainstay of antiviral treatment in leukemic patients (Table 14-30). Established indications for acyclovir are HSV infections, including encephalitis, and VZV infection.[6, 696] Infection by EBV is acyclovir sensitive. Patients with mucocutaneous or disseminated HSV infection are often unable to swallow oral preparations. Treatment with intravenous acyclovir is therefore indicated at a dosage ranging from 250 mg/m² every 8 hours for 7 days in patients with localized

TABLE 14–29. Studies with Lipid Formulations of Amphotericin B for Suspected and/or Documented Fungal Infection

Study (1st Author, Year)	Study Arms*	Total Patients	Main Results (Study Drug vs. Amphotericin B)
Prentice, 1997[689]	Amphotericin B, 1 mg/kg/day vs. AmBisome 1 vs. 3 mg/kg/day	338	AmBisome: response rate of 58% with 1 mg/kg/day vs. 64% with 3 mg/kg/day vs. 49% (P = .03 for 3 mg/kg/day) fewer severe infusion-related symptoms ($P < .01$), less renal dysfunction ($P < .01$)
Leenders, 1998[690]	Amphotericin B, 1 mg/kg/day vs. AmBisome, 5 mg/kg/day	66	AmBisome: response rate of 65% vs. 56% (P = 0.09), more complete response (P = .03), lower mortality rate (P = .03), less renal dysfunction ($P < .001$)
White, 1998[691]	Amphotericin B, 0.8 mg/kg/day vs. ABCD, 4 mg/kg/day	213	ABCD: response rate of 50% vs. 43% (P = 0.31), renal dysfunction less common ($P < 0.001$), infusion-related symptoms more common (P = .018)
Ellis, 1998[692]	AmBisome, 1 vs. 4 mg/kg/day	871	Response rate of 58% vs. 52% (P = NS), survival rate of 43% vs. 37% (P = NS)
Walsh, 1999[693]	Amphotericin B, 0.6 mg/kg/day vs. AmBisome, 3 mg/kg/day	702	AmBisome: response rate of 58% vs. 58%, fewer breakthrough fungal infections (P = .009), fewer infusion-related reactions ($P < .001$), less dysfunction ($P < .001$)
Wingard, 1999[694]	AmBisome, 3 vs. 5 mg/kg/day vs. ABLC, 5 mg/kg/day	244	AmBisome: response rate of 40% vs. 42% (P = NS), fewer infusion-related symptoms ($P < .001$), less renal dysfunction ($P < 0.001$)

* All patients are neutropenic with documented invasive aspergillosis.
ABCD, amphotericin B colloidal dispersion; ABLC, amphotericin B lipid complex.

TABLE 14–30. Treatment of Interstitial Pneumonia and Major Viral Infections in/outside the Context of HSC Transplantation

Infection	Etiology	Therapy
Interstitial pneumonia	CMV	Ganciclovir, 2.5 mg/kg IV q8h for 15 days, plus high-dose immunoglobulin (plus adrenocorticosteroids) and control of GVHD
	Pneumocystis carinii	TMP-SMX (15–20 mg/kg as TMP) PO/IV q6–12h Pentamidine (second choice), 4 mg/kg/day IV
	Legionella pneumophila	Erythromycin, other macrolide
CMV disease	CMV	As for CMV pneumonia (immunoglobulin not expected to be effective; foscarnet, 60 mg/kg IV q8h for 14–21 days, may replace ganciclovir, dual therapy possible)
HSV (simplex, visceral)	HSV	Acyclovir, 400 mg PO 5 times daily for 5–7 days (alternatives: famciclovir, valacyclovir); acyclovir, 5 mg/kg IV q8h for 14 days (severe form, unable to swallow)
VZV (zoster, visceral)	VZV	Acyclovir, 800 mg PO 5 times daily for 7–10 days (IV schedule if unable to swallow or extensive involvement)

CMV, cytomegalovirus; GVHD, graft-versus-host disease; HSC, hematopoietic stem cell; HSV, herpes simplex virus; TMP-SMX, trimethoprim-sulfamethoxazole; VZV, varicella-zoster virus.

oral or esophageal infections to 500 mg/m² every 8 hours for 10 days and longer in those with disseminated infections and multiple visceral and cerebral involvement. Disseminated VZV infection is treated similar to visceral HSV infection. Treatment of localized reactivation, herpes zoster or shingles, is accomplished with this same schedule and corresponds to 10 mg/kg/day administered in three divided doses; it is highly effective when started within 72 hours of the onset of symptoms. The absorption of oral acyclovir is erratic, so oral therapy is unlikely to result in systemic concentrations inhibiting viral replication. In the less severe forms, however, and provided that oral intake is adequate, oral administration can be attempted, with an adult patient receiving 800 mg five times per day for 7 days. Famciclovir is a new drug[193] that at 500 to 750 mg every 8 hours daily is highly effective and might reduce the duration of postherpetic neuralgia.[697] Oral valacyclovir, 1 g every 8 hours daily for 1 week, is similarly effective. Postherpetic pain could also be reduced with a concurrent prednisone course (if not contraindicated by patient age of 50 years or younger) of 60 mg/day for 7 days and then tapering over the subsequent 2 weeks.[698, 699] Management of viral infections developing in HSC transplant patients is detailed in the next paragraph.

HSC Transplant–related Infections: Interstitial Pneumonia and Viral Infections

Interstitial pneumonitis caused by CMV is a relatively frequent problem during HSC transplant procedures, although it may be significantly reduced in frequency by preemptive therapy. *P. carinii* as a causative agent is more frequent outside the transplant setting, and nosocomial outbreaks of *L. pneumophila* giving a very similar clinical picture were reported in both transplant and nontransplant patient groups.[6, 296] CMV pneumonia has been treated with a number of agents, including interferons, vidarabine, acyclovir, ganciclovir, foscarnet, and intravenous immunoglobulin, with no or poor success. When the clinical picture develops, mortality in the range of 50% or greater is expected. The results were markedly worse before the use of ganciclovir (2.5 mg/kg intravenously every 8 hours for 10 to 14 days) plus intravenous hyperimmune or polyvalent high-dose gamma globulin. Most authorities recommend the additional use of high-dose steroids to reduce interstitial inflammation and facilitate gas exchange. Response rates after combination treatment were reported to be 64% from seven recently reviewed series[433] consisting of almost only nonventilated patients. The exact mechanism of this seemingly effective synergy is unclear, and the possibility remains that the more severe cases may not be as responsive and a positive outcome might be partly due to improved prevention and treatment of GVHD. On the other hand, the use of immunoglobulin along with antiviral therapy is not effective in CMV gastrointestinal disease.[700] In summary, ganciclovir (or foscarnet or a combination) plus immunoglobulin remains the treatment of choice for CMV pneumonitis and other CMV-related syndromes[163, 433, 442, 701] (see Table 14-30). Continuous or intermittent treatment may be needed in patients showing incomplete clearing or recurrence of lung lesions. Oral ganciclovir is under evaluation for continuing maintenance therapy[31] and could be useful for prevention of late disease. The second most frequent pathogen causing interstitial pneumonia is *P. carinii*. Infection by *Pneumocystis* is possible outside the transplant setting in patients chronically treated with immunosuppressive and cytostatic agents. Treatment with intravenous TMP-SMX is usually effective, although it may take some days to document clinical improvement. If, however, clinical progression occurs after 4 to 5 days, it is appropriate to add pentamidine and to continue TMP-SMX. Because *L. pneumophila* can cause very similar lung lesions that are not always easy to differentiate, in idiopathic cases of interstitial pneumonitis and in those of uncertain etiology it is customary at many centers to empirically add erythromycin-like drugs to the former regimen. Other viruses are being recovered with increasing frequency from transplanted leukemia patients, in whom they can cause a variety of pulmonary and enteric disorders.[163, 702] These viruses are RSV, adenovirus, rotavirus, and echovirus. No effective drug therapy is available for these infections. Aerosolized ribavirin has been used in patients with RSV pneumonia.[703] As for

CMV, the use of immunoglobulin can result in improvement in some cases of enteric viral syndrome and may actually be the only treatment available.[704, 705] Infections by acyclovir-resistant HSV and VZV strains can be observed in 25% and 4% of cases, respectively, and are managed by replacing acyclovir with foscarnet (HSV infection, 71% success rate) and vidarabine (VZV).[194]

Use of Antiparasitic Drugs

Helminths and protozoa can cause infections in patients with leukemia. Treatment of *P. carinii* pneumonia was considered in the preceding section and is presented in Table 14–30. Therapy for cerebral toxoplasmosis consists of pyrimethamine, 25 to 50 mg/day for 6 weeks, plus sulfadiazine, 4 g on day 1, followed by an increased dose. Specific drugs and regimens for other less frequently encountered parasites are available.[31, 706]

Granulocyte Transfusions

In the past, granulocyte transfusions were used therapeutically in infected neutropenic patients together with standard antimicrobial therapy, but because of technical problems, toxicity, and undefined therapeutic advantage, the procedure was abandoned by many. However, positive clinical responses were observed in more than one study, as recently reviewed,[707] and more convincingly when granulocytes were obtained from compatible donors at relatively high doses.[708–711] Accordingly, this approach might have a role in selected conditions such as breakthrough septicemia or disseminated fungal infection in a severely neutropenic patient, along with the usual modifications of empiric treatment.[712] If periodic institutional review of treatment outcomes for such patients confirms a high risk of death, granulocyte transfusion can have a definite place as a lifesaving procedure. In practice, no less than 1×10^{10} and preferably more than 2×10^{10} granulocytes from donors selected on the basis of the best HLA matching or leukocyte cross-matching should be administered daily until resolution of neutropenia or infection. Administration of G-CSF to the donor before apheresis can optimize the cell yield and limit the number of donors needed.[6] G-CSF, 600 µg subcutaneously, plus dexamethasone, 8 mg, can be enough to collect 10×10^{10} granulocytes after 12 hours with a single hetastarch apheresis.[712, 713]

Miscellanea

Because infections by gram-negative microorganisms can still be lethal in a significant proportion of patients, attempts have been made to achieve passive immunization with vaccines or limit the severity of the established infection with an antiendotoxin monoclonal antibody. J-5 antiserum collected from subjects immunized against Enterobacteriaceae was tested in patients at risk for gram-negative infection. Early results were promising, but this expensive and complex approach seems to be of no value in neutropenic subjects.[6, 19, 714] The monoclonal antibody HA-1A raised against the endotoxin of gram-negative bacteria was tested in patients with sepsis. Significant activity by HA-1A was demonstrated, with reduced mortality in patients with documented gram-negative infections.[715] It is not yet known whether this approach could be profitably extended to neutropenic leukemia patients. The use of recombinant human activated protein C reduced mortality from severe sepsis in one large randomized study (1690 patients, absolute reduction of risk of death of 6.1%, $p = 0.005$).[716] Evaluation of this new drug in infected patients with leukemia appears advisable.

CONCLUSIONS

Infectious complications stand out as a major obstacle in the management of patients with leukemia. Very often,

TABLE 14–31. Major Advancements in the 1990s for the Management of Infections in Patients with Leukemia

Issues	Category	Explanatory Notes
General	Risk class	Proper context for prophylaxis and treatment application and assessment
Diagnosis	PCR, antigens, HRCT	Early demonstration of infections by certain viruses and fungi; allows preemptive therapy (confirmed)
Prophylaxis	Drugs	Application by risk category (increased efficacy, lower cost, lower emergence of drug resistance)
	Catheters	Drug impregnated
	Experimental drugs	Marrow protectants, antimucositis, cytokine modulating
Antibacterials	New drugs	β-Lactam/β-lactamase inhibitor conjugates, fourth-generation cephalosporins, new carbapenems
	Modality	Application by risk category (low risk: monotherapy, home therapy; high risk: other)
Antifungals	Fluconazole	Confirmed effective
	Itraconazole	Confirmed effective, oral solution
	Amphotericin B	New lipid formulations (AmBisome, others: confirmed effective, toxicity reduced)
Antivirals	Foscarnet	Effective (CMV)
	Preemptive therapy	Effective (ganciclovir, foscarnet: CMV)
CSFs	G-CSF, GM-CSF	Effective (shorter neutropenia: selected end points and risk category)
HSC	Circulating CD34+ cells	Effective (shorter neutropenia: after HSC transplantation)

CMV, cytomegalovirus; G/GM-CSF, granulocyte/granulocyte-macrophage colony-stimulating factor; HRCT, high-resolution computed tomography; HSC, hematopoietic stem cell; PCR, polymerase chain reaction.

when antileukemic treatment fails, death from infection occurs. Other patients who respond well to primary treatment of the disease still succumb to infections. Unfortunately, infections are closely related to the more effective (and intensive) antileukemic treatments and are therefore not fully preventable. Infections in turn markedly reduce the patient's compliance with treatment and greatly alter the quality of life. This review has emphasized the need for considering the different diagnostic, prophylactic, and therapeutic possibilities in heterogeneous risk categories and during subsequent treatment phases. In the 1990s, substantial progress occurred (Table 14-31), but the search for improved, clinically cost-effective strategies must continue.

REFERENCES

1. Johanson D: Homo sp. A.L. 666-1. In Johanson D, Edgar B, eds: From Lucy to Language. London: George Weidenfeld & Nicolson; 1996, p 168.
2. Cowen R: History of Life. Cambridge: Blackwell; 1990.
3. Gould SJ: Full House. New York: Harmony Books–Crown Publishers; 1997.
4. Bodey GP: Infectious complications in leukemic patients. Semin Hematol 1982;19:193.
5. Hughes WT: Guidelines for the use of antimicrobial agents in neutropenic patients with unexplained fever. J Infect Dis 1990;161:381.
6. Bassan R: The management of infections in patients with leukemia. In Henderson ES, Lister TA, Greaves MF, eds: Leukemia, 6th ed. Philadelphia: WB Saunders, 1996, p 257.
7. Arbo MJ: Fever of nosocomial origin: Etiology, risk factors, and outcomes. Am J Med 1993;95:505.
8. Beam TR: Patterns of infection in untreated acute leukemia: Impact of initial hospitalization. South Med J 1979;72:282.
9. Fainstein V: Patterns of oropharyngeal and fecal flora in patients with leukemia. J Infect Dis 1981;144:10.
10. Maki DG: Relation of the inanimate hospital environment to endemic nosocomial infection. N Engl J Med 1982;307:1562.
11. Walsh TJ: Nosocomial fungal infections: A classification for hospital-acquired fungal infections and mycoses arising from endogenous flora or reactivation. Annu Rev Microbiol 1988;42:517.
12. Elting LS: Outcomes of bacteremia in patients with cancer and neutropenia: Observations from two decades of epidemiological and clinical trials. Clin Infect Dis 1997;25:247.
13. Hughes WT: 1997 Guidelines for the use of antimicrobial agents in neutropenic patients with unexplained fever. Clin Infect Dis 1997;25:551.
14. Viscoli C: Planned progressive antimicrobial therapy in neutropenic patients. Br J Haematol 1998;102:879.
15. Rolston KVI: New trends in patient management: Risk-based therapy for febrile patients with neutropenia. Clin Infect Dis 1999;29:515.
16. Bodey GP: Quantitative relationships between circulating leukocytes and infection in patients with acute leukemia. Ann Intern Med 1966;64:328.
17. Bodey GP: Infection in cancer patients. A continuing association. Am J Med 1986;81(Suppl 1A):11.
18. Gerson SL: Prolonged granulocytopenia: The major risk factor for invasive pulmonary aspergillosis in patients with acute leukemia. Ann Intern Med 1984;100:345.
19. Pizzo PA: Management of fever in patients with cancer and treatment-induced neutropenia. N Engl J Med 1993;328:1323.
20. Foa R: Constitutive production of tumor necrosis factor-alpha in hairy cell leukemia: Possible role in the pathogenesis of the cytopenia(s) and effects of treatment with interferon-alpha. J Clin Oncol 1992;10:954.
21. Kipps TJ: Autoantibodies in chronic lymphocytic leukemia and related systemic autoimmune diseases. Blood 1993;81:2475.
22. Rustagi PK: Granulocyte antibodies in leukaemic chronic lymphoproliferative disorders. Br J Haematol 1987;66:461.
23. Bassan R: Large granular lymphocyte/natural killer cell proliferative disease: Clinical and laboratory heterogeneity. Scand J Haematol 1986;37:91.
24. Bassan R: Autoimmunity and B-cell dysfunction in chronic proliferative disorders of large granular lymphocytes/natural killer cells. Cancer 1989;63:90.
25. Loughran TP Jr: Clonal diseases of large granular lymphocytes. Blood 1993;82:1.
26. Gale RP: Antineoplastic chemotherapy myelosuppression: Mechanisms and new approaches. Exp Hematol 1985;13(Suppl 16):3.
27. Mac Manus M: Radiotherapy-associated neutropenia and thrombocytopenia: Analysis of risk factors and development of a predictive model. Blood 1997;89:2303.
28. Offner F: Mortality hazard functions as related to neutropenia at different times after marrow transplantation. Blood 1996;88:4058.
28a. Talcott JA, Siegel RD, Finberg R, et al. Risk assessment in cancer patients with fever and neutropenia: A prospective, two-center validation of a prediction rule. J Clin Oncol 1992;10:316.
29. Martin MV: Irradiation mucositis: A reappraisal. Eur J Cancer 1993;29B:1.
30. Spiegel RJ: The acute toxicities of chemotherapy. Cancer Treat Rep 1981;8:197.
31. Aslan T: Infections in hematological malignancies. In Freireich EJ, Kantarjian HM, eds: Medical Management of Hematological Malignant Diseases. New York: Marcel Dekker; 1998, p 321.
32. Engelhard D: Cytosine arabinoside as a major risk factor for *Streptococcus viridans* septicemia following bone marrow transplantation: A 5-year prospective study. Bone Marrow Transplant 1995;16:565.
33. Rapoport AP: Analysis of factors that correlate with mucositis in recipients of autologous and allogeneic stem-cell transplants. J Clin Oncol 1999;17:2446.
34. Ruescher TJ: The impact of mucositis on α-hemolytic streptococcal infection in patients undergoing autologous bone marrow transplantation for hematological malignancies. Cancer 1998;82:2275.
35. Eriksson KM: Nutrition and acute leukemia in adults. Relation between nutritional status and infectious complications during remission induction. Cancer 1998;82:1071.
36. Sonis ST: Validation of a new scoring system for the assessment of clinical trial research of oral mucositis induced by radiation or chemotherapy. Cancer 1999;85:2103.
37. Barber GR: Catheter-related *Malassezia furfur* fungemia in immunocompromised patients. Am J Med 1993;95:365.
38. Dugdale DC: *Staphylococcus aureus* bacteremia in patients with Hickman catheters. Am J Med 1990;89:137.
39. Lokich JJ: Complications and management of implanted venous access catheters. J Clin Oncol 1985;3:710.
40. Raad I: Low infection rate and long durability of nontunneled Silastic catheters. A safe and cost-effective alternative for long-term venous access. Arch Intern Med 1993;153:1791.
41. Raad I: Serious complications of vascular catheter-related *Staphylococcus aureus* bacteremia in cancer patients. Eur J Clin Microbiol Infect Dis 1992;11:675.
42. Tchekmedyian NS: Case report: Special studies of the Hickman catheter of a patient with recurrent bacteremia and candidemia. Am J Med Sci 1986;29:419.
43. Widmer AF: The clinical impact of culturing central venous catheters. A prospective study. Arch Intern Med 1992;152:1299.
44. Nouwen JL: Hickman catheter-related infections in neutropenic patients: Insertion in the operating theater versus insertion in the radiology suite. J Clin Oncol 1999;17:1304.
45. Lazarus HM: Contamination during in vitro processing of bone marrow for transplantation: Clinical significance. Bone Marrow Transplant 1991;7:241.
46. Boogaerts MA: Blood neutrophil function in primary myelodysplastic syndromes. Br J Haematol 1983;55:217.
47. Clarkson B: Linkage of proliferative and maturational abnormalities in chronic myelogenous leukemia and relevance to treatment. Leukemia 1993;7:1683.
48. Martin S: Defective neutrophil function and microbicidal mechanisms in the myelodysplastic disorders. J Clin Pathol 1983;36:1120.
49. Maurer AB: Restoration of impaired cytokine secretion from monocytes of patients with myelodysplastic syndromes after in vivo treatment with GM-CSF or IL-3. Leukemia 1993;7:1728.

50. Robertson MJ: Biology and clinical relevance of human natural killer cells. Blood 1990;76:2421.

51. Fernandez LA: Immunoglobulin secretory function of B cells from untreated patients with chronic lymphocytic leukemia and hypogammaglobulinemia: Role of T cells. Blood 1983;62:767.

52. Fujimiya Y: Natural killer–cell immunodeficiency in patients with chronic myelogenous leukemia. I. Analysis of the defect using the monoclonal antibodies HNK-1 (LEU-7) and B73.1. Int J Cancer 1986;37:639.

53. Kay NE: Impaired natural killer activity in patients with chronic lymphocytic leukemia is associated with a deficiency of azurophilic cytoplasmic granules in putative NK cells. Blood 1984;63:305.

54. Lotzova E: Defective NK cell in patients with leukemia. In Herberman RB, ed: Mechanisms of Cytotoxicity by NK Cells. London: Academic Press; 1985, p 507.

55. Ridgway D: Defective production of granulocyte-macrophage colony-stimulating factor and interleukin-1 by mononuclear cells from children treated for acute lymphoblastic leukemia. Leukemia 1992; 6:809.

56. Ruco LP: Severe deficiency of natural killer activity in the peripheral blood of patients with hairy cell leukemia. Blood 1983;61: 1132.

57. Zimmerli W: Neutrophil function and pyogenic infections in bone marrow transplant recipients. Blood 1991;77:393.

58. Bergmann L: Immunosuppressive effects and clinical response of fludarabine in refractory chronic lymphocytic leukemia. Ann Oncol 1993;4:371.

59. Estey E: Treatment of hairy cell leukemia with 2-chlorodeoxyadenosine (2-CdA). Blood 1992;79:882.

60. Piro LD: 2-Chlorodeoxyadenosine treatment of lymphoid malignancies. Blood 1992;79:843.

61. O'Brien S: Fludarabine and granulocyte colony-stimulating factor (G-CSF) in patients with chronic lymphocytic leukemia. Leukemia 1997;11:1631.

62. Saven A: Long-term follow-up of patients with hairy cell leukemia after cladribine treatment. Blood 1998;92:1918.

63. Cheson BD: Infectious and immunosuppressive complications of purine analog therapy. J Clin Oncol 1995;13:2431.

64. Anaissie EJ: Infections in patients with chronic lymphocytic leukemia treated with fludarabine. Ann Intern Med 1998;129:559.

65. Byrd JC: Herpes virus infections occur frequently following treatment with fludarabine: Results of a prospective natural history study. Br J Haematol 1999;105:445.

66. Lamberts SW: Corticosteroid therapy in severe illness. N Engl J Med 1997;337:1285.

67. Dannenberg AM: The antiinflammatory effects of glucocorticosteroids. Inflammation 1979;3:329.

68. Nair MPN: Immunomodulatory effects of corticosteroids on natural killer and antibody-dependent cellular cytotoxic activities of human lymphocytes. J Immunol 1984;132:2876.

69. Slade JD: Prednisone-induced alterations of circulating human lymphocyte subsets. J Lab Clin Med 1983;101:479.

70. Denning DW: Invasive aspergillosis. Clin Infect Dis 1998;26:781.

71. Kim JH: Infection and cyclosporine. Rev Infect Dis 1989;11:677.

72. Foa R: IL2 treatment for cancer: From biology to gene therapy. Br J Cancer 1992;66:992.

73. Siegel JP: Interleukin-2 toxicity. J Clin Oncol 1991;9:694.

74. Borden ES: Interferons: Rationale for clinical trials in neoplastic disease. Ann Intern Med 1979;91:472.

75. Edwards BS: Low doses of interferon alpha result in more effective clinical natural killer cell activation. J Clin Invest 1985;75:1908.

76. Neefe JR: Augmented immunity in cancer patients treated with α-interferon. Cancer Res 1985;45:874.

77. Klingemann HG: Treatment with recombinant interferon (α-2β) early after bone marrow transplantation in patients at high risk for relapse. Blood 1991;78:3306.

78. Grossbard ML: Monoclonal antibody–based therapies of leukemia and lymphoma. Blood 1992;80:863.

79. Foon KA: Effects of monoclonal antibody therapy in patients with chronic lymphocytic leukemia. Blood 1984;64:1085.

80. Grossbard ML: Serotherapy of B-cell neoplasms with anti-B4–blocked ricin: A phase I trial of daily bolus infusion. Blood 1992; 79:576.

81. Del Favero A: The new fluorinated quinolones for antimicrobial prophylaxis in neutropenic cancer patients. Eur J Cancer 1993; 29(Suppl):2.

82. Bodey GP: Infections of the gastrointestinal tract in the immunocompromised patient. Annu Rev Med 1986;37:271.

83. Cudmore MA: *Clostridium difficile* colitis associated with cancer chemotherapy. Arch Intern Med 1982;142:333.

84. Gerding DN: Disease associated with *Clostridium difficile* infection. Ann Intern Med 1989;110:255.

85. Styrt B: Recent developments in the understanding of the pathogenesis and treatment of anaerobic infections. N Engl J Med 1989; 321:240.

86. Aisner J: Invasive aspergillosis in acute leukemia: Correlation with nose culture and antibiotic use. Ann Intern Med 1979;90:4.

87. Bodey GP: Fungal infection and fever of unknown origin in neutropenic patients. Am J Med 1986;80(Suppl 5C):112.

88. Hiddeman W: Antifungal treatment by amphotericin B and 5-fluorocytosine delays the recovery of normal hematopoietic cells after intensive cytostatic therapy for acute myeloid leukemia. Cancer 1991;68:9.

89. Schimpff SC: Origin of infections in acute nonlymphocytic leukemia. Ann Intern Med 1972;77:707.

90. Champlin RE: The early complications of bone marrow transplantation. Semin Hematol 1984;21:101.

91. Deeg HJ: Bone marrow transplantation: A review of delayed complications. Br J Haematol 1984;57:185.

92. McDonald GB: Intestinal and hepatic complications of human bone marrow transplantation. Part II. Gastroenterology 1986;90: 770.

93. van der Meer JWM: Infections in bone marrow transplant recipients. Semin Hematol 1984;21:123.

94. Winston DJ: Infectious complications of bone marrow transplantation. Exp Hematol 1984;12:205.

95. Zaia JA: Infections. In Blume KG, Petz LD, eds: Clinical Bone Marrow Transplantation. New York: Churchill Livingstone; 1983, p. 131.

96. Caillot D: Improved management of invasive pulmonary aspergillosis in neutropenic patients using early thoracic computed tomographic scan and surgery. J Clin Oncol 1997;15:139.

97. Richard C: Invasive pulmonary aspergillosis prior to BMT in acute leukemia patients does not predict a poor outcome. Bone Marrow Transplant 1993;12:237.

98. Denning DW: Treatment of invasive aspergillosis. J Infect 1994; 28(Suppl 1):25.

99. Michailov G: Autologous bone marrow transplantation is feasible in patients with a prior history of invasive pulmonary aspergillosis. Bone Marrow Transplant 1996;17:569.

100. Offner F: Impact of previous aspergillosis on the outcome of bone marrow transplantation. Clin Infect Dis 1998;26:1098.

101. Ribaud P: Survival and prognostic factors of invasive aspergillosis after allogeneic bone marrow transplantation. Clin Infect Dis 1999; 28:322.

102. Pagano L: Fatal haemoptysis in pulmonary filamentous mycosis: An undervaluated cause of death in patients with acute leukaemia in haematological complete remission. A retrospective study and review of the literature. Br J Haematol 1995;89:500.

103. Bjerke JW: Hepatosplenic candidiasis—a contraindication to marrow transplantation? Blood 1994;84:2811.

104. Corbi C: Prevalence and clinical features of hepatitis G virus infection in bone marrow allograft recipients. Bone Marrow Transplant 1997;20:965.

105. Skidmore SJ: High prevalence of hepatitis G virus in bone marrow transplant recipients and patients treated for acute leukemia. Blood 1997;89:3853.

106. Ljungman P: Detection of hepatitis G virus/GB virus C after allogeneic bone marrow transplantation. Bone Marrow Transplant 1998; 22:499.

107. Kanda Y: TT virus in bone marrow transplant recipients. Blood 1999;93:2485.

108. Yamada-Osaki M: Persistence and clinical outcome of hepatitis G virus infection in pediatric bone marrow transplant recipients and children treated for hematological malignancy. Blood 1999;93:721.

109. Aach RD: Hepatitis C virus infection in post-transfusion hepatitis. N Engl J Med 1991;325:1325.

110. Gruber A: Late seroconversion and high chronicity rate of hepatitis C virus infection in patients with hematologic disorders. Ann Oncol 1993;4:229.

111. Japanese Red Cross Non-A, Non-B Hepatitis Research Group: Ef-

fects of screening for hepatitis C virus antibody and hepatitis B virus core antibody on incidence of post-transfusion hepatitis. Lancet 1991;338:1040.

112. Locasciulli A: Hepatitis C virus infection and chronic liver disease in children with leukemia in long-term remission. Blood 1991; 78:1619.

113. Liang R: Chemotherapy and bone marrow transplantation for cancer patients who are also chronic hepatitis B carriers: A review of the problem. J Clin Oncol 1999;17:394.

114. Strasser SI: Hepatitis viruses and hematopoietic cell transplantation: A guide to patient and donor management. Blood 1999; 93:1127.

115. Locasciulli A: Impact of liver disease and hepatitis infections on allogeneic bone marrow transplantation in Europe: A survey from the European Bone Marrow Transplantation (EBMT) Group–Infectious Diseases Working Party. Bone Marrow Transplant 1994; 14:833.

116. Locasciulli A: Allogeneic bone marrow transplantation from HBsAg+ donors: A multicenter study from the Gruppo Italiano Trapianto di Midollo Osseo (GITMO). Blood 1995;86:3236.

117. van Tol MJD: The origin of IgG production and homogeneous IgG components after allogeneic bone marrow transplantation. Blood 1996;87:818.

118. Dumont-Girard F: Reconstitution of the T-cell compartment after bone marrow transplantation: Restoration of the repertoire by thymic emigrants. Blood 1998;92:4464.

119. Mossad SB: Early infectious complications in autologous bone marrow transplantation: A review of 219 patients. Bone Marrow Transplant 1996;18:265.

120. Yuen KY: Unique risk factors for bacteraemia in allogeneic bone marrow transplant recipients before and after engraftment. Bone Marrow Transplant 1998;21:1137.

121. Sparrelid E: Bacteraemia during the aplastic phase after allogeneic bone marrow transplantation is associated with early death from invasive fungal infection. Bone Marrow Transplant 1998;22:795.

122. Engels EA: Early infection in bone marrow transplantation: Quantitative study of clinical factors that affect risk. Clin Infect Dis 1999; 28:256.

123. Wald A: Epidemiology of *Aspergillus* infections in a large cohort of patients undergoing bone marrow transplantation. J Infect Dis 1997;175:1459.

124. Chandrasekar PH: Autopsy-identified infections among bone marrow transplant recipients: A clinico-pathologic study of 56 patients. Bone Marrow Transplant 1995;16:675.

125. Williamson ECM: Infections in adults undergoing unrelated donor bone marrow transplantation. Br J Haematol 1999;104:560.

126. Lefrère F: Transmission of *Plasmodium falciparum* by allogenic bone marrow transplantation. Bone Marrow Transplant 1996;18:473.

127. Salutari P: *Plasmodium vivax* malaria after autologous bone marrow transplantation: An unusual complication. Bone Marrow Transplant 1996;18:805.

128. Raina V: *Plasmodium vivax* causing pancytopenia after allogeneic blood stem cell transplantation in CML. Bone Marrow Transplant 1998;22:205.

129. Harrington RD: Legionellosis in a bone marrow transplant center. Bone Marrow Transplant 1996;18:361.

130. Zomas A: Unusual infections following allogeneic bone marrow transplantation for chronic lymphocytic leukemia. Bone Marrow Transplant 1994;14:799.

131. Slavin MA: *Toxoplasma gondii* infection in marrow transplant recipients: A 20 year experience. Bone Marrow Transplant 1994; 13:549.

132. Maschke M: Opportunistic CNS infection after bone marrow transplantation. Bone Marrow Transplant 1999;23:1167.

133. Dictar M: Recipients and donors of bone marrow transplants suffering from Chagas' disease: Management and preemptive therapy of parasitemia. Bone Marrow Transplant 1998;21:391.

134. Roy V: Mycobacterial infections following bone marrow transplantation: A 20 year retrospective review. Bone Marrow Transplant 1997;19:467.

135. Aljurf M: *Mycobacterium tuberculosis* infection in allogeneic bone marrow transplantation patients. Bone Marrow Transplant 1999;24:551.

136. Childs R: High incidence of adeno- and polyomavirus-induced

137. Whimbey E: Influenza A virus infections among hospitalized adult bone marrow transplant recipients. Bone Marrow Transplant 1994; 13:437.

138. Whimbey E: Community respiratory virus infections among hospitalized adult bone marrow transplant recipients. Clin Infect Dis 1996;22:778.

139. Ghosh S: Rhinovirus infections in myelosuppressed adult blood and marrow transplant recipients. Clin Infect Dis 1999;29:528.

140. Ball ED, Mills LE, Coughlin CT, et al: Autologous bone marrow transplantation in acute myelogenous leukemia: In vitro treatment with myeloid cell-specific monoclonal antibodies. Blood 1986; 68:1311.

141. Gorin NC, Douay L: Autologous bone marrow transplantation using marrow incubated with Asta Z 7557 in adult acute leukemia. Blood 1986;67:1367.

142. Lemoli RM, Gasparetto C: Autologous bone marrow transplantation in acute myelogenous leukemia: In vitro treatment with myeloid-specific monoclonal antibodies and drugs in combination. Blood 1991;77:1829.

143. Robertson MJ, Soiffer RJ: Human bone marrow depleted of CD33-positive cells mediates delayed but durable reconstitution of hematopoiesis: Clinical trial of MY9 monoclonal antibody-purged autografts for the treatment of acute myeloid leukemia. Blood 1992; 79:2229.

144. Uckun FM, Kersey JH, Haake R, et al: Autologous bone marrow transplantation in high-risk remission B-lineage acute lymphoblastic leukemia using a cocktail of three monoclonal antibodies (BA-1/CD24, BA-2/CD9, and BA-3/CD10) plus complement and 4-hydroperoxycyclophosphamide for ex vivo bone marrow purging. Blood 1992;79:1094.

145. Yeager AM, Kaizer H: Autologous bone marrow transplantation in patients with acute nonlymphocitic leukemia, using ex vivo marrow treatment with 4-hydroperoxycyclophosphamide. N Engl J Med 1986;315:141.

146. Ault KA, Antin JH: Phenotype of recovering lymphoid cell populations after marrow transplantation. J Exp Med 1985;161:1483.

147. Lum LG. The kinetics of immune reconstitution after human marrow transplantation. Blood 1987;69:369.

148. Storek J, Saxon A: Reconstitution of B cell immunity following bone marrow transplantation. Bone Marrow Transplant 1992;9:395.

149. Witherspoon RP, Kopecky K: Immunological recovery in 48 patients following syngeneic marrow transplantation for hematological malignancy. Transplantation 1982;33:143.

150. Kalhs P, Panzer S: Functional asplenia after bone marrow transplantation: A late complication related to extensive chronic graft-versus-host disease. Ann Intern Med 1988;109:461.

151. Hoyle C, Goldman JM on behalf of 18 UK Bone Marrow Transplant Teams: Life-threatening infections occurring more than 3 months after BMT. Bone Marrow Transplant 1994;14:247.

152. Rege K, Mehta J: Fatal pneumococcal infections following allogeneic bone marrow transplant. Bone Marrow Transplant 1994; 14:903.

153. Ochs L, Shu XO: Late infections after allogeneic bone marrow transplantation: Comparison of incidence in related and unrelated donor transplant recipients. Blood 1995;86:3979.

154. Wilhelm M, Kantarjian HM: Pneumonia during remission induction chemotherapy in patients with AML or MDS. Leukemia 1996; 10:1870.

155. Zinner SH: Changing epidemiology of infections in patients with neutropenia and cancer: Emphasis on gram-positive and resistant bacteria. Clin Infect Dis 1999;29:490.

156. Rubin M, Hathorn JW: Gram-positive infections and the use of vancomycin in 550 episodes of fever and neutropenia. Ann J Med 1988;108:30.

157. Banerjee SN, Emori TG: Secular trends in nosocomial primary bloodstream infections in the United States, 1980–1989. Am J Med 1991;91:86S.

158. Anderson KC, Soiffer R: T-cell–depleted autologous bone marrow transplantation therapy: Analysis of immune deficiency and late complications. Blood 1990;76:235.

159. Radford JE, Burns CP: Adult acute lymphoblastic leukemia: Results of Iowa HOP-L Protocol. J Clin Oncol 1989;7:58.

160. Tricot G, Boogaerts MA, Vlietinck R, et al: The role of intensive remission induction and consolidation therapy in patients with acute myeloid leukemia. Br J Med 1987;66:37.

161. Weiss M, Telford P: Severe toxicity limits intensification of induction therapy for acute lymphoblastic leukemia. Leukemia 1993; 7:832.

162. Woods WG, Kobrinsky N: Intensively timed induction therapy followed by autologous or allogeneic bone marrow transplantation for children with acute myeloid leukemia or myelodysplastic syndrome: A Children Cancer Group pilot study. J Clin Oncol 1993; 11:1448.

163. Wingard JR: Advances in the management of infectious complications after bone marrow transplantation. Bone Marrow Transplant 1990;6:371.

164. Preisler HD, Davis RB: Comparison of three remission induction regimens and two postinduction strategies for the treatment of acute nonlymphocytic leukemia: A Cancer and Leukemia Group B study. Blood 1987;69:1441.

165. Preisler HD, Raza A: Intensive remission consolidation therapy in the treatment of acute nonlymphocytic leukemia. J Clin Oncol 1987;5:722.

166. Klastersky J: Empirical antibiotic therapy in neutropenic cancer patients. Eur J Cancer 1993;29:S6.

167. Jones RN: Contemporary antimicrobial susceptibility patterns of bacterial pathogens commonly associated with febrile patients with neutropenia. Clin Infect Dis 1999;29:495.

168. Buchner T, Roos N: Antifungal treatment strategy in leukemia patients. Ann Hematol 1992;65:153.

169. Lopez-Berenstein G, Bodey GP: Treatment of systemic fungal infections with liposomal amphotericin B. Arch Intern Med 1989; 149:2533.

170. De Gregorio MW, Lee WMF, Linker CA, et al: Fungal infections in patients with acute leukemia. Am J Med 1982;73:543.

171. Gorin NC, Aegerter P: Autologous bone marrow transplantation for acute myelocytic leukemia in first remission: A European survey of the role of marrow purging. Blood 1990;75:1606.

172. Verfaillie C, Weisdorf D: Candida infections in bone marrow transplant recipients. Bone Marrow Transplant 1991;8:177.

173. Bodey G, Bueltmann B: Fungal infections in cancer patients: An international autopsy survey. Eur J Clin Microbiol Infect Dis 1992; 11:99.

174. Beck-Sagué CM, Jarvis WR, National Nosocomial Infections Surveillance System: Secular trends in the epidemiology of nosocomial fungal infections in the United States, 1980–1990. J Infect Dis 1993;167:1247.

175. Jarvis WR: Epidemiology of nosocomial fungal infections, with emphasis on Candida species. Clin Infect Dis 1995;20:1526.

176. Fridkin SK, Jarvis WR: Epidemiology of nosocomial fungal infections. Clin Microb Rev 1996;9:499.

177. Wingard JR: Importance of Candida species other than C. albicans as pathogens in oncology patients. Clin Infect Dis 1995; 20:115.

178. Kataoka-Nishimura S, Akiyama H: Invasive infection due to Trichosporon cutaneum in patients with hematologic malignancies. Cancer 1998;82:484.

179. Krcmery V Jr: Emerging fungal infections in cancer patients. J Hosp Infect 1996;33:109.

180. Nguyen MH, Peacock JE: The changing face of candidemia: Emergence of non-Candida albicans species and antifungal resistance. Am J Med 1996;100:617.

181. Viscoli C, Girmenia C: Candidemia in cancer patients: A prospective, multicenter surveillance study by the invasive fungal infection group (IFIG) of the European organization for research and treatment of cancer (EORTC). Clin Infect Dis 1999;28:1071.

182. Kantarjian HM, Walters RS: Results of the vincristine, doxorubicin, and dexamethasone regimen in adults with standard- and high-risk acute lymphocytic leukemia. J Clin Oncol 1990;8:994.

183. Wang F, Dahl H: Lymphotropic herpesviruses in allogeneic bone marrow transplantation. Blood 1996;88:3615.

184. Maeda Y, Teshima T, Yamada M, et al: Monitoring of human herpesviruses after allogeneic peripheral blood stem cell transplantation and bone marrow transplantation. Br J Haematol 1999; 105:295.

185. Hale G, Waldmann H: Risk of developing Epstein-Barr virus-related lymphoproliferative disorders after T-cell–depleted marrow transplants. Blood 1998;91:3079.

186. Cone RW, Huang MW: Human hepersvirus 6 infections after bone marrow transplantation: Clinical and virologic manifestations. J Infect Dis 1999;179:311.

187. Dotti G, Fiocchi R: Primary effusion lymphoma after heart transplantation: A new entity associated with human herpesvirus-8. Leukemia 1999;13:664.

188. Drobyski WR, Knox KK, Majewski D, et al: Brief report: Fatal encephalitis due to variant B human herpesvirus-6 infection in a bone marrow-transplant recipient. N Engl J Med 1994;330:1356.

189. Gold HS, Moellering RC: Antimicrobial-drug resistance. N Engl J Med 1996;335:1445.

190. Smith TL, Pearson ML, Wilcox KR: Emergence of vancomycin resistance in Staphylococcus aureus. N Engl J Med 1999;340:493.

191. Rex JH, Rinaldi MG, Pfaller MA: Resistance of Candida species to fluconazole. Antimicrob Agents Chemother 1995;39:1.

192. Como JA, Dismukes WE: Oral azole drugs as systemic antifungal therapy. N Engl J Med 1994;330:263.

193. Balfour HH: Antiviral drugs. N Engl J Med 1999;340:1255.

194. Reusser P, Cordonnier C: European survey of herpesvirus resistance to antiviral drugs in bone marrow transplant recipients. Bone Marrow Transplant 1996;17:813.

195. Estey E, Keating MJ, McCredie KB, et al: Causes of initial remission failure in acute myelogenous leukemia. Blood 1982;60:309.

196. Harousseau JL, Milpied N: Double intensive consolidation chemotherapy in adult acute myeloid leukemia. J Clin Oncol 1991; 9:1432.

197. Schiller G, Gajewski J: A randomized study of intermediate versus conventional-dose cytarabine as intensive induction for acute myelogenous leukemia. Br J Med 1992;81:170.

198. Cassileth PA, Lynch E: Varying intensity of postremission therapy in acute myeloid leukemia. Blood 1992;79:1924.

199. Mayer RJ, Davis RB: Intensive postremission chemoterapy in adults with acute myeloid leukemia. N Engl J Med 1994;331:896.

200. Estey E, Thall P: Use of granulocyte colony-stimulating factor before, during, and after fludarabine plus cytarabine induction therapy of newly diagnosed acute myelogenous leukemia or myelodysplastic syndromes: Comparison with fludarabine plus cytarabine without granulocyte colony-stimulating factor. J Clin Oncol 1994;12:671.

201. Zittoun RA, Mandelli F: Autologous or allogeneic bone marrow transplantation compared with intensive chemotherapy in acute myelogenous leukemia. N Engl J Med 1995;332:217.

202. Bishop JF: A randomized study of high-dose cytarabine in induction in acute myeloid leukemia. Blood 1996;87:1710.

203. Weick JK: A randomized investigation of high-dose versus standard-dose cytosine arabinoside with daunorubicin in patients with previously untreated acute myeloid leukemia: A Southwest Oncology Group study. Blood 1996;88:2841.

204. Sierra J: Feasibility and results of bone marrow transplantation after remission induction and intensification chemotherapy in de novo acute myeloid leukemia. J Clin Oncol 1996;14:1353.

205. Harousseau J-L: Comparison of autologous bone marrow transplantation and intensive chemotherapy as postremission therapy in adult acute myeloid leukemia. Blood 1997;90:2978.

206. Bassan R: Outcome assessment of age group-specific (+/– 50 years) post-remission consolidation with high-dose cytarabine or bone marrow autograft for adult mylogenous leukemia. Haematologica 1998;83:627.

207. Büchner T: Double induction strategy for acute myeloid leukemia: The effect of high-dose cytarabine with mitoxantrone instead of standard-dose cytarabine with daunorubicin and 6-thioguanine: A randomized trial by the German AML Cooperative Group. Blood 1999;93:4116.

208. Mandelli F: The GIMEMA ALL 0183 trial: Analysis of 10-year follow-up. Br J Haematol 1996;92:665.

209. Rohatiner AZS: High-dose cytosine arabinoside in the initial treatment of adults with acute lymphoblastic leukaemia. Br J Cancer 1990;62:454.

210. Linker CA: Treatment of adult acute lymphoblastic leukemia with intensive cyclical chemotherapy: A follow-up report. Blood 1991; 78:2814.

211. Ellison RR: The effects of postinduction intensification treatment with cytarabine and daunorubicin in adult acute lymphocytic leukemia: A prospective randomized clinical trial by Cancer and Leukemia Group B. J Clin Oncol 1991;9:2002.

212. Bassan R: Long-term results of the HEA VD protocol for adult acute lymphoblastic leukaemia. Eur J Cancer 1991;27:441.

213. Fière D: Adult acute lymphoblastic leukaemia: A multicentric randomized trial testing bone marrow transplantation or postremission therapy. J Clin Oncol 1993;11:1990.

214. Hoelzer D: Follow-up of the first two successive German multicentre trials for adult ALL (01/81 and 02/84). Leukemia 1993;7(Suppl 2):130.

215. Durrant IJ: Results of Medical Research Council trial UKALL IX in acute lymphoblastic leukaemia in adults: Report from the Medical Research Council Working Party on adult leukemia. Br J Haematol 1993;85:84.

216. Wiernik PH: Long-term follow-up of treatment and potential cure of adult acute lymphocytic leukemia with MOAD: A non–anthracycline containing regimen. Leukemia 1993;7:1236.

217. Evensen SA: Estimated 8-year survival of more than 40% in a population-based study of 79 adult patients with acute lymphoblastic leukaemia. Br J Haematol 1994;88:88.

218. Todeschini G: Relationship between daunorubicin dosage delivered during induction therapy and outcome in adult acute lymphoblastic leukemia. Leukemia 1994;8:376.

219. Wernli M: Intensive induction/consolidation therapy without maintenance in adult acute lymphoblastic leukaemia: A pilot assessment. Br J Haematol 1994;87:39.

220. Larson RA: A five-drug remission induction regimen with intensive consolidation for adults with acute lymphoblastic leukemia: Cancer and Leukemia Group B study 8811. Blood 1995;85:2025.

221. Thomas X: Sequential induction chemotherapy with vincristine, daunorubicin, cyclophosphamide, and prednisone in adult acute lymphoblastic leukemia. Ann Hematol 1995;70:65.

222. Bosco J: Outcome of treatment in adult acute lymphoblastic leukaemia in an Asian population: Comparison with previous multicentre German study. Leukemia 1995;9:951.

223. Attal M: Consolidation treatment of adult acute lymphoblastic leukemia: A prospective, randomized trial comparing allogeneic versus autologous bone marrow transplantation and testing the impact of recombinant interleukin-2 after autologous bone marrow transplantation. Blood 1995;86:1619.

224. Dekker AW: Intensive postremission chemotherapy without maintenance therapy in adults with acute lymphoblastic leukemia. J Clin Oncol 1997;15:476.

225. Ludwig W-D: Immunophenotypic and genotypic features, clinical characteristics, and treatment outcome of adult pro-B acute lymphoblastic leukemia: Results of the German multicenter trials GMALL 03/87 and 04/89. Blood 1998;92:1998.

226. Daenen S: Improved outcome of adult acute lymphoblastic leukemia by moderately intensified chemotherapy which includes a "pre-induction" course for rapid tumour reduction: Preliminary results on 66 patients. Br J Haematol 1998;100:273.

227. Todeschini G: Estimated 6-year event-free survival of 55% in 60 consecutive adult acute lymphoblastic leukemia patients treated with an intensive phase II protocol based on high induction dose of daunorubicin. Leukemia 1998;12:144.

228. Bassan R: Induction-consolidation with an idarubicin-containing regimen, unpurged marrow autograft, and post-graft chemotherapy in adult acute lymphoblastic leukaemia. Br J Haematol 1999;104:755.

229. Bassan R: Fractioned cyclophosphamide added to the IVAP regimen (idarubicin-vincristine-L-asparaginase-prednisone) could lower the risk of primary refractory disease in T-lineage but not in B-lineage acute lymphoblastic leukemia: First results from a phase II clinical study. Haematologica 1999;84:1088.

230. Kantarjian HM: Results of treatment with hyper-CVAD, a dose-intensive regimen, in adult acute lymphocytic leukemia. J Clin Oncol 2000;18:547.

231. Goldman JM: Bone marrow transplantation for patients with chronic myeloid leukemia. N Engl J Med 1986;314:202.

232. Goldman JM: Bone marrow transplantation for chronic myelogenous leukemia in chronic phase. Increased risk for relapse associated with T-cell depletion. Ann Intern Med 1988;108:806.

233. Marks DI: Allogeneic bone marrow transplantation for chronic myeloid leukemia using sibling and volunteer unrelated donors. A comparison of complications in the first 2 years. Ann Intern Med 1993;119:207.

234. Storb R: Marrow transplantation for chronic myelocytic leukemia: A controlled trial of cyclosporine versus methotrexate for prophylaxis of graft-versus-host disease. Blood 1985;66:698.

235. Kernan NA: Analysis of 462 transplantations from unrelated donors facilitated by the national marrow donor program. N Engl J Med 1993;328:593.

236. Mackowiak PA: Infections in hairy cell leukemia. Am J Med 1980;68:718.

237. Pomeroy C: Infection in myelodysplastic syndrome. Am J MEd 1991;90:338.

238. Barbui T: Infection and hemorrhage in elderly acute myeloblastic leukemia and primary myelodysplasia. Hematol Oncol 1993;11(Suppl 1):15.

239. Burden AD: Viridans streptococcal bacteraemia in patients with haematological and solid malignancies. Eur J Cancer 1991;27:409.

240. Villablanca JG: The clinical spectrum of infections with viridans streptococci in bone marrow transplant patients. Bone Marrow Transplant 1990;6:387.

241. Bisno AL: Streptococcal infections of skin and soft tissues. N Engl J Med 1996;334:240.

242. Fainstein V: Bacteremia caused by non-sporulating anaerobes in cancer patients. A 12 year experience. Medicine (Baltimore) 1989;68:151.

243. Golomb HM: Infectious complications in 127 patients with hairy cell leukemia. Am J Hematol 1984;16:393.

244. Seshadri RS: Leukemic reticuloendotheliosis: A failure of monocyte production. N Engl J Med 1976;295:181.

245. Bross J: Risk factors for nosocomial candidemia: A case-control study in adults without leukemia. Am J Med 1989;87:614.

246. De Gregorio MW: *Candida* infections in patients with acute leukemia: Ineffectiveness of nystatin prophylaxis and relationship between oropharyngeal and systemic candidiasis. Cancer 1982;50:2780.

247. Drakos PE: Invasive fungal sinusitis in patients undergoing bone marrow transplantation. Bone Marrow Transplant 1993;12:203.

248. Tollemar J: Variables predicting deep fungal infections in bone marrow transplant recipients. Bone Marrow Transplant 1989;4:635.

249. Wingard JR: Increase in *Candida krusei* infection among patients with bone marrow transplantation and neutropenia treated prophylactically with fluconazole. N Engl J Med 1991;325:1274.

250. Pagano L: Mucormycosis in patients with haematological malignancies: A retrospective clinical study of 37 cases. Br J Haematol 1997;99:331.

251. DeShazo R: Fungal sinusitis. N Engl J Med 1997;337:254.

252. Pestalozzi BC: Hepatic lesions of chronic disseminated candidiasis may become invisible during neutropenia. Blood 1997;90:3858.

253. Girmenia C: *Fusarium* infections in patients with severe aplastic anemia: Review and implications for management. Haematologica 1999;84:114.

254. Martino P: Clinical patterns of *Fusarium* infections in immunocompromised patients. J Infect 1994;28(Suppl 1):7.

255. Riley DK: Surveillance cultures in bone marrow transplant recipients: Worthwhile or wasteful? Bone Marrow Transplant 1995;15:469.

256. Thaler M: Hepatic candidiasis in cancer patients: The evolving picture of the syndrome. Ann Intern Med 1988;108:88.

257. Fisher BD: Invasive aspergillosis. Progress in early diagnosis and treatment. Am J Med 1981;71:571.

258. Morrison VA: Mucormycosis in the BMT population. Bone Marrow Transplant 1993;11:383.

259. Bustamante CI: Herpes simplex virus infection in the immunocompromised cancer patients. J Clin Oncol 1991;9:1903.

260. Higgins JPT: Herpes lymphadenitis in association with chronic lymphocytic leukemia. Cancer 1999;86:1210.

261. Kingreen D: Herpes simplex infection of the jejunum occurring in the early post-transplantation period. Bone Marrow Transplant 1997;20:989.

262. Schuchter LM: Herpes zoster infection after autologous bone marrow transplantation. Blood 1989;74:1424.

263. Wacker P: Varicella-zoster virus infections after autologous bone marrow transplantation in children. Bone Marrow Transplant 1989;4:191.

264. Han CS: Varicella zoster infection after bone marrow transplantation: Incidence, risk factors and complications. Bone Marrow Transplant 1994;13:277.

265. Bilgrami S: Varicella zoster virus infection associated with high-dose chemotherapy and autologous stem-cell rescue. Bone Marrow Transplant 1999;23:469.

266. Reusser P: Cytomegalovirus infection after autologous bone marrow transplantation: Occurrence of cytomegalovirus disease and effect on engraftment. Blood 1990;75:1888.

267. Wingard JR: Cytomegalovirus infection after autologous bone marrow transplantation with comparison to infection after allogeneic bone marrow transplantation. Blood 1988;71:1432.

268. Maciejewski JP: Infection of hematopoietic progenitor cells by human cytomegalovirus. Blood 1992;80:170.

269. von Laer D: Detection of cytomegalovirus DNA in CD34+ cells from blood and bone marrow. Blood 1995;86:4086.

270. Zhuravskaya T: Spread of human cytomegalovirus (HCMV) after infection of human hematopoietic progenitor cells: Model of HCMV latency. Blood 1997;90:2482.

271. Taichman RS: Infection and replication of human cytomegalovirus in bone marrow stromal cells: Effects on the production of IL-6, MIP-1α, and TGF-β1. Bone Marrow Transplant 1997;19:471.

272. Link H: Cytomegalovirus infection in leucocytes after bone marrow transplantation demonstrated by mRNA in situ hybridition. Br J Haematol 1993;85:573.

273. Waldman WJ: Bidirectional transmission of infectious cytomegalovirus between monocytes and vascular endothelial cells: An in vitro model. J Infect Dis 1995;171:623.

274. Walter E: Reconstitution of cellular immunity against cytomegalovirus in recipients of allogeneic bone marrow transfer of T-cell clones from the donor. N Engl J Med 1995;333:1038.

275. Reusser P: Cytomegalovirus-specific T-cell immunity in recipients of autologous peripheral blood stem cell or bone marrow transplants. Blood 1997;89:3873.

276. Courier D: Early reactivation of cytomegalovirus and high risk of interstitial pneumonitis following T-depleted BMT for adults with hematological malignancies. Bone Marrow Transplant 1996;18:347.

277. Takenaka K: Increased incidence of cytomegalovirus (CMV) infection and CMV-associated disease after allogeneic bone marrow transplantation from unrelated donors. Bone Marrow Transplant 1997;19:241.

278. Sakuma H: Risk of cytomegalovirus after peripheral blood stem cell transplantation. Bone Marrow Transplant 1997;19:49.

279. Zaia JA: Late cytomegalovirus disease in marrow transplantation is predicted by virus load in plasma. J Infect Dis 1997;176:782.

280. Humar A: Effect of cytomegalovirus infection on 1-year mortality rates among recipients of allogeneic bone marrow transplants. Clin Infect Dis 1998;26:606.

281. Nguyen Q: Late cytomegalovirus pneumonia in adult allogeneic blood and marrow transplant recipients. Clin Infect Dis 1999;28:618.

282. Atkinson K: A comparison of the pattern of interstitial pneumonitis following allogeneic bone marrow transplantation before and after the introduction of prophylactic ganciclovir therapy in 1989. Bone Marrow Transplant 1998;21:691.

283. Ljungman P: Cytomegalovirus interstitial pneumonia in autologous bone marrow transplant recipients. Bone Marrow Transplant 1994;13:209.

284. Einsele H: Incidence of local CMV infection and acute intestinal GVHD in marrow transplant recipients with severe diarrhoea. Bone Marrow Transplant 1994;14:955.

285. Pinho Vaz C: Protein-losing gastropathy associated with cytomegalovirus: A rare and late complication of allogeneic bone marrow transplantation. Bone Marrow Transplant 1996;17:887.

286. Verdonck LF: Cytomegalovirus infection causes delayed platelet recovery after bone marrow transplantation. Blood 1991;78:844.

287. Bilgrami S: Cytomegalovirus viremia, viruria and disease after autologous peripheral blood stem cell transplantation: No need for surveillance. Bone Marrow Transplant 1999;24:69.

288. Duncombe AS: IL2 activated killer cells may contribute to cytomegalovirus induced marrow hypoplasia after bone marrow transplantation. Bone Marrow Transplant 1991;7:81.

289. Sindre H: Human cytomegalovirus suppression of and latency in early hematopoietic progenitor cells. Blood 1996;88:4526.

290. Torok-Storb B: Association of specific cytomegalovirus genotypes with death from myelosuppression after marrow transplantation. Blood 1997;90:2097.

291. Azzi A: Monitoring of polyomavirus BK viruria in bone marrow transplantation patients by DNA hybridization assay and by polymerase chain reaction: An approach to assess the relationship between BK viruria and hemorrhagic cystitis. Bone Marrow Transplant 1994;14:235.

292. Appleton AL: Human herpes virus-6 infection in marrow graft recipients: Role in pathogenesis of graft-versus-host disease. Bone Marrow Transplant 1995;16:777.

293. Chakrabarti S: Isolation of viruses from stools in stem cell transplant recipients: A prospective surveillance study. Bone Marrow Transplant 2000;25:277.

294. Benz-Lemoine E: Nosocomial legionnaires' disease in bone marrow transplant unit. Bone Marrow Transplant 1991;7:61.

295. Cone RW: Human herpesvirus 6 in lung tissue from patients with pneumonitis after bone marrow transplantation. N Engl J Med 1993;329:156.

296. Deeg HJ: Interstitial pneumonitis. In Deeg HJ, Klingemann H-G, Phillips GL, eds: A Guide to Bone Marrow Transplantation. Berlin: Springer-Verlag; 1988, p 114.

297. Granena A: Interstitial pneumonitis after BMT: 15 years experience in a single institution. Bone Marrow Transplant 1993;11:453.

298. Hamilton PJ: Bone marrow transplantation and the lung. Thorax 1986;41:497.

299. Ljungman P: Respiratory virus infection in immunocompromised patients. Bone Marrow Transplant 1989;4:35.

300. Tuan IZ: Pneumocystis carinii following bone marrow transplantation. Bone Marrow Transplant 1992;10:267.

301. Zaia JA: Human cytomegalovirus-associated pneumonitis: Pathogenesis, prevention and treatment. Transplantation 1987;19(Suppl 7):125.

302. Eden OB: Medical Research Council Childhood Leukemia Trial VIII Compared with Trial II-VII: Lessons for Future Management. Haematol Bluttransfus 1987;30:1.

303. Hughes WT: Successful intermittent chemoprophylaxis for Pneumocystis carinii pneumonitis. N Engl J Med 1987;316:1627.

304. Ruebush TK: An outbreak of Pneumocystis pneumonia in children with acute lymphocytic leukemia. Am J Dis Child 1978;132:143.

305. Greene WH: Management of infection in myelosuppressed patients: Clinical trials and common sense. Exp Hematol 1985;13(Suppl 16):80.

306. Wheeler AP: Treating patients with severe sepsis. N Engl J Med 1999;340:207.

307. O'Grady N: Practice guidelines for evaluating new fever in critically ill adult patients. Clin Infect Dis 1998;26:1042.

308. Tenholder MF: Pulmonary infiltrates in leukemia. Chest 1980;78:468.

309. Heussel CP: Pneumonia in febrile neutropenic patients and in bone marrow and blood stem-cell transplant recipients: Use of high-resolution computed tomography. J Clin Oncol 1999;17:796.

310. Kramer BS: Role of serial microbiologic surveillance and clinical evaluation in the management of cancer patients with fever and granulocytopenia. Am J Med 1982;72:561.

311. Rohatiner AZS: Infection in acute myelogenous leukaemia. An analysis of 168 patients undergoing remission induction. J Hosp Infect 1981;2:135.

312. Schots R: Monitoring of C-reactive protein after allogeneic bone marrow transplantation identifies patients at risk of severe transplant-related complications and mortality. Bone Marrow Transplant 1998;22:79.

313. Gabay C: Acute-phase proteins and other systemic responses to inflammation. N Engl J Med 1999;340:448.

314. Manabe YC: Clostridium difficile colitis: An efficient clinical approach to diagnosis. Ann Intern Med 1995;123:835.

315. Whittle AT: The safety and usefulness of routine bronchoscopy before stem cell transplantation and during neutropenia. Bone Marrow Transplant 1999;24:63.

316. Johnson TM: Detection of circulating Aspergillus fumigatus antigen in bone marrow transplant patients. J Lab Clin Med 1989;114:700.

317. Walsh TJ: Laboratory diagnosis of invasive candidias: A rationale for complementary use of culture- and nonculture-based detection system. J Infect Dis 1977;1(Suppl):11.

318. Odds FC: Chromagar candida, a new differential isolation medium for presumptive identification of clinically important Candida species. J Clin Microbiol 1994;32:1923.

319. van Belkum A: PCR-mediated genotyping of *Candida albicans* strains from bone marrow transplant patients. Bone Marrow Transplant 1994;13:811.

320. Patterson TF: *Aspergillus* antigen detection in the diagnosis of invasive aspergillosis. J Infect Dis 1995;171:1553.

321. Machetti M: Comparison of an enzyme immunoassay and a latex agglutination system for the diagnosis of invasive aspergillosis in bone marrow transplant recipients. Bone Marrow Transplant 1998; 21:917.

322. Maertens J: Autopsy-controlled prospective evaluation of serial screening for circulating galactomannan by a sandwich enzyme-linked immunosorbent assay for hematological patients at risk for invasive aspergillosis. J Clin Microb 1999;37:3223.

323. Kami M: Frequent false-positive results of *Aspergillus* latex agglutination test. Cancer 1999;86:274.

324. Ascioglu S: Analysis of definitions used in clinical research or invasive fungal infections (IFI): Consensus proposal for new, standardized definitions [abstract J92]. Paper presented at the Interscience Conference on Antimicrobial Agents and Chemotherapy, September 1999, San Francisco.

325. Denning DW: Early diagnosis of invasive aspergillosis. Lancet 2000; 355:423.

326. Aurelius E: Rapid diagnosis of herpes simplex encephalitis by nested polymerase chain reaction assay of cerebrospinal fluid. Lancet 1991;337:189.

327. Webster A: Value of routine surveillance cultures for detection of CMV pneumonitis following bone marrow transplantation. Bone Marrow Transplant 1993;12:477.

328. Cathomas G: Rapid diagnosis of cytomegalovirus pneumonia in marrow transplant recipients by bronchoalveolar lavage using the polymerase chain reaction, virus culture, and the direct immuno-staining of alveolar cells. Blood 1993;81:1909.

329. Einsele H: Polymerase chain reaction to evaluate antiviral therapy for cytomegalovirus disease. Lancet 1991;338:1170.

330. Einsele H: Early occurrence of human cytomegalovirus infection after bone marrow transplantation as demonstrated by the polymerase chain reaction technique. Blood 1991;77:1104.

331. Smith KL: PCR detection of cytomegalovirus: A review. Br J Haematol 1993;84:187.

332. Vlieger AM: Cytomegalovirus antigenemia assay or PCR can be used to monitor ganciclovir treatment in bone marrow transplant recipients. Bone Marrow Transplant 1992;9:247.

333. Fajac A: Value of cytomegalovirus detection by PCR in bronchoalveolar lavage routinely performed in asymptomatic bone marrow recipients. Bone Marrow Transplant 1997;20:581.

334. Schmidt CA: Demonstration of cytomegalovirus after bone marrow transplantation by polymerase chain reaction, virus culture and antigen detection in buffy coat leukocytes. Bone Marrow Transplant 1994;13:71.

335. Bacigalupo A: CMV-antigenemia after allogeneic bone marrow transplantation: Correlation of CMV-antigen positive cell numbers with transplant-related mortality. Bone Marrow Transplant 1995; 16:155.

336. Nicholson VA: Comparison of cytomegalovirus antigenemia and shell vial culture in allogeneic marrow transplantation recipients receiving ganciclovir prophylaxis. Bone Marrow Transplant 1997; 19:37.

337. Gor D: Longitudinal fluctuations in cytomegalovirus load in bone marrow transplant patients: Relationship between peak virus load, donor/recipient serostatus, acute GVHD and CMV disease. Bone Marrow Transplant 1998;21:597.

338. Einsele H: Polymerase chain reaction monitoring reduces the incidence of cytomegalovirus disease and the duration and side effects of antiviral therapy after bone marrow transplantation. Blood 1995;86:2815.

339. Ljungman P: Use of a semi-quantitative PCR for cytomegalovirus DNA as a basis for pre-emptive antiviral therapy in allogeneic bone marrow transplant patients. Bone Marrow Transplant 1996;17:583.

340. Boeckh M: Cytomegalovirus pp65 antigenemia-guided early treatment with ganciclovir versus ganciclovir at engraftment after allogeneic marrow transplantation: A randomized double-blind study. Blood 1996;88:4063.

341. Humar A: The clinical utility of CMV surveillance cultures and antigenemia following bone marrow transplantation. Bone Marrow Transplant 1999;23:45.

342. Talbot GH: Persistent fever after recovery from granulocytopenia in acute leukemia. Arch Intern Med 1988;148:129.

343. Karp JE: Strategies to prevent or control infections after bone marrow transplants. Bone Marrow Transplant 1991;8:1.

344. Schiffer CA: Supportive care: Issues in the use of blood products and treatment of infection. Semin Oncol 1987;14:454.

345. Barton TD: The cause of fever following resolution of neutropenia in patients with acute leukemia. Clin Infect Dis 1996;22:1064.

346. Oyen WJG: Diagnosing infection in febrile granulocytopenic patients with indium-111-labeled human immunoglobulin G. J Clin Oncol 1992;10:61.

347. Cordonnier C: Diagnostic yield of bronchoalveolar lavage in pneumonitis occurring after allogeneic bone marrow transplantation. Am Rev Respir Dis 1985;132:1118.

348. Slevin ML: The role of transtracheal aspiration in the diagnosis of respiratory infection in neutropenic patients with acute leukaemia. Leuk Res 1981;5:165.

349. Springmeyer SC: Use of bronchoalveolar lavage to diagnose acute diffuse pneumonia in the immunocompromised host. J Infect Dis 1986;154:604.

350. Albert RK: Handwashing patterns in medical intensive care units. N Engl J Med 1981;304:1465.

351. Kapur D: Incidence and outcome of vancomycin-resistant enterococcal bacteremia following autologous peripheral blood stem cell transplantation. Bone Marrow Transplant 2000;25:147.

352. Maki DG: Prevention of central venous catheter-related bloodstream infection by use of an antiseptic-impregnated catheter. Ann Intern Med 1997;127:257.

353. Raad I: Central venous catheters coated with minocycline and rifampin for the prevention of catheter-related colonization and bloodstream infections. Ann Intern Med 1997;127:267.

354. Darouiche RO: A comparison of two antimicrobial-impregnated central venous catheters. N Engl J Med 1999;340:1.

355. Hensley M: American Society of Clinical Oncology: Clinical practice guidelines for the use of chemotherapy and radiotherapy protectants. J Clin Oncol 1999;17:3333.

356. Phillips K-A: Design and interpretation of clinical trials that evaluate agents that may offer protection from the toxic effects of cancer chemotherapy. J Clin Oncol 1998;16:3179.

357. Dunlop DJ: Demonstration of stem cell inhibition and myeloprotective effects of SCI/rhMIP1α in vivo. Blood 1992;79:2221.

358. List AF: Stimulation of hematopoieis by amifostine in patients with mylodysplastic syndrome. Blood 1997;90:3364.

359. List AF: A randomized placebo-controlled trial of lisofylline in HLA-identical, sibling-donor, allogeneic bone marrow transplant recipients. Bone Marrow Transplant 2000;25:283.

360. Estey EH: Treatment of newly diagnosed AML, RAEB-t or RAEB with lisofylline or placebo in addition to chemotherapy. Leukemia 1999;13:850.

361. Ferrà C: Pentoxifylline, ciprofloxacin and prednisone failed to prevent transplant-related toxicities in bone marrow transplant recipients and were associated with an increased incidence of infectious complications. Bone Marrow Transplant 1997;20:1075.

362. Ferretti GA: Control of oral mucositis and candidiasis in marrow transplantation: A prospective, double-blind trial of chlorhexidine digluconate oral rinse. Bone Marrow Transplant 1988;3:483.

363. Mahood DJ: Inhibition of fluorouracil-induced stomatitis by oral cryotherapy. J Clin Oncol 1991;9:449.

364. Attal M: Prevention of regimen-related toxicities after bone marrow transplantation by pentoxyfilline: A prospective, randomized trial. Blood 1993;82:732.

365. Duenas-Gonzalez A: Misoprostol prophylaxis for high-dose chemotherapy-induced mucositis: A randomized double-blind study. Bone Marrow Transplant 1996;17:809.

366. Staak K: Pentoxifylline promotes replication of human cytomegalovirus in vivo and in vitro. Blood 1997;89:3682.

367. Karthaus M: Prophylaxis and treatment of chemo- and radiotherapy-induced oral mucositis—are there new strategies? Bone Marrow Transplant 1999;24:1095.

368. Sonis S: The biological basis for the attenuation of mucositis: The example of interleukin-11. Leukemia 1999;13:831.

369. Schwertschlag US: Hematopoietic, immunomodulatory and epithelial effects of interleukin-11. Leukemia 1999;13:1307.

370. Schimpff SC: Infection prevention in acute nonlymphoblastic leukemia: Laminar air flow room reverse isolation with nonabsorbable oral antibiotic prophylaxis. Ann Intern Med 1975;82:351.

371. Bodey GP: Treatment of acute leukemia in protected environment units. Cancer 1979;44:431.

372. Kurrle E: The efficiency of strict reverse isolation and antimicrobial decontamination in remission induction therapy of acute leukemia. Blut 1980;40:187.

373. Dekker AW: Infection prevention in autologous bone marrow transplantation and the role of protective isolation. Bone Marrow Transplant 1994;14:89.

374. Passweg JR, Rowlings PA, Atkinson KA, et al: Influence of protective isolation on outcome of allogeneic bone marrow transplantation for leukemia. Bone Marrow Transplant 1998;21:1231.

375. Storring RA: Oral non-absorbed antibiotics prevent infection in acute non-lymphoblastic leukemia. Lancet 1977;2:837.

376. Dekker A: Prevention of infection by trimethoprim-sulfamethoxazole plus amphotericin B in patients with acute nonlymphocytic leukemia. Ann Intern Med 1981;95:555.

377. Sleijfer DTH: Infection prevention in granulocytopenic patients by selective decontamination of the digestive tract. Eur J Cancer 1980;16:859.

378. Weiser B: Prophylactic trimethoprim-sulfamethoxazole during consolidation chemotherapy for acute leukemia: A controlled trial. Ann Intern Med 1981;95:436.

379. Clavell LA: Four agent induction and intensive asparaginase therapy for treatment of childhood acute lymphoblastic leukemia. N Engl J Med 1986;315:657.

380. Colby C: A prospective randomized trial comparing the toxicity and safety of atovaquone with trimethoprim/sulfamethoxazole as *Pneumocystis carinii* pneumonia prophylaxis following autologous peripheral blood stem cell transplantation. Bone Marrow Transplant 1999;24:897.

381. Golde DW: Trimethoprim and sulfamethoxazole inhibition of hematopoiesis in vitro. Br J Haematol 1978;40:363.

382. Lew MA: Ciprofloxacin versus trimethoprim/sulfamethoxazole for prophylaxis of bacterial infections in bone marrow transplant recipients: A randomized, controlled trial. J Clin Oncol 1995; 13:239.

383. Imrie KR: Effect of antimicrobial prophylaxis on hematopoietic recovery following autologous bone marrow transplantation: Ciprofloxacin versus co-trimoxazole. Bone Marrow Transplant 1995; 15:267.

384. Archimbaud E: Pefloxacin and vancomycin vs. gentamicin, colistin sulphate and vancomycin for prevention of infections in granulocytopenic patients: A randomised double-blind study. Eur J Cancer 1991;27:174.

385. De Pauw BE: Options and limitations of long-term oral ciprofloxacin as antibacterial prophylaxis in allogeneic bone marrow transplant recipients. Bone Marrow Transplant 1990;5:179.

386. Menichetti F: Norfloxacin prophylaxis for neutropenic patients undergoing bone marrow transplantation. Bone Marrow Transplant 1989;4:489.

387. Schmeiser T: Single-drug oral antibacterial prophylaxis with ofloxacin in BMT. Bone Marrow Transplant 1993;12:57.

388. Wimperis JZ: An assessment of the efficacy of antimicrobial prophylaxis in bone marrow autografts. Bone Marrow Transplant 1991;8:363.

389. Bow EJ: Comparison of norfloxacin with cotrimoxazole for infection prophylaxis in acute leukemia. Am J Med 1988;84:847.

390. Dekker AW: Infections prophylaxis in acute leukemia: A comparison of ciprofloxacin with trimethoprim-sulfamethoxazole and colistin. Ann Intern Med 1987;106:7.

391. Winston DJ: Norfloxacin versus vancomycin/polymixin for prevention of infections in granulocytopenic patients. Am J Med 1986; 80:884.

392. Winston DJ: Ofloxacin versus vancomycin/polymixin for prevention of infections in granulocytopenic patients. Am J Med 1990; 88:36.

393. GIMEMA Infection Group: Prevention of bacterial infection in neutropenic patients with hematologic malignancies. Ann Intern Med 1991;115:7.

394. Kletter Y: Enhanced repopulation of murine hematopoietic organs in sublethally irradiated mice after treatment with ciprofloxacin. Blood 1991;78:1685.

395. Cruciani M: Prophylaxis with fluoroquinolones for bacterial infections in neutropenic patients: A meta-analysis. Clin Infect Dis 1996;23:795.

396. Engels EA: Efficacy of quinolone prophylaxis in neutropenic cancer patients: A meta-analysis. J Clin Oncol 1998;16:1179.

397. Momin F: Antimicrobial prophylaxis in bone marrow transplantation. Ann Intern Med 1995;123:205.

398. Attal M: Prevention of gram-positive infections after bone marrow transplantation by systemic vancomycin: A prospective, randomized trial. J Clin Oncol 1991;9:865.

399. Arns da Cunha C: Early gram-positive bacteremia in BMT recipients: Impact of three different approaches to antimicrobial prophylaxis. Bone Marrow Transplant 1998;21:173.

400. Bow EJ: Quinolone-based antibacterial chemoprophylaxis in neutropenic patients: Effect of augmented gram-positive activity on infectious morbidity. Ann Intern Med 1996;125:183.

401. Beelen DW: Influence of intestinal bacterial decontamination using metronidazole and ciprofloxacin or ciprofloxacin alone on the development of acute graft-versus-host disease after marrow transplantation in patients with hematologic malignancies: Final results and long-term follow-up of an open-label prospective randomized trial. Blood 1999;93:3267.

402. Perfect JR: Antifungal prophylaxis: To prevent or not. Am J Med 1993;94:233.

403. Benhamou E: Does ketoconazole prevent fungal infection in children treated with high dose chemotherapy and bone marrow transplantation? Results of a randomized placebo-controlled trial. Bone Marrow Transplant 1991;7:127.

404. Conneally E: Nebulized amphotericin B as prophylaxis against invasive aspergillosis in granulocytopenic patients. Bone Marrow Transplant 1990;5:403.

405. Jeffery GM: Intranasal amphotericin B reduces the frequency of invasive aspergillosis in neutropenic patients. Am J Med 1991; 90:685.

406. Trigg ME: Successful program to prevent *Aspergillus* infections in children undergoing marrow transplantation: Use of nasal amphotericin. Bone Marrow Transplant 1997;19:43.

407. De Paw BE: Practical modalities for prevention of fungal infections in cancer patients. Eur J Clin Microbiol Infect Dis 1997;16:32.

408. Rousy SR: Low dose amphotericin B prophylaxis against invasive *Aspergillus* infections in allogeneic marrow transplantation. Am J Med 1991;91:484.

409. Winston DJ: Fluconazole prophylaxis of fungal infections in patients with acute leukemia. Ann J Med 1993;118:495.

410. Meunier F: Chemoprophylaxis of fungal infections in granulocytopenic patients using fluconazole vs oral amphotericin B. Drug Invest 1991;3:258.

411. Bodey GP: Antifungal prophylaxis during remission induction therapy for acute leukemia. Fluconazole versus intravenous amphotericin B. Cancer 1994;73:2099.

412. Menichetti F: Preventing fungal infection in neutropenic patients with acute leukemia: Fluconazole compared with oral amphotericin B. Ann Intern Med 1994;120:913.

413. Ellis ME: Controlled study of fluconazole in the prevention of fungal infections in neutropenic patients with haematological malignancies and bone marrow transplant recipients. Eur J Clin Microb Infect Dis 1994;13:3.

414. Goodman JL: A controlled trial of fluconazole to prevent fungal infections in patients undergoing bone marrow transplantation. N Engl J Med 1992;326:845.

415. Winston DJ: Fluconazole prophylaxis of fungal infections in patients with acute leukemia. Results of a randomized placebo-controlled, double-blind, multicenter trial. Ann Intern Med 1993; 118:495.

416. Slavin MA: Efficacy and safety of fluconazole prophylaxis for fungal infections after marrow transplantation. A prospective, randomized, double-blind study. J Infect Dis 1995;171:1545.

417. Schaffner A: Effect of prophylactic fluconazole on the frequency of fungal infections, amphotericin B use, and health care costs in patients undergoing intensive chemotherapy for hematologic neoplasia. J Infect Dis 1995;172:1035.

418. Rotstein C: Randomized placebo-controlled trial of fluconazole prophylaxis for neutropenic cancer patients: Benefit based on purpose and intensity of cytotoxic therapy. Clin Infect Dis 1999; 28:331.

419. Kern W: Failure of fluconazole prophylaxis to reduce mortality or the requirement of systemic amphotericin B therapy during treatment for refractory acute myeloid leukemia. Cancer 1998; 83:291.

420. Michallet M: Pharmacokinetics of itraconazole oral solution in allogeneic bone marrow transplant patients receiving total body irradiation. Bone Marrow Transplant 1998;21:1239.

421. Menichetti F: Itraconazole oral solution as prophylaxis for fungal infections in neutropenic patients with hematologic malignancies: A randomized, placebo-controlled, double-blind, multicenter trial. Clin Infect Dis 1999;28:250.

422. Morgenstern GR: A randomized controlled trial of itraconazole versus fluconazole for the prevention of fungal infections in patients with haematological malignancies. Br J Haematol 1999; 105:901.

423. Kelsey SM: Liposomal amphotericin (AmBisone) in the prophylaxis of fungal infections in neutropenic patients: A randomised, double-blind, placebo-controlled study. Bone Marrow Transplant 1999;23:163.

424. Gluckman E: Prophylaxis of herpes infections after bone marrow transplantation by oral acyclovir. Lancet 1983;2:706.

425. Hann IM: Acyclovir prophylaxis against herpesvirus infections in severely immunocompromised patients: Randomized double blind trial. BMJ 1983;287:384.

426. Saral R: Acyclovir prophylaxis against herpes simplex virus infection in patients with leukemia—a randomized, double-blind, placebo-controlled study. Ann Intern Med 1983;99:773.

427. Saral R: Acyclovir prophylaxis of herpes simplex virus infections: A randomized, double-blind controlled trial in bone marrow transplant recipients. N Engl J Med 1981;305:63.

428. Bergmann OJ: Acyclovir prophylaxis and fever during remission-induction therapy of patients with acute myeloid leukemia: A randomized, double-blind, placebo-controlled trial. J Clin Oncol 1997;15:2269.

429. Selby PJ: The prophylactic role of intravenous and long-term oral acyclovir after allogeneic bone marrow transplantation. Br J Cancer 1989;59:434.

430. Sempere A: Long-term acyclovir prophylaxis for prevention of varicella zoster virus infection after autologous blood stem cell transplantation in patients with acute leukemia. Bone Marrow Transplant 1992;10:495.

431. Bowden RA: Cytomegalovirus immune globulin and seronegative blood products to prevent primary cytomegalovirus infection after marrow transplantation. N Engl J Med 1986;314:1006.

432. Miller WJ: Prevention of cytomegalovirus infection following bone marrow transplantation: A randomized trial of blood product screening. Bone Marrow Transplant 1991;7:227.

433. Winston DJ: Prevention and treatment of cytomegalovirus infection and disease after bone marrow transplantation in the 1990s. Bone Marrow Transplant 1991;8:7.

434. Winston DJ: Intravenous immunoglobulin and CMV-seronegative blood products for prevention of CMV infection and disease in bone marrow transplant recipients. Bone Marrow Transplant 1993; 12:283.

435. Bowden RA: A comparison of filtered leukocyte-reduced and cytomegalovirus (CMV) seronegative blood products for the prevention of transfusion-associated CMV infection after marrow transplant. Blood 1995;86:3598.

436. Filipovich AH: Circulating cytomegalovirus (CMV) neutralizing activity in bone marrow transplant recipients: Comparison of passive immunity in a randomized study of four intravenous IgG products administered to CMV-seronegative patients. Blood 1992;80:2656.

437. Winston DJ: Intravenous immune globulin for prevention of cytomegalovirus infection and interstitial pneumonia after bone marrow transplantation. Ann Intern Med 1987;106:12.

438. Messori A: Efficacy of hyperimmune anti-cytomegalovirus immunoglobulins for the prevention of cytomegalovirus infection in recipients of allogeneic bone marrow transplantation: A meta-analysis. Bone Marrow Transplant 1994;13:163.

439. Stocchi R: Management of human cytomegalovirus infection and disease after allogeneic bone marrow transplantation. Haematologica 1998;84:71.

440. Meyers JD: Acyclovir for prevention of cytomegalovirus infection and disease after allogeneic marrow transplantation. N Engl J Med 1988;318:70.

441. Prentice HG: Long-term survival in allogeneic bone marrow transplant recipients following acyclovir prophylaxis for CMV infection. Bone Marrow Transplant 1997;19:129.

442. Prentice HG: Clinical strategies for the management of cytomega-

lovirus infection and disease in allogeneic bone marrow transplant. Bone Marrow Transplant 1997;19:135.

443. Goodrich JM: Early treatment with ganciclovir to prevent cytomegalovirus disease after allogeneic bone marrow transplantation. N Engl J Med 1991;325:1601.

444. Goodrich JM: Ganciclovir prophylaxis to prevent cytomegalovirus disease after allogeneic marrow transplant. Ann Intern Med 1993; 118:173.

445. Schmidt GM: A randomized, controlled trial of prophylactic ganciclovir for cytomegalovirus pulmonary infection in recipients of allogeneic bone marrow transplants. N Engl J Med 1991;324:1005.

446. von Bueltzingsloewen A: Prophylactic use of ganciclovir for allogeneic bone marrow transplant recipients. Bone Marrow Transplant 1993;12:197.

447. Winston DJ: Ganciclovir prophylaxis of cytomegalovirus infection and disease in allogeneic bone marrow transplant recipients. Ann Intern Med 1993;118:179.

448. Verdonck LF: A risk-adapted approach with a short course of ganciclovir to prevent cytmegalovirus (CMV) pneumonia in CMV-seropositive recipients of allogeneic bone marrow transplants. Clin Infect Dis 1997;24:901.

449. Maltzaou H: Cytomegalovirus disease in adult marrow transplant recipients receiving ganciclovir prophylaxis: A retrospective study. Bone Marrow Transplant 1999;24:665.

450. Bacigalupo A: Early treatment of CMV infections in allogeneic bone marrow transplant recipients with foscarnet or ganciclovir. Bone Marrow Transplant 1994;13:753.

451. Przepiorka D: Ganciclovir three times per week is not adequate to prevent cytomegalovirus reactivation after T cell–depleted marrow transplantation. Bone Marrow Transplant 1994;13:461.

452. Atkinson K: Prophylactic ganciclovir is more effective in HLA-identical family member marrow transplant recipients than in more heavily immune-suppressed HLA-identical unrelated donor marrow transplant recipients. Bone Marrow Transplant 1995;16: 401.

453. Salzberger B: Neutropenia in allogeneic marrow transplant recipients receiving ganciclovir for prevention of cytomegalovirus disease: Risk factors and outcome. Blood 1997;90:2502.

454. Manteiga R: Cytomegalovirus pp65 antigenemia–guided pre-emptive treatment with ganciclovir after allogeneic transplantation: A single-center experience. Bone Marrow Transplant 1998;22:899.

455. Bacigalupo A: CMV prophylaxis with foscarnet in allogeneic bone marrow transplant recipients at high risk of developing CMV infections. Bone Marrow Transplant 1994;13:783.

456. Moretti S: Foscarnet vs ganciclovir for cytomegalovirus (CMV) antigenemia after allogeneic hemopoietic stem cell transplantation (HSCT): A randomised study. Bone Marrow Transplant 1998;22: 175.

457. Stocchi R: A comparison of prophylactic vs pre-emptive ganciclovir to prevent cytomegalovirus disease after T-depleted volunteer unrelated donor bone marrow transplantation. Bone Marrow Transplant 1999;23:705.

458. Diamond DJ: Development of a candidate HLA A *0201 restricted peptide-based vaccine against human cytomegalovirus infection. Blood 1997;90:1751.

459. Foot ABM: Prophylaxis of toxoplasmosis infection with pyrimethamine/sulfadoxine (Fansidar) in bone marrow transplant recipients. Bone Marrow Transplant 1994;14:241.

460. Adams RH: Pre-emptive use of aerosolized ribavirin in the treatment of asymptomatic pediatric marrow transplant patients testing positive for RSV. Bone Marrow Transplant 1999;24:661.

461. Bass EB: Efficacy of immune globulin in preventing complications of bone marrow transplantation: A meta-analysis. Bone Marrow Transplant 1993;12:273.

462. Graham-Pole J: Intravenous immunoglobulin may lessen all forms of infection in patients receiving allogeneic bone marrow transplantation for acute lymphoblastic leukemia: A Pediatric Oncology Group study. Bone Marrow Transplant 1988;3:559.

463. Poynton CH: Use of IgM enriched intravenous immunoglobulin (Pentaglobin) in bone marrow transplantation. Bone Marrow Transplant 1992;9:451.

464. Tutschka PJ: Gammaglobulin therapy in bone marrow transplantation. In Garner RJ, Sacher RA, eds: Intravenous Gammaglobulin Therapy. Arlington, VA: American Association of Blood Banks; 1988.

465. Guglielmo BJ: Immune globulin therapy in allogeneic bone marrow transplant: A critical review. Bone Marrow Transplant 1994; 13:499.

466. Copelan EA: Alternate applications of immunoglobulin following bone marrow transplantation. Semin Hematol 1992;29(Suppl 2): 96.

467. Wolff SN: High-dose weekly intravenous immunoglobulin to prevent infections in patients undergoing autologous bone marrow transplantation or severe myelosuppressor therapy. Am J Med 1993;118:937.

468. Copelan EA: Controlled trial of orally administered immunoglobulin following bone marrow transplantation. Bone Marrow Transplant 1994;13:87.

469. Besa EC: Recent advances in the treatment of chronic lymphocytic leukemia: Defining the role of intravenous immunoglobulin. Semin Hematol 1992;29(Suppl 2):14.

470. Cooperative Group for the Study of Immunoglobulin in Chronic Lymphocytic Leukemia: Intravenous immunoglobulin for the prevention of infection in chronic lymphocytic leukemia. N Engl J Med 1988;319:902.

471. Weeks JC: Cost effectiveness of prophylactic intravenous immune globulin in chronic lymphocytic leukemia. N Engl J Med 1991; 325:81.

472. Ridgway D: Active immunization of children with leukemia and other malignancies. Leuk Lymphoma 1993;9:177.

473. Wimperis JZ: Transfer of a functioning humoral immune system in transplantation of T-lymphocyte–depleted bone marrow. Lancet 1986;1:339.

474. Molrine DC: Donor immunization with *Haemophilus influenzae* type b (HIB)-conjugate vaccine in allogeneic bone marrow transplantation. Blood 1996;87:3012.

475. King SM: Response to measles, mumps and rubella vaccine in paediatric bone marrow transplant recipients. Bone Marrow Transplant 1996;17:633.

476. Engelhard D: Immune response to polio vaccination in bone marrow recipients. Bone Marrow Transplant 1991;8:295.

477. Engelhard D: Antibody response to a two-dose regimen of influenza vaccine in allogeneic T cell–depleted and autologous BMT recipients. Bone Marrow Transplant 1993;11:1.

478. Ljungman P: Response to immunization against polio after allogeneic marrow transplantation. Bone Marrow Transplant 1991;7:89.

479. Pauksen K: Immunity to and immunization against measles, rubella and mumps in patients after autologous bone marrow transplantation. Bone Marrow Transplant 1992;9:427.

480. Ljungman P: Immunisations after bone marrow transplantation: Results of a European survey and recommendations from the Infectious Diseases Working Party of the European Group for Blood and Marrow Transplantation. Bone Marrow Transplant 1995; 15:455.

481. Somani J: Reimmunization after allogeneic bone marrow transplantation. Am J Med 1995;98:389.

482. Singhal S: Reimmunization after blood or marrow stem cell transplantation. Bone Marrow Transplant 1999;23:637.

483. Ljungman P: Immunization of transplant recipients. Bone Marrow Transplant 1999;23:635.

484. Hammarstrom V: Tetanus immunity in autologous bone marrow and blood stem cell transplant recipients. Bone Marrow Transplant 1998;22:67.

485. Sieff CA: Human recombinant granulocyte-macrophage colony-stimulating factor: A multilineage hematopoietin. Science 1985; 230:1171.

486. Strife A: Activities of four purified growth factors on highly enriched human hematopoietic progenitor cells. Blood 1987;69: 1508.

487. Rowe JM: Hematopoietic growth factors in acute leukemia. Leukemia 1997;11:328.

488. Rowe JM: Treatment of acute myeloid leukemia with cytokines: Effect on duration of neutropenia and response to infections. Clin Infect Dis 1998;26:1290.

489. Dale DC: Granulocyte colony-stimulating factor—role and relationships in infectious diseases. J Infect Dis 1995;172:1061.

490. Leavey PJ: In vivo treatment with granulocyte colony-stimulating factor results in divergent effects on neutrophil functions measured in vitro. Blood 1998;92:4366.

491. Hartung T: Effect of granulocyte colony-stimulating factor treatment on ex vivo blood cytokine response in human volunteers. Blood 1995;85:2482.

492. Held TK: Granulocyte colony-stimulating factor worsens the outcome of experimental *Klebsiella pneumoniae* pneumonia through direct interaction with the bacteria. Blood 1998;91:2525.

493. Armitage JA: Emerging applications of recombinant human granulocyte-macrophage colony-stimulating factor. Blood 1998;92:4491.

494. Blanchard DK: Production of granulocyte-macrophage colony-stimulating factor by large granular lymphocytes stimulated with *Candida albicans:* Role in activation of human neutrophil function. Blood 1991;77:2259.

495. Nemunaitis J: Phase I trial of recombinant human macrophage colony-stimulating factor in patients with invasive fungal infections. Blood 1991;78:907.

496. Nemunaitis J: Long-term follow-up of patients with invasive fungal disease who received adjunctive therapy with recombinant human macrophage colony-stimulating factor. Blood 1993;82:1422.

497. Rodriguez-Adrian LJ: The potential role of cytokine therapy for fungal infections in patients with cancer: Is recovery from neutropenia all that is needed? Clin Infect Dis 1998;26:1270.

498. Giles FJ: Monocyte-macrophages, granulocyte-macrophage colony-stimulating factor, and prolonged survival among patients with acute myeloid leukemia and stem cell transplants. Clin Infect Dis 1998;26:1282.

499. Nemunaitis J: Use of macrophage colony-stimulating factor in the treatment of fungal infections. Clin Infect Dis 1998;26:1279.

500. Cairo MS: Effect of stem cell factor with and without granulocyte colony-stimulating factor on neonatal hematopoiesis: In vivo induction of newborn myelopoiesis and reduction of mortality during experimental group B streptococcal sepsis. Blood 1992;80:96.

501. Brandt SJ: Effect of recombinant human granulocyte-macrophage colony-stimulating factor on hematopoietic reconstitution after high-dose chemotherapy and autologous bone marrow transplantation. N Engl J Med 1988;318:869.

502. American Society of Clinical Oncology: Update of recommendations for the use of hematopoietic colony-stimulating factors: Evidence-based clinical practice guidelines. J Clin Oncol 1996;14: 1957.

503. Nelson S: A randomized controlled trial of filgrastim as an adjunct to antibiotics for treatment of hospitalized patients with community-acquired pneumonia. J Infect Dis 1998;178:1075.

504. Hartmann LC: Granulocyte colony-stimulating factor in severe chemotherapy-induced afebrile neutropenia. N Engl J Med 1997;336: 1776.

505. Anaissie EJ: Randomized comparison between antibiotics alone and antibiotics plus granulocyte-macrophage colony-stimulating factor (*Escherichia coli*–derived) in cancer patients with fever and neutropenia. Am J Med 1996;100:17.

506. Blazar BR: In vivo administration of recombinant human granulocyte/macrophage colony-stimulating factor in acute lymphoblastic leukemia patients receiving purged autografts. Blood 1989;73:849.

507. Carlo-Stella C: Use of recombinant human granulocyte/macrophage colony-stimulating factor in patients with lymphoid malignancies transplanted with unpurged or adjusted-dose mafosfamide-purged autologous marrow. Blood 1992;80:2412.

508. De Witte T: Recombinant human granulocyte-macrophage colony-stimulating factor accelerates neutrophil and monocyte recovery after allogeneic T-cell–depleted bone marrow transplantation. Blood 1992;79:1359.

509. Ganser A: Sequential in vivo treatment with two recombinant human hematopoietic growth factors (interleukin-3 and granulocyte-macrophage colony-stimulating factor) as a new therapeutic modality to stimulate hematopoiesis: Results of a phase I study. Blood 1992;79:2583.

510. Kantarjian HM: Granulocyte colony stimulating factor supportive treatment following intensive chemotherapy in acute lymphocytic leukemia in first remission. Cancer 1993;72:2950.

511. Naparstek E: Enhanced marrow recovery by short preincubation of marrow allografts with human recombinant interleukin-3 and granulocyte-macrophage colony-stimulating factor. Blood 1992; 80:1673.

512. Scherrer R: Granulocyte colony-stimulating factor (G-CSF) as an adjunct to induction therapy of adult acute lymphoblastic leukemia (ALL). Ann Hematol 1993;66:283.

513. Bettelheim P: Recombinant human granulocyte-macrophage col-

ony-stimulating factor in combination with standard induction chemotherapy in de novo acute myeloid leukemia. Blood 1991; 77:700.

514. Buchner T: Recombinant human granulocyte-macrophage colony-stimulating factor after chemotherapy in patients with acute myeloid leukemia at higher age or after relapse. Blood 1991;78:1190.

515. Estey E: Effects of low doses of recombinant human granulocyte-macrophage colony-stimulating factor (GM-CSF) in patients with myelodysplastic syndromes. Br J Haematol 1991;77:291.

516. Ganser A: Recombinant human granulocyte-macrophage colony-stimulating factor in patients with myelodysplastic syndromes—a phase I/II trial. Blood 1989;73:31.

517. Gradishar WJ: Clinical and cytogenetic responses to granulocyte-macrophage colony-stimulating factor in therapy-related myelodysplasia. Blood 1992;80:2463.

518. Giralt S: Preliminary results of treatment with filgrastim for relapse of leukemia and myelodysplasia after allogeneic bone marrow transplantation. N Engl J Med 1993;329:757.

519. Vellenga E: Effects of recombinant IL-3, GM-CSF, and G-CSF on proliferation of leukemic clonogenic cells in short-term and long-term cultures. Leukemia 1987;1:584.

520. Ottmann OG: Concomitant granulocyte colony-stimulating factor and induction chemoradiotherapy in adult acute lymphoblastic leukemia: A randomized phase III trial. Blood 1995;86:444.

521. Welte K: A randomized phase-III study of the efficacy of granulocyte colony-stimulating factor in children with high-risk acute lymphoblastic leukemia. Blood 1996;87:3143.

522. Geissler K: Granulocyte colony-stimulating factor as an adjunct to induction chemotherapy for adult acute lymphoblastic leukemia. A randomized phase-III study. Blood 1997;90:590.

523. Pui C-H: Human granulocyte colony-stimulating factor after induction chemotherapy in children with acute lymphoblastic leukemia. N Engl J Med 1997;336:1781.

524. Larson RA: A randomized controlled trial of filgrastim during remission induction and consolidation chemotherapy for adults with acute lymphoblastic leukemia: CALGB study 9111. Blood 1998;92:1556.

525. Ifrah N: Intensive short term therapy with granulocyte-macrophage colony-stimulating factor support, similar to therapy for acute myeloblastic leukemia, does not improve overall results for adults with acute lymphoblastic leukemia. Cancer 1999;86:1496.

526. Chen S-H: High-dose cytarabine-containing chemotherapy with or without granulocyte colony-stimulating factor children with acute leukemia. Am J Hematol 1998;58:20.

527. Bassan R: Granulocyte colony-stimulating factor (G-CSF, filgrastim) after or during an intensive remission induction therapy for adult acute lymphoblastic leukaemia: Effects, role of patient pretreatment characteristics, and costs. Leuk Lymphoma 1996;26:153.

528. Papamichael D: Intensive chemotherapy for adult acute lymphoblastic leukemia given with or without granulocyte-macrophage colony stimulating factor. Ann Hematol 1996;73:259.

529. Saven A: Filgrastim for cladribine-induced neutropenic fever in patients with hairy cell leukemia. Blood 1999;93:2471.

530. Baer MR: Biological effects of recombinant human granulocyte colony-stimulating factor in patients with untreated acute myeloid leukemia. Blood 1996;87:1484.

531. Tomonaga M: Biosynthetic (recombinant) human granulocyte-macrophage colony-stimulating factor: Effect on normal bone marrow and leukemia cell lines. Blood 1986;67:31.

532. Cannistra SA: Granulocyte-macrophage colony-stimulating factor enhances the cytotoxic effects of cytosine arabinoside in acute myeloblastic leukemia and in the myeloid blast crisis phase of chronic myeloid leukemia. Leukemia 1989;3:328.

533. Preisler H: Effects of rhGM-CSF on myeloid clonogenic cells in acute myelogenous leukemia patients. Leuk Lymphoma 1993;10: 183.

534. Bassan R: Unexpected remission of acute myeloid leukaemia after GM-CSF. Br J Haematol 1994;87:835.

535. Jahns-Streubel G: Blast cell proliferative activity and sensitivity to GM-CSF in vitro are associated with early response to TAD-9 induction therapy in acute myeloid leukemia. Leukemia 1995; 9:1857.

536. Thomas X: Granulocyte-macrophage colony-stimulating factor (GM-CSF) to increase efficacy or intensive sequential chemotherapy with etoposide, mitoxantrone and cytarabine (EMA) in pre-

viously treated acute myeloid leukemia: A multicenter randomized placebo-controlled trial (EMA91 Trial). Leukemia 1993;13:1214.

537. Schiffer CA: Hematopoietic growth factors as adjuncts to the treatment of acute myeloid leukemia. Blood 1996;88:3675.

538. Geller RB: Use of cytokines in the treatment of acute myelocytic leukemia: A critical review. J Clin Oncol 1996;14:1371.

539. Terpstra W: Application of myeloid growth factors in the treatment of acute myeloid leukemia. Leukemia 1997;11:315.

540. Harousseau J-L: The use of GM-CSF and G-CSF in the treatment of acute leukemias. Leuk Lymphoma 1995;18:405.

541. Büchner T: Hematopoietic growth factors in acute myeloid leukemia: Supportive and priming effects. Semin Oncol 1997;24:1.

542. Ohno R: Effect of granulocyte colony-stimulating factor after intensive induction therapy in relapsed or refractory acute leukemia. N Engl J Med 1990;323:871.

543. Heil G: A randomized, double-blind, placebo-controlled, phase III study of filgrastim in remission induction and consolidation therapy for adults with de novo acute myeloid leukemia. Blood 1997; 90:4710.

544. Bernasconi C: Randomized clinical study comparing aggressive chemotherapy with or without G-CSF for high-risk myelodysplastic syndromes or secondary acute myeloid leukaemia evolving from MDS. Br J Haematol 1998;102:678.

545. Godwin JE: A double-blind placebo-controlled trial of granulocyte colony-stimulating factor in elderly patients with previously untreated acute myeloid leukemia: A Southwest Oncology Group study (9031). Blood 1998;91:3607.

546. Ossenkoppele GJ: A randomized study of granulocyte colony-stimulating factor applied during and after chemotherapy in patients with poor risk myelodysplastic syndromes: A report from the HOVON cooperative group. Leukemia 1999;13:1207.

547. Estey EH: Randomization phase II study of fludarabine + cytosine arabinoside + idarubicin ± all-trans retinoic acid ± granulocyte colony-stimulating factor in poor prognosis newly diagnosed acute myeloid leukemia and myelodysplastic syndrome. Blood 1999; 93:2478.

548. Harousseau JL: Granulocyte colony-stimulating factor after intensive consolidation chemotherapy in acute myeloid leukemia: Results of a randomized trial of the Group Ouest-Est Leucémies Aigues Myeloblastiques. J Clin Oncol 2000;18:780.

549. Dombret H: A controlled study of recombinant human granulocyte colony-stimulating factor in elderly patients after treatment for acute myelogenous leukemia. N Engl J Med 1995;332:1678.

550. Heil G: GM-CSF in a double-blind randomized, placebo controlled trial in therapy of adult patients with de novo acute myeloid leukemia (AML). Leukemia 1995;9:3.

551. Stone RM: Granulocyte-macrophage colony-stimulating factor after initial chemotherapy for elderly patients with primary acute myelogenous leukemia. N Engl J Med 1995;332:1671.

552. Zittoun R: Granulocyte-macrophage colony-stimulating factor associated with induction treatment of acute myelogenous leukemia: A randomized trial by the European Organization for Research and Treatment of Cancer Leukemia Cooperative Group. J Clin Oncol 1996;14:2150.

553. Löwenberg B: Value of different modalities of granulocyte-macrophage colony-stimulating factor applied during or after induction therapy of acute myeloid leukemia. J Clin Oncol 1997;15:3496.

554. Löwenberg B: Use of recombinant granulocyte-macrophage colony-stimulating factor during and after remission induction chemotherapy in patients aged 61 years and older with acute myeloid leukemia (AML): Final report of AML-11, a phase III randomized study of the Leukemia Cooperative Group of European Organisation for the Research and Treatment of Cancer (EORTC-LCG) and the Dutch Belgian Hemato-Oncology Cooperative Group (HOVON). Blood 1997;90:2952.

555. Witz F: A placebo-controlled study of recombinant human granulocyte-macrophage colony-stimulating factor administered during and after induction treatment for de novo acute myelogenous leukemia in elderly patients. Blood 1998;91:2722.

556. Rowe JM: A randomized placebo-controlled phase III study of granulocyte-macrophage colony-stimulating factor in adult patients (>55 to 70 years of age) with acute myelogenous leukemia: A study of the Eastern Cooperative Oncology Group (E1490). Blood 1995;86:457.

557. Ohno R: Human urinary macrophage colony-stimulating factor

reduces the incidence and duration of febrile neutropenia and shortens the period required to finish three courses of intensive consolidation therapy in acute myeloid leukemia: A double-blind controlled study. J Clin Oncol 1997;15:2954.

558. Gore SD: Granulocyte-macrophage colony stimulating factor (GM-CSF), given concurrently with induction therapy for acute myelogenous leukemia (AML), augments the syndrome of T-lymphocyte recovery. Leukemia 1994;8:409.

559. Moore JO: Granulocyte-colony stimulating factor (filgrastim) accelerates granulocyte recovery after intensive postremission chemotherapy for acute myeloid leukemia with aziridinyl benzoquinone and mitoxantrone: Cancer and Leukemia Group B study 9022. Blood 1997;89:780.

560. Richard C: Recombinant human granulocyte-macrophage colony stimulating factor (rhGM-CSF) administration after autologous bone marrow transplantation for acute myeloblastic leukemia enhances activated killer cell function and may diminish leukemia relapse. Bone Marrow Transplant 1995;15:721.

561. Weisdorf DJ: Hematopoietic growth factors for graft failure after bone marrow transplantation: A randomized trial of granulocyte-macrophage colony-stimulating factor (GM-CSF) versus sequential GM-CSF plus granulocyte-CSF. Blood 1995;85:3452.

562. Lee SJ: Efficacy and costs of granulocyte colony-stimulating factor in allogeneic T-cell depleted bone marrow transplantation. Blood 1998;92:2725.

563. San Miguel JF: A randomized study comparing the effect of GM-CSF and G-CSF on immune reconstitution after autologous bone marrow transplantation. Br J Haematol 1996;94:140.

564. Link H: A controlled trial of recombinant human granulocyte-macrophage colony-stimulating factor after total body irradiation, high-dose chemotherapy, and autologous bone marrow transplantation for acute lymphoblastic leukemia or malignant lymphoma. Blood 1992;80:2188.

565. Maiche AG: Granulocyte colony-stimulating factor (G-CSF) with or without a quinolone in the prevention of infection in cancer patients. Eur J Cancer 1993;29A:1403.

566. Körbling M: The evolution of clinical peripheral blood stem cell transplantation. Bone Marrow Transplant 1996;17(Suppl 2):4.

567. Kessinger A: Autologous peripheral hematopoietic stem cell transplantation restores hematopoietic function following marrow ablative therapy. Blood 1988;71:723.

568. Molineux G: Transplantation potential of peripheral blood stem cells induced by granulocyte colony-stimulating factor. Blood 1990;76:2153.

569. Bensinger W: Autologous transplantation with peripheral blood mononuclear cells collected after administration of recombinant granulocyte stimulating factor. Blood 1993;81:3158.

570. Berenson RJ: Antigen CD34+ marrow cells engraft lethally irradiated baboons. J Clin Invest 1988;81:951.

571. Juttner CA: Autologous blood stem cell transplantation. Transplant Proc 1989;21:2929.

572. Henon PR: Comparison of hematopoietic and immune recovery after autologous bone marrow or blood stem cell transplants. Bone Marrow Transplant 1992;9:285.

573. Roberts MM: Immune reconstitution following peripheral blood stem cell transplantation, autologous bone marrow transplantation and allogeneic bone marrow transplantation. Bone Marrow Transplant 1993;12:469.

574. To LB: Comparison of haematological recovery times and supportive care requirements of autologous recovery phase peripheral blood stem cell transplants, autologous bone marrow transplants and allogeneic bone marrow transplants. Bone Marrow Transplant 1992;9:277.

575. Guillaume T: Immune reconstitution and immunotherapy after autologous hematopoietic stem cell transplantation. Blood 1998; 92:1471.

576. Shenoy S: Immune reconstitution following allogeneic peripheral blood stem cell transplants. Bone Marrow Transplant 1999;23:335.

577. Pavletic ZS: Lymphocyte reconstitution after allogeneic blood stem cell transplantation for hematologic malignancies. Bone Marrow Transplant 1998;21:33.

578. Heitger A: Effective T cell regeneration following high-dose chemotherapy rescued with CD34+ cell enriched peripheral blood progenitor cells in children. Bone Marrow Transplant 1999;23:347.

579. Andrews RG: Precursors of colony-forming cells in humans can be distinguished from colony-forming cells by expression of the CD33 and CD34 antigens and light scatter properties. J Exp Med 1989;169:1721.

580. Scott MA: In search of the haemopoietic stem cell. Br J Haematol 1995;90:738.

581. Huang S: Lymphoid and myeloid differentiation of single human CD34+, HLA-DR+, CD38− hematopoietic stem cells. Blood 1994;83:1515.

582. Dyson PG: Increased levels of megakaryocyte progenitors in peripheral blood mobilised by chemotherapy and/or haemopoietic growth factor protocols. Bone Marrow Transplant 1996;18:705.

583. Hénon P: Primordial role of CD34+38− cells in early and late trilineage haemopoietic engraftment after autologous blood cell transplantation. Br J Haematol 1998;103:56.

584. Bensinger WI: The effects of daily recombinant human granulocyte colony stimulating factor administration on normal granulocyte donors undergoing leukapheresis. Blood 1993;81:1883.

585. Peters WP: Comparative effects of granulocyte-macrophage colony-stimulating factor (GM-CSF) and granulocyte colony-stimulating factor (G-CSF) on priming peripheral blood progenitor cells for use with autologous bone marrow after high-dose chemotherapy. Blood 1993;81:1709.

586. Sanz MA: Busulfan plus cyclophosphamide followed by autologous blood stem-cell transplantation for patients with acute myeloblastic leukemia in first complete remission: A report from a single institution. J Clin Oncol 1993;11:1661.

587. Watts MJ: Crossover study of the haematological effects and pharmacokinetics of glycosylated and non-glycosylated G-CSF in healthy volunteers. Br J Haematol 1997;98:474.

588. Hoglund M: Mobilization of CD34+ cells by glycosylated and nonglycosylated G-CSF in healthy volunteers—a comparative study. Eur J Haematol 1997;59:177.

589. Lemoli RM: Positive selection of hematopoietic CD34+ stem cells provides "indirect purging" of CD34− lymphoid cells and the purging efficiency is increased by anti-CD2 and anti-CD30 immunotoxins. Bone Marrow Transplant 1994;13:465.

590. Rambaldi A: Innovative two-step negative selection of granulocyte colony-stimulating factor–mobilized circulating progenitor cells: Adequacy for autologous and allogeneic transplantation. Blood 1998;91:2189.

591. Alcorn MJ: CD34-positive cells isolated from cryopreserved peripheral-blood progenitor cells can be expanded ex vivo and used for transplantation with little or no toxicity. J Clin Oncol 1996; 14:1839.

592. Negrin RS: Minimum number of mobilized peripheral blood CD34+ cells required for rapid trilineage engraftment. Bone Marrow Transplant 1994;14(Suppl 3):87.

593. Watts MJ: Progenitor-cell mobilization after low-dose cyclophosphamide and granulocyte colony-stimulating factor: An analysis of progenitor-cell quantity and quality and factors predicting for these parameters in 101 pretreated patients with malignant lymphoma. J Clin Oncol 1997;15:535.

594. Scheid C: Using at least 5 × 10⁶/kg CD34+ cells for autologous stem cell transplantation significantly reduces febrile complications and use of antibiotics after transplantation. Bone Marrow Transplant 1999;23:1177.

595. Weaver CH: Engraftment and outcomes of patients receiving myeloablative therapy followed by autologous peripheral blood stem cells with a low CD34+ cell content. Bone Marrow Transplant 1997;19:1103.

596. Mijovic A: Do CD34+ cell counts predict haemopoietic recovery after autologous blood stem cell transplantation (ABSCT)? Br J Haematol 1995;89:226.

597. Elliott C: When to harvest peripheral-blood stem cells after mobilization therapy: Prediction of CD34-positive cell yield by preceding day CD34-positive concentration in peripheral blood. J Clin Oncol 1996;14:970.

598. Prince HM: Microbial contamination of harvested bone marrow and peripheral blood. Bone Marrow Transplant 1995;15:87.

599. Attarian H: Microbial contamination of peripheral blood stem cell collections. Bone Marrow Transplant 1996;17:699.

600. Shea TC: Sequential cycles of high-dose carboplatin administered with recombinant human granulocyte-macrophage colony-stimulating factor and repeated infusions of autologous peripheral-blood progenitor cells: A novel and effective method for delivering multiple courses of dose-intensive therapy. J Clin Oncol 1992;10:464.

601. Shea TC: Reinfusion and serial measurements of carboplatin-mobilized peripheral-blood progenitor cells in patients receiving multiple cycles of high-dose chemotherapy. J Clin Oncol 1994;12:1012.

602. Pettengell R: Multicyclic, dose-intensive chemotherapy supported by sequential reinfusion of hematopoietic progenitors in whole blood. J Clin Oncol 1995;13:148.

603. Stoppa AM: Intensive sequential chemotherapy with repeated blood stem-cell support for untreated poor-prognosis non-Hodgkin's lymphoma. J Clin Oncol 1997;15:1722.

604. Schilder RJ: Phase I trial of multiple cycles of high-dose chemotherapy supported by autologous peripheral-blood stem cells. J Clin Oncol 1999;17:2198.

605. Wandt H: Sequential cycles of high-dose chemotherapy with dose escalation of carboplatin with or without paclitaxel supported by G-CSF mobilized peripheral blood progenitor cells: A phase I/II study in advanced ovarian cancer. Bone Marrow Transplant 1999;23:763.

606. Krüger W: Early infections in patients undergoing bone marrow or blood stem cell transplantation—a 7 year single centre investigation of 409 cases. Bone Marrow Transplant 1999;23:589.

607. Nosanchuk JD: Infectious complications of autologous bone marrow and peripheral stem cell transplantation for refractory leukemia and lymphoma. Bone Marrow Transplant 1996;18:355.

608. Lee C-K: Engraftment syndrome in autologous bone marrow and peripheral stem cell transplantation. Bone Marrow Transplant 1995;16:175.

609. Ravoet C: Clinical evidence for an engraftment syndrome associated with early and steep neutrophil recovery after autologous blood stem cell transplantation. Bone Marrow Transplant 1996;18:943.

610. Reiffers J: Is there a place for blood stem-cell transplantation for the younger adult patient with acute myelogenos leukemia? J Clin Oncol 1994;12:1100.

611. To LB: Peripheral blood stem cell autografting: A new therapeutic option for AML? Br J Haematol 1987;66:285.

612. Korbling M: Autologous blood stem cell (ABSCT) versus purged bone marrow transplantation (pABMT) in standard risk AML: Influence of source and cell composition of the autograft on hemopoietic reconstitution and disease-free survival. Bone Marrow Transplant 1991;7:343.

613. Demirer T: Rapid engraftment after autologous transplantation utilizing marrow and recombinant granulocyte colony-stimulating factor–mobilized peripheral blood stem cells in patients with acute myelogenous leukemia. Bone Marrow Transplant 1995;15:915.

614. Vellenga E: Peripheral blood stem cell transplantation as an alternative to autologous marrow transplantation in the treatment of acute myeloid leukemia? Bone Marrow Transplant 1999;23:1279.

615. Visani G: Use of peripheral blood stem cells for autologous transplantation in acute myeloid leukemia patients allows faster engraftment and equivalent disease-free survival compared with bone marrow cells. Bone Marrow Transplant 1999;24:467.

616. Demirer T: Autologous transplantation with peripheral blood stem cells collected after granulocyte colony-stimulating factor in patients with acute myelogenous leukemia. Bone Marrow Transplant 1996;18:29.

617. Gondo H: Autologous peripheral blood stem cell transplantation for acute myelogenous leukemia. Bone Marrow Transplant 1997;20:821.

618. Martìn C: Autologous peripheral blood stem cell transplantation (PBSCT) mobilized with G-CSF in AML in first complete remission. Role of intensification therapy in outcome. Bone Marrow Transplant 1998;21:375.

619. De La Rubia J: Autologous blood stem cell transplantation for acute myeloblastic leukemia in first complete remission. Intensification therapy before transplantation does not prolong disease-free survival. Haematologica 1999;84:125.

620. Archimbaud E: Multicenter randomized phase II trial of idarubicin vs mitoxantrone, combined with VP-16 and cytarabine for induction/consolidation therapy, followed by feasibility study of autologous peripheral blood stem cell transplantation in elderly patients with acute myeloid leukemia. Leukemia 1999;13:843.

621. To LB: The optimization of collection of peripheral blood stem cells for autotransplantation in acute myeloid leukaemia. Bone Marrow Transplant 1989;4:41.

622. Schlenk RF: Successful collection of peripheral blood progenitor cells in patients with acute myeloid leukaemia following early consolidation therapy with granulocyte colony-stimulating factor–supported high-dose cytarabine and mitoxantrone. Br J Haematol 1997;99:386.

623. Bilgrami S: Incidence and outcome of *Clostridium difficile* infection following autologous peripheral blood stem cell transplantation. Bone Marrow Transplant 1999;23:1039.

624. Bilgrami S: *Streptococcus viridans* bacteremia following autologous peripheral blood stem cell transplantation. Bone Marrow Transplant 1998;21:591.

625. Kolbe K: Infectious complications during neutropenia subsequent to peripheral blood stem cell transplantation. Bone Marrow Transplant 1997;19:143.

626. Powles R: Autologous bone marrow or peripheral blood stem cell transplantation followed by maintenance chemotherapy for adult acute lymphoblastic leukemia in first remission: 50 cases from a single center. Bone Marrow Transplant 1995;16:241.

627. Bensinger WI: Allogeneic peripheral blood stem cell transplantation in patients with advanced hematologic malignancies: A retrospective comparison with marrow transplantation. Blood 1996;88:2794.

628. Russell JA: Allogeneic blood cell transplants for hematological malignancy: Preliminary comparison of outcomes with bone marrow transplantation. Bone Marrow Transplant 1996;17:703.

629. Blaise D: Randomized trial of bone marrow versus lenograstim-primed blood cell allogeneic transplantation in patients with early-stage leukemia: A report from the Société Francaise de Greffe de Moelle. J Clin Oncol 2000;18:537.

630. Quagliarello VJ: Treatment of bacterial meningitis. N Engl J Med 1997;336:708.

630a. Powles R, Mehta J, Kulkarni S, et al: Allogeneic blood and bone-marrow stem cell transplantation in haematological malignant diseases: A randomised trial. Lancet 2000;355:1231.

631. Blot F: Prognostic factors for neutropenic patients in an intensive care unit: Respective roles of underlying malignancies and acute organ failures. Eur J Cancer 1997;33:1031.

632. Jackson SR: Admission of bone marrow transplant recipients to the intensive care unit: Outcome, survival and prognostic factors. Bone Marrow Transplant 1998;21:697.

633. Malik IA: Randomised comparison of oral ofloxacin alone with combination of parenteral antibiotics in neutropenic febrile patients. Lancet 1992;339:1092.

634. Rubenstein EB: Outpatient treatment of febrile episodes in low-risk neutropenic patients with cancer. Cancer 1993;71:3640.

635. Malik IA: Feasibility of outpatient management of fever in cancer patients with low-risk neutropenia: Results of a prospective randomized trial. Am J Med 1995;98:224.

636. Kern WV: Oral versus intravenous empirical antimicrobial therapy for fever in patients with granulocytopenia who are receiving cancer chemotherapy. N Engl J Med 1999;341:312.

637. Freifeld A: A double-blind comparison of empirical oral and intravenous antibiotic therapy for low-risk febrile patients with neutropenia during cancer chemotherapy. N Engl J Med 1999;341:305.

638. Mullen CA: Outpatient treatment of fever and neutropenia for low risk pediatric cancer patients. Cancer 1999;86:126.

639. Hidalgo M: Outpatient therapy with oral ofloxacin for patients with low risk neutropenia and fever. Cancer 1999;85:213.

640. Ramphal R: Is monotherapy for febrile neutropenia still a viable alternative? Clin Infect Dis 1999;29:508.

641. Winston DJ: Beta-lactam antibiotic therapy in febrile granulocytopenic patients. A randomized trial comparing cefoperazone plus piperacillin, ceftazidime plus piperacillin, and imipenem alone. Ann Intern Med 1991;115:849.

642. Freifeld AG: Monotherapy for fever and neutropenia in cancer patients: A randomized comparison of ceftazidime versus imipenem. J Clin Oncol 1995;13:165.

643. Aparicio J: Randomised comparison of ceftazidime and imipenem as initial monotherapy for febrile episodes in neutropenic cancer patients. Eur J Cancer 1996;32A:1739.

644. Raad II: How should imipenem-cilastatin be used in the treatment of fever and infection in neutropenic cancer patients? Cancer 1998;82:2449.

645. Sanders WE: Piperacilin/tazobactam: A critical review of the evolving clinical literature. Clin Infect Dis 1996;22:107.

646. Winston DJ: Randomized comparison of sulbactam/cefoperazone with imipenen as empirical monotherapy for febrile granulocytopenic patients. Clin Infect Dis 1998;26:576.

647. Gilbert DN: Outpatient parenteral antimicrobial-drug therapy. N Engl J Med 1997;337:829.

648. Rolston KVI: A comparison of imipenem to ceftazadine with or without amikacin as empiric therapy in febrile neutropenic patients. Arch Intern Med 1992;152:283.

649. EORTC International Antimicrobial Therapy Cooperative Group: Ceftazidime combined with a short or long course of amikacin for empirical therapy of gram-negative bacteremia in cancer patients with granulocytopenia. N Engl J Med 1987;317:1692.

650. Keating MJ: A randomized comparative trial of three aminoglycosides—comparison of continuous infusions of gentamicin, amikacin and sisomicin combined with carbenicillin in the treatment of infections in neutropenic patients with malignancies. Medicine (Baltimore) 1979;58:159.

651. Klastersky J: Prospective randomized comparison of three antibiotic regimens for empirical therapy of suspected bacteremic infection in febrile granulocytopenic patients. Antimicrob Agents Chemother 1986;29:263.

652. Love LJ: Randomized trial of empiric antibiotic therapy with ticarcillin in combination with gentamicin, amikacin or netilmicin in febrile patients with granulocytopenia and cancer. Am J Med 1979;66:603.

653. Pizzo PA: Empiric antibiotic and antifungal therapy for cancer patients with prolonged fever and granulocytopenia. Am J Med 1982;72:101.

654. The International Antimicrobial Therapy Cooperative Group of the European Organization for Research and Treatment of Cancer: Efficacy and toxicity of single daily doses of amikacin and ceftriaxone versus multiple daily doses of amikacin and ceftazidime for infection in patients with cancer and granulocytopenia. Ann Intern Med 1993;119:584.

655. Cordonnier C: Cefapime/amikacin versus cetazidime/amikacin as empirical therapy for febrile episodes in neutropenic patients: A comparative study. Clin Infect Dis 1997;24:41.

656. Craig WA: Continuous infusion of beta-lactam antibiotics. Antimicrob Agents Chemother 1992;36:2577.

657. Raad II: A comparison of aztreonam plus vancomycin and imipenem plus vancomycin as initial therapy for febrile neutropenia cancer patients. Cancer 1996;77:1386.

658. Karp JE: Empiric use of vancomycin during prolonged treatment-induced granulocytopenia: Randomized, double-blind, placebo-controlled trial in patients with acute leukemia. Am J Med 1986;81:237.

659. Dompeling EC: Early identification of neutropenic patients at risk of gram-positive bacteraemia and the impact of empirical administration of vancomycin. Eur J Cancer 1996;32A:1332.

660. Koya R: Analysis of the value of empiric vancomycin administration in febrile neutropenia occurring after autologous peripheral blood stem cell transplants. Bone Marrow Transplant 1998;21:923.

661. Feld R: Vancomycin as part of initial empirical antibiotic therapy for febrile neutropenia in patients with cancer: Pros and cons. Clin Infect Dis 1999;29:503.

662. Kureishi A: Double-blind comparison of teicoplanin versus vancomycin in febrile neutropenic patients receiving concomitant tobramycin and piperacillin: Effect on cyclosporin A–associated nephrotoxicity. Antimicrob Agents Chemother 1991;35:2246.

663. Fauser AA: A randomized clinical trial of ceftriaxone and teicoplanin versus ceftazidime and teicoplanin as antibiotic therapy in febrile neutropenia cancer patients and bone marrow transplant recipients. Infection 1994;22:271.

664. EORTC International Antimicrobial Therapy Cooperative Group: Empiric antifungal therapy in febrile granulocytopenic patients. Am J Med 1989;86:668.

665. Kleinfeld DI: Parenteral therapy for antibiotic-associated pseudomembranous colitis. J Infect Dis 1988;157:389.

666. Chirletti P: The surgical choice in neutropenic patients with hematological disorders and acute abdominal complications. Leuk Lymphoma 1993;9:237.

667. Martìnez E: Central venous catheter exchange by guidewire for treatment of catheter-related bacteraemia in patients undergoing BMT or intensive chemotherapy. Bone Marrow Transplant 1999;23:41.

668. Walsh TJ: Amphotericin B vs high-dose ketoconazole for empirical antifungal therapy among febrile, granulocytopenic cancer patients. Arch Intern Med 1991;151:765.

669. Viscoli C: Fluconazole versus amphotericin B as empirical antifungal therapy of unexplained fever in granulocytopenic cancer patients: A pragmatic, multicenter, prospective and randomised clinical trial. Eur J Cancer 1996;32A:814.

670. Malik IA: A randomized comparison of fluconazole with amphotericin B as empiric anti-fungal agents in cancer patients with prolonged fever and neutropenia. Am J Med 1998;105:478.

671. Rex JH: A randomized trial comparing fluconazole with amphotericin B for the treatment of candidemia in patients without neutropenia. N Engl J Med 1994;331:1325.

672. Anaissie EJ: Fluconazole versus amphotericin B in the treatment of hematogenous candidiasis: A matched cohort study. Am J Med 1996;101:170.

673. Anaissie EJ: Management of invasive candidal infections: Results of a prospective, randomized, multicenter study of fluconazole versus amphotericin B and review of the literature. Clin Infect Dis 1996;23:964.

674. Edwards JE: International conference for the development of a consensus on the management and prevention of severe candidal infections. Clin Infect Dis 1997;25:43.

675. Walsh TJ: Successful treatment of hepatosplenic candidiasis through repeated cycles of chemotherapy and neutropenia. Cancer 1995;76:2357.

676. Denning DW: Treatment of invasive aspergillosis with itraconazole. Am J Med 1989;86:791.

677. Severens JL: Two strategies for managing invasive aspergillosis: A decision analysis. Clin Infect Dis 1997;25:1148.

678. Schwartz S: Successful treatment of cerebral aspergillosis with a novel triazole (voriconazole) in a patient with acute leukaemia. Br J Haematol 1997;97:663.

679. Leenders ACAP: The use of lipid formulations of amphotericin B for systemic fungal infections. Leukemia 1996;10:1570.

680. White MH: Amphotericin B colloidal dispersion vs amphotericin B as therapy for invasive aspergillosis. Clin Infect Dis 1997;24:635.

681. Noskin G: Treatment of invasive fungal infections with amphotericin B colloidal dispersion in bone marrow transplant recipients. Bone Marrow Transplant 1999;23:697.

682. Ringden O: Severe and common side-effects of amphotericin B lipd complex (Abelcet). Bone Marrow Transplant 1998;22:733.

683. Kruger W: Experience with liposomal amphotericin-B in 60 patients undergoing high-dose therapy and bone marrow or peripheral blood stem cell transplantation. Br J Haematol 1995;91:684.

684. Mills W: Liposomal amphotericin B in the treatment of fungal infections in neutropenic patients: A single-centre experience of 133 episodes in 116 patients. Br J Haematol 1994;86:754.

685. Walsh TJ: Amphotericin B lipid complex for invasive fungal infections: Analysis of safety and efficacy in 556 cases. Clin Infect Dis 1998;26:1383.

686. Mehta J: Amphotericin B lipid complex (ABLC) for the treatment of confirmed or presumed fungal infections in immunocompromised patients with hematologic malignancies. Bone Marrow Transplant 1997;20:39.

687. Lister J: Amphotericin B lipid complex (ABELCET) in the treatment of invasive mycoses: The North American experience. Eur J Haematol 1996;56(Suppl 57):18.

688. Clark AD: A comparative analysis of lipid-complexed and liposomal amphotericin B preparations in hematological oncology. Br J Haematol 1998;103:198.

689. Prentice HG: A randomized comparison of liposomal versus conventional amphotericin B for the treatment of pyrexia of unknown origin in neutropenic patients. Br J Haematol 1997;98:711.

690. Leenders ACAP: Liposomal amphotericin B compared with amphotericin B deoxycholate in the treatment of documented and suspected neutropenia-associated invasive fungal infections. Br J Haematol 1998;103:205.

691. White MH: Randomized, double-blind clinical trial of amphotericin B colloidal dispersion vs. amphotericin B in the empirical treatment of fever and neutropenia. Clin Infect Dis 1998;27:296.

692. Ellis M: An EORTC international multicenter randomized trial (EORTC number 19923) comparing two dosages of liposomal amphotericin B for treatment of invasive aspergillosis. Clin Infect Dis 1998;27:1406.

693. Walsh TJ: Liposomal amphotericin B for empirical therapy in patients with persistent fever and neutropenia. N Engl J Med 1999;340:764.

694. Wingard JR: A randomized double blind safety study of Ambisone and Abelcet in febrile neutropenic patients. Paper presented at the 9th Focus on Fungal Infections, March 17–19, 1999, San Diego, CA.

695. Richardson MD: Antifungal therapy in "bone marrow failure." Br J Haematol 1998;100:619.

696. Whitley RJ: Acyclovir: A decade later. N Engl J Med 1992;327:782.

697. Tyring S: Famciclovir for the treatment of acute herpes zoster: Effects on acute disease and postherpetic neuralgia. Ann Intern Med 1995;123:89.

698. Whitley RJ: Acyclovir with and without prednisone for the treatment of herpes zoster. Ann Intern Med 1996;125:376.

699. Kost RG: Postherpetic neuralgia—pathogenesis, treatment, and prevention. N Engl J Med 1996;335:32.

700. Ljungman P: Use of intravenous immune globulin in addition to antiviral therapy in the treatment of CMV gastrointestinal disease in allogeneic bone marrow transplant patients: A report from the European Group of Blood and Marrow Transplantation (EBMT). Bone Marrow Transplant 1998;21:473.

701. Reed EC: Treatment of cytomegalovirus pneumonia with ganciclovir and intravenous cytomegalovirus immunoglobulin in patients with bone marrow transplant. Ann Intern Med 1988;109:783.

702. Troussard X: Virus recovery from stools of patients undergoing bone marrow transplantation. Bone Marrow Transplant 1993;12:573.

703. Fouillard L: Severe respiratory syncytial virus pneumonia after autologous bone marrow transplantation: A report of three cases and review. Bone Marrow Transplant 1992;9:97.

704. Sparrelid E: Ribavirin therapy in bone marrow transplant recipients with viral respiratory tract infections. Bone Marrow Transplant 1997;19:905.

705. Whimbey E: Combination therapy with aerosolized ribavirin and intravenous immunoglobulin for respiratory syncytial virus disease in adult bone marrow transplant recipients. Bone Marrow Transplant 1995;16:393.

706. Liu LX: Antiparasitic drugs. N Engl J Med 1996;334:1178.

707. Strauss RG: Therapeutic granulocyte transfusions in 1993. Blood 1993;81:1675.

708. Herzig RH: Successful granulocyte transfusion therapy for gram-negative septicemia. N Engl J Med 1977;296:701.

709. Higby DJ: Filtration leukapheresis for granulocytic transfusion therapy. N Engl J Med 1975;292:761.

710. Vogler WR: A controlled study of the efficacy of granulocyte transfusion in patients with neutropenia. Am J Med 1977;63:548.

711. Clarke K: Multiple granulocyte transfusions facilitating successful unrelated bone marrow transplantation in a patient with very severe aplastic anemia complicated by suspected fungal infection. Bone Marrow Transplant 1995;16:723.

712. Dale DC: Renewed interest in granulocyte transfusion therapy. Br J Haematol 1997;98:497.

713. Lee JH: A controlled comparison of the efficacy of hetastarch and pentastarch in granulocyte collections by centrifugal leukapheresis. Blood 1995;86:4662.

714. Ziegler EJ: Treatment of gram-negative bacteremia and shock with human antiserum to a mutant Escherichia coli. N Engl J Med 1982;307:1225.

715. Ziegler EJ: Treatment of gram-negative bacteremia and septic shock with HA-1A human monoclonal antibody against endotoxin. N Engl J Med 1991;324:429.

716. Bernard GR, Vincent J-L, Laterre P-F, et al: Efficacy and safety of recombinant human activated protein C for severe sepsis. N Engl J Med 2001;344:699.

15

Tiziano Barbui   Guido Finazzi   Anna Falanga

Management of Bleeding and Thrombosis in Acute Leukemia and Chronic Myeloproliferative Disorders

BLEEDING AND THROMBOSIS IN ACUTE LEUKEMIA

Bleeding in patients with untreated acute leukemia is mostly due to thrombocytopenia, almost always a direct result of bone marrow invasion by leukemic cells. After intensive remission induction chemotherapy and consolidation, a further contributory factor for the development of hemorrhagic complications is the myelosuppressive effect of most active drugs. The probability of developing life-threatening hemorrhages varies according to the types of acute leukemia and the therapy. Whereas most if not all patients with acute leukemia may have mild mucocutaneous bleeding that is responsive to platelet transfusion and chemotherapy, instances in which bleeding complications are life-threatening can develop and require separate analysis. The risk of life-threatening bleeding is critically important; with proper therapy, death can be prevented.

Thrombosis of large vessels is rarely seen in myeloblastic leukemia but is considered an emerging problem in acute lymphoblastic leukemia both in children and adults.[1]

PREVALENCE

Acute Myeloid Leukemia

During Remission Induction

A precise evaluation of the incidence of life-threatening bleeding (LTB) in acute leukemia patients is hampered by the different descriptive criteria used by clinical investigators and by incomplete reporting of data. Fatal bleeding at diagnosis and before any chemotherapy is very rare in the modern age of acute leukemia management. In a series of 305 consecutive adult patients with acute myeloid leukemia (AML),[2] we observed 4 cases of lethal bleeding on day of admission (1%), all in patients with marked hyperleukocytosis or acute promyelocytic leukemia (AML-M3). In 341 children treated in the Tenth Medical Council AML Trial, 2 deaths (0.6%) occurred before any treatment. Both children had French-American-British (FAB) subtype M4 (myelomonocytic), with a moderately high presenting white blood cell count, 92.4 and 60.7 x 10^9/L respectively, and died from pulmonary hemorrhages.[3] More substantial data are available concerning deaths after treatment has commenced. In an updated study from M.D. Anderson Hospital on the causes of initial remission induction failure in patients with AML and myelodysplastic syndromes,[4] 16 of 475 (3.3%) patients died of hemorrhage alone; in a further 31 patients (6.6%) hemorrhage was a concomitant cause of death with infection or organ failure. Thus, the overall hemorrhagic death rate was 9.9%. Pulmonary bleeding accounted for the majority of hemorrhagic deaths, being almost three times as common as fatal cerebral hemorrhage. In a report from St. Bartholomew's Hospital, hemorrhagic deaths occurred in 7% of treated cases.[5] In another study reporting hemorrhage as a contributory cause of death, as in the M.D. Anderson study, these figures increase up to 33% of all patients, or 45% of those who die within the first 40 days of treatment.[6] In the Tenth Medical Council trial, 7 children (2%) died in the early stages of treatment for pulmonary or cerebral hemorrhage.[3] Hemorrhagic deaths were associated with M4 and M5 morphology, high initial white blood cell count and, in two cases, concomitant infections. These data suggest a strong correlation between unresolved infection in the pancytopenic patient and terminal hemorrhage, either from the involved site or through a mechanism of generalized tissue damage, as in the case of septicemia. Destructive lesions from infection by *Aspergillus* species involve the vascular walls. The influence of thrombocytopenia and/or disordered hemostasis is predominant in the early treatments days, particularly in acute promyelocytic and hyperleukocytic leukemias. Later on during induction treatment, hemorrhages are often the result of a persistent pancytopenic state in conjunction with infections.

363

Infected patients at any stage of the disease are treated with antibiotics. The inhibitory effect on platelet function by penicillins and β-lactams may represent a cofactor for bleeding episodes in thrombocytopenic states.[7]

During Consolidation

Patients with acute leukemia in remission must be considered differently. Currently, postremission therapy is administered at an increased intensity; many investigators recommend allogeneic or autologous bone marrow transplantation (BMT) in first remission. Obviously, coagulation abnormalities and blast cell numbers play a minor role in this phase of treatment. Exceptions to this may be autoimmune thrombocytopenia, persistent thrombocytopenia owing to graft failure, and thrombotic thrombocytopenic purpura secondary to bone marrow transplantation. During consolidation, more commonly, thrombocytopenia is a direct consequence of myelosuppressive therapy but, again, concurrent infections may contribute to the pathogenesis of LTB. Occasionally, in patients receiving repeated myelosuppressive therapy who have been multiply transfused, LTB may follow the onset of refractoriness to platelet transfusion. The incidence of remission deaths caused specifically by hemorrhage is very low when platelet support is adequate. In AML studies dealing in detail with this aspect, the following rates were reported:1 out of 184 patients,[8] 3 (1 with sepsis) out of 123,[9] 4 out of 170,[10] 1 out 27,[11] 1 out of 67,[11] 1 out of 37,[12] and 0 out of 155.[13] The cumulative rate from these studies is 1.5%. This estimate appears reliable, given that remission deaths are not reported[5] and are not fully characterized.[2, 14, 15] Acute bleeding after BMT was specifically investigated in 1402 patients (289 with AML) receiving transplants at Johns Hopkins Hospital between 1986 and 1995.[16] Moderate and severe bleeding was seen in 23% and 32% of all and AML patients, respectively, and was more common in allogeneic (31%) and unrelated transplants (62.5%), compared with autologous BMT (18.5%) cases. Fourteen percent of patients had moderate or severe gastrointestinal hemorrhage, 6.4% had hemorrhagic cystitis, 2.8% had pulmonary hemorrhage, and 2% had intracranial hemorrhage. Bleeding was the cause of death in 13 of 258 patients (5%), who died within 100 days of transplantation, and was associated with significantly reduced survival both in the overall population and in AML patients. Another relevant problem is whether LTB and related deaths in remission are more frequent in selected risk groups. Preisler et al[15] reported an increased rate of remission deaths by any cause in older rather than younger patients. The death rates were 14% and 9% in patients aged 60 years and more and 40 to 60 years, respectively, compared with only 3% in those younger than 40 years. It may therefore be reasonable to assume that either LTB or LTB plus infection caused approximately one-third of these deaths. Thus, the higher hemorrhagic risk shared by older people must be explainable by factors other than thrombocytopenia. Natural candidates are comorbid diseases, which are more common in the elderly and favor vascular injury and/or predispose to bleeding, such as diabetes, arterial hypertension, and hepatic dysfunction. In addition, elderly patients with acute leukemia are particularly susceptible to infections during chemotherapy, which may aggravate the hemorrhagic tendency, or they may suffer from prolonged periods of thrombocytopenia following chemotherapy.[14, 17, 18] These same patients often develop acute leukemia on a background of a pre-existing myelodysplasia, a situation in which qualitative other than quantitative platelet defects have been described.[19] Table 15–1 reports the approximate frequencies of fatal bleeding in AML patients undergoing intensive treatment programs, according to the different therapeutic phases and the possible predisposing factors.

Acute Promyelocytic Leukemia

Acute promyelocytic leukemia (APL) (AML-M3) typically presents with a life-threatening hemorrhagic diathesis,[20, 21] which is particularly severe in the microgranular variant (M3v), characterized by marked hyperleukocitosis.[22, 23] Before the introduction of all-*trans* retinoic acid (ATRA) in the management of APL patients, fatal hemorrhage caused by the APL-associated coagulopathy was a major cause of induction remission failure.[24] In a prospective multicenter study of 268 consecutive APL patients treated between 1984 and 1987, the overall remission rate was 62% (167 of 268), and the incidence rate of hemorrhagic deaths in induction was 14% (37 of 268). The rate of early hemorrhagic deaths was similar among patients given heparin, antifibrinolytics, or supportive therapy alone for management of the coagulopathy.[25]

Since the first clinical experiences, ATRA has produced a high complete remission (CR) rate and a rapid resolution of the coagulopathy without causing bone marrow hypoplasia.[26, 27] ATRA promotes the terminal differentiation of leukemic promyelocytes. In these cells, the fusion of the nuclear retinoic acid receptor (RARα) gene on chromosome 17 with part of the PML gene on chromosome 15 results in the expression of a chimeric PML/RARα protein, which is involved in both the leukemogenesis and the sensitivity to myeloid differentiation induced

TABLE 15–1. Incidence, Timing, and Predisposing Factors for Lethal Bleeding in AML

Treatment Phase	Approximate Prevalence (All Patients in Study)	Predisposing Factors (In Addition to Thrombocytopenia)
Admission, pretreatment	1%	Acute promyelocytic leukemia (M3) Myelomonocytic leukemia (M4) Hyperleukocytosis >50 × 10⁹/L
Remission induction	5–7% (alone) 10%–33% (with infection)	As above, plus infection, older age Myelodysplasia
Consolidation	1.5%	Infection Drug-related cytopenia

TABLE 15–2. CR and Early Mortality in Studies with More than 100 APL Patients Treated with ATRA and Chemotherapy

Reference	Patients, n.	% CR	Deaths in Induction (%)	
			Total	Hemorrhagic
Kanamaru, 1995	109	89	8	NR
Mandelli, 1997	434	92	2	1
Tallman, 1997	172	72	11	6
Fenaux, 1999	413	92	7	2.4
Burnett, 1999	239	87 (extend ATRA)	4	NR
		70 (short ATRA)	13	NR
Sanz, 1999	123	89	10	6.5

by ATRA.[20] In nonrandomized studies compared with historical controls treated with conventional chemotherapy, APL patients administered ATRA showed a 9% to 20% improvement of the CR rate and a 5% to 6% reduction of early hemorrhagic deaths.[28-32] These preliminary findings have been confirmed by randomized clinical trials.[33-37] APL patients treated with different combination of ATRA plus chemotherapy showed a incidence rate of early hemorrhagic deaths ranging between 2.4% and 6.5%. Prognostic factors for early death were older age and higher WBC count. Current estimates of the rate of LTB in APL patients are reported in Table 15-2.

Acute Lymphoblastic Leukemia

Acute lymphoblastic leukemia (ALL), a syndrome characterized by bleeding and thrombosis, was first recognized by Priest et al[38] in 18 out of 1370 (1.2%) children, with ALL treated in eight institutions of the Children's Cancer Study Group[38] with polichemotherapeutic protocols including L-asparaginase (L-Ase). Fourteen of the 18 patients had thrombohemorrhagic events in the central nervous system, including dural sinus thrombosis and cerebral hemorrhagic infarction. In addition, some children developed deep vein thrombosis of the lower limbs, associated with cerebral hemorrhage. Subsequently, other authors confirmed these observations, reporting cerebral thrombohemorrhagic accidents and peripheral deep vein thrombosis in 2.4% to 11.5% of children with ALL.[39, 40] In

adults, hemorrhage was the main cause of early death during remission induction in 170 ALL patients treated by Hoelzer et al[41] with an intensive regimen including L-Ase. A comparable rate of vascular complications was reported in ALL patients treated without L-Ase[42] at Sloan Kettering Memorial Hospital. Out of 156 adult ALL patients, 19 (12%) had major bleeding or thrombosis, the incidence of thrombohemorrhagic events being significantly higher in the group with laboratory signs of disseminated intravascular coagulation (DIC) than in those without (34% vs 10%). To evaluate the incidence of bleeding and thrombosis, we have retrospectively reviewed our adult ALL file. From 1979 to 1991, 143 consecutive and newly diagnosed patients entered three sequential programs of varying intensity,[43-45] but with the same remission induction protocol, including Adriamycin, vincristine, prednisolone, and L-Ase. The overall CR rate was 82.5%, and the probability of being in first continous CR after 5 years was about 40%. During remission induction, major bleeding (World Health Organization grade 3–4) was observed in 16 patients (11%) and thrombotic complications in 9 (6%). Hemostatic complications were fatal in 4 cases (3%). In June 1991, idarubicin was substituted for Adriamycin,[46] and the first 16 patients were treated with idarubicin 36 mg/m² administered together with a 7-day L-Ase course, vincristine, and prednisolone. The CR rate was only 44%, because of the high incidence of toxic deaths. In 7 patients, hemorrhagic and/or thrombotic events were implicated among the complications responsible for treatment failure and death. In a second phase, the cumulative dosage of idarubicin was reduced to 20 mg/m2, and the administration of L-Ase was delayed by a week. The CR rate in 80 cases was 90%.[47] Only five major hemorrhagic complications were observed, three of which were fatal (3.7%). The types of hemorrhagic and thrombotic events, registered during remission induction in all 239 patients, are listed in Table 15-3.

PATHOGENESIS

The Physiology of the Hemostatic System

In normal hemostasis, the coagulation pathway is started at the local site of vascular injury. First, platelets adhere to the exposed subendothelium surface forming the platelet plug, which favors the interaction of clotting factors. Then, a sequence of reactions involving conversion of

TABLE 15–3. Sites of Bleeding and Thrombosis in 37 of 239 (15%) Adult ALL Patients (1979–1993)

	n.	(fatal)
Major bleeding (WHO Grade 3–4)	25	(10)
Cerebral	3	(3)
Pulmonary	3	(3)
Gastrointestinal	5	(4)
Macrohematuria	3	
Epistaxis	7	
Retinal	3	
Menometrorrhagia	1	
Thrombosis	12	(4)
Cerebral	9	(3)
Pulmonary embolism	1	(1)
Deep veins of the legs	2	

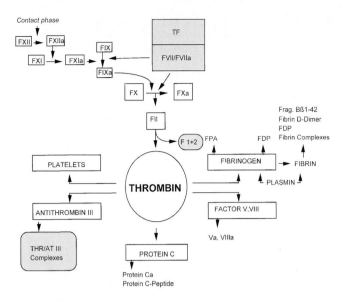

FIGURE 15–1. Schematics of blood coagulation and fibrinolysis.

proenzyme into active enzyme is started. The final product of this process is fibrin formation, which provides hemostasis and allows tissue repair.[48] The clotting cascade (Fig. 15-1) is triggered by the so-called intrinsic and extrinsic pathways of coagulation, according to old nomenclature. Such a distinction has been overcome by the demonstration that the two pathways share several reactions. At the end, both pathways lead to the activation of factor X (FX) into FXa, which plays a central role in clotting reactions. The intrinsic pathway corresponds to the contact activation that, through conversion of FXII to FXIIa and FXI to FXIa, activates FIX. FIXa, in the presence of its cofactor FVIII, converts FX to FXa. The extrinsic pathways involve the clotting reactions triggered by tissue thromboplastin or tissue factor (TF). TF is a membrane glycolipoprotein acting as a cofactor for the circulating FVII.[49] The activated TF/FVII complex promotes the proteolysis of FX to FXa. In addition, this complex also converts FIX to FIXa. Therefore, it activates both the intrinsic and the extrinsic pathways. FXa, in the presence of FVa, Ca^{2+}, and phospholipids, converts prothrombin (FII) to thrombin (FIIa), with the liberation of an inactive and stable peptide—the prothrombin fragment $1 + 2$ (F1 + 2).[50] The thrombin formed is either inactivated by its major physiologic inhibitor antithrombin (AT), thus forming the thrombin-AT complex (TAT), or it reacts with its substrate fibrinogen, with the formation of fibrin monomers and the simultaneous liberation of inactive peptides, the fibrinopeptides A and B (FP A and B).[51] In addition, thrombin can be captured and bound by thrombomodulin (TM), a highly specific thrombin receptor expressed by endothelial cells (EC).[52] The TM/thrombin complex is able to activate protein C (PCa), which acts, with its cofactor protein S (PS), as a potent inhibitor of the clotting system by degrading FVIII and FV.[53, 54] This is a mechanism by which thrombin can counteract its own prothrombotic action. The fibrin formed as the final product of clotting is stabilized by the action of FXIII, which is activated into FXIIIa by throm-

bin, and promotes the cross-linking of the fibrin monomers at the D domain site.[55] Cross-linked fibrin is a substrate for plasmin, the proteolytic enzyme produced by the activation of the fibrinolytic system. The fibrinolytic system, also named plasminogen activator system, is a highly regulated enzyme cascade that serves to generate localized proteolysis. Plasmin, the effector enzyme of this system, is the principal fibrin-degrading enzyme. It is generated from its precursor plasminogen through the actions of plasminogen activators (PA) of which two are well characterized, tissue-type PA (t-PA) and urinary-type PA (u-PA).[56, 57] t-PA, the major PA of blood vessels, has a high affinity for fibrin and therefore converts plasminogen to plasmin only within the consolidated fibrin clot and not in the fluid phase. The plasmin formed systematically proteolyzes fibrin and fibrinogen to give a series of fragments of gradually decreasing molecular size,[51] fibrinogen/fibrin degradation products (FDP X, Y, D, and E), and fragment Bβ 1–42, D-dimer. Therefore, in physiologic conditions, fibrinolysis occurs as a reactive process to activation of coagulation and fibrin formation. If primary hyperfibrinolysis occurs in pathologic conditions, plasmin is readily inactivated in the circulation by its inhibitors α_2-antiplasmin inhibitor (forming the plasmin-antiplasmin [PAP] complex) and $\alpha_2$macroglobulin.[58] t-PA and u-PA are themselves controlled by a group of plasminogen activator inhibitors (PAI-1, PAI-2, PAI-3). ECs are the major source of PAI-1, which rapidly binds PA.[59]

The Coagulopathy of Acute Leukemia

In acute leukemia, abnormalities of the blood-clotting system underlying the clinical pictures of DIC are observed in AML, especially AML-M3 subtype, less commonly in ALL.[60, 61] These abnormalities include hypofibrinogenemia, increased FDPs, and prolonged prothrombin and thrombin times.[62] These laboratory parameters often become more abnormal upon the initiation of cytotoxic chemotherapy, resulting in severe hemorrhagic complications. However, these findings are not diagnostic of any single coagulation disorder;they reflect a complex interaction of several pathophysiologic processes. Activation of coagulation, fibrinolysis, and nonspecific proteolysis may lead to similar alterations of "routine" clotting tests. The results of new and more sensitive laboratory tests to detect enzyme-inhibitor complexes and activation peptides also confirm activation of all the three systems in acute leukemia. Elevated plasma levels of F1 + 2, TAT complex, and FPA have been found and represent well-known markers of clotting activation.[21, 64] High levels of FDPs and u-PA, together with low levels of plasminogen and α_2-antiplasmin, have been described and provide evidence for hyperfibrinolysis.[65–67] Plasma levels of leukocyte elastase and fibrinogen split products of elastase have been measured and indicate nonspecific protease activity.[67] However, with new laboratory tests for hypercoagulation markers, which detect subclinical DIC, it has become clear that thrombin generation is a constant finding in acute leukemia. In this setting, particularly important is the detection of the D-dimer, the lysis product of cross-linked fibrin, which definitely demonstrates that hyperfibrinolysis occurs in response to clotting activation in leukemia.[68-70]

One of the old arguments against DIC was that the levels of the coagulation inhibitors AT and PC are often not decreased in acute leukemia with DIC. However, it must be considered that the stochiometry of the TAT complex is largely in favor of AT[71] and that thrombin can be partly protected by AT inactivation. Furthermore, both AT and PC are synthesized in the liver;their plasma levels in part reflect hepatic function. It has been demonstrated that in DIC with hepatic dysfunction, they are often decreased, whereas in DIC without hepatic dysfunction they can be normal.[72] Thus, normal AT levels do not exclude DIC in acute leukemia. Additionally, whereas reactive fibrinolysis is well documented, there is no clear definition of primary hyperfibrino(geno)lysis in acute leukemia with DIC. The findings of profound reduction of α_2-antiplasmin and plasminogen, which can be corrected with antifibrinolytic agents treatment,[73, 74] do not allow the distinction between primary and reactive hyperfibrinolysis. In a paper, Menell et al[75] described an increased (annexin II-dependent) fibrinolytic activity "in vitro" of APL cells versus non-APL blasts and claimed this activity is responsible for primary hyperfibrinolysis "in vivo." However, also in this paper, the fibrinolytic system activation in the patient's plasma was assessed by nonspecific tests, i.e., the levels of fibrinogen, FDPs, and D-dimer. Particularly, elevated D-dimer level stands for secondary hyperfibrinolysis.

The advent of ATRA for remission induction therapy of AML-M3 has opened new management perspectives. Clinicians soon noted the rapid resolution of the bleeding symptoms in patients treated with ATRA.[20, 26-27] A number of laboratory studies have confirmed the decrease or normalization of clotting and fibrinolytic variables during the first 1 or 2 weeks of ATRA therapy.[68-70] In our study,[68] plasma hemostatic variables measured at the onset of AML-M3 showed elevated hypercoagulability markers (TAT, F1 + 2, D-dimer), low mean protein C, normal AT, normal fibrinolysis proteins, and increased elastase. After starting ATRA, all markers of clotting activation and fibrin degradation dropped within 4–8 days, protein C was increased, the overall fibrinolytic balance was unchanged, and elastase remained elevated. In addition, ATRA therapy was accompanied by reduced proteolysis of the von Willebrand factor.[76] The beneficial effect on hypercoagulation/hyperfibrinolysis parameters paralleled the improvement of clinical signs of coagulopathy. The benefit persisted when ATRA was given in combination with chemotherapy.[68, 76]

Pathogenetic Factors

The major determinants for the pathogenesis of coagulopathy of acute leukemia are factors associated with leukemic cells, including the expression of procoagulant, fibrinolytic, and proteolytic properties;secretion of inflammatory cytokines, i.e., interleukin-1β (IL-1β) and tumor necrosis factor (TNF-α);cytotoxic therapy;and concomitant infectious complications.

Leukemic Cell-Related Factors

Procoagulant Activities

At least three tumor cell procoagulants have been identified (Fig. 15-2): (1) TF, which acts by forming a complex with FVII to activate FX and FIX and is the procoagulant of normal and malignant tissues[49, 77]; (2) a membrane FV receptor, which facilitates the assembly of prothrombinase complex, thus accelerating its activity up to 100,000 times[78]; and (3) cancer procoagulant (CP), a cysteine proteinase that directly activates FX, independently of the presence of FVII,[79] and has been described in fetal and malignant tissues.[80, 81]

Many studies have focused on the PCA expressed by leukemic cells. Several authors have identified TF in these cells.[77, 82-83] Our group has characterized CP in blasts of various AML phenotypes (Fig. 15-3), with the greatest expression in the AML-M3 type,[84] and also in 30% of ALL blasts.[85] In AML patients, CP levels appear to be related to the phase of the disease.[86]

We have identified CP in the NB4 cell line, the first human APL line ever isolated, with the typical t(15;17) chromosomal balance translocation. We have demonstrated that the ATRA-induced cell differentiation in these cells is associated with the loss of capacity to express CP.[87] From studies of this cell line and of cultured blast cells taken from APL patients, it has been reported that ATRA also depresses the expression of TF.[88, 89]

We have observed that ATRA exerts its inhibitory effect on the leukemic cell PCA in vivo as much as in vitro and that both TF and CP of APL marrow blasts are progressively reduced in patients given ATRA for remission-induction therapy of APL.[68] The demonstration that this effect parallels the improvement of the plasma hypercoagulation parameters provides the first evidence in vivo of a

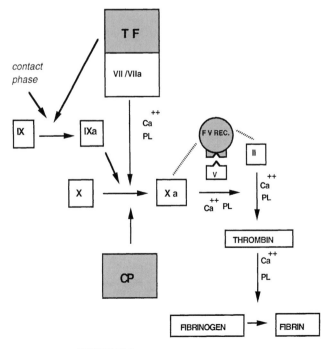

FIGURE 15-2. Tumor cell procoagulants.

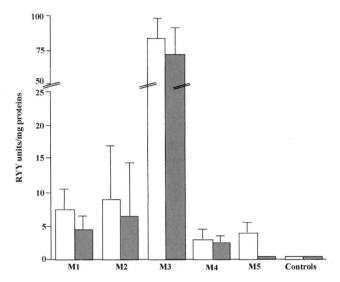

FIGURE 15–3. AML-M3 cells express high levels of procoagulant activities: total (open bars) and FVII-independent (shaded bars) procoagulant activities of AML.

Fibrinolytic and Proteolytic Properties

Fibrinolytic and proteolytic activities of leukemic cells were first described by Gralnick and Abrell.[95] Leukemic promyelocytes contain both u-PA and t-PA.[96, 97] Whereas the single chain pro-urokinase (scu-PA), which little effect on plasminogen, is predominant in cells from solid tumors, the two-chain active form (tcu-PA) is prevalent in various leukemic cells, including APL.[98] Granulocytic proteases, such as elastase and chymotrypsin, are also found in the granules of myeloid blasts. When released into the blood stream, these proteases are neutralized by their main inhibitor α1-antitrypsin. Increased plasma levels of elastase-inibitor complex have been described in acute leukemia.[16, 99] These enzymes degrade several clotting factors in vitro[100] and can enhance the fibrinolytic system by proteolysing the two plasmin inhibitors α-2-antiplasmin and C1 esterase inhibitor.[101] Further, elastase can directly break down the fibrinogen molecule, producing a pattern of peptides (FDP) different from plasmin.[102, 103]

The expression of these activities by APL cells is believed to play a major role in the pathogenesis of the bleeding syndrome. De Stefano et al[89] demonstrated that freshly isolated APL blasts express lower levels of fibrinolytic and proteolytic activities than mature neutrophils and that the granulocytic differentiation induced by ATRA is not associated with changes in these activities in vitro, except for an increase of u-PA. Similar results were obtained by others in the non-APL myeloid leukemia cell line HL60.[104] Menell et al[75] showed that APL blasts express an increased annexin II–associated fibrinolytic activity, compared with other AML subtype or ALL blast cells. However, they made no comparison with normal mature granulocytes, which makes it difficult to understand how abnormal these cells are. This activity is sensitive to ATRA treatment in NB4 cells.

A previous study of the NB4 cell fibrinolytic activity demonstrated that retinoids induce a prompt rise of u-PA activity on the cell surface, which is subsequently downregulated after 24 hours by the production of PA inhibitors.[105] Thus, various mechanisms can contribute to a reduction of APL fibrinolytic potential. These results agree with our finding that, in spite of changes in some fibrinolysis proteins, the overall plasma fibrinolytic response, as measured by the euglobulin lysis area, is unaffected in APL patients receiving ATRA.[68] In these patients, the initial signs of reactive hyperfibrinolysis (i.e., elevated D-dimer), rapidly decreased, may reflect the activation of the fibrinolytic system at a cellular site, where specific receptors favor the assembly of all the fibrinolytic components. Thereafter, ATRA-induced synthesis of PA inhibitors or annexin II reduction may down-regulate receptor-bound plasminogen activators as described in vitro.

Levels of circulating elastase are elevated at the onset of APL, possibly resulting from cell degranulation and lysis. These levels are not modified by ATRA therapy.[68] Our study found no relation between the plasma elastase concentration and the levels of the D-dimer and other hemostatic variables during treatment with ATRA. This raises the question whether this enzyme makes an important contribution to the bleeding disorders of APL.

role of tumor cell PCA in the clotting complications associated with malignancy. Reduction of leukemic cell PCA by ATRA appears to be one mechanism involved in the resolution of the coagulopathy.

Data from our group also show that, after ATRA, CP activity is virtually abolished, but only in NB4 cells sensitive to ATRA-induced cytodifferentiation, not in the resistant cells that do not differentiate, whereas TF activity is significantly reduced in all cell lines, regardless of their sensitivity to ATRA-induced differentiation.[90] These results are in agreement with known characteristics of the two procoagulants.

TF is a procoagulant of malignant cells but is also the cellular procoagulant found in normally differentiated cells that activates normal blood coagulation.[49, 91] CP has been found in extracts of neoplastic cells and in amnion-chorion tissues, but not in extracts of normally differentiated cells.[61, 92] In patients with AML, CP was detected in the bone marrow mononuclear cells at the onset of the disease but not in samples from the same subjects during complete remission.[86] All these findings support the hypothesis that CP may be expressed by undifferentiated fetal and dedifferentiated malignant cells and that, once normal differentiation occurs, the expression of this enzyme is repressed. However, TF has been shown to be down-regulated by ATRA in other subtypes of leukemic cells, not sensitive to ATRA-induced cytodifferentiation, and also in normal human ECs and monocytes.[93, 94] The different pathways of regulation of the cell procoagulants CP and TF by ATRA may have important new implications for these proteins during ATRA therapy in human malignancy. These pathways provide support for the concept that CP is a differentiation-dependent protein, which might provide a new tool (marker) to monitor leukemic cell maturation. On the other hand, the TF loss even in nondifferentiating tumor cells may be important to reduce the procoagulant potential of leukemic cells that become resistant to therapy with ATRA (which is a common condition in patients after long-term treatment).

Cytokine Release

Leukemic cells produce inflammatory cytokines, including TNF-α and IL-1β.[106] A role for the blast cytokines in the pathogenesis of the acute leukemia coagulopathy was suggested by Cozzolino et al,[107] who showed that leukemic promyelocytes from patients with DIC secrete more IL-1β than APL blasts from patients without DIC. They suggested the mechanism involves an interaction of cytokines with the hemostatic properties of the vascular endothelium. TNF-α, IL-1β, and endotoxin can induce the expression of the procoagulant TF by endothelial cells (EC).[108, 109] These cytokines also down-regulate the expression of EC thrombomodulin (TM), the surface high-affinity receptor for thrombin.[110] The TM-thrombin complex activates the protein C system, which in turn functions as a potent anticoagulant by proteolytically inactivating coagulation factors V and VIII. TF up-regulation and TM down-regulation lead to a prothrombotic condition of the vascular wall.[111] In addition TNF-α and IL-1β can stimulate the EC to produce the t-PA inhibitor PAI-1.[112] Inhibition of fibrinolysis contributes to the prothrombotic potential of EC. Although endotoxin and TNF-α can also raise t-PA levels in vivo, when administered to patients or healthy volunteers they rapidly increase t-PA, followed by a much larger increase of PAI-1.[113, 114] This demonstrates that an initial increase of fibrinolytic activity is followed by a prolonged reduction of fibrinolysis.

ATRA up-regulates the leukemic cells' ability to produce cytokines.[115, 116] In theory, this effect should favor the prothrombotic potential of the endothelium, but this does not happen because of the protective role of ATRA on EC. ATRA counteracts both the TM down-regulation and the TF up-regulation of the endothelium induced by TNF-α.[117] We have demonstrated that the TF expression induced on EC by the medium of APL NB4 cells treated with ATRA (containing IL-1β) is significantly prevented by the simultaneous presence of ATRA on the endothelium.[93] Therefore, although ATRA increases cytokine synthesis by APL cells, it is also able to protect the endothelium against the prothrombotic assault of these mediators.

The endothelium activation by IL-1β or TNF-α also leads to an increase in the expression of EC surface adhesion molecules.[118] These molecules act as counter-receptors for the tumor cell membrane adhesion molecules and are responsible for tumor cell adhesion to EC and EC matrix.[119-121] The attachment of the leukemic cell to the vessel wall is one potential mechanism of vascular complications, as it can promote localized clotting activation (through release of leukemic cell cytokines and attachment of other cells, i.e., leukocytes and platelets). ATRA treatment of APL cells increases the adhesion capacity of these cells to the endothelium.[121] However, we have observed that pretreatment of the EC monolayer with ATRA actually impairs adhesion of the APL cells to EC. ATRA can exert an antiadhesive effect by down-regulating the expression of specific counter-receptors on the endothelium surface.[122]

Chemotherapy

There has been increasing evidence that anticancer therapy can increase the risk of thromboembolic complications in this disease.[62, 123]

Among the postulated mechanisms for anticancer drug–related thrombosis are (1) release of procoagulants and cytokines from damaged malignant cells; (2) direct drug toxicity on vascular endothelium; (3) direct induction of monocyte or tumor-cell TF; and decrease in physiologic anticoagulants.[4]

The release of procoagulants and cytokines by tumor cells that have been damaged by chemotherapy is considered responsible for the exacerbation of DIC observed in laboratory and clinical data upon starting chemotherapy, particularly in acute leukemias.[27] The down-regulation of TF and CP in APL blast cells in vivo is associated with a reduction in laboratory and clinical signs of hypercoagulation in the same subjects, which provides strong evidence of a role for these activities in the pathogenesis of DIC.[68] The release of cytokines in response to chemotherapy may also have important implications for increasing the thrombotic risk. This was suggested by Bertomeu et al,[124] who demonstrated that plasma samples collected post-chemotherapy from women with breast cancer contained high levels of IL-1β, which was able to increase the reactivity of ECs to platelets, tested by an "in vitro" assay.

The second mechanism involves the direct damage exerted by chemoradiotherapy on vascular endothelium. An assay to detect the sublethal effects of drugs on endothelial integrity in tissue culture[125] identified two categories of chemotherapeutic agents:those that cause rapid binding and a reduction in the rate of EC retraction (i.e., adriamicyin); and those with no apparent effect on the rate of EC retraction (i.e., 5'-flouro-2'-deoxyuridine). These differences may depend on the different mechanisms of the drug cytotoxicity. Also, radiation therapy can cause endothelial injury, as demonstrated by the release of von Willebrand protein from human umbilical vein ECs irradiated with doses up to 40 Gy.[126] In animal studies, bleomycin has been implicated in determining morphologic damage to vascular endothelium of the lung, which may result in pulmonary thrombosis and subsequent fibrosis. Furthermore, Adriamycin, in some experimental models, directly affects glomerular cells, impairing their permeability and leading to a nephrotic syndrome, accompanied by hypercoagulation and increased thrombotic tendency.[127] The clinical counterpart of this experimental condition has not yet been completely clarified. However, profound changes of plasma markers of endothelial damage are reported in patients receiving chemotherapy.[128-130]

The third prothrombotic mechanism elicited by antitumor therapy lies in the capacity of some chemotherapeutic agents to directly stimulate the expression of TF procoagulant activity by macrophages and monocytes.[58] This activity is not the result of cell lysis because if the drug dose is increased, cell viability decreases and the drugs are less effective. Therefore, chemotherapy can induce a procoagulant response from host cells.

The fourth mechanism involves a reduction in the level of plasma anticoagulant proteins (antithrombin, protein C, and protein S) which has been reported after chemotherapy treatments.[131] This defect in naturally occurring anticoagulants is likely to be a consequence of direct hepatotoxity of radio- and chemotherapy.

In this setting, it is of particular interest to report the

case of L-Ase, a drug long regarded as the main one responsible for vascular complications during chemotherapy in ALL. L-Ase is known to be toxic for liver, pancreas, and the central nervous system and is reported to impair the hemostatic system.[132] Significant reductions in fibrinogen, plasminogen, α_2-antiplasmin, antithrombin, and protein C have been consistently described.[80, 133] These hemostatic abnormalities have been considered suggestive of a prothrombotic state, as indicated also by the significant increase of sensitive markers, such as fibrinopeptide A, TAT complexes, and F1 + 2.[134] However, the report from Memorial Hospital[42] of 12% cases of thromboembolic complications in patients not receiving L-Ase for the remission induction of ALL casts some doubts on the role of this drug in the pathogenesis of vascular events. In that study, the correlation between the hemostatic system impairment and the occurrence of vascular complications suggests that in this condition, as in APL, a systemic clotting activation with a laboratory picture of DIC is a risk factor for severe bleeding and thrombosis in patients with ALL.

Finally, one of the clinical picture of thrombosis specifically attributed to chemotherapy is hepatic veno-occlusive disease (VOD), which represents a life-threatening complication of high-dose myeloablative regimens for bone marrow or peripheral CD34 + stem cell transplantation.[135-137] VOD occurs in about 50% of patients undergoing allogeneic tranplantation, but it is also associated with autologous and syngeneic transplants, and it represents an important cause of mortality (more than 30% of cases).[138, 139] Liver VOD is characterized by hepatomegaly and ascites and results from fibrous narrowing of small hepatic venules and sinusoides rather than from occlusion of main hepatic veins. Endothelial injury, due to total body irradiation and high-dose chemotherapy, is believed to be an early event in the pathogenesis, leading to deposition of coagulation factors and platelets (fibrinogen and factor VIII) in the subendothelial space of sinusoids and hepatic venules.[140] In this context, pharmacologic treatments to prevent VOD are becoming of increasing importance. There is particular interest in those drugs that affect cellular hemostasis, i.e., at the endothelium site, without showing anticoagulant effects.[141]

Concurrent Infections

As presented in the section on the incidence of bleeding, LTB occurs much more frequently when patients with acute leukemia have concomitant infections. The mechanisms by which infection can cause bleeding include thrombocytopenia, DIC, and vascular damage.

Some infections are particularly important in the setting of acute leukemia, e.g., viral (cytomegalovirus, herpes, varicella), bacterial (sepsis due to gram-negative or gram-positive microorganisms), mycotic (*Aspergillus* species).

In some instances, thrombocytopenia is produced by suppression of hemostatic function;in other cases, the fall of platelets or the lack of recovery after platelet tranfusion can result from increased platelet distruction. The latter may occur in the setting of a worsening clinical

picture of DIC or a direct interaction between bacteria or viruses and platelets.[142-144] This interaction can produce platelet aggregation, release of platelet constituents, phagocytosis of the infectious agent and, ultimately, a shortened life span. The contribution of infection to bleeding complications is especially high in gram-negative sepsis. A unique characteristic of gram-negative bacteria is the presence of endotoxin on the cell wall. Endotoxin is a lipopolysaccharide that possesses a variety of biologic effects:pyrogenic, lethal, hypotensive, and procoagulant effects. The latter is due to the capacity of lipopolysaccharide to induce TF expression by different cells, mainly monocytes and ECs. This mechanism of blood clotting activation can trigger or worsen DIC and thrombocytopenia.[145, 146]

THERAPY

Platelet Transfusions

Prophylactic platelet transfusion therapy represents an essential part of the modern supportive care for patients with acute leukemia. This practice resulted in a marked decrease in the incidence of bleeding as well as in prolonged survival, and it also allowed for the intensification of therapy.[147, 148] However, the threshold value of the platelet count below which bleeding is significantly increased and prophylactic platelet transfusion is indicated is not firmly established.[149] Traditionally, a level of 20 × 10^9/L has been used, on the basis of a 1962 study by Gaydos et al[150] that reported an increase in hemorrhagic episodes at platelet counts below 20 × 10^9/L. However, in that report, the presence of a threshold value was not clearly demonstrated. The indication for prophylactic platelet transfusion could be modulated according to the clinical setting in which thrombocytopenia occurs, rather than the automatic administrating of platelets at a given platelet count.[151] For example, the presence of infections increases the risk of major bleeding, through a number of complex mechanisms affecting platelet number and function (described in the preceding section on Pathogenesis). Thus, febrile AL patients reasonably require a more intensive platelet transfusion support. In a study of 102 acute leukemia patients, Gmur et al[152] set the threshold for prophylactic platelet transfusion at 5 × 10^9/L in patients without fever or bleeding, at 10 × 10^9/L in patients with such signs, and at 20 × 10^9/L in those with coagulation disorders or anatomical lesions or on heparin. Deaths due to bleeding were rare, and none of them would have been prevented by prophylactic administration of platelets at the 20 x 10^9/L level. In subsequent years, the safety of a stringent prophylactic platelet transfusion policy was confirmed in comparative, nonrandomized studies[153-155] and in randomized clinical trials.[156, 157] The Italian multicenter clinical trial[156] evaluated 255 adults with acute myeloid leukemia randomly assigned to receive a transfusion when their platelet count fell below 10 × 10^9/L (or less than 20 × 10^9/L in those with fever or active bleeding, or requiring an invasive procedure) or when it was less than 20 × 10^9/L. Major bleeding occurred in 21.5% and 20% of patients in the two groups, respectively, and only one case of fatal hemorrhage was registered in a patient with a platelet count of 32×10^9/L. Use of the lower threshold reduced platelet use of 21%. Another randomized trial[158] was a single-institution study comparing the 10×10^9/L versus the 20×10^9/L trigger in 78 patients undergoing induction therapy for acute leukemia. Once again, no significant differences in the total number of bleeding episodes per patient, red blood cell transfusion requirements, remission rate, or death during induction chemotherapy were reported.

The advantages of this restrictive but safe platelet transfusion policy are relevant.[158, 159] Reducing patient exposure to blood products is expected to lower the potential risks of transmitting viral and bacterial infections as well as other potential transfusion-associated side effects such as nonhemolytic, febrile, and allergic reactions. These risks are very low, but a prudent use of allogeneic blood transfusions remains recommendable.[160, 162] One must also consider the risk of sensitization. Although the relationship between the number of units of platelets received and the development of refractoriness is controversial, the possible development of anti-HLA alloimmunization, which is a potential cause of platelet refractoriness, should be considered. Finally, platelet transfusion is an expensive procedure. In the United States, the cost of providing platelets to an average patient admitted with a hematologic or oncologic condition is more than $2000; in a patient with refractoriness to platelet transfusion who is undergoing bone marrow transplantation, the mean cost is nearly $15,000.[160] A stringent platelet transfusion policy is expected to reduce this cost by about one-third.[154]

These recommendations do not apply to patients with acute promyelocytic leukemia whose bleeding risk and platelet transfusion requirements remain higher in the retinoic acid era[27] or to patients with other cancers not yet evaluated in appropriate clinical trials.[158] Acute promyelocytic leukemia is the variety of acute leukemia in which LTB is more frequent and in which the correction of thrombocytopenia with platelet transfusion seems of special value. In a study conducted by Kantarajian et al[162] at M.D. Anderson Hospital, the incidence of fatal bleeding in patients with AML-M3 seemed related to the severity of thrombocytopenia as well as to high blast and promyelocyte count, anemia, and advanced age. Similarly, Goldberg et al[163] showed in a small group of patients that the bleeding tendency associated with AML-M3 can be successfully managed by vigorous platelet support combined with prompt introduction of chemotherapy to eradicate the cause of the coagulopathy. This was also the experience in Bergamo: in a series of 65 adults with AML-M3, CR rate was higher in patients transfused intensively with platelets and not given heparin.[65] Current recommendations for patients with AML-M3 suggest that platelets should be transfused to maintain the platelet count above 20×10^9/L in patients not actively bleeding and above 50×10^9/L in patients actively bleeding[21, 27] (Table 15-4).

A major problem of platelet transfusions in patients with acute leukemia is alloimmune refractoriness. Alloimmunization impairs the ability to provide platelet transfu-

sion support, contributes to hemorrhagic deaths and, in some cases, represents a serious limit to potentially curative treatment. Alloimmunization is defined as occurring when an adequate platelet count increment (CI) is not achieved 1 hour after transfusion,[165] calculated as follows:

$$CI = \text{observed increment (count/L) x body surface area (m}^2) \div \text{number of platelets transfused x } 10^{11}$$

After the transfusion of random donor platelets to a clinically stable adult patient, the CI should be 10 to 20 $\times 10^9$/L. For example, an improvement in count from 10 to 40×10^9/L in a 2-m^2 patient after 3×10^{11} platelets are given produces a CI of 20×10^9/L. Some clinical factors have a negative effect on CI, including fever, splenomegaly, bone marrow transplantaton, DIC, amphotericin B therapy, and anti-HLA antibodies.[160, 166] Leucocyte depletion or UVB irradiation to inactivate antigen-presenting cells significantly reduces HLA-alloimmunization rates in multitransfused patients, although unequivocal evidence of clinical benefit demonstrated by well-designed randomized controlled trials is lacking.[167] In most cases of alloimmune platelet refractoriness, successful transfusions can be obtained with the use of HLA-matched platelets or cross-match compatible platelets.[168, 169] If matched donors are not available for refractory patients, it is not recommended to continue to administer random donor platelets prophylactically. In case of bleeding, infusion of massive amount of unmatched patients can sometimes be effective.[170] Other options include intravenous immunoglobulin, plasma exchange, and acid-treated platelets (to remove HLA antigens), although good clinical evidence of benefit is lacking.[159]

Heparin and Antifibrinolytic Agents

The role of heparin therapy in the treatment of coagulopathy complicating acute leukemia, with particular reference to APL, remains uncertain. The aim of heparinization is to inhibit intravascular fibrin formation preventing microthrombus deposition and to reduce the consumption of clotting factors and platelets, hence limiting the bleeding tendency. A compilation of reported series of

TABLE 15-4. Indications for Platelet Transfusion and Dosage* in Patients with Leukemia

Acute Promyelocytic Leukemia
- If active bleeding or during chemotherapy for remission induction
  Platelets $<50 \times 10^9$/L (usually twice daily)
- If stable patient
  Platelets $<20 \times 10^9$/L

Other Acute Leukemias
If active bleeding, fever $>38°C$, or invasive procedures
  Platelets $<20 \times 10^9$/L
- If stable patient
  Platelets $<10 \times 10^9$/L

Chronic Leukemias
Major bleeding associated with severe thrombocytopenia
  ($<20 \times 10^9$/L)

*If random donor platelet concentrates: 1 U/10 kg body weight
If single donor apheresis platelets: 1 U

patients with APL reveals a statistically significant benefit for the use of the anticoagulant, with a 13% prevalence of hemorrhagic deaths being associated with the use of heparin compared with a 24% death rate without heparin.[21] However, the interpretation of these data requires caution because most studies involve small numbers of patients, are retrospective, and are not controlled. The benefit of heparin therapy has never been proved by prospective randomized trial. In several studies, the beneficial effects of heparin were demonstrated in comparison with historical series, thus not taking into account both the more intensive chemotherapy made available in recent years and the increased availability of blood products. In a large retrospective analysis,[25] 268 consecutive patients (94 received heparin, 67 received an antifibrinolytic agent, and 107 were given only supportive care) were analyzed. The results indicated no significant benefit with heparin with respect to the incidence of early hemorrhagic deaths, CR rate, or overall survival. Thus, the routine use of heparin in the management of coagulopathy in patients with acute leukemia cannot be recommended at present.

Since increased fibrinolytic[73-75] and other protease activities[27] have been implicated in the pathogenesis of coagulopathy, therapeutic regimens, including antifibrinolytic agents such as epsilon-aminocaproic acid and tranexamic acid, or protease inhibitors such as aprotinin have been suggested. However, even most recently published observations fail to demonstrate the occurrence of primary hyperfibrinolysis in vivo; thus, no clear data are available to support the use of antifibrinolytic drugs for the hemorrhagic complications of acute leukemia. The efficacy of tranexamic acid in controlling the hemorrhagic syndrome in APL with a concurrent substantial reduction of the transfusion requirements has been suggested on the basis of results obtained with small series of patients.[73] In addition, it is of great importance to also consider the clinical finding of thromboembolism, when antifibrinolytic agents are given in the course of ATRA induction therapy.[171] Previous experience with these agents[73] concerns non-ATRA-treated APL patients, so the use of ATRA for APL treatment raises new questions in this field.

Thrombopoietic Growth Factors

Thrombopoietin

Thrombopoietin (TPO), the ligand for the c-mpl cytokine receptor, is the main cytokine that regulates megakaryocytopoiesis and is the most interesting factor for the treatment of thrombocytopenia because of its lineage specificy.[172] Several recombinant c-mpl ligands were identified by purification of endogenous TPO and elucidation of its DNA sequence.[173] Intensive clinical investigation has focused on two of these molecules, recombinant human thrombopoietin (rhTPO), a glycosylated protein with an amino acid sequence identical to that of endogenous TPO, and recombinant human megakaryocyte growth and development factor (rHuMGDF), a truncated form of TPO with identical biologic activity covalently coupled to polyethylene glycol (PEG-rHuMGDF).[174]

Two phase I studies of PEG-rHuMGDF in patients with solid tumors have been completed.[175, 176] In one study, a total of 7 patients received placebo, and 16 received PEG-rHuMGDF in the absence of any chemotherapy. In the other, 22 received placebo, and 69 received PEG-rHuMGDF following chemotherapy. In both studies, the nadir platelet counts were higher and platelet counts returned to base line significantly faster in the patients given thrombopoietin than in those given placebo. However, the chemotherapeutic regimens in these two trials induced only moderate thrombocytopenia (mean nadir platelet counts in the placebo groups 11,000 and 60,000/m², respectively), not sufficient to evaluate potential effect of PEG-rHuMGDF to avoid major bleeding or platelet transfusion. These observations were consistent with those of Vadhan-Raj et al,[177] who gave a single dose of rhTPO alone before chemotherapy. They reported elevated platelet counts of up to 212%, and the kinetics of platelet recovery were similar to those found in the studies cited above.

Preliminary results of the first randomized, placebo-controlled study of PEG-rHuMGDF as an adjunct to chemotherapy in adult patients with newly diagnosed AML, excluding M3 and M7 FAB subtypes, have been reported.[178] Complete remission rate was 76% in patients who received PEG-rHuMGDF and 86% in patients who received placebo. No influence on the severity or duration of thrombocytopenia could be demonstrated. PEG-rHuMGDF has also been used after high-dose chemotherapy. In one study, 50 patients receiving high-dose chemotherapy and bone marrow support were given either placebo or PEG-rHuMGDF.[179] Platelet recovery was improved in the PEG-rHuMGDF group and was associated with a 34% reduction in the duration of severe thrombocytopenia and an almost 50% reduction in the need for platelet transfusion. In contrast, PEG-rHuMGDF did not improve platelet recovery after high-dose chemotherapy and peripheral blood progenitor cell (PBPC) support when given either after[180] or before and after[181] PBPC transfusion.

Overall, in the clinical studies whose results are available, PEG-rHuMGDF and rHuTPO were found to be biologically active, inducing intense stimulation of platelet production, without significant effect on the myeloid and erythroid lineage. Significantly, both molecules have been associated with minimal acute toxicity. No constitutional symptoms or changes in performance status, vital signs, body weight, or biochemical, renal, or liver function tests were observed. Although thromboembolic events have been reported in patients receiving PEG-rHuMGDF, the incidence was no greater than in patients given placebo and was consistent with the expected incidence in patients with advanced malignancy. However, in severely thrombocytopenic states induced by intensive regimens, the therapeutic benefit of treatment with Mpl ligands was modest or insignificant. Thus, their ability to prevent severe thrombocytopenia associated with the treatment of leukemia and bone marrow transplantation has been disappointing. In addition, subcutaneous administration of PEG-rHuMGDF has been shown to induce the formation of antibodies that neutralize native TPO and cause thrombocytopenia.[182] At present, clinical trials with PEG-rHuMGDF have been discontinued. Possibly, the greatest potential of rh-TPO in the near future may be in transfusion medicine, to collect and to store platelets from healthy donors or in an autologous setting. Mobilization of peripheral blood stem cells and megakaryocyte progenitor cells are other areas of ongoing intensive research. Finally, the potential utility of TPO for treatment of myelodysplastic syndromes or aplastic anemias, diseases in which thrombocytopenia is a leading cause of morbidity and mortality, remains to be evaluated.

Other Thrombopoietic Growth Factors

In addition to TPO, several other recombinant cytokines (including IL-1, IL-3, IL-6, IL-11, granulocyte-macrophage colony-stimulating factor and stem cell factor) have direct and indirect stimulatory effect in vitro and in vivo on cells of megakaryocytic lineage.[183, 184] However, most of these substances have not had beneficial effects on platelet recovery after myelosuppressive therapy or have had unacceptable toxic effects. In contrast, IL-11 appears to be more effective and better tolerated. Two reports outlined a role for IL-11 in the treatment of severe thrombocytopenia in patients given nonablative chemotherapy. In an initial study, eligible patients were those with solid tumors or lymphoma receiving chemotherapy who had required platelet transfusions in a previous cycle.[185] For the subsequent cycle, patients were treated with IL-11 or placebo. The number of patients who remained platelet transfusion–free was significantly higher in the IL-11 than in placebo groups (30% versus 4%, $p<0.05$). In another study, 77 women with advanced breast cancer were randomized to receive blinded treatment with IL-11 or placebo after chemotherapy.[186] IL-11 significantly reduced the need for platelet transfusion (41% versus 68%, $p = 0.04$) and enhanced platelet recovery compared to placebo. On the basis of these studies, IL-11 has been approved by the U.S. Food and Drug Administration for the secondary prevention of thrombocytopenia after chemotherapy.

ATRA

ATRA is a differentiating agent that is able to induce CR accompanied by a prompt amelioration of the acute coagulopathy in 90% of patients with APL.[27] Some of the mechanisms by which ATRA can interact with the hemostatic system have been elucidated or are under investigation.

ATRA can interfere with each of the principal hemostatic properties of the leukemic cell, including the expression of procoagulant, fibrinolytic, and proteolytic activities, and the secretion of inflammatory cytokines, i.e., IL-1β and TNF-α, which affect the hemostatic system at the vascular endothelium and leukocyte. Particularly, the profound inhibitory effect on the expression of the two major procoagulant activities, which parallels the improvement of hemostatic variables in APL patients, may propose a mechanism for the beneficial effect observed in vivo on the correction of the coagulopathy recorded within the first week of treatment with ATRA.[68]

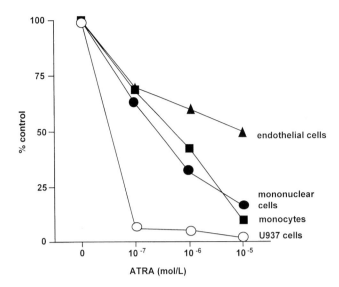

FIGURE 15–4. ATRA downregulates tissue factor in normal and transformed human cells: effect of ATRA on tissue factor expression in normal mononuclear cells (●), monocytes (■), endothelial cells (▲), and U 937 monocytic cells (○).

However, ATRA can also interfere with the hemostatic properties of normal cells, including ECs and monocytes (Fig. 15–4).

ATRA has been shown to affect the coagulant functions of ECs. ATRA is able to counteract both the downregulation of TM and the upregulation of TF induced by TNF-α and IL-1β in human EC in vitro.[187] In addition to this effect, ATRA also directly increases TM expression by cultured human ECs. Treatment with ATRA causes the elevation of TM mRNA and protein biosynthesis in ECs.[188] These effects on endothelium hemostasis provide evidence for an antithrombotic action of this drug in tumor and inflammatory diseases. ATRA can also enhance the EC fibrinolytic functions. It is known that vitamin A and other retinoids can stimulate t-PA production.[189] However, the mechanism of action is different from that of other known agonists, such as histamine, thrombin, and phorbol 12-myristate 13-acetate (PMA). These latter act through cell surface receptors, thus triggering signaling pathways that lead to the activation of gene expression. In contrast, retinoids act via intracellular receptors that belong to the family of nuclear receptors. Studies have demonstrated that ATRA potentiates the production of t-PA by ECs induced by histamine, thrombin, and PMA and that ATRA pretreatment results in the desensitization to the homologous agonist but does not affect heterologous agonist action.[190] This finding suggests that stimulation of t-PA by ATRA can involve a pathway distinct from those used by other agonists. Understanding these mechanisms of action is important as ATRA can have the potential to increase the fibrinolytic process in vivo. From these facts, it appears that ATRA induces the ECs to protect against fibrin deposition.

Concerning normal human monocyte hemostatic properties, retinoids modulate several functions of mononuclear phagocytes, such as IL-1 and IL-3 production, tumoricidal activity, phagocytosis, and Fc-receptor expression. Relevant to this review is the fact that ATRA inhibits the PCA, namely TF, of human monocytes. Like ECs, these cells do not constitutively express TF but respond to different stimuli by generating and exposing this procoagulant on their surface. Monocyte/macrophage PCA generated in vivo may be implicated in the activation of blood coagulation seen in certain pathologic conditions, including malignancy.[91] ATRA dose-dependently inhibits the procoagulant response induced by endotoxin in human peripheral mononuclear cells.[96] Our group found that the regulation of TF expression by retinoids is mediated by nuclear retinoic acid receptors and may be different from the regulation of TF in leukemic cells.[191] The inhibition of monocyte PCA generation might help explain the retinoids' anticoagulant effect.

Research insights into this field might result in an overall improved understanding of the coagulopathy mechanism in APL and might have therapeutic relevance. The use of ATRA cannot yet be recommended, alone in M3v APL, where the risk of cerebral hemorrhage is exceedingly high, and more broadly in hyperleukocytic APL as a means to induce a remission, despite reports that ATRA corrects rapidly the hemostatic disorder in vivo. This is because ATRA itself may induce transient hyperleukocytosis and signs of cerebral damage. The relationship between M3v blast cells and vascular endothelial cells should be explored more extensively with appropriate experimental studies. The best way to manage M3v APL at presentation remains to be elucidated but should probably be considered in a way different from that of classic APL.

Treatment of Thrombosis in ALL

The identification and the relative rarity of the thrombohemorrhagic syndrome in ALL patients explain the scanty data published and the difficulty of setting a randomized clinical trial of prophylaxis and therapy for thrombosis. Our patients with cerebral vein thrombosis occurring during or soon after chemotherapy induction regimen were treated with adjusted-dose heparin to maintain the APTT ratio between 1.5 and 2.0, followed by warfarin (PT International Normalized Ratio target range 2 to 3) for 30 to 45 days. A complete clinical recovery was obtained in all cases.[192] However, the duration and intensity of anticoagulant treatment should be modulated according to the extent of concomitant thrombocytopenia.

ALL patients treated with L-Ase usually show reduced levels of ATIII and other physiologic inhibitors of blood coagulation.[192, 193] Since ATIII and protein C concentrates became available, prophylactic concentrate supplementation has been suggested in order to prevent thrombotic complications. This approach is further supported by the finding that antithrombin supplementation is able to prevent the activation of blood coagulation induced by L-Ase. In fact, sensitive markers of hypercoagulability, such as plasma thrombin–antithrombin complex and D-dimer, that are significantly increased during treatment with L-Ase return to normal if ATIII concentrate is given with the goal to maintain the inhibitor concentration to normal or near-normal levels.[194] However, despite this promising laboratory finding, no clinical studies have provided evidence that ATIII supplementation may actually reduce the incidence of thrombosis in patients receiving L-Ase.

TABLE 15–5. Guidelines for Management of Bleeding in Acute Promyelocytic Leukemia

Mainstay Treatment
Platelet transfusion, twice daily, to maintain platelets $>50 \times 10^9$/L
Red blood cell transfusion to maintain Hb >8 g/dL
If cerebral bleeding is suspected:
• Perform CT scan or MRI immediately
• Avoid lumbar puncture
• Alert intensive care unit
Ancillary Therapy of Uncertain Benefit
Tranexamic acid, 6 g/day IV

Management of LTB in Acute Leukemias

LTB is usually accompanied by a fall in blood pressure and significant decrease in hemoglobin concentration if massive blood loss occurs at sites communicating with body orifices and in decreased consciousness if the central nervous system is involved. In particular, central nervous system bleeding should be suspected in every acute leukemia patient subject to intensive chemotherapy and with low platelet count who develops signs of cerebral dysfunction not explained by other causes. Recommended diagnostic procedures are computed tomography scan and magnetic resonance imaging, whereas lumbar punctures should be avoided. Immediate transfusions with platelets and packed red blood cells and antiedema medications are recommended. When cerebral or pulmonary bleeding are suspected, the intensive care unit should be alerted, bearing in mind that death due to respiratory and circulatory failure may supervene rapidly. Because of this high mortality rate, prevention of LTB with appropriate prophylactic platelet administration is mandatory. Furthermore, the identification of patients at the greatest risk may be helpful. Patients with AML-M3 are particularly prone to LTB; recommended guidelines for management are summarized in Table 15–5. In addition, LTB is especially frequent in infected patients and in those with hyperleukocytosis of more than 50×10^9/L. Thus, an effective control of infectious complications could possibly result in a decreased incidence of LTB.

BLEEDING AND THROMBOSIS IN CHRONIC MYELOPROLIFERATIVE DISORDERS

Polycythemia vera (PV) and essential thrombocythemia (ET) are chronic myeloproliferative disorders (MPD) frequently complicated by hemostatic disturbances leading to hemorrhage and thrombosis; in contrast, these complications are rarer in chronic myelogenous leukemia (CML) and essential myelofibrosis. A comprehensive description of all the biologic and clinical aspects of MPDs is beyond this chapter. Reviews of this issue have been published

(MPDs, excluding CML)[195] or are in other chapters of this book (CML).

Prevalence and Natural History

PV

PV is a clonal malignancy that arises at the level of the pluripotent stem cell and passes through three well-recognized clinical stages. The developmental phase might be insidious, and symptoms precede an overt diagnosis of PV by years. The Gruppo Italiano Studio Policitemia has shown that 14% of patients had thrombosis before diagnosis of PV and that 20% had a thrombotic event as the presenting symptom of disease.[196] Vascular complications are characteristically seen in the polycythemic phase, clearly defined by current diagnostic criteria,[197, 198] whereas the rate of events decreases during the final spent phase, characterized by anemia, leukopenia, thrombocytopenia, and a leukoerythroblastic peripheral blood picture. The most common thromboembolic symptoms, in descending order of frequency, are cerebrovascular occlusions, myocardial infarction, peripheral arterial insufficiency, pulmonary embolism, and venous thrombosis.[196, 199] Moreover, quite characteristic of PV is the development of thrombosis at unusual anatomic sites, in particular in the splenic, hepatic, portal, and mesenteric vessels.[200] The natural history of PV patients was investigated in a retrospective cohort study of 1213 patients in Italy.[196] The cumulative median duration of survival exceeded 15 years, with an overall mortality rate of 2.94 deaths/100 patients per year. The age-and sex-standardized mortality rate was 1.7 times greater than that of the general Italian population. The most frequent causes of death were thrombosis (30% of cases) and cancer (15% of patients with acute leukemia and 15% with other cancers). The overall rate of fatal and nonfatal thrombotic events was 3.4/100 patients per year. The prevalence of thrombosis increased significantly with age (younger than 40 years, 1.8%; 40 to 57 years, 2.8%; 60 to 69 years, 4.0%; older than 70 years, 5.1% per year; $p<0.001$) and with history of thrombosis (24.6% versus 17.3%; $p = 0.001$).

ET

ET is a myeloproliferative disease characterized by persistent thrombocytosis not accounted for by a reactive state or another chronic myeloid disorder.[201] In the natural history of ET, hemorrhages are reported in 13% to 63% of patients and thrombotic complications in 8% to 84% of cases.[202] The proportion of thrombohemorrhagic episodes varies in different series, depending on definition of symptoms, patient selection and, possibly, the monoclonal or polyclonal nature of the disease. If only severe (life-threatening) hemorrhages are taken into account, these are reported in 3% to 10% of cases and can be favored by concomitant plasma coagulation defects[203] or by medications inhibiting platelet function.[204] In contrast, thromboembolic events are reported to be much more frequent and include central nervous system and peripheral vascular ischemia and thrombosis of large arterial

and venous systems and at unusual sites such as the cerebral sagittal sinus and at renal, mesenteric, and subclavian vessels. The Budd-Chiari syndrome is most commonly associated with PV, but there are also several cases associated with ET.[200] Obstetric complications including recurrent spontaneous abortions, fetal growth retardation, premature deliveries, and abruptio placentae are reported with increasing frequency in ET, but the number of cases does not permit uniform recommendations about management.[205] The rate of vascular complications in ET depends on patient selection. In fact, whereas in the past the disease was diagnosed almost exclusively in middle-aged or elderly patients presenting with dramatic thrombohemorrhagic symptoms, now that platelet counts are part of routine blood count, this diagnosis is formulated with increasing frequency in completely asymptomatic cases as well as in children and young adults.[206] Many of these patients remain free of hemostatic complications during long-term follow-up. A report has shed new light on the heterogeneity of ET.[207] Forty-six females with a diagnosis of ET established according to generally accepted criteria were studied to assess the clonal nature of hemopoiesis. Ten and 13 of 23 evaluable patients had monoclonal or polyclonal myelopoiesis, respectively, and those without a clonal disorder were less likely to have experienced thrombotic events. These findings have been confirmed[208] and call for an analysis of clonality in larger series of patients to determine the natural history, in particular the incidence of thrombotic complications, of the different forms of the disease.[209]

Management

Polycythemia Vera

At present, there is no known treatment that eradicates the abnormal clone, apart deom anecdotal cases of BMT transplantation.[210] Consequently, therapy is aimed at reducing the incidence of vascular complications and limiting the progress of the myeloproliferative process. Available information for therapeutic recommendations in PV derives from a very limited number of randomized clinical trials and a series of prospective and retrospective observational studies. A landmark clinical trial carried out by the Polycythemia Vera Study Group (PVSG) in the United States[211] compared the efficacy, in terms of survival, of phlebotomy alone with that of two different myelosuppressive regimens (radiactive phosphorus and chlorambucil) supplemented by phlebotomy. Survival was significantly poorer for patients on chlorambucil than for those treated with radioactive phosphorus or phlebotomy alone; in these two latter groups, survival was comparable. Noteworthy is the fact that, with regard to thrombotic events, phlebotomy-treated patients did significantly worse during the first 5 to 7 years of the study; subsequently, however, curves of thrombosis-free cumulative survival in the treatment groups were comparable. Another fact of practical relevance was that the incidence of thrombosis was markedly increased as the phlebotomy rate increased. In subsequent investigations,[212, 213] PVSG reported that hydroxyurea (HU), supplemented by phlebotomy to maintain the Ht below 50%, significantly diminished the risk of thrombosis associated with phlebotomy alone. However, it should be stressed that the incidence of acute leukemia following myelosuppressive treatments, including HU, has not yet been fully established, and observations indicating this possibility[214, 215] have to be considered when prescribing these drugs to young people.

Recombinant interferon-α (IFN) is an active agent in PV with antiproliferative activity that is virtually devoid of mutagenic risk.[216–218] The rationale for this drug includes its myelosuppressive activity and its ability to antagonize the action of platelet-derived growth-factor (PDGF), a product of megakaryopoiesis that initiates fibroblast proliferation. This observation suggests that IFN could, theoretically, modify the natural history of PV and reduce or delay the development of myelofibrosis. IFN has been evaluated in some phase II studies, and overall results indicate that red blood cell mass can be controlled within 6 to 12 months in up to 70% of cases, as seen by a reduction in the need for phlebotomy. In addition, IFN can reverse the associated splenomegaly, leukocytosis, and thrombocytosis in the majority of patients, and it is particularly effective for the treatment of generalized pruritus. Side effects are often a major problem with this drug, causing therapy withdrawal in approximately a third of patients. Signs of chronic IFN toxicity include weakness, myalgia, weight and hair loss, severe depression, and gastrointestinal and cardiovascular toxicity.

Another drug for which a leukemogenic effect is not expected is anagrelide, a member of the imidazol-(2,1-b) quinazolin-2-1 series of compounds.[219, 220] This compound, given orally alone or in combination with HU, has been found to be highly efficacious in controlling thrombocythemia in patients with PV and other myeloproliferative disorders. The mechanism whereby anagrelide reduces platelet count without affecting leukocytes or red blood cells is not completely understood, but there are data showing that its major action is the inhibition of megakaryocyte maturation. No chromosomal damage has been reported in relation to its use. Adverse reactions including headache, fluid retention, nausea, diarrhea, and abdominal pain have been reported, and anagrelide may precipitate congestive heart failure in older people.

These new drugs are of particular interest for the treatment of younger patients with PV because their prolonged use could be theoretically devoid of leukemogenic risk. However, demonstration of their efficacy is based only on secondary end points, such as reduction of red blood cell mass and platelet count. Their capacity to prevent vascular complications and secondary malignancies and, in turn, to improve the survival of PV patients remains to be established in appropriate clinical trials.[221]

The use of aspirin or other antiplatelet agents in patients with PV and other MPDs remains controversial, and the decision rests primarily on the clinical picture.[222] In fact, laboratory tests of platelet function (e.g., bleeding time, platelet aggregation studies), which have been generally unreliable in predicting the risk of bleeding and thrombosis,[223, 224] are of little help. Aspirin is generally recommended for PV patients who have had recurrent

TABLE 15–6. Recommendations for Management of Patients with Polycythemia Vera

- Phlebotomy to maintain hematocrit level ≤45%.
- Add hydroxyurea if high rate of phlebotomy, thrombotic complications, increasing platelet counts, or splenomegaly.
- Add aspirin (100–300 mg/day) if arterial thrombosis or microcirculatory symptoms (i.e., erythromelalgia) or warfarin (PT INR 2.0–3.0) if venous thrombosis.
- Younger patients (<40 years): consider interferon or anagrelide.
- Elderly patients (>70 years): consider busulfan or radiophosphorus.

thrombotic complications, particularly those with digital or cerebrovascular occlusive syndromes. However, the risk of serious bleeding with aspirin use may be elevated in patients with prior histories of bleeding problems, especially of the gastrointestinal tract. Uncertainty reigns for those patients without a clear-cut prior history of bleeding or thrombosis in whom the benefits and risks of aspirin or related drugs have not yet been evaluated. In this setting, the Gruppo Italiano Studio Policitemia completed a pilot study aimed at assessing the safety of low-dose aspirin (40 mg/day) in PV patients.[225] In this pilot study, no differences in side effects or adverse events were apparent, showing the feasibility of a large-scale study. A multicenter, randomized clinical trial evaluating low-dose aspirin versus placebo in PV patients is being conducted in Europe (European Collaboration on Low-dose Aspirin in Polycythemia). Current recommendations for the management of PV patients are summarized in Table 15–6.

Essential Thrombocythemia

Because ET is an heterogenous disorder, treatment should be differentiated according to risk factors for thrombotic or hemorrhagic complications. Main predictors of thrombosis are advanced age (older than 60 years) and previous vascular complications.[226] Bleeding is more frequent in patients with very high platelet count (>1000 to 1500 × 10⁹/L) because extreme thrombocytosis is associated with abnormalities of von Willebrand factor.[227] Alteration of platelet function tests is frequent but should be considered as a laboratory marker of the disease rather than as a predictor of vascular symptoms.

Low-risk patients (asymptomatic, age younger than 60 years, platelets count less than 1000 to 1500 × 10⁹/L) are not generally treated with cytotoxic drugs. This prudent behavior is dictated by the fear of a second tumor, possibly arising after long-term use of myelosuppressive agents. The natural history of untreated, "lower-risk" ET patients was evaluated in a prospective, controlled study.[206] Sixty-five ET patients younger than 60 years, without a history of thrombosis or major bleeding, and having a platelet count below 1500 × 10⁹/L were compared with 65 age- and sex-matched control patients. Patients were not treated with cytoreductive therapy until the occurrence of major clinical events. After a median follow-up of 4.1 years, the prevalence of thrombosis in patients and controls was 1.91% and 1.5% patient-year, respectively. The age- and sex-adjusted risk rate ratio was 1.43 (95% c.i. 0.37 to 5.4). No major bleeding was observed. This study indicate that the thrombotic risk of young, asymptomatic ET patients is not significantly increased compared with the normal population.

In high-risk patients (age over 60 years, platelet counts greater than 1000 to 1500 $\times$ 10^9/L, or previous thrombosis), lowering platelet counts is recommended. HU is considered the first-line agent because its efficacy in reducing vascular complications has been demonstrated in a randomized clinical trial.[228] One hundred and fourteen patients (35 males and 79 females, median age 68 years [range 40 to 85 years]; median platelet count 788 $\times$ 10^9/L [range 533 to 1240]) were randomized to long-term treatment with HU (n = 56) or to no cytoreductive treatment (n = 58). During a median follow-up of 27 months, 2 thromboses were recorded in the HU-treated group (1.6%/patient-year) versus 14 in the control group (10.7%/parient-year; p = 0.003). HU was initially thought to be nonmutagenic; however, long-term follow-up studies of HU-treated patients with PV and ET revealed that some cases developed acute leukemia.[229, 230] When HU is used as a single agent in ET, the expected rate of acute leukemia is 3% to 5%, and this fatal complication is encountered 5 to 10 years after the start of treatment.[230-232] The rate of malignant events might be enhanced in patients given multiple cytotoxic drugs with different mechanisms of action (antimetabolites, alkylating agents).[230-232]

Alpha-interferon causes a decrease (within 4 weeks) of elevated platelet count in thrombocytosis secondary to MPD, but side effects or poor compliance is a frequent cause of treatment discontinuation.[233] This is particularly seen in elderly patients who are at major risk for thrombosis. Anagrelide has been used in ET,[234] but current limitations for a more extended use are the same as mentioned for PV patients. The use of antiaggregating drugs for primary prophylaxis of thrombosis in ET is still uncertain as no clinical trials have documented a benefit. On the contrary, there are special situations of microvascular arterial thrombosis and cerebrovascular or coronary disease where aspirin associated with myelosuppressive agents is indicated, as in PV patients.[235] Current recommendations for management of ET patients are summarized in Table 15-7.

TABLE 15–7. Recommendations for Management of Patients with Essential Thrombocythemia

Low-risk patients (no risk factors).
Avoid myelosuppressive therapy.
Aspirin if microcirculatory disturbances (i.e., erythromelalgia).
High-risk patients (one or more risk factors).
Hydroxyurea to maintain platelet counts <400–600 $\times 10^9$/L.
Add aspirin (100–300 mg/d) if arterial thrombosis or microcirculatory symptoms (i.e., erythromelalgia) or warfarin (PT INR 2.0–3.0) if venous thrombosis.
Younger high-risk patients (<40 years): consider interferon or anagrelide.
Elderly patients (>70 years): consider busulfan.

Risk factors: age >60 years; previous thrombosis, platelet counts >1000–1500 $\times 10^9$/L.

REFERENCES

1. Barbui T, Finazzi G, Falanga A, et al: Bleeding and thrombosis in acute lymphoblastic leukemia. Leuk Lymphoma 1993;11:43.
2. Battista R, Bassan R, D'Emilio A, et al: Short-term remission induction therapy for adult acute myelogenous leukemia. Hematol Oncol 1991;9:43.
3. Riley LC, Hahn IM, Wheatley K, et al: Treatment-related deaths during induction and first remission of acute myeloid leukemia in children treated on the Tenth Medical Research Council Acute Myeloid Leukemia Trial (MCR AML 10). Br J Haematol 1999;106:436.
4. Anderlini P, Luna M, Kantarjian HM, et al: Causes of initial remission induction failure in patients with acute myeloid leukemia and myelodysplastic syndromes. Leukemia 1996;10:600.
5. Rohatiner AZS, Gregory WM, Bassan R, et al: Short-term therapy for acute myelogenous leukemia. J Clin Oncol 1988;6:218.
6. Bishop JF, Lowenthal RM, Joshua D, et al: Etoposide in acute nonlymphocytic leukemia. Blood 1990;75:27.
7. Johnson GJ: Platelets, penicillins, and purpura: What does it all mean? J Lab Clin Med 1993;121:531.
8. Cassileth PA, Begg CB, Bennett JM, et al: A randomized study of the efficacy of consolidation therapy in adult acute nonlymphocytic leukemia. Blood 1984;63:843.
9. Preisler H, Davis RB, Kirshnerv J, et al: Comparison of three remission induction regimens and two postinduction strategies for the treatment af acute nonlymphocytic leukemia: A Cancer and Leukemia Group B study. Blood 1987;69:1441.
10. Buchner T, Urbanitz D, Hiddemann W, et al: Intensified induction and consolidation with or without maintenance chemotherapy for acute myeloid leukemia (AML): Two multicenter studies of the German AML cooperative group. J Clin Oncol 1985;3:1583.
11. Wollf SN, Herzig RH, Fay JW, et al: High-dose cytarabine and daunorubicin as consolidation therapy for acute myeloid leukemia in first remission: Long-term follow-up and results. J Clin Oncol 1989;7:1260.
12. Lowenberg B, Verdonck LJ, Dekker AW, et al: Autologous bone marrow transplantation in acute myeloid leukemia in first remission: Results of a Dutch prospective study. J Clin Oncol 1990;8:287.
13. Cassileth PA, Harrington DP, Appelbaum FR, et al: Chemotherapy compared with autologous or allogeneic bone marrow transplantation in the management of acute myeloid leukemia in first remission. N Engl J Med 1998;339:1649.
14. Mayer RJ, Schiffer CA, Peterson BA, et al: Intensive postremission therapy in adults with acute nonlymphocytic leukemia using various dose schedules of ara-C: A progress report from the CALGB. Semin Oncol 1987;14:25.
15. Preisler HD, Raza A, Early A, et al: Intensive remission consolidation therapy in the treatment of acute nonlymphocytic leukemia. J Clin Oncol 1987;5:722.
16. Nevo S, Swan V, Wojno KJ, et al: Acute bleeding after bone marrow transplantation (BMT)—incidence and effect on survival: A quantitative analysis in 1402 patients. Blood 1998;91:1469.
17. Champlin RE, Gajewski JL, Golde DW: Treatment of acute myelogenous leukemia in the elderly. Semin Oncol 1989;16:51.
18. Heinemann V, Jehn U: Acute myeloid leukemia in the elderly: Biological features and search for adequate treatment. Ann Hematol 1991;63:179.
19. Lintula R, Rasi V, Ikkala E, et al: Platelets function in preleukemia. Scand J Haematol 1981;26:65.
20. Warrell RP, de The H, Wang ZY, et al: Acute promyelocytic leukemia. N Engl J Med 1993;329:177.
21. Tallman MS, Kwaan HC: Reassessing the hemostatic disorder associated with acute promyelocytic leukemia. Blood 1992;79:543.
22. Golomb HM, Rowley JD, Vardiman JW, et al: "Microgranular" acute promyelocytic leukemia: A distinct clinical, ultrastructural and cytogenetic entity. Blood 1980;55:253.
23. Rovelli A, Biondi A, Cantù Rajnoldi A, et al: Microgranular variant of acute promyelocytic leukemia in children. J Clin Oncol 1992;10:1418.
24. Fenaux P: Management of acute promyelocytic leukemia. Eur J Haematol 1993;50:65.
25. Rodeghiero F, Avvisati G, Castaman G, et al: Early deaths and anti-hemorrhagic treatments in acute promyelocytic leukemia: A

GIMEMA retrospective study in 268 consecutive patients. Blood 1990;75:2112.

26. Castaigne S, Chomienne, Daniel MT, et al: All-trans retinoic acid as a differentiation therapy for acute promyelocytic leukemia. Blood 1990;76:1704.

27. Barbui T, Finazzi G, Falanga A: The impact of all-trans-retinoic acid on the coagulopathy of acute promyelocytic leukemia. Blood 1998;91:3093.

28. Mandelli F, Diverio D, Avvisati G, et al: Molecular remission in PML/RARa-positive acute promyelocytic leukemia by combined all-trans retinoic acid and idarubicin (AIDA) therapy. Blood 1997; 90:1014.

29. Fenaux P, Castaigne S, Dombret H, et al: All-trans retinoic acid followed by intensive chemotherapy gives a high complete remission rate and may prolong remission in newly diagnosed acute promyelocytic leukemia: A pilot study on 26 cases. Blood 1992; 80:2176.

30. Frankel SR, Eardley A, Heller G, et al: All-trans retinoic acid for acute promyelocytic leukemia. Ann Intern Med 1994;120:278.

31. Kanamaru A, Takemoto Y, Tanimoto M, et al: All-trans retinoic acid for the treatment of newly diagnosed adult acute promyelocytic leukemia. Blood 1995;85:1202.

32. Estey E, Thall P, Pierce S, et al: Treatment of newly diagnosed acute promyelocytic leukemia without cytarabine. J Clin Oncol 1997;15:483.

33. Fenaux P, Le Deley MC, Castaigne S, et al: Effect of all-trans retinoic acid in newly diagnosed acute promyelocytic leukemia: Results of a multicenter randomized trial. Blood 1993;82:3241.

34. Tallman MS, Andersen JW, Schiffer CA, et al: A prospective randomized study of all-trans-retinoic acid induction and maintenance therapy for patients with acute promyelocytic leukemia. N Engl J Med 1997;337:1021.

35. Burnett AK, Grimwade D, Solomon E, et al: Presenting white blood cell count and kinetics of molecular remission predict prognosis in acute promyelocytic leukemia treated with all-trans-retinoic acid: Results of the randomized MRC trial. Blood 1999;93:4131.

36. Fenaux P, Chastang C, Chevret S, et al: A randomized comparison of all trans-retinoic acid (ATRA) followed by chemotherapy and ATRA plus chemotherapy and the role of maintenace therapy in newly diagnosed acute promyelocytic leukemia. Blood 1999; 94:1192.

37. Sanz MA, Martin G, Rayon C, et al: A modified AIDA protocol with anthracycline-based consolidation results in high antileukemic efficacy and reduced toxicity in newly diagnosed PML/RARa-positive acute promyelocytic leukemia. Blood 1999;94:3015.

38. Priest JR, Ramsay NKC, Steinherz PG, et al: A syndrome of thrombosis and hemorrhage complicating L-asparaginase therapy for childhood acute lymphoblastic leukemia. J Pediatr 1982;100:984.

39. Pui CH, Jackson CW, Chesney C, et al: Sequential changes in platelet function and coagulation in leukemic children treated with L-asparaginase, prednisone and vincristine. J Clin Oncol 1983; 1:380.

40. Nowak-Gottl U, Wermes C, Junker R, et al: Prospective evaluation of the thrombotic risk in children with acute lymphoblastic leukemia carrying the MTHFR TT 677 genotype, the prothrombin G20210A variant, and further thrombotic risk factors. Blood 1999; 93:1595.

41. Hoelzer D, Thiel E, Loffler H, et al: Intensified therapy in acute lymphoblastic and acute undifferentiated leukemia in adults. Blood 1984;64:38.

42. Sarris AH, Kempin S, Berman E, et al: High incidence of disseminated intravascular coagulation during remission induction of adult patients with acute lymphoblastic leukemia. Blood 1992;79:1305.

43. Bassan R, Battista R, D'Emilio A, et al: Long-term results of the HEAVD protocol for adult acute lymphoblastic leukemia. Eur J Cancer 1991;27:441.

44. Bassan R, Battista R, Rohatiner AZS, et al: Treatment of adult acute lymphoblastic leukemia (ALL) over a 16-year period. Leukemia 1992;6:186.

45. Rohatiner AZS, Bassan R, Battista R, et al: High-dose cytosine arabinoside in the initial treatment of adults with acute lymphoblastic leukemia. Br J Cancer 1990;62:454.

46. Bassan R, Battista R, Corneo G, et al: Idarubicin in the initial treatment of adults with acute lymphoblastic leukemia: The effect of drug schedule on outcome. Leuk Lymphoma 1993;11:105.

47. Bassan R, Lerede T, Di Bona E, et al: Induction-consolidation with an idarubicin-containing regimen, unpurged marrow autograft, and post-graft chemotherapy in adult acute lymphoblastic leukemia. Br J Haematol 1999;104:755.

48. Mackie IJ, Bull HA: Normal hemostasis and its regulation. Blood Rev 1989;3:237.

49. Nemerson Y: The tissue factor pathway of blood coagulation. Sem Hematol 1992;29:170.

50. Bauer KA, Rosenberg RD: The pathophysiology of the prethrombotic state in humans: Insights gained from studies using markers of hemostatic system activation. Blood 1987;70:343.

51. Boisclair MD, Ireland H, Lane DA: Assessment of hypercoagulable states by measurement of activation fragments and peptides. Blood Rev 1990;4:25.

52. Dittman WA, Majerus PW: Structure and function of thrombomodulin: A natural anticoagulant. Blood 1990;75:329.

53. Esmon CT: Protein C. Semin Thromb Hemost 1984;10:109.

54. Fulcher CA, Gardiner JE, Griffin JH, et al: Proteolytic inactivation of human factor VIII procoagulant protein by activated protein C and its analogy with factor V. Blood 1984;63:486.

55. McDonagh J: Structure and function of factor XIII. In Colman RW, Hirsh J, Marder VJ, Salzman EW, eds: Hemostasis and Thrombosis. Philadelphia: Lippincott; 1982, p 164.

56. Booyse FM, Scheinbuks J, Lin PH, et al: Isolation and interrelationships of the multiple molecular tissue-type and urokinase-type plasminogen activator forms produced by cultured human umbilical vein endothelial cells. J Biol Chem 1988;263:15129.

57. Levin EG, Marzec U, Anderson J, et al: Thrombin stimulates tissue plasminogen activator release from cultured human endothelial cells. J Clin Invest 1984;74:1988.

58. Aoki N, Harpel PC: Inhibitors of the fibrinolytic enzyme system. Semin Thromb Hemost 1984;10:24.

59. Sprengers ED, Kluft C: Plasminogen activator inhibitors. Blood 1987;69:381.

60. Rodeghiero F, Castaman GC: The coagulopathy of acute leukemia. Leuk Lymphoma 1992;7:42.

61. Falanga A, Rickles FR: Pathophysiology of the thrombophilic state in the cancer patient. Semin Thromb Hemost 1999;25:173.

62. Falanga A: Mechanisms of hypercoagulation in malignancy and during chemotherapy. Haemostasis 1998;2:50.

63. Mjers TJ, Rickles FR, Barb C, et al: Fibrinopeptide A in acute leukemia: Relationship of activation of blood coagulation to disease activity. Blood 1981;57:518.

64. Bauer KA, Rosenberg RD: Thrombin generation in acute promyelocytic leukaemia. Blood 1984;64:791.

65. Booth NA, Bennett B: Plasmin-alpha-2-antiplasmin complexes in bleeding disorders characterized by primary or secondary fibrinolysis. Br J Haematol 1984;56:545.

66. Reddy VB, Kowal-vern A, Hoppensteadt DA, et al: Global and hemostatic markers in acute myeloid leukemia. Am J Clin Pathol 1990;94:397.

67. Speiser W, Pabinger-Fasching I, Kyrle PA, et al: Hemostatic and fibrinolytic parameters in patients with acute myeloid leukemia: Activation of blood coagulation, fibrinolysis and unspecific proteolysis. Blut 1990;61:298.

68. Falanga A, Iacoviello L, Evangelista V, et al: Loss of blast cell procoagulant activity and improvement of hemostatic variables in patients with acute promyelocytic leukemia given all-trans-retinoic acid. Blood 1995;86:1072.

69. Dombret H, Scroboaci ML, Ghorra P, et al: Coagulation disorders associated with acute promyelocytic leukemia: Corrective effect of all-trans-retinoic acid. Leukemia 1993;7:2.

70. Kawai Y, Watanabe K, Kizaki M, et al: Rapid improvement of coagulopathy by all-trans-retinoic acid in acute promyelocytic leukemia. Am J Hematol 1994;46:184.

71. Muller-Berghaus G, Niepoth M, Rabens Alles B, et al: Normal antithrombin III activity and concentration in experimental disseminated intravascular coagulation. Scand J Clin Lab Invest 1985; 45:107.

72. Rodeghiero F, Mannucci PM, Viganò S, et al: Liver dysfunction rather than intravascular coagulation as the main cause of low protein C, an antithrombin in acute leukaemia. Blood 1984;63:965.

73. Avvisati G, ten Cate JW, Lamping R, et al: Acquired alpha-2-antiplasmin deficiency in acute promyelocytic leukemia. Br J Haematol 1988;70:43.

74. Schwartz BS, Williams EC, Conlan MG, et al: Epsilon-aminocaproic acid in the treatment of patients with acute promyelocytic leukemia: Acquired a-2-antiplasmin inhibitor deficiency. Ann Intern Med 1986;105:873.

75. Menell JS, Cesarman GM, Jacovina AT, et al: Annexin II and bleeding in acute promyelocytic leukemia. N Engl J Med 1999;340:994.

76. Federici AB, Falanga A, Lattuada A, et al: Proteolysis of von Willebrand factor is decreased in acute promyelocytic leukemia by treatment with all-trans-retinoic acid. Br J Haematol 1996;92:733.

77. Andoh K, Kubota T, Takada M, et al: Tissue factor activity in leukemia cells: Special reference to disseminated intravascular coagulation. Cancer 1987;59:748.

78. Van de Water L, Tracy PB, Aronson D, et al: Tumor cell generation of thrombin via prothrombinase assembly. Cancer Res 1985;45:5521.

79. Falanga A, Gordon SG: Isolation and characterization of cancer procoagulant: A cysteine proteinase from malignant tissue. Biochemistry 1985;24:5558.

80. Donati MB, Gambacorti Passerini C, Casali B, et al: Cancer procoagulant in human tumor cells: Evidence from melanoma patients. Cancer Res 1986;46:6471.

81. Gordon SG, Hashiba U, Poole MA, et al: A cysteine proteinase procoagulant from amnion-chorion. Blood 1985;66:1261.

82. Gouault-Heilman M, Chardon E, Sultan E, et al: The procoagulant factor of leukemic promyelocytes: Demonstration of immunologic cross-reactivity with human brain tissue factor. Br J Haematol 1975;30:151.

83. Bauer KA, Conway EM, Bach R, et al: Tissue factor gene expression in acute myeloblastic leukemia. Thromb Res 1989; 56:425.

84. Falanga A, Alessio MG, Donati MB, et al: A new procoagulant in acute leukemia. Blood 1988;71:870.

85. Alessio MG, Falanga A, Consonni R, et al: Cancer procoagulant in acute lymphoblastic leukemia. Eur J Haematol 1990;45:78.

86. Donati MB, Falanga A, Consonni R, et al: Cancer procoagulant in acute nonlymphoid leukemia: Relationship of enzyme detection to disease activity. Thromb Haemost 1990;64:11.

87. Falanga A, Consonni R, Marchetti M, et al: Cancer procoagulant in the human promyelocytic cell line NB4 and its modulation by retinoic acid. Leukemia 1994;8:156.

88. Koyama T, Hirosawa S, Kawamata N, et al: All-trans-retinoic acid upregulates thrombomodulin and downregulates tissue factor expression in acute promyelocytic leukemia cells: Distinct expression of thrombomodulin and tissue factor in human leukemic cells. Blood 1994;84:3001.

89. De Stefano V, Teofili L, Sica S, et al: Effect of all-trans-retinoic acid on procoagulant and fibrinolytic activities of cultured blast cells from patients with acute promyelocytic leukemia. Blood 1995;86:3535.

90. Falanga A, Consonni R, Marchetti M, et al: Cancer procoagulant and tissue factor are differently modulated by all-trans-retinoic acid (ATRA) in acute promyelocytic leukemia cells. Blood 1998;92:143.

91. Semeraro N, Colucci M: Tissue factor in health and disease. Thromb Haemost 1997;78:759.

92. Gordon SG: Tumor cell procoagulants and their role in malignant disease. Semin Thromb Hemost 1992;18:424.

93. Falanga A, Marchetti M, Giovanelli S, Barbui T: All-trans-retinoic acid counteracts endothelial cell procoagulant activity induced by a human promyelocytic leukemia-derived cell line (NB4). Blood 1996;87:613.

94. Conese M, Montemurro P, Fumarulo R, et al: Inhibitory effects of retinoids on the generation of procoagulant activity by blood mononuclear phagocytes. Thromb Haemost 1991;66:662.

95. Gralnick HR, Abrell E: Studies on the procoagulant and fibrinolytic activity of promyelocytes in acute promyelocytic leukemia. Br J Haematol 1973;24:89.

96. Bennett B, Booth A, Croll A, et al: The bleeding disorder in acute promyelocytic leukemia: Fibrinolysis due to u-PA rather than defibrination. Br J Haematol 1989;71:511.

97. Francis RB, Seyfert U: Tissue plasminogen activator antigen and activity in disseminated intravascular coagulation: Clinicopathologic correlations. J Lab Clin Med 1987;110:541.

98. Stephens R, Alitalo R, Tapiovaara H, et al: Production of an active urokinase by leukemia cells: A novel distinction from cell lines of solid tumors. Leuk Res 1988;12:419.

99. Egbring R, Schmidt W, Fuchs G, et al: Demonstration of granulo-cytic proteases in plasma of patients with acute leukemia and septicemia with coagulation defects. Blood 1977;49:219.

100. Schmidt W, Egbring R, Havemann K: Effect of elastase-like and chymotrypsin-like neutral proteases from human granulocytes on isolated clotting factors. Thromb Res 1974;6:315.

101. Brower NS, Harper PC: Proteolytic cleavage and inactivation of α-2-plasmin inhibitor and C1 inactivator by human polymorphonuclear leukocyte elastase. J Biol Chem 1982;257:9849.

102. Sterrenberg L, van Liempt GJ, Nieuwenhuizen W, et al: Anticoagulant properties of purified X-like fragments of human fibrinogen produced by degradation with leukocyte elastase. Thromb Haemost 1984;51:398.

103. Sterrenberg L, Nieuwenhuizen W, Hermans J: Purification and characterization of a D-like fragment from human fibrinogen produced by human leukocyte elastase. Biochim Biophys Acta 1983;775:300.

104. Wijermans PW, Rebel VI, Ossenkoppele GJ, et al: Combined procoagulant activity and proteolytic activity of acute promyelocytic leukemic cells: Reversal of the bleeding disorder by cell differentiation. Blood 1989;73:800.

105. Tapiovaara H, Matikainen S, Hurme M, et al: Induction of differentiating therapy of promyelocytic NB4 cells by retinoic acid is associated with rapid increase in urokinase activity subsequently downregulated by production of inhibitors. Blood 1994;83:1883.

106. Griffin JD, Rambaldi A, Vellenga E, et al: Secretion of interleukin-1 by acute myeloid leukemia cells in vitro induces endothelial cells to secrete colony-stimulating factors. Blood 1987;70:1218.

107. Cozzolino F, Torcia M, Miliani A, et al: Potential role of interleukin-1 as the trigger for diffuse intravascular coagulation in acute nonlymphoblastic leukemia. Am J Med 1988;84:240.

108. Colucci M, Balconi G, Lorenzet R, et al: Cultured human endothelial cells generate tissue factor in response to endotoxin. J Clin Invest 1983;71:1893.

109. Bevilacqua MP, Pober JS, Majeau GR, et al: Recombinant tumor necrosis factor induces procoagulant activity in cultured human vascular endothelium: Characterization and comparison with the actions of interleukin-1. Proc Natl Acad Sci USA 1986;83:4533.

110. Dittman WA, Majerus PW: Structure and function of thrombomodulin: A natural anticoagulant. Blood 1990;75:329.

111. Moore KL, Esmon CT, Esmon NL: Tumor necrosis factor leads to the internalization and degradation of thrombomodulin from the surface of bovine aortic endothelial cells in culture. Blood 1989;73:159.

112. Nachman RL, Hajar KA, Silverstein RL, et al: Interleukin-1 induces endothelial cell synthesis of plasminogen activator inhibitor. J Exp Med 1993;163:1595.

113. Suffredini AF, Harpell PC, Parrillo JE: Promotion and subsequent inhibition of plasminogen activation after administration of intravenous endotoxin to normal subjects. N Engl J Med 1989;320:1165.

114. van Hinsberg VWM, Bauer KA, Kooistra T, et al: Progress of fibrinolysis during tumor necrosis factor infusion in humans: Concomitant increase of tissue-type plasminogen activator, plasminogen activator inhibitor type-1, and fibrin(ogen) degradation products. Blood 1990;76:2284.

115. Dubois C, Schlageter MH, de Gentile A, et al: Modulation of IL-8, IL-1β, and G-CSF by all-trans retinoic acid in acute promyelocytic leukemia. Leukemia 1994;8:1750.

116. Gianni M, Norio P, Terao M, et al: The effect of dexamethasone on proinflammatory cytokine expression, cell growth and maturation during granulocytic differentiation of acute promyelocytic leukemia cells. Eur Cytokine Network 1995;6:157.

117. Ishii H, Horie S, Kizaki K, et al: Retinoic acid counteracts both the downregulation of thrombomodulin and the induction of tissue factor in cultured human endothelial cells exposed to tumor necrosis factor. Blood 1992;80:2556.

118. Mantovani A, Bussolino F, Dejana E: Cytokine regulation of endothelial cell function. FASEB J 1992;6:2591.

119. Giavazzi R, Foppolo M, Dossi R, et al: Rolling and adhesion of human tumor cells on vascular endothelium under physiological flow conditions. J Clin Invest 1993;92:3038.

120. Rickles FR, Edwards RL: Leukocytes and tumor cells in thrombosis. In Colman RW, Hirsh J, Marder VJ, et al, eds: Hemostasis and Thrombosis: Basic Principles and Clinical Practice. Philadelphia: JB Lippincott; 1994, p 1164.

121. Marchetti M, Falanga A, Giovanelli S, et al: All-trans-retinoic

increases the adhesion to endothelium of the acute promyelocytic leukemia cell line NB4. Br J Haematol 1996;93:360.

122. Marchetti M, Vignoli A, Barbui T, et al: Endothelial cell/leukemic cell interaction effect of all-trans retinoic acid on cell/cell adhesion. Thromb Haemost 1999;Aug Suppl:16a.

123. Lee AY, Levine MN: The thrombophilic state induced by therapeutic agents in the cancer patient. Semin Thromb Hemost 1999; 25:137.

124. Bertomeu MC, Gallo S, Lauri D, et al: Chemotherapy enhances endothelial cell reactivity to platelets. Clin Expl Metastasis 1990; 8:511.

125. Nicolson GL, Custead SE: Effects of chemotherapeutic drugs on platelet and metastatic tumor cell–endothelial cell interactions as a model for assessing vascular endothelial intergrity. Cancer Res 1985;45:331.

126. Sporn LA, Rubin P, Marder VJ, et al: Irradiation induces release of von Willebrand protein from endothelial cells in culture. Blood 1984;64:567.

127. Poggi A, Kornblitt L, Delaini F, et al: Delayed hypercoagulability after a single dose of Adriamycin to normal rats. Thromb Res 1979;16:639.

128. Licciarello JTW, Moake JL, Rudi CK, et al: Elevated plasma von Willebrand factor levels and arterial occlusive complications associated with cisplatin-based chemotherapy. Oncology 1985;42:296.

129. Bazarbachi A, Scrobohachi ML, Gisselbracht C, et al: Changes in protein C, factor VII and endothelial markers after autologous bone marrow transplantation: Possible implications in the pathogenesis of veno-occlusive disease. Nouvelle Revue FR Haematologie 1993;35:135.

130. Catani L, Gugliotta L, Vianelli N, et al: Endothelium and bone marrow transplantation. Bone Marrow Transplant 1996;17:277.

131. Harper PL, Jarvis J, Jennings I, et al: Changes in the natural anticoagulants following bone marrow transplantation. Bone Marrow Transplant 1990;5:39.

132. Haskell CM, Canellos GP, Leventhal BG, et al: L-asparaginase: Therapeutic and toxic effects in patients with neoplastic disease. N Engl J Med 1969;281:1028.

133. Homans AC, Rybak ME, Baglini RL, et al: Effect of L-asparaginase administration on coagulation and platelet function in children with leukemia. J Clin Oncol 1987;5:811.

134. Leone G, Gugliotta L, Mazzucconi MG, et al: Evidence of a hypercoagulable state in patients with acute lymphoblastic leukemia treated with low dose of E coli L-asparaginase: A GIMEMA study. Thromb Haemost 1993;69:12.

135. Rubin P: The Franz Buschke lecture: Late effects of chemotherapy and radiation therapy—a new hypothesis. Int Rad Oncol 1983; 10:5.

136. Jirtle RL, Michaiopouious G, McLain JR, et al: Transplantation system for determining the clonogenic survival of parenchymal hepatocytes exposed to ionizing radiation. Cancer Res 1981;41: 3512.

137. Ludwig J, Axiesen R: Drug effects on the liver: An updated tabular compilation of drugs and drug-related hepatic diseases. Dig Dis Sci 1983;28:651.

138. Bearman SI: The syndrome of veno-occlusive disease after bone-marrow transplantation. Blood 1995;85:3005.

139. Bearman SI, Lee JL, Baron AE, et al: Treatment of hepatic venocclusive disease with recombinant human tissue plasminogen activator and heparin in 42 marrow transplant patients. Blood 1997;5:1501.

140. Shulman HM, Gown AM, Nugent DJ: Hepatic veno-occlusive disorder disease after bone marrow transplantation: Immunohistochemical identification of the material within occluded central venules. Am J Pathol 1987;127:549.

141. Richardson PG, Elias AD, Krishnam A, et al: Treatment of severe veno-occlusive disease with defibrotide: Compassionate use results in response without significant toxicity in a high-risk population. Blood 1998;92:737.

142. Clawson CC:Platelet inactivation with bacteria: Ultrastructure. Am J Pathol 1973;70:449.

143. Clawson CC, Rao GHR, White JG: Platelet interaction with bacteria: Stimulation of the release reaction. Am J Pathol 1975;81:411.

144. MacIntyre DE, Allen AP, Thorne KJI: Endotoxin-induced platelet aggregation and secretion: Morphological changes and pharmacological effects. J Cell Sci 1977;28:211.

145. Semeraro N, Colucci M: Changes in the coagulation-fibrinolysis

146. Shands JW Jr: The endotoxin-induced procoagulant of mouse exudate macrophages: A factor X activator. Blood 1983;62:333.

147. Chang HY, Rodriguez V, Narboni G, et al: Causes of death in adults with acute leukemia. Medicine 1976;55:259.

148. Murphy S, Litwin S, Herring LM, et al: Indications for platelet transfusion in children with acute leukemia. Am J Hematol 1982; 12:347.

149. Beutler E: Platelet transfusions: The 20,000/mL trigger. Blood 1993;81:1411.

150. Gaydos LA, Freireich EJ, Mantel N: The quantitative relation between platelet count and hemorrhage in patients with acute leukemia. N Engl J Med 1962;266:905.

151. Slichter SJ: Principles of platelet transfusion therapy. In Hoffman R, Benz EJ Jr, Shatlie SJ, et al, eds: Hematology: Basic Principles and Practice. New York: Churchill Livingstone; 1991, p 1610.

152. Gmur J, Burger J, Schanz U, et al: Safety of stringent prophylactic platelet transfusion policy for patients with acute leukemia. Lancet 1991;338:1223.

153. Gil-Fernandez JJ, Alegre A, Fernandez-Villalta MJ, et al: Clinical results of a stringent policy on prophylactic platelet transfusion: Nonrandomized comparative analysis in 190 bone marrow transplant patients from a single institution. Bone Marrow Transplant 1996;18:931.

154. Wandt H, Frank M, Ehninger G, et al: Safety and cost effectiveness of a $10 \times 10^9/L$ trigger for prophylactic platelet transfusion compared with the traditional $20 \times 10^9/L$ trigger: A prospective comparative trial in 105 patients with acute myeloid leukemia. Blood 1998;91:3601.

155. Navarro JT, Hernandez JA, Ribera JM, et al: Prophylactic platelet transfusion threshold during therapy for adult acute myeloid leukemia: 10,000/ml versus 20,000/ml. Haematologica 1998;83:998.

156. Rebulla P, Finazzi G, Marangoni F, et al: The threshold for prophylactic platelet transfusions in adults with acute myeloid leukemia. N Engl J Med 1997;337:1870.

157. Heckman KD, Weiner GJ, Davis CS, et al: Randomized study of prophylactic platelet transfusion threshold during induction therapy for adult acute leukemia: 10,000/ml versus 20,000/ml. J Clin Oncol 1997;15:1143.

158. Finazzi G: Prophylactic platelet transfusion in acute leukemia: Which threshold should be used? Haematologica 1998;83:961.

159. Norfolk DR, Ancliffe PJ, Contreras M, et al: Consensus conference on platelet transfusion: Royal College of Physicians of Edinburgh, 27–28 November 1997. Br J Haematol 1998;101:609.

160. Kruskall MS: The perils of platelet transfusions. N Engl J Med 1997;337:1914.

161. Rebulla P: Primum non nocere: Balancing allogeneic and autologous transfusion risks with a "society perspective." Haematologica 1998;83:673.

162. Kantarjian HM, Keating MJ, Walters RS, et al: Acute promyelocytic leukemia: M.D. Anderson Hospital experience. Am J Med 1986; 80:789.

163. Goldberg MA, Ginsburg D, Mayer RJ, et al: Is heparin administration necessary during induction chemotherapy for patients with acute promyelocytic leukemia? Blood 1987;69:187.

164. Bassan R, Battista R, Viero P, et al: Short-term treatment for adult hypergranular and microgranular acute promyelocytic leukemia. Leukemia 1995;9:238.

165. Daly PA, Schiffer CA, Aisner J, et al: Platelet transfusion therapy: One-hour posttransfusion increments are valuable in predicting the need for HLA-matched preparations. JAMA 1980;243:435.

166. Alcorta I, Pereira A, Ordinas A: Clinical and laboratory factors associated wth platelet transfusion refractoriness: A case-control study. Br J Haematol 1996;93:220.

167. Trial to Reduce Alloimmunization to Platelets Study Group: Leukocyte reduction and ultraviolet B irradiation of platelets to prevent alloimmunization and refractoriness to platelet transfusions. N Engl J Med 1997;337:1861.

168. Schiffer CA, Keller C, Dutcher JP, et al: Potential HLA-matched platelet donor availability for alloimmunized patients. Transfusion 1983;23:286.

169. Friedberg RC, Donnelly FF, Mintz PD: Independent roles for platelet cross-matching and HLA in the selection of platelets for alloimmunized patients. Transfusion 1994;34:215.

170. Nagasawa T, Kim BK, Baldini MG: Temporary suppression of circulating antiplatelet alloantibodies by the massive infusion of fresh, stored or lyophilized platelets. Transfusion 1978;18:429.

171. Hashimoto S, Koike T, Tatewaki W, et al: Fatal thromboembolism in acute promyelocytic leukemia during all-trans-retinoic acid therapy combined with antifibrinolytic therapy for prophylaxis of hemorrhage. Leukemia 1994;8:1113.

172. Kaushansky K: Thrombopoietin. N Engl J Med 1998;339:746.

173. Hofman WK, Ottmann OG, Hoelzer D: Megakaryocytic growth factors: Is there a new approach for management of thrombocytopenia in patients with malignancies? Leukemia 1999;13:S14.

174. Schiffer CA, Miller K, Larson RA, et al: A double-blind, placebo-controlled trial of pegylated recombinant human megakaryocyte growth and development factor as an adjunct to induction and consolidation therapy for patients with acute myeloid leukemia. Blood 2000;95:2530.

175. Basser RL, Rasko JEJ, Clarke K, et al: Randomized, blinded, placebo-controlled phase I trial of pegylated recombinant human megakaryocyte growth and development factor with filgrastim after dose-intensive chemotherapy in patients with advanced cancer. Blood 1997;89:3118.

176. Fanucchi M, Glaspy J, Crawford J, et al: Effects of polyethylene glycol-conjugated recombinant human megakaryocyte growth and development factor on platelet counts after chemotherapy for lung cancer. N Engl J Med 1997;336:404.

177. Vadhan-Raj S, Murray LJ, Bueso-Ramos C, et al: Stimulation of megakaryocyte and platelet production by a single dose of recombinant human thrombopoietin in patients with cancer. Ann Intern Med 1997;126:673.

178. Archimbaud E, Ottman O, Liu Yin, et al: A randomized, double-blind, placebo-controlled study using PEG-rHuMGDF as an adjunct to chemotherapy for adults with de novo acute myeloid leukemia: Early results. Blood 1996;88:447a.

179. Beveridge R, Schuster M, Waller E, et al: Randomized, double-blind, placebo-controlled trial of pegylated recombinant human megakaryocyte growth and development factor (PEG-rHuMGDF) in breast cancer patients following autologous bone marrow transplantation. Blood 1997;90:580a.

180. Bolwell B, Vredenburgh J, Overmoyer B, et al: Safety and biological effect of pegylated recombinant human megakaryocyte growth and development factor (PEG-rHuMGDF) in breast cancer patients following autologous peripheral blood progenitor cell transplantation. Blood 1997;90:171a.

181. Glaspy J, Vredenburgh J, Demetri GD, et al: Effects of pegylated recombinant human megakaryocyte growth and development factor (PEG-rHuMGDF) before high-dose chemotherapy with peripheral blood progenitor cell support. Blood 1997;90:580a.

182. Crawford J, Glaspy J, Belani C, et al: A randomized, placebo-controlled, blinded-dose scheduling trial of pegylated recombinant human megakaryocyte growth and development factor (PEG-rHuMGDF) with filgrastim support in non-small cell lung cancer patients treated with paclitaxel and carboplatin during multiple cycles of chemotherapy. Proc Am Soc Clin Oncol 1998;17:73a.

183. Archimbaud E, Thomas X: Thrombopoietic factors potentially useful in the treatment of acute leukemia. Leuk Res 1998;22:1155.

184. Kaushansky K: Use of thrombopoietic growth factors in acute leukemia. Leukemia 2000;14:505.

185. Tepler I, Elias L, Smith JW II, et al: A randomized placebo-controlled trial of recombinant human interleukin-11 in cancer patients with severe thrombocytopenia due to chemotherapy. Blood 1996;87:3607.

186. Isaacs C, Robert NJ, Bailey FA, et al: Randomized, placebo-controlled study of recombinant human interleukin-11 to prevent chemotherapy-induced thrombocytopenia in patients with breast cancer receiving dose-intensive cyclophosphamide and doxorubicin. J Clin Oncol 1997;15:3368.

187. Ishii H, Horie S, Kizaki K, et al: Retinoic acid counteracts both the downregulation of thrombomodulin and the induction of tissue factor in cultured endothelial cells exposed to tumor necrosis factor. Blood 1992;80:2556.

188. Horie S, Kisaki K, Ishii H, et al: Retinoic acid stimulates expression of thrombomodulin, a cell surface anticoagulant glycoprotein, on human endothelial cells: Differences between up-regulation of thrombomodulin by retinoic acid and cAMP. Biochem J 1992; 281:149.

189. Kooistra T, Opdenberg JP, Toet K, et al: Stimulation of tissue-type plasminogen activators synthesis by retinoids in cultured human endothelial cells and rat tissues in vivo. Thromb Haemost 1991; 65:565.

190. Medh RD, Santell L, Levin EG: Stimulation of tissue plasminogen activator production by retinoic acid: Synergistic effect on protein kinase C-mediated activation. Blood 1992;80:981.

191. Consonni R, Falanga A, Barbui T: PML/RARa-dependence of tissue factor (TF) regulation by retinoids in promyelocytic leukemia cells: Comparison with normal human monocytes and U937 cells. Thromb Haemost 1997;198a.

192. Barbui T, Finazzi G, Donati MB, et al: Antiblastic therapy and thrombosis. In Neri Serneri GG, Gensini GF, Abbate R, et al, eds: Thrombosis: An Update. Florence, Italy: Scientific Press; 1992, p 305.

193. Barbui T, Finazzi G, Viganò S, et al: L-asparaginase lowers protein C antigen. Thromb Haemost 1984;52:216.

194. Gugliotta L, D'Angelo A, Mattioli-Belmonte M, et al: Hypercoagulability during L-asparaginase treatment: The effect of antithrombin III supplementation in vivo. Br J Haematol 1990;74:465.

195. Barbui T, Finazzi G, Barosi G: Chronic myeloid disorders, excluding CML. In Degos L, Linch DC, and Löwenberg B, eds: Textbook of Malignant Hematology. London: Martin Dunitz Ltd; 1999, p 847.

196. Gruppo Italiano Studio Policitemia: Polycythemia vera: The natural history of 1213 patients followed over 20 years. Ann Intern Med 1995;123:656.

197. Berk PD, Goldberg JD, Donovan PB, et al: Therapeutic recommendations in polycythemia vera based on Polycythemia Vera Study Group protocols. Semin Hematol 1986;23:132.

198. Pearson TC, Messinezy M: The diagnostic criteria of polycythaemia rubra vera. Leuk Lymphoma 1996;22:87.

199. Barbui T, Finazzi G: Risk factors and prevention of vascular complications in polycythemia vera. Semin Thromb Hemost 1997;23:455.

200. Valla D, Casadevall N, Lacombe C, et al:Primary myeloproliferative disorder and hepatic vein thrombosis. Ann Intern Med 1985; 103:329.

201. Murphy S, Peterson, Iland H, et al: Experience of the Polycythemia Vera Study Group with essential thrombocythemia: A final report on diagnostic criteria, survival and leukemic transition by treatment. Semin Hematol 1997;34, 29.

202. Barbui T, Finazzi G: Management of essential thrombocythemia. Crit Rev Oncol Hematol 1999;29:257.

203. Budde U, Schaefer G, Mueller N, et al: Acquired von Willebrand's disease in the myeloproliferative syndrome. Blood 1984;64:981.

204. Barbui T, Buelli M, Cortelazzo S, et al: Aspirin and risk of bleeding in patients with thrombocythemia. Am J Med 1987;83:265.

205. Beressi AH, Tefferi A, Silverstein MN, et al: Outcome analysis of 34 pregnancies in women with essential thrombocythemia. Arch Intern Med 1995;155:1217.

206. Ruggeri M, Finazzi G, Tosetto A, et al: No treatment for low-risk thrombocythemia: Results from a prospective study. Br J Haematol 1998;103, 772.

207. Harrison CN, Gale RE, Machin SJ, et al: A large proportion of patients with a diagnosis of essential thrombocythemia do not have a clonal disorder and may be at lower risk of thrombotic complications. Blood 1999;93:417.

208. Chiusolo P, Sica S, Ortu La Barbera E, et al: Patients with essential thrombocythemia and clonal hemopoiesis detected by X-inactivation pattern are at high risk for thrombotic complications. Blood 1999;94:700a.

209. Nimer SD: Essential thrombocythemia: Another "heterogeneous" disease better understood? Blood 1999;93:415.

210. Anderson JE, Sale G, Appelbaum FR, et al: Allogeneic marrow transplantation for primary myelofibrosis and myelofibrosis secondary to polycythemia vera or essential thrombocythosis. Br J Haematol 1997;98:1010.

211. Berk PD, Goldberg JD, Donovan PD, et al: Therapeutic recommendations in polycythemia vera based on polycythemia vera study group protocols. Semin Hematol 1986;23:132.

212. Berk PD, Wasserman LR, Fruchtman SM, et al: Treatment of polycythemia vera: A summary of clinical trials conducted by the PVSG. In Wasserman LR, Berk PD, Berlin NI, eds: Polycythemia Vera and the Myeloproliferative Disorders. Philadelphia: WB Saunders; 1995, p 166.

213. Fruchtman SM, Mack K, Kaplan ME, et al: From efficacy to safety:

A polycythemia vera study group report on hydroxyurea in patients with polycythemia vera. Semin Hematol 1997;34:17.

214. Najean Y, Rain JD: Treatment of polycythemia vera: The use of hydroxyurea and pipobroman in 242 patients under the age of 65 years. Blood 1997;90, 3370.

215. Najean Y, Rain JD: Treatment of polycythemia vera: Use of 32P alone or in combination with maintenance therapy using hydroxyurea in 434 patients over the age of 65 years. Blood 1997;89, 2319.

216. Silver RT: Interferon-alpha 2b: A new treatment for polycythemia vera. Ann Intern Med 1993;119:1091.

217. Reilly JT, Vellenga E, de Wolff JTM: Interferon treatment in polycythemia vera. Leuk Lymphoma 1996; 22:143.

218. Silver RT: Interferon alfa: Effects of long-term treatment for polycythemia vera. Semin Hematol 1997;34:40.

219. Anagrelide Study Group: Anagrelide, a therapy for thrombocythemic states: Experience in 577 patients. Am J Med 1992;92:69.

220. Petitt RM, Silverstein MN, Petrone M: Anagrelide for control of thrombocythemia in polycythemia and other myeloproliferative disorders. Semin Hematol 1997;34:51.

221. Marchioli R, Landolfi R, Barbui T, et al: Feasibility of randomized trials in rare diseases: The case of polycythemia vera. Leuk Lymphoma 1996;22:121.

222. Landolfi R, Patrono C: Aspirin in polycythemia vera and essential thrombocythemia: Current facts and perspectives. Leuk Lymphoma 1996;22:83.

223. Barbui T, Cortelazzo S, Viero P, et al: Thrombohemorrhagic complications in 101 cases of myeloproliferative disorders: Relationship to platelet number and function. Eur J Cancer Clin Oncol 1883; 19:1593.

224. Finazzi G, Budde U, Michiels JJ: Bleeding time and platelet function in myeloproliferative disorders. Leuk Lymphoma 1996;22:71.

225. Gruppo Italiano Studio Policitemia: Low-dose aspirin in polycythemia vera:A pilot study. Br J Haematol 1997;97:453.

226. Cortelazzo S, Viero P, Finazzi G, et al: Incidence and risk factors for thrombotic complications in a historical cohort of 100 patients with essential thrombocythemia. J Clin Oncol 1990;8:556.

227. Van Genderen PJJ, Michiels JJ, van der Poel-van de Luytgaarde SC, et al: Acquired von Willebrand disease as a cause of recurrent mucocutaneous bleeding in primary thrombocythemia: Relationship with platelet count. Ann Hematol 1994;69:81.

228. Cortelazzo S, Finazzi G, Ruggeri M, et al:Hydroxyurea in the treatment of patients with essential thrombocythemia at high risk of thrombosis: A prospective, randomized trial. N Engl J Med 1995; 332:1132.

229. Nand S, Stock W, Godwin J, et al: Leukemogenic risk of hydroxyurea therapy in polycythemia vera, essential thrombocythemia and myeloid metaplasia with myelofibrosis. Am J Hematol 1996;52:42.

230. Sterkers Y, Preudhomme C, Lai JL, et al: Acute myeloid leukemia and myelodysplastic syndromes following essential thrombocythemia treated with hydroxyurea. Blood 1998;91:616.

231. Finazzi G, Ruggeri M, Rodeghiero F, et al: Second malignancies in patients with essential thrombocythemia treated with busulfan and hydroxyurea: Long-term follow-up of a randomized clinical trial. Br J Haematol (in press).

232. Murphy S, Iland H, Rosenthal D, et al: Essential thrombocythemia: An interim report from the Polycythemia Vera Study Group. Semin Hematol 1986;23:177.

233. Lengfelder E, Griesshammer M, Hehlmann R: Interferon-alpha in the treatment of essential thrombocythemia. Leuk Lymphoma 1996;22:135.

234. Silverstein MN, Tefferi A: Treatment of essential thrombocythemia with anagrelide. Semin Hematol 1999;36:23.

235. Griesshammer M, Bangerter M, van Vliet HHDM, et al: Aspirin in essential thrombocythemia: Status quo and quo vadis. Semin Thromb Hemost 1997;23:371.

16

Michael F. Murphy

Management of Anemia in Patients with Leukemia

INTRODUCTION

The most important aspects of supportive care for patients with leukemia are prophylaxis and treatment of infection and bleeding and management of anemia.

Anemia is an almost invariable consequence of acute leukemia due to a reduction in erythropoiesis caused by the accumulation of leukemic cells in the bone marrow and the suppressive effect of cytotoxic drug therapy. Although the ready availability of red blood cell (RBC) concentrates means that anemia can be relieved easily, there are important management considerations, such as the appropriate trigger for RBC transfusions, the avoidance of complications associated with repeated transfusions, and the use of alternative therapeutic approaches (e.g., erythropoietin).

Anemia is also common in patients with chronic leukemia. The cause is not always a reduction in erythropoiesis; for example, autoimmune hemolytic anemia may occur in chronic lymphocytic leukemia (CLL), for which steroids are the initial therapeutic option. However, RBC transfusions are frequently required in managing anemia in chronic leukemia, as they are in acute leukemia. This chapter considers the appropriate indications for their use and how to avoid complications of transfusions.

RBC TRANSFUSIONS

Indications

Responses to decreased oxygen delivery to the tissues in chronic anemia include increases in cardiac output and respiratory rate, redistribution of blood away from the kidneys and digestive system to the heart and muscles, and an increase in the unloading of oxygen from hemoglobin as a result of higher 2,3-diphosphoglycerate levels.[1] Symptoms include tiredness, dyspnea at rest or after exertion, lack of concentration, headaches, angina, and intermittent claudication. The hemoglobin level at which such symptoms begin to occur varies considerably from one patient to another, and symptoms may not appear until the hemoglobin concentration is less than 7 g/dL.

RBC transfusions are indicated in patients with chronic anemia when clinical symptoms are present or imminent;

a further consideration in patients with acute leukemia is to provide a "reserve" in case of severe hemorrhage.[2] However, an optimal schedule for RBC transfusions in acute leukemia patients has not been defined.

The usual practice in hospitals treating patients with acute leukemia is to raise the hemoglobin level by about 3 g/dL from a predetermined "trigger" level of hemoglobin, which means that transfusions are given at approximately weekly intervals during intensive therapy (one unit of RBCs increases the hemoglobin by approximately 1 g/dL). Although patients vary in their tolerance of anemia, it is convenient for each treatment center to have a standard policy for RBC transfusion, even if this results in some patients being overtransfused.

Although the trigger level varies from hospital to hospital, it is probably in the range of 8 to 10 g/dL; an audit showed that the hemoglobin level at the time of RBC transfusion was 10.7 g/dL in patients with solid tumors receiving cytotoxic chemotherapy.[3] There are no definite data from clinical studies in patients with leukemia to support the use of a trigger level as high as this. However, studies in anemic uremic patients have shown that increasing the hemoglobin level with either RBC transfusions or erythropoietin corrects the prolonged bleeding time often seen in these patients.[4, 5]

Data from an animal model showed that anemia contributed significantly to the prolongation of the bleeding time associated with thrombocytopenia and that RBC transfusions shortened the bleeding time.[6] While accepting that results obtained in an animal model cannot necessarily be extrapolated to the clinical situation and that clinical studies should be carried out, the data suggest that the trigger level of hemoglobin for RBC transfusions in anemic thrombocytopenic patients with acute leukemia should be at the upper end of the current range of 8 to 10 g/dL.

Number of Transfusions

Little has been published on the quantitative aspects of RBC transfusion therapy in the management of leukemia. Transfusion requirements clearly depend on whether the leukemia is acute or chronic and on the intensity of treatment given; requirements vary considerably among patients.

A study showed that 118 patients with acute myeloblastic leukemia (AML) undergoing remission induction and consolidation therapy received a median of 18 units (range 3 to 44 units) of RBC concentrates.[7] Patients with hemoglobin levels greater than 10 g/dL, platelets more than 100×10^9/L, and white blood cell (WBC) counts less than 5×10^9/L at initial presentation received fewer transfusions than patients with less favorable blood counts during the first cycle of chemotherapy; otherwise, the most important factors determining the number of RBC transfusions were the number of days in the hospital and the participating center within the study.[7]

More transfusions were used for patients with AML during remission induction therapy than during allogeneic bone marrow transplantation (BMT) in first remission.[8] In a later study,[9] there was no significant difference in the total requirement for RBC transfusions in patients with acute leukemia treated by remission induction therapy followed by consolidation therapy (median of 20 units) compared with patients treated by chemotherapy and radiotherapy prior to autologous BMT (median 16 units), but there was a significantly reduced requirement for RBC transfusions in patients undergoing allogeneic BMT (median 9 units). The exception to this last low requirement is ABO-incompatible BMT (see the later section on alloimmunization).

The requirement for RBC transfusions in patients with chronic leukemia is extremely variable; some patients require a considerable number of transfusions over a long time.

Complications of Multiple RBC Transfusions

Transfusion-Transmitted Infections

Patients receiving intensive treatment for leukemia will inevitably receive blood components from multiple donors and are therefore at risk of acquiring the following transfusion-transmitted infections.

Hepatitis C. Repeatedly abnormal serum transaminases are common in patients being treated for leukemia and may be due to the drug therapy, particularly cytotoxic chemotherapy, infections, graft-versus-host disease (GVHD), veno-occlusive disease, or leukemic infiltration of the liver.

Before the introduction of blood donor screening for anti-hepatitis C (HCV) in the United Kingdom in September 1991, 32 of a group of 115 patients with hematologic malignancies were found to have repeatedly elevated serum transaminase levels, and 8 were diagnosed as having acute HCV infection by the detection of HCV-RNA in the patients' serum.[10] The infection caused fulminant hepatic failure and death in one patient with AML, was associated with prolonged thrombocytopenia after autologous BMT in two patients, and was associated with cytomegalovirus pneumonitis and GVHD in a patient with acute lymphoblastic leukemia after allogeneic BMT. A follow-up study of 140 patients after the introduction of blood donor testing for anti-HCV identified no cases of HCV infection.[10a] It is currently estimated that HCV is transmitted by fewer than 1 in 200,000 donations in the United

Kingdom[11] and by fewer than 1 in 103,000 donations in the United States.[12]

Hepatitis B. Screening of blood donors to prevent hepatitis B infection has been carried out for much longer than for HCV, and since 1971 in the United Kingdom, meaning that the risk of transmission of hepatitis B is low, even in patients with leukemia receiving multiple blood components. The current risk of transmission is estimated to be 1 in 50,000 to 1 in 170,000 donations in the United Kingdom,[11] and less than 1 in 63,000 in the United States.[12]

Human Immunodeficiency Virus. The risk of contracting human immunodeficiency virus (HIV) from a blood transfusion in the United Kingdom is estimated as being less than 1 in 2 million donations[11] and less than 1 in 493,000 in the United States.[12] Routine screening of all donations for anti-HIV was introduced in 1985; prior to this, patients receiving multiple transfusions were presumably at most risk of acquiring HIV infection from blood transfusion, and there were reports of patients acquiring HIV infection after allogeneic BMT.[13, 14]

Cytomegalovirus (CMV). CMV infection causes significant morbidity and mortality in allogeneic BMT recipients; the most serious complication is interstitial pneumonia. In one study, the prevalence of infection was 69% in patients who were CMV-seropositive before transplantation as a result of reactivation of latent virus; the prevalence in CMV-seronegative patients was 36% owing to transmission from marrow and blood components from CMV-seropositive donors.[15] The probability of CMV infection is lower, but not negligible, in patients undergoing autologous BMT.[16]

Prevention of CMV infection is a major consideration in transfusion management of patients undergoing BMT. The standard method for preventing transfusion-transmitted CMV infection has been to screen blood donors for CMV antibodies. However, it may not be possible to provide sufficient quantities of CMV-seronegative blood components in some hospitals. An alternative is to use WBC-reduced blood components, prepared by filtration. This approach has been shown to be effective in reducing the risk of transfusion-transmitted CMV infection.[17-19]

Many countries, including the United Kingdom but not yet the United States, are moving to universal WBC-reduction of blood components. The main reasons for this are to improve the quality of blood components, to minimize the risk of transfusion-related complications such as febrile reactions and platelet refractoriness (see later), and to minimize the theoretical risk of transmission of variant Creutzfeldt-Jakob disease by blood transfusion.[20, 21] However, many transplant centers are not prepared to accept that WBC-reduced blood components are as safe as CMV-seronegative blood components in the prevention of transfusion-transmitted CMV infection in recipients of hemopoietic transplants; they request both WBC-reduced and CMV-seronegative blood components for high-risk situations, such as allografts involving a CMV-seronegative recipient and a CMV-seronegative donor.[22]

CMV infection is of less immediate significance during remission induction therapy for acute leukemia. However, consideration should be given to preventing primary CMV infection in patients who are candidates for allogeneic BMT and possibly also for candidates for autologous BMT.[23]

Alloimmunization

An important consequence of repeated transfusions of blood components from random donors is the development of alloimmunization to RBC, WBC, and platelet antigens.

RBCs. Patients with leukemia are sometimes believed to be at low risk of developing RBC alloantibodies. However, a study of 703 patients receiving multiple transfusions found that antibodies were detected in 20/123 (16%) of patients with myeloid leukemia (94 patients with AML and 29 with chronic myeloid leukemia). The incidence of RBC alloimmunization in patients with myeloid leukemia was similar to that in patients with aplastic anemia, hemoglobinopathy, renal failure, and gastrointestinal bleeding.[24] On the other hand, none of the 75 patients with acute lymphoblastic leukemia or the 24 patients with CLL developed RBC alloantibodies.[24]

Similar observations of a higher incidence of RBC alloimmunization in myeloproliferative disorders compared with lymphoproliferative disorders were made in another study of patients with hematologic malignancies. Patients with myeloproliferative disorders received almost three times as many units of blood in more than twice as many transfusion episodes over more than twice as long a period as patients with lymphoproliferative disorders.[25]

ABO-Incompatible Allogeneic Transplantation. There was initial concern that ABO-incompatible allogeneic transplantation might be associated with an increased risk of graft rejection and GVHD: graft rejection might occur if there were ABO antigens in the donor that were absent in the recipient (a major mismatch), and GVHD might occur if there were ABO antigens in the recipient that were absent in the donor (a minor mismatch). However, there is no evidence that ABO incompatibility increases the incidence of graft rejection or GVHD.[26, 27] The problems of ABO-incompatible allogeneic transplantation, including the prevention and management of hemolysis at the time of marrow infusion, delayed erythroid engraftment, and post-transfusion hemolysis, have been reviewed.[28–30]

Reduced survival has been reported for patients with AML receiving major ABO-incompatible transplants compared with patients receiving transplants from ABO-identical donors.[31] Suggested hypotheses to explain these results are that ABO immune complexes cause impaired cell-mediated immunity[32] or endothelial damage[31] leading to multiorgan failure and sepsis. These observations are considered to be preliminary and require further confirmation.[32]

An important syndrome of immune hemolysis occurs following minor ABO and RhD-incompatible marrow transplants and has become known as "passenger lymphocyte syndrome."[28, 33] Immune hemolytic anemia occurs because of antibodies produced by donor lymphocytes against recipient RBCs; maximum hemolysis occurs between 9 and 16 days post-transplant, and severe intravascular hemolysis may occur.

RhD Alloimmunization Following RhD-Incompatible Platelet Transfusions. Evidence provided for a low risk of RBC alloimmunization in leukemic patients includes the low incidence of anti-D (antibodies against RhD antigen) in RhD-negative leukemic patients receiving platelet concentrates from RhD-positive donors. This is an important practical issue: although it is recommended that RhD-identical platelets be administered if possible, logistic constraints sometimes dictate that RhD-negative patients be given platelet transfusions from RhD-positive donors. The question of the need to administer anti-D is raised particularly for women with childbearing potential.

Only 8 (7.8%) of 102 patients with leukemia, mainly acute leukemia, developed anti-D compared with 60% to 80% of normal volunteers receiving similar quantities of RBCs in a planned immunization program.[34] In another study, only 3 of 33 RhD-negative patients with hematologic malignancies, including 2 patients with AML, developed anti-D after RhD-positive platelet transfusions.[25]

Developments in platelet apheresis and blood component processing technology have led to considerable reduction in RBC contamination of platelet concentrates. A study using modern methods of platelet collection found that 0/24 (0%) of the hematology patients, predominantly with leukemia, formed anti-D in contrast to 8/59 (13.5%) nonhematology patients who developed detectable anti-D.[35]

It continues to be recommended that RhD-negative platelet concentrates be used where possible for RhD-negative patients, particularly for females who have not reached menopause.[36] If RhD-positive platelets are transfused to an RhD-negative female of childbearing potential, it is recommended that anti-D should be given.[36] A dose of 250 IU anti-D should be sufficient to cover 5 adult therapeutic doses of RhD-positive platelets within a 6-week period, and the dose should be given subcutaneously in thrombocytopenic patients.

WBCs and Platelets. The clinical consequences of alloimmunization to WBC and platelet antigens in leukemia patients are platelet refractoriness, nonhemolytic (febrile) transfusion reactions, and graft rejection. Table 16–1 summarizes generally accepted recommendations for the use of WBC-reduced blood components for preventing WBC-associated complications of blood transfusion.[37] As stated earlier, many countries including the United Kingdom but not yet the United States are moving to universal WBC-reduction of blood components.

When planning strategy for leukemia patients who are likely to receive multiple platelet transfusions, consider the prevention of platelet refractoriness due to HLA alloimmunization; there is considerable evidence that refractoriness may be minimized using WBC-reduced RBC and platelet concentrates.[38–40] Furthermore, it has been reported that the use of WBC-reduced blood components in patients with AML had favorable effects on the recovery of the platelet and granulocyte counts, the occurrence of serious infections, the consumption of blood components, and relapse-free survival.[41] These data still need to be confirmed in large prospective, randomized studies.

Fever and/or rigors occur in about a half hour to 2

TABLE 16–1. Recommendations for Clinical Use of WBC-reduced Blood Components*

Definition

WBC-reduced blood components must contain 5×10^6 WBC per unit (RBCs) or adult therapeutic dose (platelets).

Practical Aspects

To achieve residual WBC counts of $<5 \times 10^6$, WBC reduction should be carried out under controlled conditions, ideally within 48 hours from the collection of the donor unit.

Indications for WBC-reduced Blood Components

Recommended

Febrile nonhemolytic transfusion reactions (FNHTRs).
1. To prevent recurrent FNHTRs after RBC transfusions.
2. To prevent FNHTRs in patients likely to be dependent on long-term RBC support.
3. There is increasing evidence that the major cause of FNHTRs after platelet transfusions is the presence of pyrogenic cytokines released from WBCs during storage. FNHTRs after platelet transfusions are not reliably prevented by bedside filtration because of cytokine release during storage. The routine use of prestorage WBC-reduced platelets is associated with a low incidence of FNHTRs.

Reducing graft rejection after hemopoietic cell transplantation.

Patients with severe aplastic anemia who are potential hemopoietic cell transplant recipients should receive WBC-reduced blood components from the beginning of transfusion support. The same might apply to patients with hemoglobinopathies, but more evidence is required before a definite recommendation can be made.

Prevention of transmission of viral infections by blood transfusion.

WBC reduction of blood components is an effective alternative to the use of CMV-seronegative blood components for the prevention of transfusion-transmitted CMV infection to at-risk patients, but many hospitals prefer to use both CMV-seronegative and WBC-reduced blood components in high-risk situations; e.g., hemopoietic cell allograft when both donor and recipient are CMV-seronegative.

Fetal/neonatal transfusions.

WBC-reduced blood components should be used for intrauterine transfusions and for all transfusions to infants younger than 1 year of age.

Possible

Platelet refractoriness.

There is no definite evidence that routine WBC reduction of blood components produces clinical benefits such as a reduction in the incidence of hemorrhage or mortality in patients receiving multiple platelet transfusions, although HLA alloimmunization and platelet refractoriness are reduced.

Kidney transplants.

Pretransplant blood transfusion may confer some benefit to renal transplant recipients, although some patients will become alloimmunized, leading to difficulties in the selection of donor kidneys. Consideration should be given to the use of WBC-reduced transfusions in renal transplant patients to prevent HLA alloimmunization.

Immunomodulation.

There is insufficient evidence to recommend routine use of WBC-reduced blood components for surgical patients for the prevention of either postoperative infection or tumor recurrence.

Progression of HIV infection.

There is insufficient evidence to recommend the use of WBC-reduced blood components for reducing the progression of HIV infection.

Nonindications

A significant number of recipients of blood components receive a limited number of transfusions over a short period; e.g., most general medical and surgical patients. WBC-reduced blood components are not indicated for these recipients unless there is an additional acceptable indication.

Prevention of transfusion-associated (TA) GVHD is not an indication for receiving WBC-reduced blood components. Gamma irradiation of blood components is the standard method for avoiding TA-GVHD.

There is no need for WBC-reduced noncellular blood components such as fresh frozen plasma, cryoprecipitate, and blood products prepared from pooled plasma.

*Adapted from guidelines from the British Committee for Standards in Haematology.[37]

hours after the beginning of the transfusion in about 1% to 2% of patients receiving RBC transfusions, typically in patients who have developed HLA antibodies after pregnancies or previous transfusions.[42] The prevalence in patients with leukemia is higher because of the repeated use of transfusions; febrile reactions occurred in 7/86 (8%) of acute leukemia patients studied at St. Bartholomew's Hospital between 1983 and 1985. Most febrile reactions are mild and can be managed by slowing or stopping the transfusion or administering aspirin or paracetamol to reduce the fever; paracetamol rather than aspirin should be used for patients with thrombocytopenia. WBC-reduced RBC concentrates are recommended for patients having recurrent febrile reactions after RBC transfusions.[37] Universal WBC-reduction of blood compo-

nents, which is being adopted in some countries,[20, 21] will result in a marked decrease in nonhemolytic (febrile) transfusion reactions after RBC transfusions.

Sensitization to transplantation antigens because of previous transfusions and/or pregnancies was found to result in an increased incidence of marrow rejection in patients with aplastic anemia.[43, 44] This led to the practice of avoiding pretransplant transfusions in patients with aplastic anemia, particularly from the marrow donor and family members. Graft rejection is less of a problem in leukemia patients, but pretransplant transfusions from the marrow donor are usually avoided.[30] WBC-reduction of pretransplant transfusions has been shown to reduce the incidence of graft rejection in an animal model,[45] and irradiation of blood with ultraviolet light has a similar effect.[46, 47] However, confirmation of these results in human studies is awaited.

GVHD

Transfusion of viable donor lymphocytes may result in transfusion-associated GVHD, which usually but not always occurs in immunocompromised patients.[48, 49] The risk in leukemia patients is greatest in those undergoing allogeneic BMT. It is recommended that all BMT recipients, but not patients undergoing remission induction therapy, should receive gamma-irradiated blood components.[48, 50]

A summary of recommendations for the use of gamma-irradiated blood components (adapted from guidelines from the British Committee for Standards in Haematology[50]) is given in Table 16–2. There is some variation in practice among hospitals[51] (for example, in the length of requirement of gamma-irradiated blood for allotransplant patients), but most recommendations provided in the table are generally followed worldwide. Also see Table 16–3.

Transfusion of as few as 10^4 lymphocytes may cause fatal GVHD. Although WBC-reduction might reduce the risk, transfusion-associated GVHD has occurred in a patient with non-Hodgkin's lymphoma who received only WBC-reduced blood components.[52] Reliable prophylaxis for transfusion-associated GVHD still requires gamma-irradiated blood components.[50, 51]

How to Ensure that Patients Receive the Correct Special Blood

An important issue for hematology departments and hospital blood banks is how to ensure that patients receive special blood components, such as CMV-seronegative or gamma-irradiated, and that standard blood components not be transfused as this may have devastating consequences.

TABLE 16–2. Summary of Recommendations for Use of Gamma-irradiated Blood Components*

Prevention of Transfusion-associated Graft-versus-host Disease (TA-GVHD)

Gamma-irradiation of blood components is the only recommended method for prevention of TA-GVHD.

Practical Aspects

1. The minimum dose in the irradiation field should be 25 Gy, with no part of the component receiving >50 Gy.
2. For at-risk patients, all RBC, platelet, and granulocyte transfusions should be irradiated.
3. RBC concentrates may be irradiated at any time up to 14 days after collection and then stored for a further 14 days after gamma irradiation.
4. Platelet concentrates can be gamma-irradiated at any time during their normal 5-day shelf life.
5. Granulocytes for all recipients should be gamma-irradiated as soon as possible after collection and then transfused with the minimum of delay.

*Adapted from guidelines from the British Committee for Standards in Haematology.[50]

TABLE 16–3. Indications for Use of Gamma-irradiated Blood Components in Patients with Hematologic Disease

Acute leukemia: Only for HLA-matched platelets or donations from first- or second-degree relatives

Allogeneic bone marrow/peripheral blood progenitor cell transplantation: From the time of initiation of conditioning therapy and continuing while the patient remains on GVHD prophylaxis (usually 6 months) or until lymphocytes are greater than 1×10^9/L. It may be necessary to irradiate blood components for SCID patients for up to 2 years and for patients with chronic GVHD if there is evidence of immunosuppression. Some hospitals recommend life-long use of gamma-irradiated blood for allotransplant patients.

Donors of allogeneic bone marrow: To prevent TA-GVHD mediated by lymphocytes in donor blood transfused before or during the harvest.

Autologous bone marrow/peripheral blood progenitor cell transplantation: During and 7 days before the harvest of hemopoietic cells, and then from the initiation of conditioning therapy until 3 months post-transplant (6 months if total-body irradiation is used).

Hodgkin's disease: Life-long requirement for gamma-irradiated blood components.

Patients treated with purine analogues: Life-long requirement for gamma-irradiated blood components.

Nonindications

Aplastic anemia (even if treated with antilymphocyte globulin).

Non-Hodgkin's lymphoma (although this may be reviewed following some recent reports of TA-GVHD in patients with B-cell non-Hodgkin's lymphoma).

HIV infection.

Each hospital should establish procedures so that patients receive correct special blood components. These procedures should include the following[53]:

- Education of ward medical and nursing staff about the indications for special blood components and the importance of receiving the correct type of blood component.
- Inclusion of the patients' diagnosis and any special requirements in requests for blood components.
- Storing of individual patients' requirements for special blood components in the blood bank computer.
- Consideration of providing patients with cards indicating their special blood requirements, particularly for those patients receiving shared care between two hospitals and those with a long-term requirement for gamma-irradiated blood, such as patients with Hodgkin's disease. Examples of a patient information leaflet and card for patients requiring gamma-irradiated blood are shown in Figures 16–1 and 16–2.

Iron Overload

A major consequence of repeated RBC transfusions over a prolonged period is iron overload.[54] Symptoms and signs of iron overload do not generally occur before a total of 100 to 150 units of blood have been transfused. This number of transfusions is higher than is given to most patients with leukemia, but those patients dependent on long-term RBC transfusions should be considered for iron chelation therapy, possibly after 30 to 50 units have been transfused.

This information sheet has been prepared to answer some of your questions about why you need to have irradiated blood and why it is important to carry the card you have been given.

Your hospital will keep a record that you need irradiated blood, but the card is an additional safeguard in case your records are not available or if you are treated at another hospital. You should show the card to the doctor treating you if you need a transfusion in the future.

Why do I need irradiated blood?

You need to have irradiated blood because you might be at risk of a rare complication of transfusion called transfusion-associated graft-versus-host disease (TA-GVHD).

What is TA-GVHD?

TA-GVHD is a rare but serious complication of blood transfusion caused by white blood cells (lymphocytes) in the blood transfused to you. Even a very small number of lymphocytes may recognize the patient receiving the blood as a foreign, and cause a severe illness and even death.

Which patients are at increased risk of TA-GVHD?

Some patients are at particular risk of TA-GVHD. These include:

- patients who have undergone procedures such as bone marrow/stem cell transplantation
- patients receiving transfusions from family members or HLA-matched donors
- patients with acquired deficiencies in immunity, either because of a disease such as Hodgkin's disease or who have received treatment with 'purine analogue' drugs such as fludarabine, cladribine, or deoxycoformycin
- patients with inherited deficiencies in immunity
- babies needing exchange transfusions who have been transfused in utero

Some patients remain at increased risk of TA-GVHD for a short period, but others are at increased risk life-long, e.g. patients with inherited immune deficiencies, patients with Hodgkin's disease, and patients treated with 'purine analogue' drugs.

Some hospitals recommend that patients who have had an allogeneic bone marrow/stem cell transplant should have irradiated blood for a limited period, and some recommend that it should be used for the rest of the patient's life. Your doctor will advise you whether you will need irradiated blood for a limited period or indefinitely.

How does irradiation work?

Gamma-irradiation of blood prevents lymphocytes dividing and causing harm.

Do all types of blood need to be irradiated?

The only types of blood that need to be irradiated are red cell (blood) and platelet transfusions. These are not routinely irradiated for all patients, and need to be irradiated 'on demand' for specific patients. It is important that doctors are aware if their patients need irradiated blood as they need to order it specially.

All granulocyte (white blood cell) transfusions are routinely irradiated. Plasma products such as fresh frozen plasma, anti-D, albumin, immunoglobulin do not need to be irradiated.

Does irradiation damage the blood?

It is not thought to cause any significant damage. The blood does not become 'radioactive' and will not harm you or anyone around you.

What if I need blood in an emergency?

Although it is recommended that your blood be irradiated, the risk of TA-GVHD is very small. In emergencies, there may not be time to arrange for irradiated blood to be provided. There may be occasions when it is more important to give you blood quickly than to wait for irradiated blood to be provided. The doctor treating you will judge the balance of these risks.

If you have any further questions, please ask the doctor treating you.

FIGURE 16–1. Example of a patient information sheet for patients needing gamma-irradiated blood. (Prepared for the British Committee for Standards in Haematology by Dr. M.F. Murphy and the National Blood Service Midlands and South West Clinical Policies Group.)

NAME ....
D.O.B...../...../..... CONSULTANT................
HOSPITAL/NHS Number ....
HOSPITAL FOR ENQUIRIES ....
REASON FOR IRRADIATED BLOOD ....

....
IRRADIATED BLOOD NEEDED INDEFINITELY
OR UNTIL ...../...../.....
DATE OF ISSUE OF CARD ...../...../.....

**THIS PATIENT IS AT RISK OF
TRANSFUSION-ASSOCIATED
GRAFT-VERSUS-HOST DISEASE**

If this patient needs to have a blood transfusion,
cellular blood components
(Red Cells and Platelets) must be
GAMMA-IRRADIATED
Please inform your blood transfusion laboratory

FIGURE 16–2. Example of a patient card for patients needing gamma-irradiated blood. (Prepared for the British Committee for Standards in Haematology by Dr. M.F. Murphy and the National Blood Service Midlands and South West Clinical Policies Group.)

Exacerbation of Thrombocytopenia After RBC Transfusions

It has long been recognized that transfusions of large quantities of blood may lead to a significant decrease in the post-transfusion platelet count.[54a, 54b] Smaller transfusions of 1 to 5 units of blood have also been shown to reduce the platelet count.[55, 56] The fall in platelet count may become clinically relevant in patients who are severely thrombocytopenic at the time of their blood transfusion.

The mechanism of the worsening of thrombocytopenia is adherence of platelets to microaggregates (composed mainly of WBCs and platelets in the transfused blood) and increased sequestration of platelets in the spleen. The filtration of blood through 40-μm microaggregate filters has been shown to prevent the worsening of thrombocytopenia in thrombocytopenic patients.[55, 56] Poststorage (bedside) filtration using a more advanced filter intended to produce WBC-reduction prevented a fall in platelet count following RBC transfusions in a small number of mostly nonthrombocytopenic patients.[55] However, it remains common practice to use prophylactic platelet transfusions for severely thrombocytopenic patients immediately following RBC transfusion with the aim of preventing worsening of thrombocytopenia and hemorrhagic events.

A study found a mean reduction of 1.1×10^9/L ($p = 0.43$) in the platelet count after transfusions of 2 to 3 units of WBC-reduced RBC concentrates to 20 thrombocytopenic patients with hematologic malignancies. However, there was a mean reduction of 2.7×10^9/L ($p = 0.03$) (approximately 10%) in the platelet count after transfusions of non-WBC-reduced RBC concentrates (10 patients).[57] The findings suggest that the introduction of universal WBC-reduction of RBC concentrates[20, 21] will minimize the worsening of thrombocytopenia that occurs in severely thrombocytopenic patients receiving standard non-WBC-reduced RBC concentrates.

ERYTHROPOIETIN

Erythropoietin is a growth factor produced by the kidney in a feedback control system in which the kidney responds to changes in oxygen tension by increasing or reducing the level of the circulating hormone.[58] It activates specific receptors on erythroid progenitors in the bone marrow to enhance erythropoiesis. If levels of erythropoietin are decreased, RBC production is reduced proportionately.

Recombinant Human Erythropoietin (rHuEPO)

rHuEPO became available in 1985, and it has been used extensively in anemia due to renal disease. Administration of rHuEPO has also been used for treating anemia in patients with cancer,[59–61] myeloma, and non-Hodgkin's lymphoma.[62, 63] It has been found to be safe and effective in increasing hemoglobin levels, but an important question remains as to how to identify the patients who will most benefit.[61, 64]

There has been much recent interest in the use of rHuEPO in patients receiving intensive myelosuppression supported by BMT.

Erythropoietin Levels in BMT Patients

Studies in patients undergoing allogeneic BMT showed an immediate rise in serum erythropoietin levels after the conditioning regimen, followed by a fall to inappropriately low levels for the degree of the anemia in the early post-transplant period, with recovery to more appropriate levels after day 180.[65–67] However, serum erythropoietin levels remained lower than expected in patients with persistent anemia.[66] Active CMV infection and acute GVHD were found to have a suppressive effect on serum erythropoietin levels.[65, 66] There have been less clear-cut results in patients undergoing autologous BMT, with adequate serum erythropoietin levels reported in some series[65, 68] and subnormal levels in others.[66, 67]

The mechanism of impaired erythropoietin production after BMT is undefined, but factors such as the administration of cyclosporin and high levels of cytokines such as interleukin-1, tumor necrosis factor, and gamma-interferon may be important.[69]

Clinical Use of rHuEPO

Allogeneic BMT. The use of rHuEPO in clinical studies in allogeneic BMT has been reviewed,[64, 69] and suggested indications are shown in Table 16–4.

The accelerated erythroid reconstitution in 8 patients undergoing allogeneic BMT (58 days to reach a stable hematocrit level greater than 35%, compared with 123 days for control patients) resulted in a saving of 75% in

TABLE 16–4. Suggested Indications for Use of rHuEPO in Allogeneic Bone Marrow Transplantation*

- Hastening erythroid reconstitution.
- Treatment of patients with persistent anemia.
- PRCA† after ABO-mismatched BMT.
- Treatment of late-appearing multifactorial anemias, i.e., cyclosporin-related hemolytic uremic syndrome.
- Increasing the bone marrow donor's hematocrit level before marrow harvest.
- Increasing donations of RBCs from the bone marrow donor.

*Adapted from Rossi-Ferrini et al.[69]
†PRCA = pure red blood cell aplasia

the requirement for RBC concentrates,[70] and similar results were found in another study in which the time to platelet engraftment and the use of platelet concentrates were also reduced.[71] Other randomized controlled trials[72, 73] have confirmed that rHuEPO in high doses (200 IU/kg intravenously daily for 4 weeks and the same dose twice weekly for 4 weeks,[72] or with 150 IU/kg daily as a continuous intravenous infusion until independence from RBC transfusions or up to 42 days post-transplant[73]) reduces the RBC transfusion requirements after BMT; no effect on platelet recovery or platelet transfusion requirements was found in these two studies.

The administration of rHuEPO has also been successful in the treatment of patients with delayed erythroid regeneration and complex multifactorial anemias after allogeneic BMT and with pure RBC aplasia after major ABO-incompatible BMT.[69]

Marrow donors have been treated with rHuEPO to increase the blood available for autologous donation to avoid the need for homologous transfusions to the donor after harvesting.[74] This approach has been extended to treating both the patient and the marrow donor with rHuEPO; this allowed the marrow donor to donate RBCs to the recipient to reduce or even avoid homologous transfusion requirements.[75]

Autologous BMT and Remission Induction Therapy. Little is known about the effects of rHuEPO in patients with leukemia undergoing remission induction therapy or autologous BMT, but results so far in autologous BMT[73, 76] and peripheral blood progenitor cell transplantation[77] show little benefit of treatment.

Myelodysplasia. Patients with myelodysplasia often rely heavily on RBC transfusions, thus exposing themselves to the risks of multiple blood transfusions discussed previously. The results with rHuEPO therapy in this situation have been variable.

In a series of 46 patients with myelodysplasia, there was a variable relationship between hemoglobin concentration and serum erythropoietin, and it was suggested that serum erythropoietin was inadequate in some patients.[78] In a subsequent clinical trial by the same group, a response to rHuEPO occurred in about 20% of patients.[79] Later studies have confirmed this rate of response.[80-82]

Identification of likely responders is problematic; a diagnosis of refractory anemia, a serum erythropoietin level lower than 200 mU/mL, and no history of transfusions prior to treatment with rHuEpo are features associated with a good response.[80, 83] The combination of granulocyte colony-stimulating factor and rHuEPO increases the response rate to about 40%,[84] and about half of responders require continued treatment with both growth factors to maintain the response.[85]

Jehovah's Witnesses. The use of rHuEPO may be useful in the management of patients refusing transfusions because of their religious convictions.[86, 87]

IMMUNOSUPPRESSION

Pure Red Cell Aplasia

Pure red cell aplasia (PRCA) may occur during the course of leukemia and other hematologic malignancies, most frequently in CLL of either B- or T-cell type.[88] It may occur either at presentation of CLL or after some years, whether cytotoxic drugs have been used or not.

An immune mechanism, usually antibody-mediated suppression of erythropoiesis, is often identified in patients with PRCA, although the erythroid aplasia in CLL of both B and T types is mediated through the action of T-lymphocytes.[88]

There is debate about the most appropriate initial therapy for PRCA, but steroids are usually the first choice, and they may produce satisfactory responses in leukemia-associated PRCA.[89] Patients with CLL also have responded well to treatment with cyclosporin A,[90, 91] and a combination of steroids and cyclosporin A is probably the most effective therapy.[89]

Delayed erythroid engraftment after major ABO-incompatible allogeneic BMT is a type of PRCA; it is due to persistence in the recipient of anti-A and/or anti-B against the donor's A and/or B antigens.[28, 29] Major ABO incompatibility occurs in about 15% to 20% of HLA-matched donor-recipient pairs, and delayed erythroid engraftment occurs in about 20% following BMT. In some cases, the antibodies persist for many months, particularly in association with the use of cyclosporin as prophylaxis for GVHD.[92] Extensive plasma exchange may produce a rapid response, allowing recovery of erythropoiesis,[89] and the administration of rHuEPO has also been successful. If the anti-A and/or anti-B persists, withdrawal of cyclosporin has been suggested.[92]

Autoimmune Hemolytic Anemia

Up to 10% of patients with CLL develop a secondary autoimmune hemolytic anemia at some stage during the course of their disease, with jaundice, spherocytosis, reticulocytosis, and a positive direct antiglobulin test. A positive direct antiglobulin test without hemolytic anemia occurs in up to 20% of cases.

Management of autoimmune hemolytic anemia associated with CLL is similar to that of idiopathic autoimmune hemolytic anemia: initially, prednisolone 60 mg/day in adults, and treatment for the underlying CLL should also be given. Splenectomy may be necessary if there is no response to steroids or if the remission is not maintained when the dose of steroids is reduced. Antibiotic prophylaxis against *Pneumocystis carinii* should be routinely applied for the duration of prednisone therapy.

Blood transfusions are used only if there is fulminant hemolytic anemia or severe anemia not responding to steroids or other therapy.[93] The RBC autoantibodies on the RBCs and in the serum may cause difficulty in the identification of compatible blood. The presence of RBC alloantibodies should be excluded and an attempt made to determine the blood group specificity of the autoantibodies. When it is occasionally possible to identify the specificity of the antibodies, usually within the Rh system, blood that is negative for the relevant RBC antigen should be selected for transfusion. More often, the autoantibodies are nonspecific, and all donor RBCs show some degree of incompatibility. Transfusions of RBC concentrates may only then produce a transient increase in hemoglobin, possibly for as short a time as a few hours.[93]

THE FUTURE

Important aspects of the transfusion support of patients with leukemia will continue to be the appropriate use of blood components and the prevention of the complications associated with multiple transfusions. Although the risk of transfusion-transmitted disease may continue to decrease with improvements in donor testing, procedures to inactivate viruses in blood components and artificial oxygen-carrying blood substitutes will become available. Further studies are needed to determine the optimal use of rHuEPO and other hemopoietic growth factors to reduce transfusion requirements in patients with leukemia.

REFERENCES

1. Woodson RD, Wills RE, Lenfant C: Effect of acute and established anaemia on O_2 transport at rest, submaximal and maximal work. J Applied Physiol 1978;44:36.
2. Ho WG, Winston DJ: Infection and transfusion therapy in acute leukaemia. Clin Haematol 1986;15:873.
3. Barrett-Lee PJ, Bailey NP, O'Brien MER, et al: Large-scale UK audit of blood transfusion requirements and anaemia in patients receiving cytotoxic chemotherapy. Br J Cancer 2000;82:93.
4. Boneu B, Fernandez F: The role of the haematocrit in bleeding. Transfusion Med Rev 1987;1:182.
5. Livio M, Gotti E, Marchesi D, et al: Uraemic bleeding: Role of anaemia and beneficial effect of red cell transfusions. Lancet 1982; 1:1013.
6. Blajchman MA, Bordin JO, Bardossy L, et al: The contribution of the haematocrit to thrombocytopenic bleeding in experimental animals. Br J Haematol 1994;86:347.
7. Favre G, Fopp M, Gmur J, et al: Factors associated with transfusion requirements during treatment for acute myelogenous leukaemia. Ann Haematol 1993;67:153.
8. Watson JG, Powles RL, Clink HM, et al: Acute myeloid leukaemia: Comparison of support required during initial induction of remission and marrow transplantation in first remission. Lancet 1981; ii:957.
9. Smith OP, Prentice HG, Hazlehurst G, et al: Blood product support in patients undergoing chemotherapy and autologous or allogeneic bone marrow transplantation for haematological malignancies. Clin Lab Haematol 1991;13:107.
10. Brink NS, Chopra R, Perrons CJ, et al: Acute hepatitis C infection in patients undergoing therapy for haematological malignancies: A clinical and virological study. Br J Haematol 1993;83:498.
10a. Brink NS, Mills W, Chopra R, et al: Efficacy of donor screening for hepatitis C antibodies in preventing hepatitis C infection in multiply transfused patients. Transfusion Med 1993;3:291.
11. Regan FAM, Hewitt P, Barbara JAJ, et al: Prospective investigation of transfusion transmitted infection in recipients of over 20,000 units of blood. Br Med J 2000;320:403.
12. Schreiber GB, Busch MP, Kleinman SH, et al: The risk of transfusion-transmitted viral infections. N Engl J Med 1996;334:685.
13. Apperley JF, Rice SJ, Hewitt P, et al: HIV infection due to a platelet transfusion after allogeneic bone marrow transplantation. Eur J Haematol 1987;39:185.
14. Gluckman E, Spire B, Gluckman JC, et al: Two cases of acquired immune deficiency syndrome (AIDS) after allogeneic bone marrow transplant (BMT): Transmission of LAV by healthy marrow donors. Exp Haematol 1985;13:325.
15. Meyers JD, Flournoy N, Thomas ED: Risk factors for cytomegalovirus infection after human marrow transplantation. J Infect Dis 1986; 153:478.
16. Reusser P, Fisher LD, Buckner D, et al: Cytomegalovirus infection after autologous bone marrow transplantation: Occurrence of cytomegalovirus disease and effect on engraftment. Blood 1990;75: 1888.
17. Bowden RA, Slichter SJ, Sayers M, et al: Use of leukocyte-depleted platelets and cytomegalovirus-seronegative red blood cells for prevention of primary cytomegalovirus infection after marrow transplant. Blood 1991;78:246.
18. De Graan-Hentzen YCA, Gratama JW, Mudde GC, et al: Prevention of primary cytomegalovirus infection in patients with haematologic malignancies by intensive white cell depletion of blood products. Transfusion 1989; 29:757.
19. Murphy MF, Grint PCA, Hardiman AE, et al: Use of leucocyte-poor blood components to prevent primary cytomegalovirus (CMV) infection in patients with acute leukaemia. Br J Haematol 1988; 70:253.
20. Murphy MF: New variant Creutzfeldt-Jakob disease: The risk of transmission by blood transfusion and the potential benefit of leukocyte reduction of blood components. Transfusion Med Rev 1999; 13:1.
21. Turner M: The impact of new variant Creutzfeldt-Jakob disease on blood transfusion practice. Br J Haematol 1999;106:842.
22. Pamphilon DH, Rider JR, Barbara JAJ, et al: Prevention of transfusion-transmitted cytomegalovirus infection. Transfusion Med 1999; 9:115.
23. Sayers M, Anderson KC, Goodnough LT, et al: Reducing the risk for transfusion-transmitted cytomegalovirus infection. Ann Intern Med 1992;116:55.
24. Blumberg N, Peck K, Ross K, et al: Immune response to chronic red blood cell transfusion. Vox Sanguinis 1983;44:212.
25. Schonewille H, Haak HL, van Zijl AM: Alloimmunization after blood transfusion in patients with hematologic and oncologic diseases. Transfusion 1999;39:763.
26. Buckner CD, Clift RA, Sanders JE, et al: ABO-incompatible marrow transplants. Transplantation 1980;26:233.
27. Hershko C, Gale RP, Ho W, et al: ABH antigens and bone marrow transplantation. Br J Haematol 1980;44:65.
28. Klumpp TR: Immunohematologic complications of bone marrow transplantation. Bone Marrow Transplantation 1991;8:159.
29. Petz LD: The expanding boundaries of transfusion medicine. In Nance SJ, ed: Clinical and Basic Science Aspects of Immunohaematology. Arlington, VA: American Association of Blood Banks;1991.
30. Slichter SJ: Transfusion and bone marrow transplantation. Transfusion Med Rev 1988;2:1.
31. Benjamin RJ, McGurk S, Ralston MS, et al: ABO incompatibility as an adverse risk factor for survival after allogeneic bone marrow transplantation. Transfusion 1999;39:179.
32. Heal JM, Blumberg N: The second century of ABO: And now for something completely different. Transfusion 1999;39:1155.
33. Hows J, Beddow K, Gordon-Smith E, et al: Donor-derived red blood cell antibodies and immune haemolysis after allogeneic bone marrow transplantation. Blood 1986;67:177.
34. Goldfinger D, McGinniss MH: Rh-incompatible platelet transfusions: Risks and consequences of immunizing immunosuppressed patients. N Engl J Med 1971;284:942.
35. Atoyebi W, Mundy N, Croxton T, et al: Is it necessary to administer anti-D to prevent RhD immunisation following the transfusion of RhD-positive platelet concentrates? Br J Haematol 1999;105:103.

36. British Committee for Standards in Haematology: Guidelines for platelet transfusions. Transfusion Med 1992;2:311.

37. British Committee for Standards in Haematology: Guidelines on the clinical use of leucocyte-depleted blood components. Transfusion Med 1998;8:59.

38. Lane TA, Anderson KC, Goodnough LT, et al: Leukocyte reduction in blood component therapy. Ann Intern Med 1992;117:151.

39. Murphy MF, Waters AH: Clinical aspects of platelet transfusions. Blood Coagulation Fibrinolysis 1991;2:389.

40. The Trial to Reduce Alloimmunization to Platelets Study Group: Leukocyte reduction and ultraviolet B irradiation of platelets to prevent alloimmunization and refractoriness to platelet transfusions. N Engl J Med 1997;337:1861.

41. Oksanen K, Elonen E: Impact of leucocyte-depleted blood components on the haematological recovery and prognosis of patients with acute myeloid leukaemia. Br J Haematol 1993;84:639.

42. Mollison PL, Engelfriet CP, Contreras M: Blood Transfusion in Clinical Medicine. Oxford, UK: Blackwell Scientific Publications;1993, Chapter 15.

43. Storb R, Prentice RL, Thomas ED: Marrow transplantation for treatment of aplastic anaemia: An analysis of factors associated with graft rejection. N Engl J Med 1977;296:61.

44. Storb R, Thomas ED, Buckner CD, et al: Marrow transplantation in thirty "untransfused" patients with aplastic anaemia. Ann Intern Med 1980;92:30.

45. Storb R, Weiden PL, Deeg HJ, et al: Rejection of marrow from DLA-identical canine littermates given transfusions before grafting: Antigens involved are expressed on leukocytes and skin epithelial cells but not on platelets and red blood cells. Blood 1979;54:477.

46. Deeg HJ, Aprile J, Graham TC, et al: Ultraviolet irradiation of blood prevents transfusion-induced sensitization and marrow rejection in dogs. Blood 1986;67:537.

47. Deeg HJ: Modifications of allointeractions after blood transfusion and marrow transplantation by ultraviolet light. Semin Haemat 1992;29:95.

48. Anderson KC, Weinstein HJ: Transfusion-associated graft-versus-host disease. N Engl J Med 1990;323:315.

49. Ford JM, Lucey JJ, Cullen MH, et al: Fatal graft-versus-host disease following transfusion of granulocytes from normal donors. Lancet 1976;2:1167.

50. British Committee for Standards in Haematology: Guidelines on gamma irradiation of blood components for the prevention of transfusion-associated graft-versus-host disease. Transfusion Med 1996;6:261.

51. Anderson KC, Goodnough LT, Sayers M, et al: Variation in blood component irradiation practice: Implications for prevention of graft-versus-host disease. Blood 1991;77:2096.

52. Akahoshi M, Takanashi M, Masuda M, et al: A case of transfusion-associated graft-versus-host disease not prevented by white cell-reduction filters. Transfusion 1992;32:169.

53. Murphy MF: Clinical transfusion practice in haematological disease. In Murphy MF, Pamphilon D, eds: Practical Transfusion Medicine. Oxford, UK: Blackwell Science;2000.

54. Ley TJ, Griffith P, Nienhuis AW: Transfusion haemosiderosis and chelation therapy. Clin Haematol 1982;11:437.

54a. Mannucci PM, Federici AB, Sirchia G: Hemostasis testing during massive blood replacement: A study of 172 cases. Vox Sanguinis 1982;42:113.

54b. Miller RD, Robbins TO, Tong MJ, et al: Coagulation defects associated with massive blood transfusions. Ann Surgery 1971;174:794.

55. Bareford D, Chandler ST, Hawker RJ, et al: Splenic platelet sequestration following routine blood transfusion is reduced by filtered/washed blood products. Br J Haematol 1987;67:177.

56. Lim S, Boughton BJ, Bareford D: Thrombocytopenia following routine blood transfusion: Micro-aggregate blood filters prevent worsening thrombocytopenia in patients with low platelet counts. Vox Sanguinis 1989;56:40.

57. Schuh A, Atoyebi W, Littlewood T, et al: Prevention of worsening of severe thrombocytopenia following red cell transfusions by the use of leucocyte-depleted blood. Br J Haematol 2000;108:455.

58. Erslev AJ: Erythropoietin. N Engl J Med 1991;324:1339.

59. Oster W, Herrmann F, Gamm H, et al: Erythropoietin for the treatment of malignancy associated with neoplastic bone marrow infiltration. J Clin Oncol 1990;8:956.

60. Platanias LC, Miller CB, Mick R, et al: Treatment of chemotherapy-induced anaemia with recombinant human erythropoietin in cancer patients. J Clin Oncol 1991;9:2021.

61. Spivak JL: Recombinant human erythropoietin and the anemia of cancer. Blood 1994;84:997.

62. Ludwig H, Fritz E, Kotzman H, et al: Erythropoietin treatment of anaemia associated with multiple myeloma. N Engl J Med 1990;322:1693.

63. Osterborg A, Boogaerts MA, Cimino R, et al: Recombinant human erythropoietin in transfusion-dependent anemic patients with multiple myeloma and non-Hodgkin's lymphoma: A randomized multicenter study. Blood 1996;87:2675.

64. Cazzola M, Mercuriali F, Brugnara C: Use of recombinant human erythropoietin outside the setting of uremia. Blood 1997;89:4248.

65. Beguin Y, Clemons GK, Oris R, et al: Circulating erythropoietin levels after bone marrow transplantation: Inappropriate response to anaemia in allogeneic transplants. Blood 1991;77:868.

66. Miller CB, Jones RJ, Zahurak ML, et al: Impaired erythropoietin response to anaemia after bone marrow transplantation. Blood 1992;80:2677.

67. Schapira L, Antin JH, Ransil BJ, et al: Serum erythropoietin levels in patients receiving intensive chemotherapy and radiotherapy. Blood 1990;76:2354.

68. Lazarus HM, Goodnough LT, Goldwasser E, et al: Serum erythropoietin levels and blood component therapy after bone marrow transplantation: Implications for erythropoietin therapy in this setting. Bone Marrow Transplantation 1992;10:71.

69. Rossi-Ferrini P, Vannucchi AM, Bosi A, et al: Erythropoietin and post–bone marrow transplantation anaemia. Erythropoiesis 1993;4:48.

70. Vannucchi AM, Bosi A, Grossi A, et al: Stimulation of erythroid engraftment by recombinant human erythropoietin in ABO-compatible, HLA-identical, allogeneic bone marrow transplant patients. Leukaemia 1993;6:215.

71. Steegman JL, Lopez J, Otero MJ, et al: Erythropoietin treatment in allogeneic BMT accelerates erythroid reconstitution: Results of a prospective controlled randomized trial. Bone Marrow Transplantation 1992;10:541.

72. Klaesson S, Ringden O, Ljungman P, et al: Reduced blood transfusion requirements after allogeneic bone marrow transplantation: Results of a randomised, double-blind study with high-dose erythropoietin. Bone Marrow Transplantation 1994;13:397.

73. Link H, Boogaerts MA, Fauser AA, et al: A controlled trial of recombinant human erythropoietin after bone marrow transplantation. Blood 1994;84:3327.

74. York A, Clift RA, Sanders JE, et al: Recombinant human erythropoietin (rh-Epo) administration to normal marrow donors. Bone Marrow Transplantation 1992;10:415.

75. Mitus AJ, Antin JH, Rutherford CJ, et al: Use of recombinant human erythropoietin in allogeneic bone marrow transplant donor/recipient pairs. Blood 1994;83:1952.

76. Locatelli F, Zecca M, Pedrazolli P, et al: Use of recombinant human erythropoietin after bone marrow transplantation in pediatric patients with acute leukemia: Effect on erythroid repopulation in autologous versus allogeneic transplants. Bone Marrow Transplantation 1994;13:403.

77. Pierelli L, Scambia G, Menichella G, et al: The combination of erythroid and granulocye colony-stimulating factor increases the rate of haemopoietic recovery with clinical benefit after peripheral blood progenitor transplantation. Br J Haematol 1996;92:287.

78. Jacobs A, Janowska-Wieczorek A, Caro J, et al: Circulating erythropoietin in patients with myelodysplastic syndromes. Br J Haematol 1989;73:36.

79. Bowen D, Culligan D, Jacobs A: The treatment of anaemia in the myelodysplastic syndromes with recombinant human erythropoietin. Br J Haematol 1991;77:419.

80. Hellstrom-Lindberg E: Efficacy of erythropoietin in the myelodysplastic syndromes: A meta-analysis of 205 patients from 17 studies. Br J Haematol 1995;89:67.

81. Rose EH, Abels RI, Nelson RA, et al: The use of rHuEpo in the treatment of anemia related to myelodysplastia. Br J Haematol 1995;89:831.

82. Stenke L, Wallvik J, Celsing F, et al: Prediction of response to treatment with recombinant human erythropoietin in myelodysplastic syndromes. Leukaemia 1993;7:1324.

83. Italian Cooperative Study Group for rHuEpo in Myelodysplastic Syndromes: A randomized double-blind placebo-controlled study

with subcutaneous recombinant human erythropoietin in patients with low-risk myelodysplastic syndromes. Br J Haematol 1998;103:1070.

84. Negrin RS, Stein R, Vardiman J, et al: Treatment of the anemia of myelodysplastic syndromes using recombinant human granulocyte colony-stimulating factor in combination with erythropoietin. Blood 1993;82:737.

85. Negrin RS, Stein R, Doherty K, et al: Maintenance treatment of the anemia of myelodysplastic syndromes with recombinant human erythropoietin: Evidence for in vivo synergy. Blood 1996;87:4076.

86. Heinz R, Reisner R, Pittermann E: Erythropoietin for chemotherapy patients refusing blood transfusion. Lancet 1990;335:542.

87. Mann MC, Votto J, Kambe J, et al: Management of the severely anemic patient who refuses transfusion: Lessons learned during the care of a Jehovah's Witness. Ann Intern Med 1992;117:1042.

88. Dessypris EN: The biology of pure red cell aplasia. Semin Haematol 1991;28:275.

89. Marmont AM: Therapy of pure red cell aplasia. Semin Haematol 1991;28:285.

90. Chikappa G, Pasquale D, Phillips PG, et al: Cyclosporine A for the treatment of pure red cell aplasia in a patient with chronic lymphocytic leukaemia. Am J Haematol 1987;26:179.

91. Christen R, Morant R, Fehr J: Cyclosporin A therapy of pure red cell aplasia in a patient with B-cell chronic lymphocytic leukaemia. Eur J Haematol 1989;42:303.

92. Sniecinski IJ, Oien L, Petz LD, et al: Immunohematologic consequences of major ABO-mismatched bone marrow transplantation. Transplantation 1988;45:530.

93. Petz LD, Garratty G (1980). Acquired Immune Hemolytic Anemias. New York: Churchill Livingstone;1980.

17

Simon P. Joel   Ama Rohatiner

Pharmacology of Antileukemic Drugs

INTRODUCTION AND HISTORICAL PERSPECTIVE

Although a number of the drugs used to treat malignant disease today have been used as folk remedies for many hundreds of years, the first clinical trial of cytotoxic chemotherapy was reported only in 1946.[1] The drug involved was nitrogen mustard, a direct development of sulfur mustard (mustard gas) used during the First World War that was also noticed to produce effects in the bone marrow and gastrointestinal tract.[2] Many of the difficulties of current-day chemotherapy were encapsulated in the first patient studied—a dramatic antitumor response, profound bone marrow toxicity, but subsequent relapse.[3] At around the same time, Sidney Farber reported that certain folic acid analogues accelerated leukemic cell growth, whereas others were antagonistic and had antileukemic effects. Subsequently, aminopterin, the first antifolate, was shown to have impressive activity in childhood leukemia.[4]

This prompted much research in the area, and between 1950 and 1970, some 30 or so cytotoxic agents entered clinical practice, expanding to around 50 by the present day.[5, 6] These were discovered by a clearer understanding of the processes involved in the synthesis of DNA precursors (e.g., the antimetabolites), by synthesizing analogues of long-used folk medicines (e.g., the epipodophyllotoxins), by large screening programs (e.g., the taxanes), or by serendipity (e.g., cisplatin). Much of the success of cytotoxic chemotherapy has come from the use of these drugs in combinations that maximize their antitumor activity but limit their toxicity. However, most of these agents are fairly crude poisons that kill dividing cells by inducing damage to DNA or by damaging the mitotic spindle apparatus such that cells are unable to complete the division process, as described in more detail later. In contrast, in the past few years, a number of new compounds that target some of the specific changes that arise in cells when they become malignant have entered early clinical trials, and examples of some of these new approaches are described at the end of this chapter.

BASIC CONCEPTS
Pharmacokinetics

Pharmacokinetics, the study of drug movement, is concerned with the processes involved in determining a drug's concentration-time history or "what the body does to the drug."[7-10] It is important to distinguish this term from pharmacodynamics, which is the study of drug action or "what the drug does to the body." Knowledge of the pharmacokinetic properties of cytotoxic drugs is crucial in their initial clinical development and is increasingly being used to optimize treatment schedules and even dosing in individual patients.

Absorption

Most cytotoxic drugs are administered intravenously, so issues related to absorption are encountered less often in oncology than in other disciplines. However, some anticancer agents are administered orally, and alternative routes of administration, such as intraperitoneal delivery, have recently become more common. In addition, many of the new nonclassic anticancer agents, such as protein kinase inhibitors, may require prolonged inhibition of the target for activity; the development of such agents is often focused on oral formulations.

Absorption is a narrow term that actually includes a number of factors that influence measured drug concentration, typically in plasma. Before a drug molecule can pass through membranes, it must be in solution. This requires that the agent be liberated from the dosage form and enter or remain in solution. Many cytotoxic drugs are poorly soluble and require complex formulation with a variety of solvents and solubilizers to ensure stability. For a number of drugs, stability may be compromised when these solubilizers are diluted in the stomach contents or by the pH to which the drug is exposed.[11] This aspect of a drug's pharmacology, termed biopharmaceutics, is concerned with the influence of the drug's formulation on its activity in vivo.

Other physicochemical properties of the drug influence the site and extent of absorption. Compounds are better able to cross membranes in the unionized form in which they are less polar. Most drugs are weak acids or bases, such that local pH becomes an important factor in their absorption. Thus, acidic drugs are better absorbed from the stomach, where the pH is lower and more of the drug is unionized, whereas basic drugs are better absorbed from the small intestine, where the pH is higher and more of the drug is unionized. Depending on the drug, this may be partly offset by the large surface area of the small intestine, where most drugs are absorbed; although only a small percentage may be in the unionized, nonpolar form, the area of absorption is so large that most of the drug will eventually be absorbed.

The nature of the transport mechanism across the gut wall is also important in determining the rate and extent of absorption.[12] Most drugs cross membranes by passive diffusion; because the gut wall is well drained by the portal vasculature, there is a concentration gradient down which molecules will tend to pass until the gut concentrations become low. This process is not saturable and does not require energy. An alternative for some drugs is carrier-mediated transport by one of two processes, passive facilitated diffusion or active transport. Passive facilitated diffusion relies on a specific transport pathway; it is not energy dependent but relies on a concentration gradient that may reach a transport maximum. (Because a specific pathway is involved, this process may be inhibited by other compounds.) Active transport is able to move substances against a concentration gradient, which requires energy and can therefore be inhibited by metabolic inhibitors. (The nature of the transport process for specific drugs is often characterized by use of metabolic inhibitors such as sodium azide, 2,4-dinitrophenol, or ouabain.[13]) The intestinal absorption of 5-fluorouracil, for example, is by an active transport process.[14] All of these transport processes require the drug to be in solution, but at least some of an orally administered dose may be absorbed from the gut as solid particles by a process known as pinocytosis, or particulate absorption.[15] Finally, specific absorption processes may be influenced by the underlying disease in patients with cancer, for a number of reasons,[16] or by the co-administration of other drugs.

The contents of the stomach also influence the absorption process. The emptying time of the stomach is markedly prolonged by the presence of food, and drug absorption can be delayed depending on whether the subject is dosed on an empty stomach, after a light meal, or after a heavy meal.[17, 18] Gastric emptying time also varies according to the nature of the food, particularly its fat content, and the action of other co-administered drugs, such as opiates.[19, 20]

Successful absorption into the portal circulation requires that drug molecules are not metabolized as they cross the gut wall. Increasingly, mucosal cells in the stomach and small intestine, the major sites of drug absorption, are recognized as having metabolizing enzyme activity,[12, 21] particularly cytochrome P450 3A4 (CYP3A4).[22, 23] Changes in the activity of these enzymes, either by disease states[24] or by the ingestion of other drugs or foodstuffs,[25, 26] can markedly influence drug absorption. Finally, molecules absorbed from the gut must pass through the liver, which may metabolize drugs before they reach the systemic circulation, referred to as first-pass metabolism. Particular drugs may be completely absorbed from the gut but undergo extensive first-pass metabolism, such that their bioavailability is poor. Such low oral bioavailability does not necessarily mean that the drug is poorly absorbed.

With so many factors influencing the successful passage of drug molecules into the systemic circulation, it is not surprising that for some orally administered drugs, bioavailability shows marked interpatient and intrapatient variability.[27, 28]

Distribution

Once a drug has entered the systemic circulation, it must move into other fluid and tissue spaces within the body to exert its effects. This reversible transfer of drug between one location and another is termed distribution. Definitive information on the rate at which drugs distribute into other compartments, and the size of those compartments, requires the measurement of drug concentration in tissues, but useful estimates of these parameters can be derived from blood or plasma concentrations of drug.

The distribution of drug from the plasma into other tissues is often apparent from the concentration-time plot in plasma (Fig. 17-1A). After rapid intravenous administration, plasma drug concentration is often seen to fall rapidly initially, representing distribution of drug from the plasma, or central compartment, to a peripheral compartment, such as extracellular fluid. When the concentration of drug in these two compartments is the same, equilibrium is achieved, and plasma concentration declines more slowly, representing elimination. In many cases, elimination is principally from the central compartment, so drug must move back from the peripheral compartment for elimination to take place. The rates at which drugs move between and are eliminated from compartments can also be derived from plasma concentration-time data, as shown in Figure 17-1B. In common with most biologic processes, changes in drug concentration within and between compartments occur by a first-order process, which infers a change by a constant fractional rate rather than by a constant amount. Consequently, when plotted on a linear concentration scale, the exponential decline in plasma concentration takes the form of a curve, indicating that the *amount* of drug removed per unit time changes continuously; on a logarithmic scale, this elimination is linear (see Fig. 17-1). More complex pharmacokinetic models may include additional compartments, reflecting prolonged retention in a certain tissue, distribution into a third space (such as an effusion), or elimination from these peripheral compartments, typically by metabolism.[29]

The apparent volume of distribution can be derived from plasma concentration data, and provides useful information on the extent and possible sites of drug distribution. Many drugs have volumes of distribution at equilibrium of around 15 to 20 L, indicating distribution mainly in the extracellular fluid compartment, whereas some have high apparent distribution volumes, reflecting retention in a particular compartment, resulting in low plasma concentration. For example, mitoxantrone disappears from the systemic circulation rapidly but binds extensively to tissue proteins, giving an apparent volume of distribution of more than 500 L.[30, 31]

Metabolism

Many drugs used in oncology are prodrugs and require conversion to the active species. Therefore, metabolism

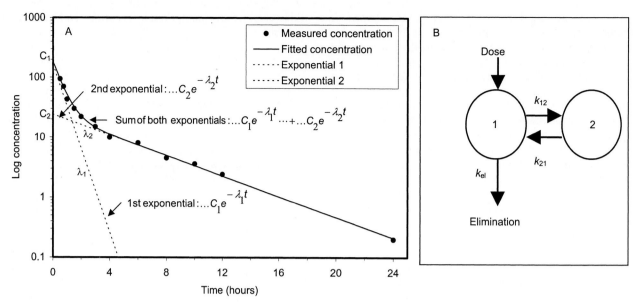

FIGURE 17–1. *A*, After intravenous bolus dosing, plasma drug concentration falls rapidly initially, representing distribution from the circulation (central compartment, 1) into other fluid spaces (peripheral compartment, 2), and then more slowly when equilibrium has been reached, representing elimination. The data shown are fitted to a two-exponential model, with the y-axis intercept denoted C_1 and C_2 for each exponential, and the slopes λ_1 and λ_2. *B*, This can be portrayed schematically. The rate (k) at which these drug movements occur (k_{12}, k_{21}, k_{el}) can be derived from plasma concentration data. Parameters that describe an overall change in drug concentration, such as the elimination rate constant (k_{el}), are referred to as macroconstants; those describing movement between compartments (k_{12}, k_{21}) are microconstants.

refers not only to a detoxification process but also the chemical modification of a drug molecule by a biologic process. It is the most complex aspect of a drug's pharmacokinetics and is influenced markedly by genetic factors, nutrition, liver function, and a range of other molecules including drugs and dietary/environmental compounds. Consequently, the metabolism of cytotoxic drugs is a major source of variability in drug plasma concentration.

The metabolism of drugs and other molecules typically takes place by two types of reaction.[32] Phase 1 biotransformations involve nonsynthetic reactions that include oxidation, reduction, and hydrolysis. The oxidation reactions are carried out by enzymes of the cytochrome P450 system, which require oxygen and reduced nicotinamide adenine dinucleotide phosphate for activity. Other phase 1 reactions involve specific enzymes relevant to oncology, such as dihydropyrimidine dehydrogenase (5-fluorouracil), cytidine deaminase (cytosine arabinoside), and carboxylesterases (irinotecan). Of the P450 enzymes, CYP3A4 is the most important in terms of the total P450-mediated oxidative capacity of the liver and is involved in the metabolism of a number of cytotoxic drugs.[33] Because the P450 enzyme superfamily can act on a wide range of substrates, there is a large potential for drug-drug interactions, including inhibition or induction of specific enzymes,[34] sometimes in association with certain dietary components such as grapefruit juice.[35] This can have a marked effect on the activity of co-administered drugs. Phase 1 reactions often result in structural alterations to a molecule that make it more liable to phase 2-type reactions.

Phase 2 biotransformations are synthetic reactions that typically involve the conjugation of the drug molecule

with another group, such as glucuronic acid, glutathione, sulfate, glycine, glutamine, or an alkyl. The products so formed are more water soluble than the drug molecule, are more easily excreted, and are often the final metabolic product of the administered drug. The conjugated metabolites of a number of drugs sometimes retain pharmacologic activity and occasionally may be more active than the parent drug.[36] Phase 2 reactions are thus not always detoxifying processes.

Because the liver is the major site of drug metabolism and patients with cancer often have deranged liver function, the pharmacokinetics of cytotoxic drugs are often altered in such patients. However, typical liver function tests give little indication of possible marked changes in phase 1 reactions in patients with liver impairment, even when phase 2 reactions are unaltered.[37] Moreover, liver disease may induce selective changes in specific P450 phase 1 enzymes that affect some oxidation reactions but not others.[38, 39] Recommendations for drug dose modification therefore require an understanding of the specific enzymes involved in the metabolism of a drug and how they are altered in liver disease. Such information is becoming available with the use of nontoxic marker compounds that are metabolized by specific P450 enzymes.[40]

Excretion

Drugs are finally eliminated from the body either as the parent compound or as a more water soluble metabolite by excretion. The most important organs involved in this process are the liver and kidneys. For both, this is a complex process with pharmacokinetic and pharmacodynamic consequences.[41] This is particularly so with cancer, when the underlying disease or the age of the patient may influence organ function and thereby drug handling.[42-46]

Excretion of drugs through the kidney involves glomerular filtration, active tubular secretion, and passive tubular reabsorption. The amount of drug that is filtered at the glomerulus depends on the degree of protein binding, with only the free fraction able to undergo filtration, and the glomerular filtration rate. A number of active tubular transport processes act to secrete endogenous compounds into the tubule, and certain cytotoxic drugs, such as methotrexate,[47] are also actively secreted by such mechanisms. More general efflux mechanisms include energy-dependent pumps such as P-glycoprotein, which is involved in the active secretion of a number of cytotoxic drugs into the tubules. Inhibition of P-glycoprotein has a marked effect on the renal clearance of such drugs.[48]

As the glomerular filtrate becomes more concentrated (because of reabsorption of water as it passes down the tubule), a concentration gradient is established between the tubular contents and the surrounding cells down which drugs can pass by passive diffusion. The degree of passive reabsorption of drugs is largely dependent on the nature of the molecule, including its molecular weight, lipid solubility, and state of ionization. Molecules that are lipophilic and unionized will be reabsorbed to a greater extent than those that are polar or ionized. The degree of ionization is determined by the urinary pH, which is typically between 5 and 8. For example, a weak acid with a pK_a of 6, at which it is 50% ionized, will be 90% unionized at pH 5 but 90% ionized at pH 7. Thus, urinary excretion of such a compound will be markedly increased by alkalinization of the urine to maintain the drug in the ionized form, thereby limiting its reabsorption. Methotrexate is such a drug.[49] Alterations in the renal excretion of cytotoxic drugs can markedly affect drug plasma concentrations, with effects on the drug's pharmacodynamics.

The liver is the other major site of drug excretion. Many compounds are actively secreted from liver cells into the bile canaliculi by transport systems similar to those found in renal tubules, such as P-glycoprotein.[50] Drugs secreted into the bile will eventually pass into the gastrointestinal tract and may again be subject to absorption processes. This is termed enterohepatic recycling.[51, 52] In addition, drug conjugates, particularly glucuronides, may be hydrolyzed back to the parent compound by bacteria in the gut and subsequently reabsorbed.

Pharmacokinetic Parameters

Pharmacokinetic studies are an important aspect of drug development and increasingly are having an impact on treatment of patients with dosing based on measurement of a pharmacokinetic parameter. A number of simple parameters can provide useful information about a drug's pharmacokinetics. Consider a typical concentration-time profile as shown in Figure 17-2.

Simple measures are the maximum measured plasma drug concentration (C_{max}), the time at which this occurs (t_{max}), the concentration at a specific time point, and the time during which the plasma concentration exceeds a certain level. This last parameter is proving to be increasingly useful in identifying maintained plasma concentrations that are associated with antitumor activity or toxicity. The decline in plasma concentration is a first-order process that occurs at a constant fractional rate, rather than at a constant amount, as shown in Figure 17-1A. The slope of each of these exponentials represents the change in concentration per unit time, or the rate of change. For example, during the terminal exponential phase, the slope of the elimination is referred to as the elimination rate constant; it is used to derive the half-life.

Half-life

During each exponential phase, the half-life represents the time taken for the drug concentration to fall by 50%. Because this is an exponential process, a fall of 50% on a

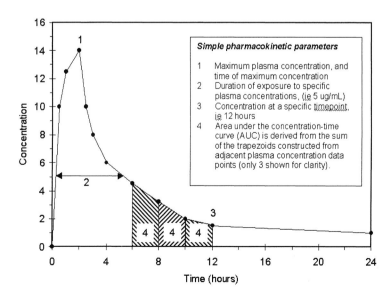

FIGURE 17-2. Typical concentration-time profile showing several simple but useful pharmacokinetic parameters.

natural logarithmic scale is equal to 0.693. The half-life can therefore be defined as

$$\text{Half-life } (t_{1/2}) = \frac{0.693}{k_{el}}$$

where k_{el} is the slope of the exponential.

Area under the Concentration-Time Curve

The area under the concentration-time curve (AUC) is a particularly useful pharmacokinetic parameter because it represents the amount of drug (or metabolite) in the compartment sampled (typically plasma) during the study period. AUC is commonly derived by dividing a concentration-time plot into trapezoids, as described by pairs of adjacent concentration-time data points (see Fig. 17-2). The total AUC to the last time point is the sum of the areas under these trapezoids, often referred to as the trapezoidal rule and can be extrapolated to infinity by dividing the concentration at the final time point by the elimination rate constant (k_{el}).

Bioavailability (F)

AUC is used to derive a number of other pharmacokinetic parameters. The bioavailability of a drug (often denoted F, the fraction absorbed) is a useful parameter that defines the proportion of an administered dose that reaches the systemic circulation relative to a test dose. The test dose is typically an intravenous (IV) administration, which has a bioavailability of 100%.

$$\text{Bioavailability (\%)} = \frac{\text{test dose AUC}}{\text{reference dose (IV) AUC}} \times 100$$

Clearance

The AUC is also used to derive clearance according to the equation

$$\text{Clearance} = \frac{\text{dose}}{\text{AUC}}$$

With continuous dosing, steady state is reached when the rate of drug elimination equals the rate of drug administration, and clearance can be derived from the formula

$$\text{Clearance} = \frac{\text{dose rate}}{\text{steady-state concentration } (C_{SS})}$$

Clearance denotes not how much of a drug is cleared but the volume of the compartment sampled that is completely cleared of drug per unit time. In this respect, it is entirely analogous to the concept of creatinine clearance and is expressed in terms of milliliters per minute or liters per hour.

Total plasma clearance is the sum of each of the clearance mechanisms relevant to a specific drug. The contribution of specific organs, such as the liver, to overall clearance can be derived from estimates of organ blood flow and measurement of drug concentrations into and out of the organ. Clearly, this is complex, and clearance estimates are more usually confined to estimates of renal clearance, derived from measured drug concentrations in urine and plasma, and the difference between this measure and total plasma clearance, referred to as nonrenal clearance. For many drugs, the two major clearance routes are renal and hepatic, such that nonrenal clearance often approximates to hepatic clearance.

Two factors that influence drug clearance are saturable metabolic pathways and protein binding. For drugs when metabolism is saturable, such as 5-fluorouracil, clearance may remain constant up to a certain concentration, or dose, but then gradually decrease with further increases in concentration as the enzyme system becomes saturated. For drugs that are highly protein bound, the amount of free drug available for clearance will be limited. The most relevant consequence of this is that changes in protein binding due to disease processes or the co-administration of other drugs can affect overall drug clearance, resulting in pharmacokinetic variability. Such variability in drug clearance is often reflected by a reciprocal change in the drug's elimination half-life, such that as clearance decreases, the elimination half-life increases.

Volume of Distribution

In a laboratory experiment, the volume of a solution in an irregular container can be derived by adding a known amount of substance and measuring the concentration of that substance in solution after thorough mixing. In pharmacokinetic studies, the volume of distribution can be determined in exactly the same way by administering a known amount of drug to a patient and determining the concentration of drug in that patient. It is complicated by the fact that elimination starts almost immediately after the drug has been administered. However, if two or more blood samples are taken and the slope of the exponential is extrapolated back to time 0, the concentration of drug at that time represents the concentration that would have resulted with immediate mixing and in the absence of any elimination. The dose of drug administered and the extrapolated concentration at time 0 can then be used to calculate the volume of distribution. This becomes more complex when drug elimination from plasma fits to a multicompartment process, in which case the extrapolated time 0 concentration would indicate the volume of distribution of the central compartment; the volume of distribution of the central and peripheral compartments together is derived from the AUC and elimination rate constant thus:

$$V_{area} = \frac{\text{dose}}{k \times \text{AUC}} \text{ or } \frac{Cl}{k}$$

One drawback with this method is that disease processes that alter the elimination rate lead to an apparent change in distribution volume. An alternative method for determining the volume of distribution at steady state is

$$V_{ss} = \text{dose} \times \text{AUMC/AUC}^2$$

where AUMC is the area under the first moment curve, namely, concentration × time versus time. Both methods require the dose to be corrected for bioavailability in cases of extravascular administration.

Pharmacodynamics

Pharmacodynamics refers to what the drug does to the body, or the drug's effects. Whereas the effect we are seeking in oncology is reduction or disappearance of the tumor, in terms of management of the patient, this often takes second place to dealing with the many other effects of cytotoxic drugs, such as myelosuppression, mucositis, diarrhea, nausea, and vomiting.

The Dose-Response Relationship

For all drugs, the relationship between the dose, or concentration of drug, and the drug's effects is a complex one. A typical dose-response curve is shown in Figure 17–3 and has a number of features worth comment. Typically, this curve starts with a lag phase in which substantial increases in dose or exposure concentration

may be required (note the log scale) with little increase in drug activity. Eventually, the effect increases more substantially with increments in dose and across a part of the dose-response curve. The relationship may appear linear. However, this increase in effect then begins to tail off, such that with the same increases in dose, the increase in effect becomes smaller and smaller. If, at a particular dose, the effect is close to the top of the linear part of the curve, substantial increases in dose may be required to bring about a significant increase in effect. This relationship may explain why high-dose trials in oncology have generally not resulted in a substantial increase in therapeutic benefit.

Drug Toxicity

A major problem in the use of anticancer drugs is drug toxicity. All drugs have side effects, but for most, the

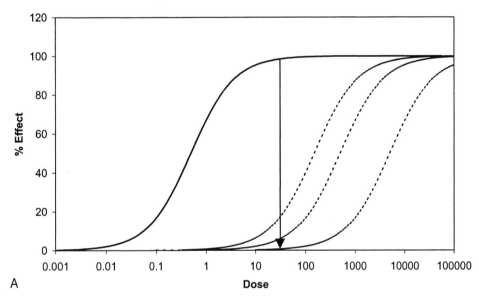

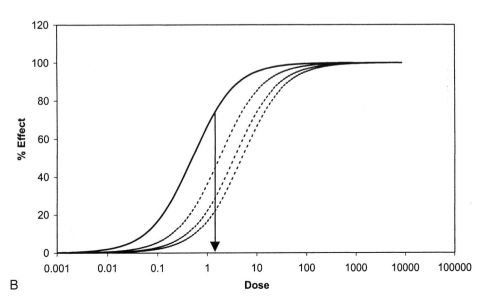

FIGURE 17–3. The relationship between dose and a desired effect *(solid line)* and side effects *(dashed lines)*. For most therapeutic agents, the difference between an active dose and a toxic dose is large *(A)*. With cytotoxic drugs, the active (antitumor) and toxic dose effects are much closer together *(B)*, such that dose is often limited by toxicity. For each situation, the recommended dose is arrowed.

difference between a therapeutic dose and a toxic dose is suitably large, such that enough drug can be administered to ensure that all patients achieve a potentially therapeutic concentration. For the same reason, variability in pharmacokinetics is less of an issue with drugs that have few side effects at therapeutic doses because, again, the dose administered can be large enough to ensure that active plasma concentrations are achieved in all patients. With cytotoxic drugs, the therapeutic and toxic dose-response curves are much closer together, with two associated problems. First, the dose that can be administered is limited by toxicity; and second but possibly more important, at doses that are tolerated by an average population of patients, individual patients may experience either excessive toxicity or low therapeutic benefit because of pharmacokinetic variability. For most drugs, this variability is large, with a coefficient of variability (standard deviation/mean) of 20% to 40%. However, around one third of patients will be outside of this range, and the extremes of AUC, for example, or steady-state plasma concentration may cover a 5- to 10-fold range.

Such variability explains in part the variability seen in the pharmacodynamic effects of cytotoxic drugs. In addition, for most cytotoxic drugs, this variability is far greater than the fairly small variation seen in body surface area, such that correcting dose on the basis of body surface area results in little change in the overall variability in a drug's pharmacodynamics and probably serves only to make dosing more complicated. Historically, dosing by body surface area has been used in oncology because this parameter is presumed to correlate with drug clearance. However, numerous studies with cytotoxic drugs have found this correlation to be poor.[53]

Although Figure 17–3B shows a typical relationship between antitumor activity and toxicity for a cytotoxic drug, the proximity of the desired and adverse effects varies between drugs, as does the proximity of the different toxicity response curves. For many drugs, this limits how much the dose can be further escalated in high-dose regimens. For instance, if the major toxicity of a specific drug is myelosuppression, it may be possible to give higher doses of the drug with bone marrow support in the form of peripheral stem cell or bone marrow transplantation. However, if the dose-response curve for the next dose-limiting toxicity, such as gastrointestinal toxicity, is close to that for myelosuppression, the increase in dose that can be realized may be relatively small and may not be large enough to achieve a real increase in antitumor activity. For example, cytosine arabinoside is used for treatment of acute leukemias at standard doses of 100 to 200 mg/m^2 daily for 7 days, but it is also used in high-dose regimens at 2 to 3 g/m^2 12-hourly for 6 days, often with bone marrow support but with little increase in nonhematologic toxicity. Vincristine, however, is used at standard doses of around 1 to 1.4 g/m^2 in adult leukemias, but neurotoxicity becomes a problem with even small increases to 2.0 g/m^2, thereby limiting further dose increases.

Pharmacokinetic-Pharmacodynamic Relationships and Individualized Dosing

An important goal in studies investigating the pharmacokinetics and pharmacodynamics of cytotoxic drugs is to identify relationships between the two. This has generally been established for a toxic effect, such as myelosuppression, rather than for antitumor activity, although such studies do exist. For instance, the clearance of teniposide in children with leukemia was greater, resulting in a decrease in steady-state plasma concentration, in patients who did not respond to treatment, even though they were treated at the same dose as those who did respond.[54]

The identification of such relationships makes it feasible to target a pharmacokinetic parameter and to optimize dose in individual patients, rather than to treat all patients with a standard dose. By reducing pharmacokinetic variability in this way, toxicity may be reduced.[55] A randomized trial in childhood acute lymphoblastic leukemia (ALL) has shown that doses of standard cytotoxic drugs can be safely increased, with resultant therapeutic benefit, by use of such an approach.[56] Although it is still at the research stage in oncology, therapeutic drug monitoring is commonly used for other classes of drug with toxicity, such as antibiotics.

At a simpler level, identification of potential sources of pharmacokinetic variability in patients before dosing allows the dose to be modified in individual patients according to factors such as organ function and previous therapy. In the future, this may be extended to include additional factors, such as drug-metabolizing enzyme activity, protein binding, and drug-drug interactions.

Finally, a number of studies have described the prognostic value of in vitro drug sensitivity testing, using peripheral blasts or bone marrow samples, in acute leukemia. Such measures of sensitivity have been reported to be predictive of the failure of induction thereby and to be independent of other prognostic factors.[57, 58] This raises the possibility of basing the choice of drug regimen in individual patients on the sensitivity of their own leukemic cells and is currently undergoing further evaluation.

Drug Resistance and Tumor Sensitivity

The biggest problem limiting the effective use of cytotoxic chemotherapy is drug resistance. Tumors differ in their initial chemosensitivity. Some, such as leukemias, are very sensitive, resulting in a relatively high percentage of responses. Others, such as small-cell lung cancer, are initially sensitive but then recur; whereas in others, such as pancreatic cancer, cytotoxic drugs have little activity. These differences reflect differences in the biology of the tumor, relating to factors such as the growth fraction, the activity of specific drug resistance mechanisms, and changes in proteins mediating apoptosis.

Resistance can be intrinsic, such that the tumor is resistant to a particular drug or drugs at presentation, or it can be acquired, such that resistance develops during treatment. Cancer is a disease that develops as a result of damage to DNA, and this damage continues to accumulate after a cancer has formed because of the genetically unstable nature of cancer cells. Consequently, alterations to genes that are involved in drug sensitivity are more likely to occur as the population of tumor cells expands.

This hypothesis, proposed by Goldie and Coldman,[59] predicts that even in a tumor with a low rate of mutation (1×10^{-6}), a population of 1×10^9 cells (a 1-cm mass) would be certain to contain at least one drug-resistant cell. With higher mutation rates, this number clearly increases. Although small in number, the resistant clone of cells is selected during cytotoxic drug treatment, when surrounding sensitive cells are killed. When this drug-resistant cell population has expanded to the point that the tumor is said to have relapsed, it will be resistant to the chemotherapy that was effective initially. This situation is often seen in medical oncology, particularly in the treatment of solid tumors.

A tumor is commonly referred to as resistant if the activity of standard chemotherapy in that patient is less than that to be expected in a typical population. However, an element of this may relate to unresponsiveness rather than to true resistance. For example, a number of cytotoxic drugs act during specific phases of the cell cycle (Fig. 17–4), and to ensure cytotoxic activity, the tumor must be exposed to the drug during that cell cycle phase. The activity is therefore referred to as being phase specific. In clinical use, the drug will exhibit schedule dependence, meaning that the antitumor activity will also vary with the duration of exposure to the drug. The influence of dose and schedule on the activity of cytotoxic drugs in experimental leukemia was well demonstrated in the studies of Skipper and colleagues[60, 61] some 40 years ago.

A patient may also be unresponsive because of pharmacokinetic variability, for instance, having a high clearance for a specific drug such that plasma drug concentrations are substantially lower than in a typical population of patients, with a resultant decrease in drug activity.[54] When the physician is faced with a patient in whom a particular treatment has failed, it can be difficult to determine whether the tumor is unresponsive or truly resistant

and what the major mechanism underlying drug resistance is.

The major mechanisms responsible for resistance to cytotoxic drugs are described in the following. Whereas overt changes in these mechanisms may mediate resistance to a particular drug or drugs, more subtle changes will alter the sensitivity of the tumor to that drug.

Cellular Mechanisms Mediating Drug Sensitivity and Resistance

TARGET-RELATED CHANGES

For many cytotoxic drugs, resistance mechanisms have been described that involve changes in the target protein itself or changes in the amount of the target protein. Changes in the structure of the target protein most often result from a mutation in the gene encoding that protein, such that the drug is no longer able to bind or binding is reduced. This has been described for most of the antimetabolites,[62-64] topoisomerase-interacting drugs,[65, 66] and tubulin-binding agents.[67] Perhaps more common are changes in the amount of the target protein. For a number of antimetabolites, which inhibit specific enzymes involved in the synthesis of DNA precursors or DNA itself, amplification or overexpression of the gene has been described, resulting in increased amounts of the protein product of that gene. For drugs of this type, such as methotrexate[68] or 5-fluorouracil,[69] this increased amount of enzyme means that inhibition is not complete, even at maximally tolerated drug doses. In the case of 5-fluorouracil, there are now good clinical data describing lower levels of tumor thymidylate synthase protein, the principal drug target, and lower thymidylate synthase in mRNA, in patients who respond to treatment.[70]

Because the antimetabolites require activation by specific enzyme systems and are often transported into cells

FIGURE 17–4. The cell cycle and cytotoxic drug activity. Schematic diagram of the cell cycle showing the two gap phases, G_1 and G_2, when cells are actively preparing for DNA synthesis or mitosis, respectively. Terminally differentiated cells that will not undergo division, such as lymphocytes, and resting cells not preparing for division are in an early subphase of G_1 referred to as G_0. A number of cytotoxic drugs act in specific phases of the cell cycle, such that the timing or duration of treatment is often critical. Other drugs, particularly those that bind to DNA, are often phase nonspecific.

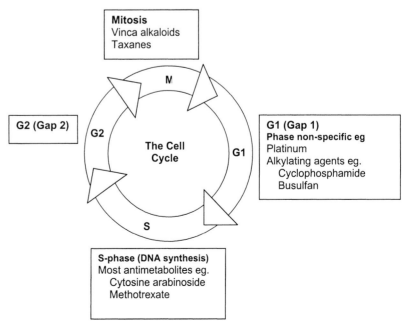

Mitosis
Vinca alkaloids
Taxanes

G2 (Gap 2)

G1 (Gap 1)
Phase non-specific eg
Platinum
Alkylating agents eg.
Cyclophosphamide
Busulfan

The Cell Cycle

M   G2   G1   S

S-phase (DNA synthesis)
Most antimetabolites eg.
Cytosine arabinoside
Methotrexate

by specific transport mechanisms, changes to proteins involved in these pathways can also result in resistance to the drug. This is perhaps best demonstrated for methotrexate.[71]

In the case of topoisomerase-acting drugs, resistance can arise by a decrease in the target enzyme[72] because initial enzyme activity is required to induce DNA strand breaks that are stabilized in the presence of drug. A decrease in the amount of specific topoisomerase protein means that adequate DNA damage to induce cell death cannot be achieved.

CHANGES IN DRUG EFFLUX MECHANISMS

P-Glycoprotein. A number of mechanisms for effluxing xenobiotics exist, their normal function being to protect the cell from potentially damaging compounds. Not surprisingly, many cytotoxic drugs are effluxed by these mechanisms, resulting in decreased intracellular drug concentrations.

The first of these pumps to be described was P-glycoprotein,[73] a member of the adenosine triphosphate (ATP)–binding cassette (ABC) superfamily of transmembrane transport proteins. This is an energy-dependent 170-kd protein with 12 transmembrane domains around a central pore through which compounds that are P-glycoprotein substrates are pumped.[74] Increased expression of this protein and activity of the pump have been described in tumors that are resistant to specific cytotoxic drugs.[75] Moreover, the selection of drug-resistant cells by prolonged exposure to specific cytotoxic drugs that are P-glycoprotein substrates results in the accumulation of cells with increased P-glycoprotein activity that are also resistant to a number of other structurally, unrelated, compounds that are also P-glycoprotein substrates. This phenomenon has been termed multidrug resistance (MDR) because resistance to one P-glycoprotein–effluxed drug is associated with resistance to multiple other agents. P-glycoprotein is commonly detected on the leukemic cells of patients with acute myelogenous leukemia (AML) in whom increased P-glycoprotein, or *MDR1* expression, is correlated with increased risk for treatment failure.[76] The influence of P-glycoprotein and *MDR1* on the outcome of patients with ALL is less clear.[77]

Drugs implicated in the MDR phenotype include the anthracyclines, vinca alkaloids, epipodophyllotoxins, and taxanes. Several noncytotoxic drugs that can inhibit P-glycoprotein have also been described, including calcium channel blockers, such as verapamil and bepridil, and immunosuppressant drugs, such as cyclosporine.[76] Clinical trials that have added such agents to standard chemotherapy in an attempt to overcome this mechanism of resistance have generally proved disappointing in solid tumors[78] (possibly because it is now clear that there are a number of other drug efflux mechanisms that may not be co-inhibited) but more successful in AML[78, 79] (see Chapters 21, 22, and 23). In addition, because P-glycoprotein is involved in the excretion of drug molecules into the bile ducts and renal tubules, P-glycoprotein inhibitors have a marked effect on clearance, and thereby AUC, of the co-administered cytotoxic agent.[48, 80, 81]

Multidrug Resistance Protein. A more recent member of the ABC superfamily associated with cytotoxic drug resistance is the multidrug resistance protein (MRP).[82] This is a 190-kd protein that shares only 15% amino acid homology with P-glycoprotein. Although most of the reports have focused on MRP1 and MRP2, six members of the MRP family have been identified to date.[83, 84] The spectrum of drugs effluxed by MRP is similar to the spectrum of drugs effluxed by P-glycoprotein but includes a number of conjugated drugs, particularly glutathione conjugates. The importance of this pump may relate to its involvement in the efflux of drugs inactivated by glutathione, although this does not include cisplatin-glutathione conjugates. Increased activity of MRP has been reported in a number of tumor types, including leukemia, although its prognostic importance in leukemia remains unclear.[85, 86]

MRP is not inhibited by agents that have been used clinically to inhibit P-glycoprotein. Agents that do specifically inhibit MRP have been reported.[87-89]

Lung Resistance Protein. A third drug efflux protein implicated in cytotoxic drug resistance is the 100-kd lung resistance protein (LRP). This is the major protein expressed on intracellular structures known as vaults, and it is involved in transporting drugs into these vaults for transport from the nucleus to the cytoplasm and then into vesicles that are exocytosed.[90] Drugs specifically implicated in LRP-mediated efflux include anthracyclines and mitoxantrone, but this efflux mechanism almost certainly extends to many other cytotoxic drugs.

The relative importance of each of these three drug efflux mechanisms is currently unclear. In a panel of 61 cell lines, LRP and MRP were expressed more commonly than P-glycoprotein, with LRP expression being the best overall predictor of sensitivity to a range of drugs.[91] Results from other studies have been contradictory. LRP expression has been associated with a poor outcome in AML[92] and multiple myeloma.[93]

DRUG DEACTIVATION

The activity of individual cytotoxic drugs is often in part dependent on the activity of metabolizing enzymes specific for that drug, but more general mechanisms exist for the detoxification of potentially DNA-damaging agents.

An important and widespread mechanism for the deactivation of reactive species, including drug molecules, carcinogens, and free radicals, involves the tripeptide glutathione in two types of reaction.[94] Reduced glutathione can inactivate free radicals and peroxides in a reaction catalyzed by glutathione peroxidase, with regeneration of reduced glutathione by glutathione reductase. This mechanism is implicated in the inactivation of free radicals generated by drugs such as doxorubicin and by ionizing radiation. A second mechanism involves the conjugation of glutathione with positively charged electrophilic molecules in a reaction catalyzed by glutathione-S-transferase (GST). These molecules are the active species of drugs such as cisplatin and alkylating agents. After conjugation in this way, drugs are effluxed from the cell by glutathione conjugate carriers, such as MRP, that appear to be specific for different conjugates.[83] MRP, for instance, does not transport cisplatin-glutathione conjugates. There are five distinct GSTs classified by their isoelectric point, and there is considerable evidence to link GST activity with drug resistance.[95, 96] In particular, the transfection of specific GSTs into drug-sensitive cell lines confers resistance to alkylating agents (GST-α), doxorubicin (GST-π), and cisplatin (GST-μ).[96]

Agents that inhibit glutathione synthesis (buthionine sulfoximine) or GSTs (ethacrynic acid and indomethacin) can increase the activity of alkylating agents in tumor cell lines, and buthionine sulfoximine has been shown to significantly decrease reduced glutathione levels in tumors in clinical trials.[97, 98]

CHANGES IN DNA REPAIR

The majority of cytotoxic drugs induce DNA damage, and a number of systems exist to repair this damage. Proteins involved in the maintenance of genome integrity that can detect DNA damage and induce either cell cycle arrest (to allow repair to take place) or apoptosis are an important component of sensitivity to such drugs. The most important factor in this pathway is the p53 protein.[99] The gene encoding p53 is mutated in around 50% of all human cancers, resulting in deactivation of the protein. These are often dominant negative mutations such that a mutation in one allele results in a protein that can inactivate the functional p53 protein from the second allele.[100] In general, tumors that are most responsive to cytotoxic chemotherapy, such as the leukemias and testicular teratomas, tend to have a much lower frequency of p53 mutations than other tumors, and this has often been attributed to the presence of functional p53.[101] However, this association may not be clear-cut, and tumors with mutations of the gene encoding p53 may have also acquired a number of other genetic abnormalities, some of which may involve genes whose products influence the activity of specific cytotoxic drugs, such that chemosensitivity may not be related directly to functional p53. Indeed, for a number of cytotoxic drugs, sensitivity may actually be increased by the loss of p53 function related to failure of p53-mediated cell cycle checkpoints.[102]

Specific pathways exist for the repair of damaged DNA, and this repair can take place at several levels.[103-105]

Damage Reversal Repair. Damage reversal repair involves the removal of DNA adducts that, if unrepaired, give rise to more profound DNA damage. Specific enzymes involved in the removal of such adducts include O^6-alkylguanine alkyltransferase (AGAT), and increased activity of AGAT has been associated with resistance or decreased sensitivity to alkylating agents because the alkyl group is removed before further DNA damage can occur. Agents that can inhibit AGAT, such as O^6-benzylguanine, have been shown to increase the activity of certain alkylating agents in preclinical models and are currently under evaluation in clinical trials. An early report has described that O^6-benzylguanine inhibited AGAT in all 56 samples of peripheral leukocytes from normal healthy donors.[106]

Base Excision Repair. Base excision repair is the removal of single damaged bases from DNA in a complex process involving a number of specific enzymes. Of particular importance are a group of enzymes called 3-methyladenine DNA glycosylases that initiate this repair by removal of the damaged base. Other enzymes then restore the damaged site using the opposite DNA strand as the template. This type of DNA repair is typically limited to one or two bases. The activity of this repair process particularly influences sensitivity to alkylating agents.

Nucleotide Excision Repair. Nucleotide excision repair is a process similar to base excision repair but involves larger sections of DNA, typically around 30 bases. This repair mechanism requires a large number of proteins in a multistep process that involves mismatch recognition, formation of a transcription factor complex that unwinds and cuts the DNA around the mismatched site, removal of the mismatch fragment, synthesis of a new nucleotide fragment, and ligation of this new fragment into the DNA strand. This is implicated in the removal of DNA cross-links formed by alkylating agents and platinum compounds, and increased activity of some of the key proteins involved results in decreased drug activity because of increased repair.

DNA Mismatch Repair. DNA mismatch repair has similarities to base and nucleotide mismatch repair processes but crucially involves a number of proteins that recognize base mismatches in DNA and initiate repair. These are hMSH2, hMLH1, hPMS1, and hPMS2, homologues of bacterial mismatch repair proteins MutL and MutS. The importance of these proteins in drug activity is that failure to detect a drug-induced base mismatch within DNA results in decreased drug activity because the DNA lesion is not recognized and the damage persists. This mechanism of resistance applies to alkylating agents, platinum compounds, and some of the antimetabolites (5-fluorouracil).[107]

CHANGES IN APOPTOSIS

Cell death after exposure to cytotoxic agents is typically by apoptosis, a complex but tightly controlled process whereby the cell contents are broken down and recycled in a highly ordered fashion.[108] A number of cellular insults, including exposure to cytotoxic drugs, can initiate this process, and a large number of proteins are involved in the apoptosis that results, many activated by a group of enzymes called caspases. Crucially, caspases are themselves activated by the release of cytochrome c from the mitochondria,[109] and this commitment to apoptosis is controlled by proteins of the Bcl-2 family. A number of these proteins are antiapoptotic and block the release of cytochrome c, including Bcl-2 (B-cell lymphoma 2) and Bcl-XL; others are proapoptotic, including Bax and Bcl-XS. Whether a cell undergoes apoptosis as a response to cytotoxic chemotherapy depends in part on the relative amounts of these proapoptotic and antiapoptotic proteins. For instance, increased levels of Bcl-2, an antiapoptotic protein, are frequently found in human cancers and are associated with resistance to cytotoxic drugs.[110, 111] Approaches that block Bcl-2, such as antisense therapy, result in increased cytotoxic drug sensitivity.[112]

Because apoptosis is the typical mechanism of cell death induced by cytotoxic drugs, changes to specific proteins in this pathway, such as Bcl-2, result in altered sensitivity or outright resistance to a wide range of agents. A number of new therapeutic approaches are aimed at modulating apoptotic proteins to improve chemosensitivity.

DRUGS USED IN THE TREATMENT OF LEUKEMIA

Overview of Leukemia Treatment

The use of chemotherapy in the treatment of leukemia has evolved remarkably during the past 30 years, particularly in childhood ALL. However, the therapies for specific leukemias differ markedly, mostly owing to the differing course of these diseases, and involve aggressive treatment with combination chemotherapy in acute leukemias but typically the use of single agents in chronic leukemias (Table 17-1).

With acute leukemias, the immediate goal is to achieve a complete remission and restore normal hematopoiesis. In ALL, early studies with vincristine and prednisone resulted in complete remissions in around 50% of patients, a figure improved to around 75% by the subsequent addition of an anthracycline and then by other drugs such as cyclophosphamide and L-asparaginase (see Chapters 26 and 27). In AML, the introduction of cytosine arabinoside (ara-C) in the 1960s resulted in complete remissions in around 20% to 30% of patients, later improved to 40% to 50% by the addition of an anthracycline and then further still by other agents such as 6-thioguanine and etoposide (see Chapter 21). These combinations now represent standard *induction therapy* for acute leukemias, with the aim of causing temporary bone marrow hypoplasia. It is therefore not surprising that they are intensely myelosuppressive and require careful support of the patient because of neutropenia or infection. The exception to this is the treatment of acute promyelocytic leukemia, which now typically involves the use of all-*trans* retinoic acid as a single agent to relieve the transcriptional block resulting from the retinoic acid receptor/PML gene translocation product.

With the chronic leukemias, the time course of the disease is different, and initial treatment often involves only a single agent, such as chlorambucil or fludarabine in chronic lymphocytic leukemia (see Chapter 28) and hydroxyurea or interferon in chronic myeloid leukemia (see Chapter 25). The use of more intensive combination chemotherapy in these chronic leukemias, like that used in acute leukemias, has not proved to be superior to single-agent treatment in terms of overall survival.

It also became apparent early in the treatment of acute leukemias that although combination chemotherapy could dramatically reduce the burden of leukemic cells, to the point at which a complete remission was achieved, this alone was not enough to result in cure of the patient because the leukemic clone was not fully eradicated. Consequently, *postremission therapy* was introduced. This takes the form of *consolidation* therapy, in which the doses used are similar to those used in induction therapy, or *intensive consolidation,* in which higher doses are employed. In some settings, more prolonged low-dose treatments are used after consolidation therapy as *maintenance.*

In AML, a number of clinical trials demonstrated that shorter, more intensive consolidation chemotherapy was superior to maintenance treatment, and today this typically comprises high-dose ara-C, often followed by a bone marrow transplantation with further high-dose chemotherapy and radiotherapy. In ALL, consolidation chemotherapy also includes ara-C, typically in combination with an anthracycline, epipodophyllotoxin, and antimetabolite. In contrast to AML, the use of maintenance chemotherapy in ALL is important to achieve a cure and typically comprises 2 years of treatment with oral methotrexate and 6-mercaptopurine in children with ALL; these drugs are given in combination with cyclophosphamide in adult ALL. A further distinctive feature in the treatment of ALL in adults and children is the use of central nervous system (CNS) prophylaxis. Within the CNS, the incidence of leukemia is only 5% to 10% at presentation in ALL but increases to a cumulative incidence of more than 30% in patients who do not receive chemotherapy specifically targeting these sanctuary sites. This typically involves intrathecally administered methotrexate.

In patients who are resistant to induction chemotherapy or who subsequently relapse, a range of established and novel combinations are employed.

Combination Chemotherapy versus Single-Agent Treatment

Whereas it is dangerous to generalize or to extrapolate from acute to chronic leukemias, treatment with a single

TABLE 17–1. Typical Roles of Specific Cytotoxic Drugs in the Treatment of the Leukemias

Acute Lymphoblastic Leukemia

Induction	Vincristine + prednisone + 2 or 3 other drugs from an anthracycline (daunorubicin or idarubicin), cyclophosphamide, L-asparaginase
Intensive consolidation	Cytarabine (ara-C), other drugs including an anthracycline (daunorubicin or idarubicin), epipodophyllotoxins (etoposide or teniposide), antimetabolite (methotrexate or 6-thioguanine)
Maintenance (2 years)	Oral methotrexate and mercaptopurine
CNS prophylaxis	Intrathecal methotrexate

Acute Myeloid Leukemia

Induction	Ara-C + an anthracycline (daunorubicin or idarubicin) + etoposide or 6-thioguanine
Intensive postremission therapy	High-dose ara-C or bone marrow/stem-cell transplantation

Acute Promyelocytic Leukemia

Induction	Retinoic acid alone or with anthracycline/ara-C combination
Postremission therapy	Anthracycline/ara-C if retinoic acid is used as a single agent in induction

Chronic Lymphold Leukemia

	Chlorambucil ± prednisone
	Cyclophosphamide, vincristine, prednisone (CVP) in relapsed or resistant patients

Chronic Myeloid Leukemia

	Hydroxyurea and/or busulfan
	Interferon-α

cytotoxic drug is typically not enough to result in cure. Consequently, in cases in which cure and increased survival are possible, drugs are used in combination. When cure or increased survival is not possible, the increased toxicity of combinations does not justify their use.

The rationale for combining specific drugs is based on several factors.[113] First, the individual drugs must clearly be active in the setting in which they are to be used, and they should be used at or close to their optimal dose and schedule. Second, individual drugs in a combination will usually have different mechanisms of action, such that if a particular tumor is resistant to one class of drugs by one or more of the resistance mechanisms described before, a drug with a different mechanism of action may still be active. Third, drugs used in combinations will generally have different toxicity profiles, thus limiting excessive toxicities of a specific type.

Finally, although cytotoxic chemotherapy is a crucial component in the treatment of leukemia, it is often used in conjunction with other modalities, such as immunotherapy or antibodies (see Chapter 18), and may require bone marrow or stem cell transplantation for complete eradication of the disease (see Chapter 20).

THE PHARMACOLOGY OF SPECIFIC ANTILEUKEMIC DRUGS

The pharmacology of drugs used in the treatment of leukemia is discussed in detail in the following sections. There is no established classification for anticancer drugs, and they have been divided into groups on the basis of their mechanism of action.

Antimetabolites

Antimetabolites interfere with the synthesis of purine and pyrimidine bases, required for the synthesis of RNA and DNA, by inhibiting key enzymes involved in these pathways. In addition, because many antimetabolites are analogues of the normal endogenous bases, some can become directly incorporated into DNA or RNA, thereby inducing direct damage.

This group of drugs includes the antifolates, which inhibit the formation of reduced folate, and drugs that act as purine or pyrimidine antagonists. Antimetabolites are prodrugs that typically require activation before they can exert their effects. With antifolates, this involves the extension of a glutamate side chain that increases activity; the other compounds require the addition of a phosphoribose sugar by specific phosphoribosyltransferases to produce a nucleoside and/or further phosphorylation by specific nucleoside kinases to the nucleotide. The triphosphorylated nucleotide can induce damage by incorporation into nucleic acid or by inhibition of key enzymes involved in DNA synthesis. Several of these analogues, including 6-thioguanine, 6-mercaptopurine, and 5-fluorouracil, require complete activation through the ribose sugar and phosphate; others, such as cytosine arabinoside, fludarabine, and 5-azacytidine, are administered as the nucleoside.

Cells can generate purine and pyrimidine nucleotides by either *de novo* or *salvage* pathways. Normal cells rely mainly on the salvage pathway and recycle partially degraded nucleotides; tumors favor the de novo pathway involving synthesis of new nucleotides. This gives a degree of selectivity to these agents in that tumor cells are likely to use more of the administered analogues in synthesizing new nucleotides.[114] Because this group of compounds is mainly involved in the inhibition of DNA synthesis, they are typically more active during the S phase of the cell cycle.[115]

Antifolates

The antifolates were among the first cytotoxic drugs described. The antileukemic activity of the first of these compounds, aminopterin, was reported in 1948.[4] An analogue of aminopterin, methotrexate (MTX), was found to be as active but less toxic and is currently the most widely used antifolate.

Folates serve an essential function as one-carbon donors in enzyme reactions that synthesize nucleotides. A crucial protein in these pathways is dihydrofolate reductase (DHFR) because folic acid can act as a coenzyme only when it is in the fully reduced state as tetrahydrofolate (Fig. 17–5). Tetrahydrofolate can act as a one-carbon carrier in two specific ways. 5,10-Methylenetetrahydrofolate provides a methyl group for the conversion of uridine to thymidine in a reaction catalyzed by thymidylate synthase; 10-formyltetrahydrofolate donates its one-carbon group to glycinamide ribonucleotide transformylase and aminoimidazole ribonucleotide transformylase in the de novo synthesis of purines. In the first of these pathways, 5,10-methylenetetrahydrofolate is hydrolyzed back to dihydrofolate, so active DHFR is required to maintain an adequate pool of reduced folate.

The presence of an amino group at the 4 position of MTX in place of the hydroxyl group in folic acid converts the molecule from an enzyme substrate to a tight binding inhibitor of DHFR. Once this inhibition occurs, reduced folate pools are rapidly depleted, resulting in inhibition of these purine and thymidine de novo pathways.[116, 117]

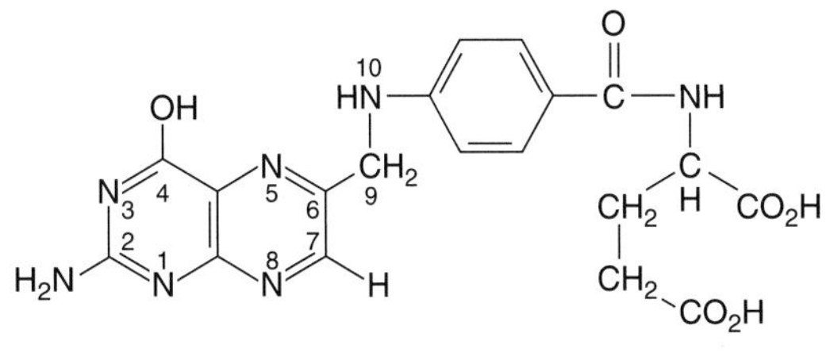

Folic acid (Pteroyl-L-Glutamic acid)

FIGURE 17–5. Structures of folic acid, reduced folates, and methotrexate (MTX). Inhibition of dihydrofolate reductase (DHFR) by MTX blocks the production of reduced folate, and existing tetrahydrofolate is soon depleted in the production of deoxythymidine monophosphate (dTMP) in a reaction catalyzed by thymidylate synthase (TS). Reduced folate can be administered as N^5-formyl tetrahydrofolate. Both MTX polyglutamates and dihydrofolate polyglutamates can also inhibit other enzymes involved in purine synthesis. (From Pratt WB, Ruddon RW, Ensminger WD, et al: The Anticancer Drugs, 2nd ed. Oxford: Oxford University Press; 1994, p. 75.)

MTX enters the cell mainly through the reduced folate carrier, a specific transmembrane energy-dependent transport system that has a higher affinity for reduced folate and MTX than for folic acid.[118, 119] Additional pathways exist that may act independently to transport folates and MTX or that may interact in some way with the reduced folate carrier. These include a specific human folate receptor that can transport folates into the cell by the formation of receptor-rich vesicles containing protein-bound folates.[120] The folate in these vesicles may then be liberated and transported into the intracellular space by the reduced folate carrier. Expression of this receptor is modulated by extracellular reduced folate concentrations, being increased in low-folate and decreased in high-folate environments.[118, 121] Although the role of this protein in MTX transport remains unclear, there is evidence that expression of such a protein in leukemic cells is associated with increased MTX transport and increased cytotoxic activity.[122] A third transport system involving passive diffusion may become more important at higher MTX concentrations (>20 μM). A number of reports have described resistance to MTX attributable to defective transport mechanisms.[121, 123, 124] This has also been reported in the leukemic blast cells of patients with recurrent ALL after initial treatment with MTX.[125]

Differences exist in the cellular transport of MTX and new antifolates. MTX has a single glutamate side chain; the new, nonglutamated analogues, including trimetrexate, piritrexim, and 10-ethyl-10-deazaaminopterin, do not require an active cellular transport system and are therefore active against cell lines resistant to MTX because of defective transport.[116, 126] The 7-hydroxy metabolite of MTX can also be transported by the reduced folate carrier and may compete with MTX for cellular uptake.[127]

MTX and its analogues are polyglutamated by folylpolyglutamyl synthetase (FPGS).[116, 128] This enzyme adds up to six glutamyl residues to folic acid, thereby effectively trapping the molecule inside cells. A different enzyme, γ-glutamyl hydrolase, acts to remove terminal glutamyl groups. The amount and extent of polyglutamated MTX within cells are determined by the relative activities of these two enzymes.[129] As much as 80% of intracellular MTX is in the polyglutamated form. Differences in the activity of FPGS have also been associated with MTX resistance.[130] Animal studies suggest that there may be selective conversion of MTX to its polyglutamate in tumor cells, rather than in normal cells, conferring a degree of selectivity in MTX cytotoxicity.[128]

MTX inhibition of DHFR results in a decrease in reduced folate pools; and the accumulation of polyglutamated species, including MTX polyglutamates, dihydrofolate polyglutamates, and 10-formyl dihydrofolate polyglutamates, in the cell. These polyglutamates can bind to folate-dependent enzymes but are not able to donate a one-carbon group, resulting in the further inhibition of thymidylate synthase, transformylase, glycinamide ribonucleotide, and aminoimidazole ribonucleotide transformylase.[131] In addition, MTX polyglutamates are as potent as MTX at inhibiting DHFR but with a slower rate of dissociation, so inhibition is prolonged.[131]

A common mechanism of resistance to MTX is increased expression of DHFR, either by amplification of the DHFR gene on chromosomal or extrachromosomal material or by increased expression of a normal gene copy number.[68] With prolonged exposure to MTX, cells also show an acute increase in the amount of DHFR protein. This is not associated with increased gene expression and is regulated by the DHFR protein, without associated folate or MTX, binding to its own mRNA and suppressing translation.[132] When the enzyme binds to either folate or MTX, it no longer binds to its mRNA, promoting increased protein synthesis. Such a response may decrease the effect of MTX on DHFR activity with time.

There is a close correlation between MTX sensitivity and the degree of DHFR binding, and resistance to MTX has been associated with decreased affinity for the enzyme.[133, 134] This may be a result of a change in the structure of the enzyme, caused by a mutation, leading to as little as a single amino acid substitution.[135]

Inhibition of the enzyme systems described starves the cell of DNA nucleotides, leading to a block in DNA synthesis and the appearance of DNA strand breaks. Some of these strand breaks may be due to incomplete DNA repair, again because of MTX-induced nucleotide depletion.

The absorption of orally administered MTX is mainly by the reduced folate carrier. Oral bioavailability is dose dependent, being 80% to 90% at doses less than 12 mg/m² but only 50% at doses higher than this.[136, 137] MTX is usually administered intravenously and rapidly distributes into extracellular fluid. It also distributes into third-space fluid compartments, such as ascites or pleural fluids, from which it is slowly absorbed back into the systemic circulation. Consequently, drug trapped in such a fluid compartment can maintain a low but prolonged plasma MTX concentration, resulting in increased toxicity,[138] and such fluid should be drained before treatment. The typical terminal elimination half-life is around 8 to 10 hours, but it may be prolonged considerably in patients with impaired renal function or a third-space compartment.[116] Most of a dose of MTX is excreted renally as unchanged drug, with a small amount excreted in the bile but subsequently reabsorbed. MTX is relatively insoluble at the slightly acidic pH of urine, and precipitation in the renal tubules results in renal toxicity with higher doses. This can be prevented by alkalinization of the urine and maintenance of an adequate urinary flow.

MTX is metabolized to the 7-hydroxy metabolite, which may have some cytotoxic activity, and to 2,4-diamino-N¹⁰-pteroic acid, which is inactive but cross-reacts in a commonly used immunoassay for MTX.[116] 7-Hydroxy MTX is less soluble than MTX, and with high-dose treatment, it may at least contribute to the renal toxicity of MTX.[139]

The major toxicities of MTX are myelosuppression, renal toxicity, and mucositis.[116] Higher doses of MTX (>100 mg/m²) are typically used with a "rescue" dose of reduced folate, N⁵-formyl-tetrahydrofolate (calcium folinate, leucovorin), with the actual dose administered determined by the MTX concentration at 24 hours. Leucovorin has a greater effect in rescuing normal tissue from the effects of MTX than tumor tissue. A likely explanation for this is that because the de novo pathway of nucleotide synthesis is much lower in normal tissue, uptake and polyglutamation of MTX are less than in tumor tissue, such that there is less active drug present for competition with folinic acid, and the inhibition of DHFR and folate-dependent enzymes is more readily overcome.

MTX is used in ALL in three different ways. It is often given as part of consolidation therapy in childhood ALL and is routinely used as part of maintenance therapy in both children and adults (see Chapters 26 and 27, respectively). Increased systemic clearance of MTX is associated with an increased risk for relapse in childhood ALL,[140] and individualization of the MTX dose on the basis of pharmacokinetic parameters has more recently permitted a dose increase resulting in improved survival in the same setting.[56]

MTX is also used as intrathecal therapy, both for CNS prophylaxis and in the treatment of established meningeal leukemia (in both ALL and AML). The drug can safely be given into the spinal fluid at a dose of 12.5 mg (see Chapter 26). In adults with ALL, it is not associated with intracranial calcification, as was originally shown to be the case in children, and it can be given either alone or as part of so-called triple therapy (in conjunction with ara-C and hydrocortisone).

NUCLEOSIDE ANALOGUES

Cytosine Arabinoside. Many antimetabolites are modified purine or pyrimidine bases that require conversion to a nucleoside by the addition of a ribose sugar, and then phosphorylation to a nucleotide, before they can interfere with RNA or DNA synthesis. During the 1950s, a nucleoside analogue, cytosine arabinoside (ara-C), isolated from the Caribbean sponge *Cryptotethya crypta,* was shown to have antitumor activity and was soon produced synthetically.[141] This compound differed from its endogenous counterpart by the presence of an arabinose rather than a ribose sugar, having a β-hydroxy group at the 2′ position. This and related compounds differ from other antimetabolites in that their activity is confined almost exclusively to DNA, having little or no RNA-directed activity. Ara-C remains the most active agent in the treatment of AML, but paradoxically, it has little activity in solid tumors. Structures of the pyrimidine antagonists are illustrated in Figure 17–6.

Ara-C is readily carried into cells by a nucleoside transporter, which becomes saturated at concentrations greater than 20 μM,[142] above which transport is by passive diffusion.[143] To exert its activity, ara-C must be converted to ara-C triphosphate (ara-CTP) by the sequential action of three phosphorylating enzymes, deoxycytidine kinase, deoxycytidine monophosphate kinase, and nucleoside-diphosphate kinase.[144] The first of these enzymes has the lowest activity and is the rate-limiting step in ara-C activation. Its activity increases markedly during the S phase of the cell cycle.[145] Competing with the first of these two anabolic enzymes are two enzymes that inactivate ara-C and ara-C monophosphate (ara-CMP) to the corresponding uridine compound (Fig. 17–7). The relative activities of these activating and deactivating pathways differ markedly between tissue types and even within similar tissues. Within leukemic cells, the ratio of

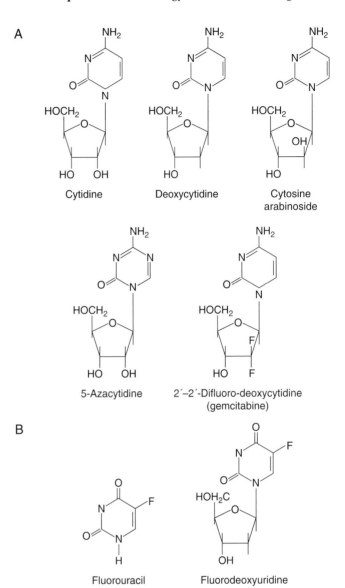

FIGURE 17–6. Structures of pyrimidine antagonists, including cytidine *(A)* and uridine *(B)* analogues.

activating to deactivating enzyme activity is markedly higher in lymphoid than in myeloid cells.[146, 147] However, this ratio may not predict the amount of final formed ara-CTP because differences between cell types with regard to activity of the nucleoside transporter contribute to ara-CTP concentration.[148]

The fully activated nucleotide of ara-C, ara-CTP, is able to compete with the natural nucleotide deoxycytidine triphosphate for incorporation into DNA by DNA polymerase. However, once incorporated into DNA, the fraudulent nucleotide is a potent inhibitor of a number of DNA polymerases involved in DNA replication and repair, resulting in termination of strand elongation.[149-151] Even in the case of limited incorporation of ara-CTP into DNA, which may be insufficient to block DNA synthesis, inhibition of DNA polymerases can occur during subsequent attempts at DNA repair or during the next round of DNA replication.[152]

Because ara-C activity is critically dependent on ongo-

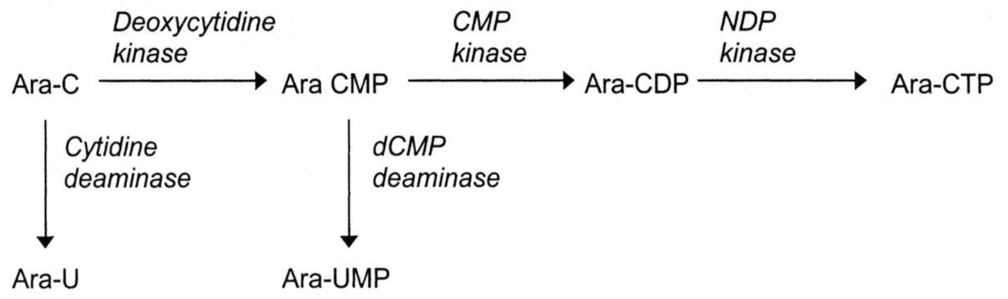

```
        Deoxycytidine              CMP              NDP
          kinase                   kinase           kinase
Ara-C ──────────────▶ Ara CMP ──────────▶ Ara-CDP ──────────▶ Ara-CTP

   │   Cytidine              │   dCMP
   │   deaminase             │   deaminase
   │                         │
   ▼                         ▼
Ara-U                    Ara-UMP
```

FIGURE 17–7. Activation and metabolism of ara-C. Ara-CTP is the active anabolite, inhibiting DNA polymerases, resulting in DNA damage.

ing DNA synthesis, cells in other phases of the cell cycle will be unresponsive to the drug. Most treatment regimens therefore involve ara-C administration during several days to maximize the chance of exposing the cell during at least one round of DNA synthesis.

In leukemic cell lines, most resistance mechanisms to ara-C relate to failure to generate sufficient ara-CTP because of decreased cellular uptake, increased deactivation, or decreased phosphorylation.[153, 154] Clinical trials have also identified a relationship between intracellular ara-CTP concentration and antileukemic activity.[155, 156] Strategies to increase ara-CTP concentration have included the use of gram doses of drug[157, 158] and, more recently, pretreatment with fludarabine (which stimulates the activity of deoxycytidine kinase) given before ara-C.[159]

The oral bioavailability of ara-C is less than 20%, mainly owing to extensive presystemic deamination in the gut and liver.[144, 160] Conventional doses of ara-C are 100 to 200 mg/m² by intravenous bolus injection twice daily over several days or by infusion, which achieves steady-state plasma concentrations of up to 1 μM. The drug distributes rapidly into total body water and is able to cross the blood-brain barrier, with steady-state cerebrospinal fluid concentration around 10% to 40% of that in plasma.[161] The elimination half-life is around 2 hours in plasma, but it is longer in the cerebrospinal fluid, probably because deaminase activity is lower.[144] Plasma pharmacokinetics are linear up to doses of 2 g/m², above which deaminase activity may be saturated and the drug's effects become more unpredictable.[162] Deamination to uracil arabinoside (ara-U) is rapid, and plasma ara-U concentrations exceed those of ara-C shortly after dose; 70% to 80% of the dose is excreted in the urine in 24 hours, predominantly as ara-U.[160]

Whereas high-dose regimens attempt to maximize ara-CTP concentrations, low-dose regimens (3 to 20 mg/m²/day) have also been used in older patients and those with myelodysplasia. Early studies suggested that this dose may induce terminal differentiation of leukemic cells,[163] but subsequent studies have been disappointing in terms of survival. These low doses may actually decrease activity by inducing cell cycle arrest,[164] such that cells pass less often through the sensitive phase of the cell cycle.

The major toxicity of ara-C is myelosuppression, manifest mostly as leukopenia and thrombocytopenia. Other toxicities include nausea and vomiting, mucositis, and diarrhea. Toxicities to other tissues, particularly neurologic, are seen with high-dose ara-C (see Chapter 21).

Ara-C is probably the single most important drug in the treatment of AML and is included in virtually all remission induction and consolidation regimens, in either conventional or gram doses. The toxicity of the ara-C

gram dose is different from that of the conventional dose; conjunctivitis and a specific rash, particularly affecting the hands and feet, are seen. The most significant toxicity of high-dose ara-C is the so-called cerebellar syndrome that in rare cases can lead to severe and permanent neurologic deficit, which is reversible in most patients.

High-dose ara-C has also been used extensively in ALL and may be particularly useful in T-cell ALL.[165, 166] It has also formed part of myeloablative regimens, particularly in the context of high-dose treatment given with autologous hematopoietic progenitor cell support, when it would seem logical to use the *best antileukemic drug* as opposed to the largely immunosuppressive cyclophosphamide.

Intrathecal ara-C is used to prevent and treat meningeal leukemia at doses of 30 mg/m², which achieves peak concentrations of up to 1 mM.[144] Intrathecal ara-C can be given alone or in combination with intrathecal MTX and hydrocortisone as CNS prophylaxis. It is also used in the not unusual situation in which cerebrospinal fluid protein is elevated after several injections of MTX in the context of known CNS leukemia.

Azacytidine. 5-Azacytidine (aza-C) differs from ara-C by the presence of a nitrogen in place of a carbon at the 5 position in the pyrimidine ring and by the presence of a ribose sugar instead of arabinose[167] (see Fig. 17–6). These small changes result in marked differences in pharmacology compared with ara-C. Aza-C enters cells by the nucleoside transporter system and is then phosphorylated by uridine-cytidine kinase rather than by deoxycytidine kinase, which catalyses the conversion of ara-C to ara-CMP.[144] Decreased activity of deoxycytidine kinase mediates resistance to ara-C, so aza-C can bypass this resistance mechanism. Further phosphorylation to aza-CTP is catalyzed by the same enzymes that phosphorylate ara-CMP. Because aza-CTP possesses a ribose sugar, it can be incorporated into RNA with effects on RNA synthesis, processing, and function.[167] Aza-CTP is also incorporated into DNA, thereby inducing termination of DNA synthesis.

The presence of a nitrogen at the 5 position in the pyrimidine ring confers an additional mechanism to aza-C.[168] The specific methylation of cytosine residues in DNA is a mechanism for switching off gene expression. This is achieved by the transfer of a methyl group to the 5 position of cytosine in a reaction catalyzed by DNA cytosine-5-methyltransferase. When the enzyme attempts this reaction with an aza-C nucleotide in the DNA strand, a covalent complex is formed that effectively traps the enzyme, resulting in its inhibition. The resultant decrease in DNA methylation permits the increased expression of a number of genes. Consequently, aza-C induces differentiation in a number of cell types.[169]

The major toxicity of aza-C is myelosuppression, although gastrointestinal toxicity, manifest as nausea, vomiting, and diarrhea, can be a problem, particularly with bolus dosing. Hepatotoxicity has also been reported,[170] and patients with impaired liver function are particularly at risk.

Gemcitabine. As mentioned, ara-C is the most active agent in the treatment of AML, but it has little or no activity in solid tumors. Gemcitabine ($2',2'$-difluoro-deoxycytidine) differs from ara-C in the presence of two fluorines in the sugar moiety of the molecule (see Fig. 17–6), resulting in marked differences in cellular pharmacology.[171] Gemcitabine is taken up by cells more avidly than is ara-C, in part because of its increased lipophilicity, and it is a better substrate for deoxycytidine kinase, both of which result in higher intracellular concentrations of gemcitabine triphosphate than of ara-CTP.[171] Gemcitabine and ara-C are cleared at similar rates by the first deaminase enzyme, cytidine deaminase, but gemcitabine is a much better substrate for deoxycytidine monophosphate deaminase. This should result in more rapid clearance of gemcitabine monophosphate, but gemcitabine triphosphate is able to inhibit this deactivating enzyme, such that gemcitabine effectively inhibits its own metabolism. Unlike ara-C diphosphate, gemcitabine diphosphate inhibits ribonucleotide reductase, an important salvage pathway for the synthesis of deoxycytidine triphosphate, which would normally compete for incorporation into DNA. These differences result in enhanced accumulation and more prolonged retention of gemcitabine nucleotides, compared with ara-C, and block the synthesis of competitive endogenous nucleotides.[172] Like ara-C, gemcitabine activity is mediated principally by incorporation into DNA.

The drug is thus considerably more active than ara-C and has shown activity in a number of solid tumors, including malignant neoplasms such as pancreatic cancer and non–small-cell lung cancer, which have previously been relatively chemoresistant.[173] In these settings, gemcitabine has been administered as a single intravenous dose once every 3 weeks, but this may be inappropriate in leukemia when the objective is to create temporary marrow aplasia. In a phase I study of patients with AML and chronic myelomonocytic leukemia treated with an infusion of gemcitabine at 10 mg/m²/min, the maximal tolerated dose was 4800 mg/m² given during 480 minutes.[174] There are currently no clinical data describing the activity of gemcitabine in hematologic malignant neoplasms, but because ara-C is such an active compound in this setting, it is likely that gemcitabine will also be active. In leukemic blast cells, depletion of endogenous deoxycytidine triphosphate pools by exposure to gemcitabine markedly increased the activity of ara-C.[175]

FLUOROPYRIMIDINES

5-Fluorouracil (5-FU) is arguably the most useful antimetabolite in the treatment of solid tumors, but it is not used in the treatment of leukemia despite preclinical data suggesting that it is effective in this setting. The drug was developed after Heiedelberger and coworkers[176] reported increased utilization of uracil by rat hepatoma cells, and attempts to modify uracil such that it would be cytotoxic resulted in a 5-fluoro–substituted compound (see Fig. 17–6).

5-FU enters cells by a facilitated uracil transport system, but like other antimetabolites, it then requires metabolic activation to exert its effects.[177] The addition of a ribose sugar results in activation down the ribose pathway to fluorouridine triphosphate. Incorporation of fluorouridine triphosphate into RNA inhibits the processing of nuclear RNA to lower molecular weight ribosomal RNA; inhibits polyadenylation of mRNA, thereby decreasing stability; and results in the production of altered proteins, suggesting translational miscoding. The nature of the RNA damage is dependent on the cell type. A number of studies have reported that these effects on RNA can be blocked by the co-administration of uridine but not thymidine, confirming that the ribose nucleotide pathway is implicated.

Activation down the deoxyribose pathway to 5-fluoro-$2'$-deoxyuridine-$5'$-monophosphate interferes with the normal function of a key enzyme, thymidylate synthase.[177] This is the only de novo mechanism for the production of deoxythymidine (deoxythymidine monophosphate) from deoxyuridine, an important step in the synthesis of deoxythymidine triphosphate (dTTP) for incorporation into DNA. This not only starves the cell of dTTP but also increases cellular levels of deoxyuridine monophosphate, which can be converted to deoxyuridine triphosphate (dUTP). Inhibition of thymidylate synthase by 5-FU can be enhanced by the co-administration of a reduced folate (a cofactor in the conversion of dUTP to dTTP), and N^5-formyl tetrahydrofolate (folinic acid, leucovorin) is now commonly used with 5-FU.[178]

5-Fluoro-$2'$-deoxyuridine-$5'$-triphosphate and dUTP that accumulate because of thymidylate synthase inhibition can be fraudulently incorporated into DNA in the absence of dTTP, resulting in inhibited DNA synthesis, altered stability, induction of DNA strand breaks, and altered DNA repair. In general, the DNA-directed effects of 5-FU can be blocked by the co-administration of thymidine.

The oral bioavailability of 5-FU is poor (25%) and saturable. Both of these are related to the main metabolic deactivator of 5-FU, dihydropyrimidine dehydrogenase, which is present in the gastrointestinal mucosa and liver. Around 80% to 90% of an intravenous dose is deactivated by dihydropyrimidine dehydrogenase.

There is no consensus on the optimal schedule of administration of 5-FU. Consequently, commonly used schedules include weekly bolus, five daily boluses repeated every 3 weeks, 5-day infusions, and continuous infusions. The toxicity profile is highly dependent on the schedule of administration and has prompted the description of 5-FU as two different drugs when it is administered as a bolus or an infusion.[179] Typically, the activity of bolus 5-FU is mediated mainly by RNA-directed effects, whereas more prolonged dosing acts mainly by DNA effects. Consequently, myelosuppression is more common with bolus dosing, whereas mucositis, diarrhea, and hand-foot syndrome are more common with infusions. Thymidylate synthase is increased during the S phase of the cell cycle, and the DNA effects of 5-FU are therefore schedule dependent.

Resistance to 5-FU can be mediated by changes in activity in metabolizing or activating enzymes. In clinical studies, resistance has most clearly been associated with increases in thymidylate synthase protein, often by gene amplification.[180]

Purine Antagonists

6-THIOPURINES

6-Thioguanine (6-TG) and 6-mercaptopurine (6-MP) are analogues of the endogenous purines hypoxanthine and guanine (Fig. 17–8). As such, they are the purine counterparts to 5-fluorouracil in that they are activated intracellularly, inhibit the synthesis of other purine nucleotides, and can be converted to nucleotides that are incorporated into RNA and DNA. A third purine antagonist, azathioprine, is rapidly converted to 6-MP in vivo.

6-MP and 6-TG are activated to the nucleosides thioinosine monophosphate and thioguanine monophosphate, respectively, by hypoxanthine phosphoribosyltransferase[181] (see Fig. 17–8). These species can inhibit the synthesis of the purine nucleotides adenine monophosphate and guanine monophosphate by their action on the key enzymes glutamate phosphoribosylpyrophosphate aminotransferase and inosine monophosphate dehydrogenase. The inhibition of purine synthesis leads to an increase in cellular levels of phosphoribosylpyrophosphate, the sugar-donating group in the conversion of

bases to nucleosides, and this increases the conversion of 6-MP and 6-TG to their respective nucleosides.

In addition, 6-MP and 6-TG can be converted to thioguanine and thiodeoxyguanosine triphosphate (thiodGTP), which can be incorporated into RNA and DNA, respectively. The relative contribution of each of these pathways is unclear, but the incorporation of 6-MP nucleotides into DNA is five times higher than incorporation into RNA.[182] Thio-dGTP is used by DNA almost as efficiently as deoxyguanosine triphosphate, and there is no specific mechanism for removing thio-dGTP from DNA. However, once it is incorporated into DNA, thio-dGTP interferes with the ability of DNA to act as a template for DNA-interacting proteins, including polymerases, ligases, and some endonucleases.[183] This is consistent with reports of the delayed appearance of DNA damage and cytotoxicity after exposure to 6-MP or 6-TG. Thio-dGTP also markedly inhibits ribonuclease H, an enzyme involved in the cleavage of RNA from RNA-DNA duplexes after gene transcription.[184]

6-MP and 6-TG are typically administered orally, although the oral bioavailability is only around 15% and 25%, respectively, and is variable.[181] This variability may have an impact on drug activity because low plasma drug concentrations are associated with an increased risk of relapse in children with ALL.[185] Low intracellular thioguanine nucleotide concentration also correlates with reduced drug activity.[186] A component of this apparently poor, erratic bioavailability may actually be attributable to poor compliance with treatment involving oral therapy for a prolonged period.[187]

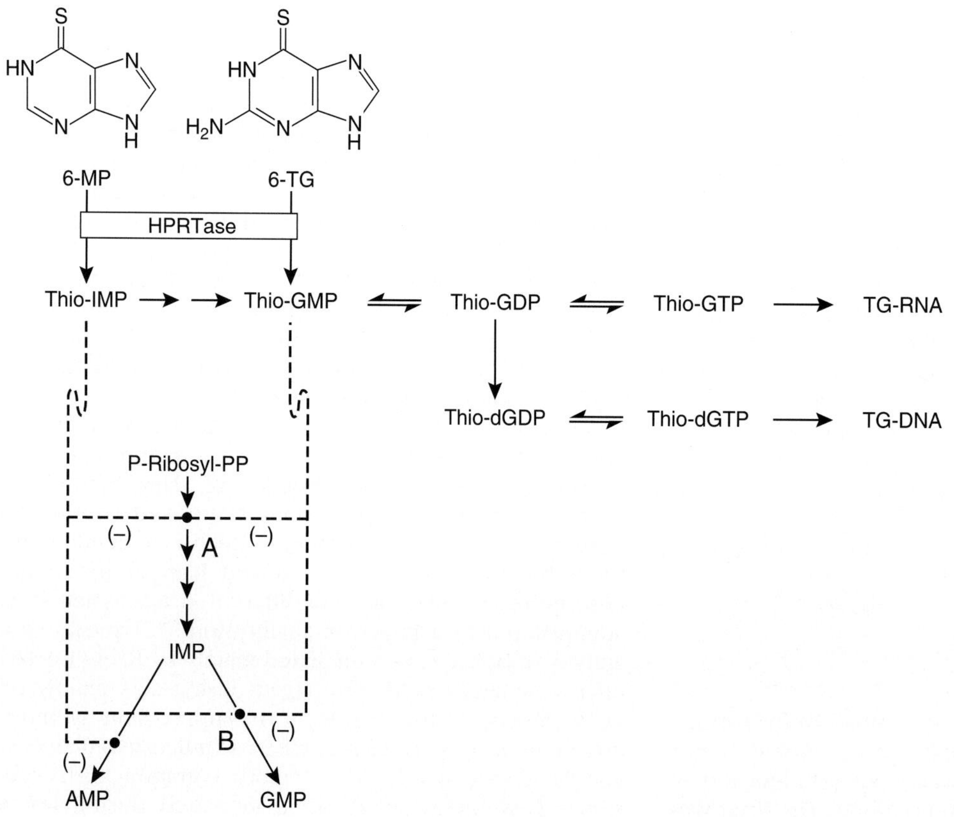

FIGURE 17–8. Structures of thioguanine (6-TG) and mercaptopurine (6-MP), showing anabolism to thio metabolites, that are incorporated into DNA and RNA, and the inhibition of PRPP aminotransferase (A), a key enzyme in the de novo purine synthesis pathway, and IMP dehydrogenase (B), involved in synthesis of guanine nucleotides. (From Pratt WB, Ruddon RW, Ensminger WD, et al: The Anticancer Drugs, 2nd ed. Oxford: Oxford University Press; 1994, p. 88.)

Clearance of 6-MP and 6-TG is mainly by catabolic metabolism. 6-MP can be inactivated by xanthine oxidase to 6-thioxanthine and 6-thiouric acid; 6-TG is inactivated by guanase to 6-thioinosine. In the case of 6-MP, xanthine oxidase is partially inhibited by allopurinol, often administered with 6-MP to prevent hyperuricemia.[188] A 6-MP dose reduction is appropriate when it is administered with allopurinol.[181] Because metabolism of 6-TG is not by xanthine oxidase, this interaction is not relevant with 6-TG.

Both 6-MP and 6-TG can be methylated by the enzyme thiopurine methyltransferase (TPMT), and these metabolites are much less active than the parent compound. TPMT activity is determined by the presence of high- or low-activity TPMT genes. Consequently, a trimodal distribution in TPMT activity is seen. Around 1 in 300 patients has low TPMT activity attributable to two low-activity alleles, 11% have intermediate activity (one high-activity and one low-activity allele), and the remainder have high activity. Patients with high TPMT activity may be at greater risk of relapse because of the increased thiopurine metabolism, which results in lower intracellular concentrations of activated thiopurine triphosphates. Conversely, those with low activity are at risk for excessive toxicity.[189, 190] Activity may also vary between racial groups.

There are currently no data to suggest which of these drugs is more useful in the maintenance phase of treatment of ALL. 6-MP has been used routinely as part of maintenance therapy for ALL in children and adults for more than 30 years (see Chapters 26 and 27). The drug is relatively devoid of toxicity, and as previously mentioned, there may be noncompliance with a treatment that continues for 2 to 3 years. 6-TG was much used as part of the DAT or TAD regimens given after anthracycline and ara-C as remission induction therapy for AML (see Chapters 21 and 22). However, no advantage was ever demonstrated in comparison with an anthracycline and ara-C alone. 6-TG is of historic interest because it was one of the first drugs to be used successfully in treatment of AML, but it is no longer widely used in this setting. It is currently being compared with 6-MP in a United Kingdom childhood ALL study.

Because of the poor and variable bioavailability and the demonstration that 6-MP activity is related to systemic exposure, reports have described high-dose and infusional 6-MP.[191, 192]

Nucleoside Purine Analogues

FLUDARABINE

In the 1960s, a series of nucleoside purine analogues was investigated for cytotoxic drug activity,[193] of which adenine arabinoside was the most potent but subject to metabolic deactivation. Modification of the purine structure by the addition of a fluorine at the 2 position made the molecule less susceptible to deamination,[194] and the monophosphate of this compound (F-ara-adenosine monophosphate, fludarabine) was much more water soluble (Fig. 17–9).

After intravenous administration, fludarabine is rapidly

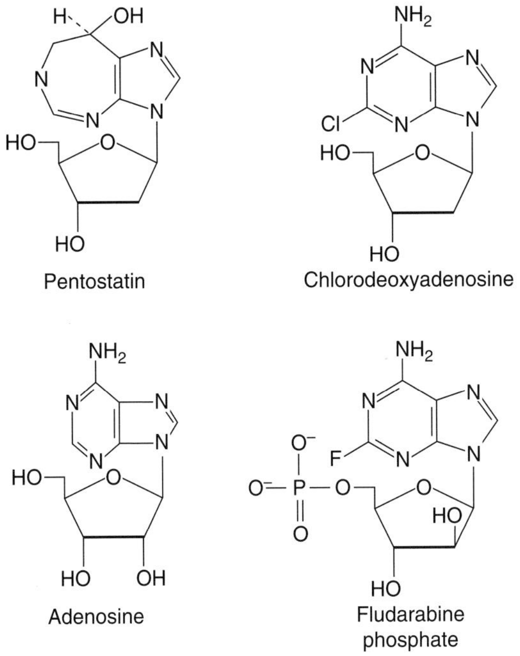

FIGURE 17–9. Structures of purine antagonists.

dephosphorylated systemically, and the nucleoside then enters cells through the nucleoside transport system. The compound is then phosphorylated, initially by deoxycytidine kinase, to the triphosphate that can be incorporated into both RNA and DNA.[181] In both RNA and DNA, incorporation of F-ara-ATP causes inhibition of polymerases and termination of chain elongation.[195, 196] In RNA, this premature termination of transcription affects protein synthesis.[197] F-ara-ADP also inhibits DNA polymerase, DNA primase, and ribonucleotide reductase, the last resulting in depletion of the endogenous adenine nucleotide that would compete for incorporation into DNA.[198] As with other antimetabolites, it is not clear which of the mechanisms described is more important for cytotoxicity. However, inhibition of DNA synthesis occurs at lower concentrations than those required for inhibition of RNA synthesis, suggesting that DNA may be the major target mediating the drug's cytotoxicity.[199] Fludarabine also has some activity in nonreplicating cells, probably in association with its RNA-mediated cytotoxicity.

Fludarabine also influences the activity of ara-C by two separate mechanisms. F-ara-ADP inhibits ribonucleotide reductase, thereby decreasing competition from the endogenous deoxynucleotide diphosphate, and F-ara-ATP stimulates the activity of deoxycytidine kinase, resulting in the increased activation of ara-C to the active ara-CTP. Consequently, fludarabine has been used in combination with ara-C.[200]

Fludarabine is typically administered intravenously over 5 days. An oral formulation has been developed with a bioavailability of 55% and with low intraindividual variability.[201]

Fludarabine is rapidly and completely dephosphorylated to fluoro-ara-A, which has an elimination half-life of around 9 hours. Although renal excretion (as F-ara-A) accounts for only 24% of an administered dose, there is a relationship between renal function and F-ara-A clearance[202] and between F-ara-A clearance and myelosuppression.[203] The influence of renal function on toxicity may in part be mediated by 2-fluoroadenine, a toxic metabolite produced by bacteria in the gut from fludarabine excreted in the bile and subsequently reabsorbed.

Fludarabine is almost totally devoid of the clinical toxicities usually associated with cytotoxic chemotherapy for leukemia. It is not associated with alopecia, nausea, or vomiting, and it can be administered entirely on an outpatient basis. It does, however, cause profound myelosuppression and is also associated with a specific T-cell dysfunction that results in an increased risk for opportunistic infection, particularly with organisms such as *Pneumocystis carinii* and *Listeria monocytogenes*, the latter presenting as septicemia, meningitis, or both. The prognosis in this situation is grave. Prophylaxis against *P. carinii* pneumonia should always be given.

Fludarabine has been used successfully with high-dose ara-C for treatment of AML. Relatively high response rates are seen in patients with AML developing on a background of myelodysplasia.

Fludarabine has most recently been used in combination with cyclophosphamide or melphalan as part of a nonmyeloablative conditioning regimen for allogeneic stem cell transplantation. The concept is based on trying to reduce the morbidity and mortality of the allogeneic transplantation procedure by reducing the toxicity of the myeloablative regimen. The T-cell effect of fludarabine can be taken advantage of to allow engraftment of donor hematopoietic progenitor cells, in most cases more slowly than with conventional myeloablative regimens. Thus, a chimeric state is achieved, allowing a graft-versus-malignancy effect to develop without the toxicity of a conventional myeloablative regimen.

This approach is being evaluated in patients with chronic myelogenous leukemia (CML) in particular and to a lesser extent in AML, typically in patients in whom a conventional allograft is considered too dangerous. Most centers are using a fludarabine-containing regimen, either with an alkylating agent and low-dose total-body irradiation or with busulfan and antithymocyte globulin.

CHLORODEOXYADENOSINE

Like fludarabine, 2-chlorodeoxyadenosine (2-CdA, cladribine) is also resistant to deamination by adenosine deaminase.[181] However, unlike fludarabine, 2-CdA contains the normal ribose sugar rather than arabinose (see Fig. 17-9). 2-CdA is rapidly phosphorylated to 2-CdA 5′-triphosphate (2-CdATP), which is incorporated into DNA, resulting in inhibition of DNA synthesis.[204, 205] 2-CdATP also inhibits ribonucleotide reductase, thereby starving cells of endogenous deoxyribonucleotides.

The use of 2-CdA is almost entirely confined to the treatment of hairy cell leukemia, for which it is now the treatment of choice. The drug is usually given by continuous intravenous infusion, although it may be given subcutaneously. It is profoundly myelosuppressive, but complete responses can usually be achieved with just one cycle of treatment.

PENTOSTATIN (DEOXYCOFORMYCIN)

Deoxycoformycin (DCF) is an adenosine analogue that inhibits adenosine deaminase, resulting in the accumulation of deoxyadenosine nucleotides and ultimately causing a lethal imbalance in nucleotide pools (see Fig. 17-9). It was originally developed for use in T-cell malignant neoplasms, but like 2-Cda, its use is now restricted almost exclusively to the treatment of hairy cell leukemia, which is almost always a B-cell disease. Indeed, it has now been largely superseded by 2-CdA (see preceding). DCF is extremely effective and can be used on more of an outpatient basis than 2-CdA can, being less myelosuppressive but requiring longer for remission to be achieved.

Hydroxyurea

Throughout the description of the pharmacology of the antimetabolites, an enzyme that appears frequently is ribonucleotide reductase. This enzyme catalyzes the conversion of ribonucleotide diphosphates to deoxyribonucleotide diphosphates, which as the subsequent triphosphate are required for DNA synthesis and repair.[206, 207]

The importance of ribonucleotide reductase lies in its involvement in the de novo synthesis of all four deoxyribonucleotides. The enzyme comprises two protein subunits, the first of which (M1) contains two binding sites, one for the nucleotide substrate and a second for a deoxyribonucleotide triphosphate, particularly dATP, which can regulate enzyme activity (a number of antimetabolites inhibit ribonucleotide reductase through this site when activated to the triphosphate form). This subunit is present at a similar level throughout the cell cycle. The second subunit (M2) contains two sites critical for activity, a free radical group located on a tyrosine residue and a neighboring nonheme iron complex that stabilizes the free radical. The concentration of this M2 subunit increases markedly during the S phase of the cell cycle.

Hydroxyurea (structure $H_2N-CO-NHOH$) inhibits ribonucleotide reductase by destabilizing the iron complex, resulting in the deactivation of the catalytic subunit,[208] thereby starving cells of deoxyribonucleotides, an effect that correlates well with decreased DNA synthesis.[209] Because this enzyme provides deoxyribonucleotides that would compete with the phosphorylated form of a number of antimetabolites, hydroxyurea is often used in combination with these drugs, most notably 5-fluorouracil,[177] to block this rescue pathway and increase drug activity.

A number of enzymes involved in the synthesis of DNA precursors, including ribonucleotide reductase, exist in a coordinated complex called a replitase complex.[210] Inhibition of one of the enzymes of this complex can result in the inhibition of other members. Inhibition of ribonucleotide reductase by hydroxyurea therefore results in the inhibition, or decreased activity, of DNA polymerase, thymidylate synthase, and thymidine kinase.[211]

The most common mechanism of resistance to hydroxyurea is increased ribonucleotide reductase activity, particularly by increased amounts of the M2 protein subunit.[212] This can be due to amplification of the gene encoding the protein or to increased translation of the protein from a normal gene copy number.

Hydroxyurea is typically administered orally, and bioavailability with oral dosing is between 80% and 100%.[206] Although hydroxyurea is known to undergo enzymatic degradation in animals, there are few data describing its metabolism in humans. Similarly, renal excretion appears to be important in plasma clearance of hydroxyurea, but this is also poorly understood. The major toxicity is myelosuppression.[206] Other side effects include nausea, vomiting, mucositis, and diarrhea, and dermatologic effects are seen in patients with prolonged dosing.

For many years, hydroxyurea was the treatment of choice for CML, having superseded busulfan because of the relative ease with which the blood count could be controlled and the less obvious leukemogenic potential of hydroxyurea. Hydroxyurea is not associated with the profound and prolonged myelosuppression that can sometimes result from the use of busulfan. Furthermore, in a randomized comparison with busulfan, hydroxyurea was shown to prolong the survival of patients with CML.[213] With the introduction of interferon, hydroxyurea now tends to be used only as initial therapy (i.e., to be followed by interferon). It is also used in essential thrombocythemia but has been shown in this context to be associated (in a small percentage of patients) with the development of secondary AML.[214, 215]

Hydroxyurea can be extremely useful for palliative treatment of patients with AML in whom the blast cell count is high. It is possible in this context, when the aim is to keep the person as well as possible for as long as possible with blood and platelet support, to use the drug in an outpatient setting. It is also used at presentation when there are clinical symptoms and signs of leukostasis, although leukapheresis is still probably the quickest and most efficient way of treating this (see Chapter 13).

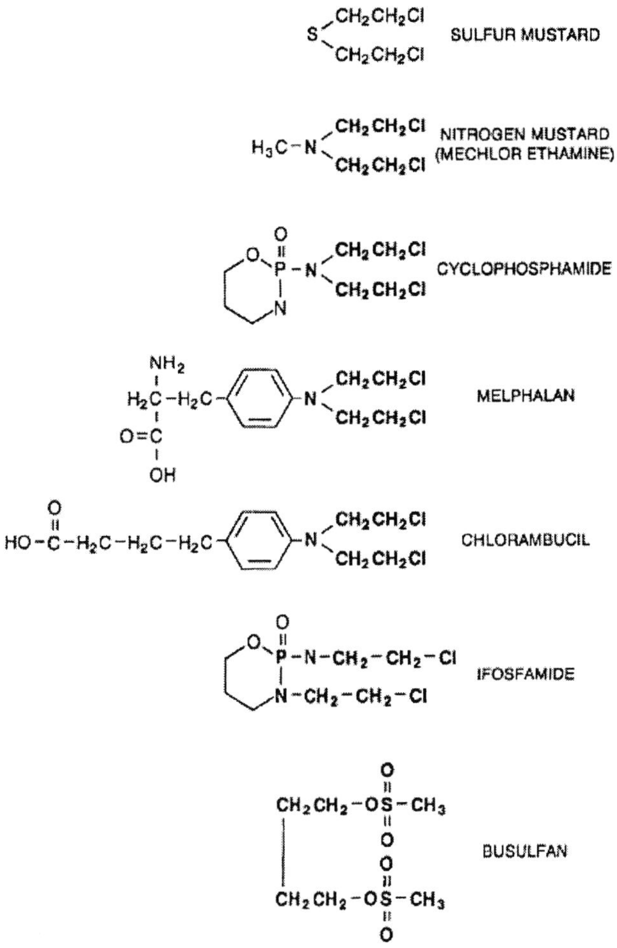

DNA-Binding Drugs

This section outlines the pharmacology of drugs that induce DNA damage by covalent bonding of reactive drug intermediates to DNA. These include the alkylating agents and platinum compounds. Drugs that exert some of their cytotoxic activity by intercalating with DNA, such as the anthracyclines, are described elsewhere.

Alkylating Agents

The alkylating agents are directly descended from the sulfur mustard gas used in the trenches during the First World War. In a review of the effects of exposure to this gas, it was noted that the acute effects to the skin, eyes, and respiratory tract were accompanied by delayed effects including myelosuppression, lymphoid aplasia, and ulceration of gastrointestinal mucosa.[2] (Similar toxicities were apparent in allied personnel exposed to mustard gas after accidental release during the Second World War.) This agent was shown to have antitumor activity but profound toxicity.[216] The related nitrogen mustard, although less reactive, also showed activity in animal models but with less toxicity, and it showed impressive activity in patients with lymphomas in subsequent clinical trials.[1]

FIGURE 17–10. Structures of alkylating agents.

The common feature of alkylating agents is the activation of the alkyl side chain (Fig. 17-10) at neutral or alkaline pH, with the loss of the chloride ions (termed leaving groups) and cyclization of the alkyl chain to the highly reactive aziridine ring ($-N-CH_2CH_2-$)$^+$ (Fig. 17-11).[217] This positively charged aziridine intermediate can react with nucleophilic molecules such as nitrogen, sulfur, and oxygen present in proteins, RNA, and DNA. However, it is the interaction with DNA that mediates the cytotoxic activity of these agents, and sites particularly susceptible to alkylation are the N^7 and O^6 positions of guanine.[217-219] Other adducts include those formed at the N^1 position of guanine; at the N^7, N^3, and N^1 positions of adenine; at the N^3 position of cytosine; and at the O^4 position of thymidine. The base preference for alkylation differs between drugs of this type. Many alkylating agents, particularly those related to nitrogen mustard, have two alkyl side chains, such that two alkylation reactions can occur, each with a different base. Alkylating agents are thus frequently referred to as monofunctional or bifunctional, depending on the presence of one or two alkyl side chains.

This alkylation of bases by monofunctional agents has a number of effects.[217] First, the alkylation of the base can result in a change in conformation such that it forms base pairs with the incorrect partner. For instance, alkyl-

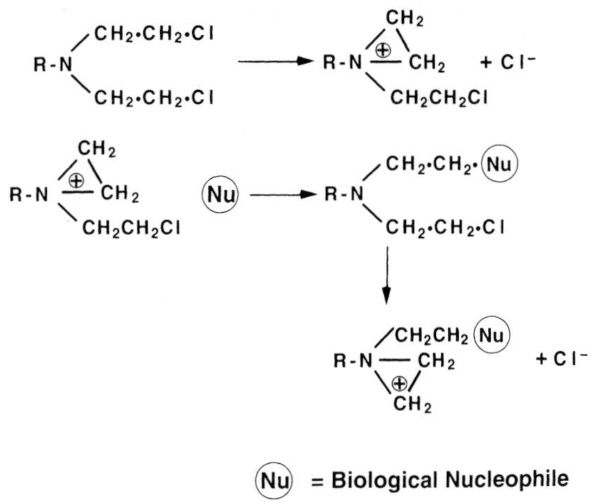

Nu = Biological Nucleophile

FIGURE 17–11. Activation of an alkylating agent by loss of the chloride ions. Reaction of the resulting aziridine ring structure with a biologic nucleophile allows the formation of a second aziridine ring and a second alkylation to take place.

ation of guanine leads to the formation of base pairs with thymidine instead of its normal partner cytidine. With subsequent DNA synthesis or repair of the alkylated adduct, this can result in translational miscoding, with substitution of a GC base pair by an AT. Alkylation can also result in opening up of the imidazole ring structure of purines, leading to DNA strand breaks due to weakening of the sugar-phosphate backbone.

In addition to these effects, bifunctional agents can alkylate two different bases, but linked by the alkylating agent. This results in the formation of interstrand cross-links between the two DNA strands or intrastrand links within the same DNA strand. The importance of these cross-links in cytotoxicity is demonstrated by the markedly increased activity of bifunctional agents compared with monofunctional agents.[220, 221] The formation of these interstrand cross-links is a particularly important mechanism of cytotoxicity, resulting in inhibition of the DNA template with an effective block in DNA synthesis. Increased understanding of the nature of the alkylation reactions with this group of compounds suggests that the interstrand cross-linking of bifunctional agents correlates with cytotoxicity, whereas a broader range of toxic events is seen with monofunctional compounds.[217]

Because these compounds bind directly to DNA, cytotoxic activity is not dependent on exposure during a particular phase of the cell cycle, that is, they are cell cycle phase nonspecific. However, their cytotoxic effect becomes apparent when the cell attempts to replicate DNA during the S phase of the cell cycle, when the presence of alkylated bases interferes with DNA synthesis. Nonproliferating cells are thus less susceptible to the activity of alkylating agents. This group of drugs is therefore described as proliferation dependent, cell cycle phase nonspecific.

General mechanisms of resistance to these agents include drug deactivation by conjugation with glutathione and increased repair of alkylated bases by a number of specific repair systems previously described.[222, 223]

NITROGEN MUSTARDS

The structure of these agents is shown in Figure 17–10. In general, the chemical activity of this group of drugs is related to the nature of the nonalkyl group because this influences the reactivity of the alkyl side chains in solution. For instance, mechlorethamine, the original nitrogen mustard, must be administered intravenously; with melphalan and chlorambucil, the presence of groups other than CH_3 slows the rate of conversion to the immonium ion sufficiently that the drug can be administered orally. Several of the nitrogen mustards were developed on the basis of differences in the activity of specific activating enzymes in tumor and normal tissue. For example, the addition of an amino acid group in melphalan (L-phenylalanine mustard) was intended to produce a compound taken up more selectively by tumor cells because of their increased proliferation and requirement for amino acids.

Chlorambucil is the phenylbutyric acid derivative of nitrogen mustard, which gives the molecule much greater stability than nitrogen mustard itself in aqueous solution. This increase in stability means that the drug can be administered orally, with a bioavailability of at least 70%.[224] The half-life of chlorambucil in plasma is only 1 to 2 hours,[225] with metabolic conversion of the phenylbutyric acid ring to phenylacetic acid mustard. Although this retains alkylating activity, it is also more toxic than the parent compound. Because chlorambucil is often administered with a steroid in the treatment of chronic lymphocytic leukemia, conjugates of the two types of compound were developed in the hope that the steroid moiety may help to localize chlorambucil to tumor tissue.[226]

Chlorambucil has been the mainstay for treatment of chronic lymphocytic leukemia for more than 30 years, at least in Europe. To a certain extent, it has been replaced by fludarabine because "complete" remission can be achieved in some patients with fludarabine. Nonetheless, many patients are still treated successfully with chlorambucil, the advantages being ease of administration because it is given orally and relative lack of toxicity. Occasional patients will have an allergic rash, in which case cyclophosphamide can be substituted. Various doses and schedules are in use for chlorambucil given alone; in some centers, it is combined with prednisolone (see Chapter 28).

The main nitrogen mustards in use clinically are cyclophosphamide and ifosfamide.[227, 228] Both are inactive as the parent compound and require metabolic activation for activity. Cyclophosphamide was also developed on the basis of targeting alkylating agent activity because tumors were reported to have increased activity of the enzyme phosphoamidase. However, the compound is actually activated in the liver, and its activation does not involve phosphoamidase but cytochrome P450 2B6, which converts the parent compound to 4-hydroxycyclophosphamide.[229] As with chlorambucil, the decreased reactivity in aqueous solution means that cyclophosphamide can be administered orally, with a bioavailability of 70% to 90%,[228] although it is more commonly given intravenously.

4-Hydroxycyclophosphamide undergoes spontaneous

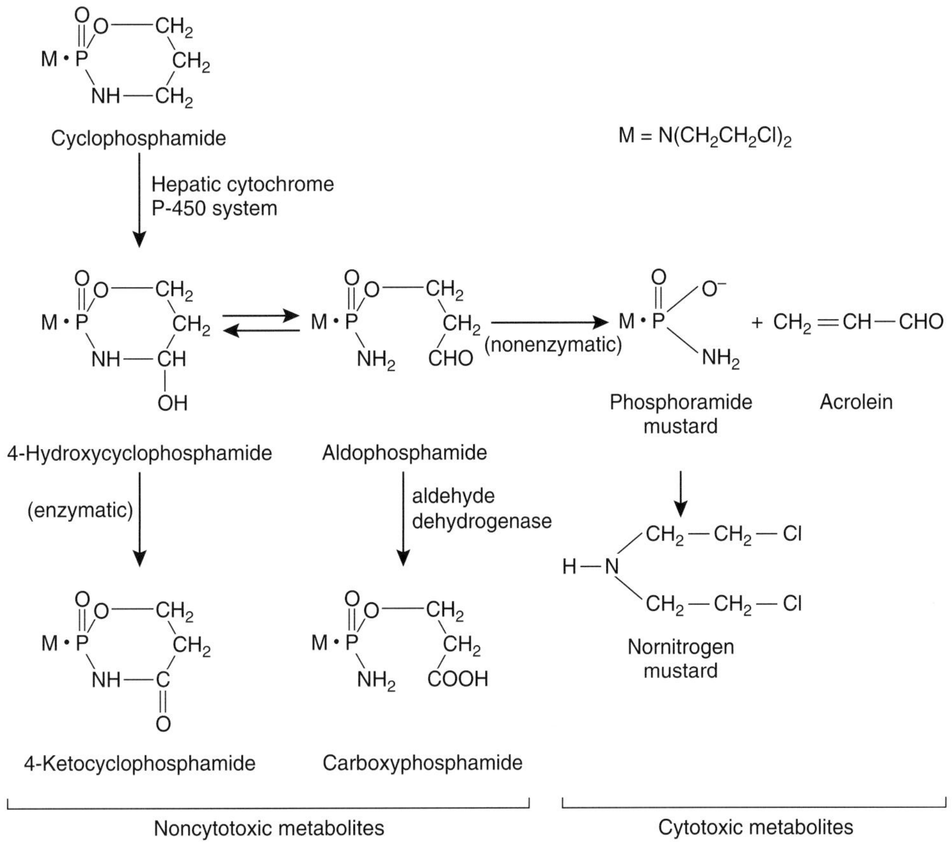

FIGURE 17–12. Activation and metabolism of cyclophosphamide. (From Pratt WB, Ruddon RW, Ensminger WD, et al: The Anticancer Drugs, 2nd ed. Oxford: Oxford University Press; 1994, p. 117.)

ring opening and exists in equilibrium with aldophospha-mide (Fig. 17-12). Both of these ring-opened and ring-closed metabolites can be inactivated by specific en-zymes, and around 80% of a dose of cyclophosphamide is recovered in the urine as 4-ketocyclophosphamide and carboxyphosphamide.[230] Aldophosphamide is taken up by tumor cells and is then converted to the active alkylat-ing species phosphoramide mustard by the elimination of acrolein.[229, 231] Although hydroxycyclophosphamide and aldophosphamide retain alkylating activity, these species are unable to alkylate directly and require conversion to the phosphoramide mustard for activity. Thus, the cytotoxic activity of cyclophosphamide is due to its con-version to phosphoramide mustard. Acrolein is excreted in the urine and is responsible for the bladder toxicity seen with cyclophosphamide.[232]

The rate-limiting step in the activation of cyclophos-phamide to phosphoramide mustard appears to be the activity of CYP2B6 because the plasma half-life of cyclo-phosphamide is 6 to 8 hours, whereas that of 4-hydroxy-cyclophosphamide is only a few minutes. CYP2B6 can be induced by cyclophosphamide (and certain other drugs that may be co-administered), whereas the rate of aldo-phosphamide deactivation can be decreased by the inhi-bition of aldehyde dehydrogenase 1 by acrolein.[233, 234] Both of these mechanisms serve to increase the AUC of hydroxycyclophosphamide with multiple doses of cyclo-phosphamide. The metabolism of cyclophosphamide is not altered at high doses of drug.

Cyclophosphamide, as the intravenous preparation, is used for ALL in both adults and children (see Chapters

26 and 27) and for chronic lymphocytic leukemia in combinations such as CAP (cyclophosphamide, doxorubi-cin, and prednisolone)[235] and, on occasion, CVP (cyclo-phosphamide, vincristine, and prednisolone).

Because it requires metabolic activation, cyclophospha-mide is not useful for purging bone marrow in vitro before reinfusion to remove morphologically undetect-able leukemic blast cells. 4-Hydroperoxycyclophospha-mide (a more stable form of 4-hydroxycyclophospha-mide) and mafosfamide (ASTA-Z), which do not require activation in the liver, are used for this purpose.

Ifosfamide is a bifunctional alkylating agent with one of the alkylating groups attached to a nitrogen in the oxazophosphorine ring structure, instead of both being linked to the same nitrogen as in cyclophosphamide (see Fig. 17-10). This change results in differences in the drug's pharmacology. Although ifosfamide is also acti-vated mainly by hepatic metabolism, the enzyme involved is the CYP3A4 isoform[236] rather than CYP2B6 with cyclo-phosphamide, and this activation pathway is saturable at clinically relevant doses. In addition, deactivation by loss of the chloroethyl side chains is much greater with ifos-famide, with the resultant urinary metabolites accounting for 50% of dose compared with only 10% with cyclophos-phamide.[228] These two factors contribute to a relative decrease in the amounts of activated species after ifosfam-ide such that the doses typically used are three to four times higher than with cyclophosphamide.[228, 237] When they are administered in this dose ratio, the toxicity profiles of the two drugs are similar, with the exception of cystitis, which occurs more frequently after ifosfamide, most likely because of increased urinary acrolein. Ifosfamide is therefore typically administered with mesna (mercaptoethane sulfonate), which is excreted in the urine and forms an acrolein-mesna conjugate.[238] Ifosfamide also enters the cerebrospinal fluid more readily than does cyclophosphamide,[239] which accounts for its increased neurotoxicity.

Busulfan differs from other alkylating agents in that the leaving groups are methane sulfonates rather than chlorides[227] (see Fig. 17-10). The loss of each of these groups activates the adjacent carbon, which then alkylates biologic molecules. Busulfan mainly targets the N^7 position of guanine in DNA[240] but also reacts with the thiol groups of amino acids and proteins more readily than do other alkylating agents. Thus, the cytotoxic activity of busulfan may be mediated by these interactions in addition to, or instead of, DNA damage. Perhaps related to this difference in mechanism, busulfan is more active in myeloid than in lymphoid cells.[241]

Busulfan used to be the standard treatment for chronic myeloid leukemia. However, with the development of hydroxyurea and more recently of interferon, and in view of the risks of protracted myelosuppression with this drug, it is now rarely used (see Chapter 25). Busulfan is, however, still extensively used (as the oral or intravenous preparation) in conjunction with gram doses of cyclophosphamide as a myeloablative conditioning regimen before allogeneic bone marrow transplantation. This has been shown to be equivalent in efficacy to total-body irradiation–containing myeloablative regimens for other hematologic malignant neoplasms (see Chapter 20). Veno-occlusive disease of the liver is perhaps more likely to occur than with total-body irradiation–containing regimens, and some centers recommend the routine prophylactic use of heparin (see Chapter 20).

NITROSOUREAS

In the 1950s, a series of novel compounds related to methylnitrosoguanidine and methylnitrosourea were shown to have antitumor activity in animal models. Activity was further improved by the modification of the methylnitrosourea structure with the addition of a chloroethyl group, resulting in a series of compounds that are used clinically: bischloroethylnitrosourea (BCNU, carmustine), cyclohexylchloroethylnitrosourea (CCNU, lomustine), and methyl CCNU (semustine).[242] These compounds are relatively lipophilic and were shown to be active against intracerebral L1210 leukemia in mice.[243] A newer member of this group of agents, streptozocin, is a methylnitrosourea isolated from *Streptomyces achromogenes*.

The nitrosoureas are unstable and decompose to two moieties, the isocyanate, which is a carbamoylating agent, and a chloroethyl diazonium or carbamonium ion, depending on the pH, each of which can act as an alkylating agent.[217] This chloroethyl group alkylates particularly at the O^6 position of guanine. With subsequent loss of the chloride ion, the reactive intermediate O^6-ethanoguanine is formed, which reacts with the nitrogen at the 3 position of cytosine to form DNA cross-links. Thus, even though these drugs possess only one alkylating group,

they act like bifunctional alkylating agents in that they form DNA intrastrand and interstrand cross-links.[221]

The isocyanate formed by the decomposition of nitrosourea is able to carbamoylate proteins, resulting in certain types of cellular damage.[244] This mechanism does not correlate well with cytotoxicity but may be related to some of the toxicities of the nitrosoureas.

The importance of alkylation at the O^6 position of guanine has been further emphasized with the identification of a specific repair enzyme, O^6-alkylguanine transferase, which can remove these alkyl adducts.[245] A number of reports describe increased activity of nitrosoureas in cells with low activity of this repair system.[246] Consequently, agents that can inhibit this enzyme, such as O^6-benzylguanine, are currently under clinical investigation as adjuncts to nitrosoureas.[247]

The lipophilicity of these agents means that they are often used for treatment of primary or metastatic brain tumors.

Platinum Compounds

This important group of compounds were discovered in the mid-1960s entirely serendipitously. Rosenberg and colleagues[248] were investigating the effect of electric current on the growth of bacteria and noticed that growth became filamentous with a block in cell division. These changes were similar to those seen after exposure to ionizing radiation or alkylating agents, and the effect was soon attributed to platinum released by electrolysis from the platinum electrode. This reacted with ammonium chloride in the media, in the presence of light, to produce an active platinum complex. Subsequent synthesis of this compound found that *cis*-diamminedichloroplatinum(II) was active in the bacterial system, but the isomer *trans*-diamminedichloroplatinum(II) was not.[249] The cisplatin complex was soon shown to exhibit marked antitumor activity in preclinical systems related to the formation of platinum-DNA (Fig. 17-13).

To interact with DNA, cisplatin must undergo aquation reactions in which the chloride ions are replaced by water to produce a hydrated intermediate[250] (see Fig. 17-13). This reaction is almost entirely dependent on the chloride environment. Cisplatin is relatively stable at chloride concentrations above 100 mM, such as saline for infusion or circulating plasma; but in lower chloride environments, such as intracellularly, aquation takes place. These aquated species can then react with nucleophilic groups in DNA, RNA, and proteins to form platinum adducts, although it is the formation of DNA adducts that best correlates with cytotoxicity, with binding preferentially to the N^7 position of guanine and adenine.[251, 252] An important component of this cytotoxicity is the presence of two leaving groups, such that platinum drugs can bind to two separate bases, resulting in the formation of intrastrand and interstrand cross-links.[251] These cross-links are crucial for activity because monofunctional platinum compounds have little cytotoxic activity.[253] Around 60% of the DNA intrastrand lesions are cross-links between adjacent guanines, 20% are cross-links between adenine and guanine, and 10% are cross-links between two guanines separated by another base.[250, 254] These intrastrand

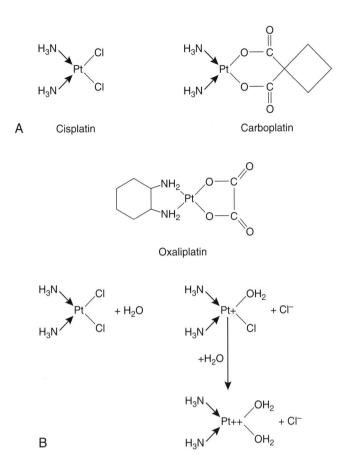

FIGURE 17–13. Structures of platinum compounds *(A)* and the aquation of cisplatin in low-chloride environments *(B).*

cross-links result in DNA distortion, leading to local kinking and separation of the two DNA strands, which inhibits key DNA enzymes and blocks DNA synthesis.

In addition to the formation of cross-links within the same DNA strand, DNA interstrand cross-links can arise, although these account for only 1% to 2% of the total DNA platination.[252] Although cisplatin cytotoxicity correlates well with the formation of intrastrand cross-links,[255] the possible contribution of interstrand cross-links to cytotoxicity is unclear. Transplatin has virtually no cytotoxic activity in mammalian cells and produces almost no interstrand cross-links (although the intrastrand links are also different from those formed by cisplatin).

A major toxicity with cisplatin is nephrotoxicity, which may be apparent as an acute or chronic effect.[250] The acute effect, due to platinum activation in the renal tubules, is manifest as a reduction in glomerular filtration, loss of magnesium, and possibly increases in serum urea and/or creatinine. Long-term renal toxicity is characterized by a reduction in creatinine clearance, often in the absence of an increase in serum creatinine. Although data are limited, cisplatin-DNA adducts are still detectable in renal tissue up to 9 months after dose, such that this chronic toxicity may be a result of long-term effects on DNA and proteins.[250]

Because of this nephrotoxicity, novel platinum compounds have been synthesized with more stable leaving

groups, resulting in reduced activity in renal tubules. The best of these compounds is carboplatin (diammine-1,1-cyclobutane-dicarboxyplatinum; see Fig. 17–13), which has a spectrum of activity broadly similar to that of cisplatin.[256] The bulkier leaving groups mean that aquation occurs more slowly than with cisplatin, and the drug takes longer to distribute into tissues such that a greater proportion of the dose is excreted in the urine in the first 24 hours. Consequently, carboplatin clearance correlates well with glomerular filtration rate, and a reliable estimate of glomerular filtration rate, for instance, by ^{51}Cr-labeled EDTA clearance, allows the dose of carboplatin to be optimized in individual patients to achieve a target AUC.[257]

Newer platinum analogues include those with a 1,2-diaminocyclohexane (DACH) ligand, particularly DACH-oxalatoplatinum (oxaliplatin; see Fig. 17–13). These compounds have a mechanism of cytotoxic activity similar to that of cisplatin but often a different spectrum of clinical activity and lack cross-resistance to cisplatin.[258, 259] This is possibly because the bulkier adducts formed by DACH-platinums are recognized by DNA repair systems different from those that detect cisplatin adducts. Consequently, failure to detect DNA adducts by decreased activity or mutation in a specific DNA repair protein may result in decreased activity with cisplatin but not necessarily with DACH platinums.[260]

The platinum compounds described are all administered intravenously, but some of the newer analogues (such as JM216) can be administered orally.[261]

Although data are limited, platinum compounds (mostly carboplatin) have been investigated in leukemias, particularly in AML. However, single-agent complete response rates are relatively low,[262] and it is unclear how much they actually contribute in a regimen such as carboplatin given with high-dose ara-C[263, 264] (see Chapter 21).

Microtubule-Acting Drugs

Microtubules form the spindle apparatus that plays a crucial role in the separation of the two sets of chromosomes during mitosis. In addition, microtubules form part of the cellular scaffold, are involved in cell movement and intracellular signaling, and are an important component of neural tissue.[265] Consequently, drugs that interact with microtubules can exert effects against both proliferating and nonproliferating cells. The assembly and disassembly of microtubules are complex, and to understand how drugs that interact with microtubules exert their effects, it is necessary to understand the normal process.

The major protein component of microtubules is tubulin, which contains two distinct 50-kd α and β subunits. These subunits combine to form heterodimers, which then assemble in a linear fashion to form protofilaments in which the α subunit of one heterodimer is associated with the β subunit of the next[266] (Fig. 17–14). Thirteen of these protofilaments, arranged in the same direction, then become aligned and close up to form a tubule, with further assembly of tubulin at one end (plus end) but little assembly or even disassembly at the other

Tubulin
heterodimer

Changes in the equilibrium between
tubulin and microtubules induced by
vinca alkaloids and taxanes

Formed microtubule
normally containing 13
protofilaments, (12 in the
presence of taxanes)

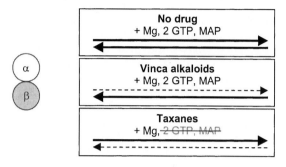

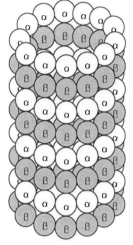

FIGURE 17–14. Schematic representation of the equilibrium between tubulin, a heterodimer of α and β subunits, and formed microtubules containing 13 protofilaments of linearly arranged tubulin dimers. Microtubules "grow" from an organizing center, such as the centrosome, with rapid changes in tubulin assembly at the free end and little change at the anchored end. Vinca alkaloids block the formation of microtubules; the taxanes promote the assembly of weakened microtubules, in the absence of GTP and microtubule-associated protein, containing only 12 protofilaments.

(minus end). Other factors required for tubulin assembly are magnesium ions and two molecules of guanosine triphosphate (GTP), one on each subunit. High calcium ion concentration inhibits the formation of microtubules. In addition, formed protofilaments, but not free tubulin, contain binding sites for microtubule-associated proteins that serve to connect protofilaments together, thus increasing rigidity, and that interact with other proteins.[267] Typically, the minus end of a microtubule is attached to an organizing center, the centrosome, which effectively prevents assembly or disassembly; further polymerization at the plus end of the microtubule is promoted by the presence of GTP.[268] The addition of a tubulin heterodimer into a microtubule results in the delayed hydrolysis of one of the GTP molecules to guanosine diphosphate (GDP); the second GTP molecule exchanges with GDP.[269] The addition of further tubulin heterodimers is promoted by the presence of GTP, which effectively lowers the critical concentration at which tubulin polymerizes. As the concentration of free tubulin decreases, further polymerization slows down, and once the end of the microtubule contains a GDP cap instead of GTP, equilibrium is shifted in favor of rapid disassembly of the microtubule. This dynamic equilibrium is an important mechanism by which the cell controls the different functions of microtubules.

Different classes of microtubule-acting drugs interfere with this process in different ways.[270] The vinca alkaloids inhibit the polymerization of tubulin and block microtubule formation. The taxanes shift the equilibrium in favor of microtubule formation.

Vinca Alkaloids

The vinca alkaloids are natural or semisynthetic compounds obtained from the periwinkle, *Catharanthus rosea* (formerly *Vinca rosea*), that have been used in folk remedies for many hundreds of years.[271] Members of this class of drugs include vincristine, vinblastine, and the more recent additions vindesine and vinorelbine. All of these molecules comprise two multiringed moieties, vindoline and catharanthine, joined by a carbon-carbon bridge[272] (Fig. 17–15).

Vincristine, vinblastine, and vindesine differ only in the vindoline ring structure, whereas vinorelbine has the same vindoline structure as vinblastine but differs in the catharanthine nucleus. Vinca alkaloids are rapidly taken up by cells, resulting in intracellular accumulation, although differences in retention between these drugs leads to differences in intracellular drug concentration.[272, 273] Once inside the cell, the vinca alkaloids can inhibit microtubule formation by binding to two distinct sites. Drug can bind to high-affinity sites at the end of formed microtubules, resulting in the inhibition of further microtubule assembly, and to low-affinity sites on the sides of protofilaments, leading to separation and disintegration of microtubules.[274] This disintegration with interaction of drug and free tubulin dimers results in the formation of drug-tubulin paracrystalline aggregates that effectively trap free tubulin, thereby shifting the equilibrium that exists between free and microtubular protein. Because of the different functions of microtubules, vinca alkaloids can have many and varied effects on a range of cellular processes. However, their most important cytotoxic effect is due to inhibition of the mitotic spindle apparatus.[275]

An important mechanism of resistance to the vinca alkaloids is increased drug efflux mediated by P-glycoprotein.[276] Differences in the ability of different vinca alkaloids to act as P-glycoprotein substrates may also contribute to their different activity profiles. Alterations to the structure of tubulin as a result of gene mutations affect alkaloid binding and can result in decreased drug activity or drug resistance.[277]

All of these agents are administered intravenously, typically by injection or short infusion. The small doses used

Vindoline nucleus

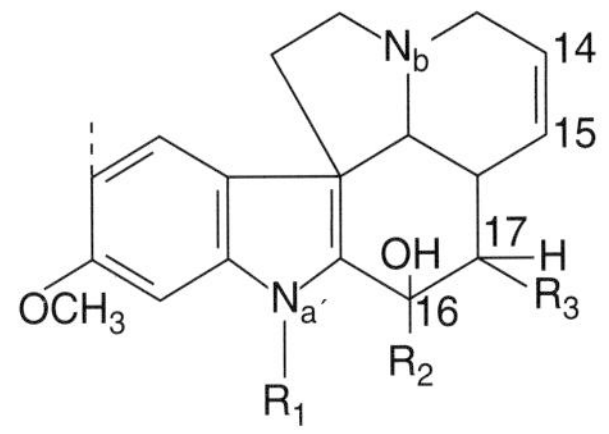

FIGURE 17–15. Structures of the vinca alkaloids.

Catharanthine nucleus

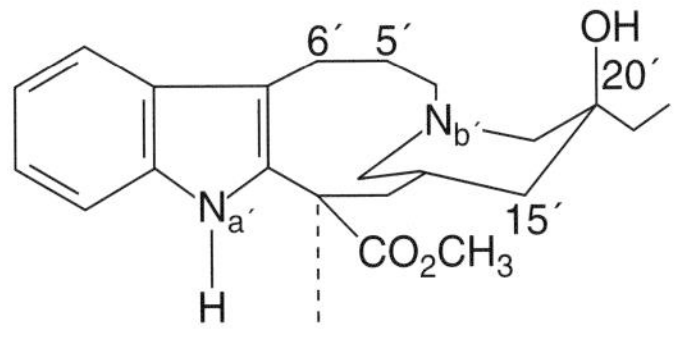

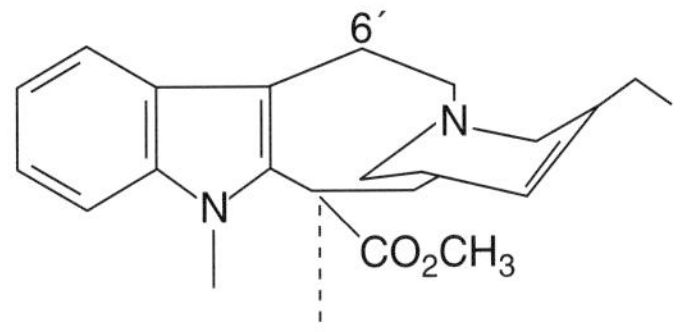

	R_1	R_2	R_3
Vindesine	$-CH_3$	$-CONH_2$	$-OH$
Vincristine	$-CHO$	$-CO_2CH_3$	$-OCOCH_3$
Vinblastine	$-CH_3$	$-CO_2CH_3$	$-OCOCH_3$
Vinorelbine	$-CH_3$	$-CO_2CH_3$	$-OCOCH_3$

for most of these agents (around 2 to 6 mg) result in low plasma concentrations, and this has hampered efforts to define their pharmacokinetics and metabolism in humans. Disappearance from plasma after intravenous dosing is rapid, reflecting extensive distribution into tissues and resulting in high volumes of distribution. The elimination half-lives are around 24 hours or longer.[278] Excretion is mainly through the bile; only small amounts of drug and metabolites are recovered in the urine.[279]

The toxicities of the vinca alkaloids vary markedly. Neurotoxicity is the major dose-limiting toxicity with vincristine, but myelosuppression is typically dose-limiting with other drugs in the class. Vincristine was one of the first drugs used for treatment of childhood ALL, and it has remained the mainstay of treatment for this illness in both adults and children (see Chapters 26 and 27). In most modern, more intensive regimens, it is given weekly as part of remission induction and then less often as consolidation therapy, the risk being peripheral neuropathy, which is more likely to occur in older than in younger patients. If symptoms of neurotoxicity are detected, doses need to be reduced. For example, patients may often complain of subtle symptoms before the development of overt signs of peripheral neuropathy, which are usually reversible; but patients should be specifically asked about symptoms at each visit because this information may not be given unprompted until a late stage. Autonomic neuropathy can also rarely occur. Vinblastine is characteristically associated with myelosuppression rather than with peripheral neuropathy, but it is not routinely used in the treatment of leukemia.

Taxanes

The first taxane to enter clinical trials, paclitaxel (Taxol), was identified in the late 1960s to be the active compo-

nent of the extract of the bark of the Pacific yew, *Taxus brevifolia*.[280] Interest in this compound was stimulated by the observation that it had a unique mechanism of action in that it altered the equilibrium between free tubulin and microtubules in favor of microtubule formation, thereby promoting microtubule assembly.[281] Taxanes bind to a specific site on β-tubulin, different from that used by vinca alkaloids, podophyllotoxins, and colchicine, and typically to β-tubulin in formed microtubules rather than to free tubulin or tubulin dimers.[282] This shift in the equilibrium between tubulin in free dimers and microtubules results in the formation of tubules at lower tubulin concentration and occurs in the absence of GTP and microtubule-associated proteins. The microtubules formed in the presence of taxanes are also characteristic in that they have only 12 protofilaments instead of the usual 13. This, and the absence of microtubule-associated protein, which cross-links the protofilaments, results in microtubules that are less rigid.

The polymerization of microtubules in the presence of taxanes results in two distinct morphologic effects. During all phases of the cell cycle, the cellular microtubule cytoskeleton reassembles to produce abundant arrays of disorganized microtubules, often aligned in parallel bundles.[283] During mitosis, taxanes induce the formation of large numbers of abnormal asters, which do not grow from centrioles as in the normal situation, resulting in cell cycle arrest. The concentrations of drug required to induce mitotic arrest are substantially lower than those that result in the appearance of bundles of microtubules during other phases of the cell cycle, and it is the mitotic effect that appears to be most important in terms of cytotoxicity.

The early clinical development of paclitaxel, the lead taxane, was somewhat slowed by two factors, drug supply and hypersensitivity reactions encountered in the first phase I trials. The yield of paclitaxel from the yew bark is extremely low, and the tree has to be felled to harvest the bark. Complete chemical synthesis of the compound is made difficult by the presence of 11 optical centers in the molecule, and although complete synthesis has now been reported, it would be extremely difficult to scale up to a commercial level. The search for alternative sources of paclitaxel resulted in the discovery of 10-deacetyl baccatin III, extracted from the needles of the European yew and hence a renewable resource.[284] This molecule can be esterified to produce paclitaxel and other active analogues, most notably docetaxel (Taxotere).[284] Clinical material is now produced by this route.

The hypersensitivity reactions are manifest as hypotension, dyspnea, urticaria, and abdominal pain, typical histamine-mediated responses, and occur within the first few minutes after dosing.[285] Because of its poor solubility, paclitaxel is formulated in Cremophor EL, which is known to cause similar reactions in other drug formulations. However, similar reactions also occurred subsequently with docetaxel, which because of its increased solubility is formulated in polysorbate 80 rather than in Cremophore, suggesting that the taxanes are at least in part responsible for this toxicity.[286] Consequently, with both paclitaxel and docetaxel, patients are given a premedication typically comprising dexamethasone, diphenhydramine, and cimetidine.

Paclitaxel is typically administered by infusion over 3 or 24 hours, although the optimal schedule remains unknown and more prolonged infusions (more than 96 hours) are also employed. Docetaxel is administered over 1 hour. The major toxicity of both drugs is myelosuppression,[286] with other side effects differing for each agent.

Topoisomerase Poisons

A number of drugs in clinical use exert their cytotoxic effects by interfering with important nuclear enzymes involved in maintaining DNA topology. The total length of DNA in eukaryotic cells is around 1 meter, and packaging this into the nucleus is clearly a complex process involving extensive twisting and knotting. However, the cell needs access to the DNA during gene transcription, DNA replication, and DNA repair, processes that require untwisting and unknotting to enable access by the protein complexes that carry out these functions. These winding/unwinding and knotting/unknotting functions are carried out by enzymes that maintain this complex topology, the topoisomerases.[287] In mammalian cells, these functions are carried out by type I and type II topoisomerase enzymes, which catalyze transient breaks in single (topoisomerase I) or double (topoisomerase II) DNA strands, thereby allowing DNA unwinding and unknotting, respectively. A large number of drugs exert at least part of their cytotoxic activity by blocking these enzymes. These compounds do not bind and inhibit free enzyme but inhibit the enzyme partway through its catalytic cycle, when the break in DNA has occurred. With normal enzyme activity, this DNA break is anchored by the enzyme in the form of a reversible cleavable complex

with DNA so that when the unwinding or unknotting step has occurred, the break is resealed. The topoisomerase-acting drugs inhibit this resealing step, resulting in the accumulation of cleavable complexes.[288, 289] Because these agents do not inhibit enzyme activity, they are often referred to as topoisomerase poisons per se inhibitors.

Topoisomerase I exists as a monomer and is not dependent on ATP for activity.[290] Topoisomerase I functions to relieve the torsional stress that builds up ahead of the DNA replication complex and transiently breaks one DNA strand in the double helix, allowing the second strand to rotate around the break to relieve this stress. Levels of the enzyme are reasonably consistent throughout the cell cycle, suggesting a role in both gene transcription and DNA replication. Drugs that act by stabilization of the topoisomerase I–DNA complex include camptothecin and its related analogues, topotecan and irinotecan.

Topoisomerase II exists as a dimer and is dependent on both magnesium and ATP for activity.[287, 291] The mechanism by which the enzyme mediates double-stranded DNA breaks has been described as a double-hinged gate, with entry and exit gates on opposite sides of the enzyme.[287] After the binding of one DNA duplex to the enzyme, a second DNA duplex can enter the in-gate (Fig. 17–16). Binding of ATP then closes the in-gate behind

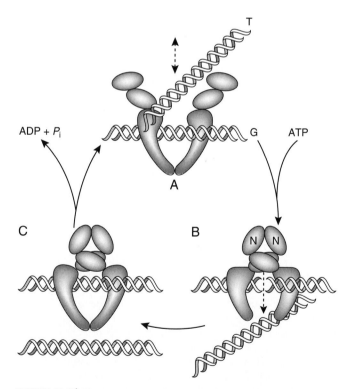

FIGURE 17–16. Topoisomerase-II as an ATP-modulated clamp with two sets of jaws mediating passage of double-stranded DNA. *A*, The enzyme is in the form of an open clamp, bound to a DNA duplex (the G segment). On binding of ATP and a second DNA duplex (the T segment), conformational changes occur *(B)* that break the G segment and cause the T segment to pass through the transiently broken strands and out of the now open exit gate. *C*, After transport, the G segment is resealed and the exit gate closed; after ATP hydrolysis, the enzyme returns to the open clamp form. N denotes the amino-terminal domains of the enzyme. (From Roca J: The mechanisms of DNA topoisomerases. Trends Biol Sci 1995;20:156.)

the second DNA duplex and cleaves the first double-stranded DNA, resulting in passage of the second duplex across this transient break and out of the gate on the opposite side of the protein. The strand break is then resealed, and the DNA is released. The breaks catalyzed by topoisomerase II in each strand of double-stranded DNA are characteristically 4 base pairs apart, and different topoisomerase II–acting drugs differ in their preference for the base adjacent to the breakpoint.[292, 293]

There are two topoisomerase II genes encoding a p170 α and p180 β isoform.[287] Topoisomerase IIβ is expressed at low levels throughout the cell cycle, suggesting a possible role in mediating DNA topologic changes during gene transcription. Topoisomerase IIα expression increases markedly during DNA synthesis and mitosis and is the pharmacologically important isoform. The induction of DNA strand breaks with topoisomerase II inhibitors therefore requires the cell to be exposed during the phase of the cell cycle during which topoisomerase IIα is active. Many topoisomerase II inhibitors, such as the anthracyclines, intercalate DNA, effectively maintaining high nuclear concentrations of active drug for a long time after dose. For drugs that do not bind to DNA, such as etoposide and teniposide, activity is dependent on exposure during these phases, that is, they are cell cycle phase–specific agents. In clinical use, this means that their activity is schedule dependent.[294] Moreover, because the epipodophyllotoxins do not bind to DNA, they are quickly effluxed from the cell when exposure to the drug is stopped, with religation of the DNA strand breaks. Cytotoxicity with these topoisomerase II agents thus requires exposure for long enough for the DNA lesions to become lethal.

Additional events subsequent to inhibition of the religation step of topoisomerase I or topoisomerase II may be important for cytotoxicity. With topoisomerase I inhibition, single-stranded DNA breaks are typically not sufficient to induce cell death, and the requirement for ongoing DNA synthesis for drug activity suggests additional events involving collision of the advancing DNA replication fork with the drug-stabilized single-stranded break.[295] This results in the conversion of a drug-stabilized single-stranded break into a double-stranded DNA break. For both topoisomerase I–acting and topoisomerase II–acting drugs, the double-stranded breaks that arise result in free DNA ends that can then recombine with other free ends, causing secondary DNA lesions,[296, 297] including deletions, insertions, and reciprocal translocations.[298] Thus, many of the topoisomerase II–acting agents are known to be mutagenic and carcinogenic in clinical use,[299, 300] and preclinical data suggest that topoisomerase I–acting drugs may have similar effects.[301]

Topoisomerase II poisons include the epipodophyllotoxins etoposide and teniposide; the anthracyclines doxorubicin, daunorubicin, and related compounds; the anthracenedione mitoxantrone; and the aminoacridine amsacrine.

Topoisomerase I–Acting Drugs

The topoisomerase I–acting drugs in current clinical use were developed from camptothecin, extracted from the Chinese willow, *Camptotheca acuminata*. Initial clinical trials with camptothecin were disappointing in terms of both antitumor activity and unpredictable toxicity, particularly bladder toxicity. However, interest in this compound was renewed in the 1980s with the demonstration that the cytotoxicity of camptothecin was mediated by inhibition of topoisomerase I, representing a unique target.[302] Subsequently, two new compounds, topotecan and irinotecan (CPT-11), were developed, and both are now licensed for clinical use (Fig. 17–17).

These molecules have the same basic 5-membered ring structure as the parent molecule, with different substituent groups at C7, C9, or C10. An important part of the molecule is the closed E ring (lactone), which is essential for activity. Opening of this ring structure to the carboxylate form (the hydroxy acid) results in loss of activity. At physiologic pH, the equilibrium between the closed and open ring forms is in favor of the inactive carboxylate; at more acidic pH, the closed lactone predominates. This in part explains the bladder toxicity of camptothecin in early trials because at urinary pH, the inactive carboxylate reverts to the active, closed-ring lactone.

Irinotecan (CPT-11) is a prodrug that requires removal of the piperidino side chain at C10 by a carboxylesterase for activity. The resulting compound, SN38, is a potent cytotoxic agent with activity in the low nanomolar range, around three to four times lower than the activity of the other licensed topoisomerase I inhibitor, topotecan, and the investigational agent 9-aminocamptothecin.[303]

Like the topoisomerase II inhibitors, topoisomerase I–acting drugs appear to have a preference, although not an absolute requirement, for a particular base, favoring a guanine adjacent to the DNA break site.[304] The activity of topoisomerase I drugs is dependent on functional enzyme, and an important mechanism of resistance is decreased cellular levels of active topoisomerase I enzyme resulting from mutations affecting gene expression or protein phosphorylation.[290, 305] The role of drug efflux pumps in resistance to topoisomerase I drugs is not clear

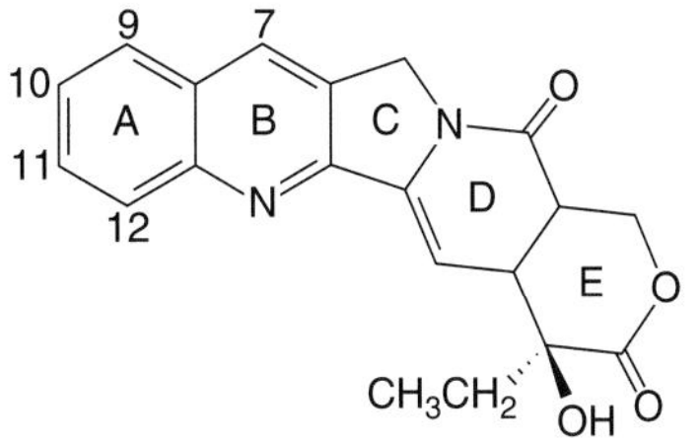

	C-10	C-9	C-7
Camptothecin	H	H	H
Topotecan	OH	(CH₃)₂NCH₂	H
9-Aminocamptothecin	H	NH2	H
SN-38	OH	H	CH₃CH₂
CPT-11	(piperidino)N—N—C(=O)—O	H	CH₃CH₂

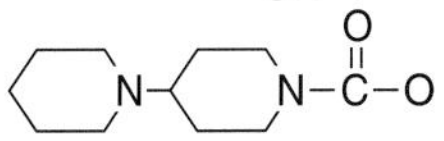

FIGURE 17–17. Structures of topoisomerase I inhibitors.

and differs for the different agents. In P-glycoprotein–overexpressing cell lines, some cross-resistance was seen between camptothecin and topotecan but not irinotecan.[306]

Topotecan and irinotecan are typically administered intravenously. The bioavailability of an oral topotecan formulation has been reported as 30%.[307] Although these agents showed marked schedule dependence in preclinical studies, irinotecan is typically administered as a single short infusion of around 350 mg/m² every 3 weeks; topotecan is most usually administered as five daily short infusions of around 1.5 mg/m². However, the optimal schedule for each of these agents is not clear, with marked differences in the toxicity profile in different schedules. It is somewhat surprising that a drug mainly active during DNA synthesis, such as irinotecan, should be administered once every 3 weeks in the clinical setting. This may be explained by the long plasma half-life (around 10 hours) of the active metabolite SN38, due in part to the high binding to albumin (98%) of the active SN38 lactone, compared with only 2 to 3 hours for topotecan.

The large difference in dose between these two agents is attributable to the lack of activity of irinotecan itself, requiring conversion to SN38, the plasma AUC of which is typically some 50 to 100 times lower than that of irinotecan. SN38 is inactivated by glucuronidation and excreted in the urine and bile, with the possibility of hydrolysis back to active SN38 and subsequent reabsorption from the gut. Plasma SN38 glucuronide AUC is several-fold higher than that of SN38. Another metabolite, 7-ethyl-10-[4-N-(5-aminopentanoic acid)-1-piperidino]-carbonyloxy campothecin, with little if any cytotoxic activity, has been described.[308]

The protein binding of irinotecan and topotecan is around 20% to 30%, resulting in significant penetration of active topotecan into the CNS, whereas the high protein binding of SN38 limits penetration into this space. Renal function is important in the clearance of topotecan, accounting for around 40% of the dose.[309] In contrast, biliary clearance is more important than renal clearance with irinotecan.[310] This results in differences in the toxicity profiles of the two agents. Although myelosuppression is the major dose-limiting toxicity with both drugs, diarrhea has been the dose-limiting toxicity with irinotecan in some studies, particularly with more frequent dosing.[311] Early-onset diarrhea has been attributed to the competitive inhibition of acetylcholinesterase by the parent molecule irinotecan, with resultant cholinergic effects. This early toxicity has been treated with atropine. Diarrhea of later onset, typically occurring 12 hours or more after the dose, is common. The severity of this diarrhea can be markedly reduced by the use of loperamide as soon as symptoms develop.

Topotecan is currently being evaluated in the treatment of leukemias, mainly at the M.D. Anderson Cancer Center.[312]

The Epipodophyllotoxins

Podophyllotoxin is a natural product extracted from the roots and rhizomes of *Podophyllum peltatum* (American

May apple) and *Podophyllum emodi* native to North America and the Himalayas and long used in folk medicines by the indigenous populations of these areas. Clinical trials with this compound in the 1940s reported antitumor activity but excessive toxicity. In the 1960s, two derivatives of podophyllotoxin, etoposide and teniposide, were described. These compounds differed from the parent in the presence of a glucoside (glucopyranoside) moiety on the C ring, a different enantiomeric configuration at C4 on the C ring, and the presence of a hydroxy in place of a methoxy group on the pendant E ring (Fig. 17–18). Etoposide and teniposide differ in the

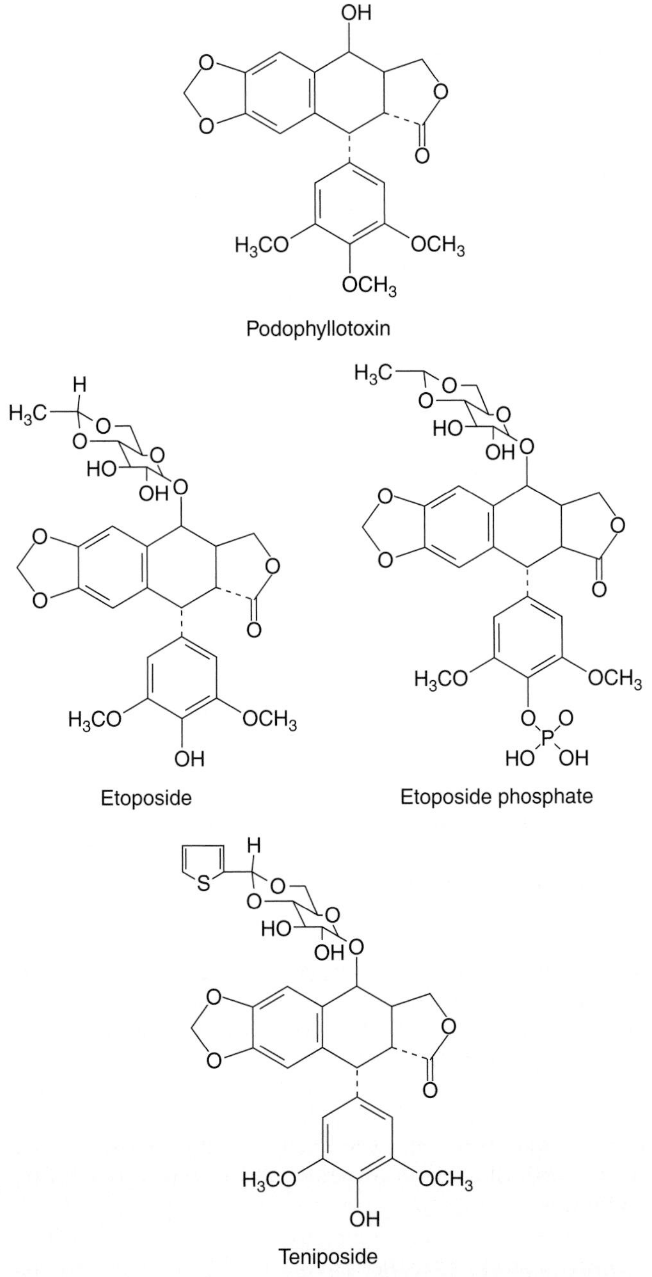

FIGURE 17–18. Structures of podophyllotoxin (the parent compound), the epipodophyllotoxins etoposide and teniposide, and etoposide phosphate.

presence of a methyl or thenylidine group, respectively, in the glucopyranoside.

For many years after these agents entered clinical trials, it was believed that their mechanism of action was the same as that of the parent compound, which inhibited the polymerization of tubulin during mitosis, thereby acting as a spindle poison. However, etoposide and teniposide have no effect on tubulin assembly but induce DNA strand breaks,[313, 314] resulting in a block in the cell cycle in late S or G_2.[315] It was soon realized that this DNA damage could not be induced with drug and isolated DNA but did occur with drug and isolated nuclei, suggesting a role for an additional nuclear factor.[316] Furthermore, the broken ends of DNA that result from exposure to etoposide and teniposide could not be end labeled, suggesting that the strand ends may be covered by a nuclear factor. This was subsequently identified as being topoisomerase II.[317] Like the other topoisomerase inhibitors, etoposide and teniposide do not inhibit free enzyme but block the religation step by interaction with the topoisomerase II–DNA cleavable complex and show a preference for cytidine at the cleaved 5′ DNA terminus.[293] The drug-induced stabilization of cleavable complexes is not itself lethal to the cell, but during ongoing DNA synthesis or chromosome segregation, these complexes become converted into double-stranded breaks. Such damage is lethal to, and these free DNA ends can also enter into illegal recombinations with other double-stranded breaks, resulting in deletions, insertions, and translocations.[298]

Resistance to etoposide and teniposide is mainly due to two mechanisms common to a number of topoisomerase II inhibitors.[318] First, increased expression of the *MDR1* gene results in increased P-glycoprotein and increased efflux of drug from the cell (classic MDR). Second, because the damage induced by these drugs is dependent on topoisomerase II activity, decreased activity of the enzyme, due to either decreased expression or changes to the protein, results in less DNA damage on exposure to the drug. Because many drugs exert at least part of their cytotoxic activity through topoisomerase II, reduced enzyme activity results in cross-resistance to these agents and is termed atypical MDR.

Uptake of teniposide by leukemic cells is more rapid than uptake of etoposide, and although intracellular concentrations of each drug reach steady state within 20 to 30 minutes, concentrations of teniposide are around 10 times higher than those of etoposide at the same exposure concentration.[319, 320] When cells are removed from the drug environment, a rapid exponential efflux is observed, with a half-life of just 3 minutes.[319]

The bioavailability of the oral formulation of etoposide is around 60% at doses of 100 mg and lower, but it decreases with doses greater than 200 mg, probably related to the poor stability of the compound in gastric fluid.[321] There is marked variability in etoposide bioavailability both within and between patients.[28] In the treatment of pediatric leukemia, the intravenous formulation of etoposide or teniposide is commonly diluted in fruit juice and given orally.

After intravenous administration, both drugs typically exhibit a biexponential decline in plasma concentration, reflecting distribution out of the plasma space into the extracellular fluid compartment, and drug elimination.[322] The terminal half-life is around 6 hours for etoposide and 10 hours for teniposide. Studies that have collected samples for several days after a dose often report triexponential decay with much longer terminal half-lives.[322]

Approximately 50% of an intravenous dose of etoposide is excreted renally, principally as the parent drug, although small amounts of etoposide glucuronide and an active catechol metabolite are also reported. The fate of the remaining dose is not clear, but a study with radiolabeled etoposide reported 44% ± 13% of the dose recovered in the feces to 120 hours.[323] Because of the importance of renal excretion in etoposide clearance, dose reductions are required in patients with abnormal renal function.[45] With teniposide, early studies suggested that nearly 50% of a radioactive dose was excreted renally, whereas subsequent studies that have measured urinary teniposide recovered less than 15% of the dose.[322] There are few data on the metabolism of teniposide, and the fate of an intravenous dose is largely unaccounted for.

In plasma, etoposide is around 95% protein bound,[45] mainly to albumin; for teniposide, this figure is around 99%.[324] Consequently, small changes in protein binding can have marked effects on free (active) drug concentrations and thereby drug effects. Dose reductions are indicated in patients with low serum albumin concentration.

A notable feature of the clinical pharmacology of these drugs is their schedule dependence, best demonstrated for etoposide. In patients with small-cell lung cancer, the response rate to single-agent etoposide was 10% in patients administered 500 mg/m² as a 24-hour infusion and 89% in patients administered the same dose as five daily 2-hour infusions of 100 mg/m².[294] As discussed earlier, this is related to the phase-specific nature of etoposide activity and the need to maintain exposure to the drug to ensure that the DNA damage induced becomes lethal.

Studies investigating pharmacodynamic-pharmacokinetic relationships have identified associations between plasma drug concentrations and tumor response and toxicity for etoposide, mainly in small-cell lung cancer,[325] and plasma clearance, steady-state drug concentrations, and tumor response for teniposide in childhood leukemia.[54] The major dose-limiting toxicity with standard doses of both drugs is myelosuppression. With high-dose etoposide, mucositis becomes dose limiting. An unpredictable toxicity with both drugs is a hypersensitivity reaction, typically manifest as flushing, respiratory problems, changes in blood pressure, and abdominal pain, often occurring soon after the start of drug administration and generally resolving rapidly if the infusion is stopped. These reactions are rare with etoposide[326] but more frequent (3% to 4% incidence) with teniposide.[327] However, other reports have described mild reactions in 34% of children receiving etoposide as part of a multiagent induction regimen for leukemia.[328]

A late complication with these agents is the appearance of therapy-related AML, with a short latency period of 2 to 3 years. These leukemias are also typically of French-American-British classification M4 or M5 morphology and commonly involve reciprocal translocations at 11q23. The overall cumulative incidence of therapy-related AML

4 to 6 years after treatment of childhood ALL is around 5%,[329, 330] but it varies with the schedule of administration, particularly the frequency of epipodophyllotoxin dose, being more common (12% incidence) with weekly or twice-weekly dosing.[329] A report from the Cancer Therapy Evaluation Program, which is monitoring 12 trials involving a range of etoposide and teniposide doses, has not found an association between the total cumulative dose and therapy-related AML.[331] The incidence may also be higher in patients treated with L-asparaginase before the epipodophyllotoxin.[332]

Teniposide has been an important feature of the so-called Total Therapy programs used at St. Jude Children's Research Hospital, Memphis, Tennessee for childhood ALL (see Chapter 26). Etoposide has also been used in ALL to some extent but has also been incorporated into the treatment of adult AML (see Chapter 21). It is currently being evaluated as part of first-line remission induction therapy, usually in combination with idarubicin and ara-C.[333] It is often used as part of second-line treatment of AML when a classic anthracycline and ara-C combination has failed.

Etoposide phosphate is a new, more water soluble prodrug of etoposide that is rapidly converted to etoposide in the systemic circulation after intravenous administration.[334] This analogue was originally developed in attempts to improve the bioavailability of oral etoposide, but trials with oral etoposide phosphate were somewhat disappointing, possibly owing to cleavage to etoposide in the acidic conditions of the stomach.

Anthracycline Antibiotics

The first anthracycline antibiotics, doxorubicin and daunorubicin, were isolated from species of *Streptomyces*[335]; the newer analogues, epirubicin and idarubicin, are produced synthetically. The structure of these compounds is remarkably similar, comprising a 4-membered chromophore ring attached to daunosamine, an amino sugar. As shown in Figure 17–19, doxorubicin and epirubicin (4-epidoxorubicin) differ only in the conformation of the hydroxyl group within the sugar moiety.

Uptake of anthracyclines into cells is by passive diffusion,[336] with rapid movement into the nucleus. The planar ring structure in all members of this group of drugs enables tight binding of the compound to DNA by intercalation of the ring chromophore between adjacent base pairs. Most of the drug is concentrated in the nucleus by binding to DNA and possibly to other nuclear components, which maintains a concentration gradient between the extracellular fluid and cytoplasm such that intracellular drug concentration can far exceed that in surrounding fluid. Intercalation of these compounds into DNA results in changes in local base interactions, with local uncoiling in the double helix. For some time it was thought that this intercalation was the cytotoxic event. However, as with the epipodophyllotoxins, the DNA strand breaks that result from exposure to anthracyclines are now known to be protein linked and to involve topoisomerase II.[337, 338] Moreover, it appears that the inhibition of DNA strand religation is not due to conformational changes in DNA resulting from intercalation; topoisomerase II inhibition occurs at concentrations much lower than

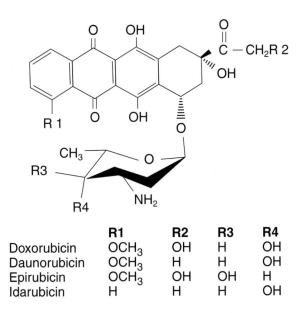

	R1	R2	R3	R4
Doxorubicin	OCH₃	OH	H	OH
Daunorubicin	OCH₃	H	H	OH
Epirubicin	OCH₃	OH	OH	H
Idarubicin	H	H	H	OH

FIGURE 17–19. Structures of the anthracyclines.

those associated with intercalation and is also seen with anthracyclines that do not intercalate DNA.[339] These agents show some sequence specificity for DNA binding, typically preferring an adenine at the cleaved 5′ DNA terminus,[340] suggesting that exposure of these sites occurs during the topoisomerase II–mediated cleavage reaction, resulting in anthracycline binding and inhibition of the subsequent religation step.

The anthracyclines can also mediate damage to cellular molecules by a separate mechanism. All members of this class possess a quinone within the chromophore moiety. The one- or two-electron reduction of this group by dehydrogenases or reductases results in the formation of semiquinones (one-electron reduction) or dihydroquinones (two-electron reduction), thereby generating reactive free radical species[341] (Fig. 17–20). In the presence of a metal ion (particularly iron), these free radicals rapidly pass on this additional electron to oxygen, resulting in the generation of a number of highly reactive species including O_2^-, H_2O_2, and OH^-. Although this can result in the generation of oxidative DNA and lipid damage, most cells have active systems for detoxifying free radicals, including glutathione peroxidase, superoxide dismutase, and catalase.[342, 343] Oxidative damage repair systems also repair DNA damage that does result from these reactive compounds. Consequently, this mechanism does not contribute substantially to anthracycline antitumor activity. However, in other tissues, the activity of these antioxidant enzyme systems varies considerably, with high activity in the liver but much lower activity in cardiac tissue.[344] Generation of anthracycline free radicals, and thereby lipid peroxidation, may also be increased in cardiac tissue. These two effects mean that free radical damage occurs more readily in cardiac tissue and is mainly responsible for the cardiotoxicity seen with these agents. Because of the importance of iron in the generation of these free radicals, the anthracyclines are often used with iron-chelating agents, most notably dexrazoxane (ICRF-187).[345]

I. One electron reduction

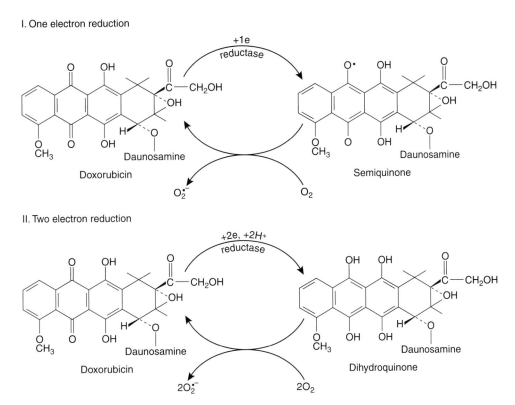

II. Two electron reduction

FIGURE 17–20. One- and two-electron reduction of doxorubicin, resulting in the formation of the semiquinone and dihydroquinone, and the resultant formation of the superoxide anion O^-_2 and hydrogen peroxide. Protective systems for mopping up these reactive species are less active in cardiac tissue, resulting in higher levels of peroxidative damage. (From Pratt WB, Ruddon RW, Ensminger WD, et al: The Anticancer Drugs, 2nd ed. Oxford: Oxford University Press; 1994.)

The importance of topoisomerase II inhibition in the cytotoxic activity of the anthracyclines is demonstrated by reports of resistance in cells with decreased topoisomerase II activity or mutations in the topoisomerase II gene.[318] Although topoisomerase II activity in AML blast cells is variable, this did not correlate with drug sensitivity in patients treated with etoposide, daunorubicin, and amsacrine.[346] Because these agents are substrates for P-glycoprotein, resistance is also reported in cells with increased *MDR1* expression, and increased P-glycoprotein is an adverse prognostic factor in anthracycline-treated leukemic patients.[347] Attempts to increase anthracycline activity by the use of P-glycoprotein reversal agents, such as cyclosporine and PSC833, have been more successful in leukemia than in solid tumors.[79]

Doxorubicin, epirubicin, and daunorubicin are administered intravenously because the chromophore ring–daunosome linkage is labile in the conditions of the gastrointestinal tract; the more lipophilic idarubicin can be administered orally, although its bioavailability is incomplete and erratic.[348] These compounds are particularly irritating to local tissues if extravasation occurs during administration, resulting in progressive ulceration that is difficult to treat. The most successful approach to treatment of this toxicity appears to be the use of local DHM3, a potent reducing agent that converts the active anthracycline to the much less active 7-deoxyaglycone.[349]

Typical doses used in AML and ALL are 45 to 60 mg/m² for doxorubicin, 30 to 45 mg/m² for daunorubicin, and 10 to 12 mg/m² for idarubicin. With doxorubicin,

the antitumor effect is not dependent on the schedule of administration but is proportional to the doxorubicin AUC achieved. This probably relates to the high intracellular drug concentrations that can be achieved and the degree of binding to nuclear components, such that once the drug is delivered to the nucleus, concentrations remain high for a long time. This is also reflected in the plasma concentration, with a terminal elimination half-life for doxorubicin of around 30 hours,[350] and concentrations exceed 10 nM for up to 1 week after a single 60 mg/m² bolus dose. Epirubicin has a similarly long terminal half-life,[351] and although the terminal half-life of idarubicin is only around 10 to 15 hours, that of the active metabolite idarubicinol is 30 to 50 hours.[348, 352]

The metabolism of the different anthracyclines is similar, differing mainly in the amounts of each metabolite produced relative to the parent drug.[353] The initial site of metabolism is the ketone at C13, which under the action of reductases is converted to the corresponding -OH metabolites (i.e., doxorubicinol), which have typically less activity than the parent drug. For daunorubicin and idarubicin, this is an important metabolic pathway, with plasma metabolite-to-AUC ratios typically greater than 2; for doxorubicin and epirubicin, the corresponding ratio is less than 0.5.[354, 355] Moreover, idarubicin differs from other anthracyclines in that idarubicinol retains cytotoxic activity.[356]

Two aglycone species (resulting from loss of the daunosamine sugar) have been reported with anthracyclines, a metabolically produced 7-deoxyaglycone from the two-electron reduction described previously and a 7-hydroxy-aglycone, which was reported in early studies but may be a degradation product produced ex vivo. These aglycones have little antitumor activity, and data suggest that the plasma concentrations of this metabolite were higher in patients with AML who failed to respond to daunorubicin-containing therapy.[357] Further metabolism by phase 2 conjugation to glucuronic acid, and possibly sulfate, has also been reported and is most important with epirubicin, for which the plasma concentrations of glucuronide are similar to those of the parent compound.[358] This is reflected in the route of clearance of an epirubicin dose, in which biliary and renal elimination are important.[358] For other anthracyclines, the biliary route predominates. Systemic clearance of the anthracyclines is reduced in patients with impaired liver function, although this is more clearly demonstrated with use of more sensitive measures, such as antipyrine clearance, rather than by standard liver biochemistry tests.[359, 360] Dosage reduction is essential in such patients.

The major dose-limiting toxicity with the anthracyclines is myelosuppression. However, the most problematic toxicity is the cardiotoxicity described previously, which presents as an acute or chronic toxicity.[353] Acute anthracycline-induced cardiotoxicity is manifest as arrhythmias, heart block, and in extreme cases pericarditis and congestive heart failure. The much more common cardiac toxicity is a cumulative dose-dependent effect on the myocardium involving specific and characteristic changes to myocytes, including dilation of the sarcoplasmic reticulum and loss of myofibrils. The frequency of these effects increases with continued dosing, and the cardiomyopathy that develops often leads to congestive heart failure.[353] With most anthracycline treatment regimens, this chronic toxicity typically becomes apparent some 2 to 3 months after the last dose, but it can arise sooner or up to several years later. The cumulative doses at which this toxicity starts to occur (1% to 10% risk) are around 500 mg/m² for doxorubicin,[353, 361] 1000 mg/m² for daunorubicin,[353, 362] 300 mg/m² for idarubicin,[363] and 900 mg/m² for epirubicin.[364] The frequency is dose dependent and increases with higher cumulative doses. Children may be particularly at risk. In adults, other risk factors include preexisting heart disease, previous radiation involving the heart, and age. Because this cardiotoxicity can be difficult to treat in some patients and indeed may be fatal, strategies to reduce occurrence include more prolonged infusions to decrease peak plasma and tissue concentrations of free radicals.[365, 366] As previously described, Dexrazoxane (ICRF-187) has been shown to reduce this late toxicity, almost certainly by chelating the iron species involved in the anthracycline-induced generation of reactive oxygen species.[345, 367]

Anthracyclines are a basic constituent of remission induction and consolidation therapy for both AML and ALL (see Chapters 21 to 23 and 26 and 27). In AML, there are really no convincing data to support the use of any one over another. Idarubicin is much favored at present.

Mitoxantrone

In the 1970s, analogues of the anthracenedione dyes (originally developed for use in the textile industry) were investigated as possible cytotoxic agents on the basis of the ability of the parent compounds to intercalate DNA. Mitoxantrone (dihydroxyanthracenedione) was the most active of a series of compounds synthesized.[368] The drug entered clinical trials in 1980 and showed activity in lymphoma, leukemia, and breast cancer.

Like the anthracyclines, mitoxantrone has a planar ring moiety that facilitates DNA intercalation (Fig. 17–21). The major mechanism of cytotoxicity is stabilization of topoisomerase II–DNA cleavable complexes, with a preference for a cytidine at the cleaved 5' terminus rather than the adenine with doxorubicin.[369] The mitoxantrone molecule is less susceptible to reduction than are the anthracyclines and therefore generates substantially less free radical damage.

Mitoxantrone is administered intravenously. The drug rapidly leaves the plasma compartment and concentrates in blood cells, from which it more slowly redistributes into other tissues. At the end of a 1-hour infusion, white blood cell mitoxantrone concentrations were 10 times higher than plasma concentrations,[370] whereas 2 to 5 hours after a dose, white blood cell or leukemic cell concentrations were 350 times higher than in plasma. The extent of tissue distribution and binding is reflected in the large apparent volume of distribution of around 500 L, an elimination half-life of around 30 hours,[30, 31, 371] and reports of significant tissue concentrations weeks or even months after a dose.[372]

Urinary excretion of a mitoxantrone dose is low (typically <10%),[30, 31] and data on metabolites are limited. Inactive monocarboxylic and dicarboxylic acid side chain derivates have been described.[373, 374] Mitoxantrone can also be oxidized to an active napthaquinoxaline metabolite that is able to bind covalently to RNA and DNA.[375, 376] Moreover, inhibition of P450 mixed function oxidases

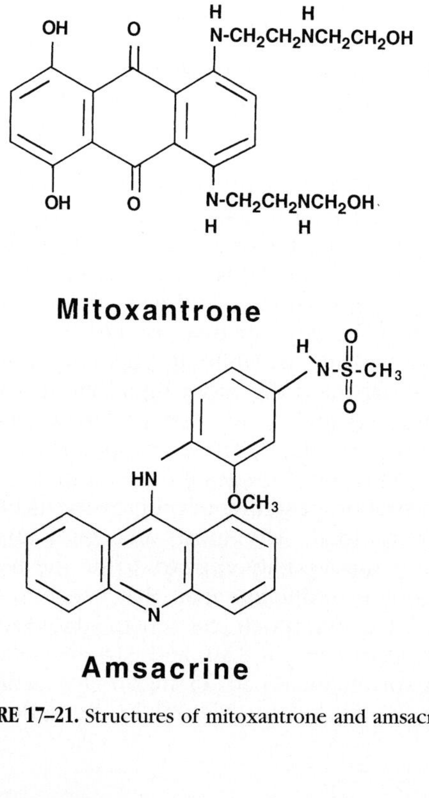

Mitoxantrone

Amsacrine

FIGURE 17–21. Structures of mitoxantrone and amsacrine.

effectively blocked the activity of mitoxantrone, suggesting that conversion to these reactive species may be important.[376] This metabolite has been identified in the urine of patients administered mitoxantrone.[377]

The major toxicity with mitoxantrone is myelosuppression. The reduction in the generation of free radicals and reactive oxygen species means that cardiac toxicity is much less of a problem with mitoxantrone than with the anthracyclines. In early phase II trials, the overall incidence was 3% and was related to previous anthracycline therapy, mediastinal radiotherapy, and history of cardiovascular disease.[378] The increase in cardiotoxic events was associated with cumulative mitoxantrone doses of greater than 120 mg/m² in patients previously treated with anthracyclines and greater than 160 mg/m² in patients not previously treated.

Amsacrine

Amsacrine contains a flat three-ring chromophore ring structure that can intercalate into DNA, but like mitoxantrone, it lacks the sugar moiety of the anthracyclines[379] (see Fig. 17–21). The cytotoxicity of amsacrine is mediated by topoisomerase II inhibition.

Like mitoxantrone, amsacrine is taken up rapidly by nucleated blood cells in vivo; peak concentrations are five times greater than peak plasma concentration and occur shortly after the end of a 3-hour infusion.[380] Over 24 hours, the mean leukemic cell amsacrine AUC was eight times that of the plasma AUC. The drug undergoes complex metabolism involving P450-mediated oxidation to reactive intermediates that are then rapidly conjugated to glutathione[381-383] (although data in humans are limited). Consequently, cardiac toxicity is much less of a problem than with the anthracyclines, with an overall incidence of just above 1% in more than 6000 patients entered into phase II trials.[384] Amsacrine has been used safely in patients with preexisting arrhythmias when serum potassium concentration was maintained above 4 mmol/L.[385]

Amsacrine has been used intravenously as part of combination chemotherapy for the treatment of leukemia in adults and children at typical intravenous doses of 90 to 120 mg/m²/day for 5 days.

Other Agents Used in Leukemia

L-Asparaginase

L-Asparaginase is unique in cancer therapy in that it acts at the amino acid level, rather than on DNA or its precursors. In most cells, L-asparagine is synthesized from L-aspartic acid and L-glutamine under the action of L-asparagine synthetase. This enzyme is notably lacking in lymphoid leukemic cells,[386] and these cells are therefore entirely dependent on circulating plasma L-asparagine. The enzyme L-asparaginase catalyzes the breakdown of L-asparagine to aspartate and glutamine, thereby depleting L-asparagine in circulating plasma. This deprives the leukemic cell of this amino acid, resulting in inhibition of protein synthesis.[387]

The discovery of L-asparaginase was entirely serendipi-

tous. In 1953, Kidd[388] reported that the growth of transplanted rat lymphomas was inhibited by the serum from guinea pigs but not by serum from other animals. Subsequently, the growth-inhibitory component in this serum was identified as L-asparaginase. The L-asparaginase in clinical use today is derived from bacterial sources, mainly *Escherichia coli*. The enzyme comprises four active subunits, each of around 34 kd (depending on the source).[387]

L-Asparaginase is administered either intravenously or intramuscularly at typical doses of 5000 to 10,000 IU/m² daily, or every other day, for between 10 and 28 days. The plasma half-life is around 0.65 days for *Erwinia*-derived asparaginase, 1.3 days for the *E. coli* preparation, and 5 days for polyethylene glycol–modified *E. coli* asparaginase.[389] The production of antibodies to L-asparaginase is not uncommon,[390] resulting in rapid disappearance from plasma.[389] Attempts to reduce immunogenicity include specific modifications to the protein, incorporating the enzyme into microspheres or into red blood cell ghosts.[387] Resistance to L-asparaginase activity is mainly by increased expression of the normally silent L-asparaginase synthetase gene in leukemic cells such that depletion of plasma L-asparagine is no longer toxic.[391]

The interaction of L-asparaginase with other cytotoxic drugs is largely understudied, but inhibition of protein synthesis typically results in a decrease in S-phase cells. Previous exposure to L-asparaginase markedly reduces methotrexate activity because of either this decrease in the number of sensitive S-phase cells or decreased methotrexate polyglutamation.[392]

The two major toxicities with L-asparaginase are hypersensitivity reactions and reductions in the concentration of important proteins due to the general inhibition of protein synthesis. Hypersensitivity reactions occur in around 10% to 15% of patients receiving L-asparaginase with other cytotoxic drugs or steroids but in possibly twice that number of patients when it is used as a single agent.[326, 393, 394] The general inhibition of protein synthesis is manifest in a range of drug effects, including alteration of clotting function, hyperglycemia due to insulin depletion, and decreases in serum albumin and lipoproteins.[387] This is associated with impairment of liver function and, in severe cases, clotting abnormalities that can lead to cerebral hemorrhage[395] (see Chapter 15). Rarely, a syndrome of acute pancreatitis can present with acute abdominal pain as in pancreatitis from any other cause. The occurrence of this pancreatitis may vary between different L-asparaginase preparations.[396, 397] Up to 70% of patients experience acute toxicities including nausea, vomiting, fever, and chills.

L-Asparaginase is still used in virtually every remission induction protocol for both children and adults with ALL. It is important to check blood glucose levels daily in patients receiving L-asparaginase.

Glucocorticoids

The glucocorticoids control a wide range of physiologic effects in an equally wide range of tissues and target cells,[398] but all of these effects are mediated through binding to the glucocorticoid receptor. The nature of the effect in different tissues is dependent on the activity of different postreceptor activation pathways in that tissue. In lymphoid tissue, high concentrations of glucocorticoids induce apoptosis through a mechanism that is not clearly understood.[399]

In the absence of hormone, the glucocorticoid receptors are complexed with heat shock proteins in the cytoplasm, thereby maintaining the receptor in an inactive state.[400] On binding of the glucocorticoid, the receptor dissociates from the complex, dimerizes, and translocates to the nucleus where it interacts with transcriptional control sequences in a number of genes, thereby altering gene expression. This binding to DNA control elements can involve either the receptor complex alone or the receptor bound to another transcription factor such as AP-1, and the nature of the transcriptional control is at least partly dependent on which other proteins are involved.[400] Resistance to prednisone has been associated with a decrease in the amount of the AP-1 protein.[401]

The important changes in gene expression on exposure to glucocorticoids at the concentrations achieved clinically are still not clear but include the altered transcription of proteins involved in signal transduction pathways involving cytokine signaling, proliferation, and apoptosis. A number of genes involved in apoptosis are upregulated by glucocorticoids, including several that encode proteins that fragment DNA, such as endonucleases.[402, 403] Whether these are direct effects or subsequent to changes in signaling pathways is not clear, but the end result of this exposure to high glucocorticoid concentrations in lymphoid cells is apoptosis.

The most widely used glucocorticoid in the treatment of lymphoid leukemias is prednisone, which can be administered orally (Fig. 17–22). This compound itself is inactive and requires activation by reduction of the ketone group at C11 to produce the 11β-hydroxy metabolite, prednisolone (see Fig. 17–22). This reaction is catalyzed by 11β-hydroxysteroid dehydrogenase, mainly in the liver. After oral administration of prednisone, plasma concentrations of prednisolone are typically several-fold higher than those of the parent drug[404, 405] and are substantially higher than concentrations that saturate steroid receptors in vitro. Prednisolone is around 90% protein bound in plasma to albumin and to specific transport proteins such as transcortin.[405] With the endogenous glucocorticoid cortisol, its activity is mediated in part by this protein binding, providing an immediate source of active compound. At pharmacologic concentrations of prednisolone, protein binding becomes saturated.[405]

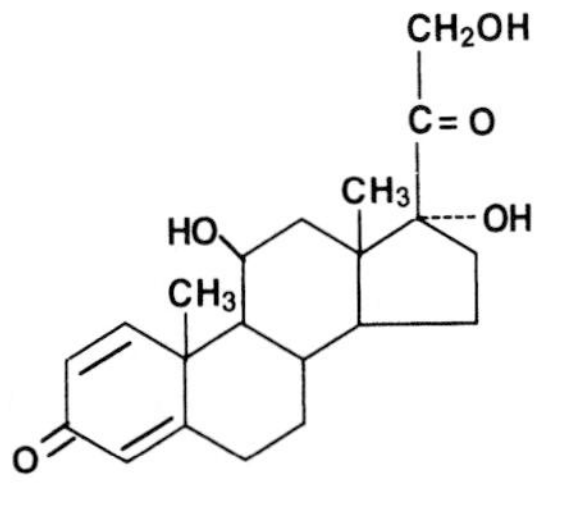

The half-life of prednisone and prednisolone is around 2 to 4 hours. Metabolic deactivation by a number of cytochrome P450 enzymes has been described. Conjugation reactions, principally with glucuronic acid, also result in inactivation.

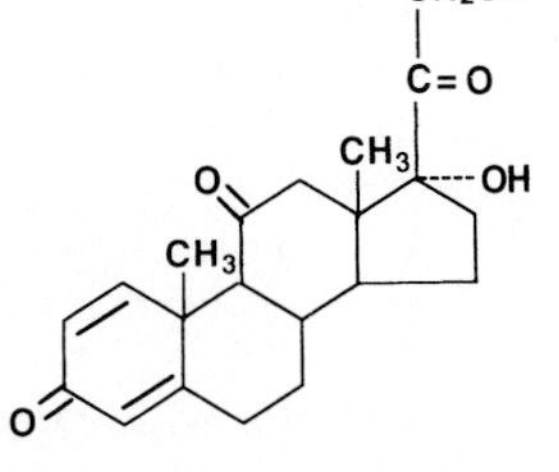

Because of the multiplicity of glucocorticoid actions, a wide variety of side effects are seen with these agents. These include direct effects attributable to prednisolone and the effect of this agent on the production of endogenous glucocorticoids. The distressing side effects of steroid therapy are well known. Weight gain and mood and sleep disturbances are common and difficult for patients to cope with. Proximal muscle weakness does not usually develop if steroids are stopped at the appropriate time, although this can be a problem in older patients, as can the development of diabetes. Prednisolone has been the mainstay for treatment of ALL since the early days of chemotherapy for this illness (see Chapters 26 and 27). It is also sometimes used in chronic lymphocytic leukemia either with chlorambucil as part of initial therapy or in the context of hemolysis (see Chapter 27).

Differentiating Agents

All-trans Retinoic Acid

The retinoic acids control the transcription of a number of genes by interaction with specific nuclear receptors.[406] These receptors include three retinoic acid receptors (RAR) and three retinoid X receptors (RXR) that dimerize on ligand binding to form RAR-RAR homodimers and RAR-RXR heterodimers. These activated dimers then bind to specific control sequences on target genes. All-trans retinoic acid (ATRA) and its isomer, 9-cis retinoic acid, are typically produced intracellularly from dietary retinol (vitamin A). ATRA binds only to RAR receptors, whereas 9-cis retinoic acid has high affinity for both the RAR and RXR subtypes and may therefore influence the transcription of different genes to ATRA. In addition, nonactivated receptors, in the absence of retinoic acid, can bind to specific DNA sequences in a number of genes and recruit nuclear co-repressor complexes that block the transcription of these genes by altering the local conformation of chromatin. On binding of retinoic acid to these receptors, interaction with these co-repressor complexes is blocked, chromatin conformation is restored, and transcription can take place.[407]

The importance of these compounds in leukemia phar-

FIGURE 17–22. Structures of steroid hormones.

macology is that the *RARA*α gene on chromosome 17 is commonly the site of a translocation in acute promyelocytic leukemia (APML).[407, 408] The partner gene in this translocation is almost always the promyelocytic leukemia gene *(PML)* on chromosome 15, but it is occasionally the promyelocytic leukemia zinc finger gene *(PLZF)* on chromosome 11. The 15;17 translocation results in a RARAα-PML fusion protein that acts as a transcriptional repressor by binding to control sequences and recruiting a co-repressor complex, as described previously. This blocks the transcription of genes involved in differentiation, giving rise to the malignant phenotype. In patients with APML with the *RARAα-PML* translocation, the administration of ATRA results in binding of ATRA to the RAR-α receptor, which then releases the co-repressor complex, allowing the transcription of these silenced genes and cell differentiation. This terminal differentiation on treatment with ATRA is apparent in the change in cell morphology and the expression of cell surface markers. After demonstration of this effect in leukemic cells, early clinical trials with oral retinoic acid were conducted mainly with the 13-*cis* retinoic acid isomer, and results were generally disappointing. However, investigators in China reported a clinical trial using oral ATRA that showed dramatic responses in APML and little toxicity. Response rates with ATRA as a single agent in APML are extremely high. Mutations in the *RARA* gene resulting in altered RARAα-PML protein have been described in resistant cell lines.

In the case of the *RARAα-PLZF* translocation, both parts of the fusion protein are able to recruit a co-repressor complex, and treatment with ATRA alone is not sufficient to lift the transcriptional repression and induce differentiation.[408] Oral ATRA has subsequently become part of initial standard treatment of this disease.[409]

Intravenous formulations of ATRA are not available, and a major difference between the pharmacokinetics of ATRA and 13-*cis* retinoic acid with oral dosing is that ATRA induces its own metabolism, resulting in a fall in plasma AUC with repeated dosing. The magnitude of this fall is substantial, with a mean reduction in plasma ATRA AUC of 70% between day 1 and day 3 in patients receiving 30 mg/m²/day orally.[410] This is due to the induction of specific metabolizing enzymes, and evidence suggests that these may be CYP2E1 and *N*-acetyltransferase.[411] This appears to be a possible mechanism of resistance to ATRA because leukemic cells from patients who relapse while receiving ATRA still show sensitivity to the drug in vitro. A new liposomal formulation of ATRA, which avoids first-pass metabolism, has been reported and does not result in enzyme induction with repeated dosing.[412]

Toxicities with ATRA include headache (which can be dose limiting and may be more common in children), dry skin, chelitis pruritus, and transient elevations of liver enzymes or serum triglycerides.[410, 413] A more serious toxicity seen in up to 25% of leukemic patients has been called the retinoic acid syndrome; it generally but not always occurs when a large population of leukemic cells is undergoing ATRA-induced differentiation.[414] The symptoms include fever and dyspnea, often with pleural or pericardial infusions, resulting in acute respiratory distress. These symptoms resolve rapidly with appropriate steroid therapy, without stopping ATRA treatment (see Chapter 23).

Although data are limited, ATRA may have a role in the treatment of other types of leukemia. Preliminary data from leukemic cell lines and blast cells suggest that ATRA can decrease Bcl-2 protein levels by effects on gene transcription and protein stability. This renders cells more sensitive to the effects of cytotoxic chemotherapy. This mechanism is distinct from that involving the RARAα-PML fusion protein and thus is not restricted to patients with promyelocytic leukemia. Data from a randomized trial in patients with a poor prognosis for AML with oral ATRA given before and during standard chemotherapy did not confirm this effect,[415] but other trials are ongoing.

NOVEL APPROACHES

Most of the drugs used to treat leukemias, and other cancers, are typically poisons that cause lethal damage to DNA or to the mitotic spindle apparatus, thereby inducing apoptosis. This approach results in substantial damage to rapidly dividing normal tissues, which can be fatal. During the last few years, a number of novel chemotherapies have entered clinical trials that differ markedly from traditional cytotoxic drugs in that they target specific proteins or processes that altered in cancer cells. These drugs have arisen from the huge increase in understanding of the altered biology of cancer cells. There is not space in this chapter to review such approaches in detail, but some of these novel agents currently at the early clinical trial stage are highlighted to give an indication of the possibilities presented by such treatments.

Farnesyltransferase Inhibitors

Ras proteins play a key role in the transduction of signals from cell surface receptors to the nucleus. Binding of appropriate ligands to growth factor receptors results in the phosphorylation of tyrosine residues on the inner surface of the receptor. This activated receptor is then able to bind proteins that in turn bind guanine nucleotide exchange factors, such as the Sos protein, that can activate Ras by promoting the formation of a Ras-GTP complex. In the GTP-bound state, Ras activates Raf, the first in a cascade of proteins resulting in transduction of the signal from the cell surface to the nucleus. These are often mitogenic signals that lead to proliferation.

Mutations in *ras* genes are the most common genetic change in human cancers and are found in both solid tumors and leukemias.[416] These mutations result in an altered protein that favors the activated state, even in the absence of receptor binding, such that the signal cascade is inappropriately activated.

An important step in the synthesis of functional Ras proteins is a prenylation reaction involving either the addition of a 15-carbon farnesyl tail or a 20-carbon geranylgeranyl tail, with which the protein is anchored to the cell membrane. This is catalyzed by the enzymes farnesyltransferase and geranylgeranyltransferase, respectively. The membrane localization of Ras resulting from this modification is essential for activity and offers a clear therapeutic target for potentially switching off inappropriately activated Ras.[417]

There are at least three different Ras proteins, including Harvey Ras (H-Ras), Kirsten Ras (K-Ras), and N-Ras, first identified in a neuroblastoma cell line. H-Ras appears to be entirely dependent on farnesylation for membrane localization; K-Ras can use either the farnesyl or the geranylgeranyl pathway. Whereas this means that certain forms of Ras are more susceptible to farnesyltransferase inhibition than others are, this pathway has been focused on therapeutically because geranylation is the more common pathway for the activation of other cellular proteins and would thus be relatively less specific for Ras.[418]

Mutations of *ras* have been reported in up to 15% of patients with ALL, 44% of patients with AML, and 65% of patients with chronic myelomonocytic leukemia, although they are rare in CML.[416] Typically, these involve K-Ras and N-Ras proteins. A number of agents have been described that inhibit farnesyltransferase, and broadly these mimic either the farnesyl group or the cysteine terminus of the Ras protein that is the site of farnesylation. These have shown impressive activity in solid tumor preclinical models. Although data are more limited, there is also evidence showing activity in hematologic malignant neoplasms. For instance, an inhibitor that mimics the Ras-cysteine terminus has shown effects on Ras prenylation and/or antiproliferative activity in leukemic cell lines, murine myeloid leukemic models, and juvenile CML blast cells.[419, 420] This compound inhibited prenylation of H-Ras but not of K-Ras or N-Ras.[420]

A phase I trial in relapsed and refractory leukemias, using a different farnesyltransferase inhibitor, described clinical responses in 7 of 22 patients with relapsed, refractory AML (2 complete responses and 5 partial responses) and in 2 of 3 patients with CML in blast crisis (2 partial responses).[421] Intriguingly, responses were seen at dose levels at which there was little toxicity but also little effect on the farnesylation of surrogate proteins (lamin A and HDJ-2), suggesting that other proteins or pathways may be implicated. Moreover, although such agents show activity when they are used alone, there is evidence that the combined use of farnesyltransferase or geranylgeranyl-transferase inhibitors with conventional cytotoxic drugs is synergistic.[422, 423] Clearly, such compounds merit further investigation in hematologic malignant disease.

Protein Kinase Inhibitors

A number of compounds that inhibit protein kinases have entered clinical trials in recent years. Protein kinases play a crucial role in the control of many cellular processes by phosphorylating and thereby activating other proteins at specific sites, typically serine/threonine or tyrosine residues. Important processes in which kinases are involved are cell surface receptors activity, signal transduction cascades, and cell cycle regulation. Because these processes are often dysregulated in cancer cells, protein kinases provide a potential target for treatment. Therapeutic approaches have particularly focused on the inhibition of kinases involved in cell cycle regulation. The

progression of cells from one phase of the cell cycle to another, such as G_1 to S or G_2 to M, is largely controlled by a number of cyclin-dependent kinases (currently at least seven) that are activated by complexing to an appropriate cyclin partner (of which there are currently 15, cyclin A to cyclin T).[424, 425] Different cyclin-dependent kinases and cyclin partners control specific phases of the cell cycle. A large number of compounds that can inhibit specific cyclin-dependent kinases have been described, of which the most advanced are flavopiridol and UCN-01. Such compounds not only induce cell cycle arrest, and thereby block proliferation, but also result in apoptosis and possibly differentiation. Flavopiridol, for instance, inhibits a number of cyclin-dependent kinases and also decreases levels of cyclin D1, often increased in cancer cells.[424] This results in arrest at the G_1/S or G_2/M boundary, depending on the cell type and possibly other factors, such as the presence of functional retinoblastoma protein, which is the target of cyclin-dependent kinases at the G_1/S checkpoint, and the induction of apoptosis.

Hematopoietic cells may be particularly sensitive to flavopiridol-induced apoptosis, and this may bypass some of the proteins involved in initiating the apoptotic response to conventional cytotoxic drugs, such as p53 and Bcl-2.[426-429] In addition, flavopiridol has shown potent antileukemic activity in a mouse xenograft HL60 model, with clear evidence of apoptosis and complete, sustained, tumor regressions in most animals after a single flavopiridol treatment.[427] Further clinical trials with these agents in leukemic patients are ongoing. Other preclinical studies have reported an antiangiogenic effect with flavopiridol, perhaps related to vascular endothelial growth factor depletion,[430, 431] and possible synergy with standard cytotoxic drugs.[432] However, some of the effects reported for flavopiridol, at least in noncycling cells, may be attributable to DNA intercalation and direct DNA effects.[433]

BCR-ABL Tyrosine Kinase Inhibitor

Whereas flavopiridol inhibits a number of protein kinases, other compounds are specific for certain cyclin-dependent kinases or other kinases. For example, reports have described the activity of signal transduction inhibitor (STI)571 (imatinib, preclinically identified as CGP 57148), a specific and potent ABL tyrosine kinase inhibitor.[434] The *BCR/ABL* fusion oncoprotein, resulting from a 9;22 translocation, is found in the leukemic cells of the majority of patients with CML and in up to 50% of patients with ALL. This results in the constitutive activation of ABL tyrosine kinase, a crucial event in the transformation of these cells, with effects on a number of critical pathways including apoptosis and Ras signaling. Early preclinical reports suggested an antiproliferative effect in cells with the *BCR-ABL* translocation treated with STI571 but little effect on normal hematopoietic cells.[434, 435] Subsequent studies in BCR-ABL leukemia–bearing mice confirmed that short exposures to the compound resulted in inhibition of BCR-ABL kinase activity and the induction of apoptosis. Prolonged exposures of 11 days resulted in cures in the majority of animals.[436]

STI571 is currently undergoing evaluation in phase III

clinical trials, and preliminary reports describe complete hematologic responses in interferon-refractory patients with CML in the absence of other cytoreductive agents.[437] Interestingly, toxicity to normal tissue was minimal, suggesting that inhibition of ABL tyrosine kinase in normal cells is well tolerated. In patients who subsequently relapse on STI571, reactivation of the BCR-ABL pathway is a common finding, due either to a single amino acid change in the protein that affects drug binding or to further amplification of the BCR-ABL gene.[437a] These data demonstrate that inhibition of a single altered protein that is driving the malignant process may be sufficient to induce tumor responses. Such an approach acts as a paradigm for what may be achieved with such novel approaches.

Antiangiogenesis

The induction of new blood vessel formation (angiogenesis) is essential for solid tumors to develop beyond a few millimeters, at both the primary and metastatic sites.[438] This is mediated by angiogenic factors released by tumor cells, such as vascular endothelial growth factor (VEGF), basic fibroblast growth factor (bFGF), and thymidine phosphorylase, that are balanced in normal tissue by antiangiogenic factors, such as endostatin and angiostatin.[439] The importance of this process in the development of solid tumors has been clear for some time, but the relevance of angiogenesis in leukemias is much less well understood despite the fact that VEGF was first cloned from the leukemic cell line HL60.[440]

Recent evidence suggests that angiogenesis also plays a role in leukemias. In bone marrow samples from 40 newly diagnosed children with acute leukemia, microvessel density was markedly increased compared with normal age-matched control subjects, and urinary concentrations of the angiogenic bFGF were increased.[441] Similar studies in patients with AML also report increased bone marrow microvessel density compared with control subjects[442, 443] and the expression of VEGF and bFGF in AML cells.[443, 444] Moreover, in patients with AML achieving a complete remission, microvessel density dropped markedly but remained elevated in those with residual blast infiltration after induction chemotherapy.[442] Increased VEGF protein was also associated with decreased survival in a retrospective study using stored, pretreatment samples from 99 patients with AML.[445]

A number of agents that target tumor angiogenesis are currently undergoing early clinical trials, including some of the endogenous agents, such as endostatin, that generated much excitement in preclinical studies.[446, 447] Other agents include those targeting specific angiogenic receptors,[448] those that decrease VEGF,[431] and others that block binding of bFGF and VEGF to their respective receptors.[449] Although there are currently few data describing the use of such approaches in leukemias, the studies reporting a relationship between VEGF and outcome, for instance, suggest that they may have a role.

Histone Deacetylase Inhibitors

The retinoic acid receptor-α (RARAα) protein can recruit a co-repressor complex that represses gene transcription by altering the local chromatin structure.[408] An important component protein in this complex is histone deacetylase. Histones are small proteins that associate closely with DNA to form chromatin, and alterations to chromatin structure are important in controlling transcription. Deacetylated histones result in the chromatin adopting a more compact, closed structure that does not permit entry of the transcription machinery. In contrast, acetylated histones open up the chromatin, thereby making the DNA more accessible and allowing transcription to take place. These changes are catalyzed by histone deacetylases and histone acetyltransferase, respectively.

A number of compounds that for many years have been known to induce differentiation in leukemic cells have recently been shown to inhibit histone deacetylase, including butyric acid, sodium phenylbutyrate, and trichostatin. The best example of this is in leukemic cells with the RARAα-PLZF fusion protein, which does not respond to ATRA because the PLZF protein can also recruit a co-repressor complex. In APML cell lines with this translocation, differentiation can be induced by treatment with ATRA and a histone deacetylase inhibitor, such as trichostatin.[450, 451] A single case report in a child with ATRA-resistant APML describes a rapid, complete clinical and cytogenetic response when sodium pheylbutyrate was added to ATRA.[452] Although very much in its infancy, this approach has been termed transcriptional therapy[450] and may be particularly relevant to the treatment of leukemias.

The introduction of these newer approaches into the treatment of leukemias holds much promise for the future. Moreover, with mapping of the human genome and the identification of the proteins encoded by these genes and their function, many more therapeutic targets will emerge. Typically, these new agents are not crude poisons, do not induce DNA damage, and do not have the same toxicity profile as the more established cytotoxic drugs. Consequently, their development is likely to involve clinical endpoints different from those employed with current agents and presents challenges of how they can best be incorporated into treatment. The investigation of such compounds in leukemic patients also offers a model system in which their molecular pharmacodynamics can be more easily evaluated than in solid tumors.

CONCLUSION

Cytotoxic chemotherapy has had a major impact on the treatment of leukemias during the last 30 to 40 years, particularly childhood ALL. With the acute leukemias, this has evolved from active single agents to a rational, evidence-driven combination of agents, often involving postremission therapy and prolonged maintenance.

However, despite these successes, most patients with leukemia, particularly of adulthood, die of their disease, and new treatments are urgently required. The best hope of major improvements in outcome in the future possibly lies in novel approaches, and because leukemias tend to have fewer transforming alterations than solid tumors do, new drugs that target one or more of these altered pathways may be particularly useful. In addition, as more information on the molecular biology of leukemias becomes available, new therapeutic targets are certain to be identified.

It is to be hoped that these novel approaches, which often act synergistically with standard treatments, will have as much of an impact on the outcome of leukemia as did the introduction of conventional cytotoxic chemotherapy in the 1950s and 1960s.

REFERENCES

1. Gilman A, Philips FS: The biologic actions and therapeutic applications of β-dichloroethyl sulfide (mustard gas). Science 1946;103:409.
2. Krumbhaar EB, Krumbhaar HD: The blood and bone marrow in yellow cross gas (mustard gas) poisoning: Changes produced in the bone marrow of fatal cases. J Med Res 1919;40:497.
3. Gilman A: The initial clinical trial of nitrogen mustard. Am J Surg 1963;105:574.
4. Farber S, Diamond LK, Mercer RD, et al: Temporary remissions in acute leukemia in children produced by folic acid antagonist, 4-aminopterotl-glutamic acid (aminopterin). N Engl J Med 1948;238:787.
5. Krakoff IH: Cancer chemotherapeutic agents. CA Cancer J Clin 1987;37:93.
6. Grever MR, Chabner BA: Cancer drug discovery and development. In DeVita VT, Hellman S, Rosenberg SA (eds): Cancer: Principles and Practice of Oncology. Philadelphia: Lipincott-Raven; 1997.
7. Benet LZ, Mitchell JR, Scheiner LB: Pharmacokinetics: The dynamics of drug absorption, distribution and elimination. In Goodman LS, Gilman A (eds): The Pharmacological Basis of Therapeutics. New York: McGraw-Hill; 1991.
8. Gibaldi M: Biopharmaceutics and Clinical Pharmacokinetics. Baltimore: Williams & Wilkins; 1990.
9. Rowland M, Tozer TN: Clinical Pharmacokinetics: Concepts and Applications. Baltimore: Williams & Wilkins; 1995.
10. Ritshcel WA, Kearns GL: Handbook of Basic Clinical Pharmacokinetics. Washington, DC: American Pharmaceutical Association; 1999.
11. Shah JC, Chen JR, Chow D: Preformulation study of etoposide: Identification of physicochemical characteristics responsible for the low and erratic oral bioavailability of etoposide. Pharm Res 1989;6:408.
12. Barthe L, Woodley J, Houin G: Gastrointestinal absorption of drugs: Methods and studies. Fundam Clin Pharmacol 1999;13:154.
13. Adair CG, McElnay JC: Studies on the mechanism of gastrointestinal absorption of melphalan and chlorambucil. Cancer Chemother Pharmacol 1986;17:95.
14. Smith P, Mirabelli C, Fondacaro J, et al: Intestinal 5-fluorouracil absorption: Use of Ussing chambers to assess transport and metabolism. Pharm Res 1988;5:598.
15. Florence AT: The oral absorption of micro- and nanoparticulates: Neither exceptional nor unusual. Pharm Res 1997;14:259.
16. Gubbins PO, Bertch KE: Drug absorption in gastrointestinal disease and surgery. Clinical pharmacokinetic and therapeutic implications. Clin Pharmacokinet 1991;21:431.
17. Singh BN: Effects of food on clinical pharmacokinetics. Clin Pharmacokinet 1999;37:213.
18. Prescott LF: Gastric emptying and drug absorption. Br J Clin Pharmacol 1974;1:189.
19. Joel SP, Clark PI, Heap L, et al: Pharmacological attempts to improve the bioavailability of oral etoposide. Cancer Chemother Pharmacol 1995;37:125.
20. Nimmo J, Heading RC, Wilson J, et al: Inhibition of gastric emptying and drug absorption by narcotic analgesics. Br J Clin Pharmacol 1975;2:509.
21. Zhang JN, Liu XG, Zhu M, et al: Assessment of presystemic factors on the oral bioavailability of rifampicin following multiple dosing. J Chemother 1998;10:354.
22. Ito K, Kusuhara H, Sugiyama Y: Effects of intestinal CYP3A4 and P-glycoprotein on oral drug absorption—theoretical approach. Pharm Res 1999;16:225.
23. Paine MF, Schmiedlin-Ren P, Watkins PB: Cytochrome P-450 1A1 expression in human small bowel: Interindividual variation and inhibition by ketoconazole. Drug Metab Dispos 1999;27:360.
24. Lang CC, Brown RM, Kinirons MT, et al: Decreased intestinal CYP3A in celiac disease: Reversal after successful gluten-free diet: A potential source of interindividual variability in first-pass drug metabolism. Clin Pharmacol Ther 1996;59:41.
25. Schmiedlin-Ren P, Edwards DJ, Fitzsimmons ME, et al: Mechanisms of enhanced oral availability of CYP3A4 substrates by grapefruit constituents. Decreased enterocyte CYP3A4 concentration and mechanism-based inactivation by furanocoumarins. Drug Metab Dispos 1997;25:1228.
26. Backman JT, Olkkola KT, Neuvonen PJ: Rifampin drastically reduces plasma concentrations and effects of oral midazolam. Clin Pharmacol Ther 1996;59:7.
27. Hahn RG, Moertel CG, Schutt AJ, et al: A double-blind comparison of intensive course 5-fluorouracil by oral vs. intravenous route in the treatment of colorectal carcinoma. Cancer 1975;35:1031.
28. Harvey VJ, Slevin ML, Joel SP, et al: Variable bioavailability following repeated oral doses of etoposide. Eur J Cancer Clin Oncol 1985;21:1315.
29. Collins JM: Pharmacokinetics and clinical monitoring. In Chabner BA, Longo DL (eds): Cancer Chemotherpy and Biotherapy, 2nd ed. Philadelphia: Lippincott-Raven; 1996, p 17.
30. Savaraj N, Lu K, Manuel V, et al: Pharmacology of mitoxantrone in cancer patients. Cancer Chemother Pharmacol 1982;8:113.
31. Alberts DS, Peng YM, Leigh S, et al: Disposition of mitoxantrone in patients. Cancer Treat Rev 1983;10:23.
32. Sitar DS: Human drug metabolism in vivo. Pharmacol Ther 1989;43:363.
33. Kivisto KT, Kroemer HK, Eichelbaum M: The role of human cytochrome P450 enzymes in the metabolism of anticancer agents: Implications for drug interactions. Br J Clin Pharmacol 1995;40:523.
34. Lin JH, Lu AY: Inhibition and induction of cytochrome P450 and the clinical implications. Clin Pharmacokinet 1998;35:361.
35. Bailey DG, Malcolm J, Arnold O, et al: Grapefruit juice–drug interactions. Br J Clin Pharmacol 1998;46:101.
36. Osborne R, Thompson P, Joel S, et al: The analgesic activity of morphine-6-glucuronide. Br J Clin Pharmacol 1992;34:130.
37. Andersen V, Sonne J, Larsen S: Antipyrine, oxazepam, and indocyanine green clearance in patients with chronic pancreatitis and healthy subjects. Scand J Gastroenterol 1999;34:813.
38. Tanaka E: Clinical importance of non-genetic and genetic cytochrome P450 function tests in liver disease. J Clin Pharm Ther 1998;23:161.
39. Adedoyin A, Arns PA, Richards WO, et al: Selective effect of liver disease on the activities of specific metabolizing enzymes: Investigation of cytochromes P450, 2C19 and 2D6. Clin Pharmacol Ther 1998;64:8.
40. Frye RF, Matzke GR, Adedoyin A, et al: Validation of the five-drug "Pittsburgh cocktail" approach for assessment of selective regulation of drug-metabolizing enzymes. Clin Pharmacol Ther 1997;62:365.
41. Canal P, Chatelut E, Guichard S: Practical treatment guide for dose individualisation in cancer chemotherapy. Drugs 1998;56:1019.
42. Lichtman SM: Physiological aspects of aging. Implications for the treatment of cancer. Drugs Aging 1995;7:212.
43. Stein BN, Petrelli NJ, Douglass HO, et al: Age and sex are independent predictors of 5-fluorouracil toxicity. Analysis of a large scale phase III trial. Cancer 1995;75:11.
44. Williams L, Lowenthal DT: Drug therapy in the elderly. South Med J 1992;85:127.
45. Joel S, Shah R, Clark P, et al: Predicting etoposide toxicity: Relationship to organ function and protein binding. J Clin Oncol 1996;14:257.
46. Kaufman D, Chabner BA: Clinical strategies for cancer treatment: The role of drugs. In Chabner BA, Longo DL (eds): Cancer Chemotherapy and Biotherapy, 2nd ed. Philadelphia: Lippincott-Raven; 1996, p 1.
47. Ferrazzini G, Sohl H, Robieux I, et al: Diurnal variation of methotrexate disposition in children with acute leukaemia. Eur J Clin Pharmacol 1991;41:425.
48. Relling MV: Are the major effects of P-glycoprotein modulators due to altered pharmacokinetics of anticancer drugs? Ther Drug Monit 1996;18:350.

49. Pitman SW, Frei E 3rd: Weekly methotrexate-calcium leucovorin rescue: Effect of alkalinization on nephrotoxicity; pharmacokinetics in the CNS; and use in CNS non-Hodgkin's lymphoma. Cancer Treat Rep 1977;61:695.

50. LeBlanc GA: Hepatic vectorial transport of xenobiotics. Chem Biol Interact 1994;90:101.

51. Rollins DE, Klaassen CD: Biliary excretion of drugs in man. Clin Pharmacokinet 1979;4:368.

52. Levine WG: Biliary excretion of drugs and other xenobiotics. Annu Rev Pharmacol Toxicol 1978;18:81.

53. Grochow LB, Baraldi C, Noe D: Is dose normalization to weight or body surface area useful in adults? J Natl Cancer Inst 1990; 82:323.

54. Rodman JH, Abromowitch M, Sinkule JA, et al: Clinical pharmacodynamics of continuous infusion teniposide: Systemic exposure as a determinant of response in a phase I trial. J Clin Oncol 1987; 5:1007.

55. Fety R, Rolland F, Barberi-Heyob M, et al: Clinical impact of pharmacokinetically-guided dose adaptation of 5-fluorouracil: Results from a multicentric randomized trial in patients with locally advanced head and neck carcinomas. Clin Cancer Res 1998;4: 2039.

56. Evans WE, Relling MV, Rodman JH, et al: Conventional compared with individualized chemotherapy for childhood acute lymphoblastic leukemia. N Engl J Med 1998;338:499.

57. Hongo T, Yajima S, Sakurai M, et al: In vitro drug sensitivity testing can predict induction failure and early relapse of childhood acute lymphoblastic leukemia. Blood 1997;89:2959.

58. Kaspers GJ, Veerman AJ, Pieters R, et al: In vitro cellular drug resistance and prognosis in newly diagnosed childhood acute lymphoblastic leukemia. Blood 1997;90:2723.

59. Goldie JH, Coldman AJ: A mathematical model for relating the drug sensitivity of tumours to their spontaneous mutation rate. Cancer Treat Rep 1979;63:1729.

60. Skipper HE: The effects of chemotherapy on the kinetics of leukemic cell behavior. Cancer Res 1965;25:1544.

61. Skipper HE, Schabel FMJ, Wilcox WS: Experimental evaluation of potential anticancer agents. XII. On the criteria and kinetics associated with the "curability" of experimental leukaemia. Cancer Chemother Rep 1964;35:1.

62. Dicker AP, Waltham MC, Volkenandt M, et al: Methotrexate resistance in an in vivo mouse tumor due to a non-active-site dihydrofolate reductase mutation. Proc Natl Acad Sci U S A 1993;90:11797.

63. Owens JK, Shewach DS, Ullman B, et al: Resistance to 1-beta-D-arabinofuranosylcytosine in human T-lymphoblasts mediated by mutations within the deoxycytidine kinase gene. Cancer Res 1992; 52:2389.

64. Kinsella AR, Smith D, Pickard M: Resistance to chemotherapeutic antimetabolites: A function of salvage pathway involvement and cellular response to DNA damage. Br J Cancer 1997;75:935.

65. Mao Y, Yu C, Hsieh TS, et al: Mutations of human topoisomerase II alpha affecting multidrug resistance and sensitivity. Biochemistry 1999;38:10793.

66. Hinds M, Deisseroth K, Mayes J, et al: Identification of a point mutation in the topoisomerase II gene from a human leukemia cell line containing an amsacrine-resistant form of topoisomerase II. Cancer Res 1991;51:4729.

67. Cabral F, Barlow SB: Resistance to antimitotic agents as genetic probes of microtubule structure and function. Pharmacol Ther 1991;52:159.

68. Banerjee D, Ercikan-Abali E, Waltham M, et al: Molecular mechanisms of resistance to antifolates: A review. Acta Biochim Pol 1995;42:457.

69. Copur S, Aiba K, Drake JC, et al: Thymidylate synthase gene amplification in human colon cancer cell lines resistant to 5-fluorouracil. Biochem Pharmacol 1995;49:1419.

70. Lenz HJ, Leichman CG, Danenberg KD, et al: Thymidylate synthase mRNA level in adenocarcinoma of the stomach: A predictor for primary tumor response and overall survival. J Clin Oncol 1996; 14:176.

71. Gorlick R, Cole P, Banerjee D, et al: Mechanisms of methotrexate resistance in acute leukemia. Decreased transport and polyglutamylation. Adv Exp Med Biol 1999;457:543.

72. Doyle L: Topoisomerase II expression in cancer cell lines and clinical samples. Cancer Chemother Pharmacol 1994;34:S32.

73. Endicott JA, Ling V: The biochemistry of P-glycoprotein-mediated multidrug resistance. Annu Rev Biochem 1989;58:137.

74. Shapiro AB, Ling V: Reconstitution of drug transport by purified P-glycoprotein. J Biol Chem 1995;270:16167.

75. Dalton WS, Grogan TM, Rybski JA: Immunohistochemical detection and quantitation of P-glycoprotein in multiple drug-resistant human myeloma cells: Association with level of drug resistance and drug accumulation. Blood 1989;73:747.

76. List AF: Role of multidrug resistance and its pharmacological modulation in acute myeloid leukemia. Leukemia 1996;10:937.

77. Marie JP, Legrand O: MDR1/P-GP expression as a prognostic factor in acute leukemias. Adv Exp Med Biol 1999;457:1.

78. Kaye SB: Multidrug resistance: Clinical relevance in solid tumors and strategies for circumvention. Curr Opin Oncol 1998;10:S15.

79. Lowenberg B, Sonneveld P: Resistance to chemotherapy in acute leukemia. Curr Opin Oncol 1998;10:31.

80. Lum BL, Kaubisch S, Yahanda AM, et al: Alteration of etoposide pharmacokinetics and pharmacodynamics by cyclosporine in a phase I trial to modulate multidrug resistance. J Clin Oncol 1992; 10:1635.

81. Giaccone G, Linn SC, Welink J, et al: A dose-finding and pharmacokinetic study of reversal of multidrug resistance with SDZ PSC 833 in combination with doxorubicin in patients with solid tumors. Clin Cancer Res 1997;3:2005.

82. Cole SP, Bhardwaj G, Gerlach JH, et al: Overexpression of a transporter gene in a multidrug-resistant human lung cancer cell line. Science 1992;258:1650.

83. Rappa G, Finch RA, Sartorelli AC, et al: New insights into the biology and pharmacology of the multidrug resistance protein (MRP) from gene knockout models. Biochem Pharmacol 1999; 58:557.

84. Borst P, Kool M, Evers R: Do cMOAT (MRP2), other MRP homologues, and LRP play a role in MDR? Semin Cancer Biol 1997; 8:205.

85. Filipits M, Stranzl T, Pohl G, et al: MRP expression in acute myeloid leukemia: An update. Adv Exp Med Biol 1999;457:141.

86. Schuurhuis GJ, Broxterman HJ, Ossenkoppele GJ, et al: Functional multidrug resistance phenotype associated with combined overexpression of Pgp/MDR1 and MRP together with 1-beta-D-arabinofuranosylcytosine sensitivity may predict clinical response in acute myeloid leukemia. Clin Cancer Res 1995;1:81.

87. Vezmar M, Georges E: Reversal of MRP-mediated doxorubicin resistance with quinoline-based drugs. Biochem Pharmacol 2000; 59:1245.

88. Curtin NJ, Turner DP: Dipyridamole-mediated reversal of multidrug resistance in MRP overexpressing human lung carcinoma cells in vitro. Eur J Cancer 1999;35:1020.

89. Payen L, Delugin L, Courtois A, et al: Reversal of MRP-mediated multidrug resistance in human lung cancer cells by the antiprogestatin drug RU486. Biochem Biophys Res Commun 1999;258:513.

90. Scheffer GL, Wijngaard PL, Flens MJ, et al: The drug resistance-related protein LRP is a major vault protein. Nat Med 1995;1:578.

91. Izquierdo MA, Scheffer GL, Flens MJ, et al: Relationship of LRP-human major vault protein to in vitro and clinical resistance to anticancer drugs. Cytotechnology 1996;19:191.

92. Pirker R, Pohl G, Stranzl T, et al: The lung resistance protein (LRP) predicts poor outcome in acute myeloid leukemia. Adv Exp Med Biol 1999;457:133.

93. Filipits M, Drach J, Pohl G, et al: Expression of the lung resistance protein predicts poor outcome in patients with multiple myeloma. Clin Cancer Res 1999;5:2426.

94. Coleman CN, Bump EA, Kramer RA: Chemical modifiers of cancer treatment. J Clin Oncol 1988;6:709.

95. Tew KD: Glutathione-associated enzymes in anticancer drug resistance. Cancer Res 1994;54:4313.

96. Salinas AE, Wong MG: Glutathione S-transferases—a review. Curr Med Chem 1999;6:279.

97. Anderson ME: Glutathione: An overview of biosynthesis and modulation. Chem Biol Interact 1998;111–112:1.

98. Calvert P, Yao KS, Hamilton TC, et al: Clinical studies of reversal of drug resistance based on glutathione. Chem Biol Interact 1998; 111–112:213.

99. Hartwell LH, Kastan MB: Cell cycle control and cancer. Science 1994;266:1821.

100. Roemer K: Mutant p53: Gain-of-function oncoproteins and wild-type p53 inactivators. Biol Chem 1999;380:879.

101. Lowe SW, Ruley HE, Jacks T, et al: p53-Dependent apoptosis modulates the cytotoxicity of anticancer agents. Cell 1993;74:957.
102. Bunz F, Hwang PM, Torrance C, et al: Disruption of p53 in human cancer cells alters the responses to therapeutic agents. J Clin Invest 1999;104:263.
103. Burt RK, Poirier MC, Link CJ Jr, et al: Antineoplastic drug resistance and DNA repair. Ann Oncol 1991;2:325.
104. Link CJ Jr, Bohr VA: DNA repair in drug resistance: Studies on the repair process at the level of the gene. Cancer Treat Res 1991; 57:209.
105. Fox M, Roberts JJ: Drug resistance and DNA repair. Cancer Metastasis Rev 1987;6:261.
106. Gerson SL, Schupp J, Liu L, et al: Leukocyte O⁶-alkylguanine-DNA alkyltransferase from human donors is uniformly sensitive to O⁶-benzylguanine. Clin Cancer Res 1999;5:521.
107. Lage H, Dietel M: Involvement of the DNA mismatch repair system in antineoplastic drug resistance. J Cancer Res Clin Oncol 1999; 125:156.
108. Reed JC: Dysregulation of apoptosis in cancer. J Clin Oncol 1999; 17:2941.
109. Kroemer G, Reed JC: Mitochondrial control of cell death. Nat Med 2000;6:513.
110. Reed JC: Bcl-2 family proteins: Regulators of apoptosis and chemoresistance in hematologic malignancies. Semin Hematol 1997; 34:9.
111. Reed JC: Bcl-2: Prevention of apoptosis as a mechanism of drug resistance. Hematol Oncol Clin North Am 1995;9:451.
112. Cotter FE: Antisense therapy for lymphomas. Hematol Oncol 1997; 15:3.
113. de Vita VT: Principles of cancer management. In de Vita VT, Hellman S, Rosenberg SA (eds): Cancer: Principles and Practice of Oncology, 5th ed. Philadelphia: Lippincott-Raven; 1997, p 333.
114. Jackson RC, Karkrader RJ: The contribution of de novo and salvage pathways of nucleotide biosynthesis in normal and malignant cells. In Tattersall MHN, Fox RM (eds): Nucleosides and Cancer Treatment. Sydney: Academic Press; 1981, p 18.
115. Pratt WB, Ruddon RW, Ensminger WD, et al: The Anticancer Drugs, 2nd ed. Oxford: Oxford University Press; 1994.
116. Allegra CJ: Antifolates. In Chabner BA, Longo DL (eds): Cancer Chemotherapy and Biotherapy: Principles and Practice. Philadelphia: Lippincott-Raven; 1996, p 109.
117. Allegra CJ, Hoang K, Yeh GC, et al: Evidence for direct inhibition of de novo purine synthesis in human MCF-7 breast cells as a principal mode of metabolic inhibition by methotrexate. J Biol Chem 1987;262:13520.
118. Antony AC: The biological chemistry of folate receptors. Blood 1992;79:2807.
119. Goldman ID, Lichtenstein NS, Oliverio VT: Carrier-mediated transport of the folic acid analogue, methotrexate, in L1210 leukemia cells. J Biol Chem 1968;243:5007.
120. Elwood PC: Molecular cloning and characterization of the human folate binding protein cDNA from placenta and malignant tissue culture (KB) cells. J Biol Chem 1989;264:14893.
121. Sirotnak FM, Moccio DM, Kelleher LE, et al: Relative frequency and kinetic properties of transport defective phenotypes among methotrexate-resistant L1210 clonal cell lines derived in vivo. Cancer Res 1981;41:4447.
122. Matherly LH, Angeles SM, Czajkowski CA: Characterization of transport-mediated methotrexate resistance in human tumor cells with antibodies to the membrane carrier for methotrexate and tetrahydrofolate cofactors. J Biol Chem 1992;267:23253.
123. Jansen G, Westerhof GR, Jarmuszewski MJ, et al: Methotrexate transport in variant human CCRF-CEM leukemia cells with elevated levels of the reduced folate carrier. J Biol Chem 1990; 265:18272.
124. Warren RD, Nichols AP, Bender RA: Membrane transport of methotrexate in human lymphoblastoid cells. Cancer Res 1978;33:668.
125. Trippett T, Schlemmer S, Elisseyeff Y, et al: Defective transport as a mechanism of acquired resistance in patients with acute lymphoblastic leukemia. Blood 1992;80:1158.
126. Mini E, Moroson BA, Franco CT, et al: Cytotoxic effects of folate antagonists against methotrexate-resistant human leukemic lymphoblast CCRF-CEM cells. Cancer Res 1985;45:325.
127. Seither RL, Rape TJ, Goldman ID: Further studies on the pharmacologic effects of the 7-hydroxy catabolite of methotrexate in L1210 murine leukemia cells. Biochem Pharmacol 1989;38:815.
128. Fabre I, Babre G, Goldman ID: Polyglutamylation, an important element in methotrexate cytotoxicity and selectivity in tumor versus murine granulocytic progenitor cells in vitro. Cancer Res 1984;44:3190.
129. Galivan J, Johnson T, Rhee M, et al: The role of folypolyglutamaote synthetase and gamma-glutamyl hydrolase in altering cellular folyl- and anti-folyl polyglutamates. Adv Enzyme Regul 1987;26:147.
130. Rodenhuis S, McGuire JJ, Narayanan R, et al: Development of an assay system for the detection and classification of methotrexate resistance in fresh human leukemic cells. Cancer Res 1986;46: 6513.
131. Allegra CJ, Drake JC, Jolivet J, et al: Inhibition of folate-dependent enzymes by methotrexate polyglutamates. In Goldman ID (ed): Proceedings of Second Workshop on Folyl and Antifolyl Polyglutamates. New York: Praeger; 1985, p 348.
132. Chu E, Takimoto CH, Voeller D, et al: Specific binding of human dihydrofolate reductase protein to dihydrofolate reductase messenger RNA in vitro. Biochemistry 1993;32:4756.
133. Jackson RC, Hart LI, Harrap KR: Intrinsic resistance to methotrexate of cultured mammalian cells in relation to the inhibition kinetics of dihydrofolate reductase. Cancer Res 1980;36:1991.
134. Dedhar S, Hartley D, Fitzgibbons D, et al: Heterogeneity in the specific activity and methotrexate sensitivity of dihydrofolate reductase from blast cells of acute myelogenous leukemia patients. J Clin Oncol 1985;3:1545.
135. Srimatkandada S, Schweitzer BI, Moroson BA, et al: Amplification of a polymorphine dihydrofolate reductase gene expressing an enzyme with decreased binding to methotrexate in a human colon carcinoma line resistant to the drug. J Biol Chem 1989;264:3524.
136. Stuart JFB, Calman KC, Watters J, et al: Bioavailability of methotrexate: Implications for clinical use. Cancer Chemother Pharmacol 1979;3:329.
137. Balis FM, Savitch JL, Bleyer WA: Pharmacokinetics of oral methotrexate in children. Cancer Res 1983;43:2342.
138. Chabner BA, Stoller RG, Hande KR, et al: Methotrexate disposition in humans: Case studies in ovarian cancer and following high-dose infusion. Drug Metab Rev 1978;8:107.
139. Jacobs SA, Stoller RG, Chabner BA, et al: 7-Hydroxy methotrexate as a urinary metabolite in human subjects and rhesus monkeys receiving high-dose methotrexate. J Clin Invest 1976;57:534.
140. Evans WE, Crom WR, Abromowitch M, et al: Clinical pharmacodynamics of high-dose methotrexate in acute lymphocytic leukemia: Identification of a relation between concentration and effect. N Engl J Med 1986;314:471.
141. Bergmann W, Feeney R: Contributions to the study of marine products. XXXII. The nucleosides of sponges. J Org Chem 1951; 16:981.
142. Plunkett W, Liliemark JO, Estey E, et al: Saturation of ara-CTP accumulation during high-dose ara-C therapy: Pharmacologic rationale for intermediate-dose ara-C. Semin Oncol 1987;14:159.
143. Jamieson GP, Snook MB, Wiley JS: Saturation of intracellular cytosine arabinoside triphosphate transport accumulation in human leukaemic blast cells. Leuk Res 1990;14:475.
144. Chabner BA: Cytidine analogues. In Chabner BA, Longo DL (eds): Cancer Chemotherapy and Biotherapy: Principles and Practice, 2nd ed. Philadelphia: Lippincott-Raven; 1996, p 213.
145. Gandhi V, Plunkett W: Cell cycle metabolism of arabinosyl nucleosides in K562 human leukaemic cells. Cancer Chemother Pharmacol 1992;31:11.
146. Chabner BA, John D, Coleman C: Purification and properties of cytidine deaminase from normal and leukemic granulocytes. J Clin Invest 1974;53:922.
147. Chou T-C, Arlin Z, Clarkson BD, et al: Metabolism of 1-beta-D-arabinofuranosylcytosine in human leukemic cells. Cancer Res 1977;37:3651.
148. White JC, Rathmell JP, Capizzi RL: Membrane trasport influences the accumulation of cytosine arabinoside in human leukemia cells. J Clin Invest 1987;79:380.
149. Townsend AJ, Cheng YC: Sequence-specific effects of ara-5-aza-CTP and ara-CTP on DNA synthesis by purified human DNA polymerases in vitro: Visualization of chain elongation on a defined template. Mol Pharmacol 1987;32:330.
150. Fram RJ, Kufe DW: DNA strand breaks caused by inhibitors of DNA synthesis: 1-beta-D-arabinofuranosylcytosine and aphidicolin. Cancer Res 1982;42:4050.

151. Ross ED, Chen SRS, Cuddy DP: Effects of 1-beta-D-arabinofuranosyl-cytosine on DNA replication intermediates monitored by pH-step alkaline elution. Cancer Res 1990;50:2658.

152. Mikita T, Beardsley GP: Functional consequences of the arabinosyl-cytosine structural lesion in DNA. Biochemistry 1988;27:4698.

153. Grem JL, Geoffroy F, Politi PM, et al: Determinants of sensitivity to 1-beta-D-arabinofuranosylcytosine in human colon carcinoma cell lines. Mol Pharmacol 1995;48:305.

154. Richel DJ, Colly LP, Arkesteijn GJA, et al: Substrate-specific deoxy-cytidine kinase deficiency in 1-beta-D-arabinofuranosylcytosine-resistant leukemic cells. Cancer Res 1990;50:6515.

155. Plunkett W, Iacoboni S, Estey E, et al: Pharmacologically directed ara-C therapy for refractory leukemia. Semin Oncol 1985;12:20.

156. Rustum UM, Riva C, Preisler HD: Pharmacokinetic parameters of 1-beta-D-arabinofuranosylcytosine (ara-C) and their relationship to intracellular metabolism of ara-C, toxicity, and response of patients with acute nonlymphocytic leukemia treated with conventional and high-dose ara-C. Semin Oncol 1987;14:141.

157. Rudnick SA, Cadman EC, Capizzi RL, et al: High dose cytosine arabinoside (HDARAC) in refractory acute leukemia. Cancer 1979;44:1189.

158. Capizzi RI, White JC, Powell BL, et al: Effect of dose on the pharmacokinetic and pharmacodynamic effects of cytarabine. Semin Hematol 1991;28:54.

159. Gandhi V, Kemena A, Keating MJ, et al: Fludarabine infusion potentiates arabinosylcytosine metabolism in lymphocytes of patients with chronic lymphocytic leukemia. Cancer Res 1992;52:897.

160. Ho DHW, Frei EI: Clinical pharmacology of 1-beta-D-arabinofuranosylcytosine. Clin Pharmacol Ther 1971;12:944.

161. Damon LE, Plunkett W, Linker CA: Plasma and cerebrospinal fluid pharmacokinetics of 1-beta-arabinofuranosylcytosine and 1-beta-D-arabinofuranosyluracil following the repeated intravenous administration of high- and intermediate-dose 1-beta-D-arabinofuranosylcytosine. Cancer Res 1991;51:4141.

162. Donehower RC, Karp JE, Burke PJ: Pharmacology and toxicity of high-dose cytarabine by 72-hour continuous infusion. Cancer Treat Rep 1986;70:1059.

163. Beran M, Hittelman WM, Anderson BS: Induction of differentiation in human myeloid leukaemic cells with cytosine arabinoside. Leuk Res 1986;10:1033.

164. Raijmakers R, de Witte T, Linssen P, et al: The relation of exposure time and drug concentration in their effect on cloning efficiency after incubation of human bone marrow with cytosine arabinoside. Br J Haematol 1986;62:447.

165. Rohatiner AZ, Bassan R, Battista R, et al: High dose cytosine arabinoside in the initial treatment of adults with acute lymphoblastic leukaemia. Br J Cancer 1990;62:454.

166. Barnett MJ, Greaves MF, Amess JA, et al: Treatment of acute lymphoblastic leukaemia in adults. Br J Haematol 1986;64:455.

167. Glover AB, Leyland Jones B: Biochemistry of azacitidine: A review. Cancer Treat Rep 1987;71:959.

168. Gabbara S, Bhagwat AS: The mechanism of inhibition of DNA (cytosine-5-)-methyltransferases by 5-azacytosine is likely to involve methyl transfer to the inhibitor. Biochem J 1995;307:87.

169. Jones PA: Effects of 5-azacytidine and its 2′-deoxyderivative on cell differentiation and DNA methylation. Pharmacol Ther 1985;28:17.

170. Bellet RE, Mastrangelo MJ, Engstrom PF, et al: Hepatotoxicity of 5-azacytidine (NSC-102816) (a clinical and pathologic study). Neoplasma 1973;20:303.

171. Heinemann V, Hertel LW, Grindey GB, et al: Comparison of the cellular pharmacokinetics and toxicity of 2′,2′-difluorodeoxycytidine and 1-beta-D-arabinofuranosylcytosine. Cancer Res 1988;48:4024.

172. Heinemann V, Xu YZ, Chubb S, et al: Cellular elimination of 2′,2′-difluorodeoxycytidine 5′-triphosphate: A mechanism of self-potentiation. Cancer Res 1992;52:533.

173. Kaye SB: Gemcitabine: Current status of phase I and II trials. J Clin Oncol 1994;12:1527.

174. Grunewald R, Kantarjian H, Du M, et al: Gemcitabine in leukemia: A phase I clinical, plasma, and cellular pharmacology study. J Clin Oncol 1992;10:406.

175. Gandhi V, Plunkett W: Modulatory activity of 2′,2′-difluorodeoxycytidine on the phosphorylation and cytotoxicity of arabinosyl nucleosides. Cancer Res 1990;50:3675.

176. Heidelberger C, Chaudhari NK, Dannenberg P, et al: Fluorinated pyrimidines: A new class of tumor inhibitory compounds. Nature 1957;179:663.

177. Grem JL: 5-Fluoropyrimidines. In Chabner BA, Longo DL (eds): Cancer Chemotherapy and Biotherapy: Principles and Practice, 2nd ed. Philadelphia: Lippincott-Raven; 1996, p 149.

178. Grem JL, Hoth D, Hamilton MJ, et al: An overview of the current status and future directions of clinical trials of 5-fluorouracil and folinic acid. Cancer Treat Rep 1987;71:1249.

179. Sobrero AF, Aschele C, Bertino JR: Fluorouracil in colorectal cancer—a tale of two drugs: Implications for biochemical modulation. J Clin Oncol 1997;15:368.

180. Johnston PG, Lenz HJ, Leichman CG, et al: Thymidylate synthase gene and protein expression correlate and are associated with response to 5-fluorouracil in human colorectal and gastric tumors. Cancer Res 1995;55:1407.

181. Hande KR, Garrow GC: Purine antimetabolites. In Chabner BA, Longo DL (eds): Cancer Chemotherapy and Biotherapy: Principles and Practice, 2nd ed. Philadelphia: Lippincott-Raven; 1996, p 235.

182. Bokkerink JP, Stet EH, De Abreu RA, et al: 6-Mercaptopurine: Cytotoxicity and biochemical pharmacology in human malignant T-lymphoblasts. Biochem Pharmacol 1993;45:1455.

183. Ling YH, Chan JY, Beattie KL, et al: Consequences of 6-thioguanine incorporation into DNA on polymerase, ligase, and endonuclease reactions. Mol Pharmacol 1992;42:802.

184. Krynetskaia NF, Krynetski EY, Evans WE: Human RNase H-mediated RNA cleavage from DNA-RNA duplexes is inhibited by 6-deoxythioguanosine incorporation into DNA. Mol Pharmacol 1999;56:841.

185. Koren G, Ferrazini G, Sulh H, et al: Systemic exposure to mercaptopurine as a prognostic factor in acute lymphocytic leukemia in children. N Engl J Med 1990;323:17.

186. Lilleyman JS, Lennard L: Mercaptopurine metabolism and risk of relapse in childhood lymphoblastic leukaemia. Lancet 1994;343:1188.

187. Davies HA, Lennard L, Lilleyman JS: Variable mercaptopurine metabolism in children with leukaemia: A problem of noncompliance? BMJ 1993;306:1239.

188. Zimm S, Collins JM, O'Neill D, et al: Chemotherapy: Inhibition of first-pass metabolism in cancer interaction of 6-mercaptopurine and allopurinol. Clin Pharmacol Ther 1983;34:810.

189. Lennard L: Clinical implications of thiopurine methyl-transferase—optimization of drug dosage and potential drug interactions. Ther Drug Monit 1998;20:527.

190. Lennard L, Lilleyman JS, Van Loon J, et al: Genetic variation in response to 6-mercaptopurine for childhood acute lymphoblastic leukaemia. Lancet 1990;336:225.

191. Lockhart S, Plunkett W, Jeha S, et al: High-dose mercaptopurine followed by intermediate-dose cytarabine in relapsed acute leukemia. J Clin Oncol 1994;12:587.

192. Pinkel D: Intravenous mercaptopurine: Life begins at 40. J Clin Oncol 1993;11:1826.

193. Montgomery JA, Hewson K: Nucleosides of 2-fluoroadenine. J Med Chem 1969;12:498.

194. Brockman RW, Schabel FM, Montgomery JA: Biological activity of 9-beta-D-arabinofuranosyl-2-fluoroadenine, a metabolically stable analog of 9-beta-D-arabinofuranosyladenine. Biochem Pharmacol 1977;26:2193.

195. Huang P, Chubb S, Plunkett W: Termination of DNA synthesis by 9-beta-D-arabinofuranosyl-2-fluoroadenine. A mechanism for cytotoxicity. J Biol Chem 1990;265:16617.

196. Plunkett W, Huang P, Gandhi V: Metabolism and action of fludarabine phosphate. Semin Oncol 1990;17:3.

197. Huang P, Plunkett W: Action of 9-beta-D-arabinofuranosyl-2-fluoroadenine on RNA metabolism. Mol Pharmacol 1991;39:449.

198. Parker WB, Bapat AR, Shen JX, et al: Interaction of 2-halogenated dATP analogues (F, Cl, and Br) with human DNA polymerases, DNA primase and ribonucleotide reductase. Mol Pharmacol 1988;34:845.

199. Plunkett W, Gandhi V: Cellular metabolism of nucleoside analogs in CLL: Implications for drug development. In Cheson BD (ed): Chronic Lymphocytic Leukemia: Scientific Advances and Clinical Developments. New York: Marcel Dekker; 1993, p 197.

200. Keating MJ, McLaughlin P, Plunkett W, et al: Fludarabine—present status and future developments in chronic lymphocytic leukemia and lymphoma. Ann Oncol 1994;5:79.

201. Foran JM, Oscier D, Orchard J, et al: Pharmacokinetic study of single doses of oral fludarabine phosphate in patients with "low-grade" non-Hodgkin's lymphoma and B-cell chronic lymphocytic leukemia. J Clin Oncol 1999;17:1574.

202. Malspeis L, Grever MR, Staubus AE, et al: Pharmacokinetics of 2-F-ara-A (9-beta-D-arabinofuranosyl-2-fluoroadenine) in cancer patients during the phase I clinical investigation of fludarabine phosphate. Semin Oncol 1990;17:18.

203. Hersh MR, Kuhn JG, Phillips JL, et al: Pharmacokinetic study of fludarabine phosphate (NSC 312887). Cancer Chemother Pharmacol 1986;17:277.

204. Plunkett W, Saunders PP: Metabolism and action of purine nucleoside analogues. Pharmacol Ther 1991;49:239.

205. Griffig J, Koob R, Blakley RL: Mechanisms of inhibition of DNA synthesis by 2-chlorodeoxyadenosine in human lymphoblastic cells. Cancer Res 1989;49:6923.

206. Donehower RC: Hydroxyurea. In Chabner BA, Longo DL (eds): Cancer Chemotherapy and Biotherapy: Principles and Practice, 2nd ed. Philadelphia: Lippincott-Raven; 1996, p 253.

207. Thelander L, Reichard P: Reduction of ribonucleotides. Annu Rev Biochem 1979;48:133.

208. Graslund A, Ehrenberg A, Thelander L: Characterization of the free radical of mammalian ribonucleotide reductase. J Biol Chem 1982;257:5711.

209. Bianchi V, Pontis E, Reichard P: Changes in deoxyribonucleoside triphosphate pools induced by hydroxyurea and their relation to DNA synthesis. J Biol Chem 1986;261:16037.

210. Reddy GP, Pardee AB: Inhibitor evidence for allosteric interaction in the replitase multienzyme complex. Nature 1983;304:86.

211. Plucinski TM, Fager RS, Reddy GP: Allosteric interaction of components of the replitase complex is responsible for enzyme cross-inhibition. Mol Pharmacol 1990;38:114.

212. Choy BK, McClarty GA, Chan AK, et al: Molecular mechanisms of drug resistance involving ribonucleotide reductase: Hydroxyurea resistance in a series of clonally related mouse cell lines selected in the presence of increasing drug concentrations. Cancer Res 1988;48:2029.

213. Hehlmann R, Heimpel H, Hasford J, et al: Randomized comparison of interferon-alpha with busulfan and hydroxyurea in chronic myelogenous leukemia. The German CML Study Group. Blood 1994;84:4064.

214. Finazzi G, Barbui T: Treatment of essential thrombocythemia with special emphasis on leukemogenic risk. Ann Hematol 1999;78:389.

215. Sterkers Y, Preudhomme C, Lai JL, et al: Acute myeloid leukemia and myelodysplastic syndromes following essential thrombocythemia treated with hydroxyurea: High proportion of cases with 17p deletion. Blood 1998;91:616.

216. Adair CPJ, Begg HJ: Experimental and clinical studies on the treatment of cancer by dichloroethylsulphide (mustard gas). Ann Surg 1931;93:193.

217. Tew KD, Colvin M, Chabner BA: Alkylating agents. In Chabner BA, Longo DL (eds): Cancer Chemotherapy and Biotherapy: Principles and Practice, 2nd ed. Philadelphia: Lippincott-Raven; 1996, p 297.

218. Hartley AJ, Gibson WN, Kohn KW, et al: DNA sequences selectivity by three antitumor chloroethylating agents. Cancer Res 1986;46:1943.

219. Bubley GJ, Ogata GK, Dupuis NP, et al: Detection of sequence-specific antitumor alkylating agent DNA damage from cells treated in culture and from a patient. Cancer Res 1994;54:6325.

220. Ewig R, Kohn KW: DNA-protein cross-linking and DNA interstrand cross-linking by haloethylnitrosoureas in L210 cells. Cancer Res 1978;38:3197.

221. Kohn KW: Interstrand cross-linking of DNA by 1,3-bis(2-chloroethyl)-1-nitrosourea and other 1-(2-haloethyl)-1-nitrosoureas. Cancer Res 1977;37:1450.

222. Hamilton TC, Lai GM, Rothenberg ML, et al: Mechanisms of resistance to alkylating agents and cisplatin. In Ozols RF (ed): Cancer Treatment and Research: Drug Resistance. Boston: Martinus Nijhoff; 1989, p 151.

223. Colvin OM: Mechanisms of resistance to alkylating agents. In Goldstein L, Ozols RF (eds): Anticancer Drug Resistance: Advances in Molecular and Clinical Research. Boston: Kluwer Academic Publishers; 1994, p 249.

224. Newell DR, Calvert AH, Harrap KR, et al: Studies on the pharmacokinetics of chlorambucil and prednimustine in man. Br J Clin Pharmacol 1983;15:253.

225. Alberts DS, Chang SY, Chen HSG: Comparative pharmacokinetics of chlorambucil and melphalan in man. Recent Results Cancer Res 1980;74:124.

226. Harrap KR, Riches PG, Gilby ED, et al: Studies on the toxicity and antitumor activity of prednimustine, a prednisolone ester of chlorambucil. Eur J Cancer 1977;13:873.

227. Colvin M: Cyclophosphamide and analogues. In Crooke ST, Prestayko AW (eds): Cancer and Chemotherapy. New York: Academic Press; 1981, p 25.

228. Colvin M: The comparative pharmacology of cyclophosphamide and ifosfamide. Semin Oncol 1982;9:2.

229. Colvin M, Padgett CA, Fenselau C: A biologically active metabolite of cyclophosphamide. Cancer Res 1973;33:915.

230. Struck RF, Kirk MC, Mellett LB, et al: Urinary metabolites of the antitumor agent cyclophosphamide. Mol Pharmacol 1971;7:519.

231. Hilton J: Role of aldehyde dehydrogenase in cyclophosphamide-resistant L1210 leukemia. Cancer Res 1984;44:5156.

232. Cox PJ: Cyclophosphamide cystitis—identification of acrolein as the causative agent. Biochem Pharmacol 1979;28:2045.

233. Ren S, Kalhorn TF, Slattery JT: Inhibition of human aldehyde dehydrogenase 1 by the 4-hydroxycyclophosphamide degradation product acrolein. Drug Metab Dispos 1999;27:133.

234. Tsukamoto N, Chen J, Yoshida A: Enhanced expressions of glucose-6-phosphate dehydrogenase and cytosolic aldehyde dehydrogenase and elevation of reduced glutathione level in cyclophosphamide-resistant human leukemia cells. Blood Cells Mol Dis 1998;24:231.

235. Johnson S, Smith AG, Loffler H, et al: Multicentre prospective randomized trial of fludarabine versus cyclophosphamide, doxorubicin, and prednisone (CAP) for treatment of advanced-stage chronic lymphocytic leukemia. The French Cooperative Group on CLL. Lancet 1996;347:1432.

236. Chang TK, Weber GF, Crespi CL, et al: Differential activation of cyclophosphamide and ifosphamide by cytochromes P-450 2B and 3A in human liver microsomes. Cancer Res 1993;53:5629.

237. Creaven PJ, Allen LM, Alford DA, et al: Clinical pharmacology of isophosphamide. Clin Pharmacol Ther 1974;16:77.

238. Andriole GL, Sandlund JT, Miser JS: The efficacy of MESNA (2-mercaptoethane sodium sulfonate) as a uroprotectant in patients with hemorrhagic cystitis receiving further oxazaphosphorine chemotherapy. J Clin Oncol 1987;5:799.

239. Yule SM, Price L, Pearson AD, et al: Cyclophosphamide and ifosfamide metabolites in the cerebrospinal fluid of children. Clin Cancer Res 1997;3:1985.

240. Tong WP, Ludlum DB: Crosslinking of DNA by busulfan formation of diguanyl derivatives. Biochim Biophys Acta 1980;608:174.

241. Friend W, Kedo A, Barone J: Effects of cyclophosphamide and busulfan on spleen colony-forming units and on hematopoietic stroma. Cancer Res 1977;37:1205.

242. Montgomery JA: The development of the nitrosoureas: A study in congener synthesis. In Prestayko AW, Crooke ST, Baker LH, et al (eds): Nitrosoureas: Current Status and New Developments. New York: Academic Press; 1981, p 3.

243. Schabel FM Jr: Experimental evaluation of potential anticancer agents. VIII. Effects of certain nitrosoureas on intracerebral L1210. Cancer Res 1963;23:725.

244. Cheng CJ, Fujimara D, Grunberger D, et al: Interaction of 1-(2-chloroethyl)-4-cyclohexyl-1-nitrosourea (NSC79037) with nucleic acids and proteins in vitro and in vivo. Cancer Res 1972;33:1921.

245. Ludlum DB: DNA alkylation by the haloethylnitrosoureas: Nature of modifications produced and their enzymatic repair or removal. Mutat Res 1990;233:117.

246. Pegg AE: Mammalian O^6-alkylguanine–DNA alkyltransferase: Regulation and importance in response to alkylating carcinogenic and therapeutic agents. Cancer Res 1990;50:6119.

247. Chae MY, McDougall MG, Dolan ME, et al: Substituted O^6-benzylguanine derivatives and their inactivation of human O^6-alkylguanine–DNA alkyltransferase. J Med Chem 1994;37:342.

248. Rosenberg B, Van Camp L, Krigas T: Inhibition of cell division in *Escherichia coli* by electrolysis products from a platinum electrode. Nature 1965;205:698.

249. Rosenberg B, Van Camp L, Grimley EB, et al: Inhibition of growth

or cell division in *Escherichia coli* by different ionic species of platinum (IV) complexes. J Biol Chem 1996;242:1347.

250. Reed E, Dabholkar M, Chabner BA: Platinum analogues. In Chabner BA, Longo DL (eds): Cancer Chemotherapy and Biotherapy: Principles and Practice, 2nd ed. Philadelphia: Lippincott-Raven; 1996, p 357.

251. Pinto AL, Lippard SJ: Binding of the antitumor drug *cis*-diammine-dichloroplatinum (II) (cisplatin) to DNA. Biochim Biophys Acta 1985;780:167.

252. Eastman A: The formation, isolation and characterization of DNA adducts produced by anticancer platinum complexes. Pharmacol Ther 1987;34:155.

253. Sherman SE, Lippard SJ: Structural aspects of platinum anticancer drug interactions with DNA. Chem Rev 1987;87:1153.

254. Plooy ACM, Fichtinger-Schepman AMJ, Schutte HH, et al: The quantitative detection of various Pt-DNA-adducts in Chinese hamster ovary cells treated with cisplatin: Application of immunochemical techniques. Carcinogenesis 1985;6:561.

255. Reed E, Ozols RF, Tarone R, et al: Platinum-DNA adducts in leukocyte DNA correlate with disease response in ovarian cancer patients receiving platinum-based chemotherapy. Proc Natl Acad Sci U S A 1987;84:5024.

256. Harrap KR: Preclinical studies identifying carboplatin as a viable cisplatin alternative. Cancer Treat Rev 1985;12:21.

257. Calvert AH, Newell DR, Gumbrell LA, et al: Carboplatin dosage: Prospect of evaluation of a simple formula based on renal function. J Clin Oncol 1989;7:1748.

258. Chaney SG: The chemistry and biology of platinum complexes with the 1,2-diaminocyclohexane carrier ligand. Int J Oncol 1995;6:1291.

259. Mathe G, Kidani Y, Sekiguchi M, et al: Oxalato-platinum or 1-OHP, a third-generation platinum complex: An experimental and clinical appraisal and preliminary comparison with *cis*-platinum and carboplatinum. Biomed Pharmacother 1989;43:237.

260. Mameata EL, Poma EE, Kaufmann WK, et al: Enhanced replicative bypass of platinum-DNA adducts in cisplatin-resistant human ovarian carcinoma cell lines. Cancer Res 1994;54:3500.

261. McKeage MJ, Mistry P, Ward J, et al: A phase I and pharmacology study of an oral platinum complex, JM216: Dose-dependent pharmacokinetics of single dose administration. Cancer Chemother Pharmacol 1995;36:451.

262. Vogler WR, Harrington DP, Winton EF, et al: Phase II clinical trial of carboplatin in relapsed and refractory leukemia. Leukemia 1992;6:1072.

263. Larrea L, Martinez JA, Sanz GF, et al: Carboplatin plus cytarabine in the treatment of high-risk acute myeloblastic leukemia. Leukemia 1999;13:161.

264. Bassan R, Lerede T, Buelli M, et al: A new combination of carboplatin, high-dose cytarabine and cross-over mitoxantrone or idarubicin for refractory and relapsed acute myeloid leukemia. Haematologica 1998;83:422.

265. Hyams JF, Lloyd CW: Microtubules. New York: Wiley Liss; 1993.

266. Amos LA, Baker TS: The three dimensional structure of tubulin protofilaments. Nature 1979;279:607.

267. Olmsted JB: Microtubule-associated proteins. Annu Rev Cell Biol 1986;2:421.

268. Erickson HP, O'Brien ET: Microtubule dynamic instability and GTP hydrolysis. Annu Rev Biophys Biomol Struct 1992;21:145.

269. Carlier MF: Role of nucleotide hydrolysis in the polymerization of actin and tubulin. Cell Biophys 1988;12:105.

270. Rowinsky K, Donehower RC: Antimicrotubule agents. In Chabner BA, Longo DL (eds): Cancer Chemotherapy and Biotherapy: Principles and Practice, 2nd ed. Philadelphia: Lippincott-Raven; 1996, p 35.

271. Johnson IS: Historical background of Vinca alkaloid research and areas of future interest. Cancer Chemother Rep 1968;52:455.

272. Rahmani R, Zhou X-J: Pharmacokinetics and metabolism of vinca alkaloids. In Workman P, Graham MA (eds): Pharmacokinetics and Cancer Chemotherapy. New York: Cold Spring Harbor Laboratory Press; 1993.

273. Ferguson PJ, Cass CE: Differential cellular retention of vincristine and vinblastine by cultured human promyelocytic leukemia HL-60/C-1 cells: The basis of differential toxicity. Cancer Res 1985;45:5480.

274. Jordan MA, Thrower D, Wilson L: Mechanism of inhibition of cell proliferation by Vinca alkaloids. Cancer Res 1991;51:2212.

275. Jordan MA, Thrower D, Wilson L: Effects of vinblastine, podophyllotoxin and nocodazole on mitotic spindles: Implications for the role of microtubule dynamics in mitosis. J Cell Sci 1992;102:401.

276. Beck WT: Cellular pharmacology of Vinca alkaloid resistance and its circumvention. Adv Enzyme Regul 1984;22:207.

277. Haber M, Burkhart CA, Regl DL, et al: Altered expression of M beta 2, the class II beta-tubulin isotype, in a murine J774.2 cell line with a high level of taxol resistance. J Biol Chem 1995;270:31269.

278. Nelson RI, Dyke RW, Root MA: Comparative pharmacokinetics of vindesine, vincristine, and vinblastine in patients with cancer. Cancer Treat Rev 1980;7:17.

279. Bender RA, Castle MC, Margileth DA, et al: The pharmacokinetics of [³H]-vincristine in man. Clin Pharmacol Ther 1977;22:430.

280. Wani MC, Taylor HL, Wall ME, et al: Plant antitumor agents. VI. The isolation and structure of taxol, a novel antileukemic and antitumor agent from *Taxus brevifolia*. J Am Chem Soc 1971;93:2525.

281. Schiff PB, Fant J, Horwitz SB: Promotion of microtubule assembly in vitro by taxol. Nature 1979;22:665.

282. Horwitz SB, Cohen D, Rao S, et al: Taxol: Mechanisms of action and resistance. Monogr Natl Cancer Inst 1993;15:63.

283. Rowinsky EK, Donehower RC, Jones RJ, et al: Microtubule changes and cytotoxicity in leukemic cell lines treated with Taxol. Cancer Res 1988;48:4093.

284. Ringel I, Horwitz SB: Studies with RP56976 (Taxotere): A semisynthetic analogue of taxol. J Natl Cancer Inst 1991;83:288.

285. Weiss R, Donehower RC, Wiernik PH, et al: Hypersensitivity reactions from Taxol. J Clin Oncol 1990;8:1263.

286. Verweij J, Clavel M, Chevalier B: Paclitaxel (Taxol) and docetaxel (Taxotere): Not simply two of a kind. Ann Oncol 1994;5:495.

287. Roca J: The mechanisms of DNA topoisomerases. Trends Biol Sci 1995;20:156.

288. Smith PJ, Soues S: Multilevel therapeutic targeting by topoisomerase inhibitors. Br J Cancer 1994;23:S47.

289. Corbett AH, Osheroff N: When good enzymes go bad: Conversion of topoisomerase II to a cellular toxin by antineoplastic drugs. Chem Res Toxicol 1993;6:585.

290. Gupta M, Fujimori A, Pommier Y: Eukaryotic DNA topoisomerases I. Biochim Biophys Acta 1995;1262:1.

291. Wigley DB: Structure and mechanism of DNA topoisomerases. Annu Rev Biophys Biomol Structure 1995;24:185.

292. Pommier Y, Capranico G, Orr A, et al: Local base sequence preferences for DNA cleavage by mammalian topoisomerase II in the presence of amsacrine or teniposide [published erratum appears in Nucleic Acids Res 1991;19:7003]. Nucleic Acids Res 1991;19:5973.

293. Freudenreich CH, Kreuzer KN: Mutational analysis of a type II topoisomerase cleavage site: Distinct requirements for enzyme and inhibitors. EMBO J 1993;12:2085.

294. Slevin ML, Clark PI, Joel SP, et al: A randomized trial to evaluate the effect of schedule on the activity of etoposide in small-cell lung cancer. J Clin Oncol 1989;7:1333.

295. Hsiang Y-H, Lihou MG, Liu LF: Arrest of replication forks by drug stabilized topoisomerase I–DNA complexes as a mechanism of cell killing by camptothecin. Cancer Res 1989;49:5077.

296. Voigt W, Matsui S, Yin MB, et al: Topoisomerase-I inhibitor SN-38 can induce DNA damage and chromosomal aberrations independent from DNA synthesis. Anticancer Res 1998;18:3499.

297. Cortes F, Pinero J, Palitti F: Cytogenetic effects of inhibition of topoisomerase I or II activities in the CHO mutant EM9 and its parental line AA8. Mutat Res 1993;288:281.

298. Maraschin J, Dutrillaux B, Aurias A: Chromosome aberrations induced by etoposide (VP-16) are not random. Int J Cancer 1990;46:808.

299. Pedersen-Bjergaard J, Rowley JD: The balanced and the unbalanced chromosome aberrations of acute myeloid leukemia may develop in different ways and may contribute differently to malignant transformation. Blood 1994;83:2780.

300. Felix CA: Secondary leukemias induced by topoisomerase-targeted drugs. Biochim Biophys Acta 1998;1400:233.

301. Hashimoto H, Chatterjee S, Berger NA: Mutagenic activity of topoisomerase I inhibitors. Clin Cancer Res 1995;1:369.

302. Hsiang Y-H, Hertzberg R, Hecht S, et al: Camptothecin induced protein-linked DNA breaks via mammalian DNA topoisomerase I. J Biol Chem 1985;260:1473.

303. Tanizawa A, Fujimori A, Fujimori Y, et al: Comparison of topoisomerase I inhibition, DNA damage, and cytotoxicity of camptothecin derivatives currently in clinical trials. J Natl Cancer Inst 1994;86:836.

304. Jaxel C, Capranico G, Kerrigan D, et al: Effect of local DNA sequence on topoisomerase I cleavage in the presence and absence of camptothecin. J Biol Chem 1991;266:20418.

305. Gupta RS, Gupta R, Eng B, et al: Camptothecin resistant mutants of Chinese hamster ovary cells containing a resistant form of topoisomerase I. Cancer Res 1988;48:6404.

306. Chen AU, Yu C, Potmesil M, et al: Camptothecin overcomes MDR1-mediated resistance in human KB carcinoma cells. Cancer Res 1991;51:6039.

307. Schellens J, Creemers G, Beijnen J, et al: Bioavailability and pharmacokinetics of oral topotecan: A new topoisomerase I inhibitor. Br J Cancer 1998;73:1268.

308. Rivory LP, Riou JF, Haaz MC, et al: Identification and properties of a major plasma metabolite of irinotecan (CPT-11) isolated from the plasma of patients. Cancer Res 1996;56:3689.

309. Herben VM, ten Bokkel Huinink WW, Beijnen JH: Clinical pharmacokinetics of topotecan. Clin Pharmacokinet 1996;31:85.

310. Chabot GG: Clinical pharmacokinetics of irinotecan. Clin Pharmacokinet 1997;33:245.

311. O'Reilly S, Rowinsky EK: The clinical status of irinotecan (CPT-11), a novel water soluble camptothecin analogue: 1996. Crit Rev Oncol Hematol 1996;24:47.

312. Kantarjian H: New developments in the treatment of acute myeloid leukemia: Focus on topotecan. Semin Hematol 1999;36:16.

313. Loike JD, Horwitz SB: Effects of podophyllotoxins and VP16-213 on microtubule assembly in vitro and nucleoside transport in HeLa cells. Biochemistry 1976;15:5435.

314. Loike JD, Horwitz SB: Effect of VP16-213 on the intracellular degradation of DNA in HeLa cells. Biochemistry 1976;15:5443.

315. Barlogie B, Drewinko B: Cell cycle stage–dependent induction of G2 arrest by different antitumor agents. Eur J Cancer 1978;14:741.

316. Glisson BS, Smallwood SE, Ross WE: Characterization of VP-16–induced DNA damage in isolated nuclei from L1210 cells. Biochim Biophys Acta 1984;783:74.

317. Chen GL, Yang L, Rowe TC, et al: Nonintercalative antitumor drugs interfere with the breakage-reunion reaction of mammalian DNA topoisomerase II. J Biol Chem 1984;259:13560.

318. Beck WT, Danks MK: Mechanisms of resistance to drugs that inhibit DNA topoisomerases. Semin Cancer Biol 1991;2:235.

319. Allen LM: Comparison of uptake and binding of two epipodophyllotoxin glucopyranosides, 4-demethyl epipodophyllotoxin thenylidene-beta-D-glucoside and 4'-demethyl epipodophyllotoxin ethylidene-beta-D-glucoside, in the L1210 leukemia cell. Cancer Res 1978;38:2549.

320. Colombo T, Broggini M, Vaghi M, et al: Comparison between VP 16 and VM 26 in Lewis lung carcinoma of the mouse. Eur J Cancer Clin Oncol 1986;22:173.

321. Joel S: The clinical pharmacology of etoposide: An update. Cancer Treat Rev 1996;22:179.

322. Clark PI, Slevin ML: The clinical pharmacology of etoposide and teniposide. Clin Pharmacokinet 1987;12:223.

323. Joel SP, Hall M, Gaver RC, et al: Complete recovery of radioactivity after administration of ¹⁴C-etoposide in man. Proc Annu Meet Am Soc Clin Oncol 1995;14.

324. Petros WP, Rodman JH, Relling MV, et al: Variability in teniposide plasma protein binding is correlated with serum albumin concentrations. Pharmacotherapy 1992;12:273.

325. Joel SP, Ellis P, O'Byrne K, et al: Therapeutic monitoring of continuous infusion etoposide in small-cell lung cancer. J Clin Oncol 1996;14:1903.

326. Weiss RB: Hypersensitivity reactions. Semin Oncol 1992;19:458.

327. O'Dwyer PJ, King SA, Fortner CL, et al: Hypersensitivity reactions to teniposide (VM-26): An analysis. J Clin Oncol 1986;4:1262.

328. Kellie SJ, Crist WM, Pui CH, et al: Hypersensitivity reactions to epipodophyllotoxins in children with acute lymphoblastic leukemia. Cancer 1991;67:1070.

329. Pui CH, Ribeiro RC, Hancock ML, et al: Acute myeloid leukemia in children treated with epipodophyllotoxins for acute lymphoblastic leukemia. N Engl J Med 1991;325:1682.

330. Winick NJ, McKenna RW, Shuster JJ, et al: Secondary acute myeloid leukemia in children with acute lymphoblastic leukemia treated with etoposide. J Clin Oncol 1993;11:209.

331. Smith MA, Rubinstein L, Anderson JR, et al: Secondary leukemia or myelodysplastic syndrome after treatment with epipodophyllotoxins. J Clin Oncol 1999;17:569.

332. Pui CH, Relling MV, Behm FG, et al: L-Asparaginase may potentiate the leukemogenic effect of the epipodophyllotoxins. Leukemia 1995;9:1680.

333. Bassan R, Barbui T: Remission induction therapy for adults with acute myelogenous leukemia: Towards the ICE age? Haematologica 1995;80:82.

334. Schacter L: Etoposide phosphate: What, why, where, and how? Semin Oncol 1996;23:1.

335. Di Marco A, Silvestrini R, Di Marco S, et al: Inhibiting effect of the new cytotoxic antibiotic daunomycin on nucleic acids and mitotic activity of HeLa cells. J Cell Biol 1965;27:545.

336. Peterson C, Trouet A: Transport and storage of daunorubicin and doxorubicin in cultured fibroblasts. Cancer Res 1978;38:4645.

337. Ross WE, Bradley MO: DNA double-strand breaks in mammalian cells after exposure to intercalating agents. Biochim Biophys Acta 1981;654:129.

338. Liu LF: DNA topoisomerase poisons as antitumor drugs. Annu Rev Biochem 1989;58:351.

339. Pommier Y: DNA topoisomerase I and II in cancer chemotherapy: Update and perspectives. Cancer Chemother Pharmacol 1993;32:103.

340. Capranico G, Kohn KW, Pommier Y: Local sequence requirements for DNA cleavage by mammalian topoisomerase II in the presence of doxorubicin. Nucleic Acids Res 1990;18:6611.

341. Bachur NR, Gordon SL, Gee MV: A general mechanism for microsomal activation of quinone anticancer agents to free radicals. Cancer Res 1978;38:1745.

342. Doroshow JH, Akman S, Chu FF, et al: Role of the glutathione-glutathione peroxidase cycle in the cytotoxicity of the anticancer quinones. Pharmacol Ther 1990;47:359.

343. Akman SA, Forrest G, Chu FF, et al: Resistance to hydrogen peroxide associated with altered catalase mRNA stability in MCF7 breast cancer cells. Biochim Biophys Acta 1989;1009:70.

344. Doroshow JH, Locker GY, Myers CE: Enzymatic defenses of the mouse heart against reactive oxygen metabolites: Alterations produced by doxorubicin. J Clin Invest 1980;65:128.

345. Speyer JL, Green MD, Kramer E, et al: Protective effect of the bispiperazinedione ICRF-187 against doxorubicin-induced cardiac toxicity in women with advanced breast cancer. N Engl J Med 1988;319:745.

346. Kaufmann SH, Karp JE, Jones RJ, et al: Topoisomerase II levels and drug sensitivity in adult acute myelogenous leukemia. Blood 1994;83:517.

347. Marie JP, Zittoun R, Sikic BI: Multidrug resistance (mdr1) gene expression in adult acute leukemias: Correlations with treatment outcome and in vitro drug sensitivity. Blood 1991;78:586.

348. Stewart DJ, Grewaal D, Green RM, et al: Bioavailability and pharmacology of oral idarubicin. Cancer Chemother Pharmacol 1991;27:308.

349. Averbuch SD, Boldt M, Gaudiano G, et al: Experimental chemotherapy-induced skin necrosis in swine. Mechanistic studies of anthracycline antibiotic toxicity and protection with a radical dimer compound. J Clin Invest 1988;81:142.

350. Eksborg S: Pharmacokinetics of anthracyclines. Acta Oncol 1989;28:873.

351. Robert J: Clinical pharmacokinetics of epirubicin. Clin Pharmacokinet 1994;26:428.

352. Robert J: Clinical pharmacokinetics of idarubicin [published erratum appears in Clin Pharmacokinet 1993;25:350]. Clin Pharmacokinet 1993;24:275.

353. Doroshow JH: Anthracyclines and anthracenediones. In Chabner BA, Longo DL (eds): Cancer Chemotherapy and Biotherapy: Principles and Practice, 2nd ed. Philadelphia: Lippincott-Raven; 1996.

354. Huffman DH, Bachur NR: Daunorubicin metabolism in acute myelocytic leukemia. Blood 1972;39:637.

355. Gil P, Favre R, Durand A, et al: Time dependency of adriamycin and adriamycinol kinetics. Cancer Chemother Pharmacol 1983;10:120.

356. Fukushima T, Kawai Y, Urasaki Y, et al: Influence of idarubicinol on the antileukemic effect of idarubicin. Leuk Res 1994;18:943.

357. Gessner T, Preisler HD, Azarnia N, et al: Plasma levels of daunorubicin metabolites and the outcome of ANLL therapy. Med Oncol Tumor Pharmacother 1987;4:23.

358. Vrignaud P, Eghbali H, Hoerni B, et al: Pharmacokinetics and metabolism of epirubicin during repetitive courses of administration in Hodgkin's patients. Eur J Cancer Clin Oncol 1985;21:1307.

359. Twelves CJ, Dobbs NA, Gillies HC, et al: Doxorubicin pharmacokinetics: The effect of abnormal liver biochemistry tests. Cancer Chemother Pharmacol 1998;42:229.

360. Gurney HP, Ackland S, Gebski V, et al: Factors affecting epirubicin pharmacokinetics and toxicity: Evidence against using body-surface area for dose calculation. J Clin Oncol 1998;16:2299.

361. Von Hoff DD, Layard MW, Basa P, et al: Risk factors for doxorubicin-induced congestive heart failure. Ann Intern Med 1979;91:710.

362. Von Hoff DD, Rozencweig M, Layard M, et al: Daunomycin-induced cardiotoxicity in children and adults. A review of 110 cases. Am J Med 1977;62:200.

363. Anderlini P, Benjamin RS, Wong FC, et al: Idarubicin cardiotoxicity: A retrospective study in acute myeloid leukemia and myelodysplasia. J Clin Oncol 1995;13:2827.

364. Ryberg M, Nielsen D, Skovsgaard T, et al: Epirubicin cardiotoxicity: An analysis of 469 patients with metastatic breast cancer. J Clin Oncol 1998;16:3502.

365. Torti FM, Bristow MR, Howes AE, et al: Reduced cardiotoxicity of doxorubicin delivered on a weekly schedule. Assessment by endomyocardial biopsy. Ann Intern Med 1983;99:745.

366. Legha SS, Benjamin RS, Mackay B, et al: Reduction of doxorubicin cardiotoxicity by prolonged continuous intravenous infusion. Ann Intern Med 1982;96:133.

367. Speyer J, Wasserheit C: Strategies for reduction of anthracycline cardiac toxicity. Semin Oncol 1998;25:525.

368. Zee-Cheng RK, Cheng CC: Antineoplastic agents. Structure-activity relationship study of bis (substituted aminoalkylamino)-anthraquinones. J Med Chem 1978;21:291.

369. Capranico G, De Isabella P, Tinelli S, et al: Similar sequence specificity of mitoxantrone and VM-26 stimulation of in vitro DNA cleavage by mammalian DNA topoisomerase II. Biochemistry 1993;32:3038.

370. Sundman-Engberg B, Tidefelt U, Gruber A, et al: Intracellular concentrations of mitoxantrone in leukemic cells in vitro vs in vivo. Leuk Res 1993;17:347.

371. Smyth JF, Macpherson JS, Warrington PS, et al: The clinical pharmacology of mitoxantrone. Cancer Chemother Pharmacol 1986; 17:149.

372. Stewart DJ, Green RM, Mikhael NZ, et al: Human autopsy tissue concentrations of mitoxantrone. Cancer Treat Rep 1986;70:1255.

373. Rentsch KM, Schwendener RA, Pestalozzi BC, et al: Pharmacokinetic studies of mitoxantrone and one of its metabolites in serum and urine in patients with advanced breast cancer. Eur J Clin Pharmacol 1998;54:83.

374. Chiccarelli FS, Morrison JA, Cosulich DB, et al: Identification of human urinary mitoxantrone metabolites. Cancer Res 1986;46:4858.

375. Panousis C, Kettle AJ, Phillips DR: Neutrophil-mediated activation of mitoxantrone to metabolites which form adducts with DNA. Cancer Lett 1997;113:173.

376. Mewes K, Blanz J, Ehninger G, et al: Cytochrome P-450–induced cytotoxicity of mitoxantrone by formation of electrophilic intermediates. Cancer Res 1993;53:5135.

377. Blanz J, Mewes K, Ehninger G, et al: Evidence for oxidative activation of mitoxantrone in human, pig, and rat. Drug Metab Dispos 1991;19:871.

378. Crossley RJ: Clinical safety and tolerance of mitoxantrone (Novantrone). Cancer Treat Rev 1983;10:29.

379. Cain BF, Atwell GJ: The experimental antitumor properties of three congeners of the acridylmethanesulphonanilide (AMSA) series. Eur J Cancer 1974;10:539.

380. Linssen P, Brons P, Knops G, et al: Plasma and cellular pharmacokinetics of m-AMSA related to in vitro toxicity towards normal and leukemic clonogenic bone marrow cells (CFU-GM, CFU-L). Eur J Haematol 1993;50:149.

381. Robertson IG, Kestell P, Dormer RA, et al: Involvement of glutathione in the metabolism of the anilinoacridine antitumor agents CI-921 and amsacrine. Drug Metabol Drug Interact 1988;6:371.

382. Robbie MA, Palmer BD, Denny WA, et al: The fate of N1′-methanesulphonyl-N4′-(9-acridinyl)-3′-methoxy-2′,5′-cyclohexa diene-1′,4′-diimine (m-AQDI), the primary oxidative metabolite of amsacrine, in transformed Chinese hamster fibroblasts. Biochem Pharmacol 1990;39:1411.

383. Shoemaker DD, Cysyk RL, Gormley PE, et al: Metabolism of 4′-(9-acridinylamino)methanesulfone-m-anisidide by rat liver microsomes. Cancer Res 1984;44:1939.

384. Weiss RB, Grillo-Lopez AJ, Marsoni S, et al: Amsacrine-associated cardiotoxicity: An analysis of 82 cases. J Clin Oncol 1986;4:918.

385. Arlin ZA, Feldman EJ, Mittelman A, et al: Amsacrine is safe and effective therapy for patients with myocardial dysfunction and acute leukemia. Cancer 1991;68:1198.

386. Haley EE, Fischer GA, Welch AD: The requirement for L-asparagine of mouse leukemic cells. Cancer Res 1961;21:532.

387. Chabner BA, Loo TL: Enzyme therapy: L-Asparaginase. In Chabner BA, Longo DL (eds): Cancer Chemotherapy and Biotherapy: Principles and Practice, 2nd ed. Philadelphia: Lippincott-Raven; 1996.

388. Kidd JG: Regression of transplanted lymphomas induced in vivo by means of normal guinea pig serum. I. Course of transplanted cancers of various kinds given guinea pig serum, horse serum or rabbit serum. J Exp Med 1953;98:565.

389. Asselin BL, Whitin JC, Coppola DJ, et al: Comparative pharmacokinetic studies of three asparaginase preparations. J Clin Oncol 1993;11:1780.

390. Woo MH, Hak LJ, Storm MC, et al: Anti-asparaginase antibodies following E. coli asparaginase therapy in pediatric acute lymphoblastic leukemia. Leukemia 1998;12:1527.

391. Haskell CM, Canellos GP: L-Asparaginase resistance in human leukemia—asparagine synthetase. Biochem Pharmacol 1969;18:2578.

392. Sur P, Fernandes DJ, Kute TE, et al: L-Asparaginase–induced modulation of methotrexate polyglutamylation in murine leukemia L5178Y. Cancer Res 1987;47:1313.

393. Oettgen HF, Stephenson PA, Schwartz MK, et al: Toxicity of E. coli L-asparaginase in man. Cancer 1970;25:253.

394. Dellinger CT, Miale TD: Comparison of anaphylactic reactions to asparaginase derived from Escherichia coli and from Erwinia cultures. Cancer 1976;38:1843.

395. Ott N, Ramsay NK, Priest JR, et al: Sequelae of thrombotic or hemorrhagic complications following L-asparaginase therapy for childhood lymphoblastic leukemia. Am J Pediatr Hematol Oncol 1988;10:191.

396. Alvarez OA, Zimmerman G: Pegaspargase-induced pancreatitis. Med Pediatr Oncol 2000;34:200.

397. Muller HJ, Boos J: Use of L-asparaginase in childhood ALL. Crit Rev Oncol Hematol 1998;28:97.

398. Swain S: Endocrine therapies of cancer. In Chabner BA, Longo DL (eds): Cancer Chemotherapy and Biotherapy: Principles and Practice, 2nd ed. Philadelphia: Lippincott-Raven; 1996.

399. Claman HN: Corticosteroids and lymphoid cells. N Engl J Med 1972;287:388.

400. Parker MG, Franks LM: Hormones and cancer. In Franks LM, Teich NM (eds): Introduction to the Cellular and Molecular Biology of Cancer. Oxford: Oxford University Press; 1997.

401. Bailey S, Hall AG, Pearson AD, et al: Glucocorticoid resistance and the AP-1 transcription factor in leukemia. Adv Exp Med Biol 1999;457:615.

402. McConkey DJ, Nicotera P, Hartzell P, et al: Glucocorticoids activate a suicide process in thymocytes through an elevation of cytosolic Ca^{2+} concentration. Arch Biochem Biophys 1989;269:365.

403. Wyllie AH: Glucocorticoid-induced thymocyte apoptosis is associated with endogenous endonuclease activation. Nature 1980;284:555.

404. Frey BM, Frey FJ: Clinical pharmacokinetics of prednisone and prednisolone. Clin Pharmacokinet 1990;19:126.

405. Rose JQ, Yurchak AM, Jusko WJ: Dose dependent pharmacokinetics of prednisone and prednisolone in man. J Pharmacokinet Biopharm 1981;9:389.

406. Minucci S, Pelicci PG: Retinoid receptors in health and disease: Co-regulators and the chromatin connection. Semin Cell Dev Biol 1999;10:215.

407. Melnick A, Licht JD: Deconstructing a disease: RAR-alpha, its fusion partners, and their roles in the pathogenesis of acute promyelocytic leukemia. Blood 1999;93:3167.

408. Lin RJ, Nagy L, Inoue S, et al: Role of the histone deacetylase complex in acute promyelocytic leukaemia. Nature 1998;391:811.

409. Tallman MS: All-trans-retinoic acid in acute promyelocytic leukemia and its potential in other hematologic malignancies. Semin Hematol 1994;31:38.

410. Adamson PC, Reaman G, Finklestein JZ, et al: Phase I trial and pharmacokinetic study of all-*trans*-retinoic acid administered on an intermittent schedule in combination with interferon-alpha2a in pediatric patients with refractory cancer. J Clin Oncol 1997; 15:3330.

411. Adedoyin A, Stiff DD, Smith DC, et al: All-*trans*-retinoic acid modulation of drug-metabolizing enzyme activities: Investigation with selective metabolic drug probes. Cancer Chemother Pharmacol 1998;41:133.

412. Estey E, Thall PF, Mehta K, et al: Alterations in tretinoin pharmacokinetics following administration of liposomal all-*trans* retinoic acid. Blood 1996;87:3650.

413. Conley BA, Egorin MJ, Sridhara R, et al: Phase I clinical trial of all-*trans*-retinoic acid with correlation of its pharmacokinetics and pharmacodynamics. Cancer Chemother Pharmacol 1997;39:291.

414. Tallman MS, Andersen JW, Schiffer CA, et al: Clinical description of 44 patients with acute promyelocytic leukemia who developed the retinoic acid syndrome. Blood 2000;95:90.

415. Estey EH, Thall PF, Pierce S, et al: Randomized phase II study of fludarabine + cytosine arabinoside + idarubicin ± all-*trans* retinoic acid ± granulocyte colony-stimulating factor in poor prognosis newly diagnosed acute myeloid leukemia and myelodysplastic syndrome. Blood 1999;93:2478.

416. Beaupre DM, Kurzrock R: RAS and leukemia: From basic mechanisms to gene-directed therapy. J Clin Oncol 1999;17:1071.

417. Gibbs JB, Oliff A: The potential of farnesyltransferase inhibitors as cancer chemotherapeutics. Annu Rev Pharmacol Toxicol 1997; 37:143.

418. Koblan KS, Kohl NE, Omer CA, et al: Farnesyltransferase inhibitors: A new class of cancer chemotherapeutics. Biochem Soc Trans 1996;24:688.

419. Emanuel PD, Snyder RC, Wiley T, et al: Inhibition of juvenile myelomonocytic leukemia cell growth in vitro by farnesyltransferase inhibitors. Blood 2000;95:639.

420. Mahgoub N, Taylor BR, Gratiot M, et al: In vitro and in vivo effects of a farnesyltransferase inhibitor on Nf1-deficient hematopoietic cells. Blood 1999;94:2469.

421. Lancet J, Rosenblatt J, Liesvold JL, et al: Use of the farnesyl transferase inhibitor R115777 in relapsed and refractory acute leukemias: Preliminary results of a phase 1 trial. J Clin Oncol 2000;19:3a.

422. Yeung SC, Xu G, Pan J, et al: Manumycin enhances the cytotoxic effect of paclitaxel on anaplastic thyroid carcinoma cells. Cancer Res 2000;60:650.

423. Agarwal B, Bhendwal S, Halmos B, et al: Lovastatin augments apoptosis induced by chemotherapeutic agents in colon cancer cells. Clin Cancer Res 1999;5:2223.

424. Senderowicz AM, Sausville EA: Preclinical and clinical development of cyclin-dependent kinase modulators. J Natl Cancer Inst 2000;92:376.

425. Scherr CJ: Cancer cell cycles. Science 1996;274:1672.

426. Konig A, Schwartz GK, Mohammad RM, et al: The novel cyclin-dependent kinase inhibitor flavopiridol downregulates Bcl-2 and induces growth arrest and apoptosis in chronic B-cell leukemia lines. Blood 1997;90:4307.

427. Arguello F, Alexander M, Sterry JA, et al: Flavopiridol induces apoptosis of normal lymphoid cells, causes immunosuppression, and has potent antitumor activity in vivo against human leukemia and lymphoma xenografts. Blood 1998;91:2482.

428. Byrd JC, Shinn C, Waselenko JK, et al: Flavopiridol induces apoptosis in chronic lymphocytic leukemia cells via activation of caspase-3 without evidence of bcl-2 modulation or dependence on functional p53. Blood 1998;92:3804.

429. Parker BW, Kaur G, Nieves-Neira W, et al: Early induction of apoptosis in hematopoietic cell lines after exposure to flavopiridol. Blood 1998;91:458.

430. Kerr JS, Wexler RS, Mousa SA, et al: Novel small molecule alpha v integrin antagonists: Comparative anti-cancer efficacy with known angiogenesis inhibitors. Anticancer Res 1999;19:959.

431. Melillo G, Sausville EA, Cloud K, et al: Flavopiridol, a protein kinase inhibitor, down-regulates hypoxic induction of vascular endothelial growth factor expression in human monocytes. Cancer Res 1999;59:5433.

432. Bible KC, Kaufmann SH: Cytotoxic synergy between flavopiridol (NSC 649890, L86–8275) and various antineoplastic agents: The importance of sequence of administration. Cancer Res 1997;57: 3375.

433. Bible KC, Bible RH Jr, Kottke TJ, et al: Flavopiridol binds to duplex DNA. Cancer Res 2000;60:2419.

434. Druker BJ, Tamura S, Buchdunger E, et al: Effects of a selective inhibitor of the Abl tyrosine kinase on the growth of Bcr-Abl positive cells. Nat Med 1996;2:561.

435. Dan S, Naito M, Tsuruo T: Selective induction of apoptosis in Philadelphia chromosome–positive chronic myelogenous leukemia cells by an inhibitor of BCR-ABL tyrosine kinase, CGP 57148. Cell Death Differ 1998;5:710.

436. le Coutre P, Mologni L, Cleris L, et al: In vivo eradication of human BCR/ABL-positive leukemia cells with an ABL kinase inhibitor. J Natl Cancer Inst 1999;91:163.

437. Druker BJ, Sawyers CL, Talpaz M, et al: Phase I trial of a specific ABL tyrosine kinase inhibitor STI 571 (CGP 57148) in interferon refractory chronic myelogenous leukemia patients. J Clin Oncol 18:7, 1999.

437a. Gorre ME, Mohammed M, Ellwood K, et al: Clinical resistance STI-571 cancer therapy caused by BCR-ABL gene mutation or amplification. Science 293:876, 2001.

438. Folkman J, Watson K, Ingber D, et al: Induction of angiogenesis during the transition from hyperplasia to neoplasia. Nature 1989; 339:58.

439. Jones A, Harris AL: New developments in angiogenesis: A major mechanism for tumor growth and target for therapy. Cancer J Sci Am 1998;4:209.

440. Leung DW, Cachianes G, Kuang WJ, et al: Vascular endothelial growth factor is a secreted angiogenic mitogen. Science 1989; 246:1306.

441. Perez-Atayde AR, Sallan SE, Tedrow U, et al: Spectrum of tumor angiogenesis in the bone marrow of children with acute lymphoblastic leukemia. Am J Pathol 1997;150:815.

442. Padro T, Ruiz S, Bieker R, et al: Increased angiogenesis in the bone marrow of patients with acute myeloid leukemia. Blood 2000; 95:2637.

443. Hussong JW, Rodgers GM, Shami PJ: Evidence of increased angiogenesis in patients with acute myeloid leukemia. Blood 2000; 95:309.

444. Fiedler W, Graeven U, Ergun S, et al: Vascular endothelial growth factor, a possible paracrine growth factor in human acute myeloid leukemia. Blood 1997;89:1870.

445. Aguayo A, Estey E, Kantarjian H, et al: Cellular vascular endothelial growth factor is a predictor of outcome in patients with acute myeloid leukemia. Blood 1999;94:3717.

446. Bergers G, Javaherian K, Lo KM, et al: Effects of angiogenesis inhibitors on multistage carcinogenesis in mice. Science 1999; 284:808.

447. O'Reilly MS, Boehm T, Shing Y, et al: Endostatin: An endogenous inhibitor of angiogenesis and tumor growth. Cell 1997;88:277.

448. Ciardiello F, Caputo R, Bianco R, et al: Antitumor effect and potentiation of cytotoxic drug activity in human cancer cells by ZD-1839 (Iressa), an epidermal growth factor receptor–selective tyrosine kinase inhibitor. Clin Cancer Res 2000;6:2053.

449. Jouan V, Canron X, Alemany M, et al: Inhibition of in vitro angiogenesis by platelet factor-4–derived peptides and mechanism of action. Blood 1999;94:984.

450. He LZ, Guidez F, Warrell RP, et al: Role of transcriptional repression and histone deacetylation in APL pathogenesis: A rationale for transcription therapy. Blood 1998;92:404a.

451. Grignani F, De Matteis S, Nervi C, et al: Fusion proteins of the retinoic acid receptor-alpha recruit histone deacetylase in promyelocytic leukaemia. Nature 1998;391:815.

452. Warrell RP Jr, He LZ, Richon V, et al: Therapeutic targeting of transcription in acute promyelocytic leukemia by use of an inhibitor of histone deacetylase. J Natl Cancer Inst 1998;90:1621.

18

Eric L. Sievers   Arthur E. Frankel

Treatment of Leukemia with Monoclonal Antibodies, Immunotoxins, and Immunoconjugates

Because of a lack of specificity for malignant cells, conventional approaches to the treatment of acute leukemias often induce noxious and sometimes life-threatening side effects. These range from disrupted mucosal integrity to more severe consequences that include central nervous system toxicity from high-dose cytarabine and veno-occlusive disease from treatment regimens that are used to prepare patients for hematopoietic stem cell transplantation (HSCT). Investigators have recently sought to target therapeutic agents more selectively to malignant and nonmalignant cells of the hematopoietic system. It is hoped that approaches using monoclonal antibodies and fusion proteins to target antigens with expression limited to the hematopoietic system specifically might spare nonhematopoietic organs from toxic effects and possibly result in greater antileukemic efficacy.

With the possible exception of the human homologue of the rat NG2 chondroitin sulfate proteoglycan molecule that is expressed by acute myelogenous leukemia (AML) blasts from many pediatric patients with *MLL* gene rearrangements,[1] leukemic cells rarely express novel cell surface antigens. For this reason, most therapeutic targeting approaches have been directed against normal hematopoietic cell surface antigens that are also expressed by leukemic blast cells. Figure 18–1 illustrates three general methods of selective targeting (see also Color Section). The first line of attack involves the use of monoclonal antibodies and a functional immune system to eliminate leukemic cells. The second approach employs monoclonal antibodies and fusion proteins as a means of delivering either chemotherapy or radiation directly to leukemic cells that express a normal hematopoietic antigen. The third tactic seeks to target increased doses of radiation more specifically to the hematopoietic system in the setting of HSCT. All three approaches are likely to result in less damage to most normal tissues. It remains to be seen whether greater antileukemic efficacy will be realized with these new therapies.

THERAPEUTIC STRATEGIES
Immune-Mediated Antileukemic Approaches

Unconjugated monoclonal antibodies can theoretically eliminate leukemic blast cells by several immune-medi-

ated mechanisms. Antibody-dependent cellular cytotoxicity works by a mechanism in which tissue macrophages clear antibody-coated target cells through binding of the antibody Fc receptor. Complement-dependent cellular cytotoxicity, which is likely to be a lesser component of antileukemic activity, results from complement fixation initiated by the Fc portion of immunoglobulin bound to tumor cells. Antibody-dependent cellular cytotoxicity has been implicated as a mechanism for the impressive non-Hodgkin's lymphoma tumor regressions seen in association with anti-CD20 antibodies.[2] However, recent evidence suggests that ligation of CD20 by antibody can interfere with normal signal transduction events and directly lead to apoptosis without a significant contribution from antibody-dependent cellular cytotoxicity.[3] Whether a cell surface antigen analogous to CD20 in myeloid leukemias can be identified and targeted in a similar manner is an approach that merits further investigation. Unconjugated antibodies to CD20 in non-Hodgkin's lymphoma and Her2-neu in breast cancer have been shown to be useful therapies; similar approaches in acute myeloid leukemia have shown some efficacy, particularly in instances of minimal tumor burden.

Delivery of Cytotoxic Agents by Use of Monoclonal Antibodies and Fusion Proteins

Antibodies have been used to deliver cytotoxic agents specifically to leukemic blast cells. Most cell surface antigens remain exterior to the cytoplasm after binding to ligand. In such instances, delivery of drug to the cytoplasm is limited. Occasional cell surface antigens are characterized by their ability to internalize on binding of an antibody or a fusion protein in a process known as modulation. This presents an opportunity to deliver a cytotoxic agent to the interior of a leukemic cell. In the instance of AML, modulating cell surface antigens expressed only on maturing myeloid cells (e.g., CD33) are particularly appealing for this approach because the pluripotent hematopoietic stem cell can be spared. Similarly, for acute lymphoblastic leukemia (ALL), CD19 is a B-cell antigen with expression that is limited to the

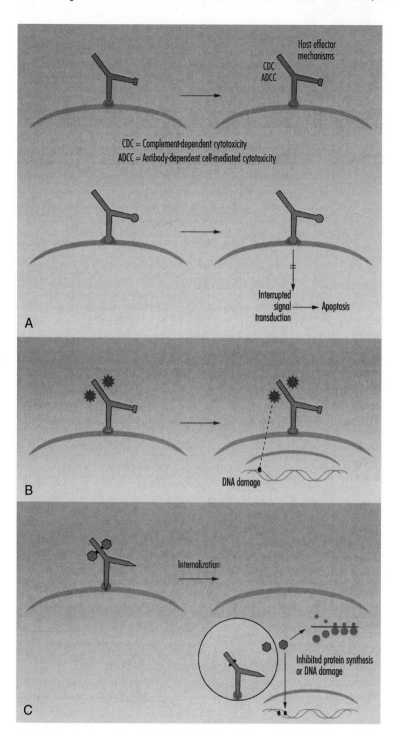

FIGURE 18–1. Antibody-targeted tumor killing, three mechanisms of action. *A,* Unconjugated monoclonal antibody: Binding of antibody initiates killing of target cells by complement-dependent cellular cytotoxicity or antibody-dependent cellular cytotoxicity in the top panel. Antibody binding (e.g., anti-CD20 antibody) interrupts cellular signal transduction, resulting in apoptosis in the lower panel. *B,* Monoclonal antibody linked with radioisotopes: Depending on the antigen targeted, radiolabeled antibody remains on the surface of the cell (CD45) or is internalized (CD33). Radiation induces DNA damage and cell death. In the instance of CD33, the radioisotope is delivered to the cell's interior. In the case of CD45, radiolabeled antibody remains on the cell surface. *C,* Both approaches damage DNA and lead to cell death. Monoclonal antibody linked with antitumor agents: Antibody-bound chemotherapy or toxin is internalized. Interaction with DNA or ribosomal protein synthesis results in cytotoxicity. (See Color Section.)

lymphoid lineage of the hematopoietic system. Elimination of CD19$^+$ cells should also spare the normal stem cell. Analogously, the receptor for granulocyte-macrophage colony-stimulating factor (GM-CSF) is expressed by most myeloid leukemias but is not, presumably, expressed by hematopoietic stem cells. As an alternative to monoclonal antibodies, fusion proteins consisting of GM-CSF ligand associated with diphtheria toxin have been proposed as a means of delivering a toxic agent to leukemic cells.[4-6] Because normal human myeloid cells, AML cells, and myeloid leukemia cell lines all express this receptor, specific tumor targeting is conceivably achievable.

Delivery of Radiation by Use of Monoclonal Antibodies

It has been hypothesized that targeted delivery of radiation to sites of leukemic involvement might effectively exploit the radiation sensitivity of leukemic blast cells and, at the same time, reduce overall systemic toxicity. Whereas the early use of radiolabeled antibodies targeting CD33 in the context of AML remission induction therapy has met with mixed results, bismuth 213–labeled and yttrium 90–labeled anti-CD33 antibody has been used with some efficacy in advanced AML (described later).

Although HSCT has long offered the best chance of long-term disease-free survival for patients with advanced leukemias, the high doses of total-body irradiation and chemotherapy required as a means of inducing durable responses can occasionally cause profound morbidity. Several studies have demonstrated that augmenting the HSCT preparative regimen might decrease the rate of subsequent leukemic recurrence. In two randomized prospective studies from the Fred Hutchinson Cancer Research Center, patients with AML in first remission[7] and chronic myelogenous leukemia (CML) in chronic phase[8] received cyclophosphamide and either 12 Gy or 15.75 Gy total-body irradiation followed by HLA-matched related marrow transplantation. The higher total-body irradiation dose was associated with a lower risk of subsequent relapse in both studies (12% versus 35% for AML, 0% versus 25% for CML). However, there was no significant difference in disease-free survival in either study because the higher total-body irradiation dose was also associated with a higher rate of transplantation-related mortality. Because a radiation dose-response effect appears to exist for myeloid leukemias, radiolabeled monoclonal antibodies have been evaluated as a means of augmenting doses of radiation to sites of leukemia, including marrow and spleen, without increasing transplantation-related mortality. In this manner, normal organs might be spared significant toxicity.

SPECIFIC HEMATOPOIETIC CELL SURFACE ANTIGENS TARGETED IN CLINICAL TRIALS

Target: Granulocyte-Macrophage Colony-Stimulating Factor

The receptor for GM-CSF has been identified on normal myeloid progenitors, mature monocytes, granulocytes, and macrophages and in malignant myeloid leukemias.[9, 10] Whereas GM-CSF receptors on leukemic blasts undergo rapid receptor-mediated endocytosis after ligand binding, this does not occur as rapidly with ligand binding to normal progenitors.[10] Thus, GM-CSF appeared to be an excellent ligand for coupling with novel cell-killing compounds that require intracellular targeting.

Diphtheria toxin (DT) is a protein synthesis–inactivating peptide toxin that is composed of a cell-binding domain, a translocation domain, and a catalytic domain[11] (Fig. 18–2) (see also Color Section). The toxin binds to heparin-binding epidermal growth factor precursors on the cell surface of many normal human tissues and undergoes receptor-mediated endocytosis. Once inside the cell in the early endosomal vesicles, the DT is cleaved and the A fragment (the catalytic domain) escapes into the cytosol. There, the toxin enzymatically ADP-ribosylates elongation factor 2, leading to irreversible protein synthesis inhibition and cell death. Murphy and coworkers[12] replaced the cell-binding domain of DT with tumor cell–directed ligands. The DT fusion toxins were found to be selectively cytotoxic to tumor cells in tissue culture. Frankel, Kreitman, and Perentesis attached GM-CSF to the DT catalytic and translocation domains, creating a GM-CSF fusion protein specific for myeloid

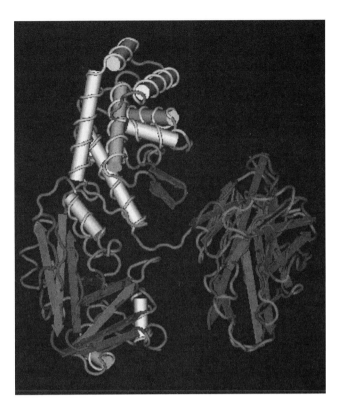

FIGURE 18–2. Ribbon drawing of α-carbon backbone of diphtheria toxin (DT) with domains in different colors. (From Choe S, Bennett MJ, Fujii G, et al: The crystal structure of diphtheria toxin. Nature 1992;357:216.) (See Color Section.)

cells.[4-6] The DT–GM-CSF fusion protein was soluble, stable, and potently cytotoxic to AML cell lines and AML progenitors, but it spared normal hematopoietic stem cells. Mice injected with leukemic cells and subsequently treated with DT–GM-CSF had prolongation of survival.[13]

Twenty-two patients with relapsed or refractory AML were treated at Wake Forest University and the University of Kentucky with escalating doses of DT-GM-CSF given by a 15-minute intravenous infusion for 5 days.[14] None of the patients had preexisting neutralizing antibodies to DT–GM-CSF, and only 4 of 20 assessable patients developed antibodies after 30 days. Five patients received a second course of DT–GM-CSF without complications. Within 4 to 8 hours after receiving the drug, most patients experienced infusion-related toxic effects that included transient fever, chills, nausea, hypoxemia, and hypotension. This reaction was preventable with steroid and antibiotic prophylaxis. Consistent with reversible liver injury, a number of patients also experienced asymptomatic, transient elevations of hepatic transaminases, creatinine kinase, and lactate dehydrogenase. Leukemic cytoreductions in the blood and marrow of more than 90% occurred at the higher dose levels by day 12. One patient had a complete remission lasting 8 months. Other patients are being treated at the same and higher doses.

Target: The Normal Myeloid Differentiation Antigen CD33

As cells mature in the myeloid lineage, pluripotent hematopoietic stem cells give rise to progenitors with lower self-renewal capacity and greater differentiation. As this process of maturation occurs, normal myeloid cells express cell surface antigens including CD33.[15-17] The myeloid cell surface antigen CD33 is an appealing target for monoclonal antibody targeting because it is expressed on AML blast cells from about 90% of patients.[16, 17] Whereas the CD33 antigen is present on maturing normal hematopoietic cells and on AML cells, normal hematopoietic stem cells lack this antigen.[18] Moreover, selective ablation of CD33+ cells from leukemic marrow aspirates from some patients with AML resulted in the growth of normal, nonclonal granulocytes and monocytes in a marrow long-term culture system.[19, 20] This suggested that selectively targeting and eliminating CD33+ cells might result in clinical remissions with reduced toxicity.

Unconjugated Anti-CD33 Antibody

Studies first reported by investigators at Memorial Sloan-Kettering Cancer Center demonstrated rapid saturation of leukemic blast cells in peripheral blood and marrow after intravenous administration of approximately 5 mg/m² of trace radioiodinated mouse anti-CD33 M195 antibody.[21] Although meaningful clinical responses were not observed with use of this approach, supersaturating doses of humanized antibody to the CD33 antigen (HuM195) have been employed with limited success.[22] In this study, patients received between 12 and 36 mg/m²/day on days 1 through 4, and the dose was then repeated on days 15 through 18. Of 10 patients with relapsed or refractory myeloid leukemias (9 AML and 1 CML) treated with supersaturating antibody concentrations, 1 achieved a complete remission, 3 had a decrease in leukemic burden, 5 had progressive disease, and 1 was not able to be evaluated for response. The patient who achieved complete remission originally had 8% blasts in his bone marrow after intensive conventional chemotherapy before receiving the anti-CD33 monoclonal antibody.

In a subsequent study, 35 patients received either 12 or 36 mg/m² of HuM195 daily for 4 consecutive days weekly for a total of four courses.[23] Two of the 35 patients achieved complete remission. Both responses occurred in patients who had less than 30% blasts in their marrow before receiving the antibody. Because some evidence of clinical efficacy was demonstrated in patients with low tumor burdens, and because the therapy appeared to be safe, this approach using an unconjugated antibody may prove to have a role in consolidation of patients with evidence of minimal residual disease.

In fact, preliminary data for use of HuM195 in patients with acute promyelocytic leukemia in complete remission suggest some clinical efficacy for those patients with minimal tumor burden.[24] Patients with acute promyelocytic leukemia who achieved complete remission after induction therapy with all-*trans* retinoic acid received HuM195 at a dose of 3 mg/m² twice weekly for 3 weeks. Subsequently, they received idarubicin and cytarabine consolidation therapy and an additional 6 months of maintenance therapy in which HuM195 was given monthly in two doses separated by 3 or 4 days. Bone marrow aspirates were evaluated serially for the promyelocytic leukemia/retinoic acid receptor-α (PML/RAR-α)

messenger RNA by reverse transcription–polymerase chain reaction (RT-PCR). Of the 27 patients treated in first remission, 25 were positive by RT-PCR before antibody treatment. Patients were considered assessable for response if adequate RNA samples were obtained for RT-PCR analysis. Whereas only 1 of 21 patients was PCR-negative after all-*trans* retinoic acid alone, 8 of 18 assessable patients (44%) became PCR-negative after receiving the first 3-week course of HuM195. After further consolidation with conventional chemotherapy, all 19 of 19 assessable patients had no evidence of disease by RT-PCR. In a historical comparison, the authors noted that only 21% of patients who continued all-*trans* retinoic acid alone for 1 month after achievement of remission experienced disappearance of the PML/RAR-α fusion gene. However, it is conceivable that the seven additional patients who became PCR-negative might have achieved PCR negativity in the absence of HuM195 treatment. For this reason, a randomized study of the antibody in patients with acute promyelocytic leukemia receiving all-*trans* retinoic acid would provide a better understanding about the contribution HuM195 makes to the achievement of molecular remission. Taken together, these early results suggest a role for antibody therapy, particularly in patients harboring a low tumor burden.

Conjugated Anti-CD33 Antibody

Administration of anti-CD33 antibody results in rapid saturation of CD33 sites throughout the body, followed by rapid modulation of the antigen-antibody complex by the cell. To exploit this behavior, a potent cytotoxic agent, calicheamicin, was linked to a humanized anti-CD33 antibody to create the experimental agent gemtuzumab ozogamicin or Mylotarg (previously named CMA-676).[25] In collaboration with Wyeth-Ayerst Research, investigators at the Fred Hutchinson Cancer Research Center and City of Hope National Medical Center conducted a phase I study of this agent. Patients with relapsed or refractory CD33+ AML were treated with escalating doses of drug every 2 weeks for three doses.[26] Leukemia was eliminated from the blood and marrow of 8 of 40 patients (20%), and blood counts normalized in 3 patients (8%). Doses up to 9 mg/m² of gemtuzumab ozogamicin were generally well tolerated, and a postinfusion syndrome of fever and chills was the most common toxic effect. Some patients who received gemtuzumab ozogamicin at high dose levels developed modest and reversible hepatic transaminase elevations and hyperbilirubinemia. At higher doses, prolonged neutropenia and thrombocytopenia were observed.

In a series of subsequent phase II studies, patients with AML in first untreated relapse after a period of at least 3 months (in most cases longer than 6 months) were treated at a dose of 9 mg/m² every 2 weeks for two doses.[27] Of the 142 patients enrolled, 30% achieved a remission characterized by less than 5% blasts in the bone marrow, more than 1500 neutrophils/mm³, and platelet transfusion independence. At the time of the report, the median overall survival was 5.9 months after receipt of gemtuzumab ozogamicin. Consistent with the drug conjugate's mechanism of action, severe neutropenia and thrombocytopenia were almost invariably observed. Mucositis of grade 3 or grade 4 was observed in 4% of patients, and infections of grade 3 or grade 4 occurred in 28% of patients. A large number of patients received the agent as outpatient therapy (38% and 41% for the first and second doses, respectively). The median time of hospitalization was 24 days, and 16% of patients required no more than 1 week of hospitalization. In contrast with findings in other studies in which frequent immune responses occurred after administration of immunoconjugates containing either murine-derived monoclonal antibodies or naturally occurring toxins, no patient in the phase II study had a positive immune response.

Radiolabeled Anti-CD33 Antibody Followed by HSCT

Two groups have investigated the combination of iodine 131–labeled anti-CD33 and conventional transplantation preparative regimens for patients with advanced AML. [131]I, with a path length of 0.8 mm and an 8-day half-life, offers the promise of eliminating antigen-negative cells as a result of a "bystander effect," whereby cells in the general vicinity of those cells binding antibody are also killed by the radiation delivered. Subsequent to initial biodistribution studies that documented localization of ^{131}I-M195 antibody in patients with advanced AML, investigators at Memorial Sloan-Kettering Cancer Center treated nine patients with AML with M195 antibody labeled with 120 to 160 mCi ^{131}I in divided doses, followed by busulfan and cyclophosphamide and matched related allogeneic marrow transplantation.[28] The transplantation procedure was reasonably well tolerated.

Investigators at the Fred Hutchinson Cancer Research Center determined the biodistribution of an alternative murine anti-CD33 antibody, p67, in nine patients with AML that was beyond first remission or refractory to conventional therapy.[29] Patients initially received a dose of trace iodine–labeled antibody to determine the biodistribution of the antibody as a means of estimating the radiation dose delivered to bone marrow and spleen in comparison with other vital organs. Patients received a therapeutic dose of ^{131}I-labeled anti-CD33 antibody combined with cyclophosphamide if the amount of radiation delivered to marrow and spleen was greater than that delivered to liver, lung, or kidney. This was followed by total-body irradiation and bone marrow infusion. Whereas this report confirmed that CD33 sites could be saturated with antibody doses of approximately 5 mg/m², favorable biodistribution was documented in only four of nine patients. This approach was well tolerated, but recurrent leukemia occurred in three of these four patients after transplantation. Moreover, after the ^{131}I-labeled anti-CD33 antibody-antigen complex internalized, ^{131}I was cleaved from the antibody and rapidly excreted into the circulation, making it difficult to deliver high doses of radiation to the marrow.

Because the expression of CD33 is somewhat limited, the best antibody dose for both p67 and M195 antibodies was low (<5 mg/m²). Higher, supersaturating antibody doses resulted in delivery of excess radiation to nonhematopoietic organs owing to prolonged circulation of unbound radiolabeled antibody. In addition, ^{131}I was rapidly excreted from target cells after internalization of the ^{131}I-labeled anti-CD33 antibody-antigen complex, and only low doses of either anti-CD33 antibody could be administered without saturating CD33 sites. For these reasons, further dose escalation was limited, and both institutions have evaluated different targeting approaches.

Radiolabeled Anti-CD33 Antibody without HSCT

Anti-CD33 antibody has been labeled with two alternative isotopes, [213]Bi and ^{90}Y, in nontransplantation studies in patients with advanced AML by investigators at Memorial Sloan-Kettering Cancer Center.[30, 31] Because [213]Bi emits an alpha particle associated with a shorter path length and briefer half-life than those of ^{131}I, it was theorized that effective tumor targeting would be achieved with minimal nonspecific cytotoxicity. Whereas a shorter path length offers the possibility of limiting nonspecific toxicity, the half-life requires rapid access to target cells for an antileukemic effect. In a phase I study, 17 patients with relapsed (n = 13) or refractory (n = 3) AML and 1 patient with chronic myelomonocytic leukemia received escalating doses of [213]Bi-HuM195 in 3 to 6 fractions during 2 to 4 days.[31] Although no acute toxic effects were observed, myelosuppression lasted 8 to 34 days. Specificity for bone marrow, liver, and spleen was documented within 10 minutes of administration by gamma camera images. Whereas 10 of 12 assessable patients had reductions in leukemic blast cell counts in peripheral blood and 12 of 17 patients had reductions in the percentages of marrow blasts, no complete remissions had been documented at the time of the report. Because myelosuppression was significant, [213]Bi-HuM195 might find a therapeutic role before hematopoietic stem cell rescue.

These investigators have also evaluated HuM195 anti-CD33 antibody labeled with the beta-emitting isotope ^{90}Y in the nontransplantation setting.[30] Although [213]Bi emits an alpha particle with a 46-minute half-life and a path length of 0.06 mm, ^{90}Y has a half-life of 2.5 days and a path length of 5.3 mm. In a phase I study, 17 patients with relapsed or refractory AML received escalating doses of ^{90}Y-HuM195. Because the absence of gamma emissions prevented direct determination of the biodistribution of ^{90}Y, the agent was combined with trace indium 111–labeled antibody in nine patients. Of 16 patients, 12 experienced decreases in the percentages of marrow blasts from pretreatment levels, and 1 patient achieved a complete remission. Myelosuppression was more profound at the highest ^{90}Y dose administered, and one patient experienced prolonged marrow aplasia and died 6 weeks after therapy. The most common acute toxic effects were rigors, fevers, and nausea. Akin to [213]Bi-labeled anti-CD33 antibody, higher doses of radiation could be delivered in the setting of HSCT, and such a study combining ^{90}Y-HuM195 antibody with etoposide followed by autologous stem cell rescue is planned.

Target: The Normal Hematopoietic Cell Antigen CD45

The CD45 cell surface antigen is densely expressed (200,000 copies per cell) by essentially all white blood cells and their precursors, including most acute myeloid and lymphoblastic leukemias. It therefore presents an appealing target for radiolabeled antibody therapy. Whereas CD33 may represent an excellent target for antibody-drug conjugates because it internalizes on antibody binding, antibody-bound CD45 antigen tends to remain on the surface of cells. For this reason, antibody-delivered ^{131}I is less likely to be cleaved and released into the general circulation. Because of ubiquitous CD45 expression by white blood cells in addition to leukemic cells, ^{131}I-labeled anti-CD45 antibody can be used in patients in remission or active relapse. Because CD45 is expressed by lymphoid as well as by myeloid cells, radiolabeled anti-CD45 antibody can deliver radiation to sites of leukemic involvement in lymph nodes in addition to the marrow and spleen.

Radiolabeled Anti-CD45 Antibody Followed by HSCT

Investigators at the Fred Hutchinson Cancer Research Center have studied the biodistribution of ^{131}I-labeled BC8 (murine anti-CD45) antibody in patients with AML, myelodysplastic syndrome, and ALL and have combined this agent with standard HSCT preparative regimens in patients with advanced disease and with AML in first remission. In a phase I study, 44 patients with high-risk acute leukemias, including 3 patients with advanced myelodysplastic syndrome, received escalating doses of ^{131}I-labeled anti-CD45 antibody in association with cyclophosphamide and total-body irradiation followed by marrow transplantation.[32] Patients received the amount of ^{131}I estimated to deliver from 3.5 Gy to a maximum of 12.25 Gy to the normal organ receiving the highest dose. Most patients had a favorable biodistribution of ^{131}I-labeled anti-CD45 antibody, and administration of a pre-clearing dose of cold antibody before the radiolabeled treatment did not significantly reduce hepatic radiation exposure. A notable improvement in biodistribution over the ^{131}I-labeled anti-CD33 approach was observed. In 84% of patients, a greater amount of radiation was delivered to marrow and spleen than to other vital organs. Among the 25 patients with AML or myelodysplastic syndrome who were treated, 7 patients remained disease-free 15 to 89 months (median of 58 months) from the time of transplantation.

Both patients who received 12.25 Gy developed life-threatening mucositis; therefore, the maximal tolerated dose of radiation delivered by ^{131}I-BC8 antibody was estimated to be 10.5 Gy (grade III veno-occlusive disease of the liver occurred in one of six patients treated at this level). Whereas engraftment was not clinically affected by estimated marrow doses of up to 28 Gy, a single patient who received an estimated marrow dose of 31 Gy experienced graft failure before her death on day 29 from fungal pneumonia. This suggests that excessive radiation to marrow stroma might impair hematopoietic growth and development.

In a similar study combining ^{131}I-labeled anti-CD45 antibody with a busulfan and cyclophosphamide preparative regimen,[33] 25 patients with AML in first or second remission or early first relapse received escalating radiation doses delivered by antibody. Favorable biodistribution

was documented in 90% of patients evaluated for protocol entry. Of the 24 patients with AML in first remission, 18 patients are surviving disease-free 10 to 63 months (median, 42 months) after transplantation. Whereas four patients died of transplantation-related causes, only two patients experienced relapse. These early data are encouraging. Historically, approximately 30% of patients with AML conditioned with busulfan and cyclophosphamide and undergoing transplantation in first remission would be expected to experience leukemic relapse. A phase III study comparing this regimen with busulfan and cyclophosphamide alone is being considered to evaluate any potential therapeutic benefit that targeted hematopoietic irradiation might provide.

Target: CD19, CD22, and Other Normal Lymphoid Cell Antigens

Most patients with ALL express the normal cell surface antigen CD19. Nonhematopoietic tissues do not express CD19, akin to the surface antigens mentioned before; hence, therapy delivered to cells expressing this antigen will be limited to the hematopoietic compartment. A protein tyrosine kinase of the *src* family linked to CD19 is normally involved in signal transduction and the regulation of apoptotic cell death. As such, it serves as an attractive target for the delivery of genistein, a naturally occurring protein tyrosine kinase inhibitor, as a means of triggering apoptotic cell death. Uckun and associates[34] evaluated the B43-genistein immunoconjugate in 15 patients aged 4 to 60 years with advanced CD19+ B-lineage ALL (and one patient with chronic lymphocytic leukemia). In a phase I study, patients received escalating doses of B43-genistein as a 1-hour intravenous infusion for 10 consecutive days or 3 consecutive days weekly for a total of nine doses. B43-genistein was generally well tolerated. Fever was the most common infusion-related adverse event, and grade 2 vascular leak syndrome was observed in one patient. Clinical efficacy was somewhat limited; only 1 of 14 assessable ALL patients achieved a complete remission of at least 19 months. However, two additional patients experienced reductions in leukemic blasts in post-treatment bone marrow aspirates. Because three of nine patients evaluated had moderately high levels of human antimouse antibodies (HAMA) that were also associated with rapid clearance of B43-genistein, immune responses might limit chronic administration of this novel agent.

Escalating doses of an immunotoxin targeting CD22, the normal adhesion molecule expressed exclusively on B cells, has been evaluated in 16 patients with hairy-cell leukemia that was resistant to treatment with purine analogues.[35] Eleven of 16 patients achieved complete remission after treatment with RFB4(dsFv)–PE38 (BL22), a recombinant immunotoxin containing an anti-CD22 variable domain (Fv) fused to truncated *Pseudomonas* exotoxin. Although therapy was reasonably well tolerated, a reversible hemolytic-uremic syndrome developed in two patients during a second cycle of treatment with BL22. Despite these potentially serious adverse events, these outstanding clinical results provide further support for antibody-directed approaches.

Target: The Interleukin-2 Receptor in Adult T-Cell and Chronic Lymphocytic Leukemias

Adult T-cell leukemia (ATL) is characterized by a malignant proliferation of mature lymphocytes induced by the retrovirus human T-lymphotropic virus type 1 (HTLV-1). Because high-affinity interleukin-2 receptors are constitutively expressed at much higher levels by ATL cells than by normal resting cells, a monoclonal antibody that blocks the interaction of interleukin-2 with its receptor might prevent continued malignant proliferation. A highly specific unconjugated anti-Tac monoclonal antibody was clinically evaluated in 19 patients with ATL.[36] The treatment was reasonably well tolerated, and two patients achieved complete remissions. Five additional patients achieved partial remissions for varying lengths of time, and several patients achieved excellent immunologic reconstitution. As a means of achieving increased cytotoxicity with this antibody-targeting approach, Waldmann and colleagues[37] clinically evaluated anti-Tac antibody conjugated with ^{90}Y in 18 patients with ATL. Patients who achieved a remission were allowed to receive up to eight additional doses of radioimmunotherapy. Of 16 assessable patients, 9 demonstrated a clinical response to ^{90}Y-labeled anti-Tac with a partial (n = 7) or complete (n = 2) remission. Although hematopoietic toxicity was observed, the treatment was otherwise well tolerated. ^{90}Y-labeled anti-Tac directed toward the interleukin-2 receptor represents a promising approach for treatment of ATL.

SUMMARY

Modest therapeutic efficacy has been observed with several antibody- or immunotoxin-targeting approaches in acute leukemias. Unconjugated humanized anti-CD33 antibody appears particularly suited to the treatment of patients with minimal residual disease. As a means of improving clinical efficacy, potent cytotoxic agents or radioisotopes have been conjugated to monoclonal antibodies to increase targeted cytotoxicity. In the non-HSCT setting, HuM195 (anti-CD33) antibody labeled with either ^{213}Bi or ^{90}Y has reduced tumor burden in patients with relapsed and refractory AML without causing significant nonhematologic toxicity. Used as a single agent, humanized anti-CD33 antibody linked to the potent antitumor antibiotic calicheamicin (gemtuzumab ozogamicin) has safely induced remission in one third of patients with AML in first relapse.

Maximal doses of radiation to leukemic cells by radiolabeled antibody require HSCT rescue. This approach offers the advantage of radiating leukemic cells even if a portion of the cells lack antigen or when the patient is in a clinical remission and the antibody is binding predominantly to normal hematopoietic cells. It is conceivable that remission induction with use of antibody-targeted chemotherapy followed by consolidation with radiolabeled antibody will achieve long-term remissions while minimizing toxic effects.

REFERENCES

1. Smith FO, Rauch C, Williams DE, et al: The human homologue of rat NG2, a chondroitin sulfate proteoglycan, is not expressed on the cell surface of normal hematopoietic cells but is expressed by acute myeloid leukemia blasts from poor-prognosis patients with abnormalities of chromosome band 11q23. Blood 1996;87:1123.
2. Buchsbaum DJ, Wahl RL, Normolle DP, et al: Therapy with unlabeled and ^{131}I-labeled pan-B-cell monoclonal antibodies in nude mice bearing Raji Burkitt's lymphoma xenografts. Cancer Res 1992; 52:6476.
3. Shan D, Ledbetter JA, Press OW: Apoptosis of malignant human B cells by ligation of CD20 with monoclonal antibodies. Blood 1998; 91:1644.
4. Hogge DE, Willman CL, Kreitman RJ, et al: Malignant progenitors from patients with acute myelogenous leukemia are sensitive to a diphtheria toxin–granulocyte-macrophage colony-stimulating factor fusion protein. Blood 1998;92:589.
5. Perentesis JP, Gunther R, Waurzyniak B, et al: In vivo biotherapy of HL-60 myeloid leukemia with a genetically engineered recombinant fusion toxin directed against the human granulocyte macrophage colony-stimulating factor receptor. Clin Cancer Res 1997;3(pt 1): 2217.
6. Kreitman RJ, Pastan I: Recombinant toxins containing human granulocyte-macrophage colony-stimulating factor and either *Pseudomonas* exotoxin or diphtheria toxin kill gastrointestinal cancer and leukemia cells. Blood 1997;90:252.
7. Clift RA, Buckner CD, Appelbaum FR, et al: Allogeneic marrow transplantation in patients with acute myeloid leukemia in first remission: A randomized trial of two irradiation regimens. Blood 1990;76:1867.
8. Clift RA, Buckner CD, Appelbaum FR, et al: Allogeneic marrow transplantation in patients with chronic myeloid leukemia in the chronic phase: A randomized trial of two irradiation regimens. Blood 1991;77:1660.
9. Park LS, Waldron PE, Friend D, et al: Interleukin-3, GM-CSF, and G-CSF receptor expression on cell lines and primary leukemia cells: Receptor heterogeneity and relationship to growth factor responsiveness. Blood 1989;74:56.
10. Cannistra SA, Groshek P, Garlick R, et al: Regulation of surface expression of the granulocyte/macrophage colony-stimulating factor receptor in normal human myeloid cells. Proc Natl Acad Sci U S A 1990;87:93.
11. Choe S, Bennett MJ, Fujii G, et al: The crystal structure of diphtheria toxin. Nature 1992;357:216.
12. Foss FM, Saleh MN, Krueger JG, et al: Diphtheria toxin fusion proteins. Curr Top Microbiol Immunol 1998;234:63.
13. Hall PD, Willingham MC, Kreitman RJ, et al: DT388–GM-CSF, a novel fusion toxin consisting of a truncated diphtheria toxin fused to human granulocyte-macrophage colony-stimulating factor, prolongs host survival in a SCID mouse model of acute myeloid leukemia. Leukemia 1999;13:629.
14. Howard D, Phillips G, Hall P, et al: Phase I trial of fusion toxin DTGM containing human GM-CSF fused to truncated diphtheria toxin in adults with relapsed or refractory acute myelogenous leukemia (AML). Proc Am Soc Clin Oncol 2000;19:26a.
15. Andrews RG, Torok-Storb B, Bernstein ID: Myeloid-associated differentiation antigens on stem cells and their progeny identified by monoclonal antibodies. Blood 1983;62:124.
16. Griffin JD, Linch D, Sabbath K, et al: A monoclonal antibody reactive with normal and leukemic human myeloid progenitor cells. Leuk Res 1984;8:521.
17. Dinndorf PA, Andrews RG, Benjamin D, et al: Expression of normal myeloid-associated antigens by acute leukemia cells. Blood 1986; 67:1048.
18. Andrews RG, Singer JW, Bernstein ID: Precursors of colony-forming cells in humans can be distinguished from colony-forming cells by expression of the CD33 and CD34 antigens and light scatter properties. J Exp Med 1989;169:1721.
19. Bernstein ID, Singer JW, Andrews RG, et al: Treatment of acute

myeloid leukemia cells in vitro with a monoclonal antibody recognizing a myeloid differentiation antigen allows normal progenitor cells to be expressed. J Clin Invest 1987;79:1153.

20. Bernstein ID, Singer JW, Smith FO, et al: Differences in the frequency of normal and clonal precursors of colony-forming cells in chronic myelogenous leukemia and acute myelogenous leukemia. Blood 1992;79:1811.

21. Scheinberg DA, Lovett D, Divgi CR, et al: A phase I trial of monoclonal antibody M195 in acute myelogenous leukemia: Specific bone marrow targeting and internalization of radionuclide. J Clin Oncol 1991;9:478.

22. Caron PC, Dumont L, Scheinberg DA: Supersaturating infusional humanized anti-CD33 monoclonal antibody HuM195 in myelogenous leukemia. Clin Cancer Res 1998;4:1421.

23. Feldman E, Kalaycio M, Schulman P, et al: Humanized monoclonal anti-CD33 antibody HuM195 in the treatment of relapsed/refractory acute myelogenous leukemia (AML): Preliminary report of a phase II study. Proc Am Soc Clin Oncol 1999;18:4a.

24. Jurcic JG, DeBlasio T, Dumont L, et al: Molecular remission induction with retinoic acid and anti-CD33 monoclonal antibody HuM195 in acute promyelocytic leukemia. Clin Cancer Res 2000;6:372.

25. Hinman LM, Hamann PR, Wallace R, et al: Preparation and characterization of monoclonal antibody conjugates of the calicheamicins: A novel and potent family of antitumor antibiotics. Cancer Res 1993;53:3336.

26. Sievers EL, Appelbaum FA, Spielberger RT, et al: Selective ablation of acute myeloid leukemia using antibody-targeted chemotherapy: A phase I study of an anti-CD33 calicheamicin immunoconjugate. Blood 1999;93:3678.

27. Sievers EL, Larson RA, Stadtmauer EA, et al: Efficacy and safety of gemtuzumab ozogamicin in patients with CD33-positive acute myeloid leukemia in first relapse. J Clin Oncol 2001;19:3244.

28. Papadopoulos E, P C, Castro-Malaspina H, et al: Results of allogeneic bone marrow transplant following ^{131}I-M195/busulfan/cyclophosphamide (Bu/Cy) in patients with advanced/refractory myeloid malignancies. Blood 1993;82:80a.

29. Appelbaum FR, Matthews DC, Eary JF, et al: The use of radiolabeled anti-CD33 antibody to augment marrow irradiation prior to marrow transplantation for acute myelogenous leukemia. Transplantation 1992;54:829.

30. Jurcic J, Divgi C, McDevitt M, et al: Potential for myeloablation with yttrium-90–HuM195 (anti-CD33) in myeloid leukemia. Proc Am Soc Clin Oncol 2000;19:8a.

31. Jurcic JG, McDevitt MR, Sgouros G, et al: Phase I trial of targeted alpha-particle therapy for myeloid leukemia with bismuth-213–HuM195 (anti-CD33). Proc Am Soc Clin Oncol 1999;18:7a.

32. Matthews DC, Appelbaum FR, Eary JF, et al: Phase I study of ^{131}I-anti-CD45 antibody plus cyclophosphamide and total body irradiation for advanced acute leukemia and myelodysplastic syndrome. Blood 1999;94:1237.

33. Matthews DC, Appelbaum FR, Eary JF, et al: [^{131}I]-anti-CD45 antibody plus busulfan/cyclophosphamide in match-related transplants for AML in first remission. Blood 1996;88:142a.

34. Uckun FM, Messinger Y, Chen CL, et al: Treatment of therapy-refractory B-lineage acute lymphoblastic leukemia with an apoptosis-inducing CD19-directed tyrosine kinase inhibitor. Clin Cancer Res 1999;5:3906.

35. Kreitman RJ, Wilson WH, Bergeron K, et al: Efficacy of the anti-CD22 recombinant immunotoxin BL22 in chemotherapy-resistant hairy-cell leukemia. N Engl J Med 2001;345:241.

36. Waldmann TA, White JD, Goldman CK, et al: The interleukin-2 receptor: A target for monoclonal antibody treatment of human T-cell lymphotrophic virus I–induced adult T-cell leukemia. Blood 1993;82:1701.

37. Waldmann TA, White JD, Carrasquillo JA, et al: Radioimmunotherapy of interleukin-2R alpha-expressing adult T-cell leukemia with yttrium-90-labeled anti-Tac. Blood 1995;86:4063.

19

Guido Marcucci   Michael A. Caligiuri

Antisense and Gene Transfer as Therapeutic Strategies in Acute and Chronic Leukemia

The explosion in innovative technologies has paved the way for establishing a better understanding of the molecular mechanisms operative in tumorigenesis and for designing strategies that target genetic differences between cancer cells and their normal counterparts.[1] "Gene therapy" is generally intended as a therapeutic approach that replaces or modifies the expression of specific genes at the DNA level and induces a selective advantage of the host normal cells over the malignant clone. Alternatively, it is possible to modify the expression of a leukemogenic gene by inhibiting translation of its messenger RNA (mRNA). Because the latter approach does not directly target a gene but, instead, its encoded transcript, or sense, it is more often referred to as "antisense therapy."[2] Chronic and acute leukemias have always been regarded as optimal targets for both gene and antisense therapy because of evidence demonstrating recurrent single abnormalities that characterize the malignant cells and directly contribute to the leukemogenic process.[1] Despite their enormous therapeutic potential, however, these strategies have left the majority of researchers' expectations unfulfilled, and their full incorporation into the management of leukemia patients remains far from being realized.[3] Much of the difficulty in translating gene-modifying approaches into the clinical setting stems from the inability of efficiently reproducing in vivo the encouraging results obtained in in vitro models. Nevertheless, recent progress in understanding the factors that govern gene expression at the level of transcription and translation, along with technical advances in transferring genomic information into normal and leukemic cells, has provided cautious optimism for the clinical development of these strategies (Table 19–1). Three major approaches are currently being developed to advantageously exploit the potentials of antisense and gene therapy in leukemia: (1) silencing genes that directly contribute to leukemogenesis, (2) transferring genomic information into leukemic cells to restore the "loss of function" of a disrupted gene, and (3) transferring genes that induce chemotherapy resistance into normal hematopoietic stem cells to produce a selective advantage of the host normal cells with respect to the leukemic counterpart. The aim of this chapter is to summarize the most recent advances achieved in therapeutic studies that use the aforementioned strategies to target populations of patients with acute or chronic leukemia and to provide a prospective overview of their applicability in future clinical trials.

ANTISENSE STRATEGIES: SILENCING LEUKEMOGENIC GENES

In leukemia, malignant clones often appear to be characterized by nonrandom chromosome rearrangements that at the molecular level induce the activation of specific oncogenes or create novel chimeric genes.[4-6] Overexpression of genes with oncogenic potential often occurs when the transcriptional regulatory elements of one gene, typically within the *Ig* or *TCR* genes, become juxtaposed to the complete reading frame of another gene. Under such control, the affected gene becomes constitutively activated and consequently overexpressed, thereby leading to malignant transformation. This mechanism of malignant transformation is most often seen in acute lymphoblastic leukemia (ALL). For example, in ALL and Burkitt's lymphoma, the t(8;14)(q24;q32) translocation results in the *MYC* gene on chromosome 8 fusing with the *IgH* promoter region on chromosome 14. Malignant proliferation is somehow driven by *MYC* overexpression.[7] In contrast, in myeloid leukemias, transformation more

TABLE 19–1. Antisense and Gene Therapy Clinical Trials in Acute and Chronic Leukemia

Strategy	Target	Disease	Number of Patients
Antisense[37]	*BCR/ABL*	CML	8
Antisense[38]	*BCR/ABL*	CML	3
Antisense[45]	*MYC*	CML	8
Antisense[2]	*MYC*	CML	18
Antisense[60]	*TP53*	Acute leukemia/MDS	16
Gene marking[79]	*neo*	Acute leukemia	12
Gene marking[81]	*neo*	CML	2

CML, chronic myelogenous leukemia; MDS, myelodysplasia.

often occurs, at least in part, as a consequence of the creation of new chimeric genes.[6] In this context, segments of two different genes are fused together to give rise to a novel structure consisting of the 5′ end of one gene and the 3′ end of another gene. The resultant fusion gene contains structural and functional domains different from their respective wild-type genes and encodes a fusion protein required (but possibly not sufficient) for malignant transformation. This situation is exemplified by the t(9;22)(p34;q11) translocation in chronic myelogenous leukemia (CML). At the molecular level, this chromosomal aberration results in fusion of the *BCR* gene on chromosome 22 with the *ABL* gene on chromosome 9, thus creating *BCR/ABL*, a fusion gene that plays a critical role in leukemogenesis.[8] In acute myeloid leukemia (AML), other examples of recurrent genomic aberrations are the t(8;21)(q22;q22) translocation resulting in the *AML1/ETO* gene fusion, the inv(16)(p13q22) inversion resulting in the *CBFβ/MYH11* gene fusion, and the t(15;17)(q22;q21) translocation resulting in the *PML/RARα* gene fusion.[9, 10] Accumulating experimental evidence, including data from transgenic animal models, strongly supports the hypothesis that these genomic aberrations play an active role in disrupting the normal programs of cell proliferation, differentiation, or survival, in addition to directly contributing to leukemogenesis.[11-15]

Because of their direct impact on malignant transformation, several investigators have focused on overexpressed oncogenes and novel chimeric oncogenes as ideal targets for therapeutic strategies that silence gene expression with antisense oligodeoxynucleotides (ODNs) or ribozyme molecules.[16-19] After many years of laboratory investigation, this approach is now being translated into the clinic.[20]

Biology and Chemistry of Antisense Oligonucleotides

The antisense or reverse complementary ODNs are sequences of 16 to 29 bases of single-stranded DNA that hybridize to specific genes or their mRNA products by Watson-Crick base pairing and disrupt their function.[2] Although certain classes of ODNs bind DNA and prevent normal gene transcription by forming DNA triple-helix structures, most of the ODNs currently in use for in vitro or in vivo studies target mRNA.[17, 21] The relatively short length of these antisense sequences is a necessary feature that facilitates cell internalization and increases hybridization efficiency by reducing base mismatch errors. Once hybridization has occurred, the ODN-mRNA complex becomes a substrate for intracellular RNAses (i.e., RNAse-H) that catalyze mRNA degradation and allow the ODN to recycle for another base pairing with the next target mRNA molecule. The net result of this process is a sustained decrease in target mRNA translation and, ultimately, a reduced rate of synthesis of the corresponding oncogenic protein. Important questions have been raised, however, regarding the specificity of the antisense strategy in providing its antitumor effect. It is becoming clear that in some cases, administration of antisense ODNs induces nonspecific activation of cytokines and other

immunologic activities, which may in turn result in suppression of malignant clones. The unmethylated dinucleotide motif CpG present in the palindromic sequence AACGTT in an ODN, for instance, may lead to activation of interferon production and augmentation of natural killer (NK) and T-cell function, and it can be a potent inhibitor of B-cell proliferation and differentiation.[22] The mechanisms leading to the immunostimulatory action of these nucleotide sequences remain unknown, although it has been hypothesized that they are mediated via the nuclear transcription factor NFκB, which activates genes involved in the proinflammatory immune response.[23]

In spite of its sound rationale, translation of the antisense strategy from the laboratory to the clinic has been unpredictably difficult. The unmodified antisense moieties used in the initial studies suffered from a variety of limitations, including an inability to cross the cell membrane, lack of resistance to intracellular catalytic enzymes, and failure to gain direct access to the target mRNA sequence.[24] Moreover, secondary conformational changes of the target, the relatively low concentration of ODNs to the target, the unknown rate of synthesis and degradation of the target, and the low ODN-to-target binding affinity have further limited the therapeutic application of these compounds. Finally, it is now clear that many of the conditions necessary to improve the specificity and therapeutic efficiency of antisense ODNs can be satisfied only at the expense of others. Therefore, the ideal conditions that would allow antisense ODNs to fully exploit their role as gene expression modifiers have been exceedingly difficult to achieve. In recent years, however, antisense research has made striking progress. By substituting a sulfur atom for an oxygen atom in the phosphodiester bound between two subsequent nucleotides of the ODN sequence, a new phosphorothioate antisense structure can be synthesized.[25] The phosphorothioate ODNs appear to have better diffusion capability across the cell membrane, improved resistance to the degrading intracellular endonucleases, and a severalfold increase in water solubility. In addition, different strategies have improved selection of the ODN-mRNA pair sequences that would most efficiently hybridize and, in turn, decrease the expression of oncogenic proteins. Some groups have used computer modeling software to predict secondary and tertiary structures of the target mRNA and, in turn, which of the mRNA sequences are more accessible to the antisense molecules.[18] Other investigators have explored the use of manufactured ODN arrays complementary to sequential radiolabeled segments of target mRNA to select the antisense sequence that forms the most efficient and strongest hybridization signal base pair with the target mRNA.[26, 27] Despite these and other sophisticated methodologies, predicting hybridization efficiency only on the basis of structural analysis of both the target mRNA and the antisense ODN continues to be difficult, and the choice of base-pairing partners still usually includes a component of empiricism.

Antisense Strategies in CML

The reciprocal translocation t(9;22)(p34.1;q11.21) is a nonrandom chromosomal rearrangement that occurs in

CML, ALL, and other myeloproliferative disorders.[28] The resultant *BCR/ABL* gene fusion is transcribed into a chimeric mRNA and translated into fusion proteins of varying size depending on the breakpoint locations of the two involved genes.[29] In CML, exon e2 or b3 of *BCR* fuses with exon a2 of *ABL* and a 210-kd fusion protein is encoded, whereas in ALL, exon e1 of *BCR* fuses with exon a2 of *ABL* and a shorter variant of the *BCR/ABL* gene fusion is produced that encodes a 190-kd chimeric protein (p190). More recently, chronic neutrophilic leukemia has been found to be associated with a variant of *BCR/ABL* fusion that spans the *BCR* exon e19 and the *ABL* exon a2 and results in a gene fusion that encodes the higher-molecular-weight BCR/ABL protein p230. Each of these *BCR/ABL* variants represents a specific tumor marker that encodes an oncogenic protein likely to play an important role in activating and sustaining leukemogenesis. Therefore, silencing of *BCR/ABL* expression has represented an ideal target and, indeed, a prototypic disease for the application of antisense strategies.[30]

Szczylik et al provided the early evidence to support the use of antisense therapy in CML.[31] In their initial experience, these authors showed that treatment of *BCR/ABL*-positive leukemic blasts with an 18-mer ODN complementary to b2a2 or b3a2 *BCR/ABL* fusion transcripts could selectively and specifically induce suppression of colony formation from leukemic clones carrying the b2a2 or b3a2 *BCR/ABL* variants, respectively. In contrast, colony formation from normal granulocyte and macrophage precursors remained intact. Similarly, when a mixture of normal and *BCR/ABL*-positive hematopoietic precursors were exposed to anti-b2a2 or anti-b3a2 *BCR/ABL* ODNs, only the *BCR/ABL*-negative cells were able to survive. The specificity of the response to the *BCR/ABL* antisense ODN treatment was, however, questioned by other groups.[32, 33] Although inhibition of *BCR/ABL*-positive cell growth could be achieved by using *BCR/ABL* antisense ODNs, the ability to selectively target cells expressing different isoforms of *BCR/ABL* fusion transcripts with the corresponding antisense ODNs could not be convincingly demonstrated. In subsequent studies, Skorski and colleagues reported that in severe combined immunodeficient (SCID) mice injected with the *BCR/ABL*-positive BV173 cell line, once the disease was established, administration of the 26-mer *BCR/ABL* antisense ODN induced a decrease in *BCR/ABL* mRNA levels, disappearance of the *BCR/ABL*-positive leukemic clones, and prolongation of the animals' survival with respect to untreated controls (18 to 23 weeks versus 8 to 13 weeks).[34] The same group also reported that when a similar population of SCID mice with established CML were treated with low-dose cyclophosphamide and *BCR/ABL* ODN antisense, a cure rate of 50% could be achieved.[35] Finally, by using a combination of the *BCR/ABL* antisense ODNs and mafosfamide to treat a 1:1 mixture of *BCR/ABL*-positive leukemic cells and normal hematopoietic precursors, it was possible to significantly decrease the number of viable *BCR/ABL*-positive elements, thus mimicking the process of ex vivo bone marrow (BM) purging.[36]

On the basis of these preliminary results, de Fabritiis et al reported the first clinical trial using *BCR/ABL* antisense ODNs for BM purging in CML patients undergoing autolo-gous BM transplantation (BMT).[37] Eight patients were selected from a pool of 35 *BCR/ABL*-positive patients on the basis of the in vitro sensitivity of their leukemic cells to the *BCR/ABL* antisense ODNs, which was defined as the ability to produce inhibition of t(9;22)-positive colony formation. Of the eight patients, seven received transplants in the accelerated phase and one in the second chronic phase. In these eight patients, three had the b2a2 *BCR/ABL* transcript and five had the b3a2 variant. BM was collected from selected patients and incubated with either a b2a2 or a b3a2 26-mer *BCR/ABL* antisense, according to the presence of the corresponding fusion variant, for 24 or 72 hours. At the completion of the purging procedure, the median recovery was 47.6% of the mononuclear cells, 48.8% of the CD34$^+$ cells, and 20.3% of the clonogenic cells. A longer incubation period with *BCR/ABL* antisense resulted in a significantly lower percentage of recovered CD34$^+$ cells ($p = .022$). Incubation of cells in culture medium that did not contain ODNs produced a recovery of CD34$^+$ and clonogenic cells similar to the values found in prepurged marrow. All eight patients showed engraftment at a median of 26.5 days for neutrophils and 45 days for platelets. No difference in hematologic recovery was seen in patients autografted with stem cells treated for 24 hours versus 72 hours. Transient disappearance of the t(9;22) cells was seen in two patients by conventional cytogenetic analysis, but not by assaying the same cells with fluorescence in situ hybridization, which showed persistence of the *BCR/ABL* fusion. With a median follow-up of 27.5 months, of the eight patients, four relapsed in chronic phase and blast crisis developed in four.

More recently, Clark and associates modified this strategy by pretreating *BCR/ABL*-positive BM with streptolysin O to permeabilize cell membranes and improve intracellular delivery of the *BCR/ABL* antisense during autograft purging.[38] BM collections from three *BCR/ABL*-positive patients with b3a2 ($n = 2$) or b2a2 ($n = 1$) *BCR/ABL* transcripts were exposed to streptolysin O, followed by treatment with the corresponding b3a2 or b2a2 breakpoint-specific antisense. After purging, BM aliquots were taken to estimate granulocyte-macrophage colony-forming unit (CFU-GM) growth. Only CFU-GM colonies from the b2a2 *BCR/ABL* patient became negative for *BCR/ABL* transcript by reverse transcription–polymerase chain reaction (RT-PCR). Of the three patients included in this study, those with b3a2 *BCR/ABL* ($n = 2$) suffered early cytogenetic relapse after the BM autograft but remained in hematologic remission 724 and 610 days after transplantation. The remaining b2a2 *BCR/ABL*-positive patient died in blastic phase 91 days after the transplant. Therefore, achieving a negative *BCR/ABL* status in the CFU-GM colony formation assay was not predictive of a better clinical outcome.

Although the *BCR/ABL* fusion transcript appears to be an obvious target for antisense strategies in CML, it might not be the ideal one.[39] It is possible that the administration of antisense ODNs induces only transient downregulation of the *BCR/ABL* protein and, in turn, only a temporary antileukemic effect. Furthermore, it is possible that despite antisense treatment, *BCR/ABL*-positive precursor cells that do not express the chimeric oncoprotein remain unperturbed and contribute to disease relapse once exposure to the *BCR/ABL* antisense is completed.[40] Thus, in searching for an alternative ideal target in CML, several groups began to silence genes downstream of *BCR/ABL* that are thought to be important in the leukemogenic pathway. Gewirtz et al proposed the *MYB* proto-oncogene as a potential therapeutic antisense target.[2, 39] The physiologic role of *MYB* has not been completely defined. Initial evidence links this gene to a regulatory function in the cell cycle and to transactivation of genes potentially important for normal hematopoiesis, such as the *c-kit* and *CD34* genes. In support of this hypothesis, it was reported that antisense down-regulation of *MYB* expression has a negative impact on normal hematopoiesis by inhibiting stem-cell multilineage colony formation.[41] Interestingly, when compared with normal hematopoietic precursors, *BCR/ABL*-positive cells appear to be more sensitive to the action of *MYB* antisense, thus suggesting that *BCR/ABL* clonal hematopoiesis may be more dependent on *MYB* expression than normal hematopoiesis is.[42] Agarwal and Gewirtz have hypothesized that down-regulation of *MYB* results in failure to transactivate *c-kit*, a gene that encodes for a tyrosine kinase receptor for the *c-kit* ligand (Steel factor), which appears to be important in preventing programmed cell death (PCD).[17, 43, 44] It is therefore conceivable that lack of *c-kit* transactivation, as a result of treatment with *MYB* antisense, induces preferential apoptosis of *BCR/ABL*-positive cells. After a series of in vitro preliminary studies, Gerwitz et al have tested this hypothesis in the clinical setting. In their initial experience, BM was harvested from eight CML patients, seven in chronic and one in accelerated phase.[2, 45] The collected products were purged with a *MYB* antisense ODN and reinfused after autograft conditioning. Seven of the eight patients showed engraftment. In four of the eight patients, 85% to 100% of marrow metaphases were *BCR/ABL* negative 3 months after transplantation. Five of the eight patients had a sustained hematologic remission for up to 2 years. These results were obtained by exposing the collected CD34+ cells to the *MYB* antisense for 24 hours. When exposure of the BM harvests to the antisense molecule was increased to 72 hours to improve purging efficiency, the engraftment rate markedly decreased. In a second study, the same group of investigators treated 18 patients with refractory CML, 13 of them in accelerated or blastic phase, by using 7-day continuous in vivo infusion of *MYB* antisense at different dose levels.[2] Of the 18, only 1 CML patient in blastic phase survived 14 months with transient restoration of the chronic phase.

Though relatively unsuccessful, these studies demonstrate the feasibility of antisense treatment in vivo and raise the question of whether differently designed therapeutic approaches could improve the clinical outcome. For instance, it is not known whether blocking the *BCR/ABL* leukemogenic pathway at different levels by using *BCR/ABL* and *MYB* antisense molecules in combination could result in better control of malignant proliferation. It is interesting that when SCID mice initially injected with blast crisis CML cells were treated with a combination of *MYB* and *BCR/ABL* antisense ODNs, they showed a significantly improved outcome when compared with those treated with only one of the two antisense ODNs or when compared with untreated controls.[46] With the recent success of the tyrosine kinase inhibitor STI571 in stable-phase CML, the combination of these molecular approaches may prove useful in accelerated-phase or blast crisis CML, where a multitude of genetic defects probably contributes to the more malignant progression of the disease.[47]

BCL-2 Antisense: A Potential Therapeutic Strategy in Acute Leukemia

The BCL-2 protein plays a major role in the prevention of apoptosis, or PCD, in normal and cancer cells.[48] The antiapoptotic activity of BCL-2 is likely to represent one of the more common mechanisms of chemotherapy resistance by preventing cancer cells from efficiently translating chemotherapy-induced damage into PCD. Initially discovered because of its involvement in t(14;18) B-cell lymphomas, BCL-2 production is found to be abnormally elevated in roughly half of human cancers, which suggests that deregulated expression of this proto-oncogene represents one of the more common events associated with human malignancies.[49] The biologic mechanisms by which BCL-2 prevents PCD are complex and remain to be fully understood. At least 10 other proteins of the BCL-2 family have been identified, all of which function as either antiapoptotic or proapoptotic factors.[50] These proteins retain the capability of homodimerization and heterodimerization with other members of the family and probably regulate the apoptotic pathway independently or by mutual antagonism. Recent data suggest that through their interaction, the BCL-2 family members regulate the mitochondrial release of cytochrome *c* and its binding to apoptotic protease-activating factor (Apaf).[49] This process, in turn, seems to modulate the caspase cascade during the terminal stages of PCD.

Initial in vitro results have suggested a direct correlation between BCL-2 expression and chemoresistance. Using gene transfer experiments, several groups have demonstrated that the dose of chemotherapy required to kill 50% of the cells induced to express a high level of BCL-2 was 5- to 10,000-fold higher than that necessary to achieve comparable results in cells with lower basal levels of BCL-2.[50] These data were subsequently confirmed in in vivo studies of patients with different hematologic malignancies, where overexpression of BCL-2 directly correlated with treatment resistance and poor clinical outcome. In a series of 348 patients with intermediate- or high-grade non-Hodgkin's lymphoma, Hermine et al found that high levels of BCL-2 expression were more frequently associated with stage III and IV disease ($p = .002$), reduced disease-free survival ($p < .01$), and decreased overall survival ($p < .05$) than were lower levels of expression.[51] Campos and colleagues analyzed 82 samples from patients with newly diagnosed AML.[52] High expression of BCL-2 was associated with a low complete remission (CR) rate (29% CR rate in patients with 20% or more BCL-2–positive cells versus an 85% CR rate in those with less than 20% BCL-2–positive cells) and significantly shorter survival after intensive chemotherapy. In multivariate analysis, the percentage of BCL-2–positive cells, age, and the percentage of CD34[+] cells were independently associated with poor survival. Banker and associates reported that expression of BCL-2 is generally lower in AML patients with the favorable t(8;21) karyotype than in AML patients with other chromosomal aberrations.[53] In the same study, it was noted that pediatric and older patients with t(8;21) AML, who generally have a poor clinical outcome despite the favorable karyotype, express higher BCL-2 levels than do young adults with t(8;21) AML, who in contrast, are expected to have a good clinical outcome. This finding was confirmed in a more recent study in which higher levels of BCL-2 had an adverse prognostic impact in AML patients with a favorable karyotype.[54]

From these kind of data, one could hypothesize that down-regulation of BCL-2 may decrease chemoresistance. The use of antisense molecules to reduce BCL-2 expression is currently being investigated in vitro and in vivo by many groups and represents an example of successful translation of an antisense strategy from the laboratory to the clinic. Initial investigative efforts have culminated in the synthesis of G3139, an 18-mer phosphorothioate antisense ODN designed to bind to the first six codons of the human BCL-2 mRNA.[55] As expected, this compound down-regulates BCL-2 expression and lowers the threshold for apoptosis of tumor cells in response to treatment with cytotoxic agents in vitro. G3139 treatment of the B-cell lymphoma cell line DoHH2, which carries the t(14;18) translocation, results in down-regulation of the overexpressed BCL-2 and a consequent 40% reduction in cell viability when compared with untreated, sense-treated, or scrambled ODN-treated controls.[56] In vivo administration of G3139 to SCID nude mice inoculated with lymphoma xenografts eliminates malignant lymphoproliferation, as measured by PCR for the t(14;18) translocation and by flow cytometry for CD45.[55] These effects appear to be related to the dose and duration of the G3139 infusion. Thus, of 60 mice treated with 100 mg of G3139 daily for 2 weeks, 83% achieved nearly complete resolution of their disease. When treatment with the same dose was extended for 3 weeks, the results improved to complete resolution of the disease in all animals, including an absence of the t(14;18) translocation by PCR assays. Similar results reported in nonobese diabetic (NOD)/SCID mice lacking NK, B-cell, or T-cell activity suggest that the G3139 antisense activity is indeed mediated by specific base-pairing hybridization to the BCL-2 mRNA and not by an NK-, B-cell–, or T-cell–immunomediated response.[57]

These intriguing preliminary results have prompted clinical application of G3139 for the treatment of hematologic malignancies and other chemoresistant neoplastic diseases such as melanoma and small-cell lung carcinoma. In a phase I dose escalation trial completed at the Royal Marsden Hospital in adults with advanced, refractory non-Hodgkin's lymphoma who were immunohistochemically or PCR positive for BCL-2 in a lymph node biopsy, G3139 was administered as a continuous subcutaneous infusion for 14 days.[58, 59] Twenty-one patients were treated at dose levels ranging from 4.6 to 195.8 mg/m²/day. Dose-limiting toxicities were observed at doses of 147.2 mg/m²/day and above and consisted of thrombocytopenia, fever, and

hypotension. These toxicities were thought to be related to the phosphothioate backbone of the ODN sequence rather than the specific BCL-2 antisense sequence itself. Pharmacokinetic analysis showed that a steady-state concentration was achieved 48 hours after the beginning of the infusion. Among 21 patients who completed at least 2 weeks of treatment, one complete and two partial remissions were observed by radiographic analysis. Of 10 patients who had lymphoma-related symptoms, 6 improved after G3139 treatment. At least a 15% reduction in BCL-2 protein levels measured by flow cytometry in peripheral mononuclear cells, BM, or lymph node needle aspirates was seen in seven patients. Lymphoma cells from lymph node specimens from one patient were inoculated into three NOD/SCID mice, which were subsequently treated with G3139, BCL-2 sense ODN, or normal saline. The two control animals treated with BCL-2 sense ODN and normal saline, euthanized at day 50, showed signs of lymphoma in the spleen and lymph nodes, whereas the mouse treated with G3139 remained well with no evidence of lymphoma at day 80 of treatment.

On the basis of these encouraging results, investigators at our institution have recently designed and initiated a phase I study that incorporates the BCL-2 antisense strategy in the treatment of refractory or relapsed acute leukemia. In this study, patients with chemoresistant disease are treated over a 10-day period with continuous infusion of G3139 and salvage chemotherapy with fludarabine, cytarabine (ara-C), and G-CSF (FLAG). During the first 5 days, patients receive only G3139, whereas G3139 infusion overlaps FLAG administration on days 6 through 10. The end point of this study is to find the maximal tolerated dose of G3139 when it is given in combination with salvage chemotherapy and to correlate disease response with down-regulation of BCL-2 in sequential BM and blood samples before, during, and after treatment with G3139. This study is ongoing, but preliminary results are encouraging (Marcucci, unpublished data).

Alternative Antisense Strategies

Other antisense ODNs are currently being tested in patients with acute leukemia. In a recent phase I trial, a total of 16 patients with AML or high-risk myelodysplasia were treated with TP53 antisense ODNs.[60] TP53 is a tumor suppressor gene that is mutated in many malignancies, including acute leukemia. In this study, continuous infusion of TP53 antisense was administered with minimal toxicity. The plasma concentration and the area under the curve linearly correlated with dose levels, and no specific toxicity directly correlated with the antisense administration was seen. Although leukemic growth in vitro was inhibited when compared with pretreatment samples, no clinical response was observed.

Ribozymes: Another Potential Approach to Silence Leukemogenesis

Ribozymes are naturally occurring RNA sequences with enzymatic activity that cause RNA cleavage by forming base pair complexes and catalyzing the hydrolysis of phosphodiester bonds within target molecules.[61] Various classes of naturally occurring ribozymes can be identified and differentiated by their structure and function. The self-splicing group I and group II introns are RNA sequences within the pre-mRNA molecules that catalyze the reactions that splice out the intronic sequences. The remaining exons are then ligated before the mRNA is transported into the cytoplasm and translated into the corresponding protein. Ribonuclease P is a ubiquitous endoribonuclease that consists of both protein and RNA components; its catalytic action cleaves target RNA bound to short complementary oligonucleotide sequences called external guide sequences. Finally, other small catalytic RNA molecules have been identified in plants, fungi, and animal virus. These molecules, whose functional domains can assume different configurations such as the hammerhead or hairpin, consist of RNA sequences that cleave their mRNA targets through base-pairing hybridization.

Several investigators have taken advantage of the catalytic activity of these molecules and have used ribozymes as a potential tool to suppress the activity of expressed leukemogenic genes.[61] Many different ribozymes have been synthesized to mimic those occurring naturally, with relative success in down-regulating target gene expression in vitro. Kobayashi et al, for instance, reported the use of ribozymes in targeting expression of the multidrug resistance gene *MRD1* in malignant cells. When MOLT-3 leukemic T cells expressing *MDR1* were treated with the corresponding ribozyme, resistance to vincristine decreased by more than 20-fold.[62] *BCR/ABL*- and *AML1/ETO*-positive leukemia cells have been used to demonstrate the value of ribozymes in down-regulating expression of their respective chimeric genes.[63, 64] The specificity of these compounds in the context of *AML1/ETO*- and *BCR/ABL*-driven leukemogenesis, however, remains to be proved. In a more recent study, Nason-Burchenal and colleagues reported the use of hammerhead ribozymes to cleave *PML/RARα* transcripts in the all-*trans*-retinoic acid (ATRA)-resistant NB4 acute promyelocytic leukemia (APL) cell line (NB4-R1).[65, 66] Exposure of this cell line to the APL1.1 ribozyme resulted in marked repression of *PML/RARα* transcription, suppression of cell growth, and an increased rate of PCD after treatment with ATRA. Despite these intriguing results, translation of ribozyme therapy to the clinic has similar limitations and hurdles as those already discussed for the antisense ODNs. Inefficient cell internalization, lack of chemical stability, and formation of secondary and tertiary structures within the ribozymes or their targets are some of the issues currently being addressed in experimental models.

GENE TRANSFER AS A THERAPEUTIC STRATEGY FOR LEUKEMIA

The concept of "gene therapy" in leukemia, or the introduction of genomic material into leukemic cells with the aim of inducing PCD or restoring regulation of cell growth and differentiation, remains an area of intensive scientific investigation. However, to date, the potential application of such an approach has yet to be realized.

Despite tremendous progress in identifying a number of critical molecular defects in many cases of leukemia, it now appears that secondary molecular "hits" are also likely to be important in initiating and maintaining the malignant phenotype.[13] Therefore, correcting the function of one disrupted gene by using gene transfer technologies so late in the disease process (i.e., at the initial clinical evaluation or at relapse) may not be sufficient to eliminate the malignant process or to restore normal hematopoiesis. In addition, many of the fusion gene products in leukemic cells induce their contribution to malignant transformation through a transdominant effect, thereby limiting the corrective action that might be offered by gene transfer of a normal allele. Finally, the methods used for the transfer of genes into hematopoietic cells are themselves still underdeveloped and relatively inefficient.[67, 68] Despite these obvious difficulties and consequent lack of clinical success, the research to target leukemia and other hematologic malignancies with gene therapy continues. Zhao et al, for instance, have recently proposed the use of gene transfer methodologies to integrate *BCR/ABL* antisense into the genome of normal and clonal hematopoietic precursors.[69] The authors will test to see whether it is possible to engineer a cell that can itself produce *BCR/ABL* antisense molecules during its own life cycle and that of its progeny. The ultimate goal is to obtain a steady level of *BCR/ABL* antisense that results in constant down-regulation of the fusion gene product responsible, at least in part, for the CML phenotype. In their initial experiments,[69] copies of the *BCR/ABL* antisense and the dihydrofolate reductase (*DHFR*) gene, which confers resistance to methotrexate, were introduced into a *BCR/ABL*-positive cell line. Cells carrying the *BCR/ABL* antisense molecule selected by methotrexate exposure were shown to have 5- to 10-fold suppression of *BCR/ABL* mRNA and protein levels, normalization of cell growth, and a 3- to 4-log reduction of tumorigenicity in vivo.

Other groups have taken a different approach. To overcome the lethal toxicity induced by dose-intensive chemotherapy on normal hematopoietic precursor cells (HPCs), investigators have introduced a multidrug resistance gene, *MDR1*, into HPCs. The feasibility of this approach was initially demonstrated in transgenic mouse models.[70, 71] With successful incorporation of *MDR1* into HPCs, mice carrying the transduced gene demonstrated markedly reduced chemotherapy-related toxicity. Similar results have been obtained by integrating the *DHFR* gene for methotrexate resistance into murine HPCs.[72] The *DHFR*-positive mice, subsequently treated with methotrexate, showed an increase in survival with respect to the *DHFR*-negative control mice. It is intriguing that the same mice had reduced chemotherapy-induced toxicity even in organs not directly targeted by the gene transduction, such as the gastrointestinal tract. This finding could imply that such toxicity might be the result of HPC injury or death inducing a cascade of events that lead to secondary injury or that rapid hematopoietic recovery significantly limits this injury. On the basis of these and other preclinical studies, a pilot clinical trial was performed.[73] In three patients undergoing autologous BMT, purified CD34+ HPCs were initially harvested and exposed to a retroviral vector carrying *MDR1*, cryopreserved, and readministered after ablative chemotherapy. After engraftment, gene transfer was documented by PCR for the vector-derived *MDR1* cDNA sequence in all three cases. Analysis of peripheral blood and BM cells 12, 15, and 18 months after the autografts, however, failed to show evidence of a persistent in vivo gene transfer effect. In a second similar study,[74] high-levels of *MDR1* expression were successfully transferred and demonstrated in erythroid burst-forming units and CFU-GMs derived from CD34+ HPCs transduced in vitro. Once reinfused into patients undergoing autologous BMT, however, only two of the five treated patients showed evidence of *MDR1* transduction in stem cells obtained from aspirated BM samples. The relatively limited success of these trials is probably related at least in part to the low level of transduction efficiency that can be obtained with the current cadre of vectors. Moreover, the benefit of this strategy in inducing protection from chemotherapy toxicity was not evaluated in these two studies and therefore remains to be demonstrated.

A recent death in a gene therapy trial using an adenovirus vector for a nonmalignant condition now mandates a more intense focus on safety and potential toxicities of the approach, along with continued careful consideration of its potential application in molecularly heterogeneous diseases such as acute leukemia and CML.[75] As a consequence, the next several years will probably be devoted to phase I studies using alternative vectors such as the adeno-associated viral vector and the lentivirus vector.[67, 68] It is thus likely that progress in evaluating the *therapeutic* efficacy of gene transfer for leukemia will advance slowly. As the technology is largely being developed for the treatment of nonmalignant genetic defects that are correctable in HPCs, several important concerns will be necessary to sort out before moving ahead with a similar strategy in leukemia, a disease whose malignant counterpart is derived from the HPC. For example, it is possible that vectors identified as ideal for transferring *MDR1* to HPCs in a disease such as ovarian cancer could be equally effective in transferring such resistance to residual leukemic cells. Alternatively, random insertion of such a gene could perturb the normal homeostasis of nonmalignant HPCs in as yet unpredictable ways. Notably, in a recent study by Bunting and colleagues, transduction of murine HPCs with an *MDR1*-carrying vector resulted in unwanted myeloproliferative syndrome.[76]

Another potential strategy is the transfer of genes encoding enzymes able to convert prodrug into active and toxic metabolites and to selectively target such therapy to malignant cells. The thymidine kinase *(tk)* gene has been used in the early studies to test this strategy.[77] Tumor cells were transfected with a vector carrying the *tk* gene and, in turn, exposed to ganciclovir. The tk product actively phosphorylates ganciclovir, which once incorporated in the cell's genome, results in its selective death. Early clinical application of this approach in cancer has been pursued in brain tumors, but attempts to efficiently transfer *tk* into HPCs have not yet met with success. However, this strategy is also being studied to control graft-versus-host disease (GVHD) after the infusion of *tk*-transduced donor lymphocytes in leukemia patients who have relapsed after allogeneic BMT, with some evidence of success.[78] Because the infused allogeneic T-cell population responsible for GVHD cannot yet be dissected from the T cells responsible for the potentially beneficial graft-versus-leukemia (GVL) effect, *tk*-transduced T cells can be quickly eliminated from the body with ganciclovir treatment if their adverse GVHD effects are found to predominate over their intended GVL effect.

Finally, gene transfer or gene "marker" strategies have been used for marking HPCs in the setting of autologous stem-cell transplantation (ASCT) for leukemia. ASCT is considered a potential useful therapeutic strategy in leukemia, but its current applicability is limited by the high rate of disease relapse in many studies. Whether relapse after ASCT is due to chemotherapy-resistant leukemic blasts residing in the host at the time of myeloablative therapy or whether relapse is due to leukemic blast contamination of the reinfused stem cells, or both, is unknown. One approach to resolve this issue is to use efficient gene transfer of a marker gene such as *neomycin* (*neo*) into harvested autologous HPCs and to assess, at the time of relapse, whether *neo* is present in the leukemic cell population. This approach assumes equivalent efficiency of gene transfer between normal HPCs and their malignant counterpart, which may or may not be present in the autologous stem-cell pool of a patient in complete remission. In the first study evaluating this approach, BM from 12 leukemic patients was harvested at the time of complete remission and marked with the *neo* gene.[79, 80] Four of the 12 patients relapsed. In three patients, leukemic colony growth from the relapsed BM tested positive for the *neo* gene by PCR and showed resistance to neomycin. One patient with t(8;21) tested positive for both the *AML1/ETO* fusion transcript and the *neo* gene. Similar results were seen in CML patients undergoing autologous BMT.[81] The results of these preliminary studies demonstrate that residual leukemic cells present in the harvested, autologous graft may contribute to disease relapse. The data do not exclude a contribution from chemoresistant cells that might reside in the host. However, the development of better methodologies for purging malignant blasts from the stem-cell product collected from a leukemic patient in remission may result in improved disease-free survival after ASCT.

CONCLUSION

The concept of gene therapy has long been pursued, and this approach has recently been used to successfully treat human disease, specifically, immune deficiency.[82] Importantly, for the purposes of malignancy, these approaches will be most useful in instances in which single-gene deficiencies or possibly single-gene mutations are responsible for the malignant phenotype. In these instances, the astounding progress with more efficient and safer vectors will probably lead to continued therapeutic success. Leukemia, unfortunately, is largely characterized by molecular heterogeneity and sequential defects that contribute to its successful malignant transformation. As an exception to this general pattern, CML has been at the center of clinically promising gene-targeting approaches with antisense, but exceptional advances in molecular targeting with the tyrosine kinase inhibitor STI571 will probably take precedence for stable-phase CML at most medical centers over the next several years. Nonetheless, as primary and secondary molecular defects continue to be unraveled in other forms of acute and chronic leukemia, antisense approaches, possibly in combination with more traditional chemotherapy and differentiation therapy, should be actively pursued. These antisense approaches will most likely be developed with ODNs, ribozymes, and gene transfer with vectors delivering antisense into the genome. The progress made in identifying good-prognosis (e.g., t[8;21] AML) and poor-prognosis (e.g., t[4;11] ALL) cytogenetics with respect to standard chemotherapy suggests that each characteristic gene fusion probably contributes to drug sensitivity or drug resistance. Therefore, antisense therapies successfully directed against these fusions, possibly given in combination with chemotherapy, might lead to enhanced efficacy, as has been demonstrated for ATRA in t(15;17) APL. In this regard, mouse models of leukemia that result at least in part from these genetic alterations will be of tremendous value in studying these gene-modifying approaches. In addition, a better understanding of the downstream targets of defects such as BCL-2 will also be critical in devising molecular therapies that target multiple pathways to prevent the induction of differentiation and/or apoptosis in leukemic cells. The last decade has provided tremendous insight into the molecular heterogeneity of leukemia. The next decade will deliver customized, molecularly targeted therapies that should have a significant impact on improving clinical outcome.

Acknowledgment

Supported by Grant P30CA16058, National Cancer Institute, Bethesda, MD, Grant KO8CA90469-01, and The Coleman Leukemia Research Foundation.

REFERENCES

1. Anderson WF: Human gene therapy. Nature 1998;392:25.
2. Gewirtz AM, Sokol DL, Ratajczak MZ: Nucleic acid therapeutics: State of the art and future prospects. Blood 1998;92:712.
3. Verma IM, Somia N: Gene therapy—promises, problems and prospects. Nature 1997;389:239.
4. Caligiuri M, Bloomfield C: Molecular biology of leukemia. In De Vita V, Hellman S, Rosemberg S, eds: Cancer: Principles and Practice of Oncology, 6th ed. Philadelphia: Lippincott-Raven; 2000.
5. Look AT: Oncogenic transcription factors in the human acute leukemias. Science 1997;278:1059.
6. Caligiuri MA, Strout MP, Gilliland DG: Molecular biology of acute myeloid leukemia. Semin Oncol 1997;24:32.
7. Dalla-Favera R, Bregni M, Erikson J, et al: Human c-myc oncogene is located on the region of chromosome 8 that is translocated in Burkitt lymphoma cells. Proc Natl Acad Sci U S A 1982;79:7824.
8. Faderl S, Talpaz M, Estrov Z, et al: Chronic myelogenous leukemia: Biology and therapy. Ann Intern Med 1999;131:207.
9. Strout MP, Marcucci G, Caligiuri MA, et al: Core-binding factor (CBF) and MLL-associated primary acute myeloid leukemia: Biology and clinical implications. Ann Hematol 1999;78:251.
10. Grignani F, Fagioli M, Alcalay M, et al: Acute promyelocytic leukemia: From genetics to treatment. Blood 1994;83:10.
11. Okuda T, Cai Z, Yang S, et al: Expression of a knocked-in AML1-ETO leukemia gene inhibits the establishment of normal definitive hematopoiesis and directly generates dysplastic hematopoietic progenitors. Blood 1998;91:3134.
12. Yergeau DA, Hetherington CJ, Wang Q, et al: Embryonic lethality and impairment of haematopoiesis in mice heterozygous for an AML1-ETO fusion gene. Nat Genet 1997;15:303.
13. Castilla LH, Garrett L, Adya N, et al: The fusion gene Cbfb-MYH11 blocks myeloid differentiation and predisposes mice to acute myelomonocytic leukaemia. Nat Genet 1999;23:144.
14. Castilla LH, Wijmenga C, Wang Q, et al: Failure of embryonic hematopoiesis and lethal hemorrhages in mouse embryos heterozygous for a knocked-in leukemia gene CBFB-MYH11. Cell 1996; 87:687.
15. He LZ, Tribioli C, Rivi R, et al: Acute leukemia with promyelocytic features in PML/RARα transgenic mice. Proc Natl Acad Sci U S A 1997;94:5302.
16. Adams SW, Emerson SG: Gene therapy for leukemia and lymphoma. Hematol Oncol Clin North Am 1998;12:631.
17. Agarwal N, Gewirtz AM: Oligonucleotide therapeutics for hematologic disorders. Biochim Biophys Acta 1999;1489:85.
18. Cotter FE: Antisense therapy of hematologic malignancies. Semin Hematol 1999;36:9.
19. Warzocha K: Antisense strategy in hematological malignancies. Cytokines Cell Mol Ther 1999;5:15.
20. Gewirtz AM: Oligonucleotide therapeutics: A step. J Clin Oncol 2000;18:1809.
21. Camerini-Otero RD, Hsieh P: Parallel DNA triplexes, homologous recombination, and other homology-dependent DNA interactions. Cell 1993;73:217.
22. Krieg AM, Matson S, Fisher E: Oligodeoxynucleotide modifications determine the magnitude of B cell stimulation by CpG motifs. Antisense Nucleic Acid Drug Dev 1996;6:133.
23. Krieg AM: Mechanisms and applications of immune stimulatory CpG oligodeoxynucleotides. Biochim Biophys Acta 1999;1489:107.
24. Crooke ST: Molecular mechanisms of action of antisense drugs. Biochim Biophys Acta 1999;1489:31.
25. Agrawal S: Importance of nucleotide sequence and chemical modifications of antisense oligonucleotides. Biochim Biophys Acta 1999; 1489:53.
26. Southern EM, Milner N, Mir KU: Discovering antisense reagents by hybridization of RNA to oligonucleotide arrays. Ciba Found Symp 1997;209:38.
27. Milner N, Mir KU, Southern EM: Selecting effective antisense reagents on combinatorial oligonucleotide arrays. Nat Biotechnol 1997;15:537.
28. Rowley JD: A new consistent chromosomal abnormality in chronic myelogenous leukaemia identified by quinacrine fluorescence and Giemsa staining [letter]. Nature 1973;243:290.
29. Sawyers CL: Chronic myeloid leukemia. N Engl J Med 1999;340: 1330.
30. Clark RE: Antisense therapeutics in chronic myeloid leukaemia: The promise, the progress and the problems. Leukemia 2000;14:347.
31. Szczylik C, Skorski T, Nicolaides NC, et al: Selective inhibition of leukemia cell proliferation by BCR-ABL antisense oligodeoxynucleotides. Science 1991;253:562.
32. Smetsers TF, van de Locht LT, Pennings AH, et al: Phosphorothioate BCR-ABL antisense oligonucleotides induce cell death, but fail to reduce cellular bcr-abl protein levels. Leukemia 1995;9:118.
33. Smetsers TF, Linders EH, van de Locht LT, et al: An antisense Bcr-Abl phosphodiester-tailed methylphosphonate oligonucleotide reduces the growth of chronic myeloid leukaemia patient cells by a non-antisense mechanism. Br J Haematol 1997;96:377.
34. Skorski T, Nieborowska-Skorska M, Nicolaides NC, et al: Suppression of Philadelphia1 leukemia cell growth in mice by BCR-ABL antisense oligodeoxynucleotide. Proc Natl Acad Sci U S A 1994; 91:4504.
35. Skorski T, Nieborowska-Skorska M, Wlodarski P, et al: Treatment of Philadelphia leukemia in severe combined immunodeficient mice by combination of cyclophosphamide and bcr/abl antisense oligodeoxynucleotides. J Natl Cancer Inst 1997;89:124.
36. Skorski T, Nieborowska-Skorska M, Barletta C, et al: Highly efficient elimination of Philadelphia leukemic cells by exposure to bcr/abl antisense oligodeoxynucleotides combined with mafosfamide. J Clin Invest 1993;92:194.
37. de Fabritiis P, Petti MC, Montefusco E, et al: BCR-ABL antisense

oligodeoxynucleotide in vitro purging and autologous bone marrow transplantation for patients with chronic myelogenous leukemia in advanced phase. Blood 1998;91:3156.

38. Clark RE, Grzybowski J, Broughton CM, et al: Clinical use of strepto-lysin-O to facilitate antisense oligodeoxyribonucleotide delivery for purging autografts in chronic myeloid leukaemia. Bone Marrow Transplant 1999;23:1303.

39. Gewirtz AM: Myb targeted therapeutics for the treatment of human malignancies. Oncogene 1999;18:3056.

40. Verfaillie CM, McIvor RS, Zhao RC: Gene therapy for chronic myelogenous leukemia. Mol Med Today 1999;5:359.

41. Gewirtz AM, Calabretta B: A c-myb antisense oligodeoxynucleotide inhibits normal human hematopoiesis in vitro. Science 1988;242: 1303.

42. Calabretta B, Sims RB, Valtieri M, et al: Normal and leukemic hematopoietic cells manifest differential sensitivity to inhibitory effects of c-myb antisense oligodeoxynucleotides: An in vitro study relevant to bone marrow purging. Proc Natl Acad Sci U S A 1991; 88:2351.

43. Yu H, Bauer B, Lipke GK, et al: Apoptosis and hematopoiesis in murine fetal liver. Blood 1993;81:373.

44. Carson WE, Haldar S, Baiocchi RA, et al: The c-kit ligand suppresses apoptosis of human natural killer cells through the upregulation of bcl-2. Proc Natl Acad Sci U S A 1994;91:7553.

45. Gewirtz A, Luger S, Sokol D, et al: Oligodeoxynucleotide therapeutics for human myelogenous leukemia: Interim results [abstract]. Blood 1996;88:270.

46. Skorski T, Nieborowska-Skorska M, Wlodarski P, et al: Antisense oligodeoxynucleotide combination therapy of primary chronic myelogenous leukemia blast crisis in SCID mice. Blood 1996;88:1005.

47. Druker BJ, Talpaz M, Resta D, et al: Clinical efficacy and safety of an abl specific tyrosine kinase inhibitor as targeted therapy for chronic myelogenous leukemia [abstract]. Blood 1999;94:368.

48. Reed J: Bcl-2 family proteins: Regulators of apoptosis and chemoresistance in hematologic malignancies. Semin Hematol 1997;34:9.

49. Reed JC: Dysregulation of apoptosis in cancer. Semin Oncol 1999; 17:2941.

50. Reed J: Molecular biology of chronic lymphocytic leukemia: Implications for therapy. Semin Hematol 1998;35:3.

51. Hermine O, Haioun C, Lepage E, et al: Prognostic significance of bcl-2 protein expression in aggressive non-Hodgkin's lymphoma. Groupe d'Etude des Lymphomes de l'Adulte (GELA). Blood 1996; 87:265.

52. Campos L, Rouault J, Sabido O, et al: High expression of bcl-2 protein in acute myeloid leukemia cells is associated with poor response to chemotherapy. Blood 1994;84:595.

53. Banker D, Radich J, Becker A, et al: The t(8;21) translocation is not consistently associated with high Bcl-2 expression in de novo acute myeloid leukemias of adults. Clin Cancer Res 1998;4:3051.

54. Kornblau S, Thall P, Estrov Z, et al: The prognostic impact of BCL2 protein expression in acute myelogenous leukemia varies with cytogenetics. Clin Cancer Res 1999;5:1758.

55. Cotter FE, Johnson P, Hall P, et al: Antisense oligonucleotides suppress B-cell lymphoma growth in a SCID-hu mouse model. Oncogene 1994;9:3049.

56. Smith MR, Abubakr Y, Mohammad R, et al: Antisense oligodeoxyribonucleotide down-regulation of bcl-2 gene expression inhibits growth of the low-grade non-Hodgkin's lymphoma cell line WSU-FSCCL. Cancer Gene Ther 1995;2:207.

57. Cotter FE, Waters J, Cunningham D: Human Bcl-2 antisense therapy for lymphomas. Biochim Biophys Acta 1999;1489:97.

58. Waters JS, Webb A, Cunningham D, et al: Phase I clinical and pharmacokinetic study of bcl-2 antisense oligonucleotide therapy in patients with non-Hodgkin's lymphoma. J Clin Oncol 2000; 18:1812.

59. Webb A, Cunningham D, Cotter F, et al: BCL-2 antisense therapy in patients with non-Hodgkin lymphoma. Lancet 1997;349:1137.

60. Bishop MR, Iversen PL, Bayever E, et al: Phase I trial of an antisense oligonucleotide OL(1)p53 in hematologic malignancies. J Clin Oncol 1996;14:1320.

61. James HA, Gibson I: The therapeutic potential of ribozymes. Blood 1998;91:371.

62. Kobayashi H, Dorai T, Holland JF, et al: Reversal of drug sensitivity in multidrug-resistant tumor cells by an MDR1 (PGY1) ribozyme. Cancer Res 1994;54:1271.

63. James H, Mills K, Gibson I: Investigating and improving the specificity of ribozymes directed against the bcr-abl translocation. Leukemia 1996;10:1054.

64. Kozu T, Sueoka E, Okabe S, et al: Designing of chimeric DNA/RNA hammerhead ribozymes to be targeted against AML1/MTG8 mRNA. J Cancer Res Clin Oncol 1996;122:254.

65. Nason-Burchenal K, Takle G, Pace U, et al: Targeting the PML/RAR alpha translocation product triggers apoptosis in promyelocytic leukemia cells. Oncogene 1998;17:1759.

66. Nason-Burchenal K, Allopenna J, Begue A, et al: Targeting of PML/RARα is lethal to retinoic acid–resistant promyelocytic leukemia cells. Blood 1998;92:1758.

67. Russell DW, Kay MA: Adeno-associated virus vectors and hematology. Blood 1999;94:864.

68. Buchschacher GL Jr, Wong-Staal F: Development of lentiviral vectors for gene therapy for human diseases. Blood 2000;95:2499.

69. Zhao RC, McIvor RS, Griffin JD, et al: Gene therapy for chronic myelogenous leukemia (CML): A retroviral vector that renders hematopoietic progenitors methotrexate-resistant and CML progenitors functionally normal and nontumorigenic in vivo. Blood 1997; 90:4687.

70. Licht T, Gottesman MM, Pastan I: Transfer of the MDR1 (multidrug resistance) gene: Protection of hematopoietic cells from cytotoxic chemotherapy, and selection of transduced cells in vivo. Cytokines Mol Ther 1995;1:11.

71. van de Vrie W, Marquet RL, Stoter G, et al: In vivo model systems in P-glycoprotein–mediated multidrug resistance. Crit Rev Clin Lab Sci 1998;35:1.

72. Allay JA, Persons DA, Galipeau J, et al: In vivo selection of retrovirally transduced hematopoietic stem cells. Nat Med 1998;4:1136.

73. Devereux S, Corney C, Macdonald C, et al: Feasibility of multidrug resistance (MDR-1) gene transfer in patients undergoing high-dose therapy and peripheral blood stem cell transplantation for lymphoma. Gene Ther 1998;5:403.

74. Hesdorffer C, Ayello J, Ward M, et al: Phase I trial of retroviral-mediated transfer of the human MDR1 gene as marrow chemoprotection in patients undergoing high-dose chemotherapy and autologous stem-cell transplantation. J Clin Oncol 1998;16:165.

75. Marshall E: Gene therapy on trial. Science 2000;288:951.

76. Bunting KD, Galipeau J, Topham D, et al: Transduction of murine bone marrow cells with an MDR1 vector enables ex vivo stem cell expansion, but these expanded grafts cause a myeloproliferative syndrome in transplanted mice. Blood 1998;92:2269.

77. Culver KW, Ram Z, Wallbridge S, et al: In vivo gene transfer with retroviral vector–producer cells for treatment of experimental brain tumors. Science 1992;256:1550.

78. Bonini C, Ferrari G, Verzeletti S, et al: HSV-TK gene transfer into donor lymphocytes for control of allogeneic graft-versus-leukemia. Science 1997;276:1719.

79. Brenner MK, Rill DR, Moen RC, et al: Gene-marking to trace origin of relapse after autologous bone-marrow transplantation. Lancet 1993;341:85.

80. Rill DR, Santana VM, Roberts WM, et al: Direct demonstration that autologous bone marrow transplantation for solid tumors can return a multiplicity of tumorigenic cells. Blood 1994;84:380.

81. Deisseroth AB, Zu Z, Claxton D, et al: Genetic marking shows that Ph+ cells present in autologous transplants of chronic myelogenous leukemia (CML) contribute to relapse after autologous bone marrow in CML. Blood 1994;83:3068.

82. Cavazzana-Calvo M, Hacein-Bey S, de Saint Basile G, et al: Gene therapy of human severe combined immunodeficiency (SCID)-X1 disease. Science 2000;288:669.

20

Robert S. Negrin   Karl G. Blume

Hematopoietic Cell Transplantation in the Leukemias

HISTORICAL DEVELOPMENTS

Bone marrow and peripheral blood progenitor cell transplantations have emerged as effective therapies for patients with a variety of hematologic malignant neoplasms. Advances in the fields of cell biology, immunology, and genetics continue to promote more successful therapies but also to suggest novel concepts. The first studies demonstrating protection of bone marrow–derived cells from the lethal effects of radiation were performed in mice. In 1949, Jacobson discovered that shielding the spleen protected animals from the otherwise fatal consequences of radiation.[1] In 1951, Lorenz demonstrated that the infusion of bone marrow cells had a similar protective effect if they were derived from an identical strain of mice.[2]

In 1957, the first bone marrow transplantations were performed in patients with advanced leukemias with limited success, but they demonstrated that large quantities of bone marrow could be infused with little toxicity.[3] Identical twin transplantations were reported in 1959; engraftment occurred in these patients promptly, indicating that the intravenous infusion of bone marrow could lead to protection against lethal irradiation.[4] Studies in dogs demonstrated the potential of storing autologous bone marrow that on reinfusion protected the animals from otherwise fatal irradiation.[5]

These studies and further important observations in immunology and genetics demonstrated that bone marrow–derived cells could be used to protect against the effects of radiation and that genetic elements are critically important to success. Understanding of these histocompatibility antigens and the development of typing methods ushered in the modern era of bone marrow transplantation.

Bone marrow transplantation was initially performed in patients with advanced leukemia with generally discouraging results; however, a subset of otherwise incurable patients attained long-term remissions, some of which have been sustained for more than 25 years.[6] A major advance was the concept that the infused bone marrow could provide not only hematopoietic support but an antileukemic effect termed graft-versus-leukemia. These studies formed the basis for successful treatment of patients with a variety of malignant and genetic diseases. With greater understanding of the cellular basis of hematopoietic cell transplantation (HCT) has come the concept that limited immunosuppression may be sufficient for engraftment and have the potential of reduced toxicity while maintaining graft-versus-leukemia effects. HCT is now being performed at numerous centers around the world. For his pioneering studies in this area, E.D. Thomas was awarded the Nobel Prize in Medicine and Physiology in 1990.

STEM CELL MODEL OF HEMATOPOIESIS

The importance of hematopoietic stem cells in the protection of lethally irradiated animals became clear in the 1950s. With the development of the Till-McCulloch spleen-colony assay, it was realized that clonotypic precursors could give rise to both erythroid and myeloid cells.[7, 8] Hematopoietic stem cells were defined as those cells that have the capacity of multilineage differentiation and are able to protect animals from otherwise lethal irradiation. With the use of cell-sorting technology, murine hematopoietic stem cells were isolated at a frequency of approximately 0.05%, and as few as 100 cells were capable of protecting lethally irradiated animals.[9]

Human hematopoietic stem cells have been more difficult to isolate because of the lack of direct assays like those employed for murine hematopoietic stem cells. However, human cells with multilineage repopulating potential express the antigen CD34, and cells enriched for CD34 expression have been shown to rescue both baboons and humans from exposure to high-dose chemotherapy and radiation.[10, 11] Further purification of human hematopoietic stem cells has been accomplished by removal of cells that express markers found on mature B, T, myeloid, and erythroid cells and of cells that either lack the expression of DR antigens[12, 13] or express Thy-1.[14, 15] Highly purified populations of hematopoietic stem cells sorted on the basis of CD34 and Thy-1 expression have been used in clinical studies, demonstrating that these cells alone are capable of rapid hematopoietic engraftment.[16]

TRANSPLANTATION PROCEDURES

Allogeneic Preparative Regimen

For a successful bone marrow transplantation (BMT), the patient is first prepared with high-dose chemotherapy with or without radiation therapy. The purpose of this is twofold: (1) to eradicate the malignant disease, and (2) to provide sufficient immunosuppression so that the transplanted graft will not be rejected. The most commonly used radiation-containing regimen combines 1200 cGy of fractionated total-body irradiation (FTBI) with 60 mg/kg of cyclophosphamide administered on each of 2 successive days (FTBI/CY).[17] Fractionation of the radiation dose and lung shielding were found to be better tolerated and more effective than single-dose irradiation.[18] It was initially thought that aggressive regimens must be used in the setting of allogeneic transplantation for sufficient immunosuppression of the recipient and to create "space." However, more modern studies using nonmyeloablative preparative regimens (see later) have demonstrated that immunosuppressive drugs can also be used and the donor marrow makes its own space.

Other chemotherapeutic agents have been used for allogeneic HCT preparation. The epipodophyllotoxin etoposide (VP-16) was introduced in 1987; the maximally tolerated dose was found to be 60 mg/kg.[19] This agent has shown excellent antileukemic activity in a large number of patients, especially patients with acute lymphoblastic leukemia (ALL).[20] Other agents, such as cytosine arabinoside, have been used with total-body irradiation (TBI) with and without cyclophosphamide.[21, 22]

Preparative regimens have also been introduced that employ chemotherapy alone. The most widely used and best tolerated of these regimens consists of busulfan and cyclophosphamide (BU/CY). Busulfan was initially administered orally at 4 mg/kg/day for 4 consecutive days (total dose of 16 mg/kg), followed by cyclophosphamide at 50 mg/kg for 4 consecutive days (total dose of 200 mg/kg). This regimen was subsequently modified by altering the cyclophosphamide dose to 60 mg/kg for 2 consecutive days (total dose of 120 mg/kg) with the same dose of busulfan.[23, 24] A randomized trial of this regimen compared with FTBI/CY in patients undergoing allogeneic matched sibling BMT for chronic myelogenous leukemia (CML) demonstrated equivalence of these two regimens.[25] Variations of this regimen have also been reported, such as the addition of VP-16 to BU/CY.[26, 27]

Other novel approaches to BMT preparation have been explored. The dose of TBI that can be safely administered has been studied in a randomized trial comparing 1220 cGy with 1575 cGy. In this study, a decrease in relapse rate was noted at the higher dose; however, there was no survival advantage owing to a higher rate of toxic deaths.[28, 29] These observations have supported the concept of attempting to deliver higher doses of radiation directly to the tumor sites by conjugation of high-emitting radionuclides to delivery vehicles such as monoclonal antibodies. This approach has led to impressive dosing to tumor sites with acceptable toxicity.[30, 31] Further follow-up is ongoing.

In another area of investigation, it has been observed that fully myeloablative preparative regimens are not required for successful allogeneic engraftment. By use of so-called mixed chimerism or nonmyeloablative transplantation, the toxicity and morbidity of the preparative regimen can be markedly reduced. With the use of immunosuppressive agents to suppress host T cells, engraftment of donor hematopoietic cells has been achieved in the majority of patients.[32-34] These regimens may be particularly effective in older patients or individuals with co-morbid conditions that preclude fully myeloablative regimens.

The goal of nonmyeloablative regimens is to achieve adequate engraftment, especially of the T-cell compartment, to capitalize on the graft-versus-leukemia effects of the donor lymphocytes. Several different regimens have been used with varying degrees of intensity. In one study, a regimen consisting of busulfan (4 mg/kg for 2 days) and fludarabine (30 mg/m² for 6 days) plus antilymphocyte globulin was followed by infusion of granulocyte colony-stimulating factor (G-CSF)–mobilized peripheral blood progenitor cells (PBPCs). Patients received only cyclosporine for prophylaxis of graft-versus-host disease (GVHD). Hematopoietic toxicity was significant, although it was less than what would be expected from standard myeloablative regimens. Additional donor leukocyte infusions could then be given to patients in whom GVHD did not develop.[32] Another group has used fludarabine and cyclophosphamide again followed by G-CSF–mobilized PBPCs.[33]

The dog model has been extremely useful in scientifically evaluating different therapeutic approaches. With this model system, a regimen has been developed using low-dose TBI (200 cGy) followed by immunosuppression with mycophenolate mofetil and cyclosporine to suppress host T cells.[34] Donor leukocyte infusion could then be administered for persisting malignant disease or to convert mixed hematopoietic chimerism into complete chimerism. Initial results from the first 45 patients have demonstrated that this regimen is extremely well tolerated; more than half of the patients never required hospital admission. Engraftment was excellent; however, 20% of patients ultimately rejected their grafts. In contrast to patients who receive myeloablative regimens, rejection was nonfatal and resulted in host hematopoiesis. GVHD remains a problem with these regimens and occurred in 47% of patients with sustained engraftment. Survival was excellent with only 6.7% transplantation-related mortality although follow-up is relatively short.[35] Modification of this regimen has included the addition of fludarabine in an effort to reduce the rate of graft rejection. The use of matched unrelated donors is under way.

Clearly, these novel concepts will require further clinical studies to evaluate the optimal application of nonmyeloablative regimens. However, there is little doubt that this approach will allow allogeneic transplantation to be used in patients who are otherwise too old or medically infirm to tolerate myeloablative combinations and thereby will extend the potential benefits of immunologic therapy to patients with indolent leukemias such as chronic lymphocytic leukemia (CLL), CML, and myelodysplastic syndromes (MDS), to name a few.

Autologous Preparative Regimen

Many of the same preparative regimens for myeloablative allogeneic transplantation are also used for autologous transplantation. The most widely used regimen for the treatment of leukemic patients has been TBI/CY. VP-16 also has excellent activity against leukemia and has been added to TBI/CY. This aggressive regimen of TBI/VP-16/CY is being explored for autologous transplantation in ALL.[36] The combination of busulfan (16 mg/kg) and VP-16 (60 mg/kg) has been promising in patients with myeloid leukemias.[37-39] Randomized studies comparing different regimens will be required to determine the optimal approach to preparation for transplantation.

A novel method of radiation therapy is to couple radioactive isotopes to monoclonal antibodies reactive against determinants found on hematopoietic cells, thereby delivering the radiation to the marrow and avoiding some of the nonhematopoietic toxicities.[31] A number of different approaches are under active investigation.

Donor Harvest and Infusion

Bone Marrow

The technique of bone marrow harvesting has now become relatively routine. Bone marrow is aspirated from the posterior iliac crests under either general or regional anesthesia. Complications of this procedure are rare and involve anesthetic, infectious, and bleeding problems.[40] Infants as young as 3 months can undergo bone marrow harvesting safely.

The administration of bone marrow is a simple procedure accomplished by infusing the cells directly into a central vein. In the allogeneic setting, this is similar to a red blood cell transfusion. The hematopoietic stem cells engraft within the bone marrow cavity by "homing" mechanisms that have not yet been fully elucidated. The role of adhesion molecules, such as vascular cell adhesion molecule-1 and heparin sulfate, has been demonstrated in this process.[41, 42] Donors with major ABO incompatibilities can be used; however, this may lead to acute hemolytic transfusion reactions, and the red blood cells need to be depleted before infusion in this setting.[43]

Peripheral Blood Progenitor Cells

A major advance in transplantation has been the use of mobilized PBPCs as the source of hematopoietic cell grafts. Hematopoietic stem cells have been detected in the peripheral blood at extremely low levels.[44] After administration of hematopoietic growth factor (e.g., granulocyte-macrophage colony-stimulating factor [GM-CSF] or G-CSF) or recovery from cytotoxic chemotherapy, there is an increase up to 1000-fold in circulating stem cells in the peripheral blood.[45, 46] After transplantation of mobilized PBPCs, recovery is much more rapid than that observed with bone marrow.[47, 48] This has resulted in a reduction in morbidity and mortality after autologous transplantation associated with lower costs.[49]

The optimal method for mobilizing PBPCs has yet to be defined. The standard method is to treat the donor with G-CSF at a dose of 10 to 16 μg/kg/day; stem cell mobilization usually occurs between days 4 and 6.[50-52] The absolute number of CD34$^+$ cells per kilogram of recipient weight has proved to be the most reliable and practical method for determining the adequacy of a PBPC product.

After infusion of the mobilized PBPCs, hematopoietic reconstitution is rapid, requiring 8 to 10 days for neutrophil recovery and 10 to 12 days for platelet recovery. The CD34$^+$ cell dose per kilogram has proved to be a useful value because patients who receive more than 2×10^6 CD34$^+$ cells per kilogram generally have rapid and sustained hematopoietic recovery.[51-53] Giving larger doses of CD34$^+$ cells per kilogram may result in slightly faster platelet recovery but has little effect on neutrophil recovery.[54-56] A randomized trial has been performed comparing mobilization of PBPCs after administration of G-CSF, GM-CSF, or a combination of both cytokines with chemotherapy. Patients who received G-CSF, either alone or in combination with GM-CSF, had higher yields of CD34$^+$ cells (median 7.1 versus 2.0×10^6/kg/apheresis; $P = .0001$), and a higher percentage of patients achieved 2.5×10^6 CD34$^+$ cells/kg (94% versus 78%; $P = .021$).[57]

G-CSF–mobilized PBPCs have also been evaluated in the allogeneic setting. The concern has been that the large numbers of T cells present in mobilized PBPCs, which are generally 50 to 100 times higher than in bone marrow, may result in an increased risk for GVHD. With use of G-CSF–mobilized PBPCs, engraftment has been rapid, similar to that observed in the autologous setting.[58, 59] Interestingly, the risk for acute GVHD has been similar to that with bone marrow, although the risk for chronic GVHD may be higher.[60] Randomized trials comparing allogeneic G-CSF–mobilized PBPCs with bone marrow are under way. Early results have confirmed the findings of rapid engraftment and equivalent acute GVHD.[58, 59] In one study, overall survival of high-risk patients was improved with the use of PBPCs owing to a reduction of transplantation-related mortality.[61, 62] In another randomized trial, an increase in the rate of chronic GVHD was observed in the PBPC recipients.[62]

Engraftment and Supportive Care

Progress in the support of immunocompromised patients has decreased the morbidity and mortality of transplantation. One of the most important advances has been the introduction of mobilized PBPCs, which has resulted in faster hematopoietic engraftment. Cloned hematopoietic growth factors such as G-CSF and GM-CSF have resulted in more rapid recovery after autologous bone marrow infusion.[63, 64]

Colony-stimulating factors have also been used to treat patients after allogeneic BMT with more rapid myeloid recovery and no impact on GVHD.[65] After PBPC transplantation, there has been less benefit, although most studies suggest that G-CSF results in faster myeloid recovery.[66, 67]

Erythropoietin has also been studied after HCT. In the autologous setting, small randomized studies have not shown reductions in red cell transfusions.[68, 69] After allogeneic transplantation, a randomized study revealed that stable hemoglobin levels were achieved more rapidly, although overall transfusional requirements were not reduced[70]; however, they were reduced in another study.[71] Erythropoietin has been used successfully at later time points for individuals who develop anemia as a result of infection, GVHD, or medications.

Thrombopoietin has generated considerable interest because of impressive in vitro and in vivo activity in animal models. So far, relatively few studies have been performed in the clinical transplantation setting. In one study of a small number of patients who had poor platelet recovery after transplantation, a dose escalation and schedule study was performed with acceptable toxicity but little apparent benefit.[72]

Other supportive care measures are critically important in the management of patients undergoing BMT. Because of high calorie needs, mucositis, and poor oral absorption in patients undergoing allogeneic BMT, parenteral nutrition is usually required. In a randomized trial of 137 patients, those who received parenteral nutrition had improved survival compared with control patients.[73] However, in another randomized study of 258 patients, those patients who received total parenteral nutrition experienced a delay in resumption of normal calorie intake, suggesting that the administration of total parenteral nutrition may suppress appetite.[74] Glutamate supplementation of parenteral nutrition has been suggested to reduce infection and microbial colonization after BMT.[75] However, a second randomized study did not confirm these findings.[76] Other supportive care measures, such as improved broad-spectrum antibiotics, protective isolation, and intravenous administration of immunoglobulins, may also decrease the risk for infection and, therefore, morbidity and possibly mortality.[77, 78] Novel strategies including the use of recombinant growth factors, such as keratinocyte growth factor, have been effective in animal models and are just entering clinical trials.[79, 80]

Donor Types

A variety of different donor types have been explored in the setting of allogeneic BMT. Identical twins would appear to be ideal donors because there is no risk for GVHD. In the first series of identical twin donors reported in 1974, infusion of aspirated bone marrow resulted in engraftment and durable remissions.[81, 82] Subsequent retrospective analyses have indicated that relapse rates are significantly higher in identical twin transplant recipients compared with HLA-identical sibling transplant recipients, although overall survival is comparable because of decreased transplantation-related complications.[83] This observation has led to the graft-versus-leukemia concept that the infused donor-derived cells are capable of recognizing and destroying host tumor cells.

Because few patients have identical twins, other sources of donor cells are required. In the majority of allogeneic transplantations, donors are matched at the A, B, C, and DR regions of the HLA loci. The chance that a given sibling will be fully matched at all of these loci is

only 25%, so alternative donors are required. One source is related donors who are mismatched at one or more of these loci. HLA incompatibility has important consequences for the clinical course of the transplant; recipients of mismatched marrow experience delayed engraftment and earlier and more severe GVHD. However, despite the increased risk for complications, patients receiving bone marrow from donors with a single-antigen mismatch appear to have survival rates similar to those of patients with matched sibling donors in some studies despite the increased risk for GVHD. Because many prospective patients do not have fully matched or single-antigen mismatched family donors, other options have been developed.[84, 85]

Alternative unrelated donor sources have been explored. HLA-matched unrelated donor transplantations have been extensively studied during the past decade. The first successful transplantations using unrelated HLA-identical bone marrow were reported approximately 20 years ago.[86, 87] Since then, a number of studies have demonstrated the feasibility of performing matched unrelated donor transplantations. In 1986, the National Marrow Donor Program (NMDP) was established in the United States to facilitate marrow procurement. Since then, more than 4 million donors have been registered and many thousands of transplantations performed with NMDP donors. Although unrelated donor transplantations are clearly complicated by more frequent and severe GVHD as well as by other complications, long-term survival has been achieved in a number of clinical settings with patients younger than 50 years.[88] With the development of improved typing, especially molecular typing at the HLA class II loci, results from matched unrelated donor transplantations rival those that can be achieved with matched sibling donors.[89] The need for several months to identify a donor limits the application of this approach to patients with relatively stable disease.

Other donor sources have also been explored. Placental cord blood is a rich source of hematopoietic stem cells.[90, 91] Furthermore, owing to the relative immaturity of cord blood stem cells, it may be possible to cross immunologic barriers. Registries have been formed that collect and characterize the cord blood under standardized procedures. These organizations can be readily accessed throughout the world. With this source of stem cells, engraftment and long-term survival have been achieved; success depends on the nature of the underlying disease.[92, 93] Engraftment has been relatively slow, and the feasibility of performing cord blood transplantations in larger children and adults is questionable. Efforts aimed at expanding the cord blood stem cells are under way in several centers.

Haploidentical or three-antigen mismatched donors have also been used in some centers. Historically, these transplantations have been complicated by graft failure and GVHD. However, the development of techniques for use of haploidentical donors is attractive because the majority of patients would have a suitable donor. The barrier to engraftment can be overcome in animal models by using high doses of hematopoietic stem cells.[94] This goal can be accomplished clinically with G-CSF–mobilized PBPCs. With use of PBPCs and highly immunosuppressive preparative regimens that include TBI, high-dose chemotherapy, and antithymocyte globulin, extensive T-cell–depleted haplotype-matched grafts have been successful in patients with advanced leukemia.[95, 96] An innovative alternative approach has been to block co-stimulation of alloreactive T cells, which theoretically may result in induction of anergy.[97] Immune reconstitution and the risk for opportunistic infections have emerged as major obstacles in the successful application of haploidentical transplantation.

CLINICAL RESULTS

Acute Myelogenous Leukemia

Allogeneic BMT. BMT for acute myelogenous leukemia (AML) was initially restricted to patients for whom all conventional therapies had failed; approximately 10% to 15% remain alive and free of disease after more than 15 years of follow-up.[6, 98] The long-term survival of at least some of these patients demonstrated the curative potential of allogeneic BMT and suggested that patients treated earlier in the course of their disease might have a more favorable outcome. Several groups then went on to perform allogeneic transplantation of patients with AML in first complete remission (CR). The first such report used preparation with TBI and cyclophosphamide, resulting in approximately 60% of patients being alive and in continued CR.[99] Similar observations were reported from the City of Hope National Medical Center, where patients having transplantations for AML while in first CR fared significantly better than did patients with more advanced disease.[100] Multiple other studies have confirmed these results, demonstrating that patients undergoing transplantation in first CR fared the best, whereas patients undergoing transplantation beyond first CR had inferior outcomes.[101–103] In all of these studies, the leading causes of failure were GVHD, interstitial pneumonitis, and leukemic relapse.

The majority of patients undergoing transplantation in these studies were prepared with TBI and cyclophosphamide (TBI/CY). VP-16 has also been studied extensively in combination with TBI. In one series of 99 patients with acute leukemia who had transplantations in first CR, 61 of whom had AML, 64% were alive and well with a median follow-up of 3 years.[104]

Considerable debate continues to center on the question of which patients should undergo allogeneic BMT and at what point in their disease. Clearly, allogeneic transplantation carries significantly more up-front risk than chemotherapy does; however, it has also resulted in lower relapse rates. To answer this question, a series of clinical trials have been performed in which patients were assigned to allogeneic BMT or continued chemotherapy on the basis of the availability of an HLA-matched sibling donor. More recently, some studies have further randomized patients who did not have sibling donors to autologous BMT or chemotherapy. The results of 17 clinical trials are presented in Table 20–1. In all of these studies, there was at least a trend toward improved disease-free survival for the patients undergoing allogeneic

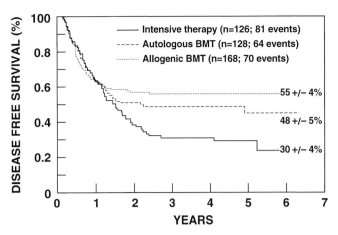

FIGURE 20–1. Disease-free survival for 422 patients randomized between intensive chemotherapy and autologous transplantation. Patients who had an HLA-matched sibling donor underwent allogeneic transplantation. (From Zittoun RA, Mandelli F, Willemze R, et al: Autologous or allogeneic bone marrow transplantation compared with intensive chemotherapy in acute myelogenous leukemia. European Organization for Research and Treatment of Cancer [EORTC] and the Gruppo Italiano Malattie Ematologiche Maligne dell'Adulto [GIMEMA] Leukemia Cooperative Groups. N Engl J Med 1995;332:217.)

BMT compared with those treated by chemotherapy. Six studies demonstrated a statistically significant advantage for the patients undergoing transplantation compared with patients receiving chemotherapy alone.[105–110] Results from one of these studies are shown in Figure 20–1. Other studies have demonstrated an equivalent outcome. In a recently completed U.S. intergroup study, actuarial disease-free survival at 4 years was 43% for patients undergoing allogeneic transplantation and 34% for patients receiving either high-dose cytarabine consolidation or autologous BMT.[111] The discrepancies among these various trials are not easy to reconcile. However, in all studies, a reduction in relapse rate could clearly be demonstrated. This benefit was offset primarily by transplantation-related complications, including GVHD, interstitial pneumonitis, and infection. With improvements in the control of these complications, for example, better prophylaxis against GVHD, effective antiviral therapies against cytomegalovirus infection, broad-spectrum antibiotics, and hematopoietic growth factors, it would be expected that disease-free survival of the patients undergoing transplantation may improve significantly because of a reduction in transplantation-related mortality.

Cytogenetic analysis has emerged as a powerful prognostic indicator in AML. Some cytogenetic abnormalities, such as t(15;17), t(8;21), and inv(16), have been associated with an excellent response to cytotoxic chemotherapy that included high-dose cytarabine.[112] Other patients can be identified who have poor outcomes with chemotherapy. On the basis of these results, most centers recommend allogeneic BMT in patients with AML in first CR who are younger than 50 years if they have genotypically matched sibling donors and have either high-risk or standard-risk cytogenetic abnormalities (Fig. 20–2).

Most of the patients in these clinical trials were prepared for transplantation with the FTBI/CY regimen. As discussed previously, a number of other regimens have

TABLE 20–1. Allogeneic Bone Marrow Transplantation versus Autologous Bone Marrow Transplantation versus Chemotherapy for AML in First Remission

	Treatment	No. of Patients	DFS (%)	P Value	OS (%)	P Value	Relapse (%)	P Value
Royal Marsden (1982)[105]	AlloBMT	53	54	P < .005				
	ChemoRx	51	21					
Seattle (1984, 1988)[107, 108]	AlloBMT	33	48	P < .05				
	ChemoRx	43	21					
	AlloBMT	43	40	P = .07				
	ChemoRx	43	21					
UCLA (1985)[336]	AlloBMT	23			40	P = NS	40	P < .01
	ChemoRx	44			27		71	
Genova (1985)[106]	AlloBMT	19	64	P < .05	70	P = NR		
	ChemoRx	18	13		21			
M.D. Anderson (1988)[337]	AlloBMT	11			36	P = NS	9	P < .01
	ChemoRx	27			15		85	
Spain (1988)[338]	AlloBMT	14	70	P = NS			10	P <.005
	ChemoRx	25	10				88	
France (1989)[109]	AlloBMT	20	66				18	
	ABMT	12	41	P < .004			50	P <.0002
	ChemoRx	20	16				83	
Netherlands (1990)[132]	AlloBMT	23	51	P = NS	66	P = .05	34	P = .03
	ABMT	32	35		37		60	
UCLA (1992)[339]	AlloBMT	42	45	P = NS	45	P = NS	32	P = .05
	ChemoRx	28	38		53		60	
ECOG (1992)[340]	AlloBMT	54	42	P = NS	43	P = NS		
	ChemoRx	29	30		42			
France (1994)[341]	AlloBMT	27	41	P = NS	41	P = NS	43	P = .1
	ChemoRx	31	27		46		67	
Boston* (1995)[139]	AlloBMT	23	62	P = NS			0	P = SGNFCT
	ABMT	27	62				38	
	AlloBMT	31	56	P = NS			20	P = .04
	ABMT	53	45				50	
SWOG (1995)[342]	AlloBMT	34	38	P = NS				
	ChemoRx	110	28					
EORTC/GIMEMA (1995)[110]	AlloBMT	168	55		59		27	
	ABMT	128	48	P = SGNFCT	56	P = NR	41	P = NR
	ChemoRx	126	30		46		57	
GOELAM (1997)[138]	AlloBMT	67	45				38	
	ABMT	67	47	P = NS			44	P = NS
	ChemoRx	61	53				43	
U.S. Intergroup (1998)[111]	AlloBMT	113	43		46	P = .04	29	
	ABMT	116	34	P = NS	43	P = .05	48	
	ChemoRx	117	34		52		62	
	AlloBMT	92	47	P = NR	45	P = NR		
	ABMT	63	48		55			
MRC AML 10 (1998)[140]	ABMT	190	53	P = .04	57	P = .2	37	P = .0007
	ChemoRx	191	40		45		58	

*Patients assigned to transplantation on the basis of availability of matched siblings or to chemotherapy and analyzed according to intent-to-treat.

AML, acute myeloid leukemia; AlloBMT, allogeneic bone marrow transplantation; ABMT, autologous bone marrow transplantation; ChemoRx, chemotherapy; SGNFCT, significant; NS, not significant; NR, not reported; DFS, disease-free survival; OS, overall survival.

been developed for preparation of patients before transplantation. Since TBI/CY has become the standard approach, randomized clinical trials have compared a given regimen with this standard. The BU/CY regimen has been compared with TBI/CY in one prospective randomized clinical trial of 101 patients with AML in first CR. Those patients who received TBI/CY had superior 2-year disease-free survival (72% versus 47%; P < .01) and a lower relapse rate (14% versus 34%; P < .04) than those patients who received BU/CY.[113] Another small randomized trial of only 63 patients with AML in first CR compared TBI/CY with TBI-melphalan and found no statistically significant difference in survival between the two groups.[114] A randomized clinical trial comparing TBI/VP-16 with BU/CY for patients with advanced hematologic malignant neoplasms demonstrated a trend toward im-

proved results with TBI/VP-16.[115] Additional randomized clinical trials comparing different preparative regimens, particularly nonmyeloablative regimens, would be of interest.

Children with high-risk AML have also been successfully treated with allogeneic BMT.[116-118] Weisdorf and colleagues[119] have analyzed the effect of age on outcome after allogeneic BMT for 149 patients treated in Minnesota. In this study, age was not predictive of outcome; approximately 50% of adults and children with AML in first CR were alive and free of disease after allogeneic BMT. Even very young patients (<2 years) who develop AML have undergone successful transplantation.[120] The upper age limit for allogeneic BMT has been rising as supportive care and prophylaxis of GVHD have improved. Patients up to 60 years of age who are in good

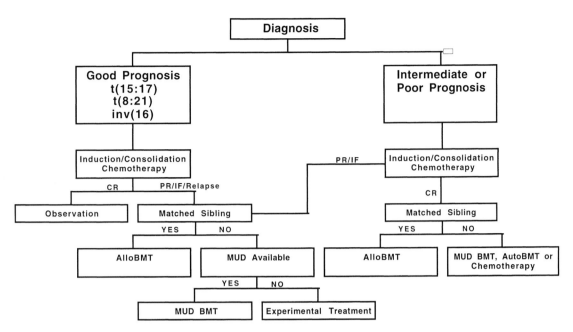

FIGURE 20–2. Algorithm for the treatment of patients with AML. (From Stockerl-Goldstein K, Blume KG: Allogeneic hematopoietic cell transplantation for adult patients with acute myeloid leukemia. In Thomas ED, Blume KG, Forman SJ, eds: Hematopoietic Cell Transplantation. Oxford, UK: Blackwell Science; 1999, pp. 823–834.)

physical condition have had successful transplantation of allogeneic marrow grafts. Nonmyeloablative transplantations, because of reduced peritransplantation toxicity, can be successfully performed in patients who are even into their seventh decade of life.[35]

Autologous BMT. The use of high-dose chemotherapy followed by autologous bone marrow or PBPCs is an attractive alternative for patients without HLA-matched sibling donors. Early studies were performed in patients who had experienced relapse after induction chemotherapy and in whom the bone marrow was collected at the time of CR. Results from these studies were encouraging; the majority of patients achieved engraftment and reentered CR. Unfortunately, virtually all of these patients relapsed and eventually died of their underlying disease.[121-123]

A central concern in the use of autologous transplantation, especially for leukemia, is the possibility that occult clonogenic tumor cells could be present in the harvested bone marrow and on reinfusion contribute to the high rate of relapse observed in these patients. Gene marking studies have demonstrated that this event does occur.[124, 125] A variety of methods have been developed in an effort to purge tumor cells from the marrow graft. The most widely used approach to purge myeloid leukemia cells from bone marrow has been the administration of the cyclophosphamide derivatives (4-hydroperoxycyclophosphamide [4-HC]) and mafosfamide. In phase I trials, it was determined that treatment of the bone marrow with 4-HC up to a concentration of 80 to 100 μg/mL resulted in delayed but acceptable engraftment. Marrow growth occurred despite the fact that virtually all of the committed hematopoietic progenitor cells (colony-forming unit–granulocyte-macrophage) were eliminated at this dose.[126] In the first report of 25 patients receiving bone marrow transplants purged with 4-HC during second or third remission, 11 patients

were free of disease with a median follow-up of more than 1 year.[127] Further follow-up of patients treated in this manner indicated that those patients who had less than 1% residual colony-forming unit–granulocyte-macrophage activity in their bone marrow after treatment with 4-HC had reduced relapse rates and improved leukemia-free survival, suggesting that the intensity of in vitro treatment with 4-HC affected outcome.[128] In addition, retrospective analyses have revealed a benefit for patients who have undergone BMT purged with mafosfamide, especially after remission induction.[129] These data continue to hold up in subsequent analyses.[130]

Encouraging results were also reported for 10 patients with AML in early relapse or second or subsequent remission whose bone marrow was purged with two monoclonal antibodies and complement.[131] The role of purging has not been directly assessed in this setting because there is no randomized trial comparing patients who received purged bone marrow with those who did not.

The role of autologous transplantation in first CR has been controversial.[130] A number of phase II studies have been performed that have reported a broad range in disease-free survival from 35% to 76% with relapse rates ranging from 22% to 60%.[38, 132-136] In studies in which allogeneic BMT has been compared directly with autologous HCT in first CR, there is either a better outcome after the allogeneic transplantation[132, 137] or no difference between the two groups.[138, 139] A European Organization for Research and Treatment of Cancer study of 623 patients indicated that the relapse rate was lower for patients who underwent autologous BMT compared with chemotherapy (41% versus 57%), with a higher proportion of patients remaining in remission (see Fig. 20–1). Disease-free survival was also superior in the autologous BMT group (48% versus 30%); however, overall survival was not different owing to the use of salvage therapy

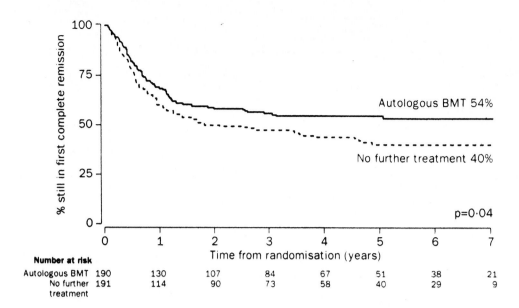

FIGURE 20–3. Disease-free survival of patients randomized between autologous transplantation and intensive chemotherapy in the Medical Research Council's AML 10 trial. (From Burnett AK, Goldstone AH, Stevens RM, et al: Randomised comparison of addition of autologous bone-marrow transplantation to intensive chemotherapy for acute myeloid leukaemia in first remission: Results of MRC AML 10 trial. UK Medical Research Council Adult and Children's Leukaemia Working Parties. Lancet 1998;351:700.)

with autologous transplantation for those patients who relapsed after chemotherapy.[110] The U.S. intergroup study used the same study design. In this smaller study of 346 patients between the ages of 16 and 55 years who achieved first remission, no significant differences in disease-free survival were noted between the three groups.[111] Surprisingly, only 54% of the patients assigned to autologous transplantation actually received the intended therapy. The Medical Research Council's AML 10 trial of 1966 patients from 163 institutions used a similar design. In this study, 381 patients were randomized between chemotherapy and autologous transplantation; of the 190 patients who were assigned to the autologous BMT arm, 126 (66%) received the intended treatment.[140] By use of an intention-to-treat analysis, those patients who underwent autologous BMT had a lower relapse rate (37% versus 58%; $P = .0007$) and superior disease-free survival at 7 years of follow-up (53% versus 40%; $P = .040$) compared with patients who received standard chemotherapy (Fig. 20–3).

In a study of 232 children with AML in first CR who were randomized between autologous BMT and chemotherapy, there were no differences in event-free survival (36% versus 38%). A lower relapse rate was observed after autologous transplantation (31% versus 58%; $P < .001$), but this benefit was offset by higher treatment-related mortality in the patients undergoing transplantation (15% versus 2.7%; $P = .005$).[141]

With the introduction of PBPCs, mortality risk after autologous transplantation has declined. In addition, immediately after recovery from chemotherapy is the optimal time for collection of PBPCs that may have a reduced tumor burden, a concept termed in vivo purging. A two-step protocol involving cytarabine and etoposide consolidation followed by collection of PBPCs has been reported. The preparative regimen included busulfan and etoposide. In this study, 128 patients were enrolled and 117 patients (91%) proceeded to transplantation. There were only two transplantation-related deaths. With a median follow-up of 30 months, 5-year disease-free survival is

projected to be 55%.[39] Patients with favorable cytogenetic abnormalities fared better (disease-free survival of 73%), whereas patients with high-risk cytogenetic abnormalities did not appear to benefit (Fig. 20–4).

Ongoing improvement in strategies for autologous transplantation, including the use of post-transplantation immune modulation as well as refinement in selection of patients, novel chemotherapy, and biologic therapies such as monoclonal antibodies, is likely to make the optimal treatment of patients with AML a source of ongoing debate well into the 21st century.

Acute Lymphoblastic Leukemia

Both allogeneic HCT and autologous HCT have been used to treat patients with ALL. As for patients with AML,

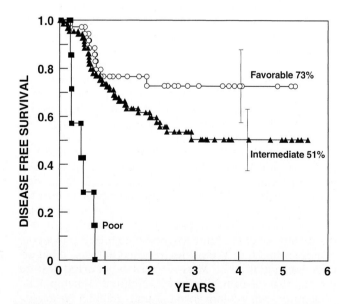

FIGURE 20–4. Disease-free survival after autologous transplantation depending on risk group. (From Linker CA, Ries CA, Damon LE, et al: Autologous stem cell transplantation for acute myeloid leukemia in first remission. Biol Blood Marrow Transplant 2000;6:50.)

results vary markedly, depending on the remission status at the time of transplantation. Advances with standard chemotherapy have resulted in effective treatment of this disease in most children. Treatment of adults with chemotherapy has steadily improved, especially for some subtypes of ALL; however, patients with high risk for recurrence can be defined. In addition, molecular diagnostic studies hold out the hope that therapeutic decisions may be based on objective determinants of disease burden rather than on risk factors. Nonetheless, risk assessment can be performed for patients, especially adults with ALL. These risk factors include advanced age; elevated white blood cell count at diagnosis; non–T-cell disease; extramedullary involvement; more than 4 weeks to achieve remission; and certain cytogenetic abnormalities, especially the Philadelphia (Ph) chromosome t(9;22) and the t(4;11) and t(8;14) translocations. Therefore, HCT studies have focused on patients with relapsed ALL or adults with high-risk disease in first CR.

Allogeneic HCT. A number of clinical trials indicate that children with ALL who suffer a relapse can be salvaged with allogeneic BMT in second CR, with 40% to 64% of patients enjoying long-term disease-free survival.[142-145] Analyses have been performed comparing results of chemotherapy with the results of HCT on the basis of registry data. In one such study, results for allogeneic HCT of 376 children in second CR reported to the International Bone Marrow Transplant Registry (IBMTR) were compared with the results of 540 children treated with chemotherapy in Pediatric Oncology Group trials. At a median follow-up of 5 years, the relapse rate was significantly lower for the patients undergoing HCT (45% versus 80%; $P < .001$), and the probability of leukemia-free survival was higher in the transplant recipients (40% versus 17%; $P < .001$).[146] Overall survival was not examined in this study.

Allogeneic BMT has also been compared with standard chemotherapy for the treatment of children in first CR with high-risk disease, defined as those patients presenting with a white blood cell count above 100,000 cells/μL. Of 198 children identified in the United Kingdom, 34 patients had an HLA-matched sibling donor and

went on to allogeneic HCT. A significant reduction in relapse rate was noted for patients who underwent transplantation (12% versus 41%; $P = .001$); however, there was also higher treatment-related mortality in the transplant recipients (18% versus 3%; $P = .0007$). The higher transplantation-related mortality offset the reduction in relapse so that no statistical difference in overall disease-free survival was observed (69% for BMT versus 52% for chemotherapy).[147]

In general, adults with ALL have a considerably worse prognosis than children do. Allogeneic BMT has been used to treat adult patients beyond first CR or patients in first CR with high-risk features. Approximately 42% to 71% of patients achieve long-term remissions.[148-152] The use of FTBI and high-dose etoposide (60 mg/kg) has been a particularly effective regimen; more than 60% of 149 adult patients with high-risk disease undergoing transplantation in first CR are alive and free of disease with follow-up exceeding 15 years[20] (Fig. 20-5).

Comparative studies using historical control subjects and registry data have been performed between allogeneic HCT and chemotherapy. Similar to studies in children, lower relapse rates have been observed for adult patients undergoing HCT compared with those patients who received chemotherapy; however, because of the increased risk for transplantation-related complications, no improvement in overall survival was observed.[153, 154] In another analysis, disease-free survival was improved for patients younger than 30 years who underwent allogeneic HCT compared with chemotherapy.[155]

Randomized studies have been performed with a design similar to that discussed previously for AML in which patients in first CR with HLA-matched sibling donors were assigned to allogeneic transplantation with or without randomization between chemotherapy and autologous HCT. In one such study, 257 eligible patients were evaluated; 116 individuals underwent allogeneic HCT, and 141 patients were treated with chemotherapy. Five-year survival rates were not statistically different between the two groups, but when patients with high-risk features were evaluated separately, there were improved disease-free survival (39% versus 14%; $P = .01$) and overall

FIGURE 20–5. Probability of event-free survival (EFS), overall survival (OS), and relapse (REL) for 149 adult patients with high-risk ALL. (Updated from Chao NJ, Forman SJ, Schmidt GM, et al: Allogeneic bone marrow transplantation for high-risk acute lymphoblastic leukemia during first complete remission. Blood 1991;78:1923.)

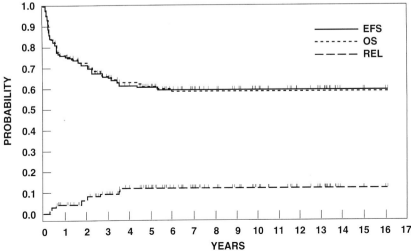

survival (44% versus 20%; $P = .03$) for the patients undergoing transplantation.[156]

Patients with the t(9;22) chromosome translocation (Philadelphia chromosome) have an extremely poor prognosis after chemotherapy; there are no or very few long-term survivors.[157, 158] In one study of 23 Ph+ ALL patients prepared with FTBI and etoposide who underwent transplantation with HLA-matched sibling bone marrow while in first CR, disease-free survival at 3 years of follow-up was 65%.[159] HCT has also been performed in this group of patients with unrelated donors with a 2-year probability of disease-free survival of 49%.[160]

Patients with remission induction failure also fare poorly. Allogeneic HCT has been attempted as salvage therapy. In one study of 21 patients, 16 with AML and 5 with ALL, the probability of disease-free survival at 10 years was 43%.[161] However, only one of the five ALL patients survived free of disease.

Autologous HCT. Autologous HCT for patients with ALL has resulted in modest success on the basis of the remission status of the patient at the time of transplantation. With advanced disease (beyond first CR), 18% to 46% of patients enjoy long-term survival.[162-168] Patients with long first remissions of greater than 24 months fared better with an event-free survival of 53% among 51 children who underwent transplantation with purged bone marrow in second CR.[169] Superior event-free survival varying from 30% to 65% has been achieved in first CR patients.[151, 163, 170, 171]

The role of purging in autologous transplants for ALL remains to be defined. Monoclonal antibody–based techniques, immunotoxins, and 4-HC have been used.[164, 172, 173] In some of these studies, polymerase chain reaction (PCR)–based methods, for example, of *BCR/ABL*, have been used to document the efficacy of the purging.[174] As in other diseases, there have been no direct comparisons between purged and unpurged stem cell grafts.

In ALL, unique chromosome rearrangements, such as the *BCR/ABL* translocation, or immunoglobulin and T-cell receptor genes, can be amplified by PCR. Molecular features serve as extremely sensitive markers for disease. *BCR/ABL* transcripts have been detected after transplantation and found to be a sensitive predictor of relapse, especially for patients with the p190 *BCR/ABL* splice variant.[175, 176] Rearrangements of immunoglobulin heavy-chain variable loci have also been used to detect minimal residual disease and found to be sensitive markers for relapse after transplantation.[176] By use of a semi-quantitative PCR technique, children and adolescent patients were grouped as having high-level disease, low-level disease, or no detectable disease by PCR amplification of immunoglobulin or T-cell receptor gene loci before allogeneic HCT performed in either first or second CR. Two-year event-free survival for these groups of patients was 0% for high-level disease, 36% for low-level disease, and 72% for those patients without PCR-detectable disease before HCT ($P < .001$).[177] This observation raises the exciting possibility that direct measurement of disease burden could be used to determine which patients should go on to high-dose therapy and which patients may already be cured of their disease.

Chronic Myelogenous Leukemia

Allogeneic HCT. Allogeneic HCT for CML has been widely used and has been established as the primary therapy for this disorder for younger patients with HLA-matched sibling donors. CML progresses from a relatively indolent disorder readily controllable with oral chemotherapy in chronic phase to a more aggressive disorder in accelerated phase to a frankly acute leukemic condition in blastic phase, which is often refractory to therapy. The results obtained with allogeneic HCT are directly related to the phase of disease at the time of transplantation, and even within the chronic phase, transplantation within the first year results in superior outcomes.[178-181] Early trials demonstrated that CML could also be effectively treated with myeloablative chemoradiotherapy followed by syngeneic transplantation.[182] However, several studies have demonstrated higher relapse rates after syngeneic than after allogeneic transplantation, which was one of the initial observations leading to the concept of a graft-versus-leukemia effect.[183-185] With the use of HLA-matched sibling donors, 50% to 75% of CML patients undergoing transplantation in the first or second chronic phase of their disease achieve long-term remissions.[179, 181, 186-188] Disease-free survival drops to 30% to 40% of patients in accelerated phase,[181, 189] and only 5% to 15% of patients in blastic phase obtain long-term disease-free survival with allogeneic HCT. The most important prognostic factor for survival after allogeneic HCT for CML is disease phase.[179, 186, 190, 191] Younger age may also influence survival,[186, 192] although patients up to 60 years have successfully undergone allogeneic transplantation. Nonmyeloablative regimens offer the possibility of allogeneic transplantations in older patients.[35]

Splenomegaly or splenectomy appears to have no impact on outcome after BMT,[186, 190] although patients with massive splenomegaly may have refractory cytopenias and may benefit from low-dose splenic irradiation. Both splenectomy and splenic irradiation have been used that have not resulted in adverse outcomes.[193] One randomized study of splenic irradiation to a total dose of 10 Gy performed in 239 patients with CML did not result in improved outcomes.[194] However, in another study of 37 patients who received splenic irradiation (2.5 to 5 Gy) within 10 days of HCT, a freedom from progression of 90% and overall survival of 82% were achieved.[195]

A number of studies have documented that early HCT during the first year after diagnosis results in superior outcomes, at least in part owing to the negative impact of previous exposure to chemotherapy, especially busulfan.[181, 190] In the subgroup of CML patients younger than 50 years who undergo allogeneic BMT during the first year of diagnosis from an HLA-matched sibling donor, 70% to 80% will be alive and free of disease 5 years later, which makes BMT the treatment of choice for younger patients.[25]

Randomized clinical trials exploring the use of non-radiation-containing preparative regimens such as BU/CY have been compared with FTBI/CY. In these studies, there were no differences in disease-free survival,[25, 196] but a decreased risk for relapse in BU/CY-treated patients was reported in one study.[196] Plasma busulfan levels below the median of 917 ng/mL were associated with a higher relapse rate in one small study of 45 transplant recipients with the BU/CY regimen.[197]

Alternative therapies for CML have emerged, such as interferon alfa and the tyrosine kinase inhibitor STI-571. Randomized studies comparing interferon with standard chemotherapy such as hydroxyurea have shown improvement in overall survival for the interferon-treated patients.[198-200] This survival benefit is primarily for patients who achieve cytogenetic remissions. A subsequent randomized study combining ara-C with interferon demonstrated a higher percentage of patients achieving a cytogenetic remission who received combined therapy, with documented improvements in long-term disease-free survival for a subset of patients.[201]

There have been no prospective trials comparing the role of allogeneic HCT with interferon, for example, by assigning patients with HLA-matched sibling donors to allogeneic transplantation and those without histocompatible donors to interferon treatment. An analysis of historical data submitted to the IBMTR has been performed comparing results obtained from allogeneic BMT (N = 548) with results obtained from the randomized trial of the German CML study group, which had accrued patients to therapy with hydroxyurea (N = 121) or interferon (N = 75).[199] In this retrospective analysis, there was a higher mortality risk in the transplantation group for the first 18 months. After approximately 3.5 years from diagnosis, the survival curves crossed such that there was significant improvement in overall survival for the transplant recipients at 4.7 years and in overall survival at 7 years (58% with transplantation and 21% with hydroxyurea or interferon; Fig. 20–6).[202] Similar results were obtained for all risk categories; however, those pa-

tients with intermediate-risk or high-risk disease benefited from the transplantation even earlier.

For patients without HLA-matched sibling donors, matched unrelated donor transplantation has been explored. Owing to the relatively indolent nature of CML, there is usually adequate time to perform a search, which may take up to 3 to 6 months. The outcome for matched unrelated donor transplantation for patients with CML in chronic phase was initially reported to be in the range of 35% to 40%, with patients with more advanced disease faring worse.[88, 203] Advances in donor-recipient typing, supportive care, GVHD prophylaxis, and infectious disease prevention have significantly improved results after matched unrelated donor transplantation such that 5-year estimates of survival for patients who are 50 years of age or younger and undergo a transplantation procedure within 1 year of diagnosis from an HLA-matched unrelated donor were reported to be 74%, which is similar to that achieved with HLA-matched sibling donors[89] (Fig. 20–7).

The decision to proceed to unrelated donor transplantation versus the use of interferon or STI-571 is often difficult for patients who lack an HLA-matched sibling donor. For younger patients with newly diagnosed CML, decision analysis has suggested that transplantation within the first year of diagnosis provides the greatest quality-adjusted expected survival and that this modality has acceptable cost-effectiveness.[204, 205] For patients without HLA-matched sibling or unrelated donors, haploidentical donors and umbilical cord blood have also been used in small numbers of patients.[96, 206, 207]

The question of whether pretreatment of patients with interferon affects outcome after BMT has generated considerable debate. Those patients who delay transplanta-

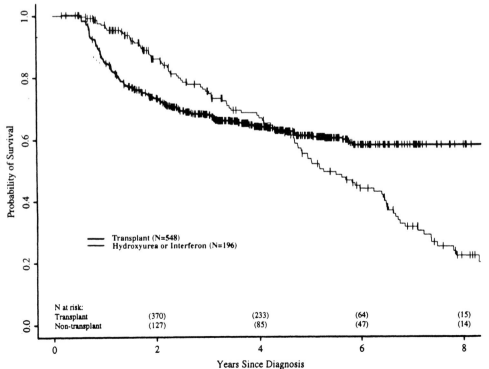

FIGURE 20–6. Retrospective analysis of survival after allogeneic transplantation for CML compared with hydroxyurea or interferon treatment. (From Gale RP, Hehlmann R, Zhang MJ, et al: Survival with bone marrow transplantation versus hydroxyurea or interferon for chronic myelogenous leukemia. The German CML Study Group. Blood 1998;91:1810.)

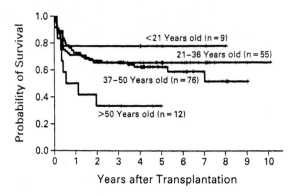

FIGURE 20–7. Overall survival of patients with CML undergoing matched unrelated donor transplantation stratified by age. (From Hansen JA, Gooley TA, Martin PJ, et al: Bone marrow transplants from unrelated donors for patients with chronic myeloid leukemia. N Engl J Med 1998;338:962.)

tion have a worse outcome independent of interferon use. Nonetheless, a number of retrospective analyses have addressed this important question. In one relatively small study, prolonged use of interferon was associated with a worse outcome mainly because of an increased risk for infection and graft failure.[208] Another study performed in the setting of unrelated transplantation supported the concept that interferon treatment of more than 6 months was associated with a worse outcome after transplantation mainly because of increased GVHD.[209] However, an IBMTR study of 873 patients in which the median length of interferon treatment was only 2 months (range, 1 to 39 months) found no adverse effect.[210]

Autologous HCT. Autologous HCT has been explored for a limited number of patients with CML. Registry data and single-institution studies have suggested that patients who undergo autologous HCT while they are in chronic phase, but not accelerated phase or blastic phase, may attain a prolonged chronic phase of their disease and possibly enjoy improved survival.[211, 212] A significant concern has been the reinfusion of clonogenic tumor cells with the stem cell inoculum. A variety of strategies have been employed in an effort to enrich for normal unaffected stem cells, including in vitro culture,[213] cell selection by fluorescence-activated cell sorting,[214] and collection of cells on recovery from chemotherapy.[215-217] Autologous transplantation may serve as a platform for subsequent immunotherapeutic interventions, for example, with interleukin (IL)-2, autologous NK cells,[218] or $CD3^+CD56^+$ effector cells.[219]

Myelodysplastic Syndromes

Allogeneic HCT. Allogeneic HCT has been used to treat patients with MDS but is limited by donor availability and the advanced age of most patients with these conditions. With improvements in supportive care and prevention of GVHD, a number of groups have extended the upper age limit for allogeneic BMT to 60 years. However, many MDS patients are older than 60 years. With the development of nonmyeloablative regimens that can safely be administered to older patients, this age limita-

tion may become less of an obstacle in the treatment of MDS with allogeneic HCT.

Results for allogeneic HCT from the Seattle group were reported in 1993.[220] In this report, 93 patients, all of whom had severe neutropenia, thrombocytopenia, or more than 5% bone marrow blasts, were prepared with either TBI/CY or BU/CY; 65 patients received grafts from HLA-matched sibling donors, whereas 28 patients received marrow grafts from other family members or unrelated donors. With a follow-up of 4 years, 41% of patients were alive and free of disease; 28% of patients relapsed, and 43% died of transplantation-related complications. Those patients who had the best overall result were younger (<40 years) or had less than 5% bone marrow blasts at the time of transplantation.

Other groups of investigators have reported similar results using TBI-based regimens that were primarily combined with cyclophosphamide.[221-224] Non–radiation-containing regimens, which have the potential advantage of less toxicity, have also been used to prepare patients for transplantation. In one report of 38 patients, BU/CY was used as the preparative regimen; the overall survival rate at 2 years was 45% with a 24% probability of relapse.[224] The BU/CY regimen has also been used in another report of 27 younger patients who underwent transplantation with HLA-matched sibling donors; the results were significantly better, with a projected 78% of patients alive and free of disease.[225]

The European Bone Marrow Transplant group reported a retrospective analysis of 131 patients with MDS who underwent allogeneic BMT with use of HLA-matched sibling donors. The 5-year disease-free survival was 34%, and overall survival of the entire group was 41%.[226] Similar variables were predictive of improved outcome, including younger age, shorter disease duration, and absence of excess marrow blasts.

Older patients have more recently been considered for allogeneic transplantation. In one study, 50 patients aged 55 to 66 years underwent this procedure with a variety of different preparative regimens. Results were similar to those achieved for younger patients, with 22 patients (44%) surviving at 9 to 80 months of follow-up.[227]

Because allogeneic transplantation is associated with significant risk, especially in elderly patients, predicting which patients are likely to benefit from HCT is important. The international MDS workshop categorization[228] could be useful. In one study, patients with high-risk disease had a much worse outcome (event-free survival of 6% versus 40% to 51% for the intermediate-risk and good-risk groups) and significantly higher relapse rate (82% versus 12% to 19%; $P = .002$).[229]

Efforts to lower transplantation-related risk have included T-cell depletion and nonmyeloablative transplantation. In one study of 35 patients in which T-cell depletion was employed, results were similar, with 24% of patients alive and free of disease at 3 years of follow-up.[230]

Rarely, children develop MDS, and a limited number of pediatric patients have undergone allogeneic HCT. This has resulted in long-term survival for a significant percentage.[231, 232]

Treatment-associated MDS and acute leukemia have an extremely poor prognosis with conventional chemotherapy. Allogeneic HCT has been used in patients with these disorders with limited success. In an analysis of 70 patients who underwent transplantation for therapy-related MDS (n = 31) or therapy-related AML (n = 39), some were treated with chemotherapy into remission (n = 24) and the others had active disease (n = 46). With a median follow-up of 7.9 years, 16 patients are alive; 19 patients died of relapse, 34 patients died of transplantation-related causes, and 1 patient died of recurrence of his primary malignancy. Patients who benefited had responsive disease and did not have poor-risk cytogenetic features.[233]

Matched unrelated donor transplantation for patients with MDS has been performed in a limited number of patients. Early reports were disappointing,[88] but with improved matching techniques and supportive care, the results have improved. In one series of 52 patients with MDS or MDS-related AML who underwent matched unrelated donor transplantation, 2-year disease-free survival was 38%.[234] The European Bone Marrow Transplant group collected data on 118 patients with MDS including 12 patients with chronic myelomonocytic leukemia. Transplantation-related mortality was high for this cohort of patients (58%), and overall survival at 2 years was 28%. Again, patients with low-risk disease had a lower relapse rate.[235]

These studies indicate that a subset of MDS patients can be cured after allogeneic HCT. This observation is in contrast to all other treatment modalities that have been evaluated for this difficult disease. However, because of the advanced age of the majority of MDS patients, only a small percentage of patients are candidates for transplantation. The development of nonmyeloablative preparative regimens or radiolabeled monoclonal antibodies may allow the treatment of older patients with this disorder, especially those patients with relatively indolent disease.

Allogeneic HCT should be considered for patients with MDS who are younger than 60 years and who have an HLA-matched sibling donor. The decision to pursue HCT depends on a number of criteria, including the risk for progression, clinical status with particular reference to underlying infections, and overall health of the patient.

Autologous HCT. Autologous HCT has been attempted in some patients with MDS, but it has been evaluated in only limited numbers of patients because of the low CR rates obtained with induction chemotherapy. Therefore, any positive results are tempered by the fact that these patients are highly selected. Nevertheless, efforts have been made to develop strategies to collect normal stem cells in these patients. The use of in vivo mobilization and purging, similar to the strategy discussed before for CML, has been attempted in small numbers of patients with defined karyotypic abnormalities; a significant percentage of patients (six of nine) had leukapheresis products that were karyotypically normal after recovery from intensive chemotherapy.[215] Results of autologous transplantation for 79 patients with MDS or secondary AML who were successfully induced into CR revealed disease-free survival at 2 years of 39%.[236] However, small numbers of patients with high-risk cytogenetic features who had progressed to AML and were induced

into remission fared poorly with autologous HCT.[39] Therefore, autologous transplantation may be considered for those unusual patients who are successfully induced into CR and who do not have an HLA-matched donor.

Myeloproliferative Disorders

Patients with myeloproliferative disorders other than CML are occasionally considered for BMT. The variability of these disorders, as well as the small number of patients who have undergone HCT, makes it difficult to come to firm conclusions about selection of patients and expected outcomes. Because of the relatively favorable prognosis for patients with polycythemia vera, there has been little role for BMT except for those patients who progress to acute leukemia. On occasion, patients with myelofibrosis are suitable candidates for HCT, although the decision of when to consider transplantation is often difficult. Interestingly, after transplantation, bone marrow fibrosis has been observed to resolve during a period of several months.[237]

Twelve patients with agnogenic myeloid metaplasia were described after transplantation, which further supports the view that allogeneic HCT can be effective in patients with this disease.[238] With a median follow-up of 25 months, the 4-year overall survival was 71% and the event-free survival was 59% despite the fact that these patients were heavily pretreated. Other reports have also documented the potential utility of allogeneic HCT for the treatment of myeloproliferative disorders other than CML.[239]

Chronic Lymphocytic Leukemia

Patients with CLL have a highly variable clinical course, and transplantation has been explored only in patients with advanced disease. Several initial trials demonstrated the potential clinical efficacy of allogeneic BMT in CLL.[240-242] A retrospective case-control analysis of patients for whom fludarabine therapy failed suggested improved survival compared with conventional chemotherapy.[243] No prospective randomized studies have been performed.

Autologous transplantation has also been explored in this population of patients. A high rate of CR has been observed, leading to cautious optimism, although longer follow-up and larger numbers of patients are clearly required.[241]

COMPLICATIONS

Graft-versus-Host Disease

GVHD remains one of the most serious and challenging complications of allogeneic HCT. GVHD results from immunologically competent donor-derived T cells that react with recipient tissue antigens. Risk factors for development of GVHD include HLA disparity between donor and recipient, age, gender disparity, type and status of underlying disease, and immunosuppressive prophylaxis used.

By definition, acute GVHD occurs before day +100 after transplantation, whereas chronic GVHD occurs beyond day +100. GVHD primarily affects the skin, gastrointestinal tract, and liver. GVHD is a clinical diagnosis, although tissue biopsy results can be helpful in making a definitive diagnosis. The severity of GVHD is based on clinical and laboratory parameters and is graded between I and IV; grades II to IV are clinically significant. However, severity on pathologic specimens must always be tempered by an assessment of the clinical condition of the patient.

Grade II to grade IV acute GVHD occurs in 9% to 50% of patients who receive an allogeneic HCT from a histocompatible sibling donor. Patients who develop moderate (grade II) to severe (grades III and IV) acute GVHD have a significantly enhanced risk for mortality. Established acute GVHD is difficult to treat, and prophylaxis is critically important. Two general approaches have been used in an effort to prevent acute GVHD, namely, immunosuppressive medications and T-cell depletion.

A number of different drugs have been used as prophylaxis against GVHD. Methotrexate (MTX), cyclosporine (CSP), and prednisone (PSE) have been the mainstays of prophylaxis and are generally used in combination. A series of randomized clinical trials from Seattle have established that CSP given over at least 6 months and MTX administered on days 1, 3, 6, and 11 after the transplantation is an effective regimen.[244, 245] Subsequent updates of these studies have documented that effective prophylaxis with CSP/MTX did not result in a significant increase in the risk for relapse, which is always a concern with any agent that prevents acute GVHD.[246]

A series of randomized clinical trials from the City of Hope National Medical Center and Stanford University have also been performed. In the initial prospective study, CSP and PSE prophylaxis resulted in a reduced rate of grade II to grade IV GVHD compared with MTX and PSE.[247] The regimen of CSP/PSE was compared with CSP/MTX/PSE, with the MTX administered on days 1, 3, and 6 in a randomized trial with all patients receiving the preparative regimen of FTBI/VP-16. Patients who received the two-drug regimen had an incidence of grade II to grade IV GVHD of 23% compared with 9% for patients who received the three-drug regimen (P = .02).[37] A subsequent randomized trial comparing CSP/MTX/PSE with CSP/MTX revealed equivalence.[248] These studies from two independent groups of investigators have confirmed CSP/MTX as an effective regimen for the prevention of acute GVHD.

Tacrolimus (FK506) has also been used to prevent acute GVHD.[249] Prospective randomized clinical trials have been performed in the setting of both HLA-matched sibling and matched unrelated donor allogeneic HCT. In the study of allogeneic HCT with HLA-matched sibling donors, 329 patients from 16 transplantation centers were randomized to receive FK506 or CSP, with both groups also receiving MTX. The incidence of grade II to grade IV acute GVHD was significantly lower in the group of patients randomized to FK506 (31.9% versus 44.4%; P = .01).[250] In addition, no differences in relapse rates

or overall survival were noted. However, paradoxically, 2-year disease-free survival was superior in the CSP arm, which was thought to be due to a larger number of patients with advanced disease who were randomized to receive FK506. FK506 has also been used with MTX for the prevention of acute GVHD in the unrelated donor setting. Phase II studies have resulted in a 42% to 50% incidence of grade II to grade IV acute GVHD, which appears promising.[251, 252] A randomized trial has been reported from Japan in which 136 patients received either an FK506- or CSP-based regimen. For those 69 patients who received unrelated donor transplants, the incidence of acute GVHD was reduced from 51.4% in the CSP group to 20.6% in the FK506 group (P < .05).[253] These results will require confirmation in a larger group of patients but are consistent with a reduction in the incidence of acute GVHD with the use of FK506 over CSP; however, this observation has not been associated with improved overall survival. With the introduction of mobilized PBPCs, studies will need to be performed comparing different regimens to prevent GVHD.

An alternative approach for the prevention of GVHD has been to deplete donor T cells from the graft before infusion. A variety of techniques have been employed, including physical separation such as elutriation or density-gradient centrifugation, monoclonal antibody–based depletion, and CD34+ cell selection. As discussed before, extensive removal of donor-derived T cells has been effective in preventing GVHD but has also been associated with an unacceptably increased risk for graft rejection and relapse.[254-258] Modifications of depletion procedures that result in only partial removal of T cells have met with more success.

Results of 39 patients with AML who underwent T-cell depletion by use of the soybean lectin agglutination and sheep red blood cell rosetting method, which results in an approximate 3-log depletion of T cells, have been encouraging. Patients were prepared with FTBI, thiotepa, and cyclophosphamide, with many also receiving additional immunosuppression with antithymocyte globulin. No cases of rejection or acute GVHD were noted. Disease-free survival at a median follow-up of 4 years or more was 77% for patients treated in first remission and 50% for patients who underwent HCT in second remission.[259]

A number of other groups have used partial T-cell depletion with monoclonal antibodies, which has resulted in significant reductions in GVHD without a high incidence of graft failure or relapse.[260-262]

An alternative approach is the use of Campath antibodies; an immunoglobulin M (Campath-IgM) is used for in vitro depletion of the graft, and an immunoglobulin G (Campath-IgG) is used for in vivo depletion of the recipient before infusion. In one report, 50 patients treated with Campath antibodies were compared with 459 historical patients reported to the IBMTR who received nondepleted grafts and conventional GVHD prophylaxis with CSP/MTX. The incidence rates of acute GVHD, chronic GVHD, and transplantation-related mortality were lower in the patients who received the Campath antibodies. Survival of the patients who were treated with the T-cell depletion approach was better at 6 months (92% versus

78%); however, at 5 years, there was no significant difference (60% versus 52%).[263]

T-cell depletion has also been employed in the unrelated donor setting with encouraging results. Clearly, the only effective way of comparing these two different prevention strategies is through a prospective randomized clinical trial. Such a trial is under way comparing T-cell depletion by use of the T10B9 monoclonal antibody and complement with unmanipulated bone marrow in the unrelated setting.

Treatment of established acute GVHD is often a difficult clinical problem. The mainstay of treatment of established GVHD is the use of corticosteroids. Dosing generally ranges between 1 and 2 mg/kg of prednisone with subsequent tapering, depending on response. In one study, the intravenous administration of 6-methylprednisolone was evaluated in low doses (2 mg/kg/day) and high doses (10 mg/kg/day) in 95 patients with acute GVHD. Responses in the two groups were similar (68% versus 71%); no differences were noted in evolution to grade III or grade IV GVHD, cytomegalovirus infection, or survival.[264] A variety of other approaches have been explored in the treatment of acute GVHD, including anti–T-cell antibodies such as antilymphocyte globulin, OKT3 directed against CD3, BT1-322 directed against CD2, and the monoclonal antibodies directed against IL-2 receptor.[239, 265] Responses have been noted in many of these studies, but these responses are often transient. The use of anti–tumor necrosis factor monoclonal antibodies has been explored in limited clinical trials of 19 patients with moderate to severe acute GVHD, of whom 14 responded.[266]

A variety of newer pharmacologic agents are under investigation for the treatment of both acute and chronic GVHD. Mycophenolate mofetil has been explored in combination with cyclosporine and prednisone. In one study, 17 patients with established acute GVHD were treated with 2 g of mycophenolate mofetil per day; improvements were observed in 11 patients (65%).[267] Myelosuppression was the most common side effect, although discontinuation of the drug was not required in any patient. The combination of cyclosporine and mycophenolate mofetil was explored in one small study of patients undergoing allogeneic HCT and was found to be well tolerated with similar rates of GVHD.[268]

Chronic GVHD

Chronic GVHD is a significant complication of allogeneic HCT. The clinical manifestations of chronic GVHD are broad and resemble those of autoimmune disorders such as scleroderma and dermatomyositis.[269, 270] Patients with extensive chronic GVHD have an increased mortality rate, especially patients with platelet counts below 100,000 cells/μL on day +100, those patients who progress from acute to chronic GVHD, patients with lichenoid changes on skin biopsy, and patients with significant liver involvement.[271] Treatment of chronic GVHD involves the use of immunosuppressive drugs; cyclosporine and prednisone are the mainstays of treatment.[272] Because of the chronic nature of the disease, long-term treatment is often required. Alternate-day dosing has been found to help re-

duce some of the toxicity of the immunosuppressive medications.[273]

Thalidomide was found to have immunosuppressive properties and has been used to treat chronic GVHD in both adults and children.[274-276] Side effects have included somnolence and constipation. Interestingly, thalidomide was not effective in preventing the onset of chronic GVHD in a small randomized trial in which there was actually a higher incidence of this complication in patients treated with the drug.[277] Psoralen plus ultraviolet radiation (PUVA) has shown encouraging results in small numbers of patients with chronic GVHD.[278] Low-dose total lymphoid irradiation (100 cGy) has also been reported to result in significant improvement in chronic GVHD in a limited number of patients.[279]

Infection, especially by gram-positive bacteria, is a common problem in patients with chronic GVHD. Monthly intravenous immunoglobulin or rotating antibiotic use is sometimes helpful in patients with recurrent infections, especially for patients who are hypogammaglobulinemic as a result of chronic GVHD. Chronic GVHD remains a significant and often debilitating clinical problem. New approaches to the prevention and treatment of this complication are urgently needed.

Infections

Patients undergoing hematopoietic stem cell transplantation are at great risk for development of infectious complications. These can occur early as a consequence of neutropenia or later from immunosuppression and immunoincompetence. Major advances in the control of opportunistic infections have resulted in improved outcomes for patients undergoing transplantation.

Broad-spectrum antibiotics are available that adequately cover the majority of infections encountered by patients, such that mortality due to bacterial sepsis is relatively rare.

Viral infections remain a major problem, especially those of herpes viruses. Herpes simplex virus type 1 and type 2 infections are common after transplantation and are effectively treated with acyclovir. Many centers preemptively treat patients who are seropositive with prophylactic antiviral therapy.[280] Later infection due to reactivation of herpes zoster is also common, occurring in 40% to 60% of patients. Although this problem is rarely life-threatening, it is annoying and often painful.

Control of cytomegalovirus infections has been one of the major advances in the treatment of patients receiving transplants. Cytomegalovirus infection was one of the most feared infectious complications. With the introduction of preemptive therapy with antivirals and intravenous immunoglobulin, this infection can be controlled in the majority of patients.[281-283] Serologic screening remains an important consideration, and seronegative patients who receive hematopoietic stem cells from a seronegative donor should always receive seronegative blood products to avoid this complication.[284] Despite effective therapy, cytomegalovirus infection remains a major clinical problem; reactivation is also common after autologous transplantation, but disease is rare. However, after extensive manipulation of the graft, cytomegalovirus infection may be more prevalent.[285]

Fungal infections remain a feared and serious complication of transplantation. Prophylaxis with antifungals such as fluconazole has reduced the risk for *Candida* infections.[286] Infection from *Aspergillus* species remains a major problem that is relatively rare (<5% of patients) but often fatal. Amphotericin is rarely effective for deep-seated *Aspergillus* infections. A number of lipid-based products are under investigation; however, more effective therapies are needed, and new drugs are under development.

Veno-occlusive Disease of the Liver

Veno-occlusive disease of the liver is characterized by unexplained weight gain, hyperbilirubinemia, abdominal pain, and ascites. Veno-occlusive disease can vary from a mild condition to a life-threatening complication.[287] Treatment, including thrombolytics and shunting, has been unsatisfactory and has generally been ineffective. Prophylaxis with low-dose heparin or ursodeoxycholic acid has been suggested to reduce the risk for development of veno-occlusive disease in some but not all studies.[288-290] Veno-occlusive disease has been found to be more common in recipients who have liver function test abnormalities at the time of transplantation and in those who receive hematopoietic stem cells from donors positive for hepatitis B or C.

Secondary Malignant Neoplasms

The success of transplantation has led to the unfortunate realization that patients who are long-term survivors are at risk for second malignant neoplasms. In one retrospective analysis of 557 patients receiving transplants from allogeneic donors, 9 patients developed 10 secondary cancers for a cumulative actuarial risk of 12% at 11 years after HCT. The age-adjusted incidence of secondary cancer was 4.2 times higher than that expected from a similar population of individuals in the general population.[291] In another large retrospective analysis of 19,229 patients who underwent allogeneic or syngeneic HCT, the risk for new solid cancers was 8.3 times higher at 10 years after transplantation compared with the risk of age-adjusted individuals.[292] Despite the higher risk, the cumulative incidence at 10 years was only 2.2%. The role of the transplantation procedure versus that of previous treatment is often difficult to resolve with clarity. Myelodysplasia and acute leukemia have also been noted after autologous HCT, which has generally ranged between 7% and 15%.[293-298] This complication generally has an extremely poor prognosis.[299]

TREATMENT AND PREVENTION OF RELAPSE AFTER TRANSPLANTATION

Relapse of the underlying disease is an unfortunate and ominous event after HCT. Patients who suffer a relapse typically do so within the first 3 years after transplantation. Once a patient relapses, the likelihood of curative therapy is remote. Patients are able to tolerate chemotherapy or radiation, which may result in responses; however, prolonged survival is rare. A number of novel therapies are under consideration in an effort to treat or preferentially prevent relapses. Second transplantations have rarely been successful because of toxicity and tumor resistance.[300-303]

A major goal is to develop therapies aimed at treating the minimal residual disease that may persist after HCT. The rationale for use of immunotherapy after HCT is based on the realization that the graft-versus-tumor effect is a major reason for success of the procedure. The cells responsible for the graft-versus-tumor effect are not known with certainty, although both T cells and NK cells have been implicated. An ideal clinical setting in which to use immunotherapy is likely to be after HCT because the majority of patients are cytoreduced to a state of minimal disease and the effector cells are readily available. A number of studies using cytokines or cell populations are in progress testing these therapeutic principles. It has been observed that after HCT, IL-2 production is impaired, yet peripheral blood lymphocytes isolated from patients retain the ability to respond to IL-2.[304, 305] A number of phase I/II clinical trials have been performed with IL-2 with and without in vitro activated cells.[306, 307] Randomized trials after autologous HCT are under way.

IL-2 therapy was not beneficial in a modestly sized randomized clinical trial after autologous HCT for ALL.[308] Other cytokines, such as IL-12 and IL-15, are also in the early stages of clinical development.

Cellular immunotherapy has been effective in the treatment of patients who have relapsed after allogeneic HCT. The use of donor leukocyte infusions for treatment of patients who have suffered a relapse after allogeneic HCT is well established, especially for CML. Since the initial reports in the 1980s, a number of studies have clearly documented that reinfusion of unmanipulated leukocytes derived from the HLA-matched donor results in significant clinical responses in relapsed patients, especially those with CML.[309-312] Responses have also been noted in other diseases, such as AML and multiple myeloma, but donor leukocyte infusion has been less effective in patients with ALL. Two large retrospective studies from Europe and North America have highlighted both the promise and the problems associated with donor leukocyte infusions. The European Group for Blood and Marrow Transplantation reported results obtained from 135 patients treated at 27 transplantation centers where 73% of patients with relapsed CML were reinduced into a durable CR with donor leukocyte infusion. Patients with AML did not respond as well; only five (29%) had a CR, and none of the ALL patients responded. Donor leukocyte infusion treatment had considerable toxicity; 42% of the patients developed clinically significant GVHD, and 34% of the patients developed myelosuppression. Seventeen (12.6%) of the patients died of causes other than their underlying malignant disease.

A second large retrospective analysis of results from donor leukocyte infusion of 140 relapsed patients after allogeneic HCT from 25 North American programs demonstrated a similar response rate of 60% among CML patients.[313] As expected, responses were superior for those patients with only cytogenetic relapses or for patients treated with donor leukocyte infusion while they were in chronic phase compared with patients who had progressed to either accelerated phase or blastic phase. Results were not favorable for patients with AML (15.4% CR) or ALL (18.2% CR). Again, complications included GVHD (60%) and pancytopenia (18.6%).

Overall, these results confirm the favorable clinical results of donor leukocyte infusion, especially for patients with CML that has not progressed beyond chronic phase. An interesting approach will be to administer donor leukocyte infusions to patients early on, for example, in those who have had only molecular relapses. Donor leukocyte infusion has also been used for patients who relapse after unrelated donor transplantation with similar response rates.[314]

As discussed before, a major complication of donor leukocyte infusion is the risk for GVHD. One approach to limiting the risk for GVHD has been to use lower doses of T cells with subsequent dose escalation if a response is not observed. In one study of patients with CML who relapsed after T-cell-depleted transplantation, a dose of 1×10^7 CD3$^+$ T cells per kilogram was defined, which resulted in excellent efficacy without causing significant GVHD.[315] However, it remains unclear whether this dose level also applies to patients who relapse after transplantation of a non–T-cell–depleted graft. Other groups have attempted to deplete CD8$^+$ cells to reduce the risk for GVHD while retaining a graft-versus-leukemia effect when patients were identified who had graft-versus-leukemia effects without GVHD.[316] An innovative approach to limit GVHD after donor leukocyte infusion has been to modify the donor leukocytes such that they are susceptible to certain drug treatments that allow their eradication if GVHD develops, for example, with the herpes simplex thymidine kinase gene, when expressing cells could then be eliminated with ganciclovir.[317] Another complication that has been observed after donor leukocyte infusion is myelosuppression and in some instances marrow aplasia, primarily in those patients who had no evidence of donor hematopoiesis at the time of donor leukocyte infusion treatment.[318]

An open question, especially in patients with relapsed CML, is what the optimal therapy is, given that excellent results have also been obtained with interferon alfa in patients who have relapsed after allogeneic HCT, especially when patients are treated early after a relapse at a time of only cytogenetic relapse.[319, 320]

Cytotoxic T lymphocytes can be generated in some instances with specific antitumor activity. The potential of this strategy has been demonstrated in pilot studies directed against defined viral targets, such as cytomegalovirus and Epstein-Barr virus.[321-323] Whether these types of results can be extended to patients with malignant neoplasms in which there are no clearly defined antigens remains to be determined.

Another approach has been to expand T cells that share functional and phenotypic properties with NK cells. One such population of cytolytic cells has been termed cytokine-induced killer (CIK) cells.[324, 325] CIK cells

have been shown to have in vivo activity in animal model systems, and clinical trials have been initiated.[219, 326]

Considerable interest has been generated by the successful isolation and expansion of professional antigen-presenting cells, such as dendritic cells, which express the molecules required for a productive immunologic reaction. The in vivo application of dendritic cells with defined experimental antigens has been explored in murine model systems with clear efficacy. Early clinical trials have been reported with antitumor cellular responses observed in vitro in some patients.[327] Clearly, clinical trials in this area are just beginning.

QUALITY OF LIFE

The success of HCT has resulted in a larger number of patients becoming long-term survivors, bringing issues of quality of life to the fore. Studies have been performed to evaluate the quality of life of HCT survivors. In these studies, the majority of individuals were employed and in good health with acceptable objective and subjective levels of functioning; however, a minority of individuals (10% to 15%) had evidence of psychosocial stress.[328-333] The major limitations in quality of life after allogeneic HCT were generally associated with chronic GVHD.[334] Similar results were obtained for patients who survived for more than 5 years after allogeneic HCT; 93% of patients were in good health, and 89% had returned to full-time work or school.[335]

CONCLUSIONS AND FUTURE DIRECTIONS

Remarkable progress continues to be made in the field of HCT. The introduction of PBPCs, which has resulted in reduced morbidity and mortality, and a number of other improvements discussed in this chapter have dramatically altered the prognosis of patients undergoing this treatment modality. HCT has grown from a "treatment of last resort" to standard up-front therapy for a variety of disorders. Randomized, prospective clinical trials have documented the benefit of HCT for a number of diseases. Major advances continue to occur in our understanding of the underlying principles and mechanisms of cancer biology, hematology, and immunology. The field of HCT is on the forefront of these developments, which predicts a rich and promising future for the benefit of our patients.

REFERENCES

1. Jacobson LO, Marks EK, Robson M, et al: Effect of spleen protection on mortality following X-irradiation. J Lab Clin Med 1949; 34:1538.
2. Lorenz E, Uphoff D, Reid TR, et al: Modification of irradiation injury in mice and guinea pigs by bone marrow injections. J Natl Cancer Inst 1951;12:197.
3. Thomas ED, Lochte HL, Lu WC, et al: Intravenous infusion of bone marrow in patients receiving radiation and chemotherapy. N Engl J Med 1957;257:491.
4. Thomas ED, Lochte HL, Cannon JH, et al: Supralethal whole body irradiation and isologous marrow transplantation in man. J Clin Invest 1959;38:1709.

5. Cavins JA, Schem SC, Thomas ED, et al: The recovery of lethally irradiated dogs given infusions of autologous leukocytes preserved at −80° C. Blood 1964;23:38.

6. Thomas ED, Buckner CD, Banaji M, et al: One hundred patients with acute leukemia treated by chemotherapy, total body irradiation, and allogeneic marrow transplantation. Blood 1977;49:511.

7. Till JE, McCulloch EA: A direct measurement of the radiation sensitivity of normal mouse bone marrow cells. Radiation Res 1961;14:213.

8. Wu AM, Till JE, Siminovitch L, et al: A cytological study of the capacity for differentiation of normal hemopoietic colony-forming cells. J Cell Physiol 1967;69:177.

9. Spangrude GJ, Heimfeld S, Weissman IL: Purification and characterization of mouse hematopoietic stem cells. Science 1988;241:58.

10. Berenson RJ, Andrews RG, Bensinger WI, et al: Antigen CD34$^+$ marrow cells engraft lethally irradiated baboons. J Clin Invest 1988;81:951.

11. Berenson RJ, Bensinger WI, Hill RS, et al: Engraftment after infusion of CD34$^+$ marrow cells in patients with breast cancer or neuroblastoma. Blood 1991;77:1717.

12. Keating A, Powell J, Takahashi M, et al: The generation of human long-term marrow cultures from marrow depleted of Ia (HLA-DR) positive cells. Blood 1984;64:1159.

13. Lu L, Walker D, Broxmeyer HE, et al: Characterization of adult human marrow hematopoietic progenitors highly enriched by two-color cell sorting with My10 and major histocompatibility class II monoclonal antibodies. J Immunol 1987;139:1823.

14. Baum CM, Weissman IL, Tsukamoto AS, et al: Isolation of a candidate human hematopoietic stem-cell population. Proc Natl Acad Sci U S A 1992; 89:2804.

15. Craig W, Kay R, Cutler RL, et al: Expression of Thy-1 on human hematopoietic progenitor cells. J Exp Med 1993;177:1331.

16. Negrin RS, Atkinson K, Leemhuis T, et al: Transplantation of highly purified CD34$^+$Thy-1$^+$ hematopoietic stem cells in patients with metastatic breast cancer. Biol Blood Marrow Transplant 2000; 6:262.

17. Thomas ED, Clift RA, Hersman J, et al: Marrow transplantation for acute nonlymphoblastic leukemia in first remission using fractionated or single-dose irradiation. Int J Radiat Oncol Biol Phys 1982; 8:817.

18. Shank B, Chu FC, Dinsmore R, et al: Hyperfractionated total body irradiation for bone marrow transplantation. Results in seventy leukemia patients with allogeneic transplants. Int J Radiat Oncol Biol Phys 1983;9:1607.

19. Blume KG, Forman SJ, O'Donnell MR, et al: Total body irradiation and high-dose etoposide: A new preparatory regimen for bone marrow transplantation in patients with advanced hematologic malignancies. Blood 1987;69:1015.

20. Chao NJ, Forman SJ, Schmidt GM, et al: Allogeneic bone marrow transplantation for high-risk acute lymphoblastic leukemia during first complete remission. Blood 1991;78:1923.

21. Riddell S, Appelbaum FR, Buckner CD, et al: High-dose cytarabine and total body irradiation with or without cyclophosphamide as a preparative regimen for marrow transplantation for acute leukemia. J Clin Oncol 1988;6:576.

22. Woods WG, Ramsay NK, Weisdorf DJ, et al: Bone marrow transplantation for acute lymphocytic leukemia utilizing total body irradiation followed by high doses of cytosine arabinoside: Lack of superiority over cyclophosphamide-containing conditioning regimens. Bone Marrow Transplant 1990;6:9.

23. Santos GW, Tutschka PJ, Brookmeyer R, et al: Marrow transplantation for acute nonlymphocytic leukemia after treatment with busulfan and cyclophosphamide. N Engl J Med 1983;309:1347.

24. Geller RB, Saral R, Piantadosi S, et al: Allogeneic bone marrow transplantation after high-dose busulfan and cyclophosphamide in patients with acute nonlymphocytic leukemia. Blood 1989; 73:2209.

25. Clift RA, Buckner CD, Thomas ED, et al: Marrow transplantation for chronic myeloid leukemia: A randomized study comparing cyclophosphamide and total body irradiation with busulfan and cyclophosphamide. Blood 1994;84:2036.

26. Spitzer TR, Cottler-Fox M, Torrisi J, et al: Escalating doses of etoposide with cyclophosphamide and fractionated total body irradiation or busulfan as conditioning for bone marrow transplantation. Bone Marrow Transplant 1989;4:559.

27. Vaughan WP, Dennison JD, Reed EC, et al: Improved results of allogeneic bone marrow transplantation for advanced hematologic malignancy using busulfan, cyclophosphamide and etoposide as cytoreductive and immunosuppressive therapy. Bone Marrow Transplant 1991;8:489.

28. Clift RA, Buckner CD, Appelbaum FR, et al: Allogeneic marrow transplantation in patients with acute myeloid leukemia in first remission: A randomized trial of two irradiation regimens. Blood 1990;76:1867.

29. Clift RA, Buckner CD, Appelbaum FR, et al: Allogeneic marrow transplantation in patients with chronic myeloid leukemia in the chronic phase: A randomized trial of two irradiation regimens. Blood 1991;77:1660.

30. Matthews DC, Appelbaum FR, Eary JF, et al: Development of a marrow transplant regimen for acute leukemia using targeted hematopoietic irradiation delivered by ^{131}I-labeled anti-CD45 antibody, combined with cyclophosphamide and total body irradiation. Blood 1995;85:1122.

31. Matthews DC, Appelbaum FR, Eary JF, et al: Phase I study of ^{131}I-anti-CD45 antibody plus cyclophosphamide and total body irradiation for advanced acute leukemia and myelodysplastic syndrome. Blood 1999;94:1237.

32. Slavin S, Nagler A, Naparstek E, et al: Nonmyeloablative stem cell transplantation and cell therapy as an alternative to conventional bone marrow transplantation with lethal cytoreduction for the treatment of malignant and nonmalignant hematologic diseases. Blood 1998;91:756.

33. Khouri IF, Keating M, Körbling M, et al: Transplant-lite: Induction of graft-versus-malignancy using fludarabine-based nonablative chemotherapy and allogeneic blood progenitor-cell transplantation as treatment for lymphoid malignancies. J Clin Oncol 1998;16:2817.

34. Storb R, Yu C, Wagner JL, et al: Stable mixed hematopoietic chimerism in DLA-identical littermate dogs given sublethal total body irradiation before and pharmacological immunosuppression after marrow transplantation. Blood 1997;89:3048.

35. McSweeney PA, Niederwieser D, Shizuru JA, et al: Hematopoietic cell transplantation in older patients with hematologic malignancies: Replacing high-dose cytotoxic therapy with graft-versus-tumor effects. Blood 2001;97:3390.

36. Linker CA, Damon LE, Ries CA, et al: Autologous stem cell transplantation for high-risk adult acute lymphocytic leukemia (ALL). Blood 1999;94:580a.

37. Chao NJ, Stein AS, Long GD, et al: Busulfan/etoposide—initial experience with a new preparatory regimen for autologous bone marrow transplantation in patients with acute nonlymphoblastic leukemia. Blood 1993;81:319.

38. Linker CA, Ries CA, Damon LE, et al: Autologous bone marrow transplantation for acute myeloid leukemia using busulfan plus etoposide as a preparative regimen. Blood 1993;81:311.

39. Linker CA, Ries CA, Damon LE, et al: Autologous stem cell transplantation for acute myeloid leukemia in first remission. Biol Blood Marrow Transplant 2000;6:50.

40. Stroncek DF, Holland PV, Bartch G, et al: Experiences of the first 493 unrelated marrow donors in the National Marrow Donor Program. Blood 1993;81:1940.

41. Siczkowski M, Clarke D, Gordon MY: Binding of primitive hematopoietic progenitor cells to marrow stromal cells involves heparan sulfate. Blood 1992;80:912.

42. Simmons PJ, Masinovsky B, Longenecker BM, et al: Vascular cell adhesion molecule-1 expressed by bone marrow stromal cells mediates the binding of hematopoietic progenitor cells. Blood 1992;80:388.

43. Sniecinski IJ, Oien L, Petz LD, et al: Immunohematologic consequences of major ABO-mismatched bone marrow transplantation. Transplantation 1988;45:530.

44. McCredie KB, Hersh EM, Freireich EJ: Cells capable of colony formation in the peripheral blood of man. Science 1972;171:293.

45. Socinski MA, Cannistra SA, Elias A, et al: Granulocyte-macrophage colony stimulating factor expands the circulating haemopoietic progenitor cell compartment in man. Lancet 1988;1:1194.

46. Siena S, Bregni M, Brando B, et al: Circulation of CD34$^+$ hematopoietic stem cells in the peripheral blood of high-dose cyclophosphamide-treated patients: Enhancement by intravenous recombinant human granulocyte-macrophage colony-stimulating factor. Blood 1989;74:1905.

47. Sheridan WP, Begley CG, Juttner CA, et al: Effect of peripheral-blood progenitor cells mobilised by filgrastim (G-CSF) on platelet recovery after high-dose chemotherapy. Lancet 1992;339:640.

48. Schmitz N, Linch DC, Dreger P, et al: Randomised trial of filgrastim-mobilised peripheral blood progenitor cell transplantation versus autologous bone-marrow transplantation in lymphoma patients. Lancet 1996;347:353.

49. Smith TJ, Hillner BE, Schmitz N, et al: Economic analysis of a randomized clinical trial to compare filgrastim-mobilized peripheral-blood progenitor-cell transplantation and autologous bone marrow transplantation in patients with Hodgkin's and non-Hodgkin's lymphoma. J Clin Oncol 1997;15:5.

50. Chao NJ, Schriber JR, Grimes K, et al: Granulocyte colony-stimulating factor "mobilized" peripheral blood progenitor cells accelerate granulocyte and platelet recovery after high-dose chemotherapy. Blood 1993;81:2031.

51. Bensinger WI, Longin K, Appelbaum F, et al: Peripheral blood stem cells (PBSCs) collected after recombinant granulocyte colony stimulating factor (rhG-CSF): An analysis of factors correlating with the tempo of engraftment after transplantation. Br J Haematol 1994;87:825.

52. Tricot G, Jagannath S, Vesole D, et al: Peripheral blood stem cell transplants for multiple myeloma: Identification of favorable variables for rapid engraftment in 225 patients. Blood 1995;85:588.

53. Negrin RS, Kusnierz-Glaz CR, Still BJ, et al: Transplantation of enriched and purged peripheral blood progenitor cells from a single apheresis product in patients with non-Hodgkin's lymphoma. Blood 1995;85:3334.

54. Glaspy JA, Shpall EJ, LeMaistre CF, et al: Peripheral blood progenitor cell mobilization using stem cell factor in combination with filgrastim in breast cancer patients. Blood 1997;90:2939.

55. Weaver CH, Hazelton B, Birch R, et al: An analysis of engraftment kinetics as a function of the CD34 content of peripheral blood progenitor cell collections in 692 patients after the administration of myeloablative chemotherapy. Blood 1995;86:3961.

56. Shpall EJ, Champlin R, Glaspy JA: Effect of CD34$^+$ peripheral blood progenitor cell dose on hematopoietic recovery. Biol Blood Marrow Transplant 1998;4:84.

57. Weaver CH, Schulman KA, Wilson-Relyea B, et al: Randomized trial of filgrastim, sargramostim, or sequential sargramostim and filgrastim after myelosuppressive chemotherapy for the harvesting of peripheral-blood stem cells. J Clin Oncol 2000;18:43.

58. Bensinger WI, Weaver CH, Appelbaum FR, et al: Transplantation of allogeneic peripheral blood stem cells mobilized by recombinant human granulocyte colony-stimulating factor. Blood 1995;85:1655.

59. Körbling M, Przepiorka D, Huh YO, et al: Allogeneic blood stem cell transplantation for refractory leukemia and lymphoma: Potential advantage of blood over marrow allografts. Blood 1995;85:1659.

60. Storek J, Gooley T, Siadak M, et al: Allogeneic peripheral blood stem cell transplantation may be associated with a high risk of chronic graft-versus-host disease. Blood 1997;90:4705.

61. Bensinger WI, Martin P, Storer B, et al: A prospective, randomized trial of transplantation of marrow vs peripheral blood cell, from HLA-identical siblings in patients treated for hematological malignancies. N Engl J Med 2001;344:175.

62. Blaise D, Kuentz M, Fortanier C, et al: Randomized trial of bone marrow versus lenograstim-primed blood cell allogeneic transplantation in patients with early-stage leukemia: A report from the Société Française de Greffe de Moelle. J Clin Oncol 2000;18:537.

63. Nemunaitis J, Rabinowe SN, Singer JW, et al: Recombinant granulocyte-macrophage colony-stimulating factor after autologous bone marrow transplantation for lymphoid cancer. N Engl J Med 1991;324:1773.

64. Advani R, Chao NJ, Horning SJ, et al: Granulocyte-macrophage colony-stimulating factor (GM-CSF) as an adjunct to autologous hemopoietic stem cell transplantation for lymphoma. Ann Intern Med 1992;116:183.

65. Powles R, Smith C, Milan S, et al: Human recombinant GM-CSF in allogeneic bone-marrow transplantation for leukaemia: Double-blind, placebo-controlled trial. Lancet 1990;336:1417.

66. Spitzer G, Adkins DR, Spencer V, et al: Randomized study of growth factors post–peripheral-blood stem-cell transplant: Neutrophil recovery is improved with modest clinical benefit. J Clin Oncol 1994;12:661.

67. Suzue T, Takaue Y, Watanabe A, et al: Effects of rhG-CSF (filgrastim) on the recovery of hematopoiesis after high-dose chemotherapy and autologous peripheral blood stem cell transplantation in children: A report from the Children's Cancer and Leukemia Study Group of Japan. Exp Hematol 1994;22:1197.

68. Chao NJ, Schriber JR, Long GD, et al: A randomized study of erythropoietin and granulocyte colony-stimulating factor (G-CSF) versus placebo and G-CSF for patients with Hodgkin's and non-Hodgkin's lymphoma undergoing autologous bone marrow transplantation. Blood 1994;83:2823.

69. Vannucchi AM, Bosi A, Ieri A, et al: Combination therapy with G-CSF and erythropoietin after autologous bone marrow transplantation for lymphoid malignancies: A randomized trial. Bone Marrow Transplant 1996;17:527.

70. Biggs JC, Atkinson KA, Booker V, et al: Prospective randomised double-blind trial of the in vivo use of recombinant human erythropoietin in bone marrow transplantation from HLA-identical sibling donors. The Australian Bone Marrow Transplant Study Group. Bone Marrow Transplant 1995;15:129.

71. Klaesson S, Ringdén O, Ljungman P, et al: Reduced blood transfusions requirements after allogeneic bone marrow transplantation: Results of a randomised, double-blind study with high-dose erythropoietin. Bone Marrow Transplant 1994;13:397.

72. Nash RA, Kuzrock R, DiPersio J: A phase I trial of recombinant human thrombopoietin (TPO) in patients with delayed platelet recovery after hematopoietic stem cell transplantation. Biol Blood Marrow Transplant 2000;6:25.

73. Weisdorf SA, Lysne J, Wind D, et al: Positive effect of prophylactic total parenteral nutrition on long-term outcome of bone marrow transplantation. Transplantation 1987;43:833.

74. Charuhas PM, Fosberg KL, Bruemmer B, et al: A double-blind randomized trial comparing outpatient parenteral nutrition with intravenous hydration: Effect on resumption of oral intake after marrow transplantation. JPEN J Parenter Enteral Nutr 1997;21:157.

75. Ziegler TR, Young LS, Benfell K, et al: Clinical and metabolic efficacy of glutamine-supplemented parenteral nutrition after bone marrow transplantation. A randomized, double-blind, controlled study. Ann Intern Med 1992;116:821.

76. Coghlin-Dickson T, Wong R, Negrin RS, et al: Effect of oral glutamine supplementation during bone marrow transplantation. JPEN J Parenter Enteral Nutr 2000;24:61.

77. Sullivan KM, Kopecky KJ, Jocom J, et al: Immunomodulatory and antimicrobial efficacy of intravenous immunoglobulin in bone marrow transplantation. N Engl J Med 1990;323:705.

78. Sullivan KM, Storek J, Kopecky KJ, et al: A controlled trial of long-term administration of intravenous immunoglobulin to prevent late infection and chronic graft-vs.-host disease after marrow transplantation: Clinical outcome and effect on subsequent immune recovery. Biol Blood Marrow Transplant 1996;2:44.

79. Playford RJ, Marchbank T, Mandir N, et al: Effects of keratinocyte growth factor (KGF) on gut growth and repair. J Pathol 1998;184:316.

80. Farrell CL, Bready JV, Rex KL, et al: Keratinocyte growth factor protects mice from chemotherapy and radiation-induced gastrointestinal injury and mortality. Cancer Res 1998;58:933.

81. Fefer A, Einstein AB, Thomas ED, et al: Bone-marrow transplantation for hematologic neoplasia in 16 patients with identical twins. N Engl J Med 1974;290:1389.

82. Fefer A, Cheever MA, Thomas ED, et al: Bone marrow transplantation for refractory acute leukemia in 34 patients with identical twins. Blood 1981;57:421.

83. Gale RP, Horowitz MM, Ash RC, et al: Identical-twin bone marrow transplants for leukemia. Ann Intern Med 1994;120:646.

84. Beatty PG, Clift RA, Mickelson EM, et al: Marrow transplantation from related donors other than HLA-identical siblings. N Engl J Med 1985;313:765.

85. Anasetti C, Amos D, Beatty PG, et al: Effect of HLA compatibility on engraftment of bone marrow transplants in patients with leukemia or lymphoma. N Engl J Med 1989;320:197.

86. O'Reilly RJ, Dupont B, Pahwa S, et al: Reconstitution in severe combined immunodeficiency by transplantation of marrow from an unrelated donor. N Engl J Med 1977;297:1311.

87. Hansen JA, Clift RA, Thomas ED, et al: Transplantation of marrow from an unrelated donor to a patient with acute leukemia. N Engl J Med 1980;303:565.

88. Kernan NA, Bartsch G, Ash RC, et al: Analysis of 462 transplantations from unrelated donors facilitated by the National Marrow Donor Program. N Engl J Med 1993;328:593.

89. Hansen JA, Gooley TA, Martin PJ, et al: Bone marrow transplants from unrelated donors for patients with chronic myeloid leukemia. N Engl J Med 1998;338:962.

90. Hogan CJ, Shpall EJ, McNulty O, et al: Engraftment and development of human CD34$^+$-enriched cells from umbilical cord blood in NOD/LtSz-scid/scid mice. Blood 1997;90:85.

91. Wang JC, Doedens M, Dick JE: Primitive human hematopoietic cells are enriched in cord blood compared with adult bone marrow or mobilized peripheral blood as measured by the quantitative in vivo SCID-repopulating cell assay. Blood 1997;89:3919.

92. Gluckman E, Rocha V, Boyer-Chammard A, et al: Outcome of cord-blood transplantation from related and unrelated donors. Eurocord Transplant Group and the European Blood and Marrow Transplantation Group. N Engl J Med 1997;337:373.

93. Rubinstein P, Carrier C, Scaradavou A, et al: Outcomes among 562 recipients of placental-blood transplants from unrelated donors. N Engl J Med 1998;339:1565.

94. Reisner Y, Martelli MF: Bone marrow transplantation across HLA barriers by increasing the number of transplanted cells. Immunol Today 1995;16:437.

95. Henslee-Downey PJ, Abhyankar SH, Parrish RS, et al: Use of partially mismatched related donors extends access to allogeneic marrow transplant. Blood 1997;89:3864.

96. Aversa F, Tabilio A, Velardi A, et al: Treatment of high-risk acute leukemia with T-cell–depleted stem cells from related donors with one fully mismatched HLA haplotype. N Engl J Med 1998;339:1186.

97. Guinan EC, Boussiotis VA, Neuberg D, et al: Transplantation of anergic histoincompatible bone marrow allografts. N Engl J Med 1999;340:1704.

98. Thomas ED: Marrow transplantation for malignant diseases. J Clin Oncol 1983;1:517.

99. Thomas ED, Buckner CD, Clift RA, et al: Marrow transplantation for acute nonlymphoblastic leukemia in first remission. N Engl J Med 1979;301:597.

100. Blume KG, Beutler E, Bross KJ, et al: Bone-marrow ablation and allogeneic marrow transplantation in acute leukemia. N Engl J Med 1980;302:1041.

101. Powles RL, Morgenstern G, Clink HM, et al: The place of bone-marrow transplantation in acute myelogenous leukaemia. Lancet 1980;1:1047.

102. Bacigalupo A, Frassoni F, Van Lint MT, et al: Bone marrow transplantation (BMT) for acute nonlymphoid leukemia (ANLL) in first remission. Acta Haematol 1985;74:23.

103. Clift RA, Buckner CD, Thomas ED, et al: The treatment of acute non-lymphoblastic leukemia by allogeneic marrow transplantation. Bone Marrow Transplant 1987;2:243.

104. Snyder DS, Chao NJ, Amylon MD, et al: Fractionated total body irradiation and high-dose etoposide as a preparatory regimen for bone marrow transplantation for 99 patients with acute leukemia in first complete remission. Blood 1993;82:2920.

105. Powles RL, Watson JG, Morgenstern GR, et al: Bone-marrow transplantation in leukaemia remission [letter]. Lancet 1982;1:336.

106. Marmont A, Bacigalupo A, Van Lint MT, et al: Bone marrow transplantation versus chemotherapy alone for acute nonlymphoblastic leukemia. Exp Hematol 1985;13(suppl 17):40.

107. Appelbaum FR, Dahlberg S, Thomas ED, et al: Bone marrow transplantation or chemotherapy after remission induction for adults with acute nonlymphoblastic leukemia. A prospective comparison. Ann Intern Med 1984;101:581.

108. Appelbaum FR, Fisher LD, Thomas ED: Chemotherapy v marrow transplantation for adults with acute nonlymphocytic leukemia: A five-year follow-up. Blood 1988;72:179.

109. Reiffers J, Gaspard MH, Maraninchi D, et al: Comparison of allogeneic or autologous bone marrow transplantation and chemotherapy in patients with acute myeloid leukemia in first remission: A prospective controlled trial. Br J Haematol 1989;72:57.

110. Zittoun RA, Mandelli F, Willemze R, et al: Autologous or allogeneic bone marrow transplantation compared with intensive chemotherapy in acute myelogenous leukemia. European Organization for Research and Treatment of Cancer (EORTC) and the Gruppo Italiano Malattie Ematologiche Maligne dell'Adulto (GIMEMA) Leukemia Cooperative Groups. N Engl J Med 1995;332:217.

111. Cassileth PA, Harrington DP, Appelbaum FR, et al: Chemotherapy compared with autologous or allogeneic bone marrow transplantation in the management of acute myeloid leukemia in first remission. N Engl J Med 1998;339:1649.

112. Bloomfield CD, Lawrence D, Byrd JC, et al: Frequency of prolonged remission duration after high-dose cytarabine intensification in acute myeloid leukemia varies by cytogenetic subtype. Cancer Res 1998;58:4173.

113. Blaise D, Maraninchi D, Archimbaud E, et al: Allogeneic bone marrow transplantation for acute myeloid leukemia in first remission: A randomized trial of a busulfan-Cytoxan versus Cytoxan-total body irradiation as preparative regimen: A report from the Group d'Etudes de la Greffe de Moelle Osseuse. Blood 1992; 79:2578.

114. Helenglass G, Powles RL, McElwain TJ, et al: Melphalan and total body irradiation (TBI) versus cyclophosphamide and TBI as conditioning for allogeneic matched sibling bone marrow transplants for acute myeloblastic leukaemia in first remission. Bone Marrow Transplant 1988;3:21.

115. Blume KG, Kopecky KJ, Henslee-Downey JP, et al: A prospective randomized comparison of total body irradiation–etoposide versus busulfan-cyclophosphamide as preparatory regimens for bone marrow transplantation in patients with leukemia who were not in first remission: A Southwest Oncology Group study. Blood 1993; 81:2187.

116. Sanders JE, Thomas ED, Buckner CD, et al: Marrow transplantation for children in first remission of acute nonlymphoblastic leukemia: An update. Blood 1985;66:460.

117. Feig SA, Nesbit ME, Buckley J, et al: Bone marrow transplantation for acute non-lymphocytic leukemia: A report from the Childrens Cancer Study Group of sixty-seven children transplanted in first remission. Bone Marrow Transplant 1987;2:365.

118. Nesbit ME Jr, Buckley JD, Feig SA, et al: Chemotherapy for induction of remission of childhood acute myeloid leukemia followed by marrow transplantation or multiagent chemotherapy: A report from the Childrens Cancer Group. J Clin Oncol 1994;12:127.

119. Weisdorf DJ, McGlave PB, Ramsay NK, et al: Allogeneic bone marrow transplantation for acute leukaemia: Comparative outcomes for adults and children. Br J Haematol 1988;69:351.

120. Johnson FL, Sanders JE, Ruggiero M, et al: Bone marrow transplantation for the treatment of acute nonlymphoblastic leukemia in children aged less than 2 years. Blood 1988;71:1277.

121. Dicke KA, Zander A, Spitzer G, et al: Autologous bone-marrow transplantation in relapsed adult acute leukaemia. Lancet 1979; 1:514.

122. Gorin NC, David R, Stachowiak J, et al: High dose chemotherapy and autologous bone marrow transplantation in acute leukemias, malignant lymphomas and solid tumors. A study of 23 patients. Eur J Cancer 1981;17:557.

123. Herve P, Rozenbaum A, Plouvier E, et al: Autologous bone marrow transplantation in acute myeloid leukemia in relapse or in complete remission. Cancer Treat Rep 1982;66:1983.

124. Brenner MK, Rill DR, Moen RC, et al: Gene-marking to trace origin of relapse after autologous bone-marrow transplantation. Lancet 1993;341:85.

125. Deisseroth AB, Zu Z, Claxton D, et al: Genetic marking shows that Ph$^+$ cells present in autologous transplants of chronic myelogenous leukemia (CML) contribute to relapse after autologous bone marrow in CML. Blood 1994;83:3068.

126. Kaizer H, Stuart RK, Brookmeyer R, et al: Autologous bone marrow transplantation in acute leukemia: A phase I study of in vitro treatment of marrow with 4-hydroperoxycyclophosphamide to purge tumor cells. Blood 1985;65:1504.

127. Yeager AM, Kaizer H, Santos GW, et al: Autologous bone marrow transplantation in patients with acute nonlymphocytic leukemia, using ex vivo marrow treatment with 4-hydroperoxycyclophosphamide. N Engl J Med 1986;315:141.

128. Miller CB, Zehnbauer BA, Piantadosi S, et al: Correlation of occult clonogenic leukemia drug sensitivity with relapse after autologous bone marrow transplantation. Blood 1991;78:1125.

129. Gorin NC, Aegerter P, Auvert B, et al: Autologous bone marrow transplantation for acute myelocytic leukemia in first remission: A European survey of the role of marrow purging. Blood 1990; 75:1606.

130. Gorin NC: Autologous stem cell transplantation in acute myelocytic leukemia. Blood 1998;92:1073.

131. Ball ED, Mills LE, Cornwell GG 3rd, et al: Autologous bone marrow transplantation for acute myeloid leukemia using monoclonal antibody–purged bone marrow. Blood 1990;75:1199.

132. Löwenberg B, Verdonck LJ, Dekker AW, et al: Autologous bone marrow transplantation in acute myeloid leukemia in first remission: Results of a Dutch prospective study. J Clin Oncol 1990; 8:287.

133. McMillan AK, Goldstone AH, Linch DC, et al: High-dose chemotherapy and autologous bone marrow transplantation in acute myeloid leukemia. Blood 1990;76:480.

134. Cassileth PA, Andersen J, Lazarus HM, et al: Autologous bone marrow transplant in acute myeloid leukemia in first remission. J Clin Oncol 1993;11:314.

135. Chao NJ, Schmidt GM, Niland JC, et al: Cyclosporine, methotrexate, and prednisone compared with cyclosporine and prednisone for prophylaxis of acute graft-versus-host disease. N Engl J Med 1993;329:1225.

136. Linker CA, Ries CA, Damon LE, et al: Autologous bone marrow transplantation for acute myeloid leukemia using 4-hydroperoxy-cyclophosphamide–purged bone marrow and the busulfan/etoposide preparative regimen: A follow-up report. Bone Marrow Transplant 1998;22:865.

137. Reiffers J, Stoppa AM, Attal M, et al: Allogeneic vs autologous stem cell transplantation vs chemotherapy in patients with acute myeloid leukemia in first remission: The BGMT 87 study. Leukemia 1996;10:1874.

138. Harousseau JL, Cahn JY, Pignon B, et al: Comparison of autologous bone marrow transplantation and intensive chemotherapy as post-remission therapy in adult acute myeloid leukemia. The Groupe Ouest Est Leucémies Aiguës Myéloblastiques (GOELAM). Blood 1997;90:2978.

139. Mitus AJ, Miller KB, Schenkein DP, et al: Improved survival for patients with acute myelogenous leukemia. J Clin Oncol 1995; 13:560.

140. Burnett AK, Goldstone AH, Stevens RM, et al: Randomised comparison of addition of autologous bone-marrow transplantation to intensive chemotherapy for acute myeloid leukaemia in first remission: Results of MRC AML 10 trial. UK Medical Research Council Adult and Children's Leukaemia Working Parties. Lancet 1998; 351:700.

141. Ravindranath Y, Yeager AM, Chang MN, et al: Autologous bone marrow transplantation versus intensive consolidation chemotherapy for acute myeloid leukemia in childhood. Pediatric Oncology Group. N Engl J Med 1996;334:1428.

142. Brochstein JA, Kernan NA, Groshen S, et al: Allogeneic bone marrow transplantation after hyperfractionated total-body irradiation and cyclophosphamide in children with acute leukemia. N Engl J Med 1987;317:1618.

143. Sanders JE, Thomas ED, Buckner CD, et al: Marrow transplantation for children with acute lymphoblastic leukemia in second remission. Blood 1987;70:324.

144. Coccia PF, Strandjord SE, Warkentin PI, et al: High-dose cytosine arabinoside and fractionated total-body irradiation: An improved preparative regimen for bone marrow transplantation of children with acute lymphoblastic leukemia in remission. Blood 1988;71:888.

145. Dopfer R, Henze G, Bender-Götze C, et al: Allogeneic bone marrow transplantation for childhood acute lymphoblastic leukemia in second remission after intensive primary and relapse therapy according to the BFM- and CoALL-protocols: Results of the German Cooperative Study. Blood 1991;78:2780.

146. Barrett AJ, Horowitz MM, Pollock BH, et al: Bone marrow transplants from HLA-identical siblings as compared with chemotherapy for children with acute lymphoblastic leukemia in a second remission. N Engl J Med 1994;331:1253.

147. Chessells JM, Bailey C, Wheeler K, et al: Bone marrow transplantation for high-risk childhood lymphoblastic leukaemia in first remission: Experience in MRC UKALL X. Lancet 1992;340:565.

148. De la Cámara R, Figuera A, Steegmann JL, et al: Allogeneic bone marrow transplantation for high risk acute lymphoblastic leukemia. Results from a single institution. Bone Marrow Transplant 1992;9:433.

149. Blume KG, Forman SJ, Snyder DS, et al: Allogeneic bone marrow transplantation for acute lymphoblastic leukemia during first complete remission. Transplantation 1987;43:389.

150. Vernant JP, Marit G, Maraninchi D, et al: Allogeneic bone marrow transplantation in adults with acute lymphoblastic leukemia in first complete remission. J Clin Oncol 1988;6:227.

151. Blaise D, Gaspard MH, Stoppa AM, et al: Allogeneic or autologous bone marrow transplantation for acute lymphoblastic leukemia in first complete remission. Bone Marrow Transplant 1990;5:7.

152. von Bueltzingsloewen A, Bélanger R, Perreault C, et al: Allogeneic bone marrow transplantation following busulfan-cyclophosphamide with or without etoposide conditioning regimen for patients with acute lymphoblastic leukaemia. Br J Haematol 1993;85:706.

153. Horowitz MM, Messerer D, Hoelzer D, et al: Chemotherapy compared with bone marrow transplantation for adults with acute lymphoblastic leukemia in first remission. Ann Intern Med 1991; 115:13.

154. Zhang MJ, Hoelzer D, Horowitz MM, et al: Long-term follow-up of adults with acute lymphoblastic leukemia in first remission treated with chemotherapy or bone marrow transplantation. The Acute Lymphoblastic Leukemia Working Committee. Ann Intern Med 1995;123:428.

155. Oh H, Gale RP, Zhang MJ, et al: Chemotherapy vs HLA-identical sibling bone marrow transplants for adults with acute lymphoblastic leukemia in first remission. Bone Marrow Transplant 1998; 22:253.

156. Sebban C, Lepage E, Vernant JP, et al: Allogeneic bone marrow transplantation in adult acute lymphoblastic leukemia in first complete remission: A comparative study. French Group of Therapy of Adult Acute Lymphoblastic Leukemia. J Clin Oncol 1994;12:2580.

157. Linker CA, Levitt LJ, O'Donnell M, et al: Treatment of adult acute lymphoblastic leukemia with intensive cyclical chemotherapy: A follow-up report. Blood 1991;78:2814.

158. Larson RA, Dodge RK, Burns CP, et al: A five-drug remission induction regimen with intensive consolidation for adults with acute lymphoblastic leukemia: Cancer and leukemia group B study 8811. Blood 1995;85:2025.

159. Snyder DS, Nademanee AP, O'Donnell MR, et al: Long-term follow-up of 23 patients with Philadelphia chromosome–positive acute lymphoblastic leukemia treated with allogeneic bone marrow transplant in first complete remission. Leukemia 1999;13:2053.

160. Sierra J, Radich J, Hansen JA, et al: Marrow transplants from unrelated donors for treatment of Philadelphia chromosome-positive acute lymphoblastic leukemia. Blood 1997;90:1410.

161. Forman SJ, Schmidt GM, Nademanee AP, et al: Allogeneic bone marrow transplantation as therapy for primary induction failure for patients with acute leukemia. J Clin Oncol 1991;9:1570.

162. Schmid H, Henze G, Schwerdtfeger R, et al: Fractionated total body irradiation and high-dose VP-16 with purged autologous bone marrow rescue for children with high risk relapsed acute lymphoblastic leukemia. Bone Marrow Transplant 1993;12:597.

163. Simonsson B, Burnett AK, Prentice HG, et al: Autologous bone marrow transplantation with monoclonal antibody purged marrow for high risk acute lymphoblastic leukemia. Leukemia 1989;3:631.

164. Ritz J, Sallan SE, Bast RC Jr, et al: Autologous bone-marrow transplantation in CALLA-positive acute lymphoblastic leukemia after in-vitro treatment with J5 monoclonal antibody and complement. Lancet 1982;2:60.

165. Sallan SE, Niemeyer CM, Billett AL, et al: Autologous bone marrow transplantation for acute lymphoblastic leukemia. J Clin Oncol 1989;7:1594.

166. Uckun FM, Kersey JH, Haake R, et al: Pretransplantation burden of leukemic progenitor cells as a predictor of relapse after bone marrow transplantation for acute lymphoblastic leukemia. N Engl J Med 1993;329:1296.

167. Messina C, Cesaro S, Rondelli R, et al: Autologous bone marrow transplantation for childhood acute lymphoblastic leukaemia in Italy. AIEOP/FONOP-TMO Group. Italian Association of Paediatric Haemato-Oncology. Bone Marrow Transplant 1998;21:1015.

168. Maldonado MS, Díaz-Heredia C, Badell I, et al: Autologous bone marrow transplantation with monoclonal antibody purged marrow for children with acute lymphoblastic leukemia in second remission. Spanish Working Party for BMT in Children. Bone Marrow Transplant 1998;22:1043.

169. Billett AL, Kornmehl E, Tarbell NJ, et al: Autologous bone marrow transplantation after a long first remission for children with recurrent acute lymphoblastic leukemia. Blood 1993;81:1651.

170. Gilmore MJ, Hamon MD, Prentice HG, et al: Failure of purged

autologous bone marrow transplantation in high risk acute lymphoblastic leukaemia in first complete remission. Bone Marrow Transplant 1991;8:19.

171. Doney K, Buckner CD, Fisher L, et al: Autologous bone marrow transplantation for acute lymphoblastic leukemia. Bone Marrow Transplant 1993;12:315.

172. Ramsay N, LeBien T, Nesbit M, et al: Autologous bone marrow transplantation for patients with acute lymphoblastic leukemia in second or subsequent remission: Results of bone marrow treated with monoclonal antibodies BA-1, BA-2, and BA-3 plus complement. Blood 1985;66:508.

173. Uckun FM, Kersey JH, Vallera DA, et al: Autologous bone marrow transplantation in high-risk remission T-lineage acute lymphoblastic leukemia using immunotoxins plus 4-hydroperoxycyclophosphamide for marrow purging. Blood 1990;76:1723.

174. Martin H, Atta J, Zumpe P, et al: Purging of peripheral blood stem cells yields BCR-ABL–negative autografts in patients with BCR-ABL–positive acute lymphoblastic leukemia. Exp Hematol 1995;23:1612.

175. Miyamura K, Tanimoto M, Morishima Y, et al: Detection of Philadelphia chromosome–positive acute lymphoblastic leukemia by polymerase chain reaction: Possible eradication of minimal residual disease by marrow transplantation. Blood 1992;79:1366.

176. Radich J, Gehly G, Lee A, et al: Detection of bcr-abl transcripts in Philadelphia chromosome–positive acute lymphoblastic leukemia after marrow transplantation. Blood 1997;89:2602.

177. Knechtli CJ, Goulden NJ, Hancock JP, et al: Minimal residual disease status before allogeneic bone marrow transplantation is an important determinant of successful outcome for children and adolescents with acute lymphoblastic leukemia. Blood 1998;92:4072.

178. Champlin R, Ho W, Arenson E, et al: Allogeneic bone marrow transplantation for chronic myelogenous leukemia in chronic or accelerated phase. Blood 1982;60:1038.

179. Goldman JM, Apperley JF, Jones L, et al: Bone marrow transplantation for patients with chronic myeloid leukemia. N Engl J Med 1986;314:202.

180. McGlave P: Bone marrow transplants in chronic myelogenous leukemia: An overview of determinants of survival. Semin Hematol 1990;27:23.

181. Biggs JC, Szer J, Crilley P, et al: Treatment of chronic myeloid leukemia with allogeneic bone marrow transplantation after preparation with BuCy2. Blood 1992;80:1352.

182. Fefer A, Cheever MA, Greenberg PD, et al: Treatment of chronic granulocytic leukemia with chemoradiotherapy and transplantation of marrow from identical twins. N Engl J Med 1982;306:63.

183. Weiden PL, Flournoy N, Thomas ED, et al: Antileukemic effect of graft-versus-host disease in human recipients of allogeneic-marrow grafts. N Engl J Med 1979;300:1068.

184. Weiden PL, Sullivan KM, Flournoy N, et al: Antileukemic effect of chronic graft-versus-host disease: Contribution to improved survival after allogeneic marrow transplantation. N Engl J Med 1981;304:1529.

185. O'Reilly RJ: Allogenic bone marrow transplantation: Current status and future directions. Blood 1983;62:941.

186. McGlave P, Arthur D, Haake R, et al: Therapy of chronic myelogenous leukemia with allogeneic bone marrow transplantation. J Clin Oncol 1987;5:1033.

187. Snyder DS, Negrin RS, O'Donnell MR, et al: Fractionated total-body irradiation and high-dose etoposide as a preparatory regimen for bone marrow transplantation for 94 patients with chronic myelogenous leukemia in chronic phase. Blood 1994;84:1672.

188. Gratwohl A, Hermans J, Niederwieser D, et al: Bone marrow transplantation for chronic myeloid leukemia: Long-term results. Chronic Leukemia Working Party of the European Group for Bone Marrow Transplantation. Bone Marrow Transplant 1993;12:509.

189. Clift RA, Buckner CD, Thomas ED, et al: Marrow transplantation for patients in accelerated phase of chronic myeloid leukemia. Blood 1994;84:4368.

190. Thomas ED, Clift RA, Fefer A, et al: Marrow transplantation for the treatment of chronic myelogenous leukemia. Ann Intern Med 1986;104:155.

191. Bacigalupo A, Gualandi F, Van Lint MT, et al: Multivariate analysis of risk factors for survival and relapse in chronic granulocytic leukemia following allogeneic marrow transplantation: Impact of

disease related variables (Sokal score). Bone Marrow Transplant 1993;12:443.

192. Clift RA, Appelbaum FR, Thomas ED: Treatment of chronic myeloid leukemia by marrow transplantation. Blood 1993;82:1954.

193. Kalhs P, Schwarzinger I, Anderson G, et al: A retrospective analysis of the long-term effect of splenectomy on late infections, graft-versus-host disease, relapse, and survival after allogeneic marrow transplantation for chronic myelogenous leukemia. Blood 1995;86:2028.

194. Gratwohl A, Hermans J, von Biezen A, et al: No advantage for patients who receive splenic irradiation before bone marrow transplantation for chronic myeloid leukaemia: Results of a prospective randomized study. Bone Marrow Transplant 1992;10:147.

195. Jabro G, Koc Y, Boyle T, et al: Role of splenic irradiation in patients with chronic myeloid leukemia undergoing allogeneic bone marrow transplantation. Biol Blood Marrow Transplant 1999;5:173.

196. Devergie A, Blaise D, Attal M, et al: Allogeneic bone marrow transplantation for chronic myeloid leukemia in first chronic phase: A randomized trial of busulfan-cytoxan versus cytoxan-total body irradiation as preparative regimen: A report from the French Society of Bone Marrow Graft (SFGM). Blood 1995;85:2263.

197. Slattery JT, Clift RA, Buckner CD, et al: Marrow transplantation for chronic myeloid leukemia: The influence of plasma busulfan levels on the outcome of transplantation. Blood 1997;89:3055.

198. Group TIC: Interferon alfa-2a as compared with conventional chemotherapy for the treatment of chronic myeloid leukemia. N Engl J Med 1994;330:820.

199. Hehlmann R, Heimpel H, Hasford J, et al: Randomized comparison of interferon-alpha with busulfan and hydroxyurea in chronic myelogenous leukemia. The German CML Study Group. Blood 1994;84:4064.

200. Ohnishi K, Ohno R, Tomonaga M, et al: A randomized trial comparing interferon-alpha with busulfan for newly diagnosed chronic myelogenous leukemia in chronic phase. Blood 1995;86:906.

201. Guilhot F, Chastang C, Michallet M, et al: Interferon alfa-2b combined with cytarabine versus interferon alone in chronic myelogenous leukemia. French Chronic Myeloid Leukemia Study Group. N Engl J Med 1997;337:223.

202. Gale RP, Hehlmann R, Zhang MJ, et al: Survival with bone marrow transplantation versus hydroxyurea or interferon for chronic myelogenous leukemia. The German CML Study Group. Blood 1998;91:1810.

203. McGlave P, Bartsch G, Anasetti C, et al: Unrelated donor marrow transplantation therapy for chronic myelogenous leukemia: Initial experience of the National Marrow Donor Program. Blood 1993;81:543.

204. Lee SJ, Kuntz KM, Horowitz MM, et al: Unrelated donor bone marrow transplantation for chronic myelogenous leukemia: A decision analysis. Ann Intern Med 1997;127:1080.

205. Lee SJ, Anasetti C, Kuntz KM, et al: The costs and cost-effectiveness of unrelated donor bone marrow transplantation for chronic phase chronic myelogenous leukemia. Blood 1998;92:4047.

206. Bogdani V, Nemet D, Kastelan A, et al: Umbilical cord blood transplantation in a patient with Philadelphia chromosome–positive chronic myeloid leukemia. Transplantation 1993;56:477.

207. Laporte JP, Gorin NC, Rubinstein P, et al: Cord-blood transplantation from an unrelated donor in an adult with chronic myelogenous leukemia. N Engl J Med 1996;335:167.

208. Beelen DW, Graeven U, Elmaagacli AH, et al: Prolonged administration of interferon-alpha in patients with chronic-phase Philadelphia chromosome–positive chronic myelogenous leukemia before allogeneic bone marrow transplantation may adversely affect transplant outcome. Blood 1995;85:2981.

209. Morton AJ, Gooley T, Hansen JA, et al: Association between pretransplant interferon-alpha and outcome after unrelated donor marrow transplantation for chronic myelogenous leukemia in chronic phase. Blood 1998;92:394.

210. Giralt S, Szydlo R, Goldman JM, et al: Effect of short-term interferon therapy on the outcome of subsequent HLA-identical sibling bone marrow transplantation for chronic myelogenous leukemia: An analysis from the international bone marrow transplant registry. Blood 2000;95:410.

211. McGlave PB, De Fabritiis P, Deisseroth A, et al: Autologous transplants for chronic myelogenous leukaemia: Results from eight transplant groups. Lancet 1994;343:1486.

212. Hoyle C, Gray R, Goldman J: Autografting for patients with CML in chronic phase: An update. Hammersmith BMT Team LRF Centre for Adult Leukaemia. Br J Haematol 1994;86:76.

213. Barnett MJ, Eaves CJ, Phillips GL, et al: Autografting with cultured marrow in chronic myeloid leukemia: Results of a pilot study. Blood 1994;84:724.

214. Verfaillie CM, Miller WJ, Boylan K, et al: Selection of benign primitive hematopoietic progenitors in chronic myelogenous leukemia on the basis of HLA-DR antigen expression. Blood 1992; 79:1003.

215. Carella AM, Chimirri F, Podestà M, et al: High-dose chemo-radiotherapy followed by autologous Philadelphia chromosome–negative blood progenitor cell transplantation in patients with chronic myelogenous leukemia. Bone Marrow Transplant 1996; 17:201.

216. Verfaillie CM, Bhatia R, Steinbuch M, et al: Comparative analysis of autografting in chronic myelogenous leukemia: Effects of priming regimen and marrow or blood origin of stem cells. Blood 1998; 92:1820.

217. Carella AM, Lerma E, Corsetti MT, et al: Autografting with Philadelphia chromosome–negative mobilized hematopoietic progenitor cells in chronic myelogenous leukemia. Blood 1999;93:1534.

218. Cervantes F, Pierson BA, McGlave PB, et al: Autologous activated natural killer cells suppress primitive chronic myelogenous leukemia progenitors in long-term culture. Blood 1996;87:2476.

219. Hoyle C, Bangs CD, Chang P, et al: Expansion of Philadelphia chromosome-negative CD3+CD56+ cytotoxic cells from chronic myeloid leukemia patients: In vitro and in vivo efficacy in severe combined immunodeficiency disease mice. Blood 1998;92:3318.

220. Anderson JE, Appelbaum FR, Fisher LD, et al: Allogeneic bone marrow transplantation for 93 patients with myelodysplastic syndrome. Blood 1993;82:677.

221. O'Donnell MR, Nademanee AP, Snyder DS, et al: Bone marrow transplantation for myelodysplastic and myeloproliferative syndromes. J Clin Oncol 1987;5:1822.

222. Bunin NJ, Casper JT, Chitambar C, et al: Partially matched bone marrow transplantation in patients with myelodysplastic syndromes. J Clin Oncol 1988;6:1851.

223. Longmore G, Guinan EC, Weinstein HJ, et al: Bone marrow transplantation for myelodysplasia and secondary acute nonlymphoblastic leukemia. J Clin Oncol 1990;8:1707.

224. O'Donnell MR, Long GD, Parker PM, et al: Busulfan/cyclophosphamide as conditioning regimen for allogeneic bone marrow transplantation for myelodysplasia. J Clin Oncol 1995;13:2973.

225. Ratanatharathorn V, Karanes C, Uberti J, et al: Busulfan-based regimens and allogeneic bone marrow transplantation in patients with myelodysplastic syndromes. Blood 1993;81:2194.

226. Runde V, de Witte T, Arnold R, et al: Bone marrow transplantation from HLA-identical siblings as first-line treatment in patients with myelodysplastic syndromes: Early transplantation is associated with improved outcome. Chronic Leukemia Working Party of the European Group for Blood and Marrow Transplantation. Bone Marrow Transplant 1998;21:255.

227. Deeg HJ, Shulman HM, Anderson JE, et al: Allogeneic and syngeneic marrow transplantation for myelodysplastic syndrome in patients 55 to 66 years of age. Blood 2000;95:1188.

228. Greenberg P, Cox C, LeBeau MM, et al: International scoring system for evaluating prognosis in myelodysplastic syndromes. Blood 1997;89:2079.

229. Nevill TJ, Fung HC, Shepherd JD, et al: Cytogenetic abnormalities in primary myelodysplastic syndrome are highly predictive of outcome after allogeneic bone marrow transplantation. Blood 1998;92:1910.

230. Ballen KK, Gilliland DG, Guinan EC, et al: Bone marrow transplantation for therapy-related myelodysplasia: Comparison with primary myelodysplasia. Bone Marrow Transplant 1997;20:737.

231. Locatelli F, Pession A, Bonetti F, et al: Busulfan, cyclophosphamide and melphalan as conditioning regimen for bone marrow transplantation in children with myelodysplastic syndromes. Leukemia 1994;8:844.

232. Rubie H, Attal M, Demur C, et al: Intensified conditioning regimen with busulfan followed by allogeneic BMT in children with myelodysplastic syndromes. Bone Marrow Transplant 1994;13:759.

233. Yakoub-Agha BI, de La Salmoniere P, Ribaud P, et al: Allogeneic bone marrow transplantation for therapy-related myelodysplastic

syndrome and acute myeloid leukemia: A long-term study of 70 patients—report of the French Society of Bone Marrow Transplantation. J Clin Oncol 2000;18:963.

234. Anderson JE, Anasetti C, Appelbaum FR, et al: Unrelated donor marrow transplantation for myelodysplasia (MDS) and MDS-related acute myeloid leukaemia. Br J Haematol 1996;93:59.

235. Arnold R, de Witte T, van Biezen A, et al: Unrelated bone marrow transplantation in patients with myelodysplastic syndromes and secondary acute myeloid leukemia: An EBMT survey. European Blood and Marrow Transplantation Group. Bone Marrow Transplant 1998;21:1213.

236. de Witte T, van Biezen A, Hermans J, et al: Autologous bone marrow transplantation for patients with myelodysplastic syndrome (MDS) or acute myeloid leukemia following MDS. Chronic and Acute Leukemia Working Parties of the European Group for Blood and Marrow Transplantation. Blood 1997;90:3853.

237. Wolf JL, Spruce WE, Bearman RM, et al: Reversal of acute ("malignant") myelosclerosis by allogeneic bone marrow transplantation. Blood 1982;59:191.

238. Guardiola P, Esperou H, Cazals-Hatem D, et al: Allogeneic bone marrow transplantation for agnogenic myeloid metaplasia. French Society of Bone Marrow Transplantation. Br J Haematol 1997; 98:1004.

239. Przepiorka D, Giralt S, Khouri I, et al: Allogeneic marrow transplantation for myeloproliferative disorders other than chronic myelogenous leukemia: Review of forty cases. Am J Hematol 1998; 57:24.

240. Michallet M, Corront B, Hollard D, et al: Allogeneic bone marrow transplantation in chronic lymphocytic leukemia: 17 cases. Report from the EBMTG. Bone Marrow Transplant 1991;7:275.

241. Rabinowe SN, Soiffer RJ, Gribben JG, et al: Autologous and allogeneic bone marrow transplantation for poor prognosis patients with B-cell chronic lymphocytic leukemia. Blood 1993;82:1366.

242. Khouri IF, Keating MJ, Vriesendorp HM, et al: Autologous and allogeneic bone marrow transplantation for chronic lymphocytic leukemia: Preliminary results. J Clin Oncol 1994;12:748.

243. Khouri I, Keating M, Lerner S, et al: Improved survival with allogeneic and autologous stem cell transplantation for chronic lymphocytic leukemia (CLL): A case-matched analysis with conventional chemotherapy. Blood 1992;92:287a.

244. Storb R, Deeg HJ, Whitehead J, et al: Methotrexate and cyclosporine compared with cyclosporine alone for prophylaxis of acute graft versus host disease after marrow transplantation for leukemia. N Engl J Med 1986;314:729.

245. Storb R, Deeg HJ, Farewell V, et al: Marrow transplantation for severe aplastic anemia: Methotrexate alone compared with a combination of methotrexate and cyclosporine for prevention of acute graft-versus-host disease. Blood 1986;68:119.

246. Storb R, Pepe M, Deeg HJ, et al: Long-term follow-up of a controlled trial comparing a combination of methotrexate plus cyclosporine with cyclosporine alone for prophylaxis of graft-versus-host disease in patients administered HLA-identical marrow grafts for leukemia [letter]. Blood 1992;80:560.

247. Forman SJ, Blume KG, Krance RA, et al: A prospective randomized study of acute graft-v-host disease in 107 patients with leukemia: Methotrexate/prednisone v cyclosporine A/prednisone. Transplant Proc 1987;19:2605.

248. Chao NJ, Snyder DS, Jain M, et al: Equivalence of two effective graft-versus-host disease prophylaxis regimens: Results of a prospective double-blind randomized trial. Biol Blood Marrow Transplant 2000;6:254.

249. Fay JW, Wingard JR, Antin JH, et al: FK506 (Tacrolimus) monotherapy for prevention of graft-versus-host disease after histocompatible sibling allogenic bone marrow transplantation. Blood 1996; 87:3514.

250. Ratanatharathorn V, Nash RA, Przepiorka D, et al: Phase III study comparing methotrexate and tacrolimus (prograf, FK506) with methotrexate and cyclosporine for graft-versus-host disease prophylaxis after HLA-identical sibling bone marrow transplantation. Blood 1998;92:2303.

251. Nash RA, Piñeiro LA, Storb R, et al: FK506 in combination with methotrexate for the prevention of graft-versus-host disease after marrow transplantation from matched unrelated donors. Blood 1996;88:3634.

252. Devine SM, Geller RB, Lin LB, et al: The outcome of unrelated

donor bone marrow transplantation in patients with hematologic malignancies using tacrolimus (FK506) and low dose methotrexate for graft-versus-host disease prophylaxis. Biol Blood Marrow Transplant 1997;3:25.

253. Hiroka A: Results of a phase III study on prophylactic use of FK506 for acute GVHD compared with cyclosporin in allogeneic bone marrow transplantation. Blood 1997;90(suppl 1):561a.

254. Prentice HG, Blacklock HA, Janossy G, et al: Use of anti–T-cell monoclonal antibody OKT3 to prevent acute graft-versus-host disease in allogeneic bone-marrow transplantation for acute leukaemia. Lancet 1982;1:700.

255. Filipovich AH, Vallera DA, Youle RJ, et al: Ex-vivo treatment of donor bone marrow with anti–T-cell immunotoxins for prevention of graft-versus-host disease. Lancet 1984;1:469.

256. Martin PJ, Hansen JA, Buckner CD, et al: Effects of in vitro depletion of T cells in HLA-identical allogeneic marrow grafts. Blood 1985;66:664.

257. Kernan NA, Flomenberg N, Dupont B, et al: Graft rejection in recipients of T-cell–depleted HLA-nonidentical marrow transplants for leukemia. Identification of host-derived antidonor allocytotoxic T lymphocytes. Transplantation 1987;43:842.

258. Racadot E, Hervé P, Beaujean F, et al: Prevention of graft-versus-host disease in HLA-matched bone marrow transplantation for malignant diseases: A multicentric study of 62 patients using 3-pan-T monoclonal antibodies and rabbit complement. J Clin Oncol 1987;5:426.

259. Papadopoulos EB, Carabasi MH, Castro-Malaspina H, et al: T-cell–depleted allogeneic bone marrow transplantation as postremission therapy for acute myelogenous leukemia: Freedom from relapse in the absence of graft-versus-host disease. Blood 1998;91:1083.

260. Hervé P, Cahn JY, Flesch M, et al: Successful graft-versus-host disease prevention without graft failure in 32 HLA-identical allogeneic bone marrow transplantations with marrow depleted of T cells by monoclonal antibodies and complement. Blood 1987;69:388.

261. Champlin R, Ho W, Gajewski J, et al: Selective depletion of CD8+ T lymphocytes for prevention of graft-versus-host disease after allogeneic bone marrow transplantation. Blood 1990;76:418.

262. Soiffer RJ, Murray C, Mauch P, et al: Prevention of graft-versus-host disease by selective depletion of CD6-positive T lymphocytes from donor bone marrow. J Clin Oncol 1992;10:1191.

263. Hale G, Zhang MJ, Bunjes D, et al: Improving the outcome of bone marrow transplantation by using CD52 monoclonal antibodies to prevent graft-versus-host disease and graft rejection. Blood 1998;92:4581.

264. Van Lint MT, Uderzo C, Locasciulli A, et al: Early treatment of acute graft-versus-host disease with high- or low-dose 6-methylprednisolone: A multicenter randomized trial from the Italian Group for Bone Marrow Transplantation. Blood 1998;92:2288.

265. Hervé P, Wijdenes J, Bergerat JP, et al: Treatment of corticosteroid resistant acute graft-versus-host disease by in vivo administration of anti–interleukin-2 receptor monoclonal antibody (B-B10). Blood 1990;75:1017.

266. Hervé P, Flesch M, Tiberghien P, et al: Phase I–II trial of a monoclonal anti-tumor necrosis factor alpha antibody for the treatment of refractory severe acute graft-versus-host disease. Blood 1992; 79:3362.

267. Basara N, Blau WI, Römer E, et al: Mycophenolate mofetil for the treatment of acute and chronic GVHD in bone marrow transplant patients. Bone Marrow Transplant 1998;22:61.

268. Bornhäuser M, Schuler U, Pörksen G, et al: Mycophenolate mofetil and cyclosporine as graft-versus-host disease prophylaxis after allogeneic blood stem cell transplantation. Transplantation 1999;67:499.

269. Shulman HM, Sale GE, Lerner KG, et al: Chronic cutaneous graft-versus-host disease in man. Am J Pathol 1978;91:545.

270. Shulman HM, Sullivan KM, Weiden PL, et al: Chronic graft-versus-host syndrome in man. A long-term clinicopathologic study of 20 Seattle patients. Am J Medicine 1980;69:204.

271. Wingard JR, Piantadosi S, Vogelsang GB, et al: Predictors of death from chronic graft-versus-host disease after bone marrow transplantation. Blood 1989;74:1428.

272. Sullivan KM, Shulman HM, Storb R, et al: Chronic graft-versus-host disease in 52 patients: Adverse natural course and successful treatment with combination immunosuppression. Blood 1981;57:267.

273. Sullivan KM, Witherspoon RP, Storb R, et al: Alternating-day cyclosporine and prednisone for treatment of high-risk chronic graft-v-host disease. Blood 1988;72:555.

274. Vogelsang GB, Farmer ER, Hess AD, et al: Thalidomide for the treatment of chronic graft-versus-host disease. N Engl J Med 1992; 326:1055.

275. Cole CH, Rogers PC, Pritchard S, et al: Thalidomide in the management of chronic graft-versus-host disease in children following bone marrow transplantation. Bone Marrow Transplant 1994;14:937.

276. Parker PM, Chao N, Nademanee A, et al: Thalidomide as salvage therapy for chronic graft-versus-host disease. Blood 1995;86:3604.

277. Chao NJ, Parker PM, Niland JC, et al: Paradoxical effect of thalidomide prophylaxis on chronic graft-vs.-host disease. Biol Blood Marrow Transplant 1996;2:86.

278. Kapoor N, Pelligrini AE, Copelan EA, et al: Psoralen plus ultraviolet A (PUVA) in the treatment of chronic graft versus host disease: Preliminary experience in standard treatment resistant patients. Semin Hematol 1992;29:108.

279. Socie G, Devergie A, Cosset JM, et al: Low-dose (one gray) total-lymphoid irradiation for extensive, drug-resistant chronic graft-versus-host disease. Transplantation 1990;49:657.

280. Saral R, Burns WH, Laskin OL, et al: Acyclovir prophylaxis of herpes-simplex-virus infections. N Engl J Med 1981;305:63.

281. Goodrich JM, Mori M, Gleaves CA, et al: Early treatment with ganciclovir to prevent cytomegalovirus disease after allogeneic bone marrow transplantation. N Engl J Med 1991;325:1601.

282. Schmidt GM, Horak DA, Niland JC, et al: A randomized, controlled trial of prophylactic ganciclovir for cytomegalovirus pulmonary infection in recipients of allogeneic bone marrow transplants; The City of Hope–Stanford-Syntex CMV Study Group [see comments]. N Engl J Med 1991;324:1005.

283. Winston DJ, Ho WG, Bartoni K, et al: Ganciclovir prophylaxis of cytomegalovirus infection and disease in allogeneic bone marrow transplant recipients. Results of a placebo-controlled, double-blind trial. Ann Intern Med 1993;118:179.

284. Bowden RA, Sayers M, Flournoy N, et al: Cytomegalovirus immune globulin and seronegative blood products to prevent primary cytomegalovirus infection after marrow transplantation. N Engl J Med 1986;314:1006.

285. Holmberg LA, Boeckh M, Hooper H, et al: Increased incidence of cytomegalovirus disease after autologous CD34-selected peripheral blood stem cell transplantation. Blood 1999;94:4029.

286. Goodman JL, Winston DJ, Greenfield RA, et al: A controlled trial of fluconazole to prevent fungal infections in patients undergoing bone marrow transplantation [see comments]. N Engl J Med 1992; 326:845.

287. Bearman SI: The syndrome of hepatic veno-occlusive disease after marrow transplantation. Blood 1995;85:3005.

288. Attal M, Huguet F, Rubie H, et al: Prevention of hepatic veno-occlusive disease after bone marrow transplantation by continuous infusion of low-dose heparin: A prospective, randomized trial [see comments]. Blood 1992;79:2834.

289. Essell JH, Schroeder MT, Harman GS, et al: Ursodiol prophylaxis against hepatic complications of allogeneic bone marrow transplantation. A randomized, double-blind, placebo-controlled trial. Ann Intern Med 1998;128:975.

290. Marsa-Vila L, Gorin NC, Laporte JP, et al: Prophylactic heparin does not prevent liver veno-occlusive disease following autologous bone marrow transplantation. Eur J Haematol 1991;47:346.

291. Lowsky R, Lipton J, Fyles G, et al: Secondary malignancies after bone marrow transplantation in adults. J Clin Oncol 1994;12:2187.

292. Curtis RE, Rowlings PA, Deeg HJ, et al: Solid cancers after bone marrow transplantation. N Engl J Med 1997;336:897.

293. Micallef INM, Lillington DM, Apostolidis J, et al: Therapy-related myelodysplasia and secondary acute myelogenous leukemia after high-dose therapy with autologous hematopoietic progenitor-cell support for lymphoid malignancies. J Clin Oncol 2000;18:947.

294. Pedersen-Bjergaard J, Pedersen M, Myhre J, et al: High risk of therapy-related leukemia after BEAM chemotherapy and autologous stem cell transplantation for previously treated lymphomas is mainly related to primary chemotherapy and not to the BEAM-transplantation procedure. Leukemia 2000;11:1654.

295. Traweek ST, Slovak ML, Nademanee AP, et al: Clonal karyotypic hematopoietic cell abnormalities occurring after autologous bone

marrow transplantation for Hodgkin's disease and non-Hodgkin's lymphoma. Blood 1994;84:957.

296. Darrington DL, Vose JM, Anderson JR, et al: Incidence and characterization of secondary myelodysplastic syndrome and acute myelogenous leukemia following high-dose chemoradiotherapy and autologous stem-cell transplantation for lymphoid malignancies. J Clin Oncol 1994;12:2527.

297. Stone RM, Neuberg D, Soiffer R, et al: Myelodysplastic syndrome as a late complication following autologous bone marrow transplantation for non-Hodgkin's lymphoma. J Clin Oncol 1994;12:2535.

298. Miller JS, Arthur DC, Litz CE, et al: Myelodysplastic syndrome after autologous bone marrow transplantation: An additional late complication of curative cancer therapy. Blood 1994;83:3780.

299. Armitage JO: Myelodysplasia and acute leukemia after autologous bone marrow transplantation. J Clin Oncol 2000;18:945.

300. Sanders JE, Buckner CD, Clift RA, et al: Second marrow transplants in patients with leukemia who relapse after allogeneic marrow transplantation. Bone Marrow Transplant 1988;3:11.

301. Wagner JE, Vogelsang GB, Zehnbauer BA, et al: Relapse of leukemia after bone marrow transplantation: Effect of second myeloablative therapy. Bone Marrow Transplant 1992;9:205.

302. Mrsíc M, Horowitz MM, Atkinson K, et al: Second HLA-identical sibling transplants for leukemia recurrence. Bone Marrow Transplant 1992;9:269.

303. Kishi K, Takahashi S, Gondo H, et al: Second allogeneic bone marrow transplantation for post-transplant leukemia relapse: Results of a survey of 66 cases in 24 Japanese institutes. Bone Marrow Transplant 1997;19:461.

304. Welte K, Ciobanu N, Moore MA, et al: Defective interleukin 2 production in patients after bone marrow transplantation and in vitro restoration of defective T lymphocyte proliferation by highly purified interleukin 2. Blood 1984;64:380.

305. Cayeux S, Meuer S, Pezzutto A, et al: T-cell ontogeny after autologous bone marrow transplantation: Failure to synthesize interleukin-2 (IL-2) and lack of CD2- and CD3-mediated proliferation by both CD4⁻ and CD8⁺ cells even in the presence of exogenous IL-2. Blood 1989;74:2270.

306. Benyunes MC, Massumoto C, York A, et al: Interleukin-2 with or without lymphokine-activated killer cells as consolidative immunotherapy after autologous bone marrow transplantation for acute myelogenous leukemia. Bone Marrow Transplant 1993;12:159.

307. Hamon MD, Prentice HG, Gottlieb DJ, et al: Immunotherapy with interleukin 2 after ABMT in AML. Bone Marrow Transplant 1993;11:399.

308. Attal M, Blaise D, Marit G, et al: Consolidation treatment of adult acute lymphoblastic leukemia: A prospective, randomized trial comparing allogeneic versus autologous bone marrow transplantation and testing the impact of recombinant interleukin-2 after autologous bone marrow transplantation. BGMT Group. Blood 1995;86:1619.

309. Kolb HJ, Mittermüller J, Clemm C, et al: Donor leukocyte transfusions for treatment of recurrent chronic myelogenous leukemia in marrow transplant patients. Blood 1990;76:2462.

310. Drobyski WR, Keever CA, Roth MS, et al: Salvage immunotherapy using donor leukocyte infusions as treatment for relapsed chronic myelogenous leukemia after allogeneic bone marrow transplantation: Efficacy and toxicity of a defined T-cell dose. Blood 1993;82:2310.

311. Porter DL, Roth MS, McGarigle C, et al: Induction of graft-versus-host disease as immunotherapy for relapsed chronic myeloid leukemia. N Engl J Med 1994;330:100.

312. Collins RH Jr, Pineiro LA, Nemunaitis JJ, et al: Transfusion of donor buffy coat cells in the treatment of persistent or recurrent malignancy after allogeneic bone marrow transplantation. Transfusion 1995;35:891.

313. Collins RH Jr, Shpilberg O, Drobyski WR, et al: Donor leukocyte infusions in 140 patients with relapsed malignancy after allogeneic bone marrow transplantation. J Clin Oncol 1997;15:433.

314. Porter DL, Collins RH Jr, Hardy C, et al: Treatment of relapsed leukemia after unrelated donor marrow transplantation with unrelated donor leukocyte infusions. Blood 2000;95:1214.

315. Mackinnon S, Papadopoulos EB, Carabasi MH, et al: Adoptive immunotherapy evaluating escalating doses of donor leukocytes for relapse of chronic myeloid leukemia after bone marrow trans-

plantation: Separation of graft-versus-leukemia responses from graft-versus-host disease. Blood 1995;86:1261.

316. Alyea EP, Soiffer RJ, Canning C, et al: Toxicity and efficacy of defined doses of CD4⁺ donor lymphocytes for treatment of relapse after allogeneic bone marrow transplant. Blood 1998;91:3671.

317. Bonini C, Ferrari G, Verzeletti S, et al: HSV-TK gene transfer into donor lymphocytes for control of allogeneic graft-versus-leukemia. Science 1997;276:1719.

318. Keil F, Haas OA, Fritsch G, et al: Donor leukocyte infusion for leukemic relapse after allogeneic marrow transplantation: Lack of residual donor hematopoiesis predicts aplasia. Blood 1997;89:3113.

319. Higano CS, Chielens D, Raskind W, et al: Use of alpha-2a-interferon to treat cytogenetic relapse of chronic myeloid leukemia after marrow transplantation. Blood 1997;90:2549.

320. Elmaagacli AH, Beelen DW, Schaefer UW: A retrospective single centre study of the outcome of five different therapy approaches in 48 patients with relapse of chronic myelogenous leukemia after allogeneic bone marrow transplantation. Bone Marrow Transplant 1997;20:1045.

321. Rooney CM, Smith CA, Ng CY, et al: Use of gene-modified virus-specific T lymphocytes to control Epstein-Barr-virus–related lymphoproliferation. Lancet 1995;345:9.

322. Walter EA, Greenberg PD, Gilbert MJ, et al: Reconstitution of cellular immunity against cytomegalovirus in recipients of allogeneic bone marrow by transfer of T-cell clones from the donor. N Engl J Med 1995;333:1038.

323. Heslop HE, Ng CY, Li C, et al: Long-term restoration of immunity against Epstein-Barr virus infection by adoptive transfer of gene-modified virus-specific T lymphocytes. Nat Med 1996;2:551.

324. Schmidt-Wolf IG, Negrin RS, Kiem HP, et al: Use of a SCID mouse/human lymphoma model to evaluate cytokine-induced killer cells with potent antitumor cell activity. J Exp Med 1991;174:139.

325. Lu PH, Negrin RS: A novel population of expanded human CD3⁺CD56⁺ cells derived from T cells with potent in vivo antitumor activity in mice with severe combined immunodeficiency. J Immunol 1994;153:1687.

326. Sweeney TJ, Mailänder V, Tucker AA, et al: Visualizing the kinetics of tumor-cell clearance in living animals. Proc Natl Acad Sci U S A 1999;96:12044.

327. Hsu FJ, Benike C, Fagnoni F, et al: Vaccination of patients with B-cell lymphoma using autologous antigen-pulsed dendritic cells. Nat Med 1996;2:52.

328. Wolcott DL, Wellisch DK, Fawzy FI, et al: Adaptation of adult bone marrow transplant recipient long-term survivors. Transplantation 1986;41:478.

329. Andrykowski MA, Altmaier EM, Barnett RL, et al: Cognitive dysfunction in adult survivors of allogeneic marrow transplantation: Relationship to dose of total body irradiation. Bone Marrow Transplant 1990;6:269.

330. Wingard JR, Curbow B, Baker F, et al: Health, functional status, and employment of adult survivors of bone marrow transplantation. Ann Intern Med 1991;114:113.

331. Chao NJ, Tierney DK, Bloom JR, et al: Dynamic assessment of quality of life after autologous bone marrow transplantation. Blood 1992;80:825.

332. Schmidt GM, Niland JC, Forman SJ, et al: Extended follow-up in 212 long-term allogeneic bone marrow transplant survivors. Issues of quality of life. Transplantation 1993;55:551.

333. Fife BL, Huster GA, Cornetta KG, et al: Longitudinal study of adaptation to the stress of bone marrow transplantation. J Clin Oncol 2000;18:1539.

334. Syrjala KL, Chapko MK, Vitaliano PP, et al: Recovery after allogeneic marrow transplantation: Prospective study of predictors of long-term physical and psychosocial functioning. Bone Marrow Transplant 1993;11:319.

335. Duell T, Van Lint MT, Ljungman P, et al: Health and functional status of long-term survivors of bone marrow transplantation. EBMT Working Party on Late Effects and EULEP Study Group on Late Effects. European Group for Blood and Marrow Transplantation. Ann Intern Med 1997;126:184.

336. Champlin RE, Ho WG, Gale RP, et al: Treatment of acute myelogenous leukemia. A prospective controlled trial of bone marrow transplantation versus consolidation chemotherapy. Ann Intern Med 1985;102:285.

337. Zander AR, Keating M, Dicke K, et al: A comparison of marrow transplantation with chemotherapy for adults with acute leukemia of poor prognosis in first complete remission. J Clin Oncol 1988; 6:1548.

338. Conde E, Iriondo A, Rayon C, et al: Allogeneic bone marrow transplantation versus intensification chemotherapy for acute myelogenous leukaemia in first remission: A prospective controlled trial. Br J Haematol 1988;68:219.

339. Schiller GJ, Nimer SD, Territo MC, et al: Bone marrow transplantation versus high-dose cytarabine-based consolidation chemotherapy for acute myelogenous leukemia in first remission. J Clin Oncol 1992;10:41.

340. Cassileth PA, Lynch E, Hines JD, et al: Varying intensity of postremission therapy in acute myeloid leukemia. Blood 1992;79:1924.

341. Archimbaud E, Thomas X, Michallet M, et al: Prospective genetically randomized comparison between intensive postinduction chemotherapy and bone marrow transplantation in adults with newly diagnosed acute myeloid leukemia. J Clin Oncol 1994; 12:262.

342. Hewlett J, Kopecky KJ, Head D, et al: A prospective evaluation of the roles of allogeneic marrow transplantation and low-dose monthly maintenance chemotherapy in the treatment of adult acute myelogenous leukemia (AML): A Southwest Oncology Group study. Leukemia 1995;9:562.

21

Acute Myelogenous Leukemia

Ama Rohatiner   T. Andrew Lister

> Nor is there any better way to advance the proper practice of medicine than to give our minds to the discovery of the visual Law of Nature by careful investigation of cases of rare forms of disease.
>
> **William Harvey, 1657,**
> **quoted by A. Garrod,**
> **The Lancet, 1928**

HISTORICAL PERSPECTIVE

In 1845, the clinical features and postmortem findings of a hitherto unacknowledged disease were independently described by Craigie[1] and Bennett[2] in Scotland and Virchow in Germany.[3] The striking features common to these reports were the description of "thick" blood, the presence of splenomegaly, and a rapidly fatal outcome, usually from infection. Virchow's remarkably prescient observations related the clinical and postmortem findings to the microscopic appearance of the blood. In 1847, in a monograph entitled "Weisses Blut," he wrote, "When I speak of white blood, I mean a blood in which the proportion between the red and the colorless corpuscles is reversed, without the addition of any chemical or morphological elements."[4] Convinced that this reversal of the normal ratio was inherent to the cause of the illness, he later used the word *Leukämie,*[5] describing the illness as the "direct cause for the increase in the number of colorless particles in the blood." Twenty years later, Neumann[6] linked the illness to changes in the bone marrow and described this form of leukemia as myelogenous.

The notion of inducing "remission" dates back to the original descriptions of short-lived regressions of childhood leukemia associated with staphylococcal infection[7, 8] and early attempts to transmit viral infections to cause leukopenia.[8] Much later, exchange blood transfusions were attempted in France, with some measure of temporary benefit termed remission.[9]

The concept of trying to cure acute myelogenous leukemia (AML) is relatively recent. In 1955, Tivey[10] eloquently described the natural history of a disease that had an inexorably progressive course and was always fatal. Only 2 years later, after the demonstration that the use of oral 6-mercaptopurine could, albeit temporarily, return the blood and bone marrow to normal, Sir Ronald Bodley Scott, concluding a lecture to the Medical Society

of London, commented, "With all humility, it may be claimed that there are at least grounds for hope and encouragement in this recently acquired ability to halt the formerly unrelenting malignant process known as acute leukaemia."[11] However, this enlightened view was shared by few physicians; more than 10 years later, there was still debate as to whether patients with AML should be treated at all.[12]

A long and careful series of observations followed. The seminal work of Skipper, Schabel, and Wilcox[13] in L1210 murine leukemia, using cytosine arabinoside (ara-C) at various doses and schedules, led in turn to the evaluation of ara-C alone and in combination with other drugs in patients,[14, 15] resulting in remissions, which, although hardly ever more than temporary, prefaced the situation today when remission can be achieved in the majority of younger adults.

In the last decade, the emphasis has therefore shifted somewhat toward intensification of treatment overall but more specifically toward trying to prevent recurrence by intensifying *postremission* therapy. Several approaches have been tested: high-dose ara-C; high-dose (i.e., myeloablative) therapy (HDT) supported by autologous bone marrow transplantation (ABMT) or, more recently, peripheral blood progenitor cells (PBPC); and, in the minority of patients for whom it is feasible, allogeneic bone marrow transplantation. Each strategy has its proponents and its advantages and disadvantages. With increasing recognition of the role played by an immunologically mediated graft-versus-leukemia effect, nonmyeloablative allogeneic stem cell transplantation is currently being evaluated in patients for whom a standard allograft is considered inappropriate (see later and Chapter 20).

This chapter focuses on the *treatment* of AML at various points in the course of the illness. To put this into perspective, etiology, incidence, and epidemiology are first addressed.

ETIOLOGY

The person who has been told the diagnosis often first asks what caused the illness. The cause of AML remains unknown in most patients. Much attention has been paid to the increased incidence of chronic myeloid leukemia in particular but also of AML in survivors of the atomic bombs detonated at Hiroshima and Nagasaki,[16-18] the highest being in people who were older than 45 years at the time of exposure. AML developed after an interval of 6 to 10 years; there is, therefore, obvious concern about the population living around Chernobyl at the time of the nuclear accident. Recent data on leukemia in the Kiev region suggest that whereas the overall pattern of acute leukemia in this area is no different from that seen previously, several specific features have been noted (i.e., the absence of an age peak in children with AML and relatively higher numbers of children with AML subtypes M4 and M5).[19] Another study from Russia looking at the incidence of acute leukemia in the Ukraine before and after the Chernobyl accident showed that the incidence of acute leukemia 4 years afterward was higher than before the accident, but since 1991, it has returned to the previous level.[20]

To clarify the mechanism of leukemogenesis in atomic bomb survivors, leukemic blast cells from patients in Japan with a history of radiation exposure were compared with cells from those in whom leukemia arose de novo by use of fluorescent in situ hybridization (FISH) analysis. A significantly higher incidence of subclones with monosomy 7 and deletion of the 20q13.2 region was found in the group exposed to radiation. Furthermore, segmental translocation of the c-*myc* gene was observed in the exposed group, suggesting that leukemic cells from patients exposed to radiation are characterized by genetic instability that may influence the development of leukemia.[21]

It has long been known that therapeutic radiation can be associated with the development of AML. Historically, the use of radiotherapy for ankylosing spondylitis[22] resulted in a fivefold increase in risk, with a latent period of 3 to 5 years. The other well-documented association is with chemotherapy (with or without radiotherapy) given for Hodgkin's disease[23-32]; leukemia occurs at 5 to 10 years, with a lower level of risk thereafter.[33-37]

The use of HDT (especially when it involves regimens containing total-body irradiation) in patients with non-Hodgkin's lymphoma has been found to be associated with secondary myelodysplasia (MDS) and secondary AML.[38-42] Results from the European Bone Marrow Transplant (EBMT) Registry show an actuarial risk for the development of secondary MDS/AML at 5 years of 3%,[40] and appreciably higher levels have now been reported.[41, 42] On multivariate analysis in the EBMT study, low-grade (versus intermediate-grade or high-grade) lymphoma, older age at the time of transplantation, total-body irradiation as part of the myeloablative regimen, interval between diagnosis and transplantation, and number of transplantation procedures (i.e., some patients had two)[40] were found to be significant risk factors. Recent data from St. Bartholomew's Hospital (using multiplex-FISH) confirm that clonal abnormalities (presumably the consequence of previous chemotherapy) not apparent on conventional G-banding were in fact present before HDT in some patients who later developed secondary MDS/AML.[43] Thus, the antecedent chemotherapy may be the critical factor, rather than the HDT itself, although HDT probably accelerates the evolution of the disease.

As mentioned before, chemotherapy can cause leuke-mia. Two classes of compound have particularly been implicated, alkylating agents[44-46] and epipodophyllotox-ins,[47-49] but it has also been suggested that the purine analogue fludarabine can lead to development of secondary AML.[42, 50] The group of patients originally recognized as being at risk for development of secondary acute leukemia were women with ovarian cancer treated with alkylating agents, specifically cyclophosphamide and melphalan.[45] Cyclophosphamide given for prolonged periods to patients with non-Hodgkin's lymphoma has likewise been shown to be associated with secondary AML,[46] as when it is used for protracted periods in patients with rheumatoid arthritis.[51] However, cisplatin and carboplatin, as used in more recent regimens for ovarian cancer, have also been reported to lead to a somewhat increased incidence of AML.[52] The drug CCNU given as adjuvant therapy for gastrointestinal tract cancer has similarly been implicated,[53] as has strontium Sr 89 for treatment of prostate cancer.[54] Alkylating agents given with topoisomerase II inhibitors for treatment of pediatric solid tumors are strongly leukemogenic.[55] The use of hydroxyurea for essential thrombocythemia has also been recognized as a cause of secondary AML in a small proportion of patients.[56]

Secondary AML that follows alkylating agent therapy is generally characterized by deletions or abnormalities of chromosomes 5 and 7.[44-46] In contrast, AML developing after exposure to etoposide is almost always associated with abnormalities of chromosome 11[47-49] (see Chapter 5). Another difference relates to the latent period, which is shorter for etoposide than that seen after exposure to alkylating agents.[47-49] Furthermore, secondary AML occurring as a late complication of alkylating agent therapy usually follows a myelodysplastic phase, often with dyserythropoiesis, with or without the presence of ring sideroblasts. Almost invariably, this progresses to overt leukemia that is generally refractory to treatment. After exposure to etoposide, AML typically occurs without preceding MDS.[47-49]

Exposure to other chemicals can also result in AML. The association between occupational exposure to benzene and other solvents[57-59] and the development of AML has led to stringent legislation relating to environmental exposure at work. Although not widely publicized, cigarette smoking has been shown to be associated with a somewhat increased risk for development of leukemia, particularly in older people[60-62] and in association with specific chromosome abnormalities such as monosomy 7.[63]

It has long been known that congenital chromosome abnormalities are associated with an increased risk for acute leukemia.[64-67] Both AML and acute lymphoblastic leukemia can occur in Down's syndrome (trisomy 21), with the incidence being approximately 18-fold that in the general population.[64, 65] Fanconi's anemia[66] and Bloom's syndrome,[67] both characterized by random chromosome breaks, are also associated with an increased risk for AML.

INCIDENCE AND EPIDEMIOLOGY

The incidence is approximately 1.75 per 100,000 in the United Kingdom[68] and approximately 2.5 in the United

States, being slightly higher in men than in women and clearly increasing with age.[69] In terms of geographic variation, the highest rates appear to be in Denmark, North America, Australia, and New Zealand (in the non-Maori population); the lowest rates are reported from India (Bombay), Latin America, and eastern Europe.[70]

Because the majority of publications about AML refer to patients younger than 60 years, AML is sometimes mistakenly thought to be a disease of younger adults. It is, in fact, a disease of older people, with a median age at presentation of 64 years.[68] The misconception has arisen because older people are often not referred for treatment at tertiary referral centers and because it may not necessarily be appropriate to treat an elderly person who has several co-morbid conditions with intensive combination chemotherapy.

CLONAL EVOLUTION

The finding of chromosome abnormalities in leukemic myeloblasts originally suggested that all the leukemic cells within a given patient are derived from a single abnormal progenitor cell. The clonal nature of AML was subsequently established in Fialkow's observations based on X chromosome inactivation.[71] Studies in younger women with AML who were heterozygous for the glucose-6-phosphate dehydrogenase (G6PD) isoenzyme showed that in a proportion in which both A- and B-types G6PD were found in the skin, only one or the other isoenzyme was present in the leukemic cells. Moreover, the red blood cells from these patients had the double-enzyme phenotype, suggesting that they and their precursors must have arisen from normal hematopoietic progenitor cells.[72-75] It has therefore been concluded that in some patients with AML, the leukemia is expressed in cells with differentiative expression restricted to the granulocyte series. In contrast, in some older patients, it appears that AML involves a multipotent progenitor that can give rise to both red blood cells and granulocytes,[76-78] and again this has been confirmed with G6PD studies. AML is thus heterogeneous in that stem-cells with different differentiative expression are involved in different individuals.

G6PD studies also suggest that there are two patterns of remission in AML. In some patients, the bone marrow returns to the double-enzyme phenotype, suggesting that normal progenitor cells were suppressed while leukemia was present. In contrast, some patients have been described as being in "clonal remission," that is, normal bone marrow morphologic features and cytogenetics but with a single-enzyme G6PD phenotype in granulocytic cells.[79-81] These findings are in keeping with the theory of multistep pathogenesis for AML; in patients with clonal remission, the cytogenetics are normal, implying that the chromosome abnormality is not essential for the clonal proliferation of bone marrow stem-cells, although it may be necessary for leukemia to become clinically manifest. It has therefore been suggested that at least two steps are involved, the first leading to proliferation of a clone of abnormal hematopoietic progenitor cells and the second inducing a chromosome change in one or more descendents of those progenitor cells. After further reports of clonal hematopoiesis in patients in first complete remission (CR), it has been documented that clonal remissions in AML are, in fact, rare.[82-84] The discrepancy in incidence (26% in the earlier studies compared with 1% more recently) can probably be explained largely by differences between the populations studied, differences in the methods, and differences in the choice of control subjects. The true significance of clonal remission for patients with AML remains to be determined.

The limitation of G6PD studies is that only women are heterozygous for G6PD. Other approaches have therefore been developed, for example, the use of X chromosome–linked DNA polymorphisms, which can be assessed with great accuracy by polymerase chain reaction (PCR)–based methods. FISH analysis, which can detect chromosome abnormalities in nondividing cells, has also been used.

CELL GROWTH AND PROLIFERATION

Contrary to the common assumption, leukemic blast cells do not proliferate particularly fast; in fact, their cell cycle is usually longer than that of normal hematopoietic cells.[85, 86] Correlations can be made, however, between treatment outcome and cell cycle times, patients with shorter cycling times tending to have a correspondingly shorter duration of remission.[87, 88]

Naturally occurring hematopoietic growth factors influence the proliferation of normal bone marrow progenitor cells. With the advent of "therapeutic" growth factors, there was concern about their theoretical potential for stimulation of myeloid blast cells[89-90] because these cells express both low- and high-affinity receptors for granulocyte colony-stimulating factor (G-CSF).[91] This has proved not to be a problem in practice (see the later section on Hematopoietic Growth Factors).

CYTOGENETICS AND PATHOPHYSIOLOGY AT THE MOLECULAR LEVEL

The cytogenetic changes in AML are of two main types, those involving activation of a proto-oncogene and those associated with disruption or lack of expression of a growth-suppressing or differentiation-inducing gene. Activation of one of the three *ras* genes (proteins involved in signal transduction) has been described in 10% to 30% of patients with AML.[92, 93] Correlations have also been described between outcome and expression of proliferation-associated proto-oncogenes such as c-*myc* and c-*myb*,[94] *BCL2*,[95] and the thrombopoietin ligand c-*mpl*,[96] *increased* expression of all of these being associated with a worse prognosis.

Conversely, *decreased* expression of tumor suppressor genes such as *TP53*[97, 98] or the retinoblastoma gene *(RB)*[99, 100] correlates with a worse outcome. These observations may have potential for therapeutic interventions (see the later section on Altering *BCL2* Expression).

MAKING THE DIAGNOSIS

Clinical Presentation

Most people with AML consult their family physician in the first instance because of symptoms associated with bone marrow failure. Symptoms have not usually been present for more than a few weeks or perhaps a month or two. The clinical findings vary from person to person, but most patients are clinically anemic; there may be bruises and petechial hemorrhages as well as conjunctival hemorrhages.

Some patients with AML have lymphadenopathy; there may also be enlargement of the liver and/or spleen. In patients with AML subtypes M4 and M5, gum infiltration is not unusual at presentation, although skin infiltration, which is also characteristically associated with AML-M5, is more often seen at recurrence.

Patients in whom the peripheral blast count at presentation is above $100 \times 10^9/L$ are at risk for development of a life-threatening clinical situation as the result of leukostasis (see Chapter 15) whereby the small vessels in the lung and the brain can thrombose because of a "sludging" phenomenon. The pathologic process shows a combination of microinfarction and hemorrhage. Patients present with shortness of breath and symptoms and signs of hypoxia, with obvious infiltrates on the chest radiograph that may appear quite white. When this process involves the cerebral vasculature, drowsiness is usually followed by loss of consciousness. The situation can be reversed. In the United Kingdom, immediate leukapheresis is favored; in the United States, hydroxyurea is usually given orally together with hydration to expand the extracellular volume. Cranial irradiation may also be useful. The prognosis is generally poor because a high circulating blast count is also itself associated with a worse prognosis.

Laboratory Investigations

Morphology

The diagnosis of acute leukemia is often suspected on the basis of the history, the clinical findings, and the appearance of the peripheral blood film. However, the definitive diagnosis requires a bone marrow aspiration (and trephine biopsy if preferred) to be performed (Table 21-1). The presence of Auer rods (in approximately 50% of patients with AML) is confirmatory, but more precise cytochemical stains are also helpful (see Chapter 11).

Until recently, AML was subclassified according to the French-American-British classification.[101] A new World Health Organization classification[102] for hematologic malignant neoplasms has now been proposed encompassing both myeloid and lymphoid neoplasms (see Chapter 11). The new classification combines morphology, immunophenotype, cytogenetic subtype, and clinical features to define distinct disease entities. Within the category of AML, four main groups are recognized:

1. AML with recurrent cytogenetic translocation.

TABLE 21–1. Mandatory Investigations at Time of Diagnosis

Complete blood count and differential	1
Bone marrow aspirate ± trephine biopsy	1
Coagulation studies	2
Electrolytes and urea	2
Liver function tests	2
Urate	2
Blood cultures (if appropriate)	2
Immunophenotyping	3
Karyotyping	2

1, mandatory for making the diagnosis; 2, required for management; 3, strictly speaking, not mandatory.

2. AML with MDS-related features.
3. Therapy-related AML and MDS.
4. AML not otherwise specified.

The other major change proposed is that 20% blast cells be adopted as the level of infiltration to define the diagnosis, whereas AML was defined by the presence of 30% myeloid blast cells in the bone marrow according to the French-American-British standard. The reason for the change is the recognition that patients with 20% to 30% blasts (previously classified as refractory anemia with excess blasts in transformation [RAEB-t]) have a prognosis similar to that of patients with more than 30% blasts. Thus, most patients in this situation would be started on treatment.

Immunocytochemistry

In general, the diagnosis of AML can be made on the basis of morphologic features alone. However, when the diagnosis is unclear (e.g., poorly differentiated AML), immunophenotyping can be helpful. In addition, the category AML-M0 can be diagnosed with certainty only by reactivity with monoclonal antibodies against myeloid-associated antigens and the absence of lymphoid antigen expression.[103] Such leukemias often express early hematopoietic progenitor cell antigens and are associated with a poor prognosis.[104]

Myeloid blast cells can also express lymphoid-associated antigens; for example, CD7 has been found in approximately 10% of patients with AML, but the significance of this is uncertain.[104] True biphenotypic acute leukemia has a poor prognosis. The natural killer (NK) cell–associated antigen CD56 has also been described in patients with AML, particularly those with AML subtypes M4 and M5.[105] The diagnosis of acute megakaryoblastic leukemia (AML-M7) is often based on immunophenotypic evidence of platelet-associated glycoproteins or the presence of factor VIII.[106, 107]

Cytogenetics

It is clear that in most patients with AML, the illness is associated with a chromosome abnormality. As new methods are developed, such changes are being described with greater definition; for example, conventional G-banding may not pick up changes demonstrable by FISH or by the more recent multiplex-FISH or spectral karyotyping technologies (see Chapter 5). Many of the cytogenetic changes in AML are closely associated with clinical findings and with a specific French-American-British subtype (see Chapter 5); some examples are discussed briefly here.

The reciprocal translocation t(15;17)(q22;q21) is pathognomonic for acute promyelocytic leukemia (AML-M3)[108]; molecular genetic studies have shown that the breakpoint on chromosome 17 occurs in the gene encoding the retinoic acid receptor[109] (see later and Chapters 5 and 23). Thirty percent of patients with AML have abnormalities of chromosome 8, the two most frequently seen being trisomy 8 and a translocation between chromosomes 8 and 21, that is, t(8;21)(q22;q22).[110] The translocation is typically associated with AML-M2 and confers a more favorable prognosis.[110]

Cytogenetic changes have been shown to correlate with prognosis (see "Prognostic Factors"), but they also afford the opportunity, by use of PCR analysis, to assess the efficacy of a treatment at the molecular level in terms of the presence or absence of morphologically undetectable, residual leukemic blast cells. So far, this method has been most useful in monitoring for the t(15; 17) in AML-M3, and treatment decisions have been based on such PCR results[111] (see Chapter 23). The future use of real-time (i.e., *quantitative*) PCR may better define which patients are at high risk for recurrence.

TREATMENT

General Aspects

The general management of the patient with leukemia is discussed in detail in Chapter 13, but certain aspects are mentioned here briefly. Once a bone marrow examination has been performed and the diagnosis confirmed, it is important to explain its implications to the person who is ill and to the person's family. People differ in the degree to which they wish to be informed of the chances of success or failure. Cultural, religious, and geographic differences relating to traditions and social mores will influence the level of explanation that is appropriate for each individual. The treatment and its side effects and risks need to be discussed together with the expectation of success. The likelihood of recurrence needs to be mentioned, both to the person and to the family. The need for such conversations continues as the situation changes, particularly if the initial treatment is failing and progressively more experimental alternatives are being considered. It is also important to be clear about the risks of infection and bleeding when the blood count is low, especially at times when the person may be at home between cycles of treatment, emphasizing the need to contact the hospital immediately in case of fever, other signs of infection, or bleeding.

Before specific treatment is started, blood and platelets may need to be given on the basis of the hematologic indices. If there are signs of infection, intravenous antibiotics should be started empirically after appropriate investigations. The treatment of infection in the immunocompromised patient is discussed fully in Chapter 14.

Renal and hepatic function need to be assessed, adequate hydration should be achieved, and the xanthine oxidase inhibitor allopurinol should be started even in the absence of hyperuricemia. The drug can be discontinued when leukemic blast cells have been cleared from the peripheral blood. Coagulation needs to be monitored carefully, especially if disseminated intravascular coagulation is present, suspected, or anticipated (in the case of patients with AML-M3, see later and Chapters 15 and 23).

The use of indwelling right atrial catheters has radically altered the management of patients with acute leukemia. Such a line should be inserted under local or general anesthetic as soon as possible to provide access for taking blood, for the administration of chemotherapy and intravenous antibiotics, and for transfusion of red blood cells and platelets. Properly placed right atrial catheters also allow easy measurement of the central venous pressure when it is required.

Side Effects

The most significant side effect of the treatment is myelosuppression, which is hardly surprising because the desired objective is to achieve temporary bone marrow aplasia. The attendant risks of potentially fatal infection and hemorrhage together with ways of preventing them are reviewed in Chapters 14 and 15, respectively.

The distressing nature of at least some of the side effects may be minimized if they are fully explained beforehand. Virtually all patients will have complete but reversible alopecia. Gastrointestinal tract toxicity varies in degree but is often manifest by nausea and vomiting. The availability of modern antiemetics has improved things considerably. The administration of cytosine arabinoside, particularly by continuous intravenous infusion and at high doses, may be associated with a syndrome of abdominal pain and distention with virtual absence of bowel sounds. A plain abdominal radiograph will show dilated loops of bowel, often with fluid levels; the symptoms usually resolve spontaneously within a few days.

High-dose ara-C (see later) is associated with a specific pattern of clinical toxicity.[112-115] Severe conjunctivitis can occur despite the use of prophylactic prednisolone eye drops, and a blistering erythematous rash, most frequently on the hands and feet, can develop; both respond to steroids. The most serious toxicity is a cerebellar ataxia that is not always reversible and is generally first manifest as nystagmus. The incidence of cerebellar toxicity is lower with somewhat lower doses (i.e., with 1 or 2 g/m² rather than 3 g/m²). If treatment is stopped when nystagmus first becomes apparent, the development of further symptoms may be prevented. Cerebellar toxicity is more likely in patients with impaired renal function.

Mucositis, manifest most frequently as mouth ulcers, is particularly associated with anthracycline treatment, being more common with doxorubicin. Antiseptic mouthwashes and the routine, prophylactic use of antifungal preparations are essential to prevent oral candidiasis. Patients specifically need to be told to continue mouth care when they go home between cycles of treatment. Impairment of liver function is rarely a major clinical problem, although transient elevations in the levels of transaminases are not infrequently seen.

Therapeutic Strategy

Most younger patients with AML are treated with curative intent. However, this is predominantly a disease of older people, and the decision to give intensive chemotherapy will depend on the person's general state of health, a history of previous illness, concurrent illnesses, the presence or absence of a preceding myelodysplastic phase, and the person's wishes. It needs to be established from the outset whether treatment is being given in the hope of cure or whether palliative therapy is being given in the form of antibiotics, blood, and platelet transfusions; in palliative care, the aim is to keep the person as well as possible for as long as possible.

The aim of treatment may change over time; for example, at first recurrence, a treatment will be given with the aim of achieving second remission to proceed to an allograft or HDT with autologous PBPC. If it becomes apparent that this and later another experimental option have failed, the person's (and the physician's) aims will alter, as will their priorities.

The strong associations between cytogenetic subtype and prognosis have been found to correlate with response to treatment, duration of remission, and survival. They hold true for conventional chemotherapy,[116-118] high-dose ara-C–containing treatment,[119] high-dose treatment supported by autologous hematopoietic progenitor cells,[118, 120, 121] and allogeneic transplantation.[122, 123] Thus, modern treatment programs are increasingly taking cytogenetic subtype into account in allocating treatment. For example, the current Medical Research Council (MRC) study (AML 12) in the United Kingdom for younger patients with AML is based on such a "risk" stratification (see "Prognostic Factors" and Chapter 22).

Treatment of AML has traditionally been divided into two parts, that given to return the morphologic bone marrow features to normal (remission induction therapy) and that given once remission has been achieved (consolidation or postremission therapy). CR is defined morphologically as the situation when there are normal numbers of red blood cells, neutrophils, and platelets in the blood; less than 5% blast cells in the marrow; and normal maturation of all bone marrow elements. These features should be present for at least 4 weeks.[124] It is important to be aware of the limitations of the definition.

It does not necessarily imply absence of leukemia for the following reasons:

1. There are situations in which all the semantic criteria are fulfilled but the "less than 5%" myeloblasts are morphologically indistinguishable from those seen at presentation.

2. It may be impossible to differentiate between leukemic myeloblasts and normal, "recovery" myeloid blast cells.

3. The definition does not take into account changes at the cytogenetic level or molecular parameters.

Nonetheless, this is the definition that is conventionally used for reporting the results of clinical trials, and it is reasonably adequate for practical purposes. Certainly, unless CR can be achieved, long-term survival is impossible.

The rationale for giving any treatment beyond CR is based on the mathematical calculation that at the time of morphologic CR, up to 10^9 morphologically undetectable leukemic blast cells may still be present.[125] The theoretical calculation is confirmed by the reality of the situation in which a person has received one or two cycles of chemotherapy and CR has been achieved, but it is obvious that to give any further treatment would incur too great a risk of life-threatening toxicity. Almost always, the patient will develop recurrent leukemia.

REMISSION INDUCTION THERAPY

The aim of the treatment is to reduce the malignant clone sufficiently to allow restoration of normal hematopoiesis. To this end, the outcome of a cycle of treatment is assessed at the time at which normal hematopoiesis is expected to have recovered. It is not the purpose of this chapter to provide a detailed historical review of the development of chemotherapy for AML. However, the interested reader is referred to the original texts describing the early studies with 6-mercaptopurine and methotrexate, which showed that it was possible, sometimes, to return the bone marrow temporarily to normal.[126-128] The subsequent development of cytosine arabinoside (ara-C) resulted in CR rates of between 9% and 33%[129-135] (Table 21-2). Although such remissions were hardly ever more than temporary, a small number of patients were cured. The introduction of the anthracycline antibiotics (daunorubicin or doxorubicin given at daily doses of 45 mg/m^2 or 25 mg/m^2, respectively, usually for 3 days) altered the whole perspective[136-143] (Table 21-3). When

TABLE 21–2. Induction of Remission: Cytosine Arabinoside—Single-Agent Activity

Schedule	Dose (mg/m²/day)	Number of Days	CR Rate (%)	References
IV bolus injection	30–450	Maximum not stated	35/169 (21)	131–134
IV infusion (4–12 hr)	30–150	To aplasia	12/53 (23)	129, 131–134
IV infusion (24 hr)	10–30	To aplasia	4/45 (9)	133
	200	5	56/175 (33)	130, 131, 135
	400	2	16/67 (24)	135

CR, complete remission; IV, intravenous.

TABLE 21–3. Induction of Remission: Anthracyclines—Single-Agent Activity

Drug	Dose (mg/m²/day)	Number of Days	CR Rate (%)	References
DNR	70	To aplasia	18/71 (25)	136
DNR	60	× 1 or 2 weeks	25/137 (18)	137
DNR	60–80	3–7	200/572 (35)	137–140
ADR	10	4	9/31 (29)	141
	20–35	2–3	1/14 (7)	142
	75	1	10/55 (18)	143

ADR, doxorubicin (Adriamycin); CR, complete remission; DNR daunorubicin.

ara-C was combined with 6-thioguanine[144] and later with daunorubicin,[145] CR could be achieved in up to 50% of patients. When this treatment was followed by relatively (by today's standards) mild consolidation and then prolonged maintenance therapy, cure became a rare but realistic possibility.

In reading the original literature (which it is worth doing at least to appreciate how much is now taken for granted), the degree to which concurrent improvements in the management of infection and prevention of bleeding have made it possible to administer doses of drugs that regularly render the bone marrow hypoplastic becomes apparent. The suggestion of synergy between daunorubicin and ara-C, which was demonstrated in the experimental mouse model L1210 leukemia,[146] led to formal clinical evaluation of the combination. The promising early results (with use of ara-C at a dose of 100 mg/m²/day for 7 days) were subsequently confirmed, leading to the classic '3 + 7' regimen, which became the most widely used remission induction regimen in the world and remained so for about 20 years. Review of the published literature shows an overall CR rate of 63% for younger patients (younger than 60 years).[147-154]

After the development of the '3 + 7' regimen, a series of studies was conducted to evaluate the combination of daunorubicin, ara-C, and 6-thioguanine (DAT).[155-167] In virtually all of them, ara-C was administered at a daily dose of 200 mg/m² (given as 100 mg/m² twice daily) by intravenous injection for 5 or 7 days. Thus, the daily dose was, in fact, twice the amount given in the '3 + 7' regimen; however, a study comparing the two regimens showed no difference in response rates. The CR rates for variations on a theme of DAT vary between 50% and 85%, but the overall CR rate with DAT (or TAD) is again approximately 60%, that is, identical to that achieved with the '3 + 7' regimen.[155-167]

The past 30 years have seen an intensification of treatment (permitted by improved supportive care), which has been paralleled by fundamental improvements in survival. The results from St. Bartholomew's Hospital in London show an increase in the proportion of people cured over time as the treatment has been intensified (Fig. 21–1). A similar analysis from Hôtel-Dieu in Paris shows improvements in both CR rate and 5-year overall survival over time.[168] A retrospective analysis based on data from 1414 patients treated according to six Eastern Cooperative Oncology Group (ECOG) protocols between 1976 and 1994 similarly shows disease-free survival to have improved as the intensity of therapy has in-

creased.[169] More, therefore, appears to be somewhat better.

Alternatives to the classic anthracyclines have since been developed and tested, originally in phase II studies in patients with recurrent or refractory AML and then in randomized studies comparing combinations of ara-C and each of these with standard DAT or '3 + 7' regimens in newly diagnosed patients. In general, equivalent results for the test combination have been observed, although there are differences in clinical toxicity. Doxorubicin (Adriamycin) was introduced in an attempt to find a less toxic analogue to daunorubicin and appears to be equivalent in efficacy, but it is associated with a greater tendency to cause mucositis and gastrointestinal tract toxicity. The anthraquinone derivative mitoxantrone has also been extensively evaluated in combination with ara-C and again is probably equivalent in efficacy to the anthracyclines.[170-176] Mitoxantrone appears to be particularly useful in older patients because it causes less mucositis and less cardiotoxicity than doxorubicin does.[174-176]

With regard to the synthetic anthracycline analogue idarubicin, the theoretical advantages are more rapid cellular uptake, more potent induction of DNA single-stranded breaks, longer plasma half-life, and increased efficacy in terms of in vitro cell kill in leukemic blast cells that express the multidrug resistance phenotype (in comparison to conventional anthracyclines).[177] Three randomized studies have compared the efficacy of idarubicin with that of daunorubicin given to patients with newly diagnosed AML in conjunction with ara-C.[178-180] All three studies show a higher CR rate in patients receiving

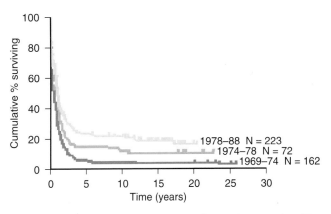

FIGURE 21–1. Overall survival of patients with AML (younger than 60 years) by era.

idarubicin; in two of the studies, this difference was statistically significant.[178, 179] However, the CR rate for patients who received the daunorubicin-containing regimen was lower than generally reported. Moreover, the duration of myelosuppression in patients receiving the idarubicin combination was longer, suggesting that the doses of the two anthracyclines being compared may not have been biologically equivalent. Studies comparing mitoxantrone with daunorubicin[175] and mitoxantrone versus idarubicin versus daunorubicin,[176] respectively, in older patients with AML have failed to show an advantage for either of the newer drugs. Thus, it is not clear that any one anthracycline is superior to any other; idarubicin is probably the one most used at present.

There was originally much excitement about the use of high-dose ara-C (1 to 3 g/m^2) in patients with recurrent, refractory, and secondary AML.[112, 113, 115, 181, 182] In view of these promising early results, there was hope that the use of high-dose ara-C might improve CR rates overall. However, this has not been the case; its use with the '3 + 7' regimen was associated with an 89% CR rate in one study, but this single center result[183] could not be confirmed in a cooperative group study.[184] Furthermore, high-dose ara-C was associated with considerable morbidity and mortality in older patients.

Thus, high-dose ara-C does not increase the proportion of patients entering CR when it is given as part of remission induction therapy to newly diagnosed patients. However, there is a tantalizing report from Australia,[185] the results of which have held up with longer follow-up.[186] Newly diagnosed, younger patients were randomized to receive either high-dose ara-C on alternate days for eight doses, with daunorubicin for 3 days and etoposide for 7 days, or standard dose ara-C by continuous intravenous infusion for 7 days, with daunorubicin and etoposide at the same dose and schedule. All patients received the same postremission therapy comprising 5 days of ara-C, 2 days of daunorubicin, and 5 days of etoposide for two cycles. At the time of publication, with a median follow-up of 4.5 years, the CR rate was the same for the two dose levels of ara-C. However, the median remission duration was nearly 4 years for the high-dose ara-C–containing regimen compared with 1 year for conventional-dose ara-C, and the estimated percentage of patients recurrence free at 5 years was 49% and 24%, respectively. There was no difference in overall survival.

Studies from the M.D. Anderson Cancer Center have focused on the use of high-dose ara-C in conjunction with fludarabine. Early studies with fludarabine in patients with acute leukemia used a high, single dose that resulted in prohibitive central nervous system (CNS) toxicity, but use of the drug in divided doses has circumvented this problem. Fludarabine, when it is given 4 hours before ara-C, can potentiate the accumulation of arabinoside cytosine triphosphate (ara-CTP).[187] Several studies have therefore been conducted using this combination with promising results,[187a] especially in patients with AML developing on a background of MDS.[188] The combination of fludarabine and ara-C with G-CSF has since been evaluated, with unexpectedly high response rates in patients with MDS and MDS/AML.[189] Fludarabine-containing remission induction therapy has also been used in Italy in similar patients and in refractory AML, with a response rate of 59% overall,[190] and with G-CSF in patients with AML who had recurrent leukemia after HDT with autologous hematopoietic progenitor cell support, a 50% CR rate being observed.[191] Thus, fludarabine does have activity as part of remission induction or consolidation therapy, but it may impair mobilization and collection of PBPC subsequently.[192]

Etoposide has also been evaluated in AML[193]; the rationale for its use comes from early in vitro studies that showed synergy with ara-C in L1210 cells.[194] When etoposide was added to "conventional" '3 + 7' remission induction therapy in newly diagnosed patients, in a randomized study, there was no difference in CR rate between the two regimens, but duration of remission was significantly longer in the patients who had received etoposide.[195] Similarly, one of the questions posed in the MRC AML 10 trial was whether the etoposide-containing regimen ADE (daunorubicin, ara-C, and etoposide) is superior to conventional DAT as remission induction; there was no difference in CR rate in patients aged up to 55 years.[165]

Thus, although there is no consensus as to what constitutes the *best* remission induction therapy, the combination of idarubicin, ara-C, and etoposide (ICE) is currently much used. CR rates on the order of 80% are achieved in younger patients.[195, 196]

Evaluation of Response

Response has traditionally been assessed by morphologic examination of a bone marrow aspirate, although some favor a trephine biopsy. Response needs to be evaluated after the first cycle of treatment has been given. The exact timing depends to some extent on local practice and on the intensity of the protocol being followed. At St. Bartholomew's Hospital, in the context of chemotherapy comprising idarubicin, ara-C, and etoposide[196] bone marrow aspiration is performed on day 21. If it is hypocellular with no leukemia, the next cycle is delayed until it is safe to give it, that is, when the neutrophil count is $1.0 \times 10^9/L$ and the platelet count is $100 \times 10^9/L$. On attainment of these counts, another bone marrow aspiration is performed (it is hoped to document CR) before proceeding to the second cycle, provided that the patient's general state of health allows it. If, on the other hand, the marrow is hypercellular with substantial amounts of leukemia still present (e.g., more than 30% blasts), the second cycle is given immediately without waiting for the counts to recover (because they will not). If CR has not been achieved with two cycles, the treatment is deemed to have failed and should be changed.

In patients known to have a cytogenetic abnormality, this serves as a further indication of disease activity if it persists. Various degrees of sophistication have been invoked in assessing cytogenetic response; PCR and reverse transcriptase–PCR analyses in particular are increasingly being used. Currently, with the advent of real-time or quantitative PCR, more precise measurement of the amount of residual disease will allow a greater degree of definition (see Chapter 12). Such studies are still experimental, but they may help to establish a biologic (rather than empirical) basis on which to formulate therapeutic decisions.

POSTREMISSION THERAPY

Because there is still morphologically undetectable leukemia present at the point of CR, it is generally accepted that some form of postremission therapy is required to prevent otherwise virtually inevitable recurrence. Two studies confirmed this a long time ago. Patients in first remission of AML were randomized to receive low doses of ara-C and 6-thioguanine as maintenance or no further treatment.[197, 198] In both studies, there was a significant advantage in remission duration and survival in favor of the patients in whom treatment was continued. Thus, even with relatively low dose maintenance therapy, some treatment is better than none. However, prolonged maintenance therapy (for 3 years) was not superior to an 8-month period of treatment.[152]

There is much debate and controversy about what constitutes the optimal postremission treatment. The following are possibilities:

- Conventional consolidation chemotherapy—a regimen the same as or different from that used to induce CR.
- Chemotherapy as described before, followed by maintenance therapy, which is defined as treatment that is less myelosuppressive than that administered during remission induction and given for a prolonged period.
- A high-dose ara-C–containing regimen.
- HDT with autologous hematopoietic progenitor cell support.
- Allogeneic transplantation.

In the early days of chemotherapy for AML, most patients received consolidation therapy that was less intensive than that given to induce remission. (It can be argued that this is illogical if one accepts that at the point of CR, there is still a substantial amount of leukemia present.) Such treatment was often followed by mildly myelosuppressive maintenance therapy. With this approach, 10% to 15% of patients in whom CR was achieved were cured.[199-202] Subsequently, most younger adults with AML were treated with more concentrated, short-term treatment without maintenance, with some improvement in

overall survival; 20% to 25% of patients in whom CR was achieved survived long term (see Fig. 21-1). Currently, most younger patients receive consolidation therapy comprising a high-dose ara-C–containing regimen (with perhaps further treatment afterward).

High-dose Ara-C

When given at conventional doses, ara-C is a cell cycle-specific drug that exerts its cytotoxic effects predominantly in S phase, functioning as an antimetabolite. At high doses (1 to 3 g/m²), it is thought to result in higher levels of ara-CTP, thus increasing inhibition of DNA synthesis.[203-205] At such doses, the drug is also thought to saturate deaminating enzymes, thus increasing entry of drug into cells.

Pharmacokinetic and intracellular studies suggest that the dose originally proposed, 3 g/m², may in fact not be necessary and that 1 g/m² or even 0.5 g/m² may be as effective.[206] On this basis, there has been a trend toward reducing individual doses from 3 g/m² to 1 g/m² with the drug being given as an infusion during 3 hours instead of 1 hour.

Several studies have now been conducted (in younger patients) with use of high-dose ara-C alone or in combination as postremission treatment. Between 30% and 40% of patients remained disease free at 4 years[184, 207-214] (Table 21-4).

Two randomized group studies in the United States have compared high-dose ara-C (3 g/m²) with lower doses of ara-C[211] or maintenance therapy.[212] In the Cancer and Leukemia Group B (CALGB) study, a conventional '3 + 7' remission induction regimen was followed by randomization to four cycles of ara-C given alone at one of three dose levels. This study is unusual in that generally speaking, when ara-C is used at standard doses (i.e., 100 or 200 mg/m²/day), it is given in combination with an anthracycline. The randomization was to high-dose ara-C (3 g/m² given during 3 hours × 6 doses), an intermediate dose (400 mg/m²/day for 5 days), or a standard dose (100 mg/m²/day for 5 days); both the intermediate and standard doses were given by continuous intravenous infusion. At the time of publication, with a median follow-up of 4.3 years in patients younger than 60 years, the probability of remaining in remission at 4 years was 44%,

TABLE 21-4. High-Dose Ara-C as Postremission Therapy

Study	No. of Patients	Median Age	Remission Induction Therapy	CR Rate (%)	Postremission Therapy	Median Duration (months) of CR	Patients in CR at 5 years (%)	Treatment-Related Deaths (%)	References
Open phase II studies	87	38	N/ST	N/ST	HD ara-C	47	49	5	207, 209
	56	47	DAT	63	HD ara-C + DNR	23	32 at 4 yr	6	
CALGB trial	187	43			HD ara-C	19	44	5	211
	206	49	3 + 7	64	ara-C:400 mg/m²	19	29	6	
	203	48			ara-C:100 mg/m²	13	24	1	
ECOG trial	99	44	DAT	68	HD ara-C + mAMSA	N/ST	28	12	212
	94	44	DAT	68	ara-C + 6-TG	N/ST	15	—	

DAT, daunorubicin + ara-C + 6-thioguanine; DNR, daunorubicin; HD, high-dose; mAMSA, amsacrine; N/ST, not stated; 6-TG, 6-thioguanine.

29%, and 24% at the three dose levels, respectively (P = .002).[211] The treatment-related mortality with high-dose ara-C was 5%.

Using a somewhat different trial design, the ECOG conducted a study in which patients with AML in first remission were randomized to receive either one cycle of high-dose ara-C (3 g/m² given during 1 hour twice daily for 6 days) in combination with amsacrine or 2 years of maintenance therapy. Again, at 4 years, for patients younger than 60 years, the probability of remaining free of disease was better for the patients receiving the high-dose ara-C–containing treatment (28%) than for patients receiving maintenance (15%; P = .05). However, the treatment-related mortality with the high-dose ara-C combination regimen was 12%.[212] A later study has also concluded that consolidation with a single course of high-dose ara-C is superior to one cycle of standard-dose ara-C given in conjunction with daunorubicin.[213]

In contrast, a Southwest Oncology Group study has investigated high-dose versus standard-dose ara-C given in conjunction with daunorubicin as both remission induction and consolidation therapy in patients with newly diagnosed AML. The high-dose ara-C–containing remission induction regimen was associated with greater toxicity, and there was no improvement in CR rate or survival. Patients in whom CR was achieved with standard-dose ara-C were then randomized to receive standard-dose or high-dose ara-C as consolidation; again, no advantage for the high-dose ara-C–containing treatment was demonstrated.[184]

As a result of the CALGB study in particular, many patients throughout the world now receive a high-dose ara-C–containing regimen as part of consolidation therapy. The data (in younger patients) confirm a dose-response relationship. High-dose ara-C is not recommended for older patients.

High-dose Therapy Supported by Autologous Hematopoietic Progenitor Cells

The limitations of allogeneic bone marrow transplantation (BMT) have led, particularly in Europe, to interest in exploiting the concept of giving more intensive postremission treatment but at the same time trying to avoid the mortality associated with graft-versus-host disease (GVHD). Thus, HDT supported by autologous bone marrow transplantation (ABMT) or, more recently, peripheral blood progenitor cells (PBPC) has now been formally evaluated in national and international comparative studies. Most asked the question, Does the *addition* of HDT plus ABMT confer additional benefit in patients who have already received intensive "conventional" consolidation therapy? For this reason, the majority of studies have compared the use of HDT plus ABMT with further conventional intensive consolidation, with the option of allogeneic transplantation in first remission if an HLA-identical sibling donor is available.

The overwhelming problem that has bedeviled all the trials has been the "attrition rate," that is, at best only half the number of patients entering CR actually proceed

to the HDT (or randomization to HDT) for the following reasons:

1. Patients (or their physicians) choose HDT because they inherently believe it to be "better," or they elect to stop treatment for fear of the potential morbidity and mortality associated with the more intensive treatment.

2. Patients are "too ill" after completing conventional consolidation, making consideration of HDT unrealistic within the time frame demanded by a protocol.

3. Even if patients are randomized to receive HDT, early recurrence precludes a substantial proportion from receiving it.

Therefore, those who reach the point of actually having the HDT are, inevitably, a highly selected group. There is, in addition, the statistical problem that event-free survival was (at least in the past) often calculated from the time of the HDT rather than from the time of CR. Also, it is only relatively recently that analyses have been performed on an intention-to-treat basis (i.e., the analysis includes all patients destined to have HDT, regardless of whether they ultimately received it). Finally, there is the philosophical dilemma that this treatment may be curing people who are already cured and is demonstrably failing to help some of those who "need it" most of all, that is, patients who develop recurrent AML too early to receive it.

High-dose Therapy plus Autologous Bone Marrow Transplantation in First Remission

In the *autologous* setting, an immunosuppressive effect is not required for engraftment (as is the case for allogeneic BMT); nonetheless, most centers have used cyclophosphamide and total-body irradiation (TBI) as the myeloablative regimen or busulfan and cyclophosphamide. Etoposide has also been substituted for cyclophosphamide, being given with TBI[215] or added to cyclophosphamide plus TBI.[216] It has also been combined with busulfan,[217, 218] but the regimen was associated with pulmonary hemorrhage, veno-occlusive disease, and reversible but severe skin toxicity.[219]

For individual studies, an advantage can be demonstrated for HDT with ABMT, disease-free survivals ranging from 34% to 70%[216-218, 220-226] (Table 21-5). In a collaborative study conducted at three European centers, patients younger than 50 years in whom a first remission was achieved with doxorubicin, ara-C, and 6-thioguanine received two further cycles of the same treatment as consolidation, followed by HDT comprising high-dose ara-C and TBI with ABMT. The marrow was not treated in vitro. With a median follow-up of now 4.5 years, the predicted actuarial survival for patients in whom CR was achieved is 58% at 3 years[226] (Fig. 21-2). Analysis by intention to treat shows both remission duration and survival to be significantly longer compared with the results for a historical control group who received identical remission induction and consolidation therapy but without HDT.

The use of high-dose ara-C–containing consolidation regimens has now, to some extent, abrogated such differences. Retrospective European Bone Marrow Transplant (EBMT) Registry data for more than 600 patients who

TABLE 21–5. HDT + ABMT in First Remission—Bone Marrow Not Treated In Vitro

Treatment	No. of Patients	Median Age (range)	Median Duration (months) of CR at Time of HDT (range)	Actuarial DFS (%)	Comments	Reference
Cy + TBI	55	37 (12–62)	5 (1–12)	51	HDT preceded by DAT	216
Bu + Cy	20	40 (16–53)	6 (2–13)	55	Various remission induction and various consolidation regimens	220
BACCT	76[a]	40 (16–57)	5 (1–12)	48, [a]67	HDT preceded by variable number of consolidation cycles	221
Cy + etoposide + TBI	60[b] 44[c]	39 (16–55)	5 (3–10)	49 61	HDT preceded by high-dose ara-C	218
Bu + Cy	51	36 (15–59)	8 (4–20)	70	Most patients received HDT "late" in first CR	222
Melphalan + TBI	74	31 (5–53)	4 (5 days–11 mo)	34	Patients who received at least 2 cycles of consolidation before HDT had the DFS	223
Cy + TBI	54	36 (15–54)	5 (2–17)	51	—	224
Cy + TBI	32	40 (16–58)	3–8	35	—	225
ara-C + TBI	106[b]	38 (15–49)	4 (3–6)	48	HDT preceded by 2 cycles of consolidation	226

ABMT, autologous bone marrow transplantation; BACCT = BCNU, adriamycin, cyclophosphamide, ara-C, 6-Ta; Bu, busulfan; CR, complete remisson; Cy, cyclophosphamide; DAT, daunorubicin + ara-C + 6-thioguanine; DFS, disease-free survival; HDT, high-dose therapy; TBI, total-body irradiation.
[a]26 patients had a double autograft.
[b]60 patients by 'intention to treat.'
[c]44 patients actually received HDT.

received high-dose treatment with ABMT in first remission show 46% disease-free survival at 2.5 years,[227] which is similar to the results now achievable with high-dose ara-C (Table 21–6; see also Table 21–4) and indeed to the results of allogeneic BMT[228–236] (see Table 21–6 and Chapter 20). An age-adapted postremission strategy has been used in Italy; patients in first CR received high-dose ara-C and TBI with ABMT if they were younger than 50 years or just intermediate-dose ara-C (1 g/m^2 twice daily for 6 days) if they were older. The long-term relapse-free survival rates for ABMT and ara-C were 53% and 54%, respectively.[237]

A number of randomized trials have now been performed to try to clarify the situation (summarized in Table 21–6). The design of these has usually been that younger patients who have an HLA-identical sibling donor are recommended to receive an allogeneic transplant, whereas the remainder are randomized between intensive consolidation chemotherapy and HDT. A study conducted

by the European Organization for Research and Treatment of Cancer (EORTC) and Gruppo Italiano Malattie Ematologiche Maligne dell'Adulto (GIMEMA) groups[238] demonstrated superiority for myeloablative therapy with ABMT or allograft over chemotherapy alone in terms of disease-free survival. However, overall survival was not significantly different in the three treatment arms because some patients who had recurrent leukemia after conventional chemotherapy were able to receive myeloablative therapy plus ABMT or an allograft in second remission. A further analysis of the data[239] compared outcome of patients who had all their treatment at a "transplant center" with outcome of patients treated at hospitals that gave only the remission induction and consolidation chemotherapy. No difference was found.

The Groupe Ouest Est Leucémies Aiguës Myéloblastique (GOELAM Group)[240] has conducted a prospective, randomized study to evaluate the three postremission treatment options, that is, allograft or HDT with ABMT and intensive consolidation chemotherapy. Patients who did not have a sibling donor received one consolidation cycle with a high-dose ara-C–containing regimen and were then randomly assigned to receive either a second cycle of intensive consolidation or the combination of busulfan and cyclophosphamide followed by ABMT. In contrast to the results of the EORTC/GIMEMA study, the type of postremission therapy had no significant impact on outcome, with no difference in 4-year disease-free survival or overall survival for the three groups. Similarly, there was no difference in outcome between ABMT and intensive chemotherapy. The reason for the discrepancy between this and the study described before probably relates to the use of more intensive (i.e., high-dose ara-C–containing) consolidation therapy as the control arm in the GOELAM study. A similar study in the United States comparing allogeneic BMT (in patients with an HLA-identical sibling donor) with ABMT or high-dose ara-C–containing consolidation therapy again showed no statisti-

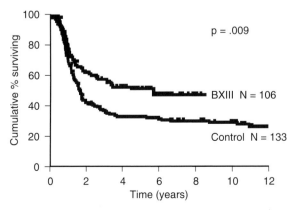

FIGURE 21–2. Survival by intention-to-treat analysis of 108 patients in whom complete remission was achieved versus a historical control group.

TABLE 21–6. Prospective Randomized Studies Comparing Chemotherapy, HDT + ABMT, and Allogeneic BMT as Consolidation of First Remission in AML

Treatment	No. of Patients	DFS (%)*	P Value	OS (%)*	P Value	Study Reference
Allogeneic BMT	168	55		59		EORTC/GIMEMA[238]
HDT+ABMT	128	48	NR†	56	NR	
CT	126	30		46		
Allogeneic BMT	67	44		53		GOELAM[240]
HDT+ABMT	67	44	NS	50		
CT	67	40		55		
Allogeneic BMT	113	43		46	.04§	U.S. Intergroup[241]
HDT+ABMT	116	35	NS	43	.05‖	
CT	117	35		52		
Allogeneic BMT	—	N/A		N/A		MRC AML 12[242]
HDT+ABMT	190	53	NS‡	57		
CT	191	40		45		

*Measured at 4 years.
†P value not stated, reported as significant.
‡No significant difference at 4 years, but significant difference in recurrence rate at 7 years.
§Comparison between allogeneic BMT and CT.
‖Comparison between HDT+ABMT and CT.
ABMT, autologous bone marrow transplantation; BMT, bone marrow transplantation; CT, chemotherapy; DFS, disease-free survival; HDT, high-dose therapy; N/A, not available; NR, not reported; NS, not significant; OS, overall survival.

cally significant difference of outcome for the three groups of patients (43%, 34%, and 34% actuarial disease-free survival at 4 years, respectively).[241]

In the MRC AML 10 study in the United Kingdom,[242] after three cycles of intensive chemotherapy, bone marrow was harvested from patients younger than 56 years in remission who lacked an HLA-matched sibling donor. These patients were then randomized to receive, after one more cycle of chemotherapy, no further treatment or HDT (cyclophosphamide and TBI) with ABMT; 381 patients were randomized (38% of those eligible). Of 190 patients allocated to HDT with ABMT, 126 patients actually received it. Outcome was then compared by intention-to-treat analysis. The number of recurrences was lower in the ABMT group than in the group assigned to no further treatment (64 of 190 [37%] versus 101 of 191 [58%]; P = .0007), resulting in superior disease-free survival at 7 years (53% versus 40%; P = .04). These results were consistent for all cytogenetic risk groups and age groups. There were (as would be expected) more treatment-related deaths in remission in the ABMT group than in the group receiving no further treatment. At 7 years, survival for the ABMT group was 57% (versus 45% for the group receiving no further treatment), although this was not statistically significant (P = .2).

Thus, in terms of *survival* (of patients in whom CR is achieved), high-dose ara-C–containing consolidation therapy is probably equivalent to HDT supported by ABMT or allogeneic BMT. In all of these studies, the results are confounded by the substantially higher treatment-related mortality of the allogeneic transplantation procedure and the appreciable although lower mortality associated with ABMT. Furthermore, there is the problem that one third of patients randomized to HDT do not actually receive the planned therapy, usually because of early recurrence.

In Vitro Treatment of Autologous Marrow

The use of autologous bone marrow is obviously associated with a potential risk of transferring morphologically undetectable leukemic blast cells within the stem-cell collection. Gene marking studies have confirmed that infusion of autologous marrow can contribute to recurrence.[243] This raises the question of the need for in vitro treatment of autologous hematopoietic progenitor cells.

Enthusiasm for in vitro treatment methods followed the original reports of use of the cyclophosphamide derivatives mafosfamide[227, 244] and 4-hydroperoxycyclophosphamide (4-HC).[245, 246] Unlike cyclophosphamide, these congeners have the advantage of not requiring oxidation by the hepatic P-450 system to become active, being activated in aqueous solution. The disadvantage is that they are also toxic to normal hematopoietic progenitor cells, the effect being dose dependent. Data from Hôpital St. Louis in Paris suggest that optimal antileukemic killing is achieved by adjusting the mafosfamide dose for each individual patient, depending on preliminary in vitro testing, the "correct" amount being that required to achieve 95% kill of normal colony-forming units–granulocyte-macrophage (CFU-GM).[247] The number of cells treated in vitro with mafosfamide and the intensity of purging have been shown to influence outcome. Patients in whom a higher stem-cell dose was submitted to in vitro treatment but who received a lower total number of cells (in terms of CFU-GM per kilogram) after mafosfamide had the lowest treatment-related mortality and a leukemia-free survival of 70% with an overall survival of 77% ± 7% at 10 years.[247] Monoclonal antibodies such as anti-CD15[248] and anti-CD33[249, 250] with complement as well as long-term marrow culture[251, 252] have also been used.

Debate continues as to the need for in vitro treatment at all because no definitive advantage has ever been demonstrated. Disease-free survivals ranging between 41% and 76% have been reported[227, 244, 246–252] for patients treated in first remission (Table 21–7), but a randomized comparison against untreated bone marrow or PBPC has never been conducted. The main problem associated with all of these methods is that blood count recovery,

TABLE 21–7. HDT + ABMT in First Remission—Bone Marrow Treated in Vitro

Treatment	No. of Patients	Median Age (range)	Median Duration (months) of CR at Time of HDT (range)	Actuarial DFS (%)	Reference
Cy + TBI	22	35 (17-50)	4 (2-6)	61	245
Bu + etoposide	32	39 (17-59)	3 (1.5-5.5)	76	217
Bu + Cy	39	36 (18-51)	2 (1.5-6)	54	241
Cy + TBI	64	36 (16-53)	5 (1.5-2 yr)	58	261
Various	24	45 (not stated)	8 (1-2 yr)	52	250
Bu + Cy	48	25 (4-56)	2.5 (1.5-15)	41	246

ABMT, autologous bone marrow transplantation; Bu, busulfan; CR, complete remission; Cy, cyclophosphamide; DFS, disease-free survival; HDT, high-dose therapy; TBI, total-body irradiation.

particularly that of platelets, is slow, superimposed on the fact that hematologic recovery after ABMT in patients with AML is slower than that for other hematologic malignant neoplasms.

The Use of Autologous Peripheral Blood Progenitor Cells

The feasibility of mobilizing autologous PBPC in newly diagnosed patients with AML has been evaluated in several studies in Europe (Table 21-8). In the majority of patients, it is possible to collect sufficient numbers of cells. The results thus far are encouraging, with blood count recovery being considerably faster than that normally seen with ABMT.[196, 253-257] There is no clear indication for the use of G-CSF after reinfusion of PBPC.[258] The number of CD34+ cells/kg correlates with CFU-GM/kg, and most centers now use the number of CD34+ cells as the main criterion for whether a collection is considered adequate.

Concern had been expressed that the use of PBPC instead of autologous marrow might be associated with earlier recurrence,[259, 260] although it has also been argued that PBPC collections might contain *fewer* leukemic blast cells. A matched-pair analysis comparing outcome of patients reported to the EBMT Registry who received HDT with PBPC with twice that number who received HDT supported by ABMT shows leukemia-free survival and recurrence rate at 2 years to be the same for the two groups.[261]

Because the use of PBPC is associated with faster hematologic recovery, it results in shorter hospital admissions, with obvious advantages in both human and economic terms. Furthermore, faster neutrophil recovery makes such a treatment safer and therefore perhaps applicable to somewhat older patients. PBPC do therefore appear to be preferable to autologous marrow.

Allogeneic Bone Marrow Transplantation

Allogeneic BMT is discussed earlier in the context of the major comparative studies of postremission therapy (see also Table 21-6) and further described in Chapter 20. The use of sibling allografting (as reported to the EBMT Registry) is increasing in parallel with an increase in matched unrelated donor transplantations[262] (see Chapter 20).

HLA–Identical Sibling Transplantation in First Remission

Outcome clearly relates to the point at which the transplantation is carried out, the patient's age, and the cytogenetic subtype. For patients receiving an HLA–identical sibling allograft in first remission, there is a 52% to 58%[263, 264] likelihood of leukemia-free survival. The treatment-related mortality predominantly relates to death from infection (especially cytomegalovirus), acute and chronic GVHD, and veno-occlusive disease of the liver. The probability for development of GVHD increases with increasing age. Because GVHD is mediated by donor T lymphocytes, T-cell depletion, popular 15 years ago, was a logical step. However, although the incidence of GVHD

TABLE 21–8. HDT + PBPC in First Remission

Treatment	No. of Patients	Median Age (range)	Median Duration (months) of CR at Time of HDT (range)	Actuarial DFS (%)	Comment	Reference
Bu + Cy	24	40 (14-62)	4 (2-5)	35	3 + 7 as consolidation before HDT	256
Cy + TBI	20	41 (5-48)	4 (2-12)	35	DNR + ara-C as consolidation before HDT	245
Cy + TBI	59	45 (18-64)	3 (1.5-7)	42	High-dose ara-C + MTR before HDT	255
Cy + etoposide + TBI	38	46 (not stated)	4 (2-12)	81	IL-2 after HDT	218
ara-C + TBI	47	45 (15-60)	3 (1-4)	48	ICE × 2 as consolidation before HDT	196

Bu, busulfan; CR, complete remission; Cy, cyclophosphamide; DFS, disease-free survival; DNR, daunorubicin; HDT, high-dose therapy; ICE, idarubicin, ara-C, etoposide; IL-2, interleukin-2; MTR, mitoxantrone; PBPC, peripheral blood progenitor cells; TBI, total-body irradiation.

was significantly reduced, the incidence of graft rejection and the probability of recurrent leukemia were substantially increased. Attention has therefore focused on selectively removing *mature* T cells while retaining those that mediate the graft-versus-leukemia effect, with some measure of success. CD6 depletion has been used at the Dana Farber Cancer Institute, resulting in only a 5% transplantation-related mortality with a disease-free survival of 63% at 4 years and an overall survival of 71%.[265] The risk for recurrence was high (25%), but the incidence of GVHD was only 15%. A similar study from Memorial Sloan-Kettering Cancer Center has shown a disease-free survival of 77% at 4 years and no episodes of grade II to grade IV GVHD.[266]

Outcome relates to age, disease status, and cytogenetic subtype, patients with "favorable" cytogenetics having a better prognosis. In a retrospective EBMT study, 500 patients who received an allogeneic BMT in first remission were retrospectively categorized according to cytogenetic risk group. Patients with good, standard, and poor cytogenetic subtypes had disease-free survivals of 67%, 57%, and 29%, respectively.[267] This study is somewhat difficult to interpret, however, because patients with a t(15;17) and hyperdiploid karyotypes were included in the standard group.

The question remains as to *which* younger patients who have an HLA sibling donor should receive an allogeneic transplant in first remission. When randomized studies have been conducted,[238-242] the recurrence rate is certainly lower than that for patients receiving combination chemotherapy or HDT supported by autologous hematopoietic progenitor cells. However, as mentioned before, the use of high-dose ara-C–containing consolidation regimens has, to some extent, abrogated any difference in *survival* between the three treatments in view of the still relatively high treatment-related mortality of an allograft.

Most people now agree that younger patients with a favorable karyotype should *not* have an allograft in first remission. Equally, there is consensus that younger patients (younger than 40 years, some would say younger than 50 years) with an unfavorable karyotype and de novo AML or AML that follows a myelodysplastic phase should have an allograft in first CR if an HLA-identical sibling donor is available. The debate continues.

Allogeneic Peripheral Blood Progenitor Cells

PBPC are now being evaluated in the allogeneic setting[268-272] (see Chapter 20). The early results were encouraging; an EBMT analysis of patients reported to the Registry for 1994 showed prompt, durable engraftment. The incidence of acute and chronic GVHD initially seemed to be comparable to that observed after allogeneic BMT.[268] In a randomized study conducted at the Royal Marsden Hospital, allogeneic PBPC resulted in significantly faster neutrophil and platelet recovery. Patients who had an allograft with PBPC also left the hospital earlier. There was no significant difference in the incidence of acute or chronic GVHD, but the probability of recurrence was higher in the bone marrow group.[273]

There has, however, been some concern about the relatively high incidence of *chronic* GVHD. A study from Canada evaluated outcome for patients receiving allogeneic bone marrow or PBPC. Whereas disease-free survival at 4 years was better after PBPC (93% vs 62%; *P* = .047), the difference relating mainly to fewer recurrences, quality of life was significantly better in patients who had received bone marrow because chronic GVHD developed in a smaller proportion of patients (*P* = .005).[270] These results notwithstanding, increasing numbers of patients are receiving allogeneic PBPC.

Matched Unrelated Donor Transplantation

With the advent of national and international marrow donor registries, matched unrelated donor transplantations have become feasible. The problem remains the high incidence of acute GVHD. This is, therefore, a contentious subject in terms of the indications for patients with AML in first CR.[274-278] There is relatively little agreement. Some argue in favor of using a matched unrelated donor in the absence of an HLA-identical sibling donor for younger patients (i.e., younger than 40 years) with unfavorable cytogenetics or AML developing on a background of MDS (see Chapter 20). For selected patients treated in first or second remission, disease-free survival of 45% at 2 years has been reported.[276] This figure falls to 19% for patients with more advanced disease.[277] However, overall, for younger patients (younger than 40 years) in whom a second CR is achieved, as prophylaxis and treatment of GVHD have improved, it is reasonable to consider a matched unrelated donor transplantation.

Nonmyeloablative Allogeneic Stem-Cell Transplantation

The conditioning regimen used before allogeneic BMT itself results in appreciable morbidity and mortality. With increasing recognition of the part played by the immune-mediated graft-versus-leukemia effect in preventing recurrence after allogeneic BMT, the feasibility and efficacy of nonmyeloablative allogeneic stem cell transplantation are being evaluated (see Chapter 20). The concept is based on using a sufficiently immunosuppressive but specifically nonmyeloablative conditioning regimen to allow engraftment of donor immunocompetent cells.

Purine analogues, in particular fludarabine, have been used, most often in combination with cyclophosphamide, although the alternative combination of intermediate-dose melphalan and fludarabine is also being evaluated. In Seattle, low-dose TBI (200 cGy) has been used alone and is now being combined with fludarabine, mycophenolate mofetil being used as the immunosuppressive agent.[279] In Israel, a different approach has been taken, fludarabine being combined with busulfan and antithymocyte globulin.[280] In some studies, donor lymphocyte infusions are given "routinely" as part of the treatment to enhance the graft-versus-malignancy effect. In others, they are given only if there is evidence of graft failure or lack of response.

In the preliminary studies to date, patients with AML

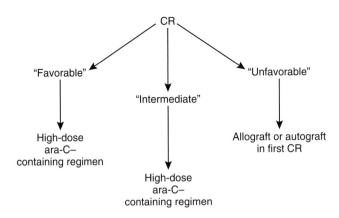

FIGURE 21–3. Algorithm of postremission therapy according to cytogenetic risk group.

have in general been those for whom a conventional allograft was considered inappropriate because of age or co-morbid conditions. In the original publication from M.D. Anderson Cancer Center, 13 patients with AML, whose median age was 59 years (range, 27 to 71 years), received a regimen containing fludarabine or 2-chlorodeoxyadenosine. Treatment was, in general, well tolerated. Blood count recovery was fast, and surprisingly (in view of the fact that 12 patients were either refractory to therapy or beyond first recurrence), CR was achieved in 8. Acute GVHD occurred in three. Chimerism analysis showed more than 90% donor cells by day 30.[281]

Thus, purine analogue–containing nonmyeloablative regimens allow engraftment of HLA-compatible hematopoietic progenitor cells, and this can be achieved without the toxicity of a conventional myeloablative regimen. Acute and, in particular, chronic GVHD continues to be a problem, and the treatment is not without morbidity and mortality. It remains to be seen whether it will prove worthwhile in the longer term.

In summary, there is little consensus regarding the best postremission therapy for younger patients with AML. However, an algorithm can be constructed in general terms according to a "risk-directed" strategy (Fig. 21-3).

WHEN TREATMENT FAILS

The treatment of AML is fraught with difficulties and disappointment. Perhaps the most difficult situation is when treatment fails, either when a person has been given chemotherapy and is found to have demonstrably resistant leukemia or when, after a time, a follow-up blood count done in the clinic reveals a more or less subtle change that immediately raises the possibility of recurrence. The two situations are different, and it is important to recognize this in reading reports of outcome to a new regimen.

Resistant Disease

When conventional first-line chemotherapy (i.e, an anthracycline plus ara-C or a variation of that basic treatment) fails, it is unfortunately most unlikely that any alternative treatment will be curative. Data from St. Bartholomew's Hospital show that for patients younger than 60 years treated between 1978 and 2000, initial treatment failed in 69 of 374 (18%) consecutive patients. Of the 69 patients, 44 received alternative therapy; there were 7 treatment-related deaths. In 28 patients, second-line treatment failed. CR was achieved in 9 of 44. Currently, only 1 of the 69 patients remains alive. The reality, therefore, is that when initial treatment fails, the prognosis is appalling (Fig. 21-4).

However, it would be wrong and in many cases inappropriate to take a totally nihilistic view. If substantial leukemic infiltration persists, it is generally agreed that to continue with the same regimen is futile. There are also patients in whom, after two cycles of treatment, the level of infiltration is relatively low (<10%) but in whom a further cycle of the same treatment has no further effect. An alternative experimental approach is justified but will, sadly, usually fail.

The decision to proceed to an alternative regimen must take into account the patient's age and general state of health, the low probability of success in anything other than the short term, and the potential toxicity of the treatment being considered. If a younger patient has an allogeneic donor, it is certainly justifiable to strive to achieve remission before an allograft. If not, one attempt at alternative, possibly curative treatment is justified in most cases. The course of action differs according to the center. Some favor dose escalation, others, a change of therapy. The rationale for the use of high-dose ara-C when conventional doses have failed is the concept that resistance to the drug is due to inadequate cellular uptake that can be circumvented by the use of higher dosages (see Chapter 17).

Various "salvage" regimens have been tested. In principle, a drug that has not been used before is more likely to be effective. Thus, mitoxantrone plus etoposide with[282] or without[283] ara-C has been used; platinum compounds,[284] high-dose etoposide plus cyclophosphamide,[285] 2-chlorodeoxyadenosine,[286] and topotecan[287] have also been used with CR rates of 20% to 35%. The EORTC Leukemia Group has conducted a pilot phase II study of idarubicin given by continuous intravenous

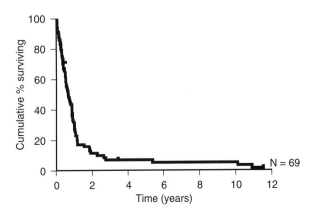

FIGURE 21–4. Overall survival of patients in whom first-line treatment failed.

TABLE 21–9. Outcome after Retreatment at First Recurrence

No. of Patients	CR Rate (%)	Overall Survival (%)	DFS at 2 Years (%)	Reference
243	33	10	25	199
54	61	15	10	289
50	68	30	25	292
114	39	19	16	290

CR, complete remission; DFS, disease-free survival.

infusion interspersed with intermediate-dose ara-C in patients with primary resistant AML. A CR rate of 52% was achieved, which compares favorably with the results usually obtained in this setting.[288]

Unfortunately, most patients in whom first-line treatment has failed will not enter CR with an alternative conventional regimen. Thus, the use of experimental strategies is entirely justified. Such remissions are hardly ever durable, unless they can be consolidated by high-dose treatment with autologous hematopoietic progenitor cell support or by an allograft.

Recurrence

Recurrent leukemia remains the main cause of treatment failure in younger patients. In younger people in whom CR is achieved, 50% to 60% will develop recurrent AML, with more than 90% of relapses involving the bone marrow; 60% of recurrences occur during the first year, with few occurring after 4 years.[289-294] With conventional therapy, the outcome is poor; overall, the 2-year survival rate is 20% at best. Second remission can be induced in between 33% and 69% of younger patients treated enthusiastically (Table 21-9), although such patients constitute a relatively selected group in that it is not necessarily appropriate to re-treat everyone.[292]

Although superficially these percentages look promising, the reality, taking a whole population of patients with recurrent AML as the denominator, is actually much worse. Using patients younger than 60 years treated at St. Bartholomew's Hospital between 1978 and 2000 as an example, it was thought appropriate to re-treat 118 of 147 patients who had recurrent AML. Second CR was achieved in 54 of 118 (46%) (this includes 9 of 11 patients with AML-M3). Of the 54 patients in whom second CR was achieved, 23 are alive without recurrence, 11 having received high-dose treatment with ABMT. Survival from first recurrence is shown in Figure 21-5.

Several factors that correlate with the probability of second CR being achieved have been identified,[288-294] that is, the length of first remission, cytogenetic risk group at presentation, age, and serum lactate dehydrogenase concentration (Table 21-10). Duration of first remission is highly significant[164, 292, 294]; the second CR rate in patients in whom the first remission lasted less than 1 year is between 10% and 30%, whereas for patients with a first remission duration of 1 to 2 years or longer than 2 years, the probability of entering second CR is between 40% and 70%.[164, 294, 295]

In most patients, the aim of inducing second CR is as a "means to an end," that is, to be followed by allogeneic transplantation or HDT with autologous hematopoietic progenitor cells, although the situation in patients with recurrent acute promyelocytic leukemia is different in that second remissions can be durable[292] (see Chapter 23). Several different approaches have been tried. Use of the same regimen that resulted in the first CR has a 30% to 50% chance of being successful.[292, 293] High-dose ara-C and mitoxantrone followed by etoposide and then further ara-C has resulted in a 61% CR rate overall (47% in patients with refractory disease and 78% in patients treated at first recurrence).[296] The MEC regimen (mitoxantrone and etoposide with ara-C at 1 g/m² daily) has been tested in Italy with a second CR rate of 68%,[297] as has the combination of mitoxantrone (or idarubicin), ara-C 1 g/m² twice daily, and carboplatin.[298]

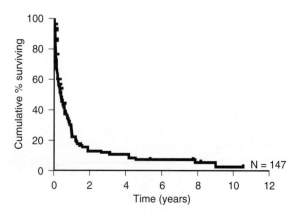

FIGURE 21–5. Survival from first relapse of patients with AML, 1978 to 2000 (censored at high-dose treatment).

TABLE 21–10. Factors Associated with a Poor Outcome to Salvage Therapy

Factor	Definition	References
Short first remission	Less than 1 year	164, 293, 295
Adverse cytogenetics	7−, 5q−, complex; not t(8;21), t(15;17), or inversion 16	295
High lactate dehydrogenase level	>600 mU/mL	290
Older age	>40 years >50 years	290, 295

TABLE 21–11. HDT in Second or Later Remission with Bone Marrow Treated In Vitro

Treatment (person)	In Vitro Treatment	No. of Patients	Median Age (range)	Remission Status at HDT	Median Duration (months) of First CR (range)	Actuarial DFS (%)	Reference
Bu + Cy or Cy + TBI	4HC	24	33 (10–61)	CR2–CR4	13 (2–51)	19	299
Cy + TBI	MAF	30	35 (17–53)	CR2–CR4	Not stated	34	245
Bu + etoposide	4HC	26	38 (15–58)	CR2–CR3	21 (1–40)	56	217
Cy + TBI	MAF	20	31 (17–53)	CR2	Not stated	34	260
Cy + TBI or Bu + Cy	A/B + C′	107	35 (not stated)	CR2 + CR3	Not stated	48	250
Bu + Cy	4HC	98	30 (1–56)	CR2–CR3	Not stated	30	246

Bu, busulfan; CR, complete remission; Cy, cyclophosphamide; DFS, disease-free survival; 4HC, 4-hydroxyperoxycyclophosphamide; HDT, high-dose therapy; MAF, mafosfamide; TBI, total-body irradiation; C′, complement.

Outcome after High-dose Therapy with an Autograft in Second Remission

Most studies have used some form of in vitro treatment with either a drug- or an antibody-based method. Disease-free survivals ranging from 19% to 56% have been reported[227, 244-246, 250, 299] (Table 21–11). Two studies in which the autologous marrow was not treated in vitro have also been reported, with disease-free survivals of 42% and 48%.[300, 301] However, in both, the patients were a somewhat selected group because the median duration of first remission was 11 and 14 months, and in one of the studies, a third of the patients had AML-M3.

A retrospective analysis has been conducted comparing HDT and ABMT with matched unrelated donor transplantation for patients in second CR treated in Seattle. With use of a matched-pair method (with matching for age and disease stage, all patients being treated at the same hospital), there was no significant difference in disease-free survival[302]; however, the recurrence rate was lower with matched unrelated donor transplantation. Thus, for somewhat older patients in whom second CR is achieved and for younger patients who do not have a suitable donor, HDT with autologous hematopoietic progenitor cell support is an appropriate alternative.

Outcome after an Allograft in Second Remission

Survival rates of between 22% and 29% have been reported in patients receiving transplants in untreated first relapse.[303-305] For those treated in second remission, disease-free survivals vary between 26% and 40%.[305, 306] The perceived wisdom is that an allograft from an HLA-identical sibling is the best therapy. To confirm or refute this assumption, 485 patients in second remission of AML were studied (the group comprising patients reported to the International Bone Marrow Transplant Registry versus those taking part in the British MRC trials, those in the ECOG studies in the United States, and patients treated at M.D. Anderson Hospital). The 3-year probability of leukemia-free survival was 17% for "chemotherapy" versus 26% for allograft.[307] A similar retrospective analysis of outcome comparing HLA-identical allografting with HDT and ABMT in second remission showed somewhat better results with allografting (43% versus 27%).[308] For patients with more advanced disease (refractory AML or beyond

second remission), the 5-year survival after an allograft was less than 10%; thus, in these situations, an allograft offers only a limited chance of cure[308] (see Chapter 20).

Recurrence after High-dose Therapy with an Autograft in First Remission

An EBMT Registry retrospective analysis[309] evaluated outcome for patients in whom disease recurred after an autograft and who subsequently had an allogeneic transplantation or second autograft. Outcome was comparable in these two situations provided that HLA-identical (related or unrelated) bone marrow was used. The treatment-related mortality was high (26% for a second autograft, 51% for a matched allograft), but the leukemia-free survival was 27% and 35% at 2 years in the two groups, respectively. The use of nonmyeloablative stem-cell transplantation is now being evaluated in this setting.

Recurrence after Allogeneic Bone Marrow Transplantation in First Remission

In some such patients, it may be inappropriate to consider further intensive therapy. Second allogeneic transplantation procedures are associated with a high mortality (25% to 50%).[310-315] It is possible that the use of less intensive (i.e., nonmyeloablative) stem-cell transplantation will be more successful.

Donor lymphocyte infusions have been used in recurrence after allogeneic BMT with complete responses in approximately 20% of selected patients. However, the use of donor lymphocyte infusions is associated with GVHD in approximately 60% of patients[316-318] (see Chapter 18).

CNS Recurrence

The incidence of CNS recurrence (see also Chapter 13) in adults with AML is about 15%.[319-321] Almost always, CNS recurrence precedes or occurs concurrently with bone marrow recurrence. Patients with AML subtypes M4 and M5 have a higher incidence of CNS involvement. Most often, the recurrence develops as myeloid blast cells in the cerebrospinal fluid. Patients usually complain of headache or back pain but may present with visual disturbance, alterations in mental state, or cranial nerve palsies. In the last situation, and when plaques of leukemic blast cells are present around cranial or spinal nerve roots or on the surface of the spinal cord itself, it is often extremely difficult to demonstrate that the symptoms are caused by CNS involvement. Even magnetic resonance scans do not necessarily help. Free-floating blast cells may be present in the cerebrospinal fluid in addition to such lesions.

Treatment of leukemic meningitis centers around the use of intrathecal methotrexate or ara-C, initially given twice weekly, together with craniospinal irradiation. The difficulty is that such treatment may be profoundly myelosuppressive, necessitating delays while the bone marrow recovers. Unfortunately, bone marrow recurrence often supervenes before treatment has been completed. In the absence of bone marrow recurrence, treatment of the CNS should be followed, nonetheless, by systemic reinduction therapy. Isolated CNS recurrence (if it is treated adequately) carries a relatively good prognosis and is a situation different from systemic recurrence. High-dose ara-C has also been shown to clear leukemic blast cells from the cerebrospinal fluid in patients with overt disease and may be useful in the context of concurrent bone marrow and CNS involvement.[322]

PROGNOSTIC FACTORS

In recent years, a considerable amount of effort has been expended in trying to identify factors that correlate with outcome. These can be divided into patient variables (such as age, performance status, blast count at presentation, and cytogenetic subtype) and treatment variables (such as the amount of consolidation therapy). However, a prognostic factor relates to the specific context in which it has been identified (although some variables, such as cytogenetic subtype, may apply to more than one type of treatment). Achievement of CR itself confers the greatest prognostic advantage, even if cure is not achieved.

Factors Relating to Achievement of First Remission

The three most important factors correlating with the probability of response to treatment are the patient's age, the cytogenetic subtype, and the presence or absence of an antecedent hematologic disorder.

Age

The most significant patient variable is age (see "The Treatment of Older People"). There is an inverse correlation with prognosis, to a large extent because a greater proportion of older people die (of infection) before CR can be achieved. Older patients tend to have other, concurrent illnesses, and there is also a higher incidence of refractory leukemia because of chromosome abnormalities associated with a poor prognosis as well as relatively higher levels of expression of genes that encode proteins mediating drug resistance (*MDR1* or gp120).[323]

TABLE 21–12. Relationship between Cytogenetic Subtype and Outcome

Cytogenetic Subtype	Karyotypic Abnormality	5-Year Survival (%)
Favorable	t(15;17)	63 ± 4
	t(8;21)	69 ± 4
	inv (16)	61 ± 7
Intermediate	Trisomy 8	48 ± 4
	Normal	45 ± 2
	11q23	45 ± 6
	Trisomy 21	47 ± 7
Unfavorable	−7	10 ± 4
	5q−	11 ± 6
	Complex (>5 abnormalities)	21 ± 4

Adapted from Grimwade D, Walker H, Oliver F, et al: The importance of diagnostic cytogenetics on outcome in AML: Analysis of 1612 patients entered into the MRC AML 10 trial. Blood 1998;92:2322.

Cytogenetics

Sakurai and Sandberg[324] first demonstrated that CR was less likely to be achieved in patients with an abnormal karyotype. These findings have subsequently been confirmed again and again. As mentioned before, a number of nonrandom clonal abnormalities have been found to correlate closely with prognosis[324-331] (Table 21–12).

In contrast to what might be assumed, a normal karyotype does not confer a better prognosis. There is, in fact, a relative benefit in having a chromosome translocation involving a core-binding factor; for example, patients with t(8;21) and inv(16) as well as those with AML-3 and the t(15;17) translocation are more likely to enter CR than are those with deletions of chromosome 5 or 7 or a rearrangement in the long arm of chromosome 11.[118, 119] In the context of the CALGB study in which three different levels of ara-C were used, patients were categorized into one of three cytogenetic groups: (1) core-binding factor type, that is, patients with a t(8;21), inv(16), t(16;16), and del(16); (2) normal; and (3) any other karyotype. With high-dose ara-C, a substantial prolongation of remission was seen in patients with core-binding factor type karyotypes but not in those with other abnormalities.[119]

Antecedent Hematologic Disorder

A favorable response to therapy is considerably less likely in patients with an antecedent hematologic disorder, for example, refractory anemia with excess blasts (RAEB), than in patients presenting with de novo AML. Patients with secondary AML (secondary to, for example, alkylating agent treatment) are also much less likely to respond to treatment.[332, 333]

Factors Correlating with Duration of First Remission and Survival

Some of the variables that have prognostic significance in terms of remission duration differ from those correlating with achievement of remission; for example, the intensity of treatment overall correlates with duration of remission.[334] Parameters relating to the "amount" of leukemia, such as hepatosplenomegaly and the height of the blast count, have also been found to be relevant, with a tendency for patients with a greater amount of disease to have a higher probability of early recurrence,[335, 336] although this is not agreed upon by all.[337]

Some variables apply both to response to therapy and to survival. As mentioned before, patients with AML-M3, that is, the t(15;17) translocation, and those with t(8;21) and inv(16) have been found to have a better prognosis.[118, 119] The Fourth International Workshop on Chromosomes in Leukemia analyzed data of 716 patients diagnosed with AML between 1980 and 1982; with a median follow-up of now more than 14 years, it is clear that for patients with de novo AML, both achievement of CR and survival correlate most significantly with cytogenetic subtype.[338]

Within the context of the MRC AML 10 trial, cytogenetic analysis of 1612 patients allowed clear definition of three prognostic groups.[118] AML associated with the t(8;21) and t(15;17) translocations or inv(16) predicted a relatively favorable outcome, whereas the presence of a complex karyotype, −5, del(5q), −7, or abnormalities of 3q defined a group with a relatively poor prognosis. The remaining patients, including those with 11q23 abnormalities, +8, +21, +22, del(9q), del(7q), or other structural or numerical defects not included in the favorable or adverse risk groups, were found to have an intermediate prognosis.

The presence of additional cytogenetic changes did not modify the outcome of patients with a favorable subtype. Subgroup analysis showed that the three prognostic groups retained their predictive value in the context of secondary as well as de novo AML. Furthermore, cytogenetic subtype determines the outcome after allogeneic or autologous BMT in first CR. Rate of response has also been shown to be a significant variable; in the MRC AML 10 trial, overall survival correlated with the percentage of blast cells present after bone marrow recovery from the first cycle.[339]

A prognostic index for use in risk-directed therapy was therefore created on the basis of these results. Two parameters, that is, cytogenetic subtype and response to the first cycle of treatment, were combined with a third, namely, AML-M3, to identify three risk groups with survivals of 70%, 48%, and 15%, respectively, and recurrence rates of 33%, 50%, and 78%.[339] The current AML 12 trial stratification is based on these parameters.

Interest has recently focused on potential "molecular" markers. Two large studies have evaluated the prognostic significance of an internal tandem duplication of the *FLT3* gene. A German study found no correlation with response, recurrence rate or survival,[339a] whereas a study of patients treated in the MRC AML10 and -12 trials reported the presence of an *FLT3* gene mutation to be the most significant prognostic factor predicting for recurrence.[339b] Consideration should probably therefore be given to analysis of the *FLT3* gene at presentation.

At Recurrence

In the last few years, there has been interest in defining additional prognostic factors that apply at recurrence. A large study from the German AML Cooperative Group in patients receiving second-line treatment comprising mitoxantrone and high-dose ara-C identified the following as having adverse significance: a first remission lasting less than 6 months and a high blast count and low neutrophil count at presentation. The probability of treatment-related mortality correlated only with age. For patients in whom karyotypic analysis was available, unfavorable chromosome abnormalities were associated with a lower second CR rate and were the only factor correlating with survival.[340]

THE TREATMENT OF OLDER PEOPLE

Most patients with AML are elderly; the incidence of AML increases with age, up to an estimated incidence of 10 per 100,000 in the elderly population.[341, 342] More than half of the notified newly diagnosed patients in England and Wales are older than 65 years at the time of diagnosis.[68] Similar figures have been reported from France[343] and the United States,[69] with a median age at presentation of 65 to 70 years. However, the proportion of patients older than 60 years reported in multicenter trials ranges from 16% to 51%.[341]

Differences of AML between Older and Younger People

AML in the older person differs from that in younger adults; there are differences in the phenotype of the leukemic blast cells and in their in vitro culture characteristics,[344, 345] and the morphologic character may be different (e.g., a lower incidence of Auer rods). Cytogenetic abnormalities also differ. Certain specific chromosome abnormalities are age related. For example, the favorable subtypes t(8;21), inv(16), and t(15;17) occur less frequently in patients older than 50 years. Aneuploidy, however, appears to be more common in older patients.[346] There is also an increased incidence of partial or full deletion of chromosome 5 or 7. Expression of multidrug resistance glycoprotein *(MDR1)* is also higher (see later).

The greatest difference of all is that disease frequently evolves on a background of MDS.[347, 348] It is now clear that trilineage MDS may be recognized in as many as 30% of older patients with de novo AML *at the time of diagnosis.*[349] In addition, the older person is less able to tolerate intensive combination chemotherapy. Older people often have concurrent illnesses so that, for example, in the context of neutropenia, an older person is much more likely to develop pneumonia and die of it before CR has ever been achieved.

Thus, there are two interrelated problems: first, the illness itself is more likely to be resistant to treatment; and second, few patients are able to receive optimal postremission treatment.

Principles of Treatment

Advanced age is in itself an adverse prognostic factor. In terms of response to treatment, CRs are achieved in at best 50% of patients.[164, 174-176, 211, 350-364] However, the results of published studies vary widely, probably reflecting greater or lesser degrees of selection of patients that occur both before referral and at the referral center. A study from Canada showed that 16% of patients who theoretically would have been eligible for a study did not actually receive any treatment, either because they did not wish to or because their physicians did not think it appropriate. This obviously affected the interpretation of results for the group that actually did receive treatment.[356] Thus, older patients enrolled in prospective randomized studies may not be representative of the total elderly AML population but may represent a group of relatively healthier patients.

There are older patients for whom anything other than palliative treatment is inappropriate from the outset. There are others who can withstand only one cycle of chemotherapy; sadly, recurrent leukemia will develop in most. However, provided that adequate remission induction and postremission treatment *can* be given, duration of remission should not inherently be different from that of younger patients.

Because most treatment-related deaths in older people receiving chemotherapy for AML are due to infection, the advent of G-CSF and GM-CSF was greeted with much enthusiasm. In phase II and phase III trials,[354, 362-366] shortening of neutropenia was certainly demonstrated (see later). However, no real benefit in terms of survival was demonstrated.

The reality is therefore that in general, the outcome of older patients with AML is different from that of younger patients for all the reasons detailed. An ECOG analysis reviewed the long-term survival of nearly 3000 patients treated between 1973 and 1996. The overall median survival was 11 months, but for patients older than 55 years, it was only 6 months, with a 5-year survival of only 7.6%.[169] Data from other studies show similarly poor long-term outcome; an update of the EORTC-HOVON data shows a median survival of 9 months and a 5-year survival of only 8%.[175] A similar analysis from the Fourth International Workshop on Chromosomes in Leukemia shows a 5-year survival for patients older than 60 years of less than 5%.[338]

Data from St. Bartholomew's Hospital for 420 consecutive patients older than 60 years referred during a 30-year-period (1969 to 1999) cogently illustrate the problem.[358, 359] Of 420 patients, 288 (60%) received treatment with curative intent. CR was achieved in 87 of 288 patients overall (31%, i.e., 21% of the entire group). Treatment-related deaths accounted for treatment failure in 50% of patients overall. Patients with a favorable or normal karyotype had significantly higher CR rates than did those with an unfavorable karyotype (71% versus 22%, $P = .05$, and 45% versus 22%, $P = .04$, respectively). The median disease-free survival for all patients in whom CR was achieved was 10 months. With a median follow-up of 11 years, actuarial survival for all patients at 1, 3, and 5 years is 20%, 7%, and 4%, respectively (Fig. 21-6).

Thus, although overall outcome of older patients with AML has improved, the prognosis is still poor. By use of prognostic factors, it may be possible to direct curative therapy more appropriately.

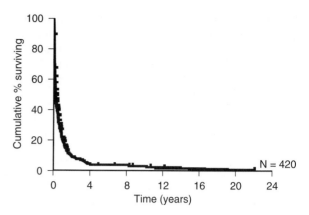

FIGURE 21-6. Overall survival of 420 consecutive older patients presenting to St. Bartholomew's Hospital between 1969 and 1999.

Intensive versus Less Intensive Therapy

Nonrandomized trials of specific antileukemic therapy consistently show an advantage over outcome with supportive care alone, as does the one prospective, randomized comparison.[357] With regard to the intensity of treatment, several studies have compared more with less intensive chemotherapy.[152, 352, 353, 360] In general, these favor the use of "full-dose" chemotherapy, although the treatment-related mortality is approximately 30%. For an individual patient, it is possible to make a decision about the advisability of using intensive chemotherapy on the basis of two facts, the cytogenetic subtype and an obvious contraindication to intensive therapy. Thus, a person *without* unfavorable cytogenetics and *no* contraindication to intensive therapy should be treated with curative intent. Conversely, patients with an unfavorable karyotype, particularly those with complex chromosome abnormalities, have such a low probability of entering CR that it is justifiable to give the best supportive care available and not incur the toxicity of intensive therapy that is destined to fail.

Remission Induction

With an anthracycline plus ara-C regimen, CR can currently be achieved in 40% to 50% of older patients.[352, 353, 357-359] Idarubicin and mitoxantrone have been substituted for daunorubicin with slightly higher CR rates.[175, 176, 179] An ECOG study[176] directly compared daunorubicin, idarubicin, and mitoxantrone, given with ara-C, with no significant difference among the groups; the overall CR rate was 42%. A "low-dose" combination of ara-C, etoposide, and mitoxantrone or 6-thioguanine has also been tried with a high response rate of 78% in patients between the ages of 60 and 84 years.[367] However, it is not known how effective such less toxic treatment will be in the longer term.

With regard to maintenance of remission, a CALGB study is currently in progress evaluating interleukin-2 as maintenance therapy for patients older than 60 years. There is also an international study using interleukin-2 and histamine as maintenance therapy.

Much attention has recently been paid to multidrug resistance (MDR) as the mechanism underlying treatment failure in older patients. The multidrug resistance gene 1 (*MDR1*) is on the long arm of chromosome 7 and encodes a 170-kd glycoprotein known as P-glycoprotein that functions as an adenosine triphosphate–dependent efflux pump. Southwest Oncology Group studies in older patients with AML have demonstrated a 71% incidence of P-glycoprotein expression in patients with AML older than 55 years, compared with a 37% incidence in younger patients.[368] The level of *MDR1* expression correlates inversely with achievement of CR (i.e., those with high *MDR1* expression have a lower probability of entering CR).[369] Modulators of multidrug resistance are therefore being evaluated. Studies are in progress with PSC833, a cyclosporine analogue, but the preliminary data, although confirming modulation of *MDR1* in vitro, have been somewhat disappointing in practice[370, 371] (see later).

ADDITIONAL THERAPIES

Hematopoietic Growth Factors

Granulocyte colony-stimulating factor (G-CSF) and granulocyte macrophage colony-stimulating factor (GM-CSF) have been used with two specific aims, to shorten duration of neutropenia and to induce cells into cycle, in the hope that cell cycle–specific drugs such as ara-C would be more effective. Both growth factors have been compared with placebo and have been given concurrently with remission induction or consolidation therapy in younger and older patients. The main problem is that although there has been a reduction in the duration of neutropenia by 4 or 5 days in some of the trials, no difference in CR rate, disease-free survival, or survival has been demonstrated (by intention-to-treat analyses).[354, 362, 366, 372-375] A large international study subsequently confirmed that G-CSF is safe and does reduce the duration of neutropenia, leading to some clinical benefit by reducing the duration of fever, the requirement for parenteral antibiotics, and the duration of hospital stay.[354] Thus, many centers still use it. In the context of high-dose ara-C–containing treatment, the German AML Cooperative Group investigated G-CSF and found a significant shortening of neutropenia together with a significant prolongation of disease-free survival in patients with primary refractory or recurrent AML.[376]

With regard to older patients who might be expected to benefit the most, all of the studies show a modest decrease in neutrophil recovery time.[354, 362-366] An analysis of cost-effectiveness and the effect on quality of life was therefore undertaken in the context of the MRC AML 11 study[377]; no survival benefit or effect on CR rate was seen.

The other reason for using G-CSF is to stimulate leukemic blast cells to enter S phase synchronously.[373, 374] This has proved possible, but again disappointingly, no real benefit has ensued. Thus, with the exception of one study, the literature does not support the use of hematopoietic growth factors during remission induction in older patients.

Reversal of Drug Resistance

It has been demonstrated that patients with resistant leukemia are more likely to express the *MDR1* gene.[369] On this basis, drugs such as cyclosporine, which inhibits the *MDR1*-mediated effect, have been given concurrently with chemotherapy. A randomized study in patients with AML deemed to have a poor prognosis showed an improvement in disease-free survival for patients who received cyclosporine.[378] Another study has shown improvements in both relapse-free and overall survival.[379] When *MDR1* modulators such as cyclosporine are used, the doses of chemotherapy may need to be adjusted.

Two phase I studies of daunorubicin given with ara-C and etoposide, with or without the multidrug resistance modulator PSC833, have been conducted by the CALGB in newly diagnosed older patients,[370] and a phase III study derived from these trials has begun. An ECOG study is also currently comparing chemotherapy comprising mitoxantrone, etoposide, and ara-C given with or without PSC833 in patients with recurrent and refractory AML.[371]

Immunotherapy

After early studies with irradiated leukemic blasts and bacille Calmette-Guérin,[154, 380, 381] interleukin-2 has been used to try to stimulate NK cell function as a means of prolonging remission after chemotherapy[382] and after hematopoietic cell transplantation.[383] However, no improvement in outcome has been demonstrated. It has been suggested that ex vivo–generated cytotoxic T lymphocytes specific for hematopoietic system–restricted minor histocompatibility antigens might be used as immunotherapy.[384] Roquinimex (Linomide), a drug that enhances NK cell function, has also been evaluated in a phase III placebo-controlled study in which patients received the drug (or placebo) for 2 years after high-dose treatment with ABMT in first remission. Again, disappointingly, there was no difference in outcome between the two groups of patients.[385] Thus, although there is a good theoretical rationale for using such immunomodulatory drugs, in practice, they have thus far failed to fulfill their promise.

Amifostine

Use of this "cytoprotective" agent has made it possible to give higher doses of chemotherapy (idarubicin) but with less oral and gastrointestinal tract toxicity.[386] In another study in which amifostine was used in older patients in conjunction with daunorubicin and ara-C, although the CR rate was not significantly different, the early mortality was lower in patients receiving amifostine, resulting in turn in better overall survival.[387]

Amifostine has also now been used to treat G-CSF–mobilized PBPC in vitro. In a preliminary laboratory study, PBPC from patients with AML were treated with mafosfamide alone or with mafosfamide and amifostine. In terms of CFU-GM results, amifostine exerted a protective effect on normal progenitors.[388] Clinical studies are planned on the basis of these preclinical results.

LEUKEMIA ARISING ON A BACKGROUND OF MYELODYSPLASIA

It has long been known that patients in whom AML arises on a background of MDS have a worse prognosis, an antecedent bone marrow disorder being one of the most important negative prognostic factors for achievement of CR[167, 347-349] (see Chapter 24). With conventional combination chemotherapy, the response rates are low, remissions are generally of short duration, and there is a high treatment-related mortality. The problems are resistant disease and prolonged aplasia, the latter resulting in a high incidence of death from infection. It has been suggested that the prolonged aplasia may be a consequence of such patients' having fewer normal stem-cells.

Allogeneic transplantation has been investigated as the initial (i.e., only) treatment of secondary AML (MDS related or therapy related).[389-392] Of 64 patients treated in Seattle, 24% were alive and disease free at 5 years, and there was no difference in outcome between these patients and another group who received remission induction chemotherapy before transplantation.[391]

Intensive chemotherapy followed by HDT with ABMT may be an alternative for younger patients with MDS (or AML after MDS) who lack a suitable donor for allografting. An EBMT study has reported outcome in 79 such patients, and the results were compared with those for a matched control group of 110 patients with de novo AML. The 2-year survival and disease-free survival were 39% and 34%, respectively, younger patients (younger than 40 years) having a significantly better disease-free survival. At 64%, the recurrence rate was significantly higher than that for patients with de novo AML ($P = .007$), but this is a treatment at least worth considering in selected patients.[393]

SECONDARY MYELODYSPLASIA /AML

The problems encountered in treating patients with secondary leukemia are similar to those seen in patients with AML arising on a background of MDS, namely, resistant disease and prolonged cytopenia after treatment. There is a suggestion that the use of high-dose ara-C can, to some degree, circumvent the resistance that is the more common experience with chemotherapy for such leukemia. However, overall, the results of treatment are still poor.

Allogeneic BMT has been used but with limited success; a series from the Dana Farber Cancer Institute in patients who had secondary MDS/AML after cyclophosphamide plus TBI plus ABMT for non-Hodgkin's lymphoma[41] reported that all 11 patients died as a consequence of multiorgan failure. A retrospective analysis from Seattle showed the probability of survival after transplantation to be only 13% overall (33% for refractory anemia and refractory anemia with ringed sideroblasts [RA/RARS], 20% for RAEB, and 8% for RAEB-t/AML). The

probability of death from treatment-related causes was extremely high (78%), death occurring from infection or organ failure. The probability of recurrence for all patients was 47% (34% for RAEB and 58% for RAEB-t/AML). However, none of the patients with RA/RARS have relapsed, suggesting that patients at risk for secondary MDS should be observed prospectively and considered for transplantation earlier rather than later.[394] Thus, this may be worthwhile in selected patients.

SPECIFIC SITUATIONS

Extramedullary Leukemia

Local collections of myeloid blast cells can occur in three situations: (1) concurrently with bone marrow infiltration; (2) as the only site of recurrence; and (3) in patients with MDS or in the context of a known myeloproliferative disorder, such as chronic myeloid leukemia or polycythemia rubra vera. In this situation, the development of such a local collection of leukemic blast cells normally precedes the development of blastic transformation in the marrow (see Chapter 25).

Previously called granulocytic sarcoma or chloroma, a localized collection of myeloid blast cells is now termed myeloblastoma. It may be difficult to diagnose because the cells are so immature; they most often occur in the skin, being associated with AML subtypes M4 and M5 in particular. However, they can also be found in the intestine or as an extradural lesion causing spinal cord compression. The approach to treatment depends on the circumstances. The lesions respond to radiotherapy, which is good palliative treatment, but they will also respond to systemic treatment given for concurrent bone marrow infiltration.

Skin Infiltration

Infiltration of the skin by myeloid blast cells is typically associated with AML subtypes M4 and M5.[395-397] The lesions may be localized or widespread and are typically red or purplish and raised. There is an association between skin involvement and meningeal leukemia.[397] Rarely, skin involvement may occur concurrently with bone marrow infiltration at the time of diagnosis or recurrence, and it may occasionally be the only site of recurrence, but in this situation, it is usually followed rapidly by bone marrow involvement.

Sweet's Syndrome

The syndrome is characterized by fevers and painful red, raised skin lesions in association with neutrophilia.[398] Sweet's syndrome has been described in the context of hematologic malignant neoplasms, most often RAEB, or AML. When it is associated with RAEB, the treatment of choice is corticosteroids. The difference between this and skin involvement with AML is that on skin biopsy in

Sweet's syndrome, there is a characteristic dermal infiltrate by *neutrophils* compared with leukemic blast cells.

AML Occurring during Pregnancy

This is a difficult situation for the patient and for the physician. If the diagnosis is made in the first trimester, most physicians would recommend termination of pregnancy to make it possible to start curative treatment for the mother. However, there are obviously patients for whom this is unacceptable. The other problem is that most of the drugs used for remission induction therapy have potential teratogenic effects when they are used in the first trimester.[399–401] When mothers are treated with chemotherapy during the second and third trimesters, there is no increase in the incidence of congenital malformations.[400, 402] Furthermore, pregnancy does not decrease the likelihood of CR being achieved. The main problems are psychologic and emotional.

For patients diagnosed in the second and third trimesters, remission induction chemotherapy should be started as soon as possible. On occasion, it is possible for patients presenting in the first trimester to be supported with blood and platelets before starting chemotherapy in the second trimester.

THE FUTURE

Antibody-Targeted Therapy for AML

The availability of monoclonal antibodies reactive with myeloid antigens provides new possibilities for treatment. Antibodies have been used in an unmodified state, conjugated with chemicals to form immunotoxins, and most recently with radionuclides. The majority of studies have used anti-CD33, directed against an antigen expressed on the surface of myeloid blast cells from more than 90% of patients with AML but not present on hematopoietic progenitor cells.

Studies with unmodified anti-CD33 resulted in only temporary reductions in the peripheral blast count. Much interest has focused on the immunoconjugate CMA-676 consisting of humanized anti-CD33 conjugated to the antitumor antibiotic calicheamicin. Phase I results in 40 patients with recurrent or refractory AML showed toxicity to be relatively modest, manifest as symptoms typically associated with administration of monoclonal antibodies (i.e., fevers and chills). A degree of pancytopenia was common, but this was temporary.[403] Phase II studies in patients with recurrent AML have recently been reported and the treatment has been associated with less clinical toxicity than that expected with chemotherapy, although prolonged thrombocytopenia has been seen in a proportion of patients.[404, 404a]

Another approach has been to use radiolabeled antibody as part of a myeloablative regimen. In a phase I study of ^{131}I-labeled anti-CD45 antibody given with cyclophosphamide and TBI to 34 patients with advanced AML and MDS, this approach was found to be feasible; 7 of 25 patients survived disease free at a median follow-up of 5 years post-transplantataion at the time of publication.[405]

Altering BCL2 Expression

BCL2 may be involved in the emergence of drug resistance by disrupting or delaying apoptosis and promoting tumor survival. To define the clinical relevance of *BCL2* expression to AML and its correlation with outcome and prognosis, a study from Germany (of 219 patients) found *BCL2* mRNA to be detectable in 84% of patients at initial diagnosis and in 95% at the time of recurrence. Patients with high expression of *BCL2* had a lower CR rate and significantly worse overall and disease-free survival.[406] Thus, therapeutic strategies aimed at modulating *BCL2* function are being tested.

All-*trans* retinoic acid (ATRA) has been found to downregulate *BCL2* in leukemic cell lines.[407] The use of *liposomal* ATRA may overcome the problem with the oral formulation whereby it induces its own metabolism, resulting in suboptimal blood levels. Preliminary studies combining chemotherapy with ATRA have been done,[408] and the combination is being investigated in an MRC trial in the UK.

Therapeutic Monitoring

Remission induction therapy for AML is associated with significant treatment-related mortality in all age groups but especially in older patients; in a proportion of patients, treatment will fail because of resistant disease. There is considerable variability in drug pharmacokinetics so that at the same dose, plasma drug concentrations may be higher in some patients, resulting in greater toxicity. Conversely, lower plasma concentrations may result in decreased toxicity but also possibly decreased antitumor activity. Therapeutic drug monitoring can abrogate such variability. This approach has been successful in children with acute lymphoblastic leukemia.[409] It is hoped that therapeutic monitoring might similarly improve results in adults with AML by decreasing toxicity and hence treatment-related mortality, with a concomitant increase in efficacy, especially in older patients.

CONCLUSION

The results of treatment of AML have improved dramatically during the last 25 years, generally as a consequence of intensification of treatment overall together with improved supportive care. The availability of new technologies for karyotyping leukemic blast cells with a greater degree of definition together with the use of PCR techniques for evaluating minimal residual disease makes it possible to test risk-directed therapy. Treatment can now be allocated on the basis of karyotype, and it may be possible to individualize postremission treatment on the basis of known fact rather than empiricism. The use of nonmyeloablative stem-cell transplantation may make allografting safer, although it is not yet clear how effective this approach will be.

The identification of other molecular parameters, such as expression of *BCL2*, may further expand the range of therapeutic intervention. New drugs and new treatment modalities, such as the use of monoclonal antibodies to target treatment, will extend the spectrum of treatment possibilities. Mouse models for acute leukemia have been described.[410, 411] The investigation of gene expression with use of microarray methodology[412] will lead to completely new laboratory and clinical correlations that, it is hoped, will identify new molecular therapeutic targets. It is an exciting time.

ACKNOWLEDGMENTS

We thank Mrs Margaret Cresswell for her patience in preparing the manuscript and Rachel Johnson for help with Virchow.

REFERENCES

1. Craigie D: Case of disease of the spleen in which death took place in consequence of the presence of purulent matter in the blood. J Surg Med 1845;64:400.
2. Bennett J: Case of hypertrophy of the spleen and liver in which death took place from suppuration of the blood. J Surg Med 1845;64:413.
3. Virchow R: Weisses Blut. Frorieps Notizen 1845;36:151.
4. Virchow R: Weisses Blut und Milztumoren II. Med Zeitung 1847;16:9.
5. Virchow R: Die Leukämie. In Gesammelte Abhandlungen zur wissenschaftlichen Medizin. Frankfurt: Meidinger; 1856, p 190.
6. Neumann E: Ein Fall von Leukämie mit Erkrankung des knochenmarkes. Arch Heilk 1870;11:1.
7. Diamond L, Luhby L: Pattern of "spontaneous" remissions in leukemia of childhood observed in 26 of 300 cases. Am J Med 1951;10:238.
8. Bierman HR, Crile DM, Dod KS, et al: Remissions in leukemia of childhood following acute infectious disease: Staphylococcus, streptococcus, varicella, and feline panleukopenia. Cancer 1953;6:591.
9. Bessis M, Bernard J: A propos du traitement de la leucemie aigue par exsanguino-transfusion. Bull Acad Med 1947:615.
10. Tivey H: The natural history of untreated acute leukemia. Ann NY Acad Sci 1955;60:322.
11. Scott R: Leukemia. Lancet 1957;1:1053.
12. Crosby W: To treat or not to treat acute granulocytic leukemia. Arch Intern Med 1968;122:79.
13. Skipper H, Schabel F, Wilcox W: Experimental evaluation of potential anticancer agents on the criteria and kinetics associated with "curability" of experimental leukemias. Cancer Chemother Rep 1964;35:1.
14. Crowther D, Bateman C, Vartan C, et al: Combination chemotherapy using L-asparaginase, daunorubicin and cytosine arabinoside in adults with acute myelogenous leukaemia. Br Med J 1970;4:513.
15. Crowther D, Powles R, Bateman C, et al: Management of adult acute myelogenous leukaemia. Br Med J 1973;1:131.
16. Beebe G, Ishida M, Jaboon F: Studies of the mortality of A-bomb survivors I. Plan of study and mortality in the medical subsample (selection 1) 1950–1958. Radiat Res 1962;16:253.
17. National Research Council Committee on the Biological Effects of Ionizing Radiations: The Effects on Populations of Exposure to Low Levels of Ionizing Radiation. Washington, DC: National Academy Press; 1980.
18. Funch S, Hoshino T, Itoga T, et al: Chronic lymphocytic leukemia in Hiroshima and Nagasaki, Japan. Blood 1969;33:79.
19. Gluzman D, Abramenko I, Sklyarenko L, et al: Acute leukemias in children from the city of Kiev and Kiev region after the Chernobyl NPP catastrophe. Pediatr Hematol Oncol 1999;16:355.
20. Mukhin V: Acute leukemia in adults: Morbidity in the Donetsk region of Ukraine before and after Chernobyl accident. Ter Arkh 2000;72:60.
21. Nakanishi M, Tanaka K, Shintani T, et al: Chromosomal instability in acute myelocytic leukemia and myelodysplastic syndrome patients among atomic bomb survivors. Radiat Res 1999;40:159.
22. Darby S, Doll R, Gill S, et al: Long term mortality after a single treatment course with x-rays in patients treated for ankylosing spondylitis. Br J Cancer 1987;55:179.
23. Aisenberg A: Acute non-lymphocytic leukemia after treatment for Hodgkin's disease. Am J Med 1983;75:449.
24. Brusamolino E, Lazzarino M, Salvameschi L, et al: Risk of leukaemia in patients treated for Hodgkin's Disease. Eur J Cancer Clin Oncol 1982;18:237.
25. Coltman C: Treatment related leukemia. In Bloomfield CD (ed): Acute Leukemia 1. The Hague: Martinus Nijhoff; 1982, p 61.
26. Glicksman A, Pajak T, Gottlieb A, et al: Second malignant neoplasms in patients successfully treated for Hodgkin's Disease. A Cancer and Leukemia Group B study. Cancer Treat Rep 1982;66:1035.
27. Henry-Amar M: Second cancers after radiotherapy and chemotherapy for early stages of Hodgkin's Disease. J Natl Cancer Inst 1983;71:911.
28. Papa G, Mauro F, Anselmo A, et al: Acute leukaemia in patients treated with Hodgkin's disease. Br J Haematol 1984;58:43.
29. Pedersen-Bjergaard J, Larsen S: Incidence of acute non-lymphocytic leukemia, preleukemia, and acute myeloproliferative syndrome up to 10 years after treatment of Hodgkin's disease. N Engl J Med 1982;307:965.
30. Tester W, Kinsella T, Waller B, et al: Second malignant neoplasms complicating Hodgkin's Disease. The National Cancer Institute experience. J Clin Oncol 1984;2:762.
31. Coltman C, Dixon D: Second malignancies complicating Hodgkin's disease: A Southwest Oncology Group 10-year follow-up. Cancer Treat Rep 1982;66:1023.
32. Valagussa P, Santoro A, Fossati-Bellani F, et al: Second acute leukemia and other malignancies following treatment for Hodgkin's disease. J Clin Oncol 1986;4:830.
33. Blayney D, Longo D, Young E, et al: Decreasing risk of leukemia with prolonged follow-up after chemotherapy and radiotherapy for Hodgkin's disease. N Engl J Med 1987;316:710.
34. Pedersen-Bjergaard J, Specht L, Larsen S, et al: Risk of therapy-related leukemia and preleukemia after Hodgkin's disease. Relation to age, cumulative dose of alkylating agents and time from chemotherapy. Lancet 1987;2:83.
35. Tucker M, Coleman C, Sox R, et al: Risk of second cancers after treatment for Hodgkin's disease. N Engl J Med 1988;318:76.
36. Andrieu J-M, Ifrah N, Payen C, et al: Increased risk of secondary acute nonlymphocytic leukemia after extended-field radiation therapy combined with MOPP chemotherapy for Hodgkin's disease. J Clin Oncol 1990;8:1148.
37. Swerdlow A, Barber J, Vaughan Hudson G, et al: Risk of second malignancy after Hodgkin's disease in a collaborative British cohort: The relation to age at treatment. J Clin Oncol 2000;18:498.
38. Darrington D, Vose J, Anderson J: Incidence and characterization of secondary myelodysplastic syndrome and acute myelogenous leukemia following high-dose chemoradiotherapy and autologous stem cell transplantation for lymphoid malignancies. J Clin Oncol 1994;12:2527.
39. Stone R, Neuberg D, Soiffer R, et al: Myelodysplastic syndrome as a late complication following autologous bone marrow transplantation for non-Hodgkin's lymphoma. J Clin Oncol 1994;12:2535.
40. Milligan D, Ruiz de Elvira M, Kolb H, et al: Secondary leukaemia and myelodysplasia after autografting for lymphoma: Results from the EBMT. EBMT Lymphoma and Late Effects Working Parties. European Group for Blood and Marrow Transplantation. Br J Haematol 1999;106:1020.
41. Friedberg J, Neuberg D, Stone R: Outcome in patients with myelodysplastic syndrome after autologous bone marrow transplantation for non-Hodgkin's lymphoma. J Clin Oncol 1999;17:3128.
42. Micallef I, Lillington D, Apostolidis J, et al: Therapy-related myelodysplasia (tMDS) and secondary acute myelogenous leukemia

(sAML) following high-dose therapy (HDT) with autologous hematopoietic progenitor cell support for lymphoid malignancies. J Clin Oncol 2000;18:947.

43. Lillington D, Micallef I, Carpenter E: Molecular cytogenetic detection of chromosome abnormalities pre-tranplantation in patients with therapy related MDS and secondary AML following high-dose treatment for non-Hodgkin's lymphoma. Proc Am Soc Clin Oncol 2000;19:14a.

44. Greene M, Harris E, Gershenson D, et al: Melphalan may be a more potent leukemogen than cyclophosphamide. Ann Intern Med 1986;105:360.

45. Kaldor J, Day N, Pettersson F, et al: Leukemia following chemotherapy for ovarian cancer. N Engl J Med 1990;322:1.

46. Pedersen-Bjergaard J, Ersboll J, Mygind H, et al: Risk of acute nonlymphocytic leukemia in patients treated with cyclophosphamide for non-Hodgkin's lymphomas. Ann Intern Med 1985;103:195.

47. Pedersen-Bjergaard J, Hansen S, Larsen S, et al: Increased risk of myelodysplasia and leukaemia after etoposide, cisplatin and bleomycin for germ cell tumours. Lancet 1991;338:359.

48. Pui C-H, Ribeiro R, Hancock M, et al: Acute myeloid leukemia in children treated with epipodophyllotoxins for acute lymphoblastic leukemia. N Engl J Med 1991;325:1682.

49. Hawkins M, Kinnier-Wilson L, Stovall M, et al: Epipodophyllotoxins, alkylating agents, and radiation and risk of secondary leukemia after childhood cancer. BMJ 1992;304:951.

50. Frewin R, Provan D, Smith A: Myelodysplasia occurring after fludarabine treatment for chronic lymphocytic leukemia. Clin Lab Haematol 1997;19:151.

51. Grunwald H, Rosner F: Acute leukemia and immunosuppressive drug use. A review of patients undergoing immunosuppressive therapy for non-neoplastic diseases. Arch Intern Med 1979;139:461.

52. Travis L, Holowaty E, Bergfeld T, et al: Risk of leukemia after platinum-based chemotherapy for ovarian cancer. N Engl J Med 1999;340:351.

53. Boice JJ, Greene M, Killen JJ, et al: Leukemia and preleukemia after adjuvant treatment of gastrointestinal cancer with semustine (methyl-CCNU). N Engl J Med 1983;309:1079.

54. Kossman S, Weiss M: Acute myelogenous leukemia after exposure to strontium-89 for the treatment of adenocarcinoma of the prostate. Cancer 2000;88:620.

55. Kushner B, Heller G, Cheung N, et al: High risk of leukemia after short-term dose-intensive chemotherapy in young patients with solid tumors. J Clin Oncol 1998;16:3016.

56. Liozon E, Brigaudeau C, Trimoreau F, et al: Is treatment with hydroxyurea leukemogenic in patients with essential thrombocythemia? An analysis of three new cases of leukemic transformation and review of the literature. Hematol Cell Ther 1997;39:11.

57. Cronkite E: Chemical leukomogenesis: Benzene as a model. Semin Hematol 1987;24:2.

58. Rinsky R, Smith A, Hornung R, et al: Benzene and leukemia. An epidemiologic risk assessment. N Engl J Med 1987;316:1044.

59. Jacobs A: Benzene and leukaemia. Br J Haematol 1989;72:119.

60. Garfinke L, Boffetto B: Association between smoking and leukemia in two American Cancer Society prospective studies. Cancer 1990;65:2356.

61. Sandler D, Shore D, Anderson J, et al: Cigarette smoking and the risk of acute leukemia: Associations with morphology and cytogenetic abnormalities in bone marrow. J Natl Cancer Inst 1994;85:1994.

62. Severson R: Cigarette smoking and leukemia. Cancer 1987;60:141.

63. Brownson R, Novotny T, Perry M: Cigarette smoking and adult leukemia. Arch Intern Med 1993;153:469.

64. Rowley J: Down's syndrome and acute leukaemia: Increased risk may be due to trisomy 21. Lancet 1981;2:1020.

65. Ganick D: Hematological changes in Down's syndrome. Crit Rev Oncol Hematol 1986;6:55.

66. Greenberg B, Wilson F, Woo L, et al: Cytogenetics and granulopoietic effects of bone marrow fibroblastic cells in Fanconi's anaemia. Br J Haematol 1981;48:85.

67. Sawitsky A, Bloom D, German J: Chromosome breakage and acute leukemia in congenital telangiectatic erythema and stunted growth. Ann Intern Med 1966;65:487.

68. Cancer Statistics Registrations. London: Her Majesty's Stationery Office, Office of Population Censuses and Surveys; 1982.

69. Ries L, Kosary C, Hankey B, et al (eds): SEER Cancer Statistics Review, 1973–1994 (NIH Publication 97-2789). Bethesda, MD: National Cancer Institute; 1997.

70. Parkin D, Muir C, Whelan S, et al: International variation in acute myeloid leukemia incidence (age-adjusted world standard) by sex, 1983 to 1987. In Cancer Incidence in Five Continents, vol 6 (IARC Scientific Publication no. 120). Lyon: International Agency for Research on Cancer; 1992.

71. Fialkow P: Use of genetic markers to study cellular origin in development of tumors in human females. Adv Cancer Res 1972;15:191.

72. Fearon E, Burke P, Schiffer C, et al: Differentiation of leukemia cells to polymorphonuclear leukocytes in patients with acute nonlymphocytic leukemia. N Engl J Med 1986;315:15.

73. Fialkow P, Singer P, Adamson J, et al: Acute non-lymphocytic leukemia: Heterogeneity of stem cell origin. Blood 1981;57:1068.

74. Fialkow P, Singer J, Adamson J, et al: Acute non-lymphocytic leukemia: Expression in cells restricted to granulocytic and monocytic differentiation. N Engl J Med 1979;301:1.

75. Fialkow P, Singer J, Raskind W, et al: Clonal development, stem cell differentiation and clinical remissions in acute non-lymphocytic leukemia. N Engl J Med 1987;317:468.

76. Fialkow P, Singer J: Tracing developing and cell lineages in human hemopoietic neoplasia. In Weissman IL (ed): Leukemia: Report of the Dahlem Workshop on Leukemia, Berlin, November 13–18, 1983. Berlin: Springer-Verlag; 1985, p 203.

77. Blackstock A, Garson O: Direct evidence for involvement of erythroid cells in acute myeloblastic leukaemia. Lancet 1974;2:1178.

78. Jenson M, Killmann S-A: Additional evidence for chromosome abnormalities in the erythroid precursors in acute leukemia. Acta Med Scand 1971;189:97.

79. Jowitt S, Yin J, Saunders M: Relapsed myelodysplastic clone differs from acute onset clone as shown by X-lined DNA polymorphism patterns in a patient with acute myeloid leukemia. Blood 1993;82:613.

80. Jacobson R, Temple M, Singer J, et al: A clonal complete remission in a patient with acute non-lymphocytic leukemia originating in a multi-potent stem cell. N Engl J Med 1984;310:1513.

81. Bartram C, Ludwig W, Hiddeman W, et al: Acute myeloid leukemia: Analysis of Ras gene mutation and clonality referred by polymorphic X-linked loci. Leukemia 1989;3:247.

82. LoCoco F, Pelicci P, D'Adamo F: Polyclonal hematopoietic reconstitution in leukemia patients at remission after suppression of specific gene rearrangements. Blood 1993;82:606.

83. Cale R, Wheadon H, Goldstone A, et al: Frequency of clonal remission in acute myeloid leukaemia. Lancet 1993;341:138.

84. Busque L, Gilliland D: Clonal evolution in acute myeloid leukemia. Blood 1993;82:337.

85. Mauer A: Cell kinetics and practical consequences for therapy of acute leukemia. N Engl J Med 1975;293:389.

86. Sjogren U: Mitotic activity in myeloid leukaemias: A study of 277 cases. Scand J Haematol 1978;20:159.

87. Raza A, Preisler H, Day R, et al: Direct relationship between remission duration in acute myeloid leukemia and cell cycle kinetics: A leukemia intergroup study. Blood 1990;76:2191.

88. Lowenberg B, Van Putten W, Touw I, et al: Autonomous proliferation of leukemic cells in vitro as a determinant of prognosis in adult acute myeloid leukemia. N Engl J Med 1993;328:614.

89. Griffin J, Young D, Herrmann F, et al: Effects of recombinant human GM-CSF on proliferation of clonogenic cells in acute myeloblastic leukemia. Blood 1986;66:1444.

90. Saeland S, Caux C, Favre C, et al: Effects of recombinant human interleukin-3 in CD34 enriched normal hematopoietic progenitors and on myeloblastic leukemia cells. Blood 1988;72:1580.

91. Lowenberg B, Touw I: Hematopoietic growth factors and their receptors in acute leukemia. Blood 1993;81:281.

92. Tokosoz D, Farr C, Marshall C: Ras genes and acute myeloid leukaemia. Br J Haematol 1989;71:1.

93. van Kamp H, de Pijper C, Verlaaen-de Vries M, et al: Longitudinal analysis of point mutations of the N-ras proto-oncogene in patients with myelodysplasia using archived blood smears. Blood 1992;79:1266.

94. Priesler H, Raza A, Larson R, et al: Proto-oncogene expression and the clinical outcome of patients with AML. Blood 1989;73:255.

95. Campos L, Rouault J-P, Sabido O, et al: High expression of bcl-2

protein in acute myeloid leukemia cells is associated with poor response to chemotherapy. Blood 1993;81:3091.

96. Bigon I, Dreyfus F, Melle J, et al: Expression of the c-mpl proto-oncogene in human hematologic malignancies. Blood 1993;82:877.

97. Sugimoto K, Hirano N, Toyoshima H, et al: Frequent mutations in the p53 gene in human myeloid leukemia cell lines. Blood 1992;79:2378.

98. Sugimoto K, Hirano N, Toyoshima H, et al: Mutations of the p53 gene in myelodysplastic syndrome (MDS) and MDS-derived leukemia. Blood 1993;81:3022.

99. Chen Y-C, Chen P-J, Yah S-H, et al: Deletion of the human retino-blastoma gene in primary leukemias. Blood 1990;76:2060.

100. Kornblau S, Xu H-J, del Giglio A, et al: Clinical implications of decreased retinoblastoma protein expression in acute myelogenous leukemia. Cancer Res 1992;52:4587.

101. Bennett J, Catovsky D, Daniel M, et al: Proposal for the recognition of minimally differentiated acute myeloid leukaemia (AML-M0). Br J Haematol 1991;78:325.

102. Harris N, Jaffe E, Diebold J, et al: World Health Organization classification of neoplastic diseases of the hematopoietic and lymphoid tissues: Report of the Clinical Advisory Committee meeting. J Clin Oncol 1999;17:3835.

103. Venditti A, Del Poeta G, Buccisano F, et al: Minimally differentiated acute myeloid leukemia (AML-M0): Comparison of 25 cases with other French-American-British subtypes. Blood 1997;89:621.

104. LoCoco F, Pasqualetti D, Lopez M, et al: Immunophenotyping of acute leukemia: Relevance of analyzing different lineage-associated markers. Blut 1989;58:235.

105. Cattei V, Carbone A, Marotta G, et al: Expression of natural killer (NK) antigens in malignant histiocytosis and a subset of acute myelomonocytic leukemias. Bone Marrow Transplant 1989;4:22.

106. Bennett J, Catovsky D, Daniel M, et al: Criteria for the diagnosis of acute leukemia of megakaryocytic lineage (M7). A report of the French-American-British Cooperative Group. Ann Intern Med 1985;103:460.

107. San Miguel J, Gonzalez M, Canizo M, et al: Leukemias with mega-karyoblastic involvement: Clinical, hematologic and immunologic characteristics. Blood 1988;72:402.

108. Larson R, Kondo K, Vardiman J, et al: Evidence for a 15;17 translocation in every patient with acute promyelocytic leukemia. Am J Med 1984;76:827.

109. Fourth International Workshop on Chromosomes in Leukemia. Cancer Genet Cytogenet 1982;11:251.

110. Li Y, Khalide C, Hayhoe F: Correlation between chromosomal pattern, cytological subtypes, response to therapy and survival in acute myeloid leukaemia. Scand J Haematol 1983;30:265.

111. Diverio D, Rossi V, Avvisati G, et al: Early detection of relapse by prospective reverse transcriptase–polymerase chain reaction analysis of the PML/RARα fusion gene in patients with acute promyelocytic leukemia enrolled in the GIMEMA-AIEOP Multicenter "AIDA" Trial. Blood 1998;92:784.

112. Capizzi R, Pool M, Cooper M, et al: Treatment of poor risk acute leukemia with sequential high-dose ara-C and L-asparaginase. Blood 1984;63:694.

113. Hertzig R, Wolff S, Lazarus H, et al: High-dose cytosine arabinoside therapy for refractory leukemia. Blood 1983;62:361.

114. Barnett M, Richards M, Ganesan T, et al: Central nervous system toxicity of high dose cytosine arabinoside. Semin Oncol 1985;2:227.

115. Rohatiner A, Gregory W, Dhaliwal H, et al: High-dose cytosine arabinoside; Response to therapy in acute leukemia and non-Hodgkin's lymphoma. Cancer Chemother Pharmacol 1984;12:90.

116. Keating M, Smith T, Kantarjian H, et al: Cytogenetic pattern in acute myelogenous leukemia: A major reproducible determinant of outcome. Leukemia 1988;2:403.

117. Dastugue N, Payen C, Lafage-Pochitaloff M, et al: Prognostic significance of karyotype in de novo adult acute myeloid leukemia. Leukemia 1995;9:1491.

118. Grimwade D, Walker H, Oliver F, et al: The importance of diagnostic cytogenetics on outcome in AML: Analysis of 1612 patients entered into the MRC AML 10 trial. Blood 1998;92:2322.

119. Bloomfield C, Lawrence D, Arthure D, et al: Curative impact of intensification with high-dose cytarabine (HiDAC) in acute myeloid leukemia (AML) varies by cytogenetic group. Blood 1994;84:111a.

120. Stein A, O'Donnell M, Slovak M, et al: Do cytogenetics predict outcome of autologous bone marrow transplantation (ABMT) for acute myelogenous leukemia (AML) in 1st remission (CR)? Blood 1996;88:485a.

121. Slater S, Bassan R, Bjorkholm M, et al: Karyotype and the outcome of high-dose treatment with autologous hematopoietic progenitor cell support in younger patients with acute myelogenous leukemia (AML). Proc Am Soc Clin Oncol 1998;17:15a.

122. Ferrant A, Doyen C, Delannoy A, et al: Karyotype in acute myeloblastic leukemia: Prognostic significance in a prospective study assessing bone marrow transplantation in first remission. Bone Marrow Transplant 1995;15:685.

123. Gale R, Horowitz M, Weiner R, et al: Impact of cytogenetic abnormalities on outcome of bone marrow transplants in acute myelogenous leukemia in first remission. Bone Marrow Transplant 1995;16:203.

124. Cheson B, Cassileth P, Head D, et al: Definition of CR. Report of the National Cancer Institute–sponsored workshop on definitions of diagnosis and response in acute myeloid leukemia. J Clin Oncol 1990;8:813.

125. Skipper H, Schabel F, Jay R, et al: Experimental evaluation of potential anti-tumour agents: On the criteria and kinetics associated with the curability of experimental leukaemia. Cancer Chemother Rep 1964;35:1.

126. Bridges J, Hawes D, Nelson M: Therapy of acute leukaemia—comparison of initial treatment with 6-mercaptopurine alone and in combination with steroids. Br J Cancer 1962;16:46.

127. Medical Research Council: Treatment of acute leukaemia in adults. Comparison of steroid therapy at high and low dosage in conjunction with 6-mercaptopurine. Br Med J 1963;1:7.

128. Vogler W, Huguley C, Rundles R: Comparison of methotrexate with 6-mercaptopurine and prednisolone in treatment of acute leukemia in adults. Cancer 1967;20:1221.

129. Armentrout S, Burns C: Cytosine arabinoside as a single agent in the therapy of adult acute leukemia. Am J Med Sci 1974;268:168.

130. Bodey G, Freireich E, Monto R, et al: Cytosine arabinoside (NSC-63879) therapy for acute leukemia in adults. Cancer Chemother Rep 1969;53:59.

131. Bodey G, Coltman C, Freireich E, et al: Chemotherapy of acute leukemia. A comparison of cytarabine alone and in combination with vincristine, prednisolone and cyclophosphamide. Arch Intern Med 1974;133:260.

132. Carey R, Ribas-Mundo M, Ellison R, et al: Comparative study of cytosine arabinoside alone and combined with thioguanine, mercaptopurine and daunorubicin in acute myelocytic leukemia. Cancer 1975;30:1560.

133. Ellison R, Holland J, Weil M, et al: Arabinoside cytosine; a useful agent in the treatment of acute leukemia in adults. Blood 1968;32:507.

134. Howard T, Albo V, Newton W: Cytosine arabinoside. Results of a comparative study in acute childhood leukemia. Cancer 1968;21:341.

135. South West Oncology Group: Cytarabine for acute leukemia in adults. Effect of schedule on therapeutic response. Arch Intern Med 1974;133:251.

136. Weil M, Glidewell O, Jacquillat D, et al: Daunorubicin in the treatment of acute granulocytic leukemia. Cancer Res 1973;33:921.

137. Weil M, Jacquillat C, Gemon-Aucler M, et al: Acute granuocytic leukemia. Treatment of the disease. Arch Intern Med 1976;136:1389.

138. Boiron M, Jacquillat C, Weil M, et al: Daunorubicin in the treatment of acute myelocytic leukemia. Lancet 1969;1:330.

139. Wiernik P, Glidewell O, Hoagland H, et al: A comparative trial of duanorubicin, cytosine arabinoside and thioguanine, and a combination of the three agents for the treatment of acute myelocytic leukemia. Med Pediatr Oncol 1979;6:261.

140. Wiernik P, Schimpff S, Schiffer C, et al: A randomised comparison of duanorubicin alone with a combination of duanorubicin, cytosine arabinoside, thioguanine and pyrimethamine for the treatment of acute non-lymphocytic leukemia. Cancer Treat Rep 1976;60:41.

141. Schwarzenberg J, Misset J, Poullart P: Adriamycin in the treatment of acute leukaemias and non-Hodgkin's lymphomas. Adriamycin Review III 1975;187.

142. Wang J, Cortes E, Sinks L, et al: Therapeutic effect and toxicity of adriamycin in patients with neoplastic disease. Cancer 1971; 28:837.

143. Wilson H, Bodey C, Moon T, et al: Adriamycin therapy in previously treated adult acute leukemia. Cancer Treat Rep 1977; 61:905.

144. Crowther D: The treatment of acute leukaemia. Br J Hosp Med 1971;6:171.

145. Cassileth P, Katz M: Chemotherapy for adult acute nonlymphocytic leukemia with daunorubicin and cytosine arabinoside. Cancer Treat Rep 1979;61:1441.

146. Edelstein M, Vietti T, Valoriote F: Schedule dependent synergism for the combination of 1-β-D-arabinofuranosyl cytosine and daunorubicin. Cancer Res 1973;33:293.

147. Yates J, Wallace J, Ellison R, et al: Cytosine arabinoside (NSC-63878) and daunorubicin (NSC-83142) therapy in acute non-lymphocytic leukemia. Cancer Treat Rep 1973;4:485.

148. Omura G, Vogler W, Lefante J, et al: Treatment of acute myelogenous leukemia: Influence of three induction regimens and maintenance chemotherapy or BCG immunotherapy. Cancer 1982;49: 1530.

149. Preisler H, Rustum Y, Henderson E, et al: Treatment of acute nonlymphocytic leukemia. Use of anthracycline–cytosine arabinoside induction therapy and comparison of 2 maintenance regimens. Blood 1979;53:455.

150. Yates J, Glidewell O, Wiernik P, et al: Cytosine arabinoside with daunorubicin or adriamycin for therapy of acute myelocytic leukemia: A CALGB study. Blood 1982;60:454.

151. Preisler H, Davis R, Krishner J, et al: Comparison of three remission induction regimens and two postinduction strategies for the treatment of acute non-lymphocytic leukemia. A Cancer and Leukemia Group B study. Blood 1987;69:1441.

152. Preisler H, Raza A, Early A, et al: Intensive remission induction and consolidation therapy in the treatment of acute nonlymphocytic leukemia. J Clin Oncol 1987;5:722.

153. Yates J, Wallace H, Ellison R, et al: Cytosine arabinoside and daunorubicin therapy in acute nonlymphocytic leukemia. Cancer Chemother Rep 1973;52:485.

154. Vogler W, Barlotini A, Omura G, et al: A randomised clinical trial of remission induction, consolidation and chemo-immunotherapy maintenance in adult acute myeloblastic leukemia. Cancer Immunol Immunother 1978;3:163.

155. Amadori S, Papa G, Meloni G, et al: Daunorubicin cytosine arabinoside and 6-thioguanine (DAT) combination therapy for the treatment of acute nonlymphocytic leukemia. Leuk Res 1979;3:147.

156. Cassileth P, Begg C, Bennett J, et al: A randomized study of the efficacy of consolidation therapy in adult acute nonlymphocytic leukemia. Blood 1984;63:843.

157. Cassileth P, Begg C, Siber R, et al: Prolonged unmaintained remission after intensive consolidation therapy in adult non-lymphocytic leukemia. Cancer Treat Rep 1987;71:137.

158. Champlin R, Jacobs A, Gale R, et al: Prolonged survival in acute myelogenous leukemia without maintenance chemotherapy. Lancet 1984;1:894.

159. Finnish Leukemia Group: The effect of thioguanine in a combination of daunorubicin, cytarabine and prednisolone in the treatment of acute leukaemia in adults. Scand J Haematol 1979;23:124.

160. Gale R, Cline M: High remission induction rate in acute myeloid leukaemia. Lancet 1977;1:497.

161. Gale R, Foon K, Cline M, et al: Intensive chemotherapy for acute myelogenous leukemia. Ann Intern Med 1981;94:753.

162. Glucksberg H, Cheever M, Farewell V, et al: High dose combination chemotherapy for acute nonlymphoblastic leukemia in adults. Cancer 1981;48:1073.

163. Rees J, Hayhoe F: DAT (daunorubicin, cytarabine, 6-thioguanine) in acute myeloid leukaemia. Lancet 1978;1:1260.

164. Rees J, Gray R, Swirsky D, et al: Principal results of the Medical Research Council's 8th acute myeloid leukaemia trial. Lancet 1986; 2:1236.

165. Hann I, Stevens R, Goldstone A, et al: Randomized comparison of DAT versus ADE as induction chemotherapy in children and younger adults with acute myeloid leukemia: Results of the Medical Research Council's 10th AML Trial (MRC AML10). Blood 1997; 89:2311.

166. Arlin S, Gee T, Fried J, et al: Rapid induction of remission in acute

non-lymphocytic leukemia (ANLL). Proc Am Assoc Cancer Res 1979;20:112.

167. Rohatiner A, Gregory W, Bassan R, et al: Short term therapy for acute myelogenous leukemia. J Clin Oncol 1988;6:218.

168. Baudard M, Beauchamp-Nicoud A, Delmer A, et al: Has the prognosis of adult patients with acute myeloid leukemia improved over years? A single institution experience of 784 consecutive patients over a 16-year period. Leukemia 1999;13:1481.

169. Mauritzson N, Johansson B, Albin M, et al: Survival time in a population-based consecutive series of adult acute myeloid leukemia—the prognostic impact of karyotype during the time period 1976–1993. Leukemia 2000;14:1039.

170. Arlin Z, Case DJ, Moore J, et al: Randomized multicenter trial of cytosine arabinoside with mitoxantrone or daunorubicin in previously untreated adult patients with acute nonlymphocytic leukemia (ANLl). Leukemia 1990;4:177.

171. Brito-Babapulle F, Catovsky D, Slocombe G, et al: Phase II study of mitoxantrone and cytarabine in acute myeloid leukemia. Cancer Treat Rep 1987;71:161.

172. MacCallum P, Davis D, Rohatiner A, et al: Mitoxantrone and cytosine arabinoside as treatment for acute myelogenous leukemia (AML) at first recurrence. Leukemia 1993;7:1496.

173. Paciucci P, Cuttner J, Holland J: Mitoxantrone as a single agent and in combination chemotherapy in patients with refractory acute leukemia. Semin Oncol 1984;11:36.

174. MacCallum P, Rohatiner A, Davis C, et al: Mitoxantrone and cytosine arabinoside as treatment for acute myeloblastic leukemia in older patients. Ann Hematol 1995;71:35.

175. Lowenberg B, Suciu S, Archimbaud E, et al: Mitoxantrone versus daunorubicin in induction-consolidation chemotherapy—the value of low-dose cytarabine for maintenance of remission, and an assessment of prognostic factors in acute myeloid leukemia in the elderly: Final report. European Organization for the Research and Treatment of Cancer and the Dutch-Belgian Hemato-Oncology Cooperative Hovon Group. J Clin Oncol 1998;16:872.

176. Rowe J, Neuberg D, Friedenberg W, et al: A phase III study of daunorubicin vs idarubicin vs mitoxantrone for older adult patients (>55 years) with acute myelogenous leukemia (AML): A study of the Eastern European Cooperative Oncology Group. Blood 1998;92:1284a.

177. Berman E, McBride M: Comparative cellular pharmacology of daunorubicin and idarubicin in human multidrug-resistant leukemia cells. Blood 1992;79:3267.

178. Vogler W, Velez-Garcia E, Weiner R, et al: A phase III trial comparing idarubicin and daunorubicin in acute myelogenous leukemia: A Southeastern Cancer Study Group study. J Clin Oncol 1992; 10:1103.

179. Berman E, Heller G, Santorsa J, et al: Results of a randomized trial comparing idarubicin and cytosine arabinoside with daunorubicin and cytosine arabinoside in adult patients with newly diagnosed acute myelogenous leukemia. Blood 1991;77:1666.

180. Wiernik P, Banks P, Case D Jr, et al: Cytarabine plus idarubicin or daunorubicin as induction and consolidation therapy for previously untreated adult patients with acute myeloid leukemia. Blood 1992;79:313.

181. Hertzig R, Lazarus H, Wolff S, et al: High-dose cytosine arabinoside therapy with and without anthracycline antibiotics for remission reinduction of acute non-lymphoblastic leukemia. J Clin Oncol 1985;3:992.

182. Preisler H, Early A, Raza A, et al: High-dose cytosine arabinoside as the initial treatment of poor-risk patients with acute non-lymphocytic leukemia—a Leukemia Intergroup study. J Clin Oncol 1987;5:75.

183. Mitus A, Miller K, Schenkein D, et al: Improved survival of patients with acute myelogenous leukemia. J Clin Oncol 1995;13:560.

184. Weick J, Kopecky K, Appelbaum F, et al: A randomized investigation of high-dose versus standard-dose cytosine arabinoside with daunorubicin in patients with previously untreated acute myeloid leukemia: A Southwest Oncology Group study. Blood 1996;88: 2841.

185. Bishop J, Matthews J, Young G, et al: A randomized study of high-dose cytarabine in induction in acute myeloid leukemia. Blood 1996;87:1710.

186. Bishop J, Matthews J, Young G, et al: Intensified induction chemotherapy with high-dose cytarabine and etoposide for acute myeloid

leukemia: A review and updated results of the Australian Leukemia Study Group. Leuk Lymphoma 1998;28:315.

187. Ghandi V, Estey E, Keating M, et al: Fludarabine potentiates metabolism of cytarabine in patients with acute myelogenous leukemia during therapy. J Clin Oncol 1993;11:116.

188. Strickland AH, Seymour C, Prince HM, et al: Fludarabine and high dose cytarabine (FLA): A well tolerated salvage regimen in acute myeloid leukemia. Aust N Z J Med 1999;29:556.

189. Estey E, Thall P, Andreef M, et al: Use of granulocyte colony stimulating factor before, during and after fludarabine plus cytarabine induction therapy of newly diagnosed acute myelogenous leukemia or myelodysplastic syndromes: Comparison with fludarabine plus cytarabine without granulocyte colony stimulating factor. J Clin Oncol 1994;12:671.

190. Clavio M, Carrara P, Miglino M, et al: High efficacy of fludarabine-containing therapy (FLAG-FLANG) in poor risk acute myeloid leukemia. Haematologica 1996;81:513.

191. Ferrara F, Melillo L, Montillo M, et al: Fludarabine, cytarabine, and G-CSF (FLAG) for the treatment of acute myeloid leukemia relapsing after autologous stem cell transplantation. Ann Hematol 1999; 78:380.

192. Visani G, Lemoli R, Tosi P, et al: Fludarabine-containing regimens severely impair peripheral blood stem cells mobilization and collection in acute myeloid leukaemia patients. Br J Haematol 1999; 105:775.

193. Ho A, Brado B, Haas R, et al: Etoposide in acute leukemia. Past experience and future perspectives. Cancer 1991;67:281.

194. Rivera G, Abery T, Roberts D: Response of L1210 to combination of cytosine arabinoside and VM-26 or VP16-213. Eur J Cancer 1975;11:639.

195. Lowenthal R, Bradstock K, Matthews J, et al: A Phase I/II study of intensive dose escalation of cytarabine in combination with idarubicin and etoposide in induction and consolidation treatment of adult acute myeloid leukemia. Leuk Lymphoma 1999;34:501.

196. Rohatiner A, Bassan R, Bjorkholm M, et al: High-dose treatment (HDT) with peripheral blood progenitor cell (PBPC) support as consolidation of first remission in younger patients (pts) with acute myelogenous leukemia (AML). Blood 1998;92:1198.

197. Embury S, Elias L, Heller P, et al: Remission maintenance therapy in acute myelogenous leukemia. West J Med 1977;126:267.

198. Cassileth P, Harrington D, Hines J, et al: Maintenance chemotherapy prolongs remission duration in adult acute nonlymphocytic leukemia. J Clin Oncol 1988;6:583.

199. Keating M, McCredia K, Bodey G, et al: Improved prospects for long-term survival in adults with acute myelogenous leukemia. JAMA 1982;248:2481.

200. Mayer R: Current chemotherapeutic treatment approaches to the management of previously untreated adults with de novo acute myeloblastic leukemia. Semin Oncol 1987;14:384.

201. Petersen B, Bloomfield C: Long term disease-free survival in acute nonlymphocytic leukemia. Blood 1981;57:1144.

202. Petersen B, Bloomfield C: Prolonged maintained remissions of adult acute nonlymphoblastic leukaemia. Lancet 1977;2:158.

203. Kufe D, Major P, Egan E, et al: Correlation of cytotoxicity with incorporation of ara-C into DNA. J Biol Chem 1980;253:8970.

204. Plunkett W, Liliemark J, Estey E, et al: Saturation of ara-CTP accumulation during high dose ara-C therapy: Pharmacologic rationale for intermediate dose ara-C. Semin Oncol 1987;14:159.

205. Rustum Y, Preisler H: Correlation between leukemic cell retention of 1-β-D-arabinosylcytosine-5′-triphosphate and response to therapy. Cancer Res 1979;39:42.

206. Plunkett W, Lacoboni S, Estey E, et al: Pharmacologically directed ara-C therapy for refractory leukemia. Semin Oncol 1985;12:20.

207. Champlin R, Gajewski J, Nimer S, et al: Post remission chemotherapy for adults with acute myelogenous leukemia: Improved survival with high-dose cytarabine and daunorubicin as consolidation treatment. J Clin Oncol 1990;8:1199.

208. Tricot G, Boogaerts M, Vlietinek R, et al: The role of intensive remission induction and consolidation therapy in patients with acute myeloid leukaemia. Br J Haematol 1987;66:37.

209. Wolff S, Herzig R, Fay J, et al: High-dose cytarabine and daunorubicin as consolidation therapy for acute myeloid leukemia in first remission: Long term follow up and results. J Clin Oncol 1989; 7:1260.

210. Phillips G, Reece D, Shepherd J, et al: High-dose cytarabine and

211. Mayer R, Davis R, Schiffer C, et al: Intensive post remission chemotherapy in adults with acute myeloid leukemia. N Engl J Med 1994;331:896.

212. Cassileth P, Lynch E, Hines J, et al: Varying intensity of post remission therapy in acute myeloid leukemia. Blood 1992;79:1924.

213. Fopp M, Fey M, Bacchi M, et al: Post-remission therapy of adult acute myeloid leukaemia: One cycle of high-dose versus standard-dose cytarabine. Leukaemia Project Group of the Swiss Group for Clinical Cancer Research (SAKK). Ann Oncol 1997;8:251.

214. Harousseau J, Milpied N, Briere J, et al: Double intensive consolidation chemotherapy in adult acute myeloid leukemia. J Clin Oncol 1991;9:1432.

215. Willemze R, Fibbe W, Kluin-Nelemans J, et al: Bone marrow transplantation or chemotherapy as post remission treatment of adult acute myelogenous leukemia. Ann Hematol 1991;62:59.

216. Carella A, Frassoni F, Van Lint M, et al: Autologous and allogeneic bone marrow transplantation in acute myeloid leukemia in first complete remission: An update of the Genoa experience with 159 patients. Ann Hematol 1992;64:128.

217. Linker C, Ries C, Damon L, et al: Autologous bone marrow transplantation for acute myeloid leukemia using busulfan plus etoposide as a preparative regimen. Blood 1993;81:311.

218. Stein A, O'Donnell M, Lee J, et al: Phase 2 study of interleukin-2 following autologous stem cell transplant for adult patients with acute myelogenous leukemia in first complete remission. Blood 1997;90:180.

219. Crilley P, Topolsky D, Styler M, et al: Extramedullary toxicity of a conditioning regimen containing busulfan, cyclophosphamide and etoposide in 84 patients undergoing autologous and allogeneic bone marrow transplantation. Bone Marrow Transplant 1995;15: 361.

220. Beelen D, Quabeck K, Graeven U, et al: Acute toxicity and first clinical results of intensive post induction therapy using a modified busulfan and cyclophosphamide regimen with autologous bone marrow rescue in first complete remission of acute myeloid leukemia. Blood 1989;74:1507.

221. McMillan A, Goldstone A, Linch D, et al: High-dose chemotherapy and autologous bone marrow transplantation in acute myeloid leukemia. Blood 1990;76:480.

222. Miggiano M, Gherlizoni F, Rossi G, et al: Autologous bone marrow transplantation in late first complete remission improves outcome in acute myelogenous leukemia. Leukemia 1996;10:402.

223. Mehta J, Powles R, Singhal S, et al: Autologous bone marrow transplantation for acute myeloid leukemia in first remission: Identification of modifiable prognostic factors. Bone Marrow Transplant 1995;16:499.

224. Burnett A, Pendry K, Rawlinson P, et al: Autograft to eliminate minimal residual disease in AML in first remission—update on the Glasgow experience. Bone Marrow Transplant 1990;6:59.

225. Lowenberg B, Verdonch L, Dekker A, et al: Autologous bone marrow transplantation in acute myeloid leukemia in first remission: Results of a Dutch prospective study. J Clin Oncol 1990; 8:287.

226. Rohatiner A, Bassan R, Raimondi R, et al: High-dose treatment with autologous bone marrow support as consolidation of first remission in younger patients with acute myelogenous leukemia. Ann Oncol 2000;11:1007.

227. Gorin N, Labopin M, Meloni G, et al: Autologous bone marrow transplantation for acute myeloblastic leukemia in Europe: Further evidence of the role of marrow purging by mafosfamide. Leukemia 1991;5:896.

228. Clift R, Buckner C, Appelbaum F, et al: Allogeneic marrow transplantation in patients with acute myeloid leukemia in first remission: A randomized trial of two irradiation regimens. Blood 1990; 76:1867.

229. Bortin M, Horowitz M, Rowlings P, et al: 1993 Progress report from the International Bone Marrow Transplant Registry. Bone Marrow Transplant 1993;12:97.

230. Forman S, Spruce W, Farbstein M, et al: Bone marrow ablation followed by allogeneic marrow grafting during first complete remission of acute nonlymphocytic leukemia. Blood 1983;61:439.

231. Bostrom B, Brunning R, McGlave P, et al: Bone marrow transplanta-

tion for acute nonlymphocytic leukemia in first remission: Analysis of prognostic factors. Blood 1985;65:1191.

232. Clift R, Buckner C, Thomas E, et al: The treatment of acute non-lymphoblastic leukemia by allogeneic marrow transplantation. Bone Marrow Transplant 1987;2:243.

233. Helenglass G, Powles R, McElwain T, et al: Melphalan and total body irradiation (TBI) versus cyclophosphamide and TBI as conditioning for allogeneic matched sibling bone marrow transplants for acute myeloblastic leukaemia in first remission. Bone Marrow Transplant 1988;3:21.

234. McGlave P, Haake R, Bostrom B, et al: Allogeneic bone marrow transplantation for acute nonlymphocytic leukemia in first remission. Blood 1988;72:1512.

235. Kim T, McGlave P, Ramsay N, et al: Comparison of two total body irradiation regimens in allogeneic bone marrow transplantation for acute non-lymphoblastic leukemia in first remission. Int J Radiat Oncol Biol Phys 1990;19:889.

236. Young J, Papadopoulos E, Cunningham I, et al: T-cell–depleted allogeneic bone marrow transplantation in adults with acute nonlymphocytic leukemia in first remission. Blood 1992;79:3380.

237. Bassan R, Raimondi R, Lerede T, et al: Outcome assessment of age group specific (± 50 years) post-remission consolidation with high-dose cytarabine or bone marrow autograft for adult acute myelogenous leukemia. Haematologica 1998;83:627.

238. Zittoun R, Mandelli F, Willemze R, et al: Autologous or allogeneic bone marrow transplantation compared with intensive chemotherapy in acute myelogenous leukemia. N Engl J Med 1995;332:217.

239. Keating S, de Witte T, Suciu S, et al: Centre effect on treatment outcome for patients with untreated acute myelogenous leukaemia? An analysis of the AML 8A study of the Leukemia Cooperative Group of the EORTC and GIMEMA. European Organisation for Research and Treatment of Cancer (EORTC), Leukemia Cooperative Group and the Gruppo Italiano Malattie Ematologiche Maligne dell'Adulto (GIMEMA). Eur J Cancer 1999;35:1440.

240. Harousseau J, Cahn J, Pignon B, et al: Comparison of autologous bone marrow transplantation and intensive chemotherapy as post remission therapy in adult acute myeloid leukemia. Blood 1997; 90:2978.

241. Cassileth P, Harrington D, Appelbaum F, et al: Chemotherapy compared with autologous or allogeneic bone marrow transplantation in the management of acute myeloid leukemia in first remission. N Engl J Med 1998;339:1649.

242. Burnett A, Goldstone A, Stevens R, et al: Randomised comparison of addition of autologous bone-marrow transplantation to intensive chemotherapy for acute myeloid leukaemia in first remission: Results of MRC AML 10 trial. Lancet 1998;351:700.

243. Brenner M, Rill D, Moen R, et al: Gene-marking to trace origin of relapse after autologous bone marrow transplantation. Lancet 1993;341:85.

244. Rizzoli V, Mangoni L, Carlo-Stella C, et al: Autologous marrow transplantation in first remission acute myeloid leukemia using marrow purged with mafosfamide. Bone Marrow Transplant 1991; 2:37.

245. Korbling M, Fliedner T, Holle R, et al: Autologous blood stem cell (ABSCT) versus purged bone marrow transplantation (pABMT) in standard risk AML: Influence of source and cell composition of the autograft on hemopoietic reconstitution and disease-free survival. Bone Marrow Transplant 1991;7:343.

246. Yeager A, Kaizer H, Santos G, et al: Autologous bone marrow transplantation in patients with acute nonlymphocytic leukemia using ex vivo marrow treatment with 4-hydroperoxycyclophosphamide. N Engl J Med 1986;315:141.

247. Gorin N, Labopin M, Laporte J, et al: Importance of marrow dose on post transplant outcome in acute leukemia: Models derived from patients autografted with mafosfamide-purged marrow at a single institution. Exp Hematol 1999;27:1822.

248. de Fabritis P, Ferrero D, Sandrelli A, et al: Monoclonal antibody purging and autologous bone marrow transplantation in acute myelogenous leukemia in complete remission. Bone Marrow Transplant 1989;4:669.

249. Robertson M, Griffin J, Soiffer R, et al: Hematologic engraftment in patients with AML after ablative therapy and reinfusion of anti-MY9 (anti-CD33) antibody purged autologous bone marrow. Blood 1989;74:283.

250. Ball E, Wilson J, Phelps V, et al: Autologous bone marrow trans-

plantation for acute myeloid leukemia in remission or first relapse using monoclonal antibody–purged marrow: Results of phase II studies with long-term follow-up. Bone Marrow Transplant 2000; 25:823.

251. Chang J, Continho L, Morganstein G, et al: Reconstitution of haematopoietic system with autologous marrow taken during relapse of acute myeloblastic leukaemia and grown in long term culture. Lancet 1986;1:294.

252. Chang J, Continho L, Morganstein G, et al: The use of bone marrow cells grown in longer term culture for autologous bone marrow transplantation in acute myeloid leukemia: An update. Bone Marrow Transplant 1989;4:5.

253. Visani G, Lemoli R, Tosi P, et al: Use of peripheral blood stem cells for autologous transplantation in acute myeloid leukemia patients allows faster engraftment and equivalent disease-free survival compared with bone marrow cells. Bone Marrow Transplant 1999; 24:467.

254. Gondo H, Harada M, Miyamoto T, et al: Autologous peripheral blood stem cell transplantation for acute myelogenous leukemia. Bone Marrow Transplant 1997;20:821.

255. Schiller G, Lee M, Paquette R, et al: Transplantation of autologous peripheral blood progenitor cells procured after high-dose cytarabine-based consolidation chemotherapy for adults with secondary acute myelogenous leukemia in first remission. Leuk Lymphoma 1999;33:475.

256. Sanz M, de la Rubia J, Sanz G, et al: Busulfan plus cyclophosphamide followed by autologous blood stem cell transplantation for patients with acute myeloblastic leukemia in first complete remission: A report from a single institution. J Clin Oncol 1993;11:1661.

257. Reiffers J, Bernard P, David B, et al: Successful autologous transplantation with peripheral blood hematopoietic cells in a patient with acute leukemia. Exp Hematol 1986;14:312.

258. Ojeda E, Garcia-Bustos J, Aguado M, et al: A prospective randomized trial of granulocyte colony-stimulating factor therapy after autologous blood stem cell transplantation in adults. Bone Marrow Transplant 1999;24:601.

259. Mehta J, Powles R, Singhal S, et al: Peripheral blood stem cells transplantation may result in increased relapse of acute myeloid leukaemia due to reinfusion of a higher number of malignant cells. Bone Marrow Transplant 1995;15:652.

260. Laporte J, Gorin N, Feuchtenbaum J, et al: Relapse after autografting with peripheral blood stem cells. Lancet 1987;2:1393.

261. Reiffers J, Labopin M, Sanz M, et al: Autologous blood cell vs marrow transplantation for acute myeloid leukemia in complete remission: An EBMT retrospective analysis. Bone Marrow Transplant 2000;25:1115.

262. Gratwohl A, Passweg J, Baldomero H, et al: Blood and marrow transplantation activity in Europe 1997. Bone Marrow Transplant 1999;24:231.

263. Weaver C, Clift R, Deeg H, et al: Effect of graft-versus-host disease prophylaxis on relapse in patients transplanted by acute myeloid leukemia. Bone Marrow Transplant 1994;14:885.

264. Nash R, Pepe M, Storb R, et al: Acute graft-versus-host disease: Analysis of risk factors after allogeneic marrow transplantation and prophylaxis with cyclosporine and methotrexate. Blood 1992; 80:1838.

265. Soiffer R, Fairclough D, Robertson M, et al: CD6-depleted allogeneic bone marrow transplantation for acute leukemia in first complete remission. Blood 1997;89:3039.

266. Papadopoulos E, Carabasi M, Castro-Malaspina H, et al: T-cell depleted allogeneic bone marrow transplantation as post remission therapy for acute myelogenous leukemia: Freedom from relapse in the absence of graft-versus-host disease. Blood 1998;91:1083.

267. Keating S, Suciu S, de Witte T, et al: Prognostic factors of patients with acute myeloid leukemia (AML) allografted in first complete remission: An analysis of the EORTC-GIMEMA AML 8A trial. The European Organization for Research and Treatment of Cancer (EORTC) and the Gruppo Italiano Malattie Ematologiche Maligne dell' Adulto (GIMEMA) Leukemia Cooperative Groups. Bone Marrow Transplant 1996;17:993.

268. Schmitz N, Bacigalupo A, Labopin M, et al: Transplantation of peripheral blood progenitor cells from HLA-identical sibling donors. European Group for Blood and Marrow Transplantation (EBMT). Br J Haematol 1996;95:715.

269. Hagglund H, Ringden O, Remberger M, et al: Faster neutrophil

and platelet engraftment, but no differences in acute GVHD or survival, using peripheral blood stem cells from related and unrelated donors, compared to bone marrow. Bone Marrow Transplant 1998;22:131.

270. Brown R, Adkins D, Khoury H, et al: Long-term follow-up of high-risk allogeneic peripheral-blood stem-cell transplant recipients: Graft-versus-host disease and transplant-related mortality. J Clin Oncol 1999;17:806.

271. Arslan O, Unstun C, Arat M, et al: Allogeneic peripheral blood stem cell transplantation in acute non-lymphoblastic leukemia. Hematol Oncol 1998;16:155.

272. Russell J, Larratt L, Brown C, et al: Allogeneic blood stem cell and bone marrow transplantation for acute myelogenous leukemia and myelodysplasia: Influence of stem cell source on outcome. Bone Marrow Transplant 1999;24:1177.

273. Powles R, Mehta J, Kulkami S, et al: Allogeneic blood and bone marrow stem cell transplantation in haematological malignant diseases: A randomised trial. Lancet 2000;355:1231.

274. Clift R, Hansen J, Thomas E, et al: Marrow transplantation from donors other than HLA-identical siblings. Transplantation 1979;28:235.

275. Howard M, Hows J, Gore S, et al: Unrelated donor marrow transplantation between 1977 and 1987 at four centres in the United Kingdom. Transplantation 1990;49:547.

276. Phillips G, Barnett M, Brain M, et al: Allogeneic bone marrow transplantation using unrelated donors. A pilot study of the Canadian Bone Marrow Transplant Group. Bone Marrow Transplant 1991;8:477.

277. Kernan N, Bartsch G, Ash R, et al: Analysis of 462 transplantations from unrelated donors facilitated by the National Marrow Donor Program. N Engl J Med 1993;328:593.

278. Schiller G, Feig S, Territo M, et al: Treatment of advanced acute leukaemia with allogeneic bone marrow transplantation from unrelated donors. Br J Haematol 1994;88:72.

279. McSweeney P, Niederwieser D, Shizuru A, et al: Outpatient allografting with minimally myelosuppressive, immunosuppressive conditioning of low-dose TBI and postgrafting cyclosporine (CSP) and mycophenolate mofetil (MMF). Blood 1999;94:1742a.

280. Slavin S, Nagler A, Naparstek G, et al: Well tolerated non-myeloablative fludarabine-based protocols for the treatment of malignant and non-malignant disorders with allogeneic bone marrow or blood stem cell transplantation. Blood 1999;94:1562.5a.

281. Giralt S, Estey E, Albitar M: Engraftment of allogeneic hematopoietic progenitor cells with purine analog–containing chemotherapy: Harnessing graft-versus-leukemia without myeloablative therapy. Blood 1997;89:4531.

282. Amadori S, Arcese W, Isacchi G, et al: Mitoxantrone, etoposide and intermediate dose cytarabine: An effective and tolerable regimen for the treatment of refractory acute myeloid leukemia. J Clin Oncol 1991;9:1210.

283. Ho A, Lipp T, Ehninger G, et al: Combination of mitoxantrone and etoposide in refractory acute myelogenous leukemia: An active and well tolerated regimen. J Clin Oncol 1988;6:213.

284. Martinez J, Martin G, Sanz G, et al: A phase II clinical trial of carboplatin infusion in high risk nonlymphoblastic leukemia. J Clin Oncol 1991;9:39.

285. Brown R, Herzig R, Wolff S, et al: High dose etoposide and cyclophosphamide without bone marrow transplantation for resistant hematologic malignancy. Blood 1990;76:473.

286. Santana V, Mirro JJ, Kearns C, et al: Chlorodeoxyadenosine produces a high rate of complete hematologic remission in relapsed acute myeloid leukemia. J Clin Oncol 1992;10:364.

287. Kantarjian H, Beran M, Ellis A, et al: Phase I study of topotecan, a new topoisomerase I inhibitor in patients with refractory or relapsed acute leukemia. Blood 1993;81:1146.

288. De Witte T, Suciu S, Selleslag D, et al: Salvage treatment for primary resistant acute myelogenous leukemia consisting of intermediate-dose cytosine arabinoside and interspaced continuous infusions of idarubicin: A phase-II study (no. 06901) of the EORTC Leukemia Cooperative Group. Ann Hematol 1996;72:119.

289. Angelov L, Brandwein J, Baker M: Results of therapy for acute myeloid leukemia in first relapse. Leuk Lymphoma 1991;6:15.

290. Thalhammer F, Geissler K, Jager U, et al: Duration of second complete remission in patients with acute myeloid leukemia treated with chemotherapy: A retrospective single-center study. Ann Hematol 1996;72:216.

291. Vey N, Keating M, Rios M, et al: Effect of CR on survival in patients with AML receiving first salvage therapy. Blood 1998;92:235a.

292. Vignetti M, Orsini E, Petti M, et al: Probability of long-term disease-free survival for acute myeloid leukemia patients after first relapse: A single-centre experience. Ann Oncol 1996;7:933.

293. Davies C, Rohatiner A, Lim J, et al: The management of recurrent acute myelogenous leukaemia at a single centre over a 15 year period. Br J Haematol 1993;83:404.

294. Whelan J, Davis C, Leahy M, et al: Etoposide in combination with intermediate cytosine arabinoside given with the intention of further myeloablative therapy for the treatment of refractory or recurrent hematological malignancy. Hematol Oncol 1992;10:87.

295. Estey E, Kornblau S, Pierce S: A stratification system for evaluating therapies in patients with relapsed or primary refractory myeloid leukemia. Blood 1996;88:756.

296. Archimbaud E, Leblond V, Fenaux P, et al: Timed sequential chemotherapy for advanced acute myeloid leukemia. Hematol Cell Ther 1996;38:161.

297. Raanani P, Shpilberg O, Gillis S, et al: Salvage therapy of refractory and relapsed acute leukemia with high-dose mitoxantrone and high-dose cytarabine. Leuk Res 1999;23:695.

298. Bassan R, Lerede T, Buelli M, et al: A new combination of carboplatin, high-dose cytarabine and cross-over mitoxantrone or idarubicin for refractory and relapsed acute myeloid leukemia. Haematologica 1998;83:422.

299. Rosenfeld C, Shadduck R, Przepiorka D, et al: Autologous bone marrow transplantation with 4-hydroperoxycyclophosphamide purged marrow for acute non-lymphocytic leukemia in late remission or early relapse. Blood 1989;74:1159.

300. Chopra R, Goldstone A, McMillan A, et al: Successful treatment of acute myeloid leukemia beyond first remission with autologous bone marrow transplantation using busulfan/cyclophosphamide and unpurged marrow. The British Autograft Group experience. J Clin Oncol 1991;9:1840.

301. Meloni G, Vignetti M, Avvisati G, et al: BAVC regimen and autograft for acute myelogenous leukemia in second complete remission. Bone Marrow Transplant 1996;18:693.

302. Busca A, Anasetti C, Anderson G, et al: Unrelated donor or autologous marrow transplantation for treatment of acute leukemia. Blood 1994;83:3077.

303. Appelbaum F, Clift R, Buckner C, et al: Allogeneic marrow transplantation for acute nonlymphoblastic leukemia after first relapse. Blood 1983;61:949.

304. Forman S, Schmidt G, Nademanee A, et al: Allogeneic bone marrow transplantation as therapy for primary induction failure for patients with acute leukemia. J Clin Oncol 1991;9:1570.

305. Grigg A, Szer J, Beresford J, et al: Factors affecting the outcome of allogeneic bone marrow transplantation for adult patients with refractory or relapsed acute leukaemia. Br J Haematol 1999;107:409.

306. Tomas F, Gomez-Garcia de Soria V, Lopez-Lorenzo J, et al: Autologous or allogeneic bone marrow transplantation for acute myeloblastic leukemia in second complete remission. Importance of duration of first complete remission in final outcome. Bone Marrow Transplant 1996;17:979.

307. Gale R, Horowitz M, Rees J, et al: Chemotherapy versus transplants for acute myelogenous leukemia in second remission. Leukemia 1996;10:13.

308. Gorin N, Labopin M, Fouillard L, et al: Retrospective evaluation of autologous bone marrow transplantation vs allogeneic bone marrow transplantation from an HLA identical related donor in acute myelocyte leukemia. A study of the European Cooperative Group for Blood and Marrow Transplantation (EBMT). Bone Marrow Transplant 1996;18:111.

309. Ringden O, Labopin M, Frassoni F, et al: Allogeneic bone marrow transplant or second autograft in patients with acute leukemia who relapse after an autograft. Bone Marrow Transplant 1999;24:389.

310. Mrsic M, Horowitz M, Atkinson K, et al: Second HLA identical transplants for leukemia recurrence. Bone Marrow Transplant 1992;9:269.

311. Barrett A, Locatelli E, Treleaven J, et al: Second transplants for leukaemic relapse after bone marrow transplantation: High early mortality but favourable effect of chronic GVHD on continued remission. A report by the EBMT Leukaemia Working Party. Br J Haematol 1991;79:567.

312. Radich J, Sanders J, Buckner C, et al: Second allogeneic marrow transplantation for patients with recurrent leukemia after initial transplant with total body irradiation containing regimens. J Clin Oncol 1993;11:304.

313. Bosi A, Bacci S, Miniero R, et al: Second allogeneic bone marrow transplantation in acute leukemia: A multicenter study from the Gruppo Italiano Trapianto di Midollo Ossen. Leukemia 1997;11:420.

314. Mehta J, Powles R, Treleaven J, et al: Outcome of acute leukaemia relapsing after bone marrow transplantation: Utility of second transplants and adoptive immunotherapy. Bone Marrow Transplant 1997;19:709.

315. Saunders J, Buckner C, Clift R, et al: Second marrow transplants in patients with leukemia who relapse after allogeneic marrow transplantation. Bone Marrow Transplant 1988;3:11.

316. Van Rhee F, Kolb H: Donor leukocyte transfusions for leukemic relapse. Curr Opin Hematol 1995;2:423.

317. Keil F, Haas O, Fritsch G, et al: Donor leukocyte infusions for leukemic relapse after allogeneic marrow transplantation: Lack of residual donor hematopoiesis predicts aplasia. Blood 1997;89:3113.

318. Falkenberg J, Swit W, Willemze R: Cytotoxic T-lymphocyte (CTL) responses against acute or chronic myeloid leukemia. Immunol Rev 1997;157:223.

319. Stewart D, Keating M, McCredie K, et al: Natural history of central nervous system acute leukemia in adults. Cancer 1981;47:184.

320. Dawson D, Rosenthal D, Moloney W: Neurological complications of acute leukemia in adults: Changing rate. Ann Intern Med 1973;79:541.

321. Meyer R, Ferriers P, Cuttner J, et al: Central nervous system involvement at presentation in acute granulocytic leukemia. A prospective cytocentrifuge study. Am J Med 1980;68:691.

322. Frick J, Ritch P, Hansen R, et al: Successful treatment of meningeal leukemia using systemic high-dose cytosine arabinoside. J Clin Oncol 1984;2:365.

323. Leith C, Kopecky K, Godwin J, et al: Acute myeloid leukemia in the elderly: Assessment of multidrug resistance (MDR1) and cytogenetics distinguishes biologic subgroups with remarkably distinct responses to standard chemotherapy. A Southwest Oncology Group study. Blood 1997;89:3323.

324. Sakurai M, Sandberg A: Prognosis of acute myeloblastic leukemia. Chromosomal correlation. Blood 1973;41:93.

325. First International Workshop on Chromosomes in Leukaemia: Chromosomes in acute nonlymphocytic leukaemia. Br J Haematol 1978;39:311.

326. Golomb H, Vardiman J, Rowley J, et al: Correlation of clinical findings with quinacrine banded chromosomes in 90 adults with acute nonlymphocytic leukemia. An eight year study (1970–1977). N Engl J Med 1978;299:613.

327. Lawler S, Summersgill B, Clink H, et al: Cytogenetic follow up study of acute nonlymphocytic leukaemia. Br J Haematol 1980;44:395.

328. Nilsson P, Brandt L, Miteeman F: Prognostic implications of chromosome analysis in acute nonlymphocytic leukaemia. Leuk Res 1977;1:31.

329. Yunis J, Brunning R, Howe R, et al: High resolution chromosomes as an independent prognostic indicator in adult acute nonlymphocytic leukemia. N Engl J Med 1984;311:812.

330. Yunis J, Brunning R: Prognostic significance of chromosomal abnormalities in acute leukemia and myelodysplastic syndromes. Clin Hematol 1986;15:597.

331. Schiffer C, Lee E, Tomiyasee T, et al: Prognostic impact of cytogenetic abnormalities in patients with de novo acute nonlymphocytic leukemia. Blood 1989;73:263.

332. Swansbury G, Lawler S, Alimena G, et al: Long term survival in acute myelogenous leukemia. Cancer Genet Cytogenet 1994;73:1.

333. Kantarjian H, Keating M, Walters R, et al: Therapy-related leukemia and myelodysplastic syndrome: Clinical, cytogenetic and prognostic features. J Clin Oncol 1986;4:1748.

334. Keating M, Smith T, Gehan E, et al: Factors related to length of complete remission in adult acute leukemia. Cancer 1980;45:2017.

335. Dutcher J, Schiffer C, Wiernick P: Hyperleukocytosis in adult acute nonlymphocytic leukemia: Impact on remission rate and duration and survival. J Clin Oncol 1987;5:1364.

336. Hug V, Keating M, McCredie K, et al: Clinical course and response to treatment of patients with acute myelogenous leukemia presenting with a high leukocyte count. Cancer 1983;52:773.

337. Passe S, Mike V, Merelsmann R, et al: Acute nonlymphoblastic leukemia. Prognostic factors in adults with long term follow up. Cancer 1982;50:1462.

338. Bloomfield C, Shuma C, Regal L, et al: Long term survival of patients with acute myeloid leukemia: A third follow-up of the Fourth International Workshop on Chromosomes in Leukemia. Cancer 1997;80:2191.

339. Wheatley K, Burnett A, Goldstone A, et al: A simple, robust, validated and highly predictive index for the determination of risk-directed therapy in acute myeloid leukaemia derived from the MRC AML 10 trial. Br J Haematol 1999;107:69.

339a. Schoch C, Kern W, Staib P, et al: FLT3 length mutations in AML: Correlation to cytogenetics, FAB-subtype, and prognosis in 652 patients. Proc Am Soc Hemat 2000;826a.

339b. Kottaridis PD, Gale RE, Frew N, et al: The presence of an FLT3 mutation in AML as important prognostic information to cytogenetic risk group and response to the first cycle of chemotherapy: Analysis of 854 patients from the MRC AML 10 and 12 trials. Proc Am Soc Hemat 2000;825a.

340. Kern W, Schoch C, Haferlach T, et al: Multivariate analysis of prognostic factors in patients with refractory and relapsed acute myeloid leukemia undergoing sequential high-dose cytosine arabinoside and mitoxantrone (S-HAM) salvage therapy: Relevance of cytogenetic abnormalities. Leukemia 2000;14:226.

341. Hiddemann W, Kern W, Schoch C, et al: Management of acute myeloid leukemia in elderly patients. J Clin Oncol 1999;17:3569.

342. Taylor P, Reid M, Stark A, et al: De novo acute myeloid leukemia in patients over 55 years old: A population-based study of incidence, treatment and outcome. Leukemia 1995;9:231.

343. Group Francais de Morphologie Hematologique: French registry of acute leukemia and myelodysplastic syndromes. Cancer 1987;60:1385.

344. Giannoulis M, Ogier C, Hast R: Difference between young and old patients in characteristics of leukemic cells. Am J Hematol 1984;16:113.

345. Beguin Y, Bury J, Fillet G, et al: Treatment of acute non-lymphocytic leukemia in young and elderly patients. Cancer 1985;5:2587.

346. Rowley J, Alimena G, Garson O, et al: A collaborative study of the relationship of the morphological type of acute nonlympocytic leukemia with patient age and karyotype. Blood 1982;59:1013.

347. Hoyle C, de Bastos M, Wheatley K, et al: AML associated with previous cytotoxic therapy, MDS or myeloproliferative disorders: Results from the MRC's 9th AML trial. Br J Haematol 1989;72:45.

348. Hamblin T: The treatment of acute myeloid leukemia preceded by the myelodysplastic syndrome. Leuk Res 1992;16:4101.

349. Brito-Babapulle F, Patovsky D, Galton D: Clinical and laboratory features of de novo acute myeloid leukaemia with trilineage myelodysplasia. Br J Haematol 1987;66:445.

350. Buchner T, Urbanitz D, Hiddemann W, et al: Intensified induction and consolidation with or without maintenance chemotherapy for acute myeloid leukemia (AML): Two multicenter studies of the German AML Cooperative Group. J Clin Oncol 1985;3:1583.

351. Rees J, Gray R, Wheatley K: Dose intensification in acute myeloid leukemia: Greater effectiveness at lower cost—principal report of the Medical Research Council's AML9 Study. Br J Haematol 1996;94:89.

352. Dillmann R, Davis R, Green M, et al: A comparative study of two different doses of cytarabine for acute myeloid leukemia: A Phase III trial of Cancer and Leukemia Group B. Blood 1991;78:2520.

353. Buchner T, Hiddemann W, Loffler H, et al: Treatment of AML in the elderly: Full dose versus reduced dose induction treatment. Blood 1995;86:434a.

354. Heil G, Hoelzer D, Sanz M, et al: A randomized double-blind, placebo-controlled, phase II study of filgrastim in remission induction and consolidation therapy for adults with de novo acute myeloid leukemia. Blood 1997;90:4710.

355. Buchner T, Hiddemann W, Loffler H, et al: Double induction strategy in AML comparing high with standard dose ara-C: Hematotoxicity and antileukemic efficacy. Blood 1994;84:232a.

356. Toronto Leukaemia Study Group: Results of chemotherapy for unselected patients with acute myeloblastic leukaemia. Effect of exclusions on the interpretation of results. Lancet 1986;1:786.

357. Lowenberg B, Zittoun R, Kerkhofs H, et al: On the value of

intensive remission-induction chemotherapy in elderly patients of 65+ years with acute myeloid leukemia: A randomized phase III study of the European Organization for Research and Treatment of Cancer Leukemia Group. J Clin Oncol 1989;7:1268.

358. Dalley C, Lillington D, Neat M, et al: Prognostic importance of cytogenetics and the application of molecular cytogenetics in elderly patients with acute myeloid leukemia treated at a single center. Proc Am Soc Hematol 1999;94:521a.

359. Dalley C, Rohatiner A, Lillington D, et al: Clinical management of acute myeloid leukemia in elderly patients at a single center (1969-1999). Abstract accepted for presentation at American Society of Hematology Meeting 2000.

360. Kahn S, Begg C, Mazza J, et al: Full dose versus attenuated dose daunorubicin, cytosine arabinoside and 6-thioguanine in the treatment of acute non-lymphocytic leukemia in the elderly. J Clin Oncol 1984;2:865.

361. Ruutu T, Almqvist A, Hallmann H, et al: Oral induction and consolidation of acute myeloid leukemia with etoposide, 6-thioguanine, and idarubicin (ETI) in elderly patients: A randomized comparison with 5-day TAD. Finnish Leukemia Group. Leukemia 1994;8:11.

362. Stone R, Berg D, George S, et al: Granulocyte-macrophage colony-stimulating factor after initial chemotherapy for elderly patients with primary acute myelogenous leukemia. N Engl J Med 1995;332:1672.

363. Witz F, Sadoun A, Perrin M, et al: A placebo-controlled study of recombinant human granulocyte-macrophage colony-stimulating factor administered during and after induction treatment for de novo acute myelogenous leukemia in elderly patients. Groupe Ouest Est Leucemies Aigues Myeloblastiques (GOELAM). Blood 1998;91:2722.

364. Rowe J, Andersen J, Mazza J, et al: A randomized placebo-controlled phase III study of granulocyte-macrophage colony-stimulating factor in adult patients (>55 to 70 years of age) with acute myelogenous leukemia. A study of the Eastern Cooperative Oncology Group (E1490). Blood 1995;86:457.

365. Dombert H, Chastang C, Fenaux P, et al: A controlled study of recombinant human granulocyte colony stimulating factor in elderly patients after treatment for acute myeloid leukemia. N Engl J Med 1995;332:1678.

366. Godwin J, Kopecky K, Head D, et al: A double blind placebo controlled trial of granulocyte colony stimulating factor in elderly patients with previously untreated acute myeloid leukemia: A Southwest Oncology Group study (9031). Blood 1998;91:3607.

367. Manoharan A, Baker R, Kyle P: Low-dose combination chemotherapy for acute myeloid leukemia in elderly patients: A novel approach. Am J Hematol 1997;55:115.

368. Leith C, Kopecky K, Chen I, et al: Frequency and clinical significance of the expression of the multidrug resistance proteins MDR1/P-glycoprotein, MRP1, and LRP in acute myeloid leukemia: A Southwest Oncology Group Study. Blood 1999;94:1086.

369. Campos L, Guyotat D, Archimbaud E, et al: Clinical significance of multidrug resistance P-glycoprotein expression on acute non-lymphoblastic leukemia cells at diagnosis. Blood 1992;79:473.

370. Lee E, George S, Caligiuri M, et al: Parallel Phase I studies of daunorubicin given with cytarabine and etoposide with or without the multidrug resistance modulator PSC-833 in previously untreated patients 60 years of age or older with acute myeloid leukemia: Results of Cancer and Leukemia Group B Study 9420. J Clin Oncol 1999;17:2831.

371. Advani R, Saba H, Tallman M, et al: Treatment of refractory and relapsed acute myelogenous leukemia with combination chemotherapy plus the multidrug resistance modulator PSC 833 (Valspodar). Blood 1999;93:787.

372. Bettelheim P, Valent P, Andreeff M, et al: Recombinant human granulocyte macrophage colony-stimulating factor in combination with standard induction chemotherapy in de novo acute myeloid leukemia. Blood 1991;77:700.

373. Cannistra S, DiCarlo J, Groshek P, et al: Simultaneous administration of granulocyte macrophage colony stimulating factor and cytosine arabinoside for the treatment of relapsed acute leukemia. Leukemia 1991;5:230.

374. Estey E, Thall P, Kantarjian H, et al: Treatment of newly diagnosed acute myelogenous leukemia with granulocyte macrophage colony stimulating factor (GM-CSF) before and during continuous infusion high-dose ara-C and daunorubicin: Comparison to patients treated without GM-CSF. Blood 1992;79:2246.

375. Ohno R, Tomonaga M, Kobayashi T, et al: Effect of granulocyte colony-stimulating factor after intensive induction therapy in relapsed or refractory acute leukemia. N Engl J Med 1990;323:871.

376. Kern W, Aul C, Maschmeyer G, et al: Granulocyte colony-stimulating factor shortens duration of critical neutropenia and prolongs disease-free survival after sequential high-dose cytosine arabinoside and mitoxantrone (S-HAM) salvage therapy for refractory and relapsed acute myeloid leukemia. German AML Cooperative Group. Ann Hematol 1998;77:115.

377. Uyl-de Groot C, Lowenberg B, Vellenga E, et al: Cost effectiveness and quality of life assessment of GM-CSF as an adjunct to intensive remission induction chemotherapy in elderly patients with acute myeloid leukaemia. Br J Haematol 1998;10:629.

378. List A, Spier C, Greer J, et al: Phase I/II trial of cyclosporine as a chemotherapy resistance modifier in acute leukemia. J Clin Oncol 1993;11:1652.

379. List A, Kopecky K, Willman C, et al: Benefit of cyclosporine (CsA) modulation of anthracycline resistance in high risk AML: A Southwest Oncology Group (SWOG) study. Blood 1998;92:1281a.

380. Powles R, Russel J, Lister T, et al: Immunotherapy for acute myelogenous leukaemia: A controlled clinical study 2 years after entry of the last patient. Br J Cancer 1977;35:265.

381. Powles R, Morgenstern G, Clink H, et al: The place of bone marrow transplantation in acute myelogenous leukaemia. Lancet 1980;1:1047.

382. Ganser A, Heil G, Seipelt G, et al: Intensive chemotherapy with idarubicin, ara-C, etoposide and M-AMSA followed by immunotherapy with interleukin-2 for myelodysplastic syndromes and high-risk acute myeloid leukemia (AML). Ann Hematol 2000;79:30.

383. Cortes J, Kantarjian H, O'Brien S, et al: A pilot study of interleukin-2 for adult patients with acute myelogenous leukemia in first complete remission. Cancer 1999;85:1506.

384. Mutis T, Verdijk R, Schrama E, et al: Feasibility of immunotherapy of relapsed leukemia with ex vivo–generated cytotoxic T lymphocytes specific for hematopoietic system–restricted minor histocompatibility antigens. Blood 1999;93:2336.

385. Simonson B, Totterman T, Hokland P, et al: Roquinimex (Linomide) vs placebo in AML after autologous bone marrow transplantation. Bone Marrow Transplant 2000;25:1121.

386. Garcia-Manero G, Grosso D, Beardell F, et al: Amifostine cytoprotection and dose escalation of idarubicin in elderly high risk patients with acute myelogenous leukemia. Blood 1998;92:3927a.

387. Schuler U, Schakel U, Wandt G, et al: Treatment of acute myelogenous leukemia in the elderly with daunorubicin + ara-C combined with amifostine—results of a pilot study. Blood 1998;92:4245a.

388. Fauth F, Martin H, Sonnhoff S, et al: Purging of G-CSF–mobilized peripheral autografts in acute leukemia with mafosfamide and amifostine to protect normal progenitor cells. Bone Marrow Transplant 2000;25:831.

389. Applebaum F, Barrall J, Storb R, et al: Bone marrow transplantation for patients with myelodysplasia. Ann Intern Med 1990;112:590.

390. O'Donnell M, Nademanee A, Synder D, et al: Bone marrow transplantation for myelodysplastic and myeloproliferative syndromes. J Clin Oncol 1987;5:1822.

391. Anderson J, Gooley T, Schoch G, et al: Stem cell transplantation for secondary acute myeloid leukemia: Evaluation of transplantation as initial therapy or following induction chemotherapy. Blood 1997;89:2578.

392. Belander R, Gyger M, Perreault C, et al: Bone marrow transplantation for myelodysplastic syndromes. Br J Haematol 1988;69:29.

393. Gorin N, Aegerter P, Auvert B, et al: Autologous bone marrow transplantation for acute myelocytic leukemia in first remission: A European survey of the role of marrow purging. Blood 1990;75:1606.

394. Witherspoon R, Deeg H: Allogeneic bone marrow transplantation for secondary leukemia or myelodsyplasia. Haematologica 1999;84:1085.

395. Krause J: Granulocytic sarcoma preceding acute leukemia. A report of six cases. Cancer 1979;44:1017.

396. Schiffer C, Sanel F, Stechmiller B, et al: Functional and morphologic characterization of the leukemic cells of patients with acute monocyte leukemia: Correlates with clinical features. Blood 1975;46:17.

397. Baer M, Barcos M, Farrell H, et al: Acute myelogenous leukemia with leukemia cutis: Eighteen cases seen between 1969 and 1986. Cancer 1989;63:2192.

398. Sheps M, Shapiro H, Ramsay C: Bullous pyoderma gangrenosum and acute leukemia. Arch Dermatol 1978;114:1842.

399. Caligiuri M, Mayer R: Pregnancy and leukemia. Semin Oncol 1989; 16:388.

400. Doll D, Riungenberg Q, Yarbro J: Anti-neoplastic agents and pregnancy. Semin Oncol 1989;16:337.

401. Caligiuri M: Leukemia and pregnancy: Effects of treatment on mother and child. Adv Oncol 1992;8:10.

402. Reynoso E, Shepherd F, Messner H, et al: Acute leukemia during pregnancy. The Toronto Leukemia Study Group experience with long-term follow-up of children exposed in utero to chemotherapeutic agents. J Clin Oncol 1987;5:1098.

403. Sievers E, Appelbaum F, Spielberger R, et al: Selective ablation of acute myeloid leukemia using antibody-targeted chemotherapy: A Phase I study of an anti-CD33 calicheamicin immunoconjugate. Blood 1999;93:3678.

404. Bernstein I: Monoclonal antibodies to the myeloid stem cells: The therapeutic implications of CMA-676, a humanized anti-CD33 antibody calicheamicin conjugate. Leukemia 2000;14:474.

404a. Sievers EL, Larson RA, Stadtmauer EA, et al: Efficacy and safety of gemtuzumab ozogamicin in patients with CD33-positive acute myeloid leukaemia in first relapse. J Clin Oncol 2001;19:3244.

405. Matthews D, Appelbaum F, Eary J, et al: Phase I study of ^{131}I-anti-CD45 antibody plus cyclophosphamide and total body irradiation for advanced acute leukemia and myelodysplastic syndrome. Blood 1999;94:1237.

406. Kornblau S, Thall P, Estrov Z, et al: The prognostic impact of BCL2 protein expression in acute myelogenous leukemia varies with cytogenetics. Clin Cancer Res 1999;5:1758.

407. Pisani F, Del Poeta G, Aronica G, et al: In vitro down-regulation of bcl-2 expression by all-*trans* retinoic acid in AML blasts. Am Hematol 1997;75:145.

408. Seiter K, Feldman E, Dorota Halicka H, et al: Clinical and laboratory evaluation of all-*trans* retinoic acid modulation of chemotherapy in patients with acute myelogenous leukaemia. Br J Haematol 2000;108:40.

409. Evans L, Jones M, Branson C: Individualization of doses improves survival of childhood acute lymphoblastic leukemia (ALL). N Engl J Med 1998;91:376.

410. Bhatia M, Bonnet D, Murdoch B, et al: A newly discovered class of human hematopoietic cells with SCID-repopulating activity. Nat Med 1998;4:1038.

411. Cuenco G, Nucifora G, Ren R: Human AML1/MDS1/EVI1 fusion protein induces an acute myelogenous leukemia (AML) in mice: A model for human AML. Proc Natl Acad Sci U S A 2000;97:1760.

412. Golub T, Slonim D, Tamayo P, et al: Molecular classification of cancer: Class discovery and class prediction by gene expression monitoring. Science 1999;286:531.

22

Beverly J. Lange

Acute Myeloid Leukemia in Children and Adolescents

Acute myeloid leukemia (AML) in children and adolescents is remarkably similar to AML in young and middle-aged adults. There are, however, important differences in demography, pathogenesis, and toxicities of therapy and outcome. In fact, it can be generalized that the younger the patient, the better the outcome,[1, 2] with spontaneous regression of congenital AML in infants with Down's syndrome (DS) being an extreme example. This chapter addresses the unique features of AML in the young. It is intended to be read in conjunction with the preceding chapter on AML in adults.

DEMOGRAPHICS

Leukemia is the most common pediatric cancer: roughly 75% to 80% is lymphoid, 15% to 20% is myeloid, and 2% is chronic, subacute, or indeterminate.[3] In the United States, the average incidence of AML is 7 per 10^6 children under age 15 years.[3] Higher rates occur in China and Japan and among the Maori in New Zealand; lower rates occur in India, Canada, Hong Kong, and Kuwait.[4] Equal numbers of males and females are affected. The incidence is higher among Hispanic Americans,[3] and in children in Latin countries, such as Italy and Peru, acute promyelocytic leukemia constitutes more than 30% of pediatric AML compared with less than 10% elsewhere.[5, 6] Orbital chloromas occur in 30% of Turkish children with AML compared with less than 5% in the United States.[7, 8] Figure 22-1 shows a peak incidence of $12/10^6$ in infancy and early childhood. This peak can be attributed to two uniquely pediatric entities: (1) myelomonocytic and monocytic AML with characteristic translocations of chromosomal band 11q23[9, 10]; and (2) acute megakaryoblastic leukemia in children with Down's syndrome (DS).[11-13]

ETIOLOGY

The cause of AML in the majority of children is unknown. Case control studies have identified an exposure to pesticides, ethanol, and inhibitors of topoisomerase II as risk factors for childhood AML. The most consistent associations are with parental exposures during gestation and patient exposure prenatally and perinatally for AML in the

first 5 years of life (Table 22-1).[3, 14-20] These associations probably reflect the extreme vulnerability of the fetus to leukemogenic agents. Previous associations with ionizing radiation[21, 22] are probably no longer relevant, and reported associations with excess fetal loss, maternal gestational marijuana use, radon, and electromagnetic fields have not been reproducible.[23]

Children exposed to cytotoxic chemotherapy during treatment of another cancer are at greatly increased risk of developing treatment-related AML (t-AML) (see Table 22-1). There are two distinct forms of t-AML. The more common form follows treatment with alkylating agents. It is characterized by poorly differentiated morphology, frequent association with -7 or del(7q), an antecedent myelodysplastic syndrome (MDS), and a latency of 5 to 7 years. The risk increases with splenectomy and in direct proportion to the cumulative dose of alkylating agent, the dose and field of irradiation, and age.[24] The highest risk reported is 23% in patients with metastatic Ewing's sarcoma treated intensively with ifosfamide, cyclophosphamide, and radiation.[25] A related form of AML occurs in children with certain constitutional disorders as described in the next section.

The second form of t-AML follows treatment with topoisomerase II poisons such as the epipodophyllotoxins and anthracyclines. It is usually myelomonocytic and monoblastic AML, often with translocations of chromosomal band 11q23 and an average latency of 2 years. This form of t-AML is not dose- or age-dependent and occurs in about 2% to 3% of exposed patients.[26] There are many similarities between this form of t-AML and de novo forms of monoblastic leukemia that occur in infancy and early childhood.[17, 18, 27]

Table 22-1 shows that the risk conferred by chemotherapy is many orders of magnitude higher than that attributed to any environmental toxin. This may be a result of very high doses and unknown leukemia predisposition genes in the population of pediatric cancer patients.

PATHOGENESIS AND PREDISPOSING CONDITIONS

AML occurs nonrandomly in children with certain constitutional disorders or a familial predisposition to leukemia

519

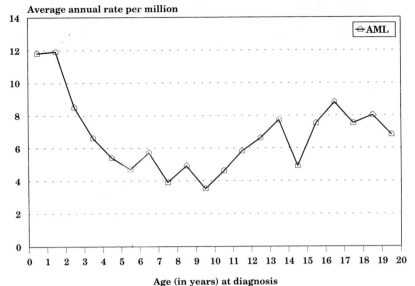

Average annual rate per million

Age (in years) at diagnosis

FIGURE 22–1. Age-specific incidence rates of AML in all races, both sexes, SEER 1976-1994. (Reproduced from Smith MA, Ries LAG, Gurney JG, et al, eds: Cancer Incidence and Survival Among Children and Adolescents: United States SEER Program 1975-1995. Washington, DC: National Cancer Institute, SEER Program, 1999; NIH Pub. No. 99-4649, p 17.)

(Table 22-2). One in 100 to 200 children with DS develop leukemia.[11, 12, 28, 29] In DS, there are two distinctive myeloid malignancies.

The first form is a congenital transient myeloproliferative disorder (TMD) that occurs at birth or in the first weeks of life. The leukemic cells are clonally derived megakaryoblasts that sometimes have acquired karyotypic abnormalities. Most often, this leukemia regresses spontaneously. Rarely do the infants succumb to overwhelming hepatic or visceral fibrosis.[30, 31] The much rarer Noonan syndrome may also be associated with a TMD.[32, 33]

The second form of AML in DS has a peak incidence at 2 years of age and is about 70% megakaryoblastic leukemia. This form of AML constitutes 10% or more of pediatric AML.[11, 12, 28, 29] At this time the gene or genes on chromosome 21 that predispose DS infants to leukemia are unknown. Paradoxically, the mechanism of leukemo-genesis may involve deletion of a tumor suppressor gene on chromosome 21 rather than increased dosage of an oncogene.[34, 35] CBFA2 (AML-1) on chromosome 21q22 may be a possible candidate gene.

Young children with neurofibromatosis type 1 (NF-1) are at increased risk of developing AML[36] or juvenile chronic myeloid leukemia (JCML) (now called juvenile myelomonocytic leukemia or JMML)[37], frequently with monosomy 7 or 7q− in the leukemic clone.[38, 39] In myeloid malignancies the NF1 gene acts as a tumor suppressor gene: there is usually loss of the normal NF1 allele in the leukemic clone and a truncating mutation in the remaining allele.[40] The NF1 gene product, neurofibromin, regulates activation of the RAS pathway, and its loss in leukemic cells leads to uncontrolled proliferation.[41-43]

TABLE 22–1. Toxic Substances Associated with Excess Risk of AML in Childhood

Toxin	Exposure	Characteristics of AML	OR	Chap. Ref.
Pesticides	Parent, >1000 days	Age <6 yr	11	14, 61
		FAB M4/5	13	
	Patient	Infancy	3	
Ethanol	Maternal (during pregnancy)	Age <2 yr	3	15, 19, 20
Topo-II inhibitors	Maternal diet (during pregnancy)	Age <2 yr M4/M5	3 9	17, 18
Chemotherapy				
Alkylating agents	Cancer patients	MDS/del(7)	100-2500	24, 25
Topo-II inhibitors	Cancer patients	M4/M5, t(11q23)	333	26

OR, odds ratio; topo-II DNA topoisomerase II for chemotherapy. OR was calculated on a risk of 9/10⁵ in children ≤15 years of age and a risk of AML of <1% to 23% after alkylating agents and 3% after exposure to topo-II inhibitors.

TABLE 22–2. Genetic Conditions Associated with AML in Children

Disorder	Approximate Incidence	Approximate Risk of AML	References
Identical twin with AML Age <6 yr	1/10⁵	1:20	55
Down's syndrome	1/150/10⁵	1:200	11, 12, 13, 28, 29
Neurofibromatosis type 1	4-5/10³ 1-9/10⁵	1:200–500 1:10	30, 40
Fanconi's anemia	Rare	Unknown	50
Bloom's syndrome			49
Kostmann's syndrome with G-CSF	Rare	1:10	44
Diamond-Blackfan	0.1/10⁵	1:250	49
Schwachman syndrome	Rare	1:20	49
Familial platelet disorder	Rare	Unknown	53
Familial monosomy 7	Rare	Unknown	39, 52
Familial 16q22	Rare	Unknown	54
Trisomy 8	Rare	Unknown	49

Only the risk of DS is firmly established. Estimates of incidence may be based on frequency of heterozygotes without considering excess fetal loss of homozygotes. Risks for the bone marrow failure syndromes are based on number of cases in literature and number of cases of AML reported. Rare is <1/10⁶ live births.

Children with NF-1 and solid tumors may be at increased risk of developing t-AML, often with −7/del(7q).[44, 45]

As granulocyte colony stimulating factor (G-CSF) has prolonged the lives of children with severe congenital neutropenia (SCN) (Kostmann's syndrome), about 10% of these children are developing t-AML, often with −7/del(7q).[46] The underlying defect in SCN patients who develop AML is truncation of the G-CSF receptor, leading to impaired receptor internalization, hyperactivity of the STAT pathway, and enhanced myeloid proliferation.[47, 48]

Other bone marrow failure syndromes associated with increased risk of AML include Fanconi's anemia (FA), Bloom's syndrome, Schwachman's syndrome, and Black-fan-Diamond syndrome.[49] FA and Bloom's syndrome are both characterized by excessive DNA breakage. One in 10 children with FA develops either MDS or AML, usually in older childhood or adolescence.[50] The magnitude of risk in most other disorders is unknown. Children with constitutional trisomy 8 and AML have been described. Although acquired trisomy 8 is the most common numerical abnormality in AML,[51] the pathophysiology of the leukemia in those with constitutional trisomy 8 is not known.

There are also rare inherited disorders of AML in which emergence of AML in a child was the event that prompted discovery of the disorder. The disorders include familial monosomy 7 with or without cerebellar ataxia,[39, 52] an autosomal familial platelet disorder with haploinsufficiency of CBFA2 on 21q22[53] and a familial form of AML mapped to 16q22.[54] The identical twin of a child with AML has a 5% chance of developing AML.[55]

CLASSIFICATION

The French-American-British (FAB) morphologic and histochemical classification system is the current international standard for pediatric and adult AML and MDS.[56-58] The FAB classification has limitations. Interobserver concordance is about only 65% in pediatric AML[59, 60]; it does not accommodate patients whose disease is myeloproliferative and myelodysplastic[61, 62]; and it does not predict treatment outcome. Classification according to well-defined, nonrandom, cytogenetic subsets seems to offer greater reproducibility and correlation with outcome[63] and a potential for targeting therapy to disease-specific macromolecules. Table 22–3 summarizes comparisons made by Raimondi et al[51] of the distribution of cytogenetic subsets among series of children with AML. Roughly 25% to 40% of patients do not have karyotyping either because of insufficient mitoses or failure to submit a specimen.[13, 51] Outcomes are similar in those with and without cytogenetics.

DIAGNOSIS AND PRESENTATION/CLINICAL MANIFESTATION

As in adults, the signs and symptoms of AML reflect the absence of normal hematopoiesis and the invasion of leukemic blasts into extramedullary sites such as skin, gingiva, orbit, brain, and spinal cord (see Chapter 21).

TABLE 22–3. Chromosomal Findings in 1992 Children with AML

Karyotype	Weighted Mean	Range
Normal	23%	(22–28)
t/inv/del(11q23)	16%	(8–18)
t(8;21)(q22;q22)	12%	(8–16)
t(15;17)(9q22;q12–21)	9%	(4–11)
+8	9%	(5–14)
+21	5%	(2–5)
Other hyperdiploid	1%	(1–3)
−7/del(7q)	5%	(4–6)
Other abnormal	20%	(19–22)

Numbers include 1404 cytogenetically characterized patients from 6 studies summarized by Raimondi et al[51] and 488 patients from CCG-2861 and CCG-2891.[13] Patients with Down's syndrome and t-AML are excluded.

Leukemia cutis is relatively more common in infants as is central nervous system disease at diagnosis.[8, 64] A hemorrhagic diathesis may be the presenting feature of acute promyelocytic leukemia (APL) (see Chapter 23) or, less frequently, monoblastic leukemia with a high tumor burden. Disorders that have been misdiagnosed as AML include metastatic alveolar rhabdomyosarcoma,[65] metastatic neuroblastoma,[66] and aplastic anemia. In the last case, a cytogenetically abnormal clone may be the only indication of the correct diagnosis. The diagnosis is made by the presence of less than 30% blasts of myeloid origin[67] or by taking a biopsy sample of a chloroma or any extramedullary collection of leukemic cells. The current World Health Organization classification has recommended a blast percentage of more than 20%, but this classification has not yet been adopted by all pediatric cooperative groups.[68] AML may also resemble FAB L2 ALL. Golub et al[69] have demonstrated their ability to distinguish pediatric AML from ALL using DNA microarrays and computer modeling to develop a molecular classification based on gene expression.

THERAPY

Figure 22–2 illustrates a generic treatment strategy for AML. In current clinical trials in children, therapy involves one or more courses of induction chemotherapy with cytosine arabinoside (ara-C) and an anthracycline and one or more courses of consolidation therapy with high-dose ara-C, followed by allogeneic or autologous bone marrow transplantation (allo-BMT or auto-BMT).[2, 70-81] Optimal dose and schedule of ara-C, choice of anthracycline, and the benefits of adding 6-thioguanine and/or etoposide in induction are under investigation in a few randomized trials.

Pediatric protocols routinely include central nervous system prophylaxis with intrathecal chemotherapy and, in the case of Berlin-Frankfurt-Muenster age-adjusted studies, cranial irradiation.[72] The Berlin-Frankfurt-Muenster protocols include 16 months of maintenance therapy,[71, 72] although both the Children's Cancer Group (CCG) 213 trial[82] and the LAME-87–91 trial[80] have shown that maintenance therapy significantly reduces event-free survival (EFS) and/or overall survival (OS). Because of excessive

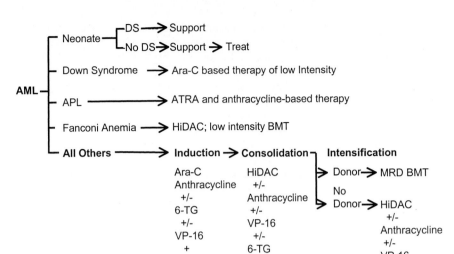

FIGURE 22–2. APL, acute promyelocytic leukemia; ATRA, all-*trans*-retinoic acid; Ara-C, cytosine arabinoside; DS, Down syndrome; 6-TG, 6 thioguanine; VP-16, etoposide; HiDAC, high-dose ara-C; MRD BMT, matched related donor bone marrow transplant. (Modified from Bleyer WA: Event-free survival of CCG patients with acute myelogenous leukemia, 1975–1995. Eur J Cancer 33;1439, 1997.)

mortality from mucositis and infection and delayed cardiomyopathy among infants younger than 3 years,[10, 14] the doses of therapy for infants are usually calculated by kilogram (m[2] dose divided by 30 times the weight in kilograms). Although much of the early success of BMT in AML in first remission used cyclophosphamide and total body irradiation (TBI) cytoreduction, today almost all cooperative groups use busulfan/cyclophosphamide. In one study, busulfan/cyclophosphamide was shown to be more effective than TBI[79] and may involve fewer serious late complications.

Five studies have achieved EFS rates more than 40% and OS rates approaching or exceeding 50% at 5 or more years from diagnosis (Table 22–4).[72, 75, 78–80, 83] These studies have in common substantial increases in dose-intensity of ara-C and anthracycline beyond that of the "standard" 7 days of ara-C at 100/mg/m[2]/day and 3 days of daunorubicin at 45 mg/m[2]/day. In most pediatric studies, biologic randomization to matched-related allo-BMT confers a significantly higher disease-free survival (DFS) and OS than does chemotherapy.[70, 76, 78–80, 84–87] However, Children's Cancer Group 2891 and Pediatric Oncology Group

8821 found no difference in DFS or OS between autologous BMT and chemotherapy.[76, 78] The Medical Research Council AML-10 study found a higher DFS with allo-BMT or auto-BMT compared with no therapy, but there was no improvement in OS because of poorer salvage after relapse in transplanted patients.[81] In contrast, in adults treated with MRC-AML-10, auto-BMT improved OS.[88] Figure 22–3 illustrates the progressive increase in EFS in CCG trials with intensification of therapy and use of allo-BMT in first remission.

There are four groups of patients that do not automatically receive standard generic AML therapy: neonates and children with DS, FA, or APL (see Fig. 22–2).

Most infants who develop congenital AML (in utero, at birth, or in the first month of life) have DS or DS mosaicism. The expectation is that their leukemia will regress spontaneously or with supportive care.[11, 12, 28, 29] Because DS mosaic patients may be phenotypically normal and because AML in a very small number of constitutionally normal neonates will also regress spontaneously,[89, 90] the recommendation is for conservative supportive management until DS has been ruled out by cytogenetics and there is clear evidence of progression. Neonatal AML outside of DS is usually fatal; however, Fernandez et al[91] reported a relatively uncomplicated course and successful outcome in a 3-day-old patient treated with CCG intensively-timed therapy.

AML in older infants with DS is highly responsive to chemotherapy involving low- or moderate-dose ara-C alone or with combination therapy of relatively low inten-

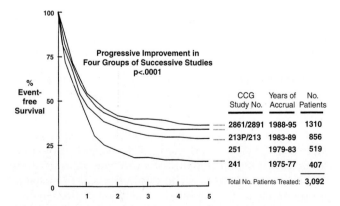

FIGURE 22–3. Event-free survival in successive Children's Cancer Group AML studies, 1972–1995. Data from 1989–1995 are for the intensive timing regimen of CCG-2891. (Courtesy of the Children's Cancer Group.)

TABLE 22–4. Event-Free Survival (EFS) and Overall Survival (OS) in Cooperative Group Trials of Pediatric AML of the Last Decade

Trial	N	EFS	OS	F/U (yr)	Chap. Ref.
MRC AML-10	341	48%	56%	7	79
BFM-92	471	53%	58%	5	72
CCG-2891 intensive	522	43%	49%	8	75, 78
POG-8821	649	34%	42%	3	74
NOPHO 88-92	118	42%	—	5	73

sity.[13, 92, 93] The more toxic, dose-intensive regimens that have improved EFS and OS in other children are of no benefit to children with DS.[13] The extreme sensitivity of DS megakaryoblasts to ara-C may be a result of three or more copies of the β-cystathionine reductase gene of chromosome 21.[94]

Patients with APL are treated with all-*trans*-retinoic acid (ATRA) and combination chemotherapy emphasizing dose-intensive anthracyclines[5] (see Chapter 23). Children and adults have a 10% risk of early mortality from coagulopathy and/or infection.[95] Children are more prone than adults to develop pseudotumor cerebri with ATRA,[96] and infants and young children are more susceptible to anthracycline-induced cardiomyopathy than adults. Outcomes are similar in children and adults.[95]

Because children with FA and aplastic anemia have a high mortality rate when treated with conventional BMT, lower-dose regimens have been used successfully.[97] However, if MDS or AML emerges, the higher doses of therapy that are needed to eradicate the malignant clone have an unacceptable mortality.[97] There is one report of success of treating MDS in FA with a reduced-intensity BMT[98] and one of successful remission induction with high-dose ara-C and mitoxantrone.[99]

Effective AML therapy is toxic. In CCG-2891, intensive timing of induction alone involves an overall mortality rate of more than 10% compared with 4% with standard timing.[77] Despite this early excess mortality, the EFS at 8 years is 15% higher in the intensive, more toxic induction.[78] MRC-AML-10 is the most effective therapy to date. In the pediatric patients, treatment involves 14 weeks of hospitalization and a treatment-related mortality rate of at least 14%,[100] and continued delayed mortality from cardiomyopathy is a distinct possibility.

Treatment of AML requires extraordinary supportive care measures involving preemptive use of antibacterial and antifungal antibiotics, high-efficiency particulate air filtration, large quantities of blood products, and nutritional support (see Chapters 13 to 16).[101-103] Children should receive treatment at centers with substantial experience with AML and BMT and with well-defined algorithms for management of hyperleukocytosis, fever, infection, shock, anemia, hemorrhage, coagulopathy, nutrition, and pain. To date, hematopoietic growth factors have reduced the duration of neutropenia by about 4 days, but in most studies in adults, these factors have had no significant impact on EFS or OS.[104, 105] In CCG-2891, the addition of G-CSF as a recruiting agent and as an adjuvant to supportive care had no impact and EFS or OS, despite a reduction in induction mortality from 13% to 9%.[78]

REFRACTORY OR RECURRENT AML

Of children with recurrent or refractory AML, 40% to 80% will experience a remission following treatment with combination chemotherapy containing high dose ara-C.[82, 106-111] Nearly a third will respond to phase I or phase II single agents.[112]

The Berlin-Frankfurt-Muenster group monitored 102 patients who received intensive therapy for first relapse.

Sixty-one percent achieved complete (51%) or partial (10%) remission. Overall survival rate at 5 years was 21% ± 5%, 40% ± 10% for those relapsing at more than 1.5 years from diagnosis, and 10% ± 5% for those with earlier relapse. Forty-three patients underwent BMT. The survival rate was 44% in 16 patients in remission who received a matched sibling donor (MSD), 0% in 7 with an MSD and residual blasts, and 20% in 5 who received a matched unrelated donor transplant.

Similar results were reported by Webb et al.[113] Of 125 children whose disease recurred during or after MRC-AML-10 therapy, 38 (30%) did not receive intensive therapy. Among those treated, 75% of those with first remission at more than 1 year and 36% of those with first remission at less than 1 year achieved a second remission. Respective survivals were 49% and 11% at 3 years.

These two studies may overestimate the outcomes in nonselected populations of pediatric AML patients. The curability of recurrent and refractory AML can be obtained by subtracting the EFS from the OS. This difference is typically between 5% and 8% (see Table 22–4); with few exceptions, most patients who are cured have received a marrow or stem cell transplant. Broadening of the donor pool to include matched unrelated donors, haplotype-matched parental donors, and cord blood increases the chances for cure for those who can arrive at that point.[86, 114-117]

PROGNOSTIC FACTORS

As the proportion of survivors of AML increases, definition of factors that predict for survival has become possible.[54, 72, 74, 113, 118-120] All prognostic factors depend on therapy. For example, t(15;17) in the pre-ATRA era was favorable in European studies, standard in the CCG, and unfavorable in a Pediatric Oncology Group study. With ATRA, outcome is favorable in all studies. The Berlin-Franfurt-Muenster and UK-AML cooperative groups are beginning to stratify patients with low-, standard-, and high-risk groups based on cytogenetics, white blood cell count, and early response.[73, 113] Table 22–5 lists the current prognostic factors defined in recent trials.

LATE COMPLICATIONS OF TREATMENT

Much of the literature on the late complications of treatment of AML focuses on comparisons of chemotherapy and BMT or the comparisons of Bu/Cy cytoreduction to TBI in BMT regimens. With the chemotherapy regimens

TABLE 22–5. Factors Predictive of Outcome in Pediatric AML

Cure >50%	Cure <25%	Variable
Down's syndrome inv 16/t(16;16) t(15;17) (q22;q12-21)	t-AML WBC >2×10⁹/L −7/del(7q) non t(9:11) 11q23 abnormality	t(9;11) (p22;11q23) t(8;21) (q22;q22) Antecedent MDS

used today, the major complication is cardiac dysfunction from anthracyclines. The magnitude of the problem is unknown, but risk factors are dose-intensity of anthracycline; cumulative dose; young age, especially infancy; and female gender.[121-123] Hearing deficits are unique to chemotherapy-treated patients, and renal impairment occurs in transplantation- and chemotherapy-treated patients.[122] Risks of infertility, neuropsychologic dysfunction, and second malignant neoplasms are negligible after chemotherapy.[122]

In contrast to BMT regimens using TBI, the combination of growth hormone deficiency and impaired skeletal growth leads to short stature in about two-thirds of those who were treated as infants or children.[124-126] Only one study[127] showed short stature in chemotherapy-treated patients. Short stature is not a problem after Bu/Cy in the absence of GVHD.[128, 129] Thyroid hormone deficiency may also contribute to short stature. Delay in sexual maturation and infertility are so common after either Cy/TBI or Bu/Cy that they have been considered universal. However, Sanders et al[130] found that among 618 female survivors, 25% recovered ovarian function, and 5.3% became pregnant. Among 708 male survivors, 15% regained testicular function, and 4.5% sired offspring. Those women who received TBI were at greater risk of spontaneous abortion, and those both with and without TBI had an increased risk of low-birth-weight infants. Congenital anomalies were not increased.[130]

Cataracts, dry eyes, and abnormal dentition are more likely after TBI.[127] Finally, both transplant cytoreduction regimens are associated with an excess risk of second malignant neoplasms, with the relative risk being three-fold greater following TBI with high-dose irradiation.[131] Patients aged less than 5 years had a relative risk of 3.7. There were 2 salivary gland mucoepidermoid carcinomas, 2 osteosarcomas, 1 malignant fibrous histiocytoma, and 3 melanomas among 1130 patients who survived more than 1 year post-transplant.[131]

CONCLUSION

Currently, more than half of pediatric patients with AML can be cured, in contrast to one-third in the last decade. Current treatment involves intensive chemotherapy with or without transplantation, aggressive supportive care, and special approaches to subsets of children such as those with DS, neonates, and those with underlying genetic disorders. With the exception of ATRA therapy for APL, treatment of AML is not leukemia-specific. It relies on subtle differences between leukemic and normal cells. Therapies that modify molecular targets are emerging, and therapies that render the AML blast amenable to immunologic recognition and destruction are the future for treatment of AML in children and adults.

REFERENCES

1. Clarke CA, Glaser SL: Acute myeloid leukemia. N Engl J Med 2000; 342:358.
2. Hann IM, Stevens RF: Randomized comparison of DAT versus ADE as induction chemotherapy in children and younger adults with acute myeloid leukemia: Results of the Medical Research Council's 10th AML trial (MRC AML 10). Adult and Childhood Leukaemia Working Parties of the Medical Research Council. Blood 1997; 89:2311.
3. Smith MA, Ries LAG, Gurney JG, et al, eds: Cancer Incidence and Survival Among Children and Adolescents: United States SEER Program 1975-1995. Washington, DC: National Cancer Institute, SEER Program, 1999; NIH Pub. No. 99-4649, p 17.
4. Bhatia S, Neglia JP: Epidemiology of childhood acute myelogenous leukemia. J Pediatr Hematol Oncol 1995;17:94.
5. Biondi A, Rovelli A, Cantu-Rajnoldi A, et al: Acute promyelocytic leukemia in children: Experience of the Italian Pediatric Hematology and Oncology Group (AIEOP). Leukemia 1994;8:1264.
6. Douer DS, Preston-Martin S: High frequency of acute promyelocytic leukemia among Latinos with acute myeloid leukemia. Blood 1996;87:308.
7. Turker A, Cadvar AO, Yavuz G, et al: Cytogenetic abnormality in Turkish children with acute myeloid leukemia (AML) and orbito-ocular granulocytic sarcoma (chloroma). Blood 1993;82:550a.
8. Dusenbery KE, Arthur DC, Howells W, et al: Granulocytic sarcomas (chloromas) in pediatric patients with newly diagnosed acute myeloid leukemia. Annual Meeting of the American Society of Clinical Oncologists, 1996, p 1096.
9. Odom LF, Lampkin BC, Tannous R, et al: Acute monoblastic leukemia: A unique subtype—a review from the Childrens Cancer Study Group. Leuk Res 1990;14:1.
10. Sorensen PH, Chen CS, Smith FO, et al: Molecular rearrangements of the *MLL* gene are present in most cases of infant acute myeloid leukemia and are strongly correlated with monocytic or myelomonocytic phenotypes. J Clin Invest 1994;93:429.
11. Fong C, Brodeur GM: Down's syndrome and leukemia: Epidemiology, genetics, cytogenetics and mechanisms of leukemogenesis. Cancer Genet Cytogenet 1987;28:55.
12. Avet-Loiseau H, Mechinaud F, Harousseau JL: Clonal hematologic disorders in Down syndrome. J Pediatr Hematol Oncol 1995;17:19.
13. Lange BJ, Kobrinsky N, Barnard DR, et al: Distinctive demography, biology and outcome of acute myeloid leukemia and myelodysplastic syndrome in children with Down syndrome: Children's Cancer Group Studies 2861 and 2891. Blood 1998;91:608.
14. Buckley JD, Robison LL, Swotinsky R, et al: Occupational exposures of parents of children with acute nonlymphocytic leukemia: A report from the Children's Cancer Study Group. Cancer Res 1989;49:4030.
15. Severson RK, Buckley JD, Woods WG, et al: Cigarette smoking and alcohol consumption by parents of children with acute myeloid leukemia: An analysis within morphological subgroups—a report from the Children's Cancer Group. Cancer Epidemiol Biomarkers Prev 1993;2:433.
16. Robison L, Ross J: Epidemiology of leukaemias and lymphomas in children. In Chessells J, Hann I, eds: Clinical Paediatrics. London: WB Saunders, 1995, p 639.
17. Ross JA: Maternal diet and infant leukemia: A role for DNA topoisomerase II inhibitors? Int J Cancer 1998;11:26.
18. Ross JA, Potter JD, Reaman GH, et al: Maternal exposure to potential inhibitors of DNA topoisomerase II and infant leukemia (United States): A report from the Children's Cancer Group. Cancer Causes Control 1996;7:581.
19. van Duijn CM, van Steensel-Moll HA, Coebergh JW, et al: Risk factors for childhood acute non-lymphocytic leukemia: An association with maternal alcohol consumption during pregnancy? Cancer Epidemiol Biomarkers Prev 1994;3:457.
20. Shu XO, Ross JA, Pendergrass TW, et al: Parental alcohol consumption, cigarette smoking, and risk of infant leukemia: A Children's Cancer Group study. J Natl Cancer Inst 1996;88:24.
21. Bithell JF, Stewart AM: Pre-natal irradiation and childhood malignancy: A review of British data from the Oxford Survey. Br J Cancer 1975;31:271.
22. Kato H, Schull WJ: Studies of the mortality of A-bomb survivors. 7. Mortality, 1950-1978: Part 1. Cancer mortality. Radiat Res 1982; 90:395.
23. Ross JA, Potter JD, Shu XO, et al: Evaluating the relationships among maternal reproductive history, birth characteristics, and infant leukemia: A report from the Children's Cancer Group. Ann Epidemiol 1997;7:172.

24. Tucker MA, Meadows AT, Boice Jr JD, et al: Leukemia after therapy with alkylating agents for childhood cancer. J Natl Cancer Inst 1987;78:459.
25. Miser J, Krailo MJ, Smith M, et al: Secondary leukemia (SL) or myelodysplastic syndrome (MDS) following therapy for Ewing's sarcoma (ES). Am Soc Clin Oncol 1997;16:518.
26. Smith MA, Rubinstein L, Anderson JR, et al: Secondary leukemia or myelodysplastic syndrome after treatment with epipodophyllotoxins. J Clin Oncol 1999;17:569.
27. Felix CA, Lange BJ: Leukemia in infants. Oncologist 1999;4:225.
28. Zipursky A, Peeters M, Poon A: Megakaryoblastic leukemia and Down's syndrome: A review. Pediatr Hematol Oncol 1987;4:211.
29. Lange B: The management of neoplastic disorders of hematopoiesis in children with Down syndrome. Br J Haematol 2000;110:512.
30. Miyauchi J, Ito Y, Kawano T, et al: Usual diffuse liver fibrosis accompanying transient myeloproliferative disorder in Down's syndrome: A report of four autopsy cases and proposal of a hypothesis. Blood 1992;80:1521.
31. Becroft DMO, Zwi LJ: Perinatal visceral fibrosis accompanying the megakaryoblastic leukemoid reaction of Down syndrome. Pediatr Pathol 1990;10:397.
32. Bader-Meunier B, Tchernia G, Mielot F, et al: Occurrence of myeloproliferative disorder in patients with Noonan syndrome. J Pediatr 1997;130:885.
33. Dinoulos J, Hawkins D, Clark B, et al: Spontaneous remission of congenital leukemia. J Pediatr 1977;131:300.
34. Cavani S, Perfumo C, Argusti A, et al: Cytogenetic and molecular study of 32 Down syndrome families: Potential leukaemia predisposing role of the most proximal segment of chromosome 21q. Br J Haematol 1998;103:213.
35. Kempski HM, Chessells JM, Reeves BR: Deletions of chromosome 21 restricted to the leukemic cells of children with Down syndrome and leukemia. Leukemia 1997;11:1973.
36. Bader JL, Miller RW: Neurofibromatosis and childhood leukemia. J Pediatr 1978;92:925.
37. Arico M, Biondi A, Pui CH: Juvenile myelomonocytic leukemia. Blood 1997;90:479.
38. Shannon KM, O'Connell P, Martin GA, et al: Loss of the normal NF1 allele from the bone marrow of children with type 1 neurofibromatosis and malignant myeloid disorders. N Engl J Med 1994;330:597.
39. Luna-Fineman S, Shannon KM, Lange BJ: Childhood monosomy 7: Epidemiology, biology, and mechanistic implications. Blood 1995;85:1985.
40. Side L, Taylor B, Cayouette M, et al: Homozygous inactivation of the NF1 gene in bone marrow cells from children with neurofibromatosis type 1 and malignant myeloid disorders. N Engl J Med 1997;336:1713.
41. Largaespada DA, Brannan CI, Jenkins NA, et al: NF1 deficiency causes *ras*-mediated granulocyte/macrophage colony stimulating factor hypersensitivity and chronic myeloid leukemia. Nat Genet 1996;12:137.
42. Largaespada DA, Brannan CI, Shaughnessy JD, et al: The neurofibromatosis type 1 (NF1) tumor suppressor gene and myeloid leukemia. Curr Top Microbiol Immunol 1996;211:233.
43. Kalra R, Paderanga DC, Olson K, et al: Genetic analysis is consistent with the hypothesis that NF1 limits myeloid cell growth through p21-*ras*. Blood 1994;84:3435.
44. Perilongo G, Felix CA, Meadows AT, et al: Sequential development of Wilms tumor, T-cell acute lymphoblastic leukemia, medulloblastoma, and myeloid leukemia in a child with type 1 neurofibromatosis: A clinical and cytogenetic case report. Leukemia 1993;7:912.
45. Maris JM, Wiersma SR, Mahgoub N, et al: Monosomy 7 myelodysplastic syndrome and other second malignant neoplasms in children with neurofibromatosis type 1. Cancer 1997;79:1438.
46. Dong F, Brynes RK: Mutations in the gene for the granulocyte colony-stimulating-factor receptor in patients with acute myeloid leukemia preceded by severe congenital neutropenia. N Engl J Med 1995;333:487.
47. Hunter MG, Avalos BR: Chromosome 21 and platelets: A gene dosage effect? Blood 1997;93:440.
48. Ward AC, van Aesch YM: Defective internalization and sustained activation of truncated granulocyte colony-stimulating factor receptor found in severe congenital neutropenia/acute myeloid leukemia. Blood 1999;93:447.
49. Alter BP, Young NS: The bone marrow failure syndrome. In Nathan DG, Orkin SH, Ginsburg D, eds: Hematology of Infancy and Childhood. Philadelphia: WB Saunders; 1998.
50. Alter BP: Franconi's anemia and malignancies. Am J Hematol 1996;53:99.
51. Raimondi SC, Chang MN, Ravindranath Y, et al: Chromosomal abnormalities in 478 children with acute myeloid leukemia: Clinical characteristics and treatment outcome in a cooperative pediataric oncology group study—POG-8821. Blood 1999;94:3707.
52. Shannon KM, Watterson J, Johnson P, et al: Monosomy 7 myeloproliferative disease in children with neurofibromatosis, type 1: Epidemiology and molecular analysis. Blood 1992;79:1311.
53. Song WJ, Sullivan MG, Legare RD, et al: Haploinsufficiency of CBFA2 causes familial thrombocytopenia with propensity to develop acute myelogenous leukaemia. Nat Genet 1999;23:166.
54. Horwitz M, Benson KF: Genetic heterogeneity in familial acute myelogenous leukemia: Evidence for a second locus at chromosome 16q21–23.2. Am J Hum Genet 1997;61:873.
55. Buckley JD, Buckley CM, Breslow NE, et al: Concordance for childhood cancer in twins. Med Pediatr Oncol 1996;26:223.
56. Bennett JM, Catovsky D, Daniel MT, et al: Proposals for the classification of the myelodysplastic syndromes. Br J Haematol 1982;51:189.
57. Bennett JM, Catovsky D., Daniel MT, et al: Proposed revised criteria for the classification of acute myeloid leukemia: A report of the French-American-British Cooperative Group. Ann Intern Med 1985;103:620.
58. Bennett JM, Catovsky D, Daniel MT, et al: Proposal for the recognition of minimally differentiated acute myeloid leukaemia (AML-MO). Br J Haematol 1991;78:325.
59. Barnard DR, Kalousek DK, Wiersma SR, et al: Morphologic, immunologic, and cytogenetic classification of acute myeloid leukemia and myelodysplastic syndrome in childhood: A report from the Childrens Cancer Group. Leukemia 1996;10:5.
60. Argyle JC, Benjamin DR, Lampkin B, et al: Acute nonlymphocytic leukemias of childhood: Inter-observer variability and problems in the use of the FAB classification. Cancer 1989;63:295.
61. Passmore SJ, Hann IM, Stiller CA, et al: Pediatric myelodysplasia: A study of 68 children and a new prognostic scoring system. Blood 1995;85:1742.
62. Luna-Fineman S, Shannon KM, Atwater SK, et al: Myelodysplastic and myeloproliferative disorders of childhood: A study of 167 patients. Blood 1999;93:459.
63. Head DR: Revised classification of acute myeloid leukemia: Debate—roundtable. Leukemia 1996;10:1826.
64. Pui CH, Dahl GV: Central nervous system leukemia in children with acute nonlymphoblastic leukemia. Blood 1985;66:1062.
65. Penchansky L, Taylor SR, Krause JR: Three infants with acute megakaryoblastic leukemia simulating metastatic tumor. Cancer 1989;64:1366.
66. Boyd JE, Parmley RT, Langevin AM, et al: Neuroblastoma presenting as acute monoblastic leukemia. J Pediatr Hematol Oncol 1996;18:206.
67. Cheson BD, Cassileth PA, Head DR, et al: Report of the National Cancer Institute–sponsored workshop on definitions of diagnosis and response in acute myeloid leukemia. J Clin Oncol 1990;8:813.
68. Harris NL, Jaffee ES, Diebold J, et al: The World Health Organization classification of hematological malignancies: Report of the clinical advisory committee meeting, Airlie House, Virginia, November 1997. Mod Pathol 2000;13:193.
69. Golub TR, Slonim DK, Tamayo P, et al: Molecular classification of cancer: Class discovery and class prediction by gene expression monitoring. Science 1999;286:531.
70. Amadori S, Testi AM, Arico M, et al: Prospective comparative study of bone marrow transplantation and postremission chemotherapy for childhood acute myelogenous leukemia: Associazione Italiano Ematologia ed Oncologia Pediatrica Cooperative Group. J Clin Oncol 1993;11:1046.
71. Creutzig U, Ritter J, Riehm H, et al: Improved treatment results in childhood acute myelogenous leukemia: A report of the German cooperative study AML-BFM-78. Blood 1985;65:298.
72. Creutzig U, Ritter J, Zimmermann M, et al: Does cranial irradiation reduce the risk for bone marrow relapse in acute myelogenous leukemia? Unexpected results of the Childhood Acute Myelogenous Leukemia Study BFM-87. J Clin Oncol 1993;11:279.

73. Creutzig U, Zimmermann M, Ritter J, et al: Definition of a standard-risk group in children with AML. Br J Haematol 1999;104:630.

74. Creutzig U, Ritter J, Zimmerman M, et al: Improved treatment results after risk-adapted intensificiaton of chemotherapy in children with AML: Results of AML BFM 1993. Blood 1999;94:628.

75. Lie SO, Jonmundsson G: A population-based study of 272 children with acute myeloid leukaemia treated on two consecutive protocols with different intensity: Best outcome in girls, infants, and children with Down's syndrome. Nordic Society of Paediatric Haematology and Oncology (NOPHO). Br J Haematol 1996; 94:82.

76. Ravindranath Y, Yeager AM: Autologous bone marrow transplantation verus intensive consolidation chemotherapy for acute myeloid leukemia in childhood. N Engl J Med 1996;334:1428.

77. Woods WG, Kobrinsky N: Timed-sequential induction therapy improves postremission outcome in acute myeloid leukemia: A report from the Children's Cancer Group. Blood 1996;87:4979.

78. Woods WG, Neudorf S, Gold S, et al: A comparison of allogeneic bone marrow transplantation, autologous bone marrow transplantation and aggressive chemotherapy in children with AML in remission: A report from the Children's Cancer Group. Blood 2001;97:56.

79. Michel G, Gluckman E, Esperou-Bourdeau H, et al: Allogeneic bone marrow transplantation for children with acute myeloblastic leukemia in first complete remission: Impact of conditioning regimen without total-body irradiation: An report from the Societe Francaise de Greffe de Moelle. J Clin Oncol 1994;12:1217.

80. Michel G, Leverger G, Leblanc T, et al: Allogeneic bone marrow transplantation vs. aggressive post-remission chemotherapy for children with acute myeloid leukemia in first complete remission: A prospective study from the French Society of Pediatric Hematology and Immunology (SHIP). Bone Marrow Transplantation 1996; 17:191.

81. Stevens RF, Hann IM, Wheatley K, et al: Marked improvement in outcome with chemotherapy alone in paediatric acute myeloid leukaemia: Results of the United Kingdom Medical Research Council's 10th AML trial. Br J Haematol 1998;101:130.

82. Wells RJ, Woods WG: Treatment of newly diagnosed children and adolescents with acute myeloid leukemia: A Children's Cancer Group Study. J Clin Oncol 1994;12:2367.

83. Creutzig U, Harbott J, Sperling C, et al: Clinical significance of surface antigen expression in children with acute myeloid leukemia: Results of study AML-BFM-87. Blood 1995;86:3097.

84. Nesbit ME Jr, Buckley JD, Feig SA, et al: Chemotherapy for induction of remission of childhood acute myeloid leukemia followed by marrow transplantation of multiagent chemotherapy: a report from the Children's Cancer Group. J Clin Oncol 1994;12:127.

85. Dahl GV, Kalwinsky DK, Mirro J Jr, et al: Allogeneic bone marrow transplantation in a program of intensive sequential chemotherapy for children and young adults with acute nonlymphocytic leukemia in first remission. J Clin Oncol 1990;8:295.

86. Dinndorf P, Bunin N: Bone marrow transplantation for children with acute myelogenous leukemia. J Pediatr Hematol Oncol 1995; 17:211.

87. Sanders JE: Bone marrow transplantation for pediatric malignancies. Pediatr Clin North Am 1997;44:1005.

88. Burnett AK, Goldstone AH, Stevens RM, et al: Randomised comparison of addition of autologous bone-marrow transplantation to intensive chemotherapy for acute myeloid leukaemia in first remission: Results of MRC AML 10 trial. UK Medical Research Council Adult and Children's Leukaemia Working Parties. Lancet 1998; 351:700.

89. Lampkin BC, Peipon JJ, Price JK, et al: Spontaneous remission of presumed congenital acute nonlymphoblastic leukemia (ANLL) in a karyotypically normal neonate. Am J Pediatr Hematol Oncol 1985;7:346.

90. Lampkin BC: The newborn infant with leukemia. J Pediatr 1997; 131:176.

91. Fernandez MD, Weiss B, Atwater S, et al: Congenital leukemia: Successful treatment of a newborn with t(5;11)(q31;q23). J Pediatr Hematol Oncol 1999;21:152.

92. Ravindranath Y, Abella E: Acute myeloid leukemia (AMLL) in Down's syndrome is highly responsive to chemotherapy: Experience on Pediatric Oncology Group AML Study 8498. Blood 1992; 80:2210.

93. Tchernia G, Lejeune F, Boccaro J-F, et al: Erythroblastic and/or megakaryoblastic leukemia in Down syndrome: Treatment with low-dose arabinosyl cytosine. J Pediatr Hematol Oncol 1996; 8:59.

94. Taub JW, Huang X, Matherly LH, et al: Expression of chromosome 21-localized genes in acute myeloid leukemia: Differences between Down syndrome and non-Down syndrome blast cells and relationship to in vitro sensitivity to cytosine arabinoside and daunorubicin. Blood 1999;94:1393.

95. Tallman MS, Anderson JW, Schiffer CA, et al: All-trans-retinoic acid in acute promyelocytic leukemia. N Engl J Med 1997;337:1021.

96. Mahmoud HH, Hurwitz CA, Roberts WM, et al: Tretinoin toxicity in children with acute promyelocytic leukaemia. Lancet 1993; 342:1394.

97. Flowers ME, Doney KC, Storb R, et al: Marrow transplantation for Fanconi anemia with or without leukemic transformation: An update of the Seattle experience. Bone Marrow Transplant 1992; 9:167.

98. Ikukshima S, Hibi S, Todo S, et al: Successful allogeneic bone marrow transplantation in a case with meylodysplastic syndrome which developed following Fanconi anemia. Bone Marrow Transplant 1995;16:621.

99. Verbeek W, Haase D, Schoch C, et al: Induction of a hematological and cytogenetic remission in a patient with a myelodysplastic syndrome secondary to Fanconi's anemia employing the S-HAM regimen. Ann Hematol 1997;74:275.

100. Riley LC, Hann IM, Wheatley K, et al: Treatment-related deaths during induction and first remission of acute myeloid leukaemia in children treated on the Tenth Medical Research Council acute myeloid leukaemia trial (MRC AML10). The MCR Childhood Leukaemia Working Party. Br J Haematol 1999;106:436.

101. Feusner JH, Hastings CA: Infections in children with acute myelogenous leukemia: Concepts of management and prevention. J Pediatr Hematol Oncol 1995;17:234.

102. Pizzo PA: Fever in immunocompromised patients. N Engl J Med 1999;341:893.

103. Sherertz RJ, Belani A, Kramer BS, et al: Impact of air filtration on nosocomial *Aspergillus* infections: Unique risk of bone marrow transplant recipients. Am J Med 19897;83:709.

104. Schiffer CA: Hematopoietic growth factors as adjuncts to the treatment of acute myeloid leukemia. Blood 1996;88:3675.

105. Estey E: Hematopoietic growth factors in the treatment of acute leukemia. Curr Opin Oncol 1998;10:23.

106. Steuber CP, Krischer J, Holbrook T, et al: Therapy of refractory or recurrent childhood acute myeloid leukemia using amsacrine and etoposide with or without azacitidine: A Pediatric Oncology Group randomized phase II study. J Clin Oncol 1996;14:1521.

107. Wells R, Feusner J, Devney R, et al: Sequential high-dose cytosine arabinoside–asparaginase treatment in advanced childhood leukemia. J Clin Oncol 1985;3:998.

108. Whitlock JA, Wells RJ, Hord JD, et al: High-dose cytosine arabinoside and etoposide: An effective regimen without anthracyclines for refractory childhood acute non-lymphocytic leukemia. Leukemia 1997;11:185.

109. Dinndorf PA, Avramis VI, Wiersma S, et al: A phase I/II study of idarubicin given with continuous infusion cytosine arabinoside in children with acute leukemia: A report from the Children's Cancer Group. J Clin Oncol 1997;15:2780.

110. Lockhart S, Plunkett W, Jeha S, et al: High-dose mercaptopurine followed by intermediate-dose cytarabine in relapsed acute leukemia. J Clin Oncol 1994;12:587.

111. Leahey A, Kelly K, Rorke L, et al: A phase I study of idarubicin (Ida) with continuous infusion fludarabine and cytarabine (Fara-A/Ara-C) for refractory or relapsed pediatric acute myeloid leukemia (AML). J Pediatr Hematol Oncol 1997;19:304.

112. Weitman S, Ochoa S, Sullivan J, et al: Pediatric phase II cancer chemotherapy trials: A Pediatric Oncology Group study. J Pediatr Hematol Oncol 1997;19:187.

113. Webb DK, Wheatley K, Harrison G, et al: Outcome for children with relapsed acute myeloid leukaemia following intial therapy in the Medical Research Council (MRC) AML 10 trial. MRC Childhood Leukaemia Working Party. Leukemia 1999;13:25.

114. Davies SM, Wagner JE, Shu XO, et al: Unrelated donor bone marrow transplantation for children with acute leukemia. J Clin Oncol 1997;15:557.

115. Wagner JE, Rosenthal J, Sweetman R, et al: Successful transplantation of HLA-matched and HLA-mismatched umbilical cord blood from unrelated donors: Analysis of engraftment and acute graft-versus-host disease. N Engl J Med 1996;88:795.

116. Gluckman E, Rocha V, Boyer-Chamnard A, et al: Outcome of cord-blood transplantation from related and unrelated. Eurocord Transplant Group and the European Blood and Marrow Transplantation Group. N Engl J Med 1997;337:373.

117. Henslee-Downey PJ, Abhyankar SH, Parrish RS, et al: Use of partially mismatched related donors extends access to allogeneic marrow transplant. Blood 1997;89:3864.

118. Grier HE, Gelber RD, Camitta BM, et al: Prognostic factors in childhood acute myelogenous leukemia. J Clin Oncol 1987; 5:1026.

119. Kalwinsky DK, Raimondi SC, Schell MJ, et al: Prognostic importance of cytogenetic subgroups in de novo pediatric acute non-lymphocytic leukemia. J Clin Oncol 1990;8:75.

120. Smith FO, Howells WB, Buckley JD, et al: Prognostic factors (PF) in children with acute myeloid leukemia (AML): Results of Children's Cancer Group (CCG) protocol 2891. Blood 1997;90: 561.

121. Steinherz LJ, Steinherz PG, Tan CT, et al: Cardiac toxicity 4 to 20 years after completing anthracycline therapy. JAMA 1991; 266:1672.

122. Liesner RJ, Leiper AD, Han IM, et al: Late effects of intensive treatment for acute myeloid leukemia and myelodysplasia in childhood. J Clin Oncol 1994;12:916.

123. Lipschultz SE, Colan SD, Gelber RD, et al: Late cardiac effects of doxorubicin therapy for acute lymphoblastic leukemia. N Engl J Med 1991;324:808.

124. Sanders JE: Late effects in children receiving total body irradiation for bone marrow transplantation. Radiother Oncol 1990;18:82.

125. Sanders JE: Endocrine problems in children after bone marrow transplant for hematologic malignancies: The long-term follow-up team. Bone Marrow Transplant 1991;8:2.

126. Shinohara O, Kato S, Yabe H, et al: Growth after bone marrow transplantation in children. Am J Pediatr Hematol Oncol 1991; 13:263.

127. Leahey AM, Teunissen H, Friedman DL, et al: Late effects of chemotherapy compared to bone marrow transplantation in the treatment of pediatric acute myeloid leukemia and myelodysplasia. Med Pediatr Oncol 1999;32:163.

128. Wingard JR, Plotnick LP, Freemer CS, et al: Growth in children after bone marrow transplantation: Busulfan plus cyclophosphamide versus cyclophosphamide plus total body irradiation. Blood 1992;79:1068.

129. Sanders JE: The impact of marrow transplant preparative regimens on subsequent growth and development: The Seattle Marrow Transplant Team. Semin Hematol 1991;28:244.

130. Sanders JE, Hawley J, Levy W, et al: Pregnancies following high-dose cyclophosphamide with or without high-dose busulfan or total-body irradiation and bone marrow transplantation. Blood 1996;87:3045.

131. Socie G, Curtis RE, Deeg J, et al: New malignant diseases after allogeneic marrow transplantation for childhood acute leukemia. J Clin Oncol 2000;18:348.

23

Alessandro Rambaldi   Andrea Biondi

Acute Promyelocytic Leukemia

Since the time of its first description,[1, 2] acute promyelocytic leukemia (APL) has been recognized for its particular morphologic features and the presence of a potentially devastating hemorrhagic syndrome related to disseminated intravascular coagulopathy and abnormal fibrinolysis. Early on it was also noted to be extremely responsive to anthracycline-containing chemotherapy.[3] Two major advances—the availability of differentiation therapy with all-*trans*-retinoic acid (ATRA) and molecular characterization of the t(15;17) translocation—have produced remarkable improvement in patient outcome in the last decade.[4-9]

DEMOGRAPHIC FEATURES

APL accounts for 10% to 15% of de novo acute myeloid leukemia (AML) in younger adults.[10] Some differences in age and ethnic distribution have been described. In particular, Latinos with AML have a higher likelihood of the APL subtype of disease.[11] Among pediatric patients as reported by cooperative groups and single oncologic centers, the incidence of APL is usually considered to be lower and is 3% to 9%.[12-17] Published data from Italian cooperative studies indicate that APL in children occurs with the same incidence generally observed in adults.[18] Several small series from different countries in Central and South America[19-21] have noted a higher than expected frequency of APL in pediatric AML. It is still unknown whether such differences may suggest a genetic predisposition to APL and/or exposure to a distinct environmental factor or factors.

ETIOLOGY AND MOLECULAR PATHOGENESIS OF APL

The cause of APL is unknown. Secondary APL, albeit less frequent than other AML subtypes, can occur in patients with cancer treated by chemotherapy and/or irradiation. Occasional cases of secondary APL have been reported in patients after treatment with alkylating agents, as well as with inhibitors of topoisomerase II.[22-26] Secondary APL is a disease with a favorable prognosis.[27] Its characteristics, response to therapy, and long-term outcome are similar to those of primary forms of APL rather than therapy-related AML.

APL is the only form of leukemia to date that responds to differentiation therapy. The explanation for this peculiar feature lies in the chromatin alteration induced by the retinoic acid receptor (RAR) fusion proteins expressed uniquely in APL cells.[28] All APL patients have a chromosomal translocation within the second intron of the *RARα* locus on chromosome 17q21 that produces a chimeric protein composed of all but the first 30 amino acids of *RARα*[29] (Fig. 23-1). The N-terminal fusion partners are *PML*[30-32] on chromosome 15q21, *PLZF* (promyelocytic leukemia zinc finger) on chromosome 11q23,[33] *NPM* (nucleolar phosphoprotein nucleophosmin) on chromosome 5q31,[34] and *NuMA* (nuclear matrix associated genes) on chromosome 11q13.[35] Recently, the *STAT5b* gene located at 17q21 has been identified as a new *RARα* partner in a der17 APL case.[36]

RARα (the three homologous RAR proteins are called α, β, and γ) is a ligand-dependent transcriptional activator that binds through its zinc finger domain, as a heterodimer with members of the RXR (retinoid X receptor) family of nuclear receptors,[37] to specific DNA sequences (called retinoic acid response elements [RAREs]) found in the promoters of retinoic acid–responsive genes.[38] The RXR/RAR heterodimer binds a nuclear co-repressor molecule, either N-CoR[39, 40] (nuclear receptor co-repressor) or SMRT[41, 42] (silencing mediator of retinoid and thyroid receptors), through specific interaction domains in the ligand-binding region of RAR. N-CoR, the better analyzed of the two, binds to many sequence-specific DNA-binding transcriptional repressor proteins. N-CoR (or SMRT) itself binds another intermediary protein, Sin3, which serves as a bridge to HDAC1, a histone deacetylase[43-45] (three homologous HDACs have been identified in human cells).[46] The PML-RARα fusion protein contains the N-terminal ring finger, a leucine zipper motif of PML joined to the RARα domains. At physiologic levels of retinoic acid, PML-RARα represses rather than activates transcription,[47-50] which is apparently the consequence of enhanced interaction between PML-RARα and the N-CoR/Sin3/HDAC1 co-repressor complex (Fig. 23-2A). PML-RARα binds N-CoR at levels of ligand that are otherwise sufficient to release the co-repressor complex from wild-type RAR. By maintaining the promoters retinoic acid–responsive genes in a repressive deacetylated configura-

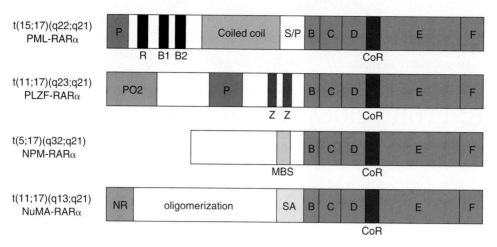

FIGURE 23–1. Chimeric fusion products arising from alternative APL associated translocations. Each of the chromosomal rearrangements disrupts *RARα* within the second intron, leading to the retention of the hormone receptor DNA-, RXR-, ligand-, and coactivator- and co-repressor-binding domain. *PML-RARα:*P: proline-rich domain; R, B1, and B2: cysteine-histidine–rich RING finger and B box domain; S/P: site of phosphorylation, nuclear localization signal. *PLZF-RARα:*POZ: repressor domain; P: proline-rich domain; Z: zinc fingers. *NPM-RARα:* MBS: potential metal binding site. *NuMA-RARα:*NR: nuclear assembly; SA: spindle association. (See Color Section.)

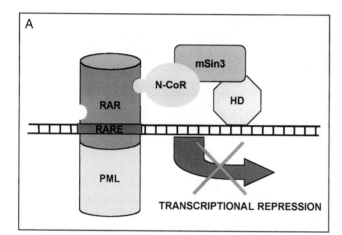

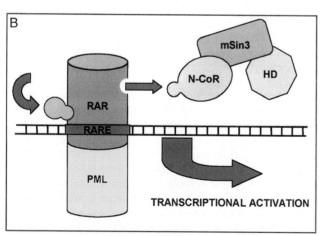

FIGURE 23–2. A schematic representation of the interaction of PML-RARα fusion protein with the N-CoR-mSin3-histone deacetylase (HD) complex. DNA-bound PML-RARα interacts with N-CoR (or SMRT) and recruits the m-Sin3-HD complex, decreasing histone acetylation and producing repressive chromatin organization and transcriptional repression (A). ATRA induces dissociation of the N-CoR-mSin3-HD complex, recruitment of coactivators with acetyltransferase activity (not shown), increased levels of histone acetylation, chromatin remodeling, and transcriptional activation (B). (See Color Section.)

tion, PML-RARα suppresses transcription and produces a phenotype identical to that experimentally produced by a dominant-negative inhibitor of RAR.[51] Only at pharmacologic levels of ligand does PML-RARα release N-CoR, recruit a co-activator complex, and allow histone acetylation and chromatin remodeling to proceed (Fig. 23–2*B*). Thus, for PML-RARα–expressing APL cells, pharmacologic levels of retinoic acid are needed to induce differentiation. The molecular mechanism underlying the strong interaction of PML-RARα with N-CoR is not yet known; apparently, no direct binding occurs between PML and N-CoR. Fusion with PML presumably inhibits the ligand-induced conformational changes necessary for release of the N-CoR complex.

If the final result of PML-RARα binding to the co-repressor complex is active repression of transcription through an HDAC1-dependent pathway, one would predict that the APL phenotype might be overcome by inhibitors of HDAC. This prediction has been validated by the finding that retinoic acid and inhibitors of HDAC1 synergize to induce differentiation of the APL cell line, NB4, or U937 cells engineered to express PML-RARα.[47, 48, 50]

Despite clinical similarity, ATRA induces differentiation of leukemic blasts and disease remission only in PML-RARα APLs, whereas PLZF/RARα APLs are ATRA resistant.[4–6, 8, 9] The t(11;17)(q23;q12) chromosomal translocation of APL fuses the same sequences of *RARα* to the N-terminus of *PLZF*.[33] PLZF is itself a DNA-binding transcription factor capable of binding N-CoR via the 120–amino acid N-terminal POZ motif[52, 53] (conserved between poxvirus and zinc finger proteins) retained in the *PLZF-RARα* fusion.[54–56] As a result, *PLZF-RARα* interacts with N-CoR through two binding sites: a ligand-dependent site in the RAR domain and a ligand-independent site in the PLZF N terminus.[47–50, 55] When retinoic acid binds to the ligand-binding domain of PLZF-RARα, the RAR domain of the fusion protein loses its attraction for N-CoR, but the PLZF ligand–independent domain continues to bind N-CoR. As a result, even in the presence of pharmacologic levels of retinoic acid, N-CoR/Sin3/HDAC1 remains bound to retinoic acid–responsive promoters and in so doing permanently suppresses transcription and blocks differentiation. In vitro ectopic expression of PML-RARα, but not PLZF/RARα, increases the ATRA sensitivity of hematopoietic cell lines and restores ATRA sensitivity to resistant cells.[57, 58] In vivo, leukemias develop in *PML-RARα* and *PLZF-RARα* transgenic mice, but only leukemias from PML-RARα mice are ATRA sensitive.[49, 59, 60]

RAR fusion proteins' biologic activity may also interfere with cell survival, and this characteristic may contribute to their leukemogenic potential. Expression of *PML-RARα* in hematopoietic cells inhibits programmed cell death, whereas in nonhematopoietic cells it induces apoptosis.[61-63] Indeed, forced expression of *PML* in a variety of cell lines induces growth arrest through apoptotic pathways,[64-67] whereas targeted disruption of the *PML* locus in mice increases the rate of spontaneous or induced carcinogenesis.[68] The molecular mechanisms by which *PML-RARα* deregulates PML intracellular pathways are not clear. *PML* localizes within distinct nuclear compartments (nuclear bodies).[69] The PML-NB structure is destroyed in APL cells and is restored after ATRA treatment as a direct consequence of PML-RARα degradation.[70] Also, *PLZF* is a growth suppressor that localizes within NBs.[71] Thus, NBs could be involved in negative growth control, and their deregulation by RAR fusion proteins might represent a critical step in promyelocytic leukemogenesis.

Therefore, in spite of extensive research, the molecular mechanism by which fusion proteins alter myeloid differentiation and growth has not been completely understood. Alternative explanations can be summarized as follows: (1) fusions behave as aberrant transcriptional repressors or activators of retinoic acid–responsive genes in the presence of physiologic levels of retinoic acid, (2) fusion inhibits the function of the normal unrearranged *RARα* gene, and (3) fusion inhibits the function of the normal unrearranged *PML,* which has been described as a potential tumor suppressor gene. More recently, other data have emerged to complicate the picture even further: normal RARα has a bidirectional function in normal granulocyte differentiation in that RARα seems to inhibit differentiation in the absence of retinoic acid whereas it stimulates differentiation in the presence of retinoic acid. These last data suggest an alternative mechanism of action for the fusion proteins in which they may mimic the normal inhibitory function of unligated RARα.

MORPHOLOGY

The initial morphologic description of APL emphasized a specific hypergranular, promyelocyte-like blast cell component in the bone marrow. Although the term *promyelocytic leukemia* has been widely accepted,[1] it is partly misleading because APL cells are morphologically different from normal promyelocytes. In 1976, the French-American-British (FAB) cooperative group revised the morphologic description of AMLs; the term M3 AML was assigned to hypergranular promyelocytic leukemia characterized by blast cells with heavy azurophilic granules, bundles of Auer rods (faggots), and a reniform or bilobed nucleus[72] (Fig. 23-3*A*).

Although the vast majority of M3 cases fit the descrip-

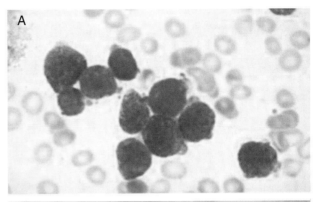

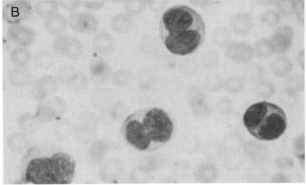

FIGURE 23–3. Representative morphology of M3-hypergranular *(A)* and M3v *(B)*. Bone marrow *(A)* and peripheral blood *(B)* smears were both stained with May-Grumwald-Giemsa × 1000-fold magnification. (Courtesy of Dr. A. Cantù-Rajnoldi, Milan, Italy.) (See Color Section.)

tion of hypergranular or classic M3, a cytologic hypogranular or microgranular variant form, M3v, has been identified (Fig. 23-3*B*). It is commonly associated with hyperleukocytosis,[73] accounts for 15% to 20% of APL cases, and shares the same t(15;17) translocation. Though less frequently observed, M3v occurs even in pediatric patients.[74] In M3v AML, the majority of blasts have a bilobed, multilobed, or reniform nucleus and, with the usual staining, are devoid of granules or contain only a few fine azurophilic granules; however, at least a few cells with all the cytoplasmic features of M3 are present.[75] Rare morphologic forms associated with t(15;17) have been reported. These cases are characterized by hyperbasophilic microgranular blast cells with cytoplasmic budding that mimics micromegakaryocytes[76-78] or by blast cells that exhibit toluidine blue–positive basophilic granules[79, 80] or eosinophilic granules.[81] Other cases have been reported to have M1- or M2-like morphology[77, 82] (Fig. 23-4). In attempts to further define the morphologic heterogeneity of APL, an European workshop has been organized in which a large series of cases with morphologically suspected APL but lacking t(15;17) were referred for central morphologic, immunophenotypic, cytogenetic, and molecular review. A novel morphologic classification system has been proposed and was found to reliably distinguish APL cases with the *PLZF-RARα* fusion gene from those with ATRA-responsive disease, including cases with underlying *PML-RARα* and *NPM-RARα* gene rearrangements.[83] When compared with control cases with the classic t(15;17) translocation, in those with

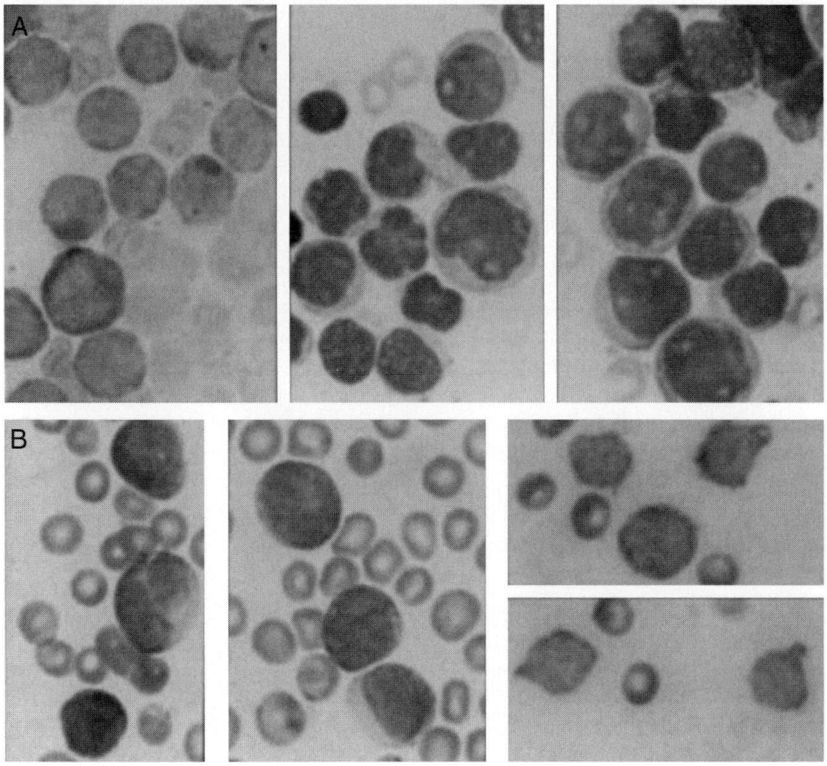

FIGURE 23-4. Representative morphology of atypical morphology in APL cases with *PML-RARα* fusion gene identified by FISH and molecular RT-PCR. Bone marrow smears were stained with May-Grumwald-Giemsa, × 1000-fold magnification. (Courtesy of Dr. D. Head, Vanderbilt University Medical School, Nashville, TN.) (See Color Section.)

PLZF-RARα rearrangements, most blasts had (1) a regular nucleus and (2) abundant cytoplasm with either coarse granules or, less frequently, fine or no granules. Faggots and Chédiak-like granules are rarely detectable (Fig. 23-5). The presence of a regular nuclear outline is a key feature of t(11;17)-associated APL. The few cases thus far described of APL with *NPM/RARα*[34, 84, 85] could be classified as M3, and the patients had hyperleukocytosis; the remaining patient[85] had M3v morphology.

IMMUNOPHENOTYPE

As with morphology and molecular genetics, the immunophenotype of APL is also very distinctive. A recent, extensive analysis performed on both adult and childhood APL showed that APL blasts have a typical surface marker expression characterized by positivity for CD33, CD13, and CD9; absence of HLA-DR; and rare expression of CD10, CD7, and CD11b. Aberrant expression of CD2 and CD34 is found in approximately 25% to 30% of patients and often coexpressed in patients with M3v morphology and a *PML/RARα* Bcr3 breakpoint.[86, 87] Aberrant expression of CD19 was also found in a minority of patients (11%) and directly correlated with white blood cell (WBC) counts.[88] Moreover, recent analysis of other markers demonstrated that CD56 expression is found in about 15% of the patients whose clinical outcome was characterized by a shorter duration of complete response and lower overall survival.[89, 90]

CYTOGENETICS

The t(15;17) translocation is the diagnostic hallmark of APL and had initially been considered to be present in all

patients with this condition.[91] Conventional cytogenetics or, more recently, fluorescence in situ hybridization (FISH) enabled identification of both derivatives chromosomes, 15q and 17q (Fig. 23-6). In addition to the classic form of the t(15;17) translocation, the existence of cryptic translocations or microinsertions has been reported.[92, 93] A recent European Working Party reported that most cases of morphologic APL lacking t(15;17) are still associated with formation of the *PML-RARα* fusion gene created by insertion events or more complex rearrangements.[94] Such mechanisms occur in approximately 4% and 2% of cases of APL, respectively, and typically lead to the formation of *PML-RARα* at its usual location on 15q (Fig. 23-7) and, less commonly, at the site of the reciprocal fusion gene on 17q or alternative chromosomal locations. These findings are highly analogous to those previously reported in chronic myeloid leukemia (CML). In this condition, 90% of cases are associated with t(9;22), which leads to rearrangement between the *BCR* and *ABL* genes. *BCR-ABL* rearrangements are also present in approximately half of the CML patients lacking the classic t(9;22) translocation. In most of these patients, chromosomes 9 and 22 have a normal appearance, with formation of the *BCR-ABL* fusion gene at its usual location on chromosome 22; more rarely, the fusion gene is located on chromosome 9 or other chromosomal sites and reflects the occurrence of more complex rearrangements.[95] The striking similarity between the frequency of the classic translocation and complex and cryptic rearrangements involving the genes disrupted by each respective translocation in CML and APL raises the possibility that similar underlying mechanisms may be involved. This possibility is supported by a recent study documenting the proximity of *BCR* and *ABL* genes and

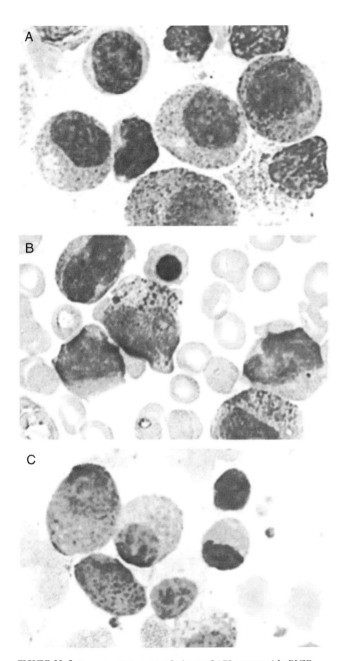

FIGURE 23–5. Representative morphology of APL cases with *PLZF-RARα*. Blasts with regular nuclei and hypergranular cytoplasm *(A)*. Blasts with irregular nuclei, hypergranular cytoplasm, and Chediak-like granules *(B)*. Blasts with regular nuclei with hypogranular cytoplasm and a Pelger-like cell *(C)* ×1000-fold magnification. (Courtesy of *Blood*.[83]) (See Color Section.)

PML and *RARα* genes at specific phases of the cell cycle in hematopoietic progenitors.[96]

DIAGNOSTIC CRITERIA FOR APL

When compared with the diagnosis of other AML subtypes, the identification of APL conveys unique therapeutic and prognostic implications. In fact, this leukemia is a medical emergency, and up to 10% of early hemorrhagic deaths are currently recorded even in patients receiving

modern state-of-the-art treatments[9, 97]; in addition, the optimized front-line approach (ATRA plus chemotherapy) is different from that used in other AMLs and is also effective in controlling the life-threatening coagulopathy.[98, 99] Although the morphologic diagnosis is straightforward in the vast majority of hypergranular cases, it appears insufficient for the identification of each and every patient who would benefit from ATRA-containing treatments.

Conventional karyotyping on banded metaphases enables documentation of the pathognomonic t(15;17) translocation in the majority (up to 90%) of morphologically defined APL cases. A recent study of patients entered in the Medical Research Council (MRC) ATRA trial showed that the translocation could be cytogenetically documented in 81 of 93 (87%) patients with polymerase chain (PCR) detectable *PML-RARα* transcripts.[100] Reasons for "false-negative" cytogenetic findings in APL include analysis of cells not belonging to the neoplastic clone (e.g., erythroblasts), which may undergo mitosis in direct or short-term preparations,[101] the existence of cryptic translocations or microinsertions, and difficulties in interpreting poor-quality preparations with few mitoses and/or fuzzy chromosomes.[100] In most of these cases, FISH analysis using specific *PML* and *RARα* probes would successfully define the genetic diagnosis. In any case, conventional karyotyping retains an important role and should always complement and not be a substitute for molecular diagnosis.

Southern blotting is laborious and time consuming (5 to 10 days). In fact, at least two probes and several enzymatic digestions are required to identify breakpoints on the *RARα* second intron in all APL cases.[102-104] Addi-

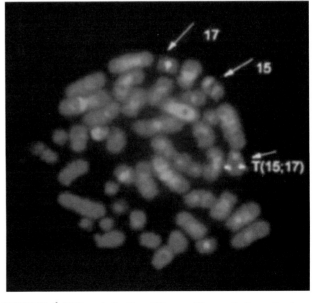

FIGURE 23–6. FISH analysis of an APL case. The result shown has been obtained by using the Vysis probe set, which is designed to detect only the *PML-RARα* fusion gene. It comprises a mixture of directly labeled probes: a *PML* probe, which begins in intron 7 and extends toward the centromere for 180 kb, and a *RARα* probe, which begins in intron 4 and extends toward the telomere for 400 kb. (Courtesy of Prof. A. Hagemeijer, Leuven, Belgium.) (See Color Section.)

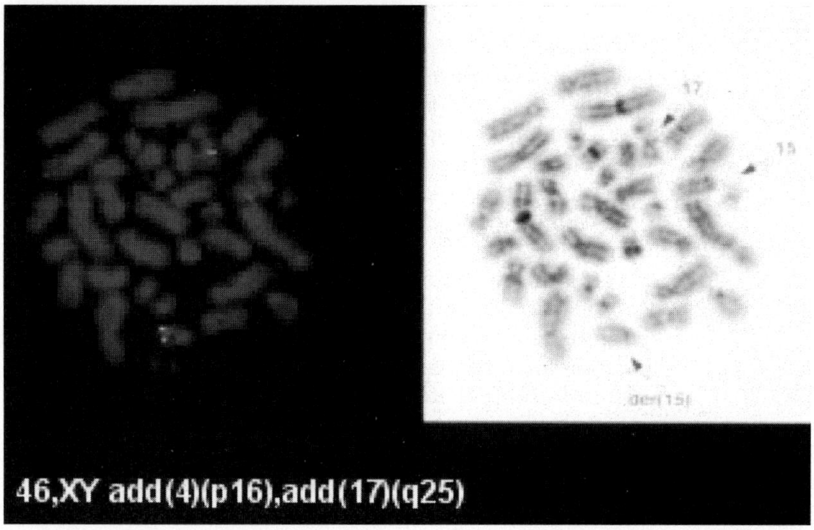

46,XY add(4)(p16),add(17)(q25)

FIGURE 23–7. FISH analysis of an APL case lacking the classic t(15;17) translocation, according to the full karyotype obtained by standard chromosomal banding techniques, but resulting positive for the presence of a *PML-RARα* fusion gene by FISH. (See Color Section.)

tional hybridizations with *PML* probes are needed to detect rearrangements on the 15q+ derivative, to determine the type of *PML* breakpoint, or to rule out a variant translocation.[104] Because of such complexity, the use of Southern blotting for the routine diagnosis of APL has been almost abandoned in specialized laboratories.

Study of the PML distribution pattern in leukemic cells provides a rapid, specific, low-cost, and relatively simple diagnostic approach.[100, 105, 106] In contrast to the wild-type (speckled) staining, which corresponds to the localization of PML into 5 to 20 discrete nuclear particles (so-called "nuclear bodies"), APL cells show a characteristic and easily distinguishable nuclear PML positivity known as "microspeckled" that results from disruption of the NBs and redistribution of the protein into more than 50 small granules per cell. Both immunocytochemistry and immunofluorescence have been successfully used as detection systems. The monoclonal antibody PG-M3[107] directed against an N-terminal PML epitope that is shared by all the known PML and PML-RAR isoforms is particularly suitable for diagnostic use.

The use of reverse transcription PCR (RT-PCR) for detection of the *PML-RARα* and *RARα-PML* fusion genes is the only technique that defines the type of PML breakpoint and allows determination of a correct strategy for subsequent monitoring of minimal residual disease. The advantage of routinely using this assay at diagnosis to better address treatment[108, 109] has subsequently been validated in prospective multicenter trials.[110–112] According to most investigators, high-quality RNA and efficient RT are the crucial determinants for successful RT-PCR of *PML-RARα*. Because of frequent leukopenia and the associated coagulopathy, the yield and quality of RNA from diagnostic samples are frequently poor.

Standardized conditions for RT-PCR analysis of fusion transcripts from chromosome aberrations in acute leukemia, including APL, have recently been reported.[113] As shown in Figure 23-8, a proper set of primers has been identified that allow detection of all the different *PML-RARα* junctions generated by the existence of different *PML* breakpoint regions in the *PML* locus and the presence of alternative *PML* splicing of *PML* transcripts.[109]

Moreover, the alternative use of two *RARα* polyadenylation sites generates extra *PML-RARα* transcripts of different size. The observation that *PML-RARα* transcripts are present in most, but not all APL cases has favored the use of *PML-RARα* transcripts as a PCR target for detection of APL cases at diagnosis and during monitoring.

Several studies have attempted to correlate the type of *PML-RARα* transcript either with clinicobiologic features at diagnosis or with treatment response and outcome.[97] The vast majority of such series compared the two major *PML-RARα* isoforms, referred to as long (L) transcripts (including *PML* bcr1 at intron 6 in 55% of cases and bcr2 at exon 6 in 5%) and short (S) transcripts (*PML* bcr3 at intron 3 in 40% of cases). Because bcr2 (also referred to as the "variant" or V form) and bcr1 are located in exon 6 and intron 6 of PML, respectively, sequencing of all L transcript cases would be needed to clearly distinguish these two isoforms. Such distinction is not usually reported in clinical studies with a large number of patients. At diagnosis, no correlation was found with respect to sex, platelet count, and the presence of coagulopathy or retinoic syndrome when comparing patients with L-type or S-type *PML-RARα* transcripts. However, patients with S-type transcripts had significantly higher WBC counts and more frequently had M3v morphology. Although S-type transcripts correlated with established adverse prognostic features (i.e., hyperleukocytosis, M3v), this association did not translate into a poorer outcome than in patients with L-type transcripts in the context of combined ATRA and chemotherapy.

Among the different methods (conventional karyotyping, FISH, and PML immunostaining with specific antibodies), RT-PCR detection of the *PML-RARα* fusion gene appears to be the only one suitable for detection of minimal residual disease.

Overall, it is generally agreed that a positive *PML-RARα* test after consolidation is a strong predictor of subsequent hematologic relapse whereas repeatedly negative results are associated with long survival in most patients. However, these correlation are not absolute in that both patients who remain PCR positive in long-term remission

A

Genes' structures :

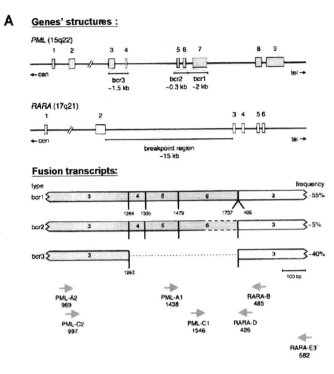

B

Primer code	5' Position^a (size)	Sequence (5'–3')
PML-A1	1438 (21)	CAGTGTACGCCTTCTCCATCA
PML-A2	969 (18)	CTGCTGGAGGCTGTGGAC
RARA-B	485 (20)	GCTTGTAGATGCGGGGTAGA
PML-C1	1546 (21)	TCAAGATGGAGTCTGAGGAGG
PML-C2	997 (19)	AGCGCGACTACGAGGAGAT
RARA-D	426 (20)	CTGCTGCTCTGGGTCTCAAT
RARA-E3'	682 (20)	GCCCACTTCAAAGCACTTCT

FIGURE 23–8. Schematic diagram of the exon/intron structure of the *PML* and *RARα* genes. The bcr1 and bcr2 breakpoint regions are juxtaposed in intron 6 and exon 6, respectively *(A)*. Schematic diagram of the three types of *PML-RARα* transcripts, related to the different *PML* breakpoint regions. The size of the bcr2 transcript is dependent on the position of the breakpoint in PML exon 6. Primers for RT-PCR analysis of the t(15;17) translocation with the *PML-RARα* fusion gene *(B)*. (Courtesy of *Leukemia*.[113]) (See Color Section.)

and, more frequently, patients who ultimately relapse after negative tests have been reported.[9, 97]

In the three large prospective studies of APL patients treated with ATRA and chemotherapy in which molecular diagnosis and monitoring have been assessed,[111, 112, 114] persistence of *PML-RARα* fusion transcripts after completion of therapy is predictive of relapse. Nevertheless, most patients who ultimately relapse test PCR negative in marrow at the end of therapy. These findings underline the notion that achievement of PCR negativity in APL cannot be equated with cure and highlight the relative insensitivity of the RT-PCR *PML-RARα* assay. In dilution experiments, we and others have been able to detect as little as 50 pg of total RNA but only 1 in 10^{-4} *PML-RARA*–positive cells, which means that this assay is approximately 1 log less sensitive than the RT-PCR applied to different chimeric genes generated by other chromo-

somal abnormalities such as *BCR/ABL* in the t(9;22) translocation.

Why do we need to molecularly monitor APL patients? The advent of ATRA has led to a dramatic improvement in survival in APL with a marked reduction in the risk of relapse to levels of only 10% to 20%. The challenge is how to identify the relatively small subgroup of patients at particular risk of relapse, who at present cannot be identified by pretreatment characteristics and who could potentially benefit from more intensive treatment in first remission.

The Italian GIMEMA (Gruppo Italiano Malattie Ematologiche Maligne Adulto) group reported that recurrence of PCR positivity, as detected by analysis of 3-month surveillance marrow after completion of therapy, was highly predictive of relapse.[115] With such a strategy, approximately 70% of relapses were successfully predicted. Clinical relapse occurred a median of 3 months after the detection of molecular relapse. These findings are of great relevance in view of data from the MRC ATRA trial that have highlighted the poor prognosis of patients relapsing after first-line therapy with ATRA and chemotherapy.[111]

A different perspective in the use of minimal residual disease to identify APL patients at higher risk for relapse has evaluated the kinetics of achievement of molecular remission. Because of the relatively low sensitivity of the *PML-RARα* assay, monitoring of the reciprocal *RARα-PML*, which is expressed in most, but not all patients, has been proposed as being at least 1 log more sensitive (i.e., 1 cell in 10^5).[116] The *RARα-PML* assay led to the detection of residual disease in an additional 20% of patients while in morphologic remission. Nevertheless, even APL patients with an informative *RARα-PML* assay who ultimately relapsed had no molecular evidence of minimal residual disease at the end of therapy.

Although molecular diagnosis plus monitoring of APL is one of the most relevant examples of the impact of molecular genetics in clinical hematology, further investigations are still needed. Whether we could benefit from a more sensitive RT-PCR assay for *PML-RARα* in the identification of patients at higher risk for relapse and whether quantitative PCR could provide further information for earlier monitoring are still unknown. Finally, even the benefit of earlier treatment at the stage of molecular relapse still has to be proved, although preliminary findings seem to support such a strategy.[117]

THERAPEUTIC STRATEGIES IN APL

Management of APL has become more successful with time because of recent advances in diagnosis and therapy. Since the early 1970s it has become clear that APL is characterized by high sensitivity to anthracycline drugs and that cure with chemotherapy alone has been achieved more frequently than in most other types of AML.[3, 118] Before the ATRA era, it also became clear that a crucial component of successful treatment of adult and childhood APL was the delivery of intensive and accurate supportive therapy, particularly daily prophylactic platelet transfusions (to >30 × 10⁹/L). Moreover, the importance of avoiding inappropriate treatment with heparin or deferring treatment in infected neutropenic patients with an atypically differentiated bone marrow pattern was recognized.[119]

Remission Induction

ATRA

In the early 1980s it was noted that in vitro, ATRA could induce granulocytic differentiation of myeloid leukemia cell lines such as HL-60 and primary cells from APL patients.[120, 121] ATRA mediates its powerful cytodifferenti-ating activity on leukemic promyelocytes by binding to a family of nuclear receptors (RARs) that regulate the expression of multiple genes, including regulators of the cell cycle, adhesion molecules, cytokines, colony-stimu-lating factors and their receptors, structural proteins, chromatin components, and transcription factors.[28] APL cells bearing the t(15;17) chromosomal translocation are uniquely sensitive to the differentiating activity of ATRA, whereas the rare APL cases harboring t(11;17) or t(5;17) show no response to this treatment and have a distinctly worse prognosis.[97] The APL-specific RARα fusion proteins PML-RARα and *PLZF-RARα* bind to and constitutively repress promoters of retinoic acid target genes via aber-rant recruitment of multi-subunit complexes containing histone deacetylase (HDAC) activities. ATRA treatment specifically relieves transcriptional repression by *PML-RARα* and triggers differentiation of APL cells. ATRA can also induce caspase-mediated degradation of the *PML-RARα* fusion protein. All in all, this pleiotropic activity played by the complex of ATRA and its receptors is followed by inhibition of growth and induction of termi-nal differentiation of leukemic promyelocytes. At the end of the 1980s, Chinese investigators provided striking evi-dence that the use of ATRA in APL patients induces complete remission in most patients, with rapid resolu-tion of the coagulopathy. The demonstration that a com-plete response can be obtained through a differentiation mechanism with ATRA opened a new age in the manage-ment of this disease.[122] These results were rapidly and largely confirmed by several other phase II clinical stud-ies, which also showed that the remission duration after

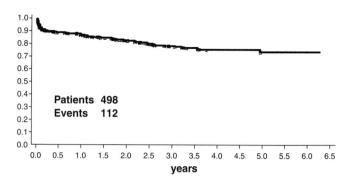

FIGURE 23–9. Overall survival of APL patients treated according to the Italian Cooperative Study protocol AIDA 0493. (Courtesy of Prof. F. Mandelli, Rome, Italy.)

ATRA alone is usually short if not consolidated by chemo-therapy.[123-128] This observation prompted several collabo-rative study groups to design phase II and phase III studies to evaluate the role of standard chemotherapy given concomitantly with or after ATRA (Table 23–1). These studies provided convincing evidence that the combination of ATRA and chemotherapy improves the prognosis of patients with APL and that the early addition of chemotherapy to ATRA during induction treatment gives better survival results than does ATRA or chemo-therapy administered alone.[111, 127, 129-131] Updated results of the Italian cooperative AIDA (ATRA plus Idarubicin) pro-tocol for newly diagnosed APL document that complete remission can be achieved in more than 90% of these pa-tients with a 5-year overall and disease-free survival rate above 70% (Figs. 23–9 and 23–10).[110] The clinical value of ATRA in APL patients (usually above 90%) has been con-firmed in most multicenter clinical studies, and it is gener-ally agreed that a synergistic rather than additive effect is played by ATRA and chemotherapy. In summary, since ATRA has become a crucial part of therapeutic protocols for APL, the outcome of this disease has changed dramati-cally, from the status of a frequently fatal leukemia to that of a highly curable disease.[132]

Postinduction Therapy

Although no consensus presently exists regarding the type and intensity of consolidation therapy, several stud-

TABLE 23–1. Main Clinical Trials in APL

Study	Treatment	Complete Remission (%)	Early Death (%)	Resistant Leukemia	Relapse Rate (%)	Overall Survival (%)	ATRA Syndrome (%)
APL 91	ATRA before CT	91	9	0	31	76	5
	CT	81	8	10	78	49	NA
ECOG (0129)	ATRA	76	11	NR	29	71	26
	CT	69	14	NR	58	50	NA
APL 93	ATRA before CT	95	7	0	16	81	20
	ATRA and CT	94	7	0	6	84	11
MRC	Short ATRA before CT	70	23	7	36	52	4
	Extended ATRA and CT	87	12	2	20	71	1
AIDA (0493)	ATRA and CT	95	5	0	20	80	2.5
PETHEMA (LPA96)	ATRA and CT	89	10	2	10	82	6

AIDA, ATRA plus idarubicin; APL, acute promyelocytic leukemia; ATRA, all-*trans*-retinoic acid; CT, chemotherapy; ECOG, Eastern Cooperative Oncology Group; MRC, Medical Research Council; NA, not available; NR, not reported; PETHEMA, Spanish cooperative group study.

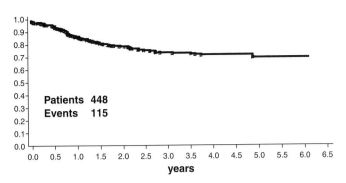

FIGURE 23–10. Disease-free survival of APL patients treated according to the Italian Cooperative Study protocol AIDA 0493. (Courtesy of Prof. F. Mandelli, Rome, Italy.)

ies have demonstrated the role of postremission therapy in preventing or deferring clinical relapse. The clinical value of intensive postremission therapy has been suggested both before and after the beginning of the ATRA era.[119] The consolidation phases of APL patients are not substantially different from those designed for the other AMLs and are usually based on a combination of anthracyclines and cytarabine. However, in a recent phase II study performed on patients with newly diagnosed leukemia, the Spanish cooperative study group (PETHEMA), after induction chemotherapy with ATRA and idarubicin, excluded the nonintercalating chemotherapy agents (cytarabine and etoposide) from consolidation treatment while maintaining the same doses and sequence of idarubicin and mitoxantrone as used in the original AIDA protocol. A preliminary report of these results showed that this protocol yielded results similar to those of the original AIDA protocol but with remarkably lower treatment-related toxicity.[133] This study and others[134] emphasize that cytarabine may not be crucial in the treatment of APL and could be omitted, particularly in low-risk patients.[135] The striking improvements in the clinical outcome of APL patients prompted several investigators to focus on detecting crucial prognostic factors that might help in the identification of high-risk patients and the design of risk-adapted therapeutic strategies. The adverse prognostic role of a high leukocyte count at diagnosis has been repeatedly reported,[111, 119, 136] and a recent joint analysis published by the PETHEMA and GIMEMA study groups[135] clearly indicates that platelet and leukocyte counts at diagnosis have strong independent prognostic value and can separate patients into low (WBC count $\leq 10 \times 10^9$/L, platelet count $> 40 \times 10^9$/L), intermediate (WBC count $\leq 10 \times 10^9$/L, platelet count $\leq 40 \times 10^9$/L) and high (WBC $\geq 10 \times 10^9$/L) risk groups. On the basis of these new findings risk-adapted protocols have been launched in Italy and Spain.

Maintenance Therapy

In contrast to other forms of AML, maintenance chemotherapy has been shown to be effective in prolonging the duration of remission in APL. During the 1980s, several studies suggested that 6-MP and methotrexate are effective in maintenance therapy for APL patients.[137] Moreover, the large clinical trials focusing on the role of ATRA in APL showed that this compound plays a crucial role when given not only for induction of a complete response but also for maintenance treatment. Indeed, in the Eastern Cooperative Oncology Group (ECOG) collaborative trial, the estimated 3-year rate of disease-free survival from the date of assignment to ATRA maintenance therapy or observation was significantly better in the ATRA group (65% and 40%, respectively), regardless of the induction regimen.[131] Similarly, the European APL 93 trial confirmed that maintenance treatment combining low-dose chemotherapy and intermittent ATRA can reduce the relapse rate, especially in patients with high WBC counts.[136]

The ATRA Syndrome

Although ATRA is generally well tolerated, fever, weight gain, musculoskeletal pain, respiratory distress, interstitial pulmonary infiltrates, pleural and pericardial effusions, skin infiltrates, hypotension, acute renal failure, and death may develop in some patients soon after the beginning of treatment.[138] These symptoms are not observed in patients receiving ATRA while in complete hematologic remission. The pathogenesis of the syndrome is probably related to heavy cytokine release (interleukin-1β, tumor necrosis factor α, interleukin-6) and to the fact that ATRA increases the expression of adhesive molecules such as CD11b, CDw65, VLA-4, and CD11a and its receptor CD54, which may allow for binding of leukemic cells to endothelial cells.[139] The reported incidence of the syndrome varied in different studies (from 3% up to 30% of patients), and the incidence seems to be higher when ATRA is given alone for induction of remission. Indeed, the concurrent administration of ATRA and chemotherapy may decrease the incidence of the syndrome. However, the mortality rate might not be different from their sum with ATRA alone if the symptoms are recognized and appropriate treatment (dexamethasone) is started early.[140, 141] Several pretreatment variables (including the WBC count at diagnosis and its increase after ATRA treatment) have been analyzed as possible predictors of the syndrome, but none were statistically correlated with the development of signs and symptoms.[136, 141, 142] Besides simultaneous administration of ATRA and chemotherapy, several strategies have been developed to prevent the syndrome, including the prophylactic administration of corticosteroids and the use of a lower dose of ATRA (25 mg/m²).[143, 144] When ATRA syndrome is definitely present or at the first sign of unexplained dyspnea, fever, or weight gain, dexamethasone should be given promptly (10 to 40 mg/day), which usually produces rapid resolution of the symptoms. However, 1% of patients continue to die of ATRA syndrome during induction of remission.

WHEN TREATMENT FAILS

Molecular and Clinical Relapse

Despite the high remission rate achieved by therapeutic protocols based on ATRA and chemotherapy, a number of patients still relapse. However, the advent of molecular monitoring of minimal residual disease has changed many aspects of leukemia relapse in APL patients. In fact, nowadays, sequential monitoring of APL patients in hematologic remission after front-line therapy permits the identification of relapsing patients with a significant time advantage. Early studies have clearly indicated that the molecular positivity seen with a relatively insensitive (10^{-4}) PCR assay almost invariably predicts overt clinical relapse and thus represents a key diagnostic tool in the follow-up management of APL patients.[115, 145] On the basis of these results, achievement of molecular remission should be considered one of the primary therapeutic objectives in the modern treatment of APL, and as a consequence, salvage therapy can be given at the time of first molecular relapse. A pilot study investigating this issue clearly suggested that early administration of salvage therapy can be advantageous for APL patients. Indeed, treatment of patients showing minimal tumor burden can be aimed at minimizing treatment-related risks such as hemorrhagic death and the ATRA syndrome and, often in an outpatient setting.[117]

The Role of Stem-Cell Transplantation

Different large cooperative clinical trials have clearly shown that combinations of chemotherapy and ATRA represent the treatment of choice of APL at diagnosis. Accordingly, it is generally agreed that nothing is to be gained in undertaking a transplant procedure in APL patients in first remission. However, despite the major advances achieved in the treatment of APL, disease relapse still occurs in about 25% of these patients, and for such patients, hematopoietic stem-cell transplantation, either autologous or allogeneic, can be a successful salvage treatment. In a retrospective study[146] it was shown that about 45% of M3 patients undergoing transplantation in second remission before the ATRA era could be cured either by an autologous or allogeneic procedure. More recent studies have confirmed that once in second remission, autologous stem-cell transplantation seems to be a highly successful procedure for reducing the risk of leukemia relapse, and disease-free survival rates exceeding 70% have been reported.[147] In this setting, an Italian study underlined the prognostic relevance of pretransplant assessment of minimal residual disease and showed that the success of autografting depends on the patient being RT-PCR negative at the time of transplantation.[148] Despite the 15% to 20% risk of transplant-related mortality, allogeneic transplantation remains an important curative option for patients in second remission or even more advanced phases of disease. Patients failing to achieve molecular remission and those of younger age should be offered this therapeutic opportunity if a donor is available.

NEW THERAPIES
Liposomal ATRA

ATRA is currently available for clinical use only in an oral form. Recently, a liposomal formulation of ATRA for intravenous infusion was developed to overcome the reduction in drug levels that occurs with oral administration and for use in patients who cannot swallow or absorb capsules and for small children. The maximal tolerated dose of liposomal ATRA was 140 mg/m².[149] Subsequent studies performed at a dosage of 90 mg/m² confirmed the safety profile of liposomal ATRA and its ability to induce molecular remission in patients with newly diagnosed and relapsed APL.[150] Therefore, although the oral formulation remains easier to administer in most patients, liposomal ATRA may be a useful and efficacious alternative in patients with low compliance to conventional treatment.[151]

New Retinoids

Prolonged treatment with ATRA results in induction of both pharmacologic[152, 153] and biologic resistance.[154] The identification of novel and more selective retinoids and their clinical use could represent a strategy to overcome this problem. In the past few years, a remarkable number of retinoic acid derivatives have been identified and studied in various cellular models, including APL-derived cell lines[155] and in some cases also in patients with ATRA-resistant relapse.[156] Another way to circumvent the mechanism of resistance could be offered by the combination of retinoids and other cytodifferentiating agents, including cytokines such as granulocyte colony-stimulating factor,[157] interferon-α,[158] and vitamin D derivatives.[159] Very recently, it has also been shown that STI571, a powerful c-Abl inhibitor used for the treatment of CML, could increase the cytodifferentiating effects of retinoids[160] in APL.

Histone Deacetylase Inhibitors

The transcriptional activity of many genes is controlled by the state of acetylation of histones, which in turn is regulated by a balance between the activity of histone acetyltransferases (HATs) and histone deacetylases (HDACs). Inhibitors of HDACs are characterized by cytodifferentiating, antiproliferative, and apoptogenic properties and include compounds such as butyrates, trichostatin, suberoylanilide hydroxamic acid (SAHA), benzamide, and cyclic peptides. Some of these compounds have shown potent antileukemic activity when combined with ATRA,[161, 162] and future laboratory and clinical research is warranted in this area.

Arsenic Trioxide

Arsenic compounds have recently been the object of renewed interest as therapeutic compounds since studies in China confirmed the efficacy of arsenic trioxide (As_2O_3) in the treatment of APL.[124, 163] These studies have been replicated in Western countries, with complete remissions achieved in most patients with refractory or relapsed APL.[164] In vitro, As_2O_3 triggers apoptosis at relatively high concentrations (0.5 to 2.0 μmol/L) and induces partial differentiation at low concentrations (0.1 to 0.5 μmol/L). Although detailed molecular mechanisms are not yet fully determined, As_2O_3 can induce partial differentiation and subsequent apoptosis of APL cells through degradation of wild-type PML and PML-RARα chimeric proteins and possible antimitochondrial effects. As_2O_3 over a wide range of concentrations (0.1 to 2.0 μmol/L) enhances the acetylation of histone, a process important for the transcriptional activation of genes. ATRA and As_2O_3 induce non–cross-resistant complete clinical remission in patients with APL and the t(15;17) translocation and target PML-RARα, the leukemogenic protein, by different pathways, thus suggesting possible therapeutic synergism. As_2O_3 at subapoptotic concentrations decreased ATRA-induced differentiation in the NB4 cell line but synergized with ATRA to induce differentiation in ATRA-resistant NB4 subclones. Severe combined immunodeficient mice bearing NB4 cells showed an additive survival effect after sequential treatment, but a toxic effect was observed after simultaneous treatment with ATRA and As_2O_3, which suggests that sequential treatment may be more effective than single agents in ATRA-resistant patients.[165] As_2O_3 effectively induces remission in relapsed APL. At Memorial Sloan-Kettering Cancer Center, patients with relapsed or refractory APL were treated with As_2O_3 for induction of remission at daily doses that ranged from 0.06 to 0.2 mg/kg, and approximately 90% of patients achieved complete remission.[164] However, as in the case of ATRA, early relapses from As_2O_3 treatment within a few months are frequently seen, thus indicating that rapidly emerging resistance to As_2O_3 can occur. Therefore, chemotherapy in combination with As_2O_3 as postremission therapy will probably yield better survival than treatment with As_2O_3 alone, which is in line with the observation that remission induction with As_2O_3 is not sufficient in most cases to obtain molecular remission as judged by RT-PCR for *PML-RARα* fusion transcripts. In summary, despite a short follow-up, the initial clinical results obtained in relapsed APL patients are very promising. Among other things, future prospective clinical trials should evaluate the role of combining As_2O_3 with ATRA in the treatment of newly diagnosed APL in patients who for are not eligible for the current therapeutic protocols based on ATRA and chemotherapy. Although most adverse reactions of As_2O_3 treatment were tolerable, certain infrequent, but severe toxicities related to As_2O_3 were observed, including renal failure, hepatic damage, cardiac arrhythmia, and chronic neuromuscular degeneration, which should be monitored carefully. Detectable polyneuropathy compatible with chronic arsenic toxicity has also been noted in patients receiving As_2O_3 as maintenance therapy. During As_2O_3 therapy, an increase in the WBC count peaking at a median of 17 days occurred in many cases, and a "retinoic acid syndrome," similar in manifestations to that noted after the administration of ATRA, has been observed.[166]

Monoclonal Antibodies

The use of monoclonal antibodies has recently been proposed for the treatment of refractory AML. HuM195 is a humanized monoclonal antibody against CD33 that has been successfully used for the treatment of minimal residual disease of PCR-positive APL patients in hematologic remission after induction therapy with ATRA and/or chemotherapy.[167] HuM195 has been also conjugated with ^{131}I, ^{90}Y, and ^{213}Bi, and these molecules are currently under investigation. Another interesting molecule has been produced by the combination of another humanized anti-CD33 antibody and calicheamicin (CMA676, Mylotarg).[168] This latter antibody has been recently approved by the Food and Drug Administration for the treatment of relapsed AML, and preliminary observations indicate its ability to control minimal residual disease in APL patients with evidence of molecular relapse.

REFERENCES

1. Hillestad LK: Acute promyelocytic leukemia. Acta Med Scand 1957;159:189.
2. Caen J, Mathe G, Xuan Chat L, et al: Étude de la fibrinolyse au cours des hémopaties malignes. Paper presented at the 6th Congress of the European Society of Hematology, Paris, 1957, p 502.
3. Bernard J, Weil M, Boiron M, et al: Acute promyelocytic leukemia: Results of treatment by daunorubicin. Blood 1973;41:489.
4. Grignani F, Fagioli M, Alcalay M, et al: Acute promyelocytic leukemia: From genetics to treatment. Blood 1994;83:10.
5. Chen SJ, Wang ZY, Chen Z: Acute promyelocytic leukemia: From clinic to molecular biology. Stem Cells 1995;13:22.
6. Warrell RP: Pathogenesis and management of acute promyelocytic leukemia. Annu Rev Med 1996;47:555.
7. Wiernik PH, Gallagher RE, Tallman MS: Diagnosis and Treatment of Acute Promyelocytic Leukemia. New York: Churchill Livingstone; 1996.
8. Fenaux P, Chomienne C, Degos L: Acute promyelocytic leukemia: Biology and treatment. Semin Oncol 1997;24:92.
9. Grimwade D: The pathogenesis of acute promyelocytic leukaemia: Evaluation of the role of molecular diagnosis and monitoring in the management of the disease. Br J Haematol 1999;106:591.
10. Stone RM, Mayer RJ: The unique aspects of acute promyelocytic leukemia. J Clin Oncol 1990;8:1913.
11. Douer D, Preston-Martin S, Chang E, et al: High frequency of acute promyelocytic leukemia among Latinos with acute myeloid leukemia. Blood 1996;87:308.
12. Chan KW, Steinherz PG, Miller DR: Acute promyelocytic leukemia in children. Med Pediatr Oncol 1981;9:5.
13. Argyle JC, Benjamin DR, Lampkin B, et al: Acute nonlymphocytic leukemias of childhood. Inter-observer variability and problems in the use of the FAB classification. Cancer 1989;63:295.
14. Carter M, Kalwinsky DK, Dahl GV, et al: Childhood acute promyelocytic leukemia: A rare variant of nonlymphoid leukemia with distinctive clinical and biologic features. Leukemia 1989;3:298.
15. Steuber CP, Civin C, Krischer J, et al: A comparison of induction and maintenance therapy for acute nonlymphocytic leukemia in childhood: Results of a Pediatric Oncology Group study. J Clin Oncol 1991;9:247.
16. Cantu-Rajnoldi A, Biondi A, Jankovic M, et al: Diagnosis and incidence of acute promyelocytic leukemia (FAB M3 and M3 variant) in childhood. Blood 1993;81:2209.
17. Creutzig U, Ritter J, Zimmermann M, et al: Does cranial irradiation reduce the risk for bone marrow relapse in acute myelogenous leukemia? Unexpected results of the Childhood Acute Myelogenous Leukemia Study BFM-87. J Clin Oncol 1993;11:279.
18. Biondi A, Rovelli A, Cantu-Rajnoldi A, et al: Acute promyelocytic leukemia in children: Experience of the Italian Pediatric Hematology and Oncology Group (AIEOP). Leukemia 1994;8:1264.
19. Malta Corea A, Pacheco Espinoza C, Cantu Rajnoldi A, et al: Childhood acute promyelocytic leukemia in Nicaragua. Ann Oncol 1993;4:892.
20. De Salvo L, Weir-Medina J, Gomez-Sanchez O, et al: Leucemia promielocitica aguda en el occidente de Venezuela [abstract]. Sangre 1989;34:329.

21. Louriero P, Azevzdo A, Maia A, et al: Acute myeloid leukemia: Presentation of the disease and response to treatment in North-East of Brasil [abstract]. Med Pediatr Oncol 1992;20:432.

22. Bhavnani M, Azzawi SA, Yin JA, et al: Therapy-related acute promyelocytic leukaemia. Br J Haematol 1994;86:231.

23. Hoffmann L, Moller P, Pedersen-Bjergaard J, et al: Therapy-related acute promyelocytic leukemia with t(15;17) (q22;q12) following chemotherapy with drugs targeting DNA topoisomerase II. A report of two cases and a review of the literature. Ann Oncol 1995; 6:781.

24. Pollicardo N, O'Brien S, Estey EH, et al: Secondary acute promyelocytic leukemia. Characteristics and prognosis of 14 patients from a single institution. Leukemia 1996;10:27.

25. Kudo K, Yoshida H, Kiyoi H, et al: Etoposide-related acute promyelocytic leukemia. Leukemia 1998;12:1171.

26. Naoe T, Kudo K, Yoshida H, et al: Molecular analysis of the t(15; 17) translocation in de novo and secondary acute promyelocytic leukemia. Leukemia 1997;11(Suppl 3):287.

27. Detourmignies L, Castaigne S, Stoppa AM, et al: Therapy-related acute promyelocytic leukemia: A report on 16 cases. J Clin Oncol 1992;10:1430.

28. Melnick A, Licht JD: Deconstructing a disease: RARα, its fusion partners, and their roles in the pathogenesis of acute promyelocytic leukemia. Blood 1999;93:3167.

29. Borrow J, Goddard AD, Sheer D, et al: Molecular analysis of acute promyelocytic leukemia breakpoint cluster region on chromosome 17. Science 1990;249:1577.

30. Kakizuka A, Miller WH, Umesono K, et al: Chromosomal translocation t(15;17) in human acute promyelocytic leukemia fuses RAR alpha with a novel putative transcription factor, PML. Cell 1991; 66:663.

31. de The H, Lavau C, Marchio A, et al: The PML-RAR alpha fusion mRNA generated by the t(15;17) translocation in acute promyelocytic leukemia encodes a functionally altered RAR. Cell 1991; 66:675.

32. Alcalay M, Zangrilli D, Pandolfi PP, et al: Translocation breakpoint of acute promyelocytic leukemia lies within the retinoic acid receptor alpha locus. Proc Natl Acad Sci U S A 1991;88:1977.

33. Chen Z, Brand NJ, Chen A, et al: Fusion between a novel Kruppel-like zinc finger gene and the retinoic acid receptor-alpha locus due to a variant t(11;17) translocation associated with acute promyelocytic leukaemia. Embo J 1993;12:1161.

34. Redner RL, Rush EA, Faas S, et al: The t(5;17) variant of acute promyelocytic leukemia expresses a nucleophosmin–retinoic acid receptor fusion. Blood 1996;87:882.

35. Wells RA, Catzavelos C, Kamel-Reid S: Fusion of retinoic acid receptor alpha to NuMA, the nuclear mitotic apparatus protein, by a variant translocation in acute promyelocytic leukaemia. Nat Genet 1997;17:109.

36. Arnould C, Philippe C, Bourdon V, et al: The signal transducer and activator of transcription STAT5b gene is a new partner of retinoic acid receptor alpha in acute promyelocytic-like leukaemia. Hum Mol Genet 1999;8:1741.

37. Yu VC, Delsert C, Andersen B, et al: RXR beta: A coregulator that enhances binding of retinoic acid, thyroid hormone, and vitamin D receptors to their cognate response elements. Cell 1991;67:1251.

38. Umesono K, Murakami KK, Thompson CC, et al: Direct repeats as selective response elements for the thyroid hormone, retinoic acid, and vitamin D_3 receptors. Cell 1991;65:1255.

39. Horlein AJ, Naar AM, Heinzel T, et al: Ligand-independent repression by the thyroid hormone receptor mediated by a nuclear receptor co-repressor. Nature 1995;377:397.

40. Kurokawa R, Soderstrom M, Horlein A, et al: Polarity-specific activities of retinoic acid receptors determined by a co-repressor. Nature 1995;377:451.

41. Chen JD, Evans RM: A transcriptional co-repressor that interacts with nuclear hormone receptors. Nature 1995;377:454.

42. Chen JD, Umesono K, Evans RM: SMRT isoforms mediate repression and anti-repression of nuclear receptor heterodimers. Proc Natl Acad Sci U S A 1996;93:7567.

43. Alland L, Muhle R, Hou H, et al: Role for N-CoR and histone deacetylase in Sin3-mediated transcriptional repression. Nature 1997;387:49.

44. Laherty CD, Yang WM, Sun JM, et al: Histone deacetylases associated with the mSin3 corepressor mediate mad transcriptional repression. Cell 1997;89:349.

45. Heinzel T, Lavinsky RM, Mullen TM, et al: A complex containing N-CoR, mSin3 and histone deacetylase mediates transcriptional repression. Nature 1997;387:43.

46. Hassig CA, Tong JK, Fleischer TC, et al: A role for histone deacetylase activity in HDAC1-mediated transcriptional repression. Proc Natl Acad Sci U S A 1998;95:3519.

47. Grignani F, De Matteis S, Nervi C, et al: Fusion proteins of the retinoic acid receptor-alpha recruit histone deacetylase in promyelocytic leukaemia. Nature 1998;391:815.

48. Lin RJ, Nagy L, Inoue S, et al: Role of the histone deacetylase complex in acute promyelocytic leukaemia. Nature 1998;391:811.

49. He LZ, Guidez F, Triboli C, et al: Distinct interactions of PML-RARα and PLZF-RARα with co-repressors determine differential responses to RA in APL. Nat Genet 1998;18:126.

50. Guidez F, Ivins S, Zhu J, et al: Reduced retinoic acid-sensitivities of nuclear receptor corepressor binding to PML- and PLZF-RARα underlie molecular pathogenesis and treatment of acute promyelocytic leukemia. Blood 1998;91:2634.

51. Tsai S, Collins SJ: A dominant negative retinoic acid receptor blocks neutrophil differentiation at the promyelocyte stage. Proc Natl Acad Sci U S A 1993;90:7153.

52. Ahmad KF, Engel CK, Prive GG: Crystal structure of the BTB domain from PLZF. Proc Natl Acad Sci U S A 1998;95:12123.

53. Li X, Lopez-Guisa JM, Ninan N, et al: Overexpression, purification, characterization, and crystallization of the BTB/POZ domain from the PLZF oncoprotein. J Biol Chem 1997;272:27324.

54. Hong SH, David G, Wong CW, et al: SMRT corepressor interacts with PLZF and with the PML–retinoic acid receptor alpha (RARα) and PLZF-RARα oncoproteins associated with acute promyelocytic leukemia. Proc Natl Acad Sci U S A 1997;94:9028.

55. David G, Alland L, Hong SH, et al: Histone deacetylase associated with mSin3A mediates repression by the acute promyelocytic leukemia–associated PLZF protein. Oncogene 1998;16:2549.

56. Dhordain P, Albagli O, Lin RJ, et al: Corepressor SMRT binds the BTB/POZ repressing domain of the LAZ3/BCL6 oncoprotein. Proc Natl Acad Sci U S A 1997;94:10762.

57. Rousselot P, Hardas B, Patel A, et al: The PML-RAR alpha gene product of the t(15;17) translocation inhibits retinoic acid-induced granulocytic differentiation and mediated transactivation in human myeloid cells. Oncogene 1994;9:545.

58. Ruthardt M, Testa U, Nervi C, et al: Opposite effects of the acute promyelocytic leukemia PML–retinoic acid receptor alpha (RAR alpha) and PLZF-RAR alpha fusion proteins on retinoic acid signalling. Mol Cell Biol 1997;17:4859.

59. He LZ, Merghoub T, Pandolfi PP: In vivo analysis of the molecular pathogenesis of acute promyelocytic leukemia in the mouse and its therapeutic implications. Oncogene 1999;18:5278.

60. Westervelt P, Ley TJ: Seed versus soil: The importance of the target cell for transgenic models of human leukemias. Blood 1999; 93:2143.

61. Grignani F, Ferrucci PF, Testa U, et al: The acute promyelocytic leukemia-specific PML-RAR alpha fusion protein inhibits differentiation and promotes survival of myeloid precursor cells. Cell 1993; 74:423.

62. Rogaia D, Grignani F, Nicoletti I, et al: The acute promyelocytic leukemia-specific PML/RAR alpha fusion protein reduces the frequency of commitment to apoptosis upon growth factor deprivation of GM-CSF–dependent myeloid cells. Leukemia 1995;9:1467.

63. Ferrucci PF, Grignani F, Pearson M, et al: Cell death induction by the acute promyelocytic leukemia-specific PML/RARα fusion protein. Proc Natl Acad Sci U S A 1997;94:10901.

64. Koken MH, Linares-Cruz G, Quignon F, et al: The PML growth-suppressor has an altered expression in human oncogenesis. Oncogene 1995;10:1315.

65. Liu JH, Mu ZM, Chang KS: PML suppresses oncogenic transformation of NIH/3T3 cells by activated neu. J Exp Med 1995;181:1965.

66. Mu ZM, Chin KV, Liu JH, et al: PML: A growth suppressor disrupted in acute promyelocytic leukemia. Mol Cell Biol 1994;14: 6858.

67. Fagioli M, Alcalay M, Tomassoni L, et al: Cooperation between the RING + B1-B2 and coiled-coil domains of PML is necessary for its effects on cell survival. Oncogene 1998;16:2905.

68. Wang ZG, Delva L, Gaboli M, et al: Role of PML in cell growth and the retinoic acid pathway. Science 1998;279:1547.

69. Hodges M, Tissot C, Howe K, et al: Structure, organization, and

dynamics of promyelocytic leukemia protein nuclear bodies. Am J Hum Genet 1998;63:297.

70. Nervi C, Ferrara FF, Fanelli M, et al: Caspases mediate retinoic acid–induced degradation of the acute promyelocytic leukemia PML/RARα fusion protein. Blood 1998;92:2244.

71. Ruthardt M, Orleth A, Tomassoni L, et al: The acute promyelocytic leukaemia specific PML and PLZF proteins localize to adjacent and functionally distinct nuclear bodies. Oncogene 1998;16:1945.

72. Bennett JM, Catovsky D, Daniel MT, et al: Proposals for the classification of the acute leukaemias. French-American-British (FAB) co-operative group. Br J Haematol 1976;33:451.

73. Golomb HM, Rowley JD, Vardiman JW, et al: "Microgranular" acute promyelocytic leukemia: A distinct clinical, ultrastructural, and cytogenetic entity. Blood 1980;55:253.

74. Rovelli A, Biondi A, Cantu Rajnoldi A, et al: Microgranular variant of acute promyelocytic leukemia in children. J Clin Oncol 1992; 10:1413.

75. Bennett JM, Catovsky D, Daniel MT, et al: A variant form of hypergranular promyelocytic leukemia (M3). Br J Haematol 1980; 44:169.

76. McKenna RW, Parkin J, Bloomfield CD, et al: Acute promyelocytic leukaemia: A study of 39 cases with identification of a hyperbasophilic microgranular variant. Br J Haematol 1982;50:201.

77. Neame PB, Soamboonsrup P, Leber B, et al: Morphology of acute promyelocytic leukemia with cytogenetic or molecular evidence for the diagnosis: Characterization of additional microgranular variants. Am J Haematol 1997;56:131.

78. Aventin A, Mateu R, Martino R, et al: A case of cryptic acute promyelocytic leukemia. Leukemia 1998;12:1490.

79. Invernizzi R, Iannone AM, Bernuzzi S, et al: Acute promyelocytic leukemia toluidine blue subtype. Leuk Lymphoma 1995;18:57.

80. Castoldi GL, Liso V, Specchia G, et al: Acute promyelocytic leukemia: Morphological aspects. Leukemia 1994;8:1441.

81. Yu RQ, Huang W, Chen SJ, et al: A case of acute eosinophilic granulocytic leukemia with PML-RAR alpha fusion gene expression and response to all-*trans* retinoic acid. Leukemia 1997;11:609.

82. Allford S, Grimwade D, Langabeer S, et al: Identification of the t(15;17) in AML FAB types other than M3: Evaluation of the role of molecular screening for the PML/RARα rearrangement in newly diagnosed AML. The Medical Research Council (MRC) Adult Leukaemia Working Party. Br J Haematol 1999;105:198.

83. Sainty D, Liso V, Cantu-Rajnoldi A, et al: A new morphologic classification system for acute promyelocytic leukemia distinguishes cases with underlying PLZF/RARA gene rearrangements. Group Francais de Cytogenetique Hematologique, UK Cancer Cytogenetics Group and BIOMED 1 European Community-Concerted Action "Molecular Cytogenetic Diagnosis in Haematological Malignancies." Blood 2000;96:1287.

84. Corey SJ, Locker J, Oliveri DR, et al: A non-classical translocation involving 17q12 (retinoic acid receptor alpha) in acute promyelocytic leukemia (APML) with atypical features. Leukemia 1994; 8:1350.

85. Hummel JL, Wells RA, Dube ID, et al: Deregulation of NPM and PLZF in a variant t(5;17) case of acute promyelocytic leukemia. Oncogene 1999;18:633.

86. Biondi A, Luciano A, Bassan R, et al: CD2 expression in acute promyelocytic leukemia is associated with microgranular morphology (FAB M3v) but not with any PML gene breakpoint. Leukemia 1995;9:1461.

87. Claxton D, Reading C, Deisseroth A: CD2 expression and the PML-RAR gene. Blood 1993;81:2210.

88. Guglielmi C, Martelli MP, Diverio D, et al: Immunophenotype of adult and childhood acute promyelocytic leukaemia: Correlation with morphology, type of PML gene breakpoint and clinical outcome. A cooperative Italian study on 196 cases. Br J Haematol 1998;102:1035.

89. Murray CK, Estey E, Paietta E, et al: CD56 expression in acute promyelocytic leukemia: A possible indicator of poor treatment outcome? J Clin Oncol 1999;17:293.

90. Ferrara F, Morabito F, Martino B, et al: CD56 expression is an indicator of poor clinical outcome in patients with acute promyelocytic leukemia treated with simultaneous all-*trans*-retinoic acid and chemotherapy. J Clin Oncol 2000;18:1295.

91. Larson RA, Kondo K, Vardiman JW, et al: Evidence for a 15;17 translocation in every patient with acute promyelocytic leukemia. Am J Med 1984;76:827.

92. Hiorns LR, Min T, Swansbury GJ, et al: Interstitial insertion of retinoic acid receptor-alpha gene in acute promyelocytic leukemia with normal chromosomes 15 and 17. Blood 1994;83:2946.

93. Grimwade D, Gorman P, Duprez E, et al: Characterization of cryptic rearrangements and variant translocations in acute promyelocytic leukemia. Blood 1997;90:4876.

94. Grimwade D, Biondi A, Mozziconacci MJ, et al: Characterization of acute promyelocytic leukemia cases lacking the classic t(15; 17): Results of the European Working Party. Groupe Francais de Cytogenetique Hematologique, Groupe de Francais d'Hematologie Cellulaire, UK Cancer Cytogenetics Group and BIOMED 1 European Community-Concerted Action "Molecular Cytogenetic Diagnosis in Haematological Malignancies." Blood 2000;96:1297.

95. Aurich J, Dastugue N, Duchayne E, et al: Location of the BCR-ABL fusion gene on the 9q34 band in two cases of Ph-positive chronic myeloid leukemia. Genes Chromosomes Cancer 1997;20:148.

96. Neves H, Ramos C, da Silva MG, et al: The nuclear topography of ABL, BCR, PML, and RARα genes: Evidence for gene proximity in specific phases of the cell cycle and stages of hematopoietic differentiation. Blood 1999;93:1197.

97. Lo Coco F, Diverio D, Falini B, et al: Genetic diagnosis and molecular monitoring in the management of acute promyelocytic leukemia. Blood 1999;94:12.

98. Tallman MS, Kwaan HC: Reassessing the hemostatic disorder associated with acute promyelocytic leukemia. Blood 1992;79:543.

99. Barbui T, Finazzi G, Falanga A: The impact of all-*trans*-retinoic acid on the coagulopathy of acute promyelocytic leukemia. Blood 1998;91:3093.

100. Grimwade D, Howe K, Langabeer S, et al: Establishing the presence of the t(15;17) in suspected acute promyelocytic leukaemia: Cytogenetic, molecular and PML immunofluorescence assessment of patients entered into the M.R.C. ATRA trial. M.R.C. Adult Leukaemia Working Party. Br J Haematol 1996;94:557.

101. Berger R, Bernheim A, Daniel MT, et al: Cytological types of mitoses and chromosome abnormalities in acute leukemia. Leuk Res 1983;7:221.

102. Biondi A, Rambaldi A, Alcalay M, et al: RAR-alpha gene rearrangements as a genetic marker for diagnosis and monitoring in acute promyelocytic leukemia. Blood 1991;77:1418.

103. Chen SJ, Zhu YJ, Tong JH, et al: Rearrangements in the second intron of the RARA gene are present in a large majority of patients with acute promyelocytic leukemia and are used as molecular marker for retinoic acid–induced leukemic cell differentiation. Blood 1991;78:2696.

104. Diverio D, Lo Coco F, D'Adamo F, et al: Identification of DNA rearrangements at the retinoic acid receptor-alpha (RAR-alpha) locus in all patients with acute promyelocytic leukemia (APL) and mapping of APL breakpoints within the RAR-alpha second intron. Italian Cooperative Study Group "GIMEMA." Blood 1992;79:3331.

105. Dyck JA, Warrell RP, Evans RM, et al: Rapid diagnosis of acute promyelocytic leukemia by immunohistochemical localization of PML/RAR-alpha protein. Blood 1995;86:862.

106. Falini B, Flenghi L, Fagioli M, et al: Immunocytochemical diagnosis of acute promyelocytic leukemia (M3) with the monoclonal antibody PG-M3 (anti-PML). Blood 1997;90:4046.

107. Flenghi L, Fagioli M, Tomassoni L, et al: Characterization of a new monoclonal antibody (PG-M3) directed against the aminoterminal portion of the PML gene product: Immunocytochemical evidence for high expression of PML proteins on activated macrophages, endothelial cells, and epithelia. Blood 1995;85:1871.

108. Miller WH, Kakizuka A, Frankel SR, et al: Reverse transcription polymerase chain reaction for the rearranged retinoic acid receptor alpha clarifies diagnosis and detects minimal residual disease in acute promyelocytic leukemia. Proc Natl Acad Sci U S A 1992; 89:2694.

109. Biondi A, Rambaldi A, Pandolfi PP, et al: Molecular monitoring of the myl/retinoic acid receptor-alpha fusion gene in acute promyelocytic leukemia by polymerase chain reaction. Blood 1992;80: 492.

110. Mandelli F, Diverio D, Avvisati G, et al: Molecular remission in PML/RAR alpha–positive acute promyelocytic leukemia by combined all-*trans* retinoic acid and idarubicin (AIDA) therapy. Gruppo Italiano-Malattie Ematologiche Maligne dell'Adulto and Associazione Italiana di Ematologia ed Oncologia Pediatrica Cooperative Groups. Blood 1997;90:1014.

111. Burnett AK, Grimwade D, Solomon E, et al: Presenting white blood cell count and kinetics of molecular remission predict prognosis in acute promyelocytic leukemia treated with all-*trans* retinoic acid: Result of the Randomized MRC Trial. Blood 1999;93:4131.

112. Sanz MA, Martin G, Diaz-Mediavilla J: All-trans-retinoic acid in acute promyelocytic leukemia. N Engl J Med 1998;338:393.

113. van Dongen JJ, Macintyre EA, Gabert JA, Delabesse E, Rossi V, Saglio G. Gottardi E, Rambaldi A, Dotti G, Griesinger F, Parreira A, Gameiro P, Diaz MG, Malec M. Langerak AW, San Miguel JF, Biondi A. Standardized RT-PCR analysis of fusion gene transcripts from chromosome aberrations in acute leukemia for detection of minimal residual disease. Report of the BIOMED-1 Concerted Action: Investigation of minimal residual disease in acute leukemia. Leukemia 1999;13:1901.

114. Mandelli F: New strategies for the treatment of acute promyelocytic leukemia. J Intern Med Suppl 1997;740:23.

115. Diverio D, Rossi V, Avvisati G, et al: Early detection of relapse by prospective reverse transcriptase–polymerase chain reaction analysis of the PML/RARα fusion gene in patients with acute promyelocytic leukemia enrolled in the GIMEMA-AIEOP multicenter "AIDA" trial. GIMEMA-AIEOP Multicenter "AIDA" Trial. Blood 1998;92:784.

116. Grimwade D, Howe K, Langabeer S, et al: Minimal residual disease detection in acute promyelocytic leukemia by reverse-transcriptase PCR: Evaluation of PML-RAR alpha and RAR alpha–PML assessment in patients who ultimately relapse. Leukemia 1996; 10:61.

117. Lo Coco F, Diverio D, Avvisati G, et al: Therapy of molecular relapse in acute promyelocytic leukemia. Blood 1999;94:2225.

118. Avvisati G, Mandelli F, Petti MC, et al: Idarubicin (4-demethoxydaunorubicin) as single agent for remission induction of previously untreated acute promyelocytic leukemia: A pilot study of the Italian cooperative group GIMEMA. Eur J Haematol 1990;44:257.

119. Bassan R, Battista R, Viero P, et al: Short-term treatment for adult hypergranular and microgranular acute promyelocytic leukemia. Leukemia 1995;9:238.

120. Breitman TR, Selonick SE, Collins SJ: Induction of differentiation of the human promyelocytic leukemia cell line (HL-60) by retinoic acid. Proc Natl Acad Sci U S A 1980;77:2936.

121. Breitman TR, Collins SJ, Keene BR: Terminal differentiation of human promyelocytic leukemic cells in primary culture in response to retinoic acid. Blood 1981;57:1000.

122. Huang ME, Ye YC, Chen SR, et al: Use of all-*trans* retinoic acid in the treatment of acute promyelocytic leukemia. Blood 1988; 72:567.

123. Castaigne S, Chomienne C, Daniel MT, et al: All-*trans* retinoic acid as a differentiation therapy for acute promyelocytic leukemia. I. Clinical results. Blood 1990;76:1704.

124. Chen Z, Chen GQ, Shen ZX, et al: Treatment of acute promyelocytic leukemia with arsenic compounds: In vitro and in vivo studies. Semin Hematol 2001;38:26.

125. Warrell RP, Frankel SR, Miller WH, et al: Differentiation therapy of acute promyelocytic leukemia with tretinoin (all-*trans*-retinoic acid). N Engl J Med 1991;324:1385.

126. Fenaux P, Castaigne S, Dombret H, et al: All-*trans* retinoic acid followed by intensive chemotherapy gives a high complete remission rate and may prolong remissions in newly diagnosed acute promyelocytic leukemia: A pilot study on 26 cases. Blood 1992; 80:2176.

127. Frankel SR, Eardley A, Heller G, et al: All-*trans* retinoic acid for acute promyelocytic leukemia. Results of the New York Study. Ann Intern Med 1994;120:278.

128. Kanamaru A, Takemoto Y, Tanimoto M, et al: All-*trans* retinoic acid for the treatment of newly diagnosed acute promyelocytic leukemia. Japan Adult Leukemia Study Group. Blood 1995;85: 1202.

129. Avvisati G, Lo Coco F, Diverio D, et al: AIDA (all-*trans* retinoic acid + idarubicin) in newly diagnosed acute promyelocytic leukemia: A Gruppo Italiano Malattie Ematologiche Maligne dell'Adulto (GIMEMA) pilot study. Blood 1996;88:1390.

130. Fenaux P, Chevret S, Guerci A, et al: Long-term follow-up confirms the benefit of all-*trans* retinoic acid in acute promyelocytic leukemia. European APL group. Leukemia 2000;14:1371.

131. Tallman MS, Andersen JW, Schiffer CA, et al: All-*trans*-retinoic acid in acute promyelocytic leukemia. N Engl J Med 1997;337:1021.

132. Lo Coco F, Nervi C, Avvisati G, et al: Acute promyelocytic leukemia: A curable disease. Leukemia 1998;12:1866.

133. Sanz M, Martinez JA, Barragan E, et al: All-*trans* retinoic acid and low-dose chemotherapy for acute promyelocytic leukaemia. Br J Haematol 2000;109:896.

134. Estey E, Thall PF, Pierce S, et al: Treatment of newly diagnosed acute promyelocytic leukemia without cytarabine. J Clin Oncol 1997;15:483.

135. Sanz MA, Lo Coco F, Martin G, et al: Definition of relapse risk and role of nonanthracycline drugs for consolidation in patients with acute promyelocytic leukemia: A joint study of the PETHEMA and GIMEMA cooperative groups. Blood 2000;96:1247.

136. Fenaux P, Chastang C, Chevret S, et al: A randomized comparison of all *trans*retinoic acid (ATRA) followed by chemotherapy and ATRA plus chemotherapy and the role of maintenance therapy in newly diagnosed acute promyelocytic leukemia. The European APL Group. Blood 1999;94:1192.

137. Kantarjian HM, Keating MJ, Walters RS, et al: Role of maintenance chemotherapy in acute promyelocytic leukemia. Cancer 1987; 59:1258.

138. Frankel SR, Eardley A, Lauwers G, et al: The "retinoic acid syndrome" in acute promyelocytic leukemia. Ann Intern Med 1992; 117:292.

139. Taraboletti G, Borsotti P, Chirivi RG, et al: Effect of all *trans*-retinoic acid (ATRA) on the adhesive and motility properties of acute promyelocytic leukemia cells. Int J Cancer 1997;70:72.

140. Asou N, Adachi K, Tamura J, et al: Analysis of prognostic factors in newly diagnosed acute promyelocytic leukemia treated with all-*trans* retinoic acid and chemotherapy. Japan Adult Leukemia Study Group. J Clin Oncol 1998;16:78.

141. Tallman MS, Andersen JW, Schiffer CA, et al: Clinical description of 44 patients with acute promyelocytic leukemia who developed the retinoic acid syndrome. Blood 2000;95:90.

142. Vahdat L, Maslak P, Miller WH, et al: Early mortality and the retinoic acid syndrome in acute promyelocytic leukemia: Impact of leukocytosis, low-dose chemotherapy, PMN/RAR-alpha isoform, and CD13 expression in patients treated with all-*trans* retinoic acid. Blood 1994;84:3843.

143. Castaigne S, Lefebvre P, Chomienne C, et al: Effectiveness and pharmacokinetics of low-dose all-*trans* retinoic acid (25 mg/m²) in acute promyelocytic leukemia. Blood 1993;82:3560.

144. Chen GQ, Shen ZX, Wu F, et al: Pharmacokinetics and efficacy of low-dose all-*trans* retinoic acid in the treatment of acute promyelocytic leukemia. Leukemia 1996;10:825.

145. Lo Coco F, Diverio D, Pandolfi PP, et al: Molecular evaluation of residual disease as a predictor of relapse in acute promyelocytic leukaemia. Lancet 1992;340:1437.

146. Mandelli F, Labopin M, Granena A, et al: European survey of bone marrow transplantation in acute promyelocytic leukemia (M3). Working Party on Acute Leukemia of the European Cooperative Group for Bone Marrow Transplantation (EMBT). Bone Marrow Transplant 1994;14:293.

147. Thomas X, Dombret H, Cordonnier C, et al: Treatment of relapsing acute promyelocytic leukemia by all-*trans* retinoic acid therapy followed by timed sequential chemotherapy and stem cell transplantation. APL Study Group. Acute promyelocytic leukemia. Leukemia 2000;14:1006.

148. Meloni G, Diverio D, Vignetti M, et al: Autologous bone marrow transplantation for acute promyelocytic leukemia in second remission: Prognostic relevance of pretransplant minimal residual disease assessment by reverse-transcription polymerase chain reaction of the PML/RAR alpha fusion gene. Blood 1997;90:1321.

149. Estey E, Thall PF, Mehta K, et al: Alterations in tretinoin pharmacokinetics following administration of liposomal all-*trans* retinoic acid. Blood 1996;87:3650.

150. Estey EH, Giles FJ, Kantarjian H, et al: Molecular remissions induced by liposomal-encapsulated all-*trans* retinoic acid in newly diagnosed acute promyelocytic leukemia. Blood 1999;94:2230.

151. Douer D, Estey E, Santillana S, et al: Treatment of newly diagnosed and relapsed acute promyelocytic leukemia with intravenous liposomal all-*trans* retinoic acid. Blood 2001;97:73.

152. Muindi JR, Frankel SR, Huselton C, et al: Clinical pharmacology of oral all-*trans* retinoic acid in patients with acute promyelocytic leukemia. Cancer Res 1992;52:2138.

153. Muindi J, Frankel SR, Miller WH, et al: Continuous treatment with

all-*trans* retinoic acid causes a progressive reduction in plasma drug concentrations: Implications for relapse and retinoid "resistance" in patients with acute promyelocytic leukemia. Blood 1992; 79:299.

154. Cote S, Zhou D, Bianchini A, et al: Altered ligand binding and transcriptional regulation by mutations in the PML/RARα ligand-binding domain arising in retinoic acid–resistant patients with acute promyelocytic leukemia. Blood 2000;96:3200.

155. Gianni M, Li Calzi M, Terao M, et al: AM580, a stable benzoic derivative of retinoic acid, has powerful and selective cyto-differentiating effects on acute promyelocytic leukemia cells. Blood 1996;87:1520.

156. Tobita T, Takeshita A, Kitamura K, et al: Treatment with a new synthetic retinoid, Am80, of acute promyelocytic leukemia relapsed from complete remission induced by all-*trans* retinoic acid. Blood 1997;90:967.

157. Gianni M, Terao M, Zanotta S, et al: Retinoic acid and granulocyte colony-stimulating factor synergistically induce leukocyte alkaline phosphatase in acute promyelocytic leukemia cells. Blood 1994; 83:1909.

158. Nason-Burchenal K, Gandini D, Botto M, et al: Interferon augments PML and PML/RAR alpha expression in normal myeloid and acute promyelocytic cells and cooperates with all-*trans* retinoic acid to induce maturation of a retinoid-resistant promyelocytic cell line. Blood 1996;88:3926.

159. Elstner E, Linker-Israeli M, Le J, et al: Synergistic decrease of clonal proliferation, induction of differentiation, and apoptosis of acute promyelocytic leukemia cells after combined treatment with novel 20-epi vitamin D₃ analogs and 9-*cis* retinoic acid. J Clin Invest 1997;99:349.

160. Gianni M, Kalac Y, Ponzanelli I, et al: Tyrosine kinase inhibitor STI571 potentiates the pharmacologic activity of retinoic acid in acute promyelocytic leukemia cells: Effects on the degradation of RARα and PML-RARα Blood 2001;97:3234.

161. Warrell RP, He LZ, Richon V, et al: Therapeutic targeting of transcription in acute promyelocytic leukemia by use of an inhibitor of histone deacetylase. J Natl Cancer Inst 1998;90:1621.

162. Kosugi H, Towatari M, Hatano S, et al: Histone deacetylase inhibitors are the potent inducer/enhancer of differentiation in acute myeloid leukemia: A new approach to anti-leukemia therapy. Leukemia 1999;13:1316.

163. Chen GQ, Zhu J, Shi XG, et al: In vitro studies on cellular and molecular mechanisms of arsenic trioxide (As₂O₃) in the treatment of acute promyelocytic leukemia: As₂O₃ induces NB4 cell apoptosis with downregulation of Bcl-2 expression and modulation of PML-RAR alpha/PML proteins. Blood 1996;88:1052.

164. Soignet SL, Maslak P, Wang ZG, et al: Complete remission after treatment of acute promyelocytic leukemia with arsenic trioxide. N Engl J Med 1998;339:1341.

165. Rego EM, Pandolfi PP: Analysis of the molecular genetics of acute promyelocytic leukemia in mouse models. Semin Hematol 2001; 38:54.

166. Camacho LH, Soignet SL, Chanel S, et al: Leukocytosis and the retinoic acid syndrome in patients with acute promyelocytic leukemia treated with arsenic trioxide. J Clin Oncol 2000;18:2620.

167. Jurcic JG, DeBlasio T, Dumont L, et al: Molecular remission induction with retinoic acid and anti-CD33 monoclonal antibody HuM195 in acute promyelocytic leukemia. Clin Cancer Res 2000; 6:372.

168. Sievers EL, Appelbaum FR, Spielberger RT, et al: Selective ablation of acute myeloid leukemia using antibody-targeted chemotherapy: A phase I study of an anti-CD33 calicheamicin immunoconjugate. Blood 1999;93:3678.

24

Jason Gotlib   Peter L. Greenberg

Myelodysplastic Syndromes

The myelodysplastic syndromes (MDS) constitute a heterogeneous group of clonal myeloid disorders characterized by refractory cytopenias, dysplastic changes in at least two of three hematopoietic cell lineages, and an increased risk of transformation to acute myeloid leukemia (AML). In addition to dysplastic changes in hemopoietic cells, a relatively indolent clinical course characterizes these patients. This indolent disease pace associated with distinctive biologic features distinguishes advanced MDS patients from those with AML. Numerous terms have been applied to the disorder since the first publication of a series of well-described patients in 1853. (Table 24-1).[1-15] The pathobiology underlying MDS is poorly understood, particularly the molecular events that initiate and promote the clonal growth of abnormal hematopoietic stem cells. A perplexing feature of MDS is the ineffective hematopoiesis that accompanies bone marrows of normal or increased cellularity. Intramedullary apoptotic cell death is recognized as an important pathogenetic mechanism underlying this apparent paradox. The heterogeneity of MDS presents a number of challenges. Diagnostically, a variety of morphologic changes occur in the peripheral blood and marrow of MDS; recognition of these changes is critical in helping clinicians and pathologists stage the disease and exclude other causes of cytopenias. The marked differences in survival among MDS patients reflect their variable potential to evolve to AML and the consequences of cytopenias—fatigue, infections, and bleeding. Patient management is further complicated by the attendant medical illnesses of the geriatric population, which MDS predominantly strikes.

CLASSIFICATION

The variable natural history of MDS prompted the development of classification methods in order to improve prognostic analysis and therapeutic decision making. In 1982, the French-American-British (FAB) Cooperative Group usefully divided MDS into five subgroups based on marrow morphology, the proportion of myeloblasts, and peripheral blood monocytosis: refractory anemia (RA), refractory anemia with ringed sideroblasts (RARS), refractory anemia with excess blasts (RAEB), refractory anemia with excess blasts in transformation (RAEB-T), and chronic myelomonocytic leukemia (CMML) (Table 24-2).[14] All of the subtypes are characterized by dysplasia in at least two hematopoietic cell lines, with RA and RARS patients having fewer than 5% blasts, RAEB patients having 5% to 20% blasts, and RAEB-T patients having 21% to 30% blasts. The diagnosis of AML is made when more than 30% marrow blasts are present. RARS defines patients with more than 15% ringed sideroblasts of their erythroid precursors. In the FAB system, CMML is defined as fewer than 20% marrow blasts and an absolute monocytosis of more than 1000/mm³. The categorization of CMML as MDS has been problematic because CMML frequently behaves as a myeloproliferative disorder (MPD). CMML patients with fewer than 13,000/mm³ white blood cells are categorized as having nonproliferative CMML, a form of MDS, whereas those with more than 13,000/mm³ white blood cells are classified as having a proliferative type of CMML, or MPD. In most cases, MDS is a primary or "de novo" acquired disorder. Secondary MDS has emerged as a significant clinical problem because of the

TABLE 24–1. Chronology and Terminology of the Myelodysplastic Syndrome

Term	Year	Author	Reference
Preleukemia	1953	Block et al	1
Refractory anemia with ringed sideroblasts	1956	Bjorkman	2
Refractory normoblastic anemia	1959	Dacie et al	3
Smoldering acute leukemia	1963	Rheingold et al	4
Chronic erythemic myelosis	1969	Dameshek	5
Preleukemic syndrome	1973	Saarni and Linman	6
Subacute myelomonocytic leukemia	1974	Sexauer et al	7
Chronic myelomonocytic leukemia	1974	Miescher and Farquet	8
Hypoplastic acute myelogenous leukemia	1975	Beard et al	9
Refractory anemia with excess myeloblasts	1976	Dreyfus	10
Hematopoietic dysplasia	1978	Linman and Bagby	11
Subacute myeloid leukemia	1979	Cohen et al	12
Dysmyelopoietic syndrome	1980	Streuli et al	13
Myelodysplastic syndromes	1982	Bennett et al	14

545

TABLE 24–2a. Myelodysplastic Syndrome Subtypes: FAB Cooperative Group Criteria

FAB Subtype	Bone Marrow Blasts (%)	Peripheral Blood Blasts (%)	Auer Rods	Monocytes >1 × 10⁹/L	Ringed Sideroblasts >15% of Nucleated Erythroid Cells
RA	<5	≤1	-	-	-
RARS	<5	<1	-	-	+
RAEB	5–20	<5	-	-	±
CMML	≤20	<5	-	+	±
RAEB-Tᵃ	21–30	≥5	±	±	±

ᵃThe diagnostic criteria for RAEB-T include 21%–30% bone marrow blasts, or ≥5 peripheral blood blasts, or the presence of Auer rods.
From Bennett et al.[14]

growing number of patients treated with chemotherapy or radiation for previous malignancies or because of exposure to environmental marrow toxins such as benzene.[16-18] Therapy-related MDS and AML (t-MDS/AML) are generally more resistant to standard induction chemotherapy and carry a worse prognosis.

In order to better characterize MDS patients, other methods are being developed to enhance their stratification by morphologic and biologic features. Such approaches could improve prognostication and treatment. Regarding morphologic approaches, a World Health Organization (WHO) panel has issued a report with proposals for reclassifying MDS (see Chapter 11),[19] although it has not been universally accepted. In this report, suggestions have been made, with limited supporting data, to modify the FAB definitions of MDS. Among several proposals, one suggestion is to exclude RAEB-T patients from MDS (proposing AML to now include patients with more than 20% blasts rather than the previously used 30% cutoff). However, as stated above, MDS is not only a disease related to blast percentage, but one that possesses a more indolent pace of disease related to distinctive biologic features that are different from de novo AML. The WHO panel also recommends that refractory anemia (RA or RARS) have abnormalities solely involving the erythroid line. However, as clinically characterized for the past 2 decades, MDS requires dysplasia in at least two hematopoietic cell lines. It is well recognized that RARS (a subtype of MDS) differs clinically from unilineage erythroid dysplasia, such as is present in pure sideroblastic anemia.[20] The latter has a markedly improved natural history, essentially lacking evolution to AML. Unilineage dysplastic changes may also occur in a number of reactive non-neoplastic conditions. The WHO panel added a new category of "refractory cytopenia with multilineage dysplasia" (RCMD). Although many patients with these findings have poorer prognoses than those lacking extensive dysplasia, data have not demonstrated independent prognostic value of these abnormalities.[21] In addition, RARS patients with multilineage dysplasia would be merged with other RCMDs, despite data indicating differences for RARS regarding certain therapeutic responses. Following the initial WHO reclassification proposal[19], dialogue regarding some of its features[19a,e] and further clarification of the categorizations have appeared.[19b-d] Table 24-2b provides a comparison of the FAB and WHO classifications. Further evidence-based studies should aid development of more comprehensive classification methods. While awaiting these data, many investigators are using both the FAB and WHO classifications systems to categorize MDS patients.

TABLE 24–2b. Comparative Categorization of MDS Patients with the FAB and WHO Classification Systems

FAB	WHO
Refractory anemia (RA)	1. RA with unilineage dysplasia¹ 2. Refractory cytopenia with multilineage dysplasia (RCMD) 3. 5q⁻ syndrome²
Refractory anemia with ringed sideroblasts (RARS)	1. RARS with unilineage dysplasia¹ 2. Refractory cytopenia with multilineage dysplasia with ringed sideroblasts
Refractory anemia with excess blasts (RAEB)	1. RAEB-I (5–9% bone marrow blasts) 2. RAEB-II (10–19% bone marrow blasts)
Refractory anemia with excess blasts in transformation	Acute myelogenous leukemia (≥20% bone marrow blasts)
Chronic myelomonocytic leukemia	Myelodysplastic Syndrome/Myeloproliferative Disorder³ (MDS)
	MDS unclassified

¹Requires 6 months of persisting anemia without other cause to establish the diagnosis.
²<5% marrow blasts, micromegakaryocytes, and thrombocytosis.
³MDS if WBC ≤13,000/mm³; MPD if WBC >13,000/mm³.

EPIDEMIOLOGY

Approximately 80% of MDS patients are older than 60 years at the time of diagnosis.[22] Ninety-one percent of the 1200 MDS cases in the Düsseldorf bone marrow registry were older than age 50 years.[23] A meta-analysis of MDS patients revealed a slightly increased male-to-female ratio of 1.2.[22]

The collection of precise epidemiologic data in MDS has been confounded by the changing nosology of the disease, disparate definitions and classification systems, and the uncertainty of diagnosis, especially in the early stages of disease.[23] Incidence rates of MDS have been published laregely by several regional cancer registries (Table 24-3).[23-26] The crude incidence of MDS in these studies ranged between 3.5 and 12.6 per 100,000 population per year. In individuals older than age 70 years, the incidence rates were 15-50 per 100,000 per year, comparable to age-related rates of chronic lymphocytic leukemia and multiple myeloma.[23-26] The incidence of MDS increases with age. In the English study, age-specific

TABLE 24–3. Crude and Age-Specific Incidences of MDS (Incidence figures per 100,000 population per year)

	Aul et al[24]	Radlund et al[25]	Williamson et al[26]
Geographic area	Düsseldorf (Germany)	Jönköping (Sweden)	East Dorset (England)
Study period	1986–1990	1988–1992	1981–1990
Age group (yr)			
≤49	0.2	0.7	0.5
50–59 } 60–69 }	4.9	1.6	5.3 15.0
70–79 } ≥80 }	22.8	15.0	49.0 89.0
All ages	4.1	3.5	12.6

From Aul C, Bowen DT, Yoshida Y: Pathogenesis, etiology, and epidemiology of myelodysplastic syndromes. Haematologica 1998;83:71.

incidence rates per 100,000 per year were 0.5 for age younger than 50 years and increased to 89 for age 80 years and older.[26] Differences in the incidence figures have been attributed to regional variations in incidence rates, patient demographics, bias due to patient referral patterns, and diagnostic expertise of the participating facilities.[23]

Although the number of MDS cases diagnosed in the last 2 decades has increased significantly, convincing data supporting a true increase in MDS incidence rates are lacking. Factors that likely contribute to the apparent rise include improved geriatric care and increased recognition of cases after the publication of widely accepted diagnostic criteria, such as the FAB classification.[23] Although increased exposure to cytotoxic chemotherapy has been cited as a contributing factor to the overall rise in the incidence of MDS, several studies have failed to document a rise in t-MDS/AML in recent years.[23]

PATHOGENESIS

Clonality Analysis

Various methods have been used to establish the possible clonal derivation of hematopoietic stem cells in MDS. Cytogenetic analysis offers clues about the location of potential MDS disease genes and provides prognostic information that has been incorporated into classification systems to guide clinical evaluation. However, karyotypic abnormalities are not diagnostic of MDS, and standard banding techniques characterize only a small fraction of bone marrow cells. Fluorescence in situ hybridization (FISH) can characterize lineage involvement in MDS cases with known cytogenetic abnormalities. In patients without detectable karyotypic abnormalities, loss of heterozygosity analysis has identified loss of genetic material from chromosomes 5q and 7q, regions that may contain critical tumor suppressor genes.[27, 28] X-inactivation clonality studies are based on restriction fragment length polymorphism (RFLP) analysis of differences in methylation patterns on inactive and active X chromosomes. The human androgen receptor assay distinguishes between X chromosomes by analyzing a highly polymorphic CAG repeat

of DNA that is informative in more than 90% of females.[29] Clonality in MDS has also been studied by RFLP analysis of the phosphoglycerate kinase and hypoxanthine phosphoribosyl transferase genes and by transcription assays of polymorphic genes such as glucose-6-phosphate dehydrogenase.[30]

These laboratory approaches have demonstrated clonality in the granulocytic, monocytic, erythroid, and megakaryocytic lineages in a high proportion of MDS patients.[31-40] Lymphoid cells are part of the abnormal clone in some but not all cases, as clonal T cells[35-39] and both monoclonal[39] and polyclonal B cells[40] have been demonstrated. Cytogenetic, FISH, and X-linked RFLP methylation analyses have been used to show recovery of either polyclonal hematopoiesis or persistent monoclonal hematopoiesis after treatment of MDS patients with chemotherapy.[41, 42]

Cytogenetics

Abnormal marrow cytogenetics are found in approximately 40% to 70% of primary and in 80% to 90% of secondary MDS cases using conventional banding techniques.[43-48] Complex chromosome abnormalities, involving at least three chromosomes, are observed in 15% to 30% of primary MDS and in approximately 50% of secondary MDS.[49-50] Cases of MDS with complex chromosomal abnormalities have an increased incidence of progression to AML and carry a relatively poor prognosis, regardless of the FAB subtype.[43, 45, 46, 48, 51-55] In contrast to AML, in which reciprocal translocations predominate, the most common abnormalities in MDS involve structural or numerical chromosomal changes.[56, 57] Unbalanced chromosomal translocations may result in hemizygosity and the inactivation of tumor suppressor genes.[58]

The most frequent clonal cytogenetic abnormalities include trisomy 8;monosomy 5 or 7;loss of Y chromosome, and interstitial deletions of the long arms of chromosomes 5, 7, 11, 13, and 20.[51, 57, 59, 60] The highest frequency of chromosomal abnormalities and complex karyotypes occurs in higher-risk RAEB and RAEB-T patients. Apart from RA, which is associated with the prognostically favorable abnormality 5q−, the other FAB subgroups are not associated with specific chromosomal changes. Monosomy 7 is rarely seen in RA patients, and 5q− is an unusual finding in CMML patients. The t(5;12) translocation, present in a small subset of CMML patients, fuses the platelet-derived growth factor β (PDGF-β) receptor to the transcription factor TEL, a member of the ETS family.[61] The PDGF-β/TEL receptor cDNA produces a chronic myeloproliferative syndrome (and lymphoid malignancies) in transgenic mice.[62, 63]

An International MDS Risk Analysis Workshop convened in order to improve the clinical utility of disparate scoring systems and to establish a consensus prognostic risk-based analysis system.[43] Cytogenetic, morphologic, and clinical data were collated from 816 untreated primary MDS patients from 7 previously reported risk-based studies that generated prognostic systems (patients with the proliferative form of CMML were excluded from the analysis). Patients with Y−, 20q− only, 5q− only, and normal karyotypes were associated with favorable prognoses.[43] Loss of the Y chromosome is relatively common in the bone marrow of elderly men, but its frequency was significantly greater in various hematologic malignancies than in a control group without evidence of disease.[64] When 20q− is associated with complex karyotypes, a poor prognosis is observed.[65] In patients who have received chemotherapy or radiation therapy, 5q− as the sole anomaly is linked to unfavorable outcomes, in contrast to de novo MDS patients with the 5q− syndrome.[48, 66] Patients with complex chromosome changes or monosomy 7 (−7/7q−) had poor outcomes. Trisomy 8 and other karyotypes not classified above had intermediate prognoses, confirming the findings of earlier studies (Fig. 24–1).

Several types of secondary MDS and AML and associated cytogenetic changes have been described. One type typically occurs after exposure to alkylating agents and presents as MDS with a high incidence of partial or total monosomy of chromosomes 5 and 7.[48] A second form occurs after treatment with topoisomerase II inhibitors and usually presents as AML with rearrangement of the mixed lineage leukemia gene at 11q23 or the *AML1* gene at 21q21.[67] Other consistent structural rearrangements

in secondary MDS involve chromosomes 3p14–21;6p23; 12p11–12;17p, and 19q13.[68] Deletion of 17p was reported in 25 cases of secondary MDS and AML and was associated with p53 mutation or overexpression.[69] In these patients, there was a long interval between use of antineoplastic drugs and the development of secondary MDS/AML, median survival was only 7 months, and −5/5q and −7/7q were frequent coexisting chromosomal anomalies.

New molecular cytogenetic techniques have been applied to MDS to more accurately characterize karyotypic abnormalities. For example, FISH investigation of 5q and 7q deletions has revealed hidden insertions, translocations, and fragmentations of these chromosomes not identified by standard karyotyping.[70, 71] Spectral karyotype analysis, which makes it possible to visualize each human chromosome with a unique color probe, is also able to uncover cryptic balanced and unbalanced translocations in MDS and has corrected several abnormalities misidentified by G-banding.[72]

Apoptosis

Apoptosis is an active process of programmed cell death with morphologic and biochemical changes distinct from those of cellular necrosis.[73] Increased intracellular ratios of proapoptotic (c-myc) to antiapoptotic (bcl-2) proteins were found in CD34+ cells and correlated with the degree of apoptosis.[74] In one series,[75] CD34+ cell apoptosis, and pro- versus antiapoptotic Bcl-2 family-protein ratios were significantly increased in MDS subtypes RA and RARS compared with advanced disease. A net balance of factors in favor of apoptosis may result in the activation of proteins called caspases, downstream effectors of the cell death signaling pathway.[76]

Intramedullary apoptotic cell death has been suggested as one basis for the finding of persistent cytopenias in spite of normal or increased bone marrow cellularity. In vitro findings that support this notion include the abortive growth pattern of marrow colony-forming unit-granulocyte-macrophage (CFU-GM), the increased

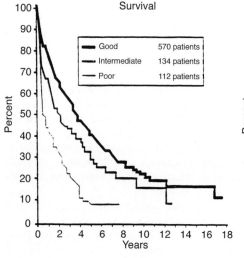
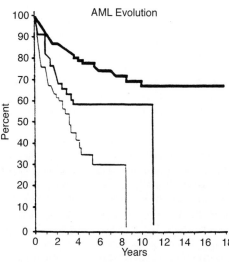

FIGURE 24–1. Survival (*left*) and freedom from AML evolution (*right*) in patients with MDS in relation to their risk-based categorical cytogenetic subgroups—good, intermediate, or poor (Kaplan-Meier curves). Good denotes normal, del(5q) only, del(20q) only, or Y− only. Poor denotes a complex karyotype (i.e., ≤3 anomalies) or chromosome 7 abnormalities. Intermediate denotes other abnormalities. (From Greenberg P, Cox C, Le Beau MM, et al: International Prognostic Scoring System for evaluating prognosis in myelodysplastic syndromes. Blood 1997;89:2079.)

incidence of apoptosis of MDS marrow cells following short-term culture, and the high proportion of cells with apoptotic nuclei in MDS bone marrow specimens.[77-79] Flow cytometry studies have shown high levels of CD34+ cell apoptosis in the early stages of MDS as compared with late stages of MDS, AML, or normal controls.[74, 75, 80] In addition to CD34+ cells, apoptosis occurs in more differentiated hematopoietic progenitors and stromal cells.[81] Although some analyses observed high levels of apoptosis only in the late stages of MDS, most studies have shown that as MDS evolves to AML, decreased apoptosis and cell proliferation occur in parallel with the accumulation of leukemic blasts.[74, 75, 80, 82, 83]

Excessive apoptosis in the marrow cells of MDS patients has been associated with marrow production of inhibitory cytokines. High levels of intramedullary TNF-α and its cellular source, macrophages, were found to correlate with high levels of apoptosis in MDS patients.[82-87] TNF-α generation is increased across all MDS risk groups and can inhibit the development of hematopoietic precursors.[82, 83, 87-89] One method by which TNF-α promotes apoptosis is via intracellular oxygen free radical production, resulting in oxidation of DNA and proteins.[90] Upregulation of other proapoptotic cytokines, such as IL-6, TGF-β, IFN-γ, and Fas ligand, has also been demonstrated in the marrow of MDS patients.[83-85, 87] Both TNF-α and IFN-γ can upregulate Fas on normal CD34+ hemopoietic precursors.[91] In a trial of erythropoietin, responders had significantly lower levels of serum TNF-α than nonresponders.[92] Treatment of MDS patients with EPO and G-CSF, alone or in combination, resulted in decreased apoptosis.[74, 93] In preclinical studies, attenuation of apoptosis and improvement of in vitro hematopoietic colony formation have been observed with the soluble recombinant Fas:Fc and TNF-α receptor:Fc fusion proteins, anti–TNF-α antibodies, and caspase inhibitors.[87, 94, 95]

Molecular Abnormalities

Accumulation of genetic lesions drives the multistep process of leukemogenesis. The activation of oncogenes coupled with the inactivation of tumor-suppressor genes may contribute to the hematopoietic failure that characterizes the clonal evolution of MDS to overt leukemia. The family of *ras* proto-oncogenes encodes 21-kd GTP-binding proteins that function as molecular switches that regulate diverse signaling pathways involved in cell growth, differentiation, and apoptosis.[96] *N-ras* mutations are frequently found in hematologic malignancies.[97] In several series of patients with MDS, the frequency of *ras* mutations ranged from 3% to 33%.[98] *Ras* mutations occur most commonly in CMML (32% to 65%) and less frequently in AML, ALL, and CML.[97] Some studies of MDS patients have associated *ras* mutations with poor survival or progression to AML, but other analyses failed to confirm this finding.[99-101]

The *FMS* proto-oncogene encodes the receptor for colony-stimulating factor (M-CSF receptor). Point mutations within the *FMS* gene can confer transforming activity to the gene.[102-104] *FMS* mutations occur at a low frequency in MDS patients (less than 20%), but like *ras,* they are preferentially observed in CMML.[101-105] The *FMS* gene maps to chromosome 5q33, a critical region containing numerous growth factor and growth factor receptor genes commonly deleted in the 5q− syndrome.

The frequency of mutations of the *p53* tumor suppressor gene in de novo MDS cases has generally been in the 5% to 20% range, with higher rates observed in t-MDS/AML patients.[106-111] In several cases, the development of a new *p53* mutation or loss of the wild-type allele was associated with progression of disease.[110, 111] Mutations of *p53* correlated with resistance to chemotherapy, evolution to leukemia, and shorter survival.[101, 112] In studies of t-MDS/AML, *p53* mutations were associated with complex karyotypes and microsatellite instability, suggesting a mutator phenotype.[113, 114] The 17p deletion is strongly correlated with the presence of *p53* mutations and has been associated with a particular type of dysgranulopoiesis that combines the pseudo–Pelger-Huët anomaly and small vacuolated neutrophils.[115]

Angiogenesis

Angiogenesis supports the growth and metastasis of solid tumors and may also play a role in hematologic malignancies.[116, 117] Two potent angiogenic peptides are vascular endothelial cell growth factor (VEGF) and basic fibroblast growth factor (bFGF).[116] VEGF is expressed by AML cells and may act as a paracrine growth factor in the development of AML.[118] Bone marrow samples from untreated AML patients have increased microvessel density (MVD) compared with samples from control patients, consistent with increased angiogenesis.[119] In addition, elevated intracellular VEGF levels in AML patients are an independent prognostic factor of shortened survival.[120] Angiogenesis may also be important in the pathogenesis of MDS. Autocrine production of VEGF has been linked to the promotion of leukemia colony formation and atypical localization of immature myeloid precursors (ALIP) in MDS.[121] MVD was significantly elevated in MDS patients, compared with control patients, but lower than AML or MPD.[122] Among MDS FAB subtypes, MVD was higher in RAEB-T and CMML and fibrosis subsets compared with RA, RARS, or RAEB, suggesting a possible link between angiogenesis and progression to leukemia.

HEMATOPOIESIS

In vitro culture systems have proved useful for analyzing the proliferative and differentiative effects of various hematopoietic growth factors (HGFs) on the hemopoietic stem/progenitor cell compartments. Such in vitro assays are particularly relevant to the study of MDS, in which defective differentiation leads to ineffective hematopoiesis.[123] The colony-forming capacities of pluripotent hemopoietic stem cells (colony-forming unit–granulocyte, erythroid, macrophage, megakaryocyte), and their progeny, committed progenitor cells (CFU-GM, burst-forming unit-erythroid [BFU-E], [CFU-E], and CFU-megakaryocyte

[CFU-Mk]), are low or absent in most MDS (and AML) patients.[123-127]

Two principal hematopoietic regulatory derangements found in MDS are diminished production and decreased responsiveness to HGFs.[1] Marrow cells and peripheral blood T cells from MDS patients produce decreased amounts of GM-CSF, IL-3, M-CSF, and IL-6.[128] Levels of monocyte-derived G-CSF are decreased in MDS patients and also in elderly control subjects.[129] In clonogenic cultures, CFU-GM stimulated with G-CSF and GM-CSF was subnormal in a majority of MDS patients.[130] In MDS, GM-CSF and IL-3 generally have greater myeloid proliferative effects in vitro than G-CSF, whereas G-CSF has more potent differentiative efects. These findings are particularly evident in RAEB/RAEB-T patients and those with normal cytogenetics.[130]

In vitro MDS erythroid progenitor cells show suboptimal responses to EPO.[131, 132] Analysis of the relationship between EPO levels in MDS and patients' erythroid progenitors indicated that the anemia in MDS was not attributable to an abnormality in the capacity of EPO to induce generation of CFU-E but was influenced by the size of the BFU-E population whose severe deficiency resulted in insufficient influx of EPO-responsive cells.[132] These findings suggested that treatment of MDS patients with EPO alone would have limited clinical benefit because the initial growth requirements and generation of BFU-E from more primitive cells are not under the regulatory influence of the hormone. These in vitro predictions have been borne out in therapeutic clinical trials where EPO has shown limited efficacy in improving the anemia of MDS patients (see later). G-CSF synergistically augments the in vitro EPO responsiveness of BFU-E in normal and MDS marrow.[132] In clinical trials of the hormone combination improved hemoglobin responses have been demonstrated, particularly in patients with RARS. Investigations using serum-free media and purified CD34+ cells with recombinant HGFs have shown decreased responsiveness of MDS hematopoietic progenitors to G-CSF and EPO.[133] The mechanisms underlying the altered responsiveness of MDS precursors to cytokines is unclear. G-CSF and IL-3 binding in MDS has not exhibited significantly different receptor numbers or affinity for the receptors.[134] Postreceptor signaling pathway abnormalities after EPO-binding have been demonstrated in precursors from some MDS patients.[135]

CLINICAL AND HEMATOLOGIC FINDINGS

Anemia is found in nearly all MDS patients at the time of diagnosis, contributing to patients' fatigue. The anemia is usually macrocytic and is associated with a low reticulocyte count, reflecting ineffective hematopoiesis. Other causes of anemia, such as vitamin B_{12} and folate deficiency, should be excluded. Additional findings associated with dyserythropoiesis may include abnormal iron metabolism,[136] disordered globin chain synthesis,[137] acquired hemoglobin H,[138, 139] reappearance of hemoglobin F,[140] changes in red blood cell antigens,[141] a positive Ham test,[142] and markers of paroxysmal nocturnal hemoglobinuria (PNH).[143] Low levels of pyruvate kinase may occur,

associated with hemolysis.[144] In the peripheral blood, red blood cell structure often consists of macrocytic and macro-ovalocytic forms, anisocytosis, poikilocytosis, nucleated forms, and stippled cells (Fig. 24-2; see also Color Section). In the bone marrow, dysplasia of erythroid precursors frequently manifests as megaloblastoid changes, with an asynchrony between maturation of the cytoplasm and nucleus. A significant number of ringed sideroblasts (more than 15% of nucleated erythroid cells), detected by Prussian blue stain, is characteristic of RARS. Macrophage iron is frequently increased, especially in multiply transfused patients. Other findings of erythroid dysplasia include multinuclear fragments, bizarre nuclear shapes, and abnormal cytoplasmic features (e.g., intense basophilia, Howell-Jolly bodies). When erythroid precursors account for more than 50% of the bone marrow cellularity in the presence of more than 30% myeloblasts, the diagnosis of erythroleukemia is made (FAB M6 variant of AML).

Neutropenia is found in a significant proportion (60%) of patients with MDS, and it is associated with a depressed inflammatory response to infection. Infections are found in 10% of patients at the time of diagnosis, and they account for approximately 20% of deaths.[145, 146] Altered granulocyte function is present in the majority of MDS patients. Granulocytes may show decreased adhesion, deficient chemotaxis and phagocytosis, and impaired microbicidal activity.[147-150] Because hematopoietic growth factors play important roles in mature neutrophil and monocyte functions, decreased production of growth factors may contribute to phagocyte abnormalities.[123] Leukocytosis characterizes the proliferative form of CMML, but qualitative impairment of monocyte function can predispose these patients to infections.[151] Hepatosplenomegaly, skin infiltrations, serous effusions, gingival hypertrophy, and lymphadenopathy occur in some CMML patients, often with high peripheral monoycte counts, but are uncommon in other subtypes of MDS.[152-157]

Morphologic abnormalities include hyposegmented neutrophils and bi-lobed chromatin condensation (pseudo–Pelger-Huët anomaly) (Fig. 24-3) (see also Color Section). Hypogranular granulocytes may be associated with cytochemical abnormalities, including reduced myeloperoxidase and low levels of leukocyte alkaline phosphatase. In the bone marrow, decreased myeloid maturation is a common finding. The proportion of marrow myeloblasts is used to determine the FAB subtype of MDS.

Thrombocytopenia occurs in 40% to 60% of patients and is found as an isolated cytopenia in fewer than 5% of cases.[158] Progressive thrombocytopenia is often a marker of evolving disease. Serious bleeding occurs in few patients at initial presentation. Giant and hypo/agranular platelets are common peripheral blood smear abnormalities (Fig. 24-4) (see also Color Section). Dysplastic megakaryocyte maturation, such as micromegakaryocytes with a single nucleus, and megakaryocytes with multiple, small separated nuclei are frequently observed. Abnormal platelet function, characterized by prolonged bleeding times or reduced platelet aggregation, may contribute to bleeding even in the setting of normal platelet counts.[159] Surgery or trauma patients with defective platelet function are at a higher risk of hemorrhage and should be given

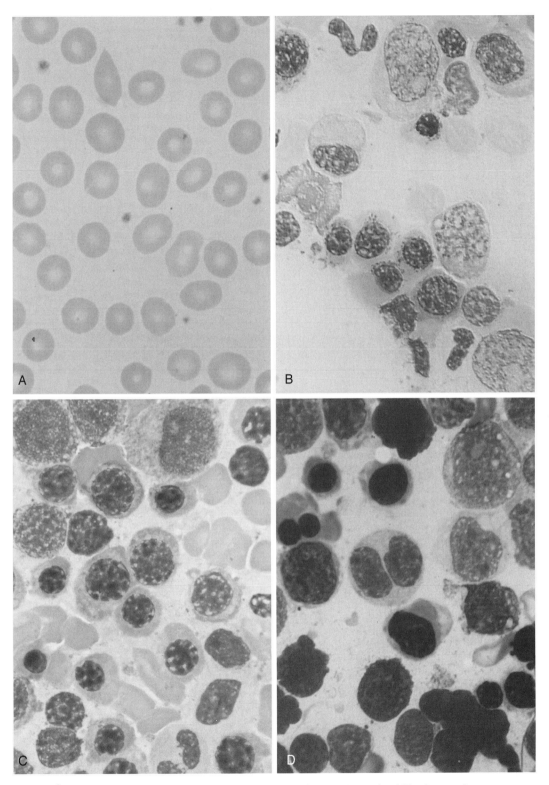

FIGURE 24–2. MDS: abnormal morphology mainly of the erythroid series. *A*, Peripheral blood smear shows macrocytic and macro-ovalocytic red blood cells in RAEB. *B*, Bone marrow aspirate shows ringed sideroblasts in RARS. *C*, Megaloblastoid dyserythropoiesis in RAEB. Atypical promyelocytes with nucleocytoplasmic asynchrony are seen here and in *D*. *D*, Bone marrow aspirate shows dyserythropoietic changes including nuclear budding (*bottom*) and a binucleate erythroid cell (*top*) in RARS. (All photographs ×64.) (See Color Section.)

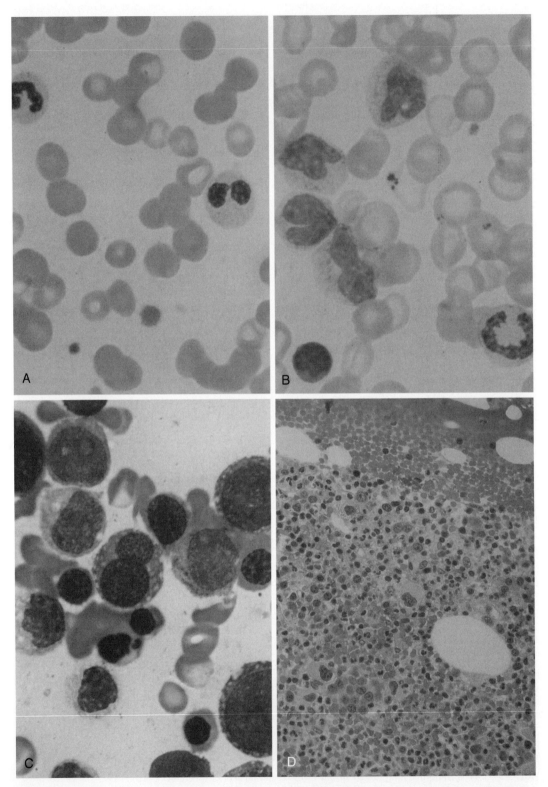

FIGURE 24–3. MDS: abnormal morphology mainly of the myeloid series. *A,* Peripheral blood smear shows dysplastic hypogranular neutrophil with a pseudo–Pelger-Huët anomaly in refractory anemia. *B,* Peripheral blood smear shows abnormal monocytes in CMML. Pappenheimer's bodies are seen in the red blood cells. *C,* Bone marrow aspirate shows a blast and atypical promyelocyte in RARS. *D,* Bone marrow biopsy shows ALIP. (All photographs ×64.) (See Color Section.)

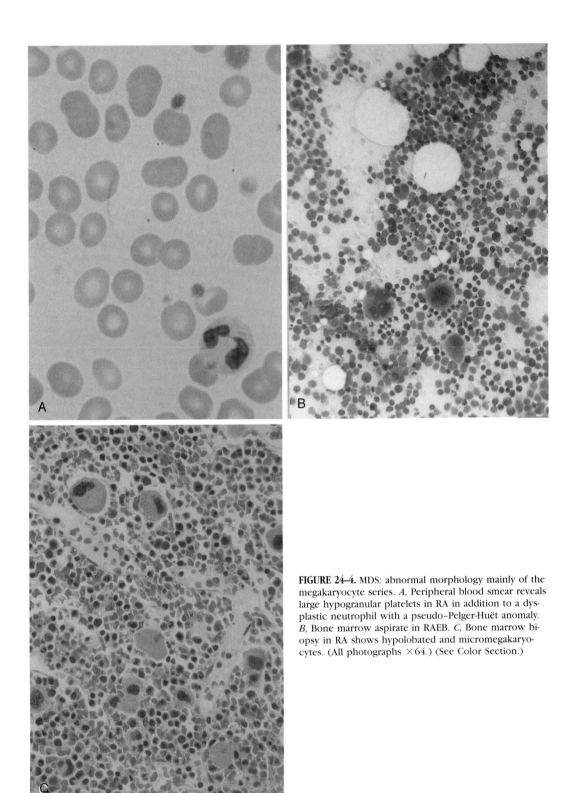

FIGURE 24–4. MDS: abnormal morphology mainly of the megakaryocyte series. *A,* Peripheral blood smear reveals large hypogranular platelets in RA in addition to a dysplastic neutrophil with a pseudo–Pelger-Huët anomaly. *B,* Bone marrow aspirate in RAEB. *C,* Bone marrow biopsy in RA shows hypolobated and micromegakaryocytes. (All photographs ×64.) (See Color Section.)

platelet transfusions if bleeding develops. Leukocyte-filtered platelet transfusions are usually provided for patients with platelet counts lower than 10,000/mm³ or for bleeding associated with higher platelet counts.

CLINICOPATHOLOGIC VARIANTS

Immunologic/Lymphoid Associations

In a low proportion of patients, MDS has been associated with lymphoproliferative diseases including CLL, hairy cell leukemia, large granular lymphocytic leukemia, monoclonal gammopathy of uncertain significance/multiple myeloma, and various types of B- and T-cell lymphomas.[160] An increased incidence of abnormalities of the immune system is found in MDS, including lymphopenia with decreased CD4+ and increased CD8+ suppressor cytotoxic T-cell populations, decreased number and function of natural killer cells, polyclonal hypergammaglobulinemia, and pure red blood cell aplasia.[160-163] The presence of a PNH clone correlates with clinical responses to immunosuppressive therapy (see later).[143] These associations suggest that lymphopoietic progenitor or effector cells may be affected during the pathogenesis of MDS. During follow-up of MDS patients, solid malignancies occur at a rate higher than expected.[164] Rheumatologic conditions associated with MDS include cutaneous vasculitis, lupus-like syndromes, and oligo/polyarthritis.[165-168]

The 5q– Syndrome

The 5q– syndrome was described in 1974 in three patients with refractory anemia and an interstitial deletion of the long arm of chromosome 5.[169] Although there is marked variability in the size of the 5q– deletion, high resolution banding has indicated that 5q12 and 5q34 are the proximal and distal breakpoints. Molecular mapping techniques have identified a minimal interval spanning 700 kb, containing nine known tumor suppressor gene candidates.[170] The 5q– syndrome is a myelodysplastic disorder characterized by a female preponderance, macrocytic anemia, modest leukopenia, a normal or high platelet count, hypolobular megakaryocytes, a low risk of transformation to acute leukemia, and a favorable prognosis.[171] The median age at diagnosis is in the mid-60s.[167] Estimates of median survival in RA patients have varied from 28 to 81 months and from 16 to 51 months in patients with RAEB or RAEB-T.[172-174] The wide range in median survival may reflect the small number of patients studied and the type of treatment received. In one study, the superior survival of 5q– syndrome patients as compared with historical MDS patients was attributed to a low incidence of deaths from infection and bleeding.[173] Nonhematologic illnesses and hemosiderosis from red blood cell transfusion dependence constitute major causes of morbidity and mortality rates in this group of patients. The presence of karyotypic abnormalities in addition to 5q– is associated with a worse prognosis.[175]

Although the WHO proposals include 5q– syndrome as a separate entity, many patients with the 5q– abnormality lack consistent clinical features, particularly if they have additional cytogenetic abnormalites or higher marrow blast percentages.[43, 176] Multivariate analyses have failed to show 5q– cytogenetic features in MDS to have independent prognostic significance.[43] Incorporating MDS patients' specific cytogenetic abnormalities with other clinical features (e.g., blast percentage, number of cytopenias), as in the IPSS categorization,[43] defines more usefully the natural history of their disease.

MDS with Fibrosis

Myelofibrosis is characterized by a focal or generalized increase in the number and thickness of reticulin fibers that is detected with a silver stain of a bone marrow core biopsy specimen.[177] Mild to moderate fibrosis has been reported in up to 50% of MDS cases, with marked fibrosis occuring in fewer than 15% of cases.[178-180] Myelofibrosis occurs in all FAB subtypes of MDS, but a higher incidence was noted in CMML cases in two large series.[176, 177] The frequency of myelofibrosis is increased in therapy-related MDS compared with primary MDS, with mild fibrosis present in up to 85% of such cases.[182] Atypical myeloproliferative disorders may closely resemble MDS with fibrosis. Other diagnoses that should be excluded include primary myelofibrosis, the accelerated phase of CML, postpolycythemia vera with myeloid metaplasia, AML (especially acute megakaryoblastic leukemia [AML-M7]), AML with trilineage dysplasia, and acute myelofibrosis.[183]

In cases of MDS and fibrosis, common bone marrow morphologic findings include hypercellularity, atypical megakaryocyte proliferation with hypolobated forms, and trilineage dysplasia. Myelofibrosis may range from 1+ to 2+ (mild to moderate) to 4+ (positive collagen stain).[184] The peripheral blood picture is characterized by varying degrees of pancytopenia, red blood cell anisopoikilocytosis and, less commonly, a leukoerythroblastic picture. Organomegaly is usually minimal or absent.

MDS with fibrosis heralds a relatively poor prognosis. In three studies, patients with myelofibrosis had a significantly shorter survival than a comparison group of MDS patients without fibrosis.[178, 181, 184] In two of these analyses, there was a high frequency of cytogenetic abnormalities in the patients with MDS and fibrosis, a possible contributing factor to the differences in survival. A higher mean survival time was found in another cohort of patients with MDS and fibrosis with predominantly low-risk FAB subtypes and normal cytogenetics.[179]

CMML

Because of the common finding of dysplasia in CMML, the disorder was classified by the FAB Cooperative Group as a subtype of MDS.[14] FAB criteria for CMML include a monocytosis of more than 1000/mm,³ a blast cell percentage of less than 5% in the peripheral blood and less than 20% in the marrow, and absence of Auer rods. Both clinically and hematologically, CMML also shares features with myeloproliferative disorders in exhibiting peripheral blood and marrow hyperleukocytosis and hepatosplenomegaly. Furthermore, the behavior of CMML marrow progenitor cells in vitro resembles that of chronic MPD, with increased colonies and clusters, rather than that of MDS, in which progenitor cells proliferate poorly in short-term cultures.[123, 185-188] In 1994, the FAB group proposed two subtypes of CMML: a dysplastic or nonproliferative type (white blood cells fewer than 13,000/mm³) and a proliferative variant (white blood cell count more than 13,000/ mm³).[189] A small subgroup of adult patients with systemic mastocytosis have an associated myelodysplastic or myeloproliferative disorder such as CMML. These patients generally have a poorer prognosis than those with isolated systemic mastocytosis.[190-192]

Median survival in CMML patients is 3 years, with a range of 8 months to more than 5 years.[152, 193, 194] In a retrospective review of 41 patients, only bone marrow blast percentage was an independent prognostic determinant in multivariate analysis.[149] The MD Anderson Cancer Center performed a retrospective review of more than 30 years' experience with 228 CMML patients.[195] The median survival was 12 months, 43 (19%) patients developed acute leukemia within a median time of 7 months, and the estimated cumulative 2-year rate of AML was 30%. Patients with a hemoglobin level greater than 12 g/ dL had superior survival (22 months). As in other studies, shorter survival in CMML was correlated with the percentage of bone marrow blasts, degree of peripheral leukocytosis (and monocytosis), anemia, thrombocytopenia, splenomegaly, immature myeloid precursors in the peripheral blood, and abnormal karyotype.[155-157, 196-200]

A retrospective study evaluated whether the refined classification of MDS-CMML versus MPD-CMML was important in terms of prognosis.[201] Hepatosplenomegaly was more common and LDH levels significantly higher in the MPD-CMML group. The percentage of bone marrow blasts and cumulative survival rates were similar in both groups. The probability of transformation to AML was higher in MDS than in MPD-CMML (32% versus 17% after 5 years), but this difference was not statistically significant. The survival of MDS-CMML patients was similar to that of other MDS patients who had similar bone marrow blasts counts. The study suggested that MDS-CMML and MPD-CMML are clinically and morphologically distinct conditions, but the grouping provides no clear prognostication.

In an attempt to diminish the heterogeneity present within MDS, the International MDS Workshop excluded the proliferative form of CMML in its analysis, including only those with a white blood cell count ≤ 12,000/ mm³.[43] The WHO proposals originally placed patients with CMML (and juvenile myelomonocytic leukemia [JMML] and atypical CML) in the new subgroup MDS/ MPD, reflecting cases that are inherently proliferative but that show dysplastic features.[19] This seems useful for proliferative forms of CMML. However, MDS patients with relatively low white blood cell counts (≤ 12,000/mm³) who have monocytosis appear to be best categorized as an MDS subgroup defined by their marrow blast percentage using FAB (or as nonproliferative CMML),[43, 202] rather than as standard CMML. The WHO proposal has subsequently been revised such that the same leukocyte count as used by the Workshop was utilized to separate MDS from MDS/MPD (the latter including proliferative CMML).[19a-c, e] Even this is not an entirely satisfactory cate-

gorization as some patients with nonproliferative CMML become proliferative over time. Additional studies are required to evaluate the clinical outcomes of the two types of CMML and their underlying biologic, cytogenetic, and molecular features.

Overlap MDS/MPD Syndrome

Increased bone marrow cellularity is a typical feature of both MDS and MPDs. In MDS, the uncoupling of proliferation and differentiation results in the finding of bone marrow hypercellularity and peripheral blood cytopenias. In MPDs, differentiation is preserved so that increased numbers of cells in at least one of the hematopoietic lineages are found in the peripheral blood. Patients with myeloproliferative disorders may evolve to MDS, heralded by increasing dysplasia and new cytopenias. The change may be due to prior drug therapy or to a shift in the natural history of the disease. Conversely, MDS patients may transform to a myeloproliferative disorder, such as proliferative-type CMML, atypical CML, myelofibrosis or, less commonly, polycythemia vera or essential thrombocythemia.[203-208] Evolution from MDS to Philadelphia chromosome–positive CML is rare and is associated with the emergence of the t(9;22) translocation and an accelerated phase of the disease.[209] Overlap syndrome is a term applied to patients displaying coexisting features of MDS as well as those of an MPD. Overlap syndrome is uncommon, with a prevalence of 4.4% in one series of 566 MDS patients.[205] Because of its rarity, the natural history of the disorder has not been well described. Some of these patients could fit into the MDS/MPD category proposed by the WHO panel.

Hypocellular MDS

The subtype of hypocellular MDS is not included in the FAB classification system for MDS.[14] The entity has not been precisely defined. Several studies have used an arbitrary bone marrow cellularity of less than 30% to distinguish hypocellular MDS from the normo/hypercellular groups.[210-212] Hypocellular cases have also been characterized by correcting the bone marrow cellularity by age.[213] The prevalence of hypocellular MDS has generally been reported to be less than 20%,[210-212, 214-216] but three series reported rates of 25% to 38%.[213, 217, 218] It may be difficult to discriminate cases of hypocellular MDS from cases of aplastic anemia, but the presence of a clonal cytogenetic abnormality and/or marrow dysplasia favors the former diagnosis. In one analysis, immunohistochemical staining for bone marrow CD34+ cells and proliferating cell nuclear antigen was significantly higher in cytogenetically characterized cases of hypoplastic MDS compared with aplastic anemia, a potentially useful method to help further distinguish the two disorders.[219] The encouraging results with immunosuppressive therapy in both aplastic anemia and hypoplastic MDS may not always make the distinction between these two diseases critical in the short term, but the eventual risk of progression to acute leukemia is greater in MDS.

Most cases of hypocellular MDS fit in the RA and RAEB categories.[210-213, 218] Controversy remains as to whether hypocellular MDS is a distinct clinicopathologic entity with its own prognostic significance. In contrast to reports linking hypocellular MDS to prolonged survival and less frequent transformation to AML,[215, 216, 218] other studies found no difference in survival and AML evolution between the cellular subsets of MDS.[211-214] Although several series showed a similar frequency of simple and complex karyotype abnormalities between the cellular forms of MDS, others analyses found that hypocellular MDS was more frequently associated with chromosome 7 abnormalities.[210, 213, 220-222] Intramedullary apoptosis, accompanied by higher levels of TNF-α and TGF-β, has been found in hypocellular MDS cases similar to the hypercellular variety.[223] In cases of hypocellular MDS not characterized by significant intramedullary apoptosis, a stem cell failure disorder may better explain the hypoplastic bone marrow phenotype.

Association of Aplastic Anemia, Paroxysmal Nocturnal Hemoglobinuria, and MDS/AML

Successful treatment of aplastic anemia (AA) with immunosuppressive therapy (IST) has resulted in long-term survival, revealing later clonal diseases such as PNH, MDS, and AML.[224] The development of these disorders may reflect the natural history of the disease, IST, or both. Longitudinal series of AA patients treated with IST, such as antithymocyte globulin (ATG), have shown that the risk of developing PNH ranges approximately 8% to 12%, 2% to 7% for MDS, and less than 2% for AML.[225-228] The actuarial probability of developing PNH appears to be increased at 5 to 15 years of follow-up.[226, 227] In a French study of AA patients treated with androgens, the probability of developing PNH at 12 years was about 10%.[229] No IST was administered to patients, suggesting that PNH may develop as part of the natural history of AA. MDS/AML may also develop from PNH.[225-228] Studies using GPI-anchored protein expression, flow cytometry, and cytogenetic analysis have shown that MDS can arise from the PNH clone[230, 231] or emerge as a separate clone.[239, 233]

In one study, flow cytometry of granulocytes was used to assess the PNH status of patients with various bone marrow failure syndromes.[143] Evidence of PNH was found in 22 of 115 (19%) AA patients and in 9 of 39 (23%) MDS patients, a higher prevalence compared with that in previous studies. AA patients had PNH clones at the time of diagnosis, and the proportion of patients who harbored PNH cells did not increase over time after ATG therapy. PNH cells do not appear to have an intrinsic growth advantage over normal stem cells.[234] Instead, they may be a surrogate marker of T-cell mediated marrow suppression, one possible mechanism underlying the pathogenesis of AA and some cases of MDS. This theory implies that PNH cells should be present in normal individuals, but studies have produced conflicting results.[143, 235] Future investigations will aim to determine which factors contribute to expansion of abnormal clones in PNH, MDS, and AML and if specific GPI-anchored proteins serve as antigenic targets of immune-mediated at-

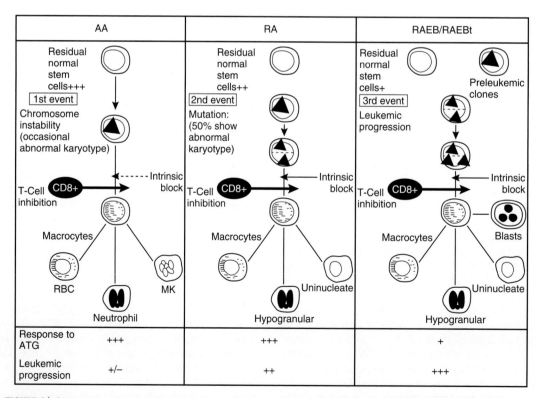

FIGURE 24–5. Hypothetical model linking etiology, pathophysiology, and response to immunosuppressive treatment in aplastic anemia and MDS. (From Barrett J, Saunthararajah Y, Molldrem J: Myelodysplastic syndrome and aplastic anemia: Distinct entities or diseases linked by a common pathophysiology? Semin Hematol 2000;37:15.)

tack. Barrett et al[236] proposed a unifying model of AA and MDS that takes into consideration the common elements of panytopenia and responsiveness to immunosuppression, differences in cellular morphology, and differences in leukemic risk (Fig. 24-5).

SECONDARY MDS/LEUKEMIA

When applied to MDS and AML, the term "secondary" denotes the development of disease after exposure to environmental or therapeutic toxins. "Therapy-related" (for example, t-MDS/AML) is attributable to the widespread use of intensive chemotherapy (conventional and high-dose chemotherapy) and radiation, the longer survival of treated cancer patients, and the advancing age of the population. Cases of therapy-related MDS/AML generally fall into two major categories, with the latency period for the development of alkylator-based t-MDS/AML being approximately 3 to 8 years, and 2 to 3 years for t-MDS/AML due to topoisomerase II therapy.[237] The risk of MDS/leukemia is related mostly to the type and duration of therapy rather than to the type of the primary neoplasm.[238]

Therapy-related MDS/leukemia following treatment of Hodgkin's disease has been extensively studied. The leukemia risk generally begins to rise 2 years after Hodgkin's disease therapy is completed, reaches a peak at approximately 4 to 6 years, with only rare cases observed after 10 years of follow-up.[237, 238] The 10-year cumulative incidence rate ranged from less than 0.3% to 10% in studies of varying size, duration of follow-up, and type of treatment administered.[239-247] Alkylator-based regimens such as MOPP are correlated with higher rates of t-MDS/AML. In contrast, treatment with radiotherapy alone or nonalkyla-

tor-containing regimens such as ABVD have very low leukemogenic potential.[239, 248, 249] Risk increases substantially when combination chemotherapy and extensive radiation therapy are used together, whereas the addition of limited-field radiation to chemotherapy probably adds a relatively small risk.[241, 243, 245, 246] As in Hodgkin's disease, the primary risk factor for t-MDS/AML in NHL is exposure to alkylator drugs, with cumulative risks of 0.6% to 8.0% up to 10 years.[242, 250-253] In multiple myeloma patients, the risk of t-MDS/AML is related to the cumulative dose of melphalan. In a cohort of 908 patients, the cumulative risk of developing t-AML was 2.8% and 10% at 5 and 10 years, respectively,[254] with a similar rate of 10% at 8 years reported in another series.[255] The risk of developing t-MDS/AML after treatment for breast cancer is low. Up to a 1.7% 10-year cumulative risk of leukemia has been reported in breast-cancer patients receiving alkylator-based adjuvant chemotherapy regimens.[256-259] The leukemic risk of modern platinum-based chemotherapy in women with ovarian cancer was evaluated in a large case-control study.[260] The risk of leukemia was significantly increased with platinum (relative risk 4.0) but considerably lower than with treatment with melphalan (relative risk 21.8). Testicular cancer patients receiving etoposide-containing chemotherapy, especially doses greater than 2 g/m², are at an increased risk of developing AML and ALL.[261-263] Cyclophosphamide-based treatment of hematologic and solid tumors has generally not been associated with an increased risk of t-MDS/AML.

Secondary MDS and leukemia have been reported in patients after high-dose therapy and autologous stem cell/ bone marrow transplantation. The crude incidence of t-MDS/AML after transplantation in lymphoma patients has ranged from 0.9% to 12% with a median latency ranging from 11 to 124 months (Table 24-4).[264-273] Factors

TABLE 24-4. Risk of MDS/AML Following High-Dose Chemoradiotherapy and Autologous Bone Marrow Transplantation for Lymphoma

Author/Center	No. Patients Transplanted	No. Patients with t-MDS/AML	Crude Incidence	Median Latency (months) from BMT (range)
Darrington et al, 1994 Nebraska	511 (NHL/HD)	12	2.3%	44 (13-74)
Traweek et al, 1994 City of Hope	275 (NHL/HD)	5	1.8%	11 (8-37)
Stone et al, 1994 Dana-Farber	262 (NHL)	20	7.6%	31 (10-31)
Miller et al, 1994 Minnesota	206 (NHL/HD)	9	4.4%	34 (5-60)
Taylor et al, 1997 Royal Victoria Infirmary, UK	114 (NHL/HD)	1	0.9%	124
Pedersen-Bjergaard et al, 1997 Rigshospitalet, Denmark	76 (NHL/HD)	6	7.9%	13 (4-43)
Andre et al, 1998 SFGM Paris	467 (HD)	8	1.7%	21 (3-43)
Milligan et al, 1999 EBMT	4998 (NHL/HD)	66	1.3%	—
Micallef et al, 2000 St. Bartholomew's, London	230 (NHL)	27	12%	4.4 yr (11 mo-8.8 yr)
Del Cañizo et al, 2000 Spain (GETH)	533 (NHL/HD)	11	2.1%	26 (1.5-63)

NHL: non-Hodgkin's lymphoma; HD: Hodgkin's disease.

Modified from Del Cañizo C, Amigo L, Hernandez J, et al: Incidence and characterization of secondary myelodysplastic syndromes following autologous transplantation. Haematologica 2000;85:403.

identified as predisposing to the development of acute leukemia include older patient age, lower dose of infused hematopoietic progenitors, prior fludarabine therapy, prior radiotherapy, increased interval from diagnosis to transplantation, bone marrow involvement, lymphoma subtype, lower platelet count before or at transplantation, slow platelet recovery, and relapse of lymphoma after transplantation.[264-267, 269, 272] Total-body radiotherapy used in transplant-preparative regimens has also been linked to t-MDS/AML after transplantation.[267, 274] In multiple myeloma, among patients who had undergone prolonged alkylator therapy before transplantation, 7 (6%) developed t-MDS after transplantation.[275] No patients who had received only one cycle of standard therapy developed t-MDS after transplantation. In a retrospective review of 864 breast cancer patients who underwent autologous bone marrow transplantation (BMT), the 4-year probability of developing t-MDS/AML was 1.6%.[276] Evidence suggests that antecedent chemotherapy, instead of the high-dose conditioning regimen or transplant procedure, is the critical factor for most cases of post-BMT t-MDS/AML.[269, 270, 275] In support of this theory, FISH could detect abnormal pretransplant clones in bone marrow and peripheral blood stem cell specimens of 9 of 12 patients who developed t-MDS after autologous transplantation.[277] In a retrospective analysis of autografted lymphoma patients, stem cell priming with VP-16 was associated with an increased risk of t-MDS/AML, particularly AML with 11q23 or 21q22 abnormalities.[278]

PEDIATRIC MDS

Population-based studies in Denmark and British Columbia have established an annual incidence of pediatric MDS of 3.2 to 4.0 cases per million, accounting for 6% to 9% of all hematologic malignancies in children.[279, 280] This incidence is approximately 10-fold less than that for MDS in adults. Classification of childhood MDS, using schemes such as the FAB system originally created for adults, has been hindered by inconsistent definitions and nomenclature and differences in the underlying pathobiology of pediatric cases. For example, childhood MDS may arise from genetically predisposing conditions such as neurofibromatosis, Down's syndrome, Schwachman-Diamond syndrome, Kostmann's agranulocytosis, familial monosomy 7, and DNA repair deficiency disorders such as Fanconi's anemia, Bloom's syndrome, and ataxia-telangiectasia.[281] Furthermore, children with MDS are often subdivided as having more adult-type MDS or as suffering from a disorder with myeloproliferative features usually observed in infancy and early childhood. Children with disorders exhibiting predominantly myeloproliferative features have been variably described as having juvenile chronic myelogenous leukemia (JCML), monosomy 7 syndrome, or CMML.[282-284] The International Juvenile Myelomonocytic Leukemia Working Group has proposed that the new term "juvenile myelomonocytic leukemia" be used to encompass the diseases JCML, monosomy 7, and CMML.[285] Monosomy 7 occurs in a heterogeneous group of myeloid disorders including MDS, JMML, and AML.[283] Data have shown that prognosis in these cases is related

to the underlying morphologic diagnosis and not to loss of chromosome 7, thus failing to support the nosology of monosomy 7 as a distinct syndrome.[286, 287] For reviews on JMML, see references 288 and 289.

A retrospective analysis was performed of childhood MDS and MPD, consisting of 167 cases from 7 institutions (101 with adult-type MDS [A-MDS], 60 with JMML, and 6 with Down's syndrome and transient myeloproliferative syndrome).[290] Clonal cytogenetic abnormalities were present in 80% of all the marrows analyzed, with monosomy 7 as an isolated finding in 51% of A-MDS cases. Median survival was 6.3 years in A-MDS. The study confirmed the prolonged survival of children with Down's syndrome and transient myeloproliferative syndrome. Evolution to AML occurred in 41% of children with A-MDS, compared with 13% with JMML. Patients with A-MDS had similar prognoses with or without BMT (e.g., 10-year actuarial survival 39% versus 43%, respectively). In contrast, another retrospective study of 340 children with MDS and JMML showed a significant survival advantage with BMT.[287] Both analyses confirmed the low response rates to intensive chemotherapy observed in previous studies.

Therapy of Pediatric MDS

When considering treatment in children, the clinician should make a distinction between A-MDS cases, which may evolve to AML over time, and the more proliferative-type disorders such as JMML, which usually result in death from complications of progressive bone marrow failure. For children with A-MDS, differentiating agents, hemopoietic growth factors, and low-dose chemotherapy with various agents have shown only modest and transient responses.[281, 289] Intensive chemotherapy has achieved prolonged remissions and survival in only a small proportion of cases.[281, 291] Children with Down's syndrome exhibit a high frequency of MDS and AML, especially of the megakaryocytic subtype. Down's syndrome children with these hematologic malignancies have better-than-expected prognoses and respond more favorably to conventional chemotherapy (see Chapter 22).[292]

Allogeneic BMT remains the only curative treatment for childhood MDS. The European Working Group on Myelodysplastic Syndrome in Childhood performed a retrospective analysis of allogeneic BMT in 29 patients with MDS other than CMML. The event-free survival rate was 58%, with transplant-related mortality and relapse rates of 21% and 26%, respectively.[293] Because of the high likelihood of death due to cytopenias or progression to AML and the lack of other satisfactory therapies, certain children with MDS and an HLA-matched donor should be offered allogeneic BMT as early as possible in the course of the disease.

PROGNOSTIC STRATIFICATION

The clinical heterogeneity of MDS makes planning therapy and predicting outcomes for individual patients a

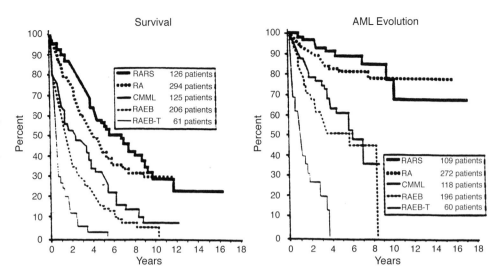

FIGURE 24–6. Survival (*left*) and freedom from AML evolution (*right*) in patients with myelodysplastic syndrome who were evaluated by the International MDS Workshop in relation to their FAB classification subgroup (Kaplan-Meier curves). RA, refractory anemia; RARS, RA with ringed sideroblasts; RAEB, RA with excess blasts; RAEB-T, RAEB in transformation; CMML, chronic myelomonocytic leukemia. (From Greenberg P, Cox C, Le Beau MM, et al: International Prognostic Scoring System for evaluating prognosis in myelodysplastic syndromes. Blood 1997;89:2079.)

difficult challenge. Since its inception in 1982, the FAB system has been relatively useful in categorizing MDS patients. There has been a moderate degree of consistency in prognostic findings in relation to survival and transformation to AML in several large studies when FAB morphologic criteria were used (Table 24–5; Fig. 24–6).[14, 43, 146, 294-299] Differences in median survival, ranging from 3 to 6 years in patients with RA or RARS and from 5 to 12 months in patients with RAEB and RAEB-T, have been delineated between these MDS subtypes. Similarly, the proportion of patients who transform to leukemia varies between an incidence of 5% to 15% in low-risk RA/RARS patients and 40% to 50% in high-risk RAEB/RAEB-T patients. In a study evaluating time to disease evolution, 25% and 55% of patients with RAEB and RAEB-T, respectively, underwent transformation to AML at 1 year and 35% and 65% at 2 years. In contrast, the incidence for RA patients was 5% and 10% at 1 and 2 years, respectively, whereas none with RARS progressed to leukemia at 2 years. In RAEB and RAEB-T patients, AML is the cause of death in 20% to 55% of patients, whereas infection and hemorrhage due to marrow failure cause approximately 36% to 50% of deaths, and nonhematologic causes account for approximately 10% to 20%.[294-299] In RA and RARS, these figures are somewhat reversed. The drawbacks of the FAB system as a prognostic tool for MDS patients include (1) the wide range of marrow blast percentages for individuals in the RAEB and CMML groups (5% to 20% and 1% to 20%, respectively) and (2) the exclusion of other important biologic criteria such as marrow cytogenetics and the number of cytopenias.

TABLE 24–5. MDS: Survival and Leukemic Evolution According to FAB Morphologic Group*

	RA	RARS	RAEB	RAEB-T	CMML
Median survival (months)	43	73	12	5	20
Transformation to AML (%)	15	5	40	50	35
Proportion of patients (%)	25	15	35	15	10

*Meta-analysis of patient results from references 146, 294–299.

These limitations may partly explain the significant differences in survival and leukemic risk observed among patients belonging to the same FAB type.

Other scoring systems that did not include karyotype as a prognostic factor were developed for predicting survival in individuals with MDS. The Bournemouth score assigned risk based on points allocated for neutropenia, anemia, thrombocytopenia, and the presence of more than 5% blasts in the marrow.[146] The Spanish scoring system by Sanz and colleagues[297] inversely related prognosis with the severity of thrombocytopenia, percentage of bone marrow blasts, and age (younger or older than 60 years). The Goasguen and Düsseldorf scoring systems used the severity of anemia, thrombocytopenia, and marrow blasts.[300, 301] The Düsseldorf score also incorporated evaluation of the serum LDH level.[301] Conflicting data exist regarding the value of LDH as an independent predictor of survival in MDS.[297, 302] In all of these scoring systems, the proportion of marrow blasts was the most useful prognostic marker of survival and progression to AML.[43, 44, 146, 155, 294-299] Studies have reported clear differences in survival for patients with more or fewer than 5% marrow blasts, with the survival curves of patients with 10% to 20% and 20% to 30% marrow blasts being similar. The percentage of marrow blasts is also a significant factor in the risk of developing AML. The addition of an extra cut-off point of 10% marrow blasts by the Spanish group added prognostic value in RAEB patients.[297]

The increasing recognition that different types of cytogenetic abnormalities have prognostic implications for patients with MDS led to the International MDS Risk Analysis Workshop.[43] A global analysis was performed on patient data and critical variables to develop a consensus system for a more refined cytogenetic classification. Using multivariate analysis, the three most significant independent variables for determining survival and AML evolution were marrow blast percentage, cytogenetic subgroup, and the number of cytopenias. In addition, age younger than 60 years and female gender were predictive of improved survival. These factors were combined to generate a model called the International Prognostic Scoring

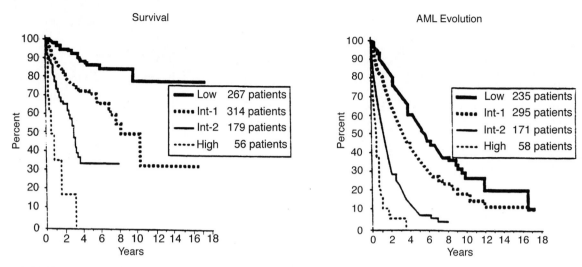

FIGURE 24–7. Survival (*left*) and freedom from AML evolution (*right*) in patients with myelodysplastic syndrome in relation to their classification by the IPSS for MDS: low, Int-1, Int-2, or high (Kaplan-Meier curves). (From Greenberg P, Cox C, Le Beau MM, et al: International Prognostic Scoring System for evaluating prognosis in myelodysplastic syndromes. Blood 1997;89: 2079.)

System (IPSS). By combining the risk scores for these three variables, patients were divided into four risk groups regarding survival and AML evolution: low = 0; intermediate 1 = 0.5-1.0; intermediate 2 = 1.5-2.0; and high = >2.5 (Table 24-6; Fig. 24-7). Stratification for age improved analysis of survival (Table 24-7; Fig. 24-8). Discrimination among the four risk groups was much less precise when either cytopenias or cytogenetic subtypes were omitted from the classification. For example, a substantial proportion of IPSS intermediate 1 and intermediate 2 patients would have been inaccurately categorized as low risk had cytogenetics not been included. Compared with the FAB, Spanish, and Lille scoring systems, the IPSS discriminated between the defined subgroups of these other categorization systems and provided an improved method for predicting survival and AML evolution.[14, 297, 303]

In Vitro Myeloid Colony Assays

In vitro MDS marrow clonal growth may be divided into leukemic and nonleukemic patterns.[123] In 6 studies of 179 MDS patients with different FAB morphologic subtypes, correlation was found between clinical outcome and in vitro marrow growth (Table 24-8).[304-309] When patients were classified according to their in vitro myeloid growth patterns, subgroups of MDS patients with nonleukemic growth patterns had a 20% to 31% incidence of transformation to AML and 20- to 47-month median survivals. In

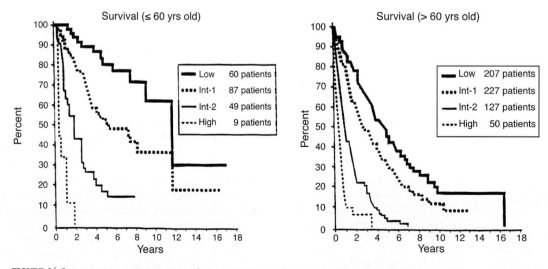

FIGURE 24–8. Survival according to age ≤60 years (*left*) or >60 years (*right*) of MDS patients in relation to their classification by the IPSS: low, Int-1, Int-2, or high (Kaplan-Meier curves). (From Greenberg P, Cox C, Le Beau MM, et al: International Prognostic Scoring System for evaluating prognosis in myelodysplastic syndromes. Blood 1997;89:2079.)

Table 24–6. International Prognostic Scoring System for MDS

Prognostic Variable	Survival and AML Evolution Score Value				
	0	*0.5*	*1.0*	*1.5*	*2.0*
Marrow blasts (%)	<5	5–10	—	11–20	21–30
Karyotype[a]	Good	Intermediate	Poor		
Cytopenias[b]	0–1	2–3			

Risk Category	Combined Score
Low	0
Int-1	0.5–1.0
Int-2	1.5–2.0
High	≥2.5

[a]Good = normal, Y−, del(5q), del(20q); poor = complex (>3 abnormalities) or chromosome 7 anomalies; intermediate = other abnormalities.
[b]Neutrophils <1800/μL, platelets <100,000/μL, hemoglobin <10 g/dL.
Modified from Greenberg P, Cox C, Le Beau MM, et al.: International Prognostic Scoring System for evaluating prognosis in myelodysplastic syndromes. Blood 1997;89:2079.

Table 24–8. Prognosis with MDS: Utility of in Vitro Marrow Myeloid Clonogenic Culture Studies

Growth Patterns	Incidence (%)	Transformation to AML (%)	Median Survival (months)
RAEB-T (n = 80)[307, 308]		51 (45–60)	9 (7–11)
Nonleukemic growth	33 (27–38)	31 (29–33)	20 (15–25)
Leukemic growth	68 (62–73)	60 (50–70)	7 (5–8)
RAEB (n = 17)[309, 310]		41	14
Nonleukemic growth	70	29	21
Leukemic growth	30	100	10
RA (n = 82)[308, 311, 312]		39 (35–44)	24 (9–20)
Nonleukemic growth	54 (30–74)	20 (21–40)	47 (9–50)
Leukemic growth	46 (26–70)	60 (50–80)	8 (4–10)

Values are means and ranges of means for cited studies.
From Greenberg PL: Biologic and clinical implications of marrow culture studies in the myelodysplastic syndromes. Semin Hematol 1996;33:163.

contrast, MDS patients with leukemic growth patterns had a 60% to 100% incidence of evolution to AML and 7- to 10-month median survivals. Factors other than in vitro growth patterns contribute to transformation as not all patients with abnormal clonal growth had poor prognoses. A correlation has been demonstrated among in vitro myeloid growth patterns, abnormal marrow cytogenetics, and poor prognoses.[123]

Other Prognostic Factors

The degree of dyshematopoiesis, especially the presence of granulocytic and megakaryocytic dysplasia, had a prog-

nostic effect in some series of MDS patients and was used to separate patients with RA and RARS into two risk groups.[53, 297, 310-313] The evaluation of dysplasia is subjective, which may limit its usefulness as a prognostic factor.[314] Using plastic-embedding techniques, several groups have described the presence of clusters of immature precursors. Instead of the usual pattern of blasts located adjacent to the cortical bone, a clustering of immature cells in the central marrow regions, called atypical localization of immature myeloid precursors, is associated with significantly shorter survival in all MDS subtypes.[43, 295-301, 315] The presence of *N-Ras, p53,* or FMS mutations has been associated with poorer outcomes in multivariate

Table 24–7. Age-Related Survival and AML Evolution in MDS Patients Within the IPSS Subgroups

	No. of Patients	Median Survival (yr)			
		Low	*Int-1*	*Int-2*	*High*
Total pts.: No. (%)	816	267 (33%)	314 (38%)	176 (22%)	59 (7%)
		5.7	3.5	1.2	0.4
Age ≤60 yr	205 (25%)	11.8	5.2	1.8	0.3
>60 yr	611	4.8	2.7	1.1	0.5
≤70 yr	445 (54%)	9.0	4.4	1.3	0.4
>70 yr	371	3.9	2.4	1.2	0.4

	No. of Patients	25% AML Evolution (yr)			
		Low	*Int-1*	*Int-2*	*High*
Total pts.: No. (%)	759	235 (31%)	295 (39%)	171 (22%)	58 (8%)
		9.4	3.3	1.1	0.2
Age ≤60 yr	187 (25%)	>9.4 (NR)	6.9	0.7	0.2
>60 yr	572	9.4	2.7	1.3	0.2
≤70 yr	414 (55%)	>9.4 (NR)	5.5	1.0	0.2
>70 yr	345	>5.8 (NR)	2.2	1.4	0.4

NR, not reached.
Modified from Greenberg P, Cox C, Le Beau MM, et al.: International Prognostic Scoring System for evaluating prognosis in myelodysplastic syndromes. Blood 1997; 89:2079.

analysis.[101] Methylation of the *p15* gene has also been linked to disease progression.[316]

THERAPY

Risk-Based Treatment

Treatment of MDS should be approached on an individual patient basis. Morbidity and mortality rates result from cytopenia-related complications and from evolution to acute leukemia. Because MDS affects predominantly the elderly, these cytopenias may aggravate nonhematologic illnesses. In turn, these co-morbid medical conditions or age-related factors may limit certain intensive forms of therapy. The FAB and IPSS classification systems have proved useful for dividing patients into prognostic risk groups. The prognostic subgroups aid selection of specific treatments.

The National Comprehensive Cancer Network (NCCN) convened a group of clinicians to establish practice guidelines for the diagnosis, evaluation, and treatment of MDS patients.[317] As shown in Figure 24-9, the initial factor in planning therapeutic options is the patient's IPSS risk category, as this feature improves outcome analysis. The patient's age and performance status are additional important determinants. The threshold of younger or older than 60 years was chosen because it is often the age of eligibility for certain intensive therapeutic options, such as BMT. Although this age is relative and arbitrary, mainly biologic rather than chronologic features are important. The therapeutic options for MDS include supportive care, low-intensity therapy, and high-intensity therapy.

Currently, supportive care is the standard community-based approach. This includes leukocyte-filtered red blood cells for symptomatic anemia and platelet-transfusions for severe thrombocytopenia or thrombocytopenia-related bleeding. In order to prevent complications related to secondary hemochromatosis, subcutaneous iron chelation therapy with desferrioxamine should be considered as the number of red blood cell transfusions approaches 20 to 30.

Low-intensity therapy includes the use of biologic response modifiers, differentiation-inducing drugs, hemopoietic growth factors, and low-intensity chemotherapy, agents that can generally be administered on an outpatient basis (Table 24-9).

High-intensity therapy includes treatments that require hospitalization, such as bone marrow transplantation (BMT) or intensive chemotherapy. Using the NCCN algo-

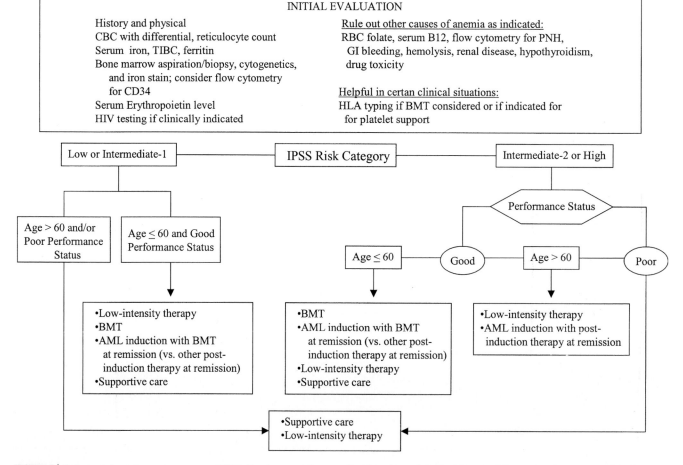

FIGURE 24-9. Approach to the management of MDS. Treatment options are listed in the order of preference. Therapy in the context of clinical trial is encouraged.

TABLE 24–9. Therapeutic Options for MDS

	Clinical Utility Shown in Selected Patients	Clinical Utility Not Demonstrated	Clinical Utility Under Preliminary Investigation	
Supportive Care	Antibiotics Transfusions Iron Chelation			
Low-Intensity Therapy				
Hemopoietic growth factors	Erythropoietin[a] G-CSF GM-CSF	Interleukin-3 Interleukin-6	Thrombopoietin Interleukin-11	
Low-intensity chemotherapy	Azacitidine Hydroxyurea[b] Etoposide[b]	Low-dose cytarabine		
Immunosuppressive agents	Anti-thymocyte globulin Cyclosporin A			
Biologic response modifiers, anti-angiogenic agents, and targeted therapy		Retinoids Sodium phenylbutyrate Hexamethylene bisacetamide Vitamin D_3 analogues	Amifostine Pentoxyfylline Vitamin K_2 Thalidomide	FTI[d] Arsenic trioxide VEGF inhibitors[e] TNFR:Fc[f]
Immunomodulatory agents Hormonal therapy		Interferon-α, -γ Glucocorticoids Androgens Danazol[c]		
High-Intensity Therapy				
Chemotherapy	AML induction chemotherapy + multi-drug resistant modulator (i.e., refractory AML therapy)		Topotecan Decitabine Gemtuzumab ozogamicin	
Marrow/peripheral blood stem cell transplant	HLA-matched sibling donor HLA-matched unrelated donor		Non-myeloablative Autologous	

[a]Utility inversely related to serum EPO levels.
[b]Demonstrated clinical efficacy in the proliferative form of CMML.
[c]May increase the platelet counts in some patients with immune-mediated thrombocytopenia.
[d]Farnesyltransferase inhibitor.
[e]VEGF: Vascular endothelial growth factor.
[f]Tumor necrosis factor-α receptor-fusion protein.

rithm, in patients younger than 60 years in IPSS intermediate 2 or high-risk categories, high-intensity therapy would be a primary consideration. The younger patients in the low-risk or intermediate 1 subgroups are candidates for low-intensity therapy. Low-intensity therapy should be offered to patients older than 60 years with good-performance status, but high-intensity treatments may be suitable for selected patients. Patients with poor-performance status should be offered predominantly low-intensity treatments or supportive care. As many of these treatments are considered experimental, enrollment of patients in clinical trials is encouraged to further define their relative efficacy and toxicities. Specific therapeutic approaches are discussed in the following sections.

LOW-INTENSITY THERAPY

Hematopoietic Growth Factors

Erythropoietin

Serum erythropoietin (EPO) levels in patients with MDS are often elevated suboptimally for the degree of anemia. The rationale of EPO therapy is to provide pharmacologic doses of the cytokine in order to increase serum and marrow EPO levels and to overcome the defective proliferation and maturation of erythroid precursors. The clinical aim is to raise hemoglobin levels and thus treat the

patient's symptomatic anemia/fatigue and to reduce transfusion requirements and the cumulative risk of secondary hemochromatosis. Although various criteria are used to define response to EPO therapy and the proportion of low- and high-risk FAB subtypes differs in each study, the average response rate of numerous published trials is approximately 20%.[318-331] A meta-analysis of 205 MDS patients from 17 published reports tallied a 16% response rate.[332] In this analysis, patients with RARS showed a significantly lower response rate (7.5%) than all other patients (21%). Other factors favoring response were the absence of transfusion need (44% versus 10%) and serum EPO concentration lower than 200 U/L. Patients without a transfusion requirement and MDS patients other than RARS patients showed a response rate greater than 50% irrespective of the serum EPO level. There was no dose-response relationship and no correlation between maximal dose and time to response. The optimal dose was relatively high and generally in the range of 450 to 1000 U/kg/week. The limited clinical efficacy of EPO in these trials partly reflects the suboptimal responsiveness of myelodysplastic BFU-E to EPO in vitro.[132, 333]

Granulocyte Colony–Stimulating Factor

In a phase I/II 6- to 8-week dose-escalation study of subcutaneous granulocyte colony–stimulating factor (G-CSF) (0.1 to 3.0 μg/kg/d), 16/18 patients experienced a rise in the absolute neutrophil count by 5- to 40-fold.[334]

Cessation of treatment resulted in return of counts to baseline values over 2 to 4 weeks. In a subsequent maintenance phase of the trial 10 of 11 patients responded with persistent improvements in neutrophil counts for up to 16 months.[335] There was a significant reduction in bacterial infection risk during periods when the absolute neutrophil count was maintained at more than 1500/mm³ with G-CSF. Enhancement of in vitro neutrophil function (phagocytosis and chemotaxis) persisted during the maintenance phase. Of 10 anemic patients, 2 nontransfusion patients had a greater than 20% impovement in hemoglobin level, and another 2 patients had decreases in their transfusion requirements.

A phase III multi-institutional randomized trial of 102 patients with high-risk MDS was performed to determine the impact of G-CSF on the natural history of the disease.[336] Fifty patients with RAEB or RAEB-T were treated with subcutaneous G-CSF 1 to 5 µg/kg daily, and 52 patients received only supportive care. G-CSF was well tolerated, with a low incidence of minor side effects. The rate and time to progression to AML were similar in RAEB and RAEB-T patients in both arms of the study. The survival of RAEB-T patients was also comparable in both arms; however, the median survival of RAEB patients was signficantly shorter in patients receiving G-CSF (10 versus 21 months) because of a higher rate of disease-related nonleukemic deaths, primarily from bleeding. A retrospective analysis found that RAEB patients receiving G-CSF had a median survival time comparable to previously reported RAEB survival data. In contrast, RAEB patients in the supportive care group had prolonged survival. An increased proportion of RAEB patients receiving G-CSF (29% versus 14%) was in the high-risk prognostic category, using a scoring system that categorizes MDS patients according to the percentage of bone marrow blasts, platelets, and age. The survival differences in RAEB patients may therefore be attributed to the increased number of high-risk patients in the G-CSF arm or to the unusually long survival of high-risk patients receiving just supportive measures. The impact of G-CSF on the rate of infections in these patients is under evaluation.

Granulocyte-Macrophage Colony-Stimulating Factor

Despite the use of different schedules and routes of administration, numerous phase I/II studies have shown that granulocyte-macrophage colony-stimulating factor (GM-CSF) produces dose-dependent increases in neutrophil counts in the majority of MDS patients.[337-348] A European Organization for Research and Treatment of Cancer (EORTC) randomized multicenter study evaluated the effects of up to 2-month GM-CSF treatment in MDS patients with fewer than 10% marrow blasts.[349] Approximately two-thirds of patients responded at dose levels of 108 or 216 µg subcutaneously daily. The small number of patients and limited duration of treatment precluded assessment of the effects of GM-CSF therapy on disease progression and rates of infection. Another multicenter study randomized MDS patients to GM-CSF 3 µg/kg subcutaneously daily for 3 months versus observation.[350] After 3 months of therapy, patients could cross over from the observation to the GM-CSF arm if infections were documented. A marked increase in neutrophils and fewer infections were observed in the GM-CSF group. GM-CSF was not associated with an increased rate of conversion to leukemia. Survival benefit could not be assessed because of the study's crossover design. These multicenter trials of GM-CSF have generally shown no clinically significant erythroid responses, and many thrombocytopenic patients developed lower platelet counts during treatment, necessitating more platelet transfusions.[349, 350] In addition, a significant proportion of patients discontinued treatment with GM-CSF because of side effects, including pulmonary infiltrates, flulike syndromes, hyperleukocytosis, and bone pain.[349-351]

G-CSF and EPO

Synergy between the hematopoietic growth factors EPO and G-CSF has been demonstrated in vitro for the production of normal and MDS marrow BFU-E numbers.[352] G-CSF enhances the development of early precursors into EPO-responsive hematopoietic progenitors.[352] Two phase II studies confirmed improved in vivo erythroid responses to combined EPO and G-CSF treatment compared with either agent alone.[334, 335] These trials initially employed G-CSF at 1 µg/kg (0.3 to 3 µg/kg) subcutaneously daily to normalize or double the neutrophil count. EPO 100 U/kg/d was then administered subcutaneously and dose-escalated to 150 to 300 U/kg/d every 4 weeks, or maintained at 120 U/kg/d in the other study, while continuing G-CSF. Ten (42%) of 24 patients in one study,[353] and 8 (38%) of 21 patients in the second study,[354] had substantial erythroid responses, characterized by increased hemoglobin values and decreased transfusion requirements. Nearly all patients had improvements in neutrophil counts. Responders had lower endogenous serum EPO levels (fewer than 200 to 500 mU/mm³), less advanced pancytopenia, less pretreatment RBC transfusion needs, and more responsive marrow BFU-E. Responses were seen in all FAB subtypes. Of interest, the best response rate (60%) was observed in RARS patients, those who generally respond poorly to EPO alone. A subsequent study of maintenance G-CSF treatment showed that approximately one-half of patients lost their response on G-CSF withdrawal and regained it when G-CSF was resumed.[355]

In a multi-institutional American-Scandinavian analysis of 98 MDS patients treated with G-CSF and EPO, a similar erythroid response rate of 36% was observed.[356] Multivariate analysis showed that baseline serum EPO levels and initial transfusion needs predicted responses to combination therapy. Using pretreatment serum EPO levels as a ternary variable (less than 100, 100 to 500, or more than 500 mU/mm²) and red blood cell transfusion requirement as a binary variable (more or fewer than 2 units per month), a scoring system was devised as a means of predicting erythroid response (Table 24–10). Patients were divided into three groups: one group with a high probability of erythroid responses (74%), one intermediate group (23%), and one group with poor responses to treatment (7%). A subsequent randomized phase II study verified the results of the American-Scandinavian analysis

Table 24–10. Model for Predicting Erythroid Responses to G-CSF and EPO in MDS Patients

Variable	Scores*					
	−3	−2	−1	0	+1	+2
Serum EPO (U/L)	>500				100–500	<100
RBC transfusions (U/month)		≥2				<2

Predictive Score	Response Group	
	Type	% Responders (pts.)
>+1	High	74 (22/29)
±1	Intermediate	23 (7/31)
<−1	Low	7 (3/34)

*Multivariate logistic regression analysis; weighted logistic coefficients.

From Hellström-Lindberg E, Negrin R, Stein R, et al: Erythroid response to treatment with G-CSF plus erythropoietin for the anemia of patients with myelodysplastic syndromes: Proposal for a predictive model. Br J Haematol 1997;99:344.

and established a durable median response time of 24 months.[357] Response rates were identical in two treatment groups primed with either G-CSF or EPO, indicating that initial treatment with G-CSF was not necessary.

GM-CSF and EPO

In small phase II trials of concurrent or sequential EPO and GM-CSF, increases in hemoglobin levels or decreased transfusion requirements occurred in 23% to 46% of patients.[358-361] A 12-week randomized, placebo-controlled trial of GM-CSF (0.3 to 5.0 μg/kg/d) and EPO therapy (150 U/kg three times a week) stratified 66 MDS patients to endogenous EPO levels of more or fewer than 500 mU/mm³.[362] As expected, combined GM-CSF and EPO therapy significantly improved neutrophil counts. Platelet counts were unaffected; and a trend toward reduced red blood cell transfusion requirements was observed in patients with EPO levels lower than 500 mU/mm³. In a study of 19 patients, sequential GM-CSF (3 μg/kg) and EPO (60 to 120 U/kg) were administered weekly for 3 months.[363] Ten of 19 patients (53%) responded, with 7 patients achieving a good response and 3 patients achieving a partial response. All responding RARS patients continued to demonstrate erythroid responses during 3 to 24 months of follow-up, whereas 1 RA and 2 RAEB patients did not have continuing responses at 2 to 12 months. Although these studies of GM-CSF and EPO treatment demonstrate some clinically important erythroid responses, the combination of G-CSF and EPO is at least as effective and is generally better tolerated because of the greater toxicity associated with GM-CSF.

Interleukin-3

Three phase I/II studies evaluated the effects of short-term treatment with recombinant human interleukin-3 (rhIL-3) in MDS patients.[364-366] These preliminary studies suggested that IL-3 could increase neutrophil counts but not as prominently as GM-CSF or G-CSF. Furthermore, it showed a role in transiently improving thrombocytopenia

in some patients, but erythropoiesis was rarely stimulated. A longer-term study of 3-month rhIL-3 therapy elicited improvements in 2 of 5 patients with initial platelet counts lower than 50,000/mm³, without notable changes in the other lineages.[367] The issue as to whether combination hematopoietic growth factor support with IL-3 and EPO could augment erythroid responses was evaluated in 22 MDS patients.[368] The combination produced a rise in reticulocyte counts in five patients, but only two patients experienced decreased red blood cell transfusion requirements. The erythroid response was comparable to that in studies of EPO alone, but rhIL-3 produced toxicity requiring dose reduction in the majority of those treated.

IL-6

The in vitro stimulatory effect of IL-6 on thrombopoiesis prompted its evaluation in a phase I study of 22 low-risk MDS patients with thrombocytopenia.[369] Eight (36%) patients experienced a transient rise in platelet counts, but only three were classified as major responders. IL-6 increased the frequency of higher ploidy megakaryocytes without increasing the number of megakaryocyte progenitors, consistent with its known maturation-inducing effect. Non–dose-dependent anemia developed in most patients, and no neutrophil responses were observed. Constitutional symptoms and anemia were seen in most patients, precluding all but three patients from receiving maintenance therapy. The marginal activity and significant therapy-related toxicity of IL-6 make it of limited value as a thrombopoietic agent in MDS.

Biologic Response Modifiers

Amifostine

Amifostine has shown efficacy in protecting bone marrow and normal tissues from cytotoxic agents, a property that may be partly attributable to antioxidant mechanisms. It is a synthetic phosphorylated aminothiol prodrug that is rapidly dephosphorylated to the active metabolite WR-1065.[370] Preclinical studies have demonstrated that amifostine promotes hematopoiesis. Brief exposure of bone marrow mononuclear cells from normal and MDS patients to amifostine in vitro stimulates the growth and the survival of multipotent and committed progenitors.[371] Hematopoietic progenitor growth is associated with reduction in the fraction of apoptotic CD34+ cells within 24 hours of drug exposure.[372]

A multicenter phase II study of amifostine has evaluated responses in more than 100 MDS patients.[373] Amifostine was administered at 200 and 400 mg/m² three times a week for 3 weeks followed by 2 weeks off therapy, allowing for dose escalation. Diagnoses were RA (13), RARS (29), RAEB (47), RAEB-T (7), and CMML (5) patients. Of the patients, 30% treated experienced a single or multilineage hematologic response (neutrophil 30%, erythroid 21%, and platelet 37% response rates). A 50% decrease in myeloblasts or ringed sideroblasts was observed in 25% of the bone marrows reviewed and was correlated with hematologic responses. Adverse events including fatigue, nausea, and vomiting occurred more frequently at the 400 mg/m² dose level. A phase II study evaluated amifostine (200 mg/m² three times a week for 4 weeks) in 26 low-risk MDS patients.[374] Hemoglobin, neutrophil, and platelet counts increased, respectively, in 6 (23%) 13 (50%), and 9 (34%) of patients. Red blood cell transfusions were reduced in only four patients and eliminated in one patient. Current trials are evaluating the clinical efficacy of varied doses and schedules of single-agent amifostine and its combination with other trophic and cytotoxic agents.

Sodium Phenylbutyrate and Hexamethylene Bisacetamide

The aromatic short-chain fatty acid sodium phenylbutyrate demonstrates an in vitro differentiating capacity in leukemia and solid tumor cell lines, inhibition of AML cell culture growth, and induction of fetal hemoglobin and differentiation antigens in normal bone marrow progenitors.[375, 376] Despite encouraging preclinical and phase I studies, a phase II study of sodium phenylbutyrate by two prolonged continuous intravenous infusion schedules showed limited clinical activity.[377-379] Hexamethylene bisacetamide is a low-molecular-weight polar-planar agent that induces differentiation of murine erythroleukemia cells and nonselectively inhibits the growth of myeloid and erythroid progenitors in MDS and normal subjects.[380, 381] In two studies evaluating different continuous infusion schedules, hexamethylene bisacetamide had minimal benefit.[382, 383] Grade 4 thrombocytopenia was the most significant toxicity, reversible with drug cessation.

Low-Intensity Chemotherapy

Chemotherapeutic options for MDS have included low-dose therapy with agents such as hydroxyurea and cytosine arabinoside (ara-C). Interest in low-dose ara-C was based on its differentiating effects in vitro on AML cell lines (clinical data also indicate cytotoxic mechanisms) and the desire to reduce the toxicity observed with conventional doses.[384] Low doses of ara-C (5 to 20 mg/m²/day), administered on an intermittent or continuous infusion schedule, have been studied in more than 350 cases of MDS and secondary AML.[385] Response rates were in the range of 15% to 20%. From these studies, the median duration of complete remission for MDS patients was 10 months, median survival was 15 months, and the treatment-related death rate was 15%. In a phase III intergroup study of low dose ara-C versus supportive care, low-dose ara-C produced complete responses in 11% of patients, and there was no difference in overall survival and transformation to AML.[386] These data show that low-dose ara-C has limited efficacy in MDS. Hyroxyurea and oral VP-16 have been used in CMML to control leukocytosis, organomegaly, and visceral involvement. A randomized trial showed that hydroxyurea gave higher response rates than those obtained with etoposide in advanced CMML, but responses were partial, and survival was generally poor with both drugs.[387]

Azacitidine

5-Azacitidine (AZA-C), a ring analogue of the pyrimidine nucleoside cytosine, acts as a DNA-hypomethylating agent by inhibiting DNA methyltransferase activity.[388] Azacitidine can induce transcription of previously quiescent genes and differentiation of leukemia cell lines in vitro. Based on promising results from phase II studies, the Cancer and Leukemia Group B performed a prospective phase III trial comparing AZA-C with supportive care in 191 patients, stratified according to FAB category (RA 19%, RAEB 42%, RAEB-T 21%) and symptomatic cytopenias.[389] Treatment with 7-day courses of subcutaneous AZA-C at 75 mg/m²/day, repeated every 28 days, led to a 63% response rate (6% CR, 10% PR, 47% improved), compared with a 7% (improved) response rate in the observation arm. The median time to leukemic transformation or death was delayed to 22 months in patients taking AZA-C, compared with 12 months in the observation group. The drug was well tolerated, with a treatment-related mortality rate of 1%. In patients taking AZA-C, quality of life assessments were significantly improved.[390] The impact of AZA-C on the natural history and overall survival of patients with MDS is encouraging, but interpretation of these endpoints is difficult because of the crossover design of the phase III study.

Retinoids/Vitamins

Retinoids (vitamin A analogues) play a critical role in numerous biologic processes, including hematopoeisis. Retinoids can induce differentiation and inhibit the proliferative capacity of several leukemia cell lines.[391, 392] All-trans-retinoic acid (ATRA) has become a well-established differentiating therapeutic agent for treatment of acute promyelocytic leukemia. Eleven studies of 13-cis-retinoic acid in more than 250 patients with MDS have shown modest response rates of 20% to 30%.[393-403] Duration of treatment extended from 4 weeks to 5 years. Maximum tolerated doses up to 100 mg/m²/day have been used. Hepatotoxicity, cheilitis, mucositis, conjunctivitis, skin erythema, and joint pains have been dose-limiting side effects. Selected studies reveal that low-risk MDS patients enjoy the best response rates, in the 50% to 60% range. Generally, no impact on rates of leukemic progression or overall survival has been observed. Five studies have evaluated ATRA as single-agent therapy in MDS.[404-408] Despite a 50% response rate in one study of 10 patients treated for 6 weeks at a dose of 45 mg/m²/day,[403] other studies have shown marginal response rates. Dose escalation up to a maximum tolerated dose of 150 mg/m²/day did not improve responses.[404-406] Based on these relatively low response rates and the lack of impact on the natural course of MDS, retinoids have not become an effective treatment modality in MDS.

Vitamin D_3 binds to intranuclear vitamin D receptors of the steroid-thyroid receptor superfamily and can induce monocyte-macrophage maturation and inhibit proliferation of several leukemia cell lines. Four trials enrolling 46 patients indicated limited responses to doses of 1 to 6 µg/day administered up to 20 weeks.[409-412] In the largest study of 18 patients treated with vitamin D$_3$ up to 2 μg/day for 12 weeks, a 44% response rate was observed, but responses were not sustained. New synthetic vitamin D$_3$ analogues that produce less hypercalcemia and that have greater differentiating and antiproliferative potential will require evaluation in MDS patients.

Vitamin K$_2$ analogues can induce apoptosis in leukemia and MDS cell lines in vitro.[413] In leukemia cells, a differentiation/maturation effect of vitamin K$_2$ analogues may also work through intracellular signaling pathways that result in cell cycle G$_1$ arrest.[414] In a pilot study, the oral vitamin K$_2$ analogue menatetrenone improved the neutropenia and thrombocytopenias of some patients, but significant increases in hemoglobin values were not observed.[415]

Combination Therapy

The low rate and lack of durable responses with monotherapy have led to evaluation of synergistic or additive drug combinations with differentiating agents, hematopoietic growth factors, and low-dose cytotoxic agents. The rationale of such therapy in MDS is to find better ways to overcome the maturation defect and complex molecular abnormalities that contribute to ineffective hematopoiesis and evolution to AML. Studies combining 13-cis-retinoic acid or ATRA with low-dose ara-C (LD-ara-C) have yielded poor response rates.[416-418] Treatment of MDS and AML patients with the combination of LD-ara-C, interferon-α (IFN-α), vitamin D$_3$, and retinoic acid produced an overall response rate of 44%, which was equivalent to that of LD-ara-C alone.[419] In a study of 69 MDS and AML patients randomized to receive LD-ara-C or LD-ara-C plus 13-cis-retinoic acid and vitamin D$_3$, only 26% of patients responded to the combination therapy, and no clinical benefit could be demonstrated on survival, remission rate, or remission duration.[420] More promising results were obtained in MDS patients treated with a 10-week course of 13-cis-retinoic acid plus vitamin D$_3$. Intermittent 6-thioguanine was added to the regimen of higher-risk patients. Although few complete responses were observed, overall response rates of 52% and 61% were observed in low- and high-risk patients, respectively. A significant difference in survival was noted between responders (25 months) and nonresponders (9 months), and red blood cell transfusion requirements were reduced by approximately 50%.[421] The EORTC evaluated the benefit of adding hematopoietic growth factor support with GM-CSF to LD-ara-C in 108 high-risk MDS patients.[422] This combination led to a complete remission rate of 14%, an overall response rate of 39%, and disease progression in 14%. Toxic death occurred in 15% of patients, and more than 50% suffered from complications related to infection and hemorrhage. Further understanding of the complex molecular pathogenesis of MDS may allow the identification of therapeutic targets to which safe drug combinations can be more effectively tailored.

Immunomodulatory Agents

IFNs

Based on the ability of human IFNs to enhance monocytic differentiation of myeloid leukemia cell lines,[423] clinical trials with MDS patients were initiated. In a study of MDS patients treated with an intermittent schedule of IFN-α (2 million units three times a week), transient improvement in blood counts were noted in some individuals, but myelosuppression was frequently observed.[424] Three-month treatment of 17 high-risk MDS patients with lymphoblastoid IFN-α (0.5 to 3 million units three times a week) elicited partial responses in 6 (35%) patients, and 4 of these 6 patients achieved a complete remission with maintenance therapy for up to 29 months.[425] Other studies of prolonged IFN-α administration with doses in the range of 3 to 21 million units/week demonstrated only limited responses and substantial toxicity at higher doses.[426-431] Despite success in small case series with IFN-γ in MDS patients,[432, 433] larger studies have not borne out these results. In a randomized, double-arm study of 30 MDS patients evaluating low- (0.1 mg/m^2/day) and high- (1 mg/m^2/day) dose IFN-γ[434] and in another study of 25 patients,[435] none achieved complete responses to IFN-γ. Cumulatively, relatively few patients have been treated with IFN-α and IFN-γ, and available data do not support their use in the treatment of MDS.

Immunosuppressive Therapy

ATG and Cyclosporin A

Immunosuppressive therapy with ATG and cyclosporin A can produce durable remissions in a high percentage of patients with aplastic anemia. Beginning in the 1980s, case reports and small case series similarly described improvement in the cytopenias of patients with hypocellular MDS treated with ATG.[436-438] An emerging pathophysiologic link between hypocellular MDS and aplastic anemia is immune destruction of hematopoietic cells resulting in pancytopenia.

In a National Institutes of Health study of 60 transfusion-dependent MDS patients treated with ATG, 40 mg/kg for 4 days, 21 (33%) patients achieved prolonged transfusion indepedence and improved neutrophil and platelet counts.[439, 440] A favorable response was predicted by RA FAB subtype, normal karyotype, age younger than 60 years, and low marrow cellularity, although patients with normo- and hypercellular marrows also responded. Responses to ATG treatment were associated with eradication of clonal CD8+ T lymphocytes, which mediated inhibition of CFU-GM progenitor cell growth in vitro and replacement by polyclonal T cells, which did not suppress CFU-GM.[440, 441] In another analysis, the presence of a PNH population was highly correlated with improvement in blood counts after ATG treatment.[143] In a pilot study of 17 MDS patients with RA FAB subtype and various marrow cellularities, cyclosporin A elicited hematologic responses in 14 (82%) patients, characterized by improvements in anemia and transfusion-independence that was maintained up to 30 months of follow-up.[442] Trilineage hematopoiesis was fully restored in 4 (23%) patients. Future studies will aim to correlate clinical responses to ATG and cyclosporin A treatment with alterations in lymphocyte and cytokine profiles and with changes in apoptosis.

Hormonal Therapy

Glucocorticoids/Androgens/Danazol

In vitro growth enhancement of MDS bone marrow cells with the addition of cortisol has been used to identify a small subset of responders to glucocorticoid therapy.[443] Two prospective studies showed that survival outcomes were no better for patients treated with androgens when compared with observation and supportive care[444] or with ara-C.[445] A retrospective review of 76 patients treated with danazol revealed no significant improvement in cytopenias and transfusion requirements.[446] In two case series, danazol or fluoxymesterone treatment led to modest improvements of variable duration in anemia, red blood cell transfusion requirements, and platelet counts.[447, 448] In some MDS patients with suspected immune-mediated thrombocytopenia and platelet-associated IgG, danazol treatment can produce a rise in platelet counts.[449, 450]

HIGH-INTENSITY THERAPY

Chemotherapy

The rationale for treating MDS with high-intensity AML-type chemotherapy is to prolong survival by eradicating the abnormal clone and restoring normal hematopoiesis. Since the early 1980s, most combination regimens have consisted of an anthracycline (daunorubicin, idarubicin, or mitoxantrone) plus conventional or large doses of ara-C, sometimes with the addition of 6-thioguanine.[451, 452] Other regimens, such as mitoxantrone, idarubicin plus etoposide, or fludarabine plus ara-C ± idarubicin, have been used. In trials enrolling more than 10 patients, the reported range of CR rates in high-risk MDS patients was quite variable: 15% to 74%.[452] The median remission duration was usually less than 12 months, and 4- to 5-year survival rates in the range of 8% to 25% have been reported.[453-455] A 19% treatment-related death rate was reported for several trials published before 1992.[456] Reviews of intensive chemotherapy trials in secondary AML have tallied CR rates of 37% to 40%.[451, 452] The average CR rate was found to be higher in series published after 1990, compared with earlier series (48% versus 38%).[452] Although convincing data are not available, the improvement in CR rates may be attributable to advances in supportive care and/or the use of hematopoietic growth factors such as GM-CSF or G-CSF. A few randomized studies have demonstrated a beneficial effect of G-CSF on either neutrophil recovery time or infection rates, but improvement in CR rates has not been a consistent finding. Also, any positive findings have not translated into prolongation of CR duration or survival.[457-460] Trials of intensive chemotherapy in MDS have established that advanced age (older than 45 to 50 years) is an unfavorable prognostic factor.[461-463] Furthermore, MDS patients with karyotypic abnormalities have lower CR and survival rates compared with patients with normal cytogenetics.[464-466] Overall, the CR rates obtained with intensive chemotherapy have been lower in high-risk

MDS patients compared with de novo AML patients. However, the higher median age and poor-risk cytogenetic features of MDS patients in these studies may partially account for the differences in CR rates. For example, in patients younger than 45 years, CR rates for MDS and de novo AML were essentially identical (71% versus 75%).[467] In addition, a retrospective Cancer and Leukemia Group B study found similar CR rates and durations for 874 de novo AML patients and for 33 RAEB/RAEB-T patients who had been misdiagnosed as having AML.[468] However, in this study, the diagnosis of RAEB-T was generally based on marrow blast count rather than on pace of disease. In a study of AML-type chemotherapy, patients with RAEB/RAEB-T had the same CR rates as those for AML patients with similar chromosome abnormalities.[469] In this analysis, patients had cytogenetics generally associated with de novo AML, and pace of disease was not considered.

Lower CR rates in high-risk MDS and secondary AML patients have also been linked to increased expression of the product of the multidrug resistance gene, P-glycoprotein (PGP).[470] In one analysis, PGP expression was found in 25 of 60 (42%) of high-risk MDS patients and in 7 of 10 patients with secondary AML.[471] Higher expression of PGP was associated with a lower CR rate (69% versus 14%) after intensive anthracycline/ara-C chemotherapy. Numerous compounds, including verapamil, amiodarone, phenothiazines, quinine, cyclosporin A, and the cyclosporin A analogue PSC-833, have been tested for their ability to reverse the MDR phenotype. The French Cooperative Leukemia Group updated the results of a phase III randomized study that showed that quinine significantly increased the CR rate and survival in PGP-positive MDS patients as compared with chemotherapy alone.[472]

Interest has developed in the activity of the topoisomerase I inhibitor, topotecan. As a single agent, topotecan can achieve complete remissions in 27% and 37% of untreated patients with RAEB/RAEB-T and CMML, respectively.[473] These response rates are similar to rates achieved with standard doses of ara-C, but topotecan may be superior to ara-C in its ability to induce higher CR rates in poor-risk cytogenetic groups. Nonhematologic toxicity, including mucositis, diarrhea, and infection, and an induction death rate of 20% have been observed. Topotecan has been evaluated in combination with other agents. Topotecan plus intermediate-dose ara-C produced an overall CR rate of 56% (61% for 59 MDS patients and 44% for 27 CMML patients).[474] Most notably, a CR rate of 70% was obtained in patients with poor-risk cytogenetics and secondary MDS. The median overall CR duration was 34 weeks. The median survival was 60 weeks for MDS patients and 44 weeks for CMML patients.

Decitabine

The hypomethylating agent decitabine (5-aza-2'-deoxycytidine) was evaluated in a phase II study of 66 high-risk MDS patients at a dose of 45 mg/m²/day for 3 days every 6 weeks.[475] Patients were classified by the IPSS as intermediate 1 (16), intermediate-2 (25), and high-risk (25). Myelosuppression was common, suggesting a cytotoxic effect, and 5 patients (7%) died during treatment, primarily because of infection. The overall response rate was 49%, with a 64% response rate in patients with a high-risk IPSS score. The actuarial median response duration was 31 weeks, and the median survival from the start of therapy was 15 months (14 months for the high-risk IPSS patients). In several patients, normalization of clonal cytogenetic abnormalities (often high-risk) was seen. A phase III study will aim to establish whether these responses translate into prolonged overall survival for high-risk patients.

Bone Marrow Transplantation

Allogeneic BMT

Allogeneic BMT is the only available potentially curative treatment for MDS. Patient age, performance status, and donor availability restrict the number of candidates who are eligible for the procedure. This treatment results in a long-term disease-free survival rate of approximately 40%.[476-479] The Fred Hutchinson Cancer Research Center has updated the largest experience of allogeneic bone marrow transplantation for MDS, comprising 251 patients between 1981 and 1996.[480] Fifty-seven percent of patients had advanced MDS (RAEB/RAEB-T/CMML), 43% had less advanced disease (RA/RARS), and 14% had therapy-related MDS. Cytogenetic IPSS categories consisted of good- (44%), intermediate- (21%), and poor- (31%) risk groups. Preparative regimens consisted primarily of cyclophosphamide plus either total body irradiation or busulfan. The 3-year actuarial disease-free survival (DFS), relapse, and nonrelapse mortality (NRM) rates were 41%, 17%, and 42%, respectively (median follow-up, 3.7 years). The European Bone Marrow Transplantation (EMBT) Group reported respective 5-year DFS and OS rates of 34% and 41% for 131 MDS patients undergoing HLA-matched sibling BMT without prior induction chemotherapy.[481] At 5 years, the actuarial probability of relapse was 39%, and the cumulative probability of transplant-related mortality was 44%. For older MDS patients (ages 55 to 66 years) undergoing allogeneic BMT, the Fred Hutchinson Cancer Research Center reported the following 3-year disease-free survival estimates: RA (53%), RAEB (46%), and RAEB-T/AML or CMML (33%).[482] Survival was highest among all FAB subgroups when levels of the conditioning agent busulfan were targeted to 600 to 900 ng/mL.

The results of allogeneic BMT for secondary MDS/ leukemia have been less favorable and may be partly explained by prior cumulative chemotherapy and radiation contributing to higher rates of treatment-related toxicity. The Fred Hutchinson Cancer Research Center reported the results of BMT for 99 consecutive patients with secondary MDS and leukemia.[483] At 6.4 years, the probability of overall survival was 13% (33% for RA/ RARS, 20% for RAEB, and 8% for RAEB-T/AML). The major barrier to long-term survival was relapse (overall 47%) and nonrelapse mortality (overall 78%), owing primarily to infections and organ failure. In a French study of 70 patients undergoing allogeneic BMT for secondary MDS/ AML, the estimated 2-year overall survival, event-free survival, relapse, and TRM rates were 30%, 28%, 42%, and 49%, respectively.[484] Poor outcomes were associated with

age older than 37 years, male gender, positive cytomegalovirus serology, absence of CR at BMT, and intensive conditioning schedules.

Prognostic Factors

In the EBMT study, multivariate analysis showed that younger age, shorter disease duration, and absence of excess blasts were associated with improved outcome. Patients with RA/RARS, RAEB, RAEB-T, and secondary AML had a 5-year DFS rate of 52%, 34% 19%, and 26%, respectively.[481] In a Vancouver study, cytogenetics were highly predictive of outcome.[485] The event-free survival rates for IPSS good-, intermediate-, and poor-risk cytogenetic subgroups were 51%, 40%, and 6%, respectively. In the Hutchinson Cancer Research Center multivariate analysis,[480] younger age, less advanced disease, and favorable cytogenetics were the three factors that predicted improved DFS rate. An increased risk of relapse was seen in patients with more rather than less advanced disease (27% versus 4% at 5 years) and poor-risk cytogenetics. The rate of relapse in less advanced MDS patients was extremely low, even with concomitant poor-risk cytogenetics. Multivariate analysis found that the adverse impact of poor-risk cytogenetics was restricted to advanced MDS patients.

When Hutchinson Cancer Research Center transplant patients were stratified according to their IPSS risk scores,[486] no significant differences in NRM were observed. However, variables such as older age, increased disease duration, mismatched donors, male gender, and therapy-related MDS significantly enhanced the likelihood of NRM. Significant differences in relapse rates were observed between IPSS risk groups, with a minimal number of relapses observed in the low- and intermediate-risk 1 patients. The IPSS risk group also influenced DFS rate. The 5-year DFS rate was 60% for the low-risk and intermediate-1 patients, 36% for intermediate-2 patients, and 28% for high-risk patients. By comparison, the median survival of nontransplanted primary MDS patients originally characterized by the IPSS scoring system was 5.7 years (low-risk), 3.5 years (intermediate-1) 1.2 years (intermediate-2), and 0.4 years (high-risk).[43] The DFS rate in the intermediate- and high-risk transplanted patients appears superior to that of nontransplanted patients. Because IPSS reflects prognosis at the time of diagnosis and not at the time of transplantation, these comparisons may not be entirely valid. Still, these findings have led to the conclusion that BMT should be considered early in the course of eligible intermediate and high-risk patients. BMT is generally not performed as a first-line treatment for low-risk patients whose relatively long median survival may be significantly compromised by the high treatment-related mortality rate, a factor that must be carefully weighed in higher-risk patients.

Other prognostic factors that have been studied include the use of various preparative regimens such as busulfan and cyclophosphamide, or cyclophosphamide and TBI. In the setting of BMT for MDS, these regimens have resulted in similar outcomes.[478, 487] Several retrospective studies have provided conflicting results regarding the value of prior cytoreductive chemotherapy in improving BMT outcomes.[484, 488-491] Prospective studies will prove useful in determining which variables impact the success of pretransplant cytoreductive therapy for MDS.

Matched Unrelated Donor

The expanding pool of HLA-typed volunteers has allowed an increasing number of matched unrelated donor (MUD) transplantations to be performed in patients with MDS. The Hutchinson Cancer Research Center reported the results of MUD transplants in 52 patients (median age 33) with MDS or MDS-related AML.[492] The 2-year DFS, relapse, and NRM rates were 38%, 28%, and 48%, respectively. Relapse rates were significantly higher in patients with RAEB-T or MDS-related AML. The EBMT Group reviewed data on 118 patients undergoing MUD transplants.[493] The actuarial 2-year probability of survival was 28%, DFS rate 28%, relapse risk 35%, and transplant-related mortality 58%. Patients with less advanced disease had a lower probability of relapse. Evidence for a graft-versus-leukemia effect was found, as patients with grade II to IV acute GVHD had a lower relapse rate, compared with patients with no acute GVHD or grade I only (26% versus 42%).

Autologous

For MDS patients not eligible for allogeneic transplantation, autologous transplantation following intensive chemotherapy may be an alternative. Chemotherapy can achieve cytogenetic remissions in patients with clonal karyotypic abnormalities.[494] In high-risk MDS or secondary/therapy-related AML patients, polyclonality of peripheral blood stem cells mobilized after chemotherapy has been demonstrated by cytogenetic analysis or PCR of X-chromosome inactivation patterns.[495, 496] Sufficient numbers of peripheral blood stem cells for rapid and stable engraftment was feasible. The EORTC, EBMT, Swiss Group for Clinical Cancer Research (SAKK), and Italian Adult Hematological Malignancy (GIMEMA) leukemia groups prospectively assessed the efficacy of intensive remission and consolidation chemotherapy, followed by autologous or allogeneic BMT, in poor-risk MDS/t-AML.[497] All patients with a donor were candidates for allogeneic BMT. An interim analysis showed that the majority of patients without a donor who achieved a CR could be treated with autologous stem cell transplantation (SCT) after intensive chemotherapy. The hematopoietic recovery after autologous BMT was slow, but the treatment-related mortality rate (14%) was much lower compared with that of allogeneic BMT (38%). The EBMT reported the results of 79 patients with MDS/secondary AML who underwent autologous BMT in first CR.[498] The 2-year survival, DFS, and relapse rates were 39%, 34%, and 64%, respectively. Patients younger than 40 years had a significantly better DFS rate than that in patients older than 40 years (39% versus 25%). The 2-year DFS rate was 28% for patients with MDS/secondary AML compared with 51% for a matched control group of patients with de novo AML. The lower DFS rate for MDS/t-AML patients compared with de novo AML patients was the result of a higher relapse rate. Another study by French investigators prospectively evaluated autologous BMT and peripheral blood SCT in MDS patients who achieved a CR.[499] Engraftment tended to be faster in the autologous SCT group. DFS and OS were 29 and 33 months, respectively. Longer follow-up is required to determine whether autologous BMT/SCT will result in longer DFS than that obtained with chemotherapy alone.

FUTURE DIRECTIONS

Publication of the FAB classification system in 1982 provided much-needed structure to the clinicopathologic assessment of MDS.[14] Although MDS patients share the common thread of chronic cytopenias and the potential to transform to AML, the heterogeneity of the disease often leads to different outcomes even within the same FAB morphologic subtypes. Additional rigor has been provided by the IPSS, which has become widely adopted as a useful prognostic scheme for evaluating survival and leukemic risk. The IPSS also helps stratify patients for clinical studies and to analyze the results of treatments. The NCCN guidelines use the patient's IPSS risk category, age, and performance status to direct evidence-based approaches to the treatment of MDS.[317]

Although further morphologic advances (e.g. degree of dysplasia, fibrosis, cellularity) should provide additive information for characterizing MDS in addition to the new proposals, such approaches will need to build upon well established forms of MDS categorization unless clear data indicate otherwise. Regarding biologic advances, as new understanding of critical molecular, immunologic, and cytogenetic features of MDS emerge, these parameters will need to be added to currently accepted methods as means to improve the characterization of MDS.

Oftentimes, the goal of low-intensity treatments, such as those outlined in the NCCN algorithm (see Fig. 24-9), is to improve blood counts and to palliate disease symptoms.[317] In these cases, hematologic responses may occur without any expected benefit in overall or progression-free survival. On the other hand, high-intensity treatments such as intensive chemotherapy or transplantation are administered with the dual objective of achieving hematologic responses and altering the natural history of the disease. Inconsistent response criteria have sometimes been used to define these responses, making the interpretation of results between published clinical trials in MDS difficult. Recently, a group of international investigators in MDS convened to establish standardized response criteria for studies involving MDS patients.[500] Proposals have been prepared for four levels of response criteria: (1) hematologic response, (2) alteration of the natural history of disease, (3) cytogenetic response, and (4) quality of life (QOL). The use of QOL measures may provide valuable insights into patients' physical, functional, emotional, social, and spiritual domains.[390, 501, 502] Uniform response criteria will help clarify the efficacy of new treatments for MDS and permit better comparisons between trials.

Novel therapies being evaluated in clinical trials of MDS include the soluble TNF-α receptor:Fc fusion protein

(TNFR:Fc) Etanercept, anti-angiogeneic drugs such as thalidomide and inhibitors of VEGF, the anti-CD33 monoclonal antibody gemtuzumab ozogamicin (Mylotarg) and arsenic trioxide. The selective tyrosine kinase inhibitor STI 571 directed against the fusion gene BCR-ABL of classical CML has shown encouraging therapeutic activity.[503] Cells expressing the activated PDGFR-β tyrosine kinase were also sensitive to this compound, suggesting that it may be useful for a subset of CMML patients with the t(5;12) translocation which results in the PDGFR-β/TEL fusion protein.[504] Given the high frequency of Ras signaling pathway abnormalities in proliferative-type hematologic disorders, drugs which inhibit Ras activity may be particularly effective in CMML and MDS/MPD.[97] Farnesyltransferase inhibitors are capable of blocking oncogenic Ras function and neoplastic cell growth in vitro and in preclinical studies.[505, 506] Clinical trials have recently begun utilizing such agents in phase I/II studies of solid tumors and hematologic malignancies.[507-509] Studies are also commencing to establish whether thrombopoietic agents, such as recombinant thrombopoietin and IL-ll (especially better-tolerated low-dose regimens) can improve the thrombocytopenia in MDS patients. The efficacy and toxicity of non-myeloablative transplantation is under investigation in MDS and other hematologic malignancies, particularly in patients who are unsuitable candidates for standard allogeneic transplantation.[510]

REFERENCES

1. Block M, Jacobsen LO, Bethard WF: Preleukemic acute human leukemia. JAMA 1953;152:1018.
2. Bjorkman SE: Chronic refractory anemia with sideroblastic bone marrow. A study of four cases. Blood 1956;11:250.
3. Dacie JV, Smith MD, White JC, et al: Refractory normoblastic anemia: A clinical and haematological study of 7 cases. Br J Haematol 1959;5:56.
4. Rheingold JJ, Kaufman R, Adelson E, et al: Smoldering acute leukemia. N Engl J Med 1963;268:812.
5. Dameshek W: The DiGuglielmo syndrome revisited. Blood 1969;34:567.
6. Saarni MI, Linman JW: Preleukemia: The hematologic syndrome preceding acute leukemia. Am J Med 1973;55:38.
7. Sexauer J, Kass L, Schnitzer B: Subacute myelomonocytic leukemia: Clinical, morphologic, and ultrastructural studies of 10 cases. Am J Med 1974;57:853.
8. Miescher PA, Farquet JJ: Chronic myelomonocytic leukemia. Semin Hematol 1974;11:129.
9. Beard MEJ, Bateman CJT, Crowther DC, et al: Hypoplastic acute myelogenous leukemia. Br J Haematol 1975;31:167.
10. Dreyfus B: Preleukemic states. I. Definition and classification. II. Refractory anemia with excess myeloblasts in the bone marrow (smoldering acute leukemia). Blood Cells 1976;2:33.
11. Linman JW, Bagby GC Jr: The preleukemic syndrome (hematopoietic dysplasia). Cancer 1978;42:852.
12. Cohen JR, Creger WP, Greenberg PL, et al: Subacute myeloid leukemia: A critical review. Am J Med 1979;66:959.
13. Streuli RA, Testa JR, Vardiman JW, et al: Dysmyelopoietic syndrome: Sequential, clinical, and cytogenetic studies. Blood 1980;55:636.
14. Bennett JM, Catovsky D, Daniel MT, et al: Proposals for the classification of the myelodysplastic syndrome. Br J Haematol 1982;51:189.
15. Doll DC, List AF: Myelodysplastic syndromes: Introduction. Semin Oncol 1992;19:1.
16. Aksoy M, Dincol K, Erdem S, et al: Acute leukemia due to chronic exposure to benzene. Am J Med 1972;52:160.
17. Travis LB, Li CY, Zhang ZN, et al: Hematopoietic malignancies and related disorders among benzene-exposed workers in China. Leuk Lymphoma 1994;14:91.
18. Yin SN, Hayes RB, Linet MS, et al: An expanded cohort study of cancer among benzene-exposed workers in China. Environ Health Persp 1996;104:1339.
19. Harris NL, Jaffe ES, Diebold J, et al: World Health Organization classification of neoplastic diseases of the hematopoietic and lymphoid tissues: Report of the clinical advisory committee meeting—Arlie House, Virginia, November 1997. J Clin Oncol 1999;17:3835.
19a. Greenberg P, Anderson J, De Witte T, et al: Problematic WHO reclassification of myelodysplastic syndromes. J Clin Oncol 2000;18:3447.
19b. Bennett JM: WHO classification of the acute leukemias and myelodysplastic syndrome. Int J Hematol 2000;72:131.
19c. Brunning R, Bennett J, Flandrin G, et al: Myelodysplastic syndromes. In Jaffe E, Harris N, Stein H, et al (eds): WHO Classification of Tumors: Pathology and Genetics of Hematopoietic and Lymphoid Tissues. IARC Press, Lyon, 2001.
19d. Vardiman J, Pierre R, Bain B, et al: Chronic myelomonocytic leukemia. In Jaffe E, Harris N, Stein H, et al (eds): WHO Classification of Tumors: Pathology and Genetics of Hematopoietic and Lymphoid Tissues. IARC Press, Lyon, 2001.
19e. Greenberg P, Anderson J, Estey E, et aal: Classifying chronic myelomonocytic leukemia. J Clin Oncol 2001;19:3791.
20. Germing U, Gatterman N, Aivado M, et al: Two types of acquired sideroblastic anemia (AISA): A time-tested distinction. Br J Haematol 2000;108:724.
21. Rosati S, Mick R, Xu F, et al: Refractory cytopenia with multilineage dysplasia: Further characterization of an "unclassifiable" myelodysplastic syndrome. Leukemia 1996;10:20.
22. Aul C, Gattermann N, Schneider W: Epidemiological and etiological aspects of myelodysplastic syndromes. Leuk Lymphoma 1995;16:247.
23. Aul C, Bowen DT, Yoshida Y: Pathogenesis, etiology, and epidemiology of myelodysplastic syndromes. Haematologica 1998;83:71.
24. Aul C, Gattermann N, Schneider W: Age-related incidence and other epidemiological aspects of myelodysplastic syndromes. Br J Haematol 1992;82:358.
25. Radlund A, Thiede T, Hansen S, et al: Incidence of myelodysplastic syndromes in a Swedish population. Eur J Haematol 1995;54:153.
26. Williamson PJ, Kruger AR, Reynolds PJ, et al: Establishing the incidence of myelodysplastic syndrome. Br J Haematol 1994;87:743.
27. Horrigan SK, Westbrook CA, Kim AH, et al: Polymerase chain reaction-based diagnosis of del (5q) in acute myeloid leukemia and myelodysplastic syndrome identifies a minimal deletion interval. Blood 1996;88:2665.
28. Liang H, Fairman J, Claxton DF, et al: Molecular anatomy of chromosome 7q deletions in myeloid neoplasms: Evidence for multiple critical loci. Proc Natl Acad Sci U S A 1998;95:3781.
29. Busque L, Zhu J, DeHart D, et al: An expression based clonality assay at the human androgen receptor locus (HUMARA) on chromosome X. Nucleic Acids Res 1994;22:697.
30. Gale RE: Evaluation of clonality in myeloid stem-cell disorders. Semin Hematol 1999;36:361.
31. Gilliland DG, Blanchard KL, Levy J, et al: Clonality in myeloproliferative disorders: analysis by means of the polymerase chain reaction. Proc Natl Acad Sci U S A 1991;88;6848.
32. Grier HE, Weinstein HJ, Revesz T, et al: Cytogenetic evidence for involvement of erythroid progenitors in a child with therapy linked myelodysplasia. Br J Haematol 1986;64:513.
33. Abrahamson G, Boultwood J, Madden J, et al: Clonality of cell populations in refractory anaemia using combined approach of gene loss and X-linked restriction fragment-length polymorphism-methylation analysis. Br J Haematol 1991;79:550.
34. Kroef MJ, Fibbe WE, Mout R, et al: Myeloid but not lymphoid cells carry the 5q deletion: Polymerase chain reaction analysis of loss of heterozygosity using mini-repeat sequences on highly purified cell fractions. Blood 1993;81:1849.
35. Kere J, Rutu T, de la Chappelle A: Monosomy 7 in granulocytes and monocytes in myelodysplastic syndrome. N Engl J Med 1987;316:499.
36. Gerritsen WR, Donohue J, Bauman J, et al: Clonal analysis of myelodysplastic syndrome: Monosomy 7 is expressed in the my-

eloid lineage but not in the lymphoid lineage as detected by fluorescent in situ hybridization. Blood 1992;80:217.

37. Tsukamoto N, Morita K, Maehara T, et al: Clonality in MDS: Demonstration of pluripotent stem cell origin using X-linked restriction fragment length polymorphisms. Br J Haematol 1993;83;589.

38. Culligan DJ, Cachai P, Whittaker J, et al: Clonal lymphocytes are detectable in only some cases of MDS. Br J Haematol 1992;81:346.

39. Anastasi J, Feng J, LeBeau MM, et al: Cytogenetic clonality in myelodysplastic syndromes studied with fluorescence in-situ hybridization: Lineage, response to growth factor therapy and clonal expansion. Blood 1993;81:1580.

40. Van Kamp H, Fibbe WE, Jansen RP, et al: Clonal involvement of granulocytes and monocytes, but not of T and B lymphocytes and natural killer cells in patients with myelodysplasia: Analysis by X-linked restriction fragment length polymorphisms and polymerase chain reaction of the phosphoglycerate kinase gene. Blood 1992;80:1774.

41. Ito T, Ohashi H, Yoshitoyo K, et al: Recovery of polyclonal hematopoiesis in patients with myelodysplastic syndromes following successful chemotherapy. Leukemia 1994;8:839.

42. Schmetzer HM, Poleck B, Mittermuller J, et al: Clonality analysis as a tool to study the biology and response to therapy in myelodysplastic syndromes. Leukemia 1997;11:660.

43. Greenberg P, Cox C, Le Beau MM, et al: International Prognostic Scoring System for evaluating prognosis in myelodysplastic syndromes. Blood 1997;89:2079.

44. Tricot G, Boogaerts MA, De Wolf-Peeters C, et al: The myelodysplastic syndromes: Different evolution patterns based on sequential morphological and cytogenetic investigations. Br J Haematol 1985;58:759.

45. Pedersen-Bjergaard J, Philip P, Larsen SO, et al: Chromosome aberrations and prognostic factors in therapy-related myelodysplasia and acute non-lymphocytic leukemia. Blood 1990;76:1083.

46. Yunis JJ, Rydell RE, Oken MM, et al: Refined chromosome analysis as an independent prognostic factor in de novo myelodysplastic syndromes. Blood 1986;67:1721.

47. Horiike S, Taniwaki M, Misawa S, et al: Chromosome abnormalities and karyotypic evolution in 83 patients with myelodysplastic syndrome and predictive value for prognosis. Cancer 1988;62:1129.

48. Le Beau MM, Albain KS, Larson RA, et al: Clinical and cytogenetic correlations in 63 patients with therapy-related myelodysplastic syndromes and acute nonlymphocytic leukemia: Further evidence for characteristic abnormalities of chromosomes no. 5 and 7. J Clin Oncol 1986;4:325.

49. Fenaux P, Morel P, Lai JL: Cytogenetics of myelodysplastic syndromes. Semin Hematol 1996;33:127.

50. Ohyashiki K, Sasao I, Ohyashiki JH, et al: Cytogenetic and clinical findings of myelodysplastic syndromes with a poor prognosis. Cancer 1992;70:1994.

51. Nowell PC, Besa EC, Stelmach T, et al: Chromosome studies in preleukemic states. V. Prognostic significance of single versus multiple abnormalities. Cancer 1986;58:2571.

52. Morel P, Hebbar M, Lai J, et al: Cytogenetic analysis has strong prognostic value in de novo myelodysplastic syndromes and can be incorporated in a new scoring system: A report on 408 cases. Leukemia 1993;7:1315.

53. Jacobs RH, Cornbleet MA, Vardiman J, et al: Prognostic implications of morphology and karyotype in primary myelodysplastic syndromes. Blood 1986;67:1765.

54. Yunis JJ, Lobell M, Arnesen MA, et al: Refined chromosome study helps define prognostic subgroups in most patients with primary myelodysplastic syndrome and acute myelogenous leukaemia. Br J Haematol 1988;68:189.

55. Toyama K, Ohyashiki K, Yoshida Y, et al: Clinical implications of chromosomal abnormalities in 401 patients with MDS: A multicentric study in Japan. Leukemia 1993;7:499.

56. Pierre RV, Catovsky D, Mufti GJ, et al: Clinical-cytogenetic correlations in myelodysplasia (preleukemia). Cancer Genet Cytogenet 1989;40:149.

57. Mufti GJ: Chromosomal deletions in myelodysplastic syndrome. Leuk Res 1992;16:35.

58. Willman CL: Molecular genetic features of myelodysplastic syndromes. Leukemia 1998;12:2.

59. Mecucci C, La Starza R: Cytogenetics of myelodysplastic syndromes: FORUM trends in experimental and clinical medicine 1999;9:4.

60. Haase D, Fonatsch C, Freund M, et al: Cytogenetic findings in 179 patients with myelodysplastic syndromes. Ann Hematol 1995;70:171.

61. Golub TR, Barker GF, Lovett M, et al: Fusion of PDGF receptor beta to a novel ets-like gene, tel, in chronic myelomonocytic leukemia with t(5;12) chromosomal translocation. Cell 1994;77:307.

62. Tomasson MH, Wiliams IR, Hasserjian R, et al: TEL-PDGFbeta-R induces hematologic malignancies in mice that respond to a specific tyrosine kinase inhibitor. Blood 1999;93:1707.

63. Ritchie K, Aprikyan A, Bowen-Pope D, et al: The Tel-PDGFbeta fusion gene produces a chronic myeloproliferative syndrome in transgenic mice. Leukemia 1999;13:1790.

64. Wiktor A, Rybicki BA, Piao ZS, et al: Clinical significance of Y chromosome loss in hematologic disease. Genes Chromosomes Cancer 2000;27:11.

65. Campbell LJ, Garson OM: The prognostic significance of deletion of the long arm of chromosome 20 in myeloid disorders. Leukemia 1994;8:67.

66. Sokal G, Michaux JL, Van den Berghe H, et al: A new hematological syndrome with a distinct karyotype: The 5q− chromosome. Blood 1975;46:519.

67. Pedersen-Bjergaard J, Philip P: Balanced translocations involving chromosome bands 11q23 and 21q22 are highly characteristic of myelodysplasia and leukemia following therapy with cytostatic agents targeting at DNA-topoisomerase II. Blood 1991;78:1147.

68. Pedersen-Bjergaard J, Philip P: Cytogenetic characteristics of therapy-related acute non-lymphocytic leukemia, preleukemia, and acute myeloproliferative syndrome: Correlation with clinical data for 61 consecutive cases. Br J Haematol 1987;66:199.

69. Merlat A, Lai JL, Sterkers Y, et al: Therapy-related myelodysplastic syndrome and acute myeloid leukemia with 17p deletion: A report on 25 cases. Leukemia 1999;13:250.

70. Lessard M, Herry A, Berthou C, et al: FISH investigation of 5q and 7q deletions in MDS/AML reveals hidden translocations, insertions and fragmentations of the same chromosomes. Leuk Res 1998;22:303.

71. Tanaka K, Arif M, Eguchi M, et al: Interphase fluorescence in situ hybridization overcomes pitfalls of G-banding analysis with special reference to underestimation of chromosomal aberration rates. Cancer Genet Cytogenet 1999;115:32.

72. Kakazu N, Taniwaki M, Horiike S, et al: Combined spectral karyotyping and DAPI banding analysis of chromosome abnormalities in myelodysplastic syndrome. Genes Chromosomes Cancer 1999;26:336.

73. Walker NI, Harmon BV, Gobe GC, et al: Patterns of cell death. Methods Achiev Exp Pathol 1988;13:18.

74. Rajapaksa R, Ginzton N, Rott L, et al: Altered oncoprotein expression and apoptosis in myelodysplastic syndrome. Blood 1996;88:4275.

75. Parker JE, Fishlock KL, Mijovic A, et al: Low-risk myelodysplastic syndrome is associated with excessive apoptosis and an increased ratio of pro- versus antiapoptotic bcl-2-related proteins. Br J Haematol 1998;103:1075.

76. Kornblau SM: The role of apoptosis in the pathogenesis, prognosis, and therapy of hematologic malignancies. Leukemia 1998;12:41.

77. Ohmori M, Ohmori S, Ueda Y, et al: Ineffective hematopoiesis in the myelodysplastic syndromes (MDS) as studied by daily in situ observation of colony-cluster formation. Int J Cell Cloning 1991;9:521.

78. Lepelley P, Campergue L, Gradel N, et al: Is apoptosis a massive process in myelodysplastic syndromes? Br J Haematol 1996;95:368.

79. Clark DM, Lampert IA: Apoptosis is a common histopathological finding in myelodysplasia: The correlate of ineffective hematopoiesis. Leuk Lymphoma 1990;2:415.

80. Ricciardi MR, Petrucci MT, Ariola C, et al: High levels of apoptosis characterize RAEB and are lost during leukemic transformation. Blood 1997;90:520.

81. Raza A, Gezer S, Mundle S, et al: Apoptosis in bone marrow biopsy samples involving stromal and hematopoietic cells in 50 patients with myelodysplastic syndromes. Blood 1995;86:268.

82. Reza S, Dar S, Andric T, et al: Biologic characteristics of 164 patients with myelodysplastic syndromes. Leuk Lymphoma 1999;33:281.

83. Alexandrakis M, Coulocheri S, Xylouri I, et al: Elevated serum TNF-alpha concentrations are predictive of shortened survival in patients with high-risk myelodysplastic syndromes. Haematologica 1998;29:13.

84. Shetty V, Mundle S, Alvi S, et al: Measurement of apoptosis, proliferation and three cytokines in 46 patients with myelodysplastic syndromes. Leuk Res 1996;20:891.

85. Kitagawa M, Saito I, Kuwata T, et al: Overexpression of tumor necrosis factor (TNF)-alpha and interferon (IFN)-gamma by bone marrow cells from patients with myelodysplastic syndromes. Leukemia 1997;11:2049.

86. Raza A, Mundle S, Shetty V, et al: Novel insights into the biology of myelodysplastic syndromes: Excessive apoptosis and the role of cytokines. Int J Hematol 1996;63:265.

87. Gersuk GM, Beckham C, Loken MR, et al: A role for tumour necrosis factor-alpha, Fas, and Fas-ligand in marrow failure associated with myelodysplastic syndrome. Br J Haematol 1998;103:176.

88. Peetre C, Gullberg U, Nilsson E, et al: Effects of recombinant tumor necrosis factor on proliferation and differentiation of leukemic and normal hemopoietic cells in vitro: Relationship to cell surface receptor. J Clin Invest 1986;78:1694.

89. Murase T, Hotta T, Saito H, et al: Effect of recombinant tumor necrosis factor on the colony growth of human leukemia progenitor cells and normal hematopoietic progenitor cells. Blood 1987;69:467.

90. Peddie CM, Wolf CR, McLellan LI, et al: Oxidative DNA damage in CD34+ myelodysplastic cells is associated with intracellular redox changes and elevated plasma tumour necrosis factor-alpha concentration. Br J Haematol 1997;99:625.

91. Maciejewski J, Selleri C, Anderson S, et al: Fas antigen expression on CD34+ human marrow cells is induced by interferon gamma and tumor necrosis factor alpha and potentiates cytokine-mediated hematopoietic suppression in vitro. Blood 1995;85:3183.

92. Stasi R, Brunetti M, Bussa S, et al: Serum levels of tumour necrosis factor-alpha predict response to recombinant human erythropoietin in patients with myelodysplastic syndrome. Clin Lab Haematol 1997;19:197.

93. Hellstrom-Lindberg E, Kanter-Lowensohn L, Ost A, et al: Morphological changes and apoptosis in bone marrow from MDS patients treated with G-CSF and erythropoietin. Leuk Res 1997;21:415.

94. Gupta P, Niehans GA, LeRoy SC, et al: Fas ligand expression in the bone marrow in myelodysplastic syndromes correlates with FAB subtype and anemia, and predicts survival. Leukemia 1999;13:44.

95. Ali A, Mundle SD, Ragasa D, et al: Sequential activation of caspase-1 and caspase-3–like proteases during apoptosis in myelodysplastic syndromes. J Hematother Stem Cell Res 1999;8:343.

96. Barbacid M: ras genes. Ann Rev Biochem 1987;56:779.

97. Beaupre DM, Kurzrock R: Ras and leukemia: From basic mechanisms to gene-directed therapy. J Clin Oncol 1999;17:1071.

98. Parker J, Mufti GJ: ras and myelodysplasia: Lessons from the last decade. Semin Hematol 1996;33:206.

99. Paquette RL, Landaw EM, Pierre RV, et al: N-ras mutations are associated with poor prognosis and increased risk of leukemia in myelodysplastic syndrome. Blood 1993;82:590.

100. Neubauer A, Greenberg P, Negrin R, et al: Mutations in the ras proto-oncogenes in patients with myelodysplasia. Leukemia 1994;8:638.

101. Padua RA, Guinn BA, Al-Sabah AI, et al: RAS, FMS, and p53 mutations and poor clinical outcome in myelodysplasias: A 10-year follow-up. Leukemia 1998;12:887.

102. Bartram CR: Molecular genetic aspects of myelodysplastic syndromes. Hematol Oncol Clin North Am 1992;6:557.

103. Ridge SA, Worwood M, Oscier D, et al: FMS mutations in myelodysplastic, leukemic, and normal subjects. Proc Natl Acad Sci U S A 1990;87:1377.

104. Tobal K, Pagliuca A, Bhatt B, et al: Mutation of the human FMS gene (M-CSF receptor) in myelodysplastic syndromes and acute myeloid leukemia. Leukemia 1990;4:486.

105. Jacobs A: Genetic lesions in preleukaemia. Leukemia 1991;5:277.

106. Kikukawa M, Aoki N, Sakamoto Y, et al: Study of p53 in elderly patients with myelodysplastic syndromes by immunohistochemistry and DNA analysis. Am J Pathol 1999;155:717.

107. Kaneko H, Misawa S, Horiike S, et al: Tp53 mutations emerge at early phase of myelodysplastic syndrome and are associated with complex chromosomal abnormalities. Blood 1995;85:2189.

108. Sugimoto K, Hirano N, Toyoshima H, et al: Mutations of the p53 gene in myelodysplastic syndrome (MDS) and MDS-derived leukemia. Blood 1993;81:3022.

109. Adamson DJ, Dawson AA, Bennett B, et al: p53 mutation in the myelodysplastic syndromes. Br J Haematol 1995;89;61.

110. Mori N, Hidai H, Yokota J, et al: Mutations of the p53 gene in myelodysplastic syndrome and overt leukemia. Leuk Res 1995;19;869.

111. Tang JL, Tien HF, Lin MT, et al: P53 mutation in advanced stage of primary myelodysplastic syndrome. Anticancer Res 1998;18:3757.

112. Wattel E, Preudhomme C, Hecquet B, et al: p53 mutations are associated with resistance to chemotherapy and short survival in hematologic malignancies. Blood 1994;84:3148.

113. Horiike S, Misawa S, Kaneko H, et al: Distinct genetic involvement of the Tp53 gene in therapy-related leukemia and myelodysplasia with chromosomal losses of nos. 5 and/or 7 and its possible relationship to replication error phenotype. Leukemia 1999;13:1235.

114. Ben-Yehuda D, Krichevsky S, Caspi O, et al: Microsatellite instability and p53 mutations in therapy-related leukemia suggest mutator phenotype. Blood 1996;88:4296.

115. Lai JL, Preudhomme C, Zandecki M, et al: Myelodysplastic syndromes and acute myeloid leukemia with 17p deletion: An entity characterized by specific dysgranulopoiesis and a high incidence of p53 mutations. Leukemia 1995;9:370.

116. Folkman J: Angiogenesis in cancer, vascular, rheumatoid, and other diseases. Nature Med 1995;1:27.

117. Perez-Atayde AR, Sallan SE, Tedrow U, et al: Spectrum of tumor angiogenesis in the bone marrow of children with acute lymphoblastic leukemia. Am J Pathol 1997;150:815.

118. Fiedler W, Graeven U, Ergun S, et al: Vascular endothelial growth factor, a possible paracrine factor in human acute myeloid leukemia. Blood 1997;89:1870.

119. Hussong JW, Rodgers GM, Shami PJ: Evidence of increased angiogenesis in patients with acute myeloid leukemia. Blood 2000;95:309.

120. Aguayo A, Estey E, Kantarjian H, et al: Cellular vascular endothelial growth factor is a predictor of outcome in patients with acute myeloid leukemia. Blood 1999;94:3717.

121. Bellamy WT, Richter L, Sirjani D, et al: Vascular endothelial cell growth factor is an autocrine promoter of abnormal localized immature myeloid precursors and leukemia progenitor formation in myelodysplastic syndromes (MDS). Blood 2001;97:1427.

122. Pruneri G, Bertolini F, Soligo D, et al: Angiogenesis in myelodysplastic syndromes. Br J Cancer 1999;81:1398.

123. Greenberg PL: Biologic and clinical implications of marrow culture studies in the myelodysplastic syndromes. Semin Hematol 1996;33:163.

124. Greenberg PL, Mara B: The preleukemic syndrome: Correlation of in vitro parameters of granulopoiesis with clinical features. Am J Med 1979;66:951.

125. Chiu DH, Clark BJ: Abnormal erythroid progenitor cells in human preleukemia. Blood 1982;60:362.

126. Juvonen E, Partanen S, Knuutila S, et al: Megakaryocyte colony formation by bone marrow progenitors in myelodysplastic syndromes. Br J Haematol 1985;64:331.

127. Nagler A, Ginzton N, Bangs C, et al: In vitro differentiative and proliferative effects of human recombinant colony-stimulating factors on marrow hemopoiesis in myelodysplastic syndromes. Leukemia 1990;4:193.

128. Schipperus MR, Sonneveld P, Lindemans J, et al: The combined effects of IL-3, GM-CSF, and G-CSF on the in vitro growth of myelodysplastic myeloid progenitor cells. Leuk Res 1990;14:1019.

129. Greenberg PL, Mackichan ML, Negrin R: Production of granulocyte colony-stimulating factor by normal and myelodysplastic syndrome peripheral blood cells. Blood 1990;76:146.

130. Nagler A, Binet C, Mackichan ML, et al: Impact of marrow cytogenetics and morphology on in vitro hemopoiesis in the myelodysplastic syndromes: Comparison between recombinant human granulocyte colony-stimulating factor and granulocyte-monocyte colony-stimulating factor. Blood 1990;76:1299.

131. Merchav S, Nielsen OJ, Rosenbaum H, et al: In vitro studies of erythropoietin-dependent regulation of erythropoiesis in myelodysplastic syndromes. Leukemia 1990;4:771.

132. Greenberg PL, Negrin RS, Ginzton N: G-CSF synergizes with eryth-

ropoietin for enhancing erythroid colony-formation in myelodysplastic syndromes. Blood 1991;78:38.

133. Sawada K, Sato N, Tarumi T, et al: Proliferation and differentiation of myelodysplastic CD34+ cells in serum-free medium: Response to individual colony-stimulating factors. Br J Haematol 1993;83: 349.

134. Budel LM, Dong F, Lowenberg B, et al: Hematopoietic growth factor receptors: Structure variations and alternatives of receptor complex formation in normal hematopoiesis and in hematopoietic disorders. Leukemia 1995;9:553.

135. Hoefsloot LH, van Amelsvoort MP, Broeders LC, et al: Erythropoietin-induced activation of STAT5 is impaired in the myelodysplastic syndrome. Blood 1997;89:1690.

136. May SJ, Smith SA, Jacobs A, et al: The myelodysplastic syndrome: Analysis of laboratory characteristics in relation to the FAB classification. Br J Haematol 1985;59:311.

137. Chalevelaski G, Karaoulis S, Yalouris AG, et al: Globin chain synthesis in myelodysplastic syndromes. J Clin Pathol 1991;44:134.

138. Annino L, Di Giovanni S, Tentori L Jr, et al: Acquired haemoglobin H disease in a case of refractory anaemia with excess of blasts (RAEB) evolving into acute nonlymphoid leukemia. Acta Haematol 1984;72:41.

139. Higgs DR, Wood WG, Barton C, et al: Clinical features and molecular analysis of acquired hemoglobin H disease. Am J Med 1983; 75:181.

140. Newman DR, Pierre RV, Linman JW: Studies on the diagnostic significance of haemoglobin F levels. Mayo Clin Proc 1973;48:199.

141. Salmon A: Blood group changes in preleukaemic states. Blood Cells 1976;2:211.

142. Hauptman GM, Sondag D, Lang JM, et al: False positive acidified serum lysis test in preleukaemic dyserythropoiesis. Acta Haematol 1978;59:73.

143. Dunn DE, Tanawattanacharuen P, Boccuni P, et al: Paroxysmal nocturnal hemoglobinuria cells in patients with bone marrow failure syndromes. Ann Intern Med 1999;131:401.

144. Lintula R: Red cell enzymes in myelodysplastic syndromes: A review. Scand J Haematol 1986;36:56.

145. Garcia S, Sanz MA, Amigo V, et al: Prognostic factors in chronic myelomonocytic syndromes. Am J Hematol 1988;27:163.

146. Mufti GJ, Stevens JR, Oscier DG, et al: Myelodysplastic syndromes: A scoring system with prognostic significance. Br J Haematol 1985;59:311.

147. Ruutu T: Granulocyte function in the myelodysplastic syndromes. Scan J Haematol 1986;36:66.

148. Boogaerts MA, Nelissen V, Roelant C, et al: Blood neutrophil function in myelodysplastic syndromes. Br J Haematol 1983;55: 217.

149. Martin S, Baldock SC, Ghoneim ATM, et al: Defective neutrophil function and microbicidal mechanisms in the myelodysplastic syndromes. J Clin Pathol 1983;36:1120.

150. Williamson PJ, Oscier DG, Mufti GJ, et al: Pyogenic abscesses in the myelodysplastic syndrome. Br J Haematol 1990;299:375.

151. Clark RE, Hoy TG, Jacobs A: Granulocyte and monocyte surface membrane markers in the myelodysplastic syndromes. J Clin Pathol 1985;38:301.

152. Tefferi A, Hoagland HC, Therneau TM, et al: Chronic myelomonocytic leukemia: Natural history and prognostic determinants. Mayo Clin Proc 1989;64:1246.

153. Mani S, Duffy TP: Pericardial tamponade in chronic myelomonocytic leukemia. Chest 1994;106:967.

154. Bourantas KL, Tsiara S, Panteli A, et al: Pleural effusion in chronic myelomonocytic leukemia. Acta Haematol 1998;99:34.

155. Fenaux P, Beuscart R, Lai JL, et al: Prognostic factors in adult chronic myelomonocytic leukemia: An analysis of 107 cases. J Clin Oncol 1988;6:1417.

156. Worsley A, Oscier DG, Stevens J, et al: Prognostic features of chronic myelomonocytic leukaemia: A modified Bournemouth score gives the best prediction of survival. Br J Haematol 1988; 68:17.

157. Solal-Celigny P, Desaint B, Herrara A, et al: Chronic myelomonocytic leukemia according to FAB classification: Analysis of 35 cases. Blood 1984;63:634.

158. Oscier D: Myelodysplastic syndromes. Ballieres Clin Haematol 1987;1:389.

159. Rasi V, Lintula R: Platelet function in the myelodysplastic syndrome. Scand J Haematol 1986;36:71.

160. Hamblin TJ: Immunological abnormalities in myelodysplastic syndromes. Semin Hematol 1996;33:150.

161. Bynoe AG, Scott CS, Ford P, et al: Decreased T-helper cells in the myelodysplastic syndrome. Br J Haematol 1983;54:97.

162. Carpani G, Rosti A, Vozzo N. T-lymphocyte subpopulations in myelodysplastic syndromes. Acta Haematol 1989;81:173.

163. Williamson PJ, Oscier DG, Bell AJ, et al: Red cell aplasia in myelodysplastic syndrome. J Clin Pathol 1991;44:431.

164. Clark RE, Payne HE, Jacobs A, et al: Primary myelodysplastic syndrome and cancer. Br Med J 1987;294:937.

165. Castro M, Conn D, Su W, et al: Rheumatic manifestations in myelodysplastic syndromes. J Rheumatol 1991;18:721.

166. Doutre MS, Beylot C, Beylot J, et al: Refractory anemia with an excess of blasts and cutaneous vasculitis. Ann Dermatol Venereol 1997;114:97.

167. Green AR, Shuttleworth D, Bowen DT, et al: Cutaneous vasculitis in patients with myelodysplasia. Br J Haematol 1990;74:364.

168. Marti JM, Cervantes F, Ribera JM, et al: Polyarthritis cutaneous vasculitis and migrant thrombophlebitis of possible immune origin associated with chronic myelomonocytic leukemia. Sangre 1987; 32:502.

169. Van den Berghe H, Cassiman JJ, David G, et al: Distinct haematological disorder with deletion of the long arm of no. 5 chromosome. Nature 1974;251:437.

170. Horrigan SK, Arbieva ZH, Xie HY, et al: Delineation of a minimal interval and identification of 9 candidates for a tumor suppressor gene in malignant myeloid disorders on 5q31. Blood 2000;95: 2372.

171. Sokal G, Michaux JL, Van den Berghe H, et al: A new hematological syndrome with a distinct karyotype: The 5q− chromosome. Blood 1975;46:519.

172. Van den Berghe H, Vermaelen K, Mecucci C, et al: The 5q− anomaly. Cancer Genet Cytogenet 1985;17:189.

173. Mathews P, Tefferi A, Dewald GW, et al: The 5q− syndrome: A single institution study of 43 consecutive patients. Blood 1993; 81:1040.

174. Lewis S, Oscier D, Boultwood J, et al: Hematological features of patients with myelodysplastic syndromes associated with a chromosome 5q deletion. Am J Hematol 1995;49:194.

175. Larripa I, Acevedo S, Paulau NM, et al: Leukemic transformation in patients with 5q− and additional abnormalities. Haematologica 1991;76:363.

176. Kantarjian H, Keating M, Walters R, et al: Therapy-related leukemia and myelodysplastic syndrome: Clinical, cytogenetic and prognostic features. J Clin Oncol 1986;4:1734.

177. Manoharan A, Horsley R, Pitney WR: The reticulin content of bone marrow in acute leukemia. Br J Haematol 1979;43:185.

178. Ohyashiki K, Sasao I, Ohyashiki JH, et al: Clinical and cytogenetic characteristics of myelodysplastic syndromes developing myelofibrosis. Cancer 1991;68:178.

179. Pagliuca A, Layton DM, Manoharan A, et al: Myelofibrosis in primary myelodysplastic syndromes: A clinico-morphological study of 10 cases. Br J Haematol 1989;71:499.

180. Ríos A, Canizo MC, Sanz MA, et al: Bone marrow biopsy in myelodysplastic syndromes: Morphological characteristics and contribution to the study of prognostic factors. Br J Haematol 1990;75:26.

181. Maschek H, Georgii A, Kaloutsi V, et al: Myelofibrosis in primary myelodysplastic syndromes: A retrospective study of 352 patients. Eur J Haematol 1992;48:208.

182. Michels SD, McKenna RW, Arthur DC, et al: Therapy-related acute myeloid leukemia and myelodysplastic syndrome: A clinical and morphologic study of 65 cases. Blood 1985;65:1364.

183. Kampmeier P, Anastasi J, Vardiman JW: Issues in the pathology of the myelodysplastic syndromes. Hematol Oncol Clin North Am 1992;6:501.

184. Lambertenghi-Deliliers G, Orazi A, Luksch R, et al: Myelodysplastic syndrome with increased marrow fibrosis: A distinct clinico-pathological entity. Br J Haematol 1991;78:161.

185. Zittoun J, Giraudier S, Jouault H, et al: Spontaneous growth of CFU-GM in myelodysplastic syndromes (MDS): Should chronic myelomonocytic leukemia (CMML) be reclassified? Blood 1999; 94:107.

186. Flores-Figueroa E, Gutierrez-Espindola G, Guerrero-Rivera S, et al: Hematopoietic progenitor cells from patients with myelodysplastic

syndromes: In vitro colony growth and long-term proliferation. Leuk Res 1999;23:385.

187. Del Canizo MC, Brufau A, Mota A, et al: The value of cell cultures for the diagnosis of mixed myelodysplastic/myeloproliferative disorders. Haematologica 1998;83:3.

188. Geissler K, Hinterberger W, Bettelheim P, et al: Colony growth characteristics in chronic myelomonocytic leukemia. Leuk Res 1988;12:373.

189. Bennett JM, Catovsky D, Daniel MT, et al: The chronic myeloid leukaemias: Guidelines for distinguishing chronic granulocytic, atypical chronic myeloid, and chronic myelomonocytic leukemia: Proposals by the French-American-British Cooperative Leukaemia Group. Br J Haematol 1994;87:746.

190. Parker RI: Hematologic aspects of mastocytosis: Management of hematologic disorders in association with systemic mast cell disease. J Invest Dermatol 1991;96:52S.

191. Smith JD, Lazarchick J: Systemic mast cell disease with marrow and splenic involvement associated with chronic myelomonocytic leukemia. Leuk Lymphoma 1998;32:391.

192. Petit A, Pulik M, Gaulier A, et al: Systemic mastocytosis associated with chronic myelomonocytic leukemia: Clinical features and response to interferon alfa therapy. J Am Acad Dermatol 1995; 32:850.

193. Ribera JM, Cervantes F, Rozman C: A multivariate analysis of prognostic factors in chronic myelomonocytic leukemia according to the FAB criteria. Br J Haematol 1987;65:307.

194. Kerkhofs H, Hermanns J, Haak HL, et al: Utility of the FAB classification for myelodysplastic syndrome: Investigation of prognostic factors in 237 cases. Br J Haematol 1987;65:73.

195. Onida F, Smith T, Shang-Ying L, et al: Prognostic factors in chronic myelomonocytic leukemia: A retrospective single institution analysis of 228 patients. Blood 1999;94:308.

196. Catalano L, Improta S, de Laurentiis M, et al: Prognosis of chronic myelomonocytic leukemia. Haematologica 1996;81:324.

197. Groupe Francais de Cytogenetique Hematologique: Chronic myelomonocytic leukemia: Single entity or heterogeneous disorder? A prospective multicenter study of 100 patients. Cancer Genet Cytogenet 1991;55:57.

198. Storniolo AM, Moloney WC, Rosenthal DS, et al: Chronic myelomonocytic leukemia. Leukemia 1990;4:766.

199. Del Canizo MC, Sanz G, San Miguel JF, et al: Chronic myelomonocytic leukemia—clinicobiological characteristics: A multivariate analysis in a series of 70 cases. Eur J Haematol 1989;42:466.

200. Stark AN, Thorogood J, Head C, et al: Prognostic factors and survival in chronic myelomonocytic leukaemia (CMML). Br J Cancer 1987;56:59.

201. Germing U, Gattermann N, Minning H, et al: Problems in the classification of CMML—dysplastic versus proliferative type. Leuk Res 1998;22:871.

202. Worsley A, Oscier D, Stevens J, et al: Prognostic features of chronic myelomonocytic leukemia. 1988;68:17.

203. Bain BJ: The relationship between the myelodysplastic syndromes and the myeloproliferative disorders. Leuk Lymphoma 1999;34:443.

204. Beris P: Primary clonal myelodysplastic syndrome. Semin Hematol 1989;26:216.

205. Neuwirtová R, Mociková K, Musilová J, et al: Mixed myelodysplastic and myeloproliferative syndromes. Leuk Res 1996;20:717.

206. Lukowicz DF, Myers TJ, Grasso JA, et al: Sideroblastic anaemia terminating in myelofibrosis. Am J Hematol 1982;13:253.

207. Williams MD, Shinton NK, Finney RD: Primary acquired sideroblastic anaemia and myeloproliferative disease: A report of three cases. Clin Lab Haematol 1985;7:113.

208. Gupta R, Abdalla SH, Bain BJ: Thrombocytosis with sideroblastic erythropoiesis: a mixed myeloproliferative/myelodysplastic syndrome. Leuk Lymphoma 1999;34:615.

209. Verhoef G, Meeus P, Stul M, et al: Cytogenetic and molecular studies of the Philadelphia translocation in the myelodysplastic syndromes. Cancer Genet Cytogenet 1992;59:161.

210. Nand S, Godwin JE: Hypoplastic myelodysplastic syndrome. Cancer 1988;62:958.

211. Yoshida Y, Oguma S, Uchino H, et al: Refractory myelodysplastic anaemias with hypocellular bone marrow. J Clin Pathol 1988; 41:763.

212. Maschek H, Kaloutsi V, Rodriguez-Kaiser M, et al: Hypoplastic

213. Tuzuner N, Cox C, Rowe, JM, et al: Hypocellular myelodysplastic syndromes (MDS): New proposals. Br J Haematol 1995;91:612.

214. Toyama K, Ohyashiki K, Yoshida Y, et al: Clinical and cytogenetic findings of myelodysplastic syndromes showing hypocellular bone marrow or minimal dysplasia, in comparison with typical myelodysplastic syndromes. Int J Hematol 1993;58:33.

215. Kitagawa M, Kamiyama R, Tekemura T, et al: Bone marrow analysis of the myelodysplastic syndromes: Histological and immunohistological features related to evolution of overt leukemia. Virchows Arch 1989;57:47.

216. Rios A, Canizo MC, Sanz MA, et al: Bone marrow biopsy in myelodysplastic syndromes: Morphological characteristics and contribution to the study of prognostic factors. Br J Haematol 1990;75:26.

217. Fohlmeister I, Fischer R, Schaefer HE. Preleukemic myelodysplastic syndromes (MDS): Pathogenetical considerations based on retrospective clinicomorphological sequential studies. Anticancer Res 1985;5:179.

218. Riccardi A, Giordano M, Girino M, et al: Refractory cytopenias: Clinical course according to bone marrow cytology and cellularity. Blut 1997;54:153.

219. Orazi A, Albitar M, Heerema NA, et al: Hypoplastic myelodysplastic syndromes can be distinguished from acquired aplastic anemia by CD34 and PCNA immunostaining of bone marrow biopsy specimens. Am J Clin Pathol 1997;107:268.

220. De Planque MM, Kluin-Nelemans HC, Van Krieken HJM, et al: Evolution of acquired severe aplastic anaemia to myelodysplasia and subsequent leukemia in adults. Br J Haematol 1988;70:55.

221. Dezza L, Caaola M, Bergamaschi G, et al: Myelodysplastic syndrome with monosomy 7 in adulthood: A distinct preleukemic disorder. Hematologica 1983;68:723.

222. Tomonaga M, Tomonaga Y, Kusano M, et al: Sequential karyotype evolutions and bone marrow aplasia preceding acute myelomonocytic transformation from myelodysplastic syndrome. Br J Haematol 1984;58:53.

223. Goyal R, Qawi H, Ali I, et al: Biologic characteristics of patients with hypocellular myelodysplastic syndromes. Leuk Res 1999; 23:357.

224. Tooze JA, Marsh JCW, Gordon-Smith EC, et al: Clonal evolution of aplastic anemia to myelodysplasia, acute myeloid leukaemia and paroxysmal nocturnal haemoglobinuria. Leuk Lymphoma 1999; 33:231.

225. Tichelli A, Gratwohl A, Würsch A, et al: Late haematological complications in severe aplastic anaemia. Br J Haematol 1988; 69:413.

226. Tichelli A, Gratwohl A, Nissen C: Late clonal complications in severe aplastic anemia. Leuk Lymphoma 1994 12:167.

227. De Planque MM, Bacigalupo A, Wursch A, et al: Long-term follow-up of severe aplastic anaemia patients treated with anti-thymocyte globulin. Br J Haematol 1989;73:121.

228. Socié G, Henry-Amar M, Bacigalupo A, et al: Malignant tumors occurring after treatment of aplastic anemia: European Bone Marrow Transplantation—Severe Aplastic Anaemia Working Party. New Engl J Med 1993;329:1152.

229. Najean Y, Haguenauer O: Long-term (5 to 20 years) evolution of nongrafted aplastic anemias: The Cooperative Group for the Study of Aplastic and Refractory Anemias. Blood 1990;76:2222.

230. Devine DV, Gluck WL, Rosse WF, et al: Acute myeloblastic leukemia in paroxysmal nocturnal hemoglobinuria: Evidence of evolution from the abnormal paroxysmal nocturnal hemoglobinuria clone. J Clin Invest 1987;79:314.

231. Longo L, Bessler M, Beris P, et al: Myelodysplasia in a patient with pre-existing paroxysmal nocturnal haemoglobinuria: A clonal disease originating from within a clonal disease. Br J Haematol 1994;87:401.

232. Van Kamp H, Smit JW, Van Den Berg E, et al: Myelodysplasia following paroxysmal nocturnal haemoglobinuria: Evidence for the emergence of a separate clone. Br J Haematol 1994;87:399.

233. Jin J-Y, Tooze JA, Marsh JCW, et al: Myelodysplasia following aplastic anaemia/paroxysmal nocturnal haemoglobinuria syndrome after immunosuppression and G-CSF: Evidence for the emergence of a separate clone. Br J Haematol 1996;94:510.

234. Maciejewski JP, Sloand EM, Sato T, et al: Impaired hematopoiesis

in paroxysmal nocturnal hemoglobinuria/aplastic anemia is not associated with a selected proliferative defect in the glycosylphosphatidylinositol-anchored protein-deficient clone. Blood 1997;89: 1173.

235. Araten DJ, Nafa K, Pakdaasuwan K, et al: Clonal populations of hematopoietic cells with paroxysmal nocturnal hemoglobinuria genotype and phenotype are present in normal individuals. Proc Natl Acad Sci U S A 1999;96:5209.

236. Barrett J, Saunthararajah Y, Molldrem J: Myelodysplastic syndrome and aplastic anemia: Distinct entities or diseases linked by a common pathophysiology? Semin Hematol 2000;37:15.

237. Leone G, Mele L, Alessandro P, et al: The incidence of secondary leukemias. Haematologica 1999;84:937.

238. Park DJ, Koeffler HP: Therapy-related myelodysplastic syndromes. Semin Hematol 1996;33:256.

239. Henry-Amar M, Dietrich PY: Acute leukemia after the treatment of Hodgkin's disease. Hematol Oncol Clin North Am 1993;7:369.

240. Blayney DW, Longo DL, Young RC, et al: Decreasing risk of leukemia with prolonged follow-up after chemotherapy and radiotherapy for Hodgkin's disease. N Engl J Med 1987;316:710.

241. Andrieu JM, Ifrah N, Payen C, et al: Increased risk of secondary acute nonlymphocytic leukemia after extended-field radiation therapy combined with MOPP chemotherapy for Hodgkin's disease. J Clin Oncol 1990;8:1148.

242. Lavey RS, Eby NL, Prosnitz LR: Impact on second malignancy risk of combined use of radiation and chemotherapy for lymphoma. Cancer 1990;66:80.

243. Van Leeuwen FE, Klokmann WJ, Hagenbeek A, et al: Second cancer risk following Hodgkin's disease: A twenty-year follow-up study. J Clin Oncol 1994;12:312.

244. Schellong G, Riepenhausen M, Creutzig U, et al: Low risk of secondary leukemias after chemotherapy without mechlorethamine in childhood Hodgkin's disease. J Clin Oncol 1997;15:2247.

245. Brusamolino E, Anselmo AP, Klersy C, et al: The risk of acute leukemia in patients treated for Hodgkin's disease is significantly higher after combined modality programs than after chemotherapy alone and is correlated with the extent of radiotherapy and type and duration of chemotherapy: A case control study. Haematologica 1998;83:812.

246. Loefler O, Brosteanu D, Hasenclever M, et al: Meta-analysis of chemotherapy versus combined modality treatment trials in Hodgkin's disease. J Clin Oncol 1998;16:818.

247. Diehl V, Franklin J, Hasenclever D, et al: BEACOPP, a new dose-escalated and accelerated regimen, is at least as effective as COPP/ABVD in patients with advanced-stage Hodgkin's lymphoma: Interim report from a trial of the German Hodgkin's lymphoma study group. J Clin Oncol 1998;16:3810.

248. Valagussa P, Santoro A, Fossati-Bellentani F, et al: Second acute leukemia and other malignancies following treatment for Hodgkin's disease. J Clin Oncol 1986;4:830.

249. Cimino G, Papa G, Tura S, et al: Primary cancer following Hodgkin's disease: Updated results of an Italian multicentric study. J Clin Oncol 1991;9:432.

250. Greene MH, Harris EL, Gershenson DM, et al: Melphalan may be a more potent leukemogen than cyclophosphamide. Ann Intern Med 1986;105:360.

251. Ingram L, Mott MG, Mann JR, et al: Second malignancies in children treated for non-Hodgkin's lymphoma and T-cell leukaemia with the UKCCSG regimens. Br J Cancer 1987;55:463.

252. Pedersen-Bjergaard J, Ersboll J, Sorensen HM, et al: Risk of acute nonlymphocytic leukemia and pre-leukemia in patients treated with cyclophosphamide for non-Hodgkin's lymphoma: Comparison with results obtained in patients treated for Hodgkin's disease and ovarian carcinoma with other alkylating agents. Ann Intern Med 1985;103:195.

253. Pui CH: Therapy-related myeloid leukaemia. Lancet 1990;336: 1130.

254. Kyle R: Second malignancies associated with chemotherapeutic agents. Prog Clin Biol Res 1983;132:45.

255. Cuzick J, Erskine S, Edelman D, et al: A comparison of the incidence of the myelodysplastic syndrome and acute myeloid leukaemia following melphalan and cyclophosphamide treatment for myelomatosis. Br J Cancer 1987;55:523.

256. Fisher B, Rockette H, Fisher ER, et al: Leukemia in breast cancer patients following adjuvant chemotherapy or postoperative radiation: The NSABP experience. J Clin Oncol 1985;3:1640.

257. Curtis RE, Boice JD Jr, Stovall M, et al: Risk of leukemia after chemotherapy and radiation treatment for breast cancer. N Engl J Med 1992;326:1745.

258. Tallman MS, Gray R, Bennett JM, et al: Leukemogenic potential of adjuvant chemotherapy for early-stage breast cancer: The Eastern Cooperative Oncology Group experience. J Clin Oncol 1995; 13:1557.

259. Diamandidou E, Buzdar AU, Smith TL, et al: Treatment-related leukemia in breast cancer patients treated with fluorouracil-doxorubicin-cyclophosphamide combination adjuvant chemotherapy: The University of Texas M.D. Anderson Cancer Center experience. J Clin Oncol 1996;14:2722.

260. Travis LB, Holowaty EJ, Bergfeldt K, et al: Risk of leukemia after platinum-based chemotherapy for ovarian cancer. New Engl J Med 1999;340:351.

261. Pedersen-Bjergaard J, Daugaard G, Hansen SW, et al: Increased risk of myelodysplasia and leukaemia after etoposide, cisplatin, and bleomycin for germ-cell tumors. Lancet 1991;338:359.

262. Kollmannsberger C, Beyer J, Droz JP, et al: Secondary leukemia following high cumulative doses of etoposide in patients treated for advanced germ cell tumors. J Clin Oncol 1998;16:3386.

263. Travis LB, Curtis RE, Storm H, et al: Risk of second malignant neoplasms among long-term survivors of testicular cancer. J Natl Cancer Inst 1997;89:1429.

264. Darrington DL, Vose JM, Anderson JR, et al: Incidence and characterization of secondary myelodysplastic syndrome and acute myelogenous leukemia following high-dose chemotherapy and autologous stem-cell transplantation for lymphoid malignancies. J Clin Oncol 1994;12:2527.

265. Traweek ST, Slovak ML, Nademanee AP, et al: Clonal karyotype hematopoietic cell abnormalities occurring after autologous bone marrow transplantation for Hodgkin's disease and non-Hodgkin's lymphoma. Blood 1994;84:957.

266. Stone MR, Neuberg D, Soiffer R, et al: Myelodysplastic syndrome as a late complication following autologous bone marrow transplantation for non-Hodgkin's lymphoma. J Clin Oncol 1994;12: 2535.

267. Miller JS, Arthur DC, Litz CE, et al: Myelodysplastic syndrome after autologous bone marrow transplantation: An additional late complication of curative cancer therapy. Blood 1994;12:3780.

268. Taylor PR, Jackson GH, Lennard AL, et al: Low incidence of myelodysplastic syndrome following transplantation using autologous non-cryopreserved bone marrow. Leukemia 1997;11:1650.

269. Pedersen-Bjergaard J, Pedersen J, Myhre C, et al: High risk of therapy-related leukemia after BEAM chemotherapy and autologous stem cell transplantation for previously treated lymphoma is mainly related to primary chemotherapy and not to the BEAM-transplantation procedure. Leukemia 1997;11:1654.

270. Andre M, Henry-Amar M, Bidier B, et al: Treatment-related deaths and second cancer risk after autologous stem-cell transplantation for Hodgkin's disease. Blood 1998;92:1933.

271. Milligan DW, Ruiz de Elvira MC, Kolb HJ: Secondary leukaemia and myelodysplasia after autografting for lymphoma: Results from the EBMT. Br J Haematol 1999;106:1020.

272. Micallef INM, Lillington DM, Apostolidis J, et al: Therapy-related myelodysplasia and secondary acute myelogenous leukemia after high-dose therapy with autologous hematopoietic progenitor-cell support for lymphoid malignancies. J Clin Oncol 2000;18:947.

273. Del Cañizo C, Amigo L, Hernandez J, et al: Incidence and characterization of secondary myelodysplastic syndromes following autologous transplantation. Haematologica 2000;85:403.

274. Ketterer N, Salles G, Dumontet C, et al: Fludarabine may increase the toxicity of peripheral blood progenitor cell transplantation. Br J Haematol 1998;102:204.

275. Govindarajan R, Jagannath S, Flick JT, et al: Preceding standard therapy is the likely cause of MDS after autologous transplants for myeloma. Br J Haematol 1996;95:349.

276. Laughlin MJ, McGaughey DS, Crews JR, et al: Secondary myelodysplasia and acute leukemia in breast cancer patients after autologous bone marrow transplant. J Clin Oncol 1998;16:1008.

277. Abruzzese E, Radford JE, Miller JS, et al: Detection of abnormal pretransplant clones in progenitor cells of patients who developed myelodysplasia after autologous transplantation. Blood 1999;94: 1814.

278. Krishnan A, Bhatia S, Slovak ML, et al: Predictors of therapy-

related leukemia and myelodysplasia following autologous transplantation for lymphoma: An assessment of risk factors. Blood 2000;95:1588.

279. Hasle H, Kerndrup G, Jacobsen BB: Childhood myelodysplastic syndrome in Denmark: Incidence and predisposing conditions. Leukemia 1995;9:1569.

280. Hasle H, Wadsworth LD, Massing BG, et al: A population-based study of childhood myelodysplastic syndrome in British Columbia, Canada. Br J Haematol 1999;106:1027.

281. Haas OA, Gadner H: Pathogenesis, biology, and management of myelodysplastic syndromes in children. Semin Hematol 1996;33: 225.

282. Hasle H: Myelodysplastic syndromes in childhood classification, epidemiology, and treatment. Leuk Lymphoma 1994;13:11.

283. Luna-Fineman S, Shannon KM, Lange BJ: Childhood monosomy 7: Epidemiology, biology, and mechanistic implications. Blood 1995; 85:1985.

284. Arico M, Biondi A, Pui C-H: Juvenile myelomonocytic leukemia. Blood 1997;90:479.

285. Castleberry RP, Freedman MH, Baruchel A, et al: Juvenile chronic myelogenous leukemia revisited: A report of the first meeting of the international juvenile myelomonocytic working group. Birmingham, AL, December 1994.

286. Hasle H, Arico M, Basso G, et al: Myelodysplastic syndrome, juvenile myelomonocytic leukemia, and acute myeloid leukemia associated with complete or partial monosomy 7. Leukemia 1999; 13:376.

287. Novitzky N: Myelodysplastic syndromes in children: A critical review of the clinical manifestations and management. Am J Hematol 2000;63:212.

288. Emanuel PD, Shannon KM, Castleberry RP: Juvenile myelomonocytic leukemia: Molecular understanding and prospects for therapy. Mol Med Today 1996;2:468.

289. Emanuel PD: Myelodysplasia and myeloproliferative disorders in childhood: An update. Br J Haematol 1999;105:852.

290. Luna-Fineman S, Shannon KM, Atwater SK, et al: Myelodysplastic and myeloproliferative disorders of childhood: A study of 167 patients. Blood 1999;93:459.

291. Hasle H, Kerndrup G, Yssing M, et al: Intensive chemotherapy in childhood myelodysplastic syndrome: A comparison with results in acute myeloid leukemia. Leukemia 1996;10:1269.

292. Lange BJ, Kobrinsky N, Barnard DR, et al: Distinctive demography, biology, and outcome of acute myeloid leukemia and myelodysplastic syndrome in children with Down syndrome: Children's Cancer Group studies 2861 and 2891. Blood 1998;91:608.

293. Locatelli F, Zecca M, Niemeyer C, et al: Role of allogeneic bone marrow transplantation for the treatment of myelodysplastic syndromes in childhood. Bone Marrow Transplant 1996;18:63.

294. Kerkhofs H, Hermans J, Haak HL, et al: Utility of the FAB classification for myelodysplastic syndromes: Investigation of prognostic factors in 237 cases. Br J Haematol 1987;65:73.

295. Tricot G, Vlietinck R, Boogaerts MA, et al: Prognostic factors in the myelodysplastic syndromes: Importance of initial data on peripheral blood counts, bone marrow cytology, trephine biopsy and chromosomal analysis. Br J Haematol 1985;60:19.

296. Vallespi T, Torrabadella M, Julia A, et al: Myelodysplastic syndromes: A study of 101 cases according to the FAB classification. Br J Haematol 1985;61:83.

297. Sanz GF, Sanz MA, Vallespi T, et al: Two regression models and a scoring system for predicting survival and planning treatment in myelodysplastic syndromes: A multivariate analysis of prognostic factors in 370 patients. Blood 1989;74:395.

298. Coiffier B, Adelaine P, Viala JJ, et al: Dysmyelopoietic syndromes: A search for prognostic factors in 193 patients. Cancer 1983;52:83.

299. Sanz GF, Sanz MA: Prognostic factors in myelodysplastic syndromes. Leuk Res 1992;16:77.

300. Goasguen JE, Garand R, Bizet M, et al: Prognostic factors of myelodysplastic syndromes: A simplified 3-D scoring system. Leuk Res 1990;14:255.

301. Aul C, Gattermann N, Heyll A, et al: Primary myelodysplastic syndromes: Analysis of prognostic factors in 235 patients and proposals for an improved scoring system. Leukemia 1992;6:52.

302. Wimazal F, Sperr WR, Kundi M, et al: The prognostic value of LDH in myelodysplastic syndromes. Blood 1999;94:288.

303. Solé F, Espinet B, Sanz GF, et al: Incidence, characterization, and prognostic significance of chromosomal abnormalities in 640 patients with primary myelodysplastic syndromes. Br J Haematol 2000;108:346.

304. Berthier R, Douady F, Metral J, et al: In vitro granulopoiesis in oligoblastic leukemia: Prognostic value, characterization, and serial cloning of bone marrow colony and cluster forming cells in agar culture. Biomedicine 1979;30:305.

305. Greenberg PL, Bax I, Mara B, et al: The myeloproliferative disorders: Correlation between clinical evolution and alteration of granulopoiesis. Am J Med 1976;61:878.

306. Faille A, Dresch C, Poirer O, et al: Prognostic value of in vitro bone marrow culture in refractory anaemia with excess of myeloblasts. Scand J Haematol 1978;20:280.

307. Milner GR, Testa NG, Geary CG, et al: Bone marrow studies in refractory cytopenia and smoldering leukaemia. Br J Haematol 1977;35:251.

308. Spitzer G, Verma D, Dicke K, et al: Subgroups of oligoleukemia as identified by in vitro agar culture. Leuk Res 1979;3:29.

309. Verma DS, Spitzer G, Dicke KA, et al: In vitro agar culture patterns in preleukemia and their clinical significance. Leuk Res 1979;3:41.

310. Gattermann N, Aul C, Schneider W, et al: Two types of acquired idiopathic sideroblastic anemia (AISA). Br J Haematol 1990; 74:45.

311. Varela BL, Chuang C, Woll JE, et al: Modifications in the classification of primary myelodysplastic syndromes: The addition of a scoring system. Hematol Oncol 1985;3:55.

312. Rosati S, Mick R, Xu F, et al: Refractory cytopenia with multilineage dysplasia: Further classification of an "unclassifiable" myelodysplastic syndrome. Leukemia 1996;10:20.

313. Matsuda A, Jinna I, Yagasaki F, et al: Refractory anemia with severe dysplasia: Clinical significance of morphological features in refractory anemia. Leukemia 1998;12:482.

314. Sanz GF, Sanz MA, Vallespi T: Two types of acquired idiopathic sideroblastic anaemia. Br J Haematol 1990;75:633.

315. Tricot G, DeWolf-Peeter C, Vlietinck R, et al: Bone marrow histology in myelodysplastic syndromes: Prognostic values of abnormal localization of immature precursors in MDS. Br J Haematol 1984; 58:217.

316. Quesnel B, Guillerm G, Vereecque R, et al: Methylation of *p15 (INK4b)* gene in myelodysplastic syndromes is frequent and acquired during disease progression. Blood 1998;91:2985.

317. Greenberg PL, Bishop M, Deeg J, et al: NCCN practice guidelines for myelodysplastic syndromes. Oncology 1998;12:53.

318. Oster W, Krumwieh D, Brune T, et al: Evaluation of erythropoietin (EPO) in the treatment of patients with myelodysplastic syndromes (MDS): Preclinical data supporting a rationale for sequential therapy with granulocyte-macrophage colony-stimulating factor (GM-CSF) and EPO. J Cancer Clin Oncol 1990;116:280.

319. Kurzrock R, Talpaz M, Estey E, et al: Erythropoietin treatment in patients with myelodysplastic syndrome and anemia. Leukemia 1991;5:985.

320. Adamson JW, Schuster M, Allen S, et al: Effectiveness of recombinant human erythropoietin therapy in myelodysplastic syndromes. Acta Haematol 1992;87:20.

321. Shepherd JD, Currie CJ, Sparling TG, et al: Erythropoietin therapy of myelodysplastic syndromes. Blood 1992;79:1891.

322. Ganser A, Hoelzer D: Treatment of myelodysplastic syndromes with hematopoietic growth factors. Hematol Oncol Clin North Am 1992;6:607.

323. Yoshida Y, Anzai N, Kawabata H, et al: Serial changes in endogenous erythropoietin levels in patients with myelodysplastic syndromes and aplastic anemia undergoing erythropoietin treatment. Ann Hematol 1993;66:175.

324. Aloe Spiriti MA, Petti MC, Latagliata R, et al: Is recombinant human erythropoietin treatment in myelodysplastic syndromes worthwhile? Leuk Lymphoma 1993;9:79.

325. Mohr B, Herrmann R, Huhn D: Recombinant human erythropoietin in patients with myelodysplastic syndromes and myelofibrosis. Acta Haematol 1993;90:65.

326. Ghio R, Balleari E, Ballestrero A, et al: Subcutaneous recombinant human erythropoietin for the treatment of anemia in myelodysplastic syndromes. Acta Haematol 1993;90:58.

327. Stone RM, Bernstein SH, Demetri G, et al: Treatment with recombinant human erythropoietin in patients with myelodysplastic syndromes. Leuk Res 1994;18:769.

328. Rose EH, Abels RI, Nelson RA, et al: The use of r-HuEPO in the treatment of anaemia related to myelodysplasia (MDS). Br J Haematol 1995;89:831.

329. DiRaimondo F, Longo G, Cacciola E Jr, et al: A good response rate to recombinant erythropoietin alone may be expected in selected myelodysplastic patients: A preliminary clinical study. Eur J Haematol 1996;56:7.

330. Stasi R, Brunetti M, Bussa S, et al: Response to recombinant human erythropoietin in patients with myelodysplastic syndromes. Clin Cancer Res 1997;3:733.

331. Italian Cooperative Study Group for rHuEpo in Myelodysplastic Syndromes: A randomized double-blind placebo-controlled study with subcutaneous recombinant human erythropoietin in patients with low-risk myelodysplastic syndromes. Br J Haematol 1998; 103:1070.

332. Hellström-Lindberg E: Efficacy of erythropoietin in the myelodysplastic syndromes: A meta-analysis of 205 patients from 17 studies. Br J Haematol 1995;89:67.

333. Merchav S, Nielsen OJ, Rosenbaum H, et al: In vitro studies of erythropoietin-dependent regulation of erythropoiesis in myelodysplastic syndromes. Leukemia 1990;4:771.

334. Negrin RS, Haeuber DH, Nagler A, et al: Treatment of myelodysplastic syndromes with recombinant human granulocyte colony-stimulating factor. Ann Intern Med 1989;110:976.

335. Negrin RS, Haeuber DH, Nagler A, et al: Maintenance treatment of patients with myelodysplastic syndromes using recombinant human granulocyte colony-stimulating factor. Blood 1990;76:36.

336. Greenberg P, Taylor K, Larson R, et al: Phase III randomized multicenter trial of recombinant human G-CSF in MDS. Blood 1993;82:196.

337. Vadhan-Raj S, Keating M, LeMaistre A, et al: Effects of recombinant human granulocyte-macrophage colony-stimulating factor in patients with myelodysplastic syndromes. N Engl J Med 1987;317:1545.

338. Antin JH, Weinberg DS, Rosenthal DS: Variable effect of recombinant human granulocyte-macrophage colony-stimulating factor on bone marrow fibrosis in patients with myelodysplasia. Exp Hematol 1990;18:266.

339. Ganser A, Volkers B, Greher J, et al: Recombinant human-granulocyte-macrophage colony-stimulating factor in patients with myelodysplastic syndromes: A phase I/II trial. Blood 1989;73:31.

340. Hermann F, Lindemann A, Klein H, et al: Effect of recombinant human granulocyte-macrophage colony-stimulating factor in patients with myelodysplastic syndrome with excess blasts. Leukemia 1989;3:335.

341. Hoelzer D, Ganser A, Greher J, et al: Phase I/II study with GM-CSF in patients with myelodysplastic syndromes. Behring Inst Mitt 1988;83:134.

342. Thompson JA, Douglas JL, Kidd P, et al: Subcutaneous granulocyte macrophage colony-stimulating factor in patients with myelodysplastic syndrome: Toxicity, pharmacokinetics, and hematological effects. J Clin Oncol 1989;7:629.

343. Dunbar CE, Smith D, Kimball J, et al: Sequential treatment with recombinant human growth factors to compare activity of GM-CSF and IL3 in the treatment of primary myelodysplasia. Blood 1990;76:141.

344. Estey EH, Kurzrock R, Talpaz M, et al: Effects of low doses of recombinant human granulocyte-macrophage colony-stimulating factor (GM-CSF) in patients with myelodysplastic syndromes. Br J Haematol 1991;77:291.

345. Rosenfeld CS, Sulecki M, Evans C, et al: Comparison of intravenous versus subcutaneous recombinant human granulocyte-macrophage colony-stimulating factor in patients with primary myelodysplasia. Exp Hematol 1991;19:273.

346. Gradishar WJ, LeBeau MM, O'Laughlin R, et al: Clinical and cytogenetic responses to granulocyte-macrophage colony-stimulating factor in therapy-related myelodysplasia. Blood 1992;80:2463.

347. Takahashi M, Yoshida Y, Kaku K, et al: Phase II study of recombinant granulocyte-macrophage colony-stimulating factor in myelodysplastic syndrome and aplastic anemia. Acta Haematol 1993;89:189.

348. Rose C, Wattel E, Bastion Y, et al: Treatment with very low-dose GM-CSF in myelodysplastic syndromes with neutropenia: A report on 28 cases. Leukemia 1994;8:1458.

349. Willemze R, Van Der Lely N, Zwierzina H, et al: A randomized

350. Schuster MW, Thompson JA, Larson R, et al: Randomized phase II study of recombinant granulocyte macrophage–colony stimulating factor (rGM-CSF) in patients with neutropenia secondary to myelodysplastic syndrome (MDS). Blood 1995;86:338.

351. Yoshida Y, Nakahata T, Shibata A, et al: Effects of long-term treatment with recombinant human granulocyte-macrophage colony-stimulating factor in patients with myelodysplastic syndrome. Leuk Lymphoma 1995;18;457.

352. Greenberg PL, Negrin RS, Ginzton N: In vitro–in vivo correlations of erythroid responses to G-CSF plus erythropoietin in myelodysplastic syndromes. Exp Hematol 1992;20:733.

353. Negrin RS, Stein R, Doherty K, et al: Treatment of the anemias of MDS using recombinant human granulocyte colony-stimulating factor in combination with erythropoietin. Blood 1993;82:737.

354. Hellström-Lindberg E, Ahlgren T, Beguin Y, et al: A combination of G-CSF plus erythropoietin for the anemia of patients with myelodysplastic syndromes. Leuk Lymphoma 1993;11:221.

355. Negrin RS, Stein R, Doherty K, et al: Maintenance treatment of the anemia of myelodysplastic syndromes with recombinant human granulocyte colony-stimulating factor and erythropoietin: Evidence for in vivo synergy. Blood 1996;87:4076.

356. Hellström-Lindberg E, Negrin R, Stein R, et al: Erythroid response to treatment with G-CSF plus erythropoietin for the anaemia of patients with myelodysplastic syndromes: Proposal for a predictive model. Br J Haematol 1997;99:344.

357. Hellström-Lindberg E, Ahlgren T, Beguin Y, et al: Treatment of anemia in myelodysplastic syndromes with granulocyte colony-stimulating factor plus erythropoietin: Results from a randomized phase II study and long-term follow-up of 71 patients. Blood 1998; 92:68.

358. Runde V, Aul C, Ebert A, et al: Sequential administration of recombinant human granulocyte-macrophage colony-stimulating factor and human erythropoietin for treatment of myelodysplastic syndromes. Eur J Haematol 1995;54:39.

359. Hansen PB, Johnsen HE, Hippe E, et al: Recombinant human granulocyte-macrophage colony-stimulting factor plus recombinant human erythropoietin may improve anemia in selected patients with myelodysplastic syndromes. Am J Hematol 1993;44:229.

360. Bernell P, Stenke L, Wallvik J, et al: A sequential erythropoietin and GM-CSF schedule offers clinical benefits in the treatment of anemia in myelodysplastic syndromes. Leuk Res 1996;20:693.

361. Stasi R, Pagano A, Terzoli E, et al: Recombinant human granulocyte-macrophage colony-stimulating factor plus erythropoietin for the treatment of cytopenias in patients with myelodysplastic syndromes. Br J Haematol 1999;105:141.

362. Thompson J, Gilliland G, Prchal J, et al: The use of GM-CSF + r-HuEPO for the treatment of cytopenias associated with myelodysplastic syndromes. Blood 1995;86:337.

363. Economopoulos T, Mellou S, Papageorgiou E, et al: Treatment of anemia in low-risk myelodysplastic syndromes with granulocyte-macrophage colony-stimulating factor plus recombinant human erythropoietin. Leukemia 1999;13:1009.

364. Ganser A, Seipelt G, Lindemann A, et al: Effects of recombinant human interleukin-3 in patients with myelodysplastic syndromes. Blood 1990;76:455.

365. Kurzrock R, Talpaz M, Estrov Z, et al: Phase I study of recombinant human interleukin-3 in patients with bone marrow failure. J Clin Oncol 1991;9:1241.

366. Nimer SD, Paquette RL, Ireland P, et al: A phase I/II study of interleukin-3 in patients with aplastic anemia and myelodysplasia. Exp Hematol 1994;22:875.

367. Ganser A, Ottmann OG, Seipelt G, et al: Effect of long-term treatment with recombinant human interleukin-3 in patients with myelodysplastic syndromes. Leukemia 1993;7:696.

368. Miller AM, Noyes WE, Taetle R, et al: Limited erythropoietic response to combined treatment with recombinant human interleukin-3 and erythropoietin in myelodysplastic syndrome. Leuk Res 1999;23:77.

369. Gordon MS, Nemunaitis J, Hoffman R, et al: A phase I trial of recombinant human interleukin-6 in patients with myelodysplastic syndromes and thrombocytopenia. Blood 1995;85:3066.

370. Calabro-Jones PM, Aguilera JA, Ward JF, et al: Uptake of WR-2721 derivatives by cells in culture: Identification of the transported form of the drug. Cancer Res 1988;48:3634.

371. List AF, Heaton R, Glinsmann-Gibson B, et al: Amifostine stimulates the formation of multipotent and erythroid hematopoietic progenitors. Leukemia 1998;12:1596.

372. Klimecki W, Heaton R, Glinsmann-Gibson B, et al: Amifostine suppresses apoptosis in myelodysplastic CD34+ cells and promotes progenitor growth via polyamine-like effects. Blood 1997; 80:520.

373. List AF, Holmes H, Greenberg PL, et al: Phase II study of amifostine in patients with myelodysplastic syndromes (MDS). Blood 1999; 94:305.

374. Grossi A, Fabbri A, Santini V, et al: Amifostine in the treatment of low-risk myelodysplastic syndromes. Haematologica 2000;85:367.

375. Perrine SP, Ginder GD, Faller GV, et al: A short-term trial of butyrate to stimulate fetal-globin-gene expression in the beta-globin disorders. N Engl J Med 1993;328:81.

376. McCaffrey PG, Newsome DA, Fibach E, et al: Induction of gamma-globin by histone-deacetylase inhibitors. Blood 1997;90:2075.

377. Gore SD, Samid D, Weng LJ: Impact of the putative differentiating agents sodium phenylbutyrate and sodium phenylacetate on proliferation, differentiation, and apoptosis of primary neoplastic myeloid cells. Clin Cancer Res 1997;3:1755.

378. Gore SD, Samid D, Weng LJ: Clinical development of sodium phenylbutyrate as a putative differentiating agent in myeloid malignancies. Anticancer Res 1997;17:3938.

379. Gore SD, Weng LJ, Griffin CA, et al: Impact of prolonged administration of the putative differentiating agent sodium phenylbutyrate (PB) on hematopoiesis in myelodysplastic syndrome (MDS) and acute myeloid leukemia (AML). Blood 1998;92:633.

380. Reuben RC, Wife RL, Breslow R, et al: A new group of potent inducers of differentiation in murine erythroleukemia cells. Proc Natl Acad Sci U S A 1976;73;862.

381. Rowinsky EK, Donehower RC, Spivak JL, et al: Effects of the differentiating agent hexamethylene bisacetamide on normal and myelodysplastic hematopoietic progenitors. J Natl Cancer Inst 1990;82:1926.

382. Rowinsky EK, Conley BA, Jones RJ, et al: Hexamethylene bisacetamide in myelodysplastic syndrome: Effect of five-day exposure to maximal therapeutic concentrations. Leukemia 1992;6:526.

383. Andreeff M, Stone R, Michaeli J, et al: Hexamethylene bisacetamide in myelodysplastic syndrome and acute myelogenous leukemia: A phase II clinical trial with a differentiation-inducing agent. Blood 1992;80:2604.

384. Lotem J, Sachs L: Potential pre-screening for therapeutic agents that induce differentiation in human myeloid leukemia cells. Int J Cancer 1980;25:561.

385. Cheson BD, Jasperse DM, Simon R, et al: A critical appraisal of low-dose cytosine arabinoside in patients with acute non-lymphocytic leukemia and myelodysplastic syndromes. J Clin Oncol 1986;4: 1857.

386. Miller KB, Kim K, Morrison FS, et al: The evaluation of low-dose cytarabine in the treatment of myelodysplastic syndromes: A phase-III intergroup study. Ann Hematol 1992;65:162.

387. Wattel E, Guerci A, Hecquet B, et al: A randomized trial of hydroxy-urea versus VP16 in adult chronic myelomonocytic leukemia. Blood 1996;88:2480.

388. List AF: Pharmacological differentiation and anti-apoptotic therapy in myelodysplastic syndromes. Forum (Genova) 1999;9:35.

389. Silverman LR, Demakos EP, Peterson R, et al: A randomized controlled trial of subcutaneous azacitidine (aza-C) in patients with the myelodysplastic syndrome (MDS): A study of the Cancer and Leukemia Group B (CALGB). Proc Am Soc Clin Oncol 1998;17:14.

390. Kornblith AB, Herndon II JE, Silverman LR, et al: The impact of 5-azacytidine on the quality of life of patients with the myelodysplastic syndrome (MDS) treated in a randomized phase III trial of the Cancer and Leukemia Group B (CALGB). Proc Am Soc Clin Oncol 1998;17:49.

391. Breitman TR, Keene B, Hemmi H: Retinoic acid–induced differentiation of fresh human leukemia cells and human myelomonocytic cell lines HL-60, U-937, and THP-1. Cancer Surv 1983;2:261.

392. Lanotte M, Martin-Thouvenin V, Najman S, et al: NB4, a maturation inducible cell line with t(15;17) marker isolated from a human acute promyelocytic leukemia (M3). Blood 1991;77:1080.

393. Abrahm J, Besa EC, Hyzinski M, et al: Disappearance of cytogenetic abnormalities and clinical remission during therapy with 13-cis retinoic acid in a patient with myelodysplastic syndrome: Inhibition of growth of the patient's malignant monocytoid clone. Blood 1986;67:1323.

394. Besa EC, Abrahm J, Bartolomew MJ, et al: Treatment with 13-cis retinoic acid in transfusion-dependent patients with myelodysplastic syndrome and decreased toxicity with addition of alpha-tocopherol. Am J Med 1990;89:739.

395. Bourantas KL, Tsiara S, Christou L: Treatment of 34 patients with myelodysplastic syndromes with 13-cis retinoic acid. Eur J Haematol 1995;55:235.

396. Clark RE, Ismail SA, Jacobs A, et al: A randomized trial of 13-cis retinoic acid with or without cytosine arabinoside in patients with myelodysplastic syndromes. Br J Haematol 1987;66:77.

397. Gold EJ, Mertelsmann RH, Itri LM, et al: Phase I clinical trial of 13-cis retinoic acid in myelodysplastic syndromes. Cancer Treat Rep 1983;67:981.

398. Greenberg BR, Durie BG, Barnett TC, et al: Phase I/II study of 13-cis retinoic acid in myelodysplastic syndrome. Cancer Treat Rep 1985;69:1369.

399. Kerndrup G, Bendix-Hansen K, Pedersen B, et al: 13-cis retinoic acid treatment of myelodysplastic syndromes. Leuk Res 1987;11:7.

400. Koeffler HP, Heijean D, Mertelsmann R, et al: Randomized study of 13-cis retinoic acid versus placebo in the myelodysplastic disorders. Blood 1988;71:703.

401. Leoni F, Ciolli S, Longo G, et al: 13-cis retinoic acid treatment in patients with myelodysplastic syndrome. Acta Haematol 1988; 80:8.

402. Picozzi VJ, Swanson GF, Morgan R, et al: 13-cis retinoic acid in the treatment of myelodysplastic syndromes. J Clin Oncol 1986; 4:589.

403. Swanson GF, Picozzi VJ, Morgan R, et al: Response of hematopoietic precursors to 13-cis retinoic acid and 1,25-dihydroxyvitamin D_3 in myelodysplastic syndromes. Blood 1986;67:1154.

404. Aul C, Runde V, Gattermann N: All-trans retinoic acid in patients with myelodysplastic syndromes: Results of a pilot study. Blood 1993;82:2967.

405. Kurzrock R, Estey E, Talpaz M: All-trans retinoic acid: Tolerance and biological effects in myelodysplastic syndrome. J Clin Oncol 1993;11:1489.

406. Ohno R: Differentiation therapy of myelodysplastic syndromes with retinoic acid. Leuk Lymphoma 1994;14:401.

407. Visani G, Cenacchi A, Tosi P, et al: All-trans retinoic acid improves erythropoiesis in myelodysplastic syndromes. Br J Haematol 1992; 81:444.

408. Visani G, Tosi P, Manfroi S, et al: All-trans retinoic acid in the treatment of myelodysplastic syndromes. Leuk Lymphoma 1995; 19:277.

409. Metha AB, Kumaran TO, Marsh GW: Treatment of myelodysplastic syndromes with alpha-calcidiol. Lancet 1984;ii:761.

410. Koeffler HP, Hirji K, Itri L: 1,25-dihydroxyvitamin D_3: In vivo and in vitro effects on human preleukemic and leukemic cells. Cancer Treat Rep 1985;69:1399.

411. Richard C, Mazo E, Cuadrado MA, et al: Treatment of myelodysplastic syndromes with 1,25-dihydroxyvitamin D_3. Am J Hematol 1986; 73:175.

412. Motomura S, Kanamori H, Maruta A, et al: The effect of 1-hydroxy-vitamin D_3 for prolongation of leukaemic transformation-free survival in myelodysplastic syndromes. Am J Hematol 1991;38:67.

413. Miyazawa K, Kawanishi Y, Yaguchi M, et al: Vitamin K_2 induces apoptosis of a novel established MDS cell line: Antagonistic effect of G-CSF. Blood 1998;92:253.

414. Yaguchi M, Miyazawa K, Kawanishi Y, et al: Vitamin K_2 induces apoptosis and cell cycle arrest in leukemia cells via distinct intracellular signaling pathways. Blood 1999;94:198.

415. Takami A, Yamauchi H, Ishiyama K, et al: Menatetrenone, a vitamin K_2 analog, ameliorates cytopenias in patients with myelodysplastic syndrome, refractory anemia (MDS-RA). Blood 1999;94:662.

416. Clark RE, Ismail SA, Jacobs A, et al: A randomized trial of 13-cis retinoic acid with or without cytosine arabinoside in patients with myelodysplastic syndromes. Br J Haematol 1987;66:77.

417. Ho AD, Marin H, Knauf W, et al: Combination of low-dose cytarabine and 13-cis retinoic acid in the treatment of myelodysplastic syndromes. Leuk Res 1987;11:1041.

418. Nair R, Nair CN, Advani SH: All-trans retinoic acid with low-dose cytosine arabinoside in the treatment of myelodysplastic syndrome. Leuk Lymphoma 1998;29:187.

419. Hellström E, Robert KH, Gahrton G, et al: Therapeutic effects of low-dose cytosine arabinoside, α-interferon, 1-α-hydroxyvitamin D₃ and retinoic acid in acute leukemic and myelodysplastic syndromes. Scand J Haematol 1988;40:449.

420. Hellström E, Robert KH, Samuelson J, et al: Treatment of myelodysplastic syndromes with retinoic acid and 1-alpha-hydroxy-vitamin D₃ in combination with low-dose ara-C is not superior to ara-C alone: Results from a randomized study. Eur J Haematol 1990;45:255.

421. Ferraro D, Bruno B, Pregno P, et al: Combined differentiating therapy for myelodysplastic syndromes: A phase II study. Leuk Res 1996;20:867.

422. Gerhartz HH, Marcus R, Delmer A, et al: A randomized phase II study of low-dose cytosine arabinoside (LD-Ara-C) plus granulocyte-macrophage colony-stimulating factor (rhGM-CSF) in myelodysplastic syndromes (MDS) with a high risk of developing leukemia. EORTC Leukemia Cooperative Group. Leukemia 1994;8:16.

423. Grant S, Bhalla K, Weinstein IB, et al: Recombinant human interferon sensitizes resistant myeloid leukemic cells to induction of terminal differentiation. Biochem Biophys Res 1985;130:379.

424. Elias L, Hoffman R, Boswell S, et al: A trial of recombinant alpha-2 interferon in the myelodysplastic syndromes: Clinical results. Leukemia 1987;1:105.

425. Galvani DW, Nethersell AB, Cawley JC: Alpha-interferon in myelodysplasia: Clinical observations and effects on NK cells. Leuk Res 1988;12:257.

426. Petti MC, Latagliata R, Avvisati G, et al: Treatment of high-risk myelodysplastic syndromes with lymphoblastoid alpha-interferon. Br J Haematol 1996;95:364.

427. Gisslinger H, Chott A, Linkesch W, et al: Long-term alpha-interferon therapy in myelodysplastic syndromes. Leukemia 1990;4:91.

428. Aul C, Gattermann N, Schneider W: Treatment of advanced myelodysplastic syndromes with recombinant interferon-alpha 2b. Eur J Haematol 1991;46:11.

429. Nand S, Ellis T, Messmore H, et al: Phase II trial of recombinant human interferon-alpha in myelodsyplastic syndromes. Leukemia 1992;6:220.

430. Holcombe RF: Mini-dose interferon alpha-2a in the treatment of myelodysplasia. Leukemia 1993;7:192.

431. Maerevoet M, Van Den Neste E, Delannoy A, et al: Limited activity of mini-dose interferon alpha-2a in the treatment of myelodysplastic syndrome. Leuk Lymphoma 1996;21:519.

432. Beran M, Andersson B, Kantarjian H, et al: Hematologic response of four patients with smoldering acute myelogenous leukemia to partially pure gamma interferon. Leukemia 1987;1:52.

433. Stone RM, Spriggs DR, Arthur KA, et al: Recombinant human gamma interferon administered by continuous intravenous infusion in acute myelogenous leukemia and myelodysplastic syndromes. Am J Clin Oncol 1993;16:159.

434. Maiolo AT, Cortelezzi A, Calori R, et al: For the Italian Study Group: Recombinant gamma-interferon as first-line therapy for high risk myelodysplastic syndromes. Leukemia 1990;4:480.

435. Ogawa M, Yoshida Y, Moriyama Y, et al: A phase II clinical trial of recombinant interferon-gamma on myelodysplastic syndromes. Blut 1988;56:21.

436. Sulecki M, Shadduck RK, Zeigler Z: Anti-thymocyte globulin for hypoplastic myelodysplastic syndrome. Blood 1988;72:229.

437. Tichelli A, Gratwohl A, Wuersch A, et al: Antilymphocyte globulin for myelodysplastic syndrome? Br J Haematol 1988;68:139.

438. Mineishi S, Filippa D, Childs B, et al: Hypoplastic myelodysplastic syndrome (MDS): Clinical, hematologic, and pathologic observations in 36 cases. Blood 1994, 84:315.

439. Molldrem JJ, Caples M, Mavroudis D, et al: Antithymocyte globulin for patients with myelodysplastic syndrome. Br J Haematol 1997;99:699.

440. Barrett AJ, Molldrem JJ, Sauntharajarian Y, et al: Prolonged transfusion independence and disease stability in patients with myelodysplastic syndrome (MDS) responding to antithymocyte globulin (ATG). Blood 1998;92:713.

441. Molldrem JJ, Jiang YZ, Stetler-Stevenson M, et al: Haematological response of patients with myelodysplastic syndrome to antithymocyte globulin is associated with a loss of lymphocyte-mediated

inhibition of CFU-GM and alterations in T-cell receptor V-beta profiles. Br J Haematol 1998;102:1314.

442. Jonasova A, Neuwirtova R, Cermak J, et al: Cyclosporin A therapy in hypoplastic MDS patients and certain refractory anaemias without hypoplastic bone marrow. Br J Haematol 1998;100:304.

443. Bagby GC Jr, Gabourel JD, Linman JW: Glucocorticoid therapy in the preleukemic syndrome (hemopoietic dysplasia): Identification of responsive patients using in vitro techniques. Ann Intern Med 1980;92:55.

444. Najean Y, Pecking A: Refractory anaemia with excess of myeloblasts in the bone marrow: A clinical trial of androgens in 90 patients. Br J Haematol 1977;37:25.

445. Najean Y, Pecking A: Refractory anemia with excess of blast cells: Prognostic factors and effect of treatment with androgens or cytosine arabinoside: Results of a prospective trial in 58 patients. Cancer 1979;44:1976.

446. Chabannon C, Molina L, Pegourie-Bandelier B, et al: A review of 76 patients with myelodysplastic syndromes treated with danazol. Cancer 1994;73:3073.

447. Marini B, Bassan R, Barbui T: Therapeutic efficacy of danazol in myelodysplastic syndromes. Eur J Cancer Clin Oncol 1988;24:1481.

448. Wattel E, Cambier N, Caulier M-T, et al: Androgen therapy in myelodysplastic syndromes with thrombocytopenia: A report on 20 cases. Br J Haematol 1994;87:205.

449. Cines DB, Cassileth PA, Kiss JE: Danazol therapy in myelodysplasia. Ann Intern Med 1985;103:58.

450. Stadtmauer EA, Cassileth PA, Edelstein M, et al: Danazol treatment of myelodysplastic syndromes. Br J Haematol 1991;77:502.

451. Gassmann W, Schmitz N, Löffler H, et al: Intensive chemotherapy and bone marrow transplantation for myelodysplastic syndromes. Semin Hematol 1996;33:196.

452. Sanz GF, Sanz MA: Progress in intensive chemotherapy for high-risk myelodysplastic syndromes. Forum (Geneva) 1999;9:63.

453. Mertelsmann R, Thaler HT, To L, et al: Morphological classification, response to therapy, and survival in 263 adult patients with acute nonlymphoblastic leukemia. Blood 1980;56:773.

454. Wattel E, De Botton S, Laï JL, et al: Long-term follow-up of de novo myelodysplastic syndromes treated with intensive chemotherapy: Incidence of long-term survivors and outcome of partial responders. Br J Haematol 1997;98:983.

455. Aul C, Runde V, Germing U, et al: Aggressive chemotherapy in MDS: The Düsseldorf experience. Leuk Res 1997;21:45.

456. San Miguel JF, Sanz GF, Vallespi T, et al: Myelodysplastic syndromes. Crit Rev Oncol Hematol 1996;23:57.

457. Estey E, Thall P, Andreeff M, et al: Use of granulocyte colony-stimulating factor before, during, and after fludarabine plus cytarabine induction therapy of newly diagnosed acute myelogenous leukemia or myelodysplastic syndromes: Comparison with fludarabine plus cytarabine without granulocyte colony-stimulating factor. J Clin Oncol 1994;12:671.

458. Bernasconi C, Alessandrino EP, Bernasconi P, et al: Randomized clinical study comparing aggressive chemotherapy with or without G-CSF support for high-risk myelodysplastic syndromes or secondary acute myeloid leukaemia evolving from MDS. Br J Haematol 1998;102:678.

459. Ossenkoppele GJ, van der Holt B, Verhoef GEG, et al: A randomized study of granulocyte colony-stimulating factor applied during and after chemotherapy in patients with poor-risk myelodysplastic syndromes: A final report from the Hovon Cooperative Group. Blood 1998;92:630.

460. Estey E, Thall PF, Pierce S, et al: Randomized phase II study of fludarabine + cytosine arabinoside + idarubicin + all-trans retinoic acid + granulocyte colony-stimulating factor in poor prognosis newly diagnosed acute myeloid leukemia and myelodysplastic syndrome. Blood 1999;93:2478.

461. Armitage JO, Dick FR, Needleman SW, et al: Effect of chemotherapy for the dysmyelopoietic syndrome. Cancer Treat Rep 1981;65:601.

462. Tricot G, Boogaerts MA: The role of aggressive chemotherapy in the treatment of myelodysplastic syndromes. Br J Haematol 1986;63:477.

463. Michels SD, Samur J, Arthur DC, et al: Refractory anemia with excess blasts in transformation: Hematologic and clinical study of 52 patients. Cancer 1989;64:2340.

464. Kantarjian HM, Keating MJ, Walters RS, et al: Therapy-related leukemia and myelodysplastic syndrome: Clinical, cytogenetic, and prognostic features. J Clin Oncol 1986;4:1748.

465. Fenaux P, Morel P, Rose C, et al: Prognostic factors in adult de novo myelodysplastic syndromes treated by intensive chemotherapy. Br J Haematol 1991;77:497.

466. De Witte T, Suciu S, Peetermans M, et al: Intensive chemotherapy for poor prognosis myelodysplasia (MDS) and secondary acute myeloid leukemia (sAML) following MDS of more than 8 months duration: A pilot study by the Leukemia Cooperative Group of the European Organisation for Research and Treatment in Cancer (EORTC-LCG). Leukemia 1995;9:1805.

467. De Witte T, Muus P, De Pauw B, et al: Intensive antileukemic treatment of patients younger than 65 years with myelodysplastic syndromes and secondary acute myelogenous leukemia. Cancer 1990;66:831.

468. Bernstein SH, Brunetto VL, Davey FR, et al: Acute myeloid leukemia-type chemotherapy for newly diagnosed patients without antecedent cytopenias having myelodysplastic syndrome as defined by French-American-British criteria: a Cancer and Leukemia Group B study. J Clin Oncol 1996;14:2486.

469. Estey E, Thall P, Beran M, et al: Effect of diagnosis (refractory anemia with excess blasts, refractory anemia with excess blasts in transformation, or acute myeloid leukemia [AML]) on outcome of AML-type chemotherapy. Blood 1997;90:2969.

470. List AF, Spier CM, Cline A, et al: Expression of the multidrug resistance gene product (P-glycoprotein) in myelodysplasia is associated with a stem cell phenotype. Br J Haematol 1991;78:28.

471. Lepelley P, Soenen V, Preudhomme C, et al: Expression of multidrug resistance P-glycoprotein and its relationship to hematological characteristics and response to treatment in myelodysplastic syndromes. Leukemia 1994;8:998.

472. Wattel E, Solary E, Hecquet B, et al: Quinine improves the results of intensive chemotherapy (IC) in myelodysplastic syndromes (MDS) expressing P-glycoprotein (PGP): Updated results of a randomized study. Groupe Français des Myelodysplasies (GFM) and Groupe GOELAMS. Adv Exp Med Biol 1999;457:35.

473. Beran M, Kantarjian H: Topotecan in the treatment of hematologic malignancies. Semin Hematol 1998;35:26.

474. Beran M, Estey E, O'Brien S, et al: Topotecan and cytarabine are an active combination regimen in myelodysplastic syndromes and chronic myelomonocytic leukemia. J Clin Oncol 1999;17:2819.

475. Wijermans P, Lubbert M, Verhoef G, et al: Low-dose 5-aza-2'-deoxycytidine, a DNA hypomethylating agent, for the treatment of high-risk myelodysplastic syndrome: A multicenter phase II study in elderly patients. J Clin Oncol 2000;18:956.

476. Nevill TJ, Shepherd JD, Reece DE, et al: Treatment of myelodysplastic syndrome with busulfan-cyclophosphamide conditioning followed by allogeneic BMT. Bone Marrow Transplant 1992;10:445.

477. Anderson JE, Appelbaum FR, Fisher LD, et al: Allogeneic bone marrow transplantation for 93 patients with myelodysplastic syndrome. Blood 1993;82:677.

478. O'Donnell MR, Long GD, Parker PM, et al: Busulfan/cyclophosphamide as conditioning regimen for allogeneic bone marrow transplantation for myelodysplasia. J Clin Onc 1995;13:2973.

479. Demuynck H, Verhoef GE, Zachee P, et al: Treatment of patients with myelodysplastic syndromes with allogeneic bone marrow transplantation from genotypically similar HLA-identical sibling and alternative donors. Bone Marrow Transplant 1996;17:745.

480. Anderson JE, Thomas ED: The Seattle experience with bone marrow transplantation for myelodysplasia (MDS). Leuk Res 1997;21:51.

481. Runde V, de Witte T, Arnold R, et al: Bone marrow transplantation from HLA-identical siblings as first-line treatment in patients with myelodysplastic syndromes: Early transplantation is associated with improved outcome. Bone Marrow Transplant 1998;21:255.

482. Deeg HJ, Shulman HM, Anderson JE, et al: Allogeneic and syngeneic marrow transplantation for myelodysplastic syndrome in patients 55 to 66 years of age. Blood 2000;95:1188.

483. Witherspoon RP, Deeg JH: Allogeneic bone marrow transplantation for secondary leukemia or myelodysplasia. Haematologica 1999;84:1085.

484. Yakoub-Agha I, De La Salmoniere P, Ribaud P, et al: Allogeneic bone marrow transplantation for therapy-related myelodysplastic syndrome and acute myeloid leukemia: A long-term study of 70

patients. Report of the French Society of Bone Marrow Transplantation. J Clin Oncol 2000;18:963.

485. Nevill TJ, Fung HC, Shepherd JD, et al: Cytogenetic abnormalities in primary myelodysplastic syndrome are highly predictive of outcome after allogeneic bone marrow transplantation. Blood 1998;92:1910.

486. Appelbaum FR, Anderson J: Allogeneic bone marrow transplantation for myelodysplastic syndrome: Outcomes analysis according to IPSS score. Leukemia 1998;12:25.

487. Anderson JE, Appelbaum FR, Schoch G, et al: Allogeneic bone marrow transplantation for refractory anemia: A comparison of two preparative regimens and analysis of prognostic factors. Blood 1996;87:51.

488. DeWitte T, Zwaan F, Hermans J, et al: Allogeneic bone marrow transplantation for secondary leukemia and myelodysplastic syndrome: A survey by the Leukaemia Working Party of the European Bone Marrow Transplantation Group (EBMTG). Br J Haematol 1990;74:151.

489. Sutton L, Chastang C, Ribaud P, et al: Factors influencing outcome in de novo myelodysplastic syndromes treated by allogeneic bone marrow transplantation: A long-term study of 71 patients. Société française de greffe de moelle. Blood 1996;88:358.

490. Anderson JE, Gooley TA, Schoch G, et al: Stem cell transplantation for secondary acute myeloid leukemia: Evaluation of transplantation as initial therapy or following induction chemotherapy. Blood 1997;89:2578.

491. Alessandrino EP, Astori C, Van Lint MT, et al: Myelodysplastic syndrome or leukemia developing after MDS treated by allogeneic bone marrow transplantation: Outcome of 90 adult patients. Leuk Res 1997;21:52.

492. Anderson JE, Anasetti C, Appelbaum FR, et al: Unrelated donor marrow transplantation for myelodysplasia (MDS) and MDS-related acute myeloid leukaemia. Br J Haematol 1996;93:59.

493. Arnold R, De Witte T, Van Biezen A, et al: Unrelated bone marrow transplantation in patients with myelodysplastic syndromes and secondary acute myeloid leukemia: An EBMT survey. Bone Marrow Transplant 1998;21:1213.

494. De Witte T, Suciu S, Peetermans M, et al: Intensive chemotherapy for poor prognosis myelodysplasia and secondary acute myelogenous leukemia following MDS of more than 6 months duration: A pilot study by the Leukemia Cooperative Group of the European Organization for Research and Treatment in Cancer (EORTC-LCG). Leukemia 1995;9:1805.

495. Carella AM, Dejana A, Lerma E, et al: In vivo mobilization of karyotypically normal peripheral blood progenitor cells in high-risk MDS, secondary or therapy-related acute myelogenous leukaemia. Br J Haematol 1996;95:127.

496. Delforge M, Demuynck H, Vandenberghe P, et al: Polyclonal primitive hematopoietic progenitors can be detected in mobilized peripheral blood from patients with high-risk myelodysplastic syndromes. Blood 1995;86:3660.

497. De Witte T, Suciu S, Verhoef G, et al: Autologous stem cell transplantation for patients with poor risk MDS and secondary AML (sAML): A joint study of the EORTC, EBMT, SAKK, and GIMEMA leukemia groups. Blood 1997;90:(Suppl 1)583a.

498. De Witte T, van Biezen A, Hermans J, et al: Autologous bone marrow transplantation for patients with myelodysplastic syndrome (MDS) or acute myeloid leukemia following MDS. Blood 1997;90:3853.

499. Wattel E, Solary E, Leleu X, et al: A prospective study of autologous bone marrow or peripheral blood stem cell transplantation after intensive chemotherapy in myelodysplastic syndromes. Leukemia 1999;13:524.

500. Cheson B, Bennett J, Kantarjian H, et al: Report of an international working group to standardize response criteria for myelodysplastic syndromes. Blood 2000;96:3671.

501. Thomas ML, Zhang J, Greenberg PL: Quality of life in individuals with myelodysplastic syndromes. Blood 1999;94:662.

502. Cella D: Quality of life outcomes: Measurement and validation. Oncology 1996;10:233.

503. Druker BJ, Talpaz M, Resta D, et al: Efficacy and safety of a specific inhibitor of the BCR-ABL tyrosine kinase in chronic myeloid leukemia. New Engl J Med 2000;344:1031.

504. Carroll M, Ohno-Jones S, Tamura S, et al: CGP 57148, a tyrosine kinase inhibitor, inhibits the growth of cells expressing BCR-ABL,

TEL-ABL, and the TEL-PDGFR fusion proteins. Blood 1997;90:
4947.

505. Rowinsky EK, Windle JJ, Von Hoff DD: Ras protein farnesyltransferase: A strategic target for anticancer therapeutic development. J
Clin Oncol 1999;17:3631.

506. Emanuel PD, Snyder RC, Wiley T, et al: Inhibition of juvenile
myelomonocytic leukemia cell growth in vitro by farnesyltransferase inhibitors. Blood 2000;95:639.

507. Zujewski J, Horak ID, Bol CJ, et al: Phase I and pharmacokinetic
study of farnesyl protein transferase inhibitor R115777 in advanced cancer. J Clin Oncol 2000;18:927.

508. Karp JE, Lancet JE, Kaufmann SH, et al: Clinical and biological
activity of the farnesyltransferase inhibitor R115777 in adults with
refractory and relapsed acute leukemias: A phase 1 clinical-labora-
tory correlative trial. Blood 2001;97:3361.

509. Johnston SR, Ellis PA, Houston S, et al: A phase II study of the
farnesyl transferase inhibitor R115777 in patients with advanced
breast cancer. Proc Am Soc Clin Oncol 2000;19:83.

510. Champlin R, Khouri I, Kornblau S, et al: Allogeneic hematopoietic
transplantation as adoptive immunotherapy: Induction of graft-
versus-malignancy as primary therapy. Hematol Oncol Clin North
Am 1999;13:1041.

25

Chronic Myeloid Leukemia

Michael J. Barnett   Connie J. Eaves

The young man, described by Bennett in 1845,[18] who after being unwell for 20 months died of "suppuration of the blood" with an enormously enlarged spleen may well have suffered from chronic myeloid leukemia (CML), as may have the patients reported by Craigie[54] and Virchow[270] in the same year. Granulocytosis and splenomegaly are characteristic features of the disease, which typically afflicts adults. Furthermore, the natural history of CML is one of inevitable progression after a few years from an initial chronic phase, which is benign, to a terminal blast phase, which is malignant and rapidly fatal.

Much of what is understood about the nature of CML was anticipated from careful clinical and laboratory studies performed in the first half of the twentieth century.[58, 229] These set the stage for the period 1960–1990, during which a remarkable series of discoveries was made about the disease, establishing it as a model for many forms of cancer. In 1960, the presence of an unusually small autosome, a shortened chromosome 22, later named the Philadelphia (Ph) chromosome, was noted in metaphase spreads from blood and marrow cells (but not skin fibroblasts) from patients with CML.[7, 197, 198, 259] This observation was followed 7 years later by the demonstration that the disease was clonal, arising from a single pluripotent hematopoietic stem cell.[82] The coexistence of Ph-positive and Ph-negative progenitor cells, the latter suggesting the persistence of normal stem cells, was reported soon thereafter.[39] With the introduction of new banding techniques in the early 1970s, it became possible to show that the Ph chromosome resulted from a reciprocal translocation between chromosomes 9 and 22.[224] The application of molecular biologic techniques in the 1980s revealed that the Ph chromosome involved a rearrangement of the *ABL* gene on chromosome 9[62] and the *BCR* (breakpoint cluster region) gene on chromosome 22,[108] leading to the creation of a *BCR-ABL* fusion gene.[231] Subsequent recognition that the *BCR-ABL* gene encodes an abnormal *ABL*-related protein (p210) with deregulated tyrosine kinase activity (in the cytoplasm)[17, 161] pointed to a molecular mechanism[177] whereby hematopoietic cells expressing this product obtain a proliferative advantage over their normal counterparts. Finally, the demonstration that hematopoietic cells transduced with *BCR-ABL* could induce a CML-like disease in mice provided more direct

evidence that the product of this gene plays a key role in the pathogenesis of the disease.[57, 78, 155]

In the last decade, considerable progress has been made in extending this basic knowledge of CML. The broad goal of such work is to define the molecular and cellular mechanisms involved in the generation, maintenance, and progression of the disease.[63, 77] In turn, it is hoped that this information will lead to the establishment of directed (i.e., targeted), rather than empiric, therapy. The pursuit of strategies to inhibit the kinase function of the *BCR-ABL* protein is an example of this endeavour.[74]

Against this background of success in the laboratory over the last 40 years, it may be argued that progress in the treatment of CML has been harder to come by. A major achievement has been the development of allogeneic stem cell transplantation. For those patients (a select minority) who can be offered this treatment, eradication of an otherwise incurable disease is a distinct possibility. For the majority, however, cure remains an elusive goal. Standard therapy of the day has involved a succession of agents: busulfan, then hydroxyurea, and then interferon. In the last few years, however, there has been a relative flurry of clinical activity, with the advent of the tyrosine kinase inhibitor STI571 and the introduction of new strategies to exploit the powerful antileukemic effect of allografting. For the physician recommending (and the patient accepting) treatment for CML, this expanding list of options should be viewed as a welcome challenge.

The management of CML is the focus of this chapter. For convenience, it will be preceded by a brief summary of basic information, most of which is covered in considerably more detail elsewhere in this volume.

TERMINOLOGY

On morphologic grounds, it has been proposed that CML be employed as a generic term for a group of leukemias that includes chronic granulocytic leukemia.[19] It is common practice, however, to use CML synonymously with chronic granulocytic leukemia to refer specifically to a leukemia that, in contrast with other myeloproliferative disorders, is characterized by the presence of a *BCR-ABL* fusion gene. In regard to this definition, it should be noted that atypical *BCR-ABL* rearrangements in CML may result in unusual disease phenotypes (i.e., clinical and laboratory features), presumably due to variations in *BCR-ABL* tyrosine kinase activity.[189, 206] In addition, *BCR-ABL* fusion genes can exist and be expressed in the blood cells of normal individuals who never show any evidence of the disease.[24, 29] This situation reflects a basal level of genetic instability during normal hematopoiesis and also shows that other events or conditions are required to produce the disease.

EPIDEMIOLOGY

The age-adjusted annual incidence of CML is approximately 1 per 100,000 population, with little variation worldwide.[207, 222] The disease is essentially one of adult life and is very uncommon in childhood. Although the largest number of cases is seen in individuals in the sixth decade of life, the age-specific incidence continues to rise with age. The incidence is also higher in males.

ETIOLOGY

The demonstration of the Ph chromosome in hematopoietic cells but not skin fibroblasts first suggested that the cytogenetic abnormality (and, by inference, the disease) is acquired.[197, 259] Studies of monozygotic twins showing a lack of concordance of CML (i.e., only one of the pair being affected) provide further support for this hypothesis.[94, 95, 137] No specific inherited features have been identified that predispose an individual to the development of CML. However, it is clear from studies of the survivors of the atomic bomb explosions in Hiroshima and Nagasaki that exposure to ionizing radiation can induce the disease; most cases were diagnosed 5-10 years after the event.[85, 133, 167, 192] It is also possible that the doses of radiation given as therapy for ankylosing spondylitis[277] or cancer of the uterus[27, 56] may place patients with these diseases at increased risk for development of CML.

NATURAL HISTORY

The disease has two distinct phases. Most patients present with a chronic (or stable) phase that is characterized by a marked expansion of the granulocytic series but with differentiation relatively unaffected. In such patients, all of the mature blood cells (except some of the B lymphocytes and most of the T lymphocytes) are leukemic but functionally normal. Although a few cases of spontaneous remission of CML have been reported,[196, 214] the natural history is one of inevitable progression. Transformation (or metamorphosis) involves the acquisition of secondary mutations, and in most cases additional cytogenetic changes (typically, duplication of the Ph chromosome, trisomy 8, and isochromosome 17) are detected.[179, 201] This results in a breakdown of the differentiation process and a rapid accumulation of nonfunctional blast cells, which, in keeping with the stem cell origin of the clone,[26, 139] may have a predominantly myeloid (most common), lymphoid, mixed, or undifferentiated pheno-

TABLE 25–1. The Phases of Chronic Myeloid Leukemia*

Chronic phase
- No significant symptoms
- None of the features of accelerated phase or blast phase

Accelerated phase
- Leukocytosis difficult to control (WBC > 50 × 10⁹/L)
- Rapid doubling of WBC (<5 days)
- ≥10% blasts in blood or marrow
- ≥20% blasts plus promyelocytes in blood or marrow
- ≥20% basophils plus eosinophils in blood
- Anemia or thrombocytopenia unresponsive to standard treatment
- Persistent thrombocytosis (platelets > 1000 × 10⁹/L)
- Clonal cytogenetic changes in addition to the Ph chromosome
- Increasing splenomegaly
- Development of chloromas
- Development of marrow fibrosis

Blast phase
- ≥30% blasts plus promyelocytes in the blood or marrow

WBC, white blood cell.
* Criteria established by the International Bone Marrow Transplant Registry.

type.[13, 22, 107, 138] Erythroblastic,[246] megakaryoblastic,[8] and T-lymphoblastic[38, 103, 106, 228] transformations have also been reported, but these are rare. The blast (or acute) phase may develop abruptly or after an accelerated phase during which clinical, hematologic, and cytogenetic changes (Table 25-1) herald its onset over a variable length of time. Occasionally, the chronic phase escapes diagnosis, and patients first present with blast-phase disease.[209]

Although it is useful to consider CML in terms of these phases, this should not be taken to imply that the chronic phase is biologically static. On the contrary, numerous subtle changes are likely to be occurring continuously over a number of years before transformation becomes apparent.

BIOLOGY

Stem Cell Origin

At the cellular level, CML represents an abnormal clone of cells that typically has expanded to dominate the entire hematopoietic system by the time the patient develops symptoms. The extent of this clonal expansion was first appreciated by the consistent finding of the Ph chromosome in most of the dividing cells (including erythroid cells and megakaryocytes) in marrow samples.[260, 278] More direct evidence that these Ph-positive cells represented expanded clonal populations was subsequently provided from studies of the product of X-linked genes (e.g., glucose-6-phosphate dehydrogenase isoenzymes) in hematopoietic cells from heterozygous females with CML as well as from other examples of mosaicism.[217] Various approaches have shown that the leukemic clone commonly includes some B lymphocytes as well as all of the myeloid lineages.[21, 182] Recent studies support the view that the initial cell transformed also has the potential to produce T lymphocytes.[111, 143] Thus, CML is a clonal disease that is maintained by a cell that has the potential to differentiate into all hematopoietic lineages.

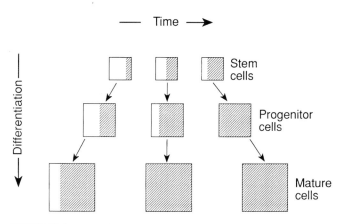

FIGURE 25–1. Expansion of the leukemic cell compartment *(hatched areas)* and suppression of the normal cell compartment *(open areas)* in CML over time and during the process of differentiation.

Leukemic Stem Cells

Leukemic (Ph-positive) stem cells in patients with chronic phase CML are characterized by increased proliferative activity[76, 77, 261] and decreased self-renewal.[210, 263] The increased turnover within the leukemic stem cell compartment, and an associated enhanced drive toward differentiation, results in the myeloid expansion that typifies the chronic phase of the disease. Recently, it has been found that an autocrine mechanism involving interleukin-3 and granulocyte colony-stimulating factor contributes to this process.[141, 142] In addition, a quiescent subset of leukemic stem cells has been identified, which may be involved in the maintenance of the disease.[129]

Normal Stem Cells

Both clinical[101, 237, 251] and laboratory[51, 263, 273] evidence indicates that Ph-negative stem cells persist in many patients. Various markers of clonality have been used to show that at least some of these cells do not belong to the leukemic clone and are presumably normal.[75, 128, 262] From a therapeutic standpoint, it is likely that this suppressed but functionally intact population of normal stem cells is of a useful size, particularly early in the course of the disease.[87, 211, 268] However, the reservoir is reduced over time (Fig. 25–1).

PRESENTATION

Clinical Features

The presenting clinical features of CML have been described in detail.[226, 229, 257] The common symptoms are fatigue or lethargy, weight loss, sweats, bleeding, abdominal discomfort, and the discovery of an abdominal mass (the spleen). There are many other less frequent complaints as well as those that are unusual, such as priapism. The most common physical finding is splenomegaly,

which may be the only abnormality on examination. Other signs include purpura, hepatomegaly, and retinal changes. Significant lymphadenopathy is uncommon and, when found, suggests that the disease is no longer in the chronic phase. Other atypical presentations involving a variety of extramedullary sites also portend an unfavorable course.

Laboratory Features

A characteristic peripheral blood film with demonstration of the Ph chromosome or *BCR-ABL* gene rearrangement in blood or marrow cells establishes the diagnosis. On infrequent occasions, it may be necessary to rely on molecular studies to reveal the *BCR-ABL* fusion gene, because a Ph chromosome is not present.[90, 164, 265] For the majority of cases, however, cytogenetic analysis is diagnostic and also offers the advantage of providing information as to the presence of cells carrying additional cytogenetic changes.

The appearance of the blood at presentation has been reviewed.[226, 245, 257] The white blood cell (WBC) count is usually in the range of 100 to 400 × 10⁹/L, although it may exceed 600 × 10⁹/L. Initial counts of 10 to 50 × 10⁹/L are more likely to be an incidental finding in asymptomatic patients who have had blood taken as part of a routine medical examination. The blood is usually found to contain a full array of granulocytic cells but with a marked predominance of myelocytes and neutrophils. Absolute numbers of basophils and eosinophils are typically elevated but usually do not exceed 5% of the WBC count. Similarly, although monocyte counts are commonly increased, a relative monocytosis (more than 4%) is unusual. Moderate anemia (normochromic and normocytic) is a characteristic of untreated CML and is usually corrected with therapy. The platelet count is typically either normal or modestly elevated but may occasionally exceed 1000 × 10⁹/L. In general, the morphology of the leukemic cells in the peripheral blood is the same as that of their counterparts in the blood and marrow of normal individuals.

The marrow is characteristically hypercellular with a considerably increased granulopoietic:erythroid ratio and numerous megakaryocytes. The presence of lipid-filled macrophages resembling Gaucher cells and sea-blue histiocytes is presumed to be a reflection of the increased cell turnover.[69] Myelofibrosis, although more commonly associated with transformed disease, may also occur in the early chronic phase.[102] In most cases, the majority of dividing marrow cells are Ph-positive,[260, 278] but their morphology appears normal.

Differential Diagnosis

A number of conditions bear a morphologic resemblance to CML.[215] These comprise other myeloproliferative disorders, including chronic neutrophilic leukemia[279] (which is extremely uncommon); some myelodysplastic syndromes, in particular chronic myelomonocytic leukemia[91]; and leukemoid reactions,[125] in which a reactive leukocytosis occurs in response to malignancy, infection, or hemolysis. All of these conditions have hematologic features that usually allow them to be distinguished from CML. Furthermore, none is associated with the presence of the Ph chromosome and, except in chronic myelomonocytic leukemia, the leukocyte alkaline phosphatase score is usually high, whereas in CML it is low.[171]

Typical CML may occur in childhood, albeit infrequently. In addition, another rare disorder, previously known as juvenile CML,[114] can afflict young children (usually less than 4 years of age). However, the term juvenile CML is a misnomer; the disease, which is distinct from both CML and chronic myelomonocytic leukemia, is more appropriately referred to as juvenile myelomonocytic leukemia.[4, 115]

MANAGEMENT OF CML

Overview with Historical Perspective

The survival of untreated patients with CML is known from a unique series reported in 1924.[190] A median survival of 32 months was calculated from the onset of symptoms by history. However, because symptoms were apparent on average approximately 12 months before diagnosis, the median survival from diagnosis was probably on the order of 20 months.[243] Therefore, it seems reasonable to use a median survival of 20 months as a general yardstick against which to compare the results of specific treatments. In doing so, however, it should be appreciated that during the last century, irrespective of advances in therapy, the median survival of patients with CML has lengthened as a consequence of an increased frequency of diagnosis earlier in the course of the disease as well as improvements in supportive care.

The first agent shown to have a therapeutic effect in CML was arsenic, which was administered as a solution of potassium arsenite (Fowler's solution)[86, 145, 165, 248] and was originally reported in 1865.[174] Radiotherapy was introduced in the early 1900s[216, 230] and remained the preferred treatment for the next 50 years. It was given mainly as irradiation to the spleen and, later, as injection of radioactive phosphorus.[221, 258] Despite being rather inconvenient and intermittent in terms of disease control, splenic irradiation was effective in resolving symptoms, shrinking the spleen, and lowering the WBC count.

Several drugs were evaluated in the middle 1900s, but it was not until the alkylating agent busulfan was introduced in the early 1950s that the next major advance occurred.[89, 110] Busulfan was the first treatment to provide continuous control of the disease. A randomized trial comparing busulfan and radiotherapy as primary therapy, conducted by the British Medical Research Council (Table 25-2), demonstrated an advantage for patients treated with busulfan (median survival 40 months) over those treated with radiotherapy (median survival 28 months).[187] Busulfan remained the treatment of choice until the 1980s, when hydroxyurea, a ribonucleotidase inhibitor of DNA synthesis first evaluated in the early 1960s,[83, 158]

TABLE 25–2. Randomized Trials in CML

Treatment	Investigators, period of trial
Busulfan versus radiotherapy	British MRC, 1959–1964[187]
Splenectomy versus no splenectomy	British MRC, 1972–1979[188] Italian CML Group, 1974–1977[136]
Hydroxyurea versus busulfan	German CML Group, 1983–1991[119]
IFN-α versus hydroxyurea versus busulfan	German CML Group, 1986–1991[120]
IFN-α versus hydroxyurea or busulfan	Italian CML Group, 1986–1988[134]
IFN-α versus hydroxyurea	British MRC, 1986–1994[1] Benelux CML Group, 1987–1992[16]
IFN-α versus busulfan	Japanese Leukemia Group, 1988–1991[203]
IFN-α + ara-C versus IFN-α	French CML Group, 1991–1996[109] Italian CML Group, 1994–1997[223]
STI571 versus IFN-α + ara-C	International CML Group, 2000–2001

CML, chronic myeloid leukemia; MRC, Medical Research Council; IFN-α, interferon-α; ara-C, cytosine arabinoside.

assumed that role. The shift to hydroxyurea was based on an appreciation that busulfan could cause serious side effects, namely marrow aplasia,[117, 274] interstitial pulmonary fibrosis,[118, 204] and a wasting syndrome resembling adrenal cortical insufficiency.[166] Later, a randomized trial carried out by the German CML Group (see Table 25-2) showed patients treated with hydroxyurea (median survival 58 months) fared significantly better than those treated with busulfan (median survival 45 months),[119] thus confirming the appropriateness of this change for standard therapy.

It might be argued that the benefits of busulfan and hydroxyurea, i.e., ease of administration (by mouth) and admirable control of myeloproliferation, obscured the fact that these drugs never prevented disease transformation and resulted in only a modest survival benefit (Fig. 25-2;

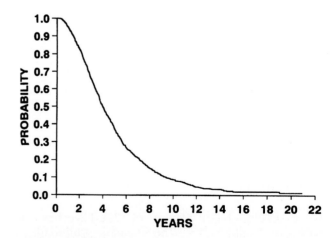

FIGURE 25–2. Survival of 813 patients presenting with CML in chronic phase and registered in the International CGL Prognosis Study. (From Cervantes F, Robertson JE, Rozman C, et al: Long-term survivors in chronic granulocytic leukaemia: A study by the International CGL Prognosis Study Group. Br J Haematol 1994; 87: 293–300. Reprinted with permission from Blackwell Science Ltd.)

TABLE 25–3. Results of Combination Chemotherapy for CML in Chronic Phase

		Cytogenetic Response*		Median Survival (months)		
Chemotherapy	*N*	*Complete*	*Partial*	*All*	*Responders*	*Nonresponders*
L-15†	42	33%	14%	50	55	46
ROAP‡	37	27%	22%	52	NR	35

CML, chronic myeloid leukemia; NR, not reached.
  * Defined by percent of Ph-negative marrow metaphases achieved: complete response = 100%; partial response = 66% to 99%.
  † Cytosine arabinoside, daunorubicin, 6-thioguanine, hydroxyurea, methotrexate, vincristine, cyclophosphamide, prednisone.[42,101]
  ‡ Rubidazone or daunorubicin, cytosine arabinoside, vincristine, prednisone.[152]

median survival 45 months).[37] In the early 1970s, however, these shortcomings of the best available therapy prompted the evaluation of four different treatments: combination chemotherapy, elective splenectomy, allogeneic bone marrow transplantation (BMT), and intensive therapy with autologous stem cell support.

In 1970, encouraged by early results in acute myelogenous leukemia, the Memorial Sloan-Kettering Cancer Center started to treat newly diagnosed patients with CML on protocols that included combination chemotherapy.[42, 55, 101] Disappointingly, this approach failed to alter the course of the disease, and the median survival of 50 months did not represent an advance. In about half of these[42, 101] and similarly treated patients,[152] however, Ph-negative hematopoiesis was restored for a brief period (Table 25–3).

Retrospective comparisons[244] and reports suggesting that transformed subclones could sometimes originate in the spleen[100, 191] led to the belief that splenectomy performed in the chronic phase might also result in improved survival benefit. This issue was formally addressed in 1972, when the British Medical Research Council organized a randomized study to determine whether elective splenectomy performed early in the chronic phase could delay the onset of transformation. The result of this trial[188] and a similar controlled study conducted by the Italian CML Group[136] (see Table 25–2) clearly demonstrated that splenectomy conferred no survival benefit.

Allogeneic BMT for the treatment of CML was introduced in 1970 by the Seattle group. Initially, only patients with disease that had transformed to an accelerated or blast phase were treated. In an attempt to eradicate the leukemia and produce enough immunosuppression to prevent rejection of the allogeneic graft, a combination of high-dose cyclophosphamide and total body irradiation (TBI) was chosen as the conditioning regimen. The patients were rescued from the marrow-ablative effects of the treatment by the transplantation of marrow from a sibling with the same human leukocyte antigen (HLA) type. Although these initial efforts were largely unsuccessful because of transplant-related mortality, the feasibility of the approach was established.[67] Recognizing the potential of these early clinical results, the Seattle group in the late 1970s went on to extend this approach to patients with chronic-phase disease,[68] including some with identical twin (i.e., syngeneic) donors.[79-81] The success of these studies[256] encouraged others, and it is now beyond doubt that, by establishing a chimeric state (i.e., hematopoiesis

is of donor origin), allogeneic BMT can result in long-term leukemia-free survival for patients with CML in any phase of the disease, although those transplanted in the chronic phase fare significantly better (Fig. 25–3). On the basis of these results, the recommended timing of BMT for CML has changed; the treatment of transformed disease has given way to the practice of treatment during the chronic phase,[232] ideally within the first year of diagnosis.[43, 99] For younger patients with chronic-phase CML who are fortunate enough to have an HLA-identical sibling donor, allogeneic BMT offers a good (50% to 60%) chance of long-term leukemia-free survival.[267] However, age and histocompatibility considerations dictate that this treatment can be offered to only a small minority of patients, even then with a significant risk of transplant-related mortality.

Evaluation of the use of intensive therapy supported by autografting was also initiated by the Seattle group in the early 1970s. As with the first allografts, the intention of these studies was to improve on the dismal prognosis of patients with blast-phase disease. Patients with transformed CML were treated with high-dose cyclophosphamide and TBI, followed by infusion of autologous marrow cells that had previously been harvested and cryopreserved during the chronic phase. Procedure-related mortality was high, but the feasibility of this strategy was established.[32, 33] Subsequently, a trial conducted at the Hammersmith Hospital in London demonstrated that cells collected from the peripheral blood by leukapheresis could also restore hematopoiesis following myeloablative

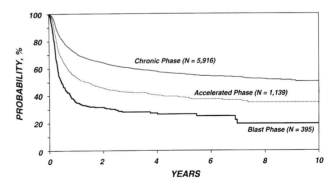

FIGURE 25–3. Leukemia-free survival after allogeneic BMT from HLA-identical sibling donors for patients with CML according to disease status at the time of transplantation. (From the International Bone Marrow Transplant Registry, with permission.)

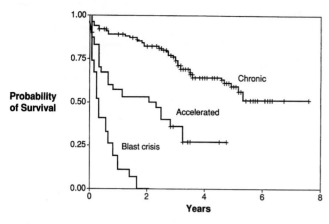

FIGURE 25–4. Survival after autografting for patients with CML according to disease status (chronic phase, n = 141; accelerated phase, n = 30; blast crisis, n = 27) at the time of autograft; combined results from 8 centers. (From Bhatia R, Verfaillie CM, Miller JS, et al: Autologous transplantation therapy for chronic myelogenous leukemia. Blood 1997; 89: 2623–2634. Copyright American Society of Hematology, used by permission.)

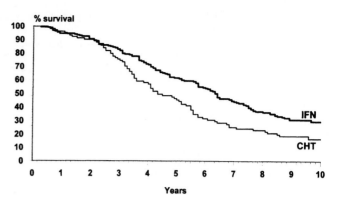

FIGURE 25–5. Survival of patients with CML assigned to interferon-α (IFN, n = 218) or chemotherapy (CHT, n = 104) in the randomized trial of the Italian CML Study Group. (From the Italian Cooperative Study Group on Chronic Myeloid Leukemia: Long-term follow-up of the Italian trial of interferon-α versus conventional chemotherapy in chronic myeloid leukemia. Blood 1998; 92: 1541–1548. Copyright American Society of Hematology, used by permission.)

therapy.[97] Although these and other studies have shown that this approach offers little benefit to the majority of patients with transformed disease,[112, 220] they were important in an historical sense because of the interest and impetus they gave to the application of this treatment in the chronic phase.[30, 131] The general rationale for intensive therapy with autologous stem cell support in chronic-phase CML is that it causes a reduction in the size of the leukemic stem cell population available for secondary mutational events. As a result, emergence of a blast-phase subclone might be delayed and survival prolonged. (Fig. 25–4).[185]

In the 1980s, continued dissatisfaction with the results of standard therapy as well as frustration that relatively few patients could undergo allogeneic BMT focused interest on three other emerging treatments: interferon, unrelated donor BMT, and intensive therapy with Ph-negative stem cell support.

In 1981, the M.D. Anderson Cancer Center initiated a study of the naturally occurring polypeptide, interferon-α, using first a partially pure form[255] and later a recombinant form.[253] The significant finding from these[251] and similar studies[205] was that unlike any other agent previously evaluated, interferon-α (given by subcutaneous injection) could result in restoration of Ph-negative hematopoiesis in some patients (Table 25–4). On the basis of these pilot studies, randomized trials to evaluate interferon-α versus hydroxyurea or busulfan were commenced in the middle/late 1980s (see Table 25–2). The CML Trialists Collaborative Group carried out a meta-analysis of the results from 7 randomized trials and showed that survival at 5 years was significantly better with interferon-α (57%) than with hydroxyurea or busulfan (42%).[41] Recently, the Italian CML group has undertaken a long-term follow-up of their trial (Fig. 25–5), in which patients treated with interferon-α (median survival 76 months) fared significantly better than those treated with hydroxyurea or busulfan (median survival 52 months).[135] These results confirmed the view that, despite significant side effects (which in some cases may be intolerable), interferon-α was a significant advance in the treatment of CML, and it became a standard therapy in the 1990s.

In the early 1980s, a few centers started to carry out allogeneic BMT with marrow from unrelated volunteers who shared the same HLA type as the patient.[14] Various registries were established worldwide, allowing such donors to be identified for a significant number of patients who lack a sibling donor. Although the feasibility and effectiveness of using such allografts have been estab-

TABLE 25–4. Results of Interferon-α Therapy for CML in Chronic Phase

| Study | N | Cytogenetic Response* | | Median Survival (months) | | |
		Complete	Partial	All	Responders	Nonresponders
MDACC†	96	19%	7%	62	NA	NA
CALGB‡	107	13%	16%	66	NA	NA

CML, chronic myeloid leukemia; MDACC, M.D. Anderson Cancer Center; CALGB, Cancer and Leukemia Group B; NA, not applicable (in view of the time to achieve a cytogenetic response).
* Defined by percent of Ph-negative marrow metaphases achieved: complete response = 100%; partial response = 66% to 99% (MDACC) or 50% to 99% (CALGB).
† Interferon-α, partially pure (n = 51) 3 to 9 × 10^6 units/day, or recombinant (n = 45) 5 × 10^6 units/m² /day.[251]
‡ Interferon-α, recombinant 5 × 10^6 units/m² /day.[205]

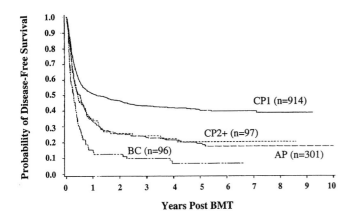

FIGURE 25–6. Disease-free survival after allogeneic BMT from unrelated donors for patients with CML according to disease status (CP, chronic phase; AP, accelerated phase; BC, blast crisis) at the time of transplantation. (From McGlave PB, Shu XO, Wen W, et al: Unrelated donor marrow transplantation for chronic myelogenous leukemia: 9 years' experience of the National Marrow Donor Program. Blood 2000; 95: 2219-2225. Copyright American Society of Hematology, used by permission.)

TABLE 25–5. Risk of Relapse after BMT for CML in Chronic Phase

	N	Relative Risk of Relapse
Allogeneic		
No GVHD	115	1.00
Acute GVHD only	267	1.15
Chronic GVHD only	45	0.28
Acute and chronic GVHD	164	0.24
Syngeneic	24	2.95
Allogeneic, T-cell depleted	154	5.14

BMT, bone marrow transplantation; CML, chronic myeloid leukemia; GVHD, graft-versus-host disease.

Data from the International Bone Marrow Transplant Registry, Horowitz MM, Gale RP, Sondel PM, et al: Graft-versus-leukemia reactions after bone marrow transplantation. Blood 1990; 75, 555.

lished (Fig. 25–6), the associated morbidity and mortality continue to pose significant challenges to their use.[113, 186] Nevertheless, with judicious selection, it is possible to identify patients for whom unrelated donor BMT is an appropriate treatment option early in the course of the disease.[113, 186]

By the late 1980s, procedures for the selective isolation of normal (i.e., Ph-negative) stem cells from patients with CML[51, 162] had advanced sufficiently to stimulate renewed interest in intensive therapy with autografting for chronic-phase disease. Accordingly, clinical studies to evaluate such autografts were undertaken. The feasibility of this approach has been established and, in some patients, Ph-negative hematopoiesis has been restored for prolonged periods.[10, 34] However, the value of the treatment in terms of effect on survival can be assessed only from the results of controlled studies. Such randomized trials were started but abandoned because of poor patient accrual. Thus, the case for autografting as a standard therapy in the management of CML remains unproved.

In the last decade, based on previous clinical studies of allogeneic BMT and interferon-α and laboratory studies of tyrosine kinase inhibition, four new treatments were introduced: infusion of donor leukocytes, a combination of interferon-α and chemotherapy, nonmyeloablative allografts, and the tyrosine kinase inhibitor STI571.

Early studies in Seattle indicated that patients who developed graft-versus-host disease (GVHD) after allogeneic BMT were less likely to have a recurrence of leukemia.[275, 276] Subsequent observations by the International Bone Marrow Transplant Registry,[130] on a large series that included patients who had received marrow depleted of donor T lymphocytes (in an attempt to prevent the severe forms of GVHD) as well as those who had syngeneic donors clearly demonstrated that the so-called graft-versus-leukemia (GVL) effect is potent in CML (Table 25–5). Against this background, in 1990 it was reported that for patients with recurrent CML after allogeneic BMT, infusion of leukocytes (obtained by leukapheresis) from the original donor could, without prior therapy, result in restoration of durable Ph-negative (i.e., donor) hematopoiesis.[159] The preliminary experience was confirmed,[160] and donor leukocyte infusion (DLI) has become a standard therapy for patients with recurrent CML after allogeneic BMT, although it can be complicated by marrow aplasia and GVHD.

Cytosine arabinoside, a pyrimidine nucleoside analogue, had been used to treat patients with CML: in the 1970s as part of combination chemotherapy regimens[55]; in the 1980s as a single agent[241] (in low dose); and later in combination with interferon-α.[146] In the early and middle 1990s, the French and Italian CML groups started randomized trials to evaluate the combination of interferon-α and cytosine arabinoside given by subcutaneous injection (see Table 25–2). Preliminary results from both trials[109, 223] showed a significantly improved survival at 3 years with interferon-α and cytosine arabinoside (French, 86%; Italian, 85%) than with interferon-α alone (French, 79%; Italian, 80%). This experience established the combination of interferon-α and cytosine arabinoside as an option for standard therapy, although side effects leading to discontinuation of treatment may be expected to occur in a substantial number of patients.

Appreciation that the GVL effect makes a significant contribution to the eradication of leukemia led to the development of a new strategy in allografting. This is based on a conditioning regimen that is sufficiently immunosuppressive to allow sustained engraftment of donor cells but does not ablate recipient myelopoiesis. After engraftment, the withdrawal of immunosuppression and, if necessary, the administration of DLI are modulated to convert mixed chimerism (i.e., recipient/donor hematopoiesis) early after allografting to a full chimeric state (i.e., exclusively donor hematopoiesis). It is hoped that these so-called nonmyeloablative allografts may significantly reduce the risk of transplant-related mortality while retaining the efficacy of the GVL effect. Pilot studies that include patients with CML began in the middle 1990s.[40, 239]

In the early 1990s, the search began for a small molecule that could inhibit the tyrosine kinase activity of BCR-ABL gene products. A process of screening identified a phenylaminopyrimidine derivative, then called CGP

57148, with a high degree of specificity for this kinase. This compound functions by competitive inhibition at the ATP-binding site of the BCR-ABL encoded kinase, thereby preventing phosphorylation of substrates involved in BCR-ABL signal transduction. After encouraging laboratory studies,[74] clinical evaluation of the now renamed signal-transduction inhibitor 571 (STI571), given by mouth, began in 1998.[73] Preliminary clinical trials included patients in chronic phase who had previously been treated with interferon-α. In these patients, it was demonstrated that STI571 could, within a matter of weeks, result in resolution of hematologic evidence of disease and, in a significant proportion, restore Ph-negative hematopoiesis. Furthermore, in addition to this impressive efficacy, STI571 was well tolerated. On the basis of this early experience, a randomized trial was started in 2000 to determine, in terms of survival, whether STI571 represents a significant advance in the primary therapy of CML (see Table 25-2).

Prognostication at Diagnosis

It is possible to classify patients with CML into different risk groups according to features of the disease at diagnosis.[147, 240, 242] The International CGL Prognosis Study Group identified age, spleen size, platelet count, and percentage of blasts in the blood as having independent prognostic significance for patients treated conventionally in the pre-interferon era.[240] A Cox model generated with these four variables was used to define risk groups. The median survival times of low- (36%), intermediate- (36%), and high- (28%) risk patients in this system (known as the Sokal classification) were 57, 44, and 34 months, respectively (Fig. 25-7).[37]

A new prognostic scoring system (based on age, spleen size, and counts of platelets, blasts, eosinophils, and basophils) has been developed by the Collaborative CML Prognostic Factors Project Group to estimate the survival

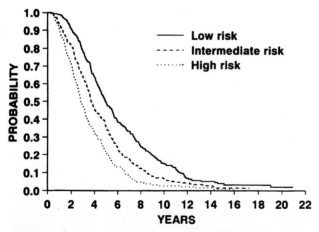

FIGURE 25-7. Survival of the low- (n = 293), intermediate- (n = 296) and high- (n = 224) risk subgroups of patients with CML according to the Sokal classification. (From Cervantes F, Robertson JE, Rozman C, et al: Long-term survivors in chronic granulocytic leukaemia: A study by the International CGL Prognosis Study Group. Br J Haematol 1994; 87: 293–300. Reprinted with permission from Blackwell Science Ltd.)

of patients treated with interferon-α. The Hasford score identifies three distinct groups of patients at low (40%), intermediate (45%), and high (15%) risk with median survival times of 98, 65, and 42 months, respectively.[116]

Thus, when large numbers of patients are monitored after therapy other than allogeneic BMT, a fairly broad range in survival times can be observed, in large part determined by the biology of the disease and predicted by clinical parameters at diagnosis. Patient selection may, therefore, be a significant confounding factor in the independent assessment of the effectiveness of a new treatment modality. In this regard, the value of carefully organized prospective randomized trials cannot be overstated.

Although at present it is common practice to use the Sokal or Hasford score to assign a risk category to patients at diagnosis, in the future biological features of CML cells may also play an important role in prognostication. For example, genetic heterogeneity in the form of large deletions adjacent to the translocation breakpoint of the derivative chromosome 9 have been reported to be associated with a poor prognosis, perhaps as a consequence of loss of one or more tumor suppressor genes.[236] In addition, the telomere length appears to be shorter in Ph-positive cells from patients in whom the clinically recognized duration of chronic phase is shorter, possibly heralding the onset of increased genetic instability.[31] Studies are under way to evaluate these predictions in prospective clinical trials.

Management of Chronic Phase Disease

Practical aspects of the treatments discussed in the preceding overview section will now be presented within the context of a strategy for the management of chronic phase disease and the development of a treatment algorithm.

Important general measures at presentation include the use of allopurinol (to avoid problems related to hyperuricemia) and adequate hydration. Also, when faced with the (unusual) situation of impending leukostasis, initial mechanical removal of cells by leukapheresis should be considered to facilitate a rapid reduction in the WBC and platelet counts.[175, 264] Leukapheresis can also be used to treat women who present during pregnancy[12, 84] when exposure to the potential teratogenic effect of chemotherapy should be avoided, if possible.

Hydroxyurea. The majority of patients with CML will receive hydroxyurea for a time, and in that sense it remains a mainstay of standard therapy.[119, 156] Although Ph-positive cells continue to predominate in the blood and marrow, hydroxyurea can usually control the overall tumor burden (as assessed by the WBC count and size of the spleen) during the chronic phase, with resolution of symptoms and restoration of the hemoglobin concentration to normal. Except for gastrointestinal symptoms (which are usually mild), stomatitis (rare), and dermatologic reactions,[157, 193] it is typically well tolerated. Furthermore, compared with busulfan, prior hydroxyurea therapy is relatively safe in terms of transplant-related mortality after allogeneic BMT[99] and does not preclude the satisfactory collection of stem cells for autografting.

For these reasons, hydroxyurea is useful at presentation of CML until a decision is made about more definitive therapy and when other treatments are poorly tolerated, ineffective, or considered inappropriate.

Interferon. Many patients with CML (including those on randomized trials [see Table 25–2]) receive interferon-α therapy.[150, 154, 173, 227, 254] Hematologic remission (resolution of clinical disease and return of peripheral counts to normal) can be achieved in the majority. In addition, varying amounts of reactivation of normal hematopoiesis may occur, with cytogenetic remission (66% to 100% Ph-negative cells in the marrow) in 10% to 35%. However, unpleasant side-effects—an influenza-like syndrome, fatigue, weakness, anorexia, depression, and others (e.g., dermatologic, hepatic, and neurologic)—are common and, although often dose-dependent, are prohibitive for about one quarter of patients. In this regard, a new formulation of interferon-α with the attachment of polyethylene glycol that prolongs the half-life (so that administration can be weekly rather than daily) may be better tolerated.[250]

Other agents have been used with interferon-α in an attempt to improve efficacy. The combination of interferon-α and cytosine arabinoside has gained acceptance, although patients are more likely to be intolerant of this than to interferon-α alone.[109] An oral preparation of cytosine arabinoside may provide a useful alternative to that given by subcutaneous injection.[163] Sequential therapy comprising the plant alkaloid homoharringtonine[199] and interferon-α has also been evaluated.[200]

Interferon-α has become a standard therapy because it offers a significant survival advantage over hydroxyurea.[41] However, this can be offset by toxicity, the extent of which may not be fully appreciated by the prescribing physician until the patient has been reviewed a few months after discontinuation of this agent. On the other hand, for patients who can tolerate interferon-α, it may be entirely appropriate treatment for prolonged periods (i.e., years) and, if necessary, it can be used during pregnancy.[6, 218] Furthermore, the achievement of cytogenetic remission (but nearly always with evidence of disease by molecular studies[126, 127]) identifies a group of patients with a favorable outlook. This has led to a strategy whereby some younger patients considering the possibility of an allogeneic BMT using an unrelated donor receive a 6–12-month trial of interferon-α early in the course of the disease. The response to interferon-α is then considered: if achievement of cytogenetic remission seems likely, continuation may be the more acceptable option; if achievement of cytogenetic remission seems unlikely, the risks of an unrelated donor BMT may be easier to accept. Relevant to this approach is the observation that a prior short trial of interferon-α is unlikely to affect adversely the outcome of allogeneic BMT.[93, 121] However, it seems reasonable to stop the interferon-α, and if necessary use hydroxyurea, for a few months before the transplant.[121]

STI571. The enthusiasm that greeted the introduction of the tyrosine kinase inhibitor STI571[73] has a number of explanations. First, it marked the advent of effective therapy based on knowledge of the molecular abnormality in CML. Second, the first trial demonstrated the unusual combination of impressive potency and mild toxicity.

Third, for the participating patients it was convenient (once-daily oral administration) and allowed freedom from the incapacitating side effects of interferon-α.

For patients with CML in chronic phase who have previously received interferon-α, STI571 can be expected to result in prompt achievement of hematologic remission for the majority and cytogenetic remission in about a third. The most common side effects are nausea, myalgias, edema, and diarrhea, but in most cases these are mild. Anemia, neutropenia, and thrombocytopenia as well as elevation of liver enzymes may necessitate a temporary interruption of therapy and/or a reduction in dose. These impressive results notwithstanding, for most patients follow-up has been short, and important information about long-term toxicity, survival benefit, and potential to cure is as yet unknown. It should, therefore, be considered a developmental (or experimental) rather than a standard therapy.

The results of the randomized trial comparing STI571 with the combination of interferon-α and cytosine arabinoside (see Table 25–2) will not be known for a few years. In the meantime, it would seem reasonable to use STI571 as a second-line therapy for patients who are intolerant of interferon-α or in whom this agent has failed to bring about a significant response. It is, however, highly likely (and understandable) that the proportion of patients deemed intolerant of interferon-α will increase if this policy is adopted. As an exception to this approach, perhaps a case could be made for using STI571 as first-line therapy in elderly patients with CML as the side effects of interferon-α can be particularly incapacitating in this group.

Allografting. Allogeneic stem cell transplantation (SCT), which includes the use of blood-[20, 235] as well as marrow-derived donor cells, is an established standard therapy for chronic-phase CML.[15, 88, 96, 183, 256, 267, 271] For younger patients (an upper age limit of 50 to 55 years being the generally accepted norm) with an HLA-identical sibling donor, the probability of long-term leukemia-free survival is about 50% to 60% (Fig. 25–8). Even for this selected group, however, the probability of transplant-related mortality is approximately 25%. The standard prescription for sibling donor SCT is: a conditioning regimen of high-dose cyclophosphamide with either TBI or high-dose busulfan[25, 44, 45, 65, 238]; an allograft that is replete with T-cells[98]; and a GVHD prophylaxis regimen of cyclosporine and methotrexate.[181] For the patient with a particularly enlarged spleen, it is reasonable to consider elective splenectomy before allografting as this may avoid delayed hematologic recovery[122] without otherwise influencing the post-transplant course.[144]

In an attempt to increase the applicability of allogeneic SCT, volunteer unrelated donors (including umbilical cord blood-derived cells[168]) have been used.[66, 70, 113, 123, 169, 170, 180, 186, 194] If all patients are considered (rather than subgroups), the probability of transplant-related mortality is double that of a sibling donor SCT, i.e., approximately 50% largely because of GVHD and associated infections. On the other hand, for patients who would otherwise not have a chance of cure and who are willing to accept these risks and the likelihood of a prolonged period of convalescence, the probability of long-term leukemia-free

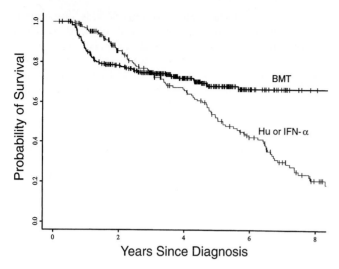

FIGURE 25–8. Survival of patients with CML who underwent allogeneic BMT from HLA-identical sibling donors within 1 year of diagnosis (BMT, n = 331, International Bone Marrow Transplant Registry) compared with those treated with hydroxyurea or interferon-α (Hu or IFN-α, n = 196, German CML Study Group). (From Gale RP, Hehlmann R, Zhang M-J, et al: Survival with bone marrow transplantation versus hydroxyurea or interferon for chronic myelogenous leukemia. Blood 1998; 91: 1810–1819. Copyright American Society of Hematology, used by permission.)

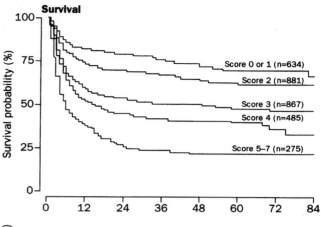

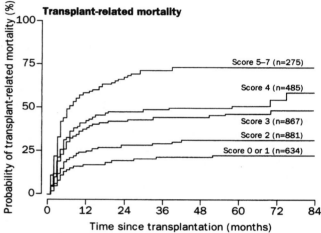

FIGURE 25–9. Survival and transplant-related mortality after allogeneic SCT for patients with CML according to pretransplant risk assessment score of the European Group for Blood and Marrow Transplantation. (From Gratwohl A, Hermans J, Goldman JM, et al: Risk assessment for patients with chronic myeloid leukaemia before allogeneic blood or marrow transplantation. Lancet 1998; 352: 1087–1092. Reprinted with permission from Elsevier Science.)

survival is about 35% to 45%. Nevertheless, an argument can be made for a more selective approach to the use of unrelated donor SCT. For younger patients (under 40 years) with closely matched donors (using high resolution histocompatibility testing[208]) transplanted early (within 1 year of diagnosis), the probability of transplant-related mortality is perhaps 25% to 30%[113, 186] and, although still significant, more acceptable.

In order to address the issue of risk assessment, the European Group for Blood and Marrow Transplantation has developed a scoring system based on five pretransplant variables (Table 25–6).[104] The risk assessment score (sum of the risk factor scores) allows the probability of transplant-related mortality and survival after allogeneic SCT to be determined for a given patient (Fig. 25-9).

TABLE 25–6. Risk Assessment before Allogeneic SCT for CML

	Risk Factor Score		
	0	1	2
Stage	CP1	AP	BP, ≥CP2
Age of patient (years)	<20	20–40	>40
Interval from diagnosis to BMT (months)	≤12	>12	
Patient/donor	Other	M/F	
Donor	SD	UD	

SCT, stem cell transplantation; CML, chronic myeloid leukemia; CP, chronic phase; AP, accelerated phase; BP, blast phase; BMT, bone marrow transplantation; other = any combination other than male patient/female donor; M, male; F, female; SD, HLA-identical sibling donor; UD, matched unrelated donor.

Developed by the European Group for Blood and Marrow Transplantation, Gratwohl A, Hermans J, Goldman JM et al; Risk assessment for patients with chronic myeloid leukaemia before allogeneic blood or marrow transplantation. Lancet 1998; 352: 1087.

This information is quite helpful when the risks and benefits of allogeneic SCT are discussed (see the algorithm).

The probability of developing recurrent disease (hematologic) after sibling donor SCT is approximately 20% to 25% (lower after unrelated donor SCT[113, 186]). For a few of these patients, it may be possible to stop immunosuppressive therapy (usually cyclosporine) abruptly and induce a GVL effect.[49] For most, however, other treatment options—hydroxyurea, interferon-α,[124, 247] second allogeneic SCT,[195] and DLI[160]—have to be considered.[3] DLI is highly effective in restoring remission[9, 11, 71, 160, 213] and has become the treatment of choice. There may be associated marrow aplasia and GVHD, although the likelihood of these complications is reduced if DLI is given at the time of (unequivocal[5, 266]) disease progression by cytogenetic and/or molecular studies[266] (i.e., before hematologic recurrence) and by the use of controlled doses[59, 178] (if necessary, escalated according to response) and selected subsets[2, 92] of donor lymphocytes. The majority of remissions are durable as assessed by molecular studies.[60] Indeed, this experience has led to the development of a new method of estimating the probability of leukemia-free survival after allografting that takes into account patients who develop recurrent disease and in whom remission is restored by DLI.[53]

Allogeneic SCT is the only treatment known to cure CML. It should be offered to suitable patients early in the course of the disease, if possible within the first year of diagnosis (Fig. 25–8).[88] New strategies[28] in allografting are directed toward making the procedure safer and applicable to a larger proportion of patients. Nonmyeloablative allografts[40, 239] are being evaluated in this context and should be regarded as developmental therapy.

Autografting. There is considerable experience of treating patients in the chronic phase with intensive therapy supported by autografting.[185] Cytogenetic remission may be achieved, but it is usually of short duration, and most patients continue with morphologic evidence of disease. The probability of procedure-related mortality is about 5% to 10%. It has been suggested that survival after such therapy is significantly longer than might be expected with conventional therapy (see Fig. 25–4).[185] However, randomized trials designed to confirm or refute this hypothesis have not been completed.

Experience with unirradiated granulocyte transfusions from donors with CML[105, 172, 176] as well as recent studies involving immunodeficient mice[273] and patients autografted with genetically marked cells[64] have provided evidence that the CML clone can be transplanted. In order to influence the genotype (i.e., leukemic or normal) of regenerating cells after grafting, in vitro[10, 35, 61, 184] and in vivo[24, 52, 219] strategies have been adopted to prepare autografts in which normal stem cells predominate. It is known that the achievement of cytogenetic remission after autografting depends on the content (i.e., Ph-positive versus Ph-negative cells) of the graft.[50, 252, 269] It seems likely, however, that the composition of the graft is influenced more by the biology of the disease, as assessed for example by the Sokal prognostic score[132] than the methodology employed for its collection. Therefore, although this approach has for some patients resulted in prolonged periods of Ph-negative hematopoiesis,[10, 34] the contribution of disease-related variables confounds an assessment of efficacy in comparison with other therapies.

The value of intensive therapy with autografting, therefore, remains unknown, and it should continue to be considered as a developmental therapy. Certainly, it comes as no surprise that the majority of patients develop recurrent disease after autografting, given that the GVL effect makes such an important contribution to eradication of CML after allografting. In this regard, new immunologic,[36] genetic,[280] and molecular[73] treatments could be used after autografting in an attempt to maintain cytogenetic remission.

Algorithm. It has become common practice to assemble expert panels to develop guidelines for the management of malignant diseases. The product of this exercise in CML[233, 249] provides a useful summary and consensus view of treatment in the late 1990s.

From the standpoint of the patient with CML, it is important to obtain a balanced overview of treatment options from a physician who is interested, knowledgeable, and experienced in the management of the disease (rather than a particular treatment). After a lengthy, inter-

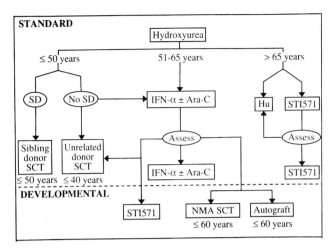

FIGURE 25–10. Proposed treatment algorithm for patients presenting with CML in chronic phase. Standard and developmental therapies are indicated as well as suggested upper age limits. SD = sibling donor (HLA-identical); IFN-α = interferon-α; Ara-C = cytosine arabinoside; Hu = hydroxyurea; NMA SCT = non-myeloablative allogeneic stem cell transplantation.

active discussion about the disease (including prognosis), as well as the risks and benefits of available therapies, the patient should receive a recommendation for treatment. In order to do this, the physician must acquire some understanding of the patient's character and circumstances as well as acknowledge the patient's opinion and ensure that it is appropriately informed. As there are a number of treatment options whose risks and benefits differ greatly, it is useful to have a framework for decision-making. One such treatment algorithm is presented in Figure 25–10.

Management of Transformed Disease

Transformation of CML to the blast phase may or may not be preceded by an accelerated phase (defined by diverse clinical and hematologic findings; see Table 25–1).

Accelerated Phase. For selected patients with accelerated-phase CML, allogeneic SCT offers a probability of long-term leukemia-free survival of about 30% to 40% for those with a sibling donor[46] (see Fig. 25–3) and 15% to 20% for those with an unrelated donor (see Fig. 25–6).[186] In patients with a sibling donor, the use of blood rather than marrow cells is preferable because of the lower probability of transplant-related mortality.[235]

For most patients, management of accelerated-phase disease should be directed toward specific problems: (1) a rising WBC or platelet count, despite increasing doses of hydroxyurea, may be controlled in the short term by the addition of or switch to another drug, such as busulfan, 6-mercaptopurine, cytosine arabinoside (given in low dose subcutaneously) or anagrelide[234] (a specific inhibitor of platelet production); (2) the patient with splenomegaly who is uncomfortable or suffering from cytopenia may benefit from splenectomy; (3) chloromas can be treated with radiotherapy; and (4) anemia and thrombocytopenia may require transfusions of blood and platelets. A relatively new agent, decitabine (a pyrimidine analogue that inhibits DNA methylation), has been shown to have activity in this phase of the disease.[149]

Blast Phase. Once the disease has transformed to a blast phase, the prognosis is dismal regardless of the therapy given, with an expected median survival of 3 to 4 months.[48, 148] An indication of the resistant nature of the blast phase subclone is that the probability of recurrence after allogeneic BMT for blast phase disease is approximately 60% (see Figs. 25–3 and 25–6). For the minority of patients eligible for allogeneic SCT, a reasonable strategy is to restrict this treatment to those in whom a second chronic phase can be achieved with appropriate combination chemotherapy (approximately 50%); for them the probability of long-term leukemia-free survival is similar to that for patients with accelerated phase disease (see Figs. 25–3 and 25–6). For the majority of patients, however, management of blast phase disease is with palliative intent.

It is important to determine the phenotype of the blast cells because this information indicates the type of chemotherapy that is likely to be most effective.[22, 107, 140] In most cases, the blasts have a myeloid phenotype, and for these patients, even with chemotherapy, the median survival is only 2 to 3 months. The presence of blasts with a lymphoid phenotype occurs in 20% to 30% of cases, and this disease is, at least in the short term, usually responsive to chemotherapy, which is reflected in the somewhat better outcome of this group, whose median survival is 6 to 8 months.

Myeloid blast phase is a highly resistant disease for which, in general, effective treatment does not exist. There is little to recommend the use of high-dose combination chemotherapy such as might be employed for de novo acute myelogenous leukemia.[151, 153, 225] Indeed, it is reasonable to give supportive care only with blood products as necessary and hydroxyurea with or without 6-mercaptopurine to control the blast count. Alternatively, cytosine arabinoside (given in low doses subcutaneously) can be useful. Preliminary experience with STI571 has been encouraging[72] and supports further evaluation in trials.

The lymphoid blast phase usually responds to the combination of vincristine and corticosteroids with or without an anthracycline.[140, 272] If a second chronic phase is achieved, further treatment with these agents can be given as consolidation therapy. Consideration should also be given to maintenance therapy with 6-mercaptopurine and, according to circumstances, central nervous system prophylaxis with intrathecal chemotherapy with or without cranial irradiation. Preliminary experience with STI571 suggests responses are common but of short duration.[72]

CONCLUSION

In the 1990s, interferon and allogeneic stem cell transplantation were the major advances in the treatment of CML. Recently a new therapy (the tyrosine kinase inhibitor STI571) and a new strategy (nonmyeloablative allografting) have been introduced. Both promise efficacy with reduced toxicity and have therefore been greeted with much enthusiasm. Preliminary experience with STI571 has been encouraging, but its effect on survival is unknown. Similarly, studies of nonmyeloablative allografting, which are the first in an iterative process to make allogeneic stem cell transplantation safer and applicable to more patients, are still at an early stage of development. Emerging novel strategies based on immunotherapy[202, 212] as well as molecular[63] and gene therapy[47] are likely to become candidates for clinical evaluation in the near future. Thus, the next decade will be an enthralling period for those involved in the management of patients with CML.

REFERENCES

1. Allan NC, Richards SM, Shepherd PCA on behalf of the UK Medical Research Council's Working Parties for Therapeutic Trials in Adult Leukaemia: UK Medical Research Council randomised, multicentre trial of interferon-αn1 for chronic myeloid leukaemia: Improved survival irrespective of cytogenetic response. Lancet 1995;345:1392.
2. Alyea EP, Soiffer RJ, Canning C, et al: Toxicity and efficacy of defined doses of CD4+ donor lymphocytes for treatment of relapse after allogeneic bone marrow transplant. Blood 1998;91:3671.
3. Arcese W, Goldman JM, D'Arcangelo E, et al: Outcome of patients who relapse after allogeneic bone marrow transplantation for chronic myeloid leukemia. Blood 1993;82:3211.
4. Aricò M, Biondi A, Pui C-H: Juvenile myelomonocytic leukemia. Blood 1997;90:479.
5. Arthur CK, Apperley JF, Guo AP, et al: Cytogenetic events after bone marrow transplantation for chronic myeloid leukemia in chronic phase. Blood 1988;71:1179.
6. Baer MR, Ozer H, Foon KA: Interferon-α therapy during pregnancy in chronic myelogenous leukaemia and hairy cell leukaemia. Br J Haematol 1992;81:167.
7. Baikie AG, Court-Brown WM, Buckton KE, et al: A possible specific chromosome abnormality in human chronic myeloid leukaemia. Nature 1960;188:1165.
8. Bain B, Catovsky D, O'Brien M, et al: Megakaryoblastic transformation of chronic granulocytic leukaemia: An electron microscopy and cytochemical study. J Clin Pathol 1977;30:235.
9. Bar BMAM, Schattenberg A, Mensink EJBM, et al: Donor leukocyte infusions for chronic myeloid leukemia relapsed after allogeneic bone marrow transplantation. J Clin Oncol 1993;11:513.
10. Barnett MJ, Eaves CJ, Phillips GL, et al: Autografting with cultured marrow in chronic myeloid leukemia: Results of a pilot study. Blood 1994;84:724.
11. Baumann H, Nagel S, Binder T, et al: Kinetics of the graft-versus-leukemia response after donor leukocyte infusions for relapsed chronic myeloid leukemia after allogeneic bone marrow transplantation. Blood 1998;92:3582.
12. Bazarbashi MS, Smith MR, Karanes C, et al: Successful management of Ph chromosome chronic myelogenous leukemia with leukapheresis during pregnancy. Am J Hematol 1991;38:235.
13. Beard MEJ, Durrant J, Catovsky D, et al: Blast crisis of chronic myeloid leukaemia (CML): Presentation simulating acute lymphoid leukaemia (ALL). Br J Haematol 1976;34:167.
14. Beatty PG, Ash R, Hows JM, et al: The use of unrelated bone marrow donors in the treatment of patients with chronic myelogenous leukemia: Experience of four marrow transplant centers. Bone Marrow Transplant 1989;4:287.
15. Beelen DW, Graeven U, Elmaagacli AH, et al: Prolonged administration of interferon-α in patients with chronic-phase Philadelphia chromosome-positive chronic myelogenous leukemia before allogeneic bone marrow transplantation may adversely affect transplant outcome. Blood 1995;85:2981.
16. Benelux CML Study Group: Randomized study on hydroxyurea

alone versus hydroxyurea combined with low-dose interferon-α2b for chronic myeloid leukemia. Blood 1998;91:2713.

17. Ben-Neriah Y, Daley GQ, Mes-Masson A-M, et al: The chronic myelogenous leukemia-specific P210 protein is the product of the *bcr/abl* hybrid gene. Science 1986;233:212.

18. Bennett JH: Case of hypertrophy of the spleen and liver, in which death took place from suppuration of the blood. Edinb Med Surg J 1845;64:413.

19. Bennett JM, Catovsky D, Daniel MT, et al: The chronic myeloid leukaemias: Guidelines for distinguishing chronic granulocytic, atypical chronic myeloid, and chronic myelomonocytic leukaemia. Br J Haematol 1994;87:746.

20. Bensinger WI, Martin PJ, Storer B, et al: Transplantation of bone marrow as compared with peripheral blood cells from HLA-identical relatives in patients with hematologic cancers. N Engl J Med 2001;344:175.

21. Bernheim A, Berger R, Preud'Homme JL, et al: Philadelphia chromosome–positive blood B lymphocytes in chronic myelocytic leukemia. Leuk Res 1981;5:331.

22. Bettelheim P, Lutz D, Majdic O, et al: Cell lineage heterogeneity in blast crisis of chronic myeloid leukaemia. Br J Haematol 1985;59:395.

23. Bhatia R, Verfaillie CM, Miller JS, et al: Autologous transplantation therapy for chronic myelogenous leukemia. Blood 1997;89:2623.

24. Biernaux C, Loos M, Sels A, et al: Detection of major *bcr-abl* gene expression at a very low level in blood cells of some healthy individuals. Blood 1995;86:3118.

25. Biggs JC, Szer J, Crilley P, et al: Treatment of chronic myeloid leukemia with allogeneic bone marrow transplantation after preparation with BuCy2. Blood 1992;80:1352.

26. Boggs DR: Hematopoietic stem cell theory in relation to possible lymphoblastic conversion of chronic myeloid leukemia. Blood 1974;44:449.

27. Boice JD Jr, Blettner M, Kleinerman RA, et al: Radiation dose and leukemia risk in patients treated for cancer of the cervix. J Natl Cancer Inst 1987;79:1295.

28. Bonini C, Ferrari G, Verzeletti S, et al: HSV-TK gene transfer into donor lymphocytes for control of allogeneic graft-versus-leukemia. Science 1997;276:1719.

29. Bose S, Deininger M, Gora-Tybor J, et al: The presence of typical and atypical bcr-abl fusion genes in leukocytes of normal individuals: Biologic significance and implications for the assessment of minimal residual disease. Blood 1998;92:3362.

30. Brito-Babapulle F, Bowcock SJ, Marcus RE, et al: Autografting for patients with chronic myeloid leukaemia in chronic phase: Peripheral blood stem cells may have a finite capacity for maintaining haemopoiesis. Br J Haematol 1989;73:76.

31. Brümmendorf TH, Holyoake TL, Rufer N, et al: Prognostic implications of differences in telomere length between normal and malignant cells from patients with chronic myeloid leukemia measured by flow cytometry. Blood 2000;95:1883.

32. Buckner CD, Clift RA, Fefer A, et al: Treatment of blastic transformation of chronic granulocytic leukemia by high dose cyclophosphamide, total body irradiation and infusion of cryopreserved autologous marrow. Exp Hematol 1974;2:138.

33. Buckner CD, Stewart P, Clift RA, et al: Treatment of blastic transformation of chronic granulocytic leukemia by chemotherapy, total body irradiation and infusion of cryopreserved autologous marrow. Exp Hematol 1978;6:96.

34. Carella AM, Lerma E, Consetti MT, et al: Autografting with Philadelphia chromosome–negative mobilized hematopoietic progenitor cells in chronic myelogenous leukemia. Blood 1999;93:1534.

35. Carlo-Stella C, Mangoni L, Almici C, et al: Autologous transplant for chronic myelogenous leukemia using marrow treated ex vivo with mafosfamide. Bone Marrow Transplant 1994;14:425.

36. Cervantes F, Pierson BA, McGlave PB, et al: Autologous activated natural killer cells suppress primitive chronic myelogenous leukemia progenitors in long-term culture. Blood 1996;87:2476.

37. Cervantes F, Robertson JE, Rozman C, et al: Long-term survivors in chronic granulocytic leukaemia: A study by the International CGL Prognosis Study Group. Br J Haematol 1994;87:293.

38. Chan LC, Furley AJ, Ford AM, et al: Clonal rearrangement and expression of the T-cell receptor β gene and involvement of the breakpoint cluster region in blast crisis of CGL. Blood 1986;67:533.

39. Chervenick PA, Ellis LD, Pan SF, et al: Human leukemic cells: In vitro growth of colonies containing the Philadelphia (Ph[1]) chromosome. Science 1971;174:1134.

40. Childs R, Clave E, Contentin N, et al: Engraftment kinetics after nonmyeloablative allogeneic peripheral blood stem cell transplantation: Full donor T-cell chimerism precedes alloimmune responses. Blood 1999;94, 3234.

41. Chronic Myeloid Leukemia Trialists' Collarborative Group: Interferon alfa versus chemotherapy for chronic myeloid leukemia: A meta-analysis of seven randomized trials. J Natl Cancer Inst 1997;89:1616.

42. Clarkson B: Chronic myelogenous leukemia: Is aggressive treatment indicated? J Clin Oncol 1985;3:135.

43. Clift RA, Appelbaum FR, Thomas ED: Treatment of chronic myeloid leukemia by marrow transplantation. Blood 1993;82:1954.

44. Clift RA, Buckner CD, Appelbaum FR, et al: Allogeneic marrow transplantation in patients with chronic myeloid leukemia in the chronic phase: A randomized trial of two irradiation regimens. Blood 1991;77:1660.

45. Clift RA, Buckner CD, Thomas ED, et al: Marrow transplantation for chronic myeloid leukemia: A randomized study comparing cyclophosphamide and total body irradiation with busulfan and cyclophosphamide. Blood 1994;84:2036.

46. Clift RA, Buckner CD, Thomas ED, et al: Marrow transplantation for patients in accelerated phase of chronic myeloid leukemia. Blood 1994;84:4368.

47. Cobaleda C, Sánchez-Garcia I: In vivo inhibition by a site-specific catalytic RNA subunit of RNase P designed against the BCR-ABL oncogenic products: A novel approach for cancer treatment. Blood 2000;95:731.

48. Coleman M, Silver RT, Pajak TF, et al: Combination chemotherapy for terminal-phase chronic granulocytic leukemia: Cancer and Leukemia Group B Studies. Blood 1980;55:29.

49. Collins RH, Rogers ZR, Bennett M, et al: Hematologic relapse of chronic myelogenous leukemia following allogeneic bone marrow transplantation: Apparent graft-versus-leukemia effect following abrupt discontinuation of immunosuppression. Bone Marrow Transplant 1992;10:391.

50. Corsetti MT, Lerma E, Dejana A, et al: Cytogenetic response to autografting in chronic myelogenous leukemia correlates with the amount of BCR-ABL positive cells in the graft. Exp Hematol 2000;28:104.

51. Coulombel L, Kalousek DK, Eaves CJ, et al: Long-term marrow culture reveals chromosomally normal hematopoietic progenitor cells in patients with Philadelphia chromosome–positive chronic myelogenous leukemia. N Engl J Med 1983;308:1493.

52. Coutinho LH, Brereton ML, Santos AMW, et al: Evaluation of cytogenetic conversion to Ph− haemopoiesis in long-term bone marrow culture for patients with chronic myeloid leukaemia on conventional hydroxyurea therapy, on pulse high-dose hydroxyurea and on interferon-alpha. Br J Haematol 1996;93:869.

53. Craddock C, Szydlo RM, Klein JP, et al: Estimating leukemia-free survival after allografting for chronic myeloid leukemia: A new method that takes into account patients who relapse and are restored to complete remission. Blood 2000;96:86.

54. Craigie D: Case of disease of the spleen, in which death took place in consequence of the presence of purulent matter in the blood. Edinb Med Surg J 1845;64:400.

55. Cunningham I, Gee T, Dowling M, et al: Results of treatment of Ph[1] + chronic myelogenous leukemia with an intensive treatment regimen (L-5 protocol). Blood 1979;53:375.

56. Curtis RE, Boice JD Jr, Stovall M, et al: Relationship of leukemia risk to radiation dose following cancer of the uterine corpus. J Natl Cancer Inst 1994;86:1315.

57. Daley GQ, Van Etten RA, Baltimore D: Induction of chronic myelogenous leukemia in mice by the P210[bcr/abl] gene of the Philadelphia chromosome. Science 1990;247:824.

58. Dameshek W: Some speculations on the myeloproliferative syndromes. Blood 1951;6:372.

59. Dazzi F, Szydlo RM, Craddock C, et al: Comparison of single-dose and escalating-dose regimens of donor lymphocyte infusion for relapse after allografting for chronic myeloid leukemia. Blood 2000;95:67.

60. Dazzi F, Szydlo RM, Cross NCP, et al: Durability of responses following donor lymphocyte infusions for patients who relapse

after allogeneic stem cell transplantation for chronic myeloid leukemia. Blood 2000;96:2712.

61. de Fabritiis P, Petti MC, Montefusco E, et al: BCR-ABL antisense oligodeoxynucleotide in vitro purging and autologous bone marrow transplantation for patients with chronic myelogenous leukemia in advanced phase. Blood 1998;91:3156.

62. de Klein A, Geurts van Kessel A, Grosveld G, et al: A cellular oncogene is translocated to the Philadelphia chromosome in chronic myelocytic leukaemia. Nature 1982;300:765.

63. Deininger MWN, Goldman JM, Melo JV: The molecular biology of chronic myeloid leukemia. Blood 2000;96:3343.

64. Deisseroth AB, Zu Z, Claxton D, et al: Genetic marking shows that Ph+ cells present in autologous transplants of chronic myelogenous leukemia (CML) contribute to relapse after autologous bone marrow in CML. Blood 1994;83:3068.

65. Devergie A, Blaise D, Attal M, et al: Allogeneic bone marrow transplantation for chronic myeloid leukemia in first chronic phase: A randomized trial of busulfan-cytoxan versus cytoxan-total body irradiation as preparative regimen: A report from the French Society of Bone Marrow Graft (SFGM). Blood 1995;85:2263.

66. Dini G, Lamparelli T, Rondelli R, et al: Unrelated donor marrow transplantation for chronic myelogenous leukaemia. Br J Haematol 1998;102:544.

67. Doney K, Buckner CD, Sale GE, et al: Treatment of chronic granulocytic leukemia by chemotherapy, total body irradiation and allogeneic bone marrow transplantation. Exp Hematol 1978;6:738.

68. Doney KC, Buckner CD, Thomas ED, et al: Allogeneic bone marrow transplantation for chronic granulocytic leukemia. Exp Hematol 1981;9:966.

69. Dosik H, Rosner F, Sawitsky A: Acquired lipidosis: Gaucher-like cells and "blue cells" in chronic granulocytic leukemia. Semin Hematol 1972;9:309.

70. Drobyski WR, Ash RC, Casper JT, et al: Effect of T-cell depletion as graft-versus-host disease prophylaxis on engraftment, relapse, and disease-free survival in unrelated marrow transplantation for chronic myelogenous leukemia. Blood 1994;83:1980.

71. Drobyski WR, Keever CA, Roth MS, et al: Salvage immunotherapy using donor leukocyte infusions as treatment for relapsed chronic myelogenous leukemia after allogeneic bone marrow transplantation: Efficacy and toxicity of a defined T-cell dose. Blood 1993; 82:2310.

72. Druker BJ, Sawyers CL, Kantarjian H, et al: Activity of a specific inhibitor of the BCR-ABL tyrosine kinase in the blast crisis of chronic myeloid leukemia and acute lymphoblastic leukemia with the Philadelphia chromsome. N Engl J Med 2001;344:1038.

73. Druker BJ, Talpaz M, Resta DJ, et al: Efficacy and safety of a specific inhibitor of the BCR-ABL tyrosine kinase in chronic myeloid leukemia. N Engl J Med 2001;344:1031.

74. Druker BJ, Tamura S, Buchdunger E, et al: Effects of a selective inhibitor of the abl tyrosine kinase on the growth of bcr-abl positive cells. Nat Med 1996;2:561.

75. Dubé ID, Arlin ZA, Kalousek DK, et al: Nonclonal hemopoietic progenitor cells detected in long-term marrow cultures from a Turner syndrome mosaic with chronic myeloid leukemia. Blood 1984;64:1284.

76. Eaves AC, Barnett MJ, Ponchio L, et al: Differences between normal and CML stem cells: Potential targets for clinical exploitation. Stem Cells 1998;16:77.

77. Eaves CJ, Eaves AC: Progenitor cell dynamics. In Carella AM, Daley GQ, Eaves CJ, Goldman JM, Hehlmann R (eds): Chronic Myeloid Leukaemia: Biology and Treatment. London, Martin Dunitz Ltd, 2001, 73.

78. Elefanty AG, Hariharan IK, Cory S: bcr-abl, the hallmark of chronic myeloid leukaemia in man, induces multiple haemopoietic neoplasms in mice. EMBO J 1990;9:1069.

79. Fefer A, Cheever MA, Greenberg PD, et al: Treatment of chronic granulocytic leukemia with chemoradiotherapy and transplantation of marrow from identical twins. N Engl J Med 1982;306:63.

80. Fefer A, Cheever MA, Thomas ED, et al: Disappearance of Ph1-positive cells in four patients with chronic granulocytic leukemia after chemotherapy, irradiation and marrow transplantation from an identical twin. N Engl J Med 1979;300:333.

81. Fefer A, Radich J, Pavletic Z, et al: Syngeneic bone marrow transplantation (BMT) for chronic myelogenous leukemia in chronic phase: Update of the original 14 Seattle patients, including PCR results. Blood 1994;84:252a.

82. Fialkow PJ, Gartler SM, Yoshida A: Clonal origin of chronic myelocytic leukemia in man. Proc Natl Acad Sci U S A 1967;58:1468.

83. Fishbein WN, Carbone PP, Freireich EJ, et al: Clinical trials of hydroxyurea in patients with cancer and leukemia. Clin Pharmacol Ther 1964; 5:574.

84. Fitzgerald D, Rowe JM, Heal J: Leukapheresis for control of chronic myelogenous leukemia during pregnancy. Am J Hematol 1986; 22:213.

85. Folley JH, Borges W, Yamawaki T: Incidence of leukemia in survivors of the atomic bomb in Hiroshima and Nagasaki, Japan. Am J Med 1952;13:311.

86. Forkner CE, McNair Scott TF: Arsenic as a therapeutic agent in chronic myelogenous leukemia. JAMA 1931;97:3.

87. Frassoni F, Podestà M, Piaggio G, et al: Normal primitive haematopoietic progenitors are more frequent than their leukaemic counterpart in newly diagnosed patients with chronic myeloid leukaemia but rapidly decline with time. Br J Haematol 1999;104:538.

88. Gale RP, Hehlmann R, Zhang M-J, et al: Survival with bone marrow transplantation versus hydroxyurea or interferon for chronic myelogenous leukemia. Blood 1998;91:1810.

89. Galton DAG: Myleran in chronic myeloid leukaemia: Results of treatment. Lancet 1953;1:208.

90. Ganesan TS, Rassool F, Guo A-P, et al: Rearrangement of the bcr gene in Philadelphia chromosome-negative chronic myeloid leukemia. Blood 1986;68:957.

91. Geary CG, Catovsky D, Wiltshaw E, et al: Chronic myelomonocytic leukaemia. Br J Haematol 1975;30:289.

92. Giralt S, Hester J, Huh Y, et al: CD8-depleted donor lymphocyte infusion as treatment for relapsed chronic myelogenous leukemia after allogeneic bone marrow transplantation. Blood 1995;86: 4337.

93. Giralt S, Szydlo R, Goldman JM, et al: Effect of short-term interferon therapy on the outcome of subsequent HLA-identical sibling bone marrow transplantation for chronic myelogenous leukemia: An analysis from the International Bone Marrow Transplant Registry. Blood 2000;95:410.

94. Goh K, Swisher SN: Identical twins and chronic myelocytic leukemia: Chromosomal studies of a patient with chronic myelocytic leukemia and his normal identical twin. Arch Intern Med 1965; 115:475.

95. Goh K, Swisher SN, Herman EC Jr: Chronic myelocytic leukemia and identical twins: Additional evidence of the Philadelphia chromosome as postzygotic abnormality. Arch Intern Med 1967;120: 214.

96. Goldman JM, Apperley JF, Jones L, et al: Bone marrow transplantation for patients with chronic myeloid leukemia. N Engl J Med 1986;314:202.

97. Goldman JM, Catovsky D, Hows J, et al: Cryopreserved peripheral blood cells functioning as autografts in patients with chronic granulocytic leukaemia in transformation. Br Med J 1979;1:1310.

98. Goldman JM, Gale RP, Horowitz MM, et al: Bone marrow transplantation for chronic myelogenous leukemia in chronic phase: Increased risk for relapse associated with T-cell depletion. Ann Intern Med 1988;108:806.

99. Goldman JM, Szydlo R, Horowitz MM, et al: Choice of pretransplant treatment and timing of transplants for chronic myelogenous leukemia in chronic phase. Blood 1993;82:2235.

100. Gomez G, Hossfeld DK, Sokal JE: Removal of abnormal clone of leukaemic cells by splenectomy. Br Med J 1975;2:421.

101. Goto T, Nishikori M, Arlin Z, et al: Growth characteristics of leukemic and normal hematopoietic cells in Ph1+ chronic myelogenous leukemia and effects of intensive treatment. Blood 1982; 59:793.

102. Gralnick HR, Harbor J, Vogel C: Myelofibrosis in chronic granulocytic leukemia. Blood 1971;37:152.

103. Gramatzki M, Bartram CR, Müller D, et al: Early T-cell differentiated chronic myeloid leukemia blast crisis with rearrangement of the breakpoint cluster region but not of the T-cell receptor β chain genes. Blood 1987;69:1082.

104. Gratwohl A, Hermans J, Goldman JM, et al: Risk assessment for patients with chronic myeloid leukaemia before allogeneic blood or marrow transplantation. Lancet 1998;352:1087.

105. Graw RG Jr, Buckner CD, Whang-Peng J, et al: Complication of bone-marrow transplantation: Graft-versus-host disease resulting from chronic-myelogenous-leukaemia leucocyte transfusions. Lancet 1970;2:338.

106. Griffin JD, Tantravahi R, Canellos GP, et al: T-cell surface antigens in a patient with blast crisis of chronic myeloid leukemia. Blood 1983;61:640.

107. Griffin JD, Todd RF III, Ritz J, et al: Differentiation patterns in the blastic phase of chronic myeloid leukemia. Blood 1983;61:85.

108. Groffen J, Stephenson JR, Heisterkamp N, et al: Philadelphia chromosomal breakpoints are clustered within a limited region, *bcr,* on chromosome 22. Cell 1984;36:93.

109. Guilhot F, Chastang C, Michallet M, et al: Interferon alfa-2b combined with cytarabine versus interferon alone in chronic myelogenous leukemia. N Engl J Med 1997;337:223.

110. Haddow A, Timmis GM: Myleran in chronic myeloid leukaemia: Chemical constitution and biological action. Lancet 1953;1:207.

111. Haferlach T, Winkemann M, Nickenig C, et al: Which compartments are involved in Philadelphia–chromosome positive chronic myeloid leukaemia? An answer at the single cell level by combining May-Grünwald-Giemsa staining and fluorescence in situ hybridization techniques. Br J Haematol 1997;97:99.

112. Haines ME, Goldman JM, Worsley AM, et al: Chemotherapy and autografting for chronic granulocytic leukaemia in transformation: Probable prolongation of survival for some patients. Br J Haematol 1984;58:711.

113. Hansen JA, Gooley TA, Martin PJ, et al: Bone marrow transplants from unrelated donors for patients with chronic myeloid leukemia. N Engl J Med 1998;338:962.

114. Hardisty RM, Speed DE, Till M: Granulocytic leukaemia in childhood. Br J Haematol 1964;10:551.

115. Harris NL, Jaffe ES, Diebold J, et al: World Health Organization classification of neoplastic diseases of the hematopoietic and lymphoid tissues: Report of the Clinical Advisory Committee meeting - Airlie House, Virginia, November 1997. J Clin Oncol 1999;17:3835.

116. Hasford J, Pfirrmann M, Hehlmann R, et al: A new prognostic score for survival of patients with chronic myeloid leukemia treated with interferon alfa. J Natl Cancer Inst 1998;90:850.

117. Hayhoe FGJ, Kok D: Medullary aplasia in chronic myeloid leukaemia during busulfan therapy. Br Med J 1957;2:1468.

118. Heard BE, Cooke RA: Busulfan lung. Thorax 1968;23:187.

119. Hehlmann R, Heimpel H, Hasford J, et al: Randomized comparison of busulfan and hydroxyurea in chronic myelogenous leukemia: Prolongation of survival by hydroxyurea. Blood 1993;82:398.

120. Hehlmann R, Heimpel H, Hasford J, et al: Randomized comparison of interferon-α with busulfan and hydroxyurea in chronic myelogenous leukemia. Blood 1994;84:4064.

121. Hehlmann R, Hochhaus A, Kolb H-J, et al: Interferon-α before allogeneic bone marrow transplantation in chronic myelogenous leukemia does not affect outcome adversely, provided it is discontinued at least 90 days before the procedure. Blood 1999;94:3668.

122. Helenglass G, Treleaven J, Parikh P, et al: Delayed engraftment associated with splenomegaly in patients undergoing bone marrow transplantation for chronic myeloid leukaemia. Bone Marrow Transplant 1990;5:247.

123. Hessner MJ, Endean DJ, Casper JT, et al: Use of unrelated marrow grafts compensates for reduced graft-versus-leukemia reactivity after T–cell-depleted allogeneic marrow transplantation for chronic myelogenous leukemia. Blood 1995;86:3987.

124. Higano CS, Raskind WH, Singer JW: Use of interferon for the treatment of relapse of chronic myelogenous leukemia in chronic phase after allogeneic bone marrow transplantation. Blood 1992;80:1437.

125. Hilts SV, Shaw CC: Leukemoid blood reactions. N Engl J Med 1953;249:434.

126. Hochhaus A, Lin F, Reiter A, et al: Quantification of residual disease in chronic myelogenous leukemia patients on interferon-α therapy by competitive polymerase chain reaction. Blood 1996;87:1549.

127. Hochhaus A, Reiter A, Saussele S, et al: Molecular heterogeneity in complete cytogenetic responders after interferon-α therapy for chronic myelogenous leukemia: Low levels of minimal residual disease are associated with continuing remission. Blood 2000;95:62.

128. Hogge DE, Coulombel L, Kalousek DK, et al: Nonclonal hemopoietic progenitors in a G6PD heterozygote with chronic myelogenous leukemia revealed after long-term marrow culture. Am J Hematol 1987;24:389.

129. Holyoake T, Jiang X, Eaves C, et al: Isolation of a highly quiescent subpopulation of primitive leukemic cells in chronic myeloid leukemia. Blood 1999;94:2056.

130. Horowitz MM, Gale RP, Sondel PM, et al: Graft-versus-leukemia reactions after bone marrow transplantation. Blood 1990;75:555.

131. Hoyle C, Gray R, Goldman J: Autografting for patients with CML in chronic phase: An update. Br J Haematol 1994;86:76.

132. Hughes TP, Grigg A, Szer J, et al: Mobilization of predominantly Philadelphia chromosome–negative blood progenitors using cyclophosphamide and rHUG-CSF in early chronic-phase chronic myeloid leukaemia: Correlation with Sokal prognostic index and haematological control. Br J Haematol 1997;96:635.

133. Ichimaru M, Ishimaru T, Mikami M, et al: Incidence of Leukemia in a Fixed Cohort of Atomic Bomb Survivors and Controls, Hiroshima and Nagasaki October 1950–December 1978. Technical Report RERF TR 13-81. Hiroshima, Radiation Effects Research Foundation, 1981.

134. Italian Cooperative Study Group on Chronic Myeloid Leukemia: Interferon alfa-2a as compared with conventional chemotherapy for the treatment of chronic myeloid leukemia. N Engl J Med 1994;330:820.

135. Italian Cooperative Study Group on Chronic Myeloid Leukemia: Long-term follow-up of the Italian trial of interferon-α versus conventional chemotherapy in chronic myeloid leukemia. Blood 1998;92:1541.

136. Italian Cooperative Study Group on Chronic Myeloid Leukemia: Results of a prospective randomized trial of early splenectomy in chronic myeloid leukemia. Cancer 1984;54:333.

137. Jacobs EM, Luce JK, Cailleau R: Chromosome abnormalities in human cancer: Report of a patient with chronic myelocytic leukemia and his nonleukemic monozygotic twin. Cancer 1966;19:869.

138. Janossy G, Greaves MF, Revesz T, et al: Blast crisis of chronic myeloid leukaemia (CML): Cell surface marker analysis of "lymphoid" and myeloid cases. Br J Haematol 1976;34:179.

139. Janossy G, Roberts M, Greaves MF: Target cell in chronic myeloid leukaemia and its relationship to acute lymphoid leukaemia. Lancet 1976;2:1058.

140. Janossy G, Woodruff RK, Pippard MJ, et al: Relation of "lymphoid" phenotype and response to chemotherapy incorporating vincristine-prednisolone in the acute phase of Ph¹-positive leukemia. Cancer 1979;43:426.

141. Jiang X, Fujisaki T, Nicolini F, et al: Autonomous multi-lineage differentiation in vitro of primitive CD34+ cells from patients with chronic myeloid leukemia. Leukemia 2000;14:1112.

142. Jiang X, Lopez A, Holyoake T, et al: Autocrine production and action of IL-3 and granulocyte colony-stimulating factor in chronic myeloid leukemia. Proc Natl Acad Sci U S A 1999;96:12804.

143. Jonas D, Lubbert M, Kawasaki ES, et al: Clonal analysis of *bcr-abl* rearrangement in T lymphocytes from patients with chronic myelogenous leukemia. Blood 1992;79:1017.

144. Kalhs P, Schwarzinger I, Anderson G, et al: A retrospective analysis of the long-term effect of splenectomy on late infections, graft-versus-host disease, relapse, and survival after allogeneic marrow transplantation for chronic myelogenous leukemia. Blood 1995;86:2028.

145. Kandel EV, LeRoy GV: Chronic arsenical poisoning during the treatment of chronic myeloid leukemia. Arch Intern Med 1937;60:846.

146. Kantarjian HM, Keating MJ, Estey EH, et al: Treatment of advanced stages of Philadelphia chromosome–positive chronic myelogenous leukemia with interferon-α and low-dose cytarabine. J Clin Oncol 1992;10:772.

147. Kantarjian HM, Keating MJ, Smith TL, et al: Proposal for a simple synthesis prognostic staging system in chronic myelogenous leukemia. Am J Med 1990;88:1.

148. Kantarjian HM, Keating MJ, Talpaz M, et al: Chronic myelogenous leukemia in blast crisis: Analysis of 242 patients. Am J Med 1987;83:445.

149. Kantarjian HM, O'Brien SM, Keating M, et al: Results of decitabine therapy in the accelerated and blastic phases of chronic myelogenous leukemia. Leukemia 1997;11:1617.

150. Kantarjian HM, Smith TL, O'Brien S, et al: Prolonged survival in chronic myelogenous leukemia after cytogenetic response to interferon-α therapy. Ann Intern Med 1995;122:254.

151. Kantarjian HM, Talpaz M, Kontoyiannis D, et al: Treatment of chronic myelogenous leukemia in accelerated and blastic phases

with daunorubicin, high-dose cytarabine, and granulocyte-macrophage colony-stimulating factor. J Clin Oncol 1992;10:398.

152. Kantarjian HM, Vellekoop L, McCredie KB, et al: Intensive combination chemotherapy (ROAP 10) and splenectomy in the management of chronic myelogenous leukemia. J Clin Oncol 1985;3:192.

153. Kantarjian HM, Walters RS, Keating MJ, et al: Treatment of the blastic phase of chronic myelogenous leukemia with mitoxantrone and high-dose cytosine arabinoside. Cancer 1988;62:672.

154. Kattan MW, Inoue Y, Giles FJ, et al: Cost-effectiveness of interferon-α and conventional chemotherapy in chronic myelogenous leukemia. Ann Intern Med 1996;125:541.

155. Kelliher MA, McLaughlin J, Witte ON, et al: Induction of a chronic myelogenous leukemia-like syndrome in mice with v-abl and BCR/ABL. Proc Natl Acad Sci U S A 1990;87:6649.

156. Kennedy BJ: Hydroxyurea therapy in chronic myelogenous leukemia. Cancer 1972;29:1052.

157. Kennedy BJ, Smith LR, Goltz RW: Skin changes secondary to hydroxyurea therapy. Arch Dermatol 1975;111:183.

158. Kennedy BJ, Yarbro JW: Metabolic and therapeutic effects of hydroxyurea in chronic myeloid leukemia. JAMA 1966;195:1038.

159. Kolb H-J, Mittermuller J, Clemm C, et al: Donor leukocyte transfusions for treatment of recurrent chronic myelogenous leukemia in marrow transplant patients. Blood 1990;76:2462.

160. Kolb H-J, Schattenberg A, Goldman JM, et al: Graft-versus-leukemia effect of donor lymphocyte transfusions in marrow grafted patients. Blood 1995;86:2041.

161. Konopka JB, Witte ON: Detection of c-abl tyrosine kinase activity in vitro permits direct comparison of normal and altered *abl* gene products. Mol Cell Biol 1985;5:3116.

162. Korbling M, Burke P, Braine H, et al: Successful engraftment of blood-derived normal hemopoietic stem cells in chronic myelogenous leukemia. Exp Hematol 1981;9:684.

163. Kühr T, Eisterer W, Apfelbeck U, et al: Treatment of patients with advanced chronic myelogenous leukemia with interferon-alpha-2b and continuous oral cytarabine ocfosfate (YNK01): A pilot study. Leuk Res 2000;24:583.

164. Kurzrock R, Blick MB, Talpaz M, et al: Rearrangement in the breakpoint cluster region and the clinical course in Philadelphia-negative chronic myelogenous leukemia. Ann Intern Med 1986;105:673.

165. Kwong YL, Todd D: Delicious poison: Arsenic trioxide for the treatment of leukemia. Blood 1997;89:3487.

166. Kyle RA, Schwartz RS, Oliner HL, et al: A syndrome resembling adrenal cortical insufficiency associated with long-term busulfan (Myleran) therapy. Blood 1961;18:497.

167. Lange RD, Moloney WC, Yamawaki T: Leukemia in atomic bomb survivors: General observations. Blood 1954;9:574.

168. Laporte J-P, Gorin N-C, Rubinstein P, et al: Cord-blood transplantation from an unrelated donor in an adult with chronic myelogenous leukemia. N Engl J Med 1996;335:167.

169. Lee SJ, Anasetti C, Kuntz KM, et al: The costs and cost-effectiveness of unrelated donor bone marrow transplantation for chronic phase chronic myelogenous leukemia. Blood 1998;92:4047.

170. Lee SJ, Kuntz KM, Horowitz MM, et al: Unrelated donor bone marrow transplantation for chronic myelogenous leukemia: A decision analysis. Ann Intern Med 1997;127:1080.

171. Leonard BJ, Israels MCG, Wilkinson JF: Alkaline phosphatase in the white cells in leukaemia and leukaemoid reactions. Lancet 1958;1:289.

172. Levin RH, Whang J, Tjio JH, et al: Persistent mitosis of transfused homologous leukocytes in children receiving antileukemic therapy. Science 1963;142:1305.

173. Liberato NL, Quaglini S, Barosi G: Cost-effectiveness of interferon alfa in chronic myelogenous leukemia. J Clin Oncol 1997;15:2673.

174. Lissauer: Zwei fälle von leucaemie. Klin Wochenschr 1865;2:403.

175. Lowenthal RM, Buskard NA, Goldman JM: Intensive leukapheresis as initial therapy for chronic granulocytic leukemia. Blood 1975;46:835.

176. Lowenthal RM, Grossman L, Goldman JM, et al: Granulocyte transfusions in treatment of infections in patients with acute leukaemia and aplastic anaemia. Lancet 1975;1:353.

177. Lugo TG, Pendergast A-M, Muller AJ, et al: Tyrosine kinase activity and transformation potency of *bcr-abl* oncogene products. Science 1990;247:1079.

178. Mackinnon S, Papadopoulos EB, Carabasi MH, et al: Adoptive

179. Majlis A, Smith TL, Talpaz M, et al: Significance of cytogenetic clonal evolution in chronic myelogenous leukemia. J Clin Oncol 1996;14:196.

180. Marks DI, Cullis JO, Ward KN, et al: Allogeneic bone marrow transplantation for chronic myeloid leukemia using sibling and volunteer unrelated donors: A comparison of complications in the first 2 years. Ann Intern Med 1993;119:207.

181. Marks DI, Hughes TP, Szydlo R, et al: HLA-identical sibling donor bone marrow transplantation for chronic myeloid leukaemia in first chronic phase: Influence of GVHD prophylaxis on outcome. Br J Haematol 1992;81:383.

182. Martin PJ, Najfeld V, Hansen JA, et al: Involvement of the B-lymphoid system in chronic myelogenous leukaemia. Nature 1980;287:49.

183. McGlave P, Arthur D, Haake R, et al: Therapy of chronic myelogenous leukemia with allogeneic bone marrow transplantation. J Clin Oncol 1987;5:1033.

184. McGlave PB, Arthur D, Miller WJ, et al: Autologous transplantation for CML using marrow treated ex vivo with recombinant human interferon gamma. Bone Marrow Transplant 1990;6:115.

185. McGlave PB, De Fabritiis P, Deisseroth A, et al: Autologous transplants for chronic myelogenous leukaemia: Results from eight transplant groups. Lancet 1994;343:1486.

186. McGlave PB, Shu XO, Wen W, et al: Unrelated donor marrow transplantation for chronic myelogenous leukemia: 9 years' experience of the National Marrow Donor Program. Blood 2000;95:2219.

187. Medical Research Council: Chronic granulocytic leukemia: Comparison of radiotherapy with busulphan therapy. Br Med J 1968;1:201.

188. Medical Research Council: Randomized trial of splenectomy in Ph^1-positive chronic granulocytic leukaemia, including an analysis of prognostic features. Br J Haematol 1983;54:415.

189. Melo JV: The diversity of *bcr-abl* fusion proteins and their relationship to leukemia phenotype. Blood 1996;88:2375.

190. Minot GR, Buckman TE, Isaacs R: Chronic myelogenous leukemia. Age incidence, duration, and benefit derived from irradiation. JAMA 1924;82:1489.

191. Mitelman F, Brandt L, Nilsson PG: Cytogenetic evidence for splenic origin of blastic transformation in chronic myeloid leukaemia. Scand J Haematol 1974;13:87.

192. Moloney WC, Lange RD: Leukemia in atomic bomb survivors: Observations on early phases of leukemia. Blood 1954;9:663.

193. Montefusco E, Alimena G, Gastaldi R, et al: Unusual dermatologic toxicity of long-term therapy with hydroxyurea in chronic myelogenous leukemia. Tumori 1986;72:317.

194. Morton AJ, Gooley T, Hansen JA, et al: Association between pretransplant interferon-α and outcome after unrelated donor marrow transplantation for chronic myelogenous leukemia in chronic phase. Blood 1998;92:394.

195. Mrsic M, Horowitz MM, Atkinson K, et al: Second HLA-identical sibling transplants for leukemia recurrence. Bone Marrow Transplant 1992;9:269.

196. Musashi M, Abe S, Yamada T, et al: Spontaneous remission in a patient with chronic myelogenous leukemia. N Eng J Med 1997;336:337.

197. Nowell PC, Hungerford DA: Chromosome studies in human leukemia: Chronic granulocytic leukemia. J Natl Cancer Inst 1961;27:1013.

198. Nowell PC, Hungerford DA: Chromosome studies on normal and leukemic human leukocytes. J Natl Cancer Inst 1960;25:85.

199. O'Brien S, Kantarjian H, Keating M, et al: Homoharringtonine therapy induces responses in patients with chronic myelogenous leukemia in late chronic phase. Blood 1995;86:3322.

200. O'Brien S, Kantarjian H, Koller C, et al: Sequential homoharringtonine and interferon-α in the treatment of early chronic phase chronic myelogenous leukemia. Blood 1999;93:4149.

201. O'Brien S, Thall PF, Siciliano MJ: Cytogenetics of chronic myelogenous leukemia. In Goldman JM (ed): Chronic Myeloid Leukaemia. Baillière's Clinical Haematology, vol 10. London, WB Saunders, 1997, 259.

202. Ohminami H, Yasukawa M, Fujita S: HLA class I-restricted lysis of

leukemia cells by a CD8+ cytotoxic T-lymphocyte clone specific for WT1 peptide. Blood 2000;95:286.

203. Ohnishi K, Ohno R, Tomonaga M, et al: A randomized trial comparing interferon-α with busulfan for newly diagnosed chronic myelogenous leukemia in chronic phase. Blood 1995;86:906.

204. Oliner H, Schwartz R, Rubio F, et al: Interstitial pulmonary fibrosis following busulfan therapy. Am J Med 1961;31:134.

205. Ozer H, George SL, Schiffer CA, et al: Prolonged subcutaneous administration of recombinant 2b interferon in patients with previously untreated Philadelphia chromosome–positive chronic-phase chronic myelogenous leukemia: Effect on remission duration and survival: Cancer and Leukemia Group B Study 8583. Blood 1993;82:2975.

206. Pane F, Frigeri F, Sindona M, et al: Neutrophilic-chronic myeloid leukemia: A distinct disease with a specific molecular marker (BCR/ABL with C3/A2 junction). Blood 1996;88:2410.

207. Parkin DM, Whelan SL, Ferlay J, et al: Cancer Incidence in Five Continents, vol. VII. International Agency for Research on Cancer, IARC Scientific Publications, No. 143. Lyon, 1997.

208. Petersdorf EW, Gooley TA, Anasetti C, et al: Optimizing outcome after unrelated marrow transplantation by comprehensive matching of HLA class I and II alleles in the donor and recipient. Blood 1998;92:3515.

209. Peterson LC, Bloomfield CD, Brunning RD: Blast crisis as an initial or terminal manifestation of chronic myeloid leukemia: A study of 28 patients. Am J Med 1976;60:209.

210. Petzer AL, Eaves CJ, Barnett MJ, et al: Selective expansion of primitive normal hematopoietic cells in cytokine-supplemented cultures of purified cells from patients with chronic myeloid leukemia. Blood 1997;90:64.

211. Petzer AL, Eaves CJ, Lansdorp PM, et al: Characterization of primitive subpopulations of normal and leukemic cells present in the blood of patients with newly diagnosed as well as established chronic myeloid leukemia. Blood 1996;88:2162.

212. Pinilla-Ibarz J, Cathcart K, Korontsvit T, et al: Vaccination of patients with chronic myelogenous leukemia with bcr-abl oncogene breakpoint fusion peptides generates specific immune responses. Blood 2000;95:1781.

213. Porter DL, Roth MS, McGarigle C, et al: Induction of graft-versus-host disease as immunotherapy for relapsed chronic myeloid leukemia. N Engl J Med 1994;330:100.

214. Provan AB, Majer RV, Herbert A, et al: Spontaneous remission of chronic myeloid leukaemia with loss of the Philadelphia chromosome. Br J Haematol 1991;78:578.

215. Pugh WC, Pearson M, Vardiman JW, et al: Philadelphia chromosome-negative chronic myelogenous leukaemia: A morphological reassessment. Br J Haematol 1985;60:457.

216. Pusey WA: Report of cases treated with roentgen rays. JAMA 1902; 38:911.

217. Raskind WH, Fialkow PJ: The use of cell markers in the study of human hematopoietic neoplasia. Adv Cancer Res 1987;49:127.

218. Reichel RP, Linkesch W, Schetitska D: Therapy with recombinant interferon alpha-2c during unexpected pregnancy in a patient with chronic myeloid leukaemia. Br J Haematol 1992;82:472.

219. Reiffers J, Taylor K, Gluckman E, et al: Collection of Ph-negative progenitor cells with granulocyte-colony-stimulating factor in patients with chronic myeloid leukaemia who respond to recombinant alpha-interferon. Br J Haematol 1998;102:639.

220. Reiffers J, Trouette R, Marit G, et al: Autologous blood stem cell transplantation for chronic granulocytic leukaemia in transformation: A report of 47 cases. Br J Haematol 1991;77:339.

221. Reinhard EH, Neely CL, Samples DM: Radioactive phosphorus in the treatment of chronic leukemias: Long-term results over a period of 15 years. Ann Intern Med 1959;50:942.

222. Ries LAG, Eisner MP, Kosary CL, et al (eds): SEER Cancer Statistics Review, 1973-1998, Bethesda, MD, 2001, National Cancer Institute.

223. Rosti G, Bonifazi F, De Vivo A, et al: Cytarabine increases karyotypic response and survival in αIFN treated chronic myelogenous leukemia patients: Results of a national prospective randomized trial of the Italian Cooperative Study Group on CML. Blood 1999; 94:600a.

224. Rowley JD: A new consistent chromosomal abnormality in chronic myelogenous leukaemia identified by quinacrine fluorescence and Giemsa staining. Nature 1973;243:290.

225. Sacchi S, Kantarjian HM, O'Brien S, et al: Chronic myelogenous leukemia in nonlymphoid blastic phase. Cancer 1999;86:2632.

226. Savage DG, Szydlo RM, Goldman JM: Clinical features at diagnosis in 430 patients with chronic myeloid leukaemia seen at a referral centre over a 16-year period. Br J Haematol 1997;96:111.

227. Schofield JR, Robinson WA, Murphy JR, et al: Low doses of interferon-α are as effective as higher doses in inducing remissions and prolonging survival in chronic myeloid leukemia. Ann Intern Med 1994;121:736.

228. Schuh AC, Sutherland DR, Horsfall W, et al: Chronic myeloid leukemia arising in a progenitor common to T-cells and myeloid cells. Leukemia 1990;4:631.

229. Scott RB: Leukaemia. Lancet 1957;1:1099.

230. Senn N: Case of splenomedullary leukaemia successfully treated by the use of the rontgen ray. Medical Record 1903;64:281.

231. Shtivelman E, Lifshitz B, Gale RP, et al: Fused transcript of abl and bcr genes in chronic myelogenous leukaemia. Nature 1985; 315:550.

232. Silberman G, Crosse MG, Peterson EA, et al: Availability and appropriateness of allogeneic bone marrow transplantation for chronic myeloid leukemia in 10 countries. N Engl J Med 1994;331:1063.

233. Silver RT, Woolf SH, Hehlmann R, et al: An evidence-based analysis of the effect of busulfan, hydroxyurea, interferon, and allogeneic bone marrow transplantation in treating the chronic phase of chronic myeloid leukemia: Developed for the American Society of Hematology. Blood 1999;94:1517.

234. Silverstein MN, Petitt RM, Solberg LA, et al: Anagrelide: A new drug for treating thrombocytosis. N Engl J Med 1988;318:1292.

235. Simpson DR, Couban S, Bredeson C, et al: A Canadian randomized study comparing peripheral blood (PB) and bone marrow (BM) in patients undergoing matched sibling transplants for myeloid malignancies. Blood 2000;96:481a.

236. Sinclair PB, Nacheva EP, Leversha M, et al: Large deletions at the t(9;22) breakpoint are common and may identify a poor-prognosis subgroup of patients with chronic myeloid leukemia. Blood 2000; 95:738.

237. Singer CRJ, McDonald GA, Douglas AS: Twenty-five year survival of chronic granulocytic leukaemia with spontaneous karyotype conversion. Br J Haematol 1984;57:309.

238. Slattery JT, Clift RA, Buckner CD, et al: Marrow transplantation for chronic myeloid leukemia: The influence of plasma busulfan levels on the outcome of transplantation. Blood 1997;89:3055.

239. Slavin S, Nagler A, Naparstek E, et al: Nonmyeloablative stem cell transplantation and cell therapy as an alternative to conventional bone marrow transplantation with lethal cytoreduction for the treatment of malignant and nonmalignant hematologic diseases. Blood 1998;91:756.

240. Sokal JE, Cox EB, Baccarani M, et al: Prognostic discrimination in "good-risk" chronic granulocytic leukemia. Blood 1984;63:789.

241. Sokal JE, Gockerman JP, Bigner SH: Evidence for a selective antileukemic effect of cytosine arabinoside in chronic granulocytic leukemia. Leuk Res 1988;12:453.

242. Sokal JE, Gomez GA, Baccarani M, et al: Prognostic significance of additional cytogenetic abnormalities at diagnosis of Philadelphia chromosome–positive chronic granulocytic leukemia. Blood 1988; 72:294.

243. Spiers ASD: The management of chronic myelocytic leukemia. In Henderson ES, Lister TA (eds): Leukemia, 5th ed. Philadelphia, WB Saunders, 1990.

244. Spiers ASD, Baikie AG, Galton DAG, et al: Chronic granulocytic leukaemia: Effect of elective splenectomy on the course of disease. Br Med J 1975;1:175.

245. Spiers ASD, Bain BJ, Turner JE: The peripheral blood in chronic granulocytic leukaemia: Study of 50 untreated Philadelphia-positive cases. Scand J Haematol 1977;18:25.

246. Srodes CH, Hyde EH, Boggs DR: Autonomous erythropoiesis during erythroblastic crisis of chronic myelocytic leukemia. J Clin Invest 1973;52:512.

247. Steegmann JL, Casado LF, Tomás JF, et al: Interferon alpha for chronic myeloid leukemia relapsing after allogeneic bone marrow transplantation. Bone Marrow Transplant 1999;23:483.

248. Stephens DJ, Lawrence JS: The therapeutic effect of solution of potassium arsenite in chronic myelogenous leukemia. Ann Intern Med 1936;9:1488.

249. Talpaz M, Berman E, Clift RA, et al: NCCN practice guidelines for chronic myelogenous leukemia. Oncology (Huntingt) 2000; 14:229.

250. Talpaz M, Cortes J, O'Brien S, et al: Phase I study of polyethylene glycol (PEG) interferon alpha-2b (intron-A) in CML patients. Blood 1998;92:251a.

251. Talpaz M, Kantarjian H, Kurzrock R, et al: Interferon-alpha produces sustained cytogenetic responses in chronic myelogenous leukemia: Philadelphia chromosome–positive patients. Ann Intern Med 1991;114:532.

252. Talpaz M, Kantarjian H, Liang J, et al: Percentage of Philadelphia chromosome (Ph)–negative and Ph-positive cells found after autologous transplantation for chronic myelogenous leukemia depends on percentage of diploid cells induced by conventional-dose chemotherapy before collection of autologous cells. Blood 1995;85:3257.

253. Talpaz M, Kantarjian HM, McCredie K: Hematologic remission and cytogenetic improvement induced by recombinant human interferon alpha-A in chronic myelogenous leukemia. N Engl J Med 1986;314:1065.

254. Talpaz M, Mavligit G, Keating M, et al: Human leukocyte interferon to control thrombocytosis in chronic myelogenous leukemia. Ann Intern Med 1983;99:789.

255. Talpaz M, McCredie K, Mavligit GM: Leukocyte interferon-induced myeloid cytoreduction in chronic myelogenous leukemia. Blood 1983;62:689.

256. Thomas ED, Clift RA, Fefer A, et al: Marrow transplantation for the treatment of chronic myelogenous leukemia. Ann Intern Med 1986;104:155.

257. Thompson RB, Stainsby D: The clinical and haematological features of chronic granulocytic leukaemia in the chronic phase. In Shaw MT (ed): Chronic Granulocytic Leukaemia, Eastbourne, UK, Praeger Publishers, 1982.

258. Tivey H: The prognosis for survival in chronic granulocytic and lymphocytic leukemia. Am J Roentgenol 1954;72:68.

259. Tough IM, Court Brown WM, Baikie AG, et al: Cytogenetic studies in chronic myeloid leukaemia and acute leukaemia associated with mongolism. Lancet 1961;1:411.

260. Tough IM, Jacobs PA, Court Brown WM, et al: Cytogenetic studies on bone marrow in chronic myeloid leukaemia. Lancet 1963;1:844.

261. Traycoff CM, Halstead B, Rice S, et al: Chronic myelogenous leukaemia CD34+ cells exit G_0/G_1 phases of cell cycle more rapidly than normal marrow CD34+ cells. Br J Haematol 1998;102:759.

262. Turhan AG, Humphries RK, Eaves CJ, et al: Detection of breakpoint cluster region–negative and nonclonal hematopoiesis in vitro and in vivo after transplantation of cells selected in cultures of chronic myeloid leukemia marrow. Blood 1990;76:2404.

263. Udomsakdi C, Eaves CJ, Swolin B, et al: Rapid decline of chronic myeloid leukemic cells in long-term culture due to a defect at the leukemic stem cell level. Proc Natl Acad Sci U S A 1992;89:6192.

264. Vallejos CS, McCredie KB, Brittin GM, et al: Biological effects of repeated leukapheresis of patients with chronic myeloid leukemia. Blood 1973;42:925.

265. van der Plas DC, Grosveld G, Hagemeijer A: Review of clinical, cytogenetic, and molecular aspects of Ph-negative CML. Cancer Genet Cytogenet 1991;52:143.

266. van Rhee F, Lin F, Cullis JO, et al: Relapse of chronic myeloid leukemia after allogeneic bone marrow transplant: The case for giving donor leukocyte transfusions before the onset of hematologic relapse. Blood 1994;83:3377.

267. van Rhee F, Szydlo RM, Hermans J, et al: Long-term results after allogeneic bone marrow transplantation for chronic myelogenous leukemia in chronic phase: A report from the Chronic Leukemia Working Party of the European Group for Blood and Marrow Transplantation. Bone Marrow Transplant 1997;20:553.

268. Verfaillie CM, Bhatia R, Miller W, et al: BCR/ABL-negative primitive progenitors suitable for transplantation can be selected from the marrow of most early-chronic phase but not accelerated-phase chronic myelogenous leukemia patients. Blood 1996;87:4770.

269. Verfaillie CM, Bhatia R, Steinbuch M, et al: Comparative analysis of autografting in chronic myelogenous leukemia: Effects of priming regimen and marrow or blood origin of stem cells. Blood 1998;92:1820.

270. Virchow R: Weisses blut. Froriep's Notizen 1845;36:151.

271. Wagner JE, Zahurak M, Piantadosi S, et al: Bone marrow transplantation of chronic myelogenous leukemia in chronic phase: Evaluation of risks and benefits. J Clin Oncol 1992;10:779.

272. Walters RS, Kantarjian HM, Keating MJ, et al: Therapy of lymphoid and undifferentiated chronic myelogenous leukemia in blast crisis with continuous vincristine and adriamycin infusions plus high-dose decadron. Cancer 1987;60:1708.

273. Wang JCY, Lapidot T, Cashman JD, et al: High level engraftment of NOD/SCID mice by primitive normal and leukemic hematopoietic cells from patients with chronic myeloid leukemia in chronic phase. Blood 1998;91:2406.

274. Weatherall DJ, Galton DAG, Kay HEM: Busulphan and bone marrow depression. Br Med J 1969;1:638.

275. Weiden PL, Flournoy N, Thomas ED, et al: Antileukemic effect of graft-versus-host disease in human recipients of allogeneic-marrow grafts. N Engl J Med 1979;300:1068.

276. Weiden PL, Sullivan KM, Flournoy N, et al: Antileukemic effect of chronic graft-versus-host disease: Contribution to improved survival after allogeneic marrow transplantation. N Engl J Med 1981;304:1529.

277. Weiss HA, Darby SC, Fearn T, et al: Leukemia mortality after x-ray treatment for ankylosing spondylitis. Radiat Res 1995;142:1.

278. Whang J, Frei E III, Tjio JH, et al: The distribution of the Philadelphia chromosome in patients with chronic myelogenous leukemia. Blood 1963;22:664.

279. You W, Weisbrot IM: Chronic neutrophilic leukemia: Report of two cases and review of the literature. J Clin Pathol 1979;72:233.

280. Zhao RCH, McIvor S, Griffin JD, et al: Gene therapy for chronic myelogenous leukemia (CML): A retroviral vector that renders hematopoietic progenitors methotrexate-resistant and CML progenitors functionally normal and nontumorigenic in vivo. Blood 1997;90:4687.

26

Paul S. Gaynon   Stuart E. Siegel

Childhood Acute Lymphoblastic Leukemia

Acute lymphoblastic leukemia (ALL), the malignant transformation of a B-lineage or T-lineage lymphocytic precursor,[1] is the most common diagnosis in pediatric oncology (Table 26-1). Among infants, children, and adolescents aged 0 to 15 years, the incidence is 31 per 10^6 per year in the United States. ALL is slightly more common in boys than girls, except for infants younger than 1 year, where girls predominate, and more common in European Americans than African Americans. Among European Americans, an incidence peak is seen between the ages of 3 and 6 years.[2, 3] The risk of ALL is markedly increased in children with Down's syndrome.[4-6]

The causes of ALL remain unclear. It is thought to represent the culmination of the evolution of an abnormal clone through successive genetic changes. The biology, etiology, genetics, and epidemiology are discussed extensively in this volume (see Chapters 2, 5, 7, 8, 9, and 10) and need not be re-reviewed here.

In the last half-century, treatment and outcomes have advanced from single agents and transient remissions, that is, temporary disappearance of microscopically identifiable leukemia and recovery of normal hematopoiesis, to multiagent therapy and a high likelihood of cure.[7, 8] The first step was the use of vincristine and prednisone for induction of remission. The next was the emergence of prolonged treatment with daily oral 6-mercaptopurine

(6-MP) and weekly oral methotrexate for prevention of marrow relapse.[9] With somewhat effective systemic therapy, central nervous system (CNS) relapse arose as a barrier to cure. The introduction of 24-Gy cranial-spinal irradiation by Pinkel and workers at St. Jude Children's Research Hospital (SJCRS), after the failure of 5 Gy and 12 Gy, resulted in the first substantial and reproducible cure rate.[10, 11] Subsequently, anthracyclines and asparaginase have been introduced,[12, 13] the use of irradiation has been limited,[14-16] and postinduction intensification has emerged as a successful strategy.[17-22] Outcomes have continued to improve. Figure 26-1 shows the improvement in event-free survival (EFS) and survival for patients treated in Children's Cancer Group (CCG) trials between 1983 and 1988 and between 1989 and 1995.[23] However, we do well to remember that relatively simple "Pinkel era" therapy was sufficient to cure half of the patients. Unfortunately, we have been unable to identify which patients these were prospectively.

Tremendous strides have been made in the primary treatment of ALL, but its relatively high incidence makes relapsed ALL more prevalent than many other common pediatric malignancies such as acute myeloblastic leuke-

TABLE 26-1. Treatment Failure in ALL Versus Incidence of Childhood Cancer Diagnoses in the United States

Diagnosis	Number in U.S. per year at Age <15 yr	Incidence in U.S. per Million, Age <15 yr
ALL	2484	30.9
Brain tumors	2205	27.6
Neuroblastoma	754	9.7
Non-Hodgkin's lymphoma	666	8.4
Wilms' tumor	638	8.3
Treatment failure in ALL	617	7.7
Hodgkin's disease	511	6.6
AML	454	5.6
Rhabdomyosarcoma	354	4.5
Retinoblastoma	309	3.9

ALL, acute lymphoblastic leukemia; AML, acute myeloblastic leukemia. Data from[2,3,23].

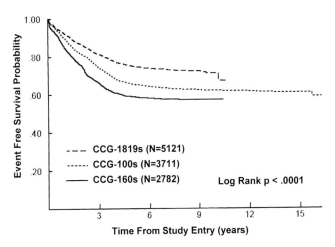

FIGURE 26-1. Event-free survival in Children's Cancer Group ALL Trials over 17 years, 1978-1995 (CCG-160s: 1978-1983; CCG-100s: 1983-1988; CCG-1819s: 1989-1995). (Courtesy Dr. Harland N. Sather and the Children's Cancer Group, Arcadia, CA.)

TABLE 26–2. Survival after Relapse on the CCG-100 Series

Location of Relapse	N	N (%)	6-yr Freedom from 2nd Adverse Event (SD) (%)
Isolated marrow	642		16 ± 2
Early		233 (36)	5 ± 2
Intermediate		194 (30)	10 ± 4
Late		215 (33)	33 ± 4
Combined marrow	120		29 ± 4
Early		34 (28)	9 ± 5
Intermediate		26 (22)	11 ± 6
Late		60 (50)	48 ± 7
Isolated CNS	220		37 ± 3
Early		102 (46)	24 ± 5
Intermediate		84 (38)	44 ± 5
Late		34 (17)	59 ± 9
Isolated testes	112		64 ± 5
Early		22 (20)	48 ± 11
Intermediate		24 (21)	44 ± 11
Late		66 (59)	76 ± 6

Early, less than 18 months; intermediate, 19 to 36 months; late, longer than 36 months.
CCG, Children's Cancer Study Group.
From[24].

mia (AML) and rhabdomyosarcoma[24] (Table 26-2). Continued poor outcome after relapse[24-26] (see Table 26-2) maintains the imperative to continue to improve initial therapy still further in order to prevent relapse even more effectively. This approach has succeeded to some extent but places an increasing burden on the growing percentage of children already cured with current therapies.

DIAGNOSIS AND COMPLICATIONS

The symptoms and signs of ALL are variable but follow from bone marrow replacement and/or organ infiltration. Pallor, bruising, and persistent bouts of fever may be attributed to aregenerative anemia, thrombobocytopenia, and neutropenia, respectively. Lymphoadenopathy, organomegaly, and bone pain may be attributed to leukemic infiltration of lymph nodes, liver and spleen, and bones, respectively. Young children may refuse to walk. Parents frequently note loss of appetite, fatigue, and abdominal pain. On occasion, patients face respiratory embarrassment from an anterior mediastinal mass, exacerbation of thrombocytopenia by a coexisting coagulopathy, and decreased kidney function from urate nephropathy.

Diagnosis requires identification of more than 25% French-American-British (FAB) L1 or L2 lymphoblasts in the bone marrow.[27] Substantial overlap exists between ALL and lymphoblastic lymphoma with bone marrow involvement (i.e., leukemic transformation). Histochemistry and flow cytometry[28] may aid in discrimination between lymphoblasts and myeloblasts. ALL is myeloperoxidase negative, although myeloperoxidase mRNA has been identified in a number of cases of ALL. FAB M0 myeloblasts may also lack myeloperoxidase. Recognition of FAB M7 megakaryoblastic leukemia may be difficult by light microscopy alone.

Perhaps 3% of patients have leukemic involvement of

the CNS at initial assessment, as defined by more than 4 cells/μL with identifiable blasts not attributable to peripheral blood contamination. The significance of blasts in the absence of pleocytosis is the subject of some controversy.[29-31] A small number of boys have overt testicular enlargement and leukemic infiltration at diagnosis.

PRIMARY TREATMENT

Determinants of Outcome

A number of initial clinical and laboratory features have been associated with better or worse outcome.[32] Conventionally, children aged 1 to 9 years with a white blood cell (WBC) count less than 50,000/μL are designated standard risk whereas adolescents older than 10 years or younger children with a WBC count greater than 50,000 are designated higher risk.[33] Infants younger than 1 year have a particularly high risk of treatment failure, and those younger than 6 months, even more so.[34-36] Some allocate patients with T-lineage immunophenotypes to more aggressive therapy.[37, 38] However, in the CCG trials, children with T-lineage disease have had an outcome as good as that of children with B-precursor disease when treated with identical age- and WBC count–defined protocols.[39, 40] Patients with T-lineage disease have had a pattern of relapse different from that of patients with B-precursor disease: a higher relapse rate early and a lower relapse rate late. However, the ultimate EFS is similar. Coexpression of both T- and B-lineage–associated membrane markers[41] or lymphoid- and myeloid-associated membrane markers[42] holds no prognostic significance with current treatments.

The risk of relapse may be modified by cytogenetic findings, and cytogenetic and molecular abnormalities are common in children with ALL.[43-46] Hyperdiploidy, especially a modal chromosome number between 51 and 63, or trisomy 10, is associated with a decreased risk of relapse.[47, 48] Pseudodiploidy and severe hypodiploidy, defined as a modal chromosome number less than 45, are associated with a poorer outcome.[49, 50] Near-tetraploidy (modal chromosome number greater than 65) is often associated with T-lineage disease and a poor outcome.[51] The translocations t(4;11) in infants[52, 53] and t(9;22)[54-56] increase the risk. The translocation t(1;19), the most common translocation in childhood ALL by conventional banded cytogenetics, carries no prognostic importance. However, about one third of such patients have a balanced translocation and probably an inferior outcome.[57, 58]

Molecular methods, fluorescent in situ hybridization (FISH)[59, 60] and reverse transcription–polymerase chain reaction (RT-PCR),[61] may increase the detection of patients with cytogenetic abnormalities. In some cases, banded cytogenetics studies are simply technically unsuccessful. The translocation t(12;21) is rarely identified by conventional banded cytogenetics, but the corresponding fusion mRNA TEL AML1 may be identified in 20% of cases by FISH or RT-PCR[60, 62, 63] (Fig. 26-2). RT-PCR increases the number of cases identified with t(4;11) and MLL-AF4, t(9;22) and BCR ABL, and t(1;19) and E2A PBX1.[61] FISH

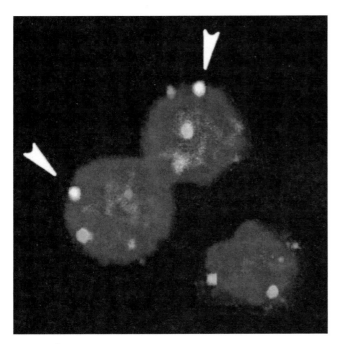

FIGURE 26–2. Fluorescence in situ hybridization (FISH) with a TEL/AML1 dual-color probe in the bone marrow cells of a child with ALL. The *TEL* gene labels with a green color, and the *AML1* gene labels with a red color. The arrows point to the *TEL/AML1* fusion gene (yellow color signals) in two interphase leukemic cells indicating the presence of t(12;21)(p13;q22). A single green signal *(TEL)* and red signal *(AML1)* from the uninvolved chromosomes may also be seen. A normal cell with two green signals (TEL genes) and two red cells (AML1 genes) is also present. (Courtesy Dr. Samual Wu, Childrens Hospital Los Angeles, Los Angeles, CA.) (See color section.)

techniques may increase the diagnosis of various specific trisomies.[64]

Importantly, single cytogenetic or molecular features fail to define homogeneous populations. National Cancer Institute (NCI)/Rome "standard-risk" trisomy 10 patients have a better outcome than "higher-risk" trisomy 10 patients do,[47] "standard-risk" t(9;22) patients by age and WBC count have a better outcome than "higher-risk" t(9;22) patients do,[54] patients with t(9;22) and a good "prednisone response" have a better outcome than do patients with t(9;22) and a poor "prednisone response,"[65] infant t(4;11) patients have a worse outcome than older t(4;11) patients do,[52, 66] and infants and children with t(4;11) and a good "prednisone response" have a better outcome than do infants and children with t(4;11) and a poor "prednisone response."[67, 68] The emergence of overt leukemia probably requires several genetic changes, and the best known or most visually obvious abnormalities may not be the most critical abnormalities.

Most chemotherapeutic drugs work through apoptosis, or programmed cell death.[69] The various proteins and functions that promote or retard apoptosis have been the subject of intense study.[70-73] Two principal pathways have been described—one is mediated by tumor necrosis factor or fas ligand and involves Fas-associated protein with death domain (FADD) and caspase 8 as the adaptor and initiator, respectively, with downstream mitochondrial release of cytochrome *c*. In a second pathway, early opening of mitochondrial megachannels leads to loss of trans-

membrane potential and release of cytochrome *c*. Cytochrome *c* binds to Apaf1. The complex in turn activates caspase 9. Ultimately, caspase 3, which is responsible for apoptotic DNA fragmentation, is activated by either pathway, along with other downstream effectors. In the fas ligand–mediated pathway, loss of Apaf1 and caspase 9 fails to prevent apoptosis.[71] Ceramide is a proximal signal for cytochrome *c* release.[74]

The cell cycle regulatory protein p53 is believed to be crucial for the translation of DNA damage into a signal for apoptosis.[75] Poor response to initial therapy has been linked to loss of p53 function through abnormalities of p53 itself or overexpression of mdm-2 in childhood ALL.[76] Stock and coworkers linked worsening outcome in adult ALL with an increasing number of abnormal cell cycle regulatory proteins, namely, p53, p15, p16, and retinoblastoma protein.[77]

In cell lines, both glutathione[78] and BCL-2[70] prevent loss of mitochondrial transmembrane potential and cytochrome *c* release. High levels of reduced glutathione depend more on faster reduction of oxidized glutathione by glutathione reductase and peroxidase than on increased synthesis by γ-glutamylcysteine synthetase.[79] A high level of glutathione in lymphoblasts is associated with in vitro resistance to chemotherapy[80] and an increased risk of relapse.[81] Better outcome is also associated with glutathione S-transferase mu-1 null, tau-1 null, or pi-1 Val105/Val105 genotypes.[82, 83] High levels of bcl-2 were linked to slow response to initial therapy but not inferior EFS in T-lineage ALL.[84] We do well to remember that gene expression is not identical to gene function. Protein function may be modulated by interaction with other proteins, and levels of gene function may change when cells are perturbed.

The risk of relapse may be altered by blast chemosensitivity. Chemosensitivity may be assessed usefully in vitro by the 3, (4,5-dimethyl-thiazol-2-yl)–2,5-diphenyltetrazolium bromide (MTT) assay[85-87] or in vivo by peripheral blood[88-90] or marrow[91-94] morphologic response in the initial days and weeks of treatment. The drug concentrations lethal for 50% of lymphoblasts (LC$_{50}$) in the MTT assay for prednisolone, dexamethasone, vincristine, L-asparaginase, and 6-thioguanine have consistent prognostic significance in univariate and multivariate analyses.[87, 95-98]

The percentage of marrow blasts on days 7 and 14 of induction therapy identifies groups with disparate treatment outcomes (Table 26–3). In one CCG study, 39% of the children had more than 5% blasts on day 7 of therapy. Almost all achieved remission by day 28, but they retained a 2.7-fold increased risk of relapse.[94] The CCG has used early marrow response for treatment allocation. Higher-risk patients with greater than 25% marrow blasts on day 7 of therapy may be "rescued" with the augmented regimen.[20, 99]

The Berlin-Frankfurt-Munster (BFM) group has used the peripheral blood response to intrathecal methotrexate and oral prednisone to identify patients at very high risk of treatment failure.[90] Examination of the peripheral blood response of patients has identified heterogeneity within cytogenetic subgroups such as t(9;22) or t(4;11).[67, 68, 100]

Residual leukemia at levels too low for detection by

TABLE 26–3. Response and Outcome

Study/Risk Measure	Proportion of Patients in Poor-Response Subset	Percentage of Total Events in Poor-Response Subset	Relative Hazard
CCG-105/AR	117/1320 (9%)	12	1.6
Day 14 marrow	M2/M3		
CCG-123/HR	30/205 (15%)	27	2.8
Day 14 marrow	M2/M3		
CCG-1881/LR	64/711 (9%)	18	2.5
Day 14 marrow	M2/M3		
CCG-123/HR	86/220 (39%)	58	2.7
Day 7 marrow	M3		
CCG-1891/AR	525/1074 (49%)	60	1.7
Day 7 marrow	M3		
CCG-1882/HR	732/1353 (54%)	62	1.5*
Day 7 marrow			
Coustan Smith et al	30/128 (23%)	49	3.1
Flow cytometry	+ End induction		
Goulden et al	38/66 (58%)		
PCR	+ End induction	82	3.4
Cave et al	63/151 (42%)	78	5.7
PCR	+ End induction		
Van Dongen	98/169 (58%)	95	14.5
PCR	+ End induction		

* Sixty percent of M3 patients received the augmented intensive regimen.

M2, marrow blasts between 55% and 25%; M3, marrow blasts 25% or greater; AR, average risk; CCG, Children's Cancer Study Group; HR, higher risk; LR, lower risk; PCR, polymerase chain reaction.

Data from[92, 103–106].

conventional microscopic techniques has been termed minimal residual disease.[101, 102] A number of flow cytometry- and PCR-based techniques are under investigation. Several have proved to have prognostic power and the potential to improve our identification of good and poor responders[103-106] (Table 26–3).

The presence of a resistant subclone concealed in the midst of a generally sensitive blast population is one potential confounder of assays of chemosensitivity and response.[107] A marrow sample might not reflect the true leukemic burden if the marrow sample is dilute or if blasts are distributed in an anatomically heterogeneous manner throughout the marrow compartment.[108] Malignant cells may be difficult to identify in day 7 or day 14 marrow by light microscopy, and multiparameter flow cytometry has been proposed as a superior strategy for blast identification.[109] However, cells may share clonotypic features or a fingerprint and not themselves be fully leukemogenic. Clonotypic features may be subject to oligoclonality or clonal evolution.[110-112] In one study, the immunophenotype changed between diagnosis and relapse in 29 of 40 cases studied.[113] In another study, changes in the immunoglobulin heavy-chain or T-cell receptor gene were found in 25 of 40 cases studied.[114] Monitoring multiple markers per patient may minimize the impact of oligoclonality or clonal evolution, for example, in PCR-based assays by focusing on downstream D-N-J junctional sequences instead of the more variable upstream V_H-D sequences.[115]

Host factors may have an important bearing on outcome. Patient and physician compliance has been discussed.[116, 117] Recent attention has turned to host factors involved in the activation and catabolism of antineoplastic agents.[118-124]

All patients with ALL require good therapy. The CCG has obtained an improved outcome for NCI/Rome standard-risk patients[33, 125] with postinduction intensification[126-128] and dexamethasone[129] in a series of randomized trials (Table 26–4). To the extent permitted by limited sample size, recent CCG data suggest that favorable trisomy 10 patients benefit from dexamethasone and postinduction intensification.[47] Favorable day 7 rapid responders may still benefit from dexamethasone.[129] The least gains have been seen for infants with ALL, especially those with t(4;11),[35, 36, 130, 131] and for children with ALL and t(9;22) or BCR ABL.[54]

Treatment is the most important prognostic factor, and allocation of treatment on the basis of estimated risk has been a common strategy to balance burden and benefit. Patients with a greater estimated risk of relapse receive more aggressive therapy, whereas patients with less risk receive less aggressive therapy. In the CCG, this practice has led to several paradoxical "flip-flops" in which putatively higher-risk patients who received more aggressive therapy achieved a better outcome than did putatively lower-risk patients who received "risk-adjusted" therapy (Table 26–5).

Induction

Current practice entails the use of three or four drugs for induction therapy in children with standard-risk disease and four to seven drugs in children with higher-risk disease.[132] Three-drug induction, vincristine, prednisone, and anthracycline, is superior to two-drug induction consisting of vincristine and prednisone.[12] Data showing an advantage for four drugs, vincristine, prednisone, L-asparaginase, and an anthracycline, over three drugs are lacking. The UKALL VIII trial found no benefit in adding

TABLE 26–4. Improved Outcome for Children with ALL in CCG Randomized Trials

Population Trial	N	Intervention 5-yr EFS (%)	Percent Change in Rate of Failure
Lower risk		± V/P pulses	36
CCG-161	631	77 vs 64	
Average risk		± DI	
CCG-105	625	77 vs 61	41
Higher risk		BFM vs CCG standard	
CCG-106	545	63 vs 40	38
		NY I vs CCG standard	
		61 vs 40	35
Higher risk		BFM vs LSA2L2	
CCG-123	694	67 vs 53	33
		NY I LSA2L2	
		67 vs 53	33
Lower risk		± DI	
CCG-1881	700	85 vs 79	29
Average risk		DI × 2 vs DI × 1	
CCG-1891	802	84 vs 77	30
Higher risk		Augmented vs standard	
CCG-1882/SER	310	BFM	44
		75 vs 55	
Standard risk		Dex vs Pred	
CCG-1922	1060	88 vs 80	40

BFM, Berlin-Frankfurt-Munster group; CCG, Children's Cancer Study Group; Dex, dexamethasone; DI, delayed intensification (protocol II); EFS, event-free survival; LSA2L2 "lymphosarcoma-2 leukemia-2" regimen; NY I, "New York I" regimen; Pred, prednisone; SER, slow early (day 7) responder; V/P, vincristine prednisone pulses.

From[23].

daunomycin in a randomized trial of over 800 patients.[133] In another randomized trial, Ekert and coworkers compared a vincristine and prednisone–based remission induction regimen with a second regimen that had been effective in obtaining second remission after marrow relapse but excluded vincristine and prednisone. For patients in the experimental arm, vincristine and prednisone were deferred to the second month. Remission induction rates were similar, but patients receiving the conventional vincristine and prednisone–containing regimen had superior EFS.[134]

Dexamethasone may be substituted for prednisone,[135, 136] and it has greater in vitro activity and better CNS penetration than prednisolone or prednisone does.[97, 137] When compared with a historical control in which patients received prednisone, the Dutch ALL VI study showed improved EFS with dexamethasone. The CCG compared dexamethasone and prednisone for induction and maintenance in more than 1000 standard-risk patients, with all patients receiving dexamethasone in intensification. Dexamethasone yielded a better 4-year EFS, 88% versus 81%.[129]

Recent trials suggest that all asparaginase preparations are not equivalent. Although native *Erwinia* asparaginase is known to have a shorter half-life than native *Escherichia coli* asparaginase, 0.7 versus 1.3 days,[138] conventional practice has been a simple unit-for-unit substitution. Several groups had reported that conventional doses and schedules of *Erwinia* asparaginase failed to provide prolonged, profound asparagine depletion in a substantial proportion of patients. This proportion increased with repeated courses of therapy.[139] The European Organization for Research on the Treatment of Cancer (EORTC) 58881 study compared *E. coli* and *Erwinia* asparaginase, both given at 10,000 IU/m² twice a week. Six hundred fifty-two patients were randomized. The 4-year EFS rate was 75% for *E. coli* and 62% for *Erwinia*.[140] Preliminary data have appeared from a Dana-Farber Cancer Institute (DFCI) study in which native *Erwinia* and *E. coli* asparaginase were compared. Again, an advantage was seen for *E. coli* asparaginase when both products were used at the same dose and schedule.[141]

Postinduction Intensification

In 1970, Riehm and coworkers in the BFM group added daunomycin to conventional vincristine, prednisone, and L-asparaginase induction and also added cyclophosphamide and cytosine arabinoside to conventional consolidation consisting of weekly intrathecal methotrexate and daily oral 6-MP to form protocol I. The impact on outcome was modest.[142] In 1976, they added a second 2-

TABLE 26–5. Impact of Therapy: Reversals of Expected Outcomes

Putative Greater Risk	Putative Lesser Risk
CCG-105: Average Risk Age 1–9 yr; WBC >10,000/μL and ≤50,000/μL Delayed intensification 10-year EFS, 74%	**CCG-104: Lower Risk** Age 1–9 yr; WBC <10,000/μL Standard/no delayed intensification 10-year EFS, 62%
CCG-1891: Average Risk Age 1–9 yr; WBC >10,000/μL and ≤50,000/μL Double delayed intensification 5-year EFS, 83%	**CCG-1881: Lower Risk** Age 1–9 yr; WBC >10,000/μL and ≤50,000/μL Standard +/− delayed intensification 5-year EFS, 79%
CCG-1882: Higher Risk Age <10 yr; WBC >50,000/μL Day 7 blasts ≥25% Augmented intensive therapy 5-year EFS, 79%	**CCG-1882: Higher Risk** Age <10 yr; WBC >50,000/μL Day 7 blasts <25% Standard intensive therapy 5-year EFS, 76%

CCG, Children's Cancer Study Group; EFS, event-free survival; WBC, white blood cell count.
From[23].

month phase of intensive therapy (protocol II) either immediately after protocol I or after an interval of 2 months (delayed intensification) [DI] for higher-risk patients. Outcomes improved markedly relative to historical controls. EFS was the same whether protocol II was administered immediately after protocol I or after a 2-month interval. DI was better tolerated than immediate intensification.[19] Two randomized CCG trials conducted between 1983 and 1988 demonstrated the superiority of the BFM approach over the then-current CCG approaches for higher-risk patients.[17, 94, 143, 144]

For average-risk patients, CCG examined the relative contribution of protocol I (intensive induction/consolidation) and protocol II (DI).[16, 128] Popular belief held that early intensive therapy was most critical as per the Goldie-Coldman hypothesis,[145] or more generally, "more was better."[146] In the CCG trial, EFS improved with DI, with or without intensive induction consolidation, 77% versus 61% (Fig. 26–3). Surprisingly, intensive induction/consolidation provided no added benefit for patients who received DI overall or in the subset of patients younger than 10 years. In the subset of patients older than 10 years, both intensive induction/consolidation and DI were required for optimal outcome.[128] However, small numbers limited the study's statistical power. The roles of intensive induction/consolidation and DI have not been studied in other higher-risk subsets. Although average-risk patients failed to benefit from intensive induction/consolidation, a subsequent trial showed a benefit for double DI over single DI, 84% versus 77%.[127] Double DI provided the backbone of the CCG 1996–2000 standard-risk study.

The CCG has omitted intensive induction/consolidation in subsequent standard-risk studies. Patients avoid 100 mg/m² of anthracycline and 2 g/m² of cyclophosphamide relative to other BFM-based protocols. Intensive induction/consolidation required an average of 10 additional hospital days per patient. More than 600 standard-risk patients are enrolled in CCG trials yearly, and omission of intensive induction/consolidation results in savings of more than 6000 hospital days per year with no decrease in EFS.

Subsequently, both BFM and CCG studies have shown that DI benefits the subset of patients at lowest risk for relapse.[18, 126] In the BFM '83 study, the 5-year EFS rate increased from 61% to 82% with application of DI. The benefit was substantial but appeared late.[18] In the CCG study, the EFS rate increased from 79% to 85%, much less than in the BFM study. The CCG trial used monthly vincristine/prednisone pulses and intrathecal methotrexate every 3 months in maintenance.[126] These interventions may have improved the outcome of children who received no DI while having less or no benefit in children who received DI. Patients need only be cured once. Interventions that are helpful individually may be redundant in whole or in part when combined. The value of vincristine and dexamethasone pulses in patients who receive BFM protocol II is currently under study in the international BFM group.

For higher risk patients, longer and stronger postinduction intensification was explored (Table 26-6). An "augmented regimen" was constructed in which patients received five pulses of Capizzi I therapy consisting of vincristine, escalating doses of intravenous methotrexate and asparaginase in place of daily oral 6-MP, and weekly oral methotrexate in the 8 weeks preceding and after DI and a second DI. Two doses of vincristine and six doses of asparaginase are administered while awaiting the recovery of peripheral counts after each of two cyclophosphamide/cytosine arabinoside/thiopurine pulses, two in consolidation and one after each DI. The regimen was tested in higher-risk patients with more than 25% marrow blasts on day 7 of therapy; in these patients the risk of relapse was believed to warrant the risk of increased toxicity with this new regimen. Patients who achieved remission were randomly assigned to the augmented intensive regimen or to the standard BFM-based intensive regimen. Nachman and coworkers reported a 5-year EFS rate of 75% for the augmented regimen versus 55% for the standard CCG-modified BFM-based regimen[20, 91] (Fig. 26-4). The individual components of this successful regimen are under study in the CCG 1997–2001 higher-risk trial.

The Medical Research Council of the United Kingdom (MRC [UK]) demonstrated the clear value of postinduction intensification in randomized trials.[147] Both EFS and survival were affected. Additional benefit was shown for extended postinduction intensification in both standard- and higher-risk patients in subsequent randomized trials.[148]

Other strategies of postinduction intensification, such as intermediate-dose methotrexate with leucovorin rescue, have been explored. Study X of the SJCRH compared rotating drug pairs, namely, 6-MP/methotrexate, cyclophosphamide/doxorubicin, and teniposide/cytosine arabinoside, with daily oral 6-MP and intermediate-dose methotrexate with leucovorin rescue (IDM). At 4 years, the DFS rate was 67% for IDM and 56% for rotating drug pairs.[149] Two CCG trials failed to show any advantage of

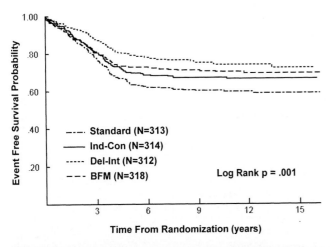

FIGURE 26–3. Impacts of intensive induction consolidation and delayed intensification on the event-free survival of children with average risk ALL (CCG-105 study; chair, Dr. David G. Tubergen). (Standard: neither intensive induction consolidation nor delayed intensification; Ind-con: intensive induction consolidation; Del-int: delayed intensification; BFM: both intensive induction consolidation and delayed intensification based on the BFM 76/79 study.) (Courtesy Dr. Harland N. Sather and the Children's Cancer Group, Arcadia, CA.)

TABLE 26–6. Augmented versus Standard CCG-Modified, BFM-Based Therapy

Consolidation (4 wk)	**Consolidation (8 wk)**
Complete prednisone taper	Complete prednisone taper
Cyclophosphamide, 1 g/m² IV days 0, 14	Cyclophosphamide, 1 g/m² IV days 0, 28
Methotrexate (dose per age) IT days 1, 8, 15, 22	Methotrexate (dose per age), IT days 1, 8, 15, 22
Cytarabine, 75 mg/m² SC/IV days 1–4, 8–11, 15–18, 22–25	Cytarabine, 75 mg/m² SC/IV days 1–4, 8–11, 29–32, 36–39
Mercaptopurine, 60 mg/m² days 0–27	Mercaptopurine, 60 mg/m² PO days 0–13, 28–41
Cranial irradiation, 18 Gy	Cranial irradiation, 18 Gy
	Vincristine, 1.5 mg/m² IV days 14, 21, 42, 49
	L-Asparaginase, 6000 IU/m² IM days 14, 16, 18, 21, 23, 25, 42, 44, 46, 49, 51, 53
Interim Maintenance (8 wk)	**Interim Maintenance #1 (8 wk)**
Mercaptopurine, 60 mg/m² PO days 0–41	Vincristine, 1.5 mg/m² IV days 0, 10, 20, 30, 40
Methotrexate, 20 mg/m² PO days 0, 7, 14, 21, 28, 35	Methotrexate, 100 mg/m² IV days 0, 10, 20, 30, 40 (escalated by 50 mg/m²/dose to tolerance)
Delayed Intensification (8 wk)	**Delayed Intensification #1 (8 wk)**
Dexamethasone, 10 mg/m² PO days 0–20 + taper	Dexamethasone, 10 mg/m² PO days 0–20 + taper
Vincristine, 1.5 mg/m² IV days 0, 7, 14	Vincristine, 1.5 mg/m² IV days 0, 7, 14, 42, 49
Doxorubicin, 25 mg/m² IV days 0, 7, 14	Doxorubicin, 25 mg/m² IV days 0, 7, 14
L-Asparaginase, 6000 IU/m² IM days 3, 5, 7, 10, 12, 14	L-Asparaginase, 6000 IU/m² IM days 3, 5, 7, 10, 12, 14, 42, 44, 46, 49, 51, 53
Cyclophosphamide, 1 g/m² IV day 28	Cyclophosphamide, 1 g/m² IV day 28
Methotrexate (dose per age) IT day 29	Methotrexate (dose per age) IT day 29
Cytarabine, 75 mg/m² SC/IV days 29–32, 36–39	Cytarabine, 75 mg/m² SC/IV days 29–32, 36–39
Thioguanine, 60 mg/m² days 28–41	Thioguanine, 60 mg/m² days 28–41
	Interim Maintenance #2 (8 wk)
	Vincristine, 1.5 mg/m² IV days 0, 10, 20, 30, 40
	Methotrexate, 100 mg/m² IV days 0, 10, 20, 30, 40 (escalated by 50 mg/m² dose to tolerance)
	Methotrexate (dose per age), IT days 0, 20, 40
	Delayed Intensification #2 (8 wk)
	Same as Delayed Intensification #1
Maintenance (12-wk Courses)	**Maintenance (12-wk Courses)**
Methotrexate (dose per age) IT day 0	Methotrexate (dose per age), IT day 0
Vincristine, 1.5 mg/m² IV days 0, 28, 56	Vincristine, 1.5 mg/m² IV days 0, 28, 56
Mercaptopurine, 75 mg/m² PO days 0–83	Mercaptopurine, 75 mg/m² PO days 0–83
Methotrexate, 20 mg/m² PO days 7, 14, 21, 28, 35, 42, 49, 56, 63, 70, 77	Methotrexate, 20 mg/m² PO days 7, 14, 21, 28, 35, 42, 49, 56, 63, 70, 77

* Standard Consolidation required 4 weeks in theory, but in practice, treatment was generally delayed 2 weeks between days 13 and 14 and between day 27 and the start of interim maintenance because of neutropenia.

BFM, Berlin-Frankfurt-Munster; CCG, Children's Cancer Study Group; IT, intrathecally.

Reprinted, by permission, from the New England Journal of Medicine, 338:1663–1671, 1998.

parenteral methotrexate at 33.6 g/m² or 0.5 g/m² with rescue over conventional weekly oral methotrexate.[150, 151] One recent British trial and one recent French trial failed to show any advantage for parenteral methotrexate at 6 to 8 g/m² with rescue over conventional weekly oral methotrexate and no leucovorin rescue.[152, 153] The Pediatric Oncology Group (POG) 9005 trial showed an advantage for parenteral methotrexate at 1 g/m² with rescue over oral methotrexate. At 3 years, the EFS rate was 89% versus 78%. However, the same leucovorin dose was given after methotrexate 1 g/m² intravenously over a 24-hour period, and methotrexate 25 mg/m² orally every 6 hours for four doses.[154] Neurotoxicity was a prohibitive when the scheduled oral methotrexate was given with no leucovorin,[155] but neurotoxicity was encountered with parenteral methotrexate also.[156, 157]

The DFCI has built a successful strategy around prolonged administration of weekly asparaginase.[13, 37, 38] A POG trial found an advantage for prolonged asparaginase administration to T-lineage patients. However, the control group received only three doses of L-asparaginase.[158] No

advantage was found in B-lineage patients for weekly asparaginase, 25,000 IU/m² intramuscularly for 24 weeks in the POG ALinC 14 study.[159]

Bone marrow transplantation (BMT) in first complete remission (CR1) has been proposed as a form of postinduction intensification for infants, children, and adolescents with ALL and very high-risk features in first remission.[26, 160] Interpretation of reported results requires identification of a control group. Comparisons of BMT and chemotherapy are regularly confounded by waiting time bias, selection bias, and violation of proportional hazards. Case-control studies may correct for waiting time bias but do not affect selection bias. Violation of proportional hazards undermines the log-rank statistic generally used in comparisons. Although the decision between a BMT and chemotherapy strategy is critical clinically, specific comparisons necessarily compare one or more BMT regimens with one or more chemotherapy regimens and cannot be extended to all BMT regimens and all chemotherapy regimens.

In general, available intent-to-treat analyses show no

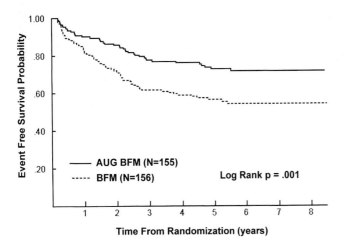

FIGURE 26–4. Benefit of longer and stronger postinduction intensification therapy on the event-free survival of children and adolescents with higher risk ALL and a poor day-7 marrow response. (BFM: standard post-induction intensification based on the BFM 76/79 study; AUG BFM: longer and stronger post-induction intensification.) (Courtesy Dr. Harland N. Sather and the Children's Cancer Group, Arcadia, CA.)

benefit for BMT approaches in very high-risk childhood ALL. CCG-1921 enrolled 111 children and adolescents with ALL and very high-risk features. In aggregate, outcomes were similar for 37 patients with donors who were to pursue a BMT approach and 64 patients with no donors who were to pursue a chemotherapy approach in the critical intent-to-treat analyses.[160] Wheeler and co-workers from the MRC (UK) identified 286 patients with very high-risk features. With a 10-year follow-up, no difference in outcome was seen between the 99 patients with family donors (76 BMTs) and 187 patients with no sibling donors (25 BMTs).[26] Overall, BMT is not a complete answer to the challenge of very high-risk ALL in children.

However, some advantage for BMT is apparent in the Philadelphia chromosome–positive (Ph[+]) group (t[9;22] or BCR ABL). Arico and coworkers gathered data for 326 children with Ph[+] ALL treated in one of seven countries around the world. Patients undergoing matched family donor BMT had two thirds fewer adverse events than did patients who received chemotherapy alone.[54] This advantage for BMT is supported by the intent-to-treat analyses in the CCG trial.[160] Subgroup data are not currently available for the MRC (UK) trial.[26]

Presymptomatic Central Nervous System Treatment

Isolated CNS relapse was a critical barrier to cure in childhood ALL. Although overt CNS leukemia occurs in less than 3% of children, more than 75% suffered isolated CNS relapse as the initial site of failure in early trials.[11] After failing with 5 Gy and 12 Gy, Pinkel and coworkers at SJCRH demonstrated the effectiveness of 24-Gy craniospinal irradiation and showed for the first time that half of these children may be cured.[11]

Subsequently, CNS treatment has evolved. Craniospinal irradiation was replaced by cranial irradiation and short-course intrathecal methotrexate.[161] The radiation dose was reduced from 24 to 18 Gy.[162] The conventional algorithm for determination of the intrathecal methotrexate dose based on body surface area was changed to a pharmacologically validated algorithm based on age, with improved efficacy and less toxicity.[163]

Concerns about secondary brain tumors[164, 165] and neurocognitive damage[166-168] led to increasing restriction of cranial irradiation. The CCG-161 study showed that cranial irradiation might be replaced by maintenance intrathecal methotrexate for lower-risk patients.[14] CCG-105 showed that irradiation might be replaced in average-risk patients who receive intensified systemic therapy,[16] and CCG-1882 showed that cranial irradiation might be replaced by additional intrathecal methotrexate for higher-risk patients with a favorable initial response to therapy. Patients who received cranial irradiation had fewer CNS relapses but had more late bone marrow relapses to obtain a similar EFS.[15] The irradiation question was never posed for the largely T-lineage, lymphomatous feature subset by the CCG. In 2000, CCG practice limits cranial irradiation to patients with overt CNS disease at diagnosis (unequivocal blasts and pleocytosis, i.e., more than 4 cells/μL[33]) and to higher-risk patients with an unfavorable day 7 response to therapy. Others recommend irradiation for patients with a high WBC count, especially those with T-lineage disease.[38]

Systemic therapy contributes to CNS control, and omission of irradiation was possible only with intensified systemic therapy in the CCG 105 study. In patients who received only standard systemic therapy, CNS relapse rates passed 20% with no cranial irradiation.[16] In CCG-1922, oral dexamethasone in induction and maintenance halved the CNS relapse rates.[129]

Maintenance intrathecal methotrexate may be excessive. In the United States, intrathecal methotrexate is generally given throughout maintenance for at least 2 years, but the BFM group limits intrathecal therapy to 11 spinal taps over the first 6 months of treatment for most patients, with excellent results. In ALL BFM '90, the cumulative rate of isolated CNS relapse was 4%.[169]

Maintenance

Childhood ALL is unique among malignancies in the role of prolonged maintenance therapy. Based on quite aggressive early therapy, a Japanese group restricted all patients to 1 year of treatment. At 4 years, the EFS rate was 60%, worse than previous trials by the same group. The greatest losses occurred in standard-risk patients.[170] The BFM group showed that 2 years of therapy is superior to 1.5 years,[22] and several groups have shown that 3 years of therapy is marginally superior to 2 years.[171] The advantage was slightly greater for boys than girls and was not reflected in a statistically significant survival advantage. Three and 5 years of therapy were equivalent.[172]

Daily oral 6-MP plus weekly oral methotrexate is the usual basic scheme for maintenance therapy. Intravenous methotrexate is no more efficacious than oral methotrexate.[173] Half-dose therapy is less effective than full-dose therapy,[174] but attempts to improve outcome by increasing dose intensity were not successful.[175] The addition of monthly vincristine and prednisone pulses increased EFS for lower-risk patients in one trial.[14] The addition of other agents—cyclophosphamide and cytosine arabinoside—to this basic combination resulted in erosion of 6-MP/methotrexate doses and a worse outcome.[174] An attempt to replace the standard daily oral 6-MP and weekly oral methotrexate with alternating pulses of cytosine arabinoside/doxorubicin (Adriamycin) and 6-MP/methotrexate resulted in an inferior outcome.[176] Curiously, one trial showed an advantage of alternating biweekly pulses of vincristine, prednisone, and 6-MP with intravenous methotrexate (no rescue) over a conventional maintenance schedule.[177] DFCI trials provide excellent outcomes with 6-MP given 3 weeks out of 4.[37, 38]

TREATMENT AFTER RELAPSE

Because ALL is so common, relapsed ALL is a relatively frequent event when compared with other pediatric malignancies[2, 3]—in spite of the signal progress to date. Our inability to treat relapse effectively[24, 25] (see Table 26-2) maintains the pressure to continue to intensify therapy to prevent relapses more effectively and imposes an increasing burden of morbidity on the growing majority of patients who would be cured with less morbid therapy.

Determinants of Outcome

Time to relapse and the site of relapse are important predictors of outcome after relapse (see Table 26-2). Later relapse is better than earlier relapse,[24, 25] testicular relapse is better than CNS relapse, and CNS relapse is better than marrow relapse (Table 26-2). Outcome may be better for combined marrow and CNS relapse than for isolated marrow relapse.[178] Outcome after relapse is better for patients with TEL AML1[179] and worse for T-cell patients[180] and t(9;22) patients,[181, 182] especially those with an initial poor peripheral blood response to intrathecal methotrexate and oral prednisone. In a multivariate analysis of more than 1000 relapses, the initial WBC count was the most important predictor of survival after relapse.[24]

Interpretation of the results of treatment after relapse is complicated by differences in previous therapy. Many trials lack internal controls and require external comparisons for evaluation. Patients who relapse with less effective primary therapy may have a better outcome with subsequent therapy than patients who relapse with more effective therapy. Conversely, patients who still relapse despite more effective previous therapy may have a worse outcome with subsequent therapy than patients who relapsed after less effective primary therapy.

Little is known about the cellular and molecular features of relapse. On a cellular level, MTT data show that relapsed ALL has a striking resistance to prednisolone and dexamethasone. The mean LC_{50} for prednisolone at relapse is more than 2 $\log_{10}$ units higher than at initial evaluation. The LC_{50} for no drug other than glucocorticosteroids increases by more than 0.5 $\log_{10}$ units.[98] This change appears to follow from the preferential relapse of patients with steroid resistance at diagnosis rather than the late emergence of steroid resistance in previously steroid-sensitive patients. LC_{50} is higher for multiple and early relapse than for late relapse.

p53 is a critical regulator of apoptosis and crucial to the activity of a variety of drugs that damage DNA.[69] Overexpression of mdm-2 may counteract p53 function and prevent apoptosis. In childhood ALL, p53 function is usually intact at diagnosis, but abnormal p53 or overexpressed mdm-2 at diagnosis is associated with induction failure or early relapse.[76] Scanty, but intriguing data suggest that p53 function may be lost at relapse, especially in patients with t(1;19)[183] or T-cell disease.[184]

Marrow Relapse

Marrow relapse may be manifested as bone pain, bruising, lymphadenopathy, hepatosplenomegaly, pallor, or persistent low-grade fever, as in primary ALL. Cytopenia and/or circulating peripheral blood blasts may provide the first hint of marrow relapse. Marrow relapse is rare in the absence of hints from the history, physical examination, and peripheral blood counts. Rogers and coworkers reviewed 1466 children treated between 1978 and 1981 and found that in the absence of signs or symptoms, about 1 bone marrow aspirate in 160 revealed relapse.[185] As primary treatment has improved and the risk of relapse decreased, this percentage may now be even lower.

Achievement of a second complete remission (CR2) is the initial goal in the treatment of ALL with marrow relapse. In a variety of trials 70% to 95% of patients may achieve a second remission with treatment similar to that used in achieving a first remission.[25] Success depends on the duration of the first remission and, perhaps, the intensity of preceding therapy. The "quality" of the second remission may be inferior to that of the first remission. In one trial using fluorescence-activated cell sorting with a leukemia progenitor cell assay system (FACS/LPC), leukemia was detectable in end-induction marrow in morphologic remission in 30% of patients in CR1 and 58% of relapsed patients in CR2.[186] Gaynon and coworkers found a link between prolonged asparagine depletion and good response to reinduction therapy.[187] Abshire and coworkers showed that weekly polyethylene glycol (PEG) asparaginase yielded a higher remission reinduction rate than did administration of PEG asparaginase every 2 weeks.[188] Poor response was associated with rapid asparaginase clearance and the appearance of high-titer antiasparaginase antibodies.[188, 189] Patients in CR2 also require presymptomatic CNS-directed retreatment.[190]

Matched sibling donor BMT has been proposed as the treatment of choice for children with ALL and bone marrow relapse. Unfortunately, some patients never achieve a second remission, some may relapse before they are able to undergo BMT or may suffer severe organ toxicity or contract a deep-seated infection and no longer be considered BMT candidates, and some patients die of the complications of BMT or graft-versus-host disease or relapse after BMT. The impact of matched sibling donor transplantation may be less than one might imagine.[191]

Several groups have compared BMT outcomes and chemotherapy outcomes in case-control trials. Barrett and coworkers examined 255 matched pairs from the International Bone Marrow Transplant Registry and found 5-year DFS rates of 40% and 17% for BMT and chemotherapy.[192] Hoogerbrugge and coworkers reported rates of 44% and 24%,[193] Uderzo and coworkers, 37% and 22%[194]; and Schroeder and coworkers, 35% and 15%.[195] A comparison of the BMT experience gathered over 20 years with the chemotherapy experience for the last several years may be misleading, however.[196] These figures exaggerate the clinical impact of BMT in that they exclude the substantial number of patients who never achieve second remission or who relapse before BMT can be performed. If one in five patients fails to achieve CR2 and one in four CR2 patients relapses before BMT can be performed, a reported 40% procedural DFS rate for BMT becomes a 24% EFS rate. Case-control analyses may allow for waiting time bias, but they cannot correct for selection bias, so even this figure is probably also an overestimate.

Only a minority of patients have matched family donors. Alternative stem-cell sources have been proposed, namely, matched unrelated marrow donor or umbilical cord stem-cell donors, haploidentical related marrow donors, and purged autologous marrow donors.[197, 198] The best results with autologous BMT have been reported for patients with longer CR1s.[199] Two trials failed to show any advantage for purged autologous BMT over conventional chemotherapy.[200, 201]

The results cited for matched unrelated donor BMT are generally similar to those reported for matched family donor BMT. Balduzzi and coworkers reported a 47% DFS rate for 15 CR1 or CR2 patients,[202] Davies and coworkers reported a 20% DFS rate for 19 CR2 patients,[203] and Oakhill and coworkers reported a 53% DFS rate for 50 patients who received transplants in CR2 with T-cell depletion.[204]

Identification of an appropriate unrelated donor and arrangement of marrow harvesting take time, so the interval from CR2 to BMT may be longer for matched unrelated donor BMT than for matched related donor BMT. More potential patients are likely to relapse or suffer major morbidity or deep-seated infection before BMT, and the clinical impact is therefore diminished. Transplant mortality remains high. Adequately controlled trials are lacking, and the generalizability of single-center series remains in doubt. In a population-based rather than center-based survey of patients with marrow and/or extramedullary relapse, Lawson and colleagues reported 5-year EFS rates of 47%, 44%, and 31% for chemotherapy, matched related donor BMT, and matched unrelated donor BMT, respectively, after adjustment for prognostic factors and time to transplant in analyses by treatment received.[191]

In summary, BMT is not a complete answer to the problem of marrow relapse because too many patients never achieve CR2, too many patients relapse before BMT can be performed, and too many patients die of BMT-related complications or relapse despite BMT. Lausen and associates note a higher post-BMT relapse rate for more recent patients who relapsed despite more recent, more intensive chemotherapy.[205] Wheeler and coworkers found

that only 2 of 16 patients survived BMT without relapse after on-therapy marrow relapse. Although substantial outcomes as high as 50% have been reported for late marrow relapse with chemotherapy, outcomes after earlier marrow relapse and for any T-cell marrow relapse are dismal.[26]

CNS Relapse

CNS relapse usually occurs between 1 and 3 years from diagnosis[24] and may be manifested by symptoms and signs of increased intracranial pressure, namely, headache, diplopia, nausea or vomiting, and/or papilledema.[206] With frequent periodic lumbar punctures and maintenance intrathecal therapy, most relapses are now asymptomatic. Pleocytosis and/or CNS symptoms may be the result of treatment as well as the consequence of disease, so relapse should not be hastily presumed in the absence of cytologic proof. In very rare cases, CNS relapse may be accompanied by cranial nerve findings or a hypothalamic syndrome of hyperphagia.[207] The cumulative incidence of isolated CNS relapse was 4.4% in the CCG-1800 series[23] and 4.0% on the BFM '90 study.[169] A substantial number of patients with an apparently isolated CNS relapse by conventional microscopic criteria have demonstrable marrow involvement by PCR or FACS/LPC.[208, 209]

Diagnosis requires pleocytosis (>4 cells/μL) and unequivocal blasts on microscopic examination of the cytospin preparation. A single, isolated cerebrospinal fluid examination with apparent blasts but without pleocytosis may not always represent relapse.[210]

Blasts may usually be cleared with weekly or twice-weekly intrathecal therapy. Intrathecal triple therapy—methotrexate, cytosine arabinoside, and hydrocortisone—has been advocated,[211] but in one trial, three-agent therapy was no more effective than two-agent therapy with methotrexate and hydrocortisone.[212]

Systemic reinduction is followed by some period of intensification and maintenance therapy. In one study, craniospinal irradiation plus intrathecal triple therapy was more effective than cranial irradiation alone.[213] Among 3712 children treated initially in CCG studies between 1983 and 1988, 220 had isolated CNS relapse. After relapse, a 6-year EFS rate of 37% was obtained.[24] A recent POG trial obtained an impressive 4-year EFS rate of 71% for 83 children with isolated CNS relapse and no previous cranial irradiation—46% and 83% for CR1 at less than 18 months and at 18 months or longer, respectively.[214] Patients received vincristine, dexamethasone, and daunomycin in induction, followed by high-dose cytosine arabinoside and asparaginase in consolidation, and then alternating intravenous methotrexate/6-MP and cyclophosphamide/etoposide for 11 weeks in intensification. After 5 months of intensive therapy, patients received vincristine, dexamethasone, and L-asparaginase with 24-Gy cranial and 15-Gy spinal irradiation and 18 months of less intensive therapy with alternating 6-week courses of daily oral 6-MP and weekly oral methotrexate and intravenous cyclophosphamide/etoposide. Patients received nine doses of intrathecal triple therapy in the first

22 weeks and no maintenance intrathecal therapy. The bone marrow was involved in 10 of 14 treatment failures.

Craniospinal irradiation therapy has been recommended[215] but may be delayed for 1 to 6 months to preserve the bone marrow reserve.[214] The usual cranial dose has been 24 Gy, but increasing success in some trials and increasing awareness of the long-term consequences of brain irradiation have spurred interest in omission of spinal irradiation, a lower dose of cranial irradiation, or omission of cranial irradiation altogether, especially for later relapse. Some have advocated low-dose extended-course irradiation therapy—150 cGy per fraction daily for 4 days, followed by craniospinal irradiation at 150 cGy per fraction per month, with an 18-Gy cumulative dose.[216] With subsequent intrathecal and intraventricular therapy, excellent results have been obtained with craniospinal doses between 6 and 9 Gy.[217]

Testicular Relapse

Testicular relapse is usually associated with painless enlargement of one or both testes. Diagnosis requires biopsy. Among boys treated in CCG protocols between 1983 and 1988, 112 suffered isolated testicular relapse with a 6-year EFS rate of 64%. Three of five relapses occurred more than 3 years after diagnosis. Again, outcomes improve with increasing duration of CR1.[24]

Therapy consists of systemic reinduction, presymptomatic CNS treatment, intensification, and maintenance. Conventionally, patients have received bilateral testicular irradiation at doses of 24 Gy.[218, 219] Provocatively, several patients have been reported in whom irradiation was omitted and replaced with intermediate-dose parenteral methotrexate.[222]

LATE EFFECTS

The expectation of cure for most children with ALL focuses attention on the quality of their survival. However, significant morbidity exists in the so-called normal population, and appropriate controls are critical for assessment of the impact of disease and treatment. McMaster University investigators compared the health status of survivors of childhood ALL with that of the general Canadian teenage population in the domains of sensation (sight and hearing), mobility, cognition, self-care, pain, and fertility.[221-224] Zero, one, and two or more deficits were found in 45%, 31%, and 24% of the normal population, and in several groups of children with ALL, zero, one, and two or more deficits were found in 30% to 60%, 32% to 47%, and 8% to 26%, respectively.[221, 224] Obvious differences are lacking, but the study populations are small and the instruments are evolving. Neither bland confidence nor wild alarm is appropriate.

Neurotoxicity

The potential neurotoxicity of brain irradiation, parenteral methotrexate, and intrathecal therapy is a continuing concern. Hill and colleagues studied 110 survivors at a mean of 14.7 years after diagnosis. Fifty-two patients had received 24-Gy cranial irradiation and 58 had received intravenous methotrexate; all received intrathecal methotrexate. Cranial irradiation was associated with poorer body image and lower academic achievement.[167] Haupt and coworkers found that leukemia survivors were more likely to enter a special education or learning disabilities program than their sibling controls were, but they had the same probability of finishing high school, entering college, and earning a bachelor's degree. Survivors in whom ALL was diagnosed before 6 years of age and those who received 24-Gy cranial irradiation were a third less likely to enter college.[225] Jankovic and coworkers studied 203 children in a multicenter European study.[168] One hundred twenty-nine received 18-Gy cranial irradiation and 74 received parenteral methotrexate and no irradiation. They found that 18-Gy cranial irradiation resulted in a gradual decline in full-scale IQ scores, first appearing 3 to 7 years after irradiation and amounting to about 10 points mean. The effect seemed confined to children younger than 3 years at diagnosis.

However, intensive oral or parenteral methotrexate causes acute neurotoxicity.[156, 157, 226, 227] Parenteral methotrexate was implicated in CNS toxicity—most commonly seizures—in 10% to 16% of cases in three recent trials.[156, 157, 226] The late neurocognitive consequences of these therapies have not yet been explored.

Others have found similar neurocognitive deficits in children treated with either 18-Gy cranial irradiation, parenteral methotrexate, or intrathecal methotrexate. Mulhern and associates note that group means may mask individual declines of greater than 15 points that may occur in 22% to 30% of children studied after cranial irradiation or no cranial irradiation.[228] Ochs and coworkers found greater than a 15-point decline in IQ in 30 of 49 patients—16 of 26 with no cranial irradiation.[229] Administration of a memory battery found losses in short-term and long-term recall. School performance was affected.[230] At a 3-year follow-up, Brown and coworkers compared children with leukemia who received intrathecal methotrexate but no intermediate-dose parenteral methotrexate with other children with cancer who received CNS-directed therapy. They found that children with leukemia scored more poorly on academic tests of spelling, reading, and arithmetic.[231] Like the dose of cranial irradiation, the frequency of parenteral methotrexate administration and the dose and timing of leucovorin rescue may affect neurotoxicity. Others have found excellent neurocognitive outcomes in infants and older patients who received very high-dose methotrexate (33.6 g/m^2) but no brain irradiation.[232, 233] Methotrexate is neurotoxic, but its effects may depend on the exact doses and schedules of both methotrexate and leucovorin.

Secondary Malignant Neoplasms

Secondary malignant neoplasms are reported in childhood ALL, especially in the context of cranial irradiation and epipodophyllotoxins (namely, etoposide or teniposide). In 1991, Neglia and coworkers found a 15-year cumulative incidence of 2.5% in 9720 children treated with CCG protocols between 1972 and 1988, a sevenfold increase in comparison to age-matched controls. Brain tumors occurred in eight children, a 22-fold increase. All had had previously undergone cranial irradiation. Two patients had secondary AML.[164] More recently, Bhatia and colleagues found a 1.5% 9-year cumulative incidence in 5118 children treated with CCG protocols between 1988 and 1995, an eightfold increased risk of cancer overall.[234] Eight children had secondary AML or myelodysplasia, a 71-fold increased incidence. Four patients had secondary lymphoma and four had soft-tissue sarcoma. Three patients had brain tumors—two after cranial irradiation. Cranial irradiation doubled the risk of secondary malignancy. The intensity of therapy increased between the two eras, and cranial irradiation was restricted to fewer patients. No patient received epipodophyllotoxins—linked to secondary AML—as a part of primary therapy. However, the incidence of secondary AML/myelodysplasia—still less than 1%—appears to be rising in recent CCG trials.

Among 5006 children treated with BFM protocols between 1979 and 1997, the cumulative incidence of secondary malignancies was 3.3%. The incidence was 3.5% in children who had received cranial irradiation and 1.2% in patients with no cranial irradiation. The incidence of AML was 0.6% in both groups.[165]

Epipodophyllotoxins have been associated with a higher incidence of secondary AML, specifically, disease involving chromosomal abnormalities at chromosome 11q23.[227, 235, 236] In one study, the incidence of secondary AML was 3.8% at 6 years—12% in patients who received weekly or semiweekly epipodophyllotoxins.[237] In another study, the incidence was 5.9% in children who received semiweekly epipodophyllotoxins.[227] In a study of T-cell ALL, the incidence reached 20%.[235]

Secondary brain tumor is strongly linked to cranial irradiation. Walter and colleagues found a cumulative incidence of 0.0%, 1.0%, 1.7%, and 3.2% in children who received 0, 10 to 21, 21 to 30, and more than 30 Gy,

respectively.[165] Host factors may play a role. Relling and coworkers found an extraordinarily high incidence of secondary brain tumors in heterozygotes for thiopurine methyltransferase who received 6-MP during cranial irradiation.[238]

Avascular Necrosis of Bone

Avascular necrosis of bone has been recognized with increasing frequency in adolescents and young adults with ALL. Loss of range of motion and pain are the usual symptoms and may appear before radiographic changes. Magnetic resonance imaging (MRI) (Fig. 26-5) or bone scans may contribute to early diagnosis.

Ojala and associates monitored 24 children and adolescents prospectively with MRI. Lesions consistent with avascular necrosis developed in nine; six had no symptoms. Lesions regressed in six cases and resolved in three. No treatment interventions were required.[239]

In a recent CCG study, the incidence of symptomatic disease was 14% in children older than 10 years and 1% in children younger than 10 years. Among older patients, avascular necrosis was more common in females than males, European Americans than African Americans, and patients receiving two courses of dexamethasone than patients receiving one course. Cases were identified within 3 years and were transient in only 16%. Disease involved the weight-bearing joints in 94% and was multifocal in 74%.[240] CCG protocols after 1995 decrease the duration of exposure to dexamethasone for patients older than 10 years. The impact of this change has yet to be evaluated.

Cardiotoxicity

Subclinical anthracycline toxicity is common. However, clinical cardiotoxicity is rare. Of 97 patients who had received at least 228 mg/m^2 of Adriamycin, Lipshultz and

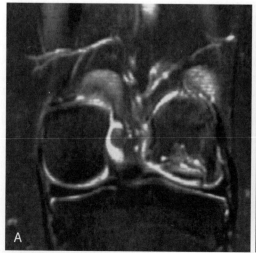
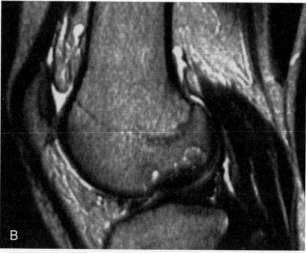

FIGURE 26–5. Coronal *(A)* and sagittal *(B)* T2 images from an MRI demonstrating corticosteroid-induced avascular necrosis of the right medial femoral condyle in a 15-year-old white woman. (Courtesy Dr. Leonard A. Mattano, Michigan State University/Kalamazoo Center for Medical Studies.)

coworkers found that 65% had increased left ventricular wall stress and 23% had a decreased stress-velocity index or both. End-systolic wall stress increased serially in 70%. A higher cumulative anthracycline dose predicted decreased contractility (stress-velocity index), and age younger than 4 years predicted increased wall stress. Eleven of 97 patients had clinical congestive heart failure within 1 year of completion of anthracycline therapy.[241] Of 120 patients who received between 90 and 270 mg/m² of daunomycin, Sorenson and colleagues found decreased mean left ventricular fractional shortening and increased left ventricular end-systolic wall stress when compared with 50 normal children. However, all values remained within the normal range, and no child had clinical cardiotoxicity. No differences were apparent between children who received 90 mg/m² and those who received 270 mg/m².[242] Krisher et al reviewed 2317 children with ALL who received anthracyclines on POG protocols between 1974 and 1990. Forty-two had clinical cardiotoxicity (1.8%). The risk of cardiotoxicity was linked to cumulative exposure of more than 550 mg/m² and a maximal bolus dose of greater than 50 mg/m². Cardiotoxicity was apparent within 1 year of completion of anthracycline therapy in about 90% of cases.[243] Persistent elevation of troponin T provides an early indication of anthracycline-induced cardiotoxicity and may provide a sensitive and cost-effective alternative to echocardiography or nuclear medicine studies.[244] Limitation of anthracycline exposure to less than 300 mg/m² is an effective strategy to avoid clinical cardiotoxicity.[245] Curiously, current practice sanctions careful screening for cardiotoxicity, which is fortunately rare, while discouraging screening for a vascular necrosis, which is relatively common in adolescents and young adults and can lead to lifelong disability.

Melanocytic Nevi

Survivors of childhood ALL and other cancers have an increased number of melanocytic nevi.[246-248] In general, the number of nevi is the most important predictor for the development of melanoma.[249, 250] Neglia and coworkers identified only one melanoma in their cohort of 9720 children, whereas Bhatia and colleagues found none in their cohort of 5181 patients.[164, 234]

FUTURE TRENDS

Treatment Allocation

More precise treatment allocation may spare many children the morbidity of unneeded intensive therapy and better identify those who need such therapy. We do well to remember that "Pinkel era" therapy cured about half of the patients. Subsequent elaborations of therapy are redundant for this near majority of patients and contribute to short-term and long-term morbidity. We just do not know who they are. Several trials have shown that certain subsets of patients derive no added benefit from elements of therapy shown to be useful in other contexts. For example, NCI/Rome standard-risk patients derive no ben-

efit from intensive induction/consolidation when they receive one DI phase.[128] Standard-risk trisomy 10 patients[47] and standard-risk patients already M1 by day 7 of therapy[127] derive no added benefit from a second DI, even though a second DI had added benefit overall.

On the other hand, some patients may be rescued with more effective therapies. For example, the augmented intensive regimen improves outcomes in higher-risk patients with a poor day 7 response.[20, 99] In the CCG experience, improvements in therapy have led to three flip-flops in which putatively higher-risk patients receiving successful novel regimens had better outcome than did putatively lower-risk patients receiving less aggressive, "risk-adjusted" therapies.[23] Standard-risk patients in CCG-105 who received DI had a better outcome than did lower-risk patients in CCG-104 who did not. Standard-risk patients in CCG-1881 who received double DI had a better outcome than did lower-risk patients in CCG-1881 who received either one or no DI. Higher-risk, slow early response patients younger than 10 years had a better outcome with the augmented intensive regimen than did higher-risk, rapid early response patients younger than 10 years who received the standard intensive regimen.

New technologies will facilitate the identification of various cytogenetic/molecular subsets and better assess response. Molecular techniques[61] will improve detection of subsets such as t(9;22), for whom specific interventions such as STI571, an ab1 tyrosine kinase inhibitor,[251-253] will be increasingly available. Patients with lower-risk trisomies and translocations such as t(12;22) may be assigned to more appropriate treatments. Preliminary CCG data suggest that standard-risk trisomy 10 patients benefit from DI and dexamethasone but not double DI, independent of early marrow response.[47] Otherwise, standard-risk patients with a rapid initial response to therapy also appear to derive no benefit from a second DI—even though the second DI is beneficial overall. We are seeking to confirm this retrospective observation in the 2000–2003 CCG standard-risk trial. Thomson and associates have identified discordance between the day 7 and day 14 blast percentages by morphology and multiparameter flow cytometry and hold out the possibility that flow cytometry might better identify residual blasts.[109] End-induction disease burden by multiparameter flow cytometry or PCR-based technologies may better detect patients needing more or less therapy.[103, 104, 106] Microarray technology will enable us to evolve from a single-marker characterization of leukemia, such as BCR ABL, to a multimarker characterization and challenge us to embrace the complexity.[254-256] Recognition of host polymorphisms will add a new layer of complexity.[82, 83, 257-259]

More Effective Antileukemia Therapy

More effective use of conventional agents and the introduction of novel agents with activity against otherwise resistant leukemic blasts may further improve cure. Gaynon et al found that poor asparagine depletion predicted a poor reinduction outcome.[187] Abshire and coworkers found that weekly PEG asparaginase yielded a better second remission rate than did PEG asparaginase every 2 weeks.[188] Much effort has been devoted to finding the best dose and schedule for methotrexate.

New agents may be divided into new old agents and new new agents. Simple substitution of dexamethasone for prednisone resulted in a 40% reduction of hazard.[129] Other glucocorticoid ligands such as cortivazol with activity against dexamethasone-resistant lymphoblasts are of interest.[260-262] Current clinical trials are comparing 6-thioguanine and 6-MP. 6-Thioguanine is more active than 6-MP in vitro[263] and provides higher levels of intracellular thioguanine nucleotides.[264, 265] Aminopterin, the original antifol, has been the subject of renewed interest.[266]

New new agents may target leukemia-specific features. The immunotoxin B43-PAP, an anti-CD19–pokeweed viral protein immunoconjugate, has entered clinical trials.[267-269] ST1571, an ab1 tyrosine kinase inhibitor, is entering evaluation. ST1571 blocks the antiapoptotic effect of BCR ABL and enhances the efficacy of other agents in this very difficult disease.[251-253] The agent 506U, a prodrug for guanine arabinoside, appears to have specific activity against T-lineage malignancies.[270-272] Recognition of the loss of sensitivity to conventional glucocorticoids and the loss of p53 function at relapse may guide therapeutic strategies.

Much effort has focused on comparisons of chemotherapy and BMT, but in reality, the value of such "apples and oranges" comparisons is limited. Such comparisons test, at best, one chemotherapy regimen against one BMT regimen and cannot be generalized to all chemotherapy regimens and all BMT regimens. A more appropriate challenge might be reasoned attempts to improve outcomes after either BMT or chemotherapy. Because so many patients never achieve a second remission or relapse too quickly to get to BMT, a focus on pre-BMT interventions may be more profitable than a focus on potential post-BMT interventions, for example, minimizing graft-versus-host disease prophylaxis or immune manipulations such as less aggressive graft-versus-host disease prophylaxis.[273]

Reduction of pre-BMT disease burden may improve outcome after BMT. Two ALL studies have linked preablation minimal residual disease with relapse after BMT.[274, 275] In AML, a recent study showed that intensively timed induction improved DFS after either marrow-ablative or conventional chemotherapy consolidation[276]—presumably through enhanced reduction of the disease burden while not affecting the remission induction rate. New technologies allowing assessment of minimal residual disease may provide a tool to compare regimens as well as monitor disease status more helpfully than has been possible with microscopy alone. More effective use of known agents and the introduction of novel agents with activity against otherwise resistant cells provide two strategies for the now measurable reduction in disease burden and improvement in outcome.

REFERENCES

1. Greaves MF: Differentiation-linked leukemogenesis in lymphocytes. Science 1986;234:697.
2. Gurney JG, Severson RK, Davis S, et al: Incidence of cancer in children in the United States. Sex-, race-, and 1-year age-specific rates by histologic type. Cancer 1995;75:2186.
3. Young JL Jr, Ries LG, Silverberg E, et al: Cancer incidence, survival, and mortality for children younger than age 15 years. Cancer 1986;58:598.
4. Dordelmann M, Schrappe M, Reiter A, et al: Down's syndrome in childhood acute lymphoblastic leukemia: Clinical characteristics and treatment outcome in four consecutive BFM trials. Berlin-Frankfurt-Munster Group. Leukemia 1998;12:645.
5. Fong CT, Brodeur GM: Down's syndrome and leukemia: Epidemiology, genetics, cytogenetics and mechanisms of leukemogenesis. Cancer Genet Cytogenet 1987;28:55.
6. Robison LL, Nesbit MEJ, Sather HN, et al: Down syndrome and acute leukemia in children: A 10-year retrospective survey from Children's Cancer Study Group. J Pediatr 1984;105:235.
7. Pui CH: Recent advances in the biology and treatment of childhood acute lymphoblastic leukemia. Curr Opin Hematol 1998; 5:292.
8. Pui CH, Boyett JM, Hancock ML, et al: Outcome of treatment for childhood cancer in black as compared with white children. The St Jude Children's Research Hospital experience, 1962 through 1992. JAMA 1995;273:633.
9. Aur R, Simone J, Verzosa M, et al: Childhood acute lymphocytic leukemia. Study VIII. Cancer 1978;42:2123.
10. Aur RJ, Simone J, Hustu HO, et al: Central nervous system therapy and combination chemotherapy of childhood lymphocytic leukemia. Blood 1971;37:272.
11. Hustu HO, Aur RJ, Verzosa MS, et al: Prevention of central nervous system leukemia by irradiation. Cancer 1973;32:585.
12. Hitchcock Bryan S, Gelber R, Cassady JR, et al: The impact of induction anthracycline on long-term failure-free survival in childhood acute lymphoblastic leukemia. Med Pediatr Oncol 1986; 14:211.
13. Sallan SE, Hitchcock Bryan S, Gelber R, et al: Influence of intensive asparaginase in the treatment of childhood non–T-cell acute lymphoblastic leukemia. Cancer Res 1983;43:5601.
14. Bleyer WA, Sather HN, Nickerson HJ, et al: Monthly pulses of vincristine and prednisone prevent bone marrow and testicular relapse in low-risk childhood acute lymphoblastic leukemia: A report of the CCG-161 study by the Children's Cancer Study Group. J Clin Oncol 1991;9:1012.
15. Nachman J, Sather HN, Cherlow JM, et al: Response of children with high-risk acute lymphoblastic leukemia treated with and without cranial irradiation: A report from the Children's Cancer Group. J Clin Oncol 1998;16:920.
16. Tubergen DG, Gilchrist GS, O'Brien RT, et al: Prevention of CNS disease in intermediate-risk acute lymphoblastic leukemia: Comparison of cranial radiation and intrathecal methotrexate and the importance of systemic therapy: A Children's Cancer Group report. J Clin Oncol 1993;11:520.
17. Gaynon PS, Steinherz PG, Bleyer WA, et al: Intensive therapy for children with acute lymphoblastic leukaemia and unfavourable presenting features. Early conclusions of study CCG-106 by the Children's Cancer Study Group. Lancet 1988;2:921.
18. Henze G, Fengler R, Reiter A, et al: Impact of early intensive reinduction therapy on event-free survival in children with low-risk acute lymphoblastic leukemia. Hamatol Bluttransfus 1990; 33:483.
19. Henze G, Langermann HJ, Bramswig J, et al: [The BFM 76/79 acute lymphoblastic leukemia therapy study]. Klin Padiatr 1981;193:145.
20. Nachman JB, Sather HN, Sensel MG, et al: Augmented post-induction therapy for children with high-risk acute lymphoblastic leukemia and a slow response to initial therapy. N Engl J Med 1998; 338:1663.
21. Riehm H, Feickert HJ, Schrappe M, et al: Therapy results in five ALL-BFM studies since 1970: Implications of risk factors for prognosis. Hamatol Bluttransfus 1987;30:139.
22. Riehm H, Gadner H, Henze G, et al: Results and significance of six randomized trials in four consecutive ALL-BFM studies. Hamatol Bluttransfus 1990;33:439.
23. Gaynon PS, Trigg ME, Heerema NA, et al: Children's Cancer Group Trials in childhood acute lymphoblastic leukemia: 1983–1995. Leukemia 2000;14:2223.
24. Gaynon PS, Qu RP, Chappell RJ, et al: Survival after relapse in childhood acute lymphoblastic leukemia: Impact of site and time to first relapse, the Children's Cancer Group experience. Cancer 1998;82:1387.

25. Chessells J: Relapsed lymphoblastic leukemia in children: A continuing challenge. Br J Haematol 1998;102:423.

26. Wheeler K, Richards S, Bailey C, et al: Comparison of bone marrow transplant and chemotherapy for relapsed childhood acute lymphoblastic leukaemia: The MRC UKALL X experience. Br J Haematol 1998;101:94.

27. Bennett JM, Catovsky D, Daniel MT, et al: The morphological classification of acute lymphoblastic leukaemia: Concordance among observers and clinical correlations. Br J Haematol 1981; 47:553.

28. Pui CH, Behm FG, Crist WM: Clinical and biologic relevance of immunologic marker studies in childhood acute lymphoblastic leukemia. Blood 1993;82:343.

29. de Graaf SS, vd Berg H, van Wering ER, et al: Lack of prognostic significance of a low number of lymphoblasts in the cerebrospinal fluid (CSF) in children with acute lymphoblastic leukemia (ALL) [meeting abstract]. Proc Am Soc Clin Oncol 1996;15:1083.

30. Gilchrist G, Sather H, Gaynon P, et al: Outcome effect of low cerebrospinal fluid (CSF) leukocyte count with blasts at diagnosis of childhood acute lymphoblastic leukemia (ALL) [abstract]. Proc Am Soc Clin Oncol 1997;16:516.

31. Mahmoud HH, Rivera GK, Hancock ML, et al: Low leukocyte counts with blast cells in cerebrospinal fluid of children with newly diagnosed acute lymphoblastic leukemia. N Engl J Med 1993;329:314.

32. Bleyer WA, Sather H, Coccia P, et al: The staging of childhood acute lymphoblastic leukemia: Strategies of the Children's Cancer Study Group and a three-dimensional technic of multivariate analysis. Med Pediatr Oncol 1986;14:271.

33. Mastrangelo R, Poplack D, Bleyer A, et al: Report and recommendations of the Rome Workshop concerning poor-prognosis acute lymphoblastic leukemia in children: Biologic bases for staging, stratification, and treatment. Med Pediatr Oncol 1986;14:191.

34. Biondi A, Cimino G, Pieters R, et al: Biologic and therapeutic aspects of infant leukemia. Blood 2000;96:24.

35. Pui CH, Kane JR, Crist WM: Biology and treatment of infant leukemias. Leukemia 1995;9:762.

36. Reaman GH, Sposto R, Sensel MG, et al: Treatment outcome and prognostic factors for infants with acute lymphoblastic leukemia treated on two consecutive trials of the Children's Cancer Group. J Clin Oncol 1999;17:445.

37. Clavell LA, Gelber RD, Cohen HJ, et al: Four-agent induction and intensive asparaginase therapy for treatment of childhood acute lymphoblastic leukemia. N Engl J Med 1986;315:657.

38. Schorin MA, Blattner S, Gelber RD, et al: Treatment of childhood acute lymphoblastic leukemia: Results of Dana-Farber Cancer Institute/Children's Hospital Acute Lymphoblastic Leukemia Consortium Protocol 85-01. J Clin Oncol 1994;12:740.

39. Uckun FM, Sensel MG, Sun L, et al: Biology and treatment of childhood T-lineage acute lymphoblastic leukemia. Blood 1998; 91:735.

40. Uckun FM, Waurzyniak BJ, Sather HN, et al: Prognostic significance of T-lineage leukemic cell growth in SCID mice: A Children's Cancer Group study. Leuk Lymphoma 1999;32:475.

41. Uckun F, Gaynon P, Sather H: Clinical features and treatment outcome of children with biphenotypic CD2+CD19+ acute lymphoblastic leukemia: A Children's Cancer Group Study. Blood 1996; 89:2488.

42. Uckun FM, Sather HN, Gaynon P, et al: Clinical features and treatment outcome of children with myeloid antigen positive acute lymphoblastic leukemia: A report from the Children's Cancer Group. Blood 1997;90:28.

43. Chessells JM, Swansbury GJ, Reeves B, et al: Cytogenetics and prognosis in childhood lymphoblastic leukaemia: Results of MRC UKALL X. Medical Research Council Working Party in Childhood Leukaemia. Br J Haematol 1997;99:93.

44. Crist WM, Pui CH: Clinical implications of cytogenetic and molecular analyses of pediatric acute lymphoblastic leukemia. Stem Cells 1993;11:81.

45. Heerema NA, Sather HN, Sensel MG, et al: Frequency and clinical significance of cytogenetic abnormalities in pediatric T-lineage acute lymphoblastic leukemia: A report from the Children's Cancer Group. J Clin Oncol 1998;16:1270.

46. Pui CH, Crist WM, Look AT: Biology and clinical significance of cytogenetic abnormalities in childhood acute lymphoblastic leukemia. Blood 1990;76:1449.

47. Heerema NA, Sather HN, Sensel MG, et al: Prognostic impact of trisomies of chromosomes 10, 17, and 5 among children with acute lymphoblastic leukemia and high hyperdiploidy (>50 chromosomes). J Clin Oncol 2000;18:1876.

48. Jackson JF, Boyett J, Pullen J, et al: Favorable prognosis associated with hyperdiploidy in children with acute lymphocytic leukemia correlates with extra chromosome 6. A Pediatric Oncology Group study. Cancer 1990;66:1183.

49. Heerema NA, Nachman JB, Sather HN, et al: Hypodiploidy with less than 45 chromosomes confers adverse risk in childhood acute lymphoblastic leukemia: A report from the Children's Cancer Group. Blood 1999;94:4036.

50. Pui CH, Williams DL, Raimondi SC, et al: Hypodiploidy is associated with a poor prognosis in childhood acute lymphoblastic leukemia. Blood 1987;70:247.

51. Pui CH, Carroll AJ, Head D, et al: Near-triploid and near-tetraploid acute lymphoblastic leukemia of childhood. Blood 1990;76:590.

52. Heerema NA, Arthur DC, Sather H, et al: Cytogenetic features of infants less than 12 months of age at diagnosis of acute lymphoblastic leukemia: Impact of the 11q23 breakpoint on outcome: A report of the Children's Cancer Group. Blood 1994;83:2274.

53. Heerema NA, Sather HN, Ge J, et al: Cytogenetic studies of infant acute lymphoblastic leukemia: Poor prognosis of infants with t(4; 11)—a report of the Children's Cancer Group. Leukemia 1999; 13:679.

54. Arico M, Valsecchi M, Camitta B, et al: Outcome of treatment in children with Philadelphia chromosome–positive acute lymphoblastic leukemia. N Engl J Med 2000;342:998.

55. Uckun FM, Nachman JB, Sather HN, et al: Clinical significance of Philadelphia chromosome positive pediatric acute lymphoblastic leukemia in the context of contemporary intensive therapies: A report from the Children's Cancer Group. Cancer 1998;83:2030.

56. Uckun FM, Nachman JB, Sather HN, et al: Poor treatment outcome of Philadelphia chromosome–positive pediatric acute lymphoblastic leukemia despite intensive chemotherapy. Leuk Lymphoma 1999;33:101.

57. Secker-Walker LM, Berger R, Fenaux P, et al: Prognostic significance of the balanced t(1;19) and unbalanced der(19)t(1;19) translocations in acute lymphoblastic leukemia. Leukemia 1992;6:363.

58. Uckun FM, Waurzyniak BJ, Sensel MG, et al: Primary blasts from infants with acute lymphoblastic leukemia cause overt leukemia in SCID mice. Leuk Lymphoma 1998;30:269.

59. Ritterbach J, Hiddemann W, Beck JD, et al: Detection of hyperdiploid karyotypes (>50 chromosomes) in childhood acute lymphoblastic leukemia (ALL) using fluorescence in situ hybridization (FISH). Leukemia 1998;12:427.

60. Romana SP, Poirel H, Leconiat M, et al: High frequency of t(12;21) in childhood B-lineage acute lymphoblastic leukemia. Blood 1995; 86:4263.

61. Gaynon PS, Crotty ML, Sather HN, et al: Expression of BCR-ABL, E2A-PBX1, and MLL-AF4 fusion transcripts in newly diagnosed children with acute lymphoblastic leukemia: A Children's Cancer Group initiative. Leuk Lymphoma 1997;26:57.

62. Borkhardt A, Cazzaniga G, Viehmann S, et al: Incidence and clinical relevance of TEL/AML1 fusion genes in children with acute lymphoblastic leukemia enrolled in the German and Italian multicenter therapy trials. Associazione Italiana Ematologia Oncologia Pediatrica and the Berlin-Frankfurt-Munster Study Group. Blood 1997;90:571.

63. Shurtleff SA, Buijs A, Behm FG, et al: TEL/AML1 fusion resulting from a cryptic t(12;21) is the most common genetic lesion in pediatric ALL and defines a subgroup of patients with an excellent prognosis. Leukemia 1995;9:1985.

64. Heinonen K, Mahlamaki E: Detection of numerical chromosome abnormalities by FISH in childhood acute lymphoblastic leukemia. Cancer Genet Cytogenet 1996;87:123.

65. Arico M, Schrappe M, Harbott J, et al: Prednisone good response (PGR) identifies a subset of t(9;22) childhood acute lymphoblastic leukemia (ALL) at lower risk for early leukemia relapse [abstract]. Blood 1997;90:560.

66. Pui CH: Acute leukemias with the t(4;11)(q21;q23). Leuk Lymphoma 1992;7:173.

67. Dordelmann M, Reiter A, Borkhardt A, et al: Prednisone response is the strongest predictor of treatment outcome in infant acute lymphoblastic leukemia. Blood 1999;94:1209.

68. Schrappe M, Viehmann S, Dordelmann M, et al: Translocation t(4; 11) (q21;q23): Is it an independent risk factor in childhood ALL [abstract]. Blood 1999;94:500.

69. Hannun Y: Apoptosis and the dilemma of cancer chemotherapy. Blood 1997;89:1845.

70. Adams J, Cory S: The BCL-2 protein family: Arbiters of cell survival. Science 1998;281:1322.

71. Ashkenazi A, Dixit V: Apoptosis control by death and decoy receptors. Curr Opin Cell Biol 1999;11:255.

72. Reed J: Dysregulation of apoptosis in cancer. J Clin Oncol 1999; 17:2941.

73. Smets L: Programmed cell death (apoptosis) and response to anticancer drugs. Anticancer Drugs 1994;5:3.

74. Green D, Reed J: Mitochondria and apoptosis. Science 1998;281: 1309.

75. Evan G, Littlewood T: A matter of life and cell death. Science 1998;281:1317.

76. Marks DI, Kurz BW, Link MP, et al: High incidence of potential p53 inactivation in poor outcome childhood acute lymphoblastic leukemia at diagnosis. Blood 1996;87:1155.

77. Stock W, Tsai T, Golden C, et al: Cell cycle regulatory gene abnormalities are important determinants of leukemogenesis and disease biology in adult acute lymphoblastic leukemia. Blood 2000;95:2364.

78. Coppola S, Ghibelli L: GSH extrusion and the mitochondrial pathway of apoptotic signalling. Biochem Soc Trans 2000;28:56.

79. Baek S, Min J, Park E, et al: Role of the small heat shock protein HSP25 in radioresistance and glutathione-redox cycle. J Cell Physiol 2000;183:100.

80. Maung ZT, Hogarth L, Reid MM, et al: Raised intracellular glutathione levels correlate with in vitro resistance to cytotoxic drugs in leukaemic cells from patients with acute lymphoblastic leukemia. Leukemia 1994;8:1487.

81. Kearns P, Pieters R, Rottier M, et al: The role of glutathione in determining prognosis in childhood acute leukaemia [abstract]. Blood 1999;94:501.

82. Anderer G, Schrappe M, Brechlin A, et al: Polymorphisms within glutathione S-transferase genes (GSTM1, GSTT1, GSTP1), initial response to prednisone and risk of relapse in childhood acute lymphoblastic leukemia [abstract]. Blood 1999;94:500.

83. Stanulla M, Schrappe M, Brechlin Am, et al: Polymorphisms within glutathione S-transferase genes (GSTM1, GSTT21, GSTP1) and risk of relapse in childhood B-precursor acute lymphoblastic leukemia: A case control study. Blood 2000;95:1222.

84. Uckun FM, Yang Z, Sather H, et al: Cellular expression of antiapoptotic BCL-2 oncoprotein in newly diagnosed childhood acute lymphoblastic leukemia: A Children's Cancer Group Study. Blood 1997;89:3769.

85. Maung ZT, Reid MM, Matheson E, et al: Corticosteroid resistance is increased in lymphoblasts from adults compared with children: Preliminary results of in vitro drug sensitivity study in adults with acute lymphoblastic leukaemia. Br J Haematol 1995;91:93.

86. Pieters R, Kaspers GJ, Klumper E, et al: Clinical relevance of in vitro drug resistance testing in childhood acute lymphoblastic leukemia: The state of the art. Med Pediatr Oncol 1994;22:299.

87. Pieters R, Loonen AH, Huismans DR, et al: In vitro drug sensitivity of cells from children with leukemia using the MTT assay with improved culture conditions. Blood 1990;76:2327.

88. Gajjar A, Ribeiro R, Hancock ML, et al: Persistence of circulating blasts after 1 week of multiagent chemotherapy confers a poor prognosis in childhood acute lymphoblastic leukemia. Blood 1995; 86:1292.

89. Rautonen J, Hovi L, Siimes MA: Slow disappearance of peripheral blast cells: An independent risk factor indicating poor prognosis in children with acute lymphoblastic leukemia. Blood 1988;71:989.

90. Riehm H, Reiter A, Schrappe M, et al: Corticosteroid-dependent reduction of leukocyte count in blood as a prognostic factor in acute lymphoblastic leukemia in childhood (therapy study ALL-BFM 83). Klin Padiatr 1987;199:151.

91. Gaynon PS, Bleyer WA, Steinherz PG, et al: Day 7 marrow response and outcome for children with acute lymphoblastic leukemia and unfavorable presenting features. Med Pediatr Oncol 1990;18:273.

92. Gaynon PS, Desai AA, Bostrom BC, et al: Early response to therapy and outcome in childhood acute lymphoblastic leukemia: A review. Cancer 1997;80:1717.

93. Miller DR, Coccia PF, Bleyer WA, et al: Early response to induction therapy as a predictor of disease-free survival and late recurrence of childhood acute lymphoblastic leukemia: A report from the Children's Cancer Study Group. J Clin Oncol 1989;7:1807.

94. Steinherz PG, Gaynon PS, Breneman JC, et al: Cytoreduction and prognosis in acute lymphoblastic leukemia—the importance of early marrow response: Report from the Children's Cancer Group. J Clin Oncol 1996;14:389.

95. Kaspers GJ, Pieters R, Van Zantwijk CH, et al: Prednisolone resistance in childhood acute lymphoblastic leukemia: Vitro-vivo correlations and cross-resistance to other drugs. Blood 1998;92:259.

96. Kaspers GJ, Pieters R, Van Zantwijk CH, et al: Clinical and cell biological features related to cellular drug resistance of childhood acute lymphoblastic leukemia cells. Leuk Lymphoma 1995;19:407.

97. Kaspers GJ, Veerman AJ, Popp Snijders C, et al: Comparison of the antileukemic activity in vitro of dexamethasone and prednisolone in childhood acute lymphoblastic leukemia. Med Pediatr Oncol 1996;27:114.

98. Klumper E, Pieters R, Veerman AJ, et al: In vitro cellular drug resistance in children with relapsed/refractory acute lymphoblastic leukemia. Blood 1995;86:3861.

99. Nachman J, Sather HN, Gaynon PS, et al: Augmented Berlin-Frankfurt-Munster therapy abrogates the adverse prognostic significance of slow early response to induction chemotherapy for children and adolescents with acute lymphoblastic leukemia and unfavorable presenting features: A report from the Children's Cancer Group. J Clin Oncol 1997;15:2222.

100. Schrappe M, Arico M, Harbott J, et al: Philadelphia chromosome-positive (Ph+) childhood acute lymphoblastic leukemia: Good initial steroid response allows early prediction of a favorable treatment outcome. Blood 1998;92:2730.

101. Campana D, Pui CH: Detection of minimal residual disease in acute leukemia: Methodologic advances and clinical significance. Blood 1995;85:1416.

102. Roberts WM, Estrov Z, Kitchingman GR, et al: The clinical significance of residual disease in childhood acute lymphoblastic leukemia as detected by polymerase chain reaction amplification by antigen-receptor gene sequences. Leuk Lymphoma 1996;20:181.

103. Cave H, van der Werff ten Bosch J, Suciu S, et al: Clinical significance of minimal residual disease in childhood acute lymphoblastic leukemia. European Organization for Research and Treatment of Cancer–Childhood Leukemia Cooperative Group. N Engl J Med 1998;339:591.

104. Coustan-Smith E, Behm FG, Sanchez J, et al: Immunological detection of minimal residual disease in children with acute lymphoblastic leukaemia. Lancet 1998;351:550.

105. Goulden NJ, Knechtli CJ, Garland RJ, et al: Minimal residual disease analysis for the prediction of relapse in children with standard-risk acute lymphoblastic leukaemia. Br J Haematol 1998;100:235.

106. van Dongen JJ, Seriu T, Panzer-Grumayer ER, et al: Prognostic value of minimal residual disease in acute lymphoblastic leukaemia in childhood. Lancet 1998;352:1731.

107. Brisco M, Hughes E, Neoh S, et al: In childhood acute lymphoblastic leukemia, a small population of highly drug-resistant cells is present at diagnosis in many patients [abstract]. Blood 1996; 88:667.

108. Martens AC, Schultz FW, Hagenbeek A: Nonhomogeneous distribution of leukemia in the bone marrow during minimal residual disease. Blood 1987;70:1073.

109. Thomson B, Green C, Loken M, et al: Minimal residual disease detection during induction therapy in pediatric acute lymphoblastic leukemia with multi-dimensional flow cytometry (MDF) [abstract]. Proc Am Soc Clin Oncol 1998;17:530.

110. Steenbergen EJ, Verhagen OJ, Nibbering CP, et al: Clonal evolution of immunoglobulin heavy chain rearrangements in childhood B-precursor acute lymphoblastic leukemia after engraftment in SCID mice. Leukemia 1996;10:1471.

111. Steenbergen EJ, Verhagen OJ, van Leeuwen EF, et al: Frequent ongoing T-cell receptor rearrangements in childhood B-precursor acute lymphoblastic leukemia: Implications for monitoring minimal residual disease. Blood 1995;86:692.

112. Steward CG, Goulden NJ, Katz F, et al: A polymerase chain reaction study of the stability of Ig heavy-chain and T-cell receptor delta gene rearrangements between presentation and relapse of childhood B-lineage acute lymphoblastic leukemia. Blood 1994;83: 1355.

113. van Wering ER, Beishuizen A, Roeffen ET, et al: Immunophenotypic changes between diagnosis and relapse in childhood acute lymphoblastic leukemia. Leukemia 1995;9:1523.

114. Beishuizen A, Verhoeven MA, Hahlen K, et al: Differences in immunoglobulin heavy chain gene rearrangement patterns between bone marrow and blood samples in childhood precursor B-acute lymphoblastic leaukemia at diagnosis [corrected and republished with original paging, article originally printed in Leukemia 1992 Jan;6(1):60-3]. Leukemia 1993;7:60.

115. Foroni L, Harrison C, Hoffbrand A, et al: Investigation of minimal residual disease in childhood and adult acute lymphoblastic leukaemia by molecular analysis. Br J Haematol 1999;105:7.

116. Davies H, Lennard L, Lilleyman J: Variable mercaptopurine metabolism in children with leukaemia: A problem in non-compliance. BMJ 1993;306:1239.

117. Peeters M, Koren G, Jakubovicz D, et al: Physician compliance and relapse rates of acute lymphoblastic leukemia in children. Clin Pharmacol Ther 1988;43:228.

118. Bostron B, Erdmann G: Cellular pharmacology of 6-mercaptopurine in acute lymphoblastic leukemia. Am J Pediatr Hematol Oncol 1993;15:80.

119. Gidding CE, Meeuwsen-de Boer GJ, Koopmans P, et al: Vincristine pharmacokinetics after repetitive dosing in children. Cancer Chemother Pharmacol 1999;44:203.

120. Lennard L: Therapeutic drug monitoring of antimetabolic cytotoxic drugs. Br J Clin Pharmacol 1999;47:131.

121. Lennard L, Van Loon JA, Lilleyman JS, et al: Thiopurine pharmacogenetics in leukemia: Correlation of erythrocyte thiopurine methyltransferase activity and 6-thioguanine nucleotide concentrations. Clin Pharmacol Ther 1987;41:18.

122. Lennard LLJS: Individualizing therapy with 6-mercaptopurine and 6-thioguanine related to the thiopurine methyltransferase genetic polymorphism. Ther Drug Monit 1996;18:328.

123. Relling MV, Yanishevski Y, Nemec J, et al: Etoposide and antimetabolite pharmacology in patients who develop secondary acute myeloid leukemia. Leukemia 1998;12:346.

124. Weinshilboum R: Thiopurine methyltransferase pharmacogenetics: Clinical implications [meeting abstract]. Proc Annu Meet Am Assoc Cancer Res 1994;35:687.

125. Smith M, Arthur D, Camitta B, et al: Uniform approach to risk classification and treatment assignment for children with acute lymphoblastic leukemia. Clin Oncol 1996;14:18.

126. Hutchinson R, Neerhout R, Bertolone S, et al: Should therapy be intensified for patients with good risk ALL [abstract]? Blood 1996;88:668.

127. Lange B, Sather H, Weetman R, et al: Double delayed intensification improves outcome in moderate risk pediatric acute lymphoblastic leukemia (ALL): A Children's Cancer Group study, CCG-1891 [abstract]. Blood 1997;90:559.

128. Tubergen D, Gilchrist G, O'Brien A, et al: Improved outcome with delayed intensification for children with acute lymphoblastic leukemia and intermediate presenting features. J Clin Oncol 1993;11:527.

129. Bostrom B, Gaynon P, Sather H, et al: Dexamethasone (DEX) decreases central nervous system (CNS) relapse and improves event-free survival (EFS) in lower risk acute lymphoblastic leukemia (ALL) [abstract]. Proc Am Soc Clin Oncol 1998;17:527.

130. Lauer S, Camitta B, Leventhal B, et al: Intensive alternating drug pairs after remission induction for treatment of infants with acute lymphoblastic leukemia: A Pediatric Oncology Group pilot study. J Pediatr Hematol Oncol 1998;20:229.

131. Silverman L, McLean T, Gelber R, et al: Intensified therapy for infants with acute lymphoblastic leukemia. Cancer 1997;80:2285.

132. O'Reilly R, Pui CH, Kernan N, et al: NCCN pediatric acute lymphoblastic leukemia practice guidelines. The National Comprehensive Cancer Network. Oncology 1996;10:1787.

133. Eden OB, Lilleyman JS, Richards S, et al: Results of Medical Research Council Childhood Leukaemia Trial UKALL VIII (report to the Medical Research Council on behalf of the Working Party on Leukaemia in Childhood). Br J Haematol 1991;78:187.

134. Ekert H, Waters K, Matthews R, et al: A randomized study of corticosteroid and noncorticosteroid containing therapy in childhood ALL. Cancer Ther Control 1990;1:87.

135. Jones B, Freeman AI, Shuster JJ, et al: Lower incidence of meningeal leukemia when prednisone is replaced by dexamethasone in the treatment of acute lymphocytic leukemia. Med Pediatr Oncol 1991;19:269.

136. Veerman AJ, Hahlen K, Kamps WA, et al: Dutch Childhood Leukemia Study Group: Early results of study All VI (1984-1988). Hamatol Bluttransfus 1990;33:473.

137. Balis FM, Lester CM, Chrousos GP, et al: Differences in cerebrospinal fluid penetration of corticosteroids: Possible relationship to the prevention of meningeal leukemia. J Clin Oncol 1987;5:202.

138. Asselin BL, Whitin JC, Coppola DJ, et al: Comparative pharmacokinetic studies of three asparaginase preparations. J Clin Oncol 1993;11:1780.

139. Rizzari C, Gentili D, D'Incalci M, et al: Inadequate L-asparagine (L-ASN) depletion after repeated courses of Erwinia L-asparaginase (L-ASP) administration in children with acute lymphoblastic leukemia (ALL). Med Pediatr Oncol 1995;25:282.

140. Otten J, Socio S, Lutz P, et al: The importance of L-asparaginase (A'ASE) in the treatment of acute lymphoblastic leukemia (ALL) in children: Results of the EORTC 58881 randomized phase III trial showing greater efficiency of Escherichia coli (E. coli) as compared to Erwinia (ERW) a'ase. Blood 1996;88:669.

141. Silverman L, Kimball Dalton V, Zou G, et al: Erwinia asparaginase is less toxic than E. coli asparaginase in children with acute lymphoblastic leukemia (ALL): Results from the Dana-Farber Cancer Institute ALL Consortium. Blood 1999;94:290.

142. Riehm H, Langermann HJ, Gadner H, et al: The Berlin Childhood Acute Lymphoblastic Leukemia Therapy Study, 1970-1976. Am J Pediatr Hematol Oncol 1980;2:299.

143. Gaynon PS, Steinherz PG, Bleyer WA, et al: Improved therapy for children with acute lymphoblastic leukemia and unfavorable presenting features: A follow-up report of the Children's Cancer Group Study CCG-106. J Clin Oncol 1993;11:2234.

144. Steinherz P, Gaynon P, Breneman J, et al: Treatment of acute lymphoblastic leukemia with bulky extramedullary disease and T-cell phenotype or other poor prognostic features: Randomized control trial from the Children's Cancer Group. Cancer 1998;82:600.

145. Goldie J, Coldman A: The genetic origin of drug resistance in neoplasms: Implications for systemic therapy. Cancer Res 1984;44:3643.

146. Sallan SE, Gelber RD, Kimball V, et al: More is better: Update of Dana-Farber Cancer Institute/Children's Hospital childhood acute lymphoblastic leukemia trials. Hamatol Bluttransfus 1990;33:459.

147. Richards S, Burrett J, Hann I, et al: Improved survival with early intensification: Combined results from the Medical Research Council childhood ALL randomised trials, UKALL X and UKALL XI. Medical Research Council Working Party on Childhood Leukaemia. Leukemia 1998;12:1031.

148. Hann I, Vora A, Richards S, et al: Benefit of intensified treatment for all children with acute lymphoblastic leukemia: Results from MRC UKALL XI and MRC ALL97 randomised trials. Leukemia 2000;14:356.

149. Abromowitch M, Ochs J, Pui CH, et al: High-dose methotrexate improves clinical outcome in children with acute lymphoblastic leukemia: St. Jude Total Therapy Study X. Med Pediatr Oncol 1988;16:297.

150. Lange BJ, Blatt J, Sather HN, et al: Randomized comparison of moderate-dose methotrexate infusions to oral methotrexate in children with intermediate risk acute lymphoblastic leukemia: A Children's Cancer Group study. Med Pediatr Oncol 1996;27:15.

151. Poplack D, Reaman G, Bleyer W, et al: Successful prevention of central nervous system (CNS) leukemia without cranial radiation in children with high risk acute lymphoblastic leukemia (ALL): A preliminary report [abstract]. Proc Am Soc Clin Oncol 1989;8:213.

152. Hill F, Gibson B, Eden T, et al: Comparison of high dose methotrexate with continuing intrathecal methotrexate versus intrathecal methotrexate alone in low white blood count childhood acute lymphoblastic leukemia: Preliminary results from the UKALLXI randomised trial [abstract]. Blood 1998;92(Suppl 1):398.

153. Leblanc T, Auclerc M-F, Landman-Parker J, et al: Impact of HD-MTX on the outcome of children with intermediate-risk ALL: Results from the FRALLE93: A randomized study [abstract]. Blood 1998;92(Suppl 1):399.

154. Mahoney DJ, Shuster J, Ruprecht R, et al: Intensification with intermediate-dose intravenous methotrexate is effective therapy for children with lower-risk B-precursor acute lymphoblastic leu-

kemia: A Pediatric Oncology Group study. J Clin Oncol 2000; 18:1285.

155. Winick NJ, Bowman WP, Kamen BA, et al: Unexpected acute neurologic toxicity in the treatment of children with acute lymphoblastic leukemia. J Natl Cancer Inst 1992;84:252.

156. Bell B, Abish S, Shuster J, et al: Neurotoxicity (NT) in children with standard-risk acute lymphoblastic lukemia (ALL) on Pediatric Oncology Group (POG) 9405 [abstract]. Blood 1997;90:559.

157. Mahoney DH Jr, Shuster JJ, Nitschke R, et al: Acute neurotoxicity in children with B-precursor acute lymphoid leukemia: An association with intermediate-dose intravenous methotrexate and intrathecal triple therapy—a Pediatric Oncology Group study. J Clin Oncol 1998;16:1712.

158. Amylon M, Shuster J, Pullen J, et al: Intensive high-dose asparaginase consolidation improves survival for pediatric patients with T cell acute lymphoblastic leukemia: A Pediatric Oncology Group study. Leukemia 1999;13:335.

159. Crist W, Shuster J, Look T, et al: Current results of studies of immunophenotype-, age- and leukocyte-based therapy for children with acute lymphoblastic leukemia. The Pediatric Oncology Group. Leukemia 1992;6(Suppl 2):162.

160. Cairo M, Sather H, Sender L, et al: Matched related allogeneic BMT (ABMT) in first remission (CR) of acute lymphoblastic leukemia with ultra high risk features. Med Pediatr Oncol 1997;29:320.

161. Nesbit ME, Sather H, Robison LL, et al: Sanctuary therapy: A randomized trial of 724 children with previously untreated acute lymphoblastic leukemia: A report from Children's Cancer Study Group. Cancer Res 1982;42:674.

162. Nesbit ME Jr, Sather HN, Robison LL, et al: Presymptomatic central nervous system therapy in previously untreated childhood acute lymphoblastic leukaemia: Comparison of 1800 rad and 2400 rad. A report for Children's Cancer Study Group. Lancet 1981;1:461.

163. Bleyer AW: Clinical pharmacology of intrathecal methotrexate. II. An improved dosage regimen derived from age-related pharmacokinetics. Cancer Treat Rep 1977;61:1419.

164. Neglia JP, Meadows AT, Robison LL, et al: Second neoplasms after acute lymphoblastic leukemia in childhood. N Engl J Med 1991; 325:1330.

165. Walter AW, Hancock ML, Pui CH, et al: Secondary brain tumors in children treated for acute lymphoblastic leukemia at St Jude Children's Research Hospital. J Clin Oncol 1998;16:3761.

166. Anderson V, Smibert E, Ekert H, et al: Intellectual, educational, and behavioural sequelae after cranial irradiation and chemotherapy. Arch Dis Child 1994;70:476.

167. Hill JM, Kornblith AB, Jones D, et al: A comparative study of the long term psychosocial functioning of childhood acute lymphoblastic leukemia survivors treated by intrathecal methotrexate with or without cranial radiation. Cancer 1998;82:208.

168. Jankovic M, Brouwers P, Valsecchi MG, et al: Association of 1800 cGy cranial irradiation with intellectual function in children with acute lymphoblastic leukaemia. ISPACC. International Study Group on Psychosocial Aspects of Childhood Cancer. Lancet 1994;344: 224.

169. Schrappe M, Reiter A, Ludwig W-D, et al: Improved outcome in childhood acute lymphoblastic leukemia despite reduced use of anthracyclines and cranial irradiation: Results of trial ALL-BFM 90. Blood 2000;95:3310.

170. Toyoda T, Manabe A, Tsuchida M, Six months maintenance chemotherapy after intensified treatment for acute lymphoblastic leukemia of childhood. J Clin Oncol 2000;18:1508.

171. Group CAC: Duration and intensity of maintenance chemotherapy in acute lymphoblastic leukaemia: Overview of 42 trials involving 12,000 randomised children. Lancet 1996;347:1783.

172. Miller DR, Leikin SL, Albo VC, et al: Three versus five years of maintenance therapy are equivalent in childhood acute lymphoblastic leukemia: A report from the Children's Cancer Study Group. J Clin Oncol 1989;7:316.

173. Chessells J, Leiper A, Tiedemann K, et al: Oral methotrexate is as effective as intramuscular methotrexate in maintenance therapy of acute lymphoblastic leukaemia. Arch Dis Child 1987;62:172.

174. Simone J: Childhood leukemia as a model for cancer research: The Richard and Hilda Rosenthal Foundation Award Lecture. Cancer 1979;39:4301.

175. van Eys J, Berry D, Crist W, et al: Treatment intensity and outcome for children with acute lymphocytic leukema of standard risk: A Pediatric Oncology Group study. Cancer 1989;63:1466.

176. Coccia P, Bleyer W, Siegel S, et al: Development and preliminary findings of Children's Cancer Study Group Protocols (161, 162 and 163) for low-, average- and high-risk acute lymphoblastic leukemia in children. In Murphy S, Gilbert J eds: Leukemia Research: Advances in Cell Biology and Treatment. Amsterdam: Elsevier; 1983.

177. Koizumi S, Fujimoto T, Takeda T, et al: Comparison of intermittent or continuous methotrexate plus 6-mercaptopurine in regimens for standard-risk acute lymphoblastic leukemia in childhood (JCCLSG-S811). The Japanese Children's Cancer and Leukemia Study Group. Cancer 1988;61:1292.

178. Buhrer C, Hartmann R, Fengler R, et al: Superior prognosis in combined compared to isolated bone marrow relapses in salvage therapy of childhood acute lymphoblastic leukemia. Med Pediatr Oncol 1993;21:470.

179. Seeger K, Adams HP, Buchwald D, et al: TEL-AML1 fusion transcript in relapsed childhood acute lymphoblastic leukemia. The Berlin-Frankfurt-Munster Study Group. Blood 1998;91:1716.

180. Henze G, Fengler R, Haertmann R, et al: Six-year experience with a comprehensive approach to the treatment of recurrent childhood acute lymphoblastic leukemia (ALL-REZ BFM 85). A relapse study of the BFM Group. Blood 1991;78:1166.

181. Beyermann B, Adams HP, Henze G: Philadelphia chromosome in relapsed childhood acute lymphoblastic leukemia: A matched-pair analysis. Berlin-Frankfurt-Munster Study Group. J Clin Oncol 1997; 15:2231.

182. Beyermann B, Agthe AG, Adams HP, et al: Clinical features and outcome of children with first marrow relapse of acute lymphoblastic leukemia expressing BCR-ABL fusion transcripts. BFM Relapse Study Group. Blood 1996;87:1532.

183. Kawamura M, Kikuchi A, Kobayashi S, et al: Mutations of the p53 and ras genes in childhood t(1;19)–acute lymphoblastic leukemia. Blood 1995;85:2546.

184. Diccianni MB, Yu J, Hsiao M, et al: Clinical significance of p53 mutations in relapsed T-cell acute lymphoblastic leukemia. Blood 1994;84:3105.

185. Rogers P, Coccia P, Siegel S, et al: Yield of unpredicted bone-marrow relapse diagnosed by routine marrow aspiration in children with acute lymphoblastic leukaemia: A report from the Children's Cancer Study Group. Lancet 1984;1:1320.

186. Gaynon P, Stork L, Sather H, et al: Leukemic progenitor cell content of pre- and post-induction chemotherapy bone marrow specimens from children with newly diagnosed or relapsed acute lymphoblastic leukemia (ALL) [abstract]. Proc Am Soc Clin Oncol 1999;18:2187.

187. Gaynon P, Harris R, Stram D, et al: Asparagine (ASN) depletion and treatment response in childhood acute lymphoblastic leukemia (ALL) after an early marrow relapse; a Children's Cancer Group trial (CCG-1941) [abstract]. Blood 1999;94:628.

188. Abshire T, Pollock B, Billett A, et al: Weekly polyethylene glycol conjugated (PEG) L-asparaginase (ASP) produces superior induction remission rates in childhood relapsed acute lymphoblastic leukemia (rALL): A Pediatric Oncology Group (POG) study 9310. Proc Am Soc Clin Oncol 1995;14:344.

189. Kurtzberg J, Asselin B, Pollack B, et al: PEG–L-asparaginase (PEG-asp) vs native E coli asparaginase (asp) for reinduction of relapsed acute lymphoblastic leukemia (ALL): Pediatric Oncology Group (POG) 8866 phase II trial [meeting abstract]. Proc Annu Meet Am Soc Clin Oncol 1993;12:1079.

190. Buhrer C, Hartmann R, Fengler R, et al: Importance of effective central nervous system therapy in isolated bone marrow relapse of childhood acute lymphoblastic leukemia. BFM (Berlin-Frankfurt-Munster) Relapse Study Group. Blood 1994;83:3468.

191. Lawson S, Harrison G, Richards S, et al: The UK experience in treating relapsed childhood acute lymphoblastic leukaemia: A report on the Medical Research Council UKALLR1 study. Br J Haematol 2000;108:531.

192. Barrett AJ, Horowitz MM, Pollock BH, et al: Bone marrow transplants from HLA-identical siblings as compared with chemotherapy for children with acute lymphoblastic leukemia in a second remission. N Engl J Med 1994;331:1253.

193. Hoogerbrugge PM, Gerritsen EJ, vd Does–van den Berg A, et al: Case-control analysis of allogeneic bone marrow transplantation versus maintenance chemotherapy for relapsed ALL in children. Bone Marrow Transplant 1995;15:255.

194. Uderzo C, Valsecchi MG, Bacigalupo A, et al: Treatment of childhood acute lymphoblastic leukemia in second remission with allogeneic bone marrow transplantation and chemotherapy: Ten-year experience of the Italian Bone Marrow Transplantation Group and the Italian Pediatric Hematology Oncology Association. J Clin Oncol 1995;13:352.

195. Schroeder H, Gustafsson G, Saarinen-Pihkala UM, et al: Allogeneic bone marrow transplantation in second remission of childhood acute lymphoblastic leukemia: A population-based case control study from the Nordic countries. Bone Marrow Transplant 1999; 23:555.

196. Boulad F, Steinherz P, Reyes B, et al: Allogeneic bone marrow transplantation versus chemotherapy for the treatment of childhood acute lymphoblastic leukemia in second remission: A single-institution study. J Clin Oncol 1999;17:197.

197. Dini G, Cornish JM, Gadner H, et al: Bone marrow transplant indications for childhood leukemias: Achieving a consensus. The EBMT Pediatric Diseases Working Party. Bone Marrow Transplant 1996;18(Suppl 2):4.

198. Sanders JE: Bone marrow transplantation for pediatric malignancies. Pediatr Clin North Am 1997;44:1005.

199. Parsons SK, Castellino SM, Lehmann LE, et al: Relapsed acute lymphoblastic leukemia: Similar outcomes for autologous and allogeneic marrow transplantation in selected children. Bone Marrow Transplant 1996;17:763.

200. Borgmann A, Schmid H, Hartmann R, et al: Autologous bone-marrow transplants compared with chemotherapy for children with acute lymphoblastic leukaemia in a second remission: A matched-pair analysis. The Berlin-Frankfurt-Munster Study Group. Lancet 1995;346:873.

201. Wheeler K, Richards S, Bailey C, et al: Comparison of bone marrow transplant and chemotherapy for relapsed childhood acute lymphoblastic leukaemia: The MRC UKALL X experience. Medical Research Council Working Party on Childhood Leukaemia. Br J Haematol 1998;101:94.

202. Balduzzi A, Gooley T, Anasetti C, et al: Unrelated donor marrow transplantation in children. Blood 1995;86:3247.

203. Davies SM, Wagner JE, Shu XO, et al: Unrelated donor bone marrow transplantation for children with acute leukemia. J Clin Oncol 1997;15:557.

204. Oakhill A, Pamphilon DH, Potter MN, et al: Unrelated donor bone marrow transplantation for children with relapsed acute lymphoblastic leukaemia in second complete remission. Br J Haematol 1996;94:574.

205. Lausen BF, Heilmann C, Vindelov L, et al: Outcome of acute lymphoblastic leukaemia in Danish children after allogeneic bone marrow transplantation. Superior survival following transplantation with matched unrelated donor grafts. Bone Marrow Transplant 1998;22:325.

206. Pinkel D, Woo S: Prevention and treatment of meningeal leukemia in children. Blood 1994;84:355.

207. Lustig R, Rose S, Burghen G, et al: Hypothalamic obesity caused by cranial insult in children: Altered glucose and insulin dynamics and reversal by a somatostatin agonist. J Pediatr 1999;135:162.

208. Neale GA, Pui CH, Mahmoud HH, et al: Molecular evidence for minimal residual bone marrow disease in children with 'isolated' extra-medullary relapse of T-cell acute lymphoblastic leukemia. Leukemia 1994;8:768.

209. Uckun FM, Gaynon PS, Stram DO, et al: Paucity of leukemic progenitor cells in the bone marrow of pediatric B-lineage acute lymphoblastic leukemia patients with an isolated extramedullary first relapse. Clin Cancer Res 1999;5:2415.

210. Tubergen DG, Cullen JW, Boyett JM: Blasts in CSF with a normal cell count do not justify alteration of therapy for acute lymphoblastic leukemia in remission: A Children's Cancer Group study. J Clin Oncol 1994;12:273.

211. Pullen J, Boyett J, Shuster J, et al: Extended triple intrathecal chemotherapy trial for prevention of CNS relapse in good-risk and poor-risk patients with B-progenitor acute lymphoblastic leukemia: A Pediatric Oncology Group study. J Clin Oncol 1993;11:839.

212. Sullivan M, Moon T, Trueworthy R, et al: Combination intrathecal therapy for meningeal leukemia: Two versus three drugs. Blood 1977;50:471.

213. Land V, Thomas P, Boyett J, et al: Comparison of maintenance treatments for first central nervous system relapse in children with acute lymphocytic leukemia. Cancer 1985;56:81.

214. Ritchey A, Pollack B, Lauer S, et al: Improved survival of children with isolated CNS relapse of acute lymphoblastic leukemia: A Pediatric Oncology Group study. J Clin Oncol 1999;17:3745.

215. Willoughby M: Treatment of overt meningeal leukaemia in children: Results of second MRC meningeal leukaemia trial. Br J Haematol 1976;1:864.

216. Belasco J, Goldwein J, Lange B, et al: Monthly low-dose craniospinal (C-S) radiotherapy (RT) to 18 Gy after CNS relapse in children with acute lymphoblastic leukemia (ALL) [meeting abstract]. Proc Annu Meet Am Soc Clin Oncol 1996;15:1089.

217. Steinherz P, Jereb B, Galicich J: Therapy of CNS leukemia with intraventricular chemotherapy and low-dose neuraxis radiotherapy. J Clin Oncol 1985;3:1217.

218. Finklestein JZ, Miller DR, Feusner J, et al: Treatment of overt isolated testicular relapse in children on therapy for acute lymphoblastic leukemia. A report from the Children's Cancer Group. Cancer 1994;73:219.

219. Wofford MM, Smith SD, Shuster JJ, et al: Treatment of occult or late overt testicular relapse in children with acute lymphoblastic leukemia: A Pediatric Oncology Group study. J Clin Oncol 1992; 10:624.

220. van den Berg H, Langeveld N, Veenhof C, et al: Treatment of isolated testicular recurrence of acute lymphoblastic leukemia without radiotherapy. Cancer 1997;79:2257.

221. Barr R, Feeny D, Furlong W, et al: A preference-based approach to health-related quality of life for children with cancer. Int J Pediatr Hematol Oncol 1995;2:305.

222. Barr R, Furlong W, Dawson S, et al: An assessment of the global health status in survivors of acute lymphoblastic leukemia in childhood. Am J Pediatr Hematol Oncol 1993;15:284.

223. Feeny D, Furlong W, Barr R, et al: A comprehensive multiattribute system of classifying the health status of survivors of childhood cancer. J Clin Oncol 1992;10:923.

224. Feeny D, Leiper A, Barr R, et al: The comprehensive assessment of health status in survivors of childhood cancer: Application to high-risk acute lymphoblastic leukemia. Br J Cancer 1993;67:1047.

225. Haupt R, Fears T, Robison L, et al: Educational attainment in long-term survivors of childhood acute lymphoblastic leukemia. JAMA 1994;272:1427.

226. Land VJ, Shuster JJ, Crist WM, et al: Comparison of two schedules of intermediate-dose methotrexate and cytarabine consolidation therapy for childhood B-precursor cell acute lymphoblastic leukemia: A Pediatric Oncology Group study. J Clin Oncol 1994;12: 1939.

227. Winick NJ, McKenna RW, Shuster JJ, et al: Secondary acute myeloid leukemia in children with acute lymphoblastic leukemia treated with etoposide. Comment in: J Clin Oncol 1993 Feb;11(2):199–201; Comment in: J Clin Oncol 1993 May;11(5):1005; Comment in: J Clin Oncol 1993 Jul;11(7):1433; Comment in: J Clin Oncol 1993 Aug;11(8):1624–5. J Clin Oncol 1993;11:209.

228. Mulhern R, Fairclough D, Ochs J: A prospective comparison of neuropsychologic performance of children surviving leukemia who received 18-Gy, 24-Gy, or no cranial irradiation. J Clin Oncol 1991;9:1348.

229. Ochs J, Mulhern R, Fairclough D, et al: Comparison of neuropsychological functioning and clinical indicators of neurotoxicity in long-term survivors of childhood leukemia given cranial radiation or parenteral methotrexate: A prospective study. J Clin Oncol 1991;9:145.

230. Mulhern R, Wasserman A, Fairclough D: Memory function in disease-free survivors of childhood acute lymphocytic leukemia given CNS prophylaxis with or without 1,800 cGy cranial irradiation. J Clin Oncol 1988;6:315.

231. Brown R, Sawyer M, Antoniou G, et al: A 3-year follow-up of the intellectual and academic functioning of children receiving central nervous system prophylactic chemotherapy for leukemia. Dev Behav Pediatr 1996;17:392.

232. Brouwers P, Moss H, Reaman G, et al: Central nervous system preventive therapy with systemic high dose methotrexate versus cranial radiation and intrathecal methotrexate: Longitudinal comparison of effects of treatment on intellectual function of children with acute lymphoblastic leukemia. Proc Am Soc Clin Oncol 1987; 6:158.

233. Kaleita TA, MacLean WE, Reaman GH, et al: Neurodevelopmental outcome of children diagnosed with ALL during infancy: A preliminary report from the Children's Cancer Study Group. Med Pediatr Oncol 1992;20:385.

234. Bhatia S, Sather H, Trigg M, et al: Second malignant neoplasms (SMN) following childhood acute lymphoblastic leukemia (ALL): Follow-up of the Children's Cancer Group (CCG) cohort [abstract]. Proc Am Assoc Clin Oncol 1998;17:528.

235. Katz JA, Shuster JJ, Ravindranath Y, et al: Secondary acute myelogenous leukemia (AML) following intensive treatment for childhood T-cell acute lymphoblastic leukemia (T-ALL) and advanced stage lymphoblastic lymphoma (LL) treated with teniposide (VM-26): A Pediatric Oncology Group (POG) study [meeting abstract]. Proc Annu Meet Am Soc Clin Oncol 1995;14:1040.

236. Sandler ES, Friedman DJ, Mustafa MM, et al: Treatment of children with epipodophyllotoxin-induced secondary acute myeloid leukemia. Cancer 1997;79:1049.

237. Pui C, Ribeiro R, Hancock M, et al: Acute myeloid leukemia in children treated with epipodophyllotoxins for acute lymphoblastic leukemia. N Engl J Med 1991;325:1882.

238. Relling MV, Rubnitz JE, Rivera GK, et al: High incidence of secondary brain tumours after radiotherapy and antimetabolites. Lancet 1999;354:34.

239. Ojala AE, Paakko E, Lanning FP, et al: Osteonecrosis during the treatment of childhood acute lymphoblastic leukemia: A prospective MRI study. Med Pediatr Oncol 1999;32:11.

240. Mattano LA Jr, Sather HN, Trigg ME, et al: Osteonecrosis as a complication of treating acute lymphoblastic leukemia in children: A report of the Children's Cancer Group. J Clin Oncol 2000; 18:3262.

241. Lipshultz S, Colan S, Gelber R, et al: Late cardiac effects of doxorubicin therapy for acute lymphoblastic leukemia in childhood. N Engl J Med 1991;324:808.

242. Sorenson K, Levitt G, Bull C, et al: Anthracycline dose in childhood acute lymphoblastic leukemia: Issues of early survival versus late cardiotoxicity. J Clin Oncol 1997;15:61.

243. Krisher J, Epstein S, Cuthbertson D, et al: Clinical cardiotoxicity following anthracycline treatment for childhood cancer: The Pediatric Oncology Group experience. J Clin Oncol 1997;15:1544.

244. Herman E, Lipshultz SE, Rifai N, et al: Use of cardiac troponin T levels as an indicator of doxorubicin induced cardiotoxicity. Cancer Res 1998;58:195.

245. Nysom K, Holm K, Lipsitz S, et al: Relationship between cumulative anthracycline dose and late cardiotoxicity in childhood acute lymphoblastic leukemia. J Clin Oncol 1998;16:545.

246. Baird E, McHenry P, MacKie R: Effect of maintenance chemotherapy in childhood on numbers of melanocytic naevi. BMJ 1992; 305:799.

247. Hughes B, Cunliffe W, Bailey C: Excess benign melanocytic naevi after chemotherapy for malignancy in childhood. BMJ 1989;299: 88.

248. Naldi L, Adamoli L, Donetella F, Number and distribution of melanocytic nevi in individuals with a history of childhood leukemia. Cancer 1996;77:1402.

249. Garbe C, Buttner P, Weiss J, et al: Risk factors for developing cutaneous melanoma and criteria for identifying persons at risk: Multicenter case-control study of the Central Malignant Melanoma Registry of the German Dermatological Society. J Invest Dermatol 1994;102:695.

250. Grob J, Gouvernet J, Aymar D, et al: Count of benign melanocytic nevi as a major indicator of risk for nonfamilial nodular and superficial spreading melanoma. Cancer 1990;66:387.

251. Druker B, Kantarjian H, Sawyers C, et al: Activity of an ABL specific tyrosine kinase inhibitor in patients with BCR-ABL positive acute leukemia including chronic myelogenous leukemia in blast crisis [abstract]. Blood 1999;94:697.

252. Druker B, Talpaz M, Resta D, et al: Clinical efficacy and safety of an ABL specific tyrosine kinase inhibitor as targeted therapy for chronic myelogenous leukemia [abstract]. Blood 1999;94:368.

253. Druker BJ, Tamura S, Buchdunger E, et al: Effects of a selective inhibitor of the Ab1 tyrosine kinase on the growth of Bcr-Ab1 positive cells. Nat Med 1996;2:561.

254. Moch H, Schraml P, Bubendorf L, et al: High-throughput tissue microarray analysis to evaluate genes uncovered by cDNA microarray screening in renal cell carcinoma. Comment in: Am J Pathol 1999 Apr;154(4):979-80. Am J Pathol 1999;154:981.

255. Ramsay G: DNA chips: State-of-the art. Nat Biotechnol 1998;16:40.

256. Welford SM, Gregg J, Chen E, et al: Detection of differentially expressed genes in primary tumor tissues using representational

differences analysis coupled to microarray hybridization. Nucleic Acids Res 1998;26:3059.

257. Alves S, Prata MJ, Ferreira F, et al: Thiopurine methyltransferase pharmacogenetics: Alternative molecular diagnosis and preliminary data from northern Portugal. Pharmacogenetics 1999;9:257.

258. Krajinovic M, Labuda D, Richer C, et al: Susceptibility to childhood acute lymphoblastic leukemia: Influence of CYP1A1, CYP2D6, GSTM1, and GSTT1 genetic polymorphisms. Blood 1999;93:1496.

259. Krynetski EY, Evans WE: Pharmacogenetics as a molecular basis for individualized drug therapy: The thiopurine S-methyltransferase paradigm. Pharm Res 1999;16:342.

260. Castillo L, Brunetto A, Conchin C, et al: Cortivazol (RU 3625) for children with acute lymphoblastic leukemia in marrow relapse. Med Pediatr Oncol 1999;33:276.

261. Juneja HS, Harvey WH, Brasher WK, et al: Successful in vitro purging of leukemic blasts from marrow by cortivazol, a pyrazolosteroid: A preclinical study for autologous transplantation in acute lymphoblastic leukemia and non-Hodgkin's lymphoma. Leukemia 1995;9:1771.

262. Schlechte J, Simons S, Lewis D, et al: Cortivazol: A unique high affinity ligand for the glucocorticoid receptor. Endocrinology 1985;117:1355.

263. Adamson PC, Poplack DG, Balis FM: The cytotoxicity of thioguanine vs mercaptopurine in acute lymphoblastic leukemia. Leuk Res 1994;18:805.

264. Lancaster D, Lennard L, Rowland K, et al: Thioguanine versus mercaptopurine for therapy of childhood lymphoblastic leukaemia. Br J Haematol 1998;102:439.

265. Lennard L, Davies HA, Lilleyman JS: Is 6-thioguanine more appropriate than 6-mercaptopurine for children with acute lymphoblastic leukaemia? Br J Cancer 1993;68:186.

266. Smith A, Hum M, Winick N, et al: A case for the use of aminopterin in treatment of patients with leukemia based on the metabolic studies of blasts in vitro. Clin Cancer Res 1996;2:69.

267. Messinger Y, Yanishevski Y, Ek O, et al: In vivo toxicity and pharmacokinetic features of B43 (anti-CD19)-genistein immunoconjugate in nonhuman primates. Clin Cancer Res 1998;4:165.

268. Myers DE, Yanishevski Y, Masson E, et al: Favorable pharmacodynamic features and superior anti-leukemic activity of B43 (anti-CD19) immunotoxins containing two pokeweed antiviral protein molecules covalently linked to each monoclonal antibody molecule. Leuk Lymphoma 1995;18:93.

269. Seibel N, Krailo M, Franklin J, et al: Phase I study of B43-PAP immunotoxin in combination with standard 4-drug induction for patients with CD19+ acute lymphoblastic leukemia in relapse: A Children's Cancer Group Study [abstract]. Blood 1998;92:400.

270. Gandhi V, Kisor D, Rodriguez CJ, et al: Pharmacokinetics of arabinosylguanine (ara-G) and its triphosphate (ara-GTP) during a phase I trial of compound 506U in refractory hematologic malignancies: Correlation with response [abstract]. Blood 1996;88:670.

271. Kurtzberg J, Keating M, Moore J, et al: 2-Amino-9-B-arabinosyl-6-methyl-9H-guanine (GW 506U) is highly active in patients with T-cell malignancies: Results of a phase I trial in pediatric and adult patients with refractory hematologic malignancies [abstract]. Blood 1996;88:669.

272. Lambe CU, Averett DR, Paff MT, et al: 2-Amino-6-methoxypurine arabinoside: An agent for T-cell malignancies. Cancer Res 1995; 55:3352.

273. Locatelli F, Zecca M, Rondelli R, et al: Graft versus host disease prophylaxis with low-dose cyclosporine-A reduces the risk of relapse in children with acute leukemia given HLA-identical sibling bone marrow transplantation: Results of a randomized study. Blood 2000;95:1572.

274. Knechtli CJ, Goulden NJ, Hancock JP, et al: Minimal residual disease status as a predictor of relapse after allogeneic bone marrow transplantation for children with acute lymphoblastic leukaemia. Br J Haematol 1998;102:860.

275. Uckun FM, Kersey JH, Haake R, et al: Pretransplantation burden of leukemic progenitor cells as a predictor of relapse after bone marrow transplantation for acute lymphoblastic leukemia. N Engl J Med 1993;329:1296.

276. Woods WG, Kobrinsky N, Buckley JD, et al: Timed-sequential induction therapy improves postremission outcome in acute myeloid leukemia: A report from the Children's Cancer Group. Blood 1996;87:4979.

27

Dieter Hoelzer   Nicola Gökbuget

Acute Lymphoblastic Leukemia in Adults

INTRODUCTION

Acute lymphoblastic leukemia (ALL) is widely perceived as a disease of childhood. There is, however, beyond the early peak of incidence a low, constant incidence increasing with advancing years after the age of 50 such that it accounts for approximately 15% of acute leukemias in adults. This chapter focuses on treatment of ALL and some features in adults that may influence or at least correlate with outcome.

The currently accepted principles of treatment of adult ALL are based on those that are successful for children:

1. Cyclical combination chemotherapy, usually including vincristine (VCR), prednisolone, and an anthracycline antibiotic with or without L-asparaginase, cytosine arabinoside (AC), and cyclophosphamide (CP), to induce complete remission (CR); the role of high-dose AC is being explored.
2. Further intensive postremission chemotherapy with or without allogeneic stem cell transplantation (SCT) or autologous SCT. Maintenance chemotherapy, based on a combination of antimetabolites with or without intensification cycles, is part of many trials but in some studies is completely omitted.
3. Prophylactic central nervous system (CNS) treatment early in CR with intrathecal (IT) chemotherapy, often with high-dose systemic therapy using drugs that penetrate the blood-brain barrier or with cranial radiation therapy (CRT).
4. Stratification according to prognostic factors based on clinical features, immunophenotype, and cytogenetic and molecular markers as a basis for risk- and subtype-adapted treatment strategies. This includes specific treatment approaches for mature B-ALL or intensive and even experimental treatment for the poor prognostic subtype Ph/*BCR-ABL*–positive ALL.
5. All this requires intensive supportive care, including hematopoietic growth factors to protect patients from infectious complications, particularly gram-negative bacteria or fungi.

The application of these principles will be successful in inducing CR in 80% or more of younger adults but considerably less in those older than 60 years and cure in approximately one-third of patients, according to the literature. Failure, manifest by inability to achieve CR or by recurrence, is extremely serious and irretrievable except in the short term with conventional strategies, unless CR can be achieved with another approach and myeloablative treatment and allogeneic transplantation can be successfully performed. There is thus room for much improvement.

DIAGNOSTIC PROCEDURE AND CRITERIA FOR CR

ALL has to be subclassified by morphologic analysis, immunophenotyping, and cytogenetic and molecular genetic analysis. The traditional definition of complete remission (CR) requires the patient to be in "normal health," manifestly not the case at the time it is usually confirmed. Hematologically, the peripheral blood count and films are required to be within normal limits, the bone marrow aspirate to be normocellular with less than 5% blast cells, none of which are leukemic. These criteria are not applied universally. The "recovery marrow with no evidence of leukemia" may be an acceptable baseline to some; the ability to recognize leukemia cells more sensitively immunologically than morphologically, and even at the level of 1 in 10^5 with molecular techniques, has encouraged others to make the definition more strict. The most important issue is to have a common policy of reporting so that like may be compared with like.

SINGLE-AGENT THERAPY

Background

The ability of cytotoxic chemicals to induce CR of ALL was first reported in 1948,[1] since which time many other agents have been discovered and proved to be effective. Despite the fact that single-agent therapy has no role in the curative treatment of ALL, an extensive knowledge of the activity of agents in various dosages and schedules is essential so that optimal combinations and sequential strategies can be planned. The results for the major drugs given and the dosage in various combinations are pre-

TABLE 27–1. Single-Drug Induction: Prednisone-Prednisolone

	Dosage, Schedule, Route	N Patients	CR Rate (%)	Reference
Children	<40 mg/d PO	100	71	3
	2 mg/kg/d PO	301	63	13
	< 1 mg/kg/d PO	11	45	13
	< 3 mg/kg/d PO	45	64	14
	≥ 3 mg/kg/d PO	62	74	14
	2 mg/kg/d PO	77	77	14
	4 mg/kg/d PO	70	73	9
	8 mg/kg/q 2 d PO	24	25	9
	16 mg/kg/q 4 d PO	16	19	9
	500–1000 mg/d IV	24 pretreated	21	15
Adults	40 mg/d PO	22	36	3
	3 mg/kg/d PO	14	45	14
	50 or 500 mg/d IV	26 pretreated	42	4
	1000 mg/d IV	11 pretreated	36	11

PO = oral; IV = intravenous; CR = complete remission.

sented in the following sections and in Tables 27-1 through 27-11.

Major Antileukemic Drugs

Adrenocorticosteroids

Of all agents currently employed in ALL treatment, the adrenocorticosteroids are the most important in initial management. Adrenocorticosteroids are lympholytic by means of mechanisms that are as yet poorly defined but that probably involve the activation of nucleases leading to internucleosomal DNA fragmentation.[2] They may in-

TABLE 27–2. Single-Drug Induction: Vinca Alkaloids

Drug, Dosage, Route	N Patients	CR Rate (%)	Reference
Vincristine			
0.1 mg/kg/wk IV	25 children	48	22
2.0–3.5 mg/m²/wk IV	103 pretreated children	57	23
0.075 mg/kg/wk IV	110 children	44	24
1.0–2.5 mg/m²/wk IV	25 children, 1ˢᵗ treatment with VCR	60	25
	16 children, 2ⁿᵈ treatment with VCR	63	
	9 children, 3ʳᵈ treatment with VCR	55	
0.05–0.075 mg/kg/wk IV	5 adults	20	25
Vinblastine			
0.15 mg/kg/biweekly IV	8 children	12	26
Vindesine			
2 mg/m² × 2 q w IV	19 children and adults	37	27
5 mg/m² q w vs 0.5 mg/m² q 12 hr IV	14 children and adults	14	28
2 mg/m² × 2 q w IV	19 children and adults	26	29
1–2 mg/m² q d IV	13 adults	0	30
4 mg/m² q w IV	35 children	8	31

TABLE 27–3. Single-Drug Induction: Methotrexate

Dosage	N Patients	CR Rate (%)	Reference
1.25–5 mg/d PO	45 untreated children	22	37
	7 untreated adults	14	
3 mg/m²/d PO	29 untreated children	31	38
30 mg/m² wk IM or PO	25 untreated children	28	38
3–6 g/m² with VCR and CF	6 adults in relapse	33	39
50 mg/m²/24-hr infusion plus CF	8 children at relapse	0	40

CF = citrovorum factor.

duce apoptosis. They affect dividing and nondividing cells. The particular susceptibility of ALL to these drugs permits rapid reduction of leukemic cell numbers with minimal myelosuppression.

The adrenocorticosteroids most commonly used are prednisone and its soluble analogue, prednisolone (see Table 27-1). These drugs are usually given daily in dosages of 40 to 80 mg/m², either orally (prednisone) or by intravenous (IV) injection (prednisolone). Given alone, they induce CR in about one-half of children at ALL's first overt appearance; they are only slightly less effective in adults with ALL.[3, 4] Other steroids, e.g, dexamethasone, have essentially identical remission induction capability. Dexamethasone has a higher antileukemic activity (5- to 16-fold compared with prednisolone)[5, 6] and is therefore administered at a lower dose level of 6 to 10 mg/m². Furthermore, dexamethasone may provide greater control of leukemia in the CNS and other extramedullary sites.[7] However, if used for a longer time, it can cause susceptibility to infections and septicemias.[8.]

The administration of prednisolone at intervals less frequent than daily, e.g., every second or fourth day, has proved less successful (see Table 27-1).[9] Higher doses of steroids have also been used; in general, they have not increased remission induction rates.[4, 10, 11]

The majority of leukemic blast cells in ALL are highly sensitive to steroids. Response to a 7-day pretreatment with prednisolone as measured by the reduction of blast cells in the peripheral blood is considered as a significant prognostic factor in childhood ALL. Approximately 10% of the patients show more than 1000/μL blast cells in peripheral blood on day 8; their prognosis is significantly

TABLE 27–4. Single-Drug Induction: Mercaptopurine

Drug and Dosage	N Patients	CR Rate (%)	Reference
2.5 mg/kg/d	45 children	33	42
3 mg/kg/d	43 children	27	43
	11 adults	9	
2.5 mg/kg/d	29 children	28	14
	12 adults	8	
2.5 mg/kg	59 children	36	44
6.6 mg/kg/d, followed by 2.5 mg/kg/d	64 children	34	44

TABLE 27–5. Fludarabine in Combination with Cytarabine and/or Idarubicin in Relapsed ALL

Drug and Dosage			N Patients	CR Rate (%)	Reference
Fludarabine	Cytarabine	Idarubicin			
30 mg/m² d 2–6	1 g/m² d 1–6	—	30 adults	30	50
30 mg/m² d 1–5	2 g/m² d 1–5	—	13 adults	67	46
30 mg/m² d 2–6	2 g/m² d 1–6	—	12 adults	83	45
25 mg/m² d 1–5	0.5 g/m² d 1–5	10 mg/m² d 1–3	6 children	50	48
30 mg/m² d 1–5	2 g/m² d 1–5	—	7 ch./adults	43	47
30 mg/m² d 1–5	2 g/m² d 1–5	8 mg/m² d 1–3	20 ch./adults	55	47

TABLE 27–6. Single-Drug Induction: New Purine Analogues

Drug and Dosage	N Patients	Response	Reference
2′-Deoxycoformycin			
10 mg/m²/d IV × 5	21 T-cell ALL 8 non-T-cell ALL	57% CR	54
5 mg/m²/d IV × 9	6 ATL	1 PR	56
4 mg/m²/wk IV × 4 (then monthly)	20 ATL	10% CR	57
3 to 9 mg/m² IV	18 ATL	3 PR	58
0.25 to 1.0 mg/kg IV × 3 d	26 childhood ALL	2 CR, 4 PR	53
2-Chlorodeoxyadenosine			
3.0–10.7 mg/m²/d CI × 5	1 adult ALL	1 response	59
	7 childhood ALL	1 response	
8.9 mg/m²/d CI × 5	7 childhood ALL	1 CR 14%	60

TABLE 27–8. Single-Drug Induction: Alkylating Agents

Drug and Dosage	N Patients	CR Rate (%)	Reference
Cyclophosphamide			
2–10 mg/kg/d PO, 5–15 mg/kg/d IV	40 children	18	83
2 mg/kg/wk	16 children + adults	0	84
10 mg/kg/wk	32 children + adults	6	84
2.5–15.0 mg/kg/wk	13 children + adults	8	84
2 mg/kg/d	45 children	40	85
Ifosfamide			
1200 mg/m²/d IV × 5 d	12 adults	33	81

TABLE 27–7. Single-Drug Induction: Cytarabine

Drug and Dosage	N Patients	CR Rate (%)	Reference
Conventional dose			
3 mg/kg/d	43 children	21	64
10–30 mg/m²/d q 12–24 h	22 adults	50	65
30–100 mg/m²/d q 12–24 h	11 adults	45	65
200 mg/m²/d 5-day infusion	36 adults	25	66
High-dose			
2–3 g/m² q 12 h × 10–12	5 adults	20	67
3 g/m² q 12 h × 4–6	4 adults	25	68
2 g/m² q 12 h × 12	8 adults	38	69
3 g/m² q 12 h × 12	12 adults	73	70
3 g/m² q 12 h × 12	16 adults	50	71
2–3 g/m² × 10–12	5 adults	20	72
3 g/m² × 12	3 adults	67	73
2–3 g/m² × 10–12	5 adults	0	74
3 g/m² × 12	15 adults	73	75
2 g/m² × 12	12 adults	42	76

TABLE 27–9. Single-Drug Induction: Anthracyclines

Drug and Dosage	N Patients	CR Rate (%)	Reference
Daunorubicin			
30 mg/m²/d × 3–7 d	38 children (ut)	58	88
1.0–1.5 mg/kg/d	25 children	48	89
30 mg/m²/d × 5 d	29 children	17	90
45 mg/m²/d × 5 d	28 children	32	90
60 mg/m²/d	39 children	38	90
Adriamycin			
0.4 mg/kg/d × 4 d	38 children	42	91
17.5 mg/m² q 2 d × 95 d	30 children	17	92
15 mg/m²/6 h × 6	39 children	37	93
75 mg/m² q 2–3 wk	30 adults	20	94
Rubidazone			
4 mg/kg/d × 5 d	44 adults	50	95
300–450 mg/m² q 21 d	19 adults	53	96
300 or 450 mg/m² q 21 d	15 adults	26	97
300 or 450 mg/m²	56 children	25	98

ut = previously untreated.

TABLE 27–10. Single-Drug Induction: Nonanthracycline DNA Intercalators

Drug and Dosage	N Patients	CR Rate (%)	Reference
m-AMSA			
60 mg/m²/d × 5 d	36 children	3 (12%)	99
90 mg/m²/d × 5 d	5 adults	2	99
75–90 mg/m²/d × 5 d	7 adults	1	100
200 mg/m²/d × 5 d	12 adults	3 (25%)	101
100–120 mg/m²/d × 5–7 d	8 adults	2	102
75–90 mg/m²/d × 7 d	10 children + adults	1 (10%)	103
50–150 mg/m²/d × 7 d	9 children + adults	2	104
120 mg/m²/d × 5 d	31 children	4 (13%)	105
60 mg/m²/d × 10 d	36 children	4 (11%)	105
Mitoxantrone			
8–16 mg/kg/d × 5 d	12 children + adults	4 (33%)	106
18–20 mg/m²/d × 5 d	24 children	5 (21%)	107
4–12 mg/m²/d × 5 d	8 adults	1	108
10–12 mg/m²/d × 5 d	13 adults	1 (8%)	109
20–32 mg/m²/d × 20 min inf. q 14 d	2 adults	0	110
10–12 mg/m²/d × 5 d	11 adults	1 (9%)	111
10–12 mg/m²/d by c.i.	3 adults	0	112
4 mg/m²/d × 5 d	28 adults	4 (14%)	113

inferior compared with those with lower blast cell count.[12]

Vinca Alkaloids

Vinca alkaloids, along with adrenocorticosteroids, are important agents for remission induction in ALL (see Table 27–2). Vincristine (VCR), although not without myelotoxicity, can be given in optimal therapeutic doses, resulting in only mild inhibition of granulopoiesis and thrombocytopoiesis in previously untreated patients. A single IV dose of 2 mg/m²/wk has become the consensus mode for VCR administration; even this dose may be too much for older patients in whom neurotoxicity with peripheral neuropathy or paralytic ileus may occur after one or two doses. More frequent injections[16] and continuous infusions[17, 18] increase the biologic effects of VCR, but unfortunately the increased toxicity of such regimens generally outweighs any increase in antileukemic action. Other vinca alkaloids such as vinblastine (VBL) and vindesine (VDS) have been employed in ALL. Of VCR-resistant

TABLE 27–11. Single-Drug Induction: Asparaginase

Dosage and Route	N Patients	CR Rate (%)	Reference
50–200 mg/kg/d biweekly IV	21 children and adults	67	119
10–500 mg/kg/d IV	95 children	42	120
200 mg/kg/d × 15 d IV	35 children	43	121
200 mg/kg/d × 14 d IV	13 children	23	122
1000 mg/kg biweekly IV	15 children	47	122
10–600 mg/m²/d IV	19 children	68	123
10–600 mg/m²/d IV	4 adults	0	123

patients, 20% to 30% have responded to VDS[19]; it showed equal activity compared with VCR in randomized trials,[20, 21] and it may be less neurotoxic compared with VCR. VDS has therefore been administered during relapse treatment or during consolidation therapy in some trials.

VCR plays a limited role in maintenance therapy; alone, it has proved to be ineffective and causes accumulating neurotoxicity. IV VCR does not enter the CNS in quantity. It has proved uniformly lethal when even small doses have been administered by error intrathecally.

Folic Acid Antimetabolites

Folic acid antagonists (see Table 27–3) initiated the revolution in treatment of ALL in children.[1] Methotrexate (M), which is the exclusively used antifolic compound, provides with 6-mercaptopurine (MP) the foundation of maintenance chemotherapy and is the key component in adjuvant chemotherapy to the CNS.

M alone is only modestly active in remission induction, with 14% to 33% of children and fewer adults responding to administration. It is more effective when coupled with simultaneous prednisolone and is highly effective when combined with L-asparaginase, the latter adding its own antileukemic effect and reducing the susceptibility of normal tissue to M cytotoxicity when scheduled appropriately.[32-34] For maintenance, M is more effective when used in combination with MP, VCR, or prednisolone, or all three.

High-dose M (HdM), championed in the 1960s by Djerassi[35] and others, provides effective antileukemic M concentration in all organ sites where leukemic cells might, through perfusion problems, escape destruction.[35] It has the potential to overcome mechanisms of resistance against M, and its efficacy is augmented by dose-dependent higher formation of M polyglutamate derivatives that confer the antileukemic effect. Thus, in childhood ALL, HdM led to a reduction of CNS and testicular relapse risk and also to a reduction of bone marrow relapse.[36]

Standard-risk childhood ALL patients have been treated successfully with regimens based mainly on antimetabolites, e.g., HdM and high-dose mercaptopurine, avoiding anthracyclines, epipodophyllotoxins, alkyating agents, and CNS irradiation.

Purine Antimetabolites

Of the numerous purine analogues tested in leukemia (see Table 27–4), MP is the traditional choice for ALL, whereas 6-thioguanine (TG) is preferred in AML. Specifically, MP and TG have not been directly compared in ALL, but they are used sequentially in induction and consolidation.[41] Nonetheless, MP is the most popular drug to combine with M in virtually all the maintenance protocols. MP is given orally either in 5-day courses or daily. Like M, and probably for the same cell-kinetic reasons, it is only slightly effective as a single-drug remission induction treatment. High-dose MP has been explored but has not achieved a role in standard treatment of ALL.

New Purine Analogues

Fludarabine is a purine analogue that exerts synergistic activity with cytarabine. It has shown modest activity as a single drug. Sequential administration of fludarabine followed by high-dose AC (HdAC) has demonstrated significant synergistic effects in leukemic cell lines, which is probably due to an increased intracellular cytosine arabinoside triphosphate (ara-CTP) level. Regimens including fludarabine and HdAC followed by granulocyte colony-stimulating factor (G-CSF)—the FLAG regimen—or in combination with additional idarubicin (IDA)—the FLAG-IDA regimen—have shown promising activity in relapsed ALL and particularly Ph/BCR-ABL–positive ALL. In five trials, the CR rate of 43 patients was 70% with FLAG or FLAG-IDA.[45-49] It is being investigated as consolidation therapy in front-line therapy in phase III studies.

2'-Deoxycoformycin (pentostatin), an adenosine deaminase inhibitor, has demonstrated activity in both T-cell and B-cell malignancies (see Table 27-6). No response was observed in one trial with pentostatin in relapsed childhood ALL,[51] but significant activity was observed in T-ALL.[52-54] Unfortunately, excessive toxicity was seen at the doses initially employed.[55] At present, 2'-deoxycoformycin is being reevaluated in relapsed and refractory T-ALL at lower dosages.

The role of 2-chlorodeoxyadenoside (cladribine) has been evaluated, preferentially in childhood ALL, and isolated single responses have been observed (see Table 27-6).

Compound GW506U78 (9-β-D-arabinosylguanine) is a prodrug of arabinosylguanine (ara-G) that is activated by intracellular phosphorylation to its triphosphate form (ara-GTP).[61] GW506U78 exerts specific cytotoxicity toward immature T cells compared with B cells. In a phase I study in adult and pediatric leukemia, 9 out of 15 patients with relapsed T-ALL achieved CR, and partial remission was observed in 3 patients.[62] Clinical phase II studies are ongoing. GW506U78 is a promising new drug for T-ALL and T-cell non-Hodgkin's lymphoma (T-NHL), but its clinical application may be limited by toxicity, particularly neurotoxicity.

Pyrimidine Antagonists

Of the pyrimidine antagonists (see Table 27-7), AC, 5-azacytidine (aza-C), and 5-fluorouracil (5-FU) have been shown to have activity in ALL. Clearly the most useful and most frequently used of these drugs is AC, which at high doses (2 to 3 g/m²) has induced remission as a single agent in up to about 70% of adults and children at relapse and has formed part of numerous successful drug combinations, including mitoxantrone, amsacrine, asparaginase, and fludarabine. HdAC yields cytotoxic drug levels in the cerebrospinal fluid (CSF) and has also been successfully used for remission induction in CNS involvement[63] and for prophylaxis of CNS relapse. In vitro studies suggest that T cells, including the blasts from patients with T-cell ALL, are especially sensitive to AC. AC is also given intrathecally in the treatment of CNS leukemia, either alone or, more often, in combination with M and adrenocorticosteroids. AC is a classic phase-specific drug, and it is more active when administered every 12 hours by injection or by continuous infusion.

Alkylating and Other DNA-Linking Agents

CP is the most commonly used alkylating agent for ALL. It has a remission induction capability similar to M, 6-MP, and AC, plus slight but definite maintenance activity when used as a single agent (see Table 27-8). It does not enter the CNS after oral or IV administration; because it is not activated within the CNS, the IT route is not useful. CP is effective in T-ALL and may act synergistically with AC.[77] In recent effective B-ALL regimens, CP is used in moderate to higher doses.[78, 79] When used in doses of 200 mg/m² × 5 in combination with prednisolone, it can induce substantial tumor mass reduction in mature B-ALL as the initial phase of treatment.[80]

Ifosfamide (IFO), another complex alkylating agent, has exhibited remission induction potential at least comparable to CP in one study.[81] IFO is now included in highly effective B-ALL regimens.[80, 82]

2'-Anthracyclines

Daunorubicin (D) was the first anthracycline antibiotic to show significant antileukemic activity (see Table 27-9). It appears equally effective in ALL and AML. It is toxic to the bone marrow but induces 25% to 50% CR in patients with ALL. It must be given intravenously, by which route it has no identifiable activity against CNS leukemia. Daunorubicin in combination adds to the effectiveness of remission induction regimens in adults.[86] There is some evidence that the application of dose-intensive anthracyclines during induction therapy may contribute to an improvement of CR rate and leukemia-free survival (LFS) as indicated in a retrospective literature analysis. Four out of 12 studies with a dose intensity (DI = total mg/m²/week over first 12 weeks) for anthracyclines lower than 20 reported LFS rates greater than 35% compared with 4 out of 5 studies with a DI greater than 20 (reviewed in Bassan et al[87]).

Adriamycin (AD) (doxorubicin) has been less extensively tested in ALL but shows similar activity and, unfortunately, similar or even higher (gastrointestinal) toxicities. As with daunorubicin, cumulative doses should not exceed 550 mg/m² especially if arrhythmia, lengthened P-R interval, or a reduced ventricular ejection fraction is noted during treatment.

Of the newer anthracyclines, both rubidazone and IDA have shown substantial antileukemic effects. Their relative value in comparison to DNR has not been established. It is assumed that IDA is an anthracycline that may circumvent P-gp-mediated drug resistance. After IV application of IDA, its breakdown product idarubidazol reaches measurable levels in the CNS. Therefore, a potential advantage for the use of IDA could be its effect in the treatment of CNS leukemia or as CNS prophylaxis, but this remains to be established.

Nonanthracycline DNA Intercalators

Two compounds of this class, 4'-[9-acridinylamino]methansulfon-m-anisidide (m-AMSA) and mitoxantrone (MI), have proved to be effective in ALL treatment.

m-AMSA, an acridine derivative, was first introduced in

1977 and has proved, alone and in combination with ara-C, to have significant antileukemic activity, particularly in AML. With recurrent ALL, remission rates varied from 0% to 40%, with an average of about 20% for both children and adults (see Table 27–10). m-AMSA is not cross-resistant with anthracyclines. Its major current role is in salvage combination chemotherapy. The compound at standard doses of 90 to 120 mg/m² does not enter the CNS in quantities sufficient for treatment of CNS leukemia, and at higher doses CNS toxicity is often limiting.

MI, a synthetic anthraquinone, is, like m-AMSA and the anthracyclines, a powerful DNA intercalator. Toxicity of the compound is largely restricted to myelosuppression, although mucositis and hepatotoxicity may be dose-limiting on occasion. CRs have been reported in up to 33% of children and adult patients in ALL relapse. The best results are obtained at 10 mg/m²/day for 5 days, but in combinations, e.g., with HdAC, it is given for 4 or 3 days only. Dosages above 10 mg/m² have proved to be toxic and less effective (see Table 27–10).

L-Asparaginase

L-Asparaginase (see Table 27–11) comes close to being the specific anti-ALL drug. Side effects abound, the result of protein synthesis inhibition and allergic reactions; however, in most cases the cytolytic effects following its administration are restricted to leukemic lymphoblasts.

L-asparaginase (A) may be given at various doses and schedules, but higher doses have been reported to increase its CR induction potential[114] and the duration of subsequent remission. The use of weekly high doses early in remission has been associated with enhanced duration of remission in children.[115, 116] The drug can be used in remission induction, but caution is required to avoid life-threatening anaphylactoid reactions. IM injection appears less liable to anaphylaxis than IV infusion. Furthermore, L-asparaginase application is frequently associated with coagulation disturbances, and careful monitoring is required.

Preparations from different origins (*Erwinia carotovora* versus *Escherichia coli*) are available. A polyethylene glycol (PEG) encapsulated L-asparaginase (*E. coli*) has been introduced. The preparations show significant differences in terms of half-time, being 5.7 days, 1.2 days, and 0.65 day for *PEG-A*, native *E. coli* A, and *Erwinia* A, respectively.[117] This has consequences for dosage schedules because *Erwinia* A has to be administered more frequently than *E. coli* A, whereas one application of PEG A substitutes a 14-day cycle of native *E. coli* A. When *Erwinia* A was administered at the same dose level as native *E. coli* A during a multidrug induction regimen for childhood ALL in a randomized comparison, its application was associated with less toxicity but also with inferior DFS.[118]

PEG-A has been explored in several pilot trials for adult and childhood ALL, mostly as part of multidrug induction therapy. In a randomized trial in de novo childhood ALL, comparing 2500 U/m² PEG-A with 6000 U/m² × 9 native *E. coli* A, the remission rate on day 28 did not differ; there was, however, more rapid response, with 63% with M1 marrow on day 7 with PEG-A compared with 47% in

patients with native *E. coli* A.[124] The addition of PEG-A to a conventional induction with VCR, prednisolone, and D yielded a high CR rate of 93% in a small cohort of adult de novo ALL patients (n = 14) with a median age of 23 years.[125]

In childhood ALL, PEG-A did not show higher toxicity compared with native *E. coli* A.[126, 127] Toxicity data for PEG-A (2000 U/m²) in adult ALL are available from the pilot study and from another trial in 26 adult patients with de novo ALL.[128] The most frequent toxicities were elevations of bilirubin (36% to 38%) or hepatic transaminases (7% to 19%), grade I to II CNS toxicity (14% to 36%), hyperglycemia (38% to 43%), fibrinogen levels lower than 100% (73%), AT III levels lower than 60% (100%), and grade III phlebitis or thrombosis (15%).[125, 128] Frequent laboratory controls particularly focusing on the coagulation system during the whole period of L-asparaginase activity are required. Reports from relapsed and de novo childhood ALL provide evidence that a dose level of 1000 U/m² PEG-A may yield sufficient asparaginase activity for at least 14 days. If similar high CR rates of 90% can be confirmed in ongoing trials in adult ALL, PEG-A would offer a promising new treatment option.

Epipodophyllotoxins

For the epipodophyllotoxins etoposide (VP16) and teniposide (VM26), data as single drugs are very scarce, but these drugs are used increasingly in combination, particularly with ara-C (see the later section on refractory or recurrent disease) or VP16 as part of a high-dose therapy conditioning regimen before SCT.

New Cytostatic Drugs Under Investigation

A variety of new cytostatic drugs, such as gemcitabine, FMdC, flavopiridol, topotecan and arsenic trioxide, showed in vitro activity against ALL blast cells. Topotecan has exhibited cytostatic activity in preclinical studies and in phase I studies in relapsed ALL, 1 CR and 1 partial remission were reported in a total of 29 patients after continuous infusion of topotecan as single-agent therapy.[129-131] In a phase II window study in adult de novo high-risk ALL, 1 CR out of 14 patients was achieved.[132] Thus, topotecan has only limited activity as a single agent in ALL; whether it might have a role in combination regimens remains to be defined.

Arsenic trioxide has been successfully administered in relapsed acute promyelocytic leukemia. It has been demonstrated that it induces apoptosis to a greater extent in *BCR-ABL*–positive than in *BCR-ABL*–negative cell lines and primary blast cells.[133] Furthermore, it led to a downregulation of *BCR-ABL* levels and Abl-kinase activity and to a higher rate of apoptosis if administered in combination with the Abl-tyrosine kinase inhibitor CGP57148.[134] These results indicate that a specific activity of arsenic trioxide may be exerted in *BCR-ABL*–positive ALL, but confirmation in clinical applications awaits.

Monoclonal Antibodies for Immunotherapy

ALL blast cells express various specific antigens, such as CD20, CD19, and leukemia-specific combinations of

TABLE 27–12. Monoclonal Antibodies with Preclinical or Clinical Activity in ALL*

Antibody	Immunotoxin	Target Cells	Clinical Activity
Anti-CD20			
Rituximab	—	B-cells (B-NHL, B-precursor ALL, B-ALL)	B-cell lymphoma High-grade NHL
Anti-CD19			
B43-Genistein	Genistein	B lymphoblasts	Relapsed B-lineage ALL
B43-PAP	PAP	B lymphoblasts	Relapsed B-lineage ALL
AntiB4-bR	Blocked ricin	B lymphoblasts	De novo B-lineage ALL B-NHL
B43-P38	P38	B lymphoblasts	—
Anti-CD52			
Campath-1H	—	Lymphoblasts (T > B cells)	Relapsed ALL
Anti-CD7			
AntiCD7-R	Ricin	T lymphoblasts	T-NHL
AntiCD7-PAP	PAP	T lymphoblasts	—
Anti-CD3			
OKT3	—	T lymphoblasts	T-ALL

*Adapted from.[135]

antigens that can serve as targets for treatment with monoclonal antibodies (Table 27–12). Antibodies can be administered in unconjugated form or conjugated to immunotoxins, to radioactive molecules, or to bispecific antibodies.

A prerequisite for antibody therapy is generally the presence of the target antigen on at least 30%, preferably 50%, of the blast cells.

B-lineage ALL and B-Cell Lymphoma

Most clinical experience has been accumulated with antibodies to CD20 and CD19. Rituximab is a mononuclear antibody to CD20 that is expressed on normal and malignant B cells, and it is already incorporated in front-line therapy for non-Hodgkin's lymphoma. CD20 (more than 30% of cells) is also expressed in one third of B-precursor ALL and the majority of mature B-ALL cells. This provides a rationale for clinical trials in B-precursor ALL, mature B-ALL, and Burkitt's lymphoma.

CD19 is expressed on more than 90% of blast cells in B-precursor and mature B-ALL. Several conjugated antibodies targeting the CD19 antigen have been developed. The conjugate of the tyrosine kinase inhibitor genistein and the antibody B43 [B43(anti-CD19)-genistein] targets the immunotoxin to CD19-positive blast cells.[136] It showed antitumor activity in children and adults with relapsed B-lineage ALL expressing CD19 (more than 50% of the leukemic blast cells). Two CRs and two partial remissions were observed in a cohort of 15 patients with heavily pretreated ALL.[137]

The B43 antibody was also conjugated to the poke-weed antiviral protein (PAP) immunotoxin [B43(anti-CD19)-PAP]. Ten out of 15 relapsed childhood ALL patients treated with 2 cycles of B43-PAP parallel to a standard 4-drug reinduction regimen achieved a CR, and 2 achieved partial remission.[138]

The protein toxin anti-B4-blocked ricin (anti-B4-bR) conjugated to the anti-CD19 mononuclear antibody was used during consolidation therapy in the CALGB 9311 trial. The median remission duration of patients treated with anti-B4-bR was similar (10.2 months) compared with those without (9.7 months).[139] Minimal residual disease (MRD) evaluations in a subset of these patients so far demonstrated little impact of anti-B4-bR on MRD levels.[140]

T-Lineage ALL

CD7 is a surface determinant of T cells. The immunotoxin ricin conjugated with an antibody to the CD7 antigen (anti-CD7-ricin) showed activity in a mouse model of primary T-cell leukemias[141] and in a phase I trial in patients with relapsed T-cell lymphoma (more than 30% CD7-positive blast cells) where two partial remissions were achieved in 11 patients.[142]

The mononuclear antibody Campath-1H is directed to the CD52 antigen, which is expressed on most lymphoblastic cells and to a higher degree in T-cell compared with B-cell lymphoblasts. It showed clinical activity in patients with relapsed adult ALL (higher than 50% expression of CD52) with reduction of white blood cells (WBCs), clearance of peripheral blast cells, and one partial remission in five patients.[143]

Antibody therapy offers new treatment options for adult ALL that deserve clinical investigation. As in NHL, the potential application could be single, or in combination with chemotherapy during induction, consolidation, or for purging. Whereas in patients with high tumor load, e.g., at overt relapse, the chance of remission induction is rather low, it would be of interest to evaluate antibody therapy as maintenance therapy, e.g., in MRD-positive patients or in patients who are not eligible for conventional chemotherapy, e.g., due to age or clinical infections.

TREATMENT STRATEGY FOR NEWLY DIAGNOSED ALL IN ADULTS

Introduction

It has been demonstrated that successful induction of remission dramatically improves survival and that the achievement of CR is essential for the chance of cure. The goals of the initial phase of treatment are (1) to prepare the patient as much as possible for cytotoxic antileukemic therapy, (2) to eliminate the inhibition of normal hematopoiesis by leukemic cells, and (3) to reduce leukemic cell numbers significantly as a first step toward eradication of the leukemic clone.

Rapid remission induction will reduce the likelihood that clinical resistance to the drugs will develop during treatment. In turn, remission induction will temporarily increase granulocytopenia and thrombocytopenia through myelotoxicity, induce further immunosuppression and, through cytolysis, increase metabolic burdens of urates, phosphates, and other intracellular organic acids and of thromboplastins. These problems must be anticipated and controlled before and throughout remission induction treatment.

Prechemotherapy Measures

Initial estimates of blood cell counts, blood sugar level, liver and renal function, serum electrolytes, and fibrinogen level must be obtained before the first administration of antileukemic drugs or irradiation. A full coagulation work-up is advisable if there is significant bleeding (other than petechiae or microscopic hematuria) on diagnosis. An analysis of potential activated protein C resistance helps identify patients with higher risk of thrombosis.[144] Bone marrow or, less desirably, peripheral blood leukemic cells should be evaluated in all cases for immunologic phenotype, for cytogenetics, and for molecular analysis, all of which can affect the choice of treatment. Adequate hydration, preferably by 24-hour IV infusion, must be ensured in order to produce a 100 mL/hour output of neutral to alkaline urine. Allopurinol usually at a dosage of no less than 300 mg/day should be started at once, increased if necessary, and continued until a CR has been achieved or at least until blast cells have been cleared from the peripheral blood. With severe thrombocytopenia and bleeding, platelet concentrates may be required. Febrile granulocytopenic patients should have thorough cultures taken and should be started on empirical antibiotic treatment. Similarly, other leukemia-related homeostatic and metabolic disturbances must be anticipated and treated.

Patients with very high circulating blast cell counts are at particular risk of blast cell thrombi (leukostasis), infiltration of vascular endothelium by leukemic cells, and massive hemorrhage from the injured vessels.[145] Significant leukostasis occurs almost exclusively in patients with more than 200×10^9 blasts/L, and chemotherapy should be started at once. Prednisolone, dexamethasone (DX) (10 mg/m^2), or VCR can reduce circulating blasts rapidly. Alternatively, peripheral blasts can be removed by leukapheresis, and chemotherapy can then be instituted. Because methods for rapid cell reduction (except leukapheresis) will further aggravate urate nephropathy and other leukemia-related metabolic problems, the most diligent attention must be given to hydration, alkalinization of the urine, and hemostasis during the phase of rapid cytoreduction.

When these conditions have been addressed, remission induction therapy can begin. The choice of induction combination should depend primarily on the patient's subtype of ALL, age and, to some extent, on the therapist's experience and preference. Although the effectiveness of remission induction is currently high, there is no unanimity among physicians when it comes to drugs, doses, or schedules.

SPECIFIC ANTILEUKEMIC THERAPY

Introduction

The currently accepted rules for treating adult ALL are (1) the use of a combination that includes prednisolone, VCR, L-asparaginase, and an anthracycline for remission induction; recent approaches also include high-dose therapy (particularly HdAC as front-line therapy); (2) postinduction therapy; in most trials, drugs such as AC, CP, or epipodophyllotoxins, or systemic high-dose therapy with AC or M, which is also CNS-active, are used; (3) SCT, allogeneic, autologous, or matched unrelated is now a major part of postinduction therapy; it is sometimes preceded by a consolidation cycle; (4) treatment of the CNS early in CR by IT-M (alone or in combination with AC and hydrocortisone or DX), with or without combination of CNS irradiation; (5) the use of combinations of antimetabolites for maintaining CR; and (6) the use of all available methods to protect patients from disease complications that might interfere with optimal therapy. In addition, clinical, immunophenotypic, cytogenetic, and molecular evaluation is needed to identify candidates for SCT in first remission.

Remission Induction

Treatment strategies for adult ALL were once very similar to those for childhood ALL, but it became evident that with mild drug combinations such as VCR and prednisolone in childhood ALL, CR rates of 85% to 95% could be obtained, whereas in adult ALL the success rate in a series of 15 studies was only 50%.[41] The median remission duration was only 3 to 8 months in spite of various consolidation and maintenance schedules. The improvement afforded by escalation in combination therapy is shown in Table 27-13, which lists conventional regimens for adult ALL used in studies of 50 or more patients who were 15 years or older. It is evident that nearly all studies employ VCR and prednisolone combined with either L-asparaginase and/or an anthracycline. Remission rates have increased to the range of 75% to 90%.

The improvement in remission rate brought by the addition of a single drug is difficult to assess. An improvement in CR rate from 41% to 85% by giving daunorubicin in addition to VCR/prednisolone was seen by Willemze and colleagues,[146] but daunorubicin was given sequentially only to patients who had not already achieved CR with VCR/prednisolone alone. The addition of daunorubicin produced a similar improvement in an Argentinian study where the CR rate rose from 33% to 50%.[115] However, clear evidence that daunorubicin does in fact increase the CR rate in adult ALL comes from a CALGB randomized trial comparing induction with VCR/prednisolone and L-asparaginase with or without daunorubicin[86]; remission rates were 79% and 47%, respectively. L-asparaginase apparently does not affect the CR rate but probably improves LFS; if not used during induction therapy, it is often included as part of the consolidation treatment. Evidence comes from pediatric studies where the addition of L-asparaginase to VCR and prednisolone

TABLE 27–13. Results of Conventional Chemotherapy in Adult ALL Studies

Group	Year	N	Age (yr)	Induction	Consolidation	Maintenance	CNS Prophylaxis	Complete Remission (%)	Probability of Continuous Remission
Gottlieb et al[86]	1984	53	37	V,P,A	V,P	M,MP	IT-M,RT	47	39% at 3 y
		46	30	V,P,A,D	V,P	M,MP	IT-M,RT	83	
		78	35	V,P,A,D	MP,M,V,P	M,MP	IT-M,RT	76	
Barnett et al[76]	1986	112	26	V,DX/P,A,AD,[C]	—	M,MP,C	IT-M/AC,RT	66	—
Marcus et al[172]	1986	36	30	V,P	V,P,A/C,AC	M,MP	IT-M,RT	75	18% at 5 y
Hussein et al[167]	1989	168	28	V,P,AD,C	M,AC,TG,A,V,P,C	M,MP,V,P,AD,DT, C,BCNU	IT-M	68	30% at 7 y
Radford et al[186]	1989	56	37	V,P,AD,A	—	V,P,AD,MP,M,DT, BCNU,C	IT-M,Rt	75	53% at 5 y
Tomonaga et al[187]	1991	117	38	V,P,AD,A,C	VP,M + other	M,M,A + other	IT-M,AC	81	30% at 4 y
Ellison et al[163]	1991	277	33	V,P,A,D	MP,M/AC,D	V,P,MP,M	IT-M,RT	64	29% at 9 y
Smedmyr et al[188]	1991	113	38	V,P,A,D,C	V,D,VP,AC,P	MP,M	IT-M [RT]	77	
Lluesma-Gonalons et al[171]	1991	137	30	V,P,D	—	M,MP,V,P	IT-M,DX	80	20% at 5 y
		145	29	V,P,D,A,C,AC,MP	AD,V,DX,A,AC,C,MP	M,MP,V,P	IT-M,DX	78	34% at 6 y
Bassan et al[153]	1992	212	28	V,AD,A,P [C]	—	MP,M	IT-M,RT	71	32% at 10 y
Hoelzer et al[189]	1993	368	25	V,P,A,D,C,AC,M,MP	V,DX,AD,AC,C,TG	MP,M	IT-M,RT	74	35% at 10 y
		562	28	V,P,A,D,C,AC,M, MP	V,DX,AD,AC,C,TG, VM, AC	MP,M	IT-M,RT	75	39% at 7 y
UKALL IX[190]	1993	266	> 14 y	V,P,A,(MP,M)/D	—	M,MP,V,P,AC	IT-M,RT	68	22% at 8 y
Fiere et al[191]	1993	581	33	V,P,D/R,C,[amsa,AC]	D/R,AC,A ± allo/ auto BMT	P,V,D/R,MP,M,DT, C,CA,M	IT-M,RT	76	17% at 5 y
Nagura et al[150]	1994	84	33	V,P,AD	V,AD,C,M,P	MP,M,V,C,P	IT-M,RT	63	24% at 7 y
		82		V,P,AD,A	V,AD,C,M,P	MP,M,V,C,MP,P	IT-M,RT	65	31% at 7 y
Todeschini et al[192]	1994	86	33	V,P,D	A	MP,M,V,P,D	IT-M,RT	79	35% at 6 y
Scherrer et al[193]	1994	61	29	V,P,A,D,C,AC,M,MP	V,DX,AD,AC,C,TG	MP,M	IT-M [RT]	85	44% at 5 y
Thomas et al[194]	1995	57	34	V,P,D,C	AC,A,Mi,V,DX	P,V,D/R,MP,M, DT,C,CA	IT-M,RT	89	44% at 2 y
Bosco et al[195]	1995	74	nr	V,P,A,D,C,AC,MP	V,AD,DX,C,AC,TG	MP,M	IT-M,RT	73	29% at 5 y
Larson et al[196]	1995	197	32	C,V,P,A,D	C,MP,AC,V,A,M,AD, DX,TG	V,P,MP,M	IT-M,RT	85	30% at 5 y
Durrant et al[176]	1997	618	nr	V,P,D,A	P,V [V,D,VP,AC, TG,P]	M,MP,V,P	IT-M,RT	82	28% at 5 y
Larson et al[197]	1998	198	35	C,D,V,P,A	C,MP,AC,V,A,M,AD, V,DX,C,TG,AC,P	MP,M,V,P	IT-M,RT	85	40% at 3 y
Bassan et al[198]	1999	80	32	IDA,V,A,P	IDA,V,A,C, ± auto SCT,V,C,VM, AC	MP,M	IT-TMX,RT	90	31% at 5 y
Bassan et al[152]	1999	61	nr	C,IDA,V,A,P	IDA,V,A,C, ± auto SCT,V,C,VM,AC	MP,M	IT-M,RT	88	nr
		4925						76%*	28%*

*Weighted mean.

leads to improved CR rates in relapsed ALL patients.[147] Further LFS was improved by the administration of L-asparaginase postinduction.[148, 149, 116] The addition of L-asparaginase to conventional induction therapy did not improve CR rate in one trial in adult ALL. There was, however, a trend toward higher LFS in patients treated with L-asparaginase.[150]

The addition of other agents such as AC, CP, 6-MP, or other cytostatic drugs does not increase CR rates substantially (see Table 27–13), although the highest remission rates have been achieved with multidrug induction regimens. The addition of CP led, however, to an improved outcome for patients with T-ALL.[151, 152]

Recent approaches to improve induction therapy include the use of HdAC, dose-intensive anthracyclines, and intensified treatment with L-asparaginase and DX instead of prednisolone.

The aim of treatment with **high-dose cytarabine** is not only to improve CR rate but even more to increase the quality of remission and to provide efficient prophylaxis of CNS relapse. That means that a lower tumor load should lead to a better LFS. HdAC (1–3 g/m^2 generally for 12 doses) was administered either after the standard induction therapy or up front. The former approach has resulted in a median CR rate of 79%,[153-157] which is not superior to conventional treatment. The only exception is the hyper-CVAD regimen, which yielded a high CR rate of 91% but also includes DX and fractionated CP.[158] Thus, it remains uncertain whether and for which subgroups HdAC during induction may be beneficial for LFS. The up-front administration of HdAC before conventional induction treatment yielded in two preliminary reports high remission rates of 85%.[159, 160]

The application of **dose-intensive anthracyclines** during induction therapy may contribute to an improvement of CR rate and LFS.[87] Todeschini et al[161] reported a trial with intensive anthracycline application (270 mg/m^2 daunorubicin as three 3-day cycles during induction), resulting in a CR rate of 93% in a patient cohort with a median age of 34 years. Thus, in most large study groups, intensification of anthracycline therapy is attempted with a dosage of 45 to 60 mg/m^2 for daunorubicin given during 2 to 3 consecutive days (repeated in some studies) instead of weekly administration.

A treatment was intensified in two pilot studies by the use of PEG-L-asparaginase.[125, 128] A high CR rate of 93% was achieved according to one report with a low patient number (14) with a low median age (23 years).[125] Thus, the data on efficacy and tolerability are still scarce, and further analyses are awaited.

DX was five to six times more cytotoxic than prednisolone in stroma-supported cultures of primary ALL blasts.[5] In an in vitro drug sensitivity assay (MTT), DX also exerted a 16-fold higher antileukemic activity compared with prednisolone,[6] which may contribute to the higher clinical activity observed in childhood ALL trials. DX also has a longer half-life in the cerebrospinal fluid compared with prednisolone.[7] In a randomized study in childhood ALL comparing DX and prednisolone during induction therapy, the rate of CNS relapses was significantly lower with DX (14% versus 26%).[162] There is, however, evidence that the extensive use of DX may increase the risk of severe septicemias and fungal infections.[8] This problem and the known risk of bone marrow necrosis may be overcome by shorter application compared with earlier trials.

Evaluation of Therapy

Assessment of CR

Comparison of CR rates among trials for newly diagnosed adult ALL is made somewhat difficult by the fact that patients are assessed at varying times after start of induction treatment. Response is usually evaluated at 4 but also after 8 weeks, when a second phase of induction therapy is applied, or even later if additional salvage regimens are used to achieve CR. The proportion of patients with disease resistant to induction is also similar in most studies at about 10%, but it is decreasing with more intensified regimens.

Morphologically defined CR bone marrow (M0 or M1) or peripheral blood is often not identical with molecular evaluation of remission, which has a much higher sensitivity of 10^{-5} to 10^{-6}. Therefore, molecular methods (e.g., PCR, TacMan PCR) or flow cytometry for detection of minimal residual disease (MRD) are increasingly employed to achieve a better definition of CR.

Death During Induction

In adult ALL, induction mortality rate is 5% to 10% and is variously referred to as "early" death or death within 2, 4, or 8 weeks, rendering a comparison of the toxicity- or therapy-related mortality of different regimens difficult. Mortality during induction is significantly higher in patients older than 50 or 60 years.[163-165]

Postinduction Therapy

Conventional Regimens

Nonrandomized trials using a variety of schedules have shown that consolidation therapy improves the outcome for adult ALL (see Table 27-13). The advantage of an intensive postinduction therapy was first demonstrated in the protocols L-2 to L-17M of the Memorial Sloan-Kettering Cancer Center in the early 1970s.[164, 166] In the L-2 protocol, a 2-month consolidation phase included conventional dose AC and TG; in the L-10 protocol with 3-month consolidation, M was given in addition; in the L-17M consolidation, M and AC were alternated with AC and TG. This consolidation in conjunction with an intensified maintenance therapy led to a promising MRD of 28 months and a survival probability of 33% at 18 years.[166] In a cooperative trial of the Southwest Oncology Group,[167] a similar protocol resulted in an MRD of 23 months and a survival rate of 30% at 7 years. Several earlier trials demonstrated in most cases an improved LFS by adding intensive consolidation without high-dose schedules (see Table 27-13).[166, 168-172]

When, however, the European Organization for Research and Treatment of Cancer Leukemia Group randomized patients to receive or not the 3 months' consolidation with M, AC, and TG, both groups had the same LFS.[173] This shows the difficulty in assessing the efficacy of specific consolidation elements. A Cancer and Leukemia Group B randomized study showed no advantage for two consolidation courses, comprising the AML regimens "7 + 3" (AC 7 days + D 3 days) and "5 + 2" over two courses of MP and M,[163] with identical continuous complete remission (CCR) rates of 29% at 9 years for the standard and intensive treatment groups. In a large randomized trial conducted by the Italian GIMEMA group comparing conventional versus intensified consolidation, no advantage for intensified treatment could be demonstrated (28% LFS at 5 years in both arms).[174] Another randomized trial also did not show any benefit in LFS for patients with late intensification (45%) compared with those without (55%).[175] In another large randomized trial, there was a reduction of relapse risk in patients receiving early and late intensification (37% LFS) versus those without (28%).[176] The great discrepancy between LFS for patients without late intensification—28% in one trial[176] compared with 55% in the other[175]—shows how difficult it is to draw conclusions about the benefit of consolidation in adult ALL.

In the German multicenter trials for adult ALL, a different approach was used for consolidation; a regimen nearly identical to the induction therapy was given after 3 months. This "reinduction" included VCR, DX, AD, AC, CP and TG and led to an MRD of 24 months and a survival rate at 10 years of 35%.[169] That this type of consolidation may be important is evident from two consecutive protocols of the Argentine Group for Treatment of Acute Leukemia. The addition of the previous consolidation therapy in the second study, but also extension of the induction regimen from 4 to 8 weeks, improved the 5-year survival rate from 22% to 35%.[171]

High-Dose Chemotherapy in Consolidation

High-dose chemotherapy—either HdAC or HdM—has been used mainly to overcome drug resistance and to achieve therapeutic drug levels in the cerebrospinal fluid.

Although there is extensive experience with HdAC for the treatment of ALL (Table 27-14), it still remains uncer-

TABLE 27–14. Results of Chemotherapy Including High-Dose Cytarabine

Group	Year	N	Age (yr)	Induction	Consolidation	Maintenance	CNS Prophylaxis	Complete Remission (%)	Probability of Continuous Remission
Clarkson et al[199]	1990	199	25	V,P,[D,A,AD,C]	V,A,AC,TG,D,P,M, C,**IdAC**,BCNU	M,MP,V,C,BCNU,TG, HU,D,P,AD,D,T	OM-M	82	33% at 18 y
Kantarjian et al[158, 200]	1990, 2000	222	30	V,AD,DX	V,AD,DX,C,M,A, **HdAC**,P,D,MP ± auto SCT	M,MP,D,P	IT-M,AC	75	32% at 3 y
Stryckmans et al[201]	1992	106	27	V,P,AD,[**HdAC**]	A,HdC,[M,TG, AC]	M,P,V,AD,BCNU, C,MP	IT-M,RT	74	40% at 8 y
Bassan et al[153]	1992	57	32	V,AD,A,P,**HdAC**	—	MP,M	IT-M	67	27% at 5 y
Cassileth et al[154]	1992	89	31	V,P,D	**HdAC**,C,AD,V, P,M,A	—	IT-M	69	13% at 4 y
		247	33	V,P,D,[AC,TG]	**HdAC**,C,AD,V, P,M,A	—	IT-M	65	17–35% at 2 y
Willemze et al[155]	1995	26	31	V,P,**HdAC**,amsa,P	V,**HdAC**,amsa,P ± BMT	No	IT-M,RT	72	35% at 5 y
Dekker et al[202]	1997	130	35	V,P,A,D	**HdAC**,amsa, Mi, VP ± alloSCT	No	IT-M,P	73	22% OS at 5 y
Daenen et al[177]	1998	66	26	[AC,VP],V,P,AD	[**HdAC**,VP], A,**IdAC**	V,P,M,MP,AC/VP,C/Mi	IT-M	88	45% at 10 y
Todeschini et al[161]	1998	60	34	V,P,D,A	**HdAC**,VP,V,D,P, C,MP,M	M,MP,V,C,P,D	IT-M,RT	93	55% at 5 y
Hallbook et al[159]	1999	120	44	**HdAC**,C,D,V,BM	AM,**HdAC**,V,BM, C,D,VP ±/− SCT	nr	nr	85	36% at 3 y
Ifrah et al[203]	1999	64	31	IDA,P,**HdAC** [IDA,AC,A]	P,**HdAC**,Mi,VP, allo or auto SCT	—	IT-M	72	24% at 4 y (S)
		1386						76%*	31%*

*Weighted mean.

tain what dose and schedule is optimal. HdAC has been included in several trials in adult de novo ALL during induction, as part of consolidation therapy, or both. Overall, the results for the LFS are not superior to trials without HdAC. Superior results have been reported only from smaller trials. A high CR rate (88%) and LFS rate (45% at 9 years) were reported, with a regimen including pretreatment with AC and etoposide followed by conventional induction and intensive rotational consolidation/ maintenance chemotherapy over a total treatment period of 3 years.[177] With a regimen including high doses of D, during induction, followed by HdAC in postremission and intensified maintenance for a total duration of 3 years, the LFS rate was 55%.[161]

It is unknown whether specific subgroups of ALL profit from HdAC treatment. Thus, excellent results are achieved for pediatric B-ALL with an LFS rate of greater than 80% with a multidrug regimen including HdAC.[178] HdAC may also play a role in the treatment of adult pro-B-ALL.[179] Furthermore, HdAC proved to be effective in the treatment of overt CNS leukemia.[75] For other adult poor-risk groups, such as late responders and Ph+ ALL and pre-T-ALL groups, the value of HdAC remains to be determined.

The use of HdM has been extensively studied for the treatment of childhood ALL and, to a lesser extent, in adult ALL (reviewed in Gökbuget and Hoelzer[180]). Intermediate doses of 0.5 g/m², high doses of 1 to 8 g/m², and doses of 33 g/m² have been used. HdM appears to be effective in preventing systemic and testicular relapses.[36] The effect of HdM on CNS leukemia may be an important factor as well. HdM at a dose of 6 g/m² resulted in an 80% CR rate in children with CNS relapse,[181] indicating that systemic application yields cytotoxic levels in the CSF.

Several studies have investigated the efficacy of HdM during consolidation and/or induction treatment (Table 27–15) in combinations with other chemotherapeutic agents in adult ALL. As for HdAC, overall the results are not superior to trials not including HdM, but more favorable results have been achieved in small trials with HdM as part of intensive multidrug consolidation regimens with LFS rates of 42% to 57%.[182-184]

The use of HdAC and HdM as consolidation therapy was reported from six trials (Table 27–16), with LFS rates ranging from 21% to 47%. The repeated application of treatment cycles including intensive D, L-asparaginase, HdAC, and HdM led to a high CR rate (92%) and improved LFS (47% at 5 years), which was particularly evident in B-lineage ALL.[185]

There is some evidence that the inclusion of HdAC and HdM as part of multidrug consolidation treatment may improve overall results in adult ALL.

Maintenance Therapy

Although remission maintenance is given for most adults with ALL, there are very few randomized trials giving information on the overall value of maintenance, the optimal drug combination, and the dosage and duration of treatment.

The most common approach for maintenance therapy in adult ALL is adopted from childhood ALL. Adult ALL studies (with few exceptions) have M and MP in their

TABLE 27–15. Results of Chemotherapy Including High-Dose Methotrexate

Group	Year	N	Median Age (yr)	Induction	Consolidation	Maintenance	CNS Prophylaxis	Complete Remission (%)	Probability of Continuous Remission
Marcus et al[172]	1986	33	30	V,P,A,[AD,C]	D,AC,TG,**HdM**	M,MP,V,P,[AD,C]	IT-M,RT	82	38% at 5 y
Linker et al[182, 185]	1991,97	109	24	V,P,D,A	V,P,A,D,**IdM**,VM,AC	MP,M	IT-M,RT	88	42% at 5 y
Elonen et al[183]	1991	76	39	V,DX,AD,AC, VP; **HdM**,V,DX	AD,C,VM,V,DX,**HdM**, D,A,MP,C	MP,M,VD,P,AC,A,C, V,ADCA	IT-M,AC,RT	82	56% at 2 y
CALGB 8513[204]	1991	164	32	V,P,Mi/D,**HdM**	V,P,Mi/D,**HdM**,AC,MP,A	—	IT-M,**IdM**	64	18% at 3 y
Elonen et al[205]	1992	51	29	V,P,AD,A,[C]	**HdM**,V,P,TG,AC, C,AD	MP,M,C,V,P,AC, TG,VM,A	IT-M,RT	82	17% at 6 y
Wiernik et al[206]	1993	38	38	V,DX,A,M	M,A,V,DX,P,**HdM**	V,DX,M,MP	—	76	30% at 14 y
Chiu et al[207]	1994	50	28	V,P,A,D,[C]	D,V,P,A,VM,AC,**IdM**	MP,M	IT-M,RT	86	13% at 5 y
Evensen et al[184]	1994	79	27	V,P,A,AD,C	D,AC,TG,**HdM**,MP	P,V,AD,C,M,MP	IT-M	82	57% at 8 y
Ribera et al[175]	1998	108	28	V,P,D,A,C	**HdM**,MP,V,D,DX,A, C,VM,AC	R: MP/M vs VD,Mi, P,A,C,VM,AC	IT-M,AC,HC	86	41% at 5 y
		708						79%*	35%*

*Weighted mean.

backbone maintenance regimen (see Tables 27-13 to 27-16). It is evident from Tables 27-12 to 27-16 that many studies intensify their maintenance by addition of drugs either in repeated single cycles or in repeated different sequences of maintenance therapy.

Although the studies are generally not randomized with regard to the value of maintenance therapy, some conclusions might be drawn from comparing larger adult ALL trials (Table 27-17).

Earlier studies without maintenance therapy yield clearly inferior overall results despite intensive induction and the application of HdAC,[154, 155, 202, 203] HdM,[204] or both,[211] unless patients are referred to an early SCT. The weighted mean for LFS for 7 studies without maintenance therapy was 22%, with only 1 study yielding an LFS above 30%.[155]

No large trial demonstrated a clear advantage for patients treated with intensive maintenance therapy. One large multicenter study addressing this question in a randomized comparison failed to demonstrate a benefit in terms of LFS for intensified (28%) versus conventional

(27%) maintenance.[210] Maintenance therapy with 6-MP and M seems beneficial if administered after intensive induction and consolidation therapy. At least in 12 studies using this approach, the weighted mean for LFS was 32%. Additional cycles with VCR and prednisolone apparently do not offer a significant advantage, with a weighted mean for LFS of 31% from 8 studies. Intensive rotational maintenance therapy with several drug combinations in addition to 6-MP and M resulted in LFS rates above 30% in 73% of the analyzed studies (see Table 27-17).

The value of maintenance therapy for specific subgroups of ALL remains open. For common ALL, it seems that in studies with intensive induction and consolidation therapy patients might benefit from reinforced maintenance when compared with those with a similarly intensive induction and consolidation but with a conventional approach using M and MP only.

This might be explained by the low proliferation rate of c-ALL blasts, which may prevent total eradication even during intensive induction and consolidation.

For the rapidly proliferating T-ALL or B-ALL cells, the

TABLE 27–16. Results of Chemotherapy Including High-Dose Methotrexate and High-Dose Cytarabine

Group	Year	N	Age (yr)	Induction	Consolidation	Maintenance	CNS Prophylaxis	Complete Remission (%)	Probability of Continuous Remission
Wernli et al[154, 208]	1994	140	31	D,V,**IdM**,A,P	**HdAC**,VP, ± allo, auto or C	No	IT-M,-HC	78	21% EFS at 5 y
Attal et al[209]	1995	135	31	V,P,A,D,C,AC,MP	**HdM**/ARAC; allo or auto BMT	[IL-2]	IT-M	93	44% at 3 y
Mandelli et al[210]	1996	767	28	V,P,A,D,R,C [**HdAC**,Mi]	P,Mi,V,HdM,IdAC, DX,VM	M,MP,V,P/ AC,Mi,VM,C,D, V,**IdAC**, **HdM**,DX	nr	82	34% at 6 y
Mandelli et al[174]	1996	358	31	V,P,A,D	D,V,**IdM**,IdAC,P,VM, AC,DX	M,MP,V,P/**IdM**,V,D,P, AC,VM,IdAC	IT-M,P	79	25% at 10 y
Linker et al[185]	1997	62	nr	V,P,D,A	**HdAC**,VP,**HdM**,MP,D, V,P,A	M,MP	IT-M,RT	92	47% at 5 y
Kantarjian et al[158]	2000	204	39	V,AD,DX,C	**HdM**,**HdAC**,P	M,MP,V,P	IT-M,-AC	91	38% at 5 y
		1666						83%*	33%*

*Weighted mean.

TABLE 27–17. Role of Maintenance Therapy in the Treatment of Adult ALL

Type of Maintenance	N Studies	N Patients	N Studies with LFS > 30%	Leukemia-free Survival (Range)
No maintenance	7	860	1 (14%)	22% (13%–35%)
6-MP/M	12	1724	7 (58%)	32% (13%–47%)
6-MP/M/V/P	8	1814	4 (50%)	31% (20%–40%)
6-MP/M + several other drugs	22	3622	16 (73%)	31% (17%–57%)

late course of disease depends mainly on whether the cells are eradicated during induction and early intensification. Therefore, in mature B-ALL there is sufficient evidence that maintenance therapy can be totally omitted if treatment is conducted according to specific B-ALL protocols.

Because the major aim of maintenance therapy is the eradication of MRD, the subsequent evaluation of MRD may provide criteria for decision making on subgroup-specific indications, intensity, and duration of maintenance therapy in ALL.

CNS Prophylaxis

Without specific CNS-directed prophylaxis, approximately 33% (29% to 40%)[212, 213] of adult ALL patients develop a meningeal recurrence. If only patients surviving more than 12 months were analyzed, the rate of CNS recurrence even reached 50%.[214]

CNS prophylaxis can be achieved in a variety of ways: CRT (18 to 24 Gy); IT administration of M or the triple combination of M, AC, and hydrocortisone; therapy via an intraventricular reservoir; and systemic high-dose chemotherapy with HdM or HdAC, whereby cytotoxic levels in the CSF can be reached (reviewed in Bleyer[215] and in Gökbuget and Hoelzer[216]). When analyzing different treatment regimens with regard to how effectively they prevent CNS relapses, most authors report only the frequency of isolated CNS relapses. In a not negligible proportion of adult ALL patients, combined CNS and bone marrow relapses occur.

With IT administration, the rate of isolated and combined CNS relapses could be reduced to 13% (8% to 19%) (Table 27–18). Intermittent application during maintenance therapy improves the efficacy compared with the application of only a few doses during induction treatment.

In most adult ALL trials, additional prophylactic CRT (24 Gy) was included (see Tables 27–13 to 27–16). This combined approach further reduces the CNS relapse rate to 12% (5% to 23%) (see Table 27–18). There is some evidence that early CRT after remission induction is superior to delayed CRT during consolidation treatment as a trial with delayed CRT reported a higher CNS relapse rate of 12% to 26%.[163, 196, 217]

Systemic high-dose treatment alone apparently does not provide sufficient prophylaxis as the CNS relapse rate is about 14% (10% to 16%) (see Table 27–18). In many recent trials, combined treatment approaches have proved to be highly efficient. With high-dose chemotherapy together with IT therapy, the rate of CNS relapses was 7% (2% to 16%). With additional CRT, CNS relapses occurred at a rate of 6% (1% to 13%). The efficacy of intensified CNS prophylaxis was also demonstrated in a retrospective analysis from the Anderson Cancer Center, where the lowest CNS relapse rate (2%) was achieved in a trial with early high-dose chemotherapy and IT therapy for all patients.[213]

Because the risk for CNS relapse is associated with other biologic features such as immunophenotype (T-ALL, B-ALL), extreme leukocytosis, high leukemia cell proliferation rate, high serum lactate dehydrogenase (LDH) levels, and extramedullary organ involvement, a risk-adapted CNS prophylaxis has been suggested.[213] This approach is, however, in contrast to that of childhood ALL not widely used in adults which may be due to the fact that long-term neuropsychologic sequelae are minimal in adult patients (older than 25 years).[218]

Hematopoietic Growth Factors in ALL Treatment

Hematopoietic growth factors, particularly granulocyte colony-stimulating factor (G-CSF) and granulocyte macrophage colony-stimulating factor (GM-CSF), have been studied extensively in ALL to shorten the regeneration time of granulocytes after chemotherapy, mainly in order to reduce morbidity and mortality due to infections and to further intensify treatment (Table 27–19). G-CSF is a

TABLE 27–18. Correlation of CNS Prophylaxis and the Rate of CNS Relapses in Adult ALL

Type of CNS Prophylaxis	N Studies	N Patients	Incidence of CNS Relapses*	References
None	2	107	31% (30%–32%)	213 219
IT therapy	3	440	13% (8%–19%)	167 171 220
IT therapy + CNS irradiation	12	2311	12% (5%–23%)	41 163 171 217 219 153 192 193 195 196 161 176
HD chemotherapy alone	2	167	14% (10%–16%)	206 213
HD chemotherapy + IT therapy	10	1489	8% (2%–16%)	153 154 184 204 213 158 177 202 210
HD chemotherapy + IT therapy + irradiation	7	662	5% (0%–12%)	155 182 190 205 221 161 207

*Weighted mean and range for isolated CNS relapses and combined bone marrow and CNS relapses.

TABLE 27–19. Application of G-CSF in Adult ALL de novo ALL

Author	Year	Chemotherapy	Growth Factor	N	Days Until ANC>500/µL >1000/µL*		Incidence Infections (%)	Early Death (%)
Kantarjian[222]	1993	Consolidation	G-CSF	14	14	<.001	2	0
			hist control	14	18		4	14
Ottmann[225]	1995	Induction	G-CSF	37	8*	.002	43	0
			rand control	39	12.5*		56	3
Geissler[226]	1997	Induction	G-CSF	23	16*	<.005	40	4
			rand control	22	24*		77	9
Larson[197]	1998	Induction	G-CSF	102	16*	<.001	nr	4
			placebo	93	22*			11

*ANC >1000 µL.

valuable component of supportive care in the treatment of ALL, and there is no evidence that it may stimulate leukemic cell growth in a clinically significant manner.

The prophylactic administration of G-CSF significantly accelerates neutrophil recovery according to the majority of clinical trials.[197, 222-226] Several prospective randomized studies also show that this is associated with a substantially reduced incidence and duration of febrile neutropenia and of severe infections[223, 225, 226] and reduced induction mortality.[197, 222, 225, 226] There may be a particular advantage in patients with intensive rotational treatment who are at high risk of infections,[223] whereas the effect may be less evident in patients at low risk for infectious complications[227]—at least in childhood ALL. Scheduling of G-CSF treatment appears to be particularly important. If administered first at the end of a 4-week chemotherapy regimen, the potential benefits are limited.[228] There is sufficient evidence that G-CSF may be given in parallel with chemotherapy without aggravating the myelotoxicity of these specific regimens[197, 224-226] and that this scheduling may be an important determinant of clinical efficacy.

A closer adherence to the dose and schedule of chemotherapeutic regimens should be made possible by the use of G-CSF. So far no trial has demonstrated a benefit of increased dose intensity as made possible by G-CSF application in terms of LFS. Cost-effectiveness has to be taken into account as the potential reduction of costs associated with a decreased rate of infection, a shortened duration of IV antibiotic use, and of hospitalization time has to be weighed against the expense of the growth factor. So far, the limited number of studies that have performed a cost-benefit analysis of G-CSF administration have demonstrated slightly decreased[229] or unchanged[228] overall treatment costs. But the authors believed that the growth factor administration contributed substantially to quality of life,[229] which is an important issue for the heavily treated ALL patient.

REFRACTORY OR RECURRENT DISEASE

The success achieved in inducing CR for the majority of adults with ALL and curing a significant proportion of them is laudable but must not disguise the fact that current strategies fail for most patients in the short or long term. The chance to achieve CR with second-line treatment when the treatment of first choice has failed is about 60% to 70%, particularly with failure after inclusion of multiple drugs from the beginning. Even if CR is achieved, it is most likely to be short without SCT and probably with it.

A variety of treatment regimens have been developed and evaluated in relapsed or refractory ALL (summarized in Welborn[230] and Bassan et al[231]) (Table 27-20). Use of single-agent HdM, HdAC, and probably the anthracycline derivatives mitoxantrone and rubidazone result in a second remission in fewer than 30% of patients, whereas other agents such as amsacrine, teniposide, and etoposide are effective in 10% to 15% (see Tables 27-1 to 27-11).

The results of different combination regimens are summarized in Table 27-20. The most widely evaluated approach was the repetition of regimens including VCR, anthracyclines, and steroids similar to standard induction treatment in earlier studies with CR rates of 29% to 69%.

HdM followed by rescue with folinic acid and combined with L-asparaginase led to response rates of 22% to 79% in resistant ALL in early studies. This combination is no longer administered in relapsed ALL but is incorporated into several regimens in de novo ALL.

The epipodophyllotoxins have been explored as single drugs in small groups of patients, and the response rate for both has been very low. However, they apparently

TABLE 27–20. Summary of Treatment Results in Relapsed/Refractory ALL

Regimen	N Studies	N Patients	CR Rate* (range) (%)
Multidrug induction	7	327	50 (29–69)
VP + other	4	54	26 (11–33)
MTX/ASP	6	131	40 (22–79)
VM26/AC ± IFO	4	93	27 (16–42)
HdAC/Mi	8	217	50 (23–84)
HdAC/Mi + other	3	98	73 (70–80)
HdAC/VP + other	4	129	49 (17–76)
HdAC/AMSA	5	143	68 (21–77)
HdAC/ASP	4	47	36 (20–45)
HdAC/IDA	7	331	56 (18–64)
HdAC/FLU ± IDA	6	87	50 (30–83)

*Weighted mean.

synergize with AC. Teniposide 165 mg/mg^2 combined with AC 200 or 300 mg/mg^2 was pioneered in several childhood ALL studies by Rivera et al[232] and resulted in CR rates of 16% to 42% in adults (see Table 27-20). Etoposide has also been explored in several combinations, resulting in remission rates of 17% to 76% if combined with HdAC and 11% to 33% if combined with conventional drugs. High-dose etoposide is apparently effective when used as part of the conditioning regimen before SCT. Only very limited data are available for the use of high-dose etoposide without SCT in adult ALL.

The most extensively studied drug in relapsed adult ALL is HdAC. From several small pilot studies consisting of 90 patients altogether, the weighted mean remission rate of the single drug was 37%.[233] Higher CR rates were achieved with combination regimens, including HdAC and mitoxantrone (23% to 84%), mitoxantrone and other drugs (70% to 80%), amsacrine (21% to 77%), etoposide (17% to 76%), L-asparaginase (20% to 45%), and IDA (18% to 64%), with a wide variation of remission rates that may be attributed to patient selection and intensity of pretreatment. Because HdAC is increasingly administered during front-line treatment, its efficacy during relapse treatment may be impaired. The synergistic combination with fludarabine has been studied in relapsed ALL, particularly Ph/*BCR-ABL*–positive ALL, and yielded CR rates of 30% to 83% (see Table 27-5).

The most significant predictive factor for treatment response in relapsed patients is the duration of first remission. Patients with longer previous remission (longer than 18 months) have a higher CR rate and longer remission duration compared with those with short previous remission (less than 18 months).[234, 235]

The selection of a treatment regimen for relapsed ALL depends on several factors, such as previously administered therapy elements, time to relapse, availability of a bone marrow donor, age, subtype, relapse localization, and so on. Patients with late bone marrow relapse often respond to the repetition of the initially effective induction regimen. In patients with early treatment failure, often new drug combinations are selected. The evaluation of drug resistance may offer additional hints for the selection of cytostatic drugs. At relapse, patients often show increased expression of MDR-1–related drug resistance[236] and increased resistance as measured by in vitro drug resistance assays.[237] Drugs with a higher chance of effectivity may be identified in individual patients with the latter method.

In patients with extramedullary relapse such as CNS or testicular relapse, treatment regimens with local effectivity and systemic retreatment are required because the majority of patients show MRD in bone marrow. Thus, in CNS relapse an effective treatment combination such as HdAC or HdM in combination with IT therapy is usually effective in inducing remission. CNS irradiation can be performed on patients who were not previously irradiated. Patients with CNS relapse and intensive CNS-directed treatment are at higher risk for neurotoxicity such as leukoencephalopathy.[238]

For all chemotherapy regimens, the duration of second remission for bone marrow as well as for extramedullary relapse is usually short (median 2 to 3 months), and the long-term survival rate with chemotherapy alone is less than 5%. Thus, the only chance of cure for adult patients with relapsed or resistant ALL is SCT. The major aim of relapse treatment is the induction of a second remission with sufficient duration in order to prepare for SCT. In patients with slow-growth dynamics of relapse, it may be preferable to perform SCT in beginning relapse with bone marrow infiltration of less than 30%[239] as any additional chemotherapy adds toxicity and may increase treatment-related mortality after SCT.

ESTIMATION OF PROGNOSTIC FACTORS

Introduction

A number of clinical and laboratory characteristics influence the response to treatment and the survival of patients with ALL. Prognostic factors are important in selecting therapy and in evaluating responses to treatments administered in clinical trials. Prognostic factors also provide a framework for explaining the probable outcome to the patients and family. The importance of these factors varies with the type and the efficacy of treatment. Before the advent of chemotherapy, all acute leukemias were lethal to a similar degree.[240] With the introduction of effective chemotherapeutics, differences in response related to leukemic cell and patient characteristics have become important.[145, 164, 169, 241-244] At present, the most important prognostic features are age, initial white blood cell count, time to achieve CR, abnormal cytogenetics or molecular genetics, immunologic subtype and, to an increasing extent, the degree of MRD.

Advanced Age: Prognostic Disadvantage and Management Problems

Treatment results in elderly patients with ALL (Table 27-21) are worse with regard to a lower CR rate, shorter remission duration, and survival. Several reasons may account for this. There is increased hematologic and nonhematologic toxicity, e.g., hepato- and cardiotoxicity, resulting in higher morbidity and mortality rates during induction therapy. Incomplete drug administration and extended intervals between cycles of therapy may lead to inferior long-term results. For example, in an early German multicenter trial, the median remission duration for patients receiving only two-thirds of the proposed treatment was 8.7 months, compared with 14.8 months for patients who received the full treatment.[41] There is a higher frequency of adverse biologic features in adults such as Ph+ ALL patients, which increase from 3% in children to 40% in patients older than 50 years.[245] Most elderly patients suffer from B-precursor ALL (40% to 59%), immature null-ALL (14% to 40%), or mature B-ALL (4% to 20%), whereas the incidence of T-ALL as a more favorable subtype is low (0% to 14%).[246-249] Biologic features, such as drug pharmacokinetics and drug resistance, depend on age. Adult ALL shows a lower accumulation of methotrexate-polyglutamates—which confer the cytostatic activity—compared with ALL in children.[250] A higher re-

TABLE 27–21. Intensive Chemotherapy and Outcome in Elderly ALL Patients

Author	Year	N Patients	Age (median)	CR Rate (%)	Median Remission Duration	Probability of CCR
Gaynor et al[164]	1988	32	>50	63	8	Nr
Delannoy et al[248]	1990	18	60–81 (70)	42	10	Nr
Ellison et al[163]	1991	10	60–79	33	14	8%
Taylor et al[247]	1992	22	60–80 (74)	37	4	Nr
Kantarjian et al[253]	1994	52	>60	58	12	22%
Späth-Schwalbe et al[249]	1994	29	60–77	43	5	3%
Todeschini et al[255]	1996	26	>60 (67)	54	14	8%
Bassan et al[256]	1996	22	60–73 (64)	59	12	12%
Delannoy et al[252]	1997	40	55–86 (67)	85	14	<10%
Legrand et al[254]	1997	46	60–87 (67)	43	11	15%
Tabata et al[257]	1998	13	>60	62	3	Nr
Nagura et al[258]	1998	20	60–88 (68)	55	7	11%
		370		50%*		13%*

*Weighted mean.

sistance to prednisolone, DX, L-asparaginase, IDA, and 6-MP was found in children older than 10 years compared with younger children.[251]

There is a continuous decline in the CR rate from 95% in children to 40% to 60% in patients older than 50 to 60 years of age. Most trials demonstrate that increasing age is also associated with shorter remission duration and survival.[164, 165] In patients older than 60 years, the remission rate is 35% to 55% (see Table 27–21) with only a few exceptions.[252] This is mainly due to a high mortality rate during remission induction of 20% to 30%[246] but also due to a higher rate of treatment failures[253] compared with younger patients.

Given poor overall results in elderly ALL patients, several studies have addressed the question whether palliative treatment, consisting mostly of VCR and prednisolone, may be preferable in elderly ALL in order to maintain quality of life. The results of these studies are inconclusive. Remission rates were clearly superior in patients treated with a curative approach and ranged between 36% to 77% compared with 16% to 53% in patients with only palliative treatment.[246, 247, 254] The median remission duration was superior (10 months) in the palliative treatment group compared with intensive treatment (4 months) in one study,[246] whereas other studies reported long-term remissions only in the curative treatment group.[247, 254] However, hospitalization time, which is an important factor for quality of life, was clearly longer in the intensive treatment group.[246]

Therefore, in elderly ALL patients, intensification of induction and consolidation therapy must be carefully weighed against the possible disadvantages of toxicity and mortality. Only limited data are available on prognostic factors in elderly ALL patients. Clearly, the "biologic"

age and the general condition of the patient should be taken into account for treatment decisions. Poor performance status and age greater than 70 years are associated with inferior remission rates. On the other hand, achievement of CR is the prerequisite for prolonged survival. Survival time is less than 1 month for patients without chemotherapy.[247] With the improving options for supportive care, it appears to be justified to administer a dose-reduced induction therapy followed by a moderate intensive consolidation therapy, e.g., including cycles with intermediate-dose methotrexate. Immunotherapy with antibodies such as anti-CD20 is a treatment option with low toxicity. STI571, a tyrosine kinase inhibitor under investigation, might be a new treatment option for the large proportion of elderly patients with Ph/BCR-ABL–positive ALL. Patients older than 50 to 55 years who have achieved a CR and good clinical condition are potential candidates for autologous SCT or for allogeneic nonmyeloablative transplants.

The development of treatment approaches for elderly ALL patients is an important challenge, given the demographic development in most Western countries and the increasing incidence of ALL in elderly population groups.

Immunophenotype

Immunologic Subtypes and Their Frequency

Table 27-22 shows the main characteristics and frequency of clinically relevant immunologic subtypes for childhood and adult ALL. The European Group for Immunological Classification of Acute Leukemias has proposed a uniform immunologic classification for ALL and for

TABLE 27–22. Immunologic Classification of Childhood and Adult ALL

	Surface Marker	Children (%)	Adults (%)
		N = 1756[263]	N = 946[263]
B-lineage	HLA-DR$^+$, TdT$^+$, CD19$^+$	**88**	**76**
• Early pre B-ALL	–	5	11
• Common-ALL	**CD10$^+$**	65	51
• Pre-B-ALL	CD10$^\pm$, **cyIgM$^+$**	15	10
• B-ALL	TdT$^\pm$, CD10$^\pm$, **sIgM$^+$**	3	4
T-lineage	TdT$^+$, cyCD3$^+$, CD7$^+$	**12**	**24**
• Pre/pro-T-ALL	CD2$^-$, sCD3$^-$, CD1a$^-$	1	7
• T-ALL	CD2$^+$, CD5$^\pm$, CD8$^\pm$, CD4$^\pm$	11	17

bilineage acute leukemia, which is roughly identical to this classification.[259] B-lineage ALL constitutes about 75% of ALL in adults, compared with 88% in children, whereas the most immature subtype, early pre-B-ALL, is more frequent in adults (11%) than in children (5%). Common ALL is the most frequent subtype in both childhood and adult ALL. The proportion of T-lineage ALL is substantially higher in adults (24%) compared with children (12%) whereby, as in B-lineage ALL, the earlier form, pre-T-ALL, is more frequent in adults (7% versus 1%). Because the various subtypes have different outcomes, their different incidence rates in childhood and adult ALL may to some extent account for the worse outcome in adults.

There have been several reports on the role of immunophenotype as an independent prognostic variable[242, 244, 260-262] However, with change in treatment strategies and improved results, e.g., for T-ALL and mature B-cell ALL, which formerly had a poor outcome, and the more elaborate marker panels, the prognostic impact of the immune phenotype has altered. Furthermore, other variables, such as the demonstration of the Philadelphia

chromosome or the corresponding *BCR-ABL* gene rearrangement, particularly in common ALL and pre-B ALL, have added information to the prognostic significance of the immunophenotype itself.

T-Lineage ALL

This subtype, usually associated with predominance of male gender (73%), younger age (75% younger than 35 years), high WBC count (more than 30,000 in 62%), initial CNS involvement (15%), and mediastinal tumor (60%),[264] formerly had a poor outcome in children as well as in adults. In early studies, the MRD was 10 months or less.[241, 265-267]

In more recent trials, results for T-ALL have improved to CR rates of greater than 80% up to 95% and LFS of 46% (Table 27–23). In a large series covering several studies of the Cancer and Leukemia Group B, the LFS in T-ALL after 3 years (62%) was clearly superior to B-lineage ALL (42%).[262]

Sufficient in vivo and in vitro evidence has accumulated that mainly CP and AC are responsible for this improvement. The inclusion of AC and CP pulses during continuation therapy was beneficial in childhood T-ALL.[77] Also, in adult ALL the combination of AC and CP, when added to the conventional drugs, improved CR rate and LFS in T-ALL.[151, 166] An increased CR rate and LFS for T-ALL was also observed in a Cancer and Leukemia Group B study by adding CP to the conventional induction with VCR, prednisolone, D, and L-asparaginase.[268] Bassan et al[152] reported a lower rate of induction failure in T-ALL patients after introduction of a prephase treatment with CP.

In childhood ALL, HdM,[269, 270] HdAC,[271] and L-asparaginase[116] contributed to a better outcome of T-ALL. For adult T-ALL, the possible benefit of these approaches remains open. In adult T-ALL, very favorable results have also been reported for allogeneic SCT.[209, 272]

Within T-ALL, an increased WBC count confers poorer prognosis but probably with a higher cut-point (greater than 100,000/µL) than in B-precursor ALL (greater than

TABLE 27–23. Treatment Results in Adult T-ALL

Author	Year	Frequency (%)	N Patients	Induction V,P +	Continuation Other +	Complete Remission (%)	Continuous Complete Remission (%)
Baccarani et al[265]	1983	19	25	D,AC,A,C,M	AC	88	26
Clarkson et al[276]	1985	20	20	AD,C,M	AC,A,D,AD	85	60
Hussein et al[167]	1989	14	10	D,A,C,M	AC,A,C	90	nr
Garand et al[277]	1990	21	76	C,AD	AD,AC,A,C	79	44
Kantarjian et al[200]	1990	19	18	AD,C	A,HdAC,HdM,VP	89	nr
Linker et al[182]	1991	21	19	A,D	A,D,VM,AC,HdM	95	59
Cuttner et al[204]	1991	17	18	D,C,Mi,HdM	D,C,A,HdM,AC	61	nr
Cassileth et al[154]	1992	11	8	D	HdAC,C,AD,A	88	nr
Hoelzer et al[170]	1993	26	302	D,A,AC,C,MP	AC,C	84	45
Fiere et al[191]	1993	28	150	C,D/Z	AC,C ± BMT	79	47
Larson et al[196]	1995	28	39	D,A,C	AC,C	97	63
Attal et al[209]	1995	26	33	D,A,AC,C,MP	HdM, BMT	97	68
Dekker et al[202]	1997	23	24	D,A	HdAC	83	30
Linker et al[185]	1997	23	14	D,A	HdAC,HdM,VP	86	30
Bassan et al[198]	1999	28	27	IDA,A	IDA,AC,C,A ± BMT	89	25

30,000/μL). Older age and late achievement of CR also exert a negative prognostic impact. The immature subtype pre- or pro-T-ALL (cyCD3 + CD2 neg) identifies a poor prognostic subgroup as well. It is associated with a lower incidence of lymphomatous features compared with mature T-ALL and thymic ALL, and the outcome is probably inferior.[273, 274] In the German Multicenter Trials, the CR rates (90% versus 71%) and the LFS (55% versus 15%) were inferior for pre/pro T-ALL compared with thymic or mature T-ALL.[275] This might be in part due to a higher expression of MDR and a higher median age (36% older than 50 years) of pre/pro-T-ALL patients.

In addition to the often increased WBC count, the higher CNS relapse rate and the presence of mediastinal tumor presents a specific treatment problem in T-ALL. Intensive CNS prophylaxis is mandatory. In two earlier trials, mediastinal irradiation was successfully administered after initial cell reduction by chemotherapy.[151] With more intensive therapy, the additional mediastinal irradiation increases toxicity, particularly neutropenia. Therefore, mediastinal irradiation should be restricted to patients with residual tumors after induction therapy. It should be administered together with CNS irradiation and directed to the remaining tumor mass and not to the whole initially involved field in order to avoid excessive hematologic toxicity.

B-Lineage ALL

B-lineage ALL comprises, according to the stage of differentiation, the subtypes early pre-B-ALL, common ALL, and pre-B-ALL.

Prognostic factors can be applied to subdivide B-precursor ALL patients into high- and low-risk subgroups. Well known adverse prognostic factors confirmed in large patient numbers are high WBC count (more than 30,000/μL), cytogenetic aberrations [t(9;22)], late achievement of CR (later than 4 weeks), and older age (range 35 to 50 years of age).[169] Overall B-precursor ALL shows an inferior outcome compared with T-lineage ALL, with a weighted mean for CR rate of 77% (71% to 91%) and CCR rates of 32% (22% to 41%).[169, 182, 193, 196, 202, 209, 278]

Common ALL (c-ALL) or CD10-positive ALL is the most frequent subtype in adults as well as in children. The outcome has not changed in recent years, and the survival rate remains 25% to 35%, in a few studies approaching 40%.[196, 279] This may be partly explained by the higher median age of c-ALL patients and by the fact that about 45% to 50% of adult patients with c-ALL are Ph/BCR-ABL–positive with extremely poor prognosis. However, also for the adult c-ALL patients who are Ph/BCR-ABL–negative, results have not greatly improved. In particular, these patients relapse in most studies over a time of up to 5 to 6 years. Thus, prolonged maintenance therapy seems to be required. Intensification with HdM or HdAC has so far not shown a substantial benefit. Higher doses of anthracyclines given in induction and reaching a certain cumulative amount may be associated with improved results.[192] In this subtype, the evaluation of MRD seems to be of particular interest, and in future trials treatment decisions may be based on MRD results.

Pre-B-ALL also includes Ph/BCR-ABL–positive cases; the outcome is similar to that for c-ALL but has not been analyzed separately in most adult ALL series.

Early pre-B-ALL, also referred to as pro-B-ALL, CALLA-negative, or pre-pre-B-ALL (CD10−, CD19+, cyIgM−, sIgM−, CD24+/−), which accounts for 11% of adult ALL, is associated with a poor outcome in children, particularly in infants, and also in adults. Early pre-B-ALL is often associated with high WBC count, coexpression of myeloid antigens (CD15/CDw65), and the translocation t(4;11) in 50% of patients.[179] Chemotherapy including HdAC and even more allogeneic SCT appear to be effective treatment strategies, with survival rates of 40% to 50%.[179] The value of HdAC in early pre-B-ALL is also confirmed by the higher sensitivity of early pre-B-ALL blast cells compared with other ALL subgroups as was demonstrated in in vitro drug resistance tests.[251]

Mature B-ALL is associated with an L3 morphology; male predominance; often lymphadenopathy; abdominal tumor masses; and renal, bone, and CNS involvement similar to the presentation of Burkitt's lymphoma.

In earlier trials, remission rates for adult B-ALL were low and remission duration and survival poor. In 9 studies (Table 27-24) with a total of 60 patients, the weighted mean CR rate was 35%, and most patients relapsed rapidly, reflected by the median remission duration of 11 months and the very low survival rate. These data are certainly incomplete as the outcome of B-ALL patients was not separately stated in most trials.

There is a dramatic change in the outcome of B-ALL and Burkitt's lymphoma in several childhood and adult studies. In childhood B-ALL, the outcome has significantly improved, with CR rates of 81% to 96% and LFS rates of up to 76%.[79, 280, 281] The drugs responsible for this improvement are fractionated CP or IFO in moderate doses, HdM (0.5 to 8 g/m²), and HdAC. In addition to CP, HdM, or HdAC, the regimens contain the cytostatic drugs AD, AC, VM26, VCR, prednisolone, D, and VP16.

The application of these childhood B-ALL protocols in original or modified amounts also brought a substantial improvement for adult patients with B-ALL. The CR rates now approach 70%, and long-term survival rates of 40% to 50% or even higher can be achieved in adult B-ALL (see Table 27-24). Maintenance treatment has been omitted. Because in childhood as well as in adult B-ALL studies, relapses occur almost exclusively within the first year, patients thereafter can be considered to be cured.

B-ALL has a higher CNS involvement rate at diagnosis, and relapses often occur. Therefore, effective measures against CNS disease, such as HdM and HdAC as well as IT therapy, are an important component of treatment regimens. Prophylactic CNS irradiation has been omitted in most of the studies.

Only few data are available on prognostic factors in B-ALL. Older age, large tumor mass as indicated by multiple organ involvement, high WBC count, increased LDH level, and clearly slow or inadequate response to therapy may be associated with inferior outcome.

Myeloid Antigen–Positive ALL

With the current more detailed immunologic analysis, increasing numbers of patients with myeloid antigen–

TABLE 27–24. Treatment Results in Adult Mature B-ALL

Author	Year	N Patients	Induction	Continuation	Complete Remission (%)	Continuous Complete Remission (%)
Conventional ALL Therapy		60	Results from 9 studies		35	0
Short Intensive Therapy						
Schaison et al[282]	1989	6	V,P,C,AD HdM 8 g/m² HdC 0.5-1 g/m²	V,P,VP,AC,AD HdM 8 g/m² HdAC 3 g/m²	83	20
Fenaux et al[78]	1989	16	V,P,D,C,VP,AD HdM 8 g/m² HdC 1 g/m²	V,P,D,C,AC,VP HdM 0.5-8 g/m² HdAC 3 g/m²	63	57
Patte et al[79]	1991	19	V,P,D,C,VP,AD HdM 0.5 g/m² HdC 0.5-1 g/m²	V,P,D,C,AC,VP HdM 8 g/m² HdAC 3 g/m²	76	58
Pees et al[283]	1992	8	C,P,VM,AC,M HdM 0.5 g/m²	AD,M,C HdM 0.5 g/m²	62	62
Hoelzer et al[80]	1996	24	C,P,VM,AC,D HdM 0.5 g/m²	C,P,VM,AC,AD HdM 0.5 g/m²	75	45
Hoelzer et al[80]	1996	35	C,P,VM,AC,V,DX HdM 1.5 g/m² HdIFO 0.8 g/m²	AD,V,C,DX HdM 1.5 g/m² HdIFO 0.8 g/m²	77	71
Lee et al[284]	1997	14	C,P,VM,AC,V,DX HdM 1.5 g/m² HdIFO 0.8 g/m²	AD,V,C,DX HdM 1.5 g/m² HdIFO 0.8 g/m²	71	7/10
Thomas et al[285]	1999	26	V,AD,DX HdM 1 g/m² HdC 0.3 g/m² HdAC 3 g/m²	V,AD,DX HdM 1 g/m² HdC 0.3 g/m² HdAC 3 g/m²	81	61
		148			75%*	59%*

*Weighted mean.

positive (My+) ALL can be detected. This has also been described as hybrid acute leukemia, biphenotypic leukemia, and acute mixed-lineage leukemia. Common to these leukemias is that in addition to the markers specific for ALL, the myeloid markers CD13, CD14, CD15, CD33, and CDw65 may be expressed. These leukemias were previously included in the subtype null-ALL.

Whether myeloid antigen expression in ALL has an adverse impact on outcome is not established. In childhood ALL, myeloid coexpression has apparently no prognostic relevance.[286] Some adult studies indicated an inferior outcome for (My+) ALL patients for CR and LFS, but recent studies do not.

Cytogenetic Aberrations

Chromosomal abnormalities are detected in more than 60% of adult ALL patients, and several aberrations are correlated with outcome, independent of other features. Due to the low incidence rate of many translocations, their prognostic value remains open (Table 27–25). Furthermore, distinct translocations are correlated with specific subtypes such as t(10;14) in T-ALL, and their prognostic value may not be independent but related to the better outcome of T-ALL.

The incidence and prognostic value of cytogenetic aberrations in adult ALL are summarized in Table 27–25 based on the reports of three large study groups with a total of 1049 patients.[287-289] All trials confirmed the poor prognosis of t(9;22) and t(4;11), whereas 7−, 9+, and hypodiploid karyotype was not identified uniformly as a poor prognostic factor. Further clonal aberrations could be grouped to intermediate- and favorable-risk groups. Patients with normal karyotype had an intermediate prog-

TABLE 27–25. Incidence and Prognostic Value of Cytogenetic Aberrations in Adult ALL

Aberration	Incidence	LFS	References
Favorable Prognosis			
12p aberrations	5% (4%-5%)	20%-76%	287 288
high hyperdiploid	8% (5%-9%)	56%-59%	287 288
t(10;14)	2% (2%-3%)	75%-100%	287 289
Intermediate Prognosis			
9p aberrations	11% (5%-15%)	22%-44%	287 288
6q aberrations	5% (4%-6%)	27%-47%	287 288
+ 21	14%	29%	288
Normal diploid	25% (15%-38%)	34%-44%	287 288
Poor Prognosis			
t(9;22)	20% (11%-29%)	5%-13%	287 288 289
t(4;11)	4% (3%-7%)	0%-24%	287 288 289
−7	6%	25%	288
+8	10%	15%	288
Hypodiploid	7% (3%-10%)	11%	287 289

nosis in all three trials, whereas 12p aberrations, t(10; 14), and high hyperdiploid karyotype—without additional aberrations—were defined as favorable prognostic subgroups.

The Cancer and Leukemia Group B suggested a stratification into three prognostic subgroups: poor—including t(9;22), t(4;11), −7, and +8; normal—diploid; and miscellaneous—all other structural aberrations. The LFS rates were 11%, 38%, and 52%, respectively. Although there was an improvement of CR rates in all subgroups in the more recent trials, no change was observed in terms of LFS for patients with unfavorable karyotype and normal karyotype, whereas LFS for the miscellaneous group improved from 30% to 57%.[287] This type of risk stratification according to cytogenetic subgroups requires further refinement, particularly with regard to the intermediate and favorable subgroup as treatment results still show a large variability depending on treatment regimen.

Philadelphia Chromosome/*BCR-ABL*–Positive ALL

Philadelphia (Ph) chromosome/*BCR-ABL*-positive ALL is the subgroup of ALL having the worst prognosis in children as well as in adults. It is detected by conventional cytogenetics but with higher sensitivity by molecular detection of the *BCR-ABL* rearrangement.[293-295] The overall incidence rate of Ph/*BCR-ABL*-positive ALL in adult ALL series is 20% to 30%. Because Ph/*BCR-ABL*-positive ALL is restricted to B-precursor ALL (c-ALL, pre-B-ALL), the incidence rate is even higher within this subgroup,[295] and it increases with age.

In 10 studies with conventional chemotherapy including a total of 306 patients, the CR rate was 68% (44% to 86%) with a median remission duration of 8 months and a survival of 0% to 15% at 2 to 3 years (Table 27-26). In 10 studies including high-dose chemotherapy cycles with HdM or HdAC, the CR rate in 402 patients was 71% (59% to 100%), the median remission duration 11 months, and the survival 0% to 30% at 2 to 3 years (see Table 27-26). The CR rate appears to be increasing in recent trials. The overall outcome in terms of median remission duration may show a slight improvement. This may be due to the more frequent incorporation of SCT in all ongoing studies for this subgroup, whereas a clear benefit of consolidation therapy with either HdM or HdAC could not be demonstrated.

The approach to using biologic response modifiers, such as interferon or interleukin-2, was initially encouraging[297, 307] but has not fulfilled its promise.

SCT in Ph/*BCR-ABL*–Positive ALL

The only chance of cure in Ph/*BCR-ABL*-positive ALL is SCT, although the results are inferior compared with Ph/*BCR-ABL*-negative patients due to a higher relapse rate and to the higher treatment-related mortality rate in this older patient cohort. According to a European Bone Marrow Transplant Group analysis, the LFS was 24% versus 61% and 20% versus 56% for allogeneic and autologous SCT, respectively, in Ph/*BCR-ABL*-positive versus –negative ALL.[308]

Allogeneic SCT from sibling donors in first CR yielded in 7 studies a median LFS rate of 49% (0% to 65%) in 92 patients.[302, 309-314] In the largest series with 33,17, and 24

TABLE 27–26. Chemotherapy Results in Ph/*BCR-ABL*–Positive ALL

Author	Year	N Patients	CR Rate (%)	Median Remission Duration	Survival
Conventional Chemotherapy					
Gaynor et al[164]	1988	18	72	7	0% at 3 y
Bloomfield et al[296]	1990	18	44	10	<10%
Secker-Walker et al[245]	1991	23	64	7	15% at 2 y
Ohyashiki et al[297]	1991	7	71	9	nr
Götz et al[298]	1992	25	76	9	6% at 3 y
Westbrook et al[299]	1992	17	71	10	nr
Hoelzer et al[189]	1993	103	75	9	10%
Fière et al 1993[300]	1993	58	57	5	0% at 4 y
Scherrer et al[193]	1994	7	86	18	0% at 5 y
Larson et al[196]	1995	30	70	9	0% at 3 y
Chemotherapy Including HdM and/or HdAC					
Cuttner et al[204]	1991	12	75	10	nr
Linker et al[182]	1991	10	70	11	nr
Kantarjian et al[301]	1991	27	56	5	nr
Cassileth et al[154]	1992	12	58	5	nr
Mandelli et al[302]	1993	29	76	11	16% at 3 y
Stryckmans et al[303]	1994	19	68		16% at 2 Y
Charrin et al[289]	1996	127	59	5	0% at 3 y
Stryckmans et al[304]	1997	125	78		30% at 2 y
Annino et al[305]	1998	12	100	44	nr
Faderl et al[306]	1998	29	90	11	nr

patients, respectively, the reported LFS rates were 38%, 46%, and 65%.[309, 312, 314]

For autologous SCT, the results are inferior, with a median LFS of 33% (0% to 100%) in 52 patients from 9 studies with mostly less than 5 patients.[302, 310, 311, 313, 315-319] In the largest series with 23 patients, the LFS was 25% at more than 2 years, giving a realistic picture of what can be achieved with autologous SCT in Ph/*BCR-ABL*–positive ALL.[318] In the latter series, it could be demonstrated that purging with immunomagnetic beads and antibodies reduced the tumor load in stem cell grafts by 2 to 3 logarithmic steps Furthermore, it was shown that the content of *BCR-ABL*–positive cell is significantly lower in peripheral stem cell compared with bone marrow grafts.[320]

For matched unrelated SCT, the results are still somewhat inferior mainly due to the higher transplant-related mortality rate compared with that for allogeneic SCT from sibling donors. In 99 patients with Ph/*BCR-ABL*–positive ALL (including children) transplanted in first or subsequent CR, the mean LFS was 37%.[319, 321-324] In one series, the LFS was 42% in 19 adult patients with a median age of 35 years (transplanted in first CR), which is a promising result.[324]

Other Molecular Aberrations

The molecular detection of *BCR-ABL* and *ALL1-AF4* fusion genes related to the translocations t(9;22) and t(4;11), respectively, is part of standard diagnosis in adult ALL. The prognostic value of other molecular aberrations is less clear and has so far been evaluated in small-patient cohorts. This applies for homozygous deletions of the p16 tumor suppressor gene, which is detected in 20% to 40% of adult and childhood ALL. [325-327] Mutations of the tumor suppressor gene p53, which have an incidence rate less than 10% in ALL, may have prognostic impact in T-ALL.[328]

Time to Response

The kinetics of blast cell reduction is measured mainly by the time required to achieve a CR. Adults with ALL not remitting within 4 or 5 weeks fare poorly. In the first German multicenter trials for adult ALL, the median remission duration was 31 months in the 220 patients achieving CR within 4 weeks, compared with only 10 months in 52 patients requiring more than 4 weeks.[169] There was a clear difference in long-term disease-free survival at 7 years with CCR rates of 42% and 23%. Similar observations have been reported by others. The worse LFS for patients with slowly induced CR may be explained by a more resistant blast cell population.

As early blast clearance is an important predictor for survival, response to chemotherapy is now evaluated earlier, e.g., 2 weeks after start of chemotherapy or in children, after 7 days of prephase therapy with prednisolone.

Minimal Residual Disease

Molecular methods have been developed that allow the quantitative measurement of residual blast cells in individual patients with high sensitivity (10^{-4} to 10^{-6}) far below the detection level of conventional morphologic analyses, with a sensitivity of 1% to 5%.

Detection of MRD is based mainly on three methods: (1) analysis of leukemia-specific phenotypes (LAIP) with multiparameter flow cytometry,[329] which is applicable in approximately 80% of ALL patients; (2) quantitative measurement of gene products from clonal gene translocations such as *BCR-ABL, E2A-PBX1, MLL-AF4,* or *TEL-AML-1,* with polymerase chain reaction; in approximately 40% to 50% of adult ALL patients, such rearrangements may be identified; and (3) quantitative measurement of individual rearrangements of the T-cell receptor (TCR-β, -δ,-λ,-γ) or immunoglobulin–heavy chain genes; one or two clonal TCR or IgH rearrangements can be identified in approximately 90% of ALL patients.[330-333] More recently, "real-time" PCR has been used for less cost-intensive and more rapid MRD detection.

For all methods of MRD detection, it is necessary to identify a patient-specific individual target—either an LAIP or a clonal rearrangement—at the time-point of diagnosis, which may be a logistical problem in some studies. From a theoretical point of view, MRD assessment is possible with either method in more than 90% of ALL patients.

MRD assessment in ALL may serve for several clinical purposes such as redefinition of CR, identification of new prognostic factors, individual treatment decisions, and evaluation of efficacy of distinct treatment elements such as consolidation cycles.

Redefinition of CR

MRD evaluation early, during, and after induction therapy shows that nearly 50% of ALL patients remain MRD-positive despite CR as defined by conventional microscopic analysis (Table 28-27). In Ph/*BCR-ABL*–positive ALL, even the majority of patients show the *BCR-ABL* transcript despite clinical remission.

Definition of New Prognostic Factors

MRD evaluation provides important new information on prognosis of individual ALL patients,[344, 347] but the following features have to be taken into account for proper risk assessment: MRD status and quantitative level of MRD after induction therapy and longitudinal course of MRD during postremission treatment.

MRD Status and Quantitative MRD Level After Induction Therapy

Overall, 47% of both childhood and adult ALL patients are MRD-positive after induction therapy, and nearly 50%

TABLE 27–27. Incidence of MRD-Positive Results at the End of Induction Therapy and Impact on Relapse Rate

Author	Year	Patients	Total	MRD + (N)	Relapse	MRD − (N)	Relapse
Wassermann et al[334]	1992	c	44	33	15 (45%)	11	3 (27%)
Nizet et al[335]	1993	c + a	25	24	8 (33%)	1	0
Knauf et al[336]	1993	a	35	5	4 (80%)	30	6 (20%)
Cavé et al[337]	1994	c	17	5	1 (20%)	12	3 (25%)
Brisco et al[338]	1994	c	88	38	26 (68%)	50	6 (12%)
Coyle et al[339]	1994	c + a	28	19	5 (26%)	9	4 (44%)
Seriu et al[340]	1995	c	30	11	1 (9%)	19	2 (11%)
Steenbergen et al[341]	1996	c	34	12	10 (83%)	22	6 (27%)
Brisco et al[342]	1996	a	22	15	11 (73%)	7	3 (43%)
Seriu et al[343]	1997	c	89	20	11 (55%)	69	3 (4%)
Cavé et al[344]	1998	c	151	63	25 (40%)	88	7 (8%)
Gruhn et al[345]	1998	c	26	7	4 (57%)	19	0
Goulden et al[346]	1998	c	59	33	23 (70%)	26	5 (19%)
van Dongen et al[347]	1998	c	169	98	40 (41%)	71	2 (3%)
			817	383 (47%*)	48%*	434	11%*

*Weighted mean.
c = children; a = adults.

of them relapse (see Table 27–27). Only few results are available in adults, but there is evidence that the relapse rate in MRD-positive patients is higher.[338, 342, 348] Further refined information arises from the quantitative evaluation of the MRD level after induction therapy.

A high MRD level at the end of induction treatment is associated with a higher relapse rate; in these patients, despite morphologic CR, a stable remission is not achieved. The relapse rate ranges from 55% to 93% in patients with an MRD level above 10^{-3}.[334, 338, 342, 344, 347, 349]

Negative MRD results depend on the sensitivity of the applied method. If no MRD is detected with a sensitive method (greater than 10^{-4}), the relapse risk appears to be low because only a few patients return to MRD-positive results during continuation therapy. There is, however, still a relapse rate of approximately 11% that may be due to (1) the detection limit, (2) false-negative results due to clonal evolution, or (3) extramedullary relapse. The relapse rate for patients with low MRD (lower than 10^{-3} to 10^{-5}) is very similar to that in patients with negative MRD status and ranged between 0% and 9% in recent studies.[344, 345, 347, 349]

For patients with intermediate MRD levels, the results are less clear; further MRD monitoring and evaluation of the further course of MRD are particularly important.

Course of MRD During Postremission Treatment

Persistent or increasing MRD is strongly correlated with relapse,[344, 347, 348, 350, 351] whereas a reduction of MRD below detection limit is a good indicator for CCR at all time-points during treatment.[344, 347] The MRD status at 12 months appeared to be highly discriminative, with a relapse rate of 9% in MRD-negative compared with 86% in MRD-positive childhood ALL patients.[347] In a report on 57 adult ALL cases in patients remaining in CCR, the incidence rate of MRD-positive results decreased rapidly (40%, 38%, 17%, and 0% at 3-month intervals from diagnosis). The prognostic significance of positive MRD results increased stepwise, being highest at 12 to 24 months

after diagnosis. Negative tests were more predictive for CCR than positive tests for relapse during the first 6 months.[352]

The MRD level after induction therapy and the longitudinal course of MRD are strongly correlated with outcome in childhood ALL. For adult ALL, results of prospective MRD evaluation are still scarce. It is not clear which time-point for MRD evaluation is most predictive, which cut-point in terms of MRD level should be selected for risk stratification, and whether subgroup-specific differences in the course of MRD have to be taken into account.

Individual Treatment Decisions

Therefore, further prospective studies are required in adult ALL in order to define criteria for individual treatment decisions based on MRD results. In patients who have repeatedly negative MRD results and a high probability of cure treatment could be stopped, for example, after 1 year in order to avoid undue toxicity and discomfort. In patients with persisting MRD despite intensive induction and consolidation therapy, further treatment approaches, e.g., SCT or experimental treatment, could be considered.

Evaluation of Single-Treatment Elements

MRD evaluation with highly sensitive methods already allows the evaluation of efficacy of single-treatment elements. Purging efficacy in *BCR-ABL*–positive ALL has been evaluated by quantitative PCR measurement of *BCR-ABL* transcripts.[320] The value of consolidation cycles, immunotherapy, and donor lymphocytes (DLI) are interesting options for MRD evaluation as well.

Definition of Risk Groups in Adult ALL

In the majority of large trials, there is agreement on the following risk factors for adult ALL: age, time to achieve

TABLE 27–28. Major Adverse Prognostic Factors in Adult ALL

Slow/incomplete response to remission induction	• Achievement of CR >3 or 4 wk • High level of MRD after induction therapy
Immunologic subtype	• Pro-B-ALL • Early T-ALL
Karyotype/molecular genetics	• t(9;22)/*BCR-ABL* • t(4;11)/*ALL1-AF4*
Older age	• >35, 50, 60 yr
High WBC count	• >20,000/μL, >30,000/μL in B-precursor ALL • >100,000/μL in T-ALL
Minimal residual disease	• persistent/increasing MRD during treatment

CR, initial WBC count, and cytogenetic and molecular aberrations (Ph/*BCR-ABL*, t(4;11)/ALL1-AF4). Other prognostic factors, such as serum LDH level, the degree of bone marrow involvement, the percentage of circulating blast cells, hepatomegaly, splenomegaly, bulky disease, and CNS involvement, have been described only in single studies. Immunologic subtypes such as pro-B-ALL and early T-ALL and the status and course of MRD have emerged as prognostic features. The adverse prognostic factors currently used in the ongoing study of the German Multicenter Study Group for Adult ALL are summarized in Table 27-28.

Prognostic factors are treatment-dependent and should therefore not be transferred from one study to another. However, within a particular study, these prognostic factors can be used to stratify adult ALL patients—as in childhood ALL—into low- and high-risk patients. This risk group classification has two major aims: (1) to allocate patients to risk group–specific treatment schedules, e.g., short intensive treatment protocols for mature B-ALL, and development of new subgroup-adjusted treatment regimens and (2) to provide for rational decisions on treatment intensity—particularly, indications for SCT—based on risk stratification.

Stem Cell Transplantation

BMT is an integral part of the treatment strategy for adult ALL. Before possible indications are discussed, the results of allogeneic sibling (allo), autologous (auto), and matched unrelated (MUD) transplantation are reviewed. As in these studies either bone marrow or peripheral blood stem cells are used, all data will be referred to as SCT.

Allogeneic SCT from Matched Sibling Donors

The largest experience in adult ALL exists for allogeneic, matched sibling transplantation. The LFS rates for adult ALL patients transplanted in first remission are 50% (21% to 71%) at 3 to 7 years (Table 27-29). The data are available from prospective studies with allo transplantation arms (for patients with available donor), compared with either chemotherapy and/or autologous SCT. Fur-

thermore there are retrospective analyses from study groups and bone marrow transplantation registries.

The survival for similarly defined cohorts of first CR patients, adjusted for differences in the disease characteristics and the time to transplant, receiving either SCT (collected by the International Bone Marrow Transplantation Registry [IBMTR]) or chemotherapy (German multicenter trials) has been compared retrospectively.[353] The 5-year LFS for chemotherapy (38%) and that for SCT in first CR (44%) was similar. A similar comparison of chemotherapy results from the Japan Adult Leukemia Study Group with IBMTR data revealed a superior LFS with SCT (53%) for patients younger than 30 years compared with chemotherapy (30%) but not in patients older than 30 years (30% and 26%, respectively). This was mainly due to the high transplant-related mortality (57%) in patients older than 30 years.[354] In the majority of larger ALL trials (see Tables 27-13 to 27-16), the median age is clearly above 30 years, whereas the median age of transplanted patients is generally below 30 years, which shows a clear selection by age and probably other conditions.

Several study groups have compared chemotherapy and allo SCT in a kind of "natural" randomization, with allo SCT for patients with matched sibling donor and chemotherapy or autologous SCT in the remaining patients. In the largest randomized trial, allo SCT was scheduled for all patients younger than 40 years with sibling donors,[300] whereas the remaining patients were randomized (control group) to receive either auto SCT or chemotherapy. The survival after allo SCT was significantly superior (46%) compared with that of the control group (31%), which was predominantly due to a higher survival rate in high-risk patients with allo SCT (37%) compared with the control group (15%), whereas in standard-risk ALL (46% versus 42%), no significant difference was observed.[355] The ongoing Eastern Cooperative Oncology Group (ECOG)/Medical Research Council (MRC) trial evaluates allo SCT in all patients with sibling donors versus auto SCT or chemotherapy in a randomized comparison (control group). The LFS after 3 years was 58% for patients who actually received allo SCT compared with 39% for the control group. Allo SCT yielded superior LFS for high-risk (57% versus 32%) and for standard-risk (71% versus 54%) ALL patients younger than 60 years.[272]

Allo SCT in second remission of adult ALL gives survival rates of 34% with a higher relapse rate of 48% (see Table 27-29). These results are superior to those obtained with chemotherapy alone, in which the survival rate at 5 years is only 5% to 10%. Allo transplants in advanced (either refractory or relapsed) ALL result in 18% LFS at 3 years (see Table 27-29). These results are clearly superior to those reported with chemotherapy, in which there are virtually no cures at this stage of the disease.

Allogeneic SCT from MUD

MUD SCT is increasingly employed in adult ALL, although only few data from adult patient cohorts are available. The LFS of 37% in published studies mostly in patients with more advanced disease (in or beyond CR2) is prom-

TABLE 27–29. Results of Allogeneic SCT in Adult ALL

Author	Year	N	Age (median)	Conditioning	LFS	TRM	Relapse Probability
In First Complete Remission							
Barrett et al[361]	1989	243	24 (16–48)	TBI ± C, ± other	39% 5 y	nr	30%
Blume et al[362]	1990	50	25 (16–41)	TBI ± VP	61%	nr	14%
Bacigalupo et al[363]	1991	40	23 (13–43)	TBI + C	52%S 10 y		25%
Doney et al[364]	1991	41	18–50	TBI + C	21% 5 y	nr	50%
Fiere et al[278]	1993	98	15–50	TBI + C	47% 5 y	18%+	34%+
Ringden et al (IBMTR)[365]	1993	106	adults	C ± TBI ± other; GVHD: M	51% 2 y	42%	12%
Ringden et al (IBMTR)[366]	1993	149	adults	C ± TBI ± other; GVHD: CSA	52% 2 y	34%	22%
de Witte et al[367]	1994	22	15–51	TBI + C ± other	63% 5 y	23%+	14%+
Vey et al[368]	1994	29	24 (16–41)	TBI + C or mel	62% 8 y	29%	10%
Attal et al[209]	1995	41	31 (15–50)	TBI + C	71% 3 y	12%	12%
Vey et al[369]	1996	36	28 (18–59)	TBI + C and/or mel	58% 7 y	nr	12%
Jiménez et al[370]	1996	33	>14	TBI + C or Bu	53% 7 y	nr	35%
Snyder et al[314]	1999	23	30 (6–44)	TBI + VP	65% 3 y	30%	12%
Rowe et al[272]	1999	173	29 (16–55)	TBI + VP	58% 3 y	21%+	
Ifrah[203]	1999	16	29 (18–46)	Various	33%	38%+	19%+
		1100			**50%***	**27%***	**24%***
In 2nd or Subsequent Complete Remission							
Doney et al[371]	1991	48	18–50	TBI + C	15% 5y	nr	64%
Copelan et al[372]	1992	12	22 (15–42)	bu + C	13% 1 y	42%+	40%
Soiffer et al[373]	1993	14	31 (19–50)	C + TBI	33% 7 y	nr	62%
Horowitz et al (IBMTR)[374]	1995	818	adults	nr	37% 5 y	nr	46%
Arnold et al[375]	1996	76	25 (15–58)	nr	22% 12 y	nr	nr
Gorin et al (EBMT)[376]	1997	nr	adults	nr	35% 5 y	nr	46%
Martino et al[377]	1997	10	adults	nr	60%+	40%	0
Kantarjian et al[200]	1990	14	adults	nr	28%	15%	75%
Przepiorka et al[378]	1998	9	adults	nr	30%	22%	62%
Jiménez et al[370]	1996	18	>14	C or Bu + TBI	18% 7 y	nr	69%
		1019			**34%***	**29%***	**48%***
Relapsed/Refractory							
Doney[364]	1991	103	23 (18–53)	TBI + C	12% 5 y	nr	76%
Arnold et al[375]	1996	63	25 (15–58)	nr	33% 12 y	nr	nr
Kantarjian et al[200]	1990	13	nr	nr	15%	46%	60%
Przepiorka et al[378]	1998	37	adults	nr	8%	47%	77%
		216			**18%***	**47%***	**75%***

*Weighted mean; + proportion not probability.

ising (Table 27–30). In adult poor-risk ALL, with a median patient age of 34 years, the results of MUD SCT were particularly favorable for patients in CR1 (42%), whereas in more advanced cases an LFS of only 7% was achieved.[324] The low relapse rate (22%) may be due to a

TABLE 27–30. Results of Matched Unrelated SCT in Childhood and Adult ALL

Author	Year	Patients	Age	LFS (%)	Follow-up
Casper[321]	1992	12	4–16 y	68	2–60 mo
Sierra[322]	1997	18	25 y	49	>2 y
Marks[323]	1998	15	nr	37	>2 y
Kröger[319]	1998	6	2–45 y	67	>1 y
Cornelissen*[324]	1998	19 CR1	35 y (18–51)	42	1 y
		29> CR1		7	1 y

*t(9;22), t(4;11), t(1;19); **weighted mean.

more pronounced graft-versus-leukemia (GvL) effect. In reports, that rate is, however, nearly outweighed by the high transplant related mortality rate (48%).[322] Results may improve with better donor selection and improved management of GVHD; MUD SCT is already a choice for high-risk patients in CR1 such as Ph/*BCR-ABL*–positive ALL patients (and probably other high-risk patients) if a sibling donor is not available.

Allogeneic SCT from Mismatched Donors

To extend the possibilities of allo SCT by increasing the bone marrow donor pool, mismatched SCT from related or unrelated donors has been attempted. In one report,[356] 31 patients were treated with mismatched SCT (3 unrelated, 28 related and genotypically identical for one haplotype but mismatched for up to 3 HLA antigens); 17 survived in remission, but the mean follow-up of 16 months is still brief.

Future Prospects for Allogeneic SCT

The outcome after allo SCT is generally better because of the GvL effect. However, many patients relapse. Further treatment in patients with persistent MRD is currently the application of donor lymphocyte infusions. GvL effects are present in ALL as evident from the fact that relapse risk is reduced in ALL patients with GVHD compared with those without GVHD,[357] and this effect is present in T- and B-lineage ALL.[358] According to several case reports of ALL patients with relapse after allo SCT, clinical responses and even remissions have been observed with the infusion of donor lymphocytes and/or the interruption of GVHD prophylaxis.

Nonmyeloablative SCT ("minitransplant") is another approach to utilizing GvL effects and may lead to an extension of the upper age limit for allo SCT. Immunosuppression with fludarabine, ATG, and busulfan is followed by the infusion of donor stem cells from siblings or matched unrelated donors with low-dose CSA to establish host tolerance.[359] In a follow-up report on 57 patients with a median age of 38 years (1 to 63 years), 10 ALL patients were included. The overall day-100 mortality was 7% for malignant diseases, and the overall DFS rate was 48%. Prospective studies are needed to evaluate whether minitransplants offer a new option in the treatment of adult ALL, particularly in patients older than 55 years or in those who are not eligible for regular allo SCT.

Intensification of conditioning regimens by increasing the dose of total-body irradiation leads to lower relapse rates but to more toxicity. Attempts have been made to target radiotherapy specifically to hematopoietic tissue with radiolabeled antibodies. Several antibodies, such as anti-CD164b and anti-CD22 in ALL patients and anti-CD20 in B-cell lymphoma, have been conjugated with radio-emitters such as ^{131}I, ^{99}Tc, and ^{90}Y. Radioimmunotherapy is administered before a conventional conditioning regimen in an allo or autologous setting. In a phase I study with ^{131}I conjugated to the murine anti-CD45 antibody explored in 44 patients with advanced leukemia, a favorable distribution with significantly higher estimated radiation doses to hematopoietic tissues compared with normal organs was achieved in 84% of the patients. Three of 9 patients with relapsed or refractory ALL survived disease-free at 19 to 66 months after SCT.[360]

Ongoing studies show that in the large cohort of Ph/*BCR-ABL*-positive patients, the Abl-tyrosine kinase inhibitor STI571 may be successful. Other modalities such as antibody, e.g., directed to CD19, have not yet been explored.

Autologous SCT

Only one third of potential transplant candidates will have an HLA-identical sibling donor. Therefore, auto SCT or, more recently, PBSC transplantation, is of increasing importance for the treatment of ALL. Auto SCT in first

CR seems promising with LFS rates of 42% (Table 27–31). There is apparently no significant difference in LFS whether PBSC (41%) or bone marrow (35%) is used as stem cell source, as evidenced by a preliminary evaluation of the EBMT data.[376]

Randomized trials comparing auto SCT with chemotherapy show contradictory results. In the French LALA87 study, the LFS after auto SCT (31%) was similar to that with chemotherapy (29%),[355] whereas in an Italian trial there was an advantage for auto SCT with a 5-year LFS of 36% compared with 17% for patients treated with chemotherapy alone.[198] These differences and also the wide range in outcome of auto SCT remain largely unexplained. The reasons might be pretreatment (that is, tumor reduction by previous chemotherapy), different patient cohorts (age, subtypes), and time to transplant as major factors.

Auto SCT in second remission ALL gives LFS rates of 24% (see Table 27–31); these results are more promising than those achieved in second remission ALL treated with chemotherapy.

The treatment-related mortality after auto SCT is low (5%), but relapse rate is high (51% for patients transplanted in CR1). This may be due to a contamination of the stem cell graft by leukemic blast cells and the lacking GvL effect. Several approaches have been made to decrease relapse rate, such as improved or different methods of conditioning, e.g., auto double transplantation[318], purging of PBSC or bone marrow graft, and maintenance therapy after auto SCT.

Purging of bone marrow or peripheral blood is one attempt to reduce tumor load and thereby reduce relapse risk. In ALL, specific markers such as measurement of *BCR-ABL* by PCR assays allow estimation of the reduction of the marrow blasts in the graft.

Two trials indicate a possible benefit of purging. In 15 adult patients with high-risk B-lineage ALL, the median for residual blast cells before purging was 8.1% of B cells compared with 0.4% after purging, which corresponds to a median 1 log reduction. The LFS was significantly higher in the patients with MRD lower than 5% in the pretreatment marrow (87%) compared with those with more than 5% (0%).[379] In a further retrospective analysis of 52 ALL patients receiving auto SCT in CR1 (children and adults), the LFS at 3 years was significantly superior with 52% for purged marrow transplants compared with 13% for unpurged marrow.[380] Studies in which an effective marrow purging by 2 to 3 log[320] was carried out in Ph/*BCR-ABL*-positive ALL showed a distinctive inferior survival of only 21%,[318] which reflects in general the poor outcome of Ph/*BCR-ABL*-positive ALL.

Maintenance therapy after auto SCT has been explored in two studies.[316, 381] Maintenance with MP/methotrexate seemed to yield an improved survival, but this was not reported from other studies.[316]

Indications for SCT in Adult ALL

Although it is agreed that SCT is one of the major approaches of postinduction therapy to improve outcome of adult ALL, it is not clear which is the most effective

TABLE 27–31. Autologous SCT in Adult ALL

Author	Year	N	Age (median)	Conditioning	LFS (%)	TRM (%)	Actuarial Relapse (%)
In First Complete Remission							
Simonsson[382]	1989	21	27 (3–55)*	TBI + C ± other	65% 2 y	nr	30% +
Durrant[383]	1991	45	>15	nr	44%	nr	49%
Carey[384]	1991	13	30 (15–50)	mel + TBI	48% 3 y	0 +	46% +
Bernasconi[385]	1992	14	adults	no	44% 3 y	nr	nr
Rizzoli[386]	1992	61	22 (16–45)	C + TBI, other	40% 8 y	nr	64%
Dicke[387]	1992	26	32 (15–49)	BCNU + VP16	54% 4 y	8% +	38% +
Gore[388]	1993	25	adults	C + TBI/Bu + C + VP16	15% 4 y		
Fiere[278]	1993	63	15–50	TBI + C	51% 5 y	6% +	56% +
Attal[209]	1995	64	31 (15–50)	C + TBI	30% 3 y	2%	62%
Nemet[389]	1995	19	28 (16–50)	C + TBI/Bu	48% 6 y		46%
EBMT[390]	1995	834	30 (18–51)	nr	42% 8 y	nr	nr
Powles[316]	1995	50	26 (15–58)	mel ± TBI	53% 5 y	nr	31%
Vey[369]	1996	52	29 (16–59)	C ± mel + TBI	28% 7 y	nr	68%
Arnold[375]	1996	27	25 (15–58)	various	48% 12 y	nr	nr
Holowiecki[391]	1997	22	29 (15–50)	AC,Eto,C	60% 3 y	nr	27% +
Sierra[392]	1999	33	Adults	nr	40% 8 y	nr	nr
		1369			**42%***	**5%***	**51%***
In 2nd or Subsequent Remission							
Arnold[375]	1996	40	25 (15–58)	various	20% 12 y		
Soiffer[373]	1993	22	28 (18–54)	C + TBI ± HdAC	20% 7 y	18% +	59% +
Holowiecki[391]	1997	12	24 (15–50)	AC,Eto,C	21% 3 y	nr	75% +
Horowitz[374]	1995	173	adults	nr	25% 5 y	nr	71%
Sierra[392]	1999	11	adults	nr	27%	nr	nr
		258			**24%***	**18%***	**70%***

*Weighted mean.

form of transplantation and in which order it should be performed.

Patients in CR1

- The indication for allogeneic transplantation is clear in all high-risk patients.
- For Ph/*BCR-ABL*–positive ALL where the outcome with chemotherapy is so poor (10%), allo sibling SCT is the first choice, the second is MUD SCT and, if no donor is available or the patient is older, an auto SCT can be performed.
- The value of allo SCT in standard-risk ALL in CR1 is being explored.

Patients in CR2

- All patients in CR2 are candidates for allo SCT, related or unrelated. Auto SCT may be successful in a low percentage of patients.

Relapsed/Refractory ALL

For these patients, there is only a minimal chance of survival with chemotherapy. They are all candidates for allo related or unrelated SCT. This approach is being performed in beginning relapse.

FUTURE ASPECTS

In the last 2 decades, substantial progress has been made in understanding and therapy of adult ALL. It is, however, likely that the limits of what may be achieved with the conventional use of the drugs presently available have almost been reached. Complete remission rates—assessed by cytomorphology, not molecular remissions—of 80% to 90% and survival rates of 30% to 35% (with better outcome for subgroups such as T-ALL and mature B-ALL, but also poorer survival in Ph/*BCR-ABL*–positive ALL) are the state of the art. Future progress seems not possible by variations of chemotherapy. New approaches are required, all of them fitting in the general concept of an individualized, subgroup-specific treatment for ALL.

Immunotherapy

Immunotherapy with monoclonal antibodies directed to ALL-specific surface antigens offers new treatment options with low toxicity that act specifically in subtypes of ALL. Immunotherapy is particularly promising if administered in combination with chemotherapy, e.g., in mature B-ALL, in CR patients with persistent MRD, in elderly patients with limited tolerance to chemotherapy, and in patients who are not eligible for intensive chemotherapy, e.g., due to previous complications. Clinical studies with a variety of unconjugated or conjugated antibodies, including antibodies conjugated to radiation isotopes, are ongoing.

Cell Therapy

New approaches in cell therapy include specific cytotoxic T cells that have been successfully generated and expanded in vitro. First clinical experiences of the value of nonmyeloablative SCT and of donor lymphocyte infusions in ALL have been reported and indicate that GvL effects in ALL may have been underestimated so far. These treatment modalities offer options particularly for patients who are ineligible for conventional SCT, e.g., due to age or for treatment of MRD in patients after allogeneic SCT.

Drug Resistance

Drug resistance may be an important factor for treatment failure in adult ALL. The data on the role of multidrug resistance measured by expression of MDR-1, MRP and other markers of drug resistance is still inconclusive in ALL. Nevertheless, treatment of relapse with drugs circumventing MDR, such as idarubicin, are being evaluated, and the exploration of drug resistance modifiers such as PSC833 may be of interest.

The overall drug resistance profile in individual patients as measured with the methylthiazoltetrazolium assay is strongly correlated with outcome in childhood ALL, and prospective data in adult ALL are awaited. Drug resistance profiles may be included in future prognostic models and may also serve for selection of active cytostatic drugs in relapse treatment.

Molecular Targeting

Molecular targeting refers to treatment approaches directed to the genes with major impact on pathogenesis of disease such as the *BCR-ABL* gene. Promising clinical experience in ALL has been accumulated with the specific Abl tyrosine kinase inhibitor STI571 in chronic myeloid leukemia and in Ph/*BCR-ABL*-positive ALL.[393] This treatment is associated with minimal side effects and induced hematologic remissions in heavily pretreated relapsed and refractory ALL patients. STI571 may soon be the treatment of choice for relapsed/refractory Ph/*BCR-ABL*-positive ALL but also for maintenance treatment in patients with persistent residual disease. Clinical trials for the incorporation in front-line therapy (in combination with chemotherapy) are expected.

REFERENCES

1. Farber S, Diamond LK, Mercer RD, et al: Temporary remission in acute leukemia produced by folic acid antagonist, 4-aminopteroylglutamic acid (aminopterin). N Engl J Med 238:787,1948.
2. Distelhorst CW: Glucocorticosteroids induce DNA fragmentation in human lymphoid leukemia cells. Blood 72:1305,1988.
3. Boggs RD, Wintrobe MM, Cartwright GE: The acute leukemias. Medicine 41:163,1962.
4. Shanbron E, Miller S: Critical evaluation of massive steroid therapy of acute leukemia. N Engl J Med 266:1354,1962.
5. Ito C, Evans WE, McNinch L, et al: Comparative cytotoxicity of dexamethasone and prednisolone in childhood acute lymphoblastic leukemia. J Clin Oncol 14:2370,1996.
6. Kaspers GJ, Veerman AJ, Popp-Snijders C, et al: Comparison of the antileukemic activity in vitro of dexamethasone and prednisolone in childhood acute lymphoblastic leukemia. Med Pediatr Oncol 27:114,1996.
7. Balis FM, Lester CM, Chrousos GP, et al: Differences in cerebrospinal fluid penetration of corticosteroids: Possible relationship to the prevention of meningeal leukemia. J Clin Oncol 5:202,1987.
8. Hurwitz CA, Silverman LB, Schorin MA, et al: Substituting dexamethasone for prednisone complicates remission induction in children with acute lymphoblastic leukemia. Cancer 88:1964,2000.
9. Leiken SL, Brubaker C, Hartmann JR, et al: Varying prednisone dosage in remission induction of previously untreated childhood leukemia. Cancer 21:346,1968.
10. Henderson ES: Combination chemotherapy of acute lymphocytic leukemia of childhood. Cancer Res 27:2570,1967.
11. Ranney HM, Gellhorn A: The effect of massive prednisone and prednisone therapy on acute leukemia and malignant lymphomas. Am J Med 22:405,1957.
12. Schrappe M, Reiter A, Ludwig WD, et al: Improved outcome in childhood acute lymphoblastic leukemia despite reduced use of anthracyclines and cranial radiotherapy: Results of trial ALL-BFM 90. German-Austrian-Swiss ALL-BFM Study Group. Blood 95:3310,2000.
13. Wolff JA, Brubaker CA, Murphy ML, et al: Prednisone therapy of acute childhood leukemia: Prognosis and duration of response in 330 treated patients. J Pediatr 70:626,1967.
14. Bernard J, Boiron M, Weil M, et al: Étude de la remission complete des leucemies aigues. Nouvelle Revue Francaise Hematolologie 2:195,1962.
15. Bouroncle BA, Doan CA, Wiseman BK: Evaluation of the effect of massive prednisone therapy in acute leukemia. Acta Haematol 22:201,1959.
16. Carbone PP, Bono V, Frei EI, et al: Clinical studies with vincristine. Blood 21:640,1963.
17. Greenberg ML, Holland J: Kinetic studies of vincristine (VCR) infusions in man. Proc Am Soc Clin Oncol 17:189,1976.
18. Weber W, Nagel GA, Nagel-Stuer E, et al: Vincristine infusion: A phase I study. Cancer Chemother Pharmacol 3:49,1979.
19. Krivit W, Anderson J, Chilcote R, et al: A study of the cross-resistance of vincristine and vindesine in reinduction therapy for acute lymphocytic leukemia in relapse: A report for Children's Cancer Study Group. Am J Pediatr Hematol Oncol 2:217,1980.
20. Vats T, Buchanan G, Mehta P, et al: A study of toxicity and comparative therapeutic efficacy of vindesine-prednisone vs. vincristine-prednisone in children with acute lymphoblastic leukemia in relapse: A Pediatric Oncology Group study. Invest New Drugs 10:231,1992.
21. Anderson J, Krivit W, Chilcote R, et al: Comparison of the therapeutic response of patients with childhood acute lymphoblastic leukemia in relapse to vindesine versus vincristine in combination with prednisone and L-asparaginase: a phase III trial. Cancer Treat Rep 65:1015,1981.
22. Storti E, Traldi A, Quaglino D: Clinical studies on the effect of imuran and vincristine in the treatment of leukemia. Acta Genet Med (Roma) 17:220,1968.
23. Karon MFEJ, Frei EI: The role of vincristine in the treatment of childhood acute leukemia. Clin Pharmacol Ther 7:332,1966.
24. Heyn RM, Beatty EC, Hammond D, et al: Vincristine in the treatment of acute leukemia in children. Pediatrics 38:83,1966.
25. Howard JP: Response of acute leukemia to repeated courses of vincristine (NSC 67574). Cancer Chemother Rep 51:465,1967.
26. Eppinger-Helft M, Garay G, Saslavsky J, et al: Adult acute lymphoblastic leukemia (ALL): 205 patients treated with standard vs. modified "BFM" protocol. Rome, Fourth International Symposium on Therapy of Acute Leukemia 174,1987.
27. Mathe G, Hulhoven R, Sokal G, et al: Phase II clinical trials with vindesine in patients with hematologic malignancies. Anticancer Res 1:1,1981.

28. Mandelli F, Amadori S, Giona F, et al: Vindesine in the treatment of refractory hematologic malignancies: A phase II study. Leuk Res 6:649,1982.

29. Baysass M, Gouveia J, Ribaud P, et al: Phase II trial with vindesine for regression induction in patients with leukemia and hematosarcomas. Cancer Chemother Pharmacol 2:247,1979.

30. Sklaroff RB, Arlin Z, Young CW: Phase II trial of vindesine in patients with acute leukemia. Cancer Treat Rep 63:2063,1979.

31. Krivit W, Hammond D: Vindesine: A phase II study by the Children's Cancer Study Group. In Siegenthaler WO, Luthy R, eds: Current Chemotherapy Proceedings. 10th International Congress of Chemotherapy. Washington, DC: American Society of Microbiology; 1978.

32. Harris RE, McCallister JA, Provisor DS, et al: Methotrexate/L-asparaginase combination chemotherapy for patients with acute leukemia in relapse: A study of 36 children. Cancer 46:2004,1980.

33. Lobel JS, O'Brien RT, McIntosh S, et al: Methotrexate and asparaginase combination chemotherapy in refractory acute lymphoblastic leukemia of childhood. Cancer 43:1089,1979.

34. Yap B-S, McCredie KB, Benjamin RS, et al: Refractory acute leukaemia in adults treated with sequential colaspase and high dose methotrexate. Br Med J 2:791,1978.

35. Djerassi I, Kim JS: Methotrexate and citrovorum factor rescue in the management of childhood lymphosarcoma and reticulum cell sarcoma (non-Hodgkin's lymphomas). Cancer 38:1043,1976.

36. Freeman AI, Weinberg V, Brecher ML, et al: Comparison of intermediate methotrexate with cranial irradiation for the post-induction treatment of acute lymphocytic leukemia in children. N Engl J Med 308:477,1983.

37. Frei EI, Freireich EJ, Gehan E, et al: Studies of sequential and combination antimetabolite therapy in acute leukemia: 6-mercaptopurine and methotrexate. Blood 18:431,1961.

38. Selawry OS, James D: Therapeutic index of methotrexate as related to dose schedule and route of administration in children with acute lymphocytic leukemia. Proc Am Soc Clin Oncol 6:57,1965.

39. Peterson BA, Bloomfield CD: High-dose methotrexate for the remission induction of refractory adult acute lymphocytic leukemia. Med Pediatr Oncol 5:79,1978.

40. Janka N, Wiesner H, Haas RJ: High-dose methotrexate therapy of relapsed acute lymphotic leukemia. Proceedings of the International Society of Hematology, Fifth Congress, European-African Section. Hamburg, 1979.

41. Hoelzer D, Thiel E, Löffler H, et al: Intensified therapy in acute lymphoblastic and acute undifferentiated leukemia in adults. Blood 64:38,1984.

42. Burchenal JM, Murphy ML, Ellison RR: Clinical evaluation of a new anti-metabolite, 6-mercaptopurine, in the treatment of leukemia and allied disease. Blood 8:965,1953.

43. Freireich EJ, Gehan EN, Sulman D: The effect of chemotherapy on acute leukemia in the human. J Chronic Dis 14:593,1961.

44. Sullivan MP, Beatty EC Jr, Hyman CG, et al: A comparison of the effectiveness of standard dose 6-mercaptopurine, combination 6-mercaptopurine and DON, and high-loading 6-mercaptopurine therapies in the treatment of acute leukemia in children: Results of a cooperative study. Cancer Chemother Rep 18:83,1962.

45. Montillo M, Tedeschi A, Centuriono R, et al: Treatment of relapsed adult acute lymphoblastic leukemia with fludarabine and cytosine arabinoside followed by granulocyte colony-stimulating factor (FLAG-GCSF). Leuk Lymphoma 25:579,1997.

46. Visani G, Tosi P, Zinzani PL, et al: FLAG (fludarabine, cytarabine, G-CSF) as a second line therapy for acute lymphoblastic leukemia with myeloid antigen expression: In vitro and in vivo effects. Eur J Haematol 56:308,1996.

47. Virchis AE, Koh MBC, Rankin P, et al: Fludarabine, ARA-C, G-CSF +/− idarubicin in the treatment of high risk acute leukemia and MDS. Blood 94:1328,1999.

48. Thyss A, Millot F, Rialland X, et al: Fludarabine, cytosine-arabinoside and idarubicin for relapsing or refractory ALL in children. Blood 92:3938,1998.

49. Byrne JL, Dasgupta E, Pallis M, et al: Early allogeneic transplantation for refractory or relapsed acute leukaemia following remission induction with FLAG. Leukemia 13:786,1999.

50. Suki S, Kantarjian H, Gandhi V, et al: Fludarabine and cytosine arabinoside in the treatment of refractory or relapsed acute lymphocytic leukemia. Cancer 72:2155,1993.

51. Miser JS, Roloff J, Blatt J, et al: Lack of significant activity of 2'-deoxycoformycin alone or in combination with adenine arabinoside in relapsed childhood acute lymphoblastic leukemia: A randomized phase II trial from the Childrens Cancer Study Group. Am J Clin Oncol 15:490,1992.

52. O'Dwyer PJ, Wagner B, Leyland-Jones B, et al: 2'-Deoxycoformycin (pentostatin) for lymphoid malignancies: Rational development of an active new drug. Ann Intern Med 108:733,1988.

53. Poplack DG, Sallan SE, Rivera G, et al: Phase I study of 2'-deoxycoformycin in acute lymphoblastic leukemia. Cancer Res 41:3343,1981.

54. Smyth JF, Prentice HG, Proctor S, et al: Deoxycoformycin in the treatment of leukemias and lymphomas. Ann N Y Acad Sci 451:123,1985.

55. Winick N, Buchanan GR, Murphy SB, et al: Deoxycoformycin treatment for childhood T-cell acute lymphoblastic leukemia early in second remission: A Pediatric Oncology Group Study. Med Pediatr Oncol 16:327,1988.

56. Lofters W, Campbell M, Gibbs WN, et al: 2'-Deoxycoformycin therapy in adult T-cell leukemia/lymphoma. Cancer 60:2605,1987.

57. Dearden C, Matutes E, Catovsky D: Deoxycoformycin in the treatment of mature T-cell leukaemias. Br J Cancer 64:903,1991.

58. Tobinai K, Shimoyama M, Inoue S, et al: Phase I study of YK-176 (2'-deoxycoformycin) in patients with adult T-cell leukemia-lymphoma: The DCF Study Group. Jpn J Clin Oncol 22:164,1992.

59. Beutler E: New chemotherapeutic agent: 2-chlorodeoxyadenosine. Semin Hematol 31:40,1994.

60. Santana VM, Mirro J Jr, Kearns C, et al: 2-Chlorodeoxyadenosine produces a high rate of complete hematologic remission in relapsed acute myeloid leukemia. J Clin Oncol 10:364,1992.

61. Lambe CU, Averett DR, Paff MT, et al: 2-Amino-6-methoxypurine arabinoside: An agent for T-cell malignancies. Cancer Res 55:3352,1995.

62. Kurtzberg J, Keating M, Moore JO, et al: 2-Amino-9-B-D-arabinosyl-6-methoxy-9H-guanine (GW506U; compound 506U) is highly active in patients with T-cell malignancies: Results of a phase I trial in pediatric and adult patients with refractory hematological malignancies. Blood 88:2666,1996.

63. Morra E, Lazzarino M, Brusamolino E, et al: The role of systemic high-dose cytarabine in the treatment of central nervous system leukemia: Clinical results in 46 patients. Cancer 72:439,1993.

64. Howard JP, Albo V, Newton WA Jr: Cytosine arabinoside—results of a cooperative study in acute childhood leukemia: Comparison of interrupted with continuous therapy. Pediatrics 24:1005,1959.

65. Ellison RR, Holland JF, Weil M, et al: Arabinosyl cytosine: A useful agent in the treatment of acute leukemia in adults. Blood 32:507,1968.

66. Bodey GP, Freireich EJ, Monro RW, et al: Cytosine arabinoside (NSC 63878) therapy for acute leukemia in adults. Cancer Chemother Rep 53:59,1969.

67. Rudnick SA, Cadman EC, Capizzi RL, et al: High dose cytosine arabinoside (HDARAC) in refractory acute leukemias. Cancer 44:1189,1979.

68. Herzig RH, Wolff SN, Lazarus HM, et al: High-dose cytosine arabinoside therapy for refractory leukemia. Blood 62:361,1983.

69. Rohatiner A, Slevin ML, Dhaliwal HS, et al: High-dose cytosine arabinoside: Response to therapy in acute leukaemia and non-Hodgkin's lymphoma. Cancer Chemother Pharmacol 12:90,1984.

70. Kantarjian HM, Estey EH, Plunkett W, et al: Phase I-II clinical and pharmacologic studies of high-dose cytosine arabinoside in refractory leukemia. Am J Med 81:387,1986.

71. Marsh RW, Wozniak A, McCarley D: Therapy of relapsed acute lymphocytic leukemia: A 5-year experience with high dose ARA-C. Proc ASCO 7:147,1987.

72. Febres S, Flessa HC, Martelo OJ: Efficacy of high dose cytosine arabinoside in refractory adult leukemia. Proc Am Soc Clin Oncol 1:128,1982.

73. Willemze R, Zwaan FE, Colpin G, et al: High-dose cytosine arabinoside in the management of refractory acute leukaemia. Scand J Haematol 29:141,1982.

74. Takaku F, Urabe A, Mizoguchi H, et al: High-dose cytosine arabinoside in the treatment of resistant acute leukemia. Semin Oncol 12:144,1985.

75. Morra E, Lazzarino M, Inverdadi D, et al: Systemic high-dose ara-C for the treatment of meningeal leukemia in adult acute lympho-

blastic leukemia and non-Hodgkin's lymphoma. J Clin Oncol 4:1207,1986.

76. Barnett MJ, Greaves MF, Amess JA, et al: Treatment of acute lymphoblastic leukemia in adults. Br J Haematol 64:455,1986.

77. Lauer SJ, Pinkel D, Buchanan GR, et al: Cytosine arabinoside/cyclophosphamide pulses during continuation therapy for childhood acute lymphoblastic leukemia. Cancer 60:2366,1987.

78. Fenaux P, Lai JL, Miaux O, et al: Burkitt cell acute leukaemia (L3 ALL) in adults: A report of 18 cases. Br J Haematol 71:371,1989.

79. Patte C, Philip T, Rodary C, et al: High survival rate in advanced-stage B-cell lymphomas and leukemias without CNS involvement with a short intensive polychemotherapy: Results from the French Pediatric Oncology Society of a randomized trial of 216 children. J Clin Oncol 9:123,1991.

80. Hoelzer D, Ludwig W-D, Thiel E, et al: Improved outcome in adult B-cell acute lymphoblastic leukemia. Blood 87:495,1996.

81. Rodriguez V, McCredie KB, Keating MJ, et al: Isophosphamide therapy for hematologic malignancies in patients refractory to prior treatment. Cancer Treat Rep 62:493,1978.

82. Reiter A, Schrappe M, Ludwig WD, et al: Intensive ALL-type therapy without local radiotherapy provides a 90% event-free survival for children with T-cell lymphoblastic lymphoma: A BFM group report. Blood 95:416,2000.

83. Tan CT, Phoa J, Plyman M: Hematological remission in acute leukemia with cyclophosphamide. Blood 18:808,1961.

84. Hoogstraten B: Cyclophosphamide (cytoxan) in acute leukemia. Cancer Chemother Rep 16:167,1962.

85. Holcomb TM: Cyclophosphamide (NCS 26271) in the treatment of acute leukemia in children. Cancer Chemother Rep 51:389,1967.

86. Gottlieb AJ, Weinberg V, Ellison RR, et al: Efficacy of daunorubicin in the therapy of adult acute lymphocytic leukemia: A prospective randomised trial by the Cancer and Leukemia Group B. Blood 64:267,1984.

87. Bassan R, Lerede T, Rambaldi A, et al: Role of anthracyclines in the treatment of adult acute lymphoblastic leukemia. Acta Haematol 95:188,1996.

88. Bernard J: Acute leukemia treatment. Cancer Res 27:2565,1964.

89. Tan CL, Tasaka H, Yu KP, et al: Daunomycin, an antitumor antibiotic in the treatment of neoplastic disease: Clinical evaluation with specific reference to childhood leukemia. Cancer 20:333,1967.

90. Jones B, Holland JF, Morrison AR, et al: Daunorubicin (NSC 82151) in the treatment of advanced childhood lymphoblastic leukemia. Cancer Res 31:84,1971.

91. Tan C, Echabanas E, Wollner N, et al: Adriamycin in children with acute leukemia and other neoplastic diseases. In Carter SK, DiMarco A, Ghione M, et al, eds: International Symposium on Adriamycin. Berlin: Springer-Verlag; 1972.

92. Wang JJ, Cortes E, Sinks LF, et al: Therapeutic effect and toxicity of adriamycin in patients with neoplastic disease. Cancer 28:837,1971.

93. Ragab AH, Sutow WW, Komp DM, et al: Adriamycin in the treatment of childhood acute leukemia: A Southwest Oncology Group study. Cancer 36:1223,1975.

94. Wilson HE, Bodey GP, Moon TE, et al: Adriamycin therapy in previously treated adult acute leukemia. Cancer Treat Rep 61:905,1977.

95. Jacquillat C, Weil M, Gnon-Auclerc MF, et al: Clinical study of rubidazone (22050RP). Cancer 37:653,1976.

96. Benjamin RS, Keating MJ, McCredie KB, et al: A phase 1 and 2 trial of rubidazone in patients with acute leukemia. Cancer Res 37:4623,1977.

97. Bickers J, Benjamin R, Wilson H, et al: Rubidazone in adults with previously treated acute leukemia and blast cell phase of chronic myelocytic leukemia: A Southwest Oncology Group Study. Cancer Treat Rep 65:427,1981.

98. Ragab AH, Boyett JM, Frankel L, et al: Rubidazone in the treatment of recurrent acute leukemia in children: A Pediatric Oncology Group Study. Cancer 57:1461,1986.

99. Winton EF, Vogler WR, Rose KL: Phase II study of acridinyl aniside (m-AMSA) (NSC-249992) in refractory adult acute leukemia. Proc Am Assoc Cancer Res/Proc Am Soc Clin Oncol 21:437,1980.

100. Legha SS, Keating MJ, McCredie KB, et al: Evaluation of AMSA in previously treated patients with acute leukemia: Results of therapy in 109 adults. Blood 60:484,1982.

101. Arlin ZA, Fanucchi MP, Gee TS, et al: Treatment of refractory adult

102. Dupont JC, Garay GE, Scaghone C, et al: Trial of AMSA in acute leukemia. Cancer Treat Rep 66:1596,1982.

103. Lawrence HJ, Ries CA, Reynolds RD, et al: AMSA—a promising new agent in refractory acute leukemia. Cancer Treat Rep 66:1475,1982.

104. Slevin ML, Shannon MS, Prentice HG, et al: A phase I and II study of m-AMSA in acute leukaemia. Cancer Chemother Pharmacol 6:137,1981.

105. Krischer J, Land VJ, Civin CI, et al: Evaluation of AMSA in children with acute leukemia: A Pediatric Oncology Group study. Cancer 54:207,1984.

106. Paciucci PA, Cuttner J, Holland JF: Mitoxantrone as a single agent and in combination chemotherapy in patients with refractory acute leukemia. Semin Oncol 11:36,1984.

107. Ungerleider RS, Pratt CB, Vietti TJ, et al: Phase I trial of mitoxantrone in children. Cancer Treat Rep 69:403,1985.

108. Estey EH, Keating MJ, McCredie KB, et al: Phase II trial of mitoxantrone in refractory acute leukemia. Cancer Treat Rep 67:389,1983.

109. Moore JO, Olsen GA: Mitoxantrone in the treatment of relapsed and refractory acute leukemia. Semin Oncol 11:41,1984.

110. Ehninger G, Ho AD, Meyer P, et al: Mitoxantrone in the treatment of relapsed and refractory acute leukemia. Onkologie 8:146,1985.

111. Arlin ZA, Silver R, Cassileth P, et al: Phase I-II trial of mitoxantrone in acute leukemia. Cancer Treat Rep 69:61,1985.

112. Capizzi RL, Cooper MR, Stuart J, et al: Continuous infusion (CI) mitoxantrone (MIT) in acute leukemia. Proc Am Assoc Cancer Res 28:210,1987.

113. Saiki J, Stuckey W, Tranum B, et al: Two dose schedules of dihydroxyanthracenedione (DHAD) in adult leukemia—a Southwest Oncology Group study. Proc Am Soc Clin Oncol 2:173,1983.

114. Keating MJ, Smith TL, Gehan EA, et al: Factors related to length of complete remission in adult acute leukemia. Cancer 45:2017,1980.

115. Sackmann-Muriel F, Svarch E, Eppinger-Helft M, et al: Evaluation of intensification and maintenance programs in the treatment of acute lymphoblastic leukemia. Cancer 42:1730,1978.

116. Amylon MD, Shuster J, Pullen J, et al: Intensive high-dose asparaginase consolidation improves survival for pediatric patients with T-cell acute lymphoblastic leukemia and advanced stage lymphoblastic lymphoma: a Pediatric Oncology Group study. Leukemia 13:335,1999.

117. Asselin BL: The three asparaginases: Comparative pharmacology and optimal use in childhood leukemia. Adv Exp Med Biol 457:621,1999.

118. Otten J, Suciu S, Lutz P, et al: The importance of L-asparaginase in the treatment of acute lymphoblastic leukemia (ALL) in children: Results of the EORTC 58881 randomized phase III trial showing greater efficiency of Escherichia coli (E.coli) as compared to Erwinia. Blood 88:669,1996.

119. Oettgen HE, Old LJ, Boyse EA, et al: Inhibition of leukemia in man by L-asparaginase. Cancer 27:2619,1967.

120. Tallal L, Tan C, Oettgen H, et al: E. coli L-asparaginase in the treatment of leukemia and solid tumors in 131 children. Cancer 25:306,1970.

121. Sutow W: L-Asparaginase therapy in children with advanced leukemia. Cancer 28:819,1971.

122. Jaffe N, Traggis D, Das L, et al: Favorable remission induction rate with twice weekly doses of asparaginase. Cancer 33:1,1973.

123. Capizzi RL, Bertino JR, Skeel RT, et al: L-Asparaginase: Clinical, biochemical, pharmacological, and immunological studies. Ann Intern Med 74:893,1971.

124. Holcenberg J, Sencer IJ, Cohen A, et al: Randomized trial of PEG vs native asparaginase in children with newly diagnosed acute lymphoblastic leukemia (ALL): CCG study 1962. Blood 94:2790a,1999.

125. Douer D, Cohen LJ, Periclou LA, et al: PEG-L-asparaginase: Pharmacokinetics and clinical response in newly diagnosed adults with acute lymphoblastic leukemia treated with multiagent chemotherapy. Blood 90:1490,1997.

126. Silverman LB, Dalton V, Gelber RD, et al: PEG-asparaginase is less toxic than E. coli L-asparaginase in children with acute lymphoblastic leukemia (ALL): Results from the Dana Farber Cancer Institute ALL Consortium. Proc ASCO 17:530,1998.

127. Patel SS, Benfield P: Pegaspargase (polyethylene glycol-L-asparaginase). Clin Immunother 5:492,1996.

128. Frankel SR, Kurtzberg J, De Oliveira D, et al: Toxicity and pharmacokinetics of PEG-asparaginase (PEG-asp) in newly diagnosed adult acute lymphoblastic leukemia (ALL): CALGB 9511. Blood 88: 88,1996.

129. Rowinsky EK, Adjei A, Donehower RC, et al: Phase I and pharmacodynamic study of the topoisomerase I-inhibitor topotecan in patients with refractory acute leukemia. J Clin Oncol 12: 2193,1994.

130. Kantarjian H, Beran M, Ellis A, et al: Phase I study of topotecan, a new topoisomerase I inhibitor in patients with refractory or relapsed acute leukemia. Blood 81:1146,1993.

131. Furman WL, Baker SD, Pratt CB, et al: Escalating systemic exposure of continuous infusion topotecan in children with recurrent acute leukemia. J Clin Oncol 14:1504,1996.

132. Gore SD, Rowinsky EK, Miller CB, et al: A phase II "window" study of topotecan in untreated patients with high-risk adult acute lymphoblastic leukemia. Clin Cancer Res 4:2677,1998.

133. Puccetti E, Guller S, Orleth A, et al: Arsenic trioxide: Rediscovery of a tumor cell–specific agent for the treatment of Ph + leukemia. Blood 94:279,1999.

134. Perkins C, Fang G, Orlando M, et al: Novel anti-bcr-abl strategy consisting of arsenic trioxide and CGP57148B lowers bcr-abl levels and tyrosine kinase activity resulting in apoptosis and differentiation of bcr-abl–positive human leukemia cells. Blood 94: 2640,1999.

135. Hoelzer D, Gökbuget N: New approaches to acute lymphoblastic leukemia in adults: Where do we go? Semin Oncol 27:540, 2000.

136. Uckun FM, Evans WE, Forsyth CJ, et al: Biotherapy of B-cell precursor leukemia by targeting genistein to CD19-associated tyrosine kinases. Science 267:886,1995.

137. Messinger Y, Levine A, Fuchs E, et al: B34 (anti-CD19)-genistein treatment of therapy refractory B-lineage acute lymphoblastic leukemia. Blood 92:2530,1998.

138. Seibel NL, Krailo M, O'Neill K, et al: Phase I study of B43-PAP immunotoxin in combination with standard 4-drug induction for patients with CD19 + acute lymphoblastic leukemia (ALL) in relapse: A Children's Cancer Group Study. Blood 92:1651,1998.

139. Szatrowski TP, Larson RA, George S, et al: Anti-B4-blocked ricin as consolidation therapy for patients with B-lineage acute lymphoblastic leukemia (ALL): A phase II trial (CALGB 9311). Blood 86:783,1995.

140. Szatrowski TP, Larson RA, Dodge R, et al: The effect of anti-B4-blocked ricin (anti-B4-BR) on minimal residual disease (MRD) in adults with B-lineage acute lymphoblastic leukemia (ALL) (CALGB 9311, 8762, 8763). Blood 88:669,1996.

141. Vallera DA, Burns LJ, Frankel AE, et al: Laboratory preparation of a deglycosylated ricin toxin A chain containing immunotoxin directed against a CD7 T-lineage differentiation antigen for phase I human clinical studies involving T-cell malignancies. J Immunol Methods 197:69,1996.

142. Frankel AE, Laver JH, Willingham MC, et al: Therapy of patients with T-cell lymphomas and leukemias using an anti-CD7 monoclonal antibody-ricin A chain immunotoxin. Leuk Lymphoma 26: 287,1997.

143. Kolitz JE, O'Mara V, Willemze R, et al: Treatment of acute lymphoblastic leukemia (ALL) with campath-1H: Initial observations. Blood 84:1191,1994.

144. Nowak-Göttl U, Aschka I, Koch HG, et al: Resistance to activated protein C (APCR) in children with acute lymphoblastic leukaemia: The need for a prospective multicenter study. Blood 6:761,1995.

145. Fritz RD, Forkner CE Jr, Freireich EJ, et al: Association of fatal intracranial hemorrhage and "blastic crisis" in patients with acute leukemia. N Engl J Med 261:59,1959.

146. Willemze R, Drenthe-Schonk AM, van Rossum J, et al: Treatment of acute lymphoblastic leukemia in adolescents and adults. Scand J Haematol 24:421,1980.

147. Ertel I, Nesbit M, Hammond D, et al: Effective dose of L-asparaginase for induction of remission in previously treated children with acute lymphocytic leukemia: A report from Childrens Cancer Study Group. Cancer Res 39:3893,1979.

148. Sallan S, Hitchcock-Bryan S, Gelber R, et al: Influence of intensive asparaginase in the treatment of childhood non-T-cell acute lymphoblastic leukemia. Cancer Res 43:5601,1983.

149. Clavell L, Gelber R, Cohen H, et al: Four-agent induction and intensive asparaginase therapy for treatment of childhood acute lymphoblastic leukemia. N Engl J Med 315:657,1986.

150. Nagura E: Nationwide randomized comparative study of doxorubicin, vincristine and prednisolone combination therapy with and without L-asparaginase for adult acute lymphoblastic leukemia. Cancer Chemother Pharmacol 33:359,1994.

151. Hoelzer D, Thiel E, Löffler H, et al: Intensified Chemotherapy and Mediastinal Irradiation in Adult T-Cell Acute Lymphoblastic Leukemia. New York: Alan R. Liss; 1990.

152. Bassan R, Pogliani E, Lerede T, et al: Fractionated cyclophosphamide added to the IVAP regimen (idarubicin-vincristine-L-asparaginase-prednisone) could lower the risk of primary refractory disease in T-lineage but not B-lineage acute lymphoblastic leukemia: First results from a phase II clinical study. Haematologica 84:1088,1999.

153. Bassan R, Battista R, Rohatiner AZS, et al: Treatment of adult acute lymphoblastic leukaemia (ALL) over a 16-year period. Leukemia 6:186,1992.

154. Cassileth PA, Andersen JW, Bennett JM, et al: Adult acute lymphocytic leukemia: the Eastern Cooperative Oncology Group experience. Leukemia 6(S2):178,1992.

155. Willemze R, Zijlmans JMJM, den Ottolander GJ, et al: High-dose ara-C for remission induction and consolidation of previously untreated adults with ALL or lymphoblastic lymphoma. Ann Hematol 70:71,1995.

156. Kaufmann SH, Karp JE, Burke PJ, et al: Addition of etoposide to initial therapy of adult acute lymphoblastic leukemia: A combined clincal and laboratory study. Leuk Lymphoma 23:71,1996.

157. Wernli M, Abt A, Bargetzi M, et al: A new therapeutic strategy in adult acute lymphoblastic leukemia: Intensive induction/consolidation, early transplant, maintenance-type therapy in relapse only. Proc Am Soc Clin Oncol 16:6,1997.

158. Kantarjian HM, O'Brien S, Smith TL, et al: Results of treatment with hyper-CVAD, a dose-intensive regimen, in adult acute lymphocytic leukemia. J Clin Oncol 18:547,2000.

159. Hallbook H, Simonsson B, Bjorkholm M, et al: High dose ara-C as upfront therapy for adult patients with acute lymphoblastic leukemia (ALL). Blood 94:1327,1999.

160. Weiss M, Maslak P, Feldman E, et al: Cytarabine with high-dose mitoxantrone induces rapid complete remission in adult acute lymphoblastic leukemia without the use of vincristine or prednisone. J Clin Oncol 14:2480,1996.

161. Todeschini G, Tecchio C, Meneghini V, et al: Estimated 6-year event-free survival of 55% in 60 consecutive adult acute lymphoblastic leukemia patients treated with an intensive phase II protocol based on high induction dose of daunorubicin. Leukemia 12:144,1998.

162. Jones B, Freeman AI, Shuster JJ, et al: Lower incidence of meningeal leukemia when prednisone is replaced by dexamethasone in the treatment of acute lymphocytic leukemia. Med Pediatr Oncol 19:269,1991.

163. Ellison RR, Mick R, Cuttner J, et al: The effects of postinduction intensification treatment with cytarabine and daunorubicin in adult acute lymphocytic leukemia: A prospective randomized clinical trial by Cancer and Leukemia Group B. J Clin Oncol 9: 2002,1991.

164. Gaynor J, Chapman D, Little C, et al: A cause-specific hazard rate analysis of prognostic factors among 199 adults with acute lymphoblastic leukemia: The Memorial Hospital experience since 1969. J Clin Oncol 6:1014,1988.

165. Hoelzer D: Aggressive chemotherapy of ALL in elderly patients. Hematol Oncol 11:12,1993.

166. Clarkson BD, Gee T, Mertelsmann R, et al: Current status of treatment of acute leukemia in adults: An overview of the Memorial experience and review of literature. Crit Rev Oncol Hematol 4:221,1986.

167. Hussein KK, Dahlberg S, Head D, et al: Treatment of acute lymphoblastic leukemia in adults with intensive induction, consolidation and maintenance chemotherapy. Blood 73:57,1989.

168. Fiere D, Archimbaud E, Extra JM, et al: Treatment of adult acute lymphoblastic leukemia: Preliminary results of a trial from the French Group. Haematol Blood Trans 30:125,1987.

169. Hoelzer D, Thiel E, Löffler H, et al: Prognostic factors in a multicenter study for treatment of acute lymphoblastic leukemia in adults. Blood 71:123,1988.

170. Hoelzer D, Thiel E, Ludwig WD, et al: Follow-up of the first two successive German multicentre trials for adult ALL (01/81 and 02/84): German Adult ALL Study Group. Leukemia 7:130,1993.

171. Lluesma-Gonalons M, Pavlovsky S, Santarelli MT, et al: Improved results of an intensified therapy in adult acute lymphocytic leukemia. Ann Oncol 2:33,1991.

172. Marcus RE, Catovsky D, Johnson SA, et al: Adult acute lymphoblastic leukaemia: A study of prognostic features and response to treatment over a ten-year period. Br J Cancer 53:175,1986.

173. Stryckmans P, de Witte T, Fillet G, et al: Treatment of adult acute lymphoblastic leukemia: ALL-2 and ALL-3 EORTC studies. Haematologica 76:109,1991.

174. Mandelli F, Annino L, Rotoli B: The GIMEMA ALL 0183 trial: Analysis of 10-year follow-up. Br J Haematol 92:665,1996.

175. Ribera JM, Ortega JJ, Oriol A, et al: Late intensification chemotherapy has not improved the results of intensive chemotherapy in adult acute lymphoblastic leukemia: Results of a prospective multicenter trial. Haematologica 83:222,1998.

176. Durrant IJ, Prentice HG, Richards SM: Intensification of treatment for adults with acute lymphoblastic leukaemia: Results of UK Medical Research Council randomized trial. Br J Haematol 99:84,1997.

177. Daenen S, van Imhoff GW, van den Berg E, et al: Improved outcome of adult acute lymphoblastic leukaemia by moderately intensified chemotherapy which includes a "pre-induction" course for rapid tumour reduction: Preliminary results on 66 patients. Br J Haematol 100:273,1998.

178. Patte C, Michon J, Frappaz D, et al: Therapy of Burkitt and other B-cell acute lymphoblastic leukaemia and lymphoma: Experience with the LMB protocols of the SFOP (French Paediatric Oncology Society) in children and adults. Bailliere Clin Haematol 7:339,1994.

179. Ludwig W-D, Rieder H, Bartram CR, et al: Immunophenotypic and genotypic features, clinical characteristics, and treatment outcome of adult pro-B acute lymphoblastic leukemia: Results of the German multicenter trials. Blood 92:1898,1998.

180. Gökbuget N, Hoelzer D: High-dose methotrexate in the treatment of adult acute lymphoblastic leukemia. Ann Hematol 72:194,1996.

181. Balis FM, Savitch JL, Bleyer WA, et al: Remission induction of meningeal leukemia with high-dose intravenous methotrexate. J Clin Oncol 3:485,1985.

182. Linker CA, Levitt LJ, O'Donnell M, et al: Treatment of adult acute lymphoblastic leukemia with intensive cyclical chemotherapy: A follow-up report. Blood 78:2814,1991.

183. Elonen E, Almqvist A, Hänninen A, et al: Intensive treatment of acute lymphatic leukaemia in adults: ALL86 protocol. Haematologica 76:133,1991.

184. Evensen SA, Brinch L, Tjonnfjord G, et al: Estimated 8-year survival of more than 40% in a population-based study of 79 adult patients with acute lymphoblastic leukaemia. Br J Haematol 88:88,1994.

185. Linker CA, Ries CA, Damon LE, et al: Intensified and shortened chemotherapy for adult acute lymphoblastic leukemia. Blood 90:1485,1997.

186. Radford JW, Burns CP, Jones MP, et al: Adult acute lymphoblastic leukemia: Results of the Iowa HOP-L protocol. J Clin Oncol 7:58,1989.

187. Tomonaga A, Omine M, Morishima Y, et al: Individualized induction therapy followed by intensive consolidation and maintenance including asparaginase in adult ALL: JALSG study. Haematologica 76:68,1991.

188. Smedmyr B, Simonsson B, Björkholm M, et al: Treatment of adult acute lymphoblastic and undifferentiated (ALL/AUL) leukemia, according to a national protocol, in Sweden. Haematologica 76:107,1991.

189. Hoelzer D, Thiel E, Ludwig WD, et al: Follow-up of the first two successive German multicenter trials for adult ALL (1/81 and 2/84). Leukemia 7(S2):130,1993.

190. Durrant IJ: Results of Medical Research Council trial UKALL IX in acute lymphoblastic leukaemia in adults: Report from the Medical Research Council Working Party on Adult Leukaemia. Br J Haematol 85:84,1993.

191. Fiere D, Lepage E, Sebban C, et al: Adult acute lymphoblastic leukemia: A multicentric randomized trial testing bone marrow transplantation as postremission therapy. J Clin Oncol 11:1990,1993.

192. Todeschini G, Meneghini V, Pizzolo G, et al: Relationship between daunorubicin dosage delivered during induction therapy and outcome in adult acute lymphoblastic leukemia. Leukemia 8:376,1994.

193. Scherrer R, Bettelheim P, Gaissler K, et al: High efficiency of the German multicenter ALL (GMALL) protocol for treatment of adult acute lymphoblastic leukemia (ALL): A single institution study. Ann Hematol 69:181,1994.

194. Thomas X, Danalla C, Bach QK, et al: Sequential induction chemotherapy with vincristine, daunorubicin, cyclophosphamide, and prednisone in adult acute lymphoblastic leukemia. Ann Hematol 70:65,1995.

195. Bosco J, Teh A: Outcome of treatment in adult acute lymphoblastic leukaemia in an Asian population: Comparison with a previous multicenter German study. Leukemia 9:951,1995.

196. Larson RA, Dodge RK, Burns CP, et al: A five-drug remission induction regimen with intensive consolidation for adults with acute lymphoblastic leukemia: Cancer and Leukemia Group B study 8811. Blood 85:2025,1995.

197. Larson RA, Dodge RK, Linker CA, et al: A randomized controlled trial of filgrastim during remission induction and consolidation chemotherapy for adults with acute lymphoblastic leukemia: CALGB study 9111. Blood 92:1556,1998.

198. Bassan R, Lerede T, Di Bona E, et al: Induction-consolidation with an idarubicin-containing regimen, unpurged marrow autograft, and post-graft chemotherapy in adult acute lymphoblastic leukaemia. Br J Haematol 104:755,1999.

199. Clarkson B, Gaynor J, Little C, et al: Importance of long-term follow-up in evaluating treatment regimens for adults with acute lymphoblastic leukemia. Haematol Blood Trans 33:397,1990.

200. Kantarjian HM, Walters RS, Keating MJ, et al: Results of the vincristine, doxorubicin, and dexamethasone regimen in adults with standard and high-risk acute lymphocytic leukemia. J Clin Oncol 8:994,1990.

201. Stryckmans P, de Witte T, Marie JP, et al: Therapy of adult ALL: Overview of 2 successive EORTC studies. Leukemia 6:199,1992.

202. Dekker AW, van't Veer MB, Sizoo W, et al: Intensive postremission chemotherapy without maintenance therapy in adults with acute lymphoblastic leukemia. J Clin Oncol 15:476,1997.

203. Ifrah N, Witz F, Jouet JP, et al: Intensive short-term therapy with granulocyte-macrophage-colony stimulating factor support, similar to therapy for acute myeloblastic leukemia, does not improve overall results for adults with acute lymphoblastic leukemia. GOELAMS Group. Cancer 86:1496,1999.

204. Cuttner J, Mick R, Budman DR, et al: Phase III trial of brief intensive treatment of adult acute lymphocytic leukemia comparing daunorubicin and mitoxantrone: A CALGB study. Leukemia 5:425,1991.

205. Elonen E: Long-term survival in acute lymphoblastic leukaemia in adults: A prospective study of 51 patients. Eur J Haematol 48:75,1992.

206. Wiernik PH, Dutcher JP, Paietta E, et al: Long-term follow-up of treatment and potential cure of adult acute lymphocytic leukemia with MOAD: A nonanthracycline-containing regimen. Leukemia 7:1236,1993.

207. Chiu EKW, Chan LC, Liang R, et al: Poor outcome of intensive chemotherapy for adult lymphoblastic leukemia: A possible dose effect. Leukemia 8:1469,1994.

208. Wernli M, Tichelli A, von Fliedner V, et al: Intensive induction/consolidation therapy without maintenance in adult acute lymphoblastic leukaemia: A pilot assessment. Br J Haematol 87:39,1994.

209. Attal M, Blaise D, Marit G, et al: Consolidation treatment of adult acute lymphoblastic leukemia: A prospective, randomized trial comparing allogeneic versus autologous bone marrow transplantation and testing the impact of recombinant interleukin-2 after autologous bone marrow transplantation. Blood 86:1619,1995.

210. Mandelli F, Annino L, Vegna ML, et al: Adult acute lymphoblastic leukemia (ALL): Results of the GIMEMA ALL 0288 trial. Br J Haematol 93:144,1996.

211. Wernli M, Fey MF, Tobler A, et al: The limit of dose-intensification in the treatment of adult acute lymphoblastic leukemia despite growth-factor therapy. Blood 84:144,1994.

212. Wolk RW, Masse SR, Conklin R, et al: The incidence of central nervous system leukemia in adults with acute leukemia. Cancer 33:863,1974.

213. Cortes J, O'Brien SM, Pierce S, et al: The value of high-dose systemic chemotherapy and intrathecal therapy for central nervous system prophylaxis in different risk groups of adult acute lymphoblastic leukemia. Blood 86:2091,1995.

214. Law IP, Blom J: Adult acute leukemia: Frequency of central system involvement in long-term survivors. Cancer 40:1304,1977.

215. Bleyer WA: Central nervous system leukemia. In Henderson ES, Lister TA, eds: Leukemia. Philadelphia: WB Saunders; 1990.

216. Gökbuget N, Hoelzer D: Meningeosis leukaemica in adult acute lymphoblastic leukaemia. J Neuro Oncol 38:167,1998.

217. Henderson ES, Scharlau C, Cooper MR, et al: Combination chemotherapy and radiotherapy for acute lymphocytic leukemia in adults: Results of CALGB protocol 7113. Leuk Res 3:395,1979.

218. Tucker J, Prior PF, Green CR, et al: Minimal neuropsychological sequelae following prophylactic treatment of the central nervous system in adult leukaemia and lymphoma. Br J Cancer 60: 775,1989.

219. Omura GA, Moffitt S, Vogler WR, et al: Combination chemotherapy of adult acute lymphoblastic leukemia with randomized central nervous prophylaxis. Blood 55:199,1980.

220. Clarkson B, Ellis S, Little C, et al: Acute lymphoblastic leukemia in adults. Semin Oncol 12:160,1984.

221. Stryckmans P, Marie JP, Suciu S, et al: Therapy for adolescent and adult acute lymphoblastic leukemia: Randomization of induction and consolidation therapies (preliminary results of EORTC Study 58791). In Buechner T, Schellong G, Hiddemann W, et al, eds: Haematology and Blood Transfusion: Acute Leukemias. Berlin: Springer-Verlag; 1987.

222. Kantarjian HM, Estey E, O'Brien S, et al: Granulocyte-stimulating factor supportive treatment following intensive chemotherapy in acute lymphocytic leukemia first remission. Cancer 72:2950,1993.

223. Welte K, Gabrilove J, Bronchud MH, et al: Filgrastim (r-metHuG-CSF): The first 10 years. Blood 88:1907,1996.

224. Scherrer R, Geissler K, Kyrle PA, et al: Granulocyte colony-stimulating factor (G-CSF) as an adjunct to induction chemotherapy of adult acute lymphoblastic leukemia (ALL). Ann Hematol 66: 283,1993.

225. Ottmann OG, Hoelzer D, Gracien E, et al: Concomitant granulocyte colony-stimulating factor and induction chemoradiotherapy in adult acute lymphoblastic leukemia: A randomized phase III trial. Blood 86:444,1995.

226. Geissler K, Koller E, Hubmann E, et al: Granulocyte colony-stimulating factor as an adjunct to induction chemotherapy for adult acute lymphoblastic leukemia: A randomized phase III study. Blood 90:590,1997.

227. Dibenedetto SP, Ragusa R, Ippolito AM, et al: Assessment of the value of treatment with granulocyte colony-stimulating factor in children with acute lymphoblastic leukemia: A randomized clinical trial. Eur J Haematol 55:93,1995.

228. Pui C-H, Boyett JM, Hughes WT, et al: Human granulocyte colony-stimulating factor after induction chemotherapy in children with acute lymphoblastic leukemia. New Engl J Med 336:1781,1997.

229. Mitchell PLR, Morland B, Stevens MCG, et al: Granulocyte colony-stimulating factor in established febrile neutropenia: A randomized study of pediatric patients. J Clin Oncol 15:1163,1997.

230. Welborn JL: Impact of reinduction regimens for relapsed and refractory acute lymphoblastic leukemia in adults. Am J Hematol 45:341,1994.

231. Bassan R, Lerede T, Barbui T: Strategies for the treatment of recurrent acute lymphoblastic leukemia in adults. Haematologica 81:20,1996.

232. Rivera G, Aur RJ, Dahl GV, et al: Combined VM-26 and cytosine arabinoside in treatment of refractory childhood lymphocytic leukemia. Cancer 45:1284,1980.

233. Hoelzer D: High-dose chemotherapy in adult acute lymphoblastic leukemia. Semin Hematol 28:84,1991.

234. Giona F, Testi AM, Moleti ML, et al: Idarubicin plus cytosine-arabinoside in advanced acute lymphoblastic leukemia: The GI-MEMA/AIEOP experience. Leuk Lymphoma 7:15,1992.

235. Freund M, Diedrich H, Ganser A, et al: Treatment of relapsed or refractory adult acute lymphocytic leukemia. Cancer 69:709,1992.

236. Goasguen JE, Dossot JM, Fardel O, et al: Expression of the multidrug resistance-associated P-glycoprotein (p170) in 59 cases of de novo acute lymphoblastic leukemia: Prognostic implications. Blood 81:2394,1993.

237. Klumper E, Pieters R, Veerman AJ, et al: In vitro cellular drug resistance in children with relapsed/refractory acute lymphoblastic leukemia. Blood 86:3861,1995.

238. Goekbuget N, Aguion-Freire E, Diedrich H, et al: Characteristics

239. Arnold R, Bunjes D, Deeg HJ, et al: BMT in refractory or relapsed adult ALL patients treated in the German Multicenter ALL studies. Bone Marrow Transplant 21:1,1998.

240. Tivey H: The natural history of untreated acute leukemia. Ann N Y Acad Sci 60:322,1954.

241. Bitran J: Prognostic value of immunological markers in adults with acute lymphoblastic leukemia. N Engl J Med 299:1317,1978.

242. Greaves MF, Lister TA: Prognostic importance of immunologic markers in adults with acute lymphoblastic leukemia. N Engl J Med 119:304,1981.

243. Miller DR, Leikin S, Albo V: Intensive therapy and prognostic factors in acute lymphoblastic leukemia of childhood CCG 141. In Neth R, Gallo RC, Graf R, et al, eds: Modern Trends in Human Leukemia IV. Berlin: Springer-Verlag; 1981.

244. Pui CH, Williams DL, Roberson PK, et al: Correlation of karyotype and immunophenotype in childhood acute lymphoblastic leukemia. J Clin Oncol 6:56,1988.

245. Secker-Walker LM, Craig JM, Hawkins JM, et al: Philadelphia positive acute lymphoblastic leukemia in adults: Age distribution, BCR breakpoint and prognostic significance. Leukemia 5:196,1991.

246. Ferrari A, Annino L, Crescenzi S, et al: Acute lymphoblastic leukemia in the elderly: Results of two different treatment approaches in 49 patients during a 25-year period. Leukemia 9:1643,1995.

247. Taylor PR, Reid MM, Bown N, et al: Acute lymphoblastic leukemia in patients aged 60 years and over: A population-based study on incidence and outcome. Blood 80:1813,1992.

248. Delannoy A, Ferrant A, Bosly A, et al: Acute lymphoblastic leukemia in the elderly. Eur J Haematol 45:90,1990.

249. Späth-Schwalbe E, Heil G, Heimpel H: Acute lymphoblastic leukemia in patients over 59 years of age: Experience in a single center over a 10-year period. Ann Hematol 69:291,1994.

250. Goker E, Lin JT, Trippett T, et al: Decreased polyglutamylation of methotrexate in acute lymphoblastic leukemia blasts in adults compared to children with this disease. Leukemia 7:1000,1993.

251. Pieters R, den Boer ML, Durian M, et al: Relation between age, immunophenotype and in vitro drug resistance in 395 children with acute lymphoblastic leukemia: Implication for treatment of infants. Leukemia 12:1344,1998.

252. Delannoy A, Sebban C, Cony-Makhoul P, et al: Age-adapted induction treatment of acute lymphoblastic leukemia in the elderly and assessment of maintenance with interferon combined with chemotherapy: A multicentric prospective study in forty patients. Leukemia 11:1429,1997.

253. Kantarjian HM, O'Brien S, Smith T, et al: Acute lymphocytic leukaemia in the elderly: Characteristics and outcome with the vincristine-adriamycin-dexamethasone (VAD) regimen. Br J Haematol 88:94,1994.

254. Legrand O, Marie J-P, Marjanovic Z, et al: Prognostic factors in elderly acute lymphoblastic leukaemia. Br J Haematol 97:596,1997.

255. Todeschini G, Scognamiglio F, Sheiban I, et al: Lack of major cardiac side effects following high-dose intensity of daunorubicin (DNM) in adult acute lymphoblastic leukemia. Blood 88:170,1996.

256. Bassan R, Di Bona E, Lerede T, et al: Age-adapted moderate-dose induction and flexible outpatients postremission therapy for elderly patients with acute lymphoblastic leukemia. Leuk Lymphoma 22:295,1996.

257. Tabata M, Yoshida M, Izumi T, et al: Retrospective analysis of elderly patients ≥60 years of age with acute leukemia. Rinsho Ketsueki 39:176,1998.

258. Nagura E, Minami S, Nagata K, et al: Acute leukemia in the elderly: A study of 179 cases in Nagoya. Blood 92:3910,1998.

259. Bene MC, Castoldi G, Knapp W, et al: Proposal for the immunological classification of acute leukemias. Leukemia 9:1783,1995.

260. Sobol RE, Royston J, LeBien TW, et al: Adult acute lymphoblastic leukemia phenotypes defined by monoclonal antibodies. Blood 65:730,1985.

261. Thiel E, Hoelzer D, Dörken B, et al: Clinical relevance of blast cell phenotype as determined with monoclonal antibodies in acute lymphoblastic leukemia of adults. Haematol Blood Transf 30: 95,1987.

262. Czuczman MS, Dodge RK, Stewart CC, et al: Value of immunophenotype in intensively treated adult acute lymphoblastic leukemia: Cancer and Leukemia Group B study 8364. Blood 93:3931,1999.

263. Ludwig WD, Raghavachar A, Thiel E: Immunophenotypic classification of acute lymphoblastic leukemia. Bailliere Clin Haematol 7:235,1994.

264. Hoelzer D, Gökbuget N, Arnold R, et al: Akute lymphatische Leukämie des Erwachsenen. Internist 37:994,1996.

265. Baccarani M, Amadori S, Willemze R, et al: E-rosette-positive acute lymphoblastic leukemia in adolescents and adults. Br J Haematol 55:295,1983.

266. Lazzarino M, Morra MJ, Allessandrino EP, et al: Adult acute lymphoblastic leukemia: Response to therapy according to presenting features in 62 patients. Eur J Cancer Clin Oncol 18:813,1982.

267. Lister TA, Roberts MM, Brearly RL, et al: Prognostic significance of cell surface phenotype in adult acute lymphoblastic leukemia. Cancer Immunol Immunother 6:227,1979.

268. Schiffer CA, Larson RA, Bloomfield CD: Cancer and Leukemia Group B studies in adult acute lymphocytic leukemia. Leukemia 6:171,1992.

269. Schorin MA, Blattner S, Gelber RD, et al: Treatment of childhood acute lymphoblastic leukemia: Results of Dana-Farber Cancer Institute/Children's Hospital acute lymphoblastic leukemia consortium protocol 85-01. J Clin Oncol 12:740,1994.

270. Feickert HJ, Bettoni C, Schrappe M, et al: Event-free survival of children with T-cell acute lymphoblastic leukemia after introduction of high dose methotrexate in multicenter trial ALL-BFM 86. Proc ASCO 12:317,1993.

271. Arico M, Basso G, Mandelli F, et al: Good steroid response in vivo predicts a favourable outcome in children with T-cell acute lymphoblastic leukemia. Cancer 75:1684,1995.

272. Rowe JM, Richards S, Wiernik PH, et al: Allogeneic bone marrow transplantation (BMT) for adults with acute lymphoblastic leukemia (ALL) in first complete remission (CR): Early results from the international ALL trial (MRC UKALL/ECOG E2993). Blood 94:732,1999.

273. Cascavilla N, Musto P, D'Arena G, et al: Are "early" and "late" T-acute lymphoblastic leukemias different diseases? A single center study of 34 patients. Leuk Lymphoma 21:437,1996.

274. Thiel E, Kranz BR, Raghavachar A, et al: Prethymic phenotype and genotype of pre-T(CD+/ER−)-cell leukemia and its clinical significance within adult acute lymphoblastic leukemia. Blood 73:1247,1989.

275. Hoelzer D, Arnold R, Freund M, et al: Characteristics, outcome and risk factors in adult T-lineage acute lymphoblastic leukemia (ALL). Blood 94:2926,1999.

276. Clarkson B, Ellis S, Little C, et al: Acute lymphoblastic leukemia in adults. Semin Oncol 12:160,1985.

277. Garand R, Vannier JP, Béné MC: Comparison of outcome, clinical, laboratory, and immunological features in 164 children and adults with T-ALL. Leukemia 4:739,1990.

278. Fiere D: Adult acute lymphoblastic leukemia: A multicentric randomized trial testing bone marrow transplantation as postremission therapy: The French Group on Therapy for Adult Acute Lymphoblastic Leukemia. J Clin Oncol 11:1990,1993.

279. Linker CA: Risk-adapted treatment of adult acute lymphoblastic leukemia (ALL). Leukemia 11:24,1997.

280. Reiter A, Schrappe M, Henze G, et al: B-cell acute lymphoblastic leukemia of childhood: Treatment strategy and results in three BFM trials. Haematologica 76:105,1991.

281. Reiter A, Schrappe M, Tiemann M, et al: Improved treatment results in childhood B-cell neoplasms with tailored intensification of therapy: A report of the Berlin-Frankfurt-Munster Group Trial NHL-BFM 90. Blood 94:3294,1999.

282. Schaison G, Patte C, Castaigne S, et al: Short and aggressive treatment (T) for B-cell lymphoblastic leukemia (B-ALL): Good results of protocol LMB 86. Blood 74:369,1989.

283. Pees HW, Radtke H, Schwamborn J, Graf N: The BFM-protocol for HIV-negative Burkitt's lymphomas and L3 ALL in adult patients: A high chance for cure. Ann Hematol 65:201,1992.

284. Lee EJ, Pettoni GR, Freter CE: Brief-duration high-intensity chemotherapy (CT) for patients (pts) with small non-cleaved lymphoma (IWF J) and FAB L3 acute lymphocytic leukemia (L3) in adults: Preliminary results of CALGB 9251. Proc ASCO 16:24,1997.

285. Thomas DA, Cortes J, O'Brien S, et al: Hyper-CVAD program in Burkitt's-type adult acute lymphoblastic leukemia. J Clin Oncol 17:2461,1999.

286. Drexler HG, Ludwig WD: Incidence and clinical relevance of myeloid antigen-positive acute lymphoblastic leukemia. Res Cancer Res 131:53,1993.

287. Wetzler M, Dodge RK, Mrozek K, et al: Prospective karyotype analysis in adult acute lymphoblastic leukemia: The Cancer and Leukemia Group B experience. Blood 93:3983,1999.

288. Secker-Walker LM, Prentice HG, Durrant J, et al: Cytogenetics adds independent prognostic information in adults with acute lymphoblastic leukaemia on MRC trial UKALL XA. Br J Haematol 96:601,1997.

289. Charrin C: Cytogenetic abnormalities in adult acute lymphoblastic leukemia: Correlations with hematologic findings and outcome—a collaborative study of the Groupe Francais de Cytogénétique Hématologique. Blood 87:3135,1996.

290. Rieder H, Fonatsch C: Cytogenetic findings in acute lymphoblastic leukemia. In Büchner T, ed: Acute Leukemias IV: Prognostic Factors. Berlin: Springer-Verlag; 1994.

291. Walters R, Kantarjian HM, Keating MJ, et al: The importance of cytogenetic studies in adult acute lymphocytic leukemia. Am J Med 89:579,1990.

292. Campbell LJ, Michael PM, White JS, et al: Prognostic implications of karyotype in 159 newly diagnosed adult patients with acute lymphoblastic leukaemia. Blood 86:173,1990.

293. Hooberman A, Westbrook C, Spino C, et al: Clinical significance of molecular detection of the BCR-ABL fusion gene in acute lymphoblastic leukemia (ALL): A Cancer and Leukemia Group B (CALGB) study. Proc ASCO 10:222,1991.

294. Janssen JWG, Fonatsch C, Ludwig WD, et al: Polymerase chain reaction analysis of BCR-ABL sequences in adult Philadelphia chromosome-negative acute lymphoblastic leukemia patients. Leukemia 6:463,1992.

295. Maurer J, Jannsen JWG, Thiel E, et al: Detection of chimeric BCR-ABL genes in acute lymphoblastic leukemia by the polymerase chain reaction. Lancet 337:1055,1991.

296. Bloomfield CD, Wurster-Hill D, Peng G, et al: Prognostic significance of the Philadelphia chromosome in adult acute lymphoblastic leukemia. In Gale RP, Hoelzer D, eds: Acute Lymphoblastic Leukemia. New York: Alan R. Liss; 1990.

297. Ohyashiki K, Ohyashiki JH, Tauchi T, et al: Treatment of Philadelphia chromosome-positive acute lymphoblastic leukemia: A pilot study which raises important questions. Leukemia 5:611,1991.

298. Götz G, Weh HJ, Walter TA, et al: Clinical and prognostic significance of the Philadelphia chromosome in adult patients with acute lymphoblastic leukemia. Ann Hematol 64:97,1992.

299. Westbrook CA, Hooberman AL, Spino C, et al: Clinical significance of the BCR-ABL fusion gene in adult acute lymphoblastic leukemia: a Cancer and Leukemia Group B study (8762). Blood 80:2983,1992.

300. Fière D, Lepage E, Sebban C, et al: Adult acute lymphoblastic leukemia: A multicentric randomized trial testing bone marrow transplantation as postremission therapy. J Clin Oncol 11:1990,1993.

301. Kantarjian HM, Talpaz M, Dhingra K, et al: Significance of the P210 versus P190 molecular abnormalities in adults with Philadelphia chromosome-positive acute leukemia. Blood 78:2411,1991.

302. Mandelli F, Annino L, Ciolli S: Philadelphia chromosome (Ph 1)-positive acute lymphoblastic leukemia (ALL) in adults: Interim results of GIMEMA ALL 0288 pilot study. Blood 82:58,1993.

303. Stryckmans P, Muus P, Marie JP, et al: Adult Ph+ acute lymphoblastic leukemia in ALL-3 EORTC study. Blood 84:144,1994.

304. Stryckmans P, Suciu S, Annino L, et al: Molecular evaluation of consolidation therapy and early allograft or autograft for BCR-ABL-positive adult acute lymphoblastic leukemia patients: A pilot study of EIGLE (European Intergroup of GIMEMA, French LALA and EORTC). Blood 90:809a,1997.

305. Annino L, Elia L, Lamanda A, et al: Clinical relevance of BCR/ABL and ALL1/AF4 molecular markers in adult acute lymphoblastic leukaemia (ALL): A retrospective study. Br J Haematol 102:227a,1998.

306. Faderl S, Kantarjian HM, Talpaz M, et al: Clinical significance of cytogenetic abnormalities in adult acute lymphoblastic leukemia. Blood 91:399,1998.

307. Haas OA, Mor W, Gadner H, et al: Treatment of Ph-positive acute lymphoblastic leukemia with α-interferon. Leukemia 2:555,1988.

308. Laport GF, Williams SF: The role of high-dose chemotherapy in patients with Hodgkin's disease and non-Hodgkin's lymphoma. Semin Oncol 25:503,1998.

309. Barrett AJ, Horowitz MM, Ash RC, et al: Bone marrow transplantation for Philadelphia chromosome–positive acute lymphoblastic leukemia. Blood 79:3067,1992.

310. Preti HA, O'Brien S, Giralt S, et al: Philadelphia chromosome-positive adult acute lymphocytic leukemia: Characteristics, treatment results, and prognosis in 41 patients. Am J Med 97:60,1994.

311. Stockschläder M, Hegewisch-Becker S, Krüger W, et al: Bone marrow transplantation for Philadelphia chromosome–positive acute lymphoblastic leukemia. Bone Marrow Transplant 16:663,1995.

312. Chao NJ, Blume KG, Forman SJ, et al: Long-term follow-up of allogeneic bone marrow recipients for Philadelphia chromosome-positive acute lymphoblastic leukemia. N Engl J Med 332:3353,1995.

313. Stryckmans P, Marie JP, Muus P, et al: Evaluation of the quality of peripheral blood progenitors (PBP) for autologous transplantation in adult Philadelphia-positive (Ph+) acute lymphoblastic leukemia (ALL): A pilot study. Blood 86:783,1995.

314. Snyder DS, Nademanee AP, O'Donnell MR, et al: Long-term follow-up of 23 patients with Philadelphia chromosome–positive acute lymphoblastic leukemia treated with allogeneic bone marrow transplant in first complete remission. Leukemia 13:2053,1999.

315. Miyamura K, Tanimoto M, Morishima Y, et al: Detection of Philadelphia chromosome–positive acute lymphoblastic leukemia by polymerase chain reaction: Possible eradication of minimal residual disease by marrow transplantation. Blood 79:1366,1992.

316. Powles R, Mehta J, Singhal S, et al: Autologous bone marrow transplantation or peripheral blood stem cell transplantation followed by maintenance chemotherapy for adult acute lymphoblastic leukemia in first remission: 50 cases from a single center. Bone Marrow Transplant 16:241,1995.

317. Mitterbauer G, Fodinger M, Scherrer R, et al: PCR monitoring of minimal residual disease after conventional chemotherapy and bone marrow transplantation in BCR-ABL–positive acute lymphoblastic leukaemia. Br J Haematol 89:937,1995.

318. Martin H, Fauth F, Atta J, et al: Single versus double autologous BMT/PBSCT in patients with BCR-ABL–positive acute lymphoblastic leukemia. Blood 94:2588,1999.

319. Kröger N, Kruger W, Wacker-Backhaus G, et al: Intensified conditioning regimen in bone marrow transplantation for Philadelphia chromosome–positive acute lymphoblastic leukemia. Bone Marrow Transplant 22:1029,1998.

320. Atta J, Fauth F, Keyser M, et al: Purging in BCR-ABL–positive lymphoblastic leukemia using immunomagnetic beads: Comparison of residual leukemia and purging efficiency in bone marrow vs. peripheral blood stem cells by semiquantitative polymerase chain reaction. Bone Marrow Transplant 25:97,2000.

321. Casper J, Camitta B, Ash R, et al: Bone marrow transplantation for Philadelphia chromosome–positive (Ph+) acute lymphocytic leukemia (ALL) using alternative donors. Blood 80:65,1992.

322. Sierra J, Radich J, Hansen JA, et al: Marrow transplants from unrelated donors for treatment of Philadelphia chromosome-positive acute lymphoblastic leukemia. Blood 90:1410,1997.

323. Marks DI, Bird JM, Cornish JM, et al: Unrelated donor bone marrow transplantation for children and adolescents with Philadelphia-positive acute lymphoblastic leukemia. J Clin Oncol 16:931,1998.

324. Cornelissen JJ, Shipp K, Kollman C, et al: Bone marrow transplantation from unrelated donors for adult patients with poor-risk acute lymphoblastic leukemia: A report from the national Marrow Donor Programme. Blood 92:114,1998.

325. Faderl S, Kantarjian H, Manshouri T, et al: The prognostic significance of p16INK4a/p14ARF and p15INK4b deletions in adult acute lymphoblastic leukemia. Clin Cancer Res 5:1855,1999.

326. Rubnitz JE, Behm FG, Pui C-H, et al: Genetic studies of childhood acute lymphoblastic leukemia with emphasis on p16, MLL, and ETV6 gene abnormalities: Results of St. Jude Total Therapy Study XII. Leukemia 15:1201,1997.

327. Stock W, Sher DA, Dodge RK, et al: High incidence of p16 deletion in adult acute lymphoblastic leukemia (ALL): Correlation with clinical features and response to treatment. Blood 86:268,1995.

328. Diccianni MB, Yu J, Hsiao M, et al: Clinical significance of p53 mutations in relapsed T-cell acute lymphoblastic leukemia. Blood 84:3105,1994.

329. Campana D: Immunophenotypic analysis in the monitoring of minimal residual disease. Rev Clin Exp Hematol 1:42,1997.

330. Campana D, Pui C-H: Detection of minimal residual disease in acute leukemia: Methodological advances and clinical significance. Blood 85:1416,1995.

331. Potter MN: The detection of minimal residual disease in acute leukemia. Blood Rev 6:68,1992.

332. Roberts M, Estrov Z, Kitchingman GR, et al: The clinical significance of residual disease in childhood acute lymphoblastic leukemia as detected by polymerase chain reaction amplification of antigen-receptor gene sequences. Leuk Lymphoma 20:181,1996.

333. Foroni L, Harrison CJ, Hoffbrand AV: Investigation of minimal residual disease in childhood and adult acute lymphoblastic leukaemia by molecular analysis. Br J Haematol 105:7,1999.

334. Wasserman R, Galili N, Ito Y, et al: Residual disease at the end of induction therapy as a predictor of relapse during therapy in childhood B-lineage acute lymphoblastic leukemia. J Clin Oncol 10:1879,1992.

335. Nizet Y, Van Daele S, Lewalle P, et al: Long-term follow-up of residual disease in acute lymphoblastic leukemia patients in complete remission using clonogeneic IgH probes and the polymerase chain reaction. Blood 82:1618,1993.

336. Knauf WU, Ho AD, Hoelzer D, et al: Detection of residual leukemic cells in adult acute lymphoblastic leukemia by analysis of gene rearrangements and correlation with early relapse. Res Cancer Res 131:197,1993.

337. Cavé H, Guidal C, Rohrlich P, et al: Prospective monitoring and quantification of residual blasts in childhood acute lymphoblastic leukemia by polymerase chain reaction study of delta and gamma T-cell receptor genes. Blood 83:1892,1994.

338. Brisco MJ, Condon J, Highes E, et al: Outcome prediction in childhood acute lymphoblastic leukaemia by molecular quantification of residual disease at the end of induction. Lancet 343:196,1994.

339. Coyle L, Yaxley JC, Cole-Sinclair M, et al: Minimal residual disease (MRD) analysis of adult and childhood ALL. Blood 84:300,1994.

340. Seriu T, Hansen-Hagge TE, Erz DHR, et al: Improved detection of minimal residual leukemia through modifications of polymerase chain reaction analyses based on clonospecific T-cell receptor junctions. Leukemia 9:316,1995.

341. Steenbergen EJ, Verhagen OJ, Nibbering CP, et al: Clonal evolution of immunoglobulin heavy chain rearrangements in childhood B-precursor acute lymphoblastic leukemia after engraftment in SCID mice. Leukemia 10:1471,1996.

342. Brisco MJ, Hughes E, Neoh SH, et al: Relationship between minimal residual disease and outcome in adult acute lymphoblastic leukemia. Blood 87:5251,1996.

343. Seriu T, Erz D, Stark Y, et al: T-cell receptor delta-2, delta-3 rearrangement: A suitable allele-specific marker for the detection of minimal residual disease in childhood acute lymphoblastic leukemia. Leukemia 11:759,1997.

344. Cavé H, Van der Werff Ten Bosch J: Clinical significance of minimal residual disease in childhood acute lymphoblastic leukemia. N Engl J Med 339:591,1998.

345. Gruhn B, Hongeng S, Yi H, et al: Minimal residual disease after intensive induction therapy in childhood acute lymphoblastic leukemia predicts outcome. Leukemia 12:675,1998.

346. Goulden NJ, Knechtli CJ, Garland RJ, et al: Minimal residual disease analysis for the prediction of relapse in children with standard-risk acute lymphoblastic leukaemia. Br J Haematol 100:235,1998.

347. van Dongen JJ, Seriu T, Panzer-Grümayer ER, et al: Prognostic value of minimal residual disease in acute lymphoblastic leukemia in childhood. Lancet 352:1731,1998.

348. Foroni L, Coyle LA, Papaioannou M, et al: Molecular detection of minimal residual disease in adult and childhood acute lymphoblastic leukaemia reveals differences in treatment response. Leukemia 11:1732,1997.

349. Jacquy C, Delepaut B, Van Daele S, et al: A prospective study of minimal residual disease in childhood B-lineage acute lymphoblastic leukaemia: MRD level at the end of induction is a strong predictive factor of relapse. Br J Haematol 98:140,1997.

350. Neale GAM, Menarguez J, Kitchingman GR, et al: Detection of minimal residual disease in T-cell acute lymphoblastic leukemia using polymerase chain reaction predicts impending relapse. Blood 78:739,1991.

351. Nizet Y, Martiat P, Vaerman JL, et al: Follow-up of residual disease (MRD) in B-lineage acute leukaemias using a simplified PCR strat-

egy: Evolution of MRD rather than its detection is correlated with clinical outcome. Br J Haematol 79:205,1991.

352. Mortuza FY, Moreira P, Gameiro M, et al: Investigation of minimal residual disease (MRD) in adult acute lymphoblastic leukemia: PCR tests show statistically significant value in predicting clinical outcome. Blood 94:1272,1999.

353. Zhang MJ, Hoelzer D, Horowitz MM, et al: Long-term follow-up of adults with acute lymphoblastic leukemia in first remission treated with chemotherapy or bone marrow transplantation: The Acute Lymphoblastic Leukemia Working Committee. Ann Intern Med 123:428,1995.

354. Oh H, Gale RP, Zhang M-J, et al: Chemotherapy vs. HLA-identical sibling bone marrow transplants for adults with acute lymphoblastic leukemia in first remission. Bone Marrow Transplant 22: 243,1998.

355. Fiere D: Long-term results of a prospective Belgium-French protocol of treatment for adult acute lymphoblastic leukemia (ALL): LALA87 study. Ann Hematol 78:32,1999.

356. Henslee-Downey PJ, Fleming D, Kryscio R, et al: Does mismatched bone marrow transplant from related or unrelated donors offer successful salvage therapy for patients with relapsed acute lymphoblastic leukemia. Haematologica 76:69,1991.

357. Ringden O, Labopin M, Gluckman E: Graft-versus-leukemia effect in allogeneic marrow transplant recipients with acute leukemia is maintained using cyclosporin A combined with methotrexate as prophylaxis. Bone Marrow Transplant 18:921,1996.

358. Passweg JR, Tiberghien P, Cahn JY, et al: Graft-versus-leukemia effects in T-lineage and B-lineage acute lymphoblastic leukemia. Bone Marrow Transplant 21:153,1998.

359. Slavin S, Nagler A, Naparstek E, et al: Nonmyeloablative stem cell transplantation and cell therapy as an alternative to conventional bone marrow transplantation with lethal cytoreduction for the treatment of malignant and nonmalignant hematologic disorders. Blood 91:756,1998.

360. Matthews DC, Appelbaum FR, Eary JF, et al: Phase I study of 131I-anti-CD45 antibody plus cyclophosphamide and total body irradiation for advanced acute leukemia and myelodysplastic syndrome. Blood 94:1237,1999.

361. Barrett AJ, Horowitz MM, Gale RP, et al: Factors affecting relapse and survival after bone marrow transplantation for acute lymphoblastic leukemia: Importance of regimens used for prophylaxis against graft-versus-host disease. Blood 74:862,1989.

362. Blume KG, Schmidt GM, Chao NJ, et al: Bone marrow transplantation for acute lymphoblastic leukemia. In Gale RP, Hoelzer D, ed: Acute Lymphoblastic Leukemia. New York: Alan R. Liss; 1990.

363. Bacigalupo A, Van Lint MT, Frassoni F, et al: Allogeneic bone marrow transplantation (BMT) for adult acute lymphoblastic leukemia (ALL) in first remission. Haematologica 76:70,1991.

364. Doney K, Fisher LD, Appelbaum FR, et al: Treatment of adult acute lymphoblastic leukemia with allogeneic bone marrow transplantation: Multivariate analysis of factors affecting acute graft-versus-host disease, relapse and relapse-free survival. Bone Marrow Transplant 7:453,1991.

365. Ringden O, Horowitz MM, Sondel P, et al: Methotrexate, cyclosporine or both to prevent graft-versus-host disease after HLA-identical sibling bone marrow transplantation. Blood 81:1094,1993.

366. Ringden O, Horowitz MM, Sondat P, et al: Methotrexate, cyclosporin, or both to prevent graft-versus-host disease after HLA-identical sibling bone marrow transplants for early leukemia? Blood 81:1094,1993.

367. de Witte T, Awwad B, Boezeman J, et al: Role of allogeneic bone marrow transplantation in adolescent or adult patients with acute lymphoblastic leukemia or lymphoblastic lymphoma in first remission. Bone Marrow Transplant 14:767,1994.

368. Vey N, Blaise D, Stoppa AM, et al: Bone marrow transplantation in 63 adult patients with acute lymphoblastic leukemia in first complete remission. Bone Marrow Transplant 14:383,1994.

369. Vey N, Stoppa AM, Faucher C, et al: Long-term results of bone marrow transplantation (BMT) as post-remission therapy in adult acute lymphoblastic leukemia: Experience of a single institution in 88 patients. Br J Haematol 93:61,1996.

370. Jiménez MA, Herrera C, Torres A, et al: Allogeneic BMT in adult acute lymphoblastic leukemia: A report of 51 cases. Br J Haematol 93:256,1996.

371. Doney K, Fisher LD, Appelbaum FR, et al: Treatment of adult acute lymphoblastic leukemia with allogeneic bone marrow transplantation: Multivariate analysis of factors affecting acute graft-versus-host disease, relapse, and relapse-free survival. Bone Marrow Transplant 7:453,1991.

372. Copelan EA, Biggs JC, Avalos BR, et al: Radiation-free preparation for allogeneic bone marrow transplantation in adults with acute lymphoblastic leukemia. J Clin Oncol 10:237,1992.

373. Soiffer RJ, Roy DC, Gonin R, et al: Monoclonal antibody-purged autologous bone marrow transplantation in adults with acute lymphoblastic leukemia at high risk of relapse. Bone Marrow Transplant 12:243,1993.

374. Horowitz MM, Hoelzer D, Klein JP: HLA-Identical sibling, unrelated donor and autologous bone marrow transplantation for acute lymphoblastic leukemia (ALL). Acta Haematol 93:3,1995.

375. Arnold R, Bunjes D, Einsele H, et al: BMT in adult ALL patients treated in the German multicenter studies. Ann Hematol 73: 91,1996.

376. Gorin N-C, Labopin M: Analysis of the acute leukemia EBMT registry. Exp Hematol 25:179,1997.

377. Martino R, Bellido M, Sureda A, et al: Salvage chemotherapy (CT) followed by allogeneic or autologous stem cell transplantation (SCT) in adults with relapsed (REL) or refractory (REF) acute lymphoblastic leukemia (ALL): Results of a prospective study. Blood 90:1997.

378. Przepiorka D, Cortes J, Folloder J, et al: Allogeneic transplantation for adult acute lymphoblastic leukemia. Blood 92:4525,1998.

379. Mizuta S, Ito Y, Miyamura K, et al: Accurate quantitation of residual tumor burden at bone marrow harvest predicts timing of subsequent relapse in patients with common ALL treated by autologous bone marrow transplantation. Bone Marrow Transplant 24: 7774,1999.

380. Granena A, Castellsague X, Badell I, et al: Autologous bone marrow transplantation for high risk acute lymphoblastic leukemia: Clinical relevance of ex vivo bone marrow purging with monoclonal antibodies and complement. Bone Marrow Transpl 24:621,1999.

381. Blaise D, Attal M, Reiffers J, et al: Randomized study of recombinant interleukin-2 after autologous bone marrow transplantation for acute leukemia (AL) in first complete remission. Blood 94: 335,1999.

382. Simonsson B, Burnett AK, Prentice HG, et al: Autologous bone marrow transplantation with monoclonal antibody purged marrow for high risk acute lymphoblastic leukemia. Leukemia 3:631,1989.

383. Durrant IJ, Richards S, Bell P, et al: Bone marrow transplantation (BMT) in first remission in adults with acute lymphoblastic leukaemia (ALL). Haematologica 76:109,1991.

384. Carey PJ, Proctor SJ, Taylor P, et al: Autologous bone marrow transplantation for high-grade lymphoid malignancy using melphalan/irradiation conditioning without purging or cryopreservation. Blood 77:1593,1991.

385. Bernasconi C, Lazzarino M, Morra E, et al: Early intensification followed by allo-BMT or auto-BMT or a second intensification in adult ALL: A randomized multicenter study. Leukemia 6:204,1992.

386. Rizzoli V, Carlo-Stella C, Almici C, et al: Autologous bone marrow transplantation for acute myeloid and lymphoid leukemia. Leukemia 6:103,1992.

387. Dicke KA, Spinolo JA: Autologous bone marrow transplantation in acute lymphocytic leukemia (ALL). Leukemia 6:136,1992.

388. Gore SD, Karp JE, Miller CB, et al: Brief intensive therapy for adult acute lymphocytic leukemia (ALL): Superiority of allogeneic bone marrow transplantation (BMT). Blood 82:56,1993.

389. Nemet D, Labar B, Bogdanic V, et al: ABMT versus chemotherapy as consolidation for acute leukemia in first remission: A prospective single center study. Bone Marrow Transplant 15:55,1995.

390. European Bone Marrow Transplant Group (EBMTG): Working party on acute leukemia. Annual report 1995.

391. Holowiecki J, Wojnar J, Krawczyk-Kulis M: Efficacy of autologous bone marrow transplantation in adult ALL: Single centre experience. Bone Marrow Transplant 19:103,1997.

392. Sierra J, Rovira M, Munoz L, et al: Autologous hematopoietic stem cell transplantation as treatment for adult acute lymphoblastic leukemia. In Dicke KA, Keating A, eds: Autologous Blood and Marrow Transplantation. Arlington, VA: Carden Jennings; 1999.

393. Druker BJ, Talpaz M, Resta D, et al: Clinical efficacy and safety of an ABL-specific tyrosine kinase inhibitor as targeted therapy for chronic myelogenous leukemia. Blood 94:1639,1999.

28

Michael J. Keating

Chronic Lymphocytic Leukemia

Chronic lymphocytic leukemia (CLL) is a hematopoietic neoplasm characterized by a clonal expansion of small lymphocytes.[108] In the earlier stages of the disease, these lymphocytes are present in bone marrow and peripheral blood; in later stages, they accumulate in lymph nodes, liver, and spleen, causing lymphadenopathy, hepatomegaly, and splenomegaly. Later in the progression of the disease, bone marrow failure occurs. In more than 95% of cases, the cells are B cells. A small proportion of cases of T-cell CLL is due to an accumulation of clonal T lymphocytes.[22, 42]

Leukemia was first defined by Virchow[381] in 1845, and one form of the disease described was probably CLL. The use of stains to differentiate myeloid and lymphoid leukemias made the differentiation between the two types possible, and in 1903, Turk[374] demonstrated the similarity between CLL and lymphoma. Minot and Isaacs,[264] in 1924, described the natural history of CLL as it was known then and for the first time discussed the role of radiation therapy in CLL. Rai[317] was the first to develop a widely accepted staging system for the disease, emphasizing the importance of bone marrow failure and high tumor burden. This simple, inexpensive classification has maintained its clinical relevance up to the present. The clonality of CLL was established by identification of restricted light-chain type immunoglobulin on the surface of B cells in 1972[310]; the association in a small proportion of cases with a monoclonal serum immunoglobulin corresponding to the immunoglobulin on the surface of the CLL cells; zygosity studies for expression of isoenzymes of glucose-6-phosphate dehydrogenase[108]; and immunoglobulin gene rearrangement studies.[227] The application of cytogenetic techniques has demonstrated that CLL has nonrandom abnormalities, with clonal evolution being identified in some cases.

DEMOGRAPHIC FEATURES

CLL is rare in patients younger than 30 years but increases exponentially with age for both men and women.[110, 388] Incidence rates are similar among whites and blacks.[239] CLL incidence rates are consistently higher in men, especially elderly men; the male-to-female ratio increases from 5:3 to 5:1 with age.[81] The incidence of CLL varies markedly from country to country. The highest rates for men appear to occur in Canada, in Denmark, and in Austra-

lia.[110] Rates for women appear highest in Canada, in Denmark, and in Israel among the Jewish population.[38,110] CLL is uncommon among Asians, especially older individuals.[276] In Los Angeles, the highest incidence rate appears to be in whites and blacks, whereas the incidence of CLL in Hispanics in Los Angeles is approximately half that of the white and black communities.[110] The Surveillance, Epidemiology and End Results data highlight the low incidence of CLL in American Indians and Chinese, Japanese, and Philippine populations living in the United States.[110] CLL accounts for 25% to 30% of all cases of leukemia in the United States and 35% to 40% in Denmark but less than 5% in Japan, China, and other Asian countries.[110] Studies conducted by Berrebi[25] in Israel have demonstrated that there is a striking prevalence of CLL in eastern European Jews compared with non-Ashkenazi Jews (ratio of 4:1).

The incidence of CLL has been increasing during the last 50 years, and this has been illustrated most clearly in studies from Olmsted County in Minnesota.[49] The increase is predominantly among men, and diagnosis has consistently been made at an earlier stage, suggesting that improved diagnostic methods are contributing to the increased incidence.

ETIOLOGY

The cause of CLL is unknown. Evidence for an association between benzene and CLL is weak despite its known role in the etiology of some cases of acute myelogenous leukemia.[4] Increased mortality rates among rubber workers,[80] workers exposed to solvents,[58] and petroleum workers are noted.[26] The associations are weak, however, and many others do not find the same associations. Slightly elevated risks have been noted in farmers in some areas.[33] Some studies have noted an excess of lymphoid leukemias in smokers.[136] There has been no association of CLL with exposure to ionizing radiation. In particular, there was no increase in the incidence of CLL after the nuclear explosions in Japan.[109]

CLL is more frequently associated with familial clustering than are other forms of leukemia,[237] and subsequent generations develop CLL at an earlier age (anticipation).[389] There is an increased likelihood of leukemia in first-degree relatives of patients with CLL,[391] and a number of twins have been reported to have CLL.[68] Familial cases appear to share haplotypes, cytogenetic abnormalities, and immunologic disturbances. Consanguinity is more common in familial cases of CLL.[237] No strong association with a particular human leukocyte antigen (HLA) type has been noted.[237, 238]

Human T-cell lymphotropic virus 1, a type C retrovirus, is associated with a variety of lymphoproliferative disorders.[34] No association of viral etiology with B-CLL, such as human herpesvirus 6, Epstein-Barr virus, or cytomegalovirus, has been established.[62, 120, 237]

As a consequence of the disturbed immune system in CLL, associations with other immunologic disorders have been sought.[64, 239] CLL has been noted to arise subsequent to other autoimmune diseases, but when it is examined more closely, the association is not supported. Coombs' test–positive autoimmune hemolytic anemia and immune-mediated thrombocytopenia are the only autoimmune disorders that appear to be more frequent in patients with CLL than in control populations.[73, 152]

IMMUNOBIOLOGY

Immunophenotyping of CLL

The earliest investigations of the cellular origin in CLL were important because they demonstrated that in most patients, CLL cells weakly expressed monoclonal cell surface immunoglobulin (sIg) but were considered to be of B-cell lineage.[3, 310] In approximately 2% to 5% of cases, CLL cells form rosettes with sheep erythrocytes, have CD3, and express CD4 or CD8, establishing a T-cell origin.[42] CLL cells are not typical B cells because they form rosettes with mouse red blood cells through receptors[53, 147]; express sIgM, often with sIgD, and rarely sIgG[162, 309]; and form rosettes only with red blood cells coated with C3d complement, not C3b.[337] These findings strongly suggest that B-cell CLL is not a neoplastic counterpart of the usual circulating peripheral blood B cell (Table 28–1; see also Table 28–4).

Freedman and colleagues[124] identified expression of CD19 and CD20 in CLL cells of all 100 patients studied; 95% expressed CD5, 90% expressed the Epstein-Barr virus/C3d receptor (CD21 antigen), and 19% expressed C3b.[370] Most pan–B-cell antigens are expressed.[15, 90, 124, 299] Pre–B-cell antigens, such as CD10, are not expressed in the majority of cases.[260] Surface immunoglobulin is present, at low intensity, in approximately 80% of patients, but cytoplasmic immunoglobulin appears in virtually all cases.[302] The cytoplasmic immunoglobulin concentration appears to be higher than in normal lymphocytes.[184] CD11A and CD54 are not present,[177, 366] whereas CD44 and L-selectin are.[288, 361] CD22 is expressed in a minority of patients.[273] Activation antigens are present in some patients with CLL.[142]

The major anomaly noted in CLL is the co-expression of CD5 (previously thought to be a pan–T-cell antigen) with typical B-cell antigens. CD5[+] B cells can be identified as a major population of fetal B cells and are present in lymph node and spleen but not in bone marrow or liver.[48, 124] These lymphocytes have been noted to express Ia, CD19, CD21, and weak sIgM/D but not CD35. It is obvious that this immunophenotype is remarkably similar

TABLE 28–1. Differentiation Stage of Surface Antigens Used in Classification of Chronic Lymphoid Leukemia

Antigen	Pan–B Cell	Mature B Cell	Activation
MHC class II	+		
CD19	+		
CD20	+		
CD22	+		
CD38	+		
CD40	+		
CD45RA	+ weak		
CD23		+	
sIg		+ * (80%)	
cIg		+ *	
CD11A		+	
CD54		+	
CD44		+	
CD25			+ (50%)
B7/BB1			+ (<25%)
CD80			+ (<25%)

*Very low density surface immunoglobulin (sIg), high-concentration cytoplasmic immunoglobulin (cIg).

to that observed in the cells of the majority of patients with CLL. CD5[+] B cells are present in small numbers in the periphery of germinal centers in normal adult lymph nodes.[48] Small numbers of CD5[+] B cells are identified in peripheral blood of normal adults and in tonsils of normal adults but not in bone marrow.[124] The other clinical situations in which CD5[+] subpopulations of B cells have been noticed to be increased are in rheumatoid arthritis, in systemic lupus erythematosus, and after allogeneic marrow transplantation.[11, 12, 306]

CD5 can be upregulated in normal B cells by stimulation with TPA (phorbol myristic acetate) but not by anti-immunoglobulin, Epstein-Barr virus, anti-CD20, interleukin (IL)-1, IL-2, IL-4, interferon-γ, and high-molecular-weight B-cell growth factor (BCGF).[125] These findings have led to the concept that Ly1 B cells are a murine counterpart of human CD5[+] B cells.[169] It is now considered that CLL may be a neoplasm specifically of the CD5[+] B cells. However, the fact that CD5 expression can be upregulated by a variety of stimuli leaves open the possibility of aberrant expression in a more common B cell.

CLL cells demonstrate several antigens, including histocompatibility antigen DR (HLA-DR), but do not contain terminal transferase and do not express common acute lymphocytic leukemia antigen (CALLA, CD10).[260] A 69-kd surface antigen named common CLL antigen (cCLLa) has been associated with the surface of leukemic cells of all patients with B-cell CLL and hairy cell leukemia (HCL); it is not present on normal lymphocytes or other B-cell or T-cell malignant neoplasms.[102] FMC7[41] and CD22 antibodies commonly react with HCL and prolymphocytic leukemia (PLL) cells, but usually not with CLL cells.

BIOLOGY OF CHRONIC LYMPHOCYTIC LEUKEMIA

The cells in B-cell CLL should no longer be regarded as autonomous resting cells. CLL cells interact with a variety of cytokines and with T cells, although frequently less well than normal B cells do.[79, 114, 174] A number of cytokines have been known to have stimulatory effects on DNA synthesis or a differentiation or both. IL-2, IL-7, IL-10, and tumor necrosis factor (TNF) appear to stimulate proliferation.[17, 182] On the other hand, IL-5,[14] interferon-α, and interferon-γ are more potent in inducing differentiation.[141] In different systems, IL-1α, IL-1β, IL-2, IL-6, low-molecular-weight BCGF, interferon-γ, and TNF-α have either a stimulatory or a differentiating effect on normal B cells.[143, 172, 245, 357, 358, 368] IL-2, IL-4, CD40 ligand (CD154), TNF-α, interferon-α, interferon-γ, low-molecular-weight BCGF, and high-molecular-weight BCGF stimulate CLL cells.[275] Thus, it is obvious that the cells in CLL express functional receptors for several cytokines.

Both high-affinity and low-affinity receptors for IL-2 have been detected on CLL cells.[384] Expression of the receptors are regulated by stimulation with phorbol esters, *Staphylococcus aureus* Cowan, and IL-2 itself.[195] Messenger RNA for IL-4, IL-8, and IL-10 is expressed, and receptors are present on CLL cells.[305] Both IL-4 and IL-8 are antiapoptotic to CLL cells. The role of IL-10 is not clear because conflicting data exist.[192] IL-4 inhibits the formation of functional high-affinity IL-2 receptor.[84] The TNF-α receptor has been demonstrated to be present in the cells of CLL, and the TNF-α pathway is a major growth-stimulatory pathway in CLL.[84] High-molecular-weight BCGF receptor is constitutively expressed in CLL.[375]

CLL clones have been demonstrated to produce IL-1α and IL-1β, IL-6, TNF-α and TNF-β, and the soluble form of CD23 (sCD23).[2, 50, 118, 349] Cytokines most regularly found to be produced in these investigations were TNF-α, TNF-β, and IL-1β.

The process of proliferation and differentiation is difficult to evaluate in CLL. Many experiments have been done without purification of the population to exclude normal T cells.[331] In addition, there appears to be marked heterogeneity in patients' cells. Thus, different factors can be stimulatory or inhibitory according to the particular set of circumstances. IL-4 is possibly related to isotype switching. TNF-α, low-molecular-weight BCGF, and anti-CD40 can induce proliferation, and high-molecular-weight BCGF can stimulate clonogenic growth of CLL cells.[275] CLL cells appear to survive better in vitro than normal B cells do. This may be related to the increased levels of Bcl-2 in CLL or other proteins inhibiting apoptosis.

TNF has been discussed in depth as a possible autocrine growth loop in CLL.[118, 173, 174] TNF has a multitude of effects in inducing cytokine and growth factor production, upregulating receptors for cytokines, and affecting transcription factors and adhesion molecules. TNF causes proliferation in a dose-dependent fashion in most cases of CLL in vitro.[85] CLL cells express TNF receptors after incubation of the cells with TNF in vitro.[84] Proliferation of CLL cells is associated with the induction of *JUN* and *FOS*.[138, 139] Others have not found proliferation of CLL cells with TNF in most cases. Levels of TNF are elevated in the serum of most patients with CLL,[118, 148] and TNF has been reported to be a possible cause of the cytopenias that occur in CLL, and serum levels increase with

stage.[118] Lindemann and colleagues[236] showed that the addition of neutralizing anti-TNF antibodies to in vitro cultures of bone marrow in patients with CLL increased the number of myeloid colonies in 11 of 15 patients.

IL-6 and IL-1 are produced by CLL cells, raising the possibility of autocrine growth loops.[2, 126, 304, 349] CLL cells constitutively express the *IL1* and *IL6* genes and secrete IL-4 and IL-6.[304, 324] In a study by Foa, 20 of 24 patients had elevated circulating levels of TNF.[118] These levels could be increased after incubation with interferon-γ or phytohemagglutinin plus phorbol myristate acetate. The cellular release was higher in patients with early-stage disease than in patients with late-stage disease. TNF was able to induce only a proliferative signal in 4 of 24 patients. Whereas the role of cytokines in CLL is undoubtedly important, the roles of each cytokine and various autocrine loops have not been clearly established.

Apoptosis in CLL

The increased interest in apoptosis as a mechanism of cell death has led to investigations into the role of failure of apoptosis in vivo as a mechanism for the long-lived nature of CLL B-cells. CLL cells are characterized by defective apoptosis. *BCL2*, a proto-oncogene, is associated with production of Bcl-2 protein in resting mantle zone B lymphocytes. Bcl-2 protein protects cells from dying through the process of apoptosis. The characteristic t(14; 18) translocation in follicular lymphomas is not present in the majority of patients with CLL.[1] *BCL2* gene hypomethylation and high levels of Bcl-2 protein have been noted in most cases studied by Hanada and associates.[163] In many patients, there is an intense expression of Bcl-2 protein. Bcl protein can be identified in the cells of the majority of patients with CLL.[163, 350] Other members of the Bcl-2 family, such as Bcl-XL, an antiapoptotic protein, and Bax, a proapoptotic protein, are present at higher levels in CLL cells, whereas Bcl-XS is present at low levels.[225] Interferon-γ has been shown to prolong the life span of CLL cells in vitro by inhibiting apoptosis. Interferon-γ inhibits the loss of Bcl-2 protein in CLL cells in vitro and has been detected in the sera of 7 of 10 CLL cases tested.[46] This suggests that interferon-γ may play a role in the survival of CLL cells. IL-4 is another cytokine capable of inhibiting apoptosis of CLL cells. Reports have shown that IL-4 inhibits apoptosis of CLL cells and causes G0 arrest.[240] IL-1, IL-2, IL-3, IL-5, IL-7, TNF, and transforming growth factor-β have no such protective effect.[71] The diminished apoptosis with IL-4 is associated with increased cellular levels of Bcl-2 protein.[71, 289] The rapid apoptosis that CLL cells demonstrate in vitro can be inhibited by culture in appropriate microenvironments. CD40 activation makes CLL cells resistant to Fas/APO1-mediated apoptosis. CLL cells are resistant to anti-Fas-induced apoptosis. The mechanism of Fas resistance is unclear. The β1 and β2 integrins on bone marrow stromal cells interact with CLL cells and prevent apoptosis.[382]

There was marked heterogeneity in the apoptosis rate demonstrated among 45 patients with CLL.[333] The spontaneous apoptosis rate was significantly greater in cells obtained from patients in earlier stages. The lowest rates were observed in patients with heavily treated refractory disease, suggesting that an apoptosis-resistant phenotype may develop with disease progression. 9β-D-Arabinofuranosyl-2-fluoroadenine (F-ara-A) and 2-chlorodeoxyadenosine induce greater DNA fragmentation than that seen with spontaneous apoptosis, and fragmentation was greater in patients with earlier stage disease. These data suggest that the purine analogues may induce apoptosis as a mechanism of action in CLL.[339]

CYTOGENETICS AND MOLECULAR GENETICS IN CLL

The cytogenetic pattern in CLL has not been evaluated to the same extent as in other leukemias because of the low mitotic index in B-CLL. A variety of mitogenic agents have been used to increase the yield of metaphases in CLL. The most frequently used mitogens have been lipopolysaccharide from *Escherichia coli*, tetradecanoylphorbol acetate, cytochalasin B, Epstein-Barr virus, and pokeweed mitogen.[333] T cells appear to be necessary to obtain sufficient numbers of mitoses.[186]

The first chromosome analyses of B-CLL were reported in 1979 and showed an 11;14 translocation now known to be associated with mantle cell leukemia.[373] Shortly after, trisomy of chromosome 12 was identified as the most frequent abnormality in B-CLL.[133] Subsequent common abnormalities identified were the deletion of the long arm of chromosome 13,[186] abnormalities in chromosome 14, and more recently, abnormalities in chromosome 11.[187, 188] The International Workshop on CLL (IWCLL) initiated a major collaborative study in different countries to evaluate CLL chromosome abnormalities. Clinical, phenotypic, and chromosome data were collected, and these were initially published in 1990.[188] The initial report of 433 patients has been expanded to 662 in a later review. Of the 662 patients, 311 were noted to have clonal abnormalities.[187] The most common numeric abnormality was trisomy 12 (36% of those with clonal abnormalities). Additional trisomies were of chromosomes 3, 18, 8, 21, 19, and 22 in decreasing frequency. Monosomies most frequently involved chromosome 17, although loss of chromosome 6 was also noted. The most common structural abnormalities noted involved chromosomes 13, 14, 11, and 6. Chromosome regions most involved were 13q14, 14q32, 13q12, 11q13, and 13q22. Although trisomy 12 was the most common abnormality, structural abnormalities in chromosome 12 were uncommon, with some breaks in both the short and long arms of chromosome 12.

The most common structural abnormality found was on chromosome 13 (13q14), close to the site of the retinoblastoma gene.[111, 186, 188] Interstitial deletions involving 13q were found in 35 patients, and in all but one patient, the site of the retinoblastoma gene was deleted.[187] By use of a variety of techniques, such as fluorescent in situ hybridization (FISH) with DNA-specific probes, deletion in 13q14 can be identified in 50% to 60% of patients.[67, 92] It is thought that a tumor suppressor gene is lost from this area of 13q14. The retinoblastoma gene *RB1* is deleted by the deletion, as is *D13S25*. With

use of similar techniques, trisomy 12 was identified in 44% of patients and *P53* deletion in 12%.[92, 365] Structural abnormalities in chromosome 14 most commonly occurred at 14q32, the site of the immunoglobulin heavy-chain genes. The most common translocation was 11q13 to 14q32.[187] The abnormality on chromosome 11 occurs at the breakpoint commonly associated with *BCL1* or *PRAD1*.[373] Deletions in chromosome 6q were noted along with abnormalities in chromosome 17, with isochromosome 17q being noted along with deletions and the complete loss of chromosome 17. FISH probes determined abnormalities in chromosome 11 in 20% of patients, 17 in 10%, and 6q deletion in 8%.[365]

Juliusson and Gharaton[187] have analyzed the likelihood of missing trisomy 12 because of lack of metaphases. By use of the technique of restriction fragment length polymorphism on genes localized to chromosome 12, chromosome 12 abnormalities were never found in patients with normal or inevaluable karyotypes.[96] However, this finding is in contradistinction to other studies using the FISH technique, in which patients with normal or insufficient metaphases have been identified to have trisomy 12.[10, 99]

An evaluation was conducted in the IWCLL study as to whether clonal evolution occurred in CLL. Forty-one patients had repeated samples, and 15% showed a change in karyotype, with 12% showing an abnormal clone only once. Others have reported a similar likelihood of karyotypic evolution.[277, 284]

Although the IWCLL and other studies have not demonstrated a high incidence of clonal evolution, other investigators have evaluated clonal evolution by a variety of techniques.[300] Immunoglobulin gene rearrangement is a fingerprint of the clone of cells present, with one or sometimes two rearranged bands being usual.[122, 241] Studies of the stability of the immunoglobulin gene rearrangement indicate that most patients have maintenance of κ or λ light-chain expression but that a number of patients either lose an initial rearranged J_H allele or gain new alleles. This may result from isotype switching or somatic hypermutation.[300] Thus, the light-chain alleles (κ and λ) appear to be stable, whereas the J_H allele showed considerable lability. In one study, 8 of 24 patients observed had change in the J_H allele pattern. Four patients developed an additional J_H allele, and another four patients lost one rearranged allele.[300] Studies of transformation to a large-cell lymphoma, which occurs in some patients with CLL (Richter's syndrome), also found some patients with similar isotypes and some others with dissimilar immunoglobulin isotypes.[363, 372, 378] However, anti-idiotype studies suggest that Richter's syndrome occurs from the same cell population in some cases.[27] One study showed similar immunoglobulin gene patterns in four patients with Richter's syndrome and different patterns in two patients.[247]

A variety of investigators have studied clonal evolution by cytogenetic analysis. Most have reported that 15% to 20% of patients had clonal evolution.[187, 277, 284] One study of 79 patients with CLL demonstrated that 11 of 28 patients drawn from the population of 79 had new or additional clonal abnormalities identified. In addition, three patients had loss of previously detected normal metaphase cells, and six had loss of previously identified clonal aberrations.[300, 301]

A number of investigators have demonstrated that complex cytogenetic abnormalities occur more frequently in patients with advanced-stage disease. It appears that additional chromosome changes occur more frequently in patients who receive therapy and may be a consequence of evolution of disease or be induced by therapy. The overall prognostic impact of cytogenetic abnormalities requires comprehensive multivariate analysis of the population of patients, including the stage, degree of previous therapy, and other defined prognostic factors. The only analysis that has included all of these factors has been the IWCLL study.

Molecular Biology

The association of the *MYC* oncogene with t(8;14) in Burkitt's lymphoma and of the *BCL2* rearrangement with t(14;18) in follicular cleaved small-cell lymphoma has led to intense interest in the possibility of proto-oncogene involvement in the pathogenesis of CLL. Rearrangements of *BCL1*, *BCL2*, or *BCL3* are rarely found in patients with CLL, being noted in less than 5% of cases.[1, 24, 176, 189, 224, 315] Because of the interest in chromosome 12, the incidence of *RAS* gene mutations was explored, and no mutations were found in 51 patients with CLL or in another series of 42 patients.[43, 274] Other candidate genes that are being evaluated include *BCL1* on chromosome 11q13. No *BCL1* or *BCL2* rearrangements were found in one series of 38 cases of B-CLL.[323] In one series, 3 of 32 patients were found to have a *BCL2* gene translocation to the κ or λ light-chain genes.[1] As well as deletion of 11q13, deletion of 11q22–23 occurs and may involve the *ATM* gene (mutated in ataxia-telangiectasia) and redoxin (a homologue of the neuroblastoma type 2 tumor suppressor gene). Germline mutations of *ATM* have been identified in CLL and confer a poor prognosis.[44, 365]

Because of the association of the *BCL2* gene with the t(14;18) chromosome translocation in follicular lymphomas, extensive investigation of this gene and gene product has been conducted in CLL. A few cases of *BCL2* gene rearrangement have been reported in CLL. In one study, none of 20 specimens had evidence of *BCL2* gene rearrangement on the basis of Southern blot analysis.[163] Studies of Bcl protein, however, demonstrated that 14 of 20 cases (70%) had levels of p26 Bcl-2 protein that were equal or greater than those found in lymphoma cell lines. In all but one case, the Bcl-2 protein was present at levels 1.7- to 25-fold higher than in normal peripheral blood lymphocytes. Cells of the patients with higher levels of Bcl protein survive longer in culture. Complete demethylation of both copies of the *BCL2* gene in a region corresponding to a 2.4-kilobase *MSP1* fragment was noted in all 20 cases. The impact of this finding in subsequent studies of the role of *BCL2* in maintaining viability of CLL cells is likely to yield significant information.

The retinoblastoma gene *(RB)* is located on the long arm of chromosome 13. None of 44 patients and 1 of 40 patients were reported to have mutations of *RB* by Southern blot analysis.[140, 315] Deletion of the gene has been demonstrated in three of seven patients with B-CLL.[283]

Studies of *RB* gene deletion occurred in 11 of 35 patients with B-CLL by use of in situ hybridization. Most of these patients did not have abnormalities in chromosome 13 documented on conventional cytogenetic analysis.[364] Somatic cell hybrids have been used to identify the 13q breakpoint in CLL. A high frequency of deletions of *D13S25*, at a locus distinct from *RB* and separated from *RB* by 530 kilobases, has been demonstrated. This deletion occurs more frequently than does the loss of *RB*.

Mutations of *p53* have been identified in 6 (15%) of 40 cases of CLL and in 3 of 7 patients with Richter's transformation.[134] In a later series, 10 of 53 patients had *p53* mutations in CLL. Patients were resistant to therapy and had a short survival time. None of 36 patients with CLL had abnormalities in the *BCL3* locus on chromosome 17q22.[386]

A high level of expression of *MDR1* and *MDR3* genes has been described in CLL.[97, 175, 263, 360, 383, 385] By use of specific probes for *MDR1* and *MDR3*, expression of both genes could be identified in 29 of 31 patients with CLL.[360] Patients with advanced-stage disease had significantly higher expression of *MDR3* than did those with early-stage disease. This difference was not noted for *MDR1*. These findings have been confirmed by other investigators who also noted an increased level of glutathione-*S*-transferase pi gene *(GST-pi)* expression in patients with CLL.[383] *GST-pi* gene is thought to be involved in cases of resistance to alkylating agents and is associated with *MDR* gene expression in some studies.[385]

Immunoglobulin Gene Utilization

During B-cell oncogeny, discontinuous genetic elements within the immunoglobulin genes for heavy chains and κ and λ light chains undergo a series of rearrangements to form the exons that will eventually encode the immunoglobulin molecule.[175] Initial gene rearrangement occurs within the heavy-chain gene complex and subsequently within the κ genes. In the heavy-chain locus, more than 20 small genes called diversity segments, which are located between the variable region genes (V_H genes), and six functional J_H minigenes rearrange and become juxtaposed with a single J_H element.[322, 325] This DJ_H complex rearranges with any one of hundreds of different V_H genes. This eventually forms a $V_H DJ_H$ exon to encode the variable part of the heavy chain of an antibody. After the heavy-chain rearrangement forms $V_H DJ_H$, the κ V genes (V_K genes), which are approximately 70 in number, undergo rearrangement to juxtapose with one of the five J_K minigenes. This rearrangement produces an exon that encodes the κ light-chain variable region.[353] Only if these gene rearrangements fail to form a functional exon do rearrangements of the λ light-chain genes occur in one of the four functional $J_\lambda C_\lambda$ complexes to elicit λ light-chain expression.[379]

Within the immunoglobulin variable regions, a number of subgroups occur. Four immunoglobulin variable region frameworks of limited amino acid sequence diversity exist between the immunoglobulin heavy- and light-chain variable regions.[193] Between these framework regions are complementarity-determining regions. The combination of the rearrangement of the immunoglobulin genes and somatic hypermutation, which occurs in the immunoglobulin V genes, creates tremendous diversity in the immunoglobulin repertoire.[244]

A variety of antibodies against immunoglobulins have been used to identify the subgroups within the immunoglobulins that are produced. Using antisera against immunoglobulins, investigators have defined cross-reactive idiotypes found initially as rheumatoid factors (IgM autoantibodies).[242, 295]

In CLL, 25% of κ light chain–expressing B cells expressed the 17.109 cross-reactive idiotype.[220] In 20% of patients with CLL, cells expressing both κ and λ light chains reacted with G6, another monoclonal antibody.[242] A third monoclonal antibody, termed Lc1, reacted with immunoglobulin-positive B cells in 13% of patients with CLL.[221] The pattern of these autoantibody-associated cross-reactive idiotypes has been tracked back to immunoglobulin V gene expression, and this has been found to be highly restricted.[223] Analysis of cases of B-CLL with the rearranged V_H1 gene demonstrated a disproportionally high use of the *51P1* gene, which encodes the G6 cross-reactive idiotype (two thirds of cases).[351] Other small V_H genes are overrepresented in the immunoglobulin heavy-chain rearrangements in CLL.[218] In a fashion similar to V_H gene expression, $V_κ$ gene rearrangement has been demonstrated to be nonrandom. The $V_κ3$ gene designated *Humkv325* leads to expression of the 17.109 cross-reactive idiotype.[223] In 24% of patients with CLL expressing λ light chain, two genes entitled *Humkv325* and *Vg* are frequently associated with abortive $V_κ$ gene rearrangements.[321] Subgroups of λ light-chain V gene have also been found to be restricted.[47]

Immunohistochemical staining with antibodies specific for major cross-reactive idiotypes demonstrates a subpopulation of B cells within the mantle zone of human lymph nodes. This is the site of the CD5$^+$ B cell. CD5$^+$ B cells spontaneously produce IgM autoantibodies with cross-reacting idiotypes.[53 167]

Anti-idiotypes have been used in therapy for CLL with impressive but short-lived responses.[6] Development of the idiotype and anti-idiotype antibodies for immunotherapy is time-consuming and complex. The possibility of using antibodies against cross-reactive idiotypes may allow the development of new immunotherapy for patients with CLL.[223]

Immune Function

Patients with CLL exhibit a diverse and extensive pattern of dysfunction of the immune system. In addition to the well-known decrease in serum immunoglobulin levels,[21] there is a relative reduction in the proportion of CD4$^+$ (T-helper) cells and an increased proportion of CD8$^+$ (T-suppressor) cells, leading to an inverted CD4$^+$/CD8$^+$ ratio in some patients, especially in those with progressive disease.[197, 230] Despite this inverted ratio, there is an increase in the absolute number of CD4$^+$ and CD8$^+$ cells through all stages of disease, but this increase is more prominent in early stages.[55, 327] The T cells that are present have reduced responsiveness to antigenic and mitogenic stimulation.[157, 328] Other studies have addressed the activity of natural killer (NK) cells, antibody-dependent cellular cytotoxicity, and lymphokine-activated killer (LAK) cell activity; these activities have been noted to be defective,[118, 307] with a decrease in autologous LAK cell activity.[113] Because of the importance of IL-2 in T-cell function, studies have led to the awareness that levels of soluble IL-2 receptor are increased and reduce IL-2 availability to CLL cells.[13, 115]

Hypogammaglobulinemia

Hypogammaglobulinemia occurs in 10% to 50% of patients with B-CLL, depending on the level set as the lower limit of normal.[21, 342] All of the three main classes of immunoglobulin, namely, IgG, IgA, and IgM, are affected, although IgA is more commonly affected than are the other types early in the disease.[342] There is a strong tendency for the hypogammaglobulinemia to worsen with progression of disease, rendering patients more susceptible to infections (Table 28–2). Early in the disease, the most common infections that are noted are bacterial, but gram-negative bacterial infections, fungal infections, and viral infections subsequently develop and are commonly associated with a fatal outcome of the disease.[226] The contribution of hypogammaglobulinemia to this changing spectrum of infections is not well understood. The levels of immunoglobulins according to the stage of disease and the extent of previous treatment in the M.D. Anderson Cancer Center (MDACC) series are illustrated in Table 28–2. PLL is also associated with hypogammaglobulinemia. Even patients with early forms of the disease have defective antibody responses to infection or immunization with specific antigens. The reason for the association of hypogammaglobulinemia with B-CLL is not well understood because it is uncommon in acute lymphocytic leukemia, B-cell lymphomas, and HCL but common in multiple myeloma.[86] Attempts to associate hypogammaglobulinemia with abnormalities in T-cell number and function, NK cell activity, and antibody-dependent cell-

TABLE 28–2. Relationship Between Incidence of Hypogammaglobulinemia, Binet Stage, and Previous Treatment Status (MDACC)

Immunoglobulin (mg²)	Untreated, Binet Stage (No. of Patients)			Previously Treated, Binet Stage		
	A (536)	B (238)	C (117)	A (214)	B (187)	C (394)
IgG <600	.14*	.22	.32	.43	.51	.55
IgA <50	.11	.21	.30	.37	.47	.54
IgM <30	.10	.24	.33	.34	.36	.39

*Proportion of patients with low levels.
MDACC, M.D. Anderson Cancer Center.

mediated cytotoxicity have not established such a relationship.[86] It is difficult to document the number of residual normal (CD5$^-$) B cells in CLL. There is a possibility that the hypogammaglobulinemia is due to a decrease in normal CD5$^-$ B cells. The murine counterpart of CD5$^-$ B cells (Ly1$^-$ B cells) responds poorly to exogenous antigens.

Monoclonal Gammopathy

Small monoclonal bands are noted in 5% to 10% of patients with B-CLL and are usually IgM.[78] If more sophisticated techniques are used to search for heavy or light immunoglobulin chains in serum or urine, up to 25% of patients with B-CLL may have circulating or excreted immunoglobulin components.[78] More sophisticated techniques, namely, high-resolution agarose gel electrophoresis and immunofixation, show a small amount of a monoclonal immunoglobulin component in more than 50% of patients.[291]

Autoimmunity

Autoimmune abnormalities are commonly noted in B-CLL. Strikingly, these autoimmune events appear largely restricted to the hematopoietic system; Coombs' test–positive autoimmune hemolytic anemia, immune thrombocytopenia, pure red blood cell aplasia, and other abnormalities are most commonly described.[152] Attempts to demonstrate a higher association of autoantibodies against other organ systems in CLL have not proved true. Thus, patients with CLL do not have a significantly higher incidence of other autoimmune diseases.[152] A positive result of the direct antiglobulin test has been reported in 10% to 35% of patients with B-CLL, varying with the stage of the disease.[86, 152] French investigators find a low incidence of Coombs' test positivity at diagnosis (1%), but between 10% and 25% of the patients developed direct antiglobulin test–positive hemolytic anemia at some stage during the course of their disease.[219] An Italian study found 52 cases (43%) of autoimmune hemolytic anemia in 1203 patients observed at a single institution.[250] The antibody was IgG in 82% of cases and IgM in 13%. High white blood cell count, advanced age, and male sex were associated. No difference was noted in patients treated with fludarabine or chlorambucil.

Most of these autoantibodies are IgG warm antibodies and are directed against the Rh system. The antibodies are not produced by the leukemic B cells.[86] It is possible that treatment with radiation therapy or chemotherapy may trigger autoimmune complications because there is often a close temporal relationship with the initiation of therapy. In one series of patients treated with fludarabine, there appeared to be no strong association with the stage of disease or whether the patients were receiving treatment, had discontinued treatment, were in remission, or had active disease.[83] It is considered that the development of the autoimmunity may be related to the dysregulation of T-cell subsets. It is well known that CD5$^+$ B cells are involved in regulation of natural autoantibodies. It is postulated that a disturbance in the idiotypic network may be involved in autoimmunity.[77, 78, 83, 86, 152,]

[166, 170, 219, 291] The inhibition of anti–factor VIII autoantibodies by injection of intravenous immune globulin suggests that anti-idiotype suppression by exogenous immunoglobulins can occur.[367]

Antibodies secreted into supernatants of CLL B lymphocytes stimulated with phorbol esters or from hybridomas demonstrate that a high proportion of CLL B cells produce natural autoantibodies.[87, 219] Half of the CLL B cells displayed rheumatoid factor activity. Kipps and colleagues[220] have demonstrated a strong association of κ light-chain variable region genes with the use of the unmutated Humkv325 gene, which is associated with a WA idiotype, a major cross-reactive idiotype (noted in cryoglobulins). Although CD5$^+$ B cells are associated with natural autoantibody production, this can also occur in CD5$^-$ B cells and in comparable animal models.[87, 219]

T-Cell Dysfunction

Because of the tremendous expansion in the neoplastic B-cell population in CLL, the percentage of T cells that are present in blood, bone marrow, lymph nodes, and spleen is decreased. However, studies have now demonstrated that the absolute number of T cells is indeed increased.[160, 197, 246] The percentage of T lymphocytes progressively decreases as the stage of the disease increases.[197, 228] T-cell subset distribution shows a progressive fall in the proportion of T-helper cells compared with T-suppressor cells as the clinical stage increases.[197, 228, 230] A number of functional studies have demonstrated a depressed or delayed response to mitogenic and antigenic stimulation,[328] a diminished mixed lymphocyte reaction,[157] and a reduced T-cell clonogenic capacity.[72] The functional activity of the T lymphocytes also decreases with disease progression.[116, 198]

NK cells and antibody-dependent cell-mediated cytotoxicity are decreased.[117] A large proportion of CD4$^+$ B cells in CLL have been reported to have granules.[380] Others have reported that the azurophilic granules in the NK cell in B-CLL may be defective.[200] LAK cell function is decreased in B-CLL, and leukemic B-CLL cells appear to be largely insensitive to the lytic action of autologous LAK cells.[113]

Various hypotheses have been generated to explain the T-cell dysfunction in CLL. Because of its importance in T-cell proliferation and function, IL-2 is being intensively studied in patients with CLL. It has been suggested that IL-2 may be absorbed by the massive neoplastic B-cell population and that the production by the residual T-cell population may be inadequate.[13, 115] Exogenous IL-2 can restore some functions of T cells in B-CLL, namely, the clonogenic potential and cytotoxic function.[8, 112] A proportion of B-CLL cells express the p55 antigen of the IL-2 receptor, and some have p75 expressed as well.[115] In addition, a proportion of patients with CLL have elevated levels of the soluble IL-2 receptor, which may play a role in quenching the activity of this important regulatory cytokine.[363] There is evidence that T cells in CLL are monoclonal in some cases. It is more likely that the decrease in T-cell number and function as the disease progresses is a secondary event. T-cell immunodeficiency may be improved by splenic irradiation and splenectomy.[252] Of concern in the use of purine analogues in the management of CLL is that these agents have an effect in decreasing $CD4^+$ and $CD8^+$ cell numbers. This decrease appears to be sustained despite discontinuation of therapy even in patients in remission.

DIAGNOSTIC CRITERIA

Ambiguity still persists as to the minimal diagnostic criteria for CLL. All recommendations require that the lower limit of the lymphocyte count in the peripheral blood of patients with CLL is greater than 4×10^9/L (the upper limit of normal) and more than 25% lymphocytes in the bone marrow.[60, 178] Increases in lymphocytes in blood and bone marrow must be sustained to differentiate them from reactive lymphocytosis due to infections and other causes. In morphologic appearance, the lymphocytes should be predominantly mature to exclude other variants, such as PLL, HCL, large granular lymphocyte leukemia, and Sézary cell leukemia. Two working groups, the National Cancer Institute Working Group (NCIWG) and IWCLL, have submitted recommendations for diagnosis and recommendations for the evaluation of patients' responses and indications for commencement of therapy[60, 178] (Table 28–3). Both require an absolute sustained lymphocytosis in the peripheral blood and the bone marrow.

A minimal threshold for blood lymphocytes is 5×10^9/L in the NCIWG study[60] and 10×10^9/L in the IWCLL study.[178] In the IWCLL study, lower lymphocyte counts are accepted if lymphocyte phenotyping demonstrates a typical pattern of $CD5^+$ B cells. The NCIWG established criteria for atypical cells as being more than 55% (PLL), and patients with a mixed PLL/CLL population of 11% to 55% were identified. Bone marrow aspiration in both studies required more than 30% lymphocytes on bone marrow differential. Bone marrow was required to be normocellular or hypercellular in the NCIWG study; this factor was not commented on in the IWCLL study. The lymphocyte immunophenotype required presence of cells positive for CD19 or CD20 and co-expression of CD5 in the absence of other pan–T-cell markers. Light-chain expression is restricted to κ or λ, and surface immunoglobulin had low cell surface density expression (Table 28-4). The French-American-British group have proposed a classification for CLL presented in Table 28-5.[23]

Most cases of CLL are easy to diagnose by clinical examination, peripheral blood analysis, and immunophenotyping of the peripheral blood. Atypical forms often require subtle testing to differentiate one from another. PLL is reported frequently by investigators in Europe, whereas it appears to be a much less common disease in the United States.[255, 256] HCL is seldom a difficult differen-

TABLE 28–3. Comparison of NCIWG and IWCLL Guidelines for CLL

	NCIWG	IWCLL
Diagnosis		
Lymphocytes × 10⁹/L	>5	• ≥10 and B phenotype or bone marrow involved
		• <10 and both of above
Atypical cells	>55%	Not stated
Duration of lymphocytosis	≥2 mo	Not stated
Bone marrow lymphocytes	≥30%	>30%
Staging	Rai, correlate with Binet	IWCLL
Eligibility for trials	Active bulky or progressive disease	A: >50 × 10⁹/L lymphocytes; doubling time <12 mo, diffuse marrow
Response criteria		B, C: all patients
Complete response (CR)		
Physical examination	Normal	Normal
Symptoms	None	None
Lymphocytes	≤4 × 10⁹/L	<4 × 10⁹/L
Neutrophils	≥1.5 × 10⁹/L	>1.5 × 10⁹/L
Platelets	>100 × 10⁹/L	>100 × 10⁹/L
Hemoglobin	>11%/dL	Not stated
Bone marrow lymphocytes	<30%	Normal
Bone marrow biopsy	No nodules or infiltrates, if present	Nodules or infiltrates permitted
Nodular partial response	CR except for bone marrow nodules or infiltrates	Not stated
Partial response (PR)		
Physical examination (nodes, liver, spleen)	≥50% decrease	Downshift in stage
Plus one or more:		
Neutrophils	≥1.5 × 10⁹/L	Duration of CR or PR
Platelets	>100 × 10⁹/L or 50% improvement	Progressive disease
Hemoglobin (g/dL)	>11	
≥2 mo	Not stated	Physical examination (nodes, liver, spleen)
Stable disease	Upshift in stage	Circulating lymphocytes
	≥50% increase or new site	Other
	≥50% increase	
	Richter's syndrome	No change in stage
	All others	

NCIWG, National Cancer Institute Working Group; IWCLL, International Workshop on Chronic Lymphocytic Leukemia.

TABLE 28–4. Surface Marker Pattern in B-CLL and Other Chronic Lymphoid Disorders

Monoclonal Antibody	B-CLL	B-PLL	NHL	HCL	T-CLL/PLL	MCL	SLVL
CD19	+ +	+ +	+ +	+ +	−	+ +	+
CD20	+	+ +	+ +	+ +	−	+ +	+ +
CD5	+ +	− (+)	− (+)	−	− (+)		− (+)
CD23	+	−	− (+)	−	−	−	−
SmIg	+ (dim)	+ +	+ +	+ +	−	+ +	+ +
CD29B	− (dim)	+ +	+ +	+	−	+ +	+ +
CD10	−	− (+)	+ +	−	−	−	−
FMC7	− (+)	+ + +	− (+)	+ +	−	+ +	+ +
CD103	−	−	−	+ +	−	−	−
CD2	−	−	−	−	+ +	−	−
CD4	−	−	−	−	− (+)	−	−
CD8	−	−	−	−	+	−	−

B-CLL, B-cell chronic lymphocytic leukemia; B-PLL, B-cell prolymphocytic leukemia; NHL, non-Hodgkin's lymphoma; HCL, hairy cell leukemia; T-CLL/PLL, T-cell chronic lymphocytic leukemia/prolymphocytic leukemia; MCL, mantle cell lymphoma; SLVL, splenic lymphoma with villous lymphocytes; +, occasionally positive; + +, usually positive; + + +, almost always positive; −, negative.

tial diagnosis, whereas splenic lymphoma with villous lymphocytes,[250, 272] leukemic phase of follicular lymphoma,[308] and intermediate or mantle zone lymphomas[308] are more difficult to differentiate. A scoring system for the diagnoses proposed by Matutes and coworkers[249] is based on expression of CD5, CD23, FMC7, surface immunoglobulin, and CD22/CD79b and should prove useful for identifying variants of CLL.

The main purpose of having an absolute lymphocyte count requirement is to differentiate patients with CLL from those with small lymphocytic lymphoma, a disease that shares immunophenotypic and morphologic features. Small lymphocytic lymphoma is differentiated from

CLL by a relative lack of involvement of the peripheral blood and less infiltration of bone marrow.[20]

Clinical Features

The majority of patients with CLL are asymptomatic at the time of initial diagnosis. Many come to see the physician because they have noted node enlargement. A few patients complain of left upper quadrant discomfort related to splenomegaly and have the symptom of early satiety. Fever, sweats, and weight loss (so-called B-symptoms) occur in less than 2% of patients at diagnosis, and

TABLE 28–5. Characteristics of Patients According to French-American-British Proposal for Classification of Chronic Lymphocytic Leukemia

	Approximate Percentage of Cases	Male/Female	Median Age at Therapy (yr)
Mature B-Cell Leukemia			
CLL—common	90–95	1.5:1	65
CLL—mixed (CLL/PLL)	1	1.5:1	65–70
PLL	1	1.5:1	70
HCL	2–5	5:1	50
HCL variant	<1	M>F	50
Splenic lymphoma with villous lymphocytes	1–2	M>F	50–60
NHL—leukemic phase of follicular or mantle zone lymphoma	<1	2:1	45–50
Lymphoplasmacytic lymphoma	1–2	1.2:1	60
Plasma cell leukemia	<1	2:1	55–60
Mature T-Cell Leukemia			
LGL	1	1.1	60
T-cell PLL	<1	M>F	65
ATL	Regional	Regional	60
Sézary's syndrome	<1	2.1	50

ATL, adult T-cell leukemia; HCL, hairy cell leukemia; LGL, large granular lymphocytes leukemia; NHL, non-Hodgkin's lymphoma; PLL, prolymphocytic leukemia.

less than 5% of patients have had a significant infection. Anemia (hemoglobin level <11 g/dL) is present in less than 5% of patients at diagnosis, causing typical symptoms of fatigue, shortness of breath, and dizziness. In many, an autoimmune mechanism is identified with a positive Coombs' test result, high reticulocyte count, and low serum haptoglobin level. Thrombocytopenia is also uncommon at diagnosis; less than 5% of patients have a platelet count below $100 \times 10^9/L$. Clinical symptoms of purpura, ecchymosis, and bleeding from other sites are rare. Nasal, labial, or genital herpetic lesions may be noted. An exaggerated reaction to insect bites is a poorly understood feature that is characteristic of CLL, occurring in 2% to 5% of patients at the time of initial diagnosis.

Increasingly, patients are being diagnosed while they are asymptomatic at an early stage of their disease because of the increased use of routine blood tests in the evaluation of other conditions or as a preoperative test.[49,88] Some patients have fever, fatigue, or malaise, of no apparent cause, that persists as an irritating feature despite a relatively low tumor burden and no other indication for therapy. As the disease progresses, treatment is initiated; with chemotherapy resistance, weakness, night sweats, fever, loss of weight, and recurrent infections of bacterial, fungal, and viral etiology are noted more frequently. Bleeding abnormalities are rare except in the uncommon circumstance in which severe thrombocytopenia has developed.

On clinical examination, the most characteristic feature is lymphadenopathy, which may involve a single area, most commonly the cervical area, but may involve all lymph node-bearing areas. Nodes tend to be firm, discrete, freely mobile, and nontender. As the disease progresses, the lymph nodes become much larger and often become confluent and matted but usually remain freely movable. Tender, hard, fixed nodes should be evaluated with fine-needle aspiration or biopsy for diagnosis of large-cell lymphomatous (Richter's) transformation, cancer metastatic from another site, or infection. Marked enlargement of the liver is uncommon, but moderate to marked splenomegaly is not. When enlargement of the spleen is present as a striking feature in the absence of lymphadenopathy, it should suggest mantle zone lymphoma,[308] splenic lymphoma with villous lymphocytes,[250, 272] or PLL.[254, 255]

Some patients will have a variety of rashes that are often nonspecific.[36] Biopsy findings may illustrate lymphocytic infiltration, but they are usually not characteristic. Infiltration of the ocular area, salivary glands, gastrointestinal tract, or lungs should raise the possibility of mucosa-associated lymphoid tissue or mantle cell lymphoma.[164, 287] Clinically significant involvement of other organs, such as the heart, lung, and kidneys, is uncommon, particularly early in the disease, and central nervous system infiltration is rare in CLL.[287, 352] As the disease progresses, lymph nodes can become massive but seldom cause obstruction of ducts or viscera. In addition, despite massive lymphadenopathy, lymphedema is an uncommon feature. Occasional patients develop ascites and pleural effusions late in their illness, a poor prognostic sign. The percentages of patients with various symptoms and signs at the time of presentation at the MDACC are presented in Table 28–6.

Laboratory Findings

The most important factor in the diagnosis of CLL is lymphocytosis in the peripheral blood and the bone mar-

TABLE 28–6. Percentage of Untreated Patients with CLL Clinical and Laboratory Features by Rai Stage*

Characteristics	Stage 0 (342 Patients)	Stages I and II (698 Patients)	Stages III and IV (210 Patients)
Clinical Features (%)			
Fever, sweats	3	3	7
Infections	20	18	25
Weight loss (≥7 lb)	7	9	17
Node groups			
0	100	6	23
1	—	28	10
2	—	29	29
3	—	37	38
Splenomegaly	0	24	55
Hepatomegaly	0	13	27
Laboratory Values (Median)			
Hemoglobin (g/dL)	14.1	13.8	10.3
White blood cell count $\times 10^3/\mu L$	23.2	30.4	51.0
Platelet count $\times 10^3/\mu L$	227	193	99
Lymphocytes (%)	74.5	80.5	88.5
IgG	906	843	775
IgA	131	106	82
IgM	62	55	46
Bone Marrow (Median)			
Cellularity	40	53	80
Lymphocytes (%)	51	68	83

*M.D. Anderson Cancer Center, 1975 to 1999, 1260 patients.

row. The minimal diagnostic criteria are described in Table 28–3. The cells appear to be morphologically mature lymphocytes. The majority of patients have marked leukocytosis. The white blood cell count increases with the clinical stage of the disease, varying from 10×10^9/L to 250×10^9/L, with the lymphocyte proportion on the white blood cell differential count being 50% to 99% (see Table 28–6). Extremely high white blood cell counts are uncommon in the early stage of disease, and a hyperviscosity syndrome due to a high white blood cell count is rare in CLL.[234] The hemoglobin level varies with the stage of disease (see Table 28–6) and degree of previous therapy, and a small percentage of patients are anemic or thrombocytopenic at diagnosis. Direct antiglobulin (Coombs') test results are positive at some stage in 15% to 20% of patients with CLL but usually in less than 5% of patients at the time of diagnosis.[73, 88, 152] Because almost all the lymphocytes in the peripheral blood are B cells, the ratio of T cells to B cells in the peripheral blood is markedly changed from normal (3:1) to 1:20 to 1:50. However, an absolute increase in T cells is found in blood and bone marrow and lymph nodes.[160, 197, 246] Patients with B-CLL characteristically express the pan–B-cell markers CD19 and CD20 and co-express CD5.[15, 121, 124, 338] The ratio of CD4$^+$ to CD8$^+$ T cells at time of diagnosis is usually normal but, in some cases, may be reversed.[197, 228] Immunophenotypic studies, in addition to confirming the pan–B-cell and CD5 expression, will usually demonstrate a clonal excess of membrane-bound κ or λ light chains.[19, 124] Low-intensity expression of surface immunoglobulin is found, and it is either sIgM or sIgD or a combination of both. Less commonly, sIgG is present.[19, 124] The cells are morphologically small with a narrow rim of cytoplasm, and the nuclear chromatin is dense. Nucleoli are not visible. Peripheral blood smears may disrupt CLL lymphocytes during preparation of the blood film and cause "smudge" cells. A bone marrow examination is not essential to establish a diagnosis of CLL because in more than 95% of patients with sustained peripheral lymphocytosis, bone marrow aspirates usually demonstrate more than 30% lymphocytes. The percentage of lymphocytes in the bone marrow increases with the stage of disease at diagnosis. The patient can have intertrabecular foci or nodules of mature lymphocytes, an interstitial infiltrate, a combination of these patterns, or diffuse infiltration. The nodular patterns are more common in early-stage disease, and the diffuse pattern becomes more prominent as the disease progresses and in patients with advanced-stage disease at diagnosis. Although lymph node biopsies are not usually performed, if they are done, the lymph node architecture is found to be effaced by small, well-differentiated lymphocytes.[232] Small foci of atypical lymphocytes may be found on occasion. Pseudonodules can also be found in the lymph node biopsy specimen.[313]

Several investigators have described different patterns of bone marrow infiltration. The most widely used classification is probably that of Rozman and colleagues,[340] which is categorized by (1) interstitial, (2) nodular, (3) mixed interstitial and nodular, and (4) diffuse patterns. In addition to the bone marrow biopsy pattern being associated with stage of disease, it is also related to the level of the white blood cell count. Rozman and colleagues[340] have reported a multivariate analysis of 329 patients with CLL in whom bone marrow biopsy had been performed. Age, lymph node involvement, hepatosplenomegaly, lymphocyte count, hemoglobin level, platelet count, and bone marrow pattern were considered. Bone marrow pattern, hemoglobin level, and hepatomegaly were considered to be independent variables. The bone marrow biopsy pattern was the strongest feature in both the previously undiagnosed and the previously diagnosed patients, and the authors considered that the bone marrow histologic pattern was the best single prognostic parameter for survival (diffuse adverse versus nondiffuse). The bone marrow pattern at the time of diagnosis will predict in which patients development of progressive disease is more likely.[293, 340]

Blood chemistry testing is not usually helpful in CLL. Occasional patients will have an increase in serum lactate dehydrogenase, bilirubin, or uric acid. These features tend to be more common as the disease progresses or if hemolysis exists. Rarely, patients are hypercalcemic at the time of diagnosis, but this condition develops in some patients as a poor prognostic feature later in the illness.[355]

Little has been written about the radiologic findings in CLL. Computed tomographic scans sometimes demonstrate marked abdominal lymph node enlargement when peripheral lymph node enlargement is not prominent. A chest x-ray study is usually an adequate method of demonstrating the degree of intrathoracic involvement at the time of initial diagnosis. Flow cytometry enables evaluation of the size of cells by use of volume histograms. These studies confirm that B-CLL lymphocytes are a uniform population of small cells, with the larger cells that predominate in B-PLL being 50% larger. The proportion of lymphocytes can be evaluated from the two cell volume curves.[273]

Ultrastructural studies demonstrate that CLL lymphocytes have condensed nuclear chromatin and scanty cytoplasm with virtually no organelles. The nucleolus is small or absent. On the other hand, prolymphocytes have more abundant cytoplasm, peripheral chromatin condensation, and prominent nucleolus.[29, 255, 256, 316]

Differential Diagnosis

A variety of monoclonal antibodies against surface antigens can be applied to the evaluation of patients with CLL. These are useful for confirmation of the diagnosis and differentiation between the less common subvarieties of the chronic lymphoid leukemias. In reactive lymphocytosis (e.g., acute infectious lymphocytosis), pertussis, and other viral infections (e.g., infectious mononucleosis, cytomegalovirus mononucleosis, and *Toxoplasma* infections), the lymphocytes are usually large, activated lymphocytes. They are mostly T cells, and B-cell populations are polyclonal. In contradistinction, the characteristic CLL cell is CD5$^+$; the lymphocytosis is sustained and can be demonstrated to be monoclonal by the use of light-chain restriction on the surface and immunoglobulin gene rearrangement patterns.

The most important differential diagnosis is between PLL, HCL, splenic lymphoma with circulating villous lymphocytes, the leukemic phase of non-Hodgkin's lymphoma, and Waldenström's macroglobulinemia. In PLL, the phenotype differs from CLL in that it has more intense expression of surface immunoglobulins, low mouse rosette formation, lower CD5 expression, and greater positivity for FMC7.[53] Some patients have a mixture of typical CLL cells and prolymphocytes (PLL/CLL).[254, 255] This combination of types is more common as the disease evolves into a prolymphocytic transformation rather than being present at diagnosis. Patients with PLL tend to have high white blood cell counts, with the degree of splenomegaly out of proportion to the degree of lymph node involvement.[254, 255] Prolymphocytes morphologically differ from typical CLL cells in that they have a larger size, a prominent nucleolus, and a lower nuclear-to-cytoplasmic ratio.

HCL is seldom a difficult diagnosis in that these patients usually present with splenomegaly and pancytopenia. In some patients, however, there is an elevated white blood cell count in the range of 10 to 30 × 10⁹/L. These cells can be morphologically differentiated by the presence of hairy cell projections and have a positive reaction to tartrate-resistant acid phosphatase staining; they are usually CD5⁻ and have a high expression of CD25, CD110, and CD103. Atypical variants of HCL have morphologic features intermediate between HCL and PLL and are often tartrate-resistant acid phosphatase negative, CD103⁻, and CD25⁻.[344] The bone marrow biopsy pattern has increased connective tissue in HCL and a lesser degree of infiltration by the lymphoid cells. Splenic lymphoma with circulating villous lymphocytes (marginal zone CLL) usually presents with massive splenomegaly, moderate leukocytosis (10 to 25 × 10⁹/L) with serum or urine monoclonal immunoglobulin bands in one half to two thirds of cases, and lymphocytes characterized by cytoplasmic villous projections. The membrane markers include moderate to strong surface immunoglobulin, usually CD5⁻, CD23⁻, CD79b⁺, FMC7⁺, and CD22⁺.[250, 272]

Some patients with non-Hodgkin's lymphoma, usually follicular or diffuse cleaved small-cell types, develop a leukemic phase (not usually a feature at that time of initial diagnosis). The cells are usually cleaved and pleomorphic. Lymph node biopsy usually demonstrates a different pattern, with follicles being prominent in most cases.[257, 362] The histologic appearance of the bone marrow is also usually follicular. The immunologic features that differentiate these patients from those with CLL are a strong surface immunoglobulin expression, FMC7⁺ and CD10⁺, and negative reaction to CD5.[257] Patients with Waldenström's macroglobulinemia usually have modest lymph node and spleen enlargement and only moderate lymphocytosis. The characteristic feature is the IgM paraprotein. The low number of circulating lymphocytes generally have plasmacytoid features. A combination of clinical features, morphologic appearance, immunophenotyping, electrophoresis evaluation, special stains, and occasionally cytogenetic information usually clearly separates these chronic lymphoid leukemias (see Tables 28–4 and 28–5).

STAGING SYSTEMS

Survival of patients with CLL varies widely. Some patients survive less than 1 year from diagnosis, and many continue to live in excellent health for more than 20 years after diagnosis. Early studies illustrated that patients with more advanced disease in terms of tumor burden, white blood cell count, and marrow failure had shorter survival.[35] Galton noted different patterns of change in the lymphocyte count. Some patients had a steady increase in the lymphocyte count, whereas others had no rise in the white blood cell count or established a new plateau after a period of increase. Other patients tended to have an oscillating pattern, with the white blood cell count alternately rising and falling. Dameshek[69] initially developed a staging system for CLL that included symptoms, size of lymph nodes, extent of splenomegaly, fever, and infections. None of these staging systems provided reproducible prognostic information.

Rai Staging System

In 1975, Rai and colleagues[317] developed a staging system (Table 28–7) that has since been prospectively found to be reproducible in independent groups of patients with a good prognostic stratification.[131, 243, 271] The Rai staging system was initially developed from a population of patients that included both previously treated and untreated patients; some had been recently diagnosed, and many had been observed for long periods. Despite these limitations, it has been amazingly robust. The staging system is based on the following categories: stage 0, lymphocytosis and bone marrow involvement; stage I, lymph node enlargement; stage II, splenomegaly or hepatomegaly; stage III, anemia; and stage IV, thrombocytopenia. The application of the Rai staging system to previously untreated patients from the date of their first presentation at the MDACC is illustrated in Figure 28–1. The median projected survival of patients in Rai's initial publication varied from a median survival time of more than 150 months for stage 0 to 19 months for stage III and stage IV. The median survival in most recent series for patients assigned to Rai stage III and stage IV is 3 to 4 years (see Fig. 28–1). The shorter survival in Rai's series presumably resulted from incorporation of patients who had received previous therapy.

Rai has reevaluated his staging system and attempted to modify it in terms of classifying patients; those assigned to stage 0 are classified as a low-risk group, those assigned to stage I and stage II combined are classified as an intermediate-risk group, and those assigned to stage III and stage IV combined are classified as a high-risk group.[316] Although this approach appears valid for stages 0, III, and IV, the difference in outcome between stage I and stage II at the MDACC and in other series is significant and should be accounted for.

Binet Staging System

Binet and colleagues[29, 31] have developed a staging system that sorts patients into three groups (see Table 28–7). Patients assigned to Binet stage A have normal marrow function with relatively modest tumor burden, those assigned to Binet stage B have no evidence of marrow

TABLE 28–7. Rai and Binet Staging Systems in CLL

Stage	Lymphocytosis	Lymphadenopathy	Hepatomegaly or Splenomegaly	Hgb (g/dL)	Platelets × 10³/μL
Rai Stage					
0	+	−	−	≥11	≥100
I	+	+	−	≥11	≥100
II	+	±	+	≥11	≥100
III	+	±	±	<11	≥100
IV	+	±	±	Any	<100
Binet Stage					
A	+	±	± (<3 lymphatic groups* positive)	≥10	≥100
B	+	±	± (<3 lymphatic groups* positive)	≥10	≥100
C	+	±	±	<10 or	<100

*Each is considered one group, whether unilateral or bilateral: cervical, axillary, and inguinal nodes; liver; and spleen.

From Keating MJ, Childs CC: Chronic Lymphocytic Leukemia: New Perspective on an Old Disease. Houston: M.D. Anderson Cancer Center; 1989, p 5. Adapted from Rai KR, Sawitsky A, Cronkite EP, et al: Clinical staging of chronic lymphocytic leukemia. Blood 1975:46:219; and Binet JL, Auguier A, Dighiero G, et al: A new prognostic class of chronic lymphocytic leukemia derived from a multivariate survival analysis. Cancer 1981:48:198.

failure with more advanced tumor burden, and those assigned to Binet stage C have anemia or thrombocytopenia. The Binet staging system includes the cervical, axillary, and inguinal lymph nodes (either unilateral or bilateral); the spleen; and the liver. Application of the Binet staging system to the MDACC patients is illustrated in Figure 28–2. Although it is obvious that there is significant stratification, the Binet A stage does not separate out the Rai stage 0 patients who appear to have an excellent prognosis. For this reason, the IWCLL recommended an integrated Binet/Rai system in which the Binet stage is further defined by providing the appropriate Rai stage in Roman numerals in parentheses.[30] The combined staging system is composed of seven stages: A(0), A(I), A(II), B(I), B(II), C(III), and C(IV). This staging system has not achieved widespread use.

Total Tumor Mass Score

Jaksic and Vitale[181] have defined total tumor mass as the sum of the square root of the number of peripheral blood lymphocytes per nanoliter, the diameter in centimeters of the largest palpable nodes, and the enlargement of the spleen in centimeters below the left coastal margin. When the sum exceeded 9, the median survival time was

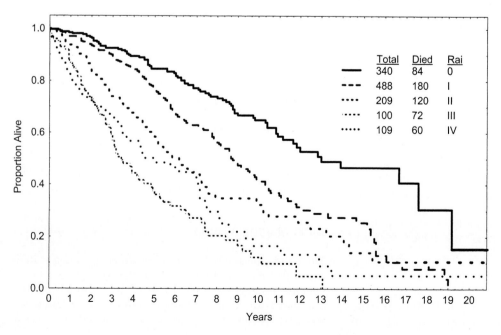

	Total	Died	Rai
——	340	84	0
- - -	488	180	I
··········	209	120	II
·–·–·	100	72	III
·······	109	60	IV

FIGURE 28–1. Survival of untreated patients with CLL (M.D. Anderson Cancer Center, 1975 to 1993) by Rai stage.

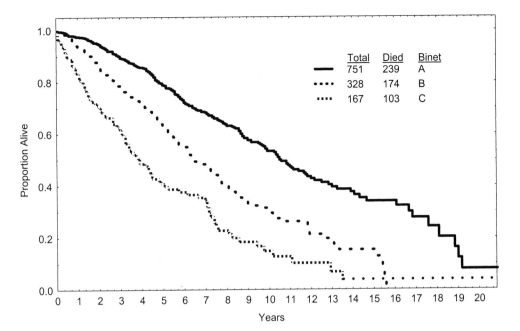

	Total	Died	Binet
——	751	239	A
····	328	174	B
····	167	103	C

FIGURE 28–2. Survival of untreated patients with CLL (M.D. Anderson Cancer Center, 1975 to 1993) by Binet stage.

short; whereas for a total tumor mass equal to or less than 9, the median survival was 101 months. The difficulty in obtaining objective measurements from a variety of series has limited the application of this scoring system to other groups of patients.

Other staging systems have not been widely adopted.[231, 243] The most widely used classification systems at present are the Rai staging system in the United States and the Binet staging system in Europe. The major advantage of these staging systems is that they give us a broad understanding of prognostic features, but they account for a relatively small proportion of the variability of the outcome of the patients. Within each stage, there is still great diversity of outcome. The systems provide a common terminology, however, so that results of one study can be compared to some degree with others. There is evidence that patients who move from one stage to another while they are under observation have an adverse outcome.

OTHER PROGNOSTIC FACTORS

Great effort has been taken to define other prognostic factors that can further define the outcome of patients with CLL. The three features that have received the most attention as prognostic factors are the lymphocyte doubling time,[265, 269] the pattern of bone marrow infiltration on bone marrow–defined biopsy,[293, 320, 340] and the chromosome karyotype analysis.[32, 159, 188]

Lymphocyte Doubling Time

Patients with CLL who are in the early stages of the disease are usually observed with no therapy (Rai stage 0 to stage II, Binet stage A). If the lymphocyte count is measured each 1 to 3 months, the rate of increase in the lymphocyte count can be determined. The prognostic impact of the doubling time was demonstrated by Montserrat and associates.[269] A median survival of 12 years was noted for patients in the early stage of the disease whose doubling time was less than 12 months, whereas the median had not been reached for those with a longer doubling times. Molica and Alberti[265] confirmed the impact of the doubling time after adjustments for age, sex, lymphocyte count, anemia, and thrombocytopenia. Thus, the lymphocyte count can be used as a measure of the "aggressiveness" of the disease. The rate of increase of the lymphocyte count is a much more powerful predictor of outcome than is the absolute lymphocyte count, which can show no increase or a slow increase in patients under observation despite a high initial count.[282, 339]

Bone Marrow Biopsy Pattern

The bone marrow biopsy pattern (diffuse versus nodular, interstitial, or mixed) provides additional information within different stages so that within all Binet stages, a diffuse pattern has a negative prognostic impact. Thus, it appears that this feature, in addition to stage, can be used to give additional prognostic information for patients.[293,340]

Staging Systems in Previously Treated Patients

One weakness of the prognostic studies is that they have been based on information from patients with previously untreated CLL. Relatively few studies have evaluated the role of stage of disease on probability of response or survival in previously treated patients with CLL. The interaction with treatment and response to treatment so far have not been well defined. In a large number of patients who were previously treated at the MDACC, the Rai and

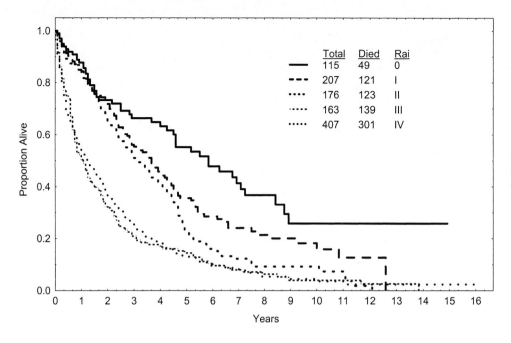

FIGURE 28-3. Survival of previously treated patients with CLL (M.D. Anderson Cancer Center, 1975 to 1993) by Rai stage.

Binet staging systems have been applied and show that the staging systems apply well to previously treated patients (Figs. 28-3 and 28-4).

Cytogenetics

The largest analysis of cytogenetic data and impact on outcome has been conducted by Juliusson and colleagues[188] in a multi-institutional study. The cytogenetic profile, particularly the percentage of abnormal metaphases, was an independent factor after accounting for the age and sex of the patients. Patients with a 13q abnormality had a normal survival, whereas those with 14q abnormalities and abnormalities of chromosome 12 had a poor survival time.[188] However, if other poor prognostic signs developed, the addition of chromosome 12 abnormality was not adverse. Patients with a normal karyotype had a better prognosis than did those with one or more chromosome abnormalities. The more cytogenetic abnormalities that were noted, the greater the likelihood of a short survival. There were too few patients with other abnormalities for conclusions to be drawn. The proportion of abnormal metaphases was a poor prognostic feature after accounting for other variables such as age, sex, and stage. Patients with 100% abnormal metaphases have the worst prognosis. Patients with insufficient metaphases appeared to have an intermediate prog-

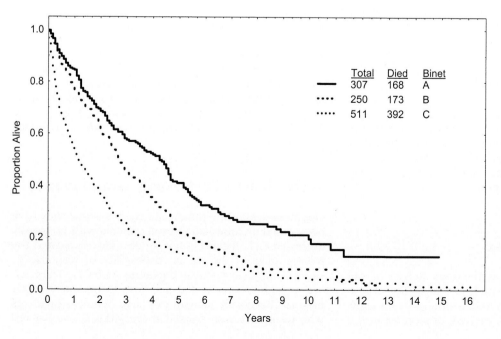

FIGURE 28-4. Survival of previously treated patients with CLL (M.D. Anderson Cancer Center, 1975 to 1993) by Binet stage.

nosis. No specific cytogenetic group assumed independent prognostic importance. Further studies using FISH probes have identified 13q14 deletion in 51% of patients with CLL, 11q22–q23 deletion in 20%, trisomy 12 in 15%, and 17p deletion in 10% to 15%. The 11q and 17p abnormalities have been identified as adverse prognostic factors associated with shorter survival times and treatment-free intervals.[93, 94] Some studies suggest that trisomy 12 is an adverse factor; there is no clear evidence that 13q deletions have prognostic significance.

Uncertain Prognostic Factors

A number of investigators have evaluated other features of the disease for their prognostic impact. A number of studies of morphologic variants, such as the number of larger lymphocytes, the number of prolymphocytes, and whether the cells are cleaved, have been evaluated with consideration of prognosis.[254, 256, 377] Melo and coworkers[254, 256] have defined a group of patients with CLL/PLL in whom the bone marrow differential revealed that 10% to 55% of the cells were prolymphocytes. These patients tended to have a course similar to that of patients with CLL, whereas those with more than 55% lymphocytes in the blood stream had a shorter survival time.

Advanced age has consistently been shown to be associated with a poor prognosis in CLL.[130, 231] In one study, the prognosis of 133 patients with CLL younger than 50 years was compared with that of 1777 older patients.[74] The younger patients had more hepatosplenomegaly and lymphadenopathy, a lower blood lymphocyte count, and higher hemoglobin and platelet levels. The hemoglobin level, white blood cell count, and bone marrow lymphocyte percentage had prognostic value in the younger group of patients. In a review of 454 patients younger than 50 years, the IWCLL obtained an overall median survival of 12 years, with a 10-year survival rate of 76% for Rai stage 0 but only 45% for stages I and II and 24% for stages III and IV.[292] Survival time has been demonstrated to be shorter for men than for women for reasons that remain unclear.[231, 243, 268]

Some reports have suggested the sIgM level on the CLL cells is characteristic of a more mature immunophenotype, and patients with a high level may have a better prognosis.[151] However, the data on this factor are conflicting.[16] Geisler and colleagues[137] reported on the prognostic importance of immunophenotyping of 514 newly diagnosed patients and found that high levels of IgM conferred a worse prognosis in a univariate analysis. Soluble IL-2 receptors shed from cells in patients with CLL are measurable in plasma. A high level of soluble IL-2 receptor correlates with clinical stage and, therefore, a worse prognosis.[354] CD23 expression has been reported to be a prognostic factor in CLL; CD23$^-$ and FMC7$^+$ cells are associated with a significantly shorter survival time.[137] These patients almost certainly have mantle cell leukemias. In addition, increased levels of serum-soluble CD23 confer a shorter survival time in patients with CLL.[40] Others have reported that the presence of so-called myelomonocytic antigens on CLL cells correlates with a diffuse bone marrow pattern and a poor prognosis.[303]

A low gamma globulin level (hypogammaglobulinemia) has not been closely correlated with survival time. Rozman and associates[342] found that the immunoglobulin levels, particularly those of IgG and IgA, worsen with progression of the disease (see Table 28–2) and had some correlation with length of survival.

Three serologic tests have been shown to have prognostic importance, namely, serum β_2-microglobulin, sCD23, and thymidine kinase. Serum β_2-microglobulin is a low-molecular-weight protein associated with the HLA complex. A shorter survival time for patients with CLL with elevated serum levels of β_2-microglobulin was noted as in lymphoma and myeloma.[82, 156] The β_2-microglobulin level is strongly correlated with stage of disease, the extent of bone marrow infiltration, and the bone marrow pattern and tumor bulk but is independently prognostic overall and within clinical stages. The independent prognostic value of the serum β_2-microglobulin level has not been demonstrated. High levels of sCD23 are associated with shorter survival[266, 345] and correlate with β_2-microglobulin levels. Identification of patients with advanced-stage disease and high levels of β_2-microglobulin and sCD23 defines a group of patients with a median survival time of less than 3 years.[267] High levels of thymidine kinase predict a shorter time to disease progression in patients with early-stage CLL.[149, 150]

Studies have demonstrated that patients whose cells have mutated immunoglobulin V_H genes have a better prognosis than do those with unmutated genes.[70, 153] The cells with mutated genes have a lower CD38 expression, which confers a better prognosis in patients with low CD38 expression.[70, 153]

SMOLDERING CHRONIC LYMPHOCYTIC LEUKEMIA

The important concept of "smoldering" CLL has evolved in recent years. Traditional clinical practice is to delay treatment in patients in the early stages of disease until there is evidence of progression. However, within early-stage disease, there are patients with a greater tendency to progression. Montserrat and coworkers[270] conducted a study of 261 patients with CLL, 134 of whom were in Binet stage A and 87 of whom were assigned to Rai stage 0. Progression and length of survival were correlated with a number of features, but a subset of patients with stage A disease, nondiffuse bone marrow histologic pattern, hemoglobin levels of 13 g/dL or greater, blood lymphocytes less than 30 × 10^9/L, and lymphocyte doubling time of more than 12 months could be defined as having smoldering CLL. Patients assigned to Binet stage A who fulfilled these criteria of smoldering CLL had a much lower rate of progression. Survival of patients with smoldering CLL was demonstrated to be similar to that of sex- and age-matched control populations. The French Cooperative Group of CLL conducted similar studies, and slightly different definitions were developed.[130] Stage A1[1] includes patients with stage A features, that is, with hemoglobin levels greater than 12 g/dL and blood lymphocytes less than 30 × 10^9/L. In stage A2[1], patients have 80% lymphocytes in the bone marrow aspirate, and the number of lymphoid areas involved is 0 to 1. Patients considered to have smoldering leukemia by use of Montserrat's definition have a 78% 10-year survival rate; only 13% of patients have disease progression at 5 years compared with a 43% 10-year survival and a 57% progression rate for more active early-stage disease.[270] These observations are of importance in giving accurate prognostic information to patients who are often concerned that no one is treating their disease.

CLINICAL COURSE IN CLL

The clinical staging systems have been useful in generally describing the outcome of patients with different stages of the disease. However, within these stages, there is marked heterogeneity. The definition of smoldering CLL suggests that there is a subset of patients who have monoclonal lymphocytosis of unknown significance, the equivalent of monoclonal gammopathy of unknown significance in association with multiple myeloma.[130, 161, 270] Although the staging systems suggest that the disease has a natural evolution, generalized lymphadenopathy never develops in some patients, and disease predominantly involves the spleen; their major complication may be the development of bone marrow failure or cytopenias, and they may progress directly from stage I to stage III or stage IV disease. In addition, some patients with stage 0 disease progress directly to stage III or stage IV disease with anemia and thrombocytopenia that is not associated with autoantibody production. Some patients with hypogammaglobulinemia have a low frequency of infection, whereas other patients have a high frequency of infection. Thus, the characteristics that are associated with disease progression are ill defined.

SPONTANEOUS REMISSION

Spontaneous remission in CLL is uncommon. Few patients had been described until Han's report in 1987, which noted 11 cases of spontaneous remission in patients with CLL seen during a 60-year period at a single institution, an incidence of less than 2%. No particular correlation with age and sex was noted, and more patients had earlier stage disease. Patients who undergo spontaneous remission tend to have a prolonged survival subsequent to this.[154] A number of the spontaneous remissions that have been reported have been preceded by viral infections and, in some patients, followed a smallpox vaccination,[387] suggesting that immunologic mechanisms are the mediators of "spontaneous" remissions.

RICHTER'S TRANSFORMATION

In contrast to chronic granulocytic leukemia, in which transformation into an acute blastic phase is the rule, such a transformation in CLL is rare.[229] Much more common is the development of a diffuse large-cell lymphoma or transformation into a more prolymphocytoid cell population.[98] Rarely, multiple myeloma develops.[105] Second-

ary myelodysplasia and acute myelogenous leukemia in CLL are uncommon considering the extensive use of alkylating agents in a population of immunosuppressed patients.

Richter[326] described the transformation to large-cell lymphoma in 1928. At that time, the disease was called reticulum cell sarcoma. A large number of cases have subsequently been reported. The frequency of Richter's transformation is uncertain. In earlier series,[123, 155, 168, 335] 3% to 10% of patients with leukemia transforming into large-cell lymphoma have been reported. Eighteen cases of Richter's transformation were reported from the Roswell Park Memorial Institute.[155] Twelve cases were diagnosed in vivo and six at autopsy. Many of these patients were reported to have complex cytogenetic changes including complex trisomy 12. Most patients who had Richter's transformation failed to respond to traditional therapy for large granular lymphocyte leukemia.

The largest report has been published from the MDACC. Of 1374 patients with CLL, 39 had Richter's transformation.[335] The clinical features associated with the condition included systemic symptoms of fever, weight loss, night sweats in more than half of the cases, progressive lymphadenopathy, extranodal involvement, elevation of the serum lactate dehydrogenase level, and monoclonal gammopathy. No specific chromosome abnormality was noted to confer an increased risk in this study, although complex abnormalities were common. Patients at all stages of disease were at risk, and cases were also reported in patients otherwise in complete remission (CR). There was no difference in the probability of development of Richter's transformation between patients receiving purine analogues and those receiving alkylating agents. The median survival time for these patients was 5 months despite vigorous treatment for large granular lymphocyte leukemia. Patients who responded to therapy for lymphoma had a prolonged survival. In some patients, Richter's transformation developed concomitantly with or shortly after the diagnosis of CLL. These patients had a better response to therapy. Comparison of surface light chains from both the CLL and the high-grade lymphoma components demonstrated isotypic light-chain expression in 12 of 15 patients. Immunoglobulin gene rearrangement analysis revealed identical rearrangement patterns in all four patients studied, suggesting that the disease evolved from the low-grade clone. The discordance of the light-chain isotopes in 3 of the 15 patients could be explained by an isotype switch. The strongest evidence to support the derivation of the large-cell lymphoma from the CLL population is the immunoglobulin gene rearrangement pattern. Some other studies have recorded different gene rearrangements that may be a consequence of somatic mutations in the immunoglobulin heavy-chain gene. Studies using anti-idiotype antibodies or nucleotide sequence analysis also support a common clonal origin of the large-cell lymphoma and CLL.[59] Gallium scanning is useful for detecting areas of transformation or uptake in the larger cells, and uptake is usually abnormal in contrast to the normal uptake in CLL generally.[294]

Less than 1% of patients undergo transformation to

acute lymphoblastic disease. In most cases reported, this is the L2 form of acute lymphocytic leukemia.

SECOND NEOPLASMS

A number of investigators have reported an increased likelihood of other malignant neoplasms in patients with CLL. This relationship has been discussed for more than 100 years, and the true relevance after adjusting for age and sex is disputed. It appears that there is a higher frequency of both melanomatous and nonmelanomatous skin cancers in patients with CLL.[371] Lung cancer is the most commonly associated neoplasm after cancer of the skin. A report of the Roswell Park Memorial Institute described 14 cases of bronchogenic carcinoma in 191 patients between 1951 and 1976.[9] The mechanisms postulated for the increase in the second neoplasms are (1) the immunodeficiency associated with the disease and (2) the use of alkylating agents in therapy for the disease. It is well known that patients receiving long-term immunosuppressive therapy have a high incidence of second or new neoplasms after organ transplantation. In a study of early versus delayed therapy for early-stage (Binet stage A) disease in France using chlorambucil, a higher incidence of epithelial neoplasms was reported.[128] Other studies have not confirmed this association. A review of second neoplasms in patients treated with purine analogues demonstrated a modestly higher incidence than would be expected in an age- and sex-matched non-CLL population.[61]

MANAGEMENT OF CLL

CLL is an unusual "malignant" disease in that the initial decision to be made is whether a patient needs therapy. The second decision that must be made is the appropriate treatment for the stage of disease. Because of the heterogeneous outcome of patients with CLL, ranging from a median of 15+ years for patients with Rai stage 0 disease to a median of 3 to 4 years for patients with Rai stage IV disease, considerable debate continues about when treatment should be initiated. Two reports from the NCIWG and the IWCLL have recommended treatment initially for patients with advanced-stage disease (Rai stage III and stage IV, Binet stage C) and those with bulky lymphadenopathy, splenomegaly, or systemic symptoms.[60, 178] The remaining patients have treatment delayed until they demonstrate evidence of progressive disease, as exhibited by increasing lymph node, liver, or spleen enlargement or rapidly rising white blood cell count or deterioration in stage. Patients with hemolytic anemia and thrombocytopenia should be treated initially with corticosteroids or splenectomy, or both, before the treatment decision to initiate chemotherapy is made. The guidelines of the NCIWG are shown in Table 28–3. The survival of newly diagnosed patients with CLL by Rai stage at the MDACC is shown in Figure 28–1.

Alkylating Agents and Corticosteroids

The two alkylating agents most widely used in the management of CLL are chlorambucil (CLB) and cyclophosphamide (CPA).[201] Both agents are bifunctional alkylating agents and form a covalent bond with DNA preferentially at DNA sites that are actively transcribing. This is thought to be the mechanism of cytotoxicity as well as of mutagenicity and carcinogenicity. Like most other chemotherapy agents, CLB and CPA have a somewhat greater effect in S phase than in other phases of the cell cycle.

CLB is usually administered orally. Peak plasma concentration occurs within 1 hour; the major metabolite is phenylacetic acid mustard. The metabolite reaches a peak 2 to 4 hours after ingestion of the tablet. CLB is protein bound, especially to albumin. Hepatic metabolism is the major route of degradation and conversion into phenylacetic acid mustard. CLB and metabolites are excreted in the urine (50% to 70% within 24 hours).[5, 63]

CPA can be given both parenterally and orally because absorption from the gastrointestinal tract is excellent. The drug is converted into the active metabolite 4-hydroxy-cyclophosphamide by liver microsomes; it crosses the cell membranes and is then converted to aldophosphamide.[5, 63] The metabolites of CPA are excreted in the urine, which is the mechanism for one of the significant toxicities of CPA, namely, hemorrhagic cystitis. Mesna (sodium 2-mercaptoethane sulfonate) is effective in diminishing the occurrence of this complication.[39]

Prednisone (PRED) is the most actively studied corticosteroid in the treatment of CLL. The drug has a predominantly glucocorticoid effect with modest mineralocorticoid activity.[101, 135] Dexamethasone has also been used but to a somewhat lesser degree. Prednisone is used in CLL because of its beneficial therapeutic effect on autoimmune acquired hemolytic anemia and immune-mediated thrombocytopenia.

CLB ± PRED have been used extensively in the treatment of CLL. First reports of the use of CLB in the treatment of CLL were presented by Galton and coworkers[135] in 1961 and Ezdinli and associates[100] in 1965. The usual dose was 4 to 8 mg/m² on a continuous basis for 4 to 8 weeks. Approximately half the patients achieved benefit for more than 6 months. The early studies noted diminishing periods of benefit as the disease progressed. A decrease in lymph node, liver, and spleen size and a fall in lymphocyte count occurred in more than half the patients, and an improvement in the hemoglobin level was noted in approximately half the patients. In the study conducted by Ezdinli and colleagues,[100] some patients also received corticosteroids. Five of seven patients who initially received CLB and PRED responded to treatment, whereas one of six responded when PRED was added after an unsatisfactory response to CLB. Knospe and colleagues[225] used a different dose schedule for CLB, giving 0.4 mg/kg of CLB as a single dose every 2 weeks. Subsequent doses were escalated according to tolerance; 25% of patients with indolent disease responded versus 58% of patients with inactive disease. The intermittent schedule produced minor responses in patients who had not responded to prolonged daily CLB therapy.

CPA has not been demonstrated to be active as a single

TABLE 28–8. Variations in Dose, Schedule, and Response Rate for Chlorambucil and Prednisone in CLL

Reference	Chlorambucil Dose and Schedule	Total 4-Week Chlorambucil Dose	Prednisone Dose and Schedule	Total 4-Week Prednisone Dose	Response Rate (%)
Keller[207]	30 mg/m² q2w	60 mg/m²	80 mg/day × 5 q2w	800 mg	74
Sawitsky[348]	0.4–0.8/kg q4w	16–32 mg/m²	0.8 mg/kg × 7 q4w	216 mg	47
	0.08/kg/day continuous	9 mg/m²	0.8 mg/kg × 7 q4w	216 mg	38
Montserrat[269]	0.4 mg/kg q2w	32 mg/m²	60 mg/m² × 5 q2w	600 mg	59
Jaksic[179]	75 mg/m² q4w	~40 mg/m²	30 mg/m² × 7 q4w	~220 mg	60
Montserrat[268]	0.4 mg/kg × 2 days q2w	64 mg/m²	60 mg/m² × 4 q2w	480 mg	75
Hansen[165]	10 mg/m² × 5 q4w	50 mg/m²	40 mg/m² × 5 q4w	200 mg	71
Raphael[319]	30 mg/m² q2w	60 mg/m²	80 mg/day × 5 q2w	800 mg	72

agent in CLL. Its major use has been in combinations with vincristine and prednisone (CVP or COP).

Galton and colleagues[135] and Ezdinli and associates[101] were also the first investigators to explore use of corticosteroids in the treatment of CLL. Different dosage schedules were used, usually on a continuous basis. Patients who were responsive to CLB also appeared to respond to corticosteroids, but none of the patients with advanced disease or those who were refractory to alkylating agents achieved a response. A third of the patients appeared to have shrinkage of lymph nodes, and approximately 45% of patients had improvement in splenomegaly. A decrease in the lymphocyte count to less than $10 \times 10^9/L$ was common, but return to a normal lymphocyte count was less common. A major concern in these initial studies was the contribution of corticosteroids to the occurrence of infections in a substantial number of patients. Ezdinli and colleagues[101] explored the outcome of corticosteroids in 60 patients. No CRs were noted. There was some improvement in organomegaly, anemia, and thrombocytopenia in one half to three quarters of patients. Approximately 6 months of therapy was required for the lymphocyte count to fall into the range of 5 to $10 \times 10^9/L$. Almost one third of the courses were associated with major infections.

Alkylating Agents plus Corticosteroids

Han and associates[158] conducted a double-blind study in which 15 patients were treated with CLB + PRED versus 11 patients who were treated with CLB alone. The small groups appeared to be comparable. CLB was given at a dose of 6 mg/day and PRED at a dose of 30 mg/day. CRs were observed in 3 of 15 patients in the combined group; another 67% achieved a partial response (PR). In the arm of the study in which CLB alone was used, one patient achieved a CR and four achieved a PR. The difference in the response rate was statistically significant, with no difference in overall survival. Han concluded that the combination was superior to CLB alone.

Sawitsky and colleagues[348] compared therapy with CLB + PRED with that of PRED alone. CLB, in two different schedules, was combined with PRED and compared with therapy with PRED alone. The PRED response rate was only 11%; response rates were 47% for the once-a-month CLB schedule and 38% for the continuous daily-dose CLB schedule. The CR rates in the two CLB + PRED arms of the study were 8% and 13%. No survival difference was noted in any of the three arms. The major complications were infectious in nature; 25% of patients had severe infectious complications, and another 30% had infections of a milder type. CLB + PRED has been administered in a variety of doses and schedules, with no evidence convincingly demonstrating superiority to CLB alone[207,262] (Tables 28–8 and 28–9).

Jaksic,[180] reporting for the International Society for Chemo-Immunotherapy CLL Cooperative Group, compared the intermittent CLB + PRED regimen of Sawitsky with CLB given at a high dose of 15 mg/day until CR or toxicity occurred. A marked difference in the overall

TABLE 28–9. Results of Randomized Clinical Trials in CLL: Alkylating Agents

Reference	Regimen	Response	P Value	Survival
Han[158]	CH v CH + P	5/11 v 13/15	.05	Similar
Sawitsky[348]	CH + P v CH + P v P	18/38 v 15/39 v 2/19	NS	Similar
Keller[207]	CH + P (a)	138/178	NS	Similar
	CH + P (b)			
	CY + ara − C			
Jaksic[179]	High Ch v CH + P	90/129 v 26/52	<.05	High Ch better (P < .01)
Jaksic[180]	High Ch v CHOP (Binet)	102/114 v 81/107	<.01	High Ch better (P < .01)
Catovsky[56]	CH v COP	38/116 v 37/60	NS	Similar
Montserrat[269]	CH + P v COP	30/51 v 14/45	<.01	Similar
Montserrat[268]	CH + P v CY, ME, P	36/48 v 26/48	.054	Similar
Raphael[319]	CH + P v COP	43/60 v 51/62	NS	Similar
Hansen[165]	CH + P v CHOP	49/80 v 55/77	CHOP higher CR (P < .01)	Similar

CH, chlorambucil; CHOP, cyclophosphamide, doxorubicin, vincristine, and prednisone; COP, cyclophosphamide, vincristine, and prednisone; CY, cyclophosphamide; high Ch, high-dose chlorambucil; ME, melphalan; P, prednisone.

response (OR) rate was noted; 70% of the patients achieved a CR and 19% achieved a PR in the high-dose CLB arm versus a CR rate of 31% and an OR rate of 50% in the CLB + PRED arm. Bone marrow criteria were not used in the evaluation of response. Survival was significantly superior in the high-dose CLB arm in earlier stage disease but not in patients with Binet stage C disease. The total dose of CLB delivered per month was five to six times higher in the high-dose arm than in the combination arm, raising the probability that the dose intensity of the alkylating agents was the significant feature in the higher response. Subsequent studies by this group compared high-dose chlorambucil with the cyclophosphamide, doxorubicin, vincristine, and prednisone (CHOP) regimen.[180] No difference in survival has been noted, although the CR rate appears to be higher in the CLB arm than in the CHOP arm.

COP or CVP (cyclophosphamide, vincristine, and prednisone) has been evaluated in patients with CLL with use of different doses and schedules. Liepman and Votaw,[235] in 1978, reported a response rate of 52% for previously untreated patients and 31% for previously treated patients. Oken and Kaplan[281] reported on the use of COP in 18 patients with advanced refractory CLL. The majority of patients had Rai stage III and stage IV disease. Two patients achieved a clinical CR. Bone marrow evaluation was not part of the study. The OR rate was 44%. Other single-arm studies that reported use of CLB and PRED are those from Michallet and associates[262] and Keller and colleagues.[207] The response in both studies was higher for patients with disease in Rai stages 0 and I than for those with disease in stages II, III, and IV. Patients with CR and PR had significantly longer survival than did nonresponders, who had a median survival of approximately 14 months.

Comparative Studies

The French Cooperative Group has mounted a series of studies of patients with Binet stage A, stage B, and stage C disease. The initial study was a randomized comparison in 612 patients (Binet stage A) with a good prognosis who received either immediate treatment with CLB at a daily dose of 0.1 mg/kg indefinitely or delayed treatment.[128] The patients who underwent delayed treatment received therapy when they had evidence of progression from stage A to stage B. Patients who progressed from stage A to stage C were treated with the COP regimen. There was no difference in the survival of the two groups, although there appeared to be a higher frequency of epithelial neoplasms in the immediate-treatment group, raising concern about the carcinogenicity of the alkylating agents. Other investigators have not been able to confirm the increased incidence of epithelial neoplasms in similar comparative studies. The immediate-treatment group had a delay in the progression to advanced stages. The survival rate was 89% at 5 years for those who achieved CR, 76% for those who had a PR, 82% for those with stable disease, and 55% for those with progressive disease. In that study, it was demonstrated that patients with a hemoglobin level of 12 g/dL and a lymphocyte count of less than 30 × 10⁹/L had a survival not signifi-

cantly different from that of an age- and sex-matched population.[128] In a subsequent study, patients receiving CLB + PRED were compared with control patients, and conclusions similar to those of the CLB-alone arm were reached.[89] Some cases of acute myelogenous leukemia were seen in the early-treatment arm. In a Medical Research Council's CLL trial, Catovsky and associates[56] conducted a similar study of patients randomized to early or delayed treatment. No difference in survival or the development of second cancers was noted in that study. Thus, the prevailing evidence is that treatment with alkylating agent regimens is not recommended for patients with early-stage disease (Binet stage A or Rai stages 0 to II) unless they have bulky disease or demonstrate evidence of progressive disease.

No difference in OR rate or survival was noted in previously treated patients, but there was a significantly higher OR in favor of CLB + PRED in untreated patients (see Table 28–9). The previously treated group had a significantly shorter survival than did the untreated group (median, 13.5 months versus 32 months). Montserrat has also conducted a trial of CLB + PRED versus CPA, melphalan, and PRED (CMP) in patients with Binet stage B and stage C. Of the group that received CLB + PRED, 75% responded with 27% CR versus 54% OR with CMP with 12.5% achieving a CR ($P < .05$). No difference in survival was noted. A large comparison was conducted by the Eastern Cooperative Oncology Group of CLB + PRED versus a more intensive CVP arm.[319] Treatment was continued for up to 18 months or until maximal response was achieved. No significant difference in survival was noted. The CR rates were 25% and 23%, respectively, for CLB + PRED versus CVP. Duration of response was 2 years for each arm of the study. The median survival of patients with Rai stage III and stage IV disease was 4.1 years. Thus, no alkylating agent regimen has been demonstrated to be superior to CLB + PRED, and the data do not show that CLB + PRED is superior to CLB alone. Indeed, Jaksic's high-dose CLB regimen appears to be at least as good as any of the regimens examined in the comparative studies.[179]

The French Cooperative Group has mounted two additional studies. In stage B, CLB was compared with COP.[369] The COP regimen used 300 mg of cyclophosphamide orally on days 1 to 5, with 1 mg/m² of vincristine intravenously on day 1 and 40 mg/m² of prednisone orally on days 1 to 5. The dose of chlorambucil was 0.1 mg/kg/day. No difference in survival (median, 5 years) was noted between the two arms of the stage B study, and there was no difference in the rate of disease progression to stage C or toxicity in either arm of the study.

In the patients assigned to Binet stage C, the COP regimen used in Binet stage B constituted one arm of the study, and doxorubicin at a dose of 25 mg/m² on day 1 was added in the other arm (Binet-CHOP or mini-CHOP regimen).[127] This study was terminated with relatively few patients being studied because of the significant improvement in survival for patients treated with the mini-CHOP regimen. Long-term follow-up publication of these data confirms the superiority of mini-CHOP.[129] The 3-year survival rates were 71% for the CHOP group and 28% for the COP group. The median survival time was 62 months in the CHOP group, compared with 22 months in the COP group. The major criticism of this study is that the median survival of patients in the COP arm was less than 2 years, whereas more recent studies of Rai stage III and stage IV disease or Binet stage B disease suggest that these patients have a survival of approximately 3 to 4 years.[319] In addition, the number of patients in each arm of the study was small. However, the study was conducted in exemplary fashion, with strict adherence to previously set rules for early stopping.

Anthracycline Combinations

Several regimens that have been used in the management of CLL include anthracyclines. No single-arm study of doxorubicin or any of the other anthracyclines used as therapy for CLL has been described. Two major studies have been conducted at the MDACC, the first being of the cyclophosphamide, doxorubicin, and prednisone (CAP) regimen (cyclophosphamide 750 mg/m² on day 1, doxorubicin 50 mg/m² intravenously on day 1, and prednisone 100 mg/day orally on days 1 to 5).[202] Courses were repeated at 3-week intervals until clinical CR and maintenance with CPA + PRED; 43% of the patients obtained a CR and 23% achieved a PR, for a total response rate of 66%. Bone marrow biopsy criteria were used to define response in addition to clinical and peripheral blood responses. The median survival of patients with Rai stage IV and Binet stage C disease was 93 and 81 months, respectively. Only 26% obtained a CR on the CAP phase of the study; additional patients obtained a CR on the maintenance phase of CPA + PRED. The study was well tolerated.

The POACH regimen (cyclophosphamide, doxorubicin, vincristine, cytosine arabinoside [ara-C], and prednisone) was studied by the MDACC group.[205] Of previously untreated patients, 56% responded, with 21% obtaining a CR. Of the 31 previously treated patients, 8 (26%) responded (6% CR). There was a highly significant difference in survival between the previously treated and untreated groups. The median survival for the untreated patients was 5 years, which was exactly that obtained with the CAP regimen (Fig. 28–5).

A number of other comparative trials have been initiated to explore the CHOP regimen. Studies comparing CHOP with CLB + PRED demonstrate a higher response rate but no difference in survival.[165, 217]

Multiple Alkylating Agents

The most notable study reporting multiple alkylating agents was from Memorial Sloan-Kettering Hospital (examining the M2 protocol).[209] This regimen used cyclophosphamide, BCNU, and melphalan together with vincristine and prednisone. The regimen was administered monthly to 63 assessable patients with advanced CLL. Rigorous criteria for response were applied. Of the 63 patients, 17% obtained a CR and 44% achieved a PR. This was the first study to report no evidence of disease when bone marrow lymphocyte subsets were analyzed by immunophenotypic evaluation. The CR rate for previously untreated patients was 32%, whereas none of 26 patients who had received previous therapy had a response. A similar study (MiNa protocol) based on the M2 protocol that used peptichemio instead of BCNU reported that 35% of patients achieved a CR.[107]

Nucleoside Analogues

The nucleoside analogues are a potent group of drugs with substantial activity in slow-growing lymphoid malignant neoplasms (Fig. 28–6). The most widely studied drug in CLL is fludarabine monophosphate (FLU), which also has documented activity in indolent lymphoma, Waldenström's macroglobulinemia, and HCL. 2-Chlorodeoxyadenosine has marked activity in HCL and substantial activity in CLL, indolent lymphoma, and Waldenström's macroglobulinemia. Pentostatin (2'-deoxycoformycin) has demonstrated activity in CLL. Both fludarabine and 2-chlorodeoxyadenosine are weak substrates for adenosine

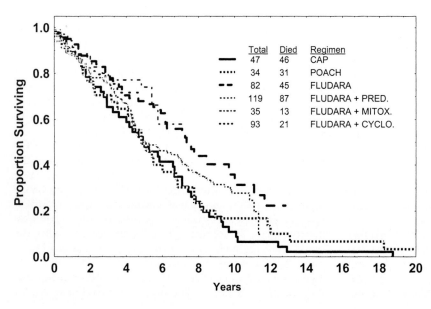

FIGURE 28–5. Survival of untreated patients with CLL categorized by regimen (M.D. Anderson Cancer Center, 1975 to 1993).

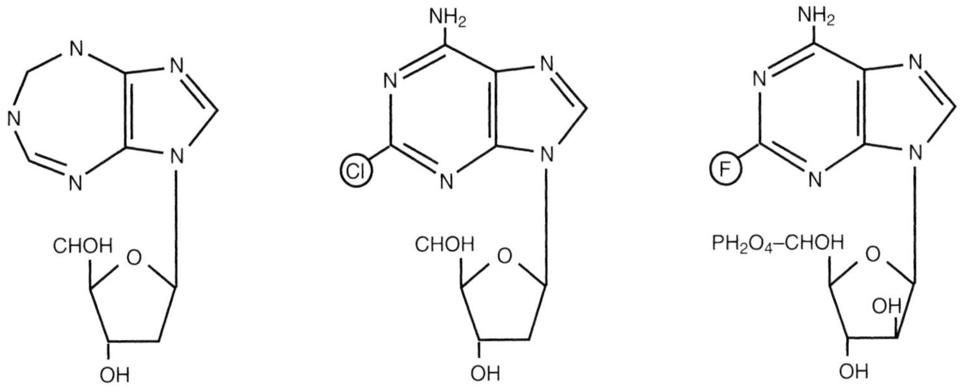

FIGURE 28–6. Chemical structures of nucleoside analogues.

DCF 2   Cl Deoxyadenosine   2 F-ARA-AMP

deaminase, whereas 2′-deoxycoformycin is a potent inhibitor of this enzyme.

Fludarabine Monophosphate

Fludarabine monophosphate (FLU) was first evaluated in CLL by Grever and associates[144] in 22 previously treated patients with good performance status. Most had advanced-stage disease. Four patients achieved a remission (one CR), and 15 others had some improvement. A study at the MDACC used FLU to treat 68 patients with previously treated CLL.[204] Ten patients (15%) achieved a CR, and 30 (44%) achieved a PR. OR rates for Rai stages 0 to II, stage III, and stage IV were 64%, 58%, and 50%, respectively. Survival was correlated with response, with CR patients having a survival superior to that of the PR group. The major morbidity was fever or infection. Myelosuppression was dose limited. Half of the courses were associated with a low neutrophil count of less than 500/μL and 25% with a low platelet count of less than 50×10^9/L. Myelosuppression was much more common in Rai stage III to stage IV. The dose used was 25 to 30 mg/m²/day for 5 days every 3 to 4 weeks. Subsequently, 33 patients with previously untreated disease were treated with the same regimen.[203] Patients with Rai stage III to stage IV disease or progressive Rai stage 0 to stage II were entered into the study. The CR rate by use of the old NCIWG guidelines was 76% (25 of 33). Fourteen of the patients with CR had residual lymphoid nodules in the bone marrow, which would now be classified as nodular PR.

Subsequent studies have evaluated the addition of PRED to FLU (FP) in both previously treated and untreated patients. Two hundred and sixty-four patients with CLL received FLU 30 mg/m² intravenously each day for 5 days with PRED 30 mg/m² orally each day for 5 days.[255] The courses were repeated every 4 weeks. One hundred and sixty-nine patients were previously treated with a median of three regimens, and 82% were refractory to therapy with alkylating agents. The OR rate for the previously treated group was 52% (12% CR). Ninety-five patients were previously untreated. The OR rate and CR rates were 82% and 28%, respectively, being 85% and 34% in Rai stage 0 to stage II and 75% and 14% in stage

III and stage IV). The survival of the patients receiving FLU and FP is updated in Figure 28–7.

The median time to development of progressive disease in previously treated patients was 22 months. In the untreated patients, the median time to progression was 30 months for patients with PR and 42 months for patients with CR. The response rates and infection rates were similar to those seen in previous studies with FLU. Multivariate analysis identified Rai stage, degree of previous therapy, older age, and low albumin levels as the characteristics most strongly associated with response to therapy.[278]

The major morbidity was infection or fever of unknown origin. The likelihood for development of major infections, such as septicemia and pneumonia, correlated significantly with the extent of previous therapy and the stage of disease. In the FP study, *Listeria monocytogenes* septicemia or *Pneumocystis carinii* pneumonia was noted in 14 patients. These infections had not been noted in the studies with FLU as a single agent. In the FP study, the CD4 levels were noted to be uniformly depressed from pretreatment levels of 1015 μL to a median of 159 μL after 3 months of FLU therapy.

A subsequent study[208] has evaluated a phase II clinical trial of FLU in previously treated patients with CLL using a once-weekly dose of 30 mg/m². Of 46 patients, only 24% responded to therapy, with 7 (15%) achieving CR. A schedule of 30 mg/m² daily for 3 days has been given to 80 patients with previously treated disease[334]; 54% were assigned to Rai stage III to stage IV. The CR and OR rates of 25% and 46%, respectively, were slightly lower than on the 5-day schedule, and the incidence of major and minor bacterial infections per treatment course (8%) was significantly lower. The rate of fall of the CD4 level was slower than in the FP study; the starting level of 975 μL fell to 556 μL at 3 months and 437 μL at 6 months. The study was effective and not associated with a shorter survival time than the 5-day regimens or the once-a-week regimen. Consideration should be given to the 3-day regimen in patients requiring less intensive therapy, namely, elderly patients or those with evidence of renal impairment. FLU is excreted solely by the kidneys, and the dose should be modified in patients with renal dysfunction.

Other small series of previously treated patients[104, 171, 312] demonstrated response rates of 52% to 55%.

FLU has also been used in the management of the prolymphocytic variant of CLL. Of 17 patients, 6 (35%) responded. Three of the six responders were previously treated. None of the patients with more than 50% prolymphocytes achieved a response. The median survival was 10 months.[194] A large Group C mechanism (National Cancer Institute) study obtained an OR of 32% in 703 patients.

2-Chlorodeoxyadenosine

The first major study that reported on therapy with 2-chlorodeoxyadenosine (2-CdA, cladribine) was conducted by a group at the Scripps Clinic and Research Foundation in La Jolla.[346] Ninety patients with advanced CLL were treated with 2-CdA by either a 7-day continuous infusion or a 2-hour bolus daily for 5 days. One patient had Binet stage A disease, 7 patients had Binet stage B disease, and 82 patients had Binet stage C disease; 70% were male, with a median age of 63 years. All patients had been previously treated and had a median of two previous therapies. The OR rate was 44%, with only 4% achieving a CR. The median duration of response was 4 months. Treatment was well tolerated, with myelosuppression being the principal form of toxicity. Twenty-four percent of patients experienced thrombocytopenia, and 18% had infections. The infections that were noted included six cases of herpes zoster, three cases of *P. carinii* pneumonia, one case of *Listeria* meningitis, one case of *Pseudomonas* pneumonia, one case of gram-negative bacteremia, and one case of disseminated cryptococcal infection.

Other studies have obtained OR rates of 31% to 68% in previously treated patients with CR rates of 0% to 31% by use of variable criteria for CR.[190, 330, 336] An initial report suggested that 2-CdA might be useful in patients who are resistant to FLU; four patients had a significant reduction in the circulating lymphocyte count.[185] A more complete study has demonstrated that in previously treated patients who were refractory to FLU, only 2 of 28 achieved a PR. Although cross-resistance between FLU and 2-CdA is not absolute, most patients do not respond, and preexisting cytopenia appears to be aggravated.[279] 2-CdA has also been used in the management of previously untreated patients with CLL. It was given at a dose of 0.1 mg/kg/day by 7-day continuous infusion every 28 to 35 days until a response or toxicity occurred. A median of four courses was administered (range, one to nine). Twenty-five percent of patients achieved a CR and an additional 60% achieved a PR for an OR rate of 85%. The major complication of therapy was myelosuppression; 20% of patients experienced grade 3 or grade 4 thrombocytopenia. Three patients, each with concomitant corticosteroid therapy, had opportunistic infections with *Mycobacteria* (two patients) and *P. carinii* (one patient). Thus, 2-CdA has substantial activity in previously untreated and treated patients with CLL.[347] 2-CdA has been given to 63 patients orally with a response rate of 91% with 16% CRs.[191]

Pentostatin (2'-Deoxycoformycin)

A number of investigators have evaluated the activity of 2'-deoxycoformycin (2-DCF) in CLL. Grever and colleagues[144, 145] tested 25 previously treated patients with a dose of 4 mg/m² every 2 weeks. An OR rate of 20% was noted (4% CR). The majority of the patients had advanced-stage disease. In this study, no correlation of response with pretreatment activity of adenosine deaminase in the leukemic cells was noted.[145] Dillman and colleagues[91] have reported on a Cancer and Leukemia Group B study of pentostatin in CLL at a dose of 4 mg/m² intravenously weekly for 3 weeks and then every 2 weeks. Twenty-six percent of patients obtained a response (3% achieved CR). The response rate was higher in the group that had no previous treatment than in the previously treated group of patients (46% versus 15%). The major complication of therapy was infection; severe life-threatening infections were noted in one third of patients. The major organisms associated with infection were herpes simplex and herpes zoster, *Candida* species, and *P. carinii*.[145]

Fludarabine Combination Studies

Purine analogues as single agents do not appear to be curative in CLL. Thus, a number of combination approaches have been evaluated. As mentioned earlier, the addition of corticosteroids to FLU and 2-CdA has not improved response rate or survival (see Fig. 28–7). FLU, 2-CdA, and 2-DCF all inhibit the repair of DNA damage associated with the use of mitoxantrone or alkylating agents. FLU, 30 mg/m²/day for 3 days, has been combined with mitoxantrone, 10 mg/m² on day 1 (FM), or cyclophosphamide, 300 mg/m² on days 1 to 3 (FC). The OR rates for FM and FC are 83% (29 of 35) and 92% (48 of 53), respectively, and are slightly superior to that for FLU. The OR rate in previously treated patients who received only alkylators is superior for FC (85%, 17 of 20) and FM (80%, 12 of 15) to for FLU (61%, 48 of 76). The survival with the different regimens in previously untreated patients is shown in Figure 28–5. Other combination programs have included fludarabine, doxorubicin, and prednisone (FLAP), and the response rate was satisfactory in a small group of patients.

Comparative Trials of Purine Analogues in CLL

The initial comparative clinical trial of FLU and CAP[132] (Table 29–10) included patients with advanced-stage CLL and patients with advanced stage B or stage C disease who had previously been treated with alkylating agents or non–anthracycline-containing regimens; 100 previously untreated patients and 96 previously treated patients were entered into the study. The OR rate was 60% for FLU versus 44% for CAP ($P < .05$). The response rate in untreated patients was 71% for FLU versus 60% for CAP; the response rate in previously treated patients was 48% versus 27% ($P < .05$). The time to progression was significantly longer for FLU than for CAP in both untreated and previously treated groups. There was no advantage in survival for the previously treated group, al-

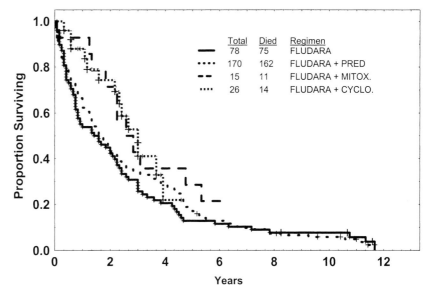

FIGURE 28–7. Survival of patients exposed to alkylator agents according to salvage regimens.

though there was a trend of survival advantage (P = .09) for FLU in untreated patients. Myelosuppression and infection were similar in the two groups. There was significantly more nausea and vomiting and hair loss in the CAP-treated group.

In North America, an intergroup study compared FLU versus CLB versus FLU + CLB.[318] The FLU + CLB arm of the study was discontinued because of excessive toxicity. The comparison, therefore, was restricted to FLU and CLB. The OR rate was 63% for FLU versus 37% for CLB (P < .01), and the CR rate was 20% versus 4% (P < .01)[318] (see Table 29–10). The duration of response was 25 months for FLU responders versus 14 months for the CLB group (P < .001). No survival advantage has been demonstrated at this time. The study was designed as a crossover study, and a higher response rate was noted for patients whose therapy with CLB failed crossing over to FLU than for patients whose therapy with FLU failed crossing over to CLB (P <.001).

The French Cooperative Group evaluated FLU versus mini-CHOP versus CAP[233] and entered 938 patients into this study. No survival advantage has been demonstrated,

but the CAP arm has been discontinued early because of a higher death rate and a lower response rate. The CR rate was higher for FLU (41%) versus mini-CHOP (30%) and CAP (15%). No difference in autoimmune complications was noted in any arm of this study.[233]

Cladribine Comparative Trial

A randomized multicenter trial compared 2-CdA + PRED versus CLB + PRED as initial therapy for CLL.[330] Patients were evaluated after 3 months with nonresponders crossing over; patients with a PR received three further courses, and patients with a CR had no further treatment. The patients who relapsed crossed over to the alternative arm. Characteristics of the patients were identical in both arms of the study apart from a significantly higher white blood cell count in the 2-CdA + PRED arm. The trial used the old NCIWG criteria for response, which allow persistent bone marrow nodules to be classified as a CR. The response rate for 2-CdA + PRED was 47% CR and 40% PR for an OR rate of 87% versus 12% CR and 45% PR for CLB + PRED. The CR and OR rates were signifi-

TABLE 28–10. Results of Randomized Clinical Trials in Frontline CLL: Purine Analogues Versus Alkylating Agents

	Reference	Previous Therapy	No. of Patients	CR (%)	OR (%)	TTP	Survival
FLU	132	—	52	—	71	34+	NR
CAP			48	—	60	7	NR
FLU	132	+	48	—	48	10	24
CAP			48	—	27	6	24
FLU	318	—	170	20	63	25	66
CLB			181	4	37	14	56
Cladribine	330	—	126	—	87	21	NR
CLB + PRED			103	—	59	18	NR
FLU	233	—	341	—	73	31	74
mini-CHOP			57	—	73	28	68
CAP			240	—	60	28	70

CAP, cyclophosphamide, doxorubicin, and prednisone; CHOP, cyclophosphamide, doxorubicin, vincristine, and prednisone; CLB, chlorambucil; CR, complete remission; FLU, fludarabine; NR, not reached; OR, overall response; PRED, prednisone; TTP, time to progression.

cantly in favor of 2-CdA + PRED ($P < .001$) (see Table 29–10). The progression-free survival was significantly superior at 24 months with 2-CdA + PRED. The event-free survival and overall survival were similar. Granulocytopenia, infections, and fevers of unknown location were significantly more common in the 2-CdA + PRED arm.

Total-Body Irradiation

Twenty years ago, Johnson[183] reported the use of total-body irradiation in the treatment of CLL; 88% of patients were reported to respond, with 39% achieving a CR. A subsequent study of total-body irradiation plus chemotherapy with cyclophosphamide was conducted. The Eastern Cooperative Oncology Group conducted a study of 26 assessable patients who were entered into total-body irradiation programs. The high-dose regimen was associated with severe thrombocytopenia and neutropenia. During that study, 26 patients were also entered into a chemotherapy arm of the study combining chlorambucil and prednisone. The OR rate was 77% (23% CR). The chemotherapy arm was associated with a longer median duration of response, although the median survival of the two treatment arms was similar.[22, 343, 362]

Monoclonal Antibody Therapy

Campath-1H is a humanized rat antibody directed against CD52. It is an IgG1 antibody.[28] The function of CD52 is unknown. A series of studies has been conducted of previously treated patients and more recently of previously untreated patients. Wide variability in response rates has been noted, depending on the population of previously treated patients chosen for study. Approximately 40% to 60% of patients who have had extensive previous therapy have responded.[210, 285] In previously untreated patients, the response rate is more likely to be approximately 80%.[253, 286]

A pivotal clinical trial (CAM-211) has been undertaken to evaluate the efficacy of Campath-1H in patients with CLL who were previously exposed to alkylating agents and refractory to fludarabine.[206] Refractoriness was defined as no response or relapse within 6 months after the last dose of a fludarabine-containing regimen. Patients were treated with *P. carinii* pneumonia prophylaxis and DNA viral prophylaxis. The OR rate was 33%, and the CR rate was 2%. Fifty-nine percent of patients achieved stable disease. The OR rate in patients with significant lymphadenopathy is substantially less than that in patients with minor or no lymphadenopathy. Campath-1H has substantial activity in T-PLL; the response rate is 77%, with 59% of patients achieving a CR.[76] The major problems associated with the use of Campath-1H are infections. The profound T-cell depletion allows the development of opportunistic infections. *P. carinii,* herpesvirus, adenovirus, and cytomegalovirus are all potential and documented pathogens.[206, 285]

Another monoclonal antibody, rituximab, binds to CD20. CD20 is tightly bound to the surface membrane and is said not to be shed. The function of CD20 is unknown, but it is involved in B-cell differentiation and calcium channel functions. The antigen density is lower in patients with CLL than in patients with follicular lymphomas.[7] The antibody is a chimeric antibody consisting of human IgG1 and κ constant regions and murine variable regions. Rituximab acts by complement lysis, antibody-dependent cellular cytotoxicity, and apoptosis pathways. Two clinical trials have used high-dose regimens in CLL; 65% of 18 patients treated by Byrd and colleagues[46] and 41% of those treated by O'Brien and coworkers[280] have obtained PRs. The latter study showed a strong dose-response relationship. These antibodies are now moving into combination studies.

Bone Marrow Transplantation

Because of the relatively advanced age of patients with CLL, no consistent efforts had been made to conduct bone marrow transplantations with use of allogeneic donors in this disease. In addition, because of the difficulty in eradicating CLL cells from the bone marrow and peripheral blood with conventional therapy, autologous bone marrow or peripheral blood stem cell replacement has not been an option. However, because CLL is presently considered incurable with use of conventional approaches to therapy, bone marrow transplantation was continually investigated.[212, 314] Thus, several studies of bone marrow transplantation have been conducted in patients with CLL (Table 28–11). Autologous stem cell transplantation has been used in several series.[211, 212, 296, 314] In most of the series of autologous stem cell transplantation, fludarabine therapy was necessary to decrease the marrow tumor burden sufficiently to use this modality of treatment. There has been marked variability in the status of the patients at the time of transplantation, from patients with minimal disease state,[311, 314] presumably a CR or OR in the Dana Farber Cancer Institute (DFCI) study, to patients with advanced refractory disease at MDACC.[214] The population of patients considered most appropriate for transplantation depends on the philosophy of the investigators.[311, 314]

The largest group of allogeneic transplant recipients has been reported by Michallet and coworkers,[261] representing the data from the European and International Bone Marrow Transplantation Groups. The most recent update of the data is presented in a study of 54 patients, reported to have B-CLL, with a median age of 41 years. All patients were HLA-identical siblings. Four patients had not received any treatment before bone marrow transplantation. Conditioning regimens varied. Of the 54 patients, 30 have died. Twenty-three of the alive patients are in hematologic remission. The most common cause of death was graft-versus-host disease. The projected survival is approximately 40% at 5 years and 33% at 6.5 years. Better results were obtained in patients still responsive to chemotherapy. Of 27 assessable patients, 16 had chronic graft-versus-host disease. Small series have also been reported from the Dana Farber Cancer Institute, Nebraska, and the MDACC.[212, 296, 314] Most patients are able to obtain stable hematologic engraftment. The risk for graft-versus-

TABLE 28–11. Transplantation in Chronic Lymphocytic Leukemia

Study	Reference	No. of Patients	TRM (%)	Relapse (%)	Stage of Therapy
Autologous					
International		107	7	50	Mixed
DFCI	Provan[311]	81	10	17	CR or PR
Kiel, Germany	Dreger[95]	36	5	10	Mostly first remission
Nebraska	Pavletic[296]	16	19	56	Sensitive relapse
MDACC	Khouri[214]	14	7	56	After second relapse
Allogeneic					
MDACC	Khouri[215]	24	13	34	Relapsed/refractory
DFCI	Gribben[146]	23	22	30	CR/PR
Nebraska	Pavletic[297]	22	36	5	Advanced

CR, complete remission; DFCI, Dana Farber Cancer Institute; MDACC, M.D. Anderson Cancer Center; PR, partial response; TRM, treatment-related mortality.

host disease is significantly less in patients treated with fludarabine regimens.[355]

The treatment-related mortality is approximately 5% to 10% in most studies, and the relapse rate is high in studies in which patients with advanced disease are treated (see Table 28–11). The largest study, which requires longer follow-up, is the Dana Farber Cancer Institute study of 81 patients; it had a low relapse rate, and a substantial number of patients achieved negativity on polymerase chain reaction analysis.[311]

Smaller series have been reported for allogeneic bone marrow transplantation with ablative regimens with variability in the status of patients going into the studies. Treatment-related mortality has been variable from a low of 8% at the MDACC versus 36% in Nebraska. The overall disease-free interval is varied from 40% to 60%.[146, 215, 297]

A new element of allogeneic bone marrow transplantation has been the use of nonablative regimens.[216, 359] The common theme of all regimens is the use of purine analogues as part of the preparative regimen along with alkylating agents and/or radiation. The largest experience has been at MDACC with 11 patients receiving nonablative stem cell transplantations.[216] The median age was 57 years. There is no difference at present in the overall survival between the nonablative and the high-dose chemotherapy transplantations,[216] suggesting that the major element of control of disease after allogeneic transplantation is the graft-versus-leukemia effect.

Biologic Response Modifiers

The most widely studied drug in this area is recombinant interferon alfa. The majority of early studies were conducted in previously treated patients and demonstrated a low response rate. Foon and associates[119] reported acceleration of some patients in their study. Later reports have evaluated recombinant interferon alfa in early-stage disease. Pangalis and coworkers[37, 290] reported response in 5 of 10 patients in one study and 10 of 26 in a second study. Approximately 10% of patients have a decrease in the size of the spleen and the lymph nodes, but the marrow infiltrate seldom changes. Others have reported more than a 50% decrease in lymphocyte count in approximately 60% of patients.[341, 390] In one study, a decrease in the pretreatment T-lymphocyte count was noted, and the serum immunoglobulin level increased by more than 3 g/L in three of seven patients studied.[390] Recombinant IL-2 has been used in the management of a small number of patients with CLL.[199] Lymphocyte counts increased in most patients with B-cell CLL, and some patients had a decrease in the size of nodes and spleen.

TREATMENT OF CLL VARIANTS

The diagnosis and treatment of diseases resembling CLL have been discussed extensively by Catovsky and colleagues.[248] Major variants considered are PLL (which is usually of the B-cell type), splenic lymphoma with villous lymphocytes, and a variety of T-CLLs, all of which are uncommon. The therapy for B-PLL with alkylating agents and corticosteroids is less satisfactory than in CLL. Responses have been noted with pentostatin[75] and fludarabine.[194] Like HCL, splenic lymphoma with villous lymphocytes is usually treated with splenectomy.[272] Treatment with alkylating agent regimens is effective in only one third of patients.[52] Treatment of follicular lymphoma in leukemic phase usually follows the approaches taken with transforming low-grade lymphoma and includes regimens such as CHOP and fludarabine.[52, 362] The situation with mantle zone lymphoma in leukemic phase is also unsatisfactory. Treatment with conventional regimens or fludarabine tends to be ineffective. Preliminary results with hyperfractionated cyclophosphamide, vincristine, doxorubicin, and dexamethasone (hyper-CVAD) are promising.[216] Large granular lymphocyte leukemia[248] is identified by a monoclonal T-cell proliferation of a T-suppressor subset that is characterized immunophenotypically as CD3+, CD8+, CD56+, and CD57+. By and large, these patients do not need therapy, but if treatment is indicated, some respond to alkylating agents or corticosteroids, or both, or use of granulocyte colony-stimulating factor or granulocyte-macrophage colony-stimulating factor for neutropenia. T-cell PLL is an uncommon diagnosis, with a predominant phenotype of CD3+, CD4+, CD7+, and CD8−. One third of patients co-express CD4 and CD8 or are characterized as being CD4− and CD8+.[248] Treatment results remain poor.[75, 248, 272] Campath-1H is active in T-cell PLL, and occasional patients respond to treatment with 2-DCF or purine analogues.

Splenectomy

In typical patients with CLL, splenectomy is used in the management of refractory or recurrent autoimmune hemolytic anemia or immune thrombocytopenia. Massive splenomegaly that produces discomfort and is associated with pancytopenia is also a cause for consideration of splenectomy as a therapeutic option. Splenectomy is recommended for patients who are considered to have reasonable bone marrow reserves.[106, 341] Ferrant and colleagues[106] performed splenectomy in 20 patients in whom ferrokinetic studies indicated that adequate erythropoiesis was still possible in the marrow. Most of the patients had an improvement in well-being and a markedly decreased transfusion requirement after splenectomy. An increase in hemoglobin and platelet count was demonstrated in most patients. No survival advantage was demonstrated compared with other patients. Pegourie and associates[298] performed splenectomy in 43 patients who were refractory to therapy with chlorambucil. Of 33 patients assigned to Rai stage IV before splenectomy, 24 became Rai stage 0 to stage II following the surgery.

An analysis of 55 patients with CLL who underwent splenectomy at MDACC was reported and compared with 55 fludarabine-treated patients matched for prognostic factors. This was the first attempt at a case-control study. The operative mortality was 9% because of infection in all cases. The only predictive factor for perioperative mortality was the preoperative performance status. Thirty days postoperatively, 81% of patients had a major platelet increment, 59% had a neutrophil increment, and one third of patients had a major hemoglobin increase. Lower spleen weight was correlated with hemoglobin and neutrophil response, but no factors predicted platelet increment because of the high probability of patients' responding. Among patients in Rai stage IV, the splenectomy group had a trend for improved survival. Laparoscopic splenectomy makes this operation more effective.

Leukapheresis

Because the white blood cell count is greatly elevated in patients with CLL, consideration has been given to the use of intensive leukapheresis in these patients. In one study, an average of 2.9×10^{11} cells could be removed at each attempt with alternate-day pheresis.[65] More than half of the patients had a significant elevation of hemoglobin and platelet levels and a decrease in the lymphocyte count. Most of the responders had a decrease in splenomegaly and lymphadenopathy. Disease control was maintained in most patients for more than 12 months. Seldom is leukapheresis necessary for leukocytosis because symptoms of leukostasis, such as dyspnea, hypoxemia, pulmonary infiltrates, and neurologic symptoms, are uncommon

unless the white blood cell count is extremely high ($>400 \times 10^9$/L).

Intravenous Immune Globulin

The majority of patients in the early stage of their disease have normal gamma globulin levels. However, as the disease progresses, the frequency of hypogammaglobulinemia increases to approximately one third in patients with advanced-stage disease and 20% to 30% for lower stage disease. Low levels of IgA and IgM are more common than are low IgG levels.[342] Hypogammaglobulinemia eventually develops in more than 50% of patients as the disease progresses and more chemotherapy is given.[103] Low levels of IgG antibodies to *E. coli*, lipopolysaccharides, and *Streptococcus pneumoniae* have been found in CLL.[57] The response to vaccination with diphtheria, typhoid, influenza, and mumps is unsatisfactory. The incidence of infection has been related to the gamma globulin level in several patients, although this is not a consistent finding. A number of anecdotal reports of reduced infection were noted in patients who received intramuscular immune globulin. The availability of preparations of monomeric IgG for intravenous administration has caused a reinvestigation of the role of prophylactic use of intravenous immune globulin (IVIG) in CLL. Delivery of high doses of IgG enables the levels of immunoglobulins to be maintained if infusions are repeated at 3- to 4-week intervals. In a randomized comparative trial of IVIG for prevention of infections, 41 patients received IVIG and 40 patients received placebo.[66] More of the patients in the placebo group had a severe decrease in IgG level below 350 mg/dL. The IVIG group had a significant decrease in moderate and trivial bacterial infections but not in major infections. No influence on the incidence of infections by fungi or viruses was noted. Consequently, the cost efficacy of such an approach is dubious at this time.

RECOMMENDATIONS FOR THE TREATMENT OF CLL

Studies, particularly those carried out by the French Cooperative Group, have demonstrated that a group of patients with smoldering CLL may never need treatment.[130] The initial evaluation of patients should, therefore, firmly establish this subset of patients with use of criteria spelled out by the French and Spanish investigators.[130, 271] Patients who do not fulfill the NCIWG and IWGCLL criteria for immediate treatment should have therapy delayed because there is no indication that early treatment with alkylating agents improves survival, although the development of aggressive disease is delayed. Patients with CLL who have marrow failure, advanced disease with bulky tumor, or systemic symptoms or those who demonstrate aggressive disease while under observation should receive therapy. There is no evidence that CHOP or CVP regimens are superior to chlorambucil regimens, especially high-dose chlorambucil therapy. Comparative studies have demonstrated that the response rate, particularly the CR rate, is higher with purine analogues than with alkylating agent regimens. Therefore, a good case can be made on scientific grounds to treat patients with fludarabine as initial therapy.

If patients have been treated with an alkylating agent regimen and are refractory or progress, the data strongly suggest that they should be treated with a purine analogue alone or in combination with alkylators. One comparative clinical trial has demonstrated a higher response rate with fludarabine than with CAP.

Many unresolved issues remain, such as the appropriate duration of treatment. Should patients continue to be treated beyond conventional CR to a molecular CR (return to germline immunoglobulin gene pattern) or at least to a pathologic CR (no residual disease by marrow biopsy or flow cytometry)? Does the higher response rate with purine analogue therapy translate into a survival advantage for the most responsive subset of patients? Should autologous and allogeneic bone marrow transplantations be used as intensification regimens or be reserved for patients who are totally refractory to alkylating agent regimens and purine analogues? These issues have not been resolved, and no strong treatment recommendations can be made. The future role of monoclonal antibodies will depend on the results of current clinical trials. Attempts to maintain remissions have not been carried out. Much work needs to be done before a clear strategy of treatment can be recommended for this long-lasting illness, especially when the diversity of patients who are afflicted with the disease is considered.

SUMMARY

The availability of a number of new biologic tests has enabled us to gain greater insights into the pathophysiologic mechanism of CLL. New treatment options, including the purine analogues and increasing use of monoclonal antibodies and bone marrow transplantation, raise a new sense of optimism that treatment will eventually change the natural history of this seductively slow-growing disease. Significant advances in diagnosis and management are predicted within the next 10 years.

REFERENCES

1. Adachi M, Tefferi A, Greipp PR, et al: Preferential linkage of BCL2 to immunoglobulin light chain gene in chronic lymphocytic leukemia. J Exp Med 1990;171:559.
2. Aguilar-Santelises M, Magnusson R, Svenson SB, et al: Expression of interleukin-1α, interleukin-1β and interleukin-6 in chronic lymphocytic leukaemia (B-CLL) cells from patients at different stages of disease progression. Clin Exp Immunol 1991;84:422.
3. Aisenberg AC, Bloch KJ: Immunoglobulins on the surface of neoplastic lymphocytes. N Engl J Med 1972;287:272.
4. Aksoy M: Benzene hematotoxicity. In Aksoy M (ed): Benzene Carcinogenicity. Boca Raton: CRC Press; 1988, p 59.
5. Alberts DS, Chang SY, Chen HSG, et al: Pharmacokinetics and metabolism of chlorambucil in man: A preliminary report. Cancer Treat Rep 1979;6:9.
6. Allebes WA, Preijers FW, Haanen C, et al: The development of nonresponsiveness to immunotherapy with monoclonal antiidiotypic antibodies in a patient with B-CLL. Br J Haematol 1988; 70:295.
7. Almasri NM, Dugue RE, Iturraspe J, et al: Reduced expression of CD20 antigen is a characteristic marker for CLL. Am J Hematol 1992;40:256.
8. Alvarez de Mon M, Casas J, Laguna R, et al: Lymphokine induction of MK-like cytotoxicity in T cells from B-CLL. Blood 1986;67:228.
9. Amamoo DG, Moayeri H, Takita H, et al: Bronchogenic carcinoma in chronic lymphocytic leukemia. Chest 1979;75:174.
10. Anastasi J, Le Beau MM, Vardiman JW, et al: Detection of trisomy 12 in chronic lymphocytic leukemia by fluorescence in situ hybridization to interphase cells: A simple and sensitive method. Blood 1992;79:1796.
11. Antin JH, Ault KA, Rappeport JM, et al: B lymphocyte reconstitution after human bone marrow transplantation. J Clin Invest 1987; 80:325.
12. Ault KA, Antin JH, Ginssburg D, et al: Phenotype of recovering lymphoid cell populations after marrow transplantation. J Exp Med 1985;161:1483.
13. Ayanlar-Batuman O, Ebert E, Hauptman SP: Defective interleukin-2 production and responsiveness by T cells in patients with chronic lymphocytic leukemia of B cell variety. Blood 1986;67:279.
14. Azuma C, Tanabe T, Konishi M, et al: Cloning of cDNA for human T-cell replacing factor (interleukin-5) and comparison with the murine homologue. Nucleic Acids Res 1986;14:149.
15. Baldini L, Cro L, Cortelezzi R, et al: Immunophenotypes in "classical" B-cell chronic lymphocytic leukemia. Correlation with normal cellular counterpart and clinical findings. Cancer 1990;66:1738.
16. Baldini L, Mozzana R, Cortelezzi A, et al: Prognostic significance of immunoglobulin phenotype in B cell chronic lymphocytic leukemia. Blood 1985;65:340.
17. Banchereau J: In Melchers F, Potter M (eds): Mechanisms of B Cell Neoplasia. Basel: Editiones Roche; 1991, p 129.
18. Bastion Y, Felman P, Dumontet C, et al: Intensive radiochemotherapy with peripheral blood stem cell transplantation in young patients with chronic lymphocytic leukemia. Bone Marrow Transplant 1992;10:467.
19. Batata A, Shen B: Immunophenotyping of subtypes of B-chronic (mature) lymphoid leukemia. A study of 242 cases. Cancer 1992; 70:2436.
20. Batata A, Shen B: Relationship between chronic lymphocytic leukemia and small lymphocytic lymphoma. A comparative study of membrane phenotypes in 270 cases. Cancer 1992;70:625.
21. Ben-Bassat I, Many A, Modan M, et al: Serum immunoglobulins in chronic lymphocytic leukemia. Am J Med Sci 1979;278:4.
22. Bennett JM, Raphael B, Moore D, et al: Comparison of chlorambucil and prednisone vs. total body irradiation and chlorambucil/prednisone vs. cytoxan, vincristine, prednisone for the therapy of active chronic lymphocytic leukemia: A long term follow-up of two ECOG studies. In Gale RP, Rai KR (eds): Chronic Lymphocytic Leukemia: Recent Progress and Future Direction. UCLA Symposium on Molecular and Cellular Biology. New series. New York: Alan R Liss; 1987, p 317.
23. Bennett JM, Catovsky D, Daniel MT, et al: The French-American-British (FAB) Cooperative Group. Proposals for the classification of chronic (mature) B and T lymphoid leukaemias. J Clin Pathol 1989;42:567.
24. Berman JE, Mellis SJ, Pollock R, et al: Content and organization of the human Ig VH locus: Definition of three new VH families and linkage to the Ig CH locus. EMBO J 1988;7:727.
25. Berrebi A: Epidemiology and ethical aspects of chronic lymphocytic leukemia. Abstracts of the 5th International Workshop on CLL. Stiges (Barcelona), Spain, April 26–28, 1991, p 36a.
26. Bertazzi PA, Zocchetti C, Pesatori AC, et al: Ten-year mortality study of the population involved in the Seveso incident in 1976. Am J Epidemiol 1989;129:1187.
27. Bertoli LF, Kubagawa H, Borzillo GV, et al: Analysis with antiidiotype antibody of a patient with chronic lymphocytic leukemia and a large cell lymphoma (Richter's syndrome). Blood 1987; 70:45.
28. Bindon CI, Hale G, Bruggemann M, et al: Human monoclonal IgG isotypes differ in complement activating function at the level of C4 binding as well as C1q. J Exp Med 1987;168:127.
29. Binet JL, Auquier A, Dighiero G, et al: A new prognostic classification of chronic lymphocytic leukemia derived from a multivariate survival analysis. Cancer 1981;48:198.
30. Binet JL, Catovsky D, Chandra P, et al: Chronic lymphocytic leukaemia: Proposals for a revised prognostic staging system. Br J Haematol 1981;48:365.

31. Binet JL, Leporrier M, Dighiero G, et al: A clinical staging system for chronic lymphocytic leukemia. Prognostic significance. Cancer 1977;40:855.

32. Bird ML, Ueshima Y, Rowley JD, et al: Chromosome abnormalities in B cell chronic lymphocytic leukemia and their clinical correlations. Leukemia 1989;3:182.

33. Blair A, Malker H, Cantor KP, et al: Cancer among farmers. A review. Scand J Work Environ Health 1985;11:397.

34. Blattner WA: Human Retrovirology: HTLV. New York: Raven Press; 1990, p 1.

35. Boggs DR, Sofferman SA, Wintrobe MM, et al: Factors influencing the duration of survival of patients with chronic lymphocytic leukemia. Am J Med 1966;40:243.

36. Bonvalet D, Foldes C, Civatte J: Cutaneous manifestations in chronic lymphocytic leukemia. J Dermatol Surg Oncol 1984; 10:278.

37. Boussiotis VA, Pangalis GA: Randomized clinical trial with alpha-2b-interferon stage A untreated B-chronic lymphocytic leukemia patients. Nouv Rev Fr Hematol 1988;30:471.

38. Brinker H: Population-based age and sex-specific incidence rates in the 4 main types of leukaemia. Scand J Haematol 1982;29:241.

39. Brock N, Pohl J, Stekar J: Detoxification of urotoxic oxazaphosphorines by sulfhydryl compounds. J Cancer Res Clin Oncol 1981; 100:311.

40. Bron D, Biron G, Leleux A, et al: Serum soluble CD23 is a prognostic marker in chronic lymphocytic leukemia (CLL). Blood 1992; 80:41a.

41. Brooks DA, Beckman IGR, Bradley J, et al: Human lymphocyte markers defined by antibodies derived from somatic cell hybrids. IV. A monoclonal antibody reacting specifically with a subpopulation of human B lymphocytes. J Immunol 1981;126:1373.

42. Brouet JC, Sasportes M, Flandrin F, et al: Chronic lymphocytic leukaemia of T cell origin. Immunologic and clinical evaluation in eleven patients. Lancet 1975;2:890.

43. Browett PJ, Yaxley JC, Norton JD: Activation of Harvey ras oncogene by mutation at codon 12 is very rare in hemopoietic malignancies. Leukemia 1989;3:86.

44. Bullrich F, Rasio D, Kitada S, et al: ATM mutations in B-cell chronic lymphocytic leukemia. Cancer Res 1999;59:24.

45. Buschle M, Campana D, Richard C, et al: Interferon gamma inhibits apoptotic cell death in B cell chronic lymphocytic leukemia. J Exp Med 1992;177:213.

46. Byrd J, Grever M, Davis B, et al: Phase I/II studies of thrice weekly rituximab in CLL/SLL. A feasible and active regimen. Blood 1999; 94:704a.

47. Cachia PG, Dewar AE, Krajweski AS, et al: Distribution of a set of idiotopes detected by a monoclonal antibody panel in 42 cases of chronic lymphocytic leukaemia: Definition of potential targets from immunotherapy. Br J Haematol 1989;72:150.

48. Caligaris-Cappio F, Gobbi M, Bofill M, et al: Infrequent normal B lymphocytes express features of B chronic lymphocytic leukemia. J Exp Med 1982;155:623.

49. Call TG, Phyliky RL, Noel P, et al: Incidence of chronic lymphocytic leukemia in Olmsted County, Minnesota, 1935–1989, with emphasis on changes in the initial stage at diagnosis. Mayo Clin Proc 1994;69:323.

50. Carlsson M, Totterman TH, Matsson P, et al: Cell cycle progression of B-chronic lymphocytic leukemia cells induced to differentiate by TPA. Blood 1988;71:415.

51. Casali P, Burastero SE, Nakamura M, et al: Human lymphocytes making rheumatoid factor and antibody to ssDNA belong to Leu-1⁺ B-cell subset. Science 1987;236:77.

52. Catovsky D: Diagnosis and treatment of CLL variants. In Cheson B (ed): Chronic Lymphocytic Leukemia: Scientific Advances and Clinical Developments. New York: Marcel Dekker; 1993, p 369.

53. Catovsky D, Cherchi M, Brooks D, et al: Heterogeneity of B-cell leukemias demonstrated by the monoclonal antibody FMC7. Blood 1981;58:406.

54. Catovsky D, Cherchi M, Okos A, et al: Mouse red blood cell rosettes in B lymphoproliferative disorders. Br J Haematol 1976; 33:173.

55. Catovsky D, Miliani E, Okos A, et al: Clinical significance of T cells in chronic lymphocytic leukaemia. Lancet 1974;2:751.

56. Catovsky D, Richards S, Fooks J, et al: CLL trials in the United Kingdom—The Medical Research Council CLL trials 1, 2, and 3. Leuk Lymphoma 1991;5:105.

57. Chapel H: Infectious complications in chronic lymphocytic leukemia. In Polliack A, Catovsky D (eds): Chronic Lymphocytic Leukemia. Chur, Switzerland: Harwood Academic Publishers; 1988, p 249.

58. Checkoway H, Wilcosky T, Wolf P, et al: An evaluation of the associations of leukemia and rubber industry solvent exposures. Am J Ind Med 1984;5:239.

59. Cherepakhin V, Baird SM, Meisenholder GW, et al: Common clonal origin of chronic lymphocytic leukemia and high-grade lymphoma of Richter's syndrome. Blood 1993;82:3141.

60. Cheson BD, Bennett JM, Rai KR, et al: Guidelines for clinical protocols for chronic lymphocytic leukemia: Recommendations of the National Cancer Institute–Sponsored Working Group. Am J Hematol 1988;29:152.

61. Cheson BD, Vena DA, Barrett J, et al: Second malignancies as a consequence of nucleoside analog therapy for chronic lymphoid leukemias. J Clin Oncol 1999;17:2454.

62. Clark DA, Alexander FE, McKinney PA, et al: The seroepidemiology of human herpes virus 6 (HHV6) from a case-control study of leukaemia and lymphoma. Int J Cancer 1990;45:829.

63. Colvin M: A review of the pharmacology and clinical use of cyclophosphamide. In Pinedo HM (ed): Clinical Pharmacology of Antineoplastic Drugs. Amsterdam: Elsevier–North Holland; 1978, p 245.

64. Conley CL, Misiti J, Laster AJ, et al: Genetic factors predisposing to CLL and to autoimmune disease. Medicine (Baltimore) 1980; 59:323.

65. Cooper IA, Ding JC, Adams PB, et al: Intensive leukapheresis in the management of cytopenias in patients with chronic lymphocytic leukemia (CLL) and lymphocytic lymphoma. Am J Hematol 1979; 6:387.

66. Cooperative Group for the Study of Immunoglobulin in Chronic Lymphocytic Leukemia: Intravenous immunoglobulin for the prevention of infection in chronic lymphocytic leukemia. N Engl J Med 1988;319:902.

67. Corcoran MM, Rasool O, Liu Y, et al: Detailed molecular delineation of 13q14.3 loss in B-cell chronic lymphocytic leukemia. Blood 1998;91:1382.

68. Cuttner J: Increased incidence of hematologic malignancies in first-degree relatives of patients with chronic lymphocytic leukemia. Cancer Invest 1992;10:103.

69. Dameshek W: Chronic lymphocytic leukemia—an accumulative disease of immunologically incompetent lymphocytes. Blood 1967;29:566.

70. Damle RN, Wasil T, Fais F, et al: Immunoglobulin V gene mutation status and CD38 expression as novel prognostic indicators in chronic lymphocytic leukemia. Blood 1999;94:1840.

71. Danescu M, Rubio-Triyillo M, Biron G, et al: Interleukin-4 protects chronic lymphocytic leukemic B-cells from death by apoptosis and upregulates BCL2 expression. J Exp Med 1992;176:1319.

72. Davis S: Characterization of the phytohemagglutinin-induced proliferating lymphocyte subpopulation in chronic lymphocytic leukemia patients using a clonogenic agar technique and monoclonal antibodies. Blood 1981;58:1053.

73. De Rossi G, Granati L, Girelli G, et al: Incidence and prognostic significance of autoantibodies against erythrocytes and platelets in chronic lymphocytic leukemia (CLL). Nouv Rev Fr Hematol 1988;30:403.

74. De Rossi G, Mandelli F, Covelli A, et al: Chronic lymphocytic leukemia (CLL) in younger adults: A retrospective study of 133 cases. Hematol Oncol 1989;7:127.

75. Dearden C, Catovsky D: Deoxycoformycin in the treatment of mature B-cell malignancies. Br J Cancer 1990;62:4.

76. Dearden CE, Matutes E, Dyer MJS, et al: Campath-1H treatment of T-prolymphocytic leukemia (T-PLL). Blood 1999;94:2929a.

77. Deegan MJ: High incidence of monoclonal proteins in the serum and urine of chronic lymphocytic leukemia patients. Blood 1984; 64:1207.

78. Deegan MJ, Abraham JP, Sawdyk M, et al: High incidence of monoclonal proteins in the serum and urine of chronic lymphocytic leukemia patients. Blood 1984;64:1207.

79. Defrance T, Fluckiger AC, Rossi JF, et al: In vitro activation of B-CLL cells. Leuk Lymphoma 1991;5:13.

80. Delzell E, Monson RR: Mortality among rubber workers. VII. Aerospace workers. Am J Ind Med 1984;6:265.

81. Diehl LF, Karnell LH, Menck HR: The American College of Surgeons Commission on Cancer and the American Cancer Society. The National Cancer Data Base report on age, gender, treatment, and outcomes of patients with chronic lymphocytic leukemia. Cancer 1999;86:2684.

82. Di Giovanni S, Valentini G, Carducci P, et al: Beta$_2$-microglobulin is a reliable tumor marker in chronic lymphocytic leukemia. Acta Haematol 1989;81:181.

83. Di Raimondo F, Giustolisi R, Cacciola E, et al: Autoimmune hemolytic anemia in chronic lymphocytic leukemia patients treated with fludarabine. Leuk Lymphoma 1993;11:63.

84. Digel W, Schoniger W, Stefanic M, et al: Receptors for tumor necrosis factor on neoplastic B cells from chronic lymphocytic leukemia are expressed in vitro but not in vivo. Blood 1990; 76:1607.

85. Digel W, Stefanic M, Sconiger W, et al: Tumor necrosis factor induces proliferation of neoplastic B cells from chronic lymphocytic leukemia. Blood 1989;73:1242.

86. Dighiero G: An attempt to explain disordered immunity and hypogammaglobulinemia in CLL. Nouv Rev Fr Hematol 1988;30:283.

87. Dighiero G, Hart S, Lim A, et al: Autoantibody activity of immunoglobulins isolated from B-cell follicular lymphomas. Blood 1991; 78:581.

88. Dighiero G, Travade P, Chevret S, et al: B-cell chronic lymphocytic leukemia: Present status and future directions. Blood 1991;78: 1901.

89. Dighiero G, Maloum K, Desablens B, et al: Chlorambucil in indolent chronic lymphocytic leukemia. N Engl J Med 1998;338:1506.

90. Dillman RO, Beauregard JL, Lea JW, et al: Chronic lymphocytic leukemia and other chronic lymphoid proliferations: Surface marker phenotypes and clinical correlations. J Clin Oncol 1983; 3:190.

91. Dillman RO, Mick R, McIntyre OR: Pentostatin in chronic lymphocytic leukemia: A phase II trial of cancer and leukemia group B. J Clin Oncol 1989;7:433.

92. Dohner H, Stilgenbauer S, Doner K, et al: Chromosome aberrations in B-cell chronic lymphocytic leukemia: Reassessment based on molecular genetic analysis. J Mol Med 1999;77:266.

93. Dohner H, Stilgenbauer S, James MR, et al: 11q deletions identify a new subset of B-cell chronic lymphocytic leukemia characterized by extensive nodal involvement and inferior prognosis. Blood 1997;89:2516.

94. Dohner H, Stilgenbauer S, Benner A, et al: Genomic aberrations and survival in chronic lymphocytic leukemia. N Engl J Med 2000; 343:1910.

95. Dreger P, Michallet M, Schmitz N: Stem-cell transplantation for chronic lymphocytic leukemia. The 1999 perspective. Ann Oncol 2000;11:S49.

96. Einhorn S, Meeker T, Juliusson G, et al: No evidence of trisomy 12 or t(11;14) by molecular genetic techniques in chronic lymphocytic leukemia cells with a normal karyotype. Cancer Genet Cytogenet 1990;48:183.

97. El Rouby S, Thomas A, Costin D, et al: p53 gene mutation in B-cell chronic lymphocytic leukemia is associated with drug resistance and is independent of MDR1/MDR3 gene expression. Blood 1993;82:3452.

98. Enno A, Catovsky D, O'Brien M, et al: "Prolymphocytoid" transformation of chronic lymphocytic leukemia. Br J Haematol 1979;41:9.

99. Escudier SM, Pereira-Leahy JM, Drach JW, et al: Fluorescent in situ hybridization and cytogenetic studies of trisomy 12 in chronic lymphocytic leukemia. Blood 1993;81:2702.

100. Ezdinli EZ, Stutzman L: Chlorambucil therapy for lymphomas and chronic lymphocytic leukemia. JAMA 1965;191:444.

101. Ezdinli EZ, Stutzman L, William Aungst C, et al: Corticosteroid therapy for lymphomas and chronic lymphocytic leukemia. Cancer 1969;23:900.

102. Faguet GB, Agee JF, DiPiro JT: Blood kinetics, tissue distribution, and radioimaging of anti-common chronic lymphatic leukemia antigen (cCLLa) monoclonal antibody CLL$_2$ in mice transplanted with cCLLa-bearing human leukemia cells. Blood 1990;75:1853.

103. Fairley GH, Scott RB: Hypogammaglobulinemia in chronic lymphocytic leukemia. Br Med J 1961;2:920.

104. Fenchel K, Bergmann L, Jahn B, et al: Fludarabine phosphate in refractory chronic lymphocytic leukemia. Onkologie 1991; 14(suppl 2):190.

105. Fermand JP, James JM, Herait P, et al: Associated chronic lymphocytic leukemia and multiple myeloma: Origin from a single clone. Blood 1985;66:291.

106. Ferrant A, Michaux JL, Sokal G: Splenectomy in advanced chronic lymphocytic leukemia. Cancer 1986;58:2130.

107. Ferrara F, Vecchio LD, Mele G, et al: A new combination chemotherapy for advanced chronic lymphocytic leukemia (vincristine, cyclophosphamide, melphalan, peptichemio, and prednisone protocol). Cancer 1989;64:789.

108. Fialkow PJ, Najfeld V, Reddy AL, et al: Chronic lymphocytic leukemia: Clonal origin in a committed B-lymphocyte progenitor. Lancet 1978;2:444.

109. Finch SC, Finch CA: Summary of the Studies at ABCC-RERF Concerning the Late Hematologic Effects of Atomic Bomb Exposure in Hiroshima and Nagasaki (RERF technical report 2388). Hiroshima, Japan: Radiation Effects Research Foundation; 1988, p 5.

110. Finch SC, Linet MS: Chronic leukaemias. Baillieres Clin Haematol 1992;5:27.

111. Fitchett M, Griffiths MJ, Oscier DG, et al: Chromosome abnormalities involving band 13q14 in hematologic malignancies. Cancer Genet Cytogenet 1987;24:143.

112. Foa R, Fierro T, Giovarelli M, et al: Immunoregulatory T-cell defects in B-cell chronic lymphocytic leukemia: Cause or consequence of the disease? The contributory role of decreased availability of interleukin 2 (IL-2). Blood Cells 1987;12:399.

113. Foa R, Fierro MT, Raspadori D, et al: Lymphokine-activated killer (LAK) cell activity in B and T chronic lymphoid leukemia: Defective LAK generation and reduced susceptibility of the leukemic cells to allogeneic and autologous LAK effectors. Blood 1990; 76:1349.

114. Foa R, Gillio Tos A, Francia di Celle P, et al: Cytokines in B-cell chronic lymphocytic leukemia. Leuk Lymphoma 1991;5:7.

115. Foa R, Giovarelli M, Jemma C, et al: Interleukin 2 (IL-2) and interferon-γ production by T lymphocytes from patients with B-chronic lymphocytic leukemia: Evidence that normally released IL-2 is absorbed by the neoplastic B cell population. Blood 1985; 66:614.

116. Foa R, Lauria F, Catovsky D, et al: Reduced T-colony forming capacity in B-chronic lymphocytic leukaemia. II. Correlation with clinical stage and findings in B-prolymphocytic leukaemia. Leuk Res 1982;6:329.

117. Foa R, Lauria F, Lusso P, et al: Discrepancy between phenotypic and functional features of natural killer T-lymphocytes in B-cell chronic lymphocytic leukaemia. Br J Haematol 1984;58:509.

118. Foa R, Massaia M, Cardona S, et al: Production of tumor necrosis factor-α by B-cell chronic lymphocytic leukemia cells: A possible regulatory role of TNF in the progression of the disease. Blood 1990;76:393.

119. Foon KA, Bottino GC, Fer MF, et al: Phase II trial of recombinant leukocyte A interferon in patients with advanced chronic lymphocytic leukemia. Am J Med 1985;78:216.

120. Foon KA, Rai KR, Gale RP: Chronic lymphocytic leukemia: New insights into biology and therapy. Ann Intern Med 1990;113:525.

121. Foon KA, Todd RF III: Immunologic classification of leukemia and lymphoma. Blood 1986;68:1.

122. Foroni L, Catovsky D, Luzzatto L: Immunoglobulin gene rearrangements in hairy cell leukemia and other chronic B cell lymphoproliferative disorders. Leukemia 1987;1:389.

123. Foucar K, Rydell RE: Richter's syndrome in chronic lymphocytic leukemia. Cancer 1980;46:118.

124. Freedman AS, Boyd AW, Bieber FR, et al: Normal cellular counterparts of B cell chronic lymphocytic leukemia. Blood 1987;70:418.

125. Freedman AS, Freeman G, Whitman J, et al: Studies on in vitro activated CD5$^+$ B cells. Blood 1989;73:202.

126. Freeman CG, Freedman AS, Rabinolowe SN, et al: Interleukin-6 gene expression in normal and neoplastic B-cells. J Clin Invest 1989;83:1512.

127. French Cooperative Group on Chronic Lymphocytic Leukaemia: Effectiveness of "CHOP" regimen in advanced untreated chronic lymphocytic leukaemia. Lancet 1986;1:1346.

128. French Cooperative Group on Chronic Lymphocytic Leukaemia: Effects of chlorambucil and therapeutic decision in initial forms of chronic lymphocytic leukaemia (stage A): Results of a randomized clinical trial in 612 patients. Blood 1990;75:1414.

129. French Cooperative Group on Chronic Lymphocytic Leukaemia:

Long-term results of the CHOP regimen in stage C chronic lymphocytic leukaemia. Br J Haematol 1989;73:334.

130. French Cooperative Group on Chronic Lymphocytic Leukaemia: Natural history of stage A chronic lymphocytic leukaemia untreated patients. Br J Haematol 1990;76:45.

131. French Cooperative Group on Chronic Lymphocytic Leukaemia: Prognostic and therapeutic advances in chronic lymphocytic leukemia management: The experience of the French Cooperative Group. Semin Hematol 1987;24:275.

132. French Cooperative Group on Chronic Lymphocytic Leukaemia, Johnson S, Smith AG, Löffler H, et al: Multicentre prospective randomised trial of fludarabine versus cyclophosphamide, doxorubicin, and prednisone (CAP) for treatment of advanced-stage chronic lymphocytic leukaemia. Lancet 1996;347:1432.

133. Gahrton G, Robert KH, Friberg K, et al: Nonrandom chromosomal aberrations in chronic lymphocytic leukemia revealed by polyclonal B-cell-mitogen stimulation. Blood 1980;56:640.

134. Gaidano G, Ballerini P, Gong JZ, et al: p53 Mutations in human lymphoid malignancies: Association with Burkitt lymphoma and chronic lymphocytic leukemia. Proc Natl Acad Sci U S A 1991; 88:5413.

135. Galton DAG, Wiltshaw E, Szur L, et al: The use of chlorambucil and steroids in the treatment of chronic lymphocytic leukaemia. Br J Haematol 1961;7:73.

136. Garfinkel L, Boffetta P: Association between smoking and leukemia in two American Cancer Society prospective studies. Cancer 1990; 65:2356.

137. Geisler CH, Larsen JK, Hansen NE, et al: Prognostic importance of flow cytometric immunophenotyping of 540 consecutive patients with B-cell chronic lymphocytic leukemia. Blood 1991;78:1795.

138. Gignac SM, Buschle M, Heslop HE, et al: Delayed activation of proto-oncogene expression in B-CLL cells by tumour necrosis factor. Leuk Lymphoma 1990;3:37.

139. Gignac SM, Buschle M, Pettit GR, et al: Expression of proto-oncogene c-jun during differentiation of B-chronic lymphocytic leukaemia. Leuk Lymphoma 1990;4:441.

140. Ginsberg AM, Raffeld M, Cossman J: Inactivation of the retinoblastoma gene in human lymphoid neoplasms. Blood 1991;77:833.

141. Goeddel DV, Yelverton E, Ullrich A, et al: Human leukocyte interferon produced by E. coli is biologically active. Nature 1980; 287:411.

142. Gordon J, Mellstedt H, Aman P, et al: Phenotypes in chronic B-lymphocytic leukemia probed by monoclonal antibodies and immunoglobulin secretion studies: Identification of stages of maturation arrest and the relation to clinical findings. Blood 1983; 62:910.

143. Gray PW, Leung DW, Pennica D, et al: Expression of human immune interferon cDNA in E. coli and monkey cells. Nature 1982;295:503.

144. Grever MR, Kopecky KJ, Coltman CA, et al: Fludarabine monophosphate: A potentially useful agent in chronic lymphocytic leukemia. Nouv Rev Fr Hematol 1988;30:457.

145. Grever MR, Leiby JM, Kraut EH, et al: Low-dose deoxycoformycin in lymphoid malignancy. J Clin Oncol 1985;3:1196.

146. Gribben JG, Neuberg D, Soiffer RJ, et al: Autologous versus allogeneic bone marrow transplantation for patients with poor-prognosis CLL. Blood 1998;92:322a.

147. Gupta S, Good RA, Siegal FP: Rosette formation with mouse erythrocytes. II. A marker for human B and non-T lymphocytes. Clin Exp Immunol 1976;25:319.

148. Hahn I, Kuminsky G, Bassous L, et al: Tumour necrosis factor production in B-cell chronic lymphocytic leukemia. Leuk Lymphoma 1991;4:117.

149. Hallek M, Langenmayer I, Nerl C, et al: Elevated serum thymidine kinase levels identify a subgroup at high risk of disease progression in early, nonsmoldering chronic lymphocytic leukemia. Blood 1999;93:1732.

150. Hallek M, Wanders L, Ostwald M, et al: Serum β_2-microglobulin and serum thymidine kinase are independent predictors of progression-free survival in chronic lymphocytic leukemia and immunocytoma. Leuk Lymphoma 1996;22:439.

151. Hamblin TJ, Oscier DG, Stevens JR, et al: Long survival in B-CLL correlates with surface IgM kappa phenotype. Br J Haematol 1987; 66:21.

152. Hamblin TJ, Oscier DJ, Young BJ: Autoimmunity in chronic lymphocytic leukemia. J Clin Pathol 1986;39:713.

153. Hamblin TJ, Davis Z, Gardiner A, et al: Unmutated immunoglobulin V_H genes are associated with a more aggressive form of chronic lymphocytic leukemia. Blood 1999;94:1848.

154. Han T: Spontaneous remission in chronic lymphocytic leukemia: An update. Blood Cells 1987;12:481.

155. Han T, Barcos M, Gomez GA, et al: Clinical, immunological and cytogenetic studies in chronic lymphocytic leukemia with large cell lymphoma transformation (Richter's syndrome) [abstract]. Proc Am Soc Clin Oncol 1988;7:714.

156. Han T, Bhargava A, Henderson ES, et al: Prognostic significance of beta$_2$microglobulin (β_2m) in chronic lymphocytic leukemia (CLL) and non-Hodgkin's lymphoma (NHL). [abstract 270]. Proc Am Soc Clin Oncol 1989;8:270.

157. Han T, Bloom ML, Dadey B, et al: Lack of autologous mixed lymphocyte reaction in patients with chronic lymphocytic leukemia: Evidence for autoreactive T-cell dysfunction not correlated with phenotype, karyotype, or clinical status. Blood 1982;60:1075.

158. Han T, Ezdinli EZ, Shimaoka K, et al: Chlorambucil vs. combined chlorambucil-corticosteroid therapy in chronic lymphocytic leukemia. Cancer 1973;31:502.

159. Han T, Henderson ES, Emrich LJ, et al: Prognostic significance of karyotypic abnormalities in B cell chronic lymphocytic leukemia: An update. Semin Hematol 1987;24:257.

160. Han T, Moayeri H, Minowada J: T- and B-lymphocytes in chronic lymphocytic leukemia: Correlation with clinical and immunologic status of the disease. J Natl Cancer Inst 1976;57:477.

161. Han T, Ozer H, Gavigan M, et al: Benign monoclonal B cell lymphocytosis—a benign variant of CLL: Clinical, immunologic, phenotypic, and cytogenetic studies in 20 patients. Blood 1984; 64:244.

162. Han T, Sadamori N, Ozer H, et al: Cytogenetic studies in 77 patients with chronic lymphocytic leukemia: Correlations with clinical, immunologic, and phenotypic data. J Clin Oncol 1984; 2:1121.

163. Hanada M, Delia D, Aiello A, et al: Bcl2 gene hypomethylation and high-level expression in B-cell chronic lymphocytic leukemia. Blood 1993;82:1820.

164. Hansen MM: Chronic lymphocytic leukaemia. Clinical studies based on 189 cases followed for a long time. Scand J Haematol 1973;18:3.

165. Hansen MM, Andersen E, Birgens H, et al: CHOP versus chlorambucil + prednisone in chronic lymphocytic leukemia. Leuk Lymphoma 1991;5:97.

166. Hardy RR, Hayakawa K: Development and physiology of Ly-1 B and its human homolog, Leu-1 B. Immunol Rev 1986;93:53.

167. Hardy RR, Hayakawa K, Shimizu K, et al: Rheumatoid factor secretion from human Leu-1$^+$ B cells. Science 1987;236:81.

168. Harousseau JL, Flandrin G, Tricot G, et al: Malignant lymphoma supervening in chronic lymphocytic leukemia and related disorders. Cancer 1981;48:1302.

169. Haughton G, Arnold LW: CD5$^+$ B cell lymphomas of mice. Leuk Lymphoma 1991;5:33.

170. Herzenberg LA, Stall AM, Lalor PA, et al: The Ly1 B cell lineage. Immunol Rev 1986;93:81.

171. Hiddeman W, Rottman R, Wormann P, et al: Treatment of advanced chronic lymphocytic leukemia by fludarabine: Results of a clinical phase II study. Ann Hematol 1991;63:1.

172. Hirano T, Yasukawa K, Harada H, et al: Complementary DNA for a novel interleukin (BSF-2) that induces B lymphocytes to produce immunoglobulin. Nature 1986;324:73.

173. Hoffbrand AV, Heslop HE, Brenner MK: Tumor necrosis factor and autocrine growth loops: Implications for therapy. In Cheson B (ed): Chronic Lymphocytic Leukemia: Scientific Advances and Clinical Developments. New York: Marcel Dekker; 1993, p 63.

174. Hoffbrand AV, Panayiotidis P, Reittie J, et al: Autocrine and paracrine growth loops in chronic lymphocytic leukemia. Semin Hematol 1993;30:306.

175. Honjo T, Habu S: Origin of immune diversity: Genetic variation and selection. Annu Rev Biochem 1985;54:803.

176. Hood L, Ein D: Immunoglobulin lambda chain structure: Two genes, one polypeptide chain. Nature 1968;220:764.

177. Inghirami G, Wieczorek R, Zhu B, et al: Differential expression of LFA1 molecules in non-Hodgkin's lymphoma and lymphoid leukemia. Blood 1988;72:1431.

178. International Workshop on Chronic Lymphocytic Leukemia:

Chronic lymphocytic leukemia: Recommendations for diagnosis, staging, and response criteria. Ann Intern Med 1989;110:236.

179. Jaksic B, Brugiatelli M: High dose continuous chlorambucil vs intermittent chlorambucil plus prednisone for treatment of B-CLL—IGCI CLL-01 trial. Nouv Rev Fr Hematol 1988;30:437.

180. Jaksic B, Brugiatelli M, Krc I, et al: High dose chlorambucil versus Binet's modified cyclophosphamide, doxorubicin, vincristine, and prednisone regimen in the treatment of patients with advanced B-cell chronic lymphocytic leukemia. Results of an international multicenter randomized trial. International Society for Chemo-Immunotherapy, Vienna. Cancer 1997;79:2107.

181. Jaksic B, Vitale B: Total tumour mass score (TIM): A new parameter in chronic lymphocytic leukemia. Br J Haematol 1981;49:405.

182. Jelinek DF, Lipsky PE: Enhancement of human B cell proliferation and differentiation by tumor necrosis factor-α and interleukin 1. J Immunol 1987;138:2970.

183. Johnson RE: Treatment of chronic lymphocytic leukemia by total body irradiation alone and combined with chemotherapy. Int J Radiat Oncol Biol Phys 1979;5:159.

184. Johnstone AP: Chronic lymphocytic leukemia and its relationship to normal B lymphopoiesis. Immunol Today 1982;3:342.

185. Juliusson G, Elmhorn-Rosenborg A, Liliemark J: Response to 2-chlorodeoxyadenosine in patients with B-cell chronic lymphocytic leukemia resistant to fludarabine. N Engl J Med 1992;327:1056.

186. Juliusson G, Gahrton G: Chromosomal aberrations in B-cell chronic lymphocytic leukemia. Pathogenetic and clinical implication. Cancer Genet Cytogenet 1990;45:143.

187. Juliusson G, Gahrton G: Chromosome abnormalities in B-cell chronic lymphocytic leukemia. In Cheson B (ed): Chronic Lymphocytic Leukemia: Scientific Advances and Clinical Developments. New York: Marcel Dekker; 1993, p 83.

188. Juliusson G, Oscier DG, Fitchett M, et al: Prognostic subgroups in B-cell chronic lymphocytic leukemia defined by specific chromosomal abnormalities. N Engl J Med 1990;323:720.

189. Juliusson G, Robert KH, Ost A, et al: Prognostic information from cytogenetic analysis in chronic B-lymphocytic leukemia and leukemic immunocytoma. Blood 1985;65:134.

190. Juliusson G, Liliemark J: Long-term survival following cladribine (2-chlorodeoxyadenosine) therapy in previously treated patients with chronic lymphocytic leukemia (CLL). Ann Oncol 1996;7:373.

191. Juliusson G, Christiansen I, Hanse MM, et al: Oral cladribine as primary therapy for patients with B-cell chronic lymphocytic leukemia. J Clin Oncol 1996;14:2160.

192. Jurlander J, Lai CF, Tan J, et al: Characterization of interleukin-10 receptor expression on B-cell chronic lymphocytic leukemia cells. Blood 1997;89:4146.

193. Kabat E, Wu TT, Reid-Miller M, et al: Sequences of Proteins of Immunological Interest. Bethesda, Md: US Government Printing Office; 1987.

194. Kantarjian HM, Redman JR, Keating MJ: Fludarabine phosphate therapy in other lymphoid malignancies. Semin Oncol 1990;17:66.

195. Karray S, Dautry-Varsat A, Tsudo M, et al: IL-4 inhibits the expression of high affinity IL-2 receptors on monoclonal human B cells. J Immunol 1990;145:1152.

196. Kaung DT, Whittington RM, Spencer HH, et al: Comparison of chlorambucil and streptonigrin (NSC45383) in the treatment of chronic lymphocytic leukemia. Cancer 1969;23:597.

197. Kay NE, Johnson JD, Stanek R, et al: T-cell subpopulations in chronic lymphocytic leukemia: Abnormalities in distribution and in in vitro receptor maturation. Blood 1979;54:540.

198. Kay NE, Kaplan ME: Defective T cell responsiveness in chronic lymphocytic leukemia. Analysis of activation events. Blood 1986;67:578.

199. Kay NE, Oken MM, Maaza JJ, et al: Evidence for tumor reduction in refractory or relapsed B-CLL patients with infusional interleukin-2. Nouv Rev Fr Hematol 1988;30:475.

200. Kay NE, Zarling JM: Impaired natural killer activity in patients with chronic lymphocytic leukemia is associated with a deficiency of azurophilic granules in putative NK cells. Blood 1984;63:305.

201. Keating MJ: Chemotherapy of chronic lymphocytic leukemia. In Cheson B (ed): Chronic Lymphocytic Leukemia: Scientific Advances and Clinical Developments. New York: Marcel Dekker; 1993, p 297.

202. Keating MJ, Hester JP, McCredie KB, et al: Long-term results of CAP therapy in chronic lymphocytic leukemia. Leuk Lymphoma 1990;2:391.

203. Keating MJ, Kantarjian H, O'Brien S, et al: Fludarabine: A new agent with marked cytoreductive activity in untreated chronic lymphocytic leukemia. J Clin Oncol 1991;9:44.

204. Keating MJ, Kantarjian H, Talpaz M, et al: Fludarabine: A new agent with major activity against chronic lymphocytic leukemia. Blood 1989;74:19.

205. Keating MJ, Scouros M, Murphy S, et al: Multiple agent chemotherapy (POACH) in previously treated and untreated patients with chronic lymphocytic leukemia. Leukemia 1988;2:157.

206. Keating MJ, Binet J-L, Brettman L, et al: Therapeutic role of Campath-1H in patients who have failed fludarabine: Results of a large international study (in press).

207. Keller JW, Knospe WH, Raney M, et al: Treatment of chronic lymphocytic leukemia using chlorambucil and prednisone with or without cycle-active consolidation chemotherapy. Cancer 1986;58:1185.

208. Kemena A, O'Brien S, Kantarjian H, et al: Phase II clinical trial of fludarabine in chronic lymphocytic leukemia on a weekly low-dose schedule. Leuk Lymphoma 1993;10:187.

209. Kempin S, Lee BH III, Thaler HT, et al: Combination chemotherapy of advanced chronic lymphocytic leukemia: The M2 protocol (vincristine, BCNU, cyclophosphamide, melphalan and prednisone). Blood 1982;60:1110.

210. Kennedy B, Rawstron AC, Evans P, et al: Campath-1H therapy in 29 patients with refractory CLL. "True" complete remission is attainable goal. Blood 1999;94:603a.

211. Khouri I, Keating M, Przepiorka D, et al: Allogeneic bone marrow transplantation for chronic lymphocytic leukemia [abstract 1540]. Blood 1993;82:389a.

212. Khouri IF, Keating MJ, Vriesendorp H, et al: Autologous and allogeneic bone marrow transplantation for chronic lymphocytic leukemia: Preliminary results. J Clin Oncol 1994;12:748.

213. Khouri I, Munsell M, Yajzi S, et al: Comparable survival for nonablative and ablative allogeneic transplantation for chronic lymphocytic leukemia (CLL): The case for early intervention [abstract 877]. Blood, 2000;96:205a.

214. Khouri IF, Keating MJ, Vriesendorp HM, et al: Autologous and allogeneic bone marrow transplantation for chronic lymphocytic leukemia: Preliminary results. J Clin Oncol 1994;12:748.

215. Khouri IF, Keating MJ, Champlin RE: Hematopoietic stem cell transplantation for chronic lymphocytic leukemia. In Armitage JO, Antman KH (eds): High-Dose Cancer Therapy: Pharmacology, Hematopoietins, Stem Cells, 3rd ed. Philadelphia: Lippincott Williams & Wilkins; 1999.

216. Khouri I, Keating MJ, Korbling M, et al: Transplant lite: Induction of graft vs. malignancy using fludarabine based nonablative chemotherapy and allogeneic progenitor-cell transplantation as treatment for lymphoid malignancies. J Clin Oncol 1998;16:2817.

217. Kimby E, Mellstedt H: Chlorambucil/prednisone versus CHOP in symptomatic chronic lymphocytic leukemias of B-cell type. A randomized trial. Leuk Lymphoma 1991;5:93.

218. Kipps T: Immunologic and therapeutic implications of anti-idiotype antibodies. In Cheson B (ed): Chronic Lymphocytic Leukemia: Scientific Advances and Clinical Developments. New York: Marcel Dekker; 1993, p 123.

219. Kipps TJ, Carson DA: Autoantibodies in chronic lymphocytic leukemia and related systemic autoimmune diseases. Blood 1993;81:2475.

220. Kipps TJ, Fong S, Tomhave E, et al: High-frequency expression of a conserved kappa light-chain variable-region gene in chronic lymphocytic leukemia. Proc Natl Acad Sci U S A 1987;84:2916.

221. Kipps TJ, Robbins BA, Tefferi A, et al: CD5-positive B-cell malignancies frequently express cross-reactive idiotypes associated with IgM autoantibodies. Am J Pathol 1990;136:809.

222. Kipps TJ, Tomhave E, Chen PP, et al: Autoantibody-associated kappa light chain variable region gene expressed in chronic lymphocytic leukemia with little or no somatic mutation. Implications for etiology and immunotherapy. J Exp Med 1988;167:840.

223. Kipps TJ, Tomhave E, Pratt LF, et al: Developmentally restricted immunoglobulin heavy chain variable region gene expressed at high frequency in chronic lymphocytic leukemia. Proc Natl Acad Sci U S A 1989;86:5913.

224. Kirsch IR, Morton CC, Nakahara K, et al: Human immunoglobulin heavy chain genes map to a region of translocations in malignant B lymphocytes. Science 1982;216:301.

225. Knospe WH, Loeb V Jr, Huguley CM Jr: Biweekly chlorambucil treatment of chronic lymphocytic leukemia. Cancer 1974;33:555.

226. Kontoyiannis DP, Anaissie EJ, Bodey GP: Infection in chronic lymphocytic leukemia: A reappraisal. In Cheson B (ed): Chronic Lymphocytic Leukemia: Scientific Advances and Clinical Developments. New York: Marcel Dekker; 1993, p 399.

227. Korsmeyer SJ: Hierarchy of immunoglobulin gene rearrangements in B-cell leukemias. In Waldmann TA (moderator): Molecular genetic analyses of human lymphoid neoplasms: Immunoglobulin genes and the c-myc oncogene. Ann Intern Med 1985;102:497.

228. Kunicka JE, Platsoucas CD: Defective helper function of purified T4 cells and excessive suppressor activity of purified T8 cells in patients with B-cell chronic lymphocytic leukemia. T4 suppressor effector cells are present in certain patients. Blood 1988;71:1551.

229. Laurent G, Gourdin MF, Flandrin G, et al: Acute blast crisis in a patient with chronic lymphocytic leukemia: Immunoperoxidase study. Acta Haematol 1981;65:60.

230. Lauria F, Foa R, Catovsky D: Increase in T gamma lymphocytes in B-cell chronic lymphocytic leukemia. Scand J Haematol 1980; 24:187.

231. Lee JS, Dixon DO, Kantarjian HM, et al: Prognosis of chronic lymphocytic leukemia: A multivariate regression analysis of 325 untreated patients. Blood 1987;69:929.

232. Lennert K, Tamm I, Wacker HH: Histopathology and immunocytochemistry of lymph node biopsies in chronic lymphocytic leukemia and immunocytoma. Leuk Lymphoma 1991;5:157.

233. Leporrier M, Chevret S, Cazin B, et al: Randomized comparison of fludarabine, CAP and ChOP, in 938 previously untreated stage B and C-chronic lymphocytic leukemia (in press).

234. Lichtman MA, Rowe JM: Hyperleukocytic leukemias: Rheological, clinical and therapeutic considerations. Blood 1982;60:279.

235. Liepman M, Votaw ML: The treatment of chronic lymphocytic leukemia with COP chemotherapy. Cancer 1978;41:1664.

236. Lindemann A, Ludwig WD, Oster W, et al: High-level secretion of tumor necrosis factor-alpha contributes to hematopoietic failure in hairy cell leukemia. Blood 1988;73:880.

237. Linet MS: The Leukemias: Epidemiologic Aspects. New York: Oxford University Press; 1985, p 14.

238. Linet MS, Bias WB, Dorgan JF, et al: HLA antigens in chronic lymphocytic leukemia. Tissue Antigens 1988a;31:71.

239. Linet MS, Blattner WA: The epidemiology of chronic lymphocytic leukemia. In Polliack A, Catovsky D (eds): Chronic Lymphocytic Leukemia. Chu, Switzerland: Harwood Academic Publishers; 1988, p 11.

240. Luo H, Rubio M, Biron G, et al: Antiproliferative effects of interleukin-4 in B-chronic lymphocytic leukemia. J Immunother 1991; 10:418.

241. Luzzatto L, Foronia L: DNA rearrangements of cell lineage specific genes in lymphoproliferative disorders. Prog Hematol 1986;14: 303.

242. Mageed RA, Dearlove M, Goodall DM, et al: Immunogenic and antigenic epitopes of immunoglobulins. XVII. Monoclonal antibodies reactive with common and restricted idiotopes to the heavy chain of human rheumatoid factors. Rheumatol Int 1986;6:179.

243. Mandelli F, DeRossi G, Mancini P, et al: Prognosis in chronic lymphocytic leukemia: A retrospective multicentric study from the GIMEMA group. J Clin Oncol 1987;5:398.

244. Manser T, Wysocki LJ, Margolies MN, et al: Evolution of antibody variable region structure during the immune response. Immunol Rev 1987;96:141.

245. March CJ, Mosley B, Larsen A, et al: Cloning, sequence and expression of two distinct human interleukin-1 complementary DNAs. Nature 1985;315:641.

246. Markey GM, Alexander HD, Agnew AND, et al: Enumeration of absolute numbers of T lymphocyte subsets in B-chronic lymphocytic leukaemia using an immunoperoxidase technique: Relation to clinical stage. Br J Haematol 1986;62:257.

247. Matolcsy A, Inghirami G, Knowles DM: Molecular genetic demonstration of the diverse evolution of Richter's syndrome (chronic lymphocytic leukemia and subsequent large cell lymphoma). Blood 1994;83:1363.

248. Matutes E, Catovsky D: Mature T-cell leukemias and leukemia/lymphoma syndromes. Review of our experience in 175 cases. Leuk Lymphoma 1991;4:81.

249. Matutes E, Owusu-Ankomah K, Morilla R, et al: The immunological profile of B-cell disorders and proposal of a scoring system for the diagnosis of CLL. Leukemia 1994;8:1640.

250. Matutes E, Morilla R, Owusu-Ankomah K, et al: The immunophenotype of splenic lymphoma with villous lymphocytes and its relevance to the differential diagnosis with other B-cell disorders. Blood 1994;83:1558.

251. Mauro FR, Foa R, Cerretti R, et al: Autoimmune hemolytic anemia in chronic lymphocytic leukemia: Clinical, therapeutic, and prognostic features. Blood 2000;95:2786.

252. McCann SR, Whelan CA, Breslin B, et al: Lymphocyte subpopulations following splenic irradiation in patients with chronic lymphocytic leukaemia. Br J Haematol 1982;50:225.

253. Mellstedt H, Osterborg A, Lundin J, et al: Campath-1H therapy of patients with previously untreated chronic lymphocytic leukemia. Blood 1998;92:490a.

254. Melo JV, Catovsky D, Galton DAG: The relationship between chronic lymphocytic leukaemia and prolymphocytic leukaemia. I. Clinical and laboratory features of 300 patients and characterization of an intermediate group. Br J Haematol 1986;63:377.

255. Melo JV, Catovsky D, Galton DAG: The relationship between chronic lymphocytic leukaemia and prolymphocytic leukaemia. II. Patterns of evolution of "prolymphocytoid" transformation. Br J Haematol 1986;64:77.

256. Melo JV, Catovsky D, Gregory WM, et al: The relationship between chronic lymphocytic leukaemia and prolymphocytic leukaemia. IV. Analysis of survival and prognostic features. Br J Haematol 1987;65:23.

257. Melo JV, Robinson DSF, de Oliveira MP, et al: Morphology and immunology of circulating cells in leukaemic phase of follicular lymphoma. J Clin Pathol 1988;41:951.

258. No reference cited.

259. Melo JV, Wardle J, Chetty M, et al: The relationship between chronic lymphocytic leukaemia and prolymphocytic leukaemia. III. Evaluation of cell size by morphology and volume measurements. Br J Haematol 1986;64:469.

260. Menon M, Drexler HG, Minowada J: Heterogeneity of marker expression on B-cell leukemias and its diagnostic significance. Leuk Res 1986;10:25.

261. Michallet M, Archimbaud E, Bandini G, et al: HLA-identical sibling bone marrow transplantation in younger patients with chronic lymphocytic leukemia [brief communications]. Ann Intern Med 1996;124:311.

262. Michallet M, Sotto JJ, Moulin JJ, et al: Management of CLL patients after chlorambucil therapy. Special value of a second Rai staging. Eur J Cancer 1980;16:511.

263. Michieli M, Raspadori D, Damiani D, et al: The expression of the multidrug resistance–associated glycoprotein in B-cell chronic lymphocytic leukaemia. Br J Haematol 1991;77:460.

264. Minot GR, Isaacs R: Lymphatic leukemia, age incidence, duration and benefit derived from irradiation. Boston Med Surg 1924;191:1.

265. Molica S, Alberti A: Prognostic value of the lymphocyte doubling time in chronic lymphocytic leukemia. Cancer 1987;60:2712.

266. Molica S, Levato D, Dell'Olio M, et al: Cellular expression and serum circulating levels of CD23 in B-cell chronic lymphocytic leukemia. Implications for prognosis. Haematologica 1996;81:28.

267. Molica S, Levato D, Cascavilla N, et al: Clinico-prognostic implications of simultaneous increased serum levels of soluble CD23 and β2-microglobulin in B-cell chronic lymphocytic leukemia. Eur J Haematol 1999;62:117.

268. Montserrat E, Gomis F, Vallespi T, et al: Presenting features and prognosis of chronic lymphocytic leukemia in younger adults. Blood 1991;78:1545.

269. Montserrat E, Sanchez-Bisono J, Vinolas N, et al: Lymphocyte doubling time in chronic lymphocytic leukaemia: Analysis of its prognostic significance. Br J Haematol 1986;62:567.

270. Montserrat E, Vinolas N, Reverter JC, et al: Natural history of chronic lymphocytic leukemia: On the progression and prognosis of early clinical stages. Nouv Rev Fr Hematol 1988;30:359.

271. Montserrat E, Virolas N, Reverter JC, et al: Natural history of chronic lymphocytic leukemia: On the progression and prognosis of early clinical stages. Nouv Rev Fr Hematol, 1988;30:359.

272. Mulligan SP, Matutes E, Dearden C, et al: Splenic lymphoma with villous lymphocytes: Natural history and response to therapy in 50 cases. Br J Haematol 1991;78:206.

273. Nadler LM: B cell/leukemia panel workshop: Summary and com-

ments in human B lymphocytes. In Reinherz EL, Haynes BF, Nadler LM, Bernstein I (eds): Leukocyte Typing II. Berlin: Springer-Verlag; 1986, p 1.

274. Neri A, Knowles DM, Greco A, et al: Analysis of RAS oncogene mutations in human lymphoid malignancies. Proc Natl Acad Sci U S A 1988;85:9268.

275. Nilsson K: The control of growth and differentiation in chronic lymphocytic leukemia (B-CLL) cells. In Cheson B (ed): Chronic Lymphocytic Leukemia: Scientific Advances and Clinical Developments. New York: Marcel Dekker; 1993, p 33.

276. Nishiyama H: Relative frequency and mortality rate of various types of leukemia in Japan. Gann 1969;60:71.

277. Nowell PC, Moreau L, Growney P, et al: Karyotypic stability in chronic B-cell leukemia. Cancer Genet Cytogenet 1988;33:155.

278. O'Brien S, Kantarjian H, Beran M, et al: Results of fludarabine and prednisone therapy in 264 patients with chronic lymphocytic leukemia with multivariate analysis–derived prognostic model for response to treatment. Blood 1993;82:1695.

279. O'Brien S, Kantarjian H, Estey E, et al: Lack of effect of 2-chloro-deoxyadenosine therapy in patients with chronic lymphocytic leukemia refractory to fludarabine therapy. N Engl J Med 1994; 330:319.

280. O'Brien SM, Thomas DA, Freireich EJ, et al: Rituximab has significant activity in patients with CLL. Blood 1999;94:603a.

281. Oken MM, Kaplan ME: Combination chemotherapy with cyclophosphamide, vincristine, and prednisone in the treatment of refractory chronic lymphocytic leukemia. Cancer Treat Rep 1979; 63:441.

282. Orfao A, Gonzalez M, San Miguel JF, et al: B-cell chronic lymphocytic leukaemia: Prognostic values of the immunophenotype and the clinico-haematological features. Am J Hematol 1989;31:26.

283. Oscier D, Chapman R, Fitchett M, et al: Deletion of a retinoblastoma gene in B cell chronic lymphocytic leukemia. Blood 1990; 76:241a.

284. Oscier D, Fitchett M, Herbert T, et al: Karyotypic evolution in B-cell chronic lymphocytic leukaemia. Genes Chromosomes Cancer 1991;3:16.

285. Osterborg A, Dyer MJS, Bunjes J, et al: Phase II multicenter study of human CD52 antibody in previously treated CLL. J Clin Oncol 1997;15:1567.

286. Osterborg A, Fassas AS, Anagnostopoulos A, et al: Humanised CD52 monoclonal antibody, Campath-1H, as first line treatment in CLL. Br J Haematol 1996;93:151.

287. Palosaari D, Colby T: Bronchiolocentric chronic lymphocytic leukemia. Cancer 1986;58:1695.

288. Pals ST, Horst E, Ossekoppels GJ, et al: Expression of lymphocyte homing receptor as a mechanism of dissemination in non-Hodgkin's lymphoma. Blood 1989;73:885.

289. Panayiotidis P, Ganeshaguru K, Jabbar SAB, et al: Interleukin-4 inhibits apoptotic cell death and loss of the bcl-2 protein in B-chronic lymphocytic leukemia cells in vitro. Br J Haematol 1993; 85:439.

290. Pangalis GA, Griva E: Recombinant alfa-2b-interferon therapy in untreated, stages A and B chronic lymphocytic leukemia. Cancer 1988;61:869.

291. Pangalis GA, Moutsopoulos HM, Papadopoulos NM, et al: Monoclonal and oligoclonal immunoglobulins in the serum of patients with B-chronic lymphocytic leukemia. Acta Haematol 1988;80:23.

292. Pangalis GA, Reverter JC, Bousiotis VA, et al: Chronic lymphocytic leukemia in younger adults: Preliminary results of a study based on 454 patients. Leuk Lymphoma 1991;5:175.

293. Pangalis GA, Roussou PA, Kittas C, et al: B-chronic lymphocytic leukemias. Prognostic implication of bone marrow histology in 120 patients. Experience from a single hematology unit. Cancer 1987;59:767.

294. Partyka S, O'Brien S, Podoloff D, et al: The usefulness of high dose (7–10 mCi) gallium (^{67}Ga) scanning to diagnose Richter's transformation. Leuk Lymphoma 1999;36:151.

295. Pasquali JL, Knapp AM, Farradji A, et al: Mapping of four light chain–associated idiotopes of a human monoclonal rheumatoid factor. J Immunol 1987;139:818.

296. Pavletic ZS, Bierman PJ, Vose JM, et al: High incidence of relapse after autologous stem-cell transplantation for B-cell chronic lymphocytic leukemia or small lymphocytic leukemia. Ann Oncol 1999;9:1023.

297. Pavletic ZS, Arrowsmith ER, Bierman P, et al: Allogeneic stem-cell transplantation for chronic lymphocytic leukemia. Blood 1998; 92:288a.

298. Pegourie B, Sotto JJ, Hollard D, et al: Splenectomy during chronic lymphocytic leukemia. Cancer 1987;59:1626.

299. Perri RT, Royston I, LeBien T, et al: Chronic lymphocytic leukemia progenitor cells carry the antigens T65, BA-1, and Ia. Blood 1983; 61:871.

300. Peterson L, Blackstadt M, Kay N: Clonal evolution in chronic lymphocytic leukemia. In Cheson B (ed): Chronic Lymphocytic Leukemia: Scientific Advances and Clinical Developments. New York: Marcel Dekker; 1993, p 181.

301. Peterson LC, Lindquist L, Kay NE: Loss of tumor suppressor genes (13q14), clonal and nonclonal cytogenetic abnormalities, and karyotypic evolution in B-chronic lymphocytic leukemia (CLL). Blood 1991;76:1223a.

302. Pianezze G, Gentilini I, Casini M, et al: Cytoplasmic immunoglobulins in chronic lymphocytic leukemia B cells. Blood 1987;69:1011.

303. Pinto A, Zagonel V, Carbone A, et al: Expression of myelomonocytic antigens (MyAgs) on chronic lymphocytic leukemia (CLL) B cells identifies a subset of patients (Pts) with a "variant" CLL phenotype and different biological and clinical features [abstract 792]. Proc Am Soc Clin Oncol 1989;8:204.

304. Pistoia V, Cozzolino F, Rubartelli M, et al: In vitro production of interleukin 1 by normal and malignant human B lymphocytes. J Immunol 1986;136:1688.

305. Pistoia V: Production of cytokines by human B cells in health and disease. Immunol Today 1997;18:343.

306. Plater-Zyberk C, Maini RN, Lam K, et al: A rheumatoid arthritis B cell subset expresses a phenotype similar to that in chronic lymphocytic leukemia. Arthritis Rheum 1985;28:971.

307. Platsoucas CD, Fernandes G, Gupta SL, et al: Defective spontaneous and antibody-dependent cytotoxicity mediated by E rosette-positive and E rosette–negative cells in untreated patients with chronic lymphocytic leukemia. Augmentation by in vitro treatment with interferon. J Immunol 1980;125:1216.

308. Pombo de Oliveira MS, Jaffe ES, Catovsky D: Leukaemic phase of mantle zone (intermediate) lymphoma: Its characterization in 11 cases. J Clin Pathol 1989;42:962.

309. Preud'homme JL, Brouet JC, Clauvel JP, et al: Surface IgD in immunoproliferative disorder. Scand J Immunol 1974;3:853.

310. Preud'homme JL, Seligmann M: Surface-bound immunoglobulins as a cell marker in human lymphoproliferative diseases. Blood 1972;40:777.

311. Provan D, Bartlett-Pandite L, Zwicky C, et al: Eradication of polymerase chain reaction–detectable chronic lymphocytic leukemia cells is associated with improved outcome after bone marrow transplantation. Blood 1996;88:2228.

312. Puccio CA, Mittelman A, Lichtman SM, et al: A loading dose/continuous infusion schedule of fludarabine phosphate in chronic lymphocytic leukemia. J Clin Oncol 1991;9:1562.

313. Pugh WC, Manning JT, Butler JJ: Paraimmunoblastic variant of small lymphocytic lymphoma/leukemia. Am J Surg Pathol 1988; 12:907.

314. Rabinowe SN, Soiffer RJ, Gribben JG, et al: Autologous and allogeneic bone marrow transplantation for poor prognosis patients with B-cell chronic lymphocytic leukemia. Blood 1993;82:1366.

315. Raghoebier S, van Krieken JH, Kluin-Nelemans JC, et al: Oncogene rearrangements in chronic B-cell leukemia. Blood 1991;77:1560.

316. Rai KR: A critical analysis of staging in CLL. In Gale RP, Rai KR (eds): Chronic Lymphocytic Leukemia. Recent Progress and Future Direction. New York: Alan R Liss; 1987, p 253.

317. Rai KR, Sawitsky A, Cronkite EP, et al: Clinical staging of chronic lymphocytic leukemia. Blood 1975;46:219.

318. Rai KR, Peterson BL, Appelbaum FR, et al: Fludarabine compared with chlorambucil as primary therapy for chronic lymphocytic leukemia. N Engl J Med 2000;343:1750.

319. Raphael B, Andersen JW, Silber R, et al: Comparison of chlorambucil and prednisone versus cyclophosphamide, vincristine, and prednisone as initial treatment for chronic lymphocytic leukemia: Long-term follow-up of an Eastern Cooperative Oncology Group randomized clinical trial. J Clin Oncol 1991;9:770.

320. Raphael M, Chastang C, Binet JL: Is bone marrow biopsy a prognostic parameter in CLL? Nouv Rev Fr Hematol 1988;30:377.

321. Rassenti LZ, Pratt LF, Chen PP, et al: Autoantibody-encoding kappa

light chain genes frequently rearranged in lambda light chain expressing chronic lymphocytic leukemia. J Immunol 1991; 147:1060.

322. Ravetch JV, Siebenlist U, Korsmeyer S, et al: Structure of the human immunoglobulin mu locus: Characterization of embryonic and rearranged J and D genes. Cell 1981;27:583.

323. Rechavi G, Katzir N, Brok-Simoni F, et al: A search for BCL1, BCL2, and c-myc oncogene rearrangements in chronic lymphocytic leukemia. Leukemia 1989;3:57.

324. Reittie JE, Ganeshaguru K, Hoffbrand AV: The effect of tumour necrosis factor (TNF), anti-TNF and alpha-interferon on interleukin-6 (IL-6) secretion in B-chronic lymphocytic leukaemia (CLL). Int Soc Haematol 1992;August:37.

325. Reth MG, Jackson S, Alt FW: VHDJH formation and DJH replacement during pre-B differentiation: Non-random usage of gene segments. EMBO J 1986;5:2131.

326. Richter MN: Generalized reticular cell sarcoma of lymph nodes associated with lymphatic leukemia. Am J Pathol 1928;6:285.

327. Roa R, Catovsky D, Brozovic M, et al: Clinical staging and immunological findings in chronic lymphocytic leukemia. Cancer 1979; 44:483.

328. Robbins JH, Lewis WR: Inherent inability of chronic lymphocytic leukaemia lymphocytes to respond to phytohaemagglutinin. Int Arch Allergy 1972;43:845.

329. Robak T, Basinska-Morawiec M, Krykowski E, et al: Intermittent 2-hour i.v. infusions of 2-chlorodeoxyadenosine in the treatment of 110 patients with refractory or previously untreated B-cell chronic lymphocytic leukemia. Leuk Lymphoma 1996;22:509.

330. Robak T, Blonski JZ, Kasznicki M, et al: Cladribine with prednisone versus chlorambucil with prednisone as first-line therapy in chronic lymphocytic leukemia: Report of a prospective, randomized, multicenter trial. Blood 2000;96:2723.

331. Robert KH, Moller E, Gahrton G, et al: B-cell activation of peripheral blood lymphocytes from patients with chronic lymphocytic leukemia. Clin Exp Immunol 1978;33:302.

332. Robertson LE, Chubb S, Meyn RE, et al: Induction of apoptotic cell death in chronic lymphocytic leukemia by 2-chloro-2'-deoxyadenosine and 9β-D-arabinosyl-2-fluoroadenine. Blood 1993;81: 143.

333. Robertson LE, Huang P, McDonnell T, et al: Apoptosis in chronic lymphocytic leukemia: Clinical correlations and in vivo evidence. Am Soc Hematol (in press).

334. Robertson LE, O'Brien S, Kantarjian H, et al: A 3-day schedule of fludarabine in previously treated chronic lymphocytic leukemia. Leukemia 1995;9:1444.

335. Robertson LE, Pugh W, O'Brien S, et al: Richter's syndrome: A report on 39 patients. J Clin Oncol 1993;11:1985.

336. Rondelli D, Lauria F, Zinzani PL, et al: 2-Chlorodeoxyadenosine in the treatment of relapsed/refractory chronic lymphoproliferative disorders. Eur J Haematol 1997;58:46.

337. Ross GD, Rabellino EM, Polley MJ, et al: Combined studies of complement receptor and surface immunoglobulin bearing cells and sheep erythrocyte rosette forming cells in normal and leukemic human lymphocytes. J Clin Invest 1973;52:377.

338. Royston I, Majda JA, Baird SM, et al: Human T cell antigens defined by monoclonal antibodies: The 65,000-dalton antigen of T cells (T65) is also found on chronic lymphocytic leukemia cells bearing surface immunoglobulins. J Immunol 1980;125:625.

339. Rozman C, Montserrat E, Feliu E, et al: Prognosis of chronic lymphocytic leukemia: A multivariate survival analysis of 150 cases. Blood 1982;59:1001.

340. Rozman C, Montserrat E, Rodriguez-Fernandez JM, et al: Bone marrow histologic pattern—the best single prognostic parameter in chronic lymphocytic leukemia: A multivariate survival analysis of 329 cases. Blood 1984;64:642.

341. Rozman C, Montserrat E, Vinolas N, et al: Recombinant alpha 2-interferon in the treatment of B chronic lymphocytic leukemia in early stages. Blood 1988;71:1295.

342. Rozman C, Montserrat E, Vinolas N: Serum immunoglobulins in B-chronic lymphocytic leukemia. Natural history and prognostic significance. Cancer 1988;61:279.

343. Rubin P, Bennett JM, Begg C, et al: The comparison of total body irradiation vs chlorambucil and prednisone for remission induction of active chronic lymphocytic leukemia: An ECOG study. Part I. Total body irradiation—response and toxicity. Int J Radiat Oncol Biol Phys 1981;7:1623.

344. Sainati L, Matutes E, Mulligan S, et al: A variant form of hairy cell leukemia resistant to α-interferon: Clinical and phenotypic characteristics of 17 patients. Blood 1990;76:157.

345. Sarfati M, Chevret S, Chastang C, et al: Prognostic importance of serum soluble CD23 level in chronic lymphocytic leukemia. Blood 1996;88:4259.

346. Saven A, Carrera CJ, Carson DA, et al: 2-Chlorodeoxyadenosine treatment of refractory chronic lymphocytic leukemia. Leuk Lymphoma 1991;5:133.

347. Saven A, Lemon RH, Kosty M, et al: 2-Chlorodeoxyadenosine activity in patients with untreated chronic lymphocytic leukemia. J Clin Oncol 1995;13:570.

348. Sawitsky A, Rai KR, Glidewell O, et al: Comparison of daily versus intermittent chlorambucil and prednisone therapy in the treatment of patients with chronic lymphocytic leukemia. Blood 1977; 50:1049.

349. Schena M, Gaidano G, Gottardi D, et al: Molecular investigation of the cytokines produced by normal and malignant B-lymphocytes. Leukemia 1992;6:120.

350. Schena M, Larsson LG, Gottardi D, et al: Growth and differentiation associated expression of BCL2 in B-chronic lymphocytic leukemia cells. Blood 1992;79:2981.

351. Schroeder HW Jr, Hillson JL, Perlmutter RM: Early restriction of the human antibody repertoire. Science 1987;238:791.

352. Scully RE, Mark EJ, McNeely WF, et al: Case records of the Massachusetts General Hospital. N Engl J Med 1988;319:1268.

353. Seidman JG, Nau MM, Norman B, et al: Immunoglobulin V/J recombination is accompanied by deletion of joining site and variable region segments. Proc Natl Acad Sci U S A 1980;77:6022.

354. Semenzato G, Foa R, Agostini C, et al: High serum levels of soluble interleukin-2 receptor in patients with B chronic lymphocytic leukemia. Blood 1987;70:396.

355. Seymour JF, Khouri IF, Champlin R, et al: Refractory chronic lymphocytic leukemia complicated by hypercalcemia treated with allogeneic bone marrow transplantation: Case report and review. Am J Clin Oncol 1994;17:360.

356. Seymour JF, Robertson LE, O'Brien S, et al: Survival of young patients with chronic lymphocytic leukemia failing fludarabine therapy: A basis for the use of myeloablative therapies. Leuk Lymphoma 1995;18:493.

357. Sharma S, Mehta S, Morgan J, et al: Molecular cloning and expression of a human B-cell growth factor gene in *Escherichia coli*. Science 1987;235:1489.

358. Shirai T, Yamaguchi H, Ito H, et al: Cloning and expression in *Escherichia coli* of the gene for human tumour necrosis factor. Nature 1985;313:803.

359. Slavin S, Nagler A, Naparstak E, et al: Nonmyeloablative stem cell transplantation and cell therapy as an alternative to conventional bone marrow transplantation with lethal cytoreduction for the treatment of malignant and non-malignant hematologic disease. Blood 1998;91:756.

360. Sonneveld P, Nooter K, Burghouts JT, et al: High expression of the mdr3 multidrug-resistance gene in advanced-stage chronic lymphocytic leukemia. Blood 1992;79:1496.

361. Spertini O, Freedman AS, Belvin MP, et al: Regulation of leukocyte adhesion molecule-1 (TQ1, Leu-8) expression and shedding by normal and malignant cells. Leukemia 1991;5:300.

362. Spiro S, Galton DAG, Wiltshaw E, et al: Follicular lymphoma: A survey of 75 cases with special reference to the syndrome resembling chronic lymphocytic leukaemia. Br J Cancer 1975;31:60.

363. Splinter TA, Noorloos BV, van Heerde P: CLL and diffuse histiocytic lymphoma in one patient. Clonal proliferation of two different B cells. Scand J Haematol 1978;20:29.

364. Stilgenbauer S, Dohner H, Bulgay-Morschel M, et al: High frequency of monoallelic retinoblastoma gene deletion in B-cell chronic lymphoid leukemia shown by interphase cytogenetics. Blood 1993;81:2118.

365. Stilgenbauer S, Lichter P, Dohner H: Genetic features of B-cell chronic lymphocytic leukemia. Rev Clin Exp Hematol 2000;4:48.

366. Stauder R, Greil R, Schulz TF, et al: Expression of leucocyte function–associated antigen-1 and 7F7-antigen, an adhesion molecule related to intercellular adhesion molecule-1 (ICAM-1) in non-Hodgkin's lymphomas and leukaemias: Possible influence on growth patterns and leukaemic behaviour. Clin Exp Immunol 1989;77:234.

367. Sultan Y, Maisonneuve P, Kazatchkine MD, et al: Anti-idiotypic suppression of autoantibodies to factor VIII (antihemophilic factor) by high-dose intravenous gamma globulin. Lancet 1984;2:765.

368. Taniguchi T, Matsui H, Fujita T, et al: Structure and expression of a cloned cDNA for human interleukin-2. Nature 1983;302:305.

369. The French Cooperative Group on Chronic Lymphocytic Leukemia: A randomized trial of chlorambucil versus COP in stage B chronic lymphocytic leukemia. Blood 1990;75:1422.

370. Tooze J, Bevan D: Decreased expression of complement receptor type 2 (CR2) on neoplastic B cells of chronic lymphocytic leukaemia. Clin Exp Immunol 1991;83:423.

371. Travis LB, Curtis RE, Hankey BF, et al: Second cancers in patients with chronic lymphocytic leukemia. J Natl Cancer Inst 1992; 84:1422.

372. Trumper L, Matthaei-Maurer DU, Knauf W, et al: Centroblastic lymphoma of the thyroid supervening long-lasting chronic lymphocytic leukemia (B-cell). Demonstration of biclonality by immunohistochemical and gene rearrangement analysis. Klin Wochenschr 1988;66:736.

373. Tsujimoto Y, Jaffe E, Cossman J, et al: Clustering of breakpoints on chromosome 11 in human B-cell neoplasms with the t(11;14) chromosome translocation. Nature 1986;315:340.

374. Turk W: Ein System der Lymphomatosen. Wien Klin Wochenschr 1903;16:1073.

375. Uckun FM, Fauci AS, Chandan-Langlie M, et al: Detection and characterization of human high molecular weight B cell growth factor receptors on leukemic B cells in chronic lymphocytic leukemia. J Clin Invest 1989;84:1595.

376. Valle A, Zuber CE, Defrance T, et al: Activation of human B lymphocytes through CD40 and interleukin 4. Eur J Immunol 1989;19:1463.

377. Vallespi T, Montserrat E, Sanz MA: Chronic lymphocytic leukaemia: Prognostic value of lymphocyte morphological subtypes. A multivariate survival analysis in 146 patients. Br J Haematol 1991; 77:478.

378. van Dongen JJM, Hooijkaas H, Michiels JJ, et al: Richter's syndrome with different immunoglobulin light chain and different heavy chain gene rearrangements. Blood 1984;64:571.

379. Vasicek TJ, Leder P: Structure and expression of the human immunoglobulin lambda genes. J Exp Med 1990;172:609.

380. Velardi A, Prchal JT, Prasthofer EF, et al: Expression of NK-lineage markers on peripheral blood lymphocytes with T-helper (Leu3$^+$/ T4$^+$) phenotype in B cell chronic lymphocytic leukemia. Blood 1985;65:149.

381. Virchow R: Weisses Blut. Froriep's Notizen 1845;36:151.

382. Wang D, Freeman GJ, Levine H, et al: Role of the CD40 and CD95 (APO-1/Fas) antigens in the apoptosis of human B-cell malignancies. Br J Haematol 1997;97:409.

383. Warr JR, Levie SE, Perkins LJ, et al: Levels of expression of mdr-3 and glutathione-S-transferase genes in chronic lymphocytic leukemia cells. Blood 1993;82:1937.

384. Yagura H, Tamaki T, Furitsu T, et al: Demonstration of high-affinity interleukin-2 receptors on B-chronic lymphocytic leukemia cells: Functional and structural characterization. Blut 1990;60:181.

385. Yang WZ, Begleiter A, Johnston JB, et al: Role of glutathione and glutathione-S-transferase in chlorambucil resistance. Mol Pharmacol 1992;41:625.

386. Yano T, Sander CA, Andrade RE, et al: Molecular analysis of the BCL3 locus at chromosome 17q22 in B-cell neoplasms. Blood 1993;82:1813.

387. Yettra M: Remission of chronic lymphocytic leukemia after smallpox vaccination. Arch Intern Med 1979;139:603.

388. Young JL, Percy CL, Asire AJ: Surveillance, Epidemiology and End Results: Incidence and Mortality Data, 1973–1977 (National Cancer Institute Monograph 57). Bethesda, Md: National Institutes of Health; 1981, p 81.

389. Yuille MR, Matutes E, Marossy A, et al: Familial chronic lymphocytic leukemia: A survey and review of published studies. Br J Haematol 2000;109:794.

390. Ziegler-Heitbrock HWL, Schlag R, Flieger D, et al: Favorable response of early stage B CLL patients to treatment with IFN-alpha 2. Blood 1989;73:1426.

391. Zuelzer WW, Cox DE: Genetic aspects of leukemia. Semin Hematol 1969;6:4.

29

Mark Hoffman   Kanti Rai

Hairy Cell Leukemia

Hairy cell leukemia (HCL) was first described as a new clinical hematologic and pathologic entity in 1958, when it was called leukemic reticuloendotheliosis.[8] The past decade has witnessed spectacular therapeutic advances in HCL, and as a result, the majority of patients with active HCL can expect to attain a durable remission. It remains to be seen, with longer follow-up, whether these durable remissions will translate into cures.

PREVALENCE

HCL is a rare, chronic lymphoproliferative disorder. It represents approximately 2% of all leukemias, with an estimated 500 to 600 new cases diagnosed in the United States each year. Men are affected more often than women are, at a ratio of 5:1. The median age at diagnosis is 52 years, with a range of 23 to 80 years.[104]

ETIOLOGY AND PATHOPHYSIOLOGY

The cause of HCL is unknown. Epstein-Barr virus messenger RNA has been detected in hairy cells with use of in situ hybridization techniques.[115] This finding was not confirmed, however, when splenic tissue from HCL was examined for evidence of Epstein-Barr virus DNA or RNA.[15]

Familial cases have been described[63, 113, 117]; it is not known whether they result from common genetic or environmental influences, but common haplotypes have been seen.[113, 117] Although the phenotype of the hairy cell is consistent with a mature B cell in the pre–plasma cell stage,[39] the normal counterpart of this cell has not been identified. In vitro bryostatin 1, a protein kinase C activator, can induce morphologic and immunophenotypic changes typical of HCL in chronic lymphocytic leukemia (CLL) cells, including coexpression of CD11c and CD22 and tartrate-resistant acid phosphatase activity.[1] However, CD5 expression is not lost, and CD25 expression is not usually induced with bryostatin.[27] Thus, the HCL phenotype may be a more mature one than the CLL phenotype, albeit one not normally appreciated in B-cell ontogeny.

Cytokines appear to play an important role in HCL. Tumor necrosis factor (TNF) prolongs the survival of HCL cells in vitro[89]; HCL cells constitutively release TNF, which may have an influence in the pathogenesis of the cytopenias in the disease by inhibiting bone marrow precursors.[26] HCL cells express CD25, the receptor for interleukin-2 on the cell surface.[5, 39] The CD25 receptor is the low-affinity p55 interleukin-2 receptor; HCL cells also express the intermediate-affinity p75 interleukin-2 receptor, which may play a physiologic role in proliferation of the HCL cells.[107]

Both the soluble CD25 molecule and TNF are found in increased quantities in serum samples from patients with HCL at diagnosis; levels also normalize with achievement of complete remission.[2, 59] It is likely that CD25 and TNF are involved in important autocrine and paracrine growth loops in HCL.

Hairy cells express specific adhesion receptors (integrins) that may be responsible for the preferential localization of these cells to the bone marrow, liver, and spleen.[73]

Cytogenetic studies of HCL have shown clonal cytogenetic abnormalities in some patients.[8, 95] One group has found abnormalities involving band 5q13 in approximately one third of patients with HCL. They postulate the existence of a tumor suppressor gene in this area that may be deleted in HCL.[116]

CLINICAL FEATURES

The most common symptoms are abdominal fullness from splenomegaly, weight loss, fatigue, bruising due to thrombocytopenia, and infection.[16, 105] Splenomegaly is found in the majority of patients, and one third have concurrent hepatomegaly. Palpable adenopathy is rare, but retroperitoneal adenopathy has been appreciated, especially with disease of long duration.[36a, 67] Involvement of lung, gastrointestinal tract, kidney, pleura, bone, and soft tissue has been reported.[16, 105]

Pancytopenia is found in most patients,[16, 105] and severe monocytopenia is often present.[46] The monocytopenia, decreased memory T-helper cells,[111] T-cell dysfunction,[110] depressed natural killer cell activity in progressive disease,[20] and lack of endogenous interferon-α production[61, 92] may contribute to the increased susceptibility to opportunistic infections, such as atypical mycobacterial infections, legionnaires' disease, and listeriosis.[16, 105]

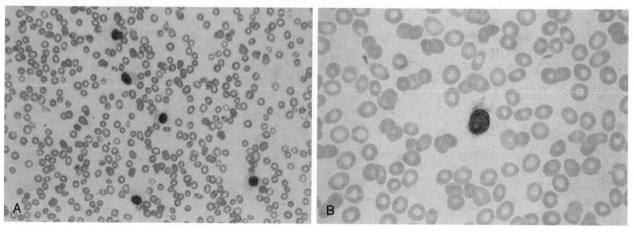

FIGURE 29–1. *A,* Light microscopy of typical hairy cells (Wright-Giemsa stain, ×200). *B,* Typical hairy cell with cytoplasmic projections (Wright-Giemsa stain, ×250). (See Color Section.)

LABORATORY DIAGNOSIS

The diagnosis of HCL is made on the basis of the morphologic features of hairy cells on the peripheral blood film, pathologic changes in the bone marrow biopsy specimen, and immunophenotypic features described later. The initial step in diagnosis is the identification of the characteristic hairy cell in the peripheral blood. The neoplastic cells have nuclei with more open, dispersed chromatin than is seen in normal lymphoid cells. The cytoplasm is pale and agranular, and it features multiple projections resembling hairs[16] (Fig. 29-1; see also Fig. 29-5*E*). These cells may be difficult to find in patients who are leukopenic, and an examination of the buffy coat smear is helpful in such cases.

Cytochemistry may aid in diagnosis in that the neoplastic cells are positive for the tartrate-resistant type 5 isoenzyme of acid phosphatase[16] (Fig. 29-2). The reaction product is seen diffusely in the cytoplasm of the cells.[16] Buffy coat smears and bone marrow imprints are helpful in increasing the number of cells for study. Tartrate-resistant acid phosphatase negativity suggests a morphologic HCL variant (see later).

By electron microscopy, the hairy cells possess extensive cytoplasmic projections. Ribosome-lamella complexes (Fig. 29-3) can be seen in approximately half of the cases.[16] These are structures with a central hollow space surrounded by parallel arrays of lamellae, with ribosome-like structures between the lamellae. These structures are not unique to hairy cells and were first described in CLL.[114]

The bone marrow in HCL is usually inaspiratable, largely owing to an increase in reticulin fibers. In the biopsy specimen, the cells have a "fried egg" appearance, featuring bland nuclei with abundant cytoplasm and interlocking cell borders[54] (Fig. 29-4). This characteristic appearance enables the pathologist to distinguish HCL from other malignant lymphoid infiltrates in which the nuclei are much more closely apposed. The bone marrow may also have a hypocellular appearance, causing confusion with aplastic anemia.[54]

The pathologic process of the spleen is characterized by exclusive involvement of the red pulp. Hairy cells can

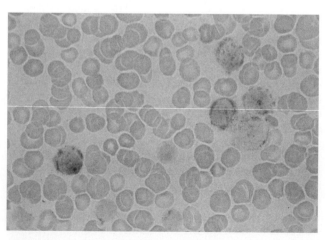

FIGURE 29–2. Tartrate-resistant acid phosphatase positivity in a case of HCL (×250). (See Color Section.)

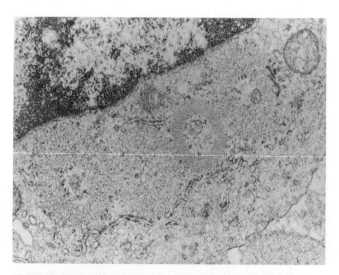

FIGURE 29–3. Ribosome-lamella complexes in the cytoplasm of a splenic hairy cell. (From Mackay B: Introduction to Diagnostic Electron Microscopy. New York: Appleton-Century-Crofts; 1981.)

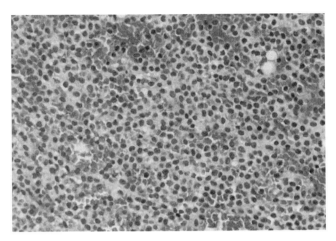

FIGURE 29–4. HCL in the bone marrow. Note the lymphoid cells with clear spaces surrounding each individual cell. (See Color Section.)

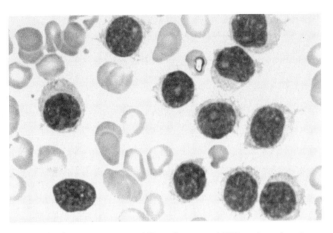

FIGURE 29–5. Peripheral blood film of a case of HCL variant showing cells with features intermediate between prolymphocytes (round nucleus and prominent nucleolus) and hairy cells (relatively abundant and villous cytoplasm).

line spaces filled with red blood cells, forming pseudosinuses.[16] In the liver, the neoplastic cells infiltrate the portal tracts as well as the sinuses.[16]

IMMUNOPHENOTYPE OF THE HAIRY CELL

Hairy cells are B lymphocytes, as demonstrated by the finding of clonal immunoglobulin heavy- and light-chain rearrangement.[16] An atypical T-cell variant of HCL has been described in association with infection by the human T-lymphotropic virus type 2.[52] One-third to one-half of patients express surface immunoglobulin.[16] Hairy cells display characteristic cell surface antigens defined by monoclonal antibodies. The cells express the B-cell markers CD19, CD20, and CD22 as well as the antigens CD11c (which is also expressed on monocytes), CD25 (the interleukin-2 receptor), and CD103 (mucosal lymphocyte antigen).[21, 69] Hairy cells may derive from a late stage of B-cell ontogeny close to the plasma cell.[39] Hairy cells can also be reliably defined by immunohistochemistry in paraffin-embedded bone marrow sections with use of monoclonal antibodies against the leukocyte common antigen (CD45) and B-cell lineage antibodies (LN2, MB2, and L26).[23, 101, 102] These findings are of relevance in detecting minimal residual disease in patients treated with modern effective therapy for HCL, as discussed subsequently.

VARIANT HAIRY CELL LEUKEMIA

Patients with a variant form of HCL have been described with a high white blood cell count and an aspirable marrow, splenomegaly, and neoplastic lymphocytes with cytoplasmic features of hairy cells but nuclear features of prolymphocytes (more condensed chromatin and a prominent nucleolus)[14, 118] (Fig. 29–5). Immunophenotypically, the cells are CD19+, CD20+, CD22+, and CD11c+ but lack CD25.[118] Variant HCL may be more common than the classic form in Japan.[55, 62] Variant HCL tends to respond less well to modern therapies for HCL (see "Treatment").

DIFFERENTIAL DIAGNOSIS

Classic morphologic features, tartrate-resistant acid phosphatase positivity, and the characteristic immunophenotype should enable one to make the diagnosis of HCL in the appropriate clinical setting. Prominent peripheral adenopathy, atypical morphologic features, lack of tartrate-resistant acid phosphatase positivity, and aberrant immunophenotype should lead one to suspect HCL variant or other lymphoproliferative disorders.

Primary splenic lymphoma with villous lymphocytes[70] is similar to variant HCL in that the cells also lack tartrate-resistant acid phosphatase staining and are CD25−. Marrow is usually aspirable, and marrow infiltration is sparse. In contrast to variant HCL, the disease predominantly involves the white pulp of the spleen, and a monoclonal gammopathy may also be present.

Monocytoid B-cell lymphoma histologically resembles HCL in that the cells also have bland nuclei with a surrounding clear rim of cytoplasm. However, patients with monocytoid B-cell lymphoma have lymphadenopathy and generally are without splenomegaly or bone marrow involvement.[92] The cells are immunophenotypically similar to HCL but lack CD25.[101]

Chronic lymphocytic leukemia (B-CLL) cells can involve the marrow extensively as in HCL and involve the spleen preferentially ("splenic CLL"), but in bone marrow biopsy specimens, the nuclei are close to one another, unlike in HCL, and B-CLL cells express CD5 and do not express CD11c or CD25.[21]

Non-Hodgkin's lymphomas can be associated with splenomegaly, bone marrow involvement, and a leukemic phase. Immunophenotypically, these cells usually have bright surface expression of immunoglobulin, may express CD5 and CD10, and lack CD11c and CD25. The involvement of the marrow is patchy and paratrabecular.[5, 16, 21]

B-prolymphocytic leukemia is distinguished by high white blood cell counts; on morphologic examination, the cells have more condensed chromatin and prominent nucleoli, and they lack CD25 and CD11c.[5, 16, 21]

TABLE 29–1. Markers in Chronic B-Cell Leukemias

Marker	CLL	B-PLL	HCL	HCL-V	NHLLP	SLVL
SmIg	Weak	Strong	Strong	Strong	Strong	Strong
CD5	+ +	±	−	−	−	−
CD19/CD20	+ +	+ +	+ +	+ +	+ +	+ +
CD22	±	+ +	+ +	+ +	+	+ +
CD10	−	±	−	−	+	−
CD25	−	−	+ +	−	−	−
CD11c	−	NT	+ +	+	NT	NT

CLL, chronic lymphocytic leukemia; B-PLL, B-prolymphocytic leukemia; HCL, hairy cell leukemia; HCL-V, hairy cell leukemia variant; NHLLP, non-Hodgkin's lymphoma in leukemic phase; SLVL, splenic lymphoma with villous lymphocytes; NT, not tested.

Table 29-1 summarizes immunophenotypic features of HCL, variant HCL, splenic lymphoma with villous lymphocytes, CLL, B-prolymphocytic leukemia, and non-Hodgkin's lymphoma in leukemic phase.

NATURAL HISTORY AND PROGNOSIS

The natural history of the disease is variable. Untreated patients are reported to have a median survival time of 5 years.[31, 108] Most patients develop significant cytopenias with disease progression and thus require therapy. Jansen and coworkers[47] formulated a clinical staging system using hemoglobin level and spleen size. Those patients with significant anemia (hemoglobin <8.5 g/dL) and with spleens greater than 10 cm below the left costal margin did poorly without therapeutic intervention. A subset of patients, who are usually older and have mild splenomegaly, may have an especially indolent course.[31] Mortality is usually due to infection, which is more common in patients with significant neutropenia (absolute neutrophil count <5 × 10^9/L).[31] Bouroncle[7] analyzed a cohort of 100 patients with HCL and found that at diagnosis, lymphadenopathy, significant cytopenias, and a marked degree of marrow infiltration were indicators of a short survival time.

TREATMENT

The last decade has seen the development of highly effective therapies for HCL. The standard indications for treatment have been significant cytopenias, life-threatening infections, and symptomatic splenomegaly, but it is likely, given the efficacy of modern therapy, that treatment will be offered to asymptomatic patients with low tumor burdens.

Splenectomy

Splenectomy was the first treatment modality to be used regularly in HCL. It can result in improvement in up to 90% of patients and normalization of blood counts in 40% to 77% of patients.[48] Splenectomy can also prolong survival.[48] One large trial demonstrated no advantage of splenectomy for patients with spleens less than 4 cm below the costal margin,[48] but other studies have not

shown a relationship between splenic size and the response to splenectomy.[32, 80] Because splenectomy does not affect cytopenias related to bone marrow infiltration, it is not surprising that the less the degree of marrow infiltration, the greater the response to splenectomy.[32] Splenectomy has now been superseded by more effective therapeutic options; however, the procedure still remains a therapeutic option in HCL in some circumstances. It may be the option of choice for management of active HCL diagnosed during pregnancy[100] when medical therapies are contraindicated.

Interferon alfa

Multiple trials have demonstrated the activity of interferon alfa in HCL.[16] (Recombinant interferon beta[30] and interferon gamma[77] are much less active, and their use is not further discussed.) The first successful use of interferon alfa in HCL was by Quesada and colleagues[78] in 1984. Of seven patients treated, three achieved a pathologic complete remission and four achieved a partial remission,[78] and these responses were maintained months after therapy was discontinued. This important study demonstrated that it was possible to return the bone marrow to a morphologically normal appearance. Criteria for complete and partial remission in HCL were defined[3] (Table 29-2). The minority of patients (8%) achieve a complete remission with interferon; the majority (74%) achieve partial remissions.[16] The usual dosage administered is 2 × 10^6 U/m^2 subcutaneously three times a week. Lower doses of interferon alfa may also be effective; a

TABLE 29–2. Criteria for Remission in Hairy Cell Leukemia

Complete Remission	Partial Remission
Regression of organomegaly to normal	Reduction in organomegaly ≥50%
Hemoglobin ≥12 g/100 mL	Normal blood counts
Platelets >100 × 10^9/L	Reduction in bone marrow hairy cells
Neutrophils >1.5 × 10^9 L	≥50%
No circulating hairy cells	<5% circulating hairy cells
Bone marrow aspirate and biopsy with no hairy cells	

Adapted from Consensus Resolution: Proposed criteria for evaluation of response to treatment in hairy cell leukemia. Leukemia 1987:1:405.

dose of 1.5 million U/day was as effective as 3 million U/day in clearing hairy cells and normalizing peripheral blood counts.[119] The platelet count returns to normal within approximately 2 months of interferon therapy, the hemoglobin level by 4 months, and the absolute granulocyte count by 4 to 6 months. Transient myelosuppression with a decrease in granulocyte and platelet counts can occur in the first few weeks of treatment. Therapy is usually administered for 12 months, but there may be a benefit to continuing interferon alfa beyond 12 months, in that prolonged therapy may recruit more patients into complete remission[71] and prevent progression of disease.[71, 119] However, for most patients, interferon alfa appears to be primarily a cytostatic treatment. Continuing administration of interferon alfa beyond 12 months was not associated with a significant reduction in relapse after discontinuation of therapy.[33] Even after 24 months of therapy, 48% of patients had disease progression at a median of 10 months after cessation of therapy.[6] Rai and colleagues[79] have published a long-term follow-up report of 52 previously untreated patients given interferon alfa, 2 million U/m² subcutaneously three times a week, for 1 year. At a median of 5 years of follow-up, 28% remained in remission, and overall survival was 86%.

Response to interferon alfa is independent of previous splenectomy.[120] A low hairy cell index (low percentage of hairy cell infiltration in the bone marrow) correlates with a favorable hematologic response.[120] Patients with the variant form of HCL do not respond to interferon alfa as well as do those with classic HCL.[85] Acquired resistance to interferon alfa-2a but not to interferon alfa-2b may be associated with the development of neutralizing anti-interferon antibodies.[99]

A randomized trial evaluated interferon alfa versus splenectomy in untreated patients with HCL. Interferon alfa achieved a response rate of 100% versus 30% for splenectomy, and the median time to treatment failure was significantly longer in the patients receiving interferon alfa (>18 months) than in the splenectomized patients (<1 month).[94]

Interferon exerts multiple effects on hairy cells.[112] Hairy cells express receptors for interferon alfa, and lack of these receptors may be associated with refractoriness to interferon.[76] Interferon alfa can modify expression of the oncogene c-fos, thus inhibiting cell proliferation, and stimulates degradation of messenger RNAs for cytokines like TNF, which, as alluded to previously, may participate in the regulation of proliferation of HCL cells.[40, 112] Interferon alfa inhibits spontaneous as well as induced DNA synthesis in HCL cells.[38] Interferon alfa also downregulates abnormal free intracytoplasmic calcium in hairy cells.[28] There is a lack of endogenous interferon-α production in HCL,[61, 93] and interferon therapy has been postulated as a "replacement" therapy in HCL.[40] The fact that variant HCL (CD25⁻) does not respond to interferon alfa suggests that CD25 expression may be an important cofactor in the response to interferon alfa.[112]

In summary, interferon alfa is an active therapeutic agent in HCL. Toxicities of interferon alfa include an influenza-like syndrome on first exposure, fatigue, dry skin, diarrhea, constipation, nausea, central nervous system depression, and loss of libido.[16]

With the advent of purine analogue therapy for HCL, as discussed subsequently, interferon alfa should no longer be considered a first-line treatment option. However, Seymour and colleagues[91] have reported responses to interferon in patients relapsing from a remission induced by 2-chlorodeoxyadenosine.

2′-Deoxycoformycin (Pentostatin)

In 1972, a congenital adenosine deaminase (ADA) deficiency syndrome was described in association with a markedly immunosuppressed state and lymphopenia.[29] The cause of profound lymphopenia in ADA deficiency syndrome was thought to be accumulation of lymphocytotoxic levels of deoxyadenosine and deoxyadenosine triphosphate (dATP). This observation led to the development of a new drug, deoxycoformycin (pentostatin, DCF) which is a potent inhibitor of ADA and therefore can induce a simulated ADA deficiency syndrome.[34] The structure of DCF and the ADA reaction are shown in Figure 29-6.

A multi-institutional trial of DCF in HCL was undertaken[97] by the Eastern Cooperative Oncology Group (ECOG) after the initial observation of remarkable activity of this drug in a small number of patients.[98] The ECOG trial[97] resulted in a 59% complete remission and 37% partial remission rate. Such a high complete remission rate was never achievable with any of the previously available therapeutic methods, including interferon alfa. The results of subsequent trials with DCF revealed a similar aggregate response rate of 86%, with a 62% complete remission rate (range, 4% to 46%).[16] Patients refractory to interferon alfa also had an 80% overall response rate with DCF therapy.[42]

A National Cancer Institute–sponsored intergroup trial compared interferon alfa and DCF in previously untreated patients with HCL. In this large multi-institutional study, more than 150 patients were assessed for response on each of the two therapeutic arms and demonstrated a complete remission rate of 76% with DCF and 11% with interferon alfa, with overall response rates of 87% and 49%, respectively.[35] With a median follow-up of 57 months, only 10 of 117 patients entering complete remission with DCF had relapsed. There was a relapse-free survival advantage for DCF over interferon alfa.[35] There are two other reports of long-term follow-up of patients treated with DCF. Deardon and associates[19] described 165 patients; 94% of patients responded (82% complete response), and 24% of patients had relapsed, with a median of 71 months of follow-up. Ribeiro and colleagues[81] described 49 patients with a median follow-up of 33 months; 5 patients (10%) had relapsed, 2 of whom died of disease progression.

DCF is usually given in an outpatient setting at a dose of 4 mg/m² intravenously by bolus injection at intervals of 2 weeks. After 3 months, the treatment interval can be extended to once a month. Intravenous hydration with 1.0 to 1.5 L is recommended at the time of each therapy. The maximally achievable response—most often a complete remission—occurs after about 4 months, after which an additional two cycles are given and then treat-

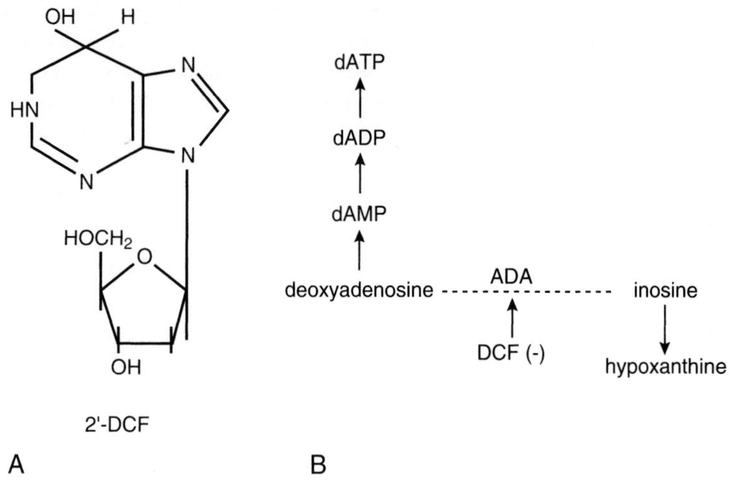

FIGURE 29–6. *A*, Structure of 2′-deoxycoformycin (DCF). *B*, Adenosine deaminase (ADA) reaction and inhibitory effect of DCF.

ment is stopped. All patients are subsequently kept under observation with return visits to the clinic at intervals of 2 to 3 months.

Retreatment with DCF or 2-chlorodeoxyadenosine (see later) is considered when there is evidence of overt clinical relapse.

When DCF was given at very high doses (up to 30 mg/m^2/day) in the initial trials, it was associated with unacceptably high levels of renal, pulmonary, and central nervous system toxicity.[72] However, DCF is well tolerated with acceptable levels of toxicity when it is given at the dosage of 4 mg/m^2 every 2 weeks. At this dosage, moderate to severe neutropenia may occur in about 20% of patients; mild nausea and vomiting and rashes have been observed, but they do not require interruption of therapy. Reversible hepatitis and keratoconjunctivitis have also been reported.[72]

By interfering with ADA in normal lymphocytes, DCF can be severely immunosuppressive. One study found profound decreases in CD4$^+$ and CD8$^+$ lymphocytes in all patients treated with DCF.[109] The lymphocytopenia was associated with a marked decrease in proliferative response to mitogens. The abnormalities continued for up to 6 months after discontinuation of treatment.[109] Because of the neutropenia from myelosuppression as well as immunosuppression, disseminated herpes zoster, *Escherichia coli, Haemophilus influenzae,* and pneumococcal infections have been seen.

In summary, DCF can induce durable complete remissions in about two thirds of patients with HCL, regardless of previous treatment. Relapses do occur after treatment with DCF, and these patients may be considered for therapy with 2-chlorodeoxyadenosine (see next section), if they have not already received it, or with interferon alfa.

2-Chlorodeoxyadenosine

Whereas DCF is a substrate inhibitor of ADA, 2-chlorodeoxyadenosine (2-CdA, cladribine) is a purine substrate analogue that is resistant to deamination by ADA.[12] The structure of 2-CdA and its similarity to the natural substrate deoxyadenosine are shown in Figure 29–7. 2-CdA

accumulates in the cell owing to lack of deamination and is phosphorylated intracellularly to its 5′-triphosphate (2-CdATP), especially in cells such as lymphocytes, which have a high deoxycytidine kinase activity.[12] 2-CdATP is most likely the active metabolite of the drug, in that accumulation of 2-CdATP results in DNA strand breaks and ATP depletion.[12] 2-CdA was found to be toxic to both resting and proliferating lymphocytes.[12] The exact mechanism of action of 2-CdA in nondividing cells has not been established. Incubation of nondividing human peripheral blood lymphocytes with 2-CdA results in the appearance of DNA strand breaks, inhibition of RNA synthesis, profound drop in nicotinamide adenosine dinucleotide levels, ATP depletion, and cell death.[90] 2-CdA induces morphologic changes of apoptosis (programmed cell death) in CLL cells.[84] The characteristic DNA strand breaks may be due to the production of an endonuclease.[41]

After their successful use of 2-CdA in two patients with HCL in 1987,[74] Piro and coworkers[75] at the Scripps Clinic in California reported dramatic results in 12 patients

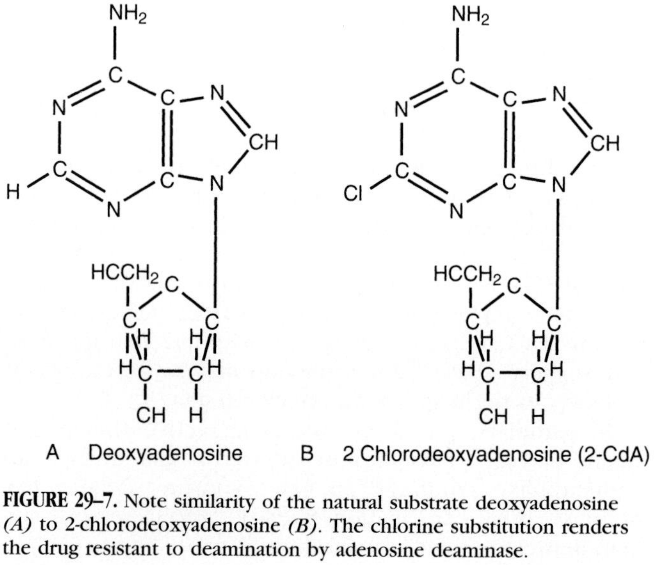

FIGURE 29–7. Note similarity of the natural substrate deoxyadenosine *(A)* to 2-chlorodeoxyadenosine *(B)*. The chlorine substitution renders the drug resistant to deamination by adenosine deaminase.

TABLE 29–3. 2-Chlorodeoxyadenosine in Hairy Cell Leukemia

Author	No. of Patients	Complete Response (%)	Partial Response (%)	Median Follow-up (months)	Relapse from Complete Response (%)
Saven et al[87]	358	91	7	52	26
Robak et al[83]	103	77	19	36	27
Jehn et al[49]	42	98	2	32	25
Cheson et al[17]	979	50	37	52	12
Lauria et al[60]	40	75	25	48	17
Hoffman et al[43]	49	76	32	55	20
Fayad et al[24]	99	81	7	78	16
Tallman et al[103]	52	80	18	24	14

treated with a single 7-day course of 2-CdA at a dosage of 0.1 mg/kg/day by continuous intravenous infusion. All patients had previously been treated with interferon alfa or by splenectomy and had active disease; 11 patients achieved a complete remission and 1 patient had a partial remission. As impressive as the response rate was the durability of the remissions obtained; at the time of publication, the median remission duration was 15.5 months, with the longest remission duration 3.8 years, and no patient had relapsed.[75] This group has since updated their experience with 358 patients, with a median follow-up of 52 months.[86] The overall response rate was 98% with 91% complete remissions; 26% of patients had relapsed at the time of the report, and the overall survival rate was 96% at 48 months.[87]

Similar impressive responses and duration of response have been described by other investigators; reported series of patients treated with 2-CdA are summarized in Table 29–3. A few common themes emerge from these data. The response to 2-CdA is not affected by previous response to interferon or splenectomy. Patients resistant to DCF may still respond to 2-CdA.[86] The majority of patients achieve a complete hematologic remission as well as a pathologic complete remission in the marrow. One group has reported inferior results in patients with abdominal adenopathy.[68] An aberrant phenotype also predicts a poorer response (see later). Approximately 20% of patients are relapsing with more mature follow-up (see Table 29–3). The majority of these relapsed patients can be induced into a second remission with a second cycle of 2-CdA.

The reason for the exquisite sensitivity of HCL cells to 2-CdA is unclear. Ratios of deoxycytidine kinase to 5′-nucleotidase, which could result in net accumulation of 2-CdA nucleotides (Fig. 29–8), were higher in six HCL 2-CdA responders than in one nonresponder.[56]

The hematologic response is characterized first by a normalization of platelet counts, followed by normalization of neutrophil counts and then of hemoglobin levels.[75] The median time required to attain a normal blood count is 61 days (range, 11 to 268 days).[75] Transient eosinophilia has been reported before the achievement of a complete remission.[82] Patients with minimal residual disease in the bone marrow at 3 months may have normal marrow at 6 months,[50] and in our experience, achievement of normal blood counts and bone marrow may take up to 9 months after one cycle of 2-CdA. Levels of serum-soluble CD25 and TNF, which are elevated in active HCL, become normal with successful therapy.[59]

2-CdA has usually been given as a continuous infusion of 0.09 mg/kg/day (3.4 mg/m²/day) for 7 days on an outpatient basis by use of a percutaneously inserted central catheter and a portable pump. Juliusson and Liliemark[51] have studied the plasma and intracellular pharmacokinetics of cladribine; the finding of a long terminal plasma half-life as well as prolonged retention of intracellular CdA-nucleotides led to the exploration of different treatment routes and schedules. As used by these authors, the regimen of 0.14 mg/kg/day intravenously over 2 hours daily for 5 days has become popular in the United States for the treatment of lymphoma. Two randomized trials in patients with HCL showed no difference in response between the continuous infusion regimen and the 5-day dosing regimen given intravenously[18] or subcutaneously.[96]

Therapy with 2-CdA is well tolerated; no nausea, vomiting, alopecia, renal dysfunction, or neurotoxicity has been encountered. Culture-negative neutropenic fever is

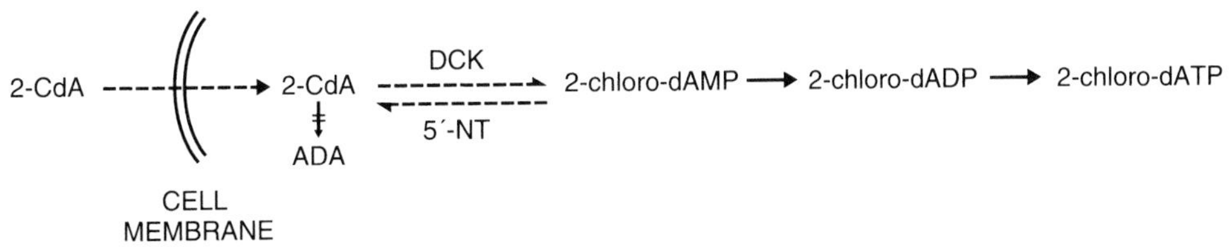

FIGURE 29–8. 2-Chlorodeoxyadenosine (2-CdA) is transported into cells and phosphorylated by deoxycytidine kinase (DCK). Conversely, 2-CdA nucleotides are dephosphorylated by 5′-nucleotidase (5′-NT). 2-CdA accumulates in the cell because it is resistant to deamination by adenosine deaminase (ADA); cells with high deoxycytidine kinase activity and low 5′-nucleotidase activity, such as lymphocytes, accumulate toxic concentrations of deoxynucleosides.

the major acute toxicity of 2-CdA therapy in HCL.[75] The fever usually occurs on the fifth to seventh day of treatment and may continue for a week or two thereafter. The use of filgrastim (granulocyte colony-stimulating factor) did not have an impact on the incidence of neutropenic fever or number of febrile days,[88] and it is not routinely recommended. However, the use of granulocyte colony-stimulating factor after the completion of treatment, to expedite neutrophil recovery, should be considered if the patient has severe neutropenia before beginning therapy. Opportunistic infections (cytomegalovirus, *Candida, Aspergillus*) have been reported but are relatively infrequent.[50]

Like DCF, 2-CdA causes a depletion of all lymphocyte subsets in the peripheral blood that lasts 6 to 12 months after one cycle of therapy.[10]

Fludarabine

Although fludarabine monophosphate, another purine analogue resistant to deamination by ADA, has proved efficacious in CLL, it has not been tested in large numbers of patients with HCL. A single institutional experience with a few patients suggests that this drug may have some efficacy in HCL.[53] At present, its use must be confined to prospective clinical trials.

Immunotherapy

Rituximab is a chimeric human/mouse antibody directed against the CD20 antigen expressed on mature B cells. The agent destroys B cells by complement-mediated lysis.[66] Clinical trials have demonstrated impressive activity of this agent in patients with low-grade B-cell lymphomas.[66]

Initial reports indicate that rituximab is an effective agent for patients with relapsed or refractory HCL, inducing remissions in the majority of patients.[36, 44, 106] The durability of these remissions remains to be determined with longer follow-up.

Kreitman and associates[57] have also recently reported on treatment of 16 cladribine-resistant patients with RFB4 (dsFv)-PE38 (BL22), an anti-CD22 antibody fused to truncated *Pseudomonas* exotoxin. Eleven patients achieved complete remission and two had a partial remission. Three of the 11 patients in CR had relapsed at the time of the report. The median followup was short (16 months).

OTHER ISSUES

Minimal Residual Disease

Some patients in morphologic complete remission are revealed to have residual hairy cells by immunohistochemistry[22, 37] and by polymerase chain reaction.[25] The implication of minimal residual disease is still unclear. Tallman and coworkers[104] analyzed the prevalence of minimal residual disease in patients in complete remission by conventional morphologic criteria, using the monoclonal

antibodies anti-CD20, DBA.44, and anti-CD45RO. The prevalence of minimal residual disease was not significantly different between patients treated with 2-CdA and patients treated with DCF. The relapse rate was much higher in patients with minimal residual disease than in those without it.[104] On the other hand, in 23 patients treated with DCF, Matutes and colleagues[64] found no difference in relapse rates between patients with and those without minimal residual disease.

Second Cancer Risk

With the majority of patients remaining in unmaintained complete remission for many years, concern has arisen about the incidence of second cancers, whether they are related to the natural history of the disease or the immunosuppressive effects of 2-CdA or DCF. Au and coworkers[4] reviewed the follow-up course of 117 patients in British Columbia and noted a statistically significant increased relative rate (2.91) of second malignant neoplasms compared with matched control subjects. Kurzrock and associates,[58] in a review of 350 patients from the M.D. Anderson database, found an overall trend to a higher rate of second malignant neoplasms overall (observed-to-expected ratio, 1.34); the incidence of second hematologic malignant neoplasms (lymphoma and myeloma) was significantly increased.

Aberrant Phenotype/Variant HCL

As discussed earlier in the differential diagnosis of HCL, variant HCL is usually clinically, morphologically, and immunophenotypically distinct from classic HCL. In our experience, lack of CD25 expression is the best discriminant in this regard. We initially reported[43] that lack of CD25 expression predicted a poorer response to 2-CdA, as had been reported for interferon alfa.[85] Robak and coworkers[83] have also published poor outcomes with cladribine in a Polish series. Matutes and colleagues[65] have reported the largest series of patients with variant HCL. Patients were resistant to alkylating agents, and only transient responses were noted with DCF and cladribine. Splenectomy resulted in improvement in the majority of patients. Overall survival was much poorer than with classic HCL, but many patients had a chronic course.[65]

SUMMARY

Therapy for the Newly Diagnosed Patient

An asymptomatic patient with mild cytopenias and minimal or no splenomegaly may be carefully observed without treatment, especially if the patient is elderly.[31] Among the various therapeutic options available today, 2-CdA is our agent of first choice for patients with active HCL because only one treatment cycle is necessary to induce a durable remission. DCF is also an option for initial therapy.

Patients with variant HCL, especially those with significant splenomegaly, should be considered for splenectomy as primary therapy because responses to purine analogue therapy have been disappointing. Rituximab should also be considered as initial therapy for these patients because they express CD20.[21]

Therapy for the Relapsed Patient

Patients relapsing after 2-CdA treatment should be considered for retreatment with the drug if there has been a long remission interval or for treatment with DCF as an alternative. The rare individuals who are primarily resistant to or have poor-quality remissions with 2-CdA should be considered for rituximab, DCF, or interferon alfa therapy. There may also be a role for splenectomy in those patients with HCL who have a massive or painfully enlarged spleen and have failed to respond to 2-CdA or DCF.

REFERENCES

1. Al Khatib A, Mohammed DM, Don M: Bryostatin 1–induced hairy cell features on chronic lymphocytic leukemia cells in vitro. Exp Hematol 1993;21:61.
2. Ambrosetti A, Nadali G, Vinante F, et al: Soluble interleukin-2 receptor in hairy cell leukemia: A reliable marker of disease. Int J Clin Lab Res 1993;23:34.
3. Anonymous: Consensus Resolution: Proposed criteria for evaluation of response to treatment in hairy cell leukemia. Leukemia 1987;1:405.
4. Au WY, Klasa RJ, Gallagher R, et al: Second malignancies in patients with hairy cell leukemia in British Columbia: A 20 year experience. Blood 1998;92:1160.
5. Bennett JM, Catovsky D, Daniel MT, et al: Proposals for the classification of chronic (mature) B and T lymphoid leukemias. J Clin Pathol 1989;42:567.
6. Berman E, Heller G, Kempin S, et al: Incidence of response and long term follow-up in patients with hairy cell leukemia treated with recombinant interferon alpha-2a. Blood 1990;75:839.
7. Bouroncle BA: The history of hairy cell leukemia: Characteristics of long term survivors. Semin Oncol 1984;11:479.
8. Bouroncle BA, Wiseman BK, Doan CA: Leukemic reticuloendotheliosis. Blood 1958;13:609.
9. Brito-Babapulle V, Pittman S, Melo JV, et al: The 14q$^+$ marker in hairy cell leukemia. A cytogenetic study of 15 cases. Leuk Res 1986;10:131.
10. Carrera CJ, Piro LD, Saven A, et al: Restoration of lymphocyte subsets following 2-chlorodeoxyadenosine remission induction in hairy cell leukemia. Blood 1990;76:260a.
11. Carson DA, Wasson DB, Esparza LM, et al: Oral antilymphocyte activity and induction of apoptosis by 2-chloro-2'-arabino-fluoro-2'-deoxyadenosine. Proc Natl Acad Sci U S A 1992;89:2970.
12. Carson DA, Watson DB, Kaye J, et al: Deoxycytidine kinase mediated toxicity of deoxyadenosine analogs toward malignant human lymphoblasts in vitro and toward murine 1210 leukemia in vivo. Proc Natl Acad Sci U S A 1980;77:6865.
13. Carson DA, Wasson DB, Taetle R, et al: Specific toxicity of 2-chlorodeoxyadenosine toward resting and proliferating human lymphocytes. Blood 1983;62:737.
14. Catovsky D, O'Brian M, Melo JV, et al: Hairy cell leukemia variant. An intermediate disease between HCL and B-prolymphocytic leukemia. Semin Oncol 1984;11:362.
15. Chang KL, Chen YY, Weiss LM: Lack of evidence of Epstein-Barr virus in hairy cell leukemia and monocytoid B-cell lymphoma. Hum Pathol 1993;24:58.
16. Chang KL, Stroup R, Weiss LM: Hairy cell leukemia. Current status. Am J Clin Pathol 1992;97:719.
17. Cheson BD, Sorenson JM, Vena DA, et al: Treatment of hairy cell leukemia with 2-chlorodeoxyadenosine via the Group C protocol mechanism of the National Cancer Institute: A report of 979 patients. J Clin Oncol 1998;16:3007.
18. Damassio EE, Resegotti L, Masoudi B, et al: Five day intermittent vs. continuous 2-chlorodeoxyadenosine infusion for the treatment of hairy cell leukemia. A study by the Italian Group for Hairy Cell Leukemia. Recenti Prog Med 1998;89:68.
19. Dearden CE, Matutes E, Hilditch BL, et al: Long term follow-up of patients with hairy cell leukaemia after treatment with pentostatin or cladribine. Br J Haematol 1999;106:515.
20. Demeter J, Paloczi K, Lehoczky D, et al: Hairy cell leukemia: Observations on natural killer activity in different clinical stages of the disease. Br J Haematol 1989;71:239.
21. DiGiuseppe JA, Borowitz MJ: Clinical utility of flow cytometry in the chronic lymphoid leukemias. Semin Oncol 1998;25:6.
22. Ellison DJ, Sharpe RW, Spinosa JC, et al: Immunomorphologic evaluation of bone marrow biopsies in patients with hairy cell leukemia following treatment with 2-chlorodeoxyadenosine. Basel: Molecular Biology of Hematopoiesis, 8th Symposium; 1993, p 163.
23. Falini B, Pileri SA, Flenghi L, et al: Selection of a panel of monoclonal antibodies for monitoring residual disease in peripheral blood and bone marrow of interferon treated hairy cell leukemia patients. Br J Haematol 1990;76:460.
24. Fayad L, Kurzrock R, Keating M, et al: Treatment of hairy cell leukemia (HCL) with 2-CdA: Long term follow-up at M.D. Anderson Cancer Center. Blood 1997;90:530a.
25. Filleul B, Delannoy A, Ferrant A: A single course of 2-chlorodeoxyadenosine (2CdA) does not eradicate leukemic cells in hairy cell leukemia (HCL) patients achieving complete remission. Blood 1993;82:142a.
26. Foa R, Guarini A, Francia di Celle P, et al: Constitutive production of tumor necrosis factor-alpha in hairy cell leukemia: Possible role in the pathogenesis of the cytopenias and effect of treatment with interferon alpha. J Clin Oncol 1992;10:954.
27. Gartenhaus R, Hoffman M, Fuchs A, et al: Differentiating agents do not induce a true hairy cell phenotype in B-CLL cells in vitro. Leuk Lymphoma 1996;22:97.
28. Genot E, Bismutin G, Degos L, et al: Interferon alpha down-regulates the abnormal intracytoplasmic free calcium concentration of tumor cells in hairy cell leukemia. Blood 1992;86:2060.
29. Giblett ER, Anderson JE, Cohen F, et al: Adenosine deaminase deficiency in two patients with severely impaired cellular immunity. Lancet 1972;2:1067.
30. Glaspy JA, Marcus SG, Amersley J, et al: Recombinant beta-serine interferon in hairy cell leukemia compared prospectively with results with recombinant alpha interferon. Cancer 1989;64:409.
31. Golomb HM, Catovsky D, Golde DW: Hairy cell leukemia: A clinical review of 71 cases. Ann Intern Med 1978;89:677.
32. Golomb HM, Vardiman JW: Response to splenectomy in 65 patients with hairy cell leukemia: An evaluation of spleen weight and bone marrow involvement. Blood 1983;69:349.
33. Golomb HM, Ratain MJ, Fefer A, et al: Randomized study of the duration of treatment with interferon alfa-2B in patients with hairy cell leukemia. J Natl Cancer Inst 1988;80:369.
34. Grever MR, Siaw MFE, Jacob WF, et al: The biochemical and clinical consequences of 2'-deoxycoformycin in refractory lymphoproliferative malignancy. Blood 1981;57:406.
35. Grever M, Kopecky K, Foucar MK, et al: Randomized comparison of pentostatin versus interferon alfa-2a in previously untreated patients with hairy cell leukemia: An intergroup study. J Clin Oncol 1995;13:974.
36. Hagberg H: Chimeric monoclonal anti-CD20 antibody (rituximab)—an effective treatment for a patient with relapsing hairy cell leukemia. Med Oncol 1999;16:221.
36a. Hakimian D, Tallman MS, Hogan D, et al: Prospective evaluation of internal adenopathy in a cohort of 43 patients with hairy cell leukemia (HCL) treated with 2-chlorodeoxyadenosine (2CdA). Basel: Molecular Biology of Hematopoiesis, 8th Symposium; 1993, p 161.
37. Hakimian D, Tallman MS, Kiley C: Detection of minimal residual disease by immunostaining of bone marrow biopsies after 2-chlorodeoxyadenosine for hairy cell leukemia. Blood 1993;82:1798.
38. Hassan IB, Gronowitz JS, Cerllson M, et al: Alpha interferon inhibits spontaneous and induced DNA synthesis in hairy cell leukemia. Leuk Lymphoma 1992;7:69.
39. Hassan IB, Hayberg H, Sordstrom C: Immunophenotype of hairy cell leukemia. Eur J Haematol 1990;45:172.

40. Heslop HE, Brenner MK, Ganeshguru K, et al: Possible mechanism of action of interferon alpha in chronic B cell malignancies. Br J Haematol 1991;79:14.
41. Hirota Y, Yoshioka A, Taraka S, et al: Imbalance of deoxyribonucleoside triphosphates, DNA double-strand breaks and cell death caused by 2-chlorodeoxyadenosine in mouse FM3A cells. Cancer Res 1989;49:915.
42. Ho AD, Thaler J, Mandelli F, et al: Response to pentostatin in hairy cell leukemia refractory to interferon alpha. The European Organization for Research and Treatment of Cancer and Leukemia Cooperative Group. J Clin Oncol 1989;7:1533.
43. Hoffman MA, Janson D, Rose E, et al: Treatment of hairy-cell leukemia with cladribine: Response, toxicity and long term follow-up. J Clin Oncol 1997;15:1138.
44. Hoffman M, Auerbach L: Bone marrow remission of hairy cell leukemia induced by rituximab (anti-CD20 antibody) in a patient refractory to cladribine. Br J Haematol 2000;109:900.
45. Hofmann V, Fehr J, Sauter C, et al: Hairy cell leukemia: An interferon deficient disease? Cancer Treat Rev 1985;12(suppl B):33.
46. Janckila AJ, Wallace JH, Yam LT: Generalized monocyte deficiency in leukaemic reticuloendotheliosis. Scand J Haematol 1982;29:153.
47. Jansen J, den Ottolander GJ, Holdrinet RSG, et al: Prognosis and therapy in hairy cell leukemia. Semin Oncol 1984;11:472.
48. Jansen J, Hermans J: Splenectomy in hairy cell leukemia: A retrospective multicenter analysis. Cancer 1981;47:2066.
49. Jehn U, Bartl R, Dietzfelbinger H, et al: Long term outcome of hairy cell leukemia treated with 2-chlorodeoxyadenosine. Ann Hematol 1999;78:139.
50. Juliusson G, Liliemark J: Rapid recovery from cytopenia in hairy cell leukemia after treatment with 2-chloro-2'-deoxyadenosine (CdA): Relation to opportunistic infections. Blood 1992;79:888.
51. Juliusson G, Liliemark J: Mechanisms of action, pharmacokinetics, and routes of administration of 2-chlorodeoxyadenosine in hairy cell leukemia. In Tallman MS, Polliack A, eds: Hairy Cell Leukemia. Amsterdam: Harwood Academic Publishers; 2000.
52. Kalyanaraman VS, Sarngadharan MG, Robert-Guroff M, et al: A new subtype of human T-cell leukemia virus (HTLVII) associated with a T-cell variant of hairy cell leukemia. Science 1982;218:571.
53. Kantarjian HM, Schacter J, Keating MJ: Fludarabine therapy in hairy cell leukemia. Cancer 1991;67:1291.
54. Katayama I: Bone marrow in hairy cell leukemia. Hematol Oncol Clin North Am 1988;2:585.
55. Katayama I, Hiroshima K, Maryuyana K, et al: Hairy cell leukemia in Japanese patients: A study with monoclonal antibodies. Leukemia 1987;1:301.
56. Kawosaki H, Carrera CJ, Piro LD, et al: Relationship of deoxycytidine kinase and cytoplasmic 5'-nucleotidase to the chemotherapeutic efficacy of 2-chlorodeoxyadenosine. Blood 1993;81:597.
57. Kreitman RJ, Wilson WH, Wyndham H, et al. Efficacy of the anti-CD22 recombinant immunotoxin BL22 in chemotherapy resistant hairy-cell leukemia. N Engl J Med 2001;345:241.
58. Kurzrock R, Strom SS, Estey E, et al: Second cancer risk in hairy cell leukemia: Analysis of 350 patients. J Clin Oncol 1997;15:1803.
59. Lauria F, Raspadori D, Benefenati D, et al: Biological markers and minimal residual disease in hairy cell leukemia. Leukemia 1992;6(suppl 4):149.
60. Lauria F, Rondelli D, Zinzani PL, et al: Long lasting complete remission in patients with hairy cell leukemia treated with 2-CdA: A 5 year survey. Leukemia 1997;11:629.
61. Lepe-Zuniga JL, Quesada JR, Baron S, et al: Alpha interferon production in patients with hairy cell leukemia: Correlations with disease activity and remission status. Hematol Pathol 1981;1:157.
62. Machii T, Tokumine Y, Inoue R, et al: Predominance of a distinct subtype of hairy cell leukemia in Japan. Leukemia 1993;7:181.
63. Mantovani G, Diso A, Santa Cruz G, et al: Familial chronic B cell malignancy. Hairy cell leukemia in mother and daughter. Haematologia (Budap) 1988;21:205.
64. Matutes E, Meeus P, McLennan K, et al: The significance of minimal residual disease in hairy cell leukemia treated with deoxycoformycin: A long term follow-up study. Br J Haematol 1997;98:375.
65. Matutes E, Wotherspoon AW, Brito-Babapulle V, et al: The variant form of hairy cell leukemia: Natural history, clinical and laboratory features in 52 patients. Blood 1999;94:301b.
66. McLaughlin P, White CA, Grillo-Lopez A, et al: Clinical status and optimal use of rituximab for B-cell lymphomas. Oncology 1998;12:1763.
67. Mercieca J, Matutes E, Moskovic E, et al: Massive abdominal adenopathy in hairy cell leukemia: A report of 12 cases. Br J Haematol 1992;82:547.
68. Mercieca J, Matutes E, Emmett E, et al: 2-Chlorodeoxyadenosine in the treatment of hairy cell leukemia: Differences in response in patients with and without abdominal adenopathy. Br J Haematol 1996;93:409.
69. Moller P, Mielke B, Moldenhauer G: Monoclonal antibody HML-1, a marker for intraepithelial T cells and lymphomas derived thereof, also recognizes hairy cell leukemia and some lymphomas. Am J Pathol 1990;136:509.
70. Mulligan SP, Matutes E, Dearden C, et al: Splenic lymphoma with villous lymphocytes: Natural history and response to therapy in 50 cases. Br J Haematol 1991;78:206.
71. Nielson B, Braide I: Three years' continuous low dose interferon-α treatment of hairy cell leukemia: Evaluation of response and maintenance dose. Eur J Haematol 1992;49:174.
72. O'Dwyer PJ, Wagner B, Leyland-Jones B, et al: 2'-Deoxycoformycin for lymphoid malignancies. Ann Intern Med 1988;108:733.
73. Pettitt AR, Zezel M, Cawley JC: Hairy cell leukemia: Biology and management. Br J Haematol 1999;106:2.
74. Piro LD, Miller WE, Carrera DA, et al: Hairy cell leukemia [letter]. N Engl J Med 1987;317:901.
75. Piro LD, Carrera CJ, Carson DA, et al: Lasting remissions in hairy cell leukemia induced by a single infusion of 2-chlorodeoxyadenosine. N Engl J Med 1990;322:1117.
76. Platanias LC, Preffer LM, Barton KP, et al: Expression of the IFN alpha receptor in hairy cell leukemia. Br J Haematol 1992;82:541.
77. Quesada JR, Alexanian R, Kurzrock R, et al: Recombinant interferon gamma in hairy cell leukemia, multiple myeloma and Waldenström's macroglobulinemia. Am J Hematol 1988;29:1.
78. Quesada JR, Reuben J, Manning JT, et al: Alpha interferon for induction of remission in hairy cell leukemia. N Engl J Med 1984;310:15.
79. Rai KR, Davey F, Peterson B, et al: Recombinant alpha-2b-interferon in therapy of previously untreated hairy cell leukemia: Long-term follow-up results of study by Cancer and Leukemia Group B. Leukemia 1995;9:1116.
80. Ratain MJ, Vardimen JW, Barker CM, et al: Prognostic variables in hairy cell leukemia after splenectomy as initial therapy. Cancer 1988;62:2420.
81. Ribeiro P, Bouaffia F, Peaud PY, et al: Long term outcome of patients with hairy cell leukemia treated with pentostatin. Cancer 1999;85:65.
82. Robak T, Basinska-Morawiec M, Krykowski E: Transient eosinophilia in a patient with hairy cell leukemia treated with 2-chlorodeoxyadenosine. Acta Hematol Pol 1992;23:285.
83. Robak T, Basinska-Morawiec M, Blonski J: 2-Chlorodeoxyadenosine (cladribine) in the treatment of hairy cell leukemia and hairy cell variant: 7 year experience in Poland. Eur J Hematol 1999;62:49.
84. Robertson LE, Chubb S, Meyn RE, et al: Induction of apoptotic cell death in chronic lymphocytic leukemia by 2-chloro-2'-deoxyadenosine and 9-beta-D-arabinosyl-2-fluoroadenine. Blood 1993;81:143.
85. Sainati L, Matutes E, Mulligan S, et al: A variant form of hairy cell leukemia resistant to alpha interferon: Clinical and phenotypic characteristics of 17 patients. Blood 1990;76:157.
86. Saven A, Piro L: Complete remissions in hairy cell leukemia with 2-chlorodeoxyadenosine after failure with 2'-deoxycoformycin. Ann Intern Med 1993;119:278.
87. Saven A, Burian C, Koziol JA, et al: Long term follow-up of patients with hairy cell leukemia after cladribine treatment. Blood 1998;92:1918.
88. Saven A, Burian C, Adusumalli J, et al: Filgrastim for cladribine-induced neutropenic fever in patients with hairy cell leukemia. Blood 1999;93:2471.
89. Schiller JH, Bittner G, Spriggs DR: Tumor necrosis factor, but not other hematopoietic growth factors, prolongs the survival of hairy cell leukemia cells. Leuk Res 1992;16:337.
90. Seto S, Carrera CJ, Kubota M, et al: Biochemical basis for deoxyadenosine and 2-chlorodeoxyadenosine toxicity to nondividing human lymphocytes. J Clin Invest 1985;75:377.
91. Seymour B, Estey EH, Keating MJ, et al: Response to interferon-α in patients with hairy cell leukemia relapsing after treatment with 2-chlorodeoxyadenosine. Leukemia 1995;9:929.

92. Shiebari K, Sohn CC, Burke JS, et al: Monocytoid B cell lymphoma: A novel B cell neoplasm. Am J Pathol 1986;124:310.

93. Siegal FP, Shodell M, Shah K, et al: Impaired interferon alpha response in hairy cell leukemia is corrected by therapy with 2-chlorodeoxyadenosine: Implications for susceptibility to opportunistic infections. Leukemia 1994;8:1474.

94. Smalley RV, Conners J, Tuttle RL, et al: Splenectomy vs. alpha interferon: A randomized study in patients with previously untreated hairy cell leukemia. Am J Hematol 1992;41:13.

95. Sole F, Woessner S, Florensa L, et al: Cytogenetic findings in five patients with hairy cell leukemia. Cancer Genet Cytogenet 1999; 110:41.

96. Sperb RA, von Rohr A, Ratschiller D, et al: 2-CDA in treatment of hairy cell leukemia: A comparison between intravenous and subcutaneous administration. Swiss Study Group of Applied Cancer Research. Schweiz Med Wochenschr 1998;128:1593.

97. Spiers ASD, Moore D, Cassileth P, et al: Remissions in hairy cell leukemia with pentostatin (2'-deoxycoformycin). N Engl J Med 1987;316:825.

98. Spiers ASD, Parekh SJ: Pentostatin (2'-deoxycoformycin, DCF) is active in hairy cell leukemia . Blood 1983;62:208a.

99. Steis RG, Smith JW, Urba WJ, et al: Resistance to recombinant interferon alfa-2a in hairy-cell leukemia associated with neutralizing anti-interferon antibodies. N Engl J Med 1988;318:1409.

100. Stiles GM, Stanco LM, Saven A, et al: Splenectomy for hairy cell leukemia in pregnancy. J Perinatol 1998;18:200.

101. Strickler JG, Schmidt CM, Wick MR: Methods in pathology. Immunophenotype of hairy cell leukemia in paraffin sections. Mod Pathol 1990;3:518.

102. Stroup R, Sheibari K: Antigenic phenotypes of hairy cell leukemia and monocytoid B-cell lymphoma: An immunohistochemical evaluation of 66 cases. Hum Pathol 1992;23:172.

103. Tallman MS, Hakimian D, Rademaker AW, et al: Relapse of hairy cell leukemia after 2-chlorodeoxyadenosine: Long term follow-up of the Northwestern University experience. Blood 1996;88:1954.

104. Tallman MS, Hakimian D, Kopecky KJ, et al: Minimal residual disease in patients with hairy cell leukemia in complete remission treated with 2-chlorodeoxyadenosine or 2-deoxycoformycin and prediction of early relapse. Clin Cancer Res 1999;5:1665.

105. Tetreault SA, Hoffman MA, Saven A: Clinical manifestations and differential diagnosis of hairy cell leukemia. In Tallman MA, Pollack A eds: Hairy Cell Leukemia. Amsterdam: Harwood Academic Publishers, 2000.

106. Thomas DA, O'Brien S, Cortes J, et al: Pilot study of rituximab in refractory or relapsed hairy cell leukemia (HCL). Blood 1999; 94:705a.

107. Trentin L, Zambello R, Benati C, et al: Expression and functional role of the p75 interleukin 2 receptor chain on leukemic hairy cells. Cancer Res 1992;5:5223.

108. Turner A, Kyeldsberg CR: Hairy cell leukemia: A review. Medicine (Baltimore) 1978;57:477.

109. Urba WJ, Baseler MV, Kopp WBC, et al: Deoxycoformycin-induced immunosuppression in patients with hairy cell leukemia. Blood 1989;73:38.

110. Van De Corput L, Falkenberg JH, Kluin-Nelemans JC: T-cell dysfunction in hairy cell leukemia: An updated review. Leuk Lymphoma 1998;30:31.

111. van der horst FA, van der Marel A, den Ottolander GJ, et al: Decrease in memory T helper cells in hairy cell leukemia. Leukemia 1993;7:46.

112. Vedenthern S, Gamliel H, Golomb HM: Mechanism of interferon action in hairy cell leukemia: A model of effective cancer biotherapy. Cancer Res 1992;52:1056.

113. Ward FT, Baker J, Krishian J: Hairy cell leukemia in two siblings. A human leukocyte antigen linked disease. Cancer 1990;65:319.

114. Woessner S, Rozman C: Ribosome-lamellae complex in CLL. Blut 1976;33:23.

115. Wolf BC, Martin AW, Neiman RS, et al: The detection of Epstein-Barr virus in hairy cell leukemia cells by in situ hybridization. Am J Pathol 1990;136:717.

116. Wu X, Ianova G, Merup M, et al: Molecular analysis of the human chromosome 5q13.3 region in patients with hairy cell leukemia and identification of tumor suppressor gene candidates. Genomics 1999;60:161.

117. Wylin RF, Greene MH, Palutke M, et al: Hairy cell leukemia in three siblings: An apparent HLA-linked disease. Cancer 1982;49:538.

118. Zinzani PL, Lauria F, Buzzi M, et al: Hairy cell leukemia variant: A morphologic, immunologic and clinical study of 7 cases. Hematologica 1990;75:54.

119. Zinzani PL, Lauria F, Raspadori D, et al: Comparison of low dose versus standard dose alpha interferon regimen in the hairy cell treatment. Acta Haematol 1991;85:161.

120. Zinzani PL, Lauria F, Raspadori D, et al: Results in hairy cell leukemia patients treated with α-interferon: Predictive prognostic factors. Eur J Haematol 1992;49:133.

30

Masao Matsuoka   Kiyoshi Takatsuki

Adult T-Cell Leukemia

Adult T-cell leukemia (ATL) was established as a distinct clinical entity in 1977 in Kyoto, Japan.[1-3] The illness is manifested by presentation in adult life: frequent rashes, skin involvement, lymphadenopathy, and hepatosplenomegaly. The peripheral white blood cell count is often elevated with abnormal lymphoid cells, but in many cases anemia or thrombocytopenia is rarely found, and limited bone marrow infiltration is observed. The abnormal ATL cells are of mature T-helper phenotype and have a characteristic appearance with especially indented nuclei. There is striking frequent hypercalcemia with increased numbers of osteoclasts. Central to the identification of the syndrome is the striking geographic clustering in southwestern Japan and the isolation of the human T-cell lymphotropic virus type-I (HTLV-I) from the cell lines of patients with ATL (HTLV-I is the causative agent for ATL and is also at least a component of other conditions; see Chapter 10).[4-6] Southwestern Japan was shown to be the major area in the world in which both HTLV-I and ATL are endemic. Both the virus and ATL were subsequently found in Caribbean migrants to the United Kingdom, the Netherlands, the United States, and parts of South America.[7, 8]

ETIOLOGY

The etiologic association of HTLV-I is based on the following observations[4, 9-11]:

1. The areas of high incidence of ATL correspond closely with those of high incidence of HTLV-I.
2. HTLV-I immortalizes human T cells in vitro.
3. Monoclonal integration of HTLV-I proviral DNA has been demonstrated in ATL cells.
4. All individuals with ATL have antibodies against HTLV-I. HTLV is therefore the first retrovirus directly associated with human malignancy.

HTLV-I belongs to the Oncovirinae subfamily of retroviruses that includes the bovine leukemia virus, the human T-cell lymphotropic virus type II, and the simian T-cell leukemia virus. Like other retroviruses, the HTLV-I proviral genome has *gag*, *pol*, and *env* genes flanked by long terminal repeat (LTR) sequences at both ends.[12] A unique structure was found between *env* and the 3'-LTR, denoted the pX region, that encodes the regulatory proteins p40[tax] (Tax), p27[rex] (Rex), p21, p12, and p13 (Fig. 30-1).[13-16] Among them, Tax protein is thought to play a central role in the leukemogenesis of ATL because of its pleiotropic actions. Tax does not bind to promoter or enhancer sequences by itself but interacts with cellular proteins that are transcriptional factors or modulators of cellular functions. By binding to various cellular factors such as NFκB, SRF, and CREB, Tax activates transcription of both viral and cellular genes. Tax can interact with IKKγ, which causes phosphorylation of IκB and NF-κB activation, resulting in transcriptional activation of cellular genes such as interleukin-2 (IL-2) and IL-2 receptor genes.[17] On the other hand, binding of Tax to CREB causes transcriptional activation of viral genes as well as cellular genes. Conversely, Tax can trans-repress the transcription of certain genes such as *lck* and *p18* and DNA polymerase-β.[18-20]

Direct interaction of Tax with cellular proteins can interrupt their functions. For example, Tax also appears to allow dysregulated cell cycling by binding and inactivating p16[INK4A], a key inhibitor of cyclin-dependent kinases 4 and 6.[21] Tax also has been reported to interact with *MAD*1, which acts as a mitotic checkpoint gene; such disturbance of checkpoint genes might be associated with chromosomal instability, which is frequently observed in ATL cells.[22] It is associated with leukemogenesis by generating chromosomal instability. In HTLV-I–transformed cell lines, the *p53* gene is highly expressed but is functionally impaired.[23] Tax interferes with recruitment of coactivator CBP/p300 on the *p53* binding site, resulting in functional inactivation of *p53*.[20] Inactivation of this major cancer suppressor gene in cooperation with inactivation of p16[INK4A] is thought to contribute to HTLV-I–related leukemogenesis and, ultimately, ATL.

The pleiotropic functions of Tax are thought to contribute to the immortalization of HTLV-I–infected cells, especially CD4-positive T lymphocytes. Indeed, the proliferation of HTLV-I–infected cells in vivo has been shown to be clonal as detected by analysis of integration sites. As described later, persistent proliferation is observed in HTLV-I carriers.[24, 25] After infection with HTLV-I, a very long latent period (about 50 years in Japan) is present before the onset of ATL. Such a long latent period indicates that multi-step tumorigenesis is necessary for the development of ATL. During this latent period, genetic

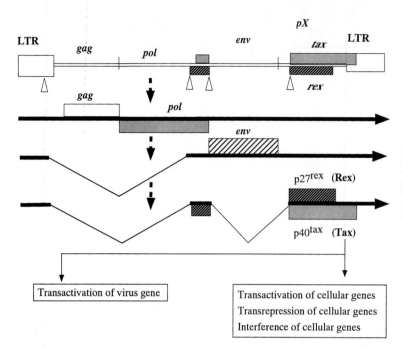

FIGURE 30–1. Structure of HTLV-I. HTLV-I proviral genome has the *gag, pol, env* genes, flanked by long terminal repeat (LTR) at both sides. The unique structure was found between *env* and 3′-LTR, which was named as pX region that encodes the regulatory proteins, p40^tax (Tax), p27^rex (Rex), and p21.

and epigenetic mutations are thought to accumulate in infected cells.

EPIDEMIOLOGY OF ATL

Both HTLV-I and ATL have been shown to be endemic in some regions of the world, especially southwest Japan,[26] the Caribbean islands, the countries surrounding the Caribbean basin, South America, and parts of Central Africa.[8, 27-29] In addition, epidemiologic studies of HTLV-I revealed high seroprevalence rates in Melanesia; Papua, New Guinea[30]; the Solomon Islands[31]; and among Australian aborigines. In the Middle East, a focus of HTLV-I was found in Iranian Jews who reside in the Mashad region.[32] HTLV-I carriers in Japan have been estimated to be approximately 1.2 million individuals,[6] and more than 800 cases of ATL have been diagnosed each year in Japan alone. The cumulative 70-year prevalence of ATL among HTLV-I carriers in Japan is estimated at about 6.6% in males and 2.1% in female.[33]

HTLV-I seroprevalence rises in a age-dependent manner, and it is higher in females than in males.[27] Three major routes of HTLV-I transmission have been identified: mother-to-infant, sexual, and parenteral. Mother-to-infant transmission occurs mainly via breast milk. HTLV-I–positive lymphocytes have been identified in the breast milk from seropositive mothers.[34] Intervention trials in Japan showed that breastfeeding accounts for most mother-to-infant transmission. Breastfed infants showed a 13% seroconversion rate, whereas bottle-fed infants experienced a 3% seroconversion rate.[35] Prolonged breastfeeding is associated with a higher rate of seroconversion among infants: 0% for less than 6 months, 28% for more than 6 months of breastfeeding. Other mechanisms of HTLV-I transmission from mother to infant remain unknown. Studies of married couples and sexually active

groups have shown that sexual transmission of HTLV-I occurs from male to female, from female to male, and from male to male. Studies in seropositive couples showed that male-to-female infection is more efficient than female-to-male infection, which may explain a part of higher HTLV-I seroprevalence among women. Transfusion with cellular components is associated with HTLV-I transmission.[36] Transfusion of plasma is not associated with transmission, showing that viable infected cells are necessary for transmission.

Evolution of ATL

The natural course of HTLV-I infection to ATL is thought to be as follows. HTLV-I transmission is mainly from mother to infant by breastfeeding or from male to female by sexual intercourse. HTLV-I can infect many kinds of cells in vivo, such as T lymphocyte, B lymphocyte, monocyte, and dendritic cells, revealing that HTLV-I may not need a cell-type specific receptor for the infection. HTLV-I provirus is detected mainly in CD4-positive memory T lymphocytes in healthy carriers.[37] Indeed, carriers with a high HTLV-I provirus load have an increased number of memory T lymphocytes, as do patients with the neurodegenerative disease HTLV-I–associated myelopathy/tropical spastic paraparesis. This suggests that viral proteins, especially Tax, promote the proliferation of CD4-positive memory T lymphocytes. HTLV-I provirus load, which is correlated with the number of HTLV-I–infected cells, differed more than 100-fold among HTLV-I carriers.[38] It was revealed that provirus loads fluctuated only two- to fourfold in most carriers, showing that provirus loads were relatively constant over time for up to 7 years in individual carriers.

The HTLV-I provirus is genetically very stable, especially compared with the other major human retrovirus, such as human immunodeficiency virus. It has been postulated that increased HTLV-I load is achieved, not by replication of virus but by clonal proliferation of infected cells. In HTLV-I carriers, HTLV-I provirus is randomly integrated in the host genome. In other words, the integration site is specific to each HTLV-I–infected cell. A part of LTR and flanking genomic DNAs were amplified by inverse polymerase chain reaction (PCR), with each detected band representing a clonal proliferation of HTLV-I–infected cells. Using this assay to analyze clonal proliferation of HTLV-I-infected cells in HTLV-I carriers, some clones persisted longer than 7 years in the same individuals.[25, 39] These persistent clones were CD4-positive lymphocytes, which is consistent with the fact that HTLV-I predominantly immortalizes CD4-positive T lymphocytes in vitro.

A latent period of about 50 years precedes the onset of ATL, suggesting the multistep mechanism of leukemogenesis. Various mutations of oncogenes and tumor-suppressor genes have been demonstrated in cancers, and it has been established that multiple changes are necessary for the appearance of malignant disease. In ATL cells, mutations of $p53$ have been detected in about 30% of patients examined.[40] Such mutations were detected in the more aggressive disease state. Deletion of the $p16^{INK4A}$ gene was also reported in ATL.[41, 42] Again, those abnormalities were observed in acute or lymphoma-type ATL, suggesting that somatic DNA changes in $p53$ or $p16^{INK4A}$ genes are associated with the progression of ATL. Epigenetic change, such as methylation of the $p16$ gene, plays an important role in the progression of ATL as well as in genetic change.[43] Such findings indicate that multistep changes are required for leukemogenesis in ATL. Other genetic and epigenetic changes remain to be analyzed.

CLINICAL FEATURES OF ATL

Takatsuki[44] studied 187 patients with ATL in Kyushu, Japan. There were 113 males and 74 females (1.5:1), whose age at onset ranged from 27 to 82 years, with a median age of 55 years.

The predominant physical findings were peripheral lymph node enlargement (72%), hepatomegaly (47%), splenomegaly (25%), and skin lesions (53%). Various skin lesions, such as papules, erythema, and nodules, were frequently observed in ATL patients. ATL cells densely infiltrate the dermis and epidermis, forming Pautrier's microabscesses in the epidermis (Fig. 30–2). Hypercalcemia (72%)[45] was frequently associated with ATL. Other findings at onset were abdominal pain, diarrhea, pleural effusion, ascites, cough, sputum, and an abnormal shadow on chest radiographs. The white blood cell count ranged from normal to 500 × 10⁹/L. Leukemic cells resembled Sézary's cells, having indented or lobulated nuclei. The typical surface phenotype of ATL cells, characterized by monoclonal antibodies, was CD3+, CD4+, CD8−, and CD25+.[46] Anemia and thrombocytopenia were rare. Eosinophilia was frequently observed in ATL patients as well as other T-cell malignancies.[47, 48]

Serum lactate dehydrogenase is elevated in most ATL patients; higher levels indicate an advanced or aggressive

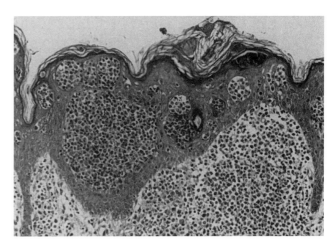

FIGURE 30–2. Skin involvement of ATL. Histology of skin invasion of an acute ATL patient. ATL cells infiltrating the dermis and epidermis form Pautrier's microabscesses.

disease state. Hypercalcemia, a frequent complication in ATL patients, can be life-threatening. Serum calcium and serum lactate dehydrogenase (LDH) levels reflect the extent of disease and are useful for monitoring the remaining tumor or disease activity. Hyperbilirubinemia, observed when ATL cells infiltrate the liver, indicates a poor prognosis. Hypergammaglobulinemia is very rare in ATL, this being consistent with the fact that ATL cells have suppressor-inducer activity to immunoglobulin synthesis in vitro. β_2-Microglobulin is a component of class I HLA antigen, and serum levels of this component are correlated with the disease activity of non-Hodgkin's lymphoma or myeloma. Serum β_2-microglobulin is also elevated in ATL patients, also being correlated with disease activity. ATL cells were shown to express IL-2 receptor alpha chain on their surfaces and secrete its soluble forms. Levels of soluble IL-2 receptors are elevated in the sera of patients with ATL, the levels of soluble IL-2 receptor being correlated with the tumor mass and clinical course.[49]

ATL cells elaborate many cytokines because they originate from activated helper T cells. Cytokines are presumed to play an important role in the pathophysiology of ATL. For example, elaborated parathyroid hormone–related protein from ATL cells activates osteoclasts and promotes the bone resorption that is thought to be a cause of hypercalcemia in ATL patients (Fig. 30–3).[50] IL-1 has multiple biologic activities, such as induction of neutrophilia and fever.[51] A high fever without overt infection and absolute neutrophilia are frequently found in ATL patients. Eosinophilia is frequently observed in patients with ATL, and IL-5 produced by ATL cells might be the causative factor.[47] Other cytokines, including TGF-β, IL-10, IL-8, and macrophage colony-stimulating factor, have been reported to be produced by ATL cells.

Familial occurrences of ATL have been reported.[52] Three sisters ranging in age from 56 to 59 years who developed lymphoma-type ATL during a 19-month period were reported.[53] The patients were born in Kumamoto Prefecture, an area where HTLV-I is endemic. As their lives and environments in adulthood were clearly differ-

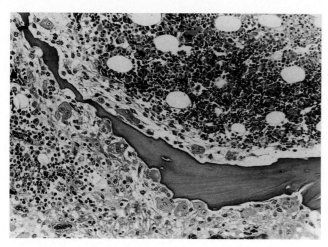

FIGURE 30–3. Marked proliferation of osteoclasts along a bone trabecula. The edge of the trabecula is serrated, displaying a saw-toothed appearance. (Courtesy of Dr. Takeya, Second Department of Pathology, Kumamoto University School of Medicine.)

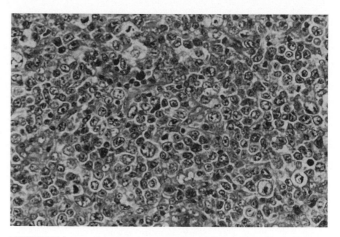

FIGURE 30–4. Histopathology of a lymph node from a patient with lymphoma-type ATL. Lymphoma cells with round-to-irregular nuclei containing multiple nucleoli are shown. Histologic findings reveal a high frequency of mitosis and pleomorphic cellular features.

ent, HTLV-I infection may have occurred in childhood. The findings suggest that genetic factors play an important role in ATL development.

Survival time in acute and lymphoma-type ATL ranged from 2 weeks to more than 1 year. The causes of death were pulmonary complications including *Pneumocystis carinii* pneumonia,[54] hypercalcemia, *Cryptococcus* meningitis, and disseminated herpes zoster. Smoldering ATL is characterized by the long duration of a few ATL cells in the peripheral blood.[55]

These features and the clinical course, ATL subtype, frequency of hypercalcemia and opportunistic infections, cell morphology, phenotypic profile, and response to treatment appear to be the same for Japanese, Caribbean, and African ATL patients. The only difference is age of onset: the Japanese patients at diagnosis are older. Blattner and Kalyanaraman[7] and Gibbs and Lofters[29] reported that the mean ages of ATL patients in the United States and Jamaica were 43 and 40 years, respectively.

DIAGNOSIS OF ATL

The diagnostic criteria for HTLV-I-associated ATL have been defined as follows:

1. Histologically and/or cytologically proven lymphoid malignancy with T-cell surface antigens.
2. Abnormal T lymphocytes always present in the peripheral blood, except in the lymphoma type. These abnormal T lymphocytes include typical ATL cells (the so-called flower cells) and the small and mature T lymphocytes with incised or lobulated nuclei that are characteristic of the chronic or smoldering type.
3. Antibody to HTLV-I present in the sera at diagnosis.
4. Demonstration of monoclonal integration of HTLV-I provirus by Southern blot method.

In addition, lymph node biopsy provides important information for diagnosis: nodal architecture is replaced by diffuse infiltration of neoplastic cells (Fig. 30–4).

Morphology of ATL Cells

Numerous abnormal lymphocytes, which vary considerably in size and cytoplasmic basophilia, are seen in acute-type ATL (Fig. 30–5A). Cells from 30% of cases of this type possess small vacuoles but lack azurophilic granules. Most of the cells characteristically exhibit lobular division of their nuclei; most are bi- or multifoliate and are separated by deep indentation. Cells with such a nuclear configuration are known as flower cells. Leukemic cells with relatively coarsely clumped nuclear chromatin are not morphologically monotonous.

Cells from chronic ATL are relatively uniform in size and nuclear configuration. Cells are smaller than those seen in either acute or smoldering ATL (see Fig. 30–5B). Chronic ATL cells rarely possess small vacuoles and do not possess azurophilic granules. Cells in this type also exhibit lobular division of their nuclei. However, most of the lobulated nuclei are bi- or trifoliate. Many cells exhibit deep indentation rather than lobulation. The nuclear chromatin is in coarse strands and is deeply stained. The

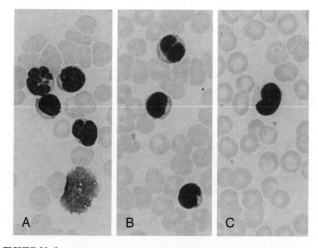

FIGURE 30–5. Cell morphology of ATL cells. Leukemic cells are shown from acute *(A)*, chronic *(B)*, and smoldering *(C)* ATL.

nucleocytoplasmic ratio is larger than that of normal lymphocytes.

Cells from smoldering type are relatively large, and they do not have cytoplasmic granules or vacuoles (see Fig. 30-5C). The lobulated nuclei are bi- or trifoliate. Some of the nuclei exhibit indentation or clefts that appear as a ridge formation. The nucleocytoplasmic ratio is large, and the nuclear chromatin is in coarse strands and is deeply stained.

Serology of HTLV-I

Anti–HTLV-I antibodies are positive in almost all patients with ATL, although seronegative ATL cases have been rarely reported.[56, 57] There is no difference between ATL patients and HTLV-I carriers in the pattern of serum antibodies. The presence of serum antibodies against HTLV-I can be demonstrated by enzyme-linked immunosorbence, gelatin particle hemagglutination, indirect immunofluorescence, and Western blotting assays.[58] Titer of antibody against HTLV-I is correlated with provirus load.[38] Carriers with high level of anti–HTLV-I antibody and low titer of anti-Tax antibody have been noted to be at high risk for ATL.[59]

Phenotypic Markers of ATL Cells

Immunophenotypic analysis of ATL cells with various monoclonal antibodies has revealed that ATL cells have the phenotype of activated helper/inducer T lymphocytes. Most ATL cells are positive for CD2, CD3, CD4, and CD25 and HLA-DR and are negative for CD7 and CD8.[46] A characteristic feature of ATL cells is the decreased expression of T-cell receptor/CD3 complex on their surfaces.[60] This is a phenomenon specific to ATL cells and is not observed in other T-cell malignancies. There are several reports of ATL cases with different leukemic cell phenotypes; e.g., CD4+ and CD8+, CD4− and CD8−, and CD4− and CD8+.[61] Most of these variant forms are observed in patients with acute ATL and indicate poor prognosis. Phenotypic changes in ATL cells have been observed in some patients during the clinical course of the disease. For example, typical CD4+, CD8− ATL cells changed into CD4+ and CD8+, perhaps indicating an exacerbation of ATL. CD95 (Fas/APO-1) antigen is highly expressed on the leukemic cells in most patients with ATL, and such ATL cells are highly susceptible to antibody against Fas antigen.[62] On the other hand, Fas-negative ATL cases were also reported, and the underlying mutations of the Fas gene were identified.[63]

HTLV-I Provirus Genome in Leukemic Cells of ATL

The definitive diagnosis of ATL requires the detection of the monoclonal integration of HTLV-I provirus in genomic DNA from peripheral blood mononuclear or lymph node cells.[64] Monoclonal integration of the HTLV-I provirus is not detected in patients with other T-cell malignancies. The detection of HTLV-I proviral DNA is essential for the diagnosis of ATL, especially in endemic areas. Monoclonal integration of HTLV-I provirus can be detected by the Southern blot method. Defective HTLV-I provirus was found in 56% of patients with ATL, and two different types of defective provirus were identified in ATL using Southern blot analysis.[65] Type 1 defective provirus retains both LTRs but lacks internal sequences such as gag, pol, or env. Type 2 defective provirus lacks 5′-LTR and 5′-internal sequences. Type 2 defective provirus is usually found in aggressive subtypes of ATL: acute and lymphoma types. This suggests that the genetic instability to generate type 2 defective provirus is associated with the progression of ATL. Because type 2 defective provirus cannot produce viral proteins including Tax, ATL cells with type 2 defective provirus can escape from immunosurveillance of the host. It is assumed that, during the early stage of leukemogenesis such as in smoldering and chronic ATL, Tax plays a critical role. Later, Tax may not be necessary as accumulated genetic or epigenetic changes cause the progression to acute or lymphoma types of ATL.

Chromosomal Abnormalities of ATL Cells

Karyotype analyses of 107 patients with ATL revealed various chromosomal abnormalities as follows[66–68]:

1. Trisomies of chromosomes 3 (21%), 7 (10%), and 21 (9%); monosomy of X chromosome (38%) in females; and loss of a Y chromosome (17%) in males were frequent numerical abnormalities.

2. Frequent structural abnormalities were translocations involving 14q32 (28%) or 14q11 (14%) and deletion of 6q (23%).

There was no chromosomal abnormality specific for ATL, but abnormalities were detected in the aggressive, acute, or lymphoma types of ATL rather than in the nonaggressive chronic or smoldering type. In situ hybridization techniques disclosed that integrated sites of provirus of HTLV-I were different in each patient and that the random pattern of Southern blot analyses of the integrated provirus also did not support the idea that HTLV-I integrated to a specific site and activated cellular (onco)-genes.[69]

CLASSIFICATION OF ATL

ATL patients can be classified into four clinical subtypes according to the clinical features: acute, chronic, smoldering, and lymphoma.[70]

The acute type is the so-called prototypic ATL in which patients exhibit increased numbers of ATL cells, skin lesions, systemic lymphadenopathy, and hepatosplenomegaly. Most of these patients are resistant to chemotherapy. Poor prognosis is indicated by elevated serum LDH, calcium, and bilirubin as well as by an increased white blood cell count.

In chronic ATL, white blood cell count is increased,

and skin lesions are exhibited. In some patients with chronic ATL, there is mild lymphadenopathy and hepatosplenomegaly, and serum LDH is sometimes elevated. However, hypercalcemia and hyperbilirubinemia are not complications in this type of ATL. In the past, chronic ATL was thought to be chronic T-lymphocytic leukemia.

Smoldering ATL is characterized by the presence of a few ATL cells in the peripheral blood over a period of years.[71] Frequent symptoms are skin or pulmonary lesions. Serum LDH levels are usually within the normal range, and serum calcium is also normal. Lymphadenopathy and hepatosplenomegaly are not so marked in smoldering ATL. Smoldering and chronic ATL often progress to acute ATL after a long period (crisis).

Lymphoma-type ATL is characterized by prominent lymphadenopathy, with few abnormal cells in the peripheral blood. This type has been diagnosed as nonleukemic malignant lymphoma.

The Lymphoma Study Group (1984–1987) in Japan proposed the following diagnostic criteria for classifying ATL into the four subtypes[70]:

1. Smoldering type: 5% or more abnormal lymphocytes of T-cell nature in the peripheral blood; normal lymphocyte level (fewer than $4 \times 10^9/L$); no hypercalcemia; LDH value of up to $1.5 \times$ normal upper limit; no lymphadenopathy; no involvement of liver, spleen, central nervous system, bone, or gastrointestinal tract; and neither ascites nor pleural effusion. Skin and pulmonary lesion(s) may be present. In patients with less than 5% abnormal T lymphocytes in peripheral blood, at least one histologically proven skin or pulmonary lesion should be present.

2. Chronic type: absolute lymphocytosis of more than $3.5 \times 10^9/L$; LDH value up to twice the normal upper limit; no hypercalcemia; no involvement of CNS bone or gastrointestinal tract; and neither ascites nor pleural effusion. There may be histologically proven lymphadenopathy with or without extranodal lesions, and there may be involvement of liver, spleen, skin, and lung and 5% or more abnormal lymphocytes.

3. Lymphoma type: no lymphocytosis, 1% or less abnormal lymphocytes, histologically proven lymphadenopathy with or without extranodal lesions.

4. Acute type: the most common form of presentation; highly aggressive malignancy that shows lymphadenopathy, hepatosplenomegaly, and skin lesions but does not meet the criteria for the other types.

TREATMENT OF ATL AND PREVENTION OF HTLV-I INFECTION

ATL is generally treated with curative intent using combination chemotherapy, although long-term success has been very limited. The acute form, with hypercalcemia, high LDH levels, and an elevated white blood cell count, carries a particularly poor prognosis. Sequential trials in Japan have resulted in the complete remission rate being increased from 16% with a four-drug combination to 43% with eight drugs.[72, 73] Unfortunately, that advance did not translate into a improvement in overall survival. In a recent study by the Lymphoma Study Group in Japan, improved survival of ATL patients was reported.[74] The overall median survival remains 13 months, and the estimated 2-year survival was 31.3%.[74] In contrast, smoldering ATL or some cases of chronic ATL may have a more protracted natural course, which may be compromised by aggressive chemotherapy. Alternative strategies for both acute and chronic forms are clearly needed.

Major obstacles in the treatment of ATL are drug resistance of ATL cells against chemotherapeutic agents and opportunistic infections due to immunodeficiency complicating in patients with ATL. The inevitable impairment of T-cell function puts the patient at high risk of fungal, protozoal, and viral infections, against which prophylactic measures should be taken.

Deoxycoformycin, the nucleotide analogue, was reported to induce long-term remission in a patient with ATL in 1985.[75] Subsequently, Yamaguchi[76] prolonged complete remission in two out of seven patients. There was profound lymphopenia but no neutropenia. Because impaired cell-mediated immunity is the major adverse effect of deoxycoformycin, which exacerbates the underlying immunodeficiency of patients with ATL, careful management is needed for prophylaxis of opportunistic infections.

α-Interferon combined with azidothymidine was administered to 19 patients with ATL, and major responses (complete plus partial remissions) were achieved in 58% (11 of 19), including complete remission in 26% (5 of 19).[77] Viral replication in ATL cells could not be detected in vivo, which means that inhibition of reverse transcriptase is not the target of AZT in this mechanism, but AZT is acting as an antileukemic drug. Other drugs, including arsenic trioxide, have been considered for treatment of ATL from data in vitro.[78] Humanized monoclonal antibody against IL-2 receptor was also used for patients with ATL.[79] Successful allogeneic bone marrow transplantation for patients with ATL was reported.[80] The authors of this chapter performed bone marrow transplantation in a patient with acute ATL who did not respond to combinational chemotherapy. The patient has been in complete remission for more than 36 months. Further studies are obviously required to show whether either of these approaches will have a major impact on ATL.

Prevention of ATL by reducing transmission of HTLV-I is obviously a more attractive goal. To prevent infection with HTLV-I by blood transfusion, all donated blood at blood centers was subjected to HTLV-I antibody testing beginning in November 1986 in Japan. None of the recipients, even patients with hematologic disorders who received multiple transfusions, were seroconverted. In Japan, absolute decline of the carrier rate among the young generation[81] was observed, possibly due to complete blood donor screening and success in preventing the majority of maternal transmission by refraining from breastfeeding. Since experiments using animal models have disclosed that vaccination against HTLV-I is possible, the generation of vaccine against HTLV-I is needed to prevent the spread of this virus among humans.

HTLV-I–RELATED DISORDERS

HTLV-I infection is both a direct cause of ATL and is associated with many other diseases, such as HTLV-I–

associated myelopathy/tropical spastic paraparesis,[82, 83] chronic lung diseases, opportunistic lung infections, strongyloidiasis,[55, 84] infective dermatits,[85] arthropathy,[86] and uveitis.[87] The association of HTLV-I infection with these diseases is considered to be due to some extent to the immunodeficiency induced by HTLV-I infection. In patients with HTLV-I–associated myelopathy/tropical spastic paraparesis and HTLV-I uveitis, increased numbers of HTLV-I–infected cells were reported,[88, 89] suggesting that inflammatory reactions, such as exceed production of cytokines, and increased expression of adhesion molecules on the surface play a critical role in pathogenesis of these diseases.

ATL patients may also have complications of other malignancies due to immunodeficiency. B lymphoma with EBV genome has been reported in an ATL patient,[90] and Kaposi's sarcoma has also occurred with ATL.[91] EBV-positive lymphoma and Kaposi's sarcoma are well known to occur in AIDS patients, and impaired cell-mediated immunity in ATL as in AIDS is an important factor in these secondary malignancies.

REFERENCES

1. Takatsuki K: Adult T-cell leukemia in Japan. In Seno S, Takaku F, Irino S, eds: Topics in Hematology. Amsterdam: Excerpta Medica; 1977, p 73.
2. Uchiyama T: Adult T-cell leukemia: Clinical and hematologic features of 16 cases. Blood 1977;50:481.
3. Yodoi J, Takatsuki K, Masuda T: Two cases of T-cell chronic lymphocytic leukemia in Japan. N Engl J Med 1974;290:572.
4. Hinuma T: Adult T-cell leukemia: Antigen in an ATL cell line and detection of antibodies to the antigen in human sera. Proc Natl Acad Sci U S A 1981;78:6476.
5. Poiesz BJ: Detection and isolation of type C retrovirus particles from fresh and cultured lymphocytes of a patient with cutaneous T-cell lymphoma. Proc Natl Acad Sci U S A 1980;77:7415.
6. Tajima K: Ethnoepidemiology of ATL in Japan with special reference to the Mongoloid dispersal. In Takatsuki K, ed: Adult T-cell Leukemia. Oxford: Oxford University Press; 1994, p 91.
7. Blattner WA, Kalyanaraman VS: The human type-C retrovirus HTLV in blacks from the Caribbean region and relationship to adult T-cell leukemia/lymphoma. Int J Cancer 1982;30:257.
8. Catovsky D: Adult T-cell lymphoma-leukaemia in blacks from the West Indies. Lancet 1982;1:639.
9. Miyoshi I: A novel T-cell line derived from adult T-cell leukemia. Gann 1980;71:155.
10. Wong-Staal F, Gallo RC: Human T-lymphotropic retroviruses. Nature 1985;317:395.
11. Yoshida M, Miyoshi I, Hinuma Y: Isolation and characterization of retrovirus from cell lines of human adult T-cell leukemia and its implication in the disease. Proc Natl Acad Sci U S A 1982;79:2031.
12. Seiki M: Human adult T-cell leukemia virus: Complete nucleotide sequence of the provirus genome integrated in leukemia cell DNA. Proc Natl Acad Sci U S A 1983;80:3618.
13. Franchini G: Molecular mechanisms of human T-cell leukemia/lymphotropic virus type I infection. Blood 1995;86:3619.
14. Seiki M: Expression of the *pX* gene of HTLV-I: General splicing mechanism in the HTLV family. Science 1985;228:1532.
15. Sodroski J: A transcriptional activator protein encoded by the x-*lor* region of the human T-cell leukemia virus. Science 1985;228:1430.
16. Yoshida M: Regulation of HTLV-I gene expression and its roles in ATL development. In Takatsuki K, ed: Adult T-cell Leukemia. Oxford: Oxford University Press; 1994, p 28.
17. Jin DY: Role of adapter function in oncoprotein-mediated activation of NF-kappa-B: Human T-cell leukemia virus type I Tax interacts directly with I-kappa-B kinase gamma. J Biol Chem 1999;274:17402.
18. Jeang KT: HTLV-I trans-activator protein Tax is a transrepressor of the human β polymerase gene. Science 1990;247:1082.
19. Lemasson I: Transrepression of *lck* gene exression by human T-cell leukemia virus type 1-encoded p40tax. J Virol 1997;71:1975.
20. Suzuki T, Uchida-Toita M, Yoshida M: Tax protein of HTLV-1 inhibits CBP/p300-mediated transcription by interfering with recruitment of CBP/p300 onto DNA element of E-box or p53 binding site. Oncogene 1999;18:4137.
21. Suzuki T: HTLV-1 Tax protein interacts with cyclin-dependent kinase inhibitor p16^{INK4A} and counteracts its inhibitory activity towards CDK4. EMBO J 1995;7:1607.
22. Jin DY, Spencer F, Jeang KT: Human T cell leukemia virus type 1 oncoprotein Tax targets the human mitotic checkpoint protein MAD1. Cell 1998;93:81.
23. Cereseto A: *p53* functional impairment and high p21waf1/cip1 expression in human T-cell lymphotropic/leukemia virus type I-transformed T cells. Blood 1996;88:1551.
24. Cavrois M: Persistent oligoclonal expansion of human T-cell leukemia virus type 1-infected circulating cells in patients with tropical spastic paraparesis/HTLV-1-associated myelopathy. Oncogene 1998; 17:77.
25. Etoh K-I: Persistent clonal proliferation of human T-lymphotropic virus type I-infected cells in vivo. Cancer Res 1997;57:4862.
26. Tajima K: Geographical features and epidemiological approach to endemic T-cell leukemia/lymphoma in Japan. Jpn J Clin Oncol 1979; 9:495.
27. Blattner WA, Gallo RC: Epidemiology of HTLV-I and HTLV-II infection. In Takatsuki K, ed: Adult T-cell Leukemia. Oxford: Oxford University Press; 1994, p 45.
28. Fleming AF: Antibodies to ATLV (HTLV) in Nigerian blood donors and patients with chronic lymphatic leukaemia or lymphoma. Lancet 1983;2:334.
29. Gibbs WN, Lofters WS: Adult T-cell leukemia/lymphoma in Jamaica and its relationship to human T-cell leukemia/lymphoma virus type I-associated lymphoproliferative disease. In Miwa M, ed: Retroviruses in Human Lymphoma/Leukemia. Tokyo: Japan Scientific Societies Press; 1985, p 77.
30. Kazura JW: Epidemiology of human T-cell leukemia virus type I infection in East Sepik province, Papua New Guinea. J Infect Dis 1987;155:1100.
31. Yanagihara R: Human T-lymphotropic virus type I infection in the Solomon Islands. Am J Trop Med Hyg 1991;44:122.
32. Meytes D, Schochat B, Lee H: Serological and molecular survey for HTLV-I infection in a high-risk Middle Eastern group. Lancet 1990; 336:1533.
33. Arisawa K: Evaluation of adult T-cell leukemia/lymphoma incidence and its impact on non-Hodgkin lymphoma incidence in southwestern Japan. Int J Cancer 2000;85:319.
34. Kinoshita K: Demonstration of adult T-cell leukemia virus antigen in milk from three seropositive mothers. Gann 1984;75:103.
35. Hino S: Maternal-infant transmission of HTLV-I: Implication for disease. In Blattner WA, ed: Human Retrovirology: HTLV. New York: Raven Press; 1990, p 363.
36. Okochi K: A retrospective study on transmission of adult T-cell leukemia virus by blood transfusion: Seroconversion in recipients. Vox Sang 1984;46:245.
37. Richardson JH: In vivo cellular tropism of human T-cell leukemia virus type 1. J Virol 1990;64:5682.
38. Etoh K-I: Rapid quantification of HTLV-I provirus load: Detection of monoclonal proliferation of HTLV-I-infected cells among blood donors. Int J Cancer 1999;81:859.
39. Mueller N: Epidemiologic perspectives of HTLV-I. In Blattner WA, ed: Human Retrovirology: HTLV. New York: Raven Press; 1990, p 281.
40. Sakashita A: Mutations of the *p53* gene in adult T-cell leukemia. Blood 1992;79:477.
41. Hatta Y: Homozygous deletions of the *p15 (MTS2)* and *p16^{INK4A} (CDKN2/MTS1)* genes in adult T-cell leukemia. Blood 1995;85: 2699.
42. Uchida T: The CDKN2 gene alterations in various types of adult T-cell leukemia. Br J Haematol 1996;94:665.
43. Nosaka K: Increasing methylation of the CDKN2A gene is associated with the progression of adult T-cell leukemia. Cancer Res 2000; 60:1043.
44. Takatsuki K: ATL and HTLV-I-related diseases. In Takatsuki K, ed: Adult T-Cell Leukemia. Oxford: Oxford University Press; 1994, p 1.
45. Kiyokawa T: Hypercalcemia and osteoclast proliferation in adult T-cell leukemia. Cancer 1987;59:1187.

46. Hattori T: Surface phenotype of Japanese adult T-cell leukemia cells characterized by monoclonal antibodies. Blood 1981;58:645.

47. Ogata M: Eosinophilia associated with adult T-cell leukemia: Role of interleukin 5 and granulocyte macrophage colony-stimulating factor. Am J Hematol 1998;59:242.

48. Vukelja SJ: Eosinophilia associated with adult T cell leukemia/lymphoma. Cancer 1988;62:1527.

49. Yasuda N: Soluble interleukin-2 receptors in sera of Japanese patients with adult T-cell leukemia mark activity of disease. Blood 1988;71:1021.

50. Watanabe T: Constitutive expression of parathyroid hormone-related protein gene in human T-cell leukemia virus type 1 (HTLV-1) carriers and adult T-cell leukemia patients that can be transactivated by HTLV-1 *tax* gene. J Exp Med 1990;172:759.

51. Wano Y: Interleukin-1 gene expression in adult T cell leukemia. J Clin Invest 1987;80:911.

52. Miyamoto Y: Familial adult T-cell leukemia. Cancer 1985;55:181.

53. Yamaguchi K: Concurrence of lymphoma-type adult T-cell leukemia in three sisters. Cancer 1985;56:1688.

54. Yoshioka R: Pulmonary complications in patients with adult T-cell leukemia. Cancer 1985;55:2491.

55. Yamaguchi K: *Strongyloides stercoralis* as candidate co-factor for HTLV-I–induced leukaemogenesis. Lancet 1987;2:94.

56. Kubota T: HTLV-I-seronegative genome-positive adult T-cell leukemia: Report of a case. Am J Hematol 1996;53:133.

57. Luo SS: Failure to detect anti-HTLV-1 antibody in a patient with adult T-cell leukemia. Br J Haematol 1998;103:1207.

58. Chosa T: Analysis of anti-HTLV-I antibodies by strip radioimmunoassay comparison with indirect immunofluorescence assay enzyme-linked immunosorbent assay and membrane immunofluorescence assay. Leuk Res 1986;10:605.

59. Hisada M: Risk factors for adult T-cell leukemia among carriers of human T-lymphotropic virus type I. Blood 1998;92:3557.

60. Matsuoka M: T3 surface molecules on adult T cell leukemia cells are modulated in vivo. Blood 1986;67:1070.

61. Kamihira S: Hemato-cytological aspects of adult T-cell leukemia. In Takasuki K, Hinuma Y, Yoshida M, eds: Advances in Adult T-Cell Leukemia and HTLV-I Research. Tokyo: Gann Monograph on Cancer Research 39, Japan Scientific Society Press 1992, p 17.

62. Debatin KM: APO-1-induced apoptosis of leukemia cells from patients with adult T-cell leukemia. Blood 1993;81:2972.

63. Tamiya S: Mutation of *CD95 (Fas/Apo-1)* gene in adult T-cell leukemia cells. Blood 1998;91:3935.

64. Yoshida M: Monoclonal integration of human T-cell leukemia provirus in all primary tumors of adult T-cell leukemia suggests causative role of human T-cell leukemia virus in disease. Proc Natl Acad Sci U S A 1984;81:2534.

65. Tamiya S: Two types of defective human T-lymphotropic virus type I provirus in adult T-cell leukemia. Blood 1996;88:3065.

66. Kamada N: Chromosome abnormalities in adult T cell leukemia/lymphoma: A karyotype review committee report. Cancer Res 1992;52:1481.

67. Sanada I: Chromosomal aberrations in adult T-cell leukemia: Relationship to the clinical severity. Blood 1985;65:649.

68. Ueshima Y: Chromosome studies in adult T-cell leukemia in Japan: Significance of trisomy 7. Blood 1981;58:420.

69. Seiki M: Nonspecific integration of the HTLV provirus genome into adult T-cell leukemia cells. Nature 1984;309:640.

70. Shimoyama M, Lymphoma Study Group: Diagnostic criteria and classification of clinical subtypes of adult T-cell leukemia-lymphoma. Br J Hematol 1991;79:428.

71. Yamaguchi K: A proposal for smoldering adult T-cell leukemia: A clinicopathologic study of five cases. Blood 1983;62:758.

72. Minato K: An interim report of LSG4 treatment for advanced peripheral T-cell lymphoma. Int J Hematol 1991;54:179.

73. Shimoyama M: Chemotherapy of ATL. In Takatsuki K, ed: Adult T-cell Leukemia. Oxford: Oxford University Press; 1994, p 221.

74. Yamada Y: A new G-CSF–supported combination chemotherapy, LSG15, for adult T-cell leukemia-lymphoma: Japan Clinical Oncology Group Study 9303. Br J Haematol 2001;113:375.

75. Daenen S: Successful chemotherapy with deoxycoformycin in adult T-cell lymphoma-leukaemia. Br J Haematol 1984;58:723.

76. Yamaguchi K: Clinical consequences of 2′-deoxycorfomycin treatment in patients with refractory adult T-cell leukemia. Leukemia Res 1986;10:989.

77. Gill PS: Treatment of adult T-cell leukemia-lymphoma with a combination of interferon alpha and zidovudine. N Engl J Med 1995;332:1744.

78. Bazarbachi A: Arsenic trioxide and interferon-alpha synergize to induce cell cycle arrest and apoptosis in human T-cell lymphotropic virus type I-transformed cells. Blood 1999;93:278.

79. Waldmann TA: The interleukin-2 receptor: A target for monoclonal antibody treatment of human T-cell lymphotrophic virus I–induced adult T-cell leukemia. Blood 1993;82:1701.

80. Borg A: Successful treatment of HTLV-1–associated acute adult T-cell leukaemia lymphoma by allogeneic bone marrow transplantation. Br J Haematol 1996;94:713.

81. Oguma S: Accelarated declining tendency of human T-cell leukemia virus type I carrier rates among younger blood donors in Kumamoto, Japan. Cancer Res 1992;52:2620.

82. Gessain A: Antibodies to human T-lymphotropic virus type I in patients with tropical spastic paraparesis. Lancet 1985;2:407.

83. Osame M: HTLV-I associated myelopathy: A new clinical entity. Lancet 1986;1:1031.

84. Nakada K: Monoclonal integration of HTLV-I proviral DNA in patients with strongyloidiasis. Int J Cancer 1987;40:145.

85. LaGrenade L: Infective dermatitis of Jamaican children: A marker for HTLV-I infection. Lancet 1990;336:1345.

86. Nishioka K: Chronic inflammatory arthropathy associated with HTLV-I. Lancet 1989;I:441.

87. Mochizuki M: HTLV-I uveitis: A distinct clinical entity caused by HTLV-I. Jpn J Cancer Res 1992;83:236.

88. Ono A: Provirus load in patients with human T-cell leukemia virus type 1 uveitis correlates with precedent Graves' disease and disease activities. Jpn J Cancer Res 1998;89:608.

89. Yoshida M: Increased replication of HTLV-I in HTLV-I–associated myelopathy. Ann Neurol 1989;26:331.

90. Tobinai K: Epstein-Barr virus (EBV) genome carrying monoclonal B-cell lymphoma in a patient with adult T-cell leukemia and lymphoma. Leuk Res 1991;15:837.

91. Greenberg SJ: Kaposi's sarcoma in human T-cell leukemia virus type I–associated adult T-cell leukemia. Blood 1990;76:971.

INDEX

Note: Page numbers followed by f indicate figures; those followed by t indicate tables.